MODERN NUTRITION
IN HEALTH AND DISEASE

ELEVENTH EDITION

EDITORS

A. Catharine Ross, Ph.D.

Benjamin Caballero, M.D., Ph.D.

Robert J. Cousins, Ph.D.

Katherine L. Tucker, Ph.D.

Thomas R. Ziegler, M.D.

Wolters Kluwer | Lippincott Williams & Wilkins
Health

Philadelphia • Baltimore • New York • London
Buenos Aires • Hong Kong • Sydney • Tokyo

Acquisitions Editor: David B. Troy
Product Manager: Matt Hauber / John Larkin
Marketing Manager: Sarah Schuessler
Creative Director: Doug Smock
Compositor: Absolute Service, Inc.

Eleventh Edition
Copyright © 2014, 2006, 1999 Lippincott Williams & Wilkins, a Wolters Kluwer business

351 West Camden Street   Two Commerce Square
Baltimore, MD 21201   2001 Market Street
                               Philadelphia, PA 19103

Printed in China

9 8 7 6 5 4 3 2 1

Library of Congress Cataloging-in-Publication Data

Modern nutrition in health and disease. — 11th ed. / editors, A. Catharine Ross ... [et al.].
    p. ; cm.
  Includes bibliographical references and index.
  ISBN 978-1-60547-461-8
  I. Ross, A. Catharine.
  [DNLM: 1. Nutritional Physiological Phenomena. 2. Micronutrients—physiology. 3. Micronutrients—therapeutic use. 4. Nutrition Therapy. QU 145]

  613.2—dc23
                                                                    2012035998

DISCLAIMER

Care has been taken to confirm the accuracy of the information present and to describe generally accepted practices. However, the authors, editors, and publisher are not responsible for errors or omissions or for any consequences from application of the information in this book and make no warranty, expressed or implied, with respect to the currency, completeness, or accuracy of the contents of the publication. Application of this information in a particular situation remains the professional responsibility of the practitioner; the clinical treatments described and recommended may not be considered absolute and universal recommendations.

The authors, editors, and publisher have exerted every effort to ensure that drug selection and dosage set forth in this text are in accordance with the current recommendations and practice at the time of publication. However, in view of ongoing research, changes in government regulations, and the constant flow of information relating to drug therapy and drug reactions, the reader is urged to check the package insert for each drug for any change in indications and dosage and for added warnings and precautions. This is particularly important when the recommended agent is a new or infrequently employed drug.

Some drugs and medical devices presented in this publication have Food and Drug Administration (FDA) clearance for limited use in restricted research settings. It is the responsibility of the health care provider to ascertain the FDA status of each drug or device planned for use in their clinical practice.

To purchase additional copies of this book, call our customer service department at **(800) 638-3030** or fax orders to **(301) 223-2320**. International customers should call **(301) 223-2300**.

Visit Lippincott Williams & Wilkins on the Internet: http://www.lww.com. Lippincott Williams & Wilkins customer service representatives are available from 8:30 a.m. to 6:00 p.m., EST.

ABOUT THE EDITORS

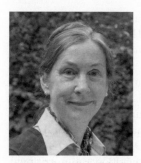

Catharine Ross is the occupant of the Dorothy Foehr Huck Chair and Professor of Nutrition at The Pennsylvania State University. She earned her B.S. degree from the University of California at Davis and a Masters of Nutrition Sciences and Ph.D. in biochemistry and molecular and cell biology from Cornell University. After postdoctoral work at Columbia University, she joined the faculty of the Medical College of Pennsylvania, where she advanced before moving to Penn State in 1994. She has served as councilor and treasurer of the American Society for Nutrition (ASN) and is currently Editor in Chief of *The Journal of Nutrition*. She received the Mead Johnson Award and the Osborne and Mendel Award from the ASN, is a fellow of the American Association for the Advancement of Science, and was elected to membership in the National Academy of Sciences in 2003. She has served on various National Institutes of Health and Institute of Medicine committees, including the Food and Nutrition Board. Her research is focused on the regulation of vitamin A transport and function, especially in the immune system. Currently, she teaches graduate courses in molecular nutrition and an undergraduate writing intensive nutrition seminar. She served as an editor for the ninth and tenth editions of *Modern Nutrition in Health and Disease*.

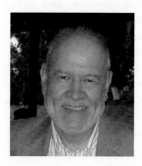

Benjamin Caballero is Professor of International Health at the Bloomberg School of Public Health, and Professor of Pediatrics at the School of Medicine, Johns Hopkins University. He received his M.D. degree from the University of Buenos Aires and his Ph.D. in neuroendocrine regulation from Massachusetts Institute of Technology. He has served on numerous national and international advisory panels, including the Food and Nutrition Board of the Institute of Medicine, the Dietary Guidelines for Americans Committee, the Food and Drug Administration Advisory Board, and several panels of the National Institutes of Health and the United States Department of Agriculture. His publications include the books *Encyclopedia of Human Nutrition*, *The Nutrition Transition*, *Obesity in China*, and *Guide to Dietary Supplements*, among others. He teaches the course Principles of Human Nutrition at the graduate program in nutrition at Johns Hopkins. He served as an editor for the tenth edition of *Modern Nutrition in Health and Disease*.

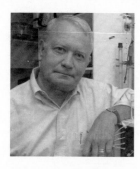

Robert J. Cousins is the Boston Family Professor of Nutrition and Eminent Scholar at the University of Florida. He has a B.A. from the University of Vermont and a Ph.D. from the University of Connecticut and was a National Institutes of Health (NIH) Postdoctoral Fellow in Biochemistry at the University of Wisconsin. He has been President and Board Chair of the Federation of American Societies for Experimental Biology and President of the American Society for Nutrition (ASN). He has received numerous awards including the Mead Johnson Award, the Osborne and Mendel Award of the ASN, the NIH MERIT Award, the United States Department of Agriculture Secretary's Honor Award, the American College of Nutrition Research Award, the Bristol-Myers Squibb/Mead Johnson Award for Distinguished Achievement in Biomedical (Nutrition) Research, the Dannon Institute Mentorship Award, and Distinguished Scientist Award from the International Society for Trace Element Research in Humans. He was elected to membership in the National Academy of Sciences in 2000. He is the editor of *The Annual Review of Nutrition*. His research is on the molecular and cell biology of zinc metabolism, nutrition, transport, and function. He teaches graduate courses in Mineral Nutrition and Analytical Techniques in Nutrition. He served as an editor for the tenth edition of *Modern Nutrition in Health and Disease*.

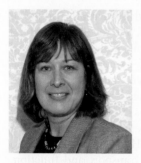

Katherine L. Tucker is Professor of Nutritional Epidemiology at Northeastern University. She received her Ph.D. from Cornell University and her B.Sc. from the University of Connecticut, both in nutritional science. She is a past Chair of the Nutritional Sciences Council and past board member of the American Society for Nutrition, and she served as an associate editor for *The Journal of Nutrition* for 8 years. Her research focuses on dietary intake, metabolism, and chronic disease (osteoporosis, diabetes, heart disease, and cognitive decline) in diverse populations. She is currently the director of the Center on Population Health and Health Disparities funded by the National Heart, Lung, and Blood Institute and is a member of the National Institutes of Health Kidney, Nutrition, Obesity and Diabetes (KNOD) study section. She teaches courses on nutrition and nutritional epidemiology.

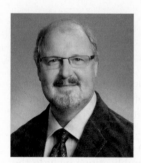

Thomas R. Ziegler is Professor of Medicine and Director of the Emory Center for Clinical and Molecular Nutrition at Emory University School of Medicine. He received his B.S. and M.S. in nutrition and his M.D. from Michigan State University, and was a postdoctoral fellow in nutrition at Harvard Medical School. He serves as Co-Program Director of the Research Education, Training and Career Development Core of the Atlanta Clinical and Translational Science Institute (ACTSI) and as a Program Director of the ACTSI Clinical Research Network. He serves on the editorial board of several nutrition-oriented research journals and performs both clinical and translational research focusing on nutritional metabolomics, nutrient/growth factor/redox regulation of intestinal cell growth, repair, and function, and metabolic and clinical effects of specialized nutrition support modalities in catabolic states. He teaches a graduate-level grant-writing course for trainees in the ACTSI Master of Science in Clinical Research program and a nutrition course for first-year medical students.

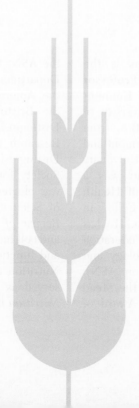

PREFACE

The eleventh edition of *Modern Nutrition in Health and Disease* follows from a long history of publishing an authoritative text related to human nutrition, from the basic science of nutrient metabolism and functions to the applications of nutrition for improving clinical outcomes and public health. The goal of this edition, like that of its predecessors, is to provide an updated, comprehensive, and authoritative text and reference source authored by experts in their fields. In this new edition, more than 190 authors have joined this effort. Nearly 60% are new authors. All authors have provided the most up-to-date view of their respective areas.

The history of *Modern Nutrition in Health and Disease* now spans more than five decades, as outlined in the following table, which lists the editions, publication year, editors, and publisher of this text.

From its outset, the book has taken a broad approach to nutritional science with a strong clinical view. The title and objectives of this work evolved from a book originally designated *Dietotherapy*, initiated by Michael G. Wohl, M.D., and Robert S. Goodhart, M.D., as Coeditors, in 1950. The second edition was the first to use the title *Modern Nutrition in Health and Disease*, subtitled *Dietotherapy*. Drs. Wohl and Goodhart continued to edit the first four editions. Beginning with the fifth edition in 1973, Maurice E. Shils, M.D., Sc.D., joined in editing the book with Dr. Goodhart. Dr. Shils became the Senior Editor beginning with the seventh edition in 1988 and continued in this role through the tenth edition. The tenth edition celebrated the 50th anniversary of *Modern Nutrition in Health and Disease*.

As planning for the eleventh edition began, Dr. Shils decided it was time to retire from this project. He and his wife, Betty, who ably assisted Maury through the organization of several editions, live in Winston-Salem, North Carolina, where they are happily taking care of two very lively Shelties as well as traveling frequently. The Editors of the eleventh edition, both those continuing and those who are new to this work, wish to extend our most sincere gratitude to Maury Shils for the guidance he has provided and for sharing his love for this book and his rigorous approach to overseeing the tasks that are involved. To many readers, *Modern Nutrition in Health and Disease* became known simply as *Goodhart & Shils* and later as *Shils*. We hope that as the book makes its most recent transition, it will continue to be the highly respected and authoritative text that this reference always has been.

The eleventh edition continues traditions and adds new ones. The basic organization remains the same as in the tenth edition, but all the topics are state of the art and some have been consolidated, with emphasis always on staying modern, as the work's title states. Beginning with this eleventh edition, the Appendices have been simplified and moved online—consistent with modern delivery of these materials—which can now be updated as needed, and it also makes the book more concise. The eleventh edition highlights many new topics that represent the most current concepts and practical concerns in nutrition and nutritional management of disease. New chapters include Functional Foods and Nutraceuticals in Health Promotion, Prebiotics and Probiotics as Modulators of the

EDITION NUMBER	PUBLICATION YEAR[a]	EDITORS	PUBLISHER
1	1950	Drs. Michael Wohl, Robert Goodhart	Lea & Febiger
2	1955	Drs. Michael Wohl, Robert Goodhart	Lea & Febiger
3	1964	Drs. Michael Wohl, Robert Goodhart	Lea & Febiger
4	1968	Drs. Michael Wohl, Robert Goodhart	Lea & Febiger
5	1973	Drs. Robert Goodhart, Maurice E. Shils	Lea & Febiger
6	1980	Drs. Robert Goodhart, Maurice E. Shils	Lea & Febiger
7	1988	Drs. Maurice E. Shils, Vernon Young	Lea & Febiger
8	1994	Drs. Maurice E. Shils, James A. Olson, Moshe Shike	Lea & Febiger[b]
9	1998	Drs. Maurice E. Shils, James A. Olson, Moshe Shike, A. Catharine Ross	Lippincott Williams & Wilkins
10	2005	Drs. Maurice E. Shils, Moshe Shike, A. Catharine Ross, Benjamin Caballero, Robert J. Cousins	Lippincott Williams & Wilkins
11	2012	Drs. A. Catharine Ross, Benjamin Caballero, Robert J. Cousins, Katherine L. Tucker, Thomas R. Ziegler	Lippincott Williams & Wilkins

[a]Year of the first printing.
[b]Lea & Febiger, Philadelphia, was purchased shortly before the publication of the eighth edition by the Waverly Company, owner of Williams & Wilkins Publishers, Baltimore. Shortly before the publication of the ninth edition, the Waverly Company was purchased by Wolters Kluwer Publishers and merged with Lippincott, the medical publisher in Philadelphia.

Gut Microbiota, Epigenetics, Mechanisms of Nutrient Sensing, Metabolic Consequences of Calorie Restriction, Bariatric Surgery, Metabolic Syndrome, Nutrition and Inflammatory Processes, Irritable Bowel Syndrome and Diverticular Disease, Food Insecurity in Children, Cancer Cachexia, Nutrition in Burn Injury, Dietary Patterns, and Approaches to Preventing Micronutrient Deficiencies.

The Editors wish to acknowledge outstanding support in the preparation, editing, and production of this extensive work. The authors who have contributed their expertise are listed alphabetically on the following pages. The Editors have worked personally with some of the staff of Lippincott Williams & Wilkins in Baltimore, whereas other members have been involved "behind the scenes" at the editorial, publication, distribution, and marketing stages. We wish to thank all of them for their support.

David Troy, Senior Acquisitions Editor, helped move the eleventh edition forward after Dr. Shils' retirement. Matt Hauber and John Larkin served as our Product Managers. The project owes an enormous thank you to Holly Lukens, chief copyeditor. She has worked with *Modern Nutrition in Health and Disease* for three editions and has consistently improved the quality of the work. We thank the various graphic artists whose illustrations are in the eleventh edition and the staff at the graphics department at Lippincott Williams & Wilkins for the special attention paid to illustrations in this new edition. We are also very indebted to those who worked closely and efficiently with us in preparing and distributing manuscripts and managing communications, and we wish to acknowledge Madeleine Stull and Carrie Guzman for their excellent staff assistance.

THE EDITORS

A. CATHARINE ROSS, Ph.D.

BENJAMIN CABALLERO, M.D., Ph.D.

ROBERT J. COUSINS, Ph.D.

KATHERINE L. TUCKER, Ph.D.

THOMAS R. ZIEGLER, M.D.

CONTRIBUTORS

Phyllis B. Acosta, M.S., Dr.P.H., R.D.
Nutrition Consultant
Medical Genetics
Emory University School of Medicine
Atlanta, Georgia

Lindsay H. Allen, Ph.D.
Center Director and Research Professor
USDA/ARS Western Human Nutrition Research Center
University of California
Davis, California

David Alpers, M.D.
William B. Kountz Professor of Medicine
Internal Medicine/Gastroenterology
Washington University School of Medicine
Physician
Internal Medicine/Gastroenterology
Barnes Jewish Hospital
St. Louis, Missouri

Aśok C. Antony, M.D., F.A.C.P.
Professor of Medicine
Department of Medicine
Indiana University School of Medicine
Attending Physician
Hematology Service
Indiana University Hospital
Staff Physician and Consultant in Hematology
Medicine Service
Roudebush Veterans Affairs Medical Center
Indianapolis, Indiana

Lawrence J. Appel, M.D., M.P.H.
Professor
Department of Medicine
Johns Hopkins University of N
Professor of Medicine
Johns Hopkins University School of Medicine
Baltimore, Maryland

Michelle Asp, Ph.D., R.D.
Postdoctoral Research Associate
College of Food, Agricultural and Natural
Resource Sciences
University of Minnesota Twin Cities Campus
St. Paul, Minnesota

David A. August, M.D.
Professor of Surgery
Chief, Division of Surgical Oncology
UMDNJ/Robert Wood Johnson Medical School and
The Cancer Institute of New Jersey
New Brunswick, New Jersey

Joseph E. Baggott, Ph.D.
Assistant Professor
Retired from Department of Nutrition Sciences
University of Alabama at Birmingham
Birmingham, Alabama

James L. Bailey, M.D.
Professor
Renal Division
Department of Medicine
Emory University School of Medicine
Atlanta, Georgia

Connie Watkins Bales, Ph.D., R.D.
Professor
Department of Medicine
Duke University Medical Center
Associate Director for Education and Evaluation
Geriatric Research, Education, and Clinical Center
Durham VA Medical Center
Durham, North Carolina

Vickie E. Baracos, Ph.D.
Professor
Palliative Care Medicine
Department of Oncology
University of Alberta
Cross Cancer Institute
Edmonton, Alberta, Canada

Joseph L. Baumert, Ph.D.
Assistant Professor
Department of Food Science and Technology
University of Nebraska–Lincoln
Lincoln, Nebraska

Juliane I. Beier, Ph.D.
Assistant Professor
Pharmacology and Toxicology
University of Louisville
Louisville, Kentucky

Chantal Bémeur, Dt.P., Ph.D.
Assistant Professor
Department of Nutrition
Université de Montréal
Researcher
Neuroscience Research Unit
Hôpital St-Luc (CHUM)
Montreal, Quebec

Stephen Robert Bloom, M.A., M.D., D.Sc., F.R.C.Path., F.R.C.P, F.Med.Sci.
Chairman of Section of Investigative Medicine
Department of Investigative Medicine
Imperial College London
Chief of Pathology Service
Department of Diabetes and Endocrinology
Hammersmith Hospital
London, United Kingdom

Rex O. Brown, Pharm.D.
Professor and Vice Chair
Director, Experiential Education
Department of Clinical Pharmacy
College of Pharmacy
University of Tennessee Health Science Center
Memphis, Tennessee

Alan L. Buchman, M.D., M.S.P.H.
Professor of Medicine and Surgery
Division of Gastroenterology and Hepatology
Feinberg School of Medicine, Northwestern University
Chicago, Illinois

Douglas G. Burrin, Ph.D.
Professor
USDA-Children's Nutrition Research Center
Section of Gastroenterology, Hepatology and Nutrition
Department of Pediatrics
Baylor College of Medicine
Houston, Texas

Nancy F. Butte, Ph.D.
Professor
Department of Pediatrics
Baylor College of Medicine
USDA/ARS Children's Nutrition Research Center
Houston, Texas

Roger F. Butterworth, Ph.D., D.Sc.
Professor
Department of Medicine
Université De Montréal
Director
Neuroscience Research Unit
Hospital St-LUC (CHUM)
Montreal, Quebec

Benjamin Caballero, M.D., Ph.D.
Professor
Center for Human Nutrition
Department of International Health
Johns Hopkins Bloomberg School of Public Health
Baltimore, Maryland

Philip C. Calder, Ph.D., D.Phil., R.Nutr.
Professor of Nutritional Immunology
Faculty of Medicine
University of Southampton
Southampton, United Kingdom

Ralph Carmel, M.D.
Director of Research
New York Methodist Hospital
Brooklyn, New York
Professor of Medicine
Weill Cornell Medical College
New York, New York

Leticia Castillo, M.D.
Thomas Fariss Marsh Jr. Chair in Pediatrics
Professor of Pediatrics
Department of Pediatrics
University of Texas Southwestern
Division of Critical Care
Children's Medical Center
Dallas, Texas

Victoria A. Catenacci, M.D.
Assistant Professor of Medicine
Anschutz Health and Wellness Center
Endocrinology, Metabolism and Diabetes
University of Colorado Anschutz Medical Campus
Aurora, Colorado

Lingtak-Neander Chan, Pharm.D., B.C.N.S.P.
Associate Professor of Pharmacy and Interdisciplinary
Faculty in Nutritional Sciences
School of Pharmacy and Graduate Program in
Nutritional Sciences
University of Washington
Seattle, Washington

Lawrence J. Cheskin, M.D.
Associate Professor
Department of Health, Behavior and Society
Johns Hopkins Bloomberg School of Public Health
Attending Staff
Department of Medicine (Gastroenterology)
Johns Hopkins Hospital
Baltimore, Maryland

Christopher R. Chitambar, M.D., F.A.C.P.
Professor of Medicine and Fellowship Program Director
Department of Medicine, Division of Hematology
and Oncology
Froedtert and Medical College of Wisconsin Clinical
Cancer Center
Medical College of Wisconsin
Milwaukee, Wisconsin

Paul M. Coates, Ph.D.
Director
Office of Dietary Supplements
National Institutes of Health
Bethesda, Maryland

James F. Collins, Ph.D.
Associate Professor
Food Science and Human Nutrition Department
University of Florida
Gainesville, Florida

Arthur Cooper, M.D., M.S.
Professor of Surgery
Columbia University College of Physicians and Surgeons
Director of Trauma and Pediatric Surgical Services
Harlem Hospital Center
New York, New York

Janelle W. Coughlin, Ph.D.
Assistant Professor
Department of Psychiatry and Behavioral Sciences
Johns Hopkins University School of Medicine
Baltimore, Maryland

Robert J. Cousins, Ph.D.
Boston Family Professor of Nutrition
Director, Center for Nutritional Sciences
Food Science and Human Nutrition Department
University of Florida
Gainesville, Florida

Susette M. Coyle, M.S.
Instructor
Department of Surgery
Robert Wood Johnson Medical School
New Brunswick, New Jersey

Vanessa R. da Silva, Ph.D.
Postdoctoral Associate and Instructor
Department of Foods and Nutrition
University of Georgia
Athens, Georgia

Akila De Silva B.Sc., M.B.B.S., M.R.C.P.
Wellcome Trust/GSK Clinical Research Fellow
Department of Investigative Medicine
Imperial College London
Honorary Specialist Registrar
Department of Diabetes and Endocrinology
Hammersmith Hospital
London, United Kingdom

Alan D. Dangour, M.Sc., Ph.D.
Senior Lecturer
Department of Population Health
London School of Hygiene and Tropical Medicine
London, United Kingdom

Cindy D. Davis, Ph.D.
Director of Grants and Extramural Activities
Office of Dietary Supplements
National Institutes of Health
Rockville, Maryland

Steven R. Davis, Ph.D.
Platform Leader
Global Discovery RBD
Abbott Nutrition
Columbus, Ohio

Teresa A. Davis, Ph.D.
Professor
USDA Children's Nutrition Research Center
Department of Pediatrics
Baylor College of Medicine
Houston, Texas

Mark H. DeLegge, M.D.
Professor of Medicine
Digestive Disease Center
Medical University of South Carolina
Charleston, South Carolina

Dominick P. DePaola, D.D.S., Ph.D.
Associate Dean, Academic Affairs
College of Dental Medicine
Nova Southeastern University
Fort Lauderdale, Florida

Nicolaas E.P. Deutz, M.D., Ph.D.
Professor, Ponder Endowed Chair
Department of Health and Kinesiology
Texas A&M University
Director Translational Research in Aging and Longevity
Department of Health and Kinesiology
College Station, Texas

John K. DiBaise, M.D.
Professor of Medicine
Division of Gastroenterology
Mayo Clinic
Scottsdale, Arizona

Adrian Dobs, M.D., M.H.S.
Professor of Medicine
Division of Endocrinology and Metabolism
Johns Hopkins University
Baltimore, Maryland

Gerald W. Dryden, M.D., M.S.P.H., M.Sc.
Associate Professor of Medicine and Bioengineering
Department of Medicine
Division of Gastroenterology, Hepatology, and Nutrition
University of Louisville School of Medicine
Louisville, Kentucky

Valerie B. Duffy, Ph.D., R.D.
Professor
Department of Allied Health Sciences
College of Agriculture and Natural Resources
University of Connecticut
Storrs, Connecticut

Curtis D. Eckhert, Ph.D.
Professor
Department of Environmental Health Sciences and
Molecular Toxicology
University of California Los Angeles
Los Angeles, California

Louis J. Elsas II, M.D., F.F.A.C.M.G.[†]
Professor of Pediatrics and Emeritus Director Center
for Medical Genetics
Department of Pediatrics and Biochemistry
Miller School of Medicine University of Miami
Chief, Medical Genetics-Emeritus
Department of Pediatrics
Jackson Memorial Hospital
Miami, Florida

Joshua Farr, Ph.D.
Postdoctoral Research Fellow
Endocrine Research Unit
Mayo Clinic
Rochester, Minnesota

Celeste C. Finnerty, Ph.D.
Associate Professor
Department of Surgery
University of Texas Medical Branch
Associate Director of Research
Shriners Hospitals for Children
Galveston, Texas

Edward A. Fisher, M.D., Ph.D.
Leon H. Charney Professor of Cardiovascular Medicine
Department of Medicine (Cardiology)
NYU School of Medicine
Director
Center for the Prevention of Cardiovascular Disease
NYU Langone Medical Center
New York, New York

Luigi Fontana, M.D., Ph.D.
Full Professor of Nutrition
Department of Medicine
Salerno University Medical School
Baronissi (Salerno), Italy
Research Professor of Medicine
Department of Medicine, Center for Human Nutrition
Washington University Medical School
St.Louis, Missouri

Harold A. Franch, M.D.
Associate Professor
Renal Division
Department of Medicine
Emory University School of Medicine
Atlanta, Georgia
Research Service
Atlanta Veterans Affairs Medical Center
Decatur, Georgia

Glenn R. Gibson, B.Sc., Ph.D.
Professor
Department of Food and Nutritional Sciences
The University of Reading
Reading, Berkshire, United Kingdom

Edward Giovannucci, M.D., Sc.D.
Professor
Department of Nutrition and Epidemiology
Harvard School of Public Health
Associate Professor of Medicine
Channing Division of Network Medicine
Brigham and Women's Hospital, Harvard Medical School
Boston, Massachusetts

Scott Going, Ph.D.
Department Head and Professor
Department of Nutritional Sciences
University of Arizona
Tucson, Arizona

Michele M. Gottschlich, Ph.D., R.D., L.D., C.N.S.D., P.S.G.T.
Adjunct Associate Professor
Department of Surgery
University of Cincinnati College of Medicine
Director of Nutrition Services
Shriners Hospitals for Children
Cincinnati, Ohio

[†]Deceased.

Jesse F. Gregory III, Ph.D.
Professor
Food Science and Human Nutrition Department
University of Florida
Gainesville, Florida

Zhenglong Gu, Ph.D.
Assistant Professor
Division of Nutritional Sciences
Cornell University
Ithaca, New York

Angela S. Guarda, M.D.
Associate Professor
Department of Psychiatry and Behavioral Sciences
Johns Hopkins University School of Medicine
Director, Johns Hopkins Eating Disorders Program
Johns Hopkins Hospital
Baltimore, Maryland

Craig Gundersen, Ph.D.
Professor
Department of Agricultural and Consumer Economics
University of Illinois
Urbana, Illinois

Paul Haggarty, B.Sc., Ph.D.
Head of Lifelong Health
Rowett Institute of Nutrition and Health
University of Aberdeen
Aberdeen, United Kingdom

Rachael A. Harrison, Ph.D.
Research Associate/cGMP Manager
Department of Biological Sciences
Sunnybrook Health Sciences Centre
Toronto, Ontario, Canada

Peter J. Havel, D.V.M., Ph.D.
Professor
Molecular Biosciences, School of Veterinary Medicine and Nutrition
University of California, Davis
Davis, California

Sophie Hawkesworth, Ph.D.
Research Fellow
Department of Population Health
London School of Hygiene and Tropical Medicine
London, United Kingdom

Robert P. Heaney, M.D.
John A. Creighton University Professor
Creighton University
Omaha, Nebraska

Robert A. Hegele, M.D., F.R.C.P.C.
Professor
Department of Medicine
University of Western Ontario
Staff Endocrinologist
London Health Sciences Center
London, Ontario, Canada

Douglas C. Heimburger, M.D., M.S.
Professor of Medicine
Vanderbilt University School of Medicine
Associate Director for Education and Training
Vanderbilt Institute for Global Health
Nashville, Tennessee

William C. Heird, M.D.
Professor Emeritus
Children's Nutritional Research Center
Baylor College of Medicine
Houston, Texas

David N. Herndon, M.D.
Chief of Staff
Shriners Hospitals for Children, Galveston
Professor of Pediatrics and Surgery
University of Texas Medical Branch
Galveston, Texas

Steve Hertzler, Ph.D., R.D.
Senior Research Scientist
Performance Nutrition
Abbott Nutrition
Columbus, Ohio

James O. Hill, Ph.D.
Professor of Pediatrics and Medicine
Anschutz Health and Wellness Center
University of Colorado Anschutz Medical Campus
Aurora, Colorado

Melanie Hingle, Ph.D., M.P.H., R.D.
Assistant Research Professor
Department of Nutritional Sciences
University of Arizona
Tucson, Arizona

L. John Hoffer, M.D., Ph.D.
Professor
Faculty of Medicine
McGill University
Senior Physician and Principal Investigator
Divisions of Internal Medicine and Endocrinology
Lady Davis Institute for Medical Research
Sir Mortimer B. Davis Jewish General Hospital
Montreal, Quebec, Canada

Maureen Huhmann, D.C.N., R.D., C.S.O.
Adjunct, Assistant Professor
Nutritional Sciences
University of Medicine and Dentistry of New Jersey
Newark, New Jersey

Gary R. Hunter, Ph.D.
Professor
Departments of Human Studies and Nutrition Sciences
University of Alabama at Birmingham
Birmingham, Alabama

Syed Sufyan Hussain, M.A., M.B. B.Chir., M.R.C.P.
Wellcome Trust Clinical Research Fellow
Department of Investigative Medicine
Imperial College London
Honorary Specialist Registrar
Department of Diabetes and Endocrinology
Hammersmith Hospital
London, United Kingdom

James K. Hyche, Ph.D.
Director, Feeding Psychology Services
Psychology
Mt. Washington Pediatric Hospital
Baltimore, Maryland

Karl L. Insogna, M.D.
Professor of Medicine (Endocrinology)
Director, Yale Bone Center
Yale University
New Haven, Connecticut

Khursheed N. Jeejeebhoy, M.B.B.S., Ph.D., F.R.C.P.C.
Professor Emeritus
Department of Medicine
Department of Nutritional Sciences
University of Toronto
Toronto, Canada

Marc G. Jeschke, M.D., Ph.D.
Director, Ross Tilley Burn Centre
Sunnybrook Health Sciences Centre
Senior Scientist
Sunnybrook Research Institute
Associate Professor
Department of Surgery, Division of Plastic Surgery
Department of Immunology
University of Toronto
Toronto, Ontario, Canada

Margaret M. Johnson, M.D.
Assistant Professor of Medicine
Division of Pulmonary Medicine
Department of Medicine
Mayo Clinic Florida
Jacksonville, Florida

Mary Ann Johnson, Ph.D.
Flatt Professor and Faculty of Gerontology
Department of Foods and Nutrition
University of Georgia
Athens, Georgia

Dean P. Jones, Ph.D.
Professor
Department of Medicine
Emory University
Atlanta, Georgia

Glenville Jones, Ph.D.
Craine Professor of Biochemistry
Biomedical and Molecular Sciences
Queen's University
Kingston, Ontario Canada

Peter J. H. Jones, Ph.D.
Professor
Department of Food Science and Human
Nutritional Sciences
Richardson Centre for Functional Foods
and Nutraceuticals
University of Manitoba
Winnipeg, Manitoba

Rita Rastogi Kalyani, M.D., M.H.S.
Assistant Professor of Medicine
Division of Endocrinology and Metabolism
Johns Hopkins University School of Medicine
Baltimore, Maryland

Richard M. Katz, M.D., M.B.A.
Associate Professor
Pediatric
Johns Hopkins University School of Medicine
Vice President Medical Affairs, Chief Medical Office
Pediatric Medicine
Mt. Washington Pediatric Hospital
Baltimore, Maryland

Nancy L. Keim, Ph.D.
Research Chemist
USDA/ARS Western Human Nutrition Research Center
University of California, Davis
Davis, California

Kathleen L. Keller, Ph.D.
Assistant Professor
Department of Nutritional Science and Food Science
Pennsylvania State University
University Park, Pennsylvania
Research Associate
New York Obesity Research Center
New York, New York

Jane E. Kerstetter, Ph.D., R.D.
Professor
Department of Allied Health Sciences
University of Connecticut
Storrs, Connecticut

Rubina Khan, M.S.
Consultant
Charlotte, North Carolina

Yeonsoo Kim, Ph.D., R.D., L.D.N.
Assistant Professor of Nutrition and Dietetics
School of Human Ecology
Louisiana Tech University
Ruston, Louisiana

Janet C. King, Ph.D.
Senior Scientist and Professor
Children's Hospital Oakland Research Institute and the
University of California at Berkeley and Davis
Oakland, California

James B. Kirkland, Ph.D.
Associate Professor
Department of Human Health and Nutritional Sciences
University of Guelph
Guelph, Ontario, Canada

Samuel Klein, M.D., M.S.
William H. Danforth Professor of Medicine and
Nutritional Science
Director, Center for Human Nutrition
Chief, Division of Geriatrics and Nutritional Science
Department of Internal Medicine
Washington University School of Medicine
St. Louis, Missouri

Joel D. Kopple, M.D.
Professor of Medicine and Public Health
David Geffen School of Medicine at UCLA and
UCLA School of Public Health
Division of Nephrology and Hypertension
Los Angeles Biomedical Research Institute at
Harbor-UCLA Medical Center
Los Angeles and Torrance, California

Kenneth A. Kudsk, M.D.
Professor of Surgery
Department of Surgery
School of Medicine
University of Wisconsin-Madison
Madison, Wisconsin

Sarah Landes, M.D.
Department of Medicine
University of Louisville
Louisville, Kentucky

Peter Laurberg, M.D., Dr. Med. Sci.
Clinical Professor
Department of Endocrinology
Aalborg University
Chief Endocrinologists
Aalborg Hospital
Aalborg, Denmark

Roy J. Levin, M.Sc., Ph.D.
Honorary Research Associate
Porterbrook Clinic
Sheffield Care Trust
Yorkshire, England

Mark Levine, M.D.
Chief, Molecular and Clinical Nutrition Section
Digestive Diseases Branch
National Institute of Diabetes and Digestive and
Kidney Diseases
Bethesda, Maryland

Louis A. Lichten, Ph.D
Application Specialist
Center of Excellence in Biological Content
Qiagen (SABiosciences)
Frederick, Maryland

Hyunjung Lim, Ph.D.
Postdoctoral Fellow
Center for Human Nutrition
Department of International Health
Johns Hopkins Bloomberg School of Public Health
Baltimore, Maryland

Stephen F. Lowry, M.D.[†]
Professor and Chair of Surgery
Robert Wood Johnson Medical School
New Brunswick, New Jersey

Yvette C. Luiking, Ph.D.
Assistant Professor
Department of Health and Kinesiology
Texas A&M University
College Station, Texas

[†]Deceased.

Amy D. Mackey, Ph.D.
Associate Director
Regulatory Science and Innovation
Abbott Nutrition
Columbus, Ohio

Thomas Magnuson, M.D., FACS
Director, Johns Hopkins Center for Bariatric Surgery
Associate Professor of Surgery
Johns Hopkins University School of Medicine
Baltimore, Maryland

Laura E. Matarese, Ph.D., R.D., L.D.N., F.A.D.A., C.N.S.C.
Associate Professor
Division of Gastroenterology, Hepatology and Nutrition
Brody School of Medicine
Department of Nutrition Science
East Carolina University
Greenville, North Carolina

Dwight E. Matthews, Ph.D.
Professor and Chair
Departments of Chemistry and Medicine
University of Vermont
Burlington, Vermont

Craig J. McClain, M.D.
Professor and Associate Vice President for Research
Division of Gastroenterology, Hepatology and Nutrition
Department of Medicine
University of Louisville School of Medicine
Chief
Division of Gastroenterology
Department of Medicine
Robley Rex VA Medical Center
Louisville, Kentucky

Linda D. Meyers, Ph.D.
Director
Food and Nutrition Board
Institute of Medicine
The National Academies
Washington, DC

John Milner, Ph.D.
Director
Beltsville Human Nutrition Research Center
USDA/ARS
Beltsville, Maryland

Gayle Minard, M.D.
Professor of Surgery
Department of Surgery
College of Medicine
University of Tennessee Health Science Center
Memphis, Tennessee

Donald M. Mock, M.D., Ph.D.
Professor
Department of Biochemistry and Molecular Biology
University of Arkansas for Medical Sciences
Professor
Department of Pediatrics
Arkansas Children's Hospital
Little Rock, Arkansas

Kris M. Mogensen, M.S., R.D., L.D.N., C.N.S.C.
Team Leader Dietitian
Department of Nutrition
Brigham and Women's Hospital and Harvard Medical School
Instructor
Sargent College of Health and Rehabilitation Sciences
Boston University
Boston, Massachusetts

Mohammad Mohammad, M.D.
Department of Medicine
University of Louisville
Louisville, Kentucky

Richard L. Mones, M.D.
Assistant Clinical Professor of Pediatrics
Columbia University College of Physicians and Surgeons
Chief of Pediatric Gastroenterology and Nutrition
Harlem Hospital Center
New York, New York

Sarah L. Morgan, M.D., M.S., R.D./L.D., F.A.D.A., F.A.C.P., C.C.D.
Professor of Nutrition Sciences and Medicine
Division of Clinical Immunology and Rheumatology
Department of Medicine
The University of Alabama at Birmingham
Birmingham, Alabama

Kimberly O. O'Brien, Ph.D.
Professor
Division of Nutritional Sciences
Cornell University
Ithaca, New York

Deborah L. O'Connor, Ph.D., R.D.
Professor of Nutritional Sciences
University of Toronto
Associate Chief, Academic and Professional Practice
The Hospital for Sick Children
Toronto, Ontario, Canada

Susan Oh, M.S., M.P.H., R.D.
Research Nutrition Manager
Institute of Clinical and Translational Research (ICTR)
Johns Hopkins University School of Medicine
Baltimore, Maryland

Stephen J. D. O'Keefe, M.D., M.Sc.
Professor of Medicine
Division of Gastroenterology
University of Pittsburgh
Pittsburgh, Pennsylvania

Sebastian J. Padayatty, M.D., Ph.D.
Staff Clinician
Molecular and Clinical Nutrition Section
Digestive Diseases Branch
National Institute of Diabetes and Digestive and
Kidney Diseases
Bethesda, Maryland

Neal M. Patel, M.D., M.P.H.
Instructor of Medicine
Department of Pulmonary Medicine
Mayo Clinic Florida
Jacksonville, Florida

Rafael Pérez-Escamilla, Ph.D.
Professor
Chronic Disease Epidemiology
Yale School of Public Health
New Haven, Connecticut

Mary Frances Picciano, Ph.D.[†]
Senior Nutrition Research Scientist
Office of Dietary Supplements
National Institutes of Health
Bethesda, Maryland

Kavita H. Poddar, Ph.D.
Postdoctoral Fellow
Health Behavior and Society
Johns Hopkins Bloomberg School of Public Health
Baltimore, Maryland

Sarit Polsky, M.D., M.P.H.
Instructor
Anschutz Health and Wellness Center
Endocrinology, Metabolism and Diabetes
University of Colorado Anschutz Medical Campus
Aurora, Colorado

Ronald L. Prior, Ph.D.
Adjunct Professor
Department of Food Science
University of Arkansas
Fayetteville, Arkansas

Diane Rigassio Radler, Ph.D., R.D.
Associate Professor
Nutritional Sciences
University of Medicine and Dentistry of New Jersey
Newark, New Jersey

Amit Raina, M.B.B.S., M.D., C.N.S.C.
Fellow in Gastroenterology
Division of Gastroenterology, Hepatology,
and Nutrition
University of Pittsburgh Medical School
Pittsburgh, Pennsylvania

Manuel Ramirez-Zea, M.D., Ph.D.
Head, INCAP Comprehensive Center for the Prevention
of Chronic Diseases (CIIPEC)
Unit of Nutrition and Chronic Diseases
Institute of Nutrition of Central America and
Panama (INCAP)
Guatemala, Guatemala

Robert Rastall, B.Sc., Ph.D.
Professor
Food and Nutritional Sciences
The University of Reading
Reading, Berkshire, United Kingdom

Charles J. Rebouche, Ph.D.
Associate Professor
Department of Pediatrics
University of Iowa
Iowa City, Iowa

Dominic N. Reeds, M.D.
Assistant Professor
Department of Internal Medicine
Washington University School of Medicine
Barnes Jewish Hospital
St. Louis, Missouri

Deborah L. Renaud, M.D.
Department of Neurology
Mayo Clinic College of Medicine
Rochester, Minnesota

[†]Deceased.

Todd Rideout, Ph.D.
Assistant Professor
Department of Exercise and Nutrition Sciences
University of Buffalo
Buffalo, New York

Malcolm K. Robinson, M.D.
Assistant Professor of Surgery
Harvard Medical School
Surgeon and Metabolic Support Physician
Brigham and Women's Hospital
Boston, Massachusetts

Gustavo C. Román, M.D.
Professor of Neurology
Department of Neurology
Weill Cornell Medical College at Methodist Hospital
Jack S. Blanton Distinguished Endowed Chair
Director, Nantz National Alzheimer Center
Methodist Neurological Institute
Houston, Texas

Clifford J. Rosen, M.D.
Director, Center for Clinical and Translational Research
Maine Medical Center Research Institute
Scarborough, Maine

A. Catharine Ross, Ph.D.
Professor, Occupant of Dorothy Foehr Huck Chair
Department of Nutritional Sciences
Pennsylvania State University
University Park, Pennsylvania

Ian R. Rowland, B.Sc., Ph.D., R. Nutr.
Professor
Food and Nutritional Sciences
The University of Reading
Reading, Berkshire, United Kingdom

Robert K. Rude, M.D.[†]
Professor Medicine
Keck School of Medicine
University of Southern California
Los Angeles, California

Hamid M. Said, Ph.D.
Professor and Vice-Chairman
Departments of Medicine and Physiology and Biophysics
University of California/VA Medical Program
Long Beach, California

Marie-Pierre St-Onge, Ph.D.
Research Associate
Department of Medicine
St. Luke's/Roosevelt Hospital
Assistant Professor
Columbia University
New York, New York

Jeff M. Sands, M.D.
Juha P. Kokko Professor of Medicine and Physiology
Director, Renal Division
Executive Vice Chair, Department of Medicine
Associate Dean for Clinical and Translational Research
Emory University
Atlanta, Georgia

Dennis Savaiano, Ph.D.
Interim Dean of the Honors College
Professor of Nutrition Science
Purdue University
West Lafayette, Indiana

F. Edward Scarbrough, Ph.D.
Former Director, Office of Food Labeling (retired)
Center for Food Safety and Applied Nutrition
Food and Drug Administration
Germantown, Maryland

Ernst J. Schaefer, M.D.
Distinguished University Professor
Senior Scientist and Director
Lipid Metabolism Laboratory
Jean Mayer USDA Human Nutrition Research Center
on Aging at Tufts University
Tufts University School of Medicine
Friedman School of Nutrition Science and Policy
Consulting Physician
Division of Endocrinology and Metabolism
Tufts Medical Center
Boston, Massachusetts

Lauren Schwartz, M.D.
Assistant Professor of Medicine
Division of Gastroenterology
Department of Medicine
Mount Sinai School of Medicine
New York, New York

Michael Schweitzer, M.D.
Associate Professor of Surgery
Johns Hopkins University School of Medicine
Director of Johns Hopkins Obesity Surgery Center
Johns Hopkins Bayview Medical Center
Baltimore, Maryland

[†]Deceased.

Margaret Seide, M.D.
Clinical Associate
Department of Psychiatry and Behavioral Sciences
Johns Hopkins University School of Medicine
Attending Physician
Johns Hopkins Hospital
Baltimore, Maryland

Douglas L. Seidner, M.D., F.A.C.G.
Associate Professor of Medicine
Division of Gastroenterology, Hepatology, and Nutrition
Department of Medicine
Director, Vanderbilt Center for Human Nutrition
Vanderbilt University School of Medicine
Nashville, Tennessee

Richard D. Semba, M.D., M.P.H.
Professor
Ophthalmology
Johns Hopkins University
Baltimore, Maryland

Carol E. Semrad, M.D.
Professor of Medicine
Section of Gastroenterology, Hepatology and Nutrition
Department of Medicine
University of Chicago Medicine
Chicago, Illinois

Rannan Shamir, M.D.
Chairman
Institute for Gastroenterology, Nutrition and
Liver Diseases
Schneider Children's Medical Center of Israel
Petah Tikva, Israel
Professor of Pediatrics
Sackler Faculty of Medicine
Tel Aviv University
Ramat Aviv, Tel Aviv, Israel

Joanne L. Slavin, Ph.D., R.D.
Professor of Food Science and Nutrition
College of Food, Agricultural, and Natural Resource
Sciences
University of Minnesota Twin Cities Campus
St. Paul, Minnesota

Ellen Smit, Ph.D., R.D.
Associate Professor
School of Biological and Population Health Sciences
College of Public Health and Human Sciences
Oregon State University
Corvallis, Oregon

Meir J. Stampfer, M.D., Dr.P.H., M.P.H.
Professor
Departments of Epidemiology and Nutrition
Harvard School of Public Health
Chief, Chronic Disease Epidemiology Unit
Channing Division of Network Medicine
Department of Medicine
Brigham and Women's Hospital
Boston, Massachusetts

Charles B. Stephensen, Ph.D.
Research Leader
U.S. Department of Agriculture
Agricultural Research Service
Western Human Nutrition Research Center
Davis, California

Martha H. Stipanuk, Ph.D.
Professor
Division of Nutritional Sciences
Cornell University
Ithaca, New York

Patrick J. Stover, Ph.D.
Professor and Director
Division of Nutritional Sciences
Cornell University
Ithaca, New York

Shelby Sullivan, M.D.
Assistant Professor
Department of Internal Medicine
Washington University School of Medicine
Assistant Professor
Division of Gastroenterology
Barnes Jewish Hospital
St. Louis, Missouri

Roger A. Sunde, Ph.D.
Professor
Department of Nutritional Sciences
University of Wisconsin-Madison
Madison, Wisconsin

John W. Suttie, Ph.D.
Professor Emeritus of Biochemistry
University of Wisconsin-Madison
Madison, Wisconsin

Christine A. Swanson, Ph.D.
Senior Nutrition Scientist
Office of Dietary Supplements
National Institutes of Health
Bethesda, Maryland

Alice M. Tang, M.S., Ph.D.
Associate Professor
Department of Public Health and Community Medicine
Tufts University School of Medicine
Boston, Massachusetts

Christine Lewis Taylor, Ph.D.
Senior Nutrition Scientist
Office of Dietary Supplements
National Institutes of Health
Bethesda, Maryland

Steve L. Taylor, Ph.D.
Professor
Department of Food Science and Technology
University of Nebraska–Lincoln
Lincoln, Nebraska

Sandra Tejero, B.Sc.
Professor
Department of Food and Nutritional Sciences
The University of Reading
Reading, Berkshire, United Kingdom

Paul R. Thomas, Ed.D.
Scientific Consultant
Office of Dietary Supplements
National Institutes of Health
Bethesda, Maryland

Cheryl Toner, M.S., R.D.
Fellow
Nutritional Science Research Group
National Cancer Institute
National Institutes of Health
Rockville, Maryland

Riva Touger-Decker, Ph.D., R.D, F.A.D.A.
Professor
Nutritional Sciences
School of Health Related Professions
Diagnostic Sciences
New Jersey Dental School
University of Medicine and Dentistry of New Jersey
Newark, New Jersey

Maret G. Traber, Ph.D.
Professor
College Of Public Health and Human Sciences
Linus Pauling Institute
Oregon State University
Corvallis, Oregon

Paula R. Trumbo, Ph.D.
Acting Director
Nutrition Programs
Office of Nutrition, Labeling, and Dietary Supplements
Center for Food Safety and Applied Nutrition
U.S. Food and Drug Administration
College Park, Maryland

Katherine L. Tucker, Ph.D.
Professor
Department of Health Sciences
Northeastern University
Boston, Massachusetts

R. Elaine Turner, Ph.D., R.D.
Professor and Associate Dean
Food Science and Human Nutrition
College of Agricultural and Life Sciences
University of Florida
Gainesville, Florida

Kevin Tymitz, M.D.
Fellow, Minimally Invasive Surgery
Johns Hopkins University School of Medicine
Baltimore, Maryland

Ricardo Uauy, M.D., Ph.D.
Professor
Human Nutrition
Institute of Nutrition INTA
University of Chile
Santiago, Chile
Nutrition for Global Health
London, United Kingdom
Attending Physician
Neonatal Medicine
Neonatology Section, Department of Pediatrics
Pontificia Universidad Católica de Chile
Santiago, Chile

Jerry Vockley, M.D., Ph.D.
Professor of Pediatrics, School of Medicine
Professor of Human Genetics
Graduate School of Public Health
University of Pittsburgh
Chief of Medical Genetics
Children's Hospital of Pittsburgh of UPMC
Pittsburgh, Pennsylvania

Xiang-Dong Wang, M.D., Ph.D.
Director
Nutrition and Cancer Biology Laboratory
Jean Mayer USDA Human Nutrition Research Center
on Aging at Tufts University
Professor
Department of Biochemical and Molecular Nutrition
Friedman School of Nutrition Science and
Policy Tufts University
Boston, Massachusetts

Youfa Wang, M.D., M.S., Ph.D.
Associate Professor
Department of International Health
Johns Hopkins Bloomberg School of Public Health
Director
Johns Hopkins Global Center on Childhood Obesity
Baltimore, Maryland

Connie M. Weaver, Ph.D.
Distinguished Professor and Department Head
Nutrition Science
Purdue University
West Lafayette, Indiana

Edward P. Weiss, Ph.D.
Associate Professor
Department of Nutrition and Dietetics
Saint Louis University
Research Assistant Professor
Division of Geriatrics and Nutritional Science
Washington University School of Medicine
Saint Louis, Missouri

Marianne Wessling-Resnick, Ph.D.
Director of the Division of Biological Sciences and
Professor of Nutritional Biochemistry
Departments of Genetics and Complex Diseases
and Nutrition
Harvard School of Public Health
Boston, Massachusetts

Walter C. Willett, M.D., Dr.P.H.
Chair, Department of Nutrition
Fredrick John Stare Professor of Epidemiology
and Nutrition
Harvard School of Public Health
Channing Laboratory, Department of Medicine
Brigham and Women's Hospital and Harvard
Medical School
Boston, Massachusetts

Melvin H. Williams, Ph. D.
Eminent Scholar Emeritus
Department of Human Movement Sciences
Old Dominion University
Norfolk, Virginia

Holly J. Willis, Ph.D., R.D.
Research Associate
Department of Food Science and Nutrition
University of Minnesota
St. Paul, Minnesota

Ellen K. Wingert, O.T.R.
Senior Occupational Therapist
Manager, Feeding Day Program
Mt. Washington Pediatric Hospital
Baltimore, Maryland

Lynne A. Wolfe, M.S. C.R.N.P., B.C.
Nurse Practitioner
Undiagnosed Diseases Program
National Institutes of Health
Bethesda, Maryland

Holly R. Wyatt, M.D.
Associate Professor of Medicine
Anschutz Health and Wellness Center
Endocrinology, Metabolism and Diabetes
University of Colorado Anschutz Medical Campus
Aurora, Colorado

Steven H. Zeisel, M.D., Ph.D.
Director
Nutrition Research Institute
School of Public Health and School of Medicine
University of North Carolina at Chapel Hill
Kannapolis, North Carolina

Thomas R. Ziegler, M.D.
Professor of Medicine
Division of Endocrinology, Metabolism, and Lipids
Emory University Hospital Nutrition and Metabolic
Support Service
Emory University School of Medicine
Atlanta, Georgia

Susan J. Zunino, Ph.D.
Research Molecular Biologist
Immunity and Disease Prevention Research Unit
USDA/ARS Western Human Nutrition Research Center
Davis, California

CONTENTS

Part V. Nutrition of Populations

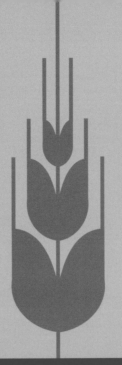

SPECIFIC DIETARY COMPONENTS

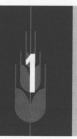

PROTEINS AND AMINO ACIDS[1]

DWIGHT E. MATTHEWS

Proteins are associated with all forms of life, and much of the effort to determine how life began has centered on how proteins were first produced. Amino acids joined together in long strings by peptide bonds form proteins that twist and fold in three-dimensional space and produce

centers to facilitate the biochemical reactions of life that either would run out of control or not run at all without them. Life could not have begun without these enzymes, thousands of different types of which are found in the body. Proteins are prepared and secreted to act as cell–cell signals in the form of hormones and cytokines. Plasma proteins produced and secreted by the liver stabilize the blood by forming a solution of the appropriate viscosity and osmolarity. These secreted proteins also transport a variety of compounds through the blood.

The largest source of protein in higher animals resides in muscle. Through complex interactions, entire sheets of proteins slide back and forth to form the basis of muscle contraction and all aspects of our mobility. Muscle contraction provides for pumping oxygen and nutrients throughout the body, for inhalation and exhalation of our lungs, and for movement. Many of the underlying causes of noninfectious diseases are the result of derangements in the sequence of proteins. The incredible advances in molecular biology provided tremendous information about DNA and RNA and introduced the field of genomics. This research is not driven to understand DNA itself, but rather to understand the purpose and function of the proteins that are translated from the genetic code. The emerging field of proteomics studies the expression, modification, and regulation of proteins.

Three major classes of substrates are used for energy: carbohydrates, fat, and protein. Protein differs from the other two primary sources of dietary energy by inclusion of nitrogen (N). Protein on average is 16% by weight N. The component amino acids of proteins contain one N in the form of an amino group and additional N, depending on the amino acid. When amino acids are oxidized to carbon dioxide (CO_2) and water to produce energy, N is also produced as a waste product that must be eliminated via incorporation into urea. Conversely, N must be available when the body synthesizes amino acids de novo. The synthetic routes of other N-containing compounds in the body (e.g., nucleic acids for DNA and RNA synthesis) obtain their N during synthesis from donation of N from amino acids. Therefore, when we think of amino acid metabolism in the body, we really mean N metabolism.

Protein and amino acids are also important to the energy metabolism of the body. As Cahill pointed out (1),

---

[1]**Abbreviations: ATP**, adenosine triphosphate; **AV**; arteriovenous; **BCAA**, branched-chain amino acid; **CO₂**, carbon dioxide; **CoA**, coenzyme A; **DAAO**, direct amino acid oxidation; **EAR**, estimated average requirement; **FAO/WHO/UNU**, Food and Agriculture Organization/World Health Organization/United Nations University; **IAAO**, indicator amino acid oxidation; **IDAA**, indispensable amino acid; **KIC**, α-ketoisocaproate; **N**, nitrogen; **NH₃**, ammonia; **PER**, protein efficiency ratio; **RDA**, recommended dietary allowance; **TCA**, tricarboxylic acid; **TML**, trimethyllysine.

TABLE 1.1	BODY COMPOSITION OF A NORMAL MAN IN TERMS OF ENERGY COMPONENTS		
COMPONENT	MASS (kg)	ENERGY (kcal)	AVAILABILITY[a] (d)
Body water and minerals	49.0	0	0
Protein	6.0	24,000	13.0
Glycogen	0.2	800	0.4
Fat	15.0	140,000	78.0
Total	70.0	164,800	91.4

[a]Availability is the duration for which the energy supply would last based on 1800 kcal/day resting energy consumption.

Data from Cahill GF. Starvation in man. N Engl J Med 1970;282:668–75, with permission.

protein is the second largest store of energy in the body after adipose tissue fat stores (Table 1.1). Carbohydrate is stored as glycogen, and although it is important for short-term energy needs, it is of very limited capacity for providing for energy needs beyond a few hours. Amino acids from protein are converted to glucose by the process called gluconeogenesis to provide a continuing supply of glucose after the glycogen is consumed during fasting. Conversely, however, protein stores must be conserved for the numerous critical roles in which protein functions in the body. Loss of more than approximately 30% of body protein results in reductions in muscle strength for breathing, immune function, organ function and, ultimately, in death. Hence, the body must adapt to fasting by conserving protein, as is seen by a dramatic decrease in N excretion within the first week of onset of starvation.

Body protein is made up of 20 different amino acids, each with different metabolic fates in the body, with diverse activities in different metabolic pathways in different organs, and with varying compositions in different proteins. When amino acids are liberated after absorption of dietary protein, the body makes a complex series of decisions concerning the fate of those amino acids: to oxidize them for energy, to incorporate them into proteins in the body, or to use them in the formation of a number of other N-containing compounds. The purpose of this chapter is to elucidate the complex pathways and roles amino acids play in the body, with a focus on nutrition.

AMINO ACIDS

Basic Definitions

The amino acids that we are familiar with and all those incorporated into mammalian protein are "α"-amino acids. By definition, they have a carboxyl-carbon group and an amino N group attached to a central α-carbon (Fig. 1.1). Amino acids differ in structure by the substitution of one of the two hydrogens on the α-carbon with another functional group. Amino acids can be characterized by their functional groups, which are often organized at neutral pH into the classes of (a) nonpolar,

(b) uncharged but polar, (c) acidic (negatively charged), and (d) basic (positively charged) groups. Within any class are considerable differences in shape and physical properties. Thus, amino acids are often grouped into other functional subgroups. For example, amino acids with an aromatic group—phenylalanine, tyrosine, tryptophan, and histidine—are often associated together, although tyrosine is clearly polar and histidine is also basic. Other common groupings are the aliphatic or neutral amino acids (glycine, alanine, isoleucine, leucine, valine, serine, threonine, and proline). Proline is different in that its functional group is also attached to the amino group, thus forming a five-membered ring. Because of the ring, proline is actually an *imino* acid, not an amino acid. Serine and threonine contain hydroxyl groups. There is also another important subgroup: the branched-chain amino acids (BCAAs: isoleucine, leucine, and valine), which share common enzymes for the first two steps of their degradation. The acidic amino acids, aspartic acid and glutamic acid, are often referred to as their ionized, salt forms: *aspartate* and *glutamate*. These amino acids become *asparagine* and *glutamine* when an amino group is added in the form of an amide group to their carboxyl tails.

The sulfur-containing amino acids are methionine and cysteine. Cysteine is often found in the body as an amino acid dimer called *cystine* in which the thiol groups (the two sulfur atoms) are connected to form a disulfide bond. Particular attention should be paid when reading the literature to note the distinction between the names *cysteine* and *cystine*, because the former is a single amino acid, and the latter is a dimer with different properties. Other amino acids that contain sulfur, such as homocysteine, are not incorporated into protein.

All amino acids exist as charged particles in solution: in water, the carboxyl group rapidly loses a hydrogen to form a carboxyl anion (negatively charged), whereas the amino group gains a hydrogen to become positively charged. The amino acids therefore become "bipolar" (often called a *zwitterion*) in solution, but without a net charge (the positive and negatively charges cancel). The attached functional group may distort that balance, however. The acidic amino acids lose the hydrogen on the second carboxyl group and become negatively charged in solution. In contrast, the basic group amino acids in part accept a hydrogen on the second N and form a molecule with a net positive charge. Although the other amino acids do not specifically accept or donate additional hydrogens in neutral solution, their functional groups do influence the relative polarity and acid–base nature of the bipolar portion of the amino acids and give each amino acid different properties in solution.

The functional groups of amino acids also vary by size. The molecular weights of the amino acids are shown in Table 1.2. Amino acids range from the smallest, glycine, to the large and bulky molecules (e.g., tryptophan). Most amino acids crystallize as uncharged molecules when they

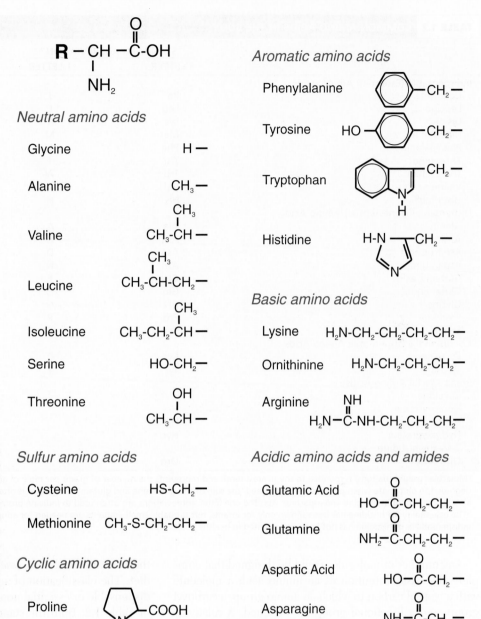

Fig. 1.1. Structural formulas of the 21 common α-amino acids. The α-amino acids all have a carboxyl group, an amino group, and a differentiating functional group attached to the α-carbon. The generic structure of amino acids is shown in the **upper left corner** with the differentiating functional group marked by *R*. The functional group for each amino acid is shown below. Amino acids have been grouped by functional class. Proline is actually an imino acid because of its cyclic structure involving its nitrogen (N).

are purified and dried. The molecular weights shown in Table 1.2 reflect their molecular weight as crystalline amino acids. The basic and acidic amino acids tend to form much more stable crystals as salts, however, rather than as free amino acids. Glutamic acid can be obtained as the free amino acid with a molecular weight of 147 and as its sodium salt, monosodium glutamate, which has a crystalline weight of 169. Lysine is typically found as a salt containing hydrogen chloride. Therefore, when amino acids are represented by weight, it is important to know whether the weight is based on the free amino acid or on its salt.

Another important property of amino acids is optical activity. Except for glycine, which has its functional group as a single hydrogen, all amino acids have at least one chiral center: the α-carbon. The term "chiral" comes from Greek for *hand* in that these molecules have a left ("*levo*" or "L") and right ("*dextro*" or "D") handedness to them around the α-carbon atom. Because of the tetrahedral structure of the carbon bonds, there are two possible arrangements of a carbon center with the same four different groups bonded to it that are not superimposable; the two configurations, called *stereoisomers*, are mirror images of each other. The body recognizes only the L-form of amino acids for most reactions in the body, although some enzymatic reactions will operate with a lower efficiency when given the D-form. Because we do encounter some D-form amino acids in the foods that we eat, the body has some mechanisms for clearing these amino acids through renal filtration.

TABLE 1.2	COMMON AMINO ACIDS IN THE BODY		
	STANDARD ABBREVIATION		
	3-LETTER	1-LETTER	MOLECULAR WEIGHT[a]
Indispensable (Essential) Amino Acids			
Isoleucine	Ile	I	131.2
Leucine	Leu	L	131.2
Lysine	Lys	K	146.2
Methionine	Met	M	149.2
Phenylalanine	Phe	F	165.2
Threonine	Thr	T	119.1
Tryptophan	Trp	W	204.2
Valine	Val	V	117.2
Histidine[b]	His	H	155.2
Dispensable (Nonessential) Amino Acids			
Alanine	Ala	A	89.1
Arginine	Arg	R	174.2
Aspartic acid	Asp	D	133.2
Asparagine	Asn	N	132.2
Glutamic acid	Glu	E	147.2
Glutamine	Gln	Q	146.2
Glycine	Gly	G	75.1
Proline	Pro	P	115.1
Serine	Ser	S	105.1
Conditionally Dispensable Amino Acids			
Cysteine	Cys	C	121.2
Tyrosine	Tyr	Y	181.2
Some Special Amino Acids			
Citrulline			175.2
Homocysteine	Hcy		135.2
Hydroxylysine	Hyl		162.2
Hydroxyproline	Hyp		131.2
3-Methylhistidine			169.2
Ornithine	Orn		132.2

[a]Molecular weight (daltons) is rounded to the nearest tenth and represents the number of grams per mole of amino acid. Because glutamine is degraded to glutamate when proteins are hydrolyzed, the sum of the glutamine and glutamate together is often abbreviated Glx. The same is true also for the sum of asparagine and aspartate: Asx. The one-letter abbreviations are often used to indicate protein sequences.
[b]The essentiality for histidine has been shown only for infants, but probably small amounts are needed for adults as well. To date, the indispensability of histidine has not been documented in healthy adults (6).

Any number of molecules could be designed that complete the basic definition of an amino acid: a molecule with a central carbon to which an amino group, a carboxyl group, and a functional group are attached. A relatively limited variety appears in nature, however, and only 20 are incorporated directly into mammalian protein. Amino acids are selected for protein synthesis when coupled to transfer RNA (tRNA). To synthesize protein, strands of DNA are transcribed into messenger RNA (mRNA). tRNA binds to mRNA in 3-base groups. Different combinations of 3 consecutive RNA molecules in the mRNA code for different tRNA molecules. However, the 3-base combinations of mRNA are recognized by only 20 different tRNA molecules, and 20 different amino acids are incorporated into protein during protein synthesis.

Of these 20 amino acids in proteins, some are synthesized de novo in the body either from other amino acids or from simpler precursors. These amino acids may be deleted from our diet without impairing health or blocking growth. These amino acids are *nonessential* and *dispensable* from the diet. No pathways exist for the synthesis of several other amino acids in humans, however, and hence

these amino acids are *essential* or *indispensable* to the diet. The classification of amino acids as nondispensable/dispensable or essential/nonessential for humans is shown in Table 1.2. Both the standard three-letter abbreviation and the one-letter abbreviation used in representing amino acid sequences in proteins are also presented in Table 1.2 for each amino acid. Some dispensable amino acids may become *conditionally indispensable* under conditions when synthesis becomes limited or when adequate amounts of precursors are unavailable to meet the needs of the body (2–4). The history and rationale of the classification of amino acids in Table 1.2 are discussed in greater detail later in this chapter.

Besides the 20 amino acids that are recognized by tRNA for incorporation into protein, other amino acids appear commonly in the body. These amino acids have important metabolic functions. Examples are ornithine and citrulline, which are linked to arginine through the urea cycle. Other amino acids appear as modifications of amino acids after they have been incorporated into proteins. Examples are hydroxyproline and hydroxylysine, which are produced when proline and lysine residues in collagen protein are hydroxylated, and 3-methylhistidine, which is produced by posttranslational methylation of select histidine residues of actin and myosin proteins. Because no tRNA exists to code for these amino acids, they cannot be reused when a protein containing them is broken down (hydrolyzed) to its individual amino acids.

Amino Acid Pools and Distribution

The distribution of amino acids is complex. Not only are different amino acids incorporated into a variety of different proteins in many different organs in the body, but also amino acids are consumed in the diet from numerous protein sources. In addition, each amino acid is maintained in part as a free amino acid in solution in blood and inside cells. Overall, a wide range of concentrations is found among amino acids across the various protein and free pools that exist. We consume protein in food that is enzymatically hydrolyzed in the alimentary tract, thus releasing free individual amino acids that are then absorbed by the gut lumen and are transported into portal blood. Amino acids then pass into the systemic circulation and are extracted by different tissues. Although the concentrations of individual amino acids vary among different free pools such as plasma and intracellular muscle, the abundance of individual amino acids is relatively constant in a variety of proteins throughout the body and nature. Table 1.3 shows

the composition of amino acids in hen egg protein, mammalian muscle and liver proteins (5), and human milk (6). The data are expressed as *moles* of amino acid. The historical expression of amino acids is on a weight basis (e.g., *grams* of amino acid). Comparing amino acids by weight skews the comparison toward the heaviest amino acids and makes them appear more abundant than they are. For example, tryptophan (molecular weight 204) appears almost three times as abundant as glycine (molecular weight 75) when quoted in terms of weight.

An even distribution of all 20 amino acids would be 5% per amino acid per protein, and the median amino acid content centers around this value for the proteins shown in Table 1.3. Tryptophan is the least common amino acid in many proteins. Considering the effect of tryptophan's large size on the conformation of proteins, it is not surprising to find less tryptophan in protein. Other amino acids of modest size and limited polarity, such as alanine, leucine, serine, and valine, are relatively abundant in protein (8% to 10% per amino acid). Although the abundance of the indispensable amino acids (IDAAs) is similar across the protein sources in Table 1.3, various vegetable proteins are deficient or low in some IDAAs. In the body, certain proteins are particularly rich in specific amino acids to produce specific functions in the protein. For example, collagen is a fibrous protein abundant in connective tissues in tendons, bone, and muscle. Collagen fibrils are arranged in different ways, depending on the functional type of collagen. Glycine comprises approximately one third of collagen, and there is also considerable proline and hydroxyproline (proline converted after it has been incorporated into collagen). The glycine and proline residues allow the collagen protein chain to turn tightly and intertwine, and the hydroxyproline residues provide for hydrogen bond crosslinking. Generally, the alterations in amino acid concentrations do not vary dramatically among proteins as they do in collagen, but such examples demonstrate the diversity and functionality of the different amino acids in proteins.

The abundance of amino acids varies among amino acids over a far wider range in the free pools of extracellular and intracellular compartments. Typical values of free amino acid concentrations in plasma and in intracellular muscle are shown in Table 1.4. The primary points of Table 1.4 are as follows: (a) amino acid concentrations vary widely among amino acids, and (b) free amino acids are generally concentrated inside cells. Although the correlation between plasma and muscle free intracellular amino acid levels is significant, the relationship is not linear (7). Concentrations of plasma amino acids range from a low of approximately 20 μM for aspartic acid and methionine to a high of approximately 500 μM for glutamine. The median level for plasma amino acids is 100 μM. No defined relationship exists between the nature of amino acids (IDAAs versus dispensable amino acids) and amino acid concentrations or type of amino acids (e.g., plasma concentrations of the three BCAAs range from 50 to 250 μM). One notable point is that the concentrations

TABLE 1.3	AMINO ACID COMPOSITION OF SEVERAL DIFFERENT PROTEIN SOURCES			
	COMPOSITION (μmol/g PROTEIN)			
		MAMMALIAN		
AMINO ACID	HEN EGG	MUSCLE	LIVER	HUMAN MILK
Alanine	810	730	750	426
Arginine	360	380	328	132
Aspartate + Asparagine	530	600	600	679
Cysteine	190	120	140	182
Glutamate + Glutamine	810	990	800	1,206
Glycine	450	670	610	306
Histidine	150	180	170	148
Isoleucine	490	360	380	434
Leucine	650	610	690	770
Lysine	425	580	510	472
Methionine	200	170	170	107
Phenylalanine	340	270	310	242
Proline	350	430	430	695
Serine	770	480	510	476
Threonine	410	390	390	395
Tryptophan	80	55	80	88
Tyrosine	220	170	200	259
Valine	600	470	520	538

Data from Block RJ, Weiss KW. Amino Acid Handbook: Methods and Results of Analysis. Springfield, IL: Charles C Thomas, 1956:343–4; and Food and Agriculture Organization/World Health Organization/United Nations University. Protein and Amino Acid Requirements in Human Nutrition. Geneva: World Health Organization, 2007:1–256, with permission.

TABLE 1.4	TYPICAL CONCENTRATIONS OF FREE AMINO ACIDS IN THE BODY		

AMINO ACID		PLASMA	CONCENTRATION (mM) INTRACELLULAR MUSCLE	GRADIENT INTRACELLULAR/ PLASMA
Aspartic acid	D	0.02		
Phenylalanine	I	0.05	0.07	1.4
Tyrosine	CI	0.05	0.10	2.0
Methionine	I	0.02	0.11	5.5
Isoleucine	I	0.06	0.11	1.8
Leucine	I	0.12	0.15	1.3
Cysteine	CI	0.11	0.18	1.6
Valine	I	0.22	0.26	1.2
Ornithine		0.06	0.30	5.0
Histidine	I	0.08	0.37	4.6
Asparagine	D	0.05	0.47	9.4
Arginine	D	0.08	0.51	6.4
Proline	D	0.17	0.83	4.9
Serine	D	0.12	0.98	8.2
Threonine	I	0.15	1.03	6.9
Lysine	I	0.18	1.15	6.4
Glycine	D	0.21	1.33	6.3
Alanine	D	0.33	2.34	7.1
Glutamic acid	D	0.06	4.38	73.0
Glutamine	D	0.57	19.45	34.1
Taurine[a]		0.07	15.44	221.0

CI, conditionally indispensable; D, dispensable; I, indispensable.

[a]Taurine is not an amino acid itself, but is highly concentrated in free form in muscle.

Data from Bergström J, Fürst P, Norée LO et al. Intracellular free amino acid concentration in human muscle tissue. J Appl Physiol 1974;36:693–7, with permission.

of the acidic amino acids, aspartate and glutamate, are very low outside cells in plasma. In contrast, the concentration of glutamate is among the highest inside cells, such as muscle (Table 1.4).

Important to bear in mind are the differences in the relative amounts of N contained in extracellular and intracellular amino acid pools and in protein itself. A physiologically normal person has approximately 55 mg of amino acid N/L outside cells in extracellular space and approximately 800 mg of amino acid N/L inside cells; this means that free amino acids are approximately 15-fold more abundant inside cells than outside cells (7). The second point is that the total pool of free amino acid N is small compared with protein-bound amino acids. Multiplying the free pools by estimates of extracellular water (0.2 L/kg) and intracellular water (0.4 L/kg) provides a measure of the total amount of N present in free amino acids: 0.33 g N/kg body weight. In contrast, body composition studies have shown that the N content of the body is 24 g N/kg body weight (8, 9). Therefore, free amino acids make up approximately 1% of the total amino N pool versus more than 99% of the amino acids that reside in proteins.

Amino Acid Transport

The gradient of amino acids within and outside cells is maintained by active transport. From a simple scan of

Table 1.4, it is clear that different transport mechanisms must exist for different amino acids to produce the range of concentration gradients observed. Many different transporters exist for different types and groups of amino acids (10–12). Amino acid transport is probably one of the more difficult areas of amino acid metabolism to quantify and characterize. The affinities of the transporters and their mechanisms of transport set the intracellular levels of the amino acids. Generally, the IDAAs have lower intracellular/extracellular gradients than do the dispensable amino acids (Table 1.4) and are transported by different carriers. The amino acid transporters are membrane-bound proteins that recognize different amino acid shapes and chemical properties (e.g., neutral, basic, or anionic). Transport occurs both into and out of cells. Transport may be thought of as a process that sets the intracellular/extracellular gradient, or the transporters may be thought of as processes that set the rates of amino acid influx into and efflux from cells, which then define the intracellular/extracellular gradients (10). Perhaps the more dynamic concept of transport defining flows of amino acids is more appropriate, but in real life the gradient (e.g., intracellular muscle amino acid levels) is measurable, not the rates.

The transporters fall into two classes: sodium-independent and sodium-dependent carriers. The sodium-dependent carriers cotransport a sodium atom into the cell along with the amino acid. The high extracellular/intracellular sodium gradient (140 mEq outside and 10 mEq inside) facilitates the inward transport of amino acids by the sodium-dependent carriers. These transporters generally produce larger gradients and accumulations of amino acids inside cells than outside them. The sodium entering the cell may be transported out via the sodium–potassium pump that transports a potassium ion in for the removal of a sodium ion.

Few of the transporter proteins have been identified; most information concerning transport has been accrued through kinetic studies of membranes using amino acids and competitive inhibitors or amino acid analogs to define and characterize individual systems. Table 1.5 lists the different amino acid transporters characterized to date and the amino acids they transport. The neutral and bulky amino acids (the BCAAs, phenylalanine, methionine, and histidine) are transported by system L. System L is sodium independent and operates with a high rate of exchange and produces small gradients. Other important transporters are systems ASC and A. These transporters use the energy available from the sodium-ion gradient as a driving force to maintain a steep gradient for the various amino acids transported (e.g., glycine, alanine, threonine, serine, and proline) (10, 11). The anionic transporter (X_{AG-}) also produces a steep gradient for the dicarboxylic amino acids, glutamate and aspartate. Other important carriers are system N and N^m for glutamine, asparagine, and histidine. System y^+ handles much of the transport

TABLE 1.5	AMINO ACID TRANSPORTERS		
SYSTEM	AMINO ACID TRANSPORTED	TISSUE LOCATION	pH DEPENDENCE
Sodium dependent			
A	Most neutrals (Ala, Ser)	Ubiquitous	Yes
ASC	Most neutrals	Ubiquitous	No
B	Most neutrals	Intestinal brush border	Yes
N	Gln, Asn, His	Hepatocytes	Yes
N^m	Gln, Asn	Muscle	No
Gly	Gly, sarcosine	Ubiquitous	
X_{AG-}	Glu, Asp	Ubiquitous	
Sodium independent			
L	Leu, Ile, Val, Met, Phe, Tyr, Trp, His	Ubiquitous	Yes
T	Trp, Phe, Tyr	Red blood cells, hepatocytes	No
y^+	Arg, Lys, Orn	Ubiquitous	No
asc	Ala, Ser, Cys, Thr	Ubiquitous	Yes

Data from references 10 to 12, with permission.

of the basic amino acids. Some overall generalizations can be made in terms of the type of amino acid transported by a given carrier, but the system is not readily simplified because individual carrier systems transport several different amino acids, whereas individual amino acids are often transported by several different carriers with different efficiencies. Thus, amino acid gradients are formed and amino acids are transported into and out of cells via a complex system of overlapping carriers.

PATHWAYS OF AMINO ACID SYNTHESIS AND DEGRADATION

Several amino acids have their metabolic pathways linked to the metabolism of other amino acids. These codependencies that link the pathways of amino acids become important when nutrient intake is limited or when metabolic requirements are increased. Two aspects of metabolism are reviewed here: (a) synthesis of amino acids and (b) amino acid degradation. Degradation serves two useful purposes: (a) production of energy from the oxidation of individual amino acids ($\approx$4 kcal/g protein, almost the same energy production as for carbohydrate) and (b) conversion of amino acids into other products. The latter is also related to amino acid synthesis: the degradation pathway of one amino acid may be the synthetic pathway of another amino acid. The other important aspect of amino acid degradation is production of other nonamino acid, N-containing compounds in the body. The need for synthesis of these compounds may also drain the pools of their amino acid precursors and thus increase the need for these amino acids in the diet. When amino acids are degraded for energy rather than converted to other compounds, the ultimate products become CO_2, water, and urea. The CO_2 and water are produced through classical pathways of intermediary metabolism involving the tricarboxylic acid (TCA) cycle. The urea is produced because other forms of waste N, such as ammonia (NH_3), are toxic if their levels rise in the blood and inside cells.

For mammals, urea production is a means of removal of waste N from the oxidation of amino acids in the form of a nontoxic, water-soluble compound.

More detailed descriptions of the amino acid pathways can be found in standard textbooks of biochemistry. Keep in mind when consulting such texts that pathways for nonmammalian systems (e.g., *Escherichia coli* and yeast) are often presented, and these pathways often have little importance to human biochemistry. When consulting reference material, the reader needs to be aware of the system of life from which the metabolic pathways and enzymes are being discussed. The discussion here is relevant to human biochemistry. Presented first is a discussion of the routes of degradation of each amino acid when the pathway is directed toward oxidation of the amino acid for energy. Next follows a discussion of pathways of amino acid synthesis, and finally the use of amino acids for other important compounds in the body is described.

Amino Acid Degradation Pathways

Complete amino acid degradation ends up with the production of N, which is removed by incorporation into urea. Carbon skeletons are eventually oxidized as CO_2 via the TCA cycle (also known as the Krebs cycle or the citric acid cycle). The inputs to the cycle are acetyl-coenzyme A (CoA) and oxaloacetate forming citrate, which is degraded to α-ketoglutarate and then to oxaloacetate. The carbon skeletons from amino acid may enter the Krebs cycle via acetate as acetyl-CoA or via oxaloacetate/α-ketoglutarate. These latter two precursors are direct metabolites of the amino acids aspartate and glutamate. An alternative to the complete oxidation of the carbon skeletons to CO_2 is the use of these carbon skeletons for the formation of fat and carbohydrate. Fat is formed from elongation of acetyl units, and so amino acids whose carbon skeletons degrade to acetyl-CoA and ketones may alternatively be used for synthesis of fatty acids. Glucose is split in glycolysis to pyruvate, and pyruvate is the immediate product of alanine. Pyruvate may be converted back to glucose by elongation to oxaloacetate. Amino acids whose degradation pathways go toward formation of pyruvate, oxaloacetate, or α-ketoglutarate may be used for synthesis of glucose. Therefore, the degradation pathways of many amino acids can be partitioned into two groups with respect to the disposal of their carbon: amino acids whose carbon skeleton may be used for synthesis of glucose (gluconeogenic amino acids) or those whose carbon skeletons degrade for potential use for fatty acid synthesis.

The amino acids that degrade directly to the primary gluconeogenic and TCA cycle precursors, pyruvate, oxaloacetate, and α-ketoglutarate, do so by rapid and reversible transamination reactions:

$$\text{L-glutamate} + \text{oxaloacetate} \leftrightarrow \alpha\text{-ketoglutarate} + \text{L-aspartate}$$

by the enzyme aspartate aminotransferase, which, of course, also can be

$$\text{L-aspartate} + \alpha\text{-ketoglutarate} \leftrightarrow \text{oxaloacetate} + \text{L-glutamate}$$

and

$$\text{L-alanine} + \alpha\text{-ketoglutarate} \leftrightarrow \text{pyruvate} + \text{L-glutamate}$$

by the enzyme alanine aminotransferase. What is quickly apparent is that the amino-N of these three amino acids may be rapidly exchanged and each amino acid rapidly converted to and from a primary compound of gluconeogenesis and the TCA cycle. As described later, compartmentation among different organ pools is the only limiting factor for complete and rapid exchange of the N of these amino acids.

The IDAAs leucine, isoleucine, and valine are grouped together under the heading of the BCAAs because the first two steps in their degradation pathway are common to all three amino acids:

$$\left.\begin{array}{l}\text{Leucine}\\\text{Isoleucine}\\\text{Valine}\end{array}\right\} + \alpha\text{-ketoglutarate} \leftrightarrow \text{glutamate} + \left\{\begin{array}{l}\alpha\text{-ketoisocaproate}\\\alpha\text{-keto-}\beta\text{-methylvalerate}\\\alpha\text{-ketovalerate}\end{array}\right.$$

The reversible transamination to keto acids is followed by irreversible decarboxylation of the carboxyl group to liberate CO_2. The BCAAs are the only IDAAs that undergo transamination and therefore are unique among IDAAs.

Together, the BCAAs, alanine, aspartate, and glutamate make up the pool of amino-N that can move among amino acids via reversible transamination. As shown in Figure 1.2, glutamic acid is central to the transamination process. In addition, N can leave the transaminating pool by removal of the glutamate N via glutamate dehydrogenase, or it can enter by the reverse process. The amino acid glutamine is intimately tied to glutamate as well: all glutamine is made from amidation of glutamate, and glutamine is degraded by removal of the amide-N to form NH_3 and glutamate.

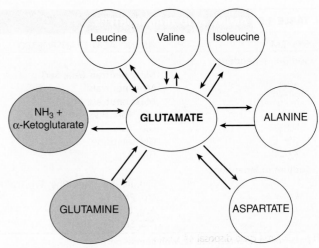

Fig. 1.2. Movement of amino-nitrogen (N) around glutamic acid. Glutamate undergoes reversible transamination with several amino acids. Nitrogen is also removed from glutamate by glutamate dehydrogenase, thus producing an α-ketoglutarate and an ammonia. In contrast, the enzyme glutamine synthetase adds an ammonia to glutamate to produce glutamine. Glutamine is degraded back to glutamate by liberation of the amide-N to release ammonia by a different enzymatic pathway (glutaminase). NH_3, ammonia.

A similar process occurs for formation and degradation of asparagine from aspartate. In terms of N metabolism, Figure 1.2 shows that the center of N flow in the body is through glutamate. This role becomes even clearer when we look at how urea is synthesized in the liver. The inputs into the urea cycle are a CO_2, adenosine triphosphate (ATP), and NH_3 to form carbamoyl phosphate, which condenses with ornithine to form citrulline (Fig. 1.3). The second N enters via aspartate to form argininosuccinate, which is then cleaved into arginine and fumarate. The arginine is hydrolyzed by arginase to ornithine, thus liberating urea. The resulting ornithine can reenter the urea cycle. As mentioned briefly later, some amino acids may liberate NH_3 directly (e.g., glutamine, asparagine, and glycine), but most transfer through glutamate first, which is then degraded to α-ketoglutarate and NH_3. The pool of aspartate is small in the body, and aspartate cannot be the primary transporter of the second N into urea synthesis. Rather, aspartate must act like arginine and ornithine as a vehicle for the introduction of the second N. If so, the second N is delivered by transamination via glutamate, again placing glutamate at another integral point in the degradative disposal of amino acid N.

An outline of the degradative pathways of the various amino acids is presented in Table 1.6. Rather than show individual reaction steps, the major pathways for degradation, including the primary end products, are presented. The individual steps may be found in current textbooks of biochemistry or in older reviews on the subject (13). Because of the importance of transamination, the majority of the N from amino acid degradation appears via N transfer to α-ketoglutarate to form glutamate. In some

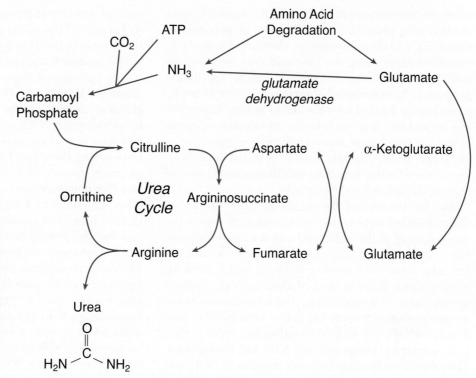

Fig. 1.3. Urea cycle disposal of amino acid nitrogen (N). Urea synthesis incorporates one N from ammonia (NH₃) and another from aspartate. Ornithine, citrulline, and arginine sit in the middle of the cycle. Glutamate is the primary source for the aspartate N; glutamate is also an important source of the ammonia into the cycle. *ATP,* adenosine triphosphate; *CO₂,* carbon dioxide; *NH₂,* amine.

TABLE 1.6	PATHWAYS OF AMINO ACID DEGRADATION		
METABOLIC PATHWAY	IMPORTANT ENZYMES	NITROGEN END PRODUCTS	CARBON END PRODUCTS
Amino acids converted to other amino acids			
Asparagine	Asparaginase	Aspartate + NH₃	
Glutamine	Glutaminase	Glutamate + NH₃	
Arginine	Arginase	Ornithine + Urea	
Phenylalanine	Phenylalanine hydroxylase	Tyrosine	
Proline		Glutamate	
Serine	Serine hydroxymethyltransferase	Glycine	
Cysteine		Taurine	
Amino acids transaminating to form glutamate			
Alanine		Glutamate	Pyruvate
Aspartate		Glutamate	Oxaloacetate
Cysteine		Glutamate	Pyruvate + SO₄⁻²
Isoleucine		Glutamate	Succinate
Leucine		Glutamate	Ketones
Ornithine		Glutamate	α-Ketoglutarate
Serine		Glutamate	3-Phosphoglycerate
Valine		Glutamate	Succinate
Tyrosine		Glutamate	Ketone + fumarate
Other pathways			
Glycine		NH₃	CO₂
Histidine		NH₃	Urocanate
Methionine		NH₃	Ketobutyrate
Serine	Serine dehydratase	NH₃	Pyruvate
Threonine	Serine dehydratase	NH₃	Ketobutyrate
Tryptophan		NH₃	Kynurenine
Lysine		2 Glutamates	Ketones

CO_2, carbon dioxide; NH_3, ammonia; SO_4^{-2}, sulfate.

cases, the aminotransferase catalyzes the transamination reaction with glutamate bidirectionally, as indicated in Figure 1.2, and these enzymes are distributed in multiple tissues. In other cases, the transamination reactions are liver specific, are compartmentalized, and act specifically to degrade N, not reversibly exchange it. For example, when leucine labeled with the stable isotope tracer ^{15}N was infused into dogs for 9 hours, considerable amounts of the ^{15}N tracer were found in circulating glutamine + glutamate, alanine, the other two BCAAs, but not in tyrosine (14)—a finding indicating that the transamination of tyrosine did not proceed backward.

Another reason that the entries in Table 1.6 do not show individual steps is that the specific pathways of the metabolism of all the amino acids are not clearly defined. For example, two pathways for cysteine are shown. Both are active, but how much cysteine is metabolized by which pathway is not as clear. Methionine is metabolized by conversion to homocysteine. The homocysteine is not directly converted to cysteine; rather, homocysteine condenses with a serine to form cystathionine, which is then broken apart to liberate cysteine, NH_3, and ketobutyrate. The original methionine molecule appears as NH_3 and ketobutyrate, however. The cysteine carbon skeleton comes from the serine. So the entry in Table 1.6 shows methionine degraded to NH_3, yet this degradation pathway is the major synthesis pathway for cysteine. Because of the importance of the sulfur-containing amino acids, a more extensive discussion of the metabolic pathways of these amino acids may be found in a later chapter.

Glycine is degraded by more than one possible pathway, depending on the text used for reference. The primary pathway, however, appears to be the glycine cleavage enzyme system that breaks glycine into CO_2 and NH_3 and transfers a methylene group to tetrahydrofolate (15). This pathway has been shown to be the prominent pathway in rat liver and in other vertebrate species (16). Although this reaction degrades glycine, its importance is the production of a methylene group that can be used in other metabolic reactions.

Synthesis of Dispensable Amino Acids

The IDAAs are those amino acids that cannot be synthesized in sufficient amounts in the body and therefore must be in the diet in sufficient amounts to meet the body's needs. Therefore, discussion of amino acid synthesis applies only to the dispensable amino acids. Dispensable amino acid synthesis falls into two groups: (a) amino acids that are synthesized by transferring an N to a carbon skeleton precursor that has come from the TCA cycle or from glycolysis of glucose and (b) amino acids that are synthesized specifically from other amino acids. Because this latter group of amino acids depends on the availability of other, specific amino acids, these amino acids are particularly vulnerable to becoming indispensable if the dietary supply of a precursor amino acid becomes limiting. In contrast, the former group is rarely rate limited in synthesis because of the ample precursor availability of carbon skeletons from the TCA cycle and from the labile amino-N pool of transaminating amino acids.

The pathways of dispensable amino acid synthesis are shown in Figure 1.4. As with amino acid degradation, glutamate is central to the synthesis of several amino acids by providing the N for synthesis. Glutamate, alanine, and aspartate may share amino-N transaminating back and forth among them (see Fig. 1.2). As Figure 1.4 is drawn, glutamate derives its N from NH_3 with α-ketoglutarate, and that glutamate goes on to promote the synthesis of other amino acids. Kitagiri and Nakamura (17) argued that we have little capacity to form glutamate from NH_3 and that the primary source of glutamate N comes from other amino acids via transamination. These amino acids ultimately result from dietary protein intake. Under circumstances of adequate dietary intake, the transaminating amino acids shown in Figure 1.2 supply more than adequate amino-N to glutamate. The transaminating amino acids act to provide a buffer pool of N that can absorb an increase in N from increased degradation or supply N when there is a drain. From this pool, glutamate provides material to maintain synthesis of ornithine and proline, of which proline is particularly important in protein synthesis of collagen and related proteins.

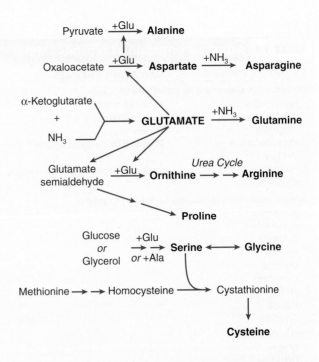

Fig. 1.4. Pathways of the synthesis of dispensable amino acids. Glutamate is produced from ammonia (NH_3) and α-ketoglutarate. That glutamate becomes the nitrogen source added to carbon precursors (pyruvate, oxaloacetate, glycolysis products of glucose, and glycerol) to form most of the other dispensable amino acids. Cysteine and tyrosine are different in that they require indispensable amino acid input for their production.

Serine is produced from 3-phosphoglycerate that comes from glycolysis of glucose. Serine may then be used to produce glycine through a process that transfers a methylene group to tetrahydrofolate. This pathway is listed in Table 1.6 as a degradative pathway for serine, but it is also a source of glycine and one-carbon unit generation (15, 16). Conversely, this pathway actively operates backward to form serine from glycine in humans. When [^{15}N]glycine is given orally, the primary transfer of ^{15}N is to serine (18). Therefore, significant reverse synthesis of serine from glycine occurs. The other major place where ^{15}N appears was in glutamate and glutamine, a finding indicating that the NH_3 released by glycine oxidation is immediately picked up and incorporated into glutamate and the transaminating N-pool via glutamate dehydrogenase.

All the amino acids shown in Figure 1.4 have *active* routes of synthesis in the body (13), in contrast to the IDAAs for which no routes of synthesis exist in humans. This statement should be a simple definition of "indispensable" versus "dispensable." In nutrition, however, we define a dispensable amino acid as an amino acid that is *dispensable* from the diet (3). This definition is different from defining the presence or absence of enzymatic pathways for an amino acid's synthesis. For example, two of the dispensable amino acids depend on the degradation of IDAAs for their production: cysteine and tyrosine. Although serine provides the carbon skeleton and amino group of cysteine, methionine provides the sulfur through condensation of homocysteine and serine to form cystathionine (19). From the foregoing discussion, neither the carbon skeleton nor the amino group of serine is likely to be in short supply, but provision of sulfur from methionine may become limiting. Therefore, cysteine synthesis depends heavily on the availability of the IDAA methionine. The same is also true for tyrosine. Tyrosine is produced by the hydroxylation of phenylalanine, which is also *the* degradative pathway of phenylalanine. The availability of tyrosine strictly depends on the availability of phenylalanine and the liver's ability to perform the hydroxylation.

Incorporation of Amino Acids into Other Compounds

Table 1.7 lists some of the compounds that amino acids are converted directly into or are used as important parts of the synthesis of other compounds in the body. The list is not inclusive, and it is meant to highlight important compounds in the body that depend on amino acids for their synthesis. Other important uses of amino acids are for the synthesis of taurine (20, 21) that is the "amino acid–like" 2-aminoethanesulfonate, found in far higher concentrations inside skeletal muscle than any amino acid (7). Another important, sulfur-containing compound is glutathione (22–24), a tripeptide composed of glycine, cysteine, and glutamate.

Carnitine (25) is important in the transport of long-chain fatty acids across the mitochondrial membrane

TABLE 1.7	IMPORTANT PRODUCTS SYNTHESIZED FROM AMINO ACIDS
AMINO ACID	**INCORPORATED INTO**
Arginine	Creatine
	Nitric oxide
Aspartate	Purines and pyrimidines
Cysteine	Glutathione
	Taurine
Glutamate	Glutathione
	Neurotransmitters
Glutamine	Purines and pyrimidines
Glycine	Creatine
	Glutathione
	Porphyrins (hemoglobin and cytochromes)
	Purines
Histidine	Histamine
Lysine	Carnitine
Methionine	One-carbon methylation/transfer reactions
	Creatine
	Choline
Serine	One-carbon methylation/transfer reactions
	Ethanolamine and choline
Tyrosine	Catecholamines
	Thyroid hormone
Tryptophan	Serotonin
	Nicotinic acid

before fatty acids can be oxidized and is synthesized from ε-N,N,N-trimethyllysine (TML) (26). TML synthesis occurs from posttranslational methylation of specific lysine residues in specific proteins. TML is liberated when the proteins containing it are broken down (26). TML can also arise from hydrolysis of ingested meats. In contrast to 3-methylhistidine, TML can be found in proteins of both muscle and other organs such as liver (27). In rat muscle, TML is approximately one eighth as abundant as 3-methylhistidine.

Amino acids are the precursors for a variety of neurotransmitters that contain N. Glutamate may be an exception in that it serves both as a precursor for neurotransmitter production and is itself a primary neurotransmitter (28). Glutamate appears important in numerous neurodegenerative diseases from amyotrophic lateral sclerosis to Alzheimer disease. (29). Tyrosine is the precursor for catecholamine synthesis. Tryptophan is the precursor for serotonin synthesis. Various studies have reported the importance of plasma concentrations of these and other amino acids on the synthesis of their neurotransmitter products. The most common putative relationship cited is the administration of tryptophan, thus increasing brain serotonin levels.

Creatine and Creatinine
Most of the creatine in the body is found in muscle, where it exists primarily as creatine phosphate (30). When muscular work is performed, creatine phosphate provides the energy through hydrolysis of its "high-energy" phosphate bond that forms creatine with transfer of the phosphate to create an ATP. The reaction is reversible and is mediated

by the enzyme ATP-creatine transphosphorylase (also known as creatine phosphokinase).

The original pathway of creatine synthesis from amino acid precursors was defined by Bloch and Schoenheimer in an elegant series of experiments using ^{15}N-labeled compounds (31). Creatine is synthesized outside muscle in a two-step process (Fig. 1.5). The first step occurs in the kidney and involves the transfer of guanidino group of arginine onto the amino group of glycine to form ornithine and guanidinoacetate. Methylation of the guanidinoacetate occurs in the liver via S-adenosylmethionine to create creatine. Although glycine donates a N and carbon backbone to creatine, arginine must be available to provide the guanidino group, as well as methionine for donation of the methyl group. Creatine is then transferred to muscle, where creatine is phosphorylated. When creatine phosphate is hydrolyzed in muscle to form creatine, most of the creatine is recycled back to the phosphate form. A nonenzymatic process forming creatinine continually dehydrates some of the muscle creatine pool, however.

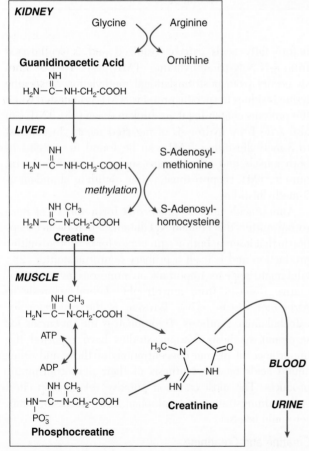

Fig. 1.5. Synthesis of creatine and creatinine. Creatine is synthesized in the liver from guanidinoacetic acid, and that is synthesized in the kidney. Creatine taken up by muscle is primarily converted to phosphocreatine. Although there is some limited direct dehydration of creatine directly to creatinine, the majority of the creatinine comes from dehydration of phosphocreatine. Creatinine is rapidly filtered by the kidney into urine. *ADP*, adenosine diphosphate; *ATP*, adenosine triphosphate.

Creatinine is not retained by muscle, but it is released into body water, is then removed by the kidney from blood, and is excreted into urine (32).

The daily rate of creatinine formation is remarkably constant ($\approx$1.7% of the total creatine pool per day) and depends on the mass of the creatine/creatine-phosphate pool, which is proportional to muscle mass (33). Thus, daily urinary output of creatinine has been used as a measure of total muscle mass in the body. Urinary creatinine excretion increases within a couple days after a creatine load has been added to the diet, and several more days are required after removal of creatine from the diet before urinary creatinine excretion returns to baseline—a finding indicating that creatine in the diet itself affects creatinine production (34). Therefore, consumption of creatine and creatinine in meat-containing foods increases urinary creatinine measurements. Although urinary creatinine measurements have been used primarily to estimate the adequacy of 24-hour urine collections, with adequate control of food composition and intake, creatinine excretion measurements are useful indices of body muscle mass (35, 36).

Purine and Pyrimidine Biosynthesis

The purines (adenine and guanine) and the pyrimidines (uracil, cytosine, and thymine) form the building blocks of DNA and RNA. Purines are heterocyclic double-ring compounds that require incorporation of two glutamine molecules (donation of the amide-N), a glycine molecule, a methylene group from tetrahydrofolate, and the amino-N of aspartic acid for their synthesis as inosine monophosphate. Adenine and guanine are formed from inosine monophosphate by the addition of another glutamine amide-N or aspartate amino-N.

Pyrimidines are synthesized after an amide-N of glutamine is condensed with a CO_2 to form carbamoyl phosphate, which is further condensed with aspartic acid to make orotic acid, the pyrimidine's heterocyclic 6-member ring. The enzyme that forms this carbamoyl phosphate is present in many tissues for pyrimidine synthesis, but it is not the enzyme found in the liver that makes urea (see Fig. 1.3). A block in the urea cycle causing a lack of adequate amounts of arginine to prime urea synthesis cycle in the liver, however, will result in diversion of unused carbamoyl phosphate to orotic acid and pyrimidine synthesis (37). Uracil is synthesized from orotic acid, and cytosine is synthesized from uracil by adding an amide group of glutamine to uridine triphosphate to form cytidine triphosphate.

TURNOVER OF PROTEINS IN THE BODY

As indicated earlier, proteins in the body are not static. Just as every protein is synthesized, it is also degraded. The concept that proteins are continually made and degraded in the body at different rates was first described by Schoenheimer and Rittenberg, who first applied isotopically labeled tracers of amino acids to the study of amino acid metabolism and protein turnover in the 1930s. We now know that the rate of turnover of proteins in the body spans a broad range and that the rate of turnover of individual proteins tends to follow their function in the body; that is, those proteins whose concentrations need to be regulated (e.g., enzymes) or that act as signals (e.g., peptide hormones) have relatively high rates of synthesis and degradation as a means of regulating concentrations. Conversely, structural proteins such as collagen and myofibrillar proteins or secreted plasma proteins have relatively long lifetimes. Overall, however, a balance must exist between synthesis and breakdown of proteins. Balance in healthy adults who are neither gaining nor losing weight will be that the amount of N consumed as protein in the diet will match the amount of N lost in urine, feces, and other routes. Considerably, more protein is mobilized in the body every day than is consumed, however (Fig. 1.6).

Although no definable entity such as "whole body protein" exists, the term is useful for understanding the amount of energy and resources spent by the body in producing and breaking down protein in the body. Several methods using isotopically labeled tracers have been defined to quantitate the whole body turnover of proteins. An important point of Figure 1.6 is that the overall turnover of protein in the body is severalfold greater than the input of new dietary amino acids (38). A physiologically normal adult may consume 90 g of protein that is hydrolyzed and absorbed as free amino acids. Those amino acids mix with amino acids entering from protein breakdown

from a variety of proteins. Approximately one third of the amino acids will appear from the large, but slowly turning over, pool of muscle protein. In contrast, considerably more amino acids will appear and disappear from proteins in the visceral and internal organs. These proteins make up a much smaller proportion of the total mass of protein in the body, but they have rapid synthesis and degradation rates. The overall result is that approximately 340 g of amino acids will enter the free pool daily, of which only 90 g will come from dietary amino acids. How do we assess in humans the turnover of protein in the body, however? These methods range from simple and noninvasive to expensive and complicated.

METHODS OF MEASURING PROTEIN TURNOVER AND AMINO ACID KINETICS

Nitrogen Balance

The oldest (and most widely used) method to follow changes in body N is the N balance method. Because of its simplicity, the N balance technique has been the standard of reference for defining minimum levels of dietary protein and IDAA intakes in humans of all ages (39). Subjects are placed for several days on a specific level of amino acid or protein intake, and their urine and feces are collected over a 24-hour period to measure N excretion. A week or more may be required before collection will reflect adaptation to a dietary change. A dramatic example of adaptation is the

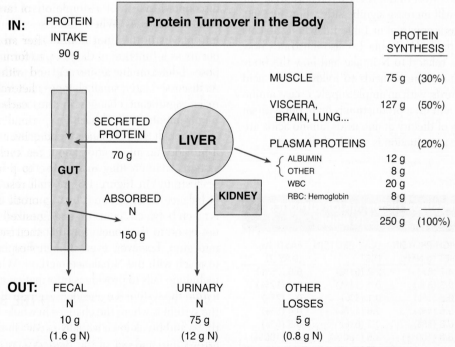

Fig. 1.6. Relative rates of protein turnover and intake in a healthy 70-kg human. Under normal circumstances, dietary intake (IN = 90 g) will match nitrogen (N) losses (OUT = 90 g). Protein breakdown will then match synthesis. Protein intake is only 90/(90 + 250) ≈ 25% of total turnover of N in the body per day. *RBC,* red blood cell; *WBC,* white blood cell. (Redrawn with permission from Hellerstein MK, Munro HN. Interaction of liver and muscle in the regulation of metabolism in response to nutritional and other factors. In: Arias IM, Jakoby WB, Popper H et al, eds. The Liver: Biology and Pathobiology. 2nd ed. New York: Raven Press, 1988:965–83.)

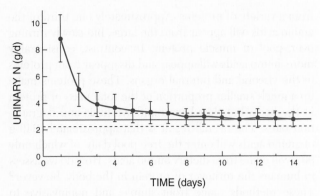

Fig. 1.7. Time required for urinary nitrogen (N) excretion to stabilize after changing from an adequate to a deficient protein intake in young men. *Horizontal solid* and *broken lines* are mean ±1 standard deviation for N excretion at the end of the measurement period. (Data from Scrimshaw NS, Hussein MA, Murray E et al. Protein requirements of man: variations in obligatory urinary and fecal nitrogen losses in young men. J Nutr 1972;102:1595–604, with permission.)

placement of healthy subjects on a diet containing a minimal amount of protein. As shown in Figure 1.7, urinary N excretion drops dramatically in response to the protein-deficient diet over the first 3 days and stabilizes at a new lower level of N excretion by day 8 (40).

The N end products excreted in the urine are end products not only of amino acid oxidation (urea and NH_3) but also of other species such as uric acid from nucleotide degradation and creatinine (Table 1.8). Fortunately, most of the nonurea, non-NH_3 N is relatively constant over a variety of situations and is a relatively small proportion of the total N in the urine. Most of the N is excreted as urea, but NH_3 N excretion will increase significantly when subjects become acidotic, as is apparent in Table 1.8, when subjects have fasted for 2 days (41). Table 1.8 also illustrates how urea production is related to N intake and how the body adapts its oxidation of amino acids to follow amino acid supply. In other words, with an ample supply, excess amino acids are oxidized and urea production is high, but with an insufficient supply of dietary amino acids, amino acids are conserved and urea production is greatly decreased.

TABLE 1.8 COMPOSITION OF THE MAJOR NITROGEN-CONTAINING SPECIES IN URINE

N SPECIES	HIGH-PROTEIN DIET (g N/d)	LOW-PROTEIN DIET	FASTING (DAY 2)
Urea	14.7 (87%)	2.2 (61%)	6.6 (75%)
Ammonia	0.5 (3%)	0.4 (11%)	1.0 (12%)
Uric acid	0.2 (1%)	0.1 (3%)	0.2 (2%)
Creatinine	0.6 (4%)	0.6 (17%)	0.4 (5%)
Undetermined	0.8 (5%)	0.3 (8%)	0.5 (6%)
Total	16.8 (100%)	3.6 (100%)	8.7 (100%)

N, nitrogen.

Data from Folin (1905) and Cathcart (1907), cited in Allison JB, Bird JWC. Elimination of nitrogen from the body. In: Munro HN, Allison JB, eds. Mammalian Protein Metabolism. New York: Academic Press, 1964:483–512, with permission.

TABLE 1.9 OBLIGATORY NITROGEN LOSSES BY MEN ON A PROTEIN-FREE DIET

	DAILY NITROGEN LOSS	
	AS NITROGEN (mg N/kg/day)	AS PROTEIN EQUIVALENT (g PROTEIN/kg/day)
Urine	38	0.23
Feces	12	0.08
Cutaneous	3	0.02
Other	2	0.01
Total	54	0.34
Upper limit (+2 standard deviations)	70	0.44

Data from Munro HN. Amino acid requirements and metabolism and their relevance to parenteral nutrition. In: Wilkinson AW, ed. Parenteral Nutrition. London: Churchill Livingstone, 1972:34–67, with permission.

N appears in the feces because the gut does not completely absorb all dietary protein and reabsorb all N secreted into the gastrointestinal tract (see Fig. 1.6). In addition, N is lost from skin via sweat as well as through shedding of dead skin cells. Moreover, additional losses occur through hair, menstrual fluid, nasal secretions, and so forth. As N excretion in the urine decreases in the case of subjects on a minimal protein diet (Fig. 1.7), it becomes increasingly important to account for N losses through nonurine, nonfecal routes (42). The loss of N by these various routes is shown in Table 1.9. Most of the losses that are not readily measurable are minimal (<10% of total N loss under conditions of a protein-free diet in which adaptation has greatly reduced urinary N excretion) and can be discounted by use of a simple offset factor for nonurine, nonfecal N losses. Where the assessment of losses comes into play is in the finer definition of where zero balance occurs as a function of dietary protein intake for the purpose of determining amino acid and protein requirements. As discussed later, small changes in N balance corrections make significant changes in the assessment of protein requirements using N balance.

Although the N balance technique is useful and simple, it provides no information about the inner workings of the system. An interesting analogy for the N balance technique is illustrated in Figure 1.8, in which the simple model of N balance is represented by a gumball machine. Balance is taken between "coins in" and "gumballs out." We should not come to the conclusion that the machine turns coins into gum, however, even though that conclusion is easy to reach with the N balance method. What the N balance technique fails to provide is information about what occurs *within* the system (i.e., inside the gumball machine). Inside the system is where the changes in whole body protein synthesis and breakdown actually occur (shown as the smaller arrows into and out of the *Body N Pool* in Figure 1.8). A further illustration of this point is made at the bottom of Figure 1.8, in which a positive increase in N balance has been observed going from zero (case 0) to positive balance (cases A to D). A positive N balance could be obtained

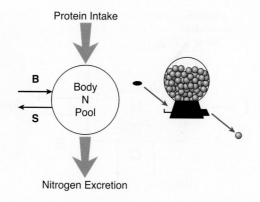

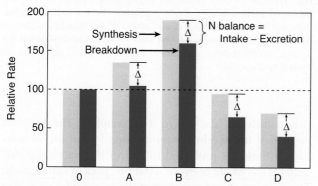

Fig. 1.8. Illustration of the nitrogen (N) balance technique. Nitrogen balance is simply the difference between input and output that is similar to the introduction of a coin into a gumball machine with the resulting release of a gumball. The perception of only the "in" and "out" observations is that the machine changes the coin directly into a gumball or the dietary intake becomes directly the N excreted without consideration of amino acid entry from protein breakdown (B) or uptake for protein synthesis (S). This point is further illustrated with four different hypothetical responses to a change from a zero N balance (case 0) to a positive N balance (cases A to D). A positive N balance can obtained by increasing protein synthesis (A), by increasing synthesis more than breakdown (B), by decreasing breakdown (C), or by decreasing breakdown more than synthesis (D). The N balance method does not distinguish among the four possibilities.

with identical increases in N balance by any of four different alterations in protein synthesis and breakdown: a simple increase in protein synthesis (case A), a decrease in protein breakdown (case C), an increase in both protein synthesis and breakdown (case B), or a decrease in both (case D). The effect is the same positive N balance for all four cases, but the energy implications are considerably different. Because protein synthesis costs energy, cases A and B are more expensive, whereas cases C and D require less energy than the starting case 0. To resolve these four cases, we have to look directly at rates of protein turnover (breakdown and synthesis) using a labeled tracer.

Arteriovenous Differences to Define Organ Balances

Just as the N balance technique can be applied across the whole body, so can the balance technique be applied across a whole organ or tissue bed. These measurements are made

from the blood delivered to the tissue and from the blood emerging from the tissue via catheters placed in an artery to define arterial blood levels and the vein draining the tissue to measure venous blood levels. This latter catheter makes the procedure particularly invasive when applied to organs such as gut and liver, kidney, or brain (43–46). Less invasive are measures of muscle metabolism inferred from measurement of arteriovenous (AV) differences across the leg or arm (45). The AV difference provides no information about the mechanism within the tissue that causes the uptake or release that is observed, however.

More information is gleaned from measurement of amino acids that are not metabolized within the tissue, such as the release of IDAAs tyrosine or lysine that are not metabolized by muscle. Their AV differences across muscle should reflect the difference between net amino acid uptake for muscle protein synthesis and release from muscle protein breakdown. 3-Methylhistidine, an amino acid that is produced by posttranslational methylation of selected histidine residues in myofibrillar protein and that cannot be reused for protein synthesis when it is released from myofibrillar protein breakdown, is quantitatively released from muscle tissue when myofibrillar protein is degraded (47, 48). Its AV difference can be used as a specific marker of myofibrillar protein breakdown (49, 50).

The limited data set of simple balance values across an organ bed is greatly enhanced when a tracer is administered and its balance is also measured across an organ bed. This approach allows for a complete solution of the various pathways operating in the tissue for each amino acid tracer used. In some cases, the measurement of tracer can become very complicated, requiring measurement of multiple metabolites to provide a true metabolite balance across the organ bed (51). Another approach using a tracer of a nonmetabolized IDAA was described by Barrett et al (52). This method requires a limited set of measurements with simplified equations to define specifically rates of protein synthesis and breakdown in muscle tissue.

Tracer Methods Defining Amino Acid Kinetics

To follow flows of *endogenous* metabolites in the body, isotopically labeled tracers are used that are identical to the endogenous metabolites in terms of chemical structure but with substitution of one or more atoms with isotopes different from those usually present. The substitution of isotopes is done to make the tracers distinguishable (measurable) from the normal metabolites. We usually think first of the radioactive isotopes (e.g., ^{3}H for hydrogen and ^{14}C for carbon) as tracers, but nonradioactive, stable isotopes can also be used. Because isotopes differ only in the number of neutrons that are contained, they can be distinguished in a compound by mass spectrometry that determines the abundance of compounds by mass. Most of the lighter elements have one *abundant* stable isotope and one or two isotopes of higher mass of *minor abundance*. The major and minor isotopes are ^{1}H and ^{2}H for hydrogen, ^{14}N and ^{15}N for N,

^{12}C and ^{13}C for carbon, and ^{16}O, ^{17}O, and ^{18}O for oxygen. Except for some isotope effects that can be significant for both the radioactive (^{3}H) and nonradioactive (^{2}H) hydrogen isotopes, a compound that is isotopically labeled is essentially indistinguishable from the corresponding unlabeled endogenous compound in the body.

Because they do not exist in nature and so little of the radioactive material is administered, radioisotopes are considered "weightless" tracers that do not add material to the system. Radioactive tracer data are expressed as counts or disintegrations per minute per unit of compound. Because the stable isotopes are naturally occurring (e.g., $\approx$1% of all carbon in the body is ^{13}C), the stable isotope tracers are administered and measured as "the excess above the naturally occurring abundance" of the isotope in the body as either the *mole ratio* of the amount of tracer isotope divided by the amount of unlabeled material (called the "tracer-to-tracee ratio" or TTR) or the *mole fraction* (usually expressed as a percentage: *mole % excess* or *atom % excess*, the latter being an older and less appropriate term in the literature) (53).

The basis of most tracer measurements to determine amino acid kinetics is the simple concept of tracer dilution. This concept is illustrated in Figure 1.9 for the determination of the flow of water in a stream. If you infuse a dye of known concentration (enrichment) into the stream, go downstream after the dye has mixed well with the stream water, and take a sample of the dye, then you can calculate from the measured dilution of the dye the rate at which water must be flowing in the stream to make that dilution. The necessary information required consists of infusion rate of dye (tracer infusion rate) and measured concentration of the dye (enrichment or specific activity of the tracer). The calculated value is the flow of water through the stream (flux of unlabeled metabolite) that causes the dilution. This simple dye-dilution analogy is the basis for almost all kinetic calculations in a wide range of formats for many different applications.

Models for Whole Body Amino Acid and Protein Metabolism

The limitations to using tracers to define amino acid and protein metabolism are largely driven by how the tracer

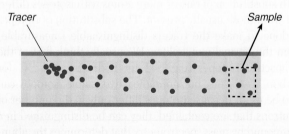

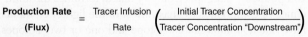

Fig. 1.9. Basic principle of the dye-dilution method of determining tracer kinetics.

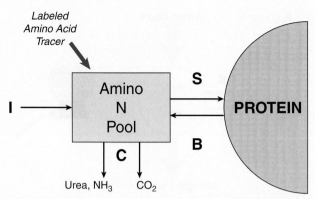

Fig. 1.10. Single-pool model of whole body protein metabolism measured using a labeled amino acid tracer. Amino acid enters the free pool from dietary intake (I) and amino acid released from protein breakdown (B) and leaves the free pool via amino acid oxidation (C) to urea, ammonia (NH_3), and carbon dioxide (CO_2) and via uptake for protein synthesis (S).

is administered and where it is sampled. The simplest method of tracer administration is orally, but intravenous administration is preferred to deliver the tracer *systemically* (to the whole body) into the free pool of amino acids. The simplest site of sampling of the tracer dilution is also from the free pool of amino acids via blood. Therefore, most approaches to measuring amino acid and protein kinetics in the whole body by using amino acid tracers have assumed a single, free pool of amino N, as shown in Figure 1.10. Amino acids enter the free pool from dietary amino acid intake (enteral or parenteral) and from amino acids released from protein breakdown. Amino acids leave the free pool by amino acid oxidation to end products (CO_2, urea, and NH_3) and from amino acid uptake for protein synthesis.

The free amino acid pool can be viewed from the standpoint of all the amino acids together (as discussed for the end-product method) or from the viewpoint of a single amino acid and its metabolism. The reason that the model in Figure 1.10 is called a single-pool model is that protein is not viewed as a pool itself, but rather as a source of entry of unlabeled amino acids into the free pool as well as a route of amino acid removal for protein synthesis. Only a small portion of the proteins in the body is assumed to turn over during the time course of the experiment. Obviously, these assumptions are not true: many proteins in the body are turning over rapidly (e.g., most enzymes). Proteins that do turn over during the time course of the experiment will become labeled and appear as part of the free amino acid pool. These proteins make up only a fraction of the total protein, however; the remainder turns over slowly (e.g., muscle protein). Most amino acids entering via protein breakdown and leaving for new protein synthesis are coming from proteins that are turning over slowly. These flows are the "B" and "S" arrows of the traditional single-pool model of whole body protein metabolism shown in Figure 1.10.

End-Product Approach

The earliest model of whole body protein metabolism in humans was applied in 1953 by San Pietro and Rittenberg, who used [^{15}N]glycine (54). Glycine was used as the first tracer because glycine is the only amino acid without an optically active α-carbon center, and it is therefore easy to synthesize with a ^{15}N label. Because measurement of the tracer in plasma glycine was very difficult at that time, San Pietro and Rittenberg (54) proposed a model based on values that could be readily measured: urinary urea and NH$_3$. The assumption was that the urinary N end products reflected the average enrichment of ^{15}N of all the free amino acids being oxidized. Although glycine ^{15}N was the tracer, the tracee was assumed to be *all* free amino acids (assumed to be a single pool). It quickly became obvious, however, that the system was more complicated and that a more sophisticated model and solution were required. In essence, the method languished until 1969, when Picou and Taylor-Roberts (55) proposed a simpler method that also followed the glycine ^{15}N tracer into urinary N. Their method dealt only with the effect of the dilution of the ^{15}N tracer in the free amino acid pool as a whole, rather than invoking solution of tracer specific equations of a specific model. Their assumptions were similar to the earlier Rittenberg approach in that the investigators presumed that the ^{15}N tracer mixed (scatters) among the free amino acids in some distribution that was not required to be known but was representative of amino acid metabolism itself. The [^{15}N]glycine tracer is administered (usually orally), and urine samples are obtained to measure the ^{15}N dilution in the free amino acid pool (56). The ^{15}N in the free amino acid pool is diluted with unlabeled amino acid entering from protein breakdown and from dietary intake. The turnover of the free pool (Q, typically expressed as mg N/kg/day) is calculated from the measured dilution of ^{15}N in the end products via the same approach illustrated in Figure 1.9:

$$Q = i/E_{UN}$$

where i is the rate of [^{15}N]glycine infusion (mg ^{15}N/kg/day), and E_{UN} is the ^{15}N enrichment in atom percent excess ^{15}N in urinary N (either urea or NH$_3$). The free pool is assumed to be in steady state (neither increasing or decreasing over time), and therefore, the turnover of amino acid will be equal to the rate of amino acids entering via whole body protein breakdown (B) and dietary intake (I) and also equal to the rate of amino acids leaving via uptake for protein synthesis (S) and via amino acid oxidation to the end products urea and NH$_3$ (C):

$$Q = I + B = C + S$$

Because dietary intake should be known and urinary N excretion is measured, the rate of whole body protein breakdown can be determined: $B = Q - I$, as well as the rate of whole body synthesis: $S = Q - C$. In these calculations, the standard value of 6.25 g protein = 1 g N is used

to interconvert protein and urinary N. Attention to the units (grams of protein versus grams of N) is important because both units are often used concurrently in the same report.

Occasionally, the term "net protein balance" or "net protein gain" appears in the literature. Net protein balance is defined as the difference between the measured protein synthesis and breakdown rates ($S-B$) that can be determined from whole body protein breakdown and synthesis measured as shown previously. As can be seen by rearranging the earlier balance equation for Q, however, $S - B = I - C$, which is simply the difference between intake and excretion (i.e., N balance). The $S-B$ term is a misnomer in that it is based solely on the N balance measurement, not on the administration of the ^{15}N tracer.

The end-product method is not without its problems. When the [^{15}N]glycine tracer is given orally at short intervals (e.g., every 3 hours) the time required to reach a plateau in urinary urea ^{15}N is approximately 60 hours, regardless of whether adults (57), children, or infants (58) are studied. The delay in attaining a plateau results from the time required for the ^{15}N tracer to equilibrate within the free glycine, serine, and urea pools (18, 56). An additional problem is plateau definition. Often, the urinary urea ^{15}N time course does not show by either visual inspection or curve-fitting regression the anticipated single exponential rise to plateau. To avoid this problem, Waterlow et al (59) suggested measuring the ^{15}N in NH$_3$ after a *single dose* of [^{15}N]glycine. The advantage is that the ^{15}N tracer passes through the body NH$_3$ pool within 24 hours. Tracer administration and urine collection are greatly simplified, and the modification does not depend on defining a plateau in urinary urea ^{15}N. The caveat here is the dependence of the single-dose end-product method on NH$_3$ metabolism. Urinary NH$_3$ ^{15}N enrichment is also usually different from urinary urea ^{15}N enrichment (60) because the amino-^{15}N precursor for NH$_3$ synthesis is of renal origin, whereas the amino-^{15}N precursor for urea synthesis is of hepatic origin. Which enrichment should be used? Probably the urea ^{15}N, but it is difficult to prove either way.

Measurement of the Kinetics of Individual Amino Acids

As an alternative to measuring the turnover of the whole amino-N pool itself, the kinetics of an individual amino acid can be followed from the dilution of an infused tracer of that amino acid. The simplest models consider only IDAAs that have no de novo synthesis components. The kinetics of IDAAs mimics the kinetics of protein turnover, as shown in Figure 1.10. The same type of model can be constructed, but cast specifically in terms of a single IDAA, and the same steady-state balance equation can be defined:

$$Q_{aa} = I_{aa} + B_{aa} = C_{aa} + S_{aa}$$

where Q_{aa} is the turnover rate (or flux) of the IDAA, I_{aa} is the rate at which the amino acid is entering the free pool from dietary intake, B_{aa} is the rate of amino acid entry from protein breakdown, C_{aa} is the rate of amino acid oxidation, and S_{aa} is the rate of amino acid uptake for protein synthesis. The most common method for defining amino acid kinetics has been a primed infusion of an amino acid tracer until isotopic steady state (constant dilution) is reached in blood. The flux for the amino acid is measured from the dilution of the tracer in the free pool. By knowing the tracer enrichment and infusion rate and by measuring the tracer dilution in blood samples taken at plateau, the rate of unlabeled metabolite appearance is determined (61–63):

$$Q_{aa} = i_{aa} \cdot [E_i/E_p - 1]$$

where i_{aa} is the infusion rate of tracer with enrichment E_i (mole % excess) and E_p is the blood amino acid enrichment.

For a carbon-labeled tracer, the amino acid oxidation rate can be measured from the rate of $^{13}CO_2$ or $^{14}CO_2$ excretion (61, 63). The choice of a carbon label that is quantitatively oxidized is critical. For example, the ^{13}C of a L-[1-^{13}C]leucine tracer is quantitatively released at the first irreversible step of leucine catabolism. In contrast, a ^{13}C label in the leucine tail will end up in acetoacetate or acetyl-CoA, which may or may not be quantitatively oxidized (64). Other amino acids, such as lysine, have even more nebulous pathways of oxidation.

Before the oxidized carbon label is recovered in exhaled air, it must pass through the body bicarbonate pool. Therefore, we must know what fraction of bicarbonate pool turnover goes to release as CO_2 into exhaled air versus retention for alternative fates in the body. In general, only approximately 80% of the bicarbonate produced is released immediately as expired CO_2, as determined from infusion of a labeled bicarbonate and measurement of the fraction infused that is recovered in exhaled CO_2 (65). The other 20% is retained in bone and metabolic pathways that "fix" carbon. The amount of bicarbonate retained is somewhat variable (ranging from 0% to 40% of its production) and needs to be determined when different metabolic situations are investigated. When retention of bicarbonate in the body may change with metabolic perturbation, parallel studies measuring the recovery of an administered dose of ^{13}C- or ^{14}C-labeled bicarbonate are indispensable in interpretation of the oxidation results (66).

The rates of amino acid release from protein breakdown and uptake for protein synthesis are calculated by subtracting dietary intake and oxidation from the flux of an IDAA, just as is done with the end-product method. The primary distinction is that the measurements are specific to a single amino acid's kinetics (micromole of amino acid per unit of time), rather than directly in terms of N itself. Flux components are then extrapolated to whole body protein kinetics by dividing the amino acid rates by the assumed concentration of the amino acid in body protein (as shown in Table 1.3).

The principal advantages in measuring the kinetics of an individual metabolite are as follows: (a) the results are specific to *that* metabolite, thus improving the confidence of the measurement; and (b) the measurements can be performed quickly because turnover time of the free pool is usually rapid (generally <4 hours using a priming dose). Drawbacks to the measurement of the kinetics of an individual amino acid are as follows: (a) an appropriately labeled tracer may not be available to follow the pathways of the amino acid being studied, especially with regard to amino acid oxidation; and (b) metabolism of amino acids occurs within cells, but the tracers are typically administered into and sampled from the blood outside cells.

α-Ketoisocaproate as a Measure of Leucine Cellular Transport. Amino acids do not freely pass through cells; they are transported. For the neutral amino acids (leucine, isoleucine, and valine, phenylalanine, and tyrosine), transport in and out of cells may be rapid, and only a small concentration gradient between plasma and intracellular milieus exists (see Table 1.4). Even that small gradient will limit exchange of intracellular and extracellular amino acids, however. For leucine, this phenomenon can be defined using α-ketoisocaproate (KIC), which is formed from leucine inside cells by transamination. Some of the KIC formed is then decarboxylated, but most of it is either reaminated to reform leucine (67) or released from cells into plasma. Thus, plasma KIC enrichment can be used as a marker of intracellular leucine enrichment from which it came (68).

Generally, plasma KIC enrichment is approximately 25% lower than plasma leucine enrichment (62, 68). If plasma KIC enrichment is substituted for the plasma leucine tracer enrichment into the calculation of leucine kinetics, then the measured leucine flux and oxidation and, similarly, estimates of protein breakdown and synthesis will be increased by approximately 25%. When protein metabolism is studied under two different conditions and the resulting leucine kinetics is compared, however, the same relative response will be obtained regardless of whether leucine or KIC enrichment is used for the calculation of kinetics (68).

Most amino acids do not have a convenient metabolite that can be readily measured in plasma to define aspects of their intracellular metabolism, but an intracellular marker for leucine does not necessarily authenticate leucine as the tracer for defining whole body protein metabolism. Numerous investigators have measured the turnover rate of many of the amino acids, both indispensable and dispensable, in humans for purposes of defining aspects of the metabolism of these amino acids. The general trend of the amino acid kinetic data from these studies was reviewed by Bier (62). The fluxes of IDAAs should represent their release rates from whole body protein breakdown for postabsorptive humans who have no dietary intake. Therefore, if the Waterlow model of Figure 1.10 is a reasonable representation of whole body protein turnover, the individual rates of IDAA turnover should be proportional to each amino acid's content in body protein, and a linear relationship of amino acid flux and amino acid abundance in body protein should exist. That relationship is shown in Figure 1.11 for data gleaned from a variety of studies in humans measured in the postabsorptive state (without dietary intake during the infusion studies) who were previously consuming diets of adequate N and energy intake. A correlation of amino acid flux and amino acid composition in protein exists across various amino acid tracers and studies. This correlation suggests that even if there are problems defining intracellular/extracellular concentration gradients of tracers to assess true intracellular events, changes in fluxes measured for the various IDAAs still reflect changes in breakdown in general.

Because dispensable amino acids are synthesized in the body, their fluxes are anticipated to be higher than their expected flux based on the regression line in Figure 1.11 by the amount of de novo synthesis that occurs. Because de novo synthesis and disposal of the dispensable amino acids would be expected to be based on the metabolic pathways of individual amino acids, the degree to which individual dispensable amino acids lie above the line should also be variable. For example, tyrosine is a dispensable amino acid because it is made from the hydroxylation of phenylalanine, which is also the pathway of phenylalanine disposal. The rate of tyrosine de novo synthesis *is* the rate of phenylalanine disposal. In the postabsorptive state, 10% to 20% of an IDAA's turnover will go to oxidative disposal. For phenylalanine with a flux of approximately 40 μmol/kg/hour, phenylalanine disposal produces approximately 6 μmol/kg/hour of tyrosine. We would predict from the tyrosine content of body protein that tyrosine release from protein breakdown would be 21 μmol/kg/hour and that

the flux of tyrosine (tyrosine release from protein breakdown plus tyrosine production from phenylalanine) would be 21 + 6 = 27 μmol/kg/hour. The measured tyrosine flux approximates this prediction (Fig. 1.11) (69).

Compared with tyrosine, which has a de novo synthesis component limited by phenylalanine oxidation, most dispensable amino acids have very large de novo synthesis components because of their corresponding metabolic pathways. For example, arginine is at the center of the urea cycle (see Fig. 1.3). Normal synthesis for urea is 8 to 12 g of N/day. That amount of urea production translates into an arginine de novo synthesis of approximately 250 μmol/kg/hour, which is four times the expected approximately 60 μmol/kg/hour of arginine released from protein breakdown. As can be seen in Figure 1.11, however, the *measured* arginine flux approximates the arginine release from protein breakdown (70). The large de novo synthesis component does not exist in the measured flux. The explanation for this low flux is that the arginine in urea synthesis is very highly compartmentalized in the liver, and this arginine does not exchange with the tracer arginine infused intravenously.

Similar disparities are seen between the measured fluxes of glutamine and glutamate determined with intravenously infused tracers and their anticipated fluxes from their expected de novo synthesis components. The predicted flux for glutamate should include transamination with the BCAAs, alanine and aspartate, as well as glutamate's contribution to the production and degradation of glutamine. The glutamate flux measured in postabsorptive adult subjects infused with [^{15}N]glutamate was 80 μmol/kg/hour, however, barely higher than anticipated rate of glutamate release from protein breakdown (Fig. 1.11). The size of free glutamate pool was also determined in this study from the tracer dilution. The tracer determined pool of glutamate was very small and approximated only the pool size predicted for extracellular water. The much larger intracellular pool that exists in muscle (see Table 1.4) was not seen with the intravenously administered tracer. The flux measured for glutamine is considerably larger (350 μmol/kg/hour), reflecting a large de novo synthesis component (Fig. 1.11). The pool size determined with the [^{15}N]glutamine tracer also was a small pool, however, one not much larger than glutamine in extracellular water. The large intracellular muscle free pool of glutamine was not found (71). Thus, the large intracellular pools (especially those in muscle) are tightly compartmentalized and do not readily mix with extracellular glutamine and glutamate. The glutamine and glutamate tracers, administered intravenously, define pools of glutamine and glutamate that reflect primarily extracellular free glutamine and glutamate. The glutamate tracer does not detect intracellular events such as glutamate transamination. The prominent role of glutamine in the body *is interorgan transport* (i.e., production by muscle and release for use by other tissues [72]), however, and that event is measured by the

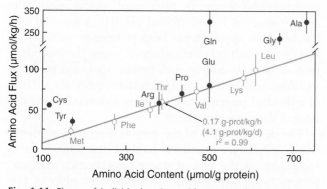

Fig. 1.11. Fluxes of individual amino acids measured in postabsorptive humans plotted against amino acid concentration in protein. The *closed circles* are for dispensable amino acids, and the *open circles* represent indispensable amino acids. The *regression line* is for the flux of the indispensable amino acids versus their content in protein. *Error bars* represent the range of reported values that were taken from various reports in the literature of studies of amino acid kinetics in healthy humans eating adequate diets of nitrogen and energy intake studied in the postabsorptive state. The amino acid content of protein data are taken for muscle values from Table 1.3. The regression line slope of 4.1-g protein/kg/day is similar to other estimates of whole body protein turnover. (Redrawn with permission from Bier DM. Intrinsically difficult problems: the kinetics of body proteins and amino acids in man. Diabetes Metab Rev 1989;5:111–32, with additional data.)

glutamine tracer (as is obvious from Figure 1.11, in which the tracer-determined glutamine flux shows the highest flux measured of any amino acid).

Splanchnic Bed Metabolism of Dietary Amino Acids. The model in Figure 1.10 does not consider the potential first-pass effect of the splanchnic bed (gut and liver) on regulating the delivery of nutrients from the oral route. Under normal circumstances, the amino acid tracer is infused intravenously to measure whole body systemic kinetics. Enterally delivered amino acids pass through the gut and liver before entering the systemic circulation, however. Any metabolism of these amino acids by gut or liver on the first pass during absorption will not be "seen" by an intravenously infused tracer in terms of systemic kinetics. Therefore, another pool with a second arrow showing the first-pass removal by gut and liver should precede the input arrow for "I" (Fig. 1.12) to indicate the role of the splanchnic bed. A fraction "f" of the dietary intake ($I \cdot f$) is sequestered on the first pass, and only $I \cdot (1 - f)$ enters systemic circulation.

Two approaches to addressing this problem are used. The first does not evaluate the fraction sequestered explicitly, but rather it builds the tracer administration scheme into the first-pass losses. Simply add the amino acid tracer to the dietary intake so that the tracer administration *is* the oral route (I_{gi}) and enrichments in blood (E_{gi}) come after any first-pass metabolism by the splanchnic bed (73, 74). This approach is especially useful for studying the effect of varying levels of amino acid intake, but it does not evaluate itself the amount of material sequestered by the splanchnic bed.

The second approach applies the tracer both by the intravenous route and by the enteral route. Intravenous tracer infusion (I_{iv}) and plasma enrichment (E_{iv}) are used to determine systemic kinetics, and the enteral tracer infusion and its plasma enrichment determine systemic kinetics plus the effect of the first pass. By the difference, the fraction, f, is readily calculated (75). This approach can be applied even in the postabsorptive state to determine basal

uptake of amino acid tracers by the splanchnic bed. Several IDAAs and dispensable amino acids have been studied, and first-pass fractional uptake values for these different amino acids have been determined. In general, the splanchnic bed extracts between 20% and 50% of the IDAAs leucine (75), phenylalanine (75, 76), and lysine (77, 78). More than half of the dispensable amino acids are extracted by the splanchnic bed on the first pass, including alanine (79), arginine (80), and glutamine (76, 81), but the splanchnic bed extracts almost all enteral glutamate (81, 82).

Synthesis of Specific Proteins

The foregoing methods deal with measurements at the whole body level, but they do not address specific proteins and their rates of synthesis and degradation. To do so requires obtaining samples of the proteins that can be purified. Some proteins are readily sampled, such as lipoproteins, albumin, fibrinogen, and other proteins secreted into blood. Other proteins require tissue sampling, such as by obtaining a muscle biopsy. If a protein or group of proteins can be sampled and purified, then their synthetic rates can be determined directly from the rate of tracer incorporation into the proteins. Proteins that turn over slowly (e.g., muscle protein or albumin) incorporate only a small amount of tracer during a tracer infusion. Because the incorporation rate of tracer is approximately linear during this time, protein synthesis can be measured by obtaining only two samples. This technique has been especially useful for evaluating protein synthesis of myofibrillar protein with a limited number of muscle biopsies (53). Once a tissue biopsy has been obtained, the sample may be fractionated into cellular components, and the synthetic rate of proteins in organelles (e.g., mitochondria) or specific proteins of muscle (e.g., actin and myosin) can be determined (83, 84). A more recent, but laborious approach has been to separate proteins by two-dimensional gel electrophoresis, excise the individual protein spots, hydrolyze each protein spot, and measure its amino acid enrichment to determine rates of synthesis of individual proteins (85) and even individual modifications of the same protein (86).

The determination of the protein fractional synthetic rate is a "precursor-product" method that requires both knowledge of the rate of tracer incorporation into the protein being synthesized and an understanding of the enrichment of the amino acid precursor used for synthesis. For muscle, L-[1-^{13}C]leucine is often used as the tracer, and plasma KIC ^{13}C enrichment is used to approximate the intracellular muscle leucine enrichment (87). Alternatively, intracellular amino acid enrichment of free amino acids has been measured, and some researchers have measured tracer enrichment in tRNA, the direct site of the precursor enrichment for protein synthesis (88). For proteins that turn over at a faster rate, the tracer concentration rises exponentially in these proteins during the course of the tracer infusion toward a plateau value of enrichment that matches that of the precursor amino

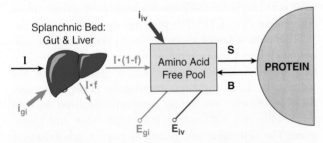

Fig. 1.12. Model of whole body protein metabolism for the fed state in which the first-pass uptake of dietary intake is considered. A labeled amino acid tracer is administered by the gastrointestinal route (i_{gi}) to follow dietary amino acid intake (I). The fraction of dietary amino acid sequestered on the first pass by the splanchnic bed (f) can be determined by administering the tracer by both the gastrointestinal and the intravenous route (i_{iv}) and comparing the enrichments in blood for the two tracers (E_{gi} and E_{iv}, respectively). *B*, protein breakdown; *S*, protein synthesis.

acids used for its synthesis (i.e., intracellular amino acid enrichment). The types of protein that have been measured under these conditions have been the lipoproteins, especially apolipoprotein-B in very-low-density lipoprotein (89, 90).

Degradation of Specific Proteins

Measurement of protein degradation is much more limited in terms of the methods available. To measure protein degradation, the protein must be prelabeled. Three methods have been used: (a) removal of plasma proteins, followed by iodination with radioactive iodine and reinjection back into the body to follow the disappearance of the labeled protein (91, 92); (b) administration of a labeled amino acid to label proteins by incorporation of the tracer via protein synthesis, followed by measurement of labeled amino acid release from degradation of the protein; and (c) use of posttranslational amino acids such as 3-methylhistidine.

Slow-turnover proteins may be labeled by long infusions of amino acid tracer or by long-term administration of deuterated water. The deuterium becomes incorporated into several IDAAs (e.g., alanine), and these amino acids become incorporated into protein. This approach has largely been used to measure rates of protein synthesis (93, 94), but it can also be used to label proteins for measurement of protein degradation (95). After the tracer infusion is stopped, the tracer enrichment will disappear quickly from plasma. At that point, serial sampling of the protein and measurement of the decrease in tracer enrichment with time will give its degradation rate. Another problem occurs, however: 80% or more of the amino acids released from protein breakdown will be reused for synthesis of new proteins. Therefore, amino acid tracer from protein degradation is recycled back into the new proteins. Because the starting enrichment in the proteins being measured is generally not large, recycling of low enrichments of tracer becomes an important and greatly complicating problem in the interpretation of the labeled protein data by this method (95).

3-Methylhistidine and Other Posttranslationally Modified Amino Acids. In the body, several enzymes can modify the structure of proteins after they have been synthesized. The posttranslational changes are generally modest, occur in specific amino acids, and often consist of the addition of a hydroxyl group (e.g., conversion of proline to hydroxyproline in collagen [96]) or methylation of N-moieties of amino acid residues such as histidine or lysine. Because tRNAs do not code for these hydroxylated or methylated amino acids, they are not reused for protein synthesis once the protein containing them is degraded, and their release and collection in urine can be used as a measure of the degradation rate of the proteins that contained them.

Because of the quantitative importance of muscle to whole body protein metabolism, measurement of the release of 3-methylhistidine is a valuable tool for following myosin and actin breakdown, which are both primary proteins in skeletal muscle and the primary proteins containing 3-methylhistidine (48, 97). Caveats exist regarding the use of 3-methylhistidine excretion for measurement of myofibrillar protein breakdown, however. Dietary meat distorts urinary 3-methylhistidine collection (98). As much as 5% of the 3-methylhistidine released in the urine may be acetylated in the liver first (a pathway that is much more predominant in the rat), and the urinary samples may have to by hydrolyzed before measurement of the 3-methylhistidine.

Myofibrillar protein and 3-methylhistidine are not specific to skeletal muscle (99). Although skin and gut only contain a small pool of myofibrillar protein (compared with the large mass of myofibrillar protein found in skeletal muscle), skin and gut protein turn over rapidly and therefore can contribute a significant amount of 3-methylhistidine to the urine. Some work suggests that skin and gut contributions, although noticeable, can be accommodated in the calculation of human skeletal muscle turnover from urinary 3-methylhistidine excretion (100).

A more specific approach to 3-methylhistidine measurement of skeletal muscle myofibrillar protein breakdown is to measure the specific release of 3-methylhistidine from skeletal muscle via AV blood measurements across a muscle bed, such as leg or arm (101). This measurement of protein breakdown from the 3-methylhistidine AV difference can be combined with the AV difference measurement of an IDAA that is not metabolized in muscle, such as tyrosine. The AV difference of tyrosine across an arm or leg defines net protein balance, that is, the difference between protein breakdown and synthesis. If we subtract this protein balance measurement from the myofibrillar protein breakdown measurement from the AV difference of 3-methylhistidine, we obtain an estimate of muscle protein synthesis (102, 103). A final twist is to include coinfusion of an isotopically labeled 3-methylhistidine tracer and measure the AV difference of the tracer in conjunction with the concentration of 3-methylhistidine to provide the most complete and detailed kinetic picture of 3-methylhistidine and myofibrillar protein breakdown (104, 105).

CONTRIBUTION OF SPECIFIC ORGANS TO PROTEIN METABOLISM

Whole Body Metabolism of Protein

From the preceding discussion of tracers of amino acid and protein metabolism, it is clear that the body is not static and that all compounds are being made and degraded over time. A general balance of the processes occurring is shown in Figure 1.6 for an average adult. Approximately 250 g of protein will turn over in a day, of which muscle protein turnover accounts for approximately 75 g/day. The proportion of skeletal muscle mass in the body is consistent with skeletal muscle's contribution to whole body protein turnover: skeletal muscle comprises about one third of the protein in the body (8) and accounts for about one fourth of the turnover. Visceral and other organ protein turnover accounts for an additional 127 g/day. White and red blood cell synthesis accounts for approximately 28 g/day of protein, and proteins are synthesized and secreted by liver into plasma (≈20 g/day).

Protein is also added directly into the gut lumen in the form of secreted proteins, and the small intestine is continually being remodeled as cells formed in the crypts migrate toward the villus tips, where cells are sloughed off the tips. A reasonable estimate is that 20 g/day of secreted proteins and 50 g/day protein from sloughed cells contribute 70 g/day of protein into the gut, which then very efficiently reabsorbs the protein.

If amino acids could be completely conserved, that is, if none were oxidized for energy or synthesized into other compounds, then all amino acids released from proteolysis could be completely reincorporated into new protein synthesis. Obviously, that is not the case, and when no dietary intake occurs, whole body protein breakdown must be greater than protein synthesis by an amount equal to net disposal of amino acids by oxidative and other routes. Therefore, we need to consume enough amino acids during the day to make up for the losses that occur both during this period and during the nonfed period. This concept becomes the basis for methods defining amino acid and protein requirements discussed later.

As shown in Figure 1.6, if someone eats 90 g of protein in a day, of which 10 g will be lost to the feces, the net absorption will be 80 g. At the same time, considerably more protein is synthesized and degraded in the body. The total turnover of protein in the body, including both dietary intake and endogenous metabolism, is 90 + 250 = 340 g/day, of which oxidation of dietary protein accounts for (75 + 5)/340 = 24% of the turnover of protein in the body per day. When dietary protein intake is restricted, adaptation occurs whereby the body reduces N losses (e.g., see Fig. 1.7) and protein intake/oxidation becomes a much smaller proportion of total protein turnover.

The preceding discussion defines turnover of protein in various parts of the body, but it does not integrate flows of material itself or highlight the relationship of amino acids to metabolites that are used for energy, such as glucose and

fatty acids. Clearly, there must be interorgan cooperation to maintain protein homeostasis simply because tissues such as muscle have large amino acid reservoirs, yet all tissues have amino acid needs. A regular feeding schedule means that part of the day is a fasting period when endogenous protein is used for energy and gluconeogenesis. The fed period then supplies amino acids from dietary protein to replenish these losses and provide additional amino acids that can be used for energy during the feeding portion as well. Such a normal diurnal feeding and fasting pattern causes movement of amino acids among organs. Such movement takes on particular importance in situations of trauma and stress in which adaptation, or rather lack of adaptation, of amino acid metabolism to physiologic insults or pathophysiologic states occurs.

As Cahill emphasized (1, 106), the primary consideration of the body is to maintain and distribute energy supplies (oxygen and oxidative substrates). The caloric needs of different tissues in the body are shown in Table 1.10. As can be seen from the table, the brain makes up only approximately 2% of body weight yet has 20% of the energy needs (107). The brain also lacks the ability to store energy (e.g., glycogen depots), so it depends continually on delivery of energy substrates via the blood from other organs (Fig. 1.13A). In the postabsorptive state, the primary energy substrate for the brain is glucose. In infancy and early childhood, when the brain makes up a significantly greater proportion of body mass, glucose production and utilization rates are proportionately higher (108). The pioneering studies of Cahill, Felig, and Wahren and their colleagues provided us with a wealth of data concerning flows of amino acids and glucose from organ balance studies in humans studied over a range of nutritional states (44, 45, 109–111). Some basic concepts may be defined from these studies.

As shown in Figure 1.13A, in the postabsorptive state, the body provides energy for the brain in the form of glucose primarily from hepatic glycogenolysis and secondarily from glucose synthesis (gluconeogenesis) from amino acids. Other substrates, such as glycerol released from triglyceride lipolysis, may also be used for gluconeogenesis, but amino acids provide the bulk of the gluconeogenic substrate. The pathways of conversion are discussed

TABLE 1.10   CONTRIBUTION OF DIFFERENT ORGANS AND TISSUES TO ENERGY EXPENDITURE

ORGAN OR TISSUE	WEIGHT kg	(% OF TOTAL)	METABOLIC RATE kcal/kg TISSUE/d	(% OF TOTAL)
Kidneys	0.3	(0.5)	440	(8)
Brain	1.4	(2.0)	240	(20)
Liver	1.8	(2.6)	200	(21)
Heart	0.3	(0.5)	440	(9)
Muscle	28.0	(40.0)	14	(22)
Adipose tissue	15.0	(40.0)	4	(4)
Other (e.g., skin, gut, bone)	23.2	(33.0)	12	(16)
Total	70.0	(100.0)		(100)

Data for a 70-kg man from Elia M. Organ and tissue contribution to metabolic rate. In: Kinney JM, Tucker HN, eds. Energy Metabolism: Determinants and Cellular Corollaries. New York: Raven Press, 1992:61–79, with permission.

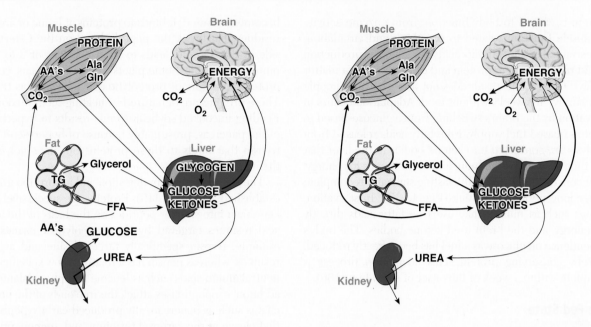

A Postabsorptive state   **B** Starvation

Fig. 1.13. Interorgan flow of substrates in the body to maintain energy balance in the postabsorptive state **(A)** and after adaptation to starvation **(B)**. The schematic diagrams are patterned after the work of Cahill. In all states, energy needs of the brain must be satisfied. In the postabsorptive state, glucose from liver glycogenolysis provides the majority of the glucose needed by the brain. After liver glycogen stores have been depleted (fasting state), gluconeogenesis from amino acids from muscle stores predominates as the glucose source. Eventually, the body adapts to starvation by production and utilization of ketone bodies instead of glucose, thereby sparing amino acid loss for gluconeogenesis. *AA's,* amino acids; *Ala,* alanine; *CO₂,* carbon dioxide; *FFA,* free fatty acids; *Gln,* glutamine; *O₂,* oxygen; *TG,* triglycerides. (Redrawn with permission from Cahill GF Jr, Aoki TT. Partial and total starvation. In: Kinney JM, ed. Assessment of Energy Metabolism in Health and Disease. Report of the First Ross Conference on Medical Research. Columbus, OH: Ross Laboratories, 1980:129–34.)

previously for those amino acids for which their carbon skeletons can be easily rearranged to form gluconeogenic precursors. The remaining amino acids released from protein breakdown and not used for gluconeogenesis may be oxidized. The amino acid N released by this process is removed from the body by incorporation into urea via synthesis in the liver and excretion into urine via the kidney. Gluconeogenesis also occurs in the kidney, but the effect and magnitude are masked from AV measurements because the kidney is also a glucose consumer (112, 113).

Role of Skeletal Muscle in Whole Body Amino Acid Metabolism

An interesting observation from the early AV difference studies across the human leg and arm was that more than 50% of the amino acids released from skeletal muscle was in the form of alanine and glutamine (114), yet alanine and glutamine comprise less than 20% of amino acids in protein (see Table 1.3). Several possible reasons exist for the release of alanine and glutamine from muscle in such large amounts. First, skeletal muscle oxidizes dispensable amino acids and the BCAAs in situ for energy. Because amino acid oxidation produces waste N and because NH_3 is neurotoxic, release of waste N as NH_3 must be avoided. Given that both alanine and glutamine are readily synthesized from intermediates derived from glucose (alanine from transamination of pyruvate from glycolysis,

and glutamine from α-ketoglutarate), they are excellent vehicles to remove waste N from muscle while avoiding NH_3 release. Alanine removes one and glutamine removes two Ns per amino acid. These observations led to the proposal of a glucose-alanine cycle in which glucose made by the liver is taken up by muscle where glycolysis liberates pyruvate. The pyruvate is then transaminated to alanine and is released from muscle. That alanine is extracted by the liver and is transaminated to pyruvate, which is then used for glucose synthesis (114). This scheme has been expanded to explain the utilization of BCAAs by muscle for energy and disposal through alanine of their amino-N groups. Such a scheme resolves a problem related to the BCAAs. In contrast to the other IDAAs that are metabolized only in liver, the BCAAs are readily oxidized in other tissues, especially muscle.

Metabolic Adaptation to Fasting and Starvation

As indicated in Figure 1.13A, lipolysis (breakdown of adipose triglyceride to free fatty acids and glycerol) plays a lesser role in postabsorptive energy supply, especially to the brain. Glycogen stores are limited, however, and become depleted in less than 24 hours. That point in time when liver glycogen stores are exhausted is by definition the beginning of the *fasting* state. Now glucose needs of the brain must be met completely by gluconeogenesis, which means sacrificing amino acids from protein. Because protein is critical to body function, from enzyme activity to muscle function related to breathing and circulation, unrestrained use of amino acids for glucose production would rapidly deplete protein and cause death in a matter of days. Clearly, this result does not occur because people may survive for weeks without food. Adaptation occurs in starvation by the brain's switching from a glucose-based to a ketone-based fuel supply. Free fatty acids released from lipolysis are converted into ketone bodies in the liver that can then be used by the brain and other tissues for energy. That conversion begins in the fasting state and is complete under long periods of fasting (Fig. 1.13B). In starvation, tissues such as muscle may use free fatty acids directly for energy, and the brain used ketone bodies. The body's dependence on glucose as a fuel has been greatly reduced, thereby conserving protein. This adaptation process is complete within a week of the onset of starvation (106).

The Fed State

Although the body can accommodate to starvation, it is not a normal occurrence in our lives. The adaptations that are seen in everyday life evolve around the postabsorptive period and the fed period. Basically, we go through our nights after completing absorption of the last meal by using nutrient stores of glycogen and protein, as depicted in Figure 1.13A. During the fed portion of the day, three things occur to the dietary intake of amino acids and glucose: (a) they are used to replete protein and glycogen that were lost during the postabsorptive period; and intake in amounts greater than what is needed to replete nighttime losses is either (b) oxidized or (c) stored to increase protein, glycogen, or fat for growth or for storage of excess calories. Although muscle contains the bulk of body protein, all organs are expected to lose protein during the postabsorptive period and therefore need repletion during the fed period. What is poorly understood is how the individual amino acids that enter through the diet are distributed among the various tissues in the amounts needed for each tissue. Just as each amino acid has its own separate metabolic pathways, the rates and fates of absorption and utilization are expected to be different among amino acid. Thus, dietary protein requirements cannot be discussed without also considering the requirements of individual amino acids.

Digestion and Absorption of Protein

All dietary intake passes first through the gut and then through the liver via portal blood flow. Digestion of protein begins with pepsin secretion in gastric juice and with proteolytic enzymes secreted from pancreas and mucosa of the small intestine (115). These enzymes are secreted in their "pro" (or zymogen) form and become activated by cleavage of a small peptide portion. The pancreatic proenzymes become activated by intestinal enterokinase secreted into the intestinal juice to cleave trypsinogen to trypsin. The presence of dietary protein in the gut appears to signal the secretion of the enzymes. As trypsin

becomes activated, it binds to proteins at lysine or arginine residues that break the peptide bond on the C-terminus side of these amino acids to form peptides of 2 to 20 or more amino acids. Some plants, such as soybeans, contain protein inhibitors of proteolytic enzymes such as trypsin. These proteins are denatured by heating (i.e., by cooking). Feeding uncooked soybean to rats results in hypertrophy of the pancreas, presumably because of hypersecretion of trypsin that binds to these proteins but does not cleave them (116).

The events of protein digestion and absorption are well established (115, 117–119). Proteins are successively broken down into smaller peptides on the basis of the amino acid residues targeted by the proteolytic enzymes. For example, trypsin specifically targets lysine and arginine residues, whereas pepsin has a relatively low specificity for neutral amino acids such as leucine and phenylalanine. In addition, exopeptidases attack the free ends of the peptide chains such as pancreatically produced carboxypeptidases that cleave at the carboxyl terminus and aminopeptidases secreted in intestinal juice that cleave at the amino terminus of proteins.

The free amino acids are absorbed from gut lumen by active transport into the mucosa by transporters specific to different types of amino acids (117, 118). At the same time, dipeptides and tripeptides are also absorbed by the luminal side intact that are then hydrolyzed by peptide hydrolases present in the brush border and cytosol of the mucosal cells. Specific transport systems for peptide uptake into mucosal cells are separate from the transporters for amino acids. Investigators believe that one fourth of dietary protein is absorbed as dipeptides and tripeptides (120). For example, patients with the rare genetic Hartnup disease who have a defect in renal and gut transport of selected amino acids cannot transport free tryptophan into mucosal cells, but they do indeed absorb tryptophan when it is administered as a dipeptide (121).

To a limited but important extent, some proteins and large peptides pass from the gut intact into the basolateral blood. Absorption of intact proteins or large portions of proteins is a tenable physiologic explanation for diseases involving food allergies. The gut is generally viewed as an impermeable barrier where nutrients cross by active transport or where a break in the barrier occurs through cell injury. Small amounts of some proteins may pass this barrier by several possible mechanisms, such as through "leaks" between epithelial cell junctions or possibly by transport through uptake into vesicles from the lumen to the submucosal side of the epithelial cells (122). Again, the amount of protein entering intact is small, but it may be important in situations of immune response to the proteins or in delivery of some peptide drugs.

PROTEIN AND AMINO ACID REQUIREMENTS

A fundamental question in nutrition is this: *What amount of protein is required in the diets of humans to maintain health?* This question has several subparts. First, we must evaluate the intake of both protein and the amounts of the individual amino acids in that protein. Second, we need to evaluate requirements across (a) the complete range of life and development, (b) in sickness and in health, and (c) under different conditions of work and environment. For these reasons, protein requirement has been defined as "the lowest level of dietary protein intake that will balance the losses of N from the body, and thus maintain the body protein mass, in persons at energy balance with modest levels of physical activity, plus, in children or in pregnant or lactating women, the needs associated with the deposition of tissues or the secretion of milk at rates consistent with good health" (6).

When we discuss the amino acid composition of a specific protein source, we generally focus on IDAA content because this is by definition the *indispensable* portion in our diet. Which amino acids are dispensable and which are indispensable were originally determined by testing whether a diet deficient in a particular amino acid would support growth in a rat. Important species differences between rats and humans limit this comparison, however. Furthermore, the growth retardation model, which is effective with the rat, is not applicable to humans.

A technique for studying amino acid requirements in humans is the N balance method. A diet that is adequate in total N, but deficient in any IDAA, cannot produce a positive N balance because protein can be synthesized only if every amino acid is present in adequate amounts, and adequate intake of every IDAA is required for protein to be synthesized. The body is then faced with a dietary excess of the other *nonlimiting* IDAAs and dispensable amino acids that it cannot put into protein. Therefore, these amino acids must be oxidized to urea, and a negative N balance results.

The classic studies of Rose et al measured N balance in humans fed diets deficient in individual amino acids. These investigators determined that eight amino acids produced a negative N balance when they were deficient in the diet of adult humans (123, 124). Although the synthetic pathways are missing for the IDAAs, several of these amino acids have a catabolic pathway in which the first step in their catabolism is reversible transamination. For example, the BCAAs transaminate to form branched-chain keto acids, but this process is equally reversible (125). For example, growth can be supported in rats by replacing the IDAAs that transaminate with their keto acid analogs, and various formulations have been proposed for supplying the carbon skeleton of several IDAAs without adding N, which is detrimental in disease states such as renal disease (126).

Do dispensable amino acids ever become indispensable? If a dispensable amino acid is used in the body faster than it can be synthesized, it becomes indispensable for that *condition* (2). For example, tyrosine and cysteine are made from phenylalanine and methionine, respectively. If phenylalanine or methionine is consumed in insufficient amounts,

tyrosine and cysteine will become deficient and *indispensable*. This question must be evaluated across the range of life from infancy to the elderly as well as in sickness and health. For example, enzymes for amino acid metabolism mature at different rates in the growing fetus and newborn infant. Histidine is indispensable in infants, but not necessarily in healthy children or adults (6, 127). Therefore, the classification of "indispensable" or "dispensable" depends on (a) species, (b) maturation (i.e., infant, growing child, or adult), (c) diet, (d) nutritional status, and (e) pathophysiologic condition. Also to be considered is whether a particular amino acid *given in excess of requirement* has properties that may ameliorate or improve a clinical condition. These considerations must somehow be evaluated for each population group where they are important.

Protein Requirements

Determination of protein requirement must consider both the amount of amino acid N as well as its quality, that is, the ability to be digest and absorb protein and its IDAA content (6). The simplest approach to the measurement of the nutritional quality of a protein is to measure the ability of that protein to promote growth in young, growing animals, such as rats. Their growth depends on synthesis of new protein that, in turn, depends on IDAA intake. Because alterations in rat growth can be measured in several days, the growing rat has been often used as the model to compare differences in quality (composition) of protein and amino acid diets. Because this approach cannot ethically be applied to humans, other approaches for assessing *human* requirements have been applied.

Factorial Method

When a person is placed on a protein-free diet, rates of amino acid oxidation and urea production will decrease over a several day period as the body tries to conserve its resources, but amino acid oxidation and urea production do not drop to zero (see Fig. 1.7). Some *obligatory* oxidation of amino acids and urea formation and miscellaneous losses of N will always occur (see Table 1.9). The factorial method assesses all routes of losses possible for adult humans on an N-free diet. The minimum daily requirement of protein is assumed to be that amount that matches the sum of the various obligatory N losses.

Various studies were performed to assess these losses, and the results were tabulated and used as a basis for determining protein requirements as late as the 1985 Food and Agriculture Organization/World Health Organization (FAO/WHO) report (128). At that time, a total obligatory daily loss of endogenous loss of N of 54 mg/kg/day was assumed for men in a temperate climate, which corresponds to a protein intake of 0.34 g/kg/day (where 1 g N = 6.25 g protein). Additional obligatory N losses for people living in a tropical climate must be included for this group, however. Then these values are adjusted upward to account for inefficiency of utilization of dietary protein and for the quality (amino acid composition and digestibility) of the source of protein consumed. For children and pregnant or lactating women, an additional (theoretically determined) amount of protein is added to this recommendation to account for growth and milk formation. Clearly, this approach is based on extrapolation of N losses from protein-starvation conditions and may reflect an adaptation to N deprivation that may not reflect normal metabolism and N requirements of healthy humans near the actual requirement level. Rand and Young (129) also pointed out that the relationship between protein intake and N retention is curvilinear, making it troublesome to extrapolate obligatory N loss to a protein requirement. Hence, the most recent reports from 2002 have put much less weight on the factorial method in assessing protein requirements and more weight on the balance method (6, 130).

Balance Method

In the balance method, subjects are fed varying amounts of protein or amino acids, and the *balance* of a particular parameter, usually *N balance*, is measured. An adequate amount of dietary protein is that level of intake that will maintain a neutral or slightly positive N balance. The balance method can be used to titrate N intake in infants, children, and women during pregnancy, in whom the end point in this case is a balance positive enough to allow for appropriate accretion of new tissue. The balance method is also useful for testing the validity of the factorial method estimates. In general, N balance studies in which dietary protein intake is titrated give higher measures of protein requirements than predicted by the factorial method.

The N balance method has important errors associated with it that are not minor (6, 42, 129, 131). Urine collections tend to underestimate N losses, and intake tends to be overestimated. Miscellaneous losses are best guesses and may contain small but substantial errors. Although these factors affect both methods, the problem with the balance method is that it "titrates" dietary intake to determine zero balance, and that response is nonlinear as protein intake is increased from a grossly deficient status toward an adequate status (129, 131). In a meta-analysis, Rand et al (6, 131) systematically reviewed all N balance studies related to determining protein requirements. Through a very careful analysis of all factors, the 2002 Food and Nutrition Board report adopted the results of this study and set the median estimated average requirement (EAR) to be 0.66 g/kg/day for protein for men and women 19 years old and older (130). This recommendation considers that most studies of N balance have been performed at presumably adequate levels of energy intake, and N balance is affected by energy intake. Decreasing energy intake to less than requirements causes the N balance measurement to go from zero to negative when the protein intake is near the requirement. In addition, the recommendation considers protein quality and digestibility of the protein being consumed. Generally, it is assumed that protein of lesser quality and digestibility than egg white will be consumed, and a correction factor is added.

Recommended Dietary Allowances for Protein

In 1989, the Food and Nutrition Board subcommittee of the US Institute of Medicine, National Research Council updated their recommended dietary allowances (RDAs) for protein and amino acids (132) that were largely based on the 1985 FAO/WHO/United Nations University (UNU) committee report (128). In 2002, the Food and Nutrition Board prepared a report that was released in 2005 on dietary reference intakes for a range of macronutrients, including protein and amino acids (130). The RDA values for protein shown in Table 1.11 are based on the 2002 report and reflect N balance data (rather than factorial method data) from studies that used a high-quality, highly digestible source of protein. Data are presented for the EAR for protein. The EAR represents a protein intake that produced zero N balance in half of the population. That value was then increased by two standard deviations to encompass 97.5% of the population to obtain the RDA for the reference protein. For example, from studies of young men, the EAR value of 0.66 g/kg/day was increased to 0.80 g/kg/day for the RDA (130).

Special cases occur in which growth and accretion of tissue must be accounted for in the RDAs: during pregnancy, during lactation, and in infants and children. In pregnancy, total protein deposited was estimated to be 925 g based on maternal weight gain and an average birth weight at term. The rates of protein accretion were then divided by trimesters with adjustments for variation in birth weight (+15%) and an assumed efficiency of conversion of dietary protein to fetal, placental, and maternal tissues (+70%) to produce increments in reference protein intake of +1.0, +6.3, and +10.6 g protein/day for the first, second, and third

TABLE 1.11	RECOMMENDED INTAKES OF HIGH-QUALITY REFERENCE PROTEIN FOR NORMAL HUMANS			
AGE (y)	WEIGHT (kg)		EAR[a] (g/kg/d)	RDA[b] (g/kg/d)
0–0.5	6			1.52[c]
0.5–1	9		1.10	1.50
1–3	13		0.88	1.10
4–8	20		0.76	0.95
9–13	36		0.76	0.95
	Male	Female		
14–18	61	54	0.72	0.85
>18	70	57	0.66	0.80

[a]EAR, estimated average requirement: the intake that meets the estimated nutrient needs of half of the individuals in a group.
[b]RDA, recommended dietary allowance: the intake that meets the nutrient need of almost all (97.5%) of individuals in a group.
[c]Value for infants in the first half-year of life is the adequate intake estimate determined in that population that appears to sustain a defined nutritional status, including growth rate, normal circulating nutrient values, and other functional indicators of health. This value is not equivalent to an RDA.

Data from Food and Nutrition Board, Institute of Medicine. Proteins and amino acids. In: Dietary Reference Intakes for Energy, Carbohydrate, Fiber, Fat, Fatty Acids, Cholesterol, Protein, and Amino Acids. Washington, DC: National Academy Press, 2002, with permission.

trimesters, respectively (130). The amount of additional protein needed to be added to the diet during the last two trimesters to compensate for uncertainties about rates of tissue deposition and maintenance of those increases is estimated to be an EAR of +21 g protein/day or an RDA of +25 g/day additional protein over prepregnancy needs (130).

Women who are lactating also require additional protein intake. Using the factorial method and data for the protein content of human milk, volume of milk produced, and adjustment for the estimated 50% conversion efficiency of dietary protein into newly synthesized milk protein, an increase of +23.4 g protein/day needs to be added to the EAR of women in their first month of lactation. The EAR drops to +22 g/day in month 2 and to +18.3 g/day for months 4 to 6 of lactation (130). To compensate for variance among women, the EAR value is increased to an RDA of +25 g/day additional protein for women in their first month of lactation.

Amino Acid Requirements

The recommendations for the intake of individual amino acids are largely based on the pioneering work of W. C. Rose et al in the 1950s (123). Irwin and Hegsted (133) reviewed these and other studies of amino acid requirement levels published before 1971. Rose's studies are N balance measurements in which young male subjects were placed on diets with a N intake consisting of a mixture of crystalline amino acids. The intake of a single amino acid could be altered, and the N balance was measured. Because of the expense of crystalline amino acid diets and the great difficulty in performing serial N balance studies at different intakes, Rose et al were able to study only a very limited number of subjects per amino acid. Problems with interpreting the N balance data for a limited number of subjects cloud the extrapolation of these data to populations (134–136), yet the data of Rose et al have formed the primary basis for amino acid recommendations in adults for years.

Direct Amino Acid Oxidation Method

An alternative approach was taken by Young et al (135, 137, 138). Their approach, the direct amino acid oxidation (DAAO) method, is based on the method of Harper and other investigators to assess amino acid requirements in growing animals by using amino acid oxidation as an index of dietary sufficiency. Animals fed an insufficient amount of a specific individual amino acid reduce their oxidation of the deficient amino acid to obligatory levels. The oxidation of the dietary deficient amino acid will remain at obligatory oxidation levels until the requirement level is met. As dietary amino acid intake rises to more than the requirement, the excess amino acid from the diet will be oxidized. Therefore, a two-line curve of amino acid oxidation should appear when plotted against amino acid intake: a flat line below requirement (indicating obligatory oxidation) and a rising curve above the requirement (indicating oxidation of excess amino acid intake). The requirement level for the amino acid should

be the intersection of the two curves (i.e., where oxidation of excess amino acid begins).

The DAAO method uses the breakpoint in amino acid oxidation as a function of the intake of the test amino acid to determine requirement. Amino acid oxidation is determined by administering a ^{13}C- or ^{14}C-labeled amino acid tracer of the test amino acid being manipulated in the diet. The tracer amino acid is administered at the end of each diet period. The DAAO method was used by Young et al to estimate amino acid requirements for isoleucine, leucine, lysine, phenylalanine and tyrosine, and valine in healthy adults (137, 138).

Indicator Amino Acid Oxidation Method

Zello et al (139) took a different approach, the indicator amino acid oxidation (IAAO) method, to measure amino acid requirements. Rather than administer and measure the oxidation of a tracer of the same amino acid that is being manipulated in the diet, they use the oxidation of a tracer of another IDAA tracer as an *indicator* of N balance. N balance becomes negative when a single amino acid is deficient in the diet because of increased urea production resulting from oxidation of excess amino acids that cannot be incorporated into protein when the one test amino acid is deficient. Because measurement of the increase in urea production is fraught with problems, the oxidation of the indicator amino acid is measured instead, by using a carbon-labeled amino acid tracer. As the dietary intake of the test amino acid is decreased to less than requirement levels, the oxidation of the indicator amino acid will increase as excess amino acids are wasted (140). An example of this method is shown in Figure 1.14,

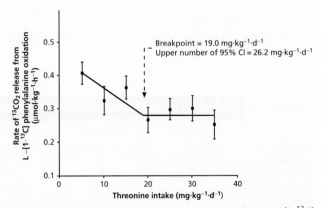

Fig. 1.14. Oxidation of the indicator amino acid tracer [1-^{13}C] phenylalanine to $^{13}CO_2$ in young men fed different dietary intakes of threonine. Phenylalanine oxidation is constant above the dietary requirement threonine, but it progressively increases as threonine intake drops below requirement because limitation of threonine intake limits the body's ability to synthesize protein and causes the excess amino acids to be oxidized, including the indicator amino acid, phenylalanine. Thus, the breakpoint between the two lines indicates the threonine requirement in these subjects. *CI,* confidence interval. (Reprinted with permission from Wilson DC, Rafii M, Ball RO et al. Threonine requirement of young men determined by indicator amino acid oxidation with use of L-[1-(13)C] phenylalanine. Am J Clin Nutr 2000;71:757–64. Copyright American Society for Clinical Nutrition.)

in which [1-^{13}C]phenylalanine is infused as the indicator amino acid in young men consuming different levels of dietary threonine intake (141). The intake of all other amino acids is held constant (including that of the indicator, phenylalanine). At threonine intakes greater than the requirement, phenylalanine oxidation is constant, but phenylalanine oxidation progressively increases as threonine intake is decreased to less than the threonine requirement. The breakpoint between the two curves in Figure 1.14 indicates the mean EAR for threonine intake. The RDA for threonine intake would be set two confidence intervals above the EAR.

The key to this method is the availability of an indicator amino acid tracer whose oxidation can be accurately and precisely measured that is different from the test amino acid being manipulated in the diet. Using this approach and [1-^{13}C]phenylalanine as the indicator amino acid, Elango et al redetermined the requirement levels for several different amino acids (142, 143). These estimates are largely in agreement with estimates by the DAAO method. A concern about the IAAO method is that relatively short (e.g., 3 days) adaptation periods are used for the different dietary intakes tested, however. Classical N balance studies require 7 to 10 days for equilibration to occur in urinary N output, but this constraint is not required when using the indicator tracer to measure oxidation directly. Thus, short adaptation periods can and are typically used with the IAAO method. The impact of these short adaptation periods has not been fully defined.

Twenty-Four Hour Tracer Balance Method

A final twist has been added to the DAAO and IAAO methods to account for the fact that we oxidize amino acids 24 hours a day, not just during periods of feeding. El-Khoury et al (144, 145) infused a [1-^{13}C]leucine tracer for 24 hours into subjects receiving different intakes of leucine to determine leucine requirements by the DAAO

method. Borgonha et al (146) infused [1-^{13}C]leucine for 24 hours as an IAAO tracer into subjects receiving different intakes of threonine to determine threonine requirements. Several similar studies, such as two from Young and Borgonha's group (147), were performed to redefine amino acid requirements in humans and were used to put together recommendations for amino acid intakes that are considerably greater for several IDAAs than determined previously, largely by the N balance method.

Both the Food and Nutrition Board and the FAO/WHO/UNU reports on RDAs of IDAAs from meetings in 2002 considered the myriad of new data from stable isotope tracer studies in making their current recommendations (6, 130). Their current recommendations are shown in Table 1.12 for infants, children, and adults. The RDAs for infants decreased with the 2002 report for most amino acids. The RDAs for children were reduced primarily for the BCAAs, but the RDAs for amino acids for which DAAO and IAAO method data were available increased significantly (Table 1.12).

Histidine

Although histidine has been shown to be indispensable to the diet of the rat, it has been difficult to define as indispensable to the diet of adult humans (134). The limited studies of adults indicate that the requirement for histidine may be less than 2 mg/kg/day (148). This requirement has not been clearly documented in physiologically normal subjects, however (124). Proving histidine to be indispensable in adults has largely been restricted to studies of renal failure (4). Currently, the EAR for histidine is 10 to 14 mg/kg/day (Table 1.12), and this recommendation is largely based on histidine content of protein and the RDA for protein.

Why is it so difficult to define whether histidine is indispensable in adults when there is little evidence that a metabolic pathway for histidine synthesis exists in humans

TABLE 1.12	ESTIMATES OF RECOMMENDED DIETARY AMINO ACID ALLOWANCES (MG/KG/D) BY AGE GROUP				
	INFANTS[a]	CHILDREN[a]		ADULTS (>18 y)	
AMINO ACID	7–12 mo	1–3 y	4–13 y	FNB[a]	FAO/WHO[b]
Histidine[c]	32	21	16	14	10
Isoleucine	43	28	22	19	20
Leucine	96	62	48	42	39
Lysine	89	58	45	38	30
Methionine + cysteine	43	28	22	19	15
Phenylalanine + tyrosine	84	54	41	33	25
Threonine	49	32	24	20	15
Tryptophan	13	8	6	5	4
Valine	58	37	28	24	26

FNB, Food and Nutrition Board; FAO/WHO, Food and Agriculture Organization/World Health Organization.

[a]Data from Food and Nutrition Board, Institute of Medicine. Proteins and amino acids. In: Dietary Reference Intakes for Energy, Carbohydrate, Fiber, Fat, Fatty Acids, Cholesterol, Protein, and Amino Acids. Washington, DC: National Academy Press, 2002.
[b]Data from Food and Agriculture Organization/World Health Organization/United Nations University. Protein and Amino Acid Requirements in Human Nutrition. Geneva: World Health Organization, 2007.
[c]Although no requirement for histidine has been quantified beyond infancy, histidine has been recommended for children and adults based on the histidine content of the recommended dietary allowance for protein of each of these age groups.

(13)? The difficulties occur because the requirement for histidine is small and the stores of histidine in the body are large (4, 124). Histidine is particularly abundant in hemoglobin and carnosine (the dipeptide β-alanylhistidine that is present in large quantities in muscle). Furthermore, gut flora synthesizes an unknown amount of histidine, which may be absorbed and used. Histidine must be removed from the diet for more than a month to observe effects, and those effects are indirect measures of histidine insufficiency (a fall in hemoglobin and a rise in serum iron), rather than an alteration in conventional indices (N balance). Kriengsinyos et al (127) of the Pencharz group placed four adults on a histidine-free diet for 48 days and periodically measured protein turnover by using $[1\text{-}^{13}C]$ phenylalanine. The investigators noted a small, significant fall in protein turnover over time, but urinary excretion of N or 3-methylhistidine was unaffected. No direct effect of histidine requirement could be determined in adults in this study. Thus, even though little direct evidence for histidine synthesis in humans exists, our estimates for the necessity of dietary histidine intake in adults are still largely inferential.

Assessment of Protein Quality

The "quality" of a protein is defined by its ability to support growth in animals. High-quality protein produces a faster growth rate. Such growth rate measurements evaluate the actual factors important in a protein: (a) pattern and abundance of IDAAs, (b) relative amounts of dispensable amino acids versus IDAAs in the mixture, (c) digestibility when eaten, and (d) presence of toxic materials such as trypsin inhibitors or allergenic stimuli. Methods to define the quality of a formula or protein source generally fall into two categories: empiric biologic assays and scoring systems.

Biologic Assays

It is assumed that the "highest-quality protein" is protein that supports maximal growth in a young animal. Because rats grow quickly, have limited protein stores, and a high metabolic rate, it is easy to detect deficiencies and imbalances in amino acid patterns in young growing rats in a short period of time. The *protein efficiency ratio (PER)* has been defined as the weight gained (in grams) divided by the amount of test protein consumed (in grams) by a young growing rat over a several day period. Obviously, duration of diet, age, starting body weight, and species of rat employed are important variables. Typically, 21-day old male rats fed 9% to 10% protein (by weight) for 10 days to 4 weeks have been used. For example, in one series of tests, casein produced a PER of 2.8, soy protein 2.4, and wheat gluten 0.4, findings indicating what we already know, that gluten is a poor-quality protein. Such an approach has been useful in defining the relative efficacy of clinical formulas used in enteral and parenteral nutrition (149). The formula that provides the optimal mixture of IDAAs and dispensable amino acids should induce the most rapid growth. This method's results will be skewed in application to humans, however, depending on the extent to which human requirements for individual amino acids do not mimic those of the rat. Nonetheless, the method has been very useful in comparing a new protein source against reference proteins, such as egg protein, and it does evaluate other factors such as relative digestibility.

Scoring Systems

Rather than using growth in an animal species as an indicator of protein quality, various methods have been developed to assign a quantitative value to the pattern of amino acids in a nutritional formula or to a particular dietary protein source. Thus, assignment is based on the amounts and importance of the individual amino acids in a formula. These scoring methods can be applied to define protein quality in terms of amino acid content for any species. Block and Mitchell (150) pointed out in 1946 that all amino acids must be provided simultaneously at the sites of protein synthesis in the body in the same proportions that go into protein. Assuming that dispensable amino acids would not be limiting, these investigators proposed that the value of a protein could be determined from the IDAA most limiting in abundance relative to the optimum amount needed. From this idea of "most limiting amino acid" came the concept of chemical scoring that has been incorporated into reports assessing dietary needs of humans (6, 130). The key to the method is that the test protein is defined "against" a reference protein, deemed to be of the "highest quality" in terms of amino acid composition. Historically, proteins that support maximal growth in animals were considered the proteins of the highest quality. Those proteins from the most available sources for human consumption (eggs and cow milk) were consequently used as reference proteins.

The scoring system is easy to apply because no animal studies or clinical studies are required to compare different nutritional formulations. The *chemical score* of a protein is calculated in two steps. First, a score is calculated for each IDAA in the protein against the reference protein or a reference pattern of IDAA amino acids:

$$\text{IDAA score} = \frac{\left(\text{content of the IDAA in the } test \frac{\text{protein}}{\text{mixture}}\right)}{\left(\text{content of the IDAA in the } reference \frac{\text{protein}}{\text{mixture}}\right)} \cdot 100$$

Next, the lowest IDAA score is selected. The amino acid with the lowest score is defined as the *limiting amino acid* and is the test protein is assigned that score.

Typically, the most common limiting amino acid is lysine, which is particularly low in cereal proteins, then the sulfur-containing amino acids, threonine and tryptophan. The BCAAs and phenylalanine/tyrosine are not usually limiting. The scoring method points out the obvious: proteins not balanced among the IDAAs are not as good as those that are, and this method is a useful tool for assessing the quality of individual proteins or protein from a particular food source.

Ratio of Indispensable to Dispensable Amino Acids in Protein

Protein requirements diminish from infancy onward (see Table 1.11) because rates of accretion of new protein diminish with maturity. When the changes in requirements for IDAAs in Table 1.12 are compared with the total protein requirements in Table 1.11 with age, however, a greater drop with age is seen in IDAA requirements than in protein requirements. IDAAs make up more than 30% of protein requirements in infancy and early childhood and then drop to 20% in later childhood and to 11% in adulthood. As IDAAs become a decreasingly important part of the amino acid requirements with age, dispensable amino acid intake could increase and become an increasingly greater proportion of our intake. Such substitution does not necessarily happen, however. Except for possibly changing the type of protein eaten (e.g., decreased intake of milk proteins), we continue to eat protein presumably at or higher than the RDA. If that protein is of high quality, it will provide about half of its amino acids as IDAAs. Therefore, consumption of high-quality protein by adults at levels appropriate to meet the RDA for protein will provide an excess of individual IDAAs beyond requirements. In general, it is not difficult for adults to meet the minimum for IDAA intake, as recommended (6, 130), when protein is consumed at or higher than the requirement.

Protein and Amino Acid Needs in Disease

Most of the discussion up to this point has centered around amino acid and protein metabolism in physiologically normal individuals. Although the effect of disease on amino acid and protein requirements is beyond the limits of this chapter, a few important general points need to be made. The first is that energy and protein needs are tied together as illustrated in Figure 1.13. When metabolic rate rises, body protein is mobilized for use as a fuel (amino acid oxidation) and for supply of carbon for gluconeogenesis. Several disease states produce an increase in metabolic rate. The first is infection, in which the onset of fever is a hallmark of increased metabolic rate. The second is injury, be it trauma, burn injury, or surgery. Along with onset of a hypermetabolic state comes a characteristic increase in the loss of protein measured by increased urea production. In 1930, Sir David Cuthbertson observed that a simple bone fracture causes significant loss of N in the urine (151). Since then, numerous studies of the hypermetabolic state of injury and infection have been performed.

For most people, the injuries we suffer are minimal and self-limiting: the fever goes away in a couple of days or the injury heals. In physiologically normal, healthy people, the impact of the injury on overall protein metabolism is as minimal as would be a bout of fasting. In chronic, long-term illness or in patients otherwise weakened by age or other factors, however, the onset of a hypermetabolic state may produce a significant and dangerous loss of body N.

The second point is that although the diagnosis of a metabolic condition that needs correcting may be straightforward (e.g., finding an increased loss of N and wasting of body protein), correcting the problem by administration of nutritional support is not as simple. The underlying illness usually resists or complicates simple nutritional replacement of amino acids. Trauma and infection are classic problems for which prevention of N loss is very difficult. Supplying additional nutrients either enterally (by mouth or feeding tube) or parenterally (by intravenous administration) may blunt, but will not reverse, the N loss seen in injury (see the chapters on hypercatabolic states, on surgery, infection, trauma, and on burn and wound healing).

Simple tools have been used to identify the hypermetabolic state: indirect calorimetry to measure energy expenditure and N balance to follow protein loss. These measurement methods have shown that blunting the N loss in such patients is not as simple as supplying more calories, more amino acids, or different formulations of amino acids. What becomes clear is that, although a nutritional problem exists, nutritional replacement will not correct the problem; instead, the metabolic factors that cause the condition must be identified and corrected. Wilmore (152) categorized the factors that produce the hypermetabolic state into three groups: stress hormones (cortisol, catecholamines, glucagon), cytokines (e.g., tumor necrosis factor, interleukins), and lipid mediators (e.g., prostaglandins, thromboxanes). Strategies have been developed to address these various components. For example, insulin and growth hormone have been administered to provide anabolic hormonal stimuli to improve N balance. Alternatively, studies have been conducted in healthy individuals in whom one or more of the potential mediators are administered to define the effect of the mediator on amino acid and protein metabolism (153).

In some situations, administration of a specific amino acid may produce a pharmacologic effect in ameliorating the disease state. Examples are the administration of glutamine and arginine or the limiting of sulfur amino acid intake. Glutamine is the most highly concentrated amino acid inside muscle cells and in plasma (154). Glutamine is an important nutrient to many cells, especially the gut and white blood cells, where the glutamine may be used as a source of energy and also for critical processes such as the synthesis of nucleotides. Glutamine is an essential nutrient for cell culture media. Because a hallmark of injury is a drop in the intracellular level of muscle glutamine, presumably as a result of increased utilization by other tissues, glutamine has been proposed as a nutrient that becomes conditionally indispensable in trauma and infection (152, 155).

Arginine is another dispensable amino acid with important properties for promoting immune system function. Arginine is the precursor for nitric oxide synthesis (156), and it has been proposed as a nutrient for altering immune function and improving wound healing (157, 158). We believe that adequate ornithine is synthesized to maintain arginine supplies under normal conditions, but we do not know whether additional demands for arginine can be met endogenously or whether arginine becomes a conditionally indispensable nutrient. For example, Yu et al (159) measured arginine kinetics by using stable isotope tracers in pediatric patients with burn injury and determined little net de novo arginine synthesis. This finding suggests that under conditions of burn injury, insufficient arginine is made to meet the body's presumed increased need for arginine when the immune system is under challenge.

Although supplementation of specific amino acids or cofactors may produce beneficial responses, on some occasions supplementation may produce undesirable effects on the disease state. Supplementing glutamine in the diets of patients with cancer may be counterproductive because the glutamine (which is essential for fast growing cell lines in culture) may promote accelerated tumor growth (160). Similarly, arginine supplementation may stimulate nitric oxide synthesis because of the increased availability of the precursor for its formation. Nitric oxide production has both helpful and detrimental effects, however (156). In these and other applications of specific nutrients, the use of isotopically labeled tracers is particularly helpful because the metabolic fate of the administered nutrient may be followed (labeled nitrate production from nitric oxide synthesis from ^{15}N-labeled arginine), and the promotion or suppression of protein synthesis and proteolysis in specific tissues may be measured. Definition of amino acid and protein requirements in various diseases is difficult to assess and requires a multifactorial approach.

REFERENCES

1. Cahill GF. N Engl J Med 1970;282:668–75.
2. Chipponi JX, Bleier JC, Santi MT et al. Am J Clin Nutr 1982;35:1112–6.
3. Harper AE. Dispensable and indispensable amino acid interrelationships. In: Blackburn GL, Grant JP, Young VR, eds. Amino Acids: Metabolism and Medical Applications. Boston: John Wright, 1983:105–21.
4. Laidlaw SA, Kopple JD. Am J Clin Nutr 1987;46:593–605.
5. Block RJ, Weiss KW. Amino Acid Handbook: Methods and Results of Analysis. Springfield, IL: Charles C Thomas, 1956.
6. Food and Agriculture Organization/World Health Organization/United Nations University. Protein and Amino Acid Requirements in Human Nutrition. Geneva: World Health Organization, 2007:1–256.
7. Bergström J, Fürst P, Norée LO et al. J Appl Physiol 1974; 36:693–7.
8. Cohn SH, Vartsky D, Yasumura S et al. Am J Physiol 1980; 239:E524–30.
9. Heymsfield SB, Waki M, Kehayias J et al. Am J Physiol 1991;261:E190–8.
10. Christensen HN. Physiol Rev 1990;70:43–77.
11. Souba WW, Pacitti AJ. JPEN J Parenter Enteral Nutr 1992;16:569–78.
12. Rennie MJ, Tadros L, Khogali S et al. J Nutr 1994;124(Suppl): 1503S–8S.
13. Krebs HA. The metabolic fate of amino acids. In: Munro HN, Allison JB, eds. Mammalian Protein Metabolism, vol 1. New York: Academic Press, 1964:125–76.
14. Ben Galim E, Hruska K, Bier DM et al. J Clin Invest 1980;66:1295–304.
15. Yoshida T, Kikuchi G. Arch Biochem Biophys 1970;139:380–92.
16. Yoshida T, Kikuchi G. J Biochem (Tokyo) 1972;72:1503–16.
17. Katagiri M, Nakamura M. Biochem Biophys Res Commun 2003;312:205–8.
18. Matthews DE, Conway JM, Young VR et al. Metabolism 1981;30:886–93.
19. Stipanuk MH. Annu Rev Nutr 1986;6:179–209.
20. Jacobsen JG, Smith LH Jr. Physiol Rev 1968;48:424–511.
21. Hayes KC. Nutr Rev 1985;43:65–70.
22. Beutler E. Annu Rev Nutr 1989;9:287–302.
23. Griffith OW. Free Radic Biol Med 1999;27:922–35.
24. Wu G, Fang YZ, Yang S et al. J Nutr 2004;134:489–92.
25. Rebouche CJ, Seim H. Annu Rev Nutr 1998;18:39–61.
26. Rebouche CJ. Fed Proc 1982;41:2848–52.
27. Watkins CA, Morgan HE. J Biol Chem 1979;254:693–701.
28. Meldrum BS. J Nutr 2000;130(Suppl):1007S–15S.
29. Rothstein JD, Martin LJ, Kuncl RW. N Engl J Med 1992;326:1464–8.
30. Wyss M, Kaddurah-Daouk R. Physiol Rev 2000;80:1107–213.
31. Bloch K, Schoenheimer R. J Biol Chem 1941;138:167–94.
32. Heymsfield SB, Arteaga C, McManus C et al. Am J Clin Nutr 1983;37:478–94.
33. Walser M. JPEN J Parenter Enteral Nutr 1987;11(Suppl):73S–8S.
34. Crim MC, Calloway DH, Margen S. J Nutr 1975;105:428–38.
35. Welle S, Thornton C, Totterman S et al. Am J Clin Nutr 1996; 63:151–6.
36. Wang Z, Gallagher D, Nelson M et al. Am J Clin Nutr 1996;63: 863–9.
37. Milner JA, Visek WJ. Nature 1973;245:211–2.
38. Hellerstein MK, Munro HN. Interaction of liver and muscle in the regulation of metabolism in response to nutritional and other factors. In: Arias IM, Jakoby WB, Popper H et al, eds. The Liver: Biology and Pathobiology. 2nd ed. New York: Raven Press, 1988:965–83.
39. Harper AE. Am J Clin Nutr 1985;41:140–8.
40. Scrimshaw NS, Hussein MA, Murray E et al. J Nutr 1972;102: 1595–604.
41. Allison JB, Bird JWC. Elimination of nitrogen from the body. In: Munro HN, Allison JB, eds. Mammalian Protein Metabolism. New York: Academic Press, 1964:483–512.
42. Munro HN. Amino acid requirements and metabolism and their relevance to parenteral nutrition. In: Wilkinson AW, ed. Parenteral Nutrition. London: Churchill Livingstone, 1972: 34–67.
43. Owen OE, Reichle FA, Mozzoli MA et al. J Clin Invest 1981; 68:240–52.
44. Owen OE, Morgan AP, Kemp HG et al. J Clin Invest 1967; 46:1589–95.
45. Wahren J, Felig P, Hagenfeldt L. J Clin Invest 1976;57:987–99.
46. Brundin T, Wahren J. Am J Physiol 1994;267:E648–55.
47. Young VR, Haverberg LN, Bilmazes C et al. Metabolism 1973;23:1429–36.
48. Young VR, Munro HN. Fed Proc 1978;37:2291–2300.
49. Pisters PWT, Pearlstone DB. Crit Rev Clin Lab Sci 1993; 30:223–72.
50. Louard RJ, Bhushan R, Gelfand RA et al. J Clin Endocrinol Metab 1994;79:278–84.
51. Cheng KN, Dworzak F, Ford GC et al. Eur J Clin Invest 1985;15:349–54.

52. Barrett EJ, Revkin JH, Young LH et al. Biochem J 1987; 245:223–8.
53. Wolfe RR, Chinkes DL. Isotope Tracers in Metabolic Research: Principles and Practice of Kinetic Analysis. 2nd ed. Hoboken, NJ: Wiley-Liss, 2004:1–488.
54. San Pietro A, Rittenberg D. J Biol Chem 1953;201:457–73.
55. Picou D, Taylor-Roberts T. Clin Sci 1969;36:283–96.
56. Bier DM, Matthews DE. Fed Proc 1982;41:2679–85.
57. Steffee WP, Goldsmith RS, Pencharz PB et al. Metabolism 1976;25:281–97.
58. Yudkoff M, Nissim I, McNellis W et al. Pediatr Res 1987; 21:49–53.
59. Waterlow JC, Golden MHN, Garlick PJ. Am J Physiol 1978; 235:E165–74.
60. Fern EB, Garlick PJ, McNurlan MA et al. Clin Sci 1981; 61:217–28.
61. Matthews DE, Motil KJ, Rohrbaugh DK et al. Am J Physiol 1980;238:E473–9.
62. Bier DM. Diabetes Metab Rev 1989;5:111–32.
63. Wolfe RR. Radioactive and Stable Isotope Tracers in Biomedicine: Principles and Practice of Kinetic Analysis. New York: Wiley-Liss, 1992:1–471.
64. Toth MJ, MacCoss MJ, Poehlman ET et al. Am J Physiol 2001;281:E233–41.
65. Allsop JR, Wolfe RR, Burke JF. J Appl Physiol 1978;45:137–9.
66. El-Khoury AE, Sánchez M, Fukagawa NK et al. J Nutr 1994; 124:1615–27.
67. Matthews DE, Bier DM, Rennie MJ et al. Science 1981; 214:1129–31.
68. Matthews DE, Schwarz HP, Yang RD et al. Metabolism 1982;31:1105–12.
69. Tessari P, Barazzoni R, Zanetti M et al. Am J Physiol 1996; 271:E733–41.
70. Castillo L, Sánchez M, Vogt J et al. Am J Physiol 1995;268: E360–67.
71. Darmaun D, Matthews DE, Bier DM. Am J Physiol 1986; 251:E117–26.
72. Souba WW. Annu Rev Nutr 1991;11:285–308.
73. Cortiella J, Matthews DE, Hoerr RA et al. Am J Clin Nutr 1988;48:988–1009.
74. Tessari P, Pehling G, Nissen SL et al. Diabetes 1988;37: 512–9.
75. Matthews DE, Marano MA, Campbell RG. Am J Physiol 1993;264:E109–18.
76. Haisch M, Fukagawa NK, Matthews DE. Am J Physiol 2000; 278:E593–602.
77. Hoerr RA, Matthews DE, Bier DM et al. Am J Physiol 1993;264:E567–75.
78. Metges CC, El Khoury AE, Henneman L et al. Am J Physiol 1999;277:E597–607.
79. Battezzati A, Haisch M, Brillon DJ et al. Metabolism 1999; 48:915–21.
80. Castillo L, Chapman TE, Yu YM et al. Am J Physiol 1993; 265:E532–9.
81. Matthews DE, Marano MA, Campbell RG. Am J Physiol 1993;264:E848–54.
82. Battezzati A, Brillon DJ, Matthews DE. Am J Physiol 1995; 269:E269–76.
83. Rooyackers OE, Adey DB, Ades PA et al. Proc Natl Acad Sci U S A 1996;93:15364–9.
84. Rooyackers OE, Balagopal P, Nair KS. Muscle Nerve Suppl 1997;5:S93–6.
85. Jaleel A, Short KR, Asmann YW et al. Am J Physiol 2008; 295:E1255–68.
86. Jaleel A, Henderson GC, Madden BJ et al. Diabetes 2010; 59:2366–74.
87. Nair KS, Halliday D, Griggs RC. Am J Physiol 1988;254: E208–13.
88. Toffolo G, Albright R, Joyner M et al. Am J Physiol 2003; 285:E1142–9.
89. Cryer DR, Matsushima T, Marsh JB et al. J Lipid Res 1986; 27:508–6.
90. Reeds PJ, Hachey DL, Patterson BW et al. J Nutr 1992; 122:457–66.
91. Brinton EA, Eisenberg S, Breslow JL. Arterioscler Thromb 1994;14:707–20.
92. Ikewaki K, Zech LA, Brewer HB Jr et al. J Lab Clin Med 2002;140:369–74.
93. Busch R, Kim YK, Neese RA et al. Biochim Biophys Acta 2006;1760:730–44.
94. Dufner D, Previs SF. Curr Opin Clin Nutr Metab Care 2003; 6:511–7.
95. Holm L, Kjaer M. Curr Opin Clin Nutr Metab Care 2010; 13:526–31.
96. Laurent GJ. Am J Physiol 1987;252:C1–9.
97. Long CL, Dillard DR, Bodzin JH et al. Metabolism 1988;37: 844–9.
98. Elia M, Carter A, Bacon S et al. Clin Sci 1980;59:509–11.
99. Rennie MJ, Millward DJ. Clin Sci 1983;65:217–25.
100. Rathmacher JA, Flakoll PJ, Nissen SL. Am J Physiol 1995; 269:E193–8.
101. Lundholm K, Bennegård K, Edén E et al. Cancer Res 1982;42:4807–11.
102. Morrison WL, Gibson JNA, Rennie MJ. Eur J Clin Invest 1988;18:648–54.
103. Möller-Loswick A-C, Zachrisson H, Hyltander A et al. Am J Physiol 1994;266:E645–52.
104. Vissers YL, Von Meyenfeldt MF, Braulio VB et al. Clin Sci 2003;104:585–90.
105. Vesali RF, Klaude M, Thunblad L et al. Metabolism 2004; 53:1076–80.
106. Cahill GF Jr, Aoki TT. Partial and total starvation. In: Kinney JM, ed. Assessment of Energy Metabolism in Health and Disease. Report of the First Ross Conference on Medical Research. Columbus, OH: Ross Laboratories, 1980: 129–34.
107. Elia M. Organ and tissue contribution to metabolic rate. In: Kinney JM, Tucker HN, eds. Energy Metabolism: Determinants and Cellular Corollaries. New York: Raven Press, 1992:61–79.
108. Bier DM, Leake RD, Haymond MW et al. Diabetes 1977;26:1016–23.
109. Owen OE, Felig P, Morgan AP et al. J Clin Invest 1969;48: 574–83.
110. Pozefsky T, Felig P, Tobin JD et al. J Clin Invest 1969;48: 2273–82.
111. Felig P, Owen OE, Wahren J et al. J Clin Invest 1969;48: 584–94.
112. Stumvoll M, Chintalapudi U, Perriello G et al. J Clin Invest 1995;96:2528–33.
113. Cersosimo E, Judd RL, Miles JM. J Clin Invest 1994;93:2584–9.
114. Felig P. Annu Rev Biochem 1975;44:933–55.
115. Alpers DH. Digestion and absorption of carbohydrates and proteins. In: Johnson LR, Alpers DH, Christensen J et al, eds. Physiology of the Gastrointestinal Tract. 3rd ed. New York: Raven Press, 1994:1723–49.
116. Green GM, Olds BA, Matthews G et al. Proc Soc Exp Biol Med 1973;142:1162–7.

117. Matthews DM. Protein Absorption: Development and Present State of the Subject. New York: Wiley-Liss, 1991:1–414.

118. Ganapathy V, Brandsch M, Leibach FH. Intestinal transport of amino acids and peptides. In: Johnson LR, Alpers DH, Christensen J et al, eds. Physiology of the Gastrointestinal Tract. 3rd ed. New York: Raven Press, 1994:1773–94.

119. Freeman HJ, Kim YS. Annu Rev Med 1978;29:99–116.

120. Alpers DH. Fed Proc 1986;45:2261–7.

121. Asatoor AM, Cheng B, Edwards KDG et al. Gut 1970;11:380–7.

122. Gardner ML. Absorption of intact proteins and peptides. In: Johnson LR, Alpers DH, Christensen J et al, eds. Physiology of the Gastrointestinal Tract. 3rd ed. New York: Raven Press, 1994:1795–820.

123. Rose WC. Nutr Abstr Rev 1957;27:631–47.

124. Visek WJ. Annu Rev Nutr 1984;4:137–55.

125. Matthews DE, Harkin R, Battezzati A et al. Metabolism 1999;48:1555–63.

126. Walser M. Clin Sci 1984;66:1–15.

127. Kriengsinyos W, Rafii M, Wykes LJ et al. J Nutr 2002;132:3340–8.

128. Food and Agriculture Organization/World Health Organization/United Nations University. Energy and Protein Requirements. Technical series no. 724. Geneva: World Health Organization, 1985:1–206.

129. Rand WM, Young VR. J Nutr 1999;129:1920–6.

130. Food and Nutrition Board, Institute of Medicine. Proteins and amino acids. In: Dietary Reference Intakes for Energy, Carbohydrate, Fiber, Fat, Fatty Acids, Cholesterol, Protein, and Amino Acids. Washington, DC: National Academy Press, 2002:589–768.

131. Rand WM, Pellett PL, Young VR. Am J Clin Nutr 2003;77:109–27.

132. Food and Nutrition Board, National Research Council. Recommended Dietary Allowances. 10th ed. Washington, DC: National Academy Press, 1989:52–77.

133. Irwin MI, Hegsted DM. J Nutr 1971;101:539–66.

134. Millward DJ, Price GM, Pacy PJH et al. Proc Nutr Soc 1990;49:473–87.

135. Young VR, Bier DM, Pellett PL. Am J Clin Nutr 1989;50:80–92.

136. Young VR. Am J Clin Nutr 1987;46:709–25.

137. Young VR. J Nutr 1994;124(Suppl):1517S–23S.

138. Young VR, El-Khoury AE. Proc Natl Acad Sci U S A 1995;92:300–4.

139. Zello GA, Wykes LJ, Ball RO et al. J Nutr 1995;125:2907–15.

140. Elango R, Ball RO, Pencharz PB. J Nutr 2008;138:243–6.

141. Wilson DC, Rafii M, Ball RO et al. Am J Clin Nutr 2000;71:757–64.

142. Elango R, Ball RO, Pencharz PB. Curr Opin Clin Nutr Metab Care 2008;11:34–9.

143. Elango R, Ball RO, Pencharz PB. Amino Acids 2009;37:19–27.

144. El-Khoury AE, Fukagawa NK, Sánchez M et al. Am J Clin Nutr 1994;59:1000–11.

145. El-Khoury AE, Fukagawa NK, Sánchez M et al. Am J Clin Nutr 1994;59:1012–20.

146. Borgonha S, Regan MM, Oh SH et al. Am J Clin Nutr 2002;75:698–704.

147. Young VR, Borgonha S. J Nutr 2000;130(Suppl):1841S–9S.

148. Kopple JD, Swendseid ME. J Nutr 1981;111:931–942.

149. Bjelton L, Sandberg G, Wennberg A et al. Assessment of biological quality of amino acid solutions for intravenous nutrition. In: Kinney JM, Borum PR, eds. Perspectives in Clinical Nutrition. Baltimore: Urban & Schwarzenberg, 1989:31–41.

150. Block RJ, Mitchell HH. Nutr Abstr Rev 1946;16:249–278.

151. Cuthbertson DP. Injury 1980;11:175–89.

152. Wilmore DW. N Engl J Med 1991;325:695–702.

153. Lowry SF. Proc Nutr Soc 1992;51:267–77.

154. Souba WW, Herskowitz K, Austgen TR et al. JPEN J Parenter Enteral Nutr 1990;14(Suppl):237S–43S.

155. Labow BI, Souba WW. World J Surg 2000;24:1503–13.

156. Griffith OW, Stuehr DJ. Annu Rev Physiol 1995;57:707–36.

157. Brittenden J, Heys SD, Ross J et al. Clin Sci 1994;86:123–32.

158. Ziegler TR, Gatzen C, Wilmore DW. Annu Rev Med 1994;45:459–80.

159. Yu YM, Sheridan RL, Burke JF et al. Am J Clin Nutr 1996;64:60–6.

160. Souba WW. Ann Surg 1993;218:715–28.

SUGGESTED READINGS

Food and Agriculture Organization/World Health Organization/United Nations University. Protein and Amino Acid Requirements in Human Nutrition. Geneva: World Health Organization, 2007:1–256.

Food and Nutrition Board, Institute of Medicine. Dietary Reference Intakes for Energy, Carbohydrate, Fiber, Fat, Fatty Acids, Cholesterol, Protein, and Amino Acids (Macronutrients). Washington, DC: National Academy Press, 2002.

Munro HN, Allison JB. Mammalian Protein Metabolism, vol 1. New York: Academic Press, 1964.

Wolfe RR, Chinkes DL. Isotope Tracers in Metabolic Research: Principles and Practice of Kinetic Analysis. 2nd ed. Hoboken, NJ: Wiley-Liss, 2004:1–488.

2 CARBOHYDRATES[1]

NANCY L. KEIM, ROY J. LEVIN, AND PETER J. HAVEL

[1]**Abbreviations: ACC**, acetyl-coenzyme A carboxylase; **AI**, adequate intake; **ATP**, adenosine triphosphate; **Ca^{2+}**, calcium; **ChoRE**, carbohydrate response element; **ChREBP**, carbohydrate-responsive element binding protein; **GIP**, glucose-dependent insulinotropic polypeptide; **GLP-1**, glucagon-like peptide-1; **GLUT**, glucose transporter; **HFCS**, high-fructose corn syrup; **IRS**, insulin receptor substrate; **K^+**, potassium; **K_{IR}**, inward rectifier potassium channel; **K_m**, Michaelis-Menten constant; **LDL**, low-density lipoprotein; **Na^+**, sodium; **PYY**, peptide-YY; **RDA**, recommended dietary allowance; **RS**, resistant starch; **SGLT**, sodium-linked glucose transporter; **SRE**, sterol regulatory element; **SREBP**, sterol regulatory element binding protein; **VLDL**, very-low-density lipoprotein.

HISTORICAL HIGHLIGHTS

Modern humans began consuming domesticated grains approximately 10,000 years ago as agrarian societies emerged. Before this time, humans were hunter-gatherers, and their diets consisted mainly of meats and wild plants. Relative to the history of *Homo sapiens*, consumption of diets high in grains is a fairly recent event in human evolution. Rice grown in the Near East is the oldest domesticated grain, and the cultivation of oats in Europe occurred about 3000 years ago. The origin of sugar cane is thought to be Papua New Guinea, where it was likely cultivated from wild plants, also at the time of the global Neolithic agricultural revolution. The slow diffusion of migrants brought sugar cane to India, Southeast Asia, and China. After the Arabs defeated the Romans, they brought sugar cane from Persia to Europe and the Mediterranean, where it failed to thrive, apart from the Moroccan coast. The returning crusaders brought sugar to the European courts, where it became an important and desirable luxury dietary constituent. Sugar cane was introduced to the Caribbean by Christopher Columbus on his second voyage in 1493. These plants thrived and were dispersed to Central and South America and throughout the Caribbean. By the early seventeenth century, raw sugar was being handled by refineries in England and France.

The chemistry of carbohydrates was launched in 1812 when Kirchoff, a Russian chemist, reported that starch, when boiled with dilute acid, produced a free sugar known to be contained in grapes (glucose). Schmidt, in 1844, designated carbohydrates as compounds that contained carbon, hydrogen, and oxygen and showed that sugar was found in the blood. Glycogen, the animal storage form of carbohydrate in liver and muscle, was discovered by the accomplished French physiologist Claude Bernard in 1856.

Today, sugar is produced and consumed worldwide, along with eight major cereal grains: wheat, rye, barley, oats, corn, rice, sorghum, and millet. Wheat and corn are the two major grains consumed in the Western countries. Technologic advances in harvesting techniques and plant breeding to produce disease-resistant plants since the early 1960s have yielded plants that are very different genetically from their ancient counterparts. Further, the refinement of grains to produce palatable, inexpensive foods coincided with a 48% increase in grain consumption (wheat and corn) from the 1970s to the new millennium. As awareness around the inverse relationship between whole grain consumption and chronic disease grows, there has been a resurgence of efforts to increase consumption of whole grains. Better accessibility to products and information through technology has spurred increased public demand for whole grains such as high-fiber wheat products, gluten-free products (quinoa, rice, amaranth), and other diverse grains (bulgur, Kamut [Khorasan wheat], rye).

DEFINITION

What are carbohydrates? The formal definition is a class of compounds having the formula $C_n(H_2O)_n$; that is, the molar ratio of carbon to hydrogen to oxygen is 1:2:1. Simple carbohydrates include the hexose monosaccharides (e.g., glucose, galactose, and fructose) and the disaccharides: maltose (glucose-glucose), sucrose (glucose-fructose), and lactose (glucose-galactose). Complex carbohydrates include the oligosaccharides that yield 3 to 10 monosaccharides on hydrolysis; examples include trioses (glycerose, $C_3H_6O_3$), tetroses (erythrose, $C_4H_8O_4$), and pentoses (ribose, $C_5H_{10}O_5$). Pentoses are important constituents of nucleic acids. Polysaccharides are larger complex carbohydrates containing more than 10 monosaccharide units. Common polysaccharides include starch, glycogen, pectins, cellulose, and gums. The polysaccharides serve both energy storage and structural functions. Chitin is a modified polysaccharide containing nitrogen as N-acetylglucosamine that forms the exoskeleton of arthropods such as insects and crustaceans. Starch is the storage form carbohydrate of plants, whereas animals store carbohydrate as glycogen (liver contains up to 6% and muscle ~1% glycogen by weight). Many different types of starch exist depending on the plant source. Inulin, for example, is a starch found in the tubers and roots of dahlias, artichokes, and dandelions and, when hydrolyzed, yields only fructose; hence it is a fructosan. Cellulose consists of glucose units linked by β (1–4) bonds to form long, straight chains strengthened by hydrogen bonding. It is the chief structural framework of plants and cannot be digested by humans because we do not produce an intestinal carbohydrase that hydrolyzes the β (1–4) linkage. Thus, cellulose is considered to be a dietary fiber that provides bulk to plant-based foods. Bacterial enzymes, however, can break down cellulose. A small amount of fiber or cellulose is hydrolyzed by this process in the human colon, although microbial digestion of cellulose provides only negligible amounts of energy for humans.

DIETARY CARBOHYDRATES

As discussed earlier, carbohydrates represent a large family of naturally occurring compounds and derivatives of these compounds (Fig. 2.1). Only relatively small numbers of carbohydrates are produced commercially and used in the food industry or are of significant metabolic importance, however. Dietary carbohydrate is a major macronutrient for both humans and omnivorous animals. Human adults in the Western countries obtain approximately half their daily caloric requirements from dietary carbohydrate; in other countries, carbohydrate has been the major source of energy, at least until the more recent introduction of Western foods—with higher proportions of fat and protein—to many developing countries. Of ingested carbohydrate, approximately 60% is in the form of polysaccharides, mainly starch; but the disaccharides sucrose and lactose contribute 30% and 10%, respectively (Table 2.1). Monosaccharides (glucose and fructose) are naturally present in fruits and also are found in manufactured foods and drinks, primarily in the form of high-fructose corn syrup (HFCS). Some oligosaccharides, such as raffinose and stachyose, are found in small amounts in various legumes. They cannot be digested by pancreatic and intestinal enzymes (Table 2.2), but they are digested by bacterial enzymes, especially in the colon.

Digestible polysaccharides need to be broken down into their constituent monosaccharides before they can be absorbed and metabolized. This breakdown is initiated during mastication and gastric passage by the carbohydrase α-amylase secreted by the salivary glands, continued by pancreatic amylase in the duodenum, and completed by disaccharidases located in the brush-border membrane of the enterocytes in the small intestine (see Table 2.2 for the major intestinal glycosidases) (1).

Starch

Starch, the predominant dietary polysaccharide, consists only of glucose units and is thus a homopolysaccharide

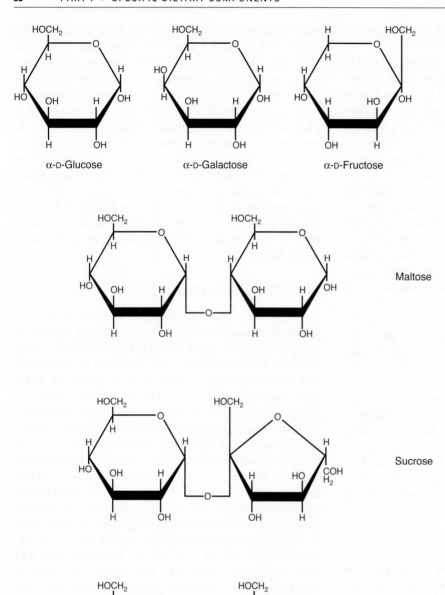

α-D-Glucose   α-D-Galactose   α-D-Fructose

Maltose

Sucrose

Lactose

Fig. 2.1. Structures of the common dietary monosaccharides and disaccharides in perspective. Haworth representation.

and is designated a glucosan or glucan. It is actually composed of two such homopolymers (Fig. 2.2): amylose, which has linear (1–4) linked α-D-glucose, and amylopectin, a highly branched form containing both (1–4) and (1–6) linkages at the branch points. Plants contain both forms as insoluble, semicrystalline granules and differing ratios of amylopectin and amylose, depending on the plant source (Table 2.3). The salivary and pancreatic amylases act on the interior (1–4) linkages but cannot break the outer glucose-glucose links. Thus, the final breakdown products formed by the

amylases are α-(1–4)–linked disaccharides (maltose) and trisaccharides (maltotriose).

Starch Breakdown

The breakdown of starch begins in the mouth with salivary amylase. It is often assumed that as this enzyme is swallowed into an acid stomach, the enzymatic carbohydrate breakdown is stopped (although acid hydrolysis may still occur) because salivary amylase is inhibited by a pH lower than 4. Starch and its end products and the proteins and

TABLE 2.1	PRINCIPAL DIETARY CARBOHYDRATES					
FOOD SOURCE	GRAINS	STARCHY VEGETABLES	LEGUMES	FRUITS	SUGARS AND SWEETENERS	MILK
	Rice	Yam	Soybeans	Apple	Cane sugar	
	Wheat	Potato	Dried peas	Orange	Beet sugar	
	Oats	Sweet corn	Lima beans	Grapes	Sorghum	
	Barley	Cassava		Peach	Honey	
	Rye			Pineapple	Corn syrup	
	Maize			Banana		
Polysaccharide	Starch	Starch	Starch			
Oligosaccharide			Raffinose, stachyose			
Disaccharide	Maltose			Sucrose	Sucrose	Lactose
Monosaccharide				Fructose	Fructose	
				Glucose	Glucose	

amino acids present in a mixed meal all buffer the acid of the stomach and allow some amount of hydrolysis to continue, however. Thus, the quantitative involvement of salivary amylase in the breakdown of starch may be underestimated. Pancreatic α-amylase added to the emptying gastric contents (chyme) in the duodenum cannot hydrolyze the (1–6) branching links and has little specificity for the (1–4) links adjacent to the branching points. Amylase action produces large oligosaccharides (α-limit dextrins) containing on average approximately eight glucose units with one or more (1–6) links. These α-limit dextrins are split by the enzymatic action of glucoamylase (α-limit dextrinase), which sequentially removes a single glucose unit from the nonreducing end of a linear α-(l–4)-glucosyl oligosaccharide. Maltose and maltotriose are then broken down by secreted and brush-border disaccharidases, especially sucrase-isomaltase, into free glucose, which is then transported into and across the enterocytes by hexose transporters (Table 2.4).

The initial breakdown of starch into α-limit dextrins, the intraluminal or cavital digestion phase, occurs mainly in the bulk fluid phase of the intestinal contents. In humans, there appears to be little of the so-called contact or membrane digestion in which adsorption of amylase onto the brush-border surface of enterocytes facilitates its enzymatic activity (2).

Normally, α-amylase is not a limiting factor in the assimilation of starches in humans; but newborn babies, and especially premature ones, cannot assimilate starch because the pancreas secretes insufficient α-amylase to digest it. Within a month, however, the secretion of α-amylase is usually sufficient for full digestion (3).

Resistant Starch

Starch is most frequently eaten after cooking. The heat of cooking gelatinizes the starch granules and thus increases their susceptibility to enzymatic (α-amylase) digestion. A proportion of the starch, however, known as resistant starch (RS), is indigestible even after prolonged incubation with amylase. In cereals, RS represents 0.4% to 2% of the dry matter; in potatoes, it is 1% to 3.5%; and in legumes, it is 3.5% to 5.7%. RS has been categorized as the sum of the starch and degradation products not absorbed in the small intestine of a healthy person (4). Three main categories are recognized: RS1, physically enclosed starch (partially milled grains and seeds); RS2, ungelatinized crystalline granules of the B-type x-ray pattern (as found in bananas and potatoes); and RS3, retrograded amylose (formed during the cooling of starch gelatinized by moist heating). The RSs escape digestion in the small intestine, but then they enter the colon where they can be fermented by the local resident bacteria (>400 different types). In this respect, RS is somewhat similar to dietary fiber. Estimates of the RS and unabsorbed starch represent approximately 2% to 5% of the total starch ingested in the average Western diet, approximately 10 g/day (5). The end products of the fermentation of the RS in the colon are short-chain fatty

TABLE 2.2	MAJOR GLYCOSIDASES OF THE MAMMALIAN ENTEROCYTE BRUSH BORDER	
GLYCOSIDASE	ENZYME COMPLEX	ENZYME ACTIVITY
Maltase-sucrase Maltase-isomaltase	Sucrase-isomaltase	80% of maltase; some α-limit dextrinase; all of sucrase; most of isomaltase
Maltase-glucomylase (2)	Glucoamylase	All glucoamylase; most of α-limit dextrinase; 20% maltase; small percentage of isomaltase
Trehalase		All trehalase
Lactase	β-glycosidase	All neutral lactase and cellobiose
Glycosyl-ceramidase (phlorizin hydrolase)		Most of aryl-β-glycosidase

Adapted with permission from Dahlquist A, Semenza G. Disaccharidases of small-intestinal mucosa. J Pediatr Gastroenterol 1988;4:857–65.

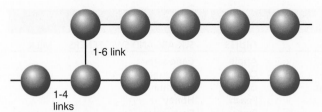

Fig. 2.2. Starch is composed of amylose (15% to 20%) and amylopectin (80% to 85%). Amylose is a nonbranching helical chain structure of glucose residues, whereas amylopectin (a portion shown here) has branched chains of 24 to 30 glucose residues *(blue)* joined by *(1→4)* glucosidic linkages with *(1–6)* linkages creating the branching points.

TABLE 2.3	AMYLOSE AND AMYLOPECTIN CONTENT OF VARIOUS PLANT STARCHES	
PLANT	AMYLOSE (%)	AMYLOPECTIN (%)
Maize (standard)	24	76
Potato	20	80
Rice	18.5	81.5
Tapioca	16.7	83.3
Wheat	25	75

acids (e.g., acetate, butyrate, propionate), carbon dioxide, hydrogen, and methane (released as flatus).

RSs stimulate bacterial growth in the colon. Short-chain fatty acids stimulate crypt cell mitosis in animals and humans (6). If the human colon is bypassed surgically, however, colonocytes lose their absorptive function, and ionic absorption is reduced. Luminal short-chain fatty acids from bacterial fermentation are used by colonocytes as metabolic substrates and appear to be required for normal colonic function (7). The volatile fatty acids such as butyrate and propionate produced by the microbial digestion of RSs and oligosaccharides (such as inulin and oligofructose) and dietary fiber (see later) can stimulate the expression and production of hormones produced by the distal gastrointestinal tract, including glucagon-like peptide-1 (GLP-1) and peptide-YY (PYY). GLP-1 and PYY can contribute to satiety in part by inhibiting gastric emptying, and GLP-1 in particular has beneficial effects on insulin secretion and carbohydrate and lipid metabolism (8, 9).

Dietary Fiber

Dietary fiber was originally defined as "the remnants of plant cell walls not hydrolyzed by the alimentary enzymes of man," but the definition was subsequently modified to include "all plant polysaccharides and lignins, which are resistant to hydrolysis by the digestive enzymes of man" (10). Soluble dietary fiber includes pectin and hydrocolloids, and insoluble fiber includes cellulose and hemicellulose (11). Soluble and insoluble fibers are fermented by the luminal bacteria of the colon. High-fiber diets maintained for the long term reduce the incidence of colon cancer, but the mechanisms involved are not well understood. Investigators have suggested that the bulk action of fiber speeds colonic transit and reduces the absorption of luminal chemicals or that fiber absorbs the carcinogenic agents (6) (see also the chapter on fiber).

Sugars: Functions and Properties

Sugars, unlike starch, have an obvious impact on human taste because they are sweet. Sweet is one of five distinct tastes linked to specific receptors, and all other taste sensations are considered mixtures of these. The prevailing thought is that sweetness is not a unitary quality, and individual variation exists in the ability to "taste" different sweetness qualities for different sweeteners. Human neonates recognize and like sweetness—a finding that is not surprising because the lactose in their major food, human milk, gives it a sweet taste. Estimates of relative sweetness of various carbohydrates by humans are usually made against the standard, sucrose (100%). On this scale, glucose is less sweet (sweetness rating = 61 to 70), whereas fructose is sweeter, with a fruity taste (sweetness rating = 130 to 180). The sweetness of maltose is 43 to 50 and that of lactose is between 15 and 40. The sweetness ratings of the HFCS sweeteners are 128 for HFCS-55 (55% fructose) and 116 for HFCS-42 (42% fructose). Investigators have speculated that during human evolution, the quest for foods containing maximal energy caused primitive

TABLE 2.4	HUMAN FACILITATED-DIFFUSION GLUCOSE TRANSPORTER FAMILY (GLUT1 TO GLUT5)			
TYPE	AMINO ACIDS (N)	CHROMOSOME LOCATION	K_m (mmol/L) FOR HEXOSE UPTAKE[a]	MAJOR EXPRESSION SITES
GLUT1 (red cell)	492	1	1–2 (red blood cells)	Placenta, brain, kidney, colon
GLUT2 (liver)	524	3	15–20 (hepatocytes)	Liver, β cell, kidney, small intestine
GLUT3 (brain)	496	12	10 (*Xenopus* oocytes)	Brain, testis
GLUT4 (muscle/fat)	509	17	5 (adipocytes)	Skeletal and heart muscle, brown and white fat
GLUT5 (small intestine)	501	1	6–11(fructose) (*Xenopus* oocytes)	Small intestine, sperm

K_m, Michaelis-Menten constant.

[a]The approximate K_m values refer to the uptake of glucose (fructose in the case of GLUT5) in the designated tissue or cells in parentheses and are shown to give an approximate index of the affinity of the transporter for glucose.

humans to acquire the ability to recognize that sweetness indicated safety and energy.

Today, sugars (primarily sucrose, glucose, and fructose) are used extensively in foods to provide sweetness, energy, texture, and bulk and also for appearance, preservation (by raising the osmotic pressure), and fermentation (in bread, alcoholic beverages). The palatability, appearance, and shelf life of a huge variety of foods and drinks are enhanced by adding sucrose; examples are as follows: breads, cakes, and biscuits; preserves and jellies; confectionery; dairy products; cured, dried, and preserved meats; breakfast cereals; and frozen and canned vegetables. As a result of the addition of sugars to so many food products, sugar consumption has increased by 20% overall since the 1970s, and corn-based sweetener use has increased by 277% (12). In certain Western countries, soft drinks, "juice" drinks, and other beverages—sweetened with sucrose or HFCS—are major sources of dietary sugar. Incorporation of sweeteners into beverages and many other commonly consumed foods makes accurate assessment of dietary sugar intake difficult.

GETTING GLUCOSE INTO CELLS: THE TRANSPORTERS

A major source of metabolic energy for most, if not all, mammalian cells is the oxidation of D-glucose. The lipid-rich membranes of such cells, however, are relatively impermeable to hydrophilic polar molecules such as glucose. Specific transport processes have evolved to allow the cellular entry and exit of glucose. Carrier proteins located in the plasma membranes of cells can bind glucose and allow it to traverse the lipid membrane barrier, thus releasing the hexose into the cellular cytoplasm or body fluids.

Two distinct classes have been described: (a) a family of facilitative glucose transporters (see Table 2.4) and (b) sodium (Na^+)-glucose cotransporters (symporters). The former class consists of membrane integral proteins found on the surface of all cells. They transport D-glucose down its concentration gradient (from high to low), a process described as *facilitative diffusion*. The energy for the transfer is derived from the concentration gradient of glucose across plasma membranes. Glucose transporters allow glucose to enter cells readily, but they can also allow it to exit from cells according to the prevailing concentration gradient. In contrast, the Na^+-glucose cotransporters participate in the "uphill" movement of D-glucose against its concentration gradient; that is, they perform *active transport*. They are especially expressed in the specialized brush borders of the enterocytes of the small intestine and the epithelial cells of the kidney (proximal) tubule. They occur at lower levels in the epithelial cells lining the lung and in the liver (13). Cooperation between the two classes of glucose transporters, together with the hormones involved in carbohydrate metabolism, allows fine control of glucose concentration in the plasma and thus maintains a continuous supply of the body's main source of cellular energy.

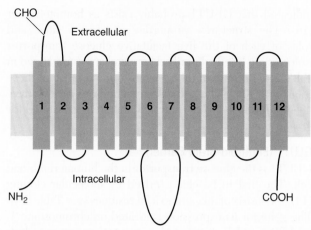

Fig. 2.3. Highly schematic diagram illustrating the predicted secondary structure model of the glucose transporter molecule (GLUT1) in the cell membrane *(gray shaded)*. The putative membrane-spanning α-helices are shown as rectangles numbered *1* to *12* connected by chains *(lines)* of linked amino acids. (Adapted with permission from Mueckler M, Caruso C, Baldwin SA et al. Sequence and structure of a human glucose transporter. Science 1985;229:941–5.)

Human Facilitative-Diffusion Glucose Transporter Family

Several major hexose transporters have been identified and cloned since the characterization of the first, glucose transporter 1 (GLUT1), by molecular cloning (14). The classical glucose transporters, GLUT1 to GLUT4, are well-characterized proteins with similar molecular structures containing between 492 and 524 amino acid residues. Mueckler et al (14), using hydropathic and secondary structure predictions, proposed a two-dimensional orientation model of GLUT1 in the plasma membrane (Fig. 2.3). The molecule has three major domains: (a) 12 α-spanning the membrane with the N and C termini of the protein on the cytoplasmic side of the cell membrane, (b) an intracellular domain of 65 hydrophilic amino acids (between membrane [M] regions 6 and M7 of Fig. 2.3), and (c) an extracellular 33-amino acid segment (between M1 and M2) containing the site for an asparagine-linked oligosaccharide at asparagine 45.

The prediction was that the polypeptide backbone of the molecule traverses or spans the plasma membrane 12 times. Both the amino- and carboxy-terminal ends of the molecule are on the cytoplasmic side of the membrane, whereas an N-glycosylation site is present on the first extracytoplasmic loop (M1 and M2). These basic topologic features have been confirmed by studies using proteolytic digestion and sequence-specific antibodies. GLUT1, purified from human red blood cells and reconstituted in liposomes, appears to be predominant in the α-helical form, and the transmembrane segments form α-helices at right angles to the plane of the lipid membrane (15). The molecular structure of GLUT1, shown in Figure 2.3, is, of course, a two-dimensional model. Studies using radiation inactivation of the carrier in intact red blood cells have indicated that GLUT1 probably exists as homotetramer (16). The structures, properties, expression sites, and roles of each of the five facilitative glucose transporter isoforms are briefly described here and are summarized in Table 2.4. Because of the recognized importance of these transporters in health and disease, numerous reviews have been published (17–21), and they should be consulted for greater detail.

GLUT1 (Erythroid-Brain Carrier)

GLUT1 is the glucose transporter in the human red blood cell. The first to be characterized by molecular cloning (14), it consists of 492 amino acid residues (see Table 2.4). The gene for its expression is located on chromosome 1. GLUT1 is widely distributed in many other tissues including heart, kidney, adipose cells, fibroblasts, placenta, retina, and brain, but little is expressed in muscle or liver. There is particularly high expression in the endothelial cells of the microvessels of the brain, where GLUT1 forms part of the blood–brain barrier (22). The transport process for D-glucose in the red blood cell is asymmetric, because the affinity (Michaelis-Menten constant $[K_m]$) for D-glucose uptake is approximately 1 to 2 mmol/L, whereas the K_m for the exit of glucose is 20 to 30 mmol/L. This asymmetry appears to be allosterically regulated by the binding of intracellular metabolites and inhibited by adenosine triphosphate (ATP) (23). The asymmetry allows the transporter to be effective when the extracellular glucose is low and the intracellular demand is high.

GLUT2 (Hepatic Glucose Transporter)

Many biochemical studies indicated that the glucose transporter in liver cells was distinct from that of the red blood cells. Moreover, adult liver cells had only very low levels of GLUT1 mRNA. Cloning of the second glucose carrier, GLUT2, was accomplished by screening rat and human cDNA libraries with a cDNA probe for GLUT1. GLUT2 has 55% identity in amino acid sequence with GLUT1, and it displays the same topologic organization in the cell membrane as predicted for GLUT1. Human GLUT2 contains 524 amino acids (see Table 2.4) compared with rat GLUT1 of 522 residues, and they show 82% identity in amino acid sequences—an excellent example of conservation of structure among species. GLUT2 is preferentially expressed in liver (sinusoidal membranes), kidney (tubule cells), small intestine (enterocytes), and the insulin-secreting β cells of the pancreas.

In the liver cell, GLUT2 has a low affinity for glucose ($K_m = 17$ mmol/L) and shows symmetric transport, that is, a similar K_m for influx and efflux. This high-capacity, low-affinity transporter is useful for rapid glucose efflux following gluconeogenesis. GLUT2 can also transport galactose, mannose, and fructose (24).

GLUT3 (Brain Glucose Transporter)

GLUT3 was originally cloned from a human fetal muscle cDNA library (25). It contains 496 amino acid residues (see Table 2.4) and shows 64% identity with GLUT1 and 52% identity with GLUT2. Its amino acid sequence again suggests that its membrane topology is similar to that of GLUT1 (see Fig. 2.3). GLUT3 mRNA appears to be present in all tissues, but its highest expression is in adult brain, kidney, and placenta. Adult muscle, however, shows only very low levels. In the brain, it is mainly expressed in neurons. GLUT3 mRNA is found in fibroblasts and in smooth muscle. Because both these cell types are found in practically all tissues, the ubiquitous expression of GLUT3 is understandable. Its affinity for glucose transport is relatively low ($K_m \approx 10$ mmol/L) but significantly higher than that of GLUT1 (17 mmol/L). GLUT3 is also found in spermatozoa. Such cells undertake glycolysis in the male genital tract and take up glucose from epididymal fluid.

GLUT4 (Insulin-Responsive Glucose Transporter)

Glucose is transported across the cell membranes of adipocytes (fat cells), and its rate of transport can be speeded up 20- to 30-fold within 2 or 3 minutes by addition of insulin, without evidence of protein synthesis. Studies showed that this stimulation of glucose transport resulted in part from translocation of GLUT1 from an intracellular pool into the membrane. Careful quantitative measurements showed, however, that this could account for only a 12- to 15-fold increase in glucose transport. It became obvious that another transporter would have to be involved to account for the much larger insulin-stimulated transport. This new transporter, GLUT4, was first identified in rat adipocytes by use of a monoclonal antibody. Subsequently, GLUT4 has been cloned from rat, mouse, and human DNA (24). It is a protein with 509 amino acid residues (see Table 2.4), with 65% identity with GLUT1, 54% identity with GLUT2, and 58% identity with GLUT3. Rat and mouse GLUT4s have 95% and 96% identity, respectively, with human GLUT4. As with the previous GLUT transporters, the two-dimensional orientation of the structure in the cell membrane is similar to that proposed for GLUT1 (see Fig. 2.3).

GLUT4 is the major glucose transporter of the insulin-sensitive tissues, brown and white fat, and skeletal and cardiac muscle. It occurs primarily in intracellular vesicles in the cells of these tissues. Insulin stimulation causes a rapid increase in the number of glucose transporters on the membranes of these cells because the vesicles are translocated toward the membrane and then fuse with it, thereby releasing the molecule. This process ensures a high density of glucose transporters and enhances the ability to move glucose from the surrounding cellular fluid into the interior of the cell, that is, increased maximal velocity for glucose uptake. Because of this mechanism, the position of GLUT4 and its regulation are important components of glucose homeostasis, and the role of GLUT4 in diabetes has been and continues to be the subject of intense investigation.

GLUT5 (The Fructose Transporter)

GLUT5 was isolated from human (26), rat, and rabbit enterocyte cDNA libraries. It consists of 501 amino acid residues (see Table 2.4), and it has only 42%, 40%, 39%, and 42% identity with GLUTs 1, 2, 3, and 4, respectively. It is said to be primarily expressed in the jejunum (both in the brush border and basolateral membrane); but its mRNA has been detected, albeit at low levels, in human kidney, skeletal muscle and adipocytes, microglial cells, and the blood–brain barrier. GLUT5 appears to transport glucose poorly and is really the transporter for fructose. It is found in high concentrations in mature human spermatozoa (27), which are known to use fructose as an energy source (human seminal fluid contains high concentrations of fructose, which is manufactured by the seminal vesicles). The K_m for fructose uptake by expressed GLUT5 was 6 to 11 mmol/L. With importance to the regulation of energy homeostasis, the expression of GLUT5 in pancreatic β cells is very low (28), and consequently fructose has little if any effect on stimulation of insulin secretion (29).

Other Transporters

Currently, 14 isoforms in the family of sugar transport proteins have been recognized, including GLUT6 to GLUT14 (30–32). Thus, the list of both Na^+-dependent and facilitative carbohydrate transport proteins identified continues to grow. Because these transporters exhibit a wide range of properties with variable combinations of these proteins distributed across different cell and tissue types (33, 34), the capacity exists for far greater complexity in sugar transport, storage, and metabolism than originally considered at the time the first transporters were initially identified.

Study of Glucose Transporters by Use of Transgenic and Knockout Mice

Although many metabolic inhibitors are available for use in examining metabolic pathways, the specificity of these agents is often questionable. With molecular techniques, however, metabolic pathways can be altered in quite specific ways, even in intact animals. A protein (e.g., enzyme/ carrier) can be overexpressed, expressed in a tissue that normally does not contain it, or eliminated in a particular cell type. Site-directed mutations allow a molecule to be dissected and particular component groups removed or altered so their role in the molecule's functioning can be studied. Application of these techniques to the investigation of metabolic pathways is yielding interesting insights into the biologic roles of glucose transport proteins.

Transgenic mice were established that expressed high levels of human GLUT1, properly located in the muscle sarcolemma. The increase in GLUT1 expression resulted in a three- to fourfold increase in glucose transport into specific muscles—a finding confirming that GLUT1 plays a major role in controlling glucose entry into resting muscle. Strangely, insulin did not increase the entry of glucose into the transgenic mice muscles even though GLUT4 levels in these mice were the same as those of control mice. Possibly, the GLUT1 levels were elevated in the transgenic animals to a degree that glucose transport was not limited by transporter activity. Muscle glucose concentrations were 4- to 5-fold and glycogen 10-fold higher in the transgenic mice, even though they showed 18% (fed) to 30% (fasted) decreases in plasma glucose concentration. Oral glucose loads did not increase plasma levels as much as in normal mice, and glucose disposal was enhanced. Thus, increasing the number of GLUT1 transporters affected not only muscle metabolism but also whole body glucose homeostasis.

Selective overexpression of GLUT4 in muscle or adipose tissue protects against the development of diabetes in several rodent models (35). Mice with genetic ablation of GLUT4 in all tissues exhibit impaired glucose tolerance despite postprandial hyperinsulinemia and decreased glucose lowering after insulin injection—a finding indicating that they are insulin resistant; however, these animals do not develop overt diabetes (36). Investigators showed that glucose disposal in rodents, and mice in particular, has a large insulin-independent component that may protect against diabetes induced by ablation of GLUT4. In addition, the background strain of the animals used for genetic manipulations can have major influence on the phenotypic outcome. For example, overt diabetes and glucose toxicity were observed in mice with muscle-specific inactivation of GLUT4 (37). Finally, adipose-specific GLUT4 ablation not only markedly impairs glucose uptake in isolated adipocytes from these animals but also induces insulin resistance in skeletal muscle and liver, despite preservation of GLUT4 expression in these tissues (38). These results suggest that some factors regulated by adipose glucose transport are involved in the control of insulin action in extra-adipose tissue and thus whole body insulin sensitivity.

Because increased expression of the insulin-responsive transporter GLUT4 occurs in human and rodent adipocytes and is associated with obesity, the question arises whether increasing the GLUT4 levels in adipocytes plays a role in obesity. Transgenic mice were produced that expressed human GLUT4 in their adipocytes. Basal-level glucose transport into adipocytes was increased approximately 20-fold compared with wild-type animals, but insulin stimulated glucose uptake only by a factor of 2.5 rather than the 15-fold increase of controls. Again, the possible explanation is that glucose transport is already so high in the adipocytes of transgenic animals that the number of transporters activated by insulin has a reduced relative contribution to the overall transport. Although the fat cell size was unchanged in the transgenic mice, the number of fat cells was more than doubled, and total body lipid nearly tripled, reflecting the increase in cell number. The results suggest that a specific increase in GLUT4 in adipocytes can contribute to obesity.

One major limitation of using transgenic and knockout mice is that the induced genetic alterations often occur very early in the developing animal. Thus, observed phenotypic outcomes in these animals may result from the presence or absence of the transgene at the time of the laboratory measurements, or, alternatively, the genetic alteration could initiate a plethora of other events contributing to the observed phenotype. The development of conditional transgenic or knockout models in which transgenic manipulations allow temporal expression or inactivation of specific genes will help to overcome this limitation (39).

Sodium-Glucose Cotransporters and Transepithelial Hexose Transport: Intestine and Kidney

The intestine and the kidney are two major organs that have epithelia with the specific function of transferring hexoses across their cells into the bloodstream. In the intestine, the transporters of the mature enterocytes capture the hexoses from the lumen after breakdown of dietary polysaccharides into simple hexoses, D-glucose, D-galactose, and D-fructose. In the kidney, the cells of the proximal tubule capture the glucose from the glomerular filtrate to return it to the blood. These glucose transporters, localized in the brush-border membranes of the epithelial cells, differ from the GLUT1 to GLUT5 types and share no sequence homology. They are thus members of quite a different protein family.

Moreover, they transport glucose across the cell membrane by having both hexose and Na^+ binding sites, hence the name Na^+-glucose cotransporters. They couple cellular glucose transfer to the inwardly directed electrochemical gradient of Na^+. The low intracellular concentration of Na^+ ions, maintained by Na^+-potassium (K^+)/ATPase or the Na^+ pump at the basolateral borders of the cells, powers the uphill transfer of glucose through the agency of

the cotransporter. The affinity of the sugar molecule for its cotransporter binding site is greater when the Na^+ ions are attached to the transporter than when they are removed. Thus, the external binding of Na^+ and its subsequent intracellular dissociation (because of the lower intracellular Na^+ ion concentration) cause the binding and then release of glucose, that allow it to be transported uphill against its concentration gradient. Glucose is then transported across the basolateral membranes of the cells of the small intestine and kidney usually by GLUT2, but in the S3 segments of straight kidney tubules, GLUT1 is found. In this part of the kidney, GLUT1 is probably involved both in the transepithelial transfer of glucose and in its uptake from the blood to provide energy for cellular glycolysis.

The low concentration of the cotransporters in cell membranes (0.05% to 0.7%), their hydrophobic nature, and their sensitivity to proteolysis and denaturation made them nearly impossible to prepare by normal biochemical extraction and purification techniques. The first to be cloned and sequenced was Na^+-linked glucose transporter-1 (SGLT-1), the form found in the rabbit small intestine (40). Poly(A)$^+$ mRNA isolated from the rabbit small intestinal mucosa and microinjected into *Xenopus* oocytes stimulated Na^+-dependent uptake of the hexose analog α-methyl glucoside that could be blocked by the plant glycoside phlorizin, a high-affinity competitor for the sugar site of the transporter (19). Phlorizin has no effect on the GLUT1 to GLUT5 transporters; they are inhibited by the mold metabolite phloretin, which is the aglycone of phlorizin. Phloretin has no effect on the Na^+-glucose transporter but blocks the GLUT1 to GLUT5 transporters. The predicted topologic organization of SGLT-1 in the cell membranes was surmised from its amino acids, and, like the glucose transporter family, it is a large polypeptide with 12 putative membrane-spanning α-helices (Fig. 2.4). The polypeptide

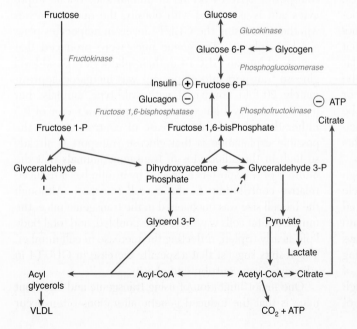

Fig. 2.4. Fructose and glucose utilization in the liver. Hepatic fructose metabolism begins with phosphorylation by fructokinase. Fructose carbon enters the glycolytic pathway at the triose phosphate level (dihydroxyacetone phosphate to and glyceraldehyde-3-phosphate [P]). Thus, fructose bypasses the major control point by which glucose carbon enters glycolysis (phosphofructokinase) where glucose metabolism is limited by feedback inhibition by citrate and adenosine triphosphate (ATP). This allows fructose to serve as an unregulated source of both glycerol-3-phosphate and acetyl-coenzyme A (CoA) for hepatic lipogenesis. *VLDL*, very-low-density lipoprotein. (Adapted with permission from Havel PJ. Dietary fructose: implication for dysregulation of energy homeostasis and lipid/carbohydrate metabolism. Nutr Rev 2005;63:133–7.)

is glycosylated at one site, but this has little effect on its function (41). Radiation inactivation analysis of SGLT-1 suggests that the functional form in the membrane is a tetramer. It is composed of 664 amino acids.

More recently, investigators showed that three different isoforms of the SGLT cotransporters exist, designated SGLT-1, SGLT-2 (672 amino acids), and SGLT-3 (18). The cotransporters SGLT-1 and SGLT-2 have different glucose-Na^+ coupling ratios; the former high-affinity cotransporter ($K_m \approx 0.8$ mmol glucose/L), primarily expressed in the small intestine, transports each glucose molecule with two Na^+ ions, whereas the latter, lower-affinity ($K_m \approx 1.6$ mmol glucose/L) cotransporter, expressed in the kidney tubules, transports glucose with one Na^+. SGLT-3, isolated from pig intestine, is a low-affinity cotransporter. It has approximately 60% homology in amino acid sequence to SGLT-2 (42). Inhibitors of SGLT-2 that prevent renal tubular glucose reabsorption are currently being explored as a method for markedly increasing urine glucose spillover to reduce hyperglycemia in diabetes mellitus (43).

Glucose-Galactose Malabsorption

The importance of human SGLT-1 for intestinal glucose absorption is exemplified in glucose-galactose malabsorption, a rare inborn error of glucose transport. This condition gives rise to severe watery diarrhea in neonates that is lethal unless glucose- and galactose-containing foods are removed from the diet. The diarrhea occurs because the unabsorbed hexoses enter the colon and are fermented into compounds that promote diarrhea. The lack of hexose absorption in two sisters identified with this condition appeared to result from a single base change at nucleotide position 92, where a guanine was replaced by adenine. The mutation changed amino acid 28 of SGLT-1 from aspartate to asparagine and rendered the SGLT-1 cotransporter inactive. Thus, single amino acid alteration in the 664 that comprise the molecule results in an inability to function as a cotransporter (44), and humans who lack a functional SGLT-1 cannot absorb glucose and galactose. Experimental studies measuring the absorption of glucose in human jejunum in vivo showed that more than 95% of glucose absorption occurs through a carrier-mediated process—a finding that agrees with the described pathophysiology of glucose-galactose malabsorption (45, 46).

Electrogenic Glucose-Linked Sodium Transfer

Because SGLT cotransporters transport both glucose and Na^+ ions across cell membranes without countercharged ions, movement of the charged Na^+ ions creates an electrical potential difference across the cell membrane and subsequently across the epithelium. The transfer of glucose (or galactose) across the intestine or kidney tubule is called *electrogenic* (potential generating) or *rheogenic* (current generating). This electrical activity has been of inestimable value in the assessment of the kinetics of active hexose transport in native tissues and injected *Xenopus* eggs. This linking of the electrogenic Na^+ ion transfer with the hexose also enhances the net absorption of fluid across the small intestine. It is so effective that it overcomes the terrible excessive fluid secretory consequences of cholera toxin action in the small bowel. The application of this principle—oral rehydration therapy—is a highly effective and inexpensive treatment to keep patients hydrated and alive. A simple solution of Na chloride (NaCl) and glucose (or even rice water) has very likely saved more lives than many drugs.

BLOOD GLUCOSE: METABOLIC, HORMONAL, AND TRANSCRIPTIONAL REGULATION

Metabolic Regulation of Carbohydrate Metabolism

Glucose is among the most highly regulated circulating substrates. The concentration of glucose in the blood after an overnight fast has a normal range of 3.9 to 5.8 mmol/L (70 to 105 mg/dL). When a carbohydrate-containing meal is ingested, the level may temporarily rise to 6.5 to 7.4 mmol/L, and during prolonged fasting it can fall to 3.3 to 3.9 mmol/L. One of the major reasons that blood glucose levels are so tightly regulated is that the brain normally depends on a continuous supply of glucose for its energy needs, although it can adapt to lower levels and use ketone bodies from fat breakdown if the adaptation occurs slowly during prolonged fasting or starvation (47). The adaptation to use ketones becomes essential during starvation, because the adult human brain uses approximately 140 g/day of glucose (48), and only approximately 130 g/day of glucose can be obtained from noncarbohydrate sources. The importance of maintaining blood glucose concentrations within the physiologic range is underscored by the finding that an acute reduction in blood glucose resulting from an overdose of insulin can rapidly lead to convulsions, coma, and even death if it is not promptly treated.

Glucose enters the circulating pool from both exogenous (diet) and endogenous (hepatic production through glycogenolysis and gluconeogenesis) sources. In physiologically normal postabsorptive humans, the plasma appearance rate is 8 to 10 g/hour, with the circulating pool replaced every 2 hours. At normal blood glucose levels, the liver is a net producer of glucose. After digestion of dietary carbohydrates, the absorbed monosaccharides are transported through the portal vein to the liver. The rising levels of glucose and insulin, as well as the indirect effect of insulin to inhibit lipolysis from adipose tissue to reduce the systemic and portal delivery of free fatty acids to the liver, lead to a decrease of hepatic glucose production. As glucose arrives at the liver and peripheral tissues, the first metabolic step is phosphorylation by hexokinase. Hexokinase has tissue-specific isoforms that catalyze the same reaction but with different kinetics and regulatory mechanisms. Hexokinase I, found in skeletal muscle, has a low K_m and is coordinated with the low K_m of GLUT4.

Together, hexokinase I and GLUT4 work to balance glucose uptake and phosphorylation. Hexokinase I is subject to feedback inhibition by its product, glucose-6-phosphate. The liver enzyme glucokinase (hexokinase IV) is not inhibited by glucose-6-phosphate and has a lower affinity for glucose. Glucokinase activity is coordinated with the high K_m GLUT2, such that both are active when portal glucose delivery is elevated. Thus, glucokinase can increase its activity over the relatively larger range of glucose concentrations in the portal blood. The hexokinases, coupled with the effects of increases of circulating insulin and translocation of GLUT4, possess the characteristics required for the efficient uptake of the substantial amounts of glucose arriving at the liver and peripheral tissues following consumption of a carbohydrate-containing meal.

Gluconeogenesis and the Cori Cycle

As discussed earlier, in the postabsorptive state, the normal plasma appearance rate of glucose in humans is 8 to 10 g/hour; and at normal blood glucose levels, the liver is a net producer of glucose, with the circulating glucose pool replaced approximately every 2 hours. In addition to the liver, gluconeogenesis also occurs in the kidney and, to a lesser extent, the small intestine. Metabolic precursors for the formation of glucose include the glucogenic amino acids (especially alanine during starvation), glycerol, and propionate. Both muscle and red blood cells metabolize glucose to form lactate, which on entering the liver can be resynthesized into glucose. This newly formed glucose is then available for recirculation back to the tissue, a process known as the Cori, or lactic acid, cycle. During exercise, the Cori cycle may account for approximately 40% of the normal plasma glucose turnover.

Hormonal Regulation of Carbohydrate Metabolism

The level of glucose in the blood is regulated by both hormonal and metabolic mechanisms. The major hormones involved in the acute control of circulating glucose concentrations are insulin, glucagon, and epinephrine (adrenaline); but other hormones including thyroid hormone, glucocorticoids, growth hormone, leptin, and adiponectin also play a role.

Insulin and Diabetes Mellitus (Type 1 and Type 2)

Insulin has a central role in regulating glucose metabolism. It is secreted by the β cells of the islets of Langerhans in the pancreas. The daily output of insulin by the human pancreas is approximately 40 to 50 U, or 15% to 20% of pancreatic insulin stores. Circulating glucose concentrations are the major signals controlling insulin secretion. Increasing blood glucose concentrations (hyperglycemia) stimulate the secretion of insulin, whereas low glucose levels (hypoglycemia) result in reduced insulin secretion. When the pancreas is unable to secrete insulin or to secrete sufficient insulin to compensate for insulin resistance, the medical condition is known as diabetes mellitus. This disease, the third most prevalent in the Western world, is normally classified as type 1, insulin-dependent diabetes mellitus or type 2, non–insulin-dependent diabetes mellitus. Type 2 diabetes is strongly associated with obesity and accounts for more than 90% of all diabetes cases. Type 1 diabetes is caused by autoimmune-mediated destruction of pancreatic β cells that results in an absolute inability to produce insulin and the need for daily injections of the hormone to prevent severe hyperglycemia that can progress to diabetic ketoacidosis and death. The onset of insulin-dependent diabetes mellitus occurs in children and younger adults predominantly and manifests when more than 80% to 90% of the β cells are destroyed.

Most cases of type 2 diabetes occur in adults, although the number of cases reported in adolescents and children has increased dramatically since the mid-1990s in association with the increase of childhood obesity in many countries. A form of type 2 diabetes occurs in pregnancy and is termed *gestational diabetes*. In type 2 diabetes, patients have reduced secretion of insulin accompanied by reduced metabolic responses to insulin in certain key insulin-sensitive tissues including liver and skeletal muscle (i.e., peripheral insulin resistance). The precise molecular mechanisms underlying insulin resistance are yet to be fully identified; however, ectopic fat (triglyceride) deposition in liver and muscle is strongly associated with insulin resistance.

Findings about the role of GLUT4 in insulin insensitivity are conflicting. Some researchers have reported no changes in GLUT4 mRNA expression or protein levels (49), but others have found a small (18%) decrease (50). Thus, a defect in translocation of GLUT4 to the muscle membrane could contribute to insulin resistance (24). In addition, defects at numerous control points in insulin receptor function, including impaired phosphorylation of tyrosine and increased phosphorylation of serine residues in the insulin receptor and postreceptor signal transduction cascade, such as insulin receptor substrate-1 (IRS-1), have been implicated in the etiology of insulin resistance. Inflammation and oxidative stress are now considered likely to have causal roles in the development of insulin resistance (40).

Mechanism of Insulin Secretion

The mechanism of the regulation of insulin secretion by the external glucose level has been studied using patch clamp techniques to control the ionic channels in the β cell membrane. The resting membrane potential of the β cells is maintained by the Na^+-K^+/ATPase and ATP-sensitive K^+ channels (K_{ATP} channels). Normally, these channels are open, but they close in response to events triggered by the metabolism of glucose, when there is a concomitant increase in the ratio of ATP to adenosine diphosphate (51). This depolarizes the cell membrane and opens voltage-gated calcium (Ca^{2+}) channels. The resulting increase in the intracellular free Ca^{2+} concentration activates secretion of insulin through exocytosis, the fusion of insulin-containing granules with the plasma membrane and the release of their contents (52). Certain drugs (sulfonylureas), such as tolbutamide and glibenclamide, induce insulin secretion by inhibiting the K_{ATP} channels of the β cells and are used medically in the treatment of type 2 diabetes. K_{ATP} channels are a heteromultimeric complex of the inward rectifier K^+ channel (K_{IR} 6.2) and a receptor for sulfonylureas, SUR1, a member of the ATP-binding cassette or traffic family of plasma membrane proteins (53).

In addition to glucose, other nutrients, including certain amino acids and fatty acids, can contribute to increased insulin secretion. Gastrointestinal hormones, including glucagon, secretin, and the known incretin hormones, GLP-1, and glucose-dependent insulinotropic polypeptide (GIP), augment meal-induced insulin secretion (54). The pancreatic islet is well innervated by the autonomic nervous system; and the classic neurotransmitters, including acetylcholine and norepinephrine, as well as neuropeptides including galanin, vasoactive intestinal polypeptide, and pituitary adenylate cyclase-activating polypeptide, modulate insulin secretion (55). Neural regulation by the parasympathetic nervous system augments insulin responses to meal ingestion and improves postprandial glucose tolerance (56, 57), whereas the sympathetic nervous system inhibits insulin secretion during periods of stress to increase glucose availability for the central nervous system (58). In pregnancy, the hormones placental lactogen, estrogens, and progestin all increase insulin secretion. For a detailed overview of the biology of insulin secretion, see Taborsky and Ahren (59).

Insulin lowers blood glucose levels by facilitating its entrance into insulin-sensitive tissues and uptake by the liver. It does this by increasing GLUT4 translocation in tissues such as muscle and adipose tissue. In the liver, however, insulin stimulates the storage of glucose as glycogen or enhances its metabolism through the glycolytic pathway. Glucose entry into liver cells is not mediated by changes in glucose transporter function, even though these transporters are present in hepatocyte membranes (60). The liver has functional specialization with regard to the disposition of GLUT1 and GLUT2. GLUT2 has higher expression in the periportal hepatocytes than in the perivenous hepatocytes. In the perivenous region, however, GLUT1 is also present in the sinusoidal membranes of the hepatocytes, which form rows around the terminal hepatic venules. Periportal hepatocytes are more gluconeogenic than the more glycolytic perivenous cells (61). Why hepatocytes have GLUT2 in their membranes is an enigma, because it is certainly not necessary for the entrance or release of glucose. Investigators have suggested that GLUT2 may be involved in transporting fructose, because GLUT5, the fructose transporter, is not well expressed in the liver. GLUT1 expression correlates well with the glycolytic activity of cells, however; in general, the higher the activity, the greater the concentration of GLUT1. Thus, the presence of GLUT1 in the perivenous liver cells may aid the efficient functioning of glucose entry into the glycolytic pathway.

TABLE 2.5	INFLUENCE OF GLUCOSE VIA INSULIN	
POSITIVE EFFECTS		**NEGATIVE EFFECTS**
Glucose uptake		Pyruvate→glucose
Amino acid uptake		Apoptosis
Acetyl-coenzyme A→fatty acid		Gene expression
Glucose→glycogen		
Protein synthesis		
DNA synthesis		
Sodium-potassium pump		
Gene expression		

Although insulin has a primary influence on glucose homeostasis, it also influences many other cellular functions (Table 2.5). Glucose has a profound effect on the secretion of insulin, and insulin strongly affects the normal storage of ingested fuels, including fatty acid and amino acid and protein metabolism as well as cellular growth and differentiation (as exemplified in Table 2.5). Thus, indirectly, glucose also influences these cellular events—a finding that underscores the crucial role of glucose in influencing metabolism and catabolism, both directly and indirectly.

Glucagon

Glucagon is secreted by the α cells of the pancreatic islets of Langerhans. A major stimulus for its secretion is hypoglycemia (low blood glucose concentrations). Glucagon acts on the liver to activate glycogenolysis, the breakdown of glycogen, by activating the enzyme phosphorylase. It also enhances gluconeogenesis (formation of glucose) from amino acids and lactate. Thus, the major actions of glucagon oppose those of insulin. Pancreatic α and β cells in the islets have a close anatomic and functional relationship with intraislet regulation of glucagon by insulin and of insulin by glucagon (62). The suppression of glucagon secretion by glucose during hyperglycemia is mediated in part by the actions of increased intraislet insulin release and by the islet hormone, somatostatin (63).

Glucagon binds to its specific receptor in the plasma membrane to activate cellular responses. This glucagon receptor is a member of a superfamily of G-protein–coupled receptors, and it is also a member of a smaller subfamily of homologous receptors for GLP-1 peptides, which is a product of the proglucagon gene produced by endocrine L cells in the distal small intestine, as well as other peptides including GIP, vasoactive intestinal peptide, secretin, growth hormone–releasing factor, and pituitary adenylate cyclase–activating polypeptide. Using specific glucagon receptor mRNA expression in rat tissues, glucagon receptor mRNA was observed to be relatively abundant in liver, adipose tissue, and pancreatic islets, as expected, but it was also present in heart, kidney, spleen, thymus, and stomach. Low levels were found in adrenal glands, small intestine, thyroid, and skeletal muscle. No expression was observed in testes, lung, large intestine, or brain (64). Increased glucagon secretion is the first line of defense against low blood glucose levels (hypoglycemia). Activation of the autonomic nervous system (both parasympathetic and sympathoadrenal divisions) is an important mediator of increased glucagon secretion during hypoglycemia, and this mechanism becomes impaired in people with diabetes and thus leaves these patients at increased risk of hypoglycemia during insulin treatment (65).

Other Counterregulatory Hormones

Epinephrine. Epinephrine is secreted by the chromaffin cells of the adrenal medulla. It is often called the "fight-or-flight" hormone because adrenal epinephrine release is triggered in response to many types of stress, such as fear, excitement, hypoglycemia, hypoxia, and blood loss (hypotension). Epinephrine acts in the liver, along with norepinephrine released from hepatic sympathetic nerves, to increase glycogenolysis directly by activating glycogen phosphorylase and indirectly by stimulating glucagon secretion and inhibiting insulin secretion, thereby releasing glucose for use by muscle and the central nervous system.

Thyroid Hormone. In humans, fasting blood glucose levels are elevated in hyperthyroid patients and are lower than normal in hypothyroid patients. Thyroid hormones enhance the action of epinephrine in increasing glycolysis and gluconeogenesis and can potentiate the actions of insulin on glycogen synthesis and glucose utilization. Thyroid hormones have a biphasic action in animals by enhancing glycogen synthesis in the presence of insulin at low doses but increasing glycogenolysis at higher doses.

Glucocorticoids. Glucocorticoids (cortisol and corticosterone) are secreted by the adrenal cortex in response to adrenocorticotrophic hormone (ACTH) released from the anterior pituitary. Glucocorticoids increase gluconeogenesis and inhibit the use of glucose in the extrahepatic tissues and thus are antagonistic to insulin's actions. The increased gluconeogenesis stimulated by the glucocorticoids is enhanced by increased protein catabolism, leading to increased availability of glucogenic amino acids to the liver and increased activity of transaminases and other enzymes involved with hepatic gluconeogenesis.

Growth Hormone. Growth hormone is secreted by the anterior pituitary. Its secretion is enhanced by hypoglycemia. It has direct and indirect effects on decreasing glucose uptake in specific tissues such as muscle. Part of this effect may be the result of the liberation of fatty acids from adipose tissue, which then inhibits glucose metabolism. If growth hormone is administered on a long-term basis or is released from a pituitary tumor, it results in a persistent modest elevation of circulating glucose levels. If the capacity of the pancreatic β cells to secrete insulin becomes exhausted, however, overt diabetes will ensue.

Transcriptional Regulation of Carbohydrate Metabolism

Excess blood glucose can have pathologic consequences. Control of blood glucose requires that surplus glucose be converted into and stored as fat after liver and muscle glycogen stores have been repleted. The conversion of carbon from carbohydrate (mainly glucose or fructose) into fatty acids is known as *de novo lipogenesis*. Homeostatic control of blood glucose is essential to prevent pathologic processes associated with diabetes. This control is achieved either through hormonal and intermediate regulation of constitutive enzymes (as discussed earlier) or by inducing transcription of enzymes either through direct actions of glucose itself or indirectly by hormonal mechanisms (e.g., insulin).

Integration of Carbohydrate and Lipid Metabolism

Excess dietary carbohydrate is lipogenic. In the liver, surplus pyruvate derived from carbohydrates is converted to triglycerides. Unlike synthesis of other lipids, such as cholesterol, that is highly controlled, hepatic triglyceride synthesis is primarily driven by the presence of excess carbon produced from the glycolytic metabolism of dietary carbohydrates glucose and fructose (66). The lipogenic characteristics of fructose are discussed in more detail later. Numerous nuclear and membrane-bound factors involved in transcriptional regulation of substrate metabolism have been identified (67). There appear to be several factors involved with lipid and a few with carbohydrate metabolism. Specific transcription factors that play a key role in lipogenesis following excess carbohydrate consumption are sterol regulatory element binding protein 1-c (SREBP1-c) and carbohydrate-responsive element binding protein (ChREBP).

SREBPs are a family of membrane-bound protein factors that bind to sterol regulatory element (SRE), present in the transcription domain of key genes that regulate lipid metabolism, and induce transcription of target proteins (68). Three isoforms of SREBPs (1a, 1c, and 2) have been identified. SREBP-1a and SREBP-1c are primarily involved in transcription of proteins involved in glucose and lipid metabolic homeostasis, whereas SREBP-2 is involved in cholesterol synthesis (66). Hepatic and adipose tissues have been known to express threefold and ninefold higher abundance of SREBP1-c gene as opposed to SREBP-2 (68).

SREBP1-c, bound to the nuclear membrane, homodimerizes on activation, is cleaved from the membrane, and binds to SRE-1 (5′-ATC-ACCCCAC-3′) (69), to activate transcription of target proteins. These include enzymes involved in fatty acid synthesis such as acetyl-coenzyme A carboxylase (ACC), fatty acid synthase, and glycerol-3-phosphate acyl transferase (66). Insulin-mediated activation of SREBP1-c occurs through IRS-1. Activation of IRS-1 has been shown to induce activation of SREBP1-c at several diverse steps. Primary among these involves IRS-1 activation of Akt, which is directly involved in mobilizing nascent SREBP from endoplasmic reticulum to Golgi bodies, where it undergoes final transcriptional activation (70–72).

When a high-carbohydrate diet is consumed, hepatic glucose uptake through GLUT2 occurs concomitant with activation of SREBP1-c through IRS-1, thereby promoting lipogenesis, particularly when dietary carbohydrate is consumed in excess of energy requirements. Excess glucose is converted to triglycerides and is either stored or oxidized; thus normal blood glucose concentrations are maintained. This insulin-mediated lipogenic response acts in conjunction with glucose-induced lipogenesis (73, 74). Glucose regulates transcription through a ChREBP-mediated pathway. ChREBP is a nuclear transcription factor that is activated by intracellular glucose. Once activated, ChREBP translocates into the nucleus to bind to and activate carbohydrate response elements (ChoREs) on target genes (75, 76). ChoREs have been found in genes responsible for liver pyruvate kinase, glucose-6-phosphate dehydrogenase, and, importantly, fatty acid synthase and ACC (74). ChREBP activation results in induction of both glycolysis and lipogenesis. ChREBP knockout mice exhibit reductions in both pathways (77). Hence, the combined activation of ChREBP and SREBP1-c mediated by glucose and insulin results in de novo lipogenesis, particularly following excess carbohydrate consumption.

GALACTOSE AND FRUCTOSE METABOLISM

Galactose Metabolism and Transport

Galactose is a hexose monosaccharide whose dietary intake is usually in the form of the disaccharide lactose (milk sugar). Lactose is hydrolyzed by the digestive enzyme lactase into its hexose moieties, glucose and galactose. Galactose shares the same transport mechanisms as glucose in enterocytes, specifically, apical SGLT cotransporters and the basolateral GLUT2. It enters the portal blood and is practically cleared in its passage through the liver, so little or no galactose greater than 1 mmol/L is seen in the systemic blood even after ingestion of as much as 100 g of lactose. Ingestion of galactose without glucose, however, induces higher plasma concentrations. Alcohol has been shown to decrease galactose uptake and metabolism by the liver, thus leading to increased circulating galactose concentrations (galactosemia). In the liver cells, galactose is converted by the enzyme galactokinase into galactose-1-phosphate. This, in turn, is converted by a two-stage enzymatic transformation into glucose-1-phosphate, which can be converted into glycogen. Although in theory glucose-1-phosphate can enter the glycolytic pathway, it does not normally do so to any large extent. Most tissues have enzymes that can metabolize galactose. Even in the complete absence of dietary galactose, however, glucose can be converted into galactose and supply cellular needs for galactose when required. Many structural elements of cells and tissues (glycoproteins and mucopolysaccharides) contain galactose, and in mammals endogenously synthesized galactose is produced and secreted into breast milk.

Cataracts and Inborn Errors of Galactose Metabolism

Galactose concentrations in peripheral blood normally do not exceed 1 mmol/L. When concentrations are higher than this (considered galactosemia), several tissues can remove galactose from the blood and convert it into galactitol (dulcitol) through the actions of the enzyme aldehyde reductase. Because it is not metabolized, galactitol can accumulate in tissues, with resulting pathologic changes caused by increased osmotic pressure. In the lens of the eye, the result is cataract formation (78). Cataracts are also observed in two inborn errors of galactose metabolism resulting from deficiencies of the enzymes galactose-1-phosphate uridyltransferase and galactokinase. The former enzyme deficiency produces classic galactosemia. Unless it is treated promptly in the neonate by withdrawing galactose from the diet (from the lactose component of milk), either death or severe mental retardation can occur. Cataracts can also occur as a complication of diabetes mellitus when high blood glucose concentrations result in excess glucose transport into the lens, where glucose is metabolized to sorbitol and thus causes the lens to swell and become opaque.

Fructose Absorption and Metabolism

Fructose, a monosaccharide ketohexose, is present as the free hexose naturally occurring in honey and fruit or produced by isomerization of glucose from corn and added to soft drinks and many other sweetened beverages and foods as HFCS. Fructose is also produced from hydrolysis of the dietary disaccharide sucrose (yielding glucose and fructose). Fruits contain various combinations of free fructose, free glucose, and sucrose usually yielding between 45% and 70% fructose. Although fructose is absorbed across the enterocytes of the small intestine, it is not a substrate for the SGLT cotransporters. The evidence for this is threefold: (a) fructose absorption is normal in those with glucose-galactose malabsorption, who have defective SGLT-1 cotransporters; (b) fructose absorption is not reduced by phlorizin, the classic inhibitor of SGLT 1 cotransporters; and (c) fructose absorption is neither Na^+ sensitive nor electrogenic like that of glucose or galactose. Studies on the expression of human GLUT5 transporter in *Xenopus* oocytes showed that the transporter exhibited selectivity for high-affinity fructose transport that was not blocked by cytochalasin B, a potent inhibitor of facilitative glucose transport by glucose transporters (27). Because GLUT5 is also expressed in high levels in the brush border of enterocytes in the small intestine (79), this isoform is likely to be the major fructose transporter of the small intestine. Indirect evidence for the likelihood of fructose transport by GLUT5 is the finding that it is expressed in high concentration in human spermatids and spermatozoa (79)—gamete cells known to metabolize fructose. Although GLUT2, localized to the basolateral membrane of enterocytes, has a much lower affinity for fructose transport than GLUT5, it probably mediates the exit of the absorbed fructose from the enterocytes into the portal circulation. Investigators have reported that GLUT5 is also localized on the basolateral membrane in the human jejunum (80), so fructose could also exit from the enterocytes through this transporter. In humans, absorption of fructose from sucrose ingestion is more rapid than that from equimolar amounts of fructose ingestion. The explanations for this phenomenon include differences in gastric emptying, the close association of sucrase activity with proximity to the intestinal brush-border membrane-enhanced fluid absorption initiated by the glucose entraining fructose, and cotransport of fructose and glucose by a disaccharidase-related transport system (81, 82).

The majority of fructose absorbed and entering into the portal circulation is cleared in a single passage through the liver, although a substantial amount of ingested fructose can be metabolized through glycolysis to lactate and released. Thus, low concentrations of fructose (>0.25 mmol/L) can be measured in the systemic circulation after consumption of substantial amounts of fructose with meals (83). After a large oral dose of 1 g free fructose/kg body weight, the plasma concentration increases to 0.5 mmol/L in 30 minutes and then slowly decreases during the next 90 minutes. In the liver, fructose is phosphorylated by the abundant enzyme fructokinase into fructose-1-phosphate, which is cleaved by hepatic aldolase into glyceraldehyde and dihydroxyacetone phosphate. Dihydroxyacetone phosphate is an intermediary metabolite in both the glycolytic and gluconeogenic pathways. Glyceraldehyde, although not an intermediary in either pathway, can be converted by various liver enzymes into glycolytic intermediary metabolites, ultimately to produce glycogen. This glycogen can then be broken down into glucose by glycogenolysis. Thus, a relatively small but measurable amount of ingested fructose is converted to glucose by the liver. In addition, small "catalytic" amounts of fructose appear to enhance hepatic glucose uptake, perhaps by activation of glucokinase (84–86), and this has led to the idea that including limited amounts of dietary fructose may be beneficial in the management of postprandial blood glucose excursions in patients with diabetes mellitus (87, 88). Caution should be exercised in recommending fructose in the dietary management of diabetes, however, because larger amounts could contribute to weight gain and visceral adipose deposition and could exacerbate hyperlipidemia or insulin resistance (see later) or induce protein fructosylation or oxidative damage (89–91) involved in the pathogenesis of diabetic complications.

When large amounts of fructose are ingested, such as occurs when a large serving of beverage sweetened with sucrose (50% fructose) or HFCS (55% fructose) is rapidly consumed, the glycolytic pathway becomes saturated with intermediates that can be used for the glycerol moiety of triglyceride synthesis or can enter the pathway of de novo lipogenesis to form fatty acids that are then esterified to triglycerides, packaged with apolipoprotein-B, and exported as very-low-density lipoproteins (VLDLs). The preferential increase of lipogenic precursors after fructose ingestion occurs in large part because, unlike glucose metabolism through phosphofructokinase, fructokinase is not subject to allosteric negative feedback inhibition by ATP and citrate (92) (Fig. 2.4). Thus, although only a small percentage (1% to 3%) of ingested glucose-containing carbohydrate enters de novo lipogenesis and is incorporated into triglyceride in normal-weight insulin-sensitive individuals, a proportionally much greater amount of carbon from ingested fructose is metabolized to form triglycerides. This is thought to be a major reason that ingestion of fructose increases circulating triglyceride levels, particularly in the postprandial state (see later).

Inborn Errors of Fructose Metabolism

Six genetically determined abnormalities in the metabolism of fructose have been described in humans (93). These abnormalities are caused by deficiencies in fructokinase, aldolase A and B, fructose-1,6-diphosphatase, glycerate kinase, and by fructose malabsorption. Limiting dietary fructose produces a favorable result in each of these conditions except aldolase A deficiency. Fructokinase deficiency, manifests in the liver, causes fructosemia (elevated blood fructose concentrations) and fructosuria (fructose excretion in urine). In contrast to the low levels of fructose observed in the blood of physiologically normal persons after ingestion of 1 g of free fructose/kg, the concentration in fructokinase-deficient subjects approaches 3 mmol/L and is sustained for many hours. Despite the sustained high levels of fructose in the blood, cataracts do not develop—in sharp contrast to cases of galactokinase deficiency and diabetes mellitus (see specific sections).

The three aldolases, A, B, and C, catalyze the reversible conversion of fructose-1,6-diphosphate into glyceraldehyde-3-phosphate and dihydroxyacetone phosphate. Each aldolase is coded for by a different gene: A is on chromosome 16, B is on chromosome 9, and C is on chromosome 17. Expression of the enzymes is regulated during development, so A is produced in embryonic tissues and adult muscle; B is produced in adult liver, kidney, and intestine; and C is produced in adult nervous tissue. Deficiency of aldolase A causes a syndrome of mental retardation, short stature, hemolytic anemia, and abnormal facial appearance. Deficiency of aldolase A probably results in these defects because it is involved in fetal glycolysis. No treatment exists for the condition. Deficiency of aldolase B (hereditary fructose intolerance), the most frequent of the three deficiencies, was first described in the early 1950s (94). When fructose is ingested, vomiting, failure to thrive, and liver dysfunction occur.

Deficiency of fructose-1,6-diphosphatase was first described in 1970. Patients exhibit hypoglycemia, acidosis, ketonuria, and hyperventilation. Urinalysis shows many changes in organic acids, but excretion of glycerol is diagnostic. The treatment is to avoid dietary fructose. D-Glyceric aciduria is rare and is caused by D-glycerate kinase deficiency. The presentation of the disease is highly variable, from no clinical symptoms to severe metabolic acidosis and psychomotor retardation—findings that suggest that among the 10 described cases, other enzyme deficiencies are also present.

In fructose malabsorption, ingestion of moderate to large quantities of fructose produces abdominal bloating, flatulence, and diarrhea. Persons with this condition appear to have a defect in fructose absorption. No assessments of intestinal GLUT5 or its controlling gene have yet been made in any of these patients. If either glucose or galactose is ingested with fructose, fructose absorption is enhanced, and often symptoms of malabsorption do not occur (82, 93).

CARBOHYDRATES AND ATHLETIC PERFORMANCE

Carbohydrate present in limited amounts in muscle (300 g glycogen), liver (90 g glycogen), and body fluids (30 g glucose) is a major fuel for physical performance. The ATP stored in muscle cells can provide energy for high-power output for only a few seconds. It can be resynthesized anaerobically for a further few seconds (5 to 8 seconds) by using the phosphate from creatinine phosphate. These short, intense bursts of muscular activity occur in sprints (100 m), track-and-field events, and sports such as tennis, hockey, football, gymnastics, and weightlifting. If the maximum effort lasts for 30 seconds or longer, then muscle glycogenolysis can supply the energy for physical activity, with concurrent buildup of lactic acid in muscle. Most physical activity, however, requires an energy source that can power muscles for longer periods.

Both duration and intensity of exercise determine the mix of fuel used. At light to moderate activity levels, as duration of exercise lengthens, the contribution of fat to energy used for physical activity increases. In contrast, as the intensity of activity increases from rest to light to moderate to intense, the contribution of carbohydrate to energy production increases. The change to using carbohydrate is not a linear response but accelerates with the intensity of the work. At higher exercise intensities, the versatility of carbohydrate as a fuel source is demonstrated, because it can produce energy under conditions of limited oxygen supply. Endurance athletes use more fat and so conserve the carbohydrate stored in muscle and liver and maintain blood glucose concentrations for longer periods. Ultimately, the amount of carbohydrate stored sets the limits for continued performance, and fatigue arises when the glycogen stores becomes depleted. The store of carbohydrate usually suffices for just 1 to 3 hours of physical exertion, depending on the intensity of effort.

Dietary Manipulation of Glycogen Stores: Carbohydrate Loading

Dietary manipulation can be used to increase the stores of glycogen in muscle and liver. Glycogen increases when more carbohydrate is consumed. The practice is known as *carbohydrate loading*. The traditional protocol called for 3 days of exhausting physical exercise on a low-carbohydrate diet followed by 3 days of rest on a high-carbohydrate diet. In general, athletes dislike both phases; in the first, they often feel both mentally and physically exhausted and are at increased risk of injury; and in the second, they may feel bloated because the glycogen is stored with water. For these reasons, the traditional protocol has been modified. One protocol calls for the elimination of the initial carbohydrate depletion phase and relies solely on the tapering of exercise with a high-carbohydrate diet several days before the event to augment glycogen stores. Another protocol shortens the process of glycogen depletion and loading into a 1-day time frame by having the athletes perform a short-duration (~3 minutes), high-intensity (supramaximal) workout and then consume a high-carbohydrate diet during the next 24 hours. For athletes in general, it makes sense to eat plenty of carbohydrate to maximize glycogen storage, because the usual training periods of several hours per day can deplete it. Little doubt exists that a high-carbohydrate diet increases glycogen storage and can improve athletic performance.

What to advise athletes to ingest just before an event is still debated and constantly evolving. A meal or snack taken 3 to 4 hours before exercise should include about 200 to 300 g of carbohydrate, or about 1 hour before exercise, approximately 13 to 60 g of carbohydrate can be taken to maximize maintenance of blood glucose, but consumption of solid food is not advisable immediately before strenuous exercise. During endurance events, beverages containing simple carbohydrates (solutions of glucose, fructose, or sweetened fruit juices) can be provided to aid in the maintenance of blood glucose. Fructose ingestion has been proposed to result in smaller increases of blood glucose and insulin levels and thus a slower loss of muscle glycogen (95). After glycogen-depleting exercise, carbohydrate intake of approximately 200 to 400 g spaced over 4 to 6 hours after exercise will aid in the restoration of muscle glycogen.

OTHER DISORDERS OF CARBOHYDRATE DIGESTION, ABSORPTION, OR METABOLISM

Carbohydrate Intolerance

In several clinical disorders, sugar digestion or absorption is disturbed and gives rise to sugar intolerance, creating symptoms as a result of undigested or unabsorbed sugar and water that enters the intestine, activates peristalsis, and induces passage of frequent fluid stools. The undigested carbohydrate can also enter the colon and undergo fermentation by colonic microflora into products that promote diarrhea. These disorders are classified as either congenital or secondary to some other disease, to impaired digestion of disaccharides, or to impaired absorption of the monosaccharides. The congenital deficiencies, although relatively rare, can be life threatening: examples are sucrase-maltase deficiency (watery diarrhea after ingesting sucrose-containing foods), alactasia (absence of lactase, diarrhea from ingestion of milk), glucose-galactose malabsorption (diarrhea from ingestion of glucose, galactose, or lactose), and the rare trehalase deficiency (intolerance to trehalose contained in mushrooms). Sugar intolerance secondary to underlying gastrointestinal disease is more common, especially in pediatric patients. Infections of the gastrointestinal tract, for example, often result in temporary intolerance to lactose.

Lactose Intolerance

Adult mammals and most human groups after weaning retain only a fraction of the intestinal lactase activity of neonates (who need it to digest the lactose from breast milk). The persistence of lactase activity in Europeans has been regarded as the exception to the rule, because most human populations are hypolactasic and therefore malabsorb lactose (96). Small amounts of dietary lactose, however, as in up to 250 mL of milk, can be tolerated by most adults who do not fully digest lactose. The decrease in lactase in adults is a developmentally programmed event, and feeding high-lactose diets does not prevent the decrease. The mechanisms of the decline in activity have been studied in rats. As the animal matures, more and more mRNA message for lactase is needed to maintain the decreasing lactase activity in the enterocytes—a finding suggesting that translational or posttranslational events are of greater importance than decreased lactase gene expression (97).

Diagnostic Tests to Evaluate Carbohydrate Digestion, Absorption, or Metabolism

Breath Hydrogen Tests

Carbohydrates that have not been digested or absorbed reach the colon and undergo fermentation by the resident bacteria. Hydrogen gas is produced, and some of this is absorbed by the colon, enters the bloodstream, and is excreted in the breath as it reaches the lungs. Measuring breath hydrogen thus provides an estimate of sugar or carbohydrate malabsorption. This test was first used to detect lactose intolerance and has since been used in numerous studies of carbohydrate intolerance (98). The test has certain weaknesses; for example, it gives no indication of the amount of carbohydrate absorbed before the sugar reached the colon, and the hydrogen in the breath is only a fraction of that formed.

Sugar Tolerance Tests

Clinical quantitative assessment of the efficiency of the digestion and absorption of carbohydrates in humans rests mainly on relatively simple tests in which carbohydrate loads (≥50 g) are ingested and blood samples are collected to estimate the sugar levels attained at various time intervals after ingestion. The levels are then compared with those obtained in physiologically normal subjects. The most commonly used test is the oral glucose tolerance test. Typically, nonpregnant adults consume 75 g of glucose as a liquid solution over 5 minutes, and the glucose is measured in serum or blood at 0, 30, 60, 90, and 120 minutes. For assessment of glucose intolerance and gestation diabetes in pregnancy, women consume 75 to 100 g of glucose, and samples for blood glucose measurement are obtained. In children, the test consists of 1.75 g/kg of glucose up to the maximum of 75 g (99). Values greater than normal indicate impaired glucose tolerance or diabetes. Often the criteria are glucose concentrations greater than 2000 mg/dL 2 hours after glucose ingestion. The reproducibility of the oral glucose tolerance test has been claimed to be poor, even when the test is repeated in the same individual (100). An oral glucose tolerance test is sometimes also performed with galactose. Because the liver is a major site of galactose metabolism, the test has been used to assess liver function. Similar oral tolerance tests exist for fructose and the disaccharides lactose (lactase deficiency) and sucrose (sucrase deficiency).

The Glycemic Index

A form of oral tolerance test is used to assess the glycemic potential of different carbohydrate-containing foods. For each food item under evaluation, a measured quantity containing 50 g of carbohydrate is ingested, and blood glucose concentrations are measured usually over a period of 2 hours. The glycemic response, typically the incremental area under the curve over 2 hours, is compared with that obtained by ingesting a reference food, usually a 50-g glucose load or a portion of white bread containing 50 g of carbohydrate. This normalized value, expressed as a percentage of the value obtained with the reference food, is designated as the *glycemic index* of the food (101). Several factors are known to affect the glycemic index of a given food, including the nature of the starch structure, the particle size, pH, content of fiber, fat, and protein in the food matrix, as well as the cooking methods and time. The average glycemic index of a meal can be calculated by summing the products of the glycemic index for each food multiplied by the amount of carbohydrate in the food portion and dividing by the total amount of carbohydrate in the meal.

Another concept, the *glycemic load*, combines the glycemic index with the total amount of carbohydrate consumed to characterize the full glycemic potential of a mixed meal or diet plan. The glycemic load is determined by calculating the sum of the products of the glycemic index for each constituent food multiplied by the amount of carbohydrate in the each food. These classifications have been useful for the dietetic management of diabetes and hypoglycemia.

More recently, epidemiologic evidence has linked the glycemic index and the glycemic load with the risk of developing chronic diseases such as type 2 diabetes (102, 103), cardiovascular disease (104), and diet-related cancers of the colon and breast (105–107), thus raising the issue of whether restricting foods with a high glycemic index and the overall glycemic load may be potentially useful in disease prevention. Investigators have shown considerable interest in applying the concept of glycemic index to the management of body weight. Some of the current evidence suggests that under free-living conditions, when food intake is not controlled, diets with lower glycemic loads are associated with weight reduction, whereas higher glycemic loads are associated with weight gain. It is not clear, however, whether this relationship is driven by the glycemic index itself, or by other differences between high– and low–glycemic index diets, particularly dietary fiber, which lowers the glycemic index of foods (108).

Dietary fructose is another potential contributing factor to the inconsistent effects of dietary glycemic index and load. In one study, when a lower glycemic index diet containing fructose-sweetened beverages (glycemic index = 38) was consumed by overweight to obese men and women, several adverse changes were noted in lipid profiles, including increases of low-density lipoprotein (LDL) cholesterol and apolipoprotein-B, and insulin sensitivity decreased over 10 weeks compared with a moderate glycemic index baseline diet (glycemic index = 64) (109, 110). In contrast, in subjects consuming higher glycemic index diets with glucose-sweetened beverages (glycemic index = 83), these adverse effects of plasma lipids and insulin sensitivity were not observed. Another study in which diets with high versus low glycemic indices were compared in overweight men and women for 11 weeks reported no differences in fasting glucose or insulin, lipids, or several inflammatory markers between the diets (111). These and other results lend support to the suggestion that a dietary fructose index may be more relevant than the glycemic index (112).

Before public health recommendations can be made, well-controlled long-term clinical trials, in which the effects of the diets on postprandial circulating glucose and insulin concentrations are assessed over the course of the study, are needed to determine that the glycemic index and load of a diet has a role in body weight regulation or directly influences risk factors for chronic diseases such as type 2 diabetes and cardiovascular disease. The value of the glycemic index remains controversial; there are arguments in support of (113) and opposed to (114) the use of the glycemic index in health and disease. In addition, foods are not consumed in isolation (as when they are tested for their glycemic indices) but generally in the form of meals containing a mixture of macronutrients and carbohydrate types, including fiber. Thus, the glycemic effects of any particular food in the context of a mixed meal may be quite different from the effects when a food is tested as the sole ingested food item. The glycemic index does illustrate that carbohydrate foods can differ widely in their effects on blood glucose and hormonal responses after a meal, however (see later).

DIETARY REFERENCE INTAKES FOR CARBOHYDRATE

The recommended dietary allowance (RDA) for carbohydrate is set at 130 g/day for adults and children ages 1 through 18 years (115). This value is based on the amount of available carbohydrate that can provide an adequate supply of glucose for brain and central nervous system cells without the need for glucose production from ingested proteins or triacylglycerols. It also assumes that energy intake is sufficient, and the central nervous system is not relying on a partial replacement of glucose fuel by ketones. For infants, an RDA value has not been established, but the adequate intake (AI) is set at 60 g/day for infants 0 to 6 months of age. This value is equal to the amount of carbohydrate consumed in human milk and is considered optimal for growth and development during the first 6 months of life. For infants 7 to 12 months of age, the AI is set at 95 g/day. This value is based on the amount of carbohydrate consumed from human milk and complementary foods in the diets of infants of this age group. No gender differences exist for the RDA or AI values for recommended amounts of carbohydrate.

The amount of dietary carbohydrate that supports optimal health is unknown, but an acceptable macronutrient distribution range has been set, with carbohydrate contributing between 45% and 65% of energy intake. The potential for adverse effects of overconsumption of carbohydrate was considered. Specifically, the potential effects of glycemic index, total sugar intake, and added sugar intake on increasing the risk for coronary heart disease, cancer, diabetes, or obesity were examined. Currently, available evidence is insufficient to support an upper limit of carbohydrate intake based on the glycemic index of the diet. The World Health Organization recommended that added sugar intake should not exceed 10% of total energy intake (116). Recommendations from the American Heart Association set an upper daily limit of energy intake from added sugar at 100 kcal for women and 150 kcal for men (117).

CARBOHYDRATES AND CHRONIC DISEASE

Sugar and Dental Caries

Dental caries is a disease created by bacterial plaque on the enamel of teeth. Gradual and progressive demineralization of the enamel, dentin, and cementum occurs. Many studies have suggested that carbohydrates, especially sugars and in particular sucrose, are important dietary components that promote dental caries. Despite a large amount of laboratory and clinical research, however, the relationship between sugar and caries is still poorly characterized. A major reason for this is the complexity of the problem because the formation of caries involves interactions such as nutrients and food components of diet, plaque bacteria, salivary flow and composition, minerals and fluoride status, genetics, age, and even race. The most common organism in dental plaque associated with caries is *Streptococcus mutans*, but other bacteria also appear to contribute. Most studies have focused on the acids (lactic and acetic) generated from sugars (sucrose) by the bacteria, but the complex formation and accumulation of plaque from the insoluble dextran made from sucrose may also be important features (118, 119). A role for acids such as phosphoric acid added to many soft drinks in the demineralization in dental caries is possible.

Health Impact of Fructose Consumption

The consumption of simple sugars comprises a significant portion of dietary energy intake and has increased significantly since the 1980s. The mean annual consumption of sucrose plus fructose in developed countries is approximately 25% of the caloric intake. The proceedings of a workshop on the health aspects of dietary sugars summarized this topic (120). Although precise data on total fructose intake are not available, mean per capita intake in the United States from the combined consumption of sucrose and HFCS is probably in the range of 25 to 35 kg/year/person. Fructose has been proposed to contribute to metabolic diseases including hyperlipidemia, insulin resistance, and obesity (92). The idea that fructose has these adverse metabolic effects is based on a substantial number of studies reporting that feeding high-sucrose and high-fructose diets to experimental animals induces weight gain, hyperlipidemia, insulin resistance, hypertension, and an accelerated onset of diabetes (121)—findings supported by data from a smaller number of human studies (92).

Because of the differences in the hepatic metabolism of fructose and glucose discussed earlier, fructose is more lipogenic than glucose and is therefore more readily converted in the liver to triglyceride, which can be exported as VLDL containing apolipoprotein-B and stored in adipose tissue. In addition, several studies have demonstrated that fructose increases circulating triglyceride levels in the postprandial period (122–124), and evidence indicates that this effect is more pronounced in persons with existing hyperlipidemia or insulin resistance (83, 125, 126). Thus, long-term consumption of a diet high in fructose may increase the risk of atherosclerosis or other cardiovascular disease. In addition, data indicate that compared with glucose, consuming fructose with meals, which does not stimulate insulin secretion, results in a reduction of circulating leptin concentrations and an attenuated postprandial suppression of ghrelin, a hormone produced by the stomach that stimulates hunger and increases food intake (124). Thus, with respect to the hormones insulin, leptin, and ghrelin

that are involved in the long-term endocrine regulation of food intake, energy balance, and body adiposity (127, 128), dietary fructose behaves more like dietary fat than do other types of carbohydrate that are composed of glucose (Fig. 2.5). The lack of effect of fructose on these hormones suggests that long-term consumption of a diet high in fructose could contribute, along with dietary fat and inactivity, to increased energy intake, weight gain, and obesity.

In a study designed to address and compare the metabolic effects of fructose and glucose consumption on body composition and lipid and carbohydrate metabolism, glucose or fructose-sweetened beverages were consumed for

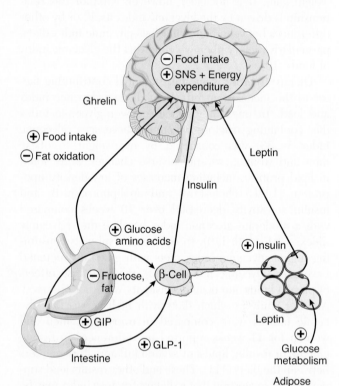

Fig. 2.5. Long-term signals regulating food intake and energy homeostasis. Insulin and leptin are important long-term regulators of food intake and energy balance. Both insulin and leptin act in the central nervous system to inhibit food intake and to increase energy expenditure, most likely by activating the sympathetic nervous system (SNS). Insulin is secreted from the β cells in the endocrine pancreas in response to circulating nutrients (glucose and amino acids) and to the incretin hormones, glucose-dependent insulinotropic polypeptide (GIP) and glucagon-like peptide-1 (GLP-1), which are released during meal ingestion and absorption. Insulin can also act indirectly by stimulating leptin production from adipose tissue through increased glucose metabolism. In contrast, dietary fat and fructose do not stimulate insulin secretion and therefore do not increase leptin production. Ghrelin, a hormone produced by endocrine cells in the stomach, increases food intake and decreases fat oxidation and appears to have an anabolic role in long-term regulation of energy balance. Ghrelin secretion is normally suppressed after meals, but it is not suppressed by fat or fructose consumption. The long-term signals interact with the short-term signals in the regulation of energy homeostasis and appear to set sensitivity to the satiety-producing effects of short-term signals such as cholecystokinin. (Adapted with permission from Havel PJ. Peripheral signals conveying metabolic information to the brain: short-term and long-term regulation of food intake and energy homeostasis. Exp Biol Med [Maywood] 2001;226:963–77.)

10 weeks at 25% of energy requirements by older (aged 40 to 72 years) overweight to obese men and women (110). During the first 8 weeks of the intervention, when the subjects consumed the sweetened beverages along with their usual diets ad libitum, both groups of subjects gained approximately 1.5 kg. In the subjects consuming fructose-sweetened beverages, however, investigators noted a significant increase in intra-abdominal (visceral) fat that was not observed in the group of subjects consuming glucose-sweetened beverages in which the increase of fat in the abdominal area was primarily in the subcutaneous compartment. In addition, subjects consuming fructose-sweetened beverages had increases of isotopically determined de novo lipogenesis, 24-hour postprandial triglyceride profiles, LDL cholesterol, apolipoprotein-B, small-dense LDL cholesterol, oxidized LDL, remnant lipoproteins, and a 20% decrease of insulin sensitivity that did not occur in the subjects consuming glucose-sweetened beverages. Important differences are seen in the effects of fructose and fructose-containing sweeteners between men and women on lipid and carbohydrate metabolism (110, 129–131). The metabolic effects of effects of dietary fructose and the mechanisms by which fructose consumption increases visceral adiposity and adversely alters lipid profiles and insulin sensitivity have been the subjects of several reviews (109, 123, 132–134).

ACKNOWLEDGMENTS

Dr. Havel acknowledges research support from National Institutes of Health Grants HL-075675, HL-091333, and DK-087307 and the American Diabetes Association.

Dr. Keim acknowledges research funding from US Department of Agriculture CRIS 5306-51530-019-00D.

REFERENCES

1. Dahlquist A, Semenza G. J Pediatr Gastroenterol Nutr 1985;4:857–65.
2. Ugolev AM, De Laey P. Biochim Biophys Acta 1973;300:105–28.
3. Gray GM. J Nutr 1992;122:172–7.
4. Asp NG. Am J Clin Nutr 1994;59(Suppl):679S–81S.
5. Wursch P. World Rev Nutr Diet 1989;60:199–256.
6. Wursch P. Dietary fibre and unabsorbed carbohydrates. In: Gracey M, Kretchmer N, Rossi E, eds. Sugars in Nutrition. Nestle Nutrition Workshop series. New York: Raven Press, 1991;25:153–68.
7. Roediger WE. Dis Colon Rectum 1990;33:858–62.
8. Cani PD, Delzenne NM. Curr Pharm Des 2009;15:1546–58.
9. Delzenne NM, Cani PD, Neyrinck AM. J Nutr 2007;137(Suppl):2547S–51S.
10. Trowell H, Southgate DA, Wolever TM et al. Lancet 1976;1:967.
11. Marlett JA. J Am Diet Assoc 1992;92:175–86.
12. Drewnowski A. Epidemiol Rev 2007;29:160–71.
13. Lee WS, Kanai Y, Wells RG et al. J Biol Chem 1994;269:12032–9.
14. Mueckler M, Caruso C, Baldwin SA et al. Science 1985;229:941–5.
15. Alvarez J, Lee DC, Baldwin SA et al. J Biol Chem 1987;262:3502–9.
16. Cuppoletti J, Jung CY, Green FA. J Biol Chem 1981;256:1305–6.
17. Bell GI, Kayano T, Buse JB et al. Diabetes Care 1990;13:198–208.
18. Hediger MA, Kanai Y, You G et al. J Physiol 1995;482(Suppl):7S–17S.
19. Hediger MA, Rhoads DB. Physiol Rev 1994;74:993–1026.
20. Silverman M. Annu Rev Biochem 1991;60:757–94.
21. Thorens B. Annu Rev Physiol 1993;55:591–608.
22. Maher F, Vannucci SJ, Simpson IA. FASEB J 1994;8:1003–11.
23. Diamond DL, Carruthers A. J Biol Chem 1993;268:6437–44.
24. Gould GW, Holman GD. Biochem J 1993;295:329–41.
25. Kayano T, Fukumoto H, Eddy RL et al. J Biol Chem 1988;263:15245–8.
26. Kayano T, Burant CF, Fukumoto H et al. J Biol Chem 1990;265:13276–82.
27. Burant CF, Takeda J, Brot-Laroche E et al. J Biol Chem 1992;267:14523–6.
28. Sato Y, Ito T, Udaka N et al. Tissue Cell 1996;28:637–43.
29. Curry DL. Pancreas 1989;4:2–9.
30. Augustin R. IUBMB Life 2010;62:315–33.
31. Joost HG, Bell GI, Best JD et al. Am J Physiol 2002;282:E974–6.
32. Joost HG, Thorens B. Mol Membr Biol 2001;18:247–56.
33. Uldry M, Thorens B. Pflugers Arch 2004;447:480–9.
34. Wood IS, Trayhurn P. Br J Nutr 2003;89:3–9.
35. Wallberg-Henriksson H, Zierath JR. Mol Membr Biol 2001;18:205–11.
36. Katz EB, Stenbit AE, Hatton K et al. Nature 1995;377:151–5.
37. Kim JK, Zisman A, Fillmore JJ et al. J Clin Invest 2001;108:153–60.
38. Abel ED, Peroni O, Kim JK et al. Nature 2001;409:729–33.
39. Misra RP, Duncan SA. Endocrine 2002;19:229–38.
40. Hediger MA, Coady MJ, Ikeda TS et al. Nature 1987;330:379–81.
41. Wright EM, Turk E, Zabel B et al. J Clin Invest 1991;88:1435–40.
42. Mackenzie B, Panayotova-Heiermann M, Loo DD et al. J Biol Chem 1994;269:22488–91.
43. Bays H. Curr Med Res Opin 2009;25:671–81.
44. Turk E, Zabel B, Mundlos S et al. Nature 1991;350:354–6.
45. Fine KD, Santa Ana CA, Porter JL et al. Gastroenterology 1993;105:1117–25.
46. Levin RJ. Am J Clin Nutr 1994;59(Suppl):690S–98S.
47. Owen OE, Morgan AP, Kemp HG et al. J Clin Invest 1967;46:1589–95.
48. Cahill GF Jr, Owen OE, Felig P. Physiologist 1968;11:97–102.
49. Pedersen O, Bak JF, Andersen PH et al. Diabetes 1990;39:865–70.
50. Dohm GL, Elton CW, Friedman JE et al. Am J Physiol 1991;260:E459–63.
51. Ashcroft FM, Harrison DE, Ashcroft SJ. Nature 1984;312:446–8.
52. Dunne MJ, Petersen OH. Biochim Biophys Acta 1991;1071:67–82.
53. Inagaki N, Gonoi T, Clement JP et al. Science 1995;270:1166–70.
54. Vahl T, D'Alessio D. Curr Opin Clin Nutr Metab Care 2003;6:461–8.
55. Ahren B. Diabetologia 2000;43:393–410.
56. Ahren B, Holst JJ. Diabetes 2001;50:1030–8.
57. D'Alessio DA, Kieffer TJ, Taborsky GJ Jr et al. J Clin Endocrinol Metab 2001;86:1253–9.
58. Havel PJ, Taborsky GJ Jr. Stress-induced activation of the neuroendocrine system and its effects on carbohydrate metabolism. In: Porte D Jr, Sherwin R, Baron AD, eds. Ellenberg and Rifkin's Diabetes Mellitus. 6th ed. New York: McGraw-Hill, 2003:127–49.

59. Taborsky GJ Jr, Ahren B. Beta-cell function and insulin secretion. In: Porte D Jr, Sherwin R, Baron AD, eds. Ellenberg and Rifkin's Diabetes Mellitus. 6th ed. New York: McGraw-Hill, 2003:43–66.

60. Thorens B, Cheng ZQ, Brown D et al. Am J Physiol 1990;259:C279–85.

61. Jungermann K, Katz N. Physiol Rev 1989;69:708–64.

62. Pipeleers D. Diabetologia 1987;30:277–91.

63. Greenbaum CJ, Havel PJ, Taborsky GJ Jr et al. J Clin Invest 1991;88:767–73.

64. Hansen LH, Abrahamsen N, Nishimura E. Peptides 1995;16:1163–6.

65. Taborsky GJ Jr, Ahren B, Havel PJ. Diabetes 1998;47:995–1005.

66. Shimano H. Prog Lipid Res 2001;40:439–52.

67. Chawla A, Repa JJ, Evans RM et al. Science 2001;294:1866–70.

68. Osborne TF. J Biol Chem 2000;275:32379–82.

69. Yokoyama C, Wang X, Briggs MR et al. Cell 1993;75:187–97.

70. Matsumoto M, Ogawa W, Teshigawara K et al. Diabetes 2002;51:1672–80.

71. Osborne TF, Espenshade PJ. Genes Dev 2009;23:2578–91.

72. Yellaturu CR, Deng X, Cagen LM et al. J Biol Chem 2009;284:7518–32.

73. Dentin R, Girard J, Postic C. Biochimie 2005;87:81–6.

74. Iizuka K, Horikawa Y. Endocr J 2008;55:617–24.

75. Fukasawa M, Ge Q, Wynn RM et al. Biochem Biophys Res Commun 2010;391:1166–9.

76. Kawaguchi T, Takenoshita M, Kabashima T et al. Proc Natl Acad Sci U S A 2001;98:13710–5.

77. Iizuka K, Bruick RK, Liang G et al. Proc Natl Acad Sci U S A 2004;101:7281–6.

78. Van Heyningen R. Exp Eye Res 1971;11:415–28.

79. Davidson NO, Hausman AM, Ifkovits CA et al. Am J Physiol 1992;262:C795–800.

80. Blakemore SJ, Aledo JC, James J et al. Biochem J 1995;309:7–12.

81. Fujisawa T, Riby J, Kretchmer N. Gastroenterology 1991;101:360–7.

82. Riby JE, Fujisawa T, Kretchmer N. Am J Clin Nutr 1993;58(Suppl):748S–53S.

83. Teff KL, Grudziak J, Townsend RR et al. J Clin Endocrinol Metab 2009;94:1562–9.

84. Moore MC, Cherrington AD, Mann SL et al. J Clin Endocrinol Metab 2000;85:4515–9.

85. Petersen KF, Laurent D, Yu C et al. Diabetes 2001;50:1263–8.

86. Shiota M, Galassetti P, Monohan M et al. Diabetes 1998;47:867–73.

87. McGuinness OP, Cherrington AD. Curr Opin Clin Nutr Metab Care 2003;6:441–8.

88. Moore MC, Davis SN, Mann SL et al. Diabetes Care 2001;24:1882–7.

89. Bell RC, Carlson JC, Storr KC et al. Br J Nutr 2000;84:575–82.

90. Dills WL Jr. Am J Clin Nutr 1993;58(Suppl):779S–87S.

91. Levi B, Werman MJ. J Nutr 1998;128:1442–9.

92. Elliott SS, Keim NL, Stern JS et al. Am J Clin Nutr 2002;76:911–22.

93. Hommes FA. Am J Clin Nutr 1993;58(Suppl):788S–95S.

94. Cori GT. Harvey Lect 1952–1953;48:148–71.

95. Stanton R. Sugars in the diet of athletes. In: Gracey M, Kretchmer N, Rossi E, eds. Sugars in Nutrition. Nestle Nutrition Workshop series. New York: Raven Press, 1991;25;267–78.

96. Kretchmer N. Gastroenterology 1971;61:805–13.

97. Nudell DM, Santiago NA, Zhu JS et al. Am J Physiol 1993;265:G1108–15.

98. Levitt MD, Donaldson RM. J Lab Clin Med 1970;75:937–45.

99. Potparic O, Gibson J, eds. A Dictionary of Clinical Tests. Lancashire, UK: Parthenon Publishing, 1993.

100. McDonald GW, Fisher GF, Burnham C. Diabetes 1965;14:473–80.

101. Jenkins DJ, Wolever TM, Taylor RH et al. Am J Clin Nutr 1981;34:362–6.

102. Salmeron J, Ascherio A, Rimm EB et al. Diabetes Care 1997;20:545–50.

103. Salmeron J, Manson JE, Stampfer MJ et al. JAMA 1997;277:472–7.

104. Liu S, Willett WC, Stampfer MJ et al. Am J Clin Nutr 2000;71:1455–61.

105. Augustin LS, Dal Maso L, La Vecchia C et al. Ann Oncol 2001;12:1533–8.

106. Franceschi S, Dal Maso L, Augustin L et al. Ann Oncol 2001;12:173–8.

107. Hu FB, Manson JE, Liu S et al. J Natl Cancer Inst 1999;91:542–7.

108. Mann J. Eur J Clin Nutr 2007;87(Suppl):258S–68S.

109. Stanhope KL, Havel PJ. Ann N Y Acad Sci 2010;1190:15–24.

110. Stanhope KL, Schwarz JM, Keim NL et al. J Clin Invest 2009;119:1322–34.

111. Vrolix R, Mensink RP. Am J Clin Nutr 2010;61(Suppl 1):S100–11.

112. Johnson RJ, Segal MS, Sautin Y et al. Am J Clin Nutr 2007;86:899–906.

113. Jenkins DJ, Kendall CW, Augustin LS et al. Am J Clin Nutr 2002;76(Suppl):266S–73S.

114. Pi-Sunyer FX. Am J Clin Nutr 2002;76(Suppl):290S–8S.

115. Food and Nutrition Board, Institute of Medicine. Dietary Reference Intakes for Energy, Carbohydrate, Fiber, Fat, Fatty Acids, Cholesterol, Protein, and Amino Acids (Macronutrients). Washington, DC: National Academy Press, 2002. Available at: http://www.nap.edu.

116. Nishida C, Uauy R, Kumanyika S et al. Public Health Nutr 2004;7:245–50.

117. Johnson RK, Appel LJ, Brands M et al. Circulation 2009;120:1011–20.

118. Bowen W. Simple carbohydrates as microbiological substrates. In: Conning D, eds. Biological Functions of Carbohydrates: Proceedings of the British Nutrition Foundation/World Sugar Research Organisation International Symposium. London: British Nutrition Foundation, 1993:64–7.

119. Navia JM. Am J Clin Nutr 1994;59(Suppl):719S–27S.

120. Lineback DR, Jones JM. Am J Clin Nutr 2003;78(Suppl):893S–97S.

121. Cummings BP, Stanhope KL, Graham JL et al. Am J Physiol 2010;298:R1343–50.

122. Bantle JP, Raatz SK, Thomas W et al. Am J Clin Nutr 2000;72:1128–34.

123. Stanhope KL, Havel PJ. Am J Clin Nutr 2008;88(Suppl):1733S–37S.

124. Teff KL, Elliott SS, Tschop M et al. J Clin Endocrinol Metab 2004;89:2963–72.

125. Abraha A, Humphreys SM, Clark ML et al. Br J Nutr 1998;80:169–75.

126. Jeppesen J, Chen YI, Zhou MY et al. Am J Clin Nutr 1995;61:787–91.

127. Havel PJ. Exp Biol Med (Maywood) 2001;226:963–77.

128. Havel PJ. Diabetes 2004;53(Suppl 1):S143–51.

129. Bantle JP, Raatz SK, Thomas W et al. Am J Clin Nutr 2000;72:1128–34.

130. Stanhope KL, Griffen SC, Bair BR et al. Am J Clin Nutr 2008;87:1194–203.

131. Tran C, Jacot-Descombes D, Lecoultre V et al. Br J Nutr 2010;104:1–9.
132. Le KA, Ith M, Kreis R et al. Am J Clin Nutr 2009;89:1760–5.
133. Stanhope KL, Havel PJ. J Nutr 2009;119(Suppl):1236S–41S.
134. Stanhope KL, Havel PJ. Curr Opin Lipidol 2008;19:16–24.

SUGGESTED READINGS

Havel PJ. Peripheral signals conveying metabolic information to the brain: short-term and long-term regulation of food intake and energy homeostasis. Exp Biol Med (Maywood) 2001;226:963–77.

Havel PJ. Dietary fructose: implication for dysregulation of energy homeostasis and lipid/carbohydrate metabolism. Nutr Rev 2005;63: 133–57.

Johnson RK, Appel LJ, Brands M et al. American Heart Association Nutrition Committee of the Council on Nutrition, Physical Activity, and Metabolism and the Council on Epidemiology and Prevention. Dietary sugars intake and cardiovascular health: a scientific statement from the American Heart Association. Circulation 2009;120:1011–20.

Joost HG, Thorens B. The extended GLUT-family of sugar/polyol transport facilitators: nomenclature, sequence characteristics, and potential function of its novel members. Mol Membr Biol 2001;18:247–56.

Lineback DR, Jones JM. Sugars and health workshop. Am J Clin Nutr 2003;78(Suppl):814S–97S.

Stanhope KL, Havel PJ. Fructose consumption: potential mechanisms for its effects to increase visceral adiposity and induce dyslipidemia and insulin resistance. Curr Opin Lipidol 2008;19:16–24.

Stanhope KL, Havel PJ. Fructose consumption: recent results and their potential implications. N Y Acad Sci 2010;1190:15–24.

Wood IS, Trayhurn P. Glucose transporters (GLUT and SGLT): expanded families of sugar transport proteins. Br J Nutr 2003;89:3–9.

3 DIETARY FIBER[1]

HOLLY J. WILLIS AND JOANNE L. SLAVIN

WHAT IS THE DEFINITION OF FIBER?

In the 1950s, fiber was described as any nondigestible portion of a plant cell wall (1). Fast forward more than half a century, and not much has changed. In 2002, the Institute of Medicine (IOM) stated that *total fiber* is the sum of *dietary fiber* plus *functional fiber* (2). Dietary fiber consists of nondigestible carbohydrates and lignin that are intrinsic and intact in plants, whereas functional fiber consists of isolated, nondigestible carbohydrates that have beneficial physiologic effects in humans. Similar fiber definitions have been described by governments and organizations worldwide.

A globally accepted fiber definition was proposed by the Codex Alimentarius Commission (part of the Food and Agriculture Organization and the World Health Organization) in mid-2009. This definition has not yet been approved by the US Food and Drug Administration (FDA), however. Despite nuanced differences, all definitions agree that fiber is mostly carbohydrate that is not completely digested or absorbed in the small intestine but that may be fermented in the large intestine.

WHAT ARE THE CHARACTERISTICS OF FIBER?

No matter which definition one chooses to accept, many different types of fiber exist, and each is unique. In the United States, fiber must be included on the Nutrition Facts panel on food packaging, but soluble and insoluble fiber can also be specifically identified (3). These fiber values are measured by methods accepted by the Association of Official Analytical Chemists. Fiber is undeniably a complex substance, so to characterize a fiber by solubility alone would be remiss. In fact, in 2001 the IOM Fiber Panel recommended that this practice be abandoned because the solubility of fiber was not a predictor of physiologic effects. Characteristics such as viscosity and fermentability may be more important in predicting the health benefits of fiber in humans.

Viscosity is similar to solubility and is often (but not always) associated with the fiber's water-holding properties (4). Determining the viscosity of a liquid product is relatively simple, but the methods used to determine the viscosity of fiber as part of a food or diet are difficult, and the results are inconsistent among methods. For example, a particular fiber may be extremely viscous in water, but when it is baked into bread with other ingredients, the same fiber may behave quite differently. Animal studies attempted to determine intestinal content viscosity after an animal ate various fibers (5). However, it is unreasonable to extrapolate the results of viscosity at a set point in the digestive process because viscosity likely changes at different points in the digestive tract and at different times throughout the digestive process.

The fermentability of fiber is also important yet difficult to assess. Because fiber is not digested in the small intestine, it arrives in the large intestine intact and available for fermentation by the resident microflora (6). The fermentation process yields short-chain fatty acids (SCFAs), which are available for uptake by colonocytes. Fiber fermentation is believed to play a key role in colonic health. Neither in vitro nor in vivo assessments clarify

---

[1]**Abbreviations: ADA**, American Dietetic Association; **AI**, adequate intake; **CHD**, coronary heart disease; **CVD**, cardiovascular disease; **FDA**, Food and Drug Administration; **GI**, gastrointestinal; **HDL**, high-density lipoprotein; **IOM**, Institute of Medicine; **LDL**, low-density lipoprotein; **PPT**, Polyp Prevention Trial; **SCFA**, short-chain fatty acid

the way in which a specific fiber would be fermented in a specific individual, however. In vitro methods attempt to determine fermentability by inoculating various fibers with human fecal samples, but this closed, static system does not represent the dynamic and changing environment of the human colon (7). In vivo measurements of fiber fermentation are impossible to extrapolate to the in vivo situation because the large intestine of every individual is colonized with different types and amounts of microflora.

The dilemma is that viscosity and fermentability are two important characteristics of fiber, but no "gold standards" exist for measuring either property. Ultimately, this limitation makes discussions of fiber challenging and should be considered when one interprets research on fiber and health.

WHAT FOODS CONTAIN FIBER, AND HOW MUCH?

Most commonly consumed foods are low in dietary fiber (Table 3.1). In general, standard food portions only contain approximately 1 to 3 g of fiber per serving. Higher fiber contents are found in drier foods such as whole grain cereals, legumes, and dried fruits. Other fiber sources include over-the-counter laxatives containing fiber, fiber supplements, and fiber-fortified foods.

According to the FDA, the official method for reporting the calorie content of fiber is to assume that soluble fibers provide 4 kcal/g; this assumption is surprising to

some people because 4 kcal/g is the same number of calories as fully digestible carbohydrate. Also notable, insoluble fiber is reported to provide 0 kcal/g. Some insoluble fibers, however, are fermented in the large intestine and produce SCFAs. SCFAs are absorbed in the colon; therefore, the concept that insoluble fiber contributes 0 kcal/g is not always true. Assigning a caloric value to fiber is difficult, however, because each type of fiber is not fermented to the same extent across individuals. The best estimate of calories supplied by fiber fermentation is probably between 1.5 and 2.5 kcal/g of fiber (8), compared with 4 kcal/g for digestible carbohydrates.

WHAT ARE THE RECOMMENDATIONS FOR FIBER INTAKE?

The Nutrition Facts panel recommends 25 g of dietary fiber for a 2000-kcal diet. The IOM recommends an adequate intake (AI) level of 14 g of fiber per 1000 kcal of energy consumed for all people who are more than 1 year old. Based on average energy intakes across the United States, this equates to approximately 25 g/day for women and 38 g/day for men ages 19 to 50 years. The recommendation for adults older than 51 years of age is 21 g/day for women and 30 g/day for men. The recommended amount of fiber decreases for older adults because average energy intakes tend to decrease with age.

No data suggest that pregnant or lactating women would benefit from increased fiber intake. Because energy intakes increase for these two groups, however, the recommended AIs are 28 g/day for pregnant women and 29 g/day for lactating women.

In addition, given that fiber recommendations are linked to calorie recommendations, 1- to 3-year-old children have an AI for fiber of 14 g/day. This value is unrealistically high. The fiber guide of "age plus 5" is more useful. This means that a 2-year-old child would be expected to consume approximately 7 g of fiber daily (9).

HOW MUCH AND WHAT TYPE OF FIBER DO MOST PEOPLE IN THE UNITED STATES CONSUME?

Residents of the United States typically consume less than half of the recommended amounts of fiber each day (approximately 15 g/day) (8). Flours, grains, and potatoes are the most popular sources of fiber in the US diet, whereas fruits, legumes, and nuts are the sources consumed in the least quantities (10). Many food manufacturers add fiber to foods that would not normally contain fiber (this is called *functional fiber*). Whether functional fiber actually increases the amount of fiber consumed or whether these products merely become a substitute for other fiber-containing foods in the diet is unclear, however (10). The American Dietetic Association (ADA) suggests that the addition of functional fiber to foods is likely less beneficial to health than is the consumption of whole foods that are naturally high in fiber (9).

TABLE 3.1	**TOTAL DIETARY FIBER IN COMMON FOODS**	
FOOD	QUANTITY	FIBER (g)
White bread	1 slice	0.6
Whole wheat bread	1 slice	1.9
Brown rice	½ cup	1.7
White rice	½ cup	0.3
Kellogg's All Bran Original	½ cup	8.8
Kellogg's Product 19	1 cup	1.0
Kellogg's Raisin Bran	1 cup	7.3
Wheat Chex (General Mills)	1 cup	3.3
Rice Chex (General Mills)	1 cup	0.2
Oatmeal, cooked	1 cup	4.0
Apple, with skin	1 medium	3.3
Orange	1 medium	3.1
Prunes, dried	5	3.0
Raspberries	½ cup	4.0
Broccoli, raw	½ cup	1.1
Cauliflower, raw	½ cup	1.2
Sweet corn	½ cup	2.1
Iceberg lettuce, raw	½ cup	0.35
Kidney beans	½ cup	6.6
Peas	½ cup	4.4
Pinto beans	½ cup	7.7
Baked potato	1 small	2.3
Yellow squash, cooked	½ cup	1.25

Data from US Department of Agriculture, Agricultural Research Service, Nutrient Database for Standard Reference, Release 22. Washington, DC: US Department of Agriculture, 2009. Available at: http://www.ars.usda.gov/ba/bhnrc/ndl. Accessed August 1, 2010, with permission.

Meeting recommended fiber intake levels without drastically altering food choices is possible. In fact, the 2005 dietary reference intake book provides specific examples of omnivorous diets that provide adequate fiber (and other nutrients) within reasonable calorie limits (8). The US Department of Agriculture Nutrient Data Laboratory website provides a comprehensive listing of the fiber content of commonly consumed foods (11).

WHAT HAPPENS TO FIBER IN THE GASTROINTESTINAL TRACT?

In general, an average meal empties from the stomach in approximately 2 to 5 hours, clears through the small intestine in approximately 3 to 6 hours, and then resides in the colon for anywhere from 12 to 42 hours (12). Fiber may speed up or delay the process at any point throughout the digestive tract. The role of fiber in the digestive tract is specific to each fiber's unique physical and chemical properties. For example, certain viscous fibers (e.g., β-glucan) may absorb large quantities of water and form gels, which can increase gastric distension and slow gastric emptying time (13). Other fibers (e.g., wheat bran and resistant starch), however, may not influence gastric distension or emptying time (14). Regardless of the time it takes fiber to empty from the stomach, most fiber remains intact and is resistant to degradation in the stomach.

In the small intestine, certain fibers may slow the digestion and absorption of all nutrients, including digestible carbohydrates, protein, and fat (15, 16). The delayed or reduced absorption of carbohydrate explains the potential for certain fibers to blunt the glycemic response. Although many studies provided evidence that fiber-containing foods can reduce glucose or insulin levels compared with fiber-free foods (17), other studies implied that these relationships are more complex than previously believed. Several randomized controlled trials suggested that the glycemic response to fiber-containing foods likely depends on fiber viscosity, fiber dose, and food matrix (18).

The function of fiber in the large intestine depends on two key factors: the fermentability of the specific fiber and the microflora residing in an individual's large intestine. Fibers such as pectin and fructooligosaccharides are extensively fermented, whereas cellulose and wheat bran are slowly fermented or are not fermented at all (19). The degree of fermentation affects fecal bulk, such that less fermentable fibers may increase fecal bulk and contribute to a laxative effect. Fermentable fibers also have the potential to create fecal bulk, but this effect does not stem from the fiber itself. Instead, fermentable fibers may lead to an increase in bacterial mass, which can attract water and increase stool size.

WHAT ARE THE HEALTH BENEFITS OF FIBER?

Summarizing the conclusions of fiber and health research is difficult because it is often impossible to determine whether health outcomes are a result of consuming fiber itself or a result of changes in nutrient density and nutrient intake that occur when fiber is present in a food. Specifically, high-fiber diets often increase the intake of biologically active compounds such as phytochemicals and antioxidants that are not present in lower-fiber diets. That said, many epidemiologic and intervention studies do suggest that regular fiber intake is associated with various beneficial health outcomes. These benefits, however, largely depend on the type of fiber consumed, as well as on the individual person.

Cardiovascular Disease

The AI level of 14 g of fiber per 1000 kcal of energy consumed, established by the IOM, is based on protection against cardiovascular disease (CVD). Thus, the data for this relationship are strong. Epidemiologic studies suggest that adequate fiber intake consistently lowers the risk of CVD and coronary heart disease (CHD) primarily through a reduction in low-density lipoprotein (LDL) levels. For example, one review reported that the prevalence of CHD was 29% lower in individuals in the highest quintile of dietary fiber intake compared with those in the lowest quintile (20).

Although the epidemiology literature is convincing, this type of data cannot be used to imply cause and effect. The results of randomized clinical trials are inconsistent, but they seem to suggest that fiber may play a beneficial role in reducing C-reactive protein levels, apolipoprotein levels, and blood pressure—all of which are biomarkers for heart disease. One review of well-controlled intervention studies found that water-soluble fibers (specifically, β-glucan, psyllium, pectin, and guar gum) were most effective for lowering serum LDL cholesterol concentrations without affecting high-density lipoprotein (HDL) concentrations (21). In the United States, health claims for the ability of oats, barley, and psyllium to lower blood lipid concentrations are accepted (9).

Although it would be helpful to identify the most beneficial types and doses of fiber needed to prevent CVD, this type of data is not available. Table 3.2 summarizes various types and doses of fiber that have been shown to reduce LDL cholesterol concentrations (20), however.

Type 2 Diabetes and Glycemic Control

Many theories of the relationship between fiber intake and type 2 diabetes have been proposed. For example, regular consumption of the recommended amount of fiber has the potential to attenuate glucose absorption rate, prevent weight gain, and increase the load of beneficial nutrients and antioxidants in the diet, all of which may help to prevent diabetes (9).

Numerous large-scale cohort studies supported a strong inverse relationship between fiber consumption and the development of type 2 diabetes. In a multiethnic cohort study, which followed 75,000 people for 14 years, people

TABLE 3.2	EFFECTS OF SOLUBLE FIBER INTAKE ON SERUM LOW-DENSITY LIPOPROTEIN CHOLESTEROL VALUES			
TYPE OF FIBER	NO. OF TRIALS	NO. OF SUBJECTS	AVERAGE GRAMS OF ADDED FIBER PER DAY	CHANGES IN LDL (REPORTED AS TREATMENT CHANGE MINUS PLACEBO CHANGE)
Pectin	5	71	15	−13.0
Barley β-glucan	9	129	5	−11.1
Guar gum	4	79	15	−10.6
Hydroxypropyl methylcellulose	2	59	5	−8.5
Psyllium	9	494	6	−5.5

LDL, low-density lipoprotein.

Adapted from Anderson JW, Baird P, Davis RH Jr et al. Health benefits of dietary fiber. Nutr Rev 2009;67:188–205.

who ate more than 15 g/day of fiber had a significantly lower diabetes risk (22). Specifically, high cereal-fiber intake reduced diabetes risk by 10% in men and women, whereas high vegetable-fiber intake reduced risk by 22% in men, but not in women. In another study, people who ate high amounts of insoluble fiber (more than 17 g/day) or cereal fiber (more than 8 g/day) had a lower risk of developing type 2 diabetes than did people who had lower fiber intakes (23). In the same study, soluble fiber intake was not associated with diabetes risk.

It would take many years (and be too costly) for an intervention study to assess the impact of a long-term, controlled-fiber diet on diabetes development. Thus, the most common way to assess this relationship is through interventions that evaluate glycemic response after fiber intake. Intervention studies provide inconsistent results. For instance, compared with a 5-week control diet, 5 weeks of oat β-glucan (5 g) significantly reduced postprandial glucose and insulin responses, whereas 5 weeks of barley β-glucan (5 or 10 g) did not (24). Many acute intervention trials have failed to find a relationship between fiber intake and postprandial glucose response (25–27).

Nonetheless, the ADA stated that serum glucose levels are generally lower when diets provide 30 to 50 g/day of fiber from whole food sources, as compared with low-fiber diets (9). The ADA also suggested that fiber supplements providing an additional 10 to 29 g/day of fiber may have some benefits in terms of glycemic control.

Appetite Control

Fiber intake and satiety are related, but different fibers are more likely to alter satiety (28–31). The relationship probably depends on many factors, including the type of fiber consumed (soluble, insoluble, viscous, or fermentable), the dose of fiber (1 g versus 25 g), the individual person (man, woman, obese, lean, young, old), and the duration of fiber intake (one dose at lunch or daily consumption for years).

Multiple mechanisms have been used to describe how fiber influences satiation and satiety. Greater satiation may be a product of the increased time required to chew certain fiber-rich foods (29, 30). Increased time chewing promotes saliva and gastric acid production, which may increase gastric distension. Some soluble or viscous fibers bind water, and this also may increase distension. Stomach distension is believed to trigger afferent vagal signals of fullness, which likely contribute to satiation during meals and satiety in the postmeal period (32). Furthermore, certain fibers may slow gastric emptying and decrease the rate of glucose absorption in the small intestine. When glucose is released slowly, the insulin response may also be blunted. Slow, steady postprandial glucose and insulin responses are sometimes correlated with satiation and satiety, although not always (33).

As food moves through the upper and lower gastrointestinal (GI) tract, various satiety-related hormones are released, and signals are sent to the brain (see also the chapter on control of food intake and appetite). Many of these gut hormones (i.e., ghrelin, polypeptide YY, glucagon-like peptide) are thought to regulate satiety, food intake, and overall energy balance (34).

The ileal brake may also influence satiety. This inhibitory feedback mechanism controls transit of a meal through the GI tract (35). As food is pushed out of the stomach by contraction and into the small intestine, distal messengers dictate how quickly food will traverse the digestive tract. By controlling the speed and movement of an ingested food, nutrient digestion and absorption are optimized. The types and amounts of nutrients consumed influence ileal brake action; the role of fiber in ileal brake activation is not clear, however (36). Finally, certain types of fiber are largely fermentable in the colon. The fermentation process has been described as a potential satiety modifier (37–39).

Fiber and satiety intervention studies provided conflicting results. It is clear that not all fibers are equal when it comes to satiety. Viscous fibers, such as oat bran and psyllium, may be more effective, although insoluble fibers that survive gut transit, such as wheat bran and cellulose, may also positively alter satiety. In addition, fibers from whole foods may increase satiety more than processed or isolated fibers from the same food (40, 41).

Body Weight

In 1973, Heaton described how fiber intake may reduce energy intake, which theoretically could lead to weight loss (42). Today, prospective cohort studies consistently report that people who consume higher amounts of fiber weigh less than people who consume lesser amounts (43). In fact, one study reported that in a 20-month period, every 1-g increase in total fiber consumed per day decreased body weight by 0.25 kg (44).

In most large-scale research, fiber intake usually covaries with other beneficial lifestyle factors, such as fruit and vegetable intake and exercise habits. Moreover, diets that are high in fiber are typically lower in fat and energy density, both of which are helpful for maintaining a healthy body weight. This factor is important to consider because merely adding fiber supplements to the diet may not yield the same results.

When considering the clinical data, Howarth et al. (29) summarized the results of more than 50 intervention studies that assessed relationships among energy intake, body weight, and fiber intake. These investigators estimated that increasing fiber intake by 14 g/day was associated with a 10% decrease in energy intake and a 2-kg weight loss over approximately 4 months. The observed changes in energy intake and body weight occurred without regard to the fiber's source as a naturally high-fiber food or a functional fiber supplement.

Cancer

Colon Cancer

In the 1970s, many reports suggested that the increased prevalence of colorectal cancer was a result of low-fiber diets (45). These assumptions were predominantly based on differences in colorectal cancer rates among nations and regions with high- and low-fiber intakes; this type of data clearly lacks causal evidence.

Since 2005, the results of several large-scale studies, including some intervention trials, have suggested that fiber intake is not associated with an overall risk for colorectal cancer (46–48). For example, the 8-year Polyp Prevention Trial (PPT) evaluated the effects of a high-fiber (18 g/1000 kcal), high-fruit and high-vegetable, and low-fat diet on the recurrence of adenomatous polyps in the colon (49). This study failed to show an effect of diet on adenoma recurrence after 8 years of follow-up. Possibly, recurrent adenomas were not an appropriate marker for colon cancer development. This study is the largest and most comprehensive intervention trial to date, however. The lack of relationship between high-fiber diet interventions and colorectal cancer risk may be authentic, or it may reflect the long latency period for colorectal cancer development. Poor adherence to dietary interventions among study participants may also have diluted the strength of this relationship. When the PPT "supercompliers" (study participants who reported exceeding all dietary goals over a 4-year period) were put into subgroup analysis, researchers found a 35% reduction in colorectal adenoma recurrence compared with controls (50). These supercompliers, however, also had a collection of statistically different lifestyle factors.

Thus, whether fiber intake is protective against colorectal cancer remains unclear. However, novel study designs hope to reveal better options for understanding colonic changes during colon cancer development and specifically how these changes may relate to fiber intake (51).

Breast Cancer

Reproductive factors and body fatness can affect estrogen, progesterone, and insulin levels; each of these values has been identified as a potential risk factor for breast cancer development. Fiber intake has been hypothesized to lower the risk of breast cancer development specifically by modulating hormonal metabolism. This hypothesis is largely based on research showing that vegetarian women excrete more fecal estrogens and have decreased estrogen concentrations in plasma compared with women who consume animal protein (52). Many prospective cohort studies have failed to find an association between fiber intake and breast cancer risk in women, however (53, 54).

Conversely, a more recent study reported that postmenopausal women who consumed more than 26 g/day of fiber had a 13% lower risk of breast cancer than did women who consumed less than 11 g/day of fiber (55). The risk reduction was stronger for lobular tumors than for ductal tumors and for estrogen and progesterone receptor–negative tumors than for estrogen and progesterone receptor–positive tumors. Fiber from grains, fruit, vegetables, and beans was not related to breast cancer risk, whereas soluble (but not insoluble) fiber intake was inversely associated with breast cancer risk. This finding confirms that breast cancer is a complex disease and that dietary factors, such as fiber intake, probably do not play a consistent role across specific subtypes of cancer or menopausal status.

Immunity

Some evidence suggests improved immune function with fiber intake. The mechanism of action often involves the presence or absence of certain gut microflora. Probiotics and prebiotics are often used in discussions of fiber and immune function. Probiotics are live microorganisms that, when consumed, survive transit through the GI tract and benefit the host (56). Prebiotics are the nondigestible food ingredients that stimulate the growth or activity of beneficial bacteria in the colon (56) (see also the chapter on prebiotics and probiotics). Probiotics are commonly added to foods and products that contain fiber, whereas prebiotics are often a type of fiber (i.e., fructooligosaccharides). Research on the potential health benefits of probiotics and prebiotics has been ongoing for many years, although research studies of the effects of these substances on the immune system and inflammatory processes are sparse. The effects of probiotics on immune function, infection, and inflammation were reviewed in 2009 (57). Overall, the data suggested that the relationships depend largely on the type of species and strains evaluated. *Lactobacillus* and *Bifidobacterium* are the two species most likely to be studied and deemed beneficial for various conditions. A similar review was also conducted on prebiotics (58). The results of human trials are mixed. Ten prebiotics trials involving infants and children reported beneficial effects on infectious outcomes, whereas 15 adult trials showed little effect.

Laxation and Constipation

A review of nearly 100 studies evaluated the effect of fiber intake on bowel habits (59). The review suggested that all sources of fiber may lead to an increase in fecal output. Not all fibers contributed equally, however. For example, pectin (the type of fiber found in the flesh of fruits such as apples) increased stool weight only by 1.3 g/g of fiber consumed, whereas wheat bran increased stool weight by 5.7 g/g of fiber consumed. The explanation of these stool weight differences is largely based on the distinctive properties of each fiber. Contributors to stool size are as follows: certain fibers may hold more water than others, some fibers may be less susceptible to degradation throughout the digestive tract, and fermentable fibers may increase bacterial mass. In general, larger stools are associated with more rapid transit through the colon and thus less constipation (60).

IF FIBER IS BENEFICIAL FOR HEALTH, IS IT HARMFUL TO EAT TOO MUCH?

Although a tolerable upper intake level (UL) for fiber intake has not been established, certain types of fiber may cause gas, bloating, abdominal discomfort, or undesirable changes in bowel movements. However, these effects are merely "symptoms" of fiber consumption and are not an indication of fiber toxicity. Tolerance varies widely among individuals. For example, in a study in which subjects consumed 10 g of inulin, some subjects described no effects, whereas others reported multiple symptoms continuously for 48 hours; this finding confirmed the wide range in individual tolerance (61).

Moreover, some research suggests that diets high in fiber are significantly associated with decreased hormone concentrations and a higher probability of anovulation (62). High-fiber diets are also a concern because of links to decreased absorption of minerals including calcium, iron, and zinc (9). For Western populations consuming a typical low-fiber diet, however, decreased mineral absorption is not a clinical problem. Additionally, research suggests that certain fibers (e.g., inulin) may actually enhance calcium absorption in certain populations (63).

REFERENCES

1. Hipsley EH. Br Med J 1953;2:420–2.
2. Food and Nutrition Board, Institute of Medicine. Dietary Reference Intakes. Dietary, Functional, and Total Fiber. Washington, DC: National Academy Press, 2002.
3. Jones JR, Lineback DM, Levine MJ. Nutr Rev 2006;64:31–8.
4. Dikeman CL, Fahey GC. Crit Rev Food Sci Nutr 2006;46: 649–63.
5. Gallaher DD, Wood KJ, Gallaher CM et al. Cereal Chem 1999; 76:21–24.
6. Barry JL, Hoebler C, Macfarlane GT et al. Br J Nutr 1995;74: 303–22.
7. Rose DJ, DeMeo MT, Keshavarzian A et al. Nutr Rev 2007;65: 51–62.
8. Food and Nutrition Board, Institute of Medicine. Dietary Reference Intakes for Energy, Carbohydrate, Fiber, Fat, Fatty Acids, Cholesterol, Protein, and Amino Acids. Washington, DC: National Academy Press, 2005.
9. Slavin JL. J Am Diet Assoc 2008;108:1716–31.
10. US Department of Agriculture, Center for Nutrition Policy and Promotion. Trends in Dietary Fiber in the US Food Supply: Sales of Grain Products. Alexandria, VA: US Department of Agriculture Center for Nutrition Policy and Promotion, 2007.
11. US Department of Agriculture, Agricultural Research Service, Nutrient Database for Standard Reference, Release 22. Washington, DC: US Department of Agriculture, 2009. Available at: http://www.ars.usda.gov/ba/bhnrc/ndl. Accessed August 1, 2010.
12. Maqbool S, Parkman HP, Friedenberg FK. Dig Dis Sci 2009; 54:2167–74.
13. Juvonen KR, Purhonen AK, Salmenkallio-Marttila M et al. J Nutr 2009;139:461–6.
14. De Peter V, Cloetens L, Rutgeerts P et al. Scand J Gastroenterol 2007;42:1187–93.
15. Ganji V, Kies CV. Eur J Clin Nutr 1994;48:595–7.
16. Aman P, Pettersson D, Zhang JX et al. J Nutr 1995;125:2341–7.
17. Juvonen KR, Salmenkallio-Marttila M, Lyly M et al. Nutr Metab Cardiovasc Dis. 2011;21(9):748–56.
18. Brand-Miller JC, Stockmann K, Atkinson F et al. Am J Clin Nutr 2009;89:97–105.
19. Klosterbuer A, Roughead ZF, Slavin JL. Nutr Clin Pract 2011;26(5):625–35.
20. Anderson JW, Baird P, Davis RH Jr et al. Nutr Rev 2009;67: 188–205.
21. Theuwissen E, Mensink RP. Physiol Behav 2008;94:285–92.
22. Hopping BN, Erber E, Grandinetti A et al. J Nutr 2010;140: 68–74.
23. Meyer KA, Kushi LH, Jacobs DR et al. Am J Clin Nutr 2000; 71:921–30.
24. Biorklund M, van Rees A, Mensink RP et al. Eur J Clin Nutr 2005;59:1272–81.
25. Kim H, Stote KS, Behall KM et al. Eur J Nutr 2009;48:170–5.
26. Hlebowicz J, Wickenberg J, Fahlstrom R et al. Nutr J 2007;6:22.
27. Mathern JR, Raatz SK, Thomas W et al. Phytother Res 2009; 23:1543–8.
28. Slavin J, Green H. 2007;32:32–42.
29. Howarth NC, Saltzman E, Roberts SB. Nutr Rev 2001;59: 129–39.
30. Burton-Freeman B. J Nutr 2000;130:272S–5S.
31. Willis HJ, Eldridge AL, Beiseigel J et al. Nutr Res 2009; 29:100–5.
32. de Graaf C, Blom WA, Smeets PA et al. Am J Clin Nutr 2004; 79:946–61.
33. Flint A, Gregersen NT, Gluud LL et al. Br J Nutr 2007; 98:17–25.
34. Chaudhri OB, Salem V, Murphy KG et al. Annu Rev Physiol 2008;70:239–55.

35. Van Citters GW, Lin HC. Curr Gastroenterol Rep 1999;1: 404–9.

36. Van Citters GW, Lin HC. Curr Gastroenterol Rep 2006;8: 367–73.

37. Wong JM, de Souza R, Kendall CW et al. J Clin Gastroenterol 2006;40:235–43.

38. Nilsson AC, Ostman EM, Holst JJ et al. J Nutr 2008;138: 732–9.

39. Zhou J, Martin RJ, Tulley RT et al. Am J Physiol Endocrinol Metab 2008;295:E1160–6.

40. Flood-Obbagy JE, Rolls BJ. Appetite 2009;52:416–22.

41. Anne Moorhead S, Welch RW, Barbara M et al. Br J Nutr 2006;96:587–95.

42. Heaton KW. Lancet 1973;2:1418–21.

43. Maskarinec G, Takata Y, Pagano I et al. Obesity 2006;14: 717–26.

44. Tucker LA, Thomas KS. J Nutr 2009;139:576–81.

45. Walker AR. Am J Clin Nutr 1976;29:1417–26.

46. Uchida K, Kono S, Yin G et al. Scand J Gastroenterol 2010; 45:1223–31.

47. Schatzkin A, Mouw T, Park Y et al. Am J Clin Nutr 2007; 85:1353–60.

48. Michels KB, Fuchs CS, Giovannucci E et al. Cancer Epidemiol Biomarkers Prev 2005;14:842–9.

49. Lanza E, Yu B, Murphy G et al. Cancer Epidemiol Biomarkers Prev 2007;16:1745–52.

50. Sansbury LB, Wanke K, Albert PS et al. Am J Epidemiol 2009; 170:576–84.

51. Corfe BM, Williams EA, Bury JP et al. BMC Cancer 2009; 9:332.

52. Goldin BR, Adlercreutz H, Gorbach SL et al. N Engl J Med 1982;307:1542–7.

53. Lajous M, Boutron-Ruault MC, Fabre A et al. Am J Clin Nutr 2008;87:1384–91.

54. Cade JE, Burley VJ, Greenwood DC et al. Int J Epidemiol 2007;36:431–8.

55. Park Y, Brinton LA, Subar AF et al. Am J Clin Nutr 2009;90: 664–71.

56. Douglas LC, Sanders ME. J Am Diet Assoc 2008;108: 510–21.

57. Lomax AR, Calder PC. Curr Pharm Des 2009;15:1428–518.

58. Lomax AR, Calder PC. Br J Nutr 2009;101:633–58.

59. Cummings JH. The effect of dietary fiber on fecal weight and composition. In: CRC Handbook of Dietary Fiber in Human Nutrition. 3rd ed. Boca Raton, FL: CRC Press, 2001.

60. Birkett AM, Jones GP, de Silva AM et al. Eur J Clin Nutr 1997; 51:625–32.

61. Bonnema AL, Kolberg LW, Thomas W et al. J Am Diet Assoc 2010;110:865–8.

62. Gaskins AJ, Mumford SL, Zhang C et al. Am J Clin Nutr 2009; 90:1061–9.

63. Holloway L, Moynihan S, Abrams SA et al. Br J Nutr 2007; 97:365–72.

SUGGESTED READINGS

Food and Nutrition Board, Institute of Medicine. Dietary Reference Intakes for Energy, Carbohydrate, Fiber, Fat, Fatty Acids, Cholesterol, Protein, and Amino Acids. Washington, DC: National Academy Press, 2005.

Gray J. Dietary Fibre: Definition, Analysis, Recommendations, and Health Benefits. Brussels: ILSI Europe, 2006.

Slavin JL. Position of the American Dietetic Association: health implications of dietary fiber. J Am Diet Assoc 2008;108:1716–31.

Intestinal Digestion

Intestinal digestion requires bile salts (BSs) and pancreatic lipase. BSs, PLs, and sterols are the three principal lipid components of bile—the emulsifying fluid produced by the liver. Primary BSs, defined as those synthesized directly from hepatic CH, include the trihydroxy and dihydroxy BSs, namely cholate and chenodeoxycholate, respectively. Secondary BSs, including deoxycholate and lithocholate, are produced from primary BSs via bacterial conversion on cholate and chenodeoxycholate in the large intestine.

Pancreatic lipase, the principal enzyme of TG digestion, acts to hydrolyze ester bonds at sn-1 and sn-3 positions (Fig. 4.2). BSs inhibit lipase activity through displacement of the enzyme from its substrate at the surface of the lipid droplet. Colipase, also a pancreatic protein, reverses BS inhibition on pancreatic lipase by binding lipase and ensuring its adhesion to the lipid droplet. Then, through its affinity to BSs, PLs, and CH, colipase facilitates shuttling of hydrolysis products monoglycerides (MGs) and free FAs from the lipid droplet into the BS-containing micelle. FAs linked at the sn-2 position of MGs, PLs, and cholesteryl ester (CE) are resistant to hydrolysis by lipase. The action of pancreatic lipase is extremely rapid, and MGs and free FAs are produced faster than their subsequent incorporation into micelles (15).

Micellar solubilization of the products of fat hydrolysis results from the amphipathic actions of BSs and PLs, which are secreted in bile at a ratio of approximately 1:3. CH is present in bile only in the unesterified form, which is the major sterol form (16). The polar terminus of BSs orients itself toward the water milieu of the chyme, whereas the nonpolar ends containing hydrocarbon groups face the center of the micelle. BSs and PLs naturally aggregate such that the nonpolar termini form a hydrophobic core. The incorporation of MGs into the micelle increases the ability of the particle to solubilize free FAs and CH. BS micelles generally possess the highest affinity for MGs and unsaturated long-chain FAs (LCFAs) (17). Both diglycerides (DGs) and TGs have limited incorporation into micelles. On formation, mixed micelles containing FAs, MGs, CH, PLs, and BSs migrate to the unstirred water layer adjacent to the surface of the enterocyte brush-border membrane.

Absorption

The process of lipid absorption appears to occur in large part through passive diffusion. Micelles containing fat digestion products exist in dynamic equilibrium with each other; the peristaltic, churning action of the intestine maintains a high frequency of intermicellar contact. This contact results in partitioning of constituents from more highly populated micelles to less populated micelles, with consequent equalization of the overall micellar concentration of digestion products. Thus, during digestion of a bolus of fat, micelles evenly accrue digestion products. The 2-MGs and free FAs are released through the action of pancreatic lipase until the saturation capacity of the micelles is reached.

The penetration of micelles across the unstirred water layer bordering the intestinal mucosal cells represents the first stage of absorption. Micelles, but not lipid droplets,

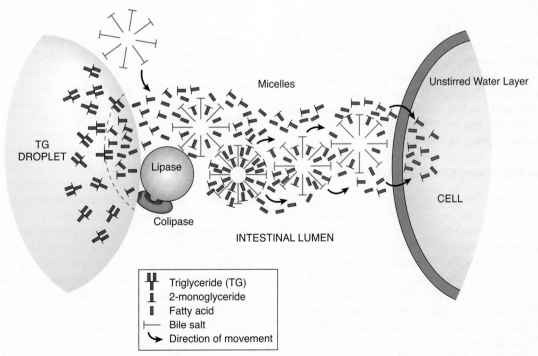

Fig. 4.2. Transport hypothesis of fatty acids and 2-monoglycerides through lipase-mediated hydrolysis, micellar transfer, and cellular uptake stages.

approach and enter this water layer selectively for two reasons: first, micelles are much smaller (30 to 100 Å) particles than emulsified droplets of fat (25,000 + 20,000 Å); and second, the hydrophobic nature of the larger lipid droplet results in reduced solubilization at the site of the unstirred water layer.

Transport of micellar products across the unstirred water layer into the enterocyte occurs as illustrated in Figure 4.2. The digestion products shuttle from the micelles across the unstirred water layer and create a chain reaction effect. This action hinges on the lower cellular concentration of digestion products at the enterocyte. Intestinal FA-binding proteins (FABPs) assist in transmucosal shunting of digestion product FAs, and possibly MGs and BSs. Elevated FABP activity in the distal bowel has been shown to be associated with higher FA absorption (18).

The overall efficiency of fat absorption in human adults is approximately 95%. However, the qualitative nature of the dietary fat influences overall efficiency (19). Evidence also suggests that as FA chain length increases, absorption efficiency decreases. Similarly, the positional distribution of FAs on dietary TGs is an important determinant of the eventual efficiency of absorption. When octanoate, palmitate, or linoleate were substituted at different sn positions on a TG molecule, the positional distribution altered characteristics of digestion, absorption, and lymphatic transport of these two FAs (20, 21). The natural tendency of C16:0 to be present in the sn-2 position in breast milk may therefore explain the high digestibility of this milk fat. FAs with chain lengths less than 12 carbon atoms are also absorbed passively by the gastric mucosal boundary and taken up by the portal vein (22).

Micellar BSs are not absorbed with fat digestion products, but rather are taken up further along the gastrointestinal tract. Passive intestinal absorption of unconjugated BSs occurs throughout the small intestine and colon. Active transport components predominate in the ileum and include the brush-border membrane receptor, cytosolic bile acid binding proteins, and basolateral anion exchange proteins. The enterohepatic recirculation of BSs is approximately 98% efficient (23).

Digestion and Absorption of Phospholipids

Dietary PLs comprise only a small portion of ingested lipid; however, PLs are secreted in large quantities in bile. PLs assist in emulsification of TG droplets, as well as in micellar solubilization of CH. In particular, phosphatidylcholine (PC) is also essential in the stabilization of the micelle within the unstirred water layer. PLs of both dietary and biliary origins are digested through cleavage by phospholipase A_2, a pancreatic enzyme secreted in bile. In contrast to pancreatic lipase, phospholipase A_2 cleaves FAs at the sn-2 position of PLs, thus yielding lysophosphoglycerides and free FAs. These products undergo absorption through a similar process, as described earlier.

Digestion and Absorption of Sterols

CH within the intestine originates from both diet and bile. The amount of CH in the diet varies markedly depending on the degree of inclusion of foods from nonplant sources, whereas biliary CH secretion is more consistent. Dietary CH and biliary CH differ in several ways. Biliary CH is also absorbed at a site more proximal than diet-derived CH within the small intestine.

Being hydrophobic, CH requires a specialized system for digestion and absorption to occur within a water-soluble environment. Notably, absorption efficiency for CH is much less than for TG, and the major rate-limiting factor is the poor micellar solubility of CH. Using various methodologies, investigators have demonstrated that only 40% to 65% of CH is absorbed over the physiologic range of CH intakes in humans (24). The digestion of dietary CE involves release of the esterified FAs through the action of a BS-dependent CE hydrolase secreted by the pancreas. Removal of esterified FAs does not appear to be rate limiting, because mixtures of free and esterified CH are absorbed with equal efficiency in rats (25). Free sterol then undergoes solubilization within mixed micelles in the upper small intestine. It is now recognized that the uptake of dietary and endogenous CH into intestinal enterocytes is tightly controlled by apical membrane-bound proteins that serve as gatekeepers of intestinal CH absorption. Niemann-Pick-C1–like 1 (NPC1L1) was characterized in an attempt to identify proteins involved in intracellular CH trafficking (26). Shortly thereafter, NPC1L1 was singled out as the putative intestinal CH transporter using a genomics-bioinformatics approach that identified possible transporter candidates based on anticipated structural characteristics including a transmembrane sequence and a sterol sensing domain (27).

Alternatively, adenosine triphosphate (ATP)–binding cassette transporters ABCG5 and ABCG8 exist as CH efflux proteins on the apical surface of the intestinal enterocyte. Mutations in intestinal ABCG5 and ABCG8 cause sitosterolemia, a rare inherited disease characterized by the hyperabsorption of plant sterols and premature atherosclerosis (28). Studies have greatly advanced our knowledge of the structure and function of these genes and have demonstrated that ABCG5 and ABCG8 have the following characteristics: (a) each contains 13 exons organized in head-to-head conformation and separated by a small (<160 bases) intergenic region; (b) these are half-transporters that must heterodimerize in the endoplasmic reticulum (ER) to become a functional export pump; (c) they are expressed on the apical surface of intestinal enterocytes and the canalicular membrane of hepatocytes; and (d) they function in the efflux of neutral sterols from the enterocyte into the intestinal lumen and to promote biliary secretion of neutral sterols from the liver (27).

The amount of CH in circulatory lipoproteins appears to be marginally responsive to the amount of dietary CH within the normal, physiologic range. Likely, compensatory

TABLE 4.3	PHYSICAL–CHEMICAL CHARACTERISTICS OF THE MAJOR LIPOPROTEIN CLASSES					
LIPOPROTEIN	DENSITY (g/dL)	MOLECULAR MASS (DALTONS)	DIAMETER (nm)	LIPID (%)[a]		
				TRIGLYCERIDE	CHOLESTEROL	PHOSPHOLIPID
Chylomicrons	0.95	1400×10^6	75–1200	80–95	2–7	3–9
VLDL	0.95–1.006	$10–80 \times 10^6$	30–80	55–80	5–15	10–20
IDL	1.006–1.019	$5–10 \times 10^6$	25–35	20–50	20–40	15–25
LDL	1.019–1.063	2.3×10^6	18–25	5–15	40–50	20–25
HDL	1.063–1.21	$1.7–3.6 \times 10^5$	5–12	5–10	15–25	20–30

HDL, high-density lipoprotein; IDL, intermediate-density lipoprotein; LDL, low-density lipoprotein; VLDL, very-low-density lipoprotein.

[a]Percentage composition of lipids; apolipoproteins make up the rest.

Reprinted with permission from WB Saunders from Ginsberg HN. Lipoprotein metabolism and its relationship to atherosclerosis. Med Clin North Am 1994;78:1–20.

changes in CH absorption and biosynthesis serve to protect circulatory CH levels from shifting greatly in response to changes in dietary intake (29). In contrast to CH, plant sterol absorption is very limited and differs across dietary phytosterols. For the major plant sterol β-sitosterol, typical absorption efficiency is 4% to 5%, approximately one tenth that of CH. Absorption efficiency is higher for campesterol; approximately 10%, and almost nonexistent for sitostanol (30, 31). This structure-specific discrimination depends on both the number of carbon atoms at the C24 side-chain position and the degree of hydrogenation of the sterol nucleus. Differences in absorption across phytosterols are reflected in their circulating concentrations. Plasma campesterol levels are usually higher than those of sitosterol, whereas highly saturated sitostanol is almost undetectable (14).

Reasons for the low absorption efficiency of phytosterols are twofold. First, apical ABCG5 and ABCG8 transporters possess high affinity for phytosterols and preferentially excrete them back into the intestinal lumen. Second, inadequate esterification of phytosterols may occur within enterocyte membranes. Acyl coenzyme A (CoA):CH acyltransferase (ACAT)–dependent esterification of CH exceeds that of β-sitosterol (32).

Dietary phytosterols appear to compete with each other and with CH for absorption. Sitosterol consumption results in reduced absorption of CH, and that, in turn, lowers circulating CH levels. Addition of sitostanol to diets causes a depression in circulating levels of both CH and unsaturated plant sterols (11) apparently through a reduction in intestinal absorption of both types of sterols. Saturated and unsaturated plant sterols and their esters are useful in lowering serum total lipoprotein and low-density lipoprotein (LDL) CH levels (32).

TRANSPORT AND METABOLISM

Solubility of Lipids

Transport of largely hydrophobic lipids through the circulation is achieved in large part using aggregates of lipids and protein called lipoproteins. Principal lipid components of lipoproteins are TGs, CH, CE, and PLs. Protein constituents termed *apolipoproteins*, or *apoproteins*, serve to increase both particle solubility and recognition by enzymes and receptors located at the outer surface of lipoproteins. The major lipoprotein classes are listed in Table 4.3. Lipoproteins differ in composition; however, all types feature hydrophilic apolipoproteins, PL polar headgroups, and CH hydroxyl groups facing outward at the water interface, with PL acyl tails and CH steroid nuclei oriented toward the interior of the lipoprotein particle. Hydrophobic CE and TG molecules form the core of the lipoprotein particle. In this manner, hydrophobic lipids can be internally solubilized and transported within the aqueous media of lymph, plasma, and extracellular fluids. Although lipoproteins discussed here and in later chapters are characterized into subclasses, they represent a continuous spectrum of lipoprotein particles varying in size, density, composition, and function. Internal transport of lipids can be divided into exogenous and endogenous systems that reflect lipids of dietary and internal origins, respectively.

Exogenous Transport System

The exogenous transport system transfers lipids of intestinal origin to peripheral and hepatic tissues (Fig. 4.3). The exogenous system commences with reorganization in the enterocyte of absorbed FAs, 2-MGs, lysophospholipids, PLs, smaller amounts of glycerol, and CH into chylomicrons. Chylomicron TGs are reassembled predominantly using the monoacylglycerol pathway. Absorbed FAs are activated by microsomal FA-CoA synthase to yield acyl-CoA and are then combined sequentially with 2-MGs through the action of MG and DG acyltransferases.

Chylomicron assembly within the intestinal enterocyte is tightly regulated by the production of apolipoprotein-B (Apo-B) and the activity of microsomal TG transfer protein (MTP), which transfers lipids onto nascent Apo-B particles (33). Furthermore, the synthesis of new lipid appears to be a driving force in assembly and secretion of lipoproteins. Uptake of dietary LCFAs, incorporation into TGs by the glycerol-3-phosphate pathway, and assembly of lipoproteins all require FABP (34).

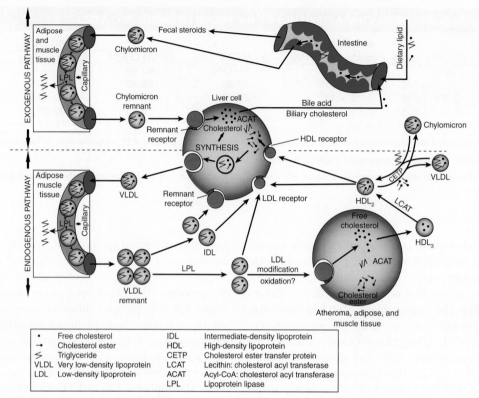

Fig. 4.3. Exogenous and endogenous pathways of lipid transport.

Not all FAs must be incorporated into chylomicrons for transport. FAs less than 14 carbons in length and those containing several double bonds undergo, to a variable degree, direct internal transport via the portal circulation that may be either as lipoprotein-bound TGs or as albumin-bound free (unesterified) FAs. Portal transfer results in more immediate delivery of FAs to the liver compared with chylomicron transit. Chylomicrons released from mucosal cells circulate first through the intestinal lymphatic system and the thoracic duct and then enter the superior vena cava. Release into the circulation is followed by TG hydrolysis at the capillary surface of tissues by lipoprotein lipase (LPL). Hydrolysis of TGs within the core of the chylomicron results in movement of FAs into tissues and subsequent production of TG-depleted chylomicron remnant particles. Chylomicron remnants then pick up CE from high-density lipoproteins (HDLs) and are rapidly taken up by liver.

Endogenous Transport System

The endogenous shuttle for lipids and their metabolites consists of three interrelated components. The first, involving very-low-density lipoproteins (VLDLs), intermediate-density lipoproteins (IDLs), and LDLs, coordinates movement of lipids from liver to peripheral tissues. The second, involving HDLs, encompasses a series of events that returns CH from peripheral tissues to liver, termed *reverse CH transport*. The third component of the system, not involving lipoproteins, affects the free

FA-mediated transfer of lipids from storage reservoirs to metabolizing organs.

Components of the endogenous lipoprotein system are illustrated in Figure 4.3. The system begins with assembly of VLDL particles, mostly in the liver but to a lesser extent in the small intestine. Assembly of nascent hepatic VLDL starts in the ER and depends on the presence of adequate core lipids, CE, and TGs. Using stable isotope tracers, investigators have estimated that the majority of TG FA within VLDL is preformed (35, 36). Addition of surface lipids, mainly PLs and free CH, occurs in the Golgi apparatus before the particle is secreted.

Following secretion of VLDL particles into the circulation, certain interchanges with tissues and lipoproteins occur. A major event is deposition of lipids into peripheral tissues. Hydrolysis of VLDL TGs occurs through the action of LPL, an enzyme located on the endothelial side of vessel tissue that mediates hydrolysis of chylomicron TGs. Lipase-generated free FAs can be used as energy sources, as a structural component for lipids including PLs, leukotrienes (LTs), and thromboxanes (TXAs), or converted back to TGs and stored. TGs and PLs from both chylomicron remnants and LDL also undergo hydrolysis by the enzyme hepatic lipase. When hepatic lipase is absent, accumulation of large LDL particles and TG-rich lipoproteins (TRLs) occurs. Through TG depletion, the VLDL particle is converted to a denser, smaller CH and TRL remnant, structurally analogous to the chylomicron remnant. High circulatory levels of TRL remnants are associated with progression of coronary artery disease. TRL remnants themselves can be cleared from plasma through hepatic lipoprotein receptors or converted to smaller LDLs. LDL is the major CH-carrying lipoprotein. Although LDL levels are associated with heart disease risk in general, evidence suggests that a predominance of smaller, denser LDL particles in the circulation confers an elevated risk of coronary heart disease (37). The classically defined LDL receptor allows for the efficient hepatic uptake and catabolism of LDL (38). Modified or oxidized LDL can also be taken up by a scavenger receptor on macrophages in various tissues, including the arterial wall.

The second component of the endogenous transport system, often termed reverse CH transport, involves movement of CH from peripheral tissues to the liver. Since 1975, when Miller and Miller (39) described the protective effect of HDL on atherosclerosis, much work has been undertaken to understand the structure and function of HDL more clearly. HDL particles are highly heterogeneous, with subcomponents originating from both the intestinal tract and the liver. Investigators have proposed that HDL particles participate in reverse CH transport by acquiring CH from tissues and other lipoproteins and transporting it to the liver for excretion. Numerous receptors are involved in the efflux of CH from peripheral tissues to HDL. Membrane receptors of the ABCA1 and ABCG1 family mediate unidirectional efflux of cellular CH and PLs to lipid-poor HDL and lipid-rich HDL particles, respectively. The hepatic scavenger receptor, SR-B1, mediates the uptake of HDL-derived CH into the liver (40). Because elevated HDL levels are associated with reduced coronary risk in humans, much interest exists in dietary and pharmacologic strategies to increase circulating HDL concentrations (41). The third component of the endogenous lipid transport system involves non–lipoprotein-associated movement of free FAs through the circulation. These FAs, derived largely as products of cellular TG hydrolysis, are secreted by adipose tissue into plasma where they bind with albumin. Albumin-bound FAs are removed in a concentration gradient-dependent manner by metabolically active tissues and are used largely as energy sources.

Apolipoproteins, Lipid Transfer Proteins, and Lipoprotein Metabolism

The interorgan movement of exogenous and endogenous lipids within lipoproteins is not incidental but rather is orchestrated by a series of apolipoproteins. Apolipoproteins confer greater water solubility, coordinate the movement and activities of lipoproteins by modulating enzyme activity, and mediate lipoprotein removal from the circulation by specific receptors. Indeed, rates of synthesis and catabolism of the major lipoproteins are regulated to a large extent by surface apolipoproteins that are recognized by specific cellular receptors.

Lipoproteins vary in apoprotein content. Apo-B is the major protein contained in chylomicrons and in VLDL, IDL, and LDL particles. A larger Apo-B-100 is associated with VLDL and LDL of hepatic origin, whereas a lesser molecular weight Apo-B-48 species is found in chylomicrons and intestinally derived VLDL. Apo-B-48 is thought to be generated from the same mRNA as is Apo-B-100. Within the intestine, however, only about one half of the length of the Apo-B-100 protein is translated because of the presence of a stop sequence. Apo-E is synthesized in liver and is present on all forms of lipoproteins. Apo-E binds both heparin-like molecules present on all cells and the LDL receptor. The Apo-E gene is polymorphic with three alleles (ε2, ε3, and ε4) that code for isoforms E2, E3, and E4; at least three alleles of the Apo-E gene produce six or more possible genotypes that differ in their ability to bind the LDL receptor. Apo-E genotype associates with plasma total and LDL-CH and may be correlated with the incidence of cardiovascular disease (42). Most HDL particles contain Apo-A-I, the crucial structural protein for HDL, as well as Apo-A-II, Apo-A-IV, and Apo-C. Apo-A-I and Apo-A-IV function as activators of lecithin: CH acyltransferase (LCAT), an enzyme that esterifies CH in plasma. Three C apolipoproteins, Apo-C-I, Apo-C-II, and Apo-C-III, possess distinct functions and all are synthesized in the liver. Apo-C-II, present in chylomicrons, VLDL, IDL, and HDL, is important in activation of LPL along with Apo-E. Apo-C-III, present in chylomicrons, IDL, and HDL, may inhibit PL action.

Apolipoproteins play a role in interorgan lipid movement and distribution at several levels. For instance, VLDL undergoes modification through LPL action in peripheral tissues, thus resulting in formation of LDL particles. Apo-C-II, activating LPL, hydrolyzes VLDL and chylomicron TG. Investigators believe that HDL exchanges Apo-E and Apo-C for Apo-A-I and Apo-A-IV on chylomicrons in the circulation. Apo-E is important in the hepatic clearance of TG-depleted chylomicron remnants.

Apolipoproteins are critical in the removal of particles from the circulation. LDL is cleared not only from the plasma into liver cells, but also in adipocytes, smooth muscle cells, and fibroblasts through the LDL receptor. The first process is receptor dependent and involves the interaction of Apo-B-100 and LDL with specific LDL receptors on cell surfaces. Quantitatively, most LDL receptors are present in the liver (Fig. 4.3). Postcontact events involve clustering of these receptors in coated pits and LDL internalization.

The activity of the LDL receptor is sensitive to both the total amount and the unesterified fraction of CH within the cell. Individuals with genetically inherited abnormalities in their LDL receptors have greatly elevated LDL levels as a result of faulty receptor-apoprotein interactions (43). Similarly, genetic problems with apoprotein structure can result in similar elevations of LDL. CH in LDL particles can undergo oxidative modification within the arterial wall and can be taken up by macrophage LDL scavenger receptors in an unregulated fashion—potentially resulting in foam cell production and atherogenesis. Formation of HDL also critically depends on apolipoproteins. Coalescence of PL-apoprotein complexes results in aggregation of Apo-A-I, Apo-A-II, Apo-A-IV, and possibly Apo-E, to form nascent HDL particles. These CH-poor, smaller Apo-A-I–containing forms of HDL are heterogeneous in size and can be classified overall as pre-β or discoidal HDL. Subsequently, discoidal HDL undergoes changes in size and composition in plasma and extracellular spaces as a result of acquiring free CH from cell membranes of peripheral tissues. Free CH taken up by HDL undergoes esterification by the enzyme LCAT and moves to the core of the HDL particle. As HDL becomes enriched with CE, Apo-C-II and Apo-C-III are picked up from other proteins to form three spherical categories of spherical HDL, termed, in order of increasing size and lipid content, HDL_3, HDL_{2a}, and HDL_{2b}. Spherical HDL is likely to go through repeated cycles of size increase and to decrease over a circulatory lifespan of 2 to 3 days.

Removal of spherical HDL from the circulation and metabolism can proceed via two routes. First, HDL_2 can transfer CE molecules to either Apo-B–containing lipoproteins or directly to cells. Movement of CH from HDL_2 occurs through CE transfer protein (CETP) that mediates the transfer of CE from HDL_2 to VLDL and chylomicrons in exchange for TG, after which Apo-B containing particles transport CE to liver. CETP is produced in liver and associates with HDL. As a result of CETP's action, HDL_2 reconverts to the HDL_3 form. Other apolipoproteins on HDL that play a role in reverse CH transport and can activate LCAT include Apo-A-IV, Apo-C-1, and Apo-E. Second, entire particles of HDL_2 can be taken up by LDL receptors and possibly by a separate Apo-E receptor on hepatocytes. The CH content of HDL particles can be transferred to the liver through the scavenger receptor B1 (SR-B1) that creates a lipophilic channel through which HDL can offload its CH core.

Dietary Factors Influencing Plasma Lipoproteins

Dietary factors profoundly influence lipoprotein levels and metabolism, which, in turn, alter an individual's susceptibility to atherosclerosis. Several major dietary factors have been identified including fat, CH, fiber, phytosterols, protein, alcohol consumption, and energy balance. Classic studies originally revealed that consumption of saturated fats produce an elevation in circulating total lipoprotein and LDL CH levels in humans (44). Plasma CH-raising effects of saturated FAs (SAFAs), particularly myristic (C14:0) and palmitic (C16:0) acids, have been well established. The CH-raising effect is believed to result from the regulatory pool of liver CH shifting from CE to free CH under dietary conditions in which hepatocytes become enriched with C14:0 and C16:0 FAs. Higher levels of free CH in the liver suppress LDL receptor activity and drive

up circulatory levels. Postmeal accumulation of VLDL is more prolonged in individuals consuming diets rich in SAFAs versus MUFA-containing diets (45).

Conversely, metabolic studies showed that consumption of n-6 PUFAs lowers circulatory CH values, although epidemiologic data failed to demonstrate any direct protective effect of dietary PUFAs on coronary heart disease risk (46). Alternatively, consumption of n-3 PUFAs from fish oil is strongly inversely correlated with the incidence of heart disease and is associated with potent TG-lowering and anti-inflammatory actions. The anti-inflammatory effects of n-3 FAs have been shown to be mediated by binding to the G-protein–coupled receptor 120.

n-3 PUFAs, which lower circulating TG levels, have only a minor impact on lipoprotein CH levels in humans. The role of n-3 FAs in reducing heart disease risk through their antiarrhythmic action is also becoming increasingly recognized (47). As an alternative to marine-based n-3 FAs, plant-based oils engineered to contain significant quantities of stearidonic acid 18:4(n-3)—a metabolic intermediate in the conversion of 18:3n-3 to 20:5n-3—have been shown reduce multiple biomarkers of cardiovascular disease risk.

Consumption of fats rich in MUFAs also results in lower CH levels, although to no greater extent than for fats rich in n-6 PUFAs. Consumption of *trans* FAs has also been shown to raise LDL and to lower HDL levels in a dose-dependent fashion. Investigators have suggested that dietary *trans* fat consumption may increase CETP activity, thus explaining the higher circulatory LDL levels associated with *trans* fat consumption (48). The role of dietary CH in hyperlipidemia has engendered considerable debate. Within the range of CH intakes normally consumed, changing dietary CH content seems to produce little alteration in circulating CH levels or subsequent metabolism (49). Certain individuals demonstrate a hypersensitivity to dietary CH that may result in a misleading perception of the response to dietary CH within a population overall.

Dietary fiber is an additional factor influencing CH levels (50). In general, insoluble fibers such as cellulose, hemicellulose, and lignin from grain and vegetables have limited effects on CH levels, whereas more soluble forms such as gums and pectins found in legumes and fruit possess greater CH-lowering properties. Fiber exhibits CH-lowering action by at least three mechanisms other than simple replacement of hypercholesterolemic dietary ingredients. First, fiber may act as a CH and bile acid sequestering agent within the small intestine; second, fiber likely reduces the rate of insulin rise by slowing carbohydrate absorption, thus slowing CH synthesis; and third, fiber fermentation in the large intestine may produce SCFAs, which are absorbed by the portal circulation and inhibit CH synthesis.

Phytosterols, as discussed earlier, are plant-based sterols similar in structure to mammalian CH. North American phytosterol consumption is comparable to that of CH at approximately 300 to 400 mg/day, mainly from vegetable oils, nuts, and seeds. Plant sterols have a long-standing history as effective CH-lowering agents; the first reported animal and clinical interventions occurred in the early 1950s. Cytellin, the first phytosterol-based CH-lowering pharmaceutical, showed effective CH-lowering effects at high doses of 6 to 18 g/day. Since the early 1990s, many different phytosterol-fortified food products including spreads, juices, salad dressings, and soymilk have steadily become available in more than 35 countries worldwide. Metaanalyses suggest that consumption of phytosterols at the recommended intake of 2 g/day reduces plasma CH concentrations by 10% by interfering with intestinal CH absorption (32).

The quality of protein intake is an additional factor that may influence circulating CH levels because consumption of animal versus plant protein increases circulating CH levels. Alcohol intake is another, albeit controversial, dietary factor associated with heart disease risk. The relationship between alcohol consumption and CH levels is "J" shaped. At lower levels of intake, wine and spirits, but not beer, produce a more favorable lipid profile by lowering LDL and raising HDL CH values. Further, consumption of excess calories resulting in obesity is associated with higher circulating CH levels. Studies have shown that both CH and TG levels fall during weight loss (51). The distribution of excess weight appears to have a stronger association with circulating lipid levels than the amount of weight (52). In summary, these dietary factors suggest that substitution of energy-dense and saturated fat–rich, animal-based foods by those obtained from plant sources is warranted to maintain a desirable profile of circulating lipids.

OXIDATION AND CONVERSION OF LIPIDS TO OTHER METABOLITES

Fatty Acid Oxidation

FAs are the most energy dense compared with other macronutrients because of their high content in carbon-hydrogen bonds, which are stronger bonds, and therefore contain more oxidizable energy than the bonds between carbon and other atoms, as found in carbohydrates, protein, and alcohol. For FAs to be used for energy, they must pass through several stages including transport to oxidative tissues, transcellular uptake, mitochondrial transfer, and subsequent β-oxidation.

FAs partitioned for oxidation undergo activation to fatty acyl-CoA, which then must pass into mitochondria to be oxidized. However, LCFAs and their CoA derivatives cannot cross the mitochondrial membrane without transferase-mediated binding to carnitine, synthesized in humans from lysine and methionine. After transmission of the fatty acyl-carnitine across the mitochondrial membrane, FAs

are reactivated with CoA, whereas carnitine recycles to the cytoplasmic surface.

Mitochondrial β-oxidation of FAs entails the consecutive release of 2-carbon acetyl-CoA units from the carboxyl terminus of the acyl chain. Before release of each 2-carbon unit, the β-carbon atoms of the acyl chain undergo cyclic degradation through four stages including dehydrogenation (removal of hydrogen), hydration (addition of water), dehydrogenation (removal of hydrogens), and cleavage. Completion through these four reactions represents one cycle of β-oxidation. For unsaturated bonds within FAs, the initial dehydrogenation reaction is omitted. The entire cycle is repeated until the fatty acyl chain is completely degraded.

Peroxisomal FA β-oxidation also occurs, yet several differences exist between FA oxidation in peroxisomes and that in mitochondria. First, peroxisomes, and the ER, contain very long acyl-CoA synthetase, the enzyme responsible for the activation of VLCFAs, but mitochondria do not, likely explaining why VLCFAs are oxidized predominantly in peroxisomes. Second, the initial reaction in peroxisomal β-oxidation (desaturation of acyl-CoA) is catalyzed by a flavin adenine dinucleotide (FAD)-containing fatty acyl-CoA oxidase, presumed to be the rate-limiting enzyme, whereas an acyl-CoA dehydrogenase is the first enzyme in the mitochondrial pathway. Additionally, peroxisomal β-oxidation is not directly coupled to the electron transfer chain that conserves energy by means of oxidative phosphorylation. In peroxisomes, electrons generated in the first oxidation step are transferred directly to molecular oxygen yielding hydrogen peroxide that is disposed of by catalase, whereas energy produced in the second oxidation step (nicotinamide adenine dinucleotide [NAD^+] reduction) is conserved in the form of high-energy-level electrons of reduced NAD (NADH).

Dietary Modulation of Fatty Acid Oxidation

Considerable interest has surrounded differential partitioning, based on chemical structure of dietary fat, for oxidation versus retention for storage and structural use. This issue is relevant to human health for at least two reasons: first, consumption of fats associated with greater retention in storage tissues may result in an increased tendency toward obesity; and, second, the greater accumulation in cells of less preferentially oxidized FAs may confer structural or functional changes resulting from shifts in membrane PL FA patterns or in prostaglandin (PG)/TXA ratios. The influence of tissue FA composition on functional ability such as insulin sensitivity has been well defined (53).

Discriminative oxidation of certain FAs has been established. For instance, short- and medium-chain TGs are associated with increased energy production in humans, possibly because of direct portal transfer of SCFAs and medium-chain FAs from gut to liver. The lack of requirement for carnitine in mitochondrial membrane transit by SCFAs may also be responsible for their more rapid oxidation. For LCFAs, evidence suggests that n-6 and n-3 PUFAs are more rapidly oxidized for energy compared with SAFAs. Labeled PUFAs are more readily converted to carbon dioxide than are SAFAs (54, 55), whereas PUFA consumption exhibits greater thermogenic effect (56), oxygen consumption (57), and sympathetic nervous system stimulation (58). Whole body FA balance data also support the concept that C18:2 n-6 is more readily used for energy than are SAFAs (59). Other studies support the preferential contribution to whole body oxidation of n-9 monounsaturated fats (60). Although these findings have yet to be confirmed in humans, consumption of fats containing PUFAs or MUFAs appear to enhance the contribution of dietary fat to total energy production in healthy individuals (61) and influence the use of other FAs for energy (62). Rates of portal venous transfer, release of FAs from adipose tissue, hepatic FA oxidation, and mitochondrial entry of FAs generally increase with the degree of acyl chain unsaturation.

Oxidative Processes. Cellular membrane PLs are highly vulnerable to oxidative damage because of the susceptibility of their PUFA side chains to peroxidation. Membrane lipid peroxidation results in loss of PUFAs, decreased membrane fluidity, and increased permeability of the membrane to substances such as calcium (Ca^{2+}) ions. Lipid peroxidation can lead to loss of enzyme and receptor activity and can have deleterious effects on membrane secretory functions. Continued lipid peroxidation can lead to complete loss of membrane integrity, as can be observed from the hemolysis associated with lipid peroxidation of erythrocyte membranes.

Many different dietary components have been reported to influence membrane susceptibility to oxidative damage. Cellular lipid peroxidation strongly depends on PUFA intake as well as on intake of vitamin E and other lipid antioxidants. In isolated erythrocytes from human subjects, the production of lipid peroxidation products following hydrogen peroxide–induced oxidative stress has been measured as thiobarbituric acid reactive substances (TBARS). Multivariate analysis has shown that the unsaturation index was the best predictor of erythrocyte-TBARS variability (63). A relatively stable C18:2 n-6 to vitamin E ratio in vegetable oils provides protection from risk of excessive lipid peroxidation and vitamin E deficiency at high PUFA intakes. Fish oils are an exception to the observation of a natural association between PUFAs and vitamin E in edible fats and oils and the stability of PUFAs to oxidation in the diet and body. The highly unsaturated n-3 pentaenoic and hexaenoic FAs, found in high concentrations in fish and marine oils with relatively low vitamin E contents, markedly increase the in vivo susceptibility of these oils to peroxidation (64). TBARS increase with higher concentrations of total n-3 PUFA in isolated human erythrocytes, whereas TBARS decrease with higher concentrations of total MUFA (63).

Numerous studies have suggested that oxidized lipids may exert atherogenic effects (65, 66). Oxidized free FAs exert effects on cell proliferation and survival, cell signaling, and chemotaxis, which have been indicated to be important mediators of atherogenesis. Oxidized PLs that contain oxidized FAs have also been shown to exert adverse effects on vascular cells (67). Cells are exposed regularly to oxidized FAs through endogenous metabolism by products produced by lipoxygenase (LO) and cyclooxygenase (CO) action as well as by absorption of end products of lipolysis of dietary oxidized lipids. Dietary oxidized lipids may contribute to the atherogenicity of lipoproteins by increasing oxidative stress and oxidized LDL in the plasma and arterial walls (65). The typical Western diet contains large quantities of PUFAs that are exposed to heating or processing generating oxidized FAs (67). Oxidized FAs, such as 13-hydroxylinoleic acid, share structural similarities with the monohydroxy bile acid, lithocholic acid, which is required for intestinal absorption of CH. Such dietary oxidized FAs may thus act as BS enhancers to increase the solubilization and absorption of dietary CH and may thereby lead to higher plasma CH concentrations (65).

The actions of oxygen free radicals on membrane CH may be as important as the effects observed on membrane PLs FAs because oxidized CH derivatives, the oxysterols or CH oxides, have been suggested to play key roles in the development of atherosclerosis (68). This concept has been fostered by increasing evidence of the role of oxidatively modified lipoproteins in atherogenesis. CH readily undergoes oxidation (69), and the metabolites derived display a wide variety of actions on cellular metabolism including angiotoxic, mutagenic, and carcinogenic effects (68). Common CH oxidation products include the following: CH-5α,6α-epoxide; CH-5β,6β-epoxide; and cholestane-3β,5α,6β triol. CH oxides disturb endothelial integrity by perturbing vascular permeability, whereas purified CH has no effect. CH oxidation products have been detected in human serum lipoproteins and human atheromatous plaques (70). Substantial amounts of oxidized CH are detected in a variety of foods of animal origin exposed to oxidizing conditions (69). These highly atherogenic oxysterols may also be ingested and absorbed from processed foods or generated by free radical oxidation of lipoproteins. To date, however, it is unclear whether CH oxides merely serve as markers for oxidatively modified lipoproteins or whether they contribute to the toxicity of oxidized lipoproteins.

LDL oxidation has been implicated as a causal factor in the development of human atherosclerosis (71). Unsaturated LDL lipids are subject to peroxidative degradation, and the susceptibility of LDL to oxidation has been correlated with the degree of coronary atherosclerosis (72). Oxidized LDL is present in atherosclerotic plaque (73). Possible sources of LDL lipid oxidation include endothelial cells, smooth muscle cells, monocytes and macrophages, and other inflammatory cells. In the presence of the peroxidative promoter copper, peroxidation of LDL results in the formation of hydroxyalkenals such as 4-hydroxynonenal and malondialdehyde (MDA) that modify Apo-B by reacting with its amino lysine groups. This chemical modification of Apo-B could, in turn, impair its uptake by the LDL receptor. Oxidatively modified LDL may exert atherogenic effects via its cytotoxic and chemotactic properties or through the promotion of LDL uptake by the scavenger receptors on macrophages, thus leading to the formation of lipid-enriched foam cells.

Nutritional and biochemical studies suggest that diet can modulate the susceptibility of plasma LDL to oxidative degradation by altering the concentration of PUFAs and antioxidants in the lipoprotein particle. The first targets of peroxidation in the oxidation of LDL are the PUFAs of PLs on the LDL surface. In studies of LDL isolated from healthy humans and animals, a diet rich in C18:2 n-6 increases the susceptibility of plasma LDL to copper-induced oxidation and to in vitro macrophage uptake, as compared with a diet high in C18:1 n-9 (74). C18:1 n-9 and other MUFAs do not contain the easily oxidized conjugated double bonds found in PUFAs. In addition, C18:1 n-9 has a high affinity for transition metals that renders them unavailable for LDL peroxidation. Studies have shown consistently that MUFA-rich diets induce

an increased resistance of LDL to oxidative modification (75). Depending on the dose used, subjects treated with n-3 PUFAs showed either an increase or no change in LDL oxidation (76).

BIOSYNTHESIS OF LIPIDS

Fatty Acids

Biosynthesis of FAs occurs in the extramitochondrial compartment by a group of enzymes known as FA synthetases. Compared with other species, human FA synthesis occurs predominantly in the liver and appears to be much less active in adipose tissue. The FA biosynthetic pathway is almost identical in all organisms examined to date. The process involves acetyl-CoA combining sequentially with a succession of malonyl-CoA molecules.

In mammals, complete de novo synthesis results in C16:0, with other FAs formed from C16:0 by chain elongation via a microsomal malonyl-CoA–dependent elongase enzyme. Mammals also possess a series of desaturases and elongases to generate long-chain PUFAs from C16:0, C18:0, C18:2n-6, and C18:3n-3 (Fig. 4.4). These reactions take place predominantly in ER membranes. Desaturase reactions are catalyzed by membrane-bound desaturases with broad chain-length specificity that includes Δ^9, Δ^6, Δ^5, and Δ^4 fatty acyl-CoA desaturases. These enzymes are involved in desaturation of C16:1n-7, C18:1n-9, C18:2n-6,

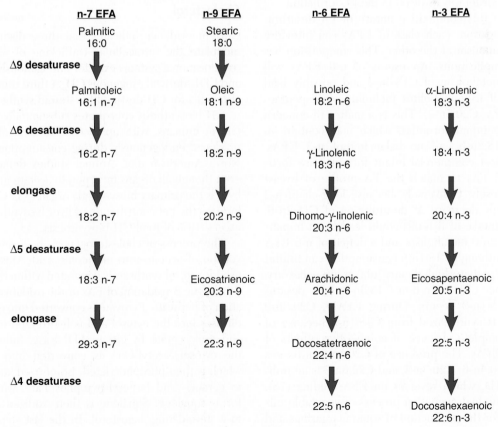

Fig. 4.4. Effects of desaturase and elongase on essential fatty acids (EFAs).

and C18:3n-3 FA families. Δ^4 desaturation is required for the formation of C22:6n-3 from C22:5n-3 and for the formation of C22:5n-6 from C22:4n-6.

Precursors for the n-7 and n-9 families of PUFAs are MUFAs that are synthesized via microsomal Δ^9 oxidative desaturation of C16:0 and C18:0 to form C16:ln-7 and C18:1n-9, respectively (Fig. 4.4). Additional double bonds can be introduced into existing MUFAs C16:1n-7 and C18:1n-9 and also into C18:2n-6 via Δ^6 desaturase (Fig. 4.4). Until relatively recently, humans and other mammals were thought incapable of synthesizing long-chain n-3 (C18:3n-3) and n-6 (C18:2n-6) EFAs. Previous work suggested that C18:2n-6 and C18:3n-3 could be synthesized in humans and other mammals via elongation of the dietary precursors C16:2n-6 and C16:3n-3, respectively (77). Edible green plants can contain amounts of up to 14% of C16:2n-6 and C16:3n-3 (77). In a practical sense, a dietary supply of 18C EFA is still important because humans likely do not obtain sufficient quantities of 16-carbon precursors.

The n-3, n-6, and n-9 family of FAs compete with each other, especially at the rate-limiting Δ^6 desaturase step. In general, the desaturase enzymes display highest affinity for the most unsaturated substrate, with the order of preference being α-linolenic family (n-3) > linoleic family (n-6) > oleic acid family (n-9) > palmitoleic acid family (n-7) > elaidic acid family (n-9, *trans*). Competition also exists among the PUFA families for the elongase enzymes and the acyltransferases involved in the PL formation.

Because of this competitive nature of FA desaturation and elongation, each class of EFAs can interfere with the metabolism of the other. This competition has nutritional implications. An excess of n-6 EFAs will reduce the metabolism of C18:3n-3 and possibly lead to a deficit of its metabolites including eicosapentaenoic acid (EPA; C20:5n-3). This is a matter of concern in relation to infant formulas, which may contain an excess of C18:2n-6 and no balancing of n-3 EFAs. Therefore, most commercial infant formulas are fortified with n-3 FAs to match the FA profile of breast milk more closely. Conversely, because long-chain n-3 EFAs markedly decrease Δ^6 desaturation of C18:2n-6, an excessive intake of fish oils could lead to an impairment of C18:2n-6 metabolism and a deficit of n-6 EFA derivatives. Although C18:1n-9 consumption can inhibit Δ^6 desaturase activity, high dietary intakes are necessary. In the presence of C18:2n-6 or C18:3n-3, little desaturation of C18:1n-9 occurs. During EFAD, C20:3n-9 (Mead acid) is synthesized from C18:1n-9 because of the nearly complete absence of competitive effects of n-3 and n-6 EFAs. The presence of C20:3n-9 in tissues instead of C20:4n-6, C20:5n-3, and C22:6n-3 is an indicator of EFAD, which reverses on EFA feeding (78). In the catalytic hydrogenation process of vegetable oils and fish oils for the production of some margarines and shortenings, various geometric and positional isomers of

unsaturated FAs are formed in varying amounts. After absorption, these *trans* FA isomers may compete with the EFAs and endogenously synthesized FAs for desaturation and chain elongation.

In a phenomenon called *retroversion*, very-long-chain C22 PUFAs, present in marine oils, may be shortened by two carbons with concomitant saturation of a double bond. For example, C22:6n-3 is converted to C22:5n-3 and to C20:5n-3 (79). This peroxisomal pathway is also active in converting C22:5n-6 into C20:4n-6 (80). As a result of competition among various PUFA families for desaturases, elongases, and acyltransferases, and because of retroversion, a characteristic pattern of end products accumulates in tissue lipids for each family. Hence, the major PUFA product for the palmitoleate n-7 family is C20:3n-7, the oleate n-9 is C20:3n-9, and linoleate is C20:4n-6 and some C20:3n-6. The most common products for the n-3 FA family are C20:5n-3 and C22:6n-3.

The efficiency of the multistage synthesis of PUFAs is unclear in humans. Stable isotope studies have indicated that in healthy subjects, the conversion of dietary C18:3n-3 to C20:5n-3 appears to be limited, and the conversion to C22:6n-3 is even more minor (81, 82). Whole body conversion of 18:3n-3 to 22:6n-3 in humans has generally been shown to be less than 5% with substantial variability, and it appears to depend on dietary concentration of n-6 FAs and long-chain PUFAs (82).

Cholesterol

Current evidence indicates that three distinct pathways modulate the intracellular trafficking of CH. Separate translocational systems exist for endogenously synthesized and LDL-derived exogenous CH. A third transport system also exists for CH destined for steroid synthesis.

CH biosynthesis contributes substantially to total body CH in humans, with up to 60% to 80% of body pools produced endogenously during consumption of a typical North American diet. Animal studies demonstrate that even though all organs incorporate acetate into sterol, the liver is the primary biosynthetic organ (83). Conversely, in humans the net contribution of liver biosynthesis does not exceed 10% of total CH biosynthesis.

The process of cholesterogenesis begins with the conversion of acetate into mevalonic acid. Most acetyl-CoA used for sterol synthesis is generated within the mitochondria by the β-oxidation of FAs or the oxidative decarboxylation of pyruvate. Pyruvate is converted into citrate, which diffuses into the cytosol and is hydrolyzed to acetyl-CoA and oxaloacetate by citrate-ATP lyase. Subsequently, in the cytosol, acetyl-CoA is converted into mevalonate, which is then phosphorylated, isomerized, and converted to geranyl- and farnesyl-pyrophosphate, which, in turn, forms squalene. Squalene is then oxidized and cyclized to a steroid ring, lanosterol. In the last steps, lanosterol is converted into CH by the loss of three methyl groups, saturation of the side chain, and a shift of the double bond from Δ^8 to Δ^5.

Control of CH biosynthesis in humans is sensitive to several dietary factors. Adding CH to the diet at physiologic levels results in modest increases in circulating CH levels, with a mild reciprocal inhibition of synthesis (84, 85). Dietary fat selection exhibits a more pronounced influence on human cholesterogenesis because consumption of PUFA-rich fats is associated with enhanced biosynthesis compared with other plant or animal fats. Both differences in FA composition and plant sterol levels may be contributing factors (35). Higher meal frequency has been shown to reduce human CH biosynthesis rates, which may explain the lower circulating CH synthesis rates observed with consumption of more numerous smaller meals (86). Insulin, which is associated with hepatic CH synthesis in animals, may be released in greater amounts when less frequent but larger meals are consumed. In considering dietary factors capable of modifying CH synthesis, energy restriction exhibits the greatest effect. Humans fasted for 24 hours exhibit complete cessation of CH biosynthesis (19). CH synthesis appears to act both passively and actively in relation to circulatory CH levels, depending on dietary perturbation. Passively, the liver responds to high CH levels through LDL receptor–mediated suppression of synthesis; the modest suppression in the presence of increasing dietary and circulating levels reflects the limited hepatic contribution to total body production of CH (84). Substitution of PUFAs in place of other fats results in a decrease in the ratio of hepatic intracellular free to esterified CH that, in turn, up-regulates both LDL receptor number and cholesterogenesis. In both ways, CH synthesis responds passively to external stimuli. In contrast, nonhepatic synthesis is less sensitive to dietary CH level and fat type, whereas hepatic synthesis is actively more responsive to synthesis pathway substrate availability (87). In this manner, several dietary factors actively modify CH synthesis and levels. Such differential sensitivity may explain the more pronounced decrement in CH synthesis and levels occurring after energy deficit in humans.

CH serves as a required precursor for important steroid compounds including sex hormones, adrenocorticoid hormones, and vitamin D. Production of steroidal sex hormones, including estrogen, androgen, and progesterone, and corticosteroid hormone synthesis, involves removal of the CH side chain at C-17 and rearrangement of the double bonds in the steroid nucleus. 7-Dehydrocholesterol is the precursor of cholecalciferol (vitamin D) formed at the skin surface through the action of ultraviolet irradiation. Steroid hormone metabolites are excreted principally through the urine. Investigators have estimated that in humans, approximately 50 mg/day of CH is converted to steroid hormones.

Vertebrates are incapable of converting plant sterols to CH. Insects and prawns have been shown capable of transforming phytosterols into steroid hormones or bile acids through a CH intermediate, however.

FUNCTIONS OF ESSENTIAL FATTY ACIDS

After ingestion of EFAs, C18:2n-6 and C18:3n-3 are distributed between adipose TGs, other tissue stores, and tissue structural lipids. A proportion of C18:2n-6 and C18:3n-3 contributes to provide energy, with these PUFAs apparently oxidized more rapidly than SAFAs or MUFAs. In contrast, long-chain PUFAs derived from EFAs (i.e., C20:3n-6, C20:4n-6, C20:5n-3, and C22:6n-3) are less readily oxidized. These FAs, when present preformed in the diet, are incorporated into structural lipids approximately 20 times more efficiently than after synthesis from dietary C18:2n-6 and C18:3n-3. The liver is the site of most of the PUFA metabolism that transforms dietary C18 EFAs into 20–22C PUFAs. Long-chain PUFAs are transported to extrahepatic tissues for incorporation into cell lipids, even though differential uptake and acylation of PUFAs occurs among different tissues. The final tissue composition of long-chain PUFAs is an outcome of the foregoing complex processes along with the influence of dietary factors. The major elements in the diet that determine the final distribution of long-chain PUFAs in cell PLs include the relative proportions of n-3, n-6, and n-9 FA families and the amounts of preformed long-chain PUFAs versus their shorter chain precursors (88).

Membrane structural PLs contain high concentrations of PUFAs and the 20- and 22-carbon PUFAs that predominate from the two families of EFAs. C20:4n-6 is the most important and abundant long-chain PUFA found in membrane PLs; it is the primary precursor of eicosanoids. The concentration of free C20:4n-6 is strictly regulated by phospholipases and acyltransferases. In terms of EFAs from the n-3 PUFA series, C20:5n-3 and C22:6n-3 are most prevalent in membrane PLs. The long-chain PUFAs derived from EFAs are incorporated primarily in the 2-acyl position in bilayer PLs of mammalian plasma, mitochondrial, and nuclear membranes. The 20-carbon FAs, when released from their PLs, can be transformed into intracellular metabolites (i.e., inositol triphosphate [IP$_3$], as well as diacylglycerol [DAG]) and extracellular metabolites (i.e., platelet-activating factor [PAF] and eicosanoids), which participate in many important cell signaling responses. The relative proportions in tissue PLs of C20:4n-6 and other long-chain PUFAs (C18:3n-6, C20:4n-6, and C20:5n-3) are important because these PUFAs can compete for or inhibit enzymes involved with the generation of intracellular and extracellular biologically active products. Moreover, dietary C18:1n-9, C18:2n-6, C18:2n-6 *trans*, C18:3n-6, C18:3n-3, and long-chain n-3 PUFAs (C20:5n-3 and C22:6n-3) can compete with C20:4n-6 for the acyltransferases for esterification into PL pools and can thereby inhibit C20:4n-6–mediated membrane functions (Fig. 4.4).

FAs and eicosanoids have the capacity to regulate gene transcription through peroxisome proliferator-activated receptors (PPARs), which are nuclear hormone receptors that play an important role in the genetic regulation of FA oxidation and lipogenesis. Chawla et al (89) reviewed the various families of nuclear receptors with important functions in lipid physiology, including the PPARs, which act as FA sensors. Four PPAR isotypes have been identified: α, β (also known as δ), and γ. PPARs are ligand-dependent transcription factors and act such that activation of target gene transcription depends on the binding of the ligand to the receptor. Certain ligands such as PUFAs and oxidized FAs are shared by all three isotypes. Several eicosanoids and FAs bind with high affinity to PPAR-α, including long C18:2n-6, conjugated linoleic acid, and eicosanoids such as LT-B$_4$ (90). PPAR-α operates in the catabolism of FAs in the liver because it promotes FA oxidation under conditions of lipid catabolism such as fasting (91). Hepatic oxidation of FAs to acetyl-CoA and subsequent metabolism to ketone bodies are strongly stimulated by PPAR-α, whose expression is elevated with fasting. PPAR-β regulates the expression of acyl-CoA synthetase 2 in brain tissue (91). PPAR-γ promotes lipogenesis in adipose tissue under anabolic conditions, because PPAR-γ target genes in adipose tissue include FA transport protein (FATP), acyl-CoA synthase, LPL, and adipocyte FABP (A-FABP) (91, 92). PPAR-γ could participate in the development of atherosclerosis by stimulating the cellular uptake of oxidized LDL. Oxidized FAs entering cells via oxidized LDL can activate PPAR-γ to stimulate cellular uptake of oxidized LDL further (91). PPAR-δ has been characterized as a mediator of lipoprotein signaling in macrophages (93).

Membrane Functions and Integrity

Because fragile membranes in erythrocytes and mitochondria are typically present in EFAD, an early function attributed to EFAs was their role as integral components of PLs required for plasma and intracellular membrane integrity. EFAD results in a progressive decrease in C20:4n-6 in membrane PLs, with a concomitant increase in C18:1n-9 and its product, C20:3n-9. The fluidity and other physical properties of membrane PLs are largely determined by the chain length and degree of unsaturation of their component FAs. These physical properties, in turn, affect the ability of PLs to perform structural functions such as the maintenance of normal activities of membrane bound enzymes. Dietary SAFAs, MUFAs, and PUFAs, the major determinants of the composition of stored and structural lipids, have been shown to alter the activity and affinity of receptors, membrane permeability, and transport properties (94).

The heterogeneity and selectivity of PUFAs with respect to their tissue membrane distribution among different organs may be related to their structural and functional roles (94). For example, long-chain derivatives of n-3 PUFAs are concentrated in biologic structures involved in fast movement as required in transport mechanisms in brain and its synaptic junction, as well as retina (95). Approximately 50% of the PL in the disc membrane of the retinal rod outer segment in which rhodopsin resides contains C22:6n-3 (96). The C22:6n-3 is concentrated in the major PL classes (i.e., PC, phosphatidylethanolamine [PE], and phosphatidylserine [PS] in the disc membrane), whereas C20:4n-6 is found in the minor PL components such as phosphatidylinositol (PI). This observation has led to speculation that C22:6n-3 is important as a structural component in these membranes, whereas C20:4n-6 may play more of a functional role (97).

BIOSYNTHESIS AND FUNCTION OF EICOSANOIDS

Some of the most potent effects of PUFAs are related to their enzymatic conversion into a series of oxygenated metabolites termed eicosanoids, so called because their precursors are PUFAs with chain lengths of 20 carbon units. Eicosanoids include PG, TXA, LTs, hydroxy FAs, and lipoxins. PG and TXA are generated via CO enzymes, whereas LT, hydroxy FAs, and lipoxins are produced from LO metabolism. Under stimulation, a rapid and transient synthesis of active eicosanoids activates specific receptors locally in the tissues in which they are formed. Eicosanoids modulate cardiovascular, pulmonary, immune, reproductive, and secretory functions in many cells. These regulators are rapidly converted to their inactive forms via selective catabolic enzymes. Humans depend on the dietary presence of the n-3 and n-6 structural families of PUFAs for adequate biosynthesis of eicosanoids. Three direct precursor FAs are reused to form eicosanoids by the action of membrane-bound CO or specific LO enzyme systems, including C20:3n-6, C20:4n-6, and C20:5n-3. A series of prostanoids and LTs, containing different biologic properties, is generated from each of these FAs (Fig. 4.5). The first irreversible, committed step in the synthesis of PG and LT is a hydroperoxide-activated FA oxygenase action exerted by either PG H synthase (PGHS) or LO enzymes on the nonesterified precursor PUFA (Fig. 4.6).

Stimulation of normal cells via specific physiologic or pathologic stimuli such as thrombin, adenosine diphosphate (ADP), or collagen initiates a calcium-mediated cascade. This cascade involves phospholipase A$_2$ activation that releases PUFAs on position 2 of the cell membrane. The greatest proportion of PUFAs available to phospholipase A$_2$ action contains C20:4n-6. Hydrolytic release from PL esters appears to occur indiscriminately with n-3 and n-6 types of PUFAs involving all major classes of PLs including PC, PE, and PI. These FAs serve as direct precursors for generation of eicosanoid products via CO and LO enzymatic action (Fig. 4.6). Enzymatic biotransformation of PUFA precursors to PG is catalyzed via two PG synthase isozymes designated PGHS-1 and PGHS-2 (98). PGHS-1 is located in the ER, and PGHS-2

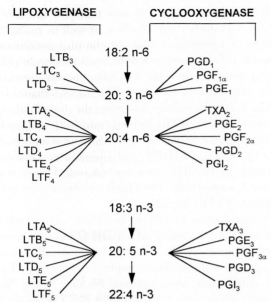

Fig. 4.5. Formation of prostaglandin (PG), thromboxane (TXA), and leukotriene (LT) from dihomo-γ-linolenic acid (DHGA) (C20:3n-6), arachidonic acid (C20:4n-6), and eicosapentaenoic acid (C20:5n-3) via cyclooxygenase and lipoxygenase pathways.

is located in the nuclear envelope. Both forms are bifunctional enzymes that catalyze the oxygenation of C20:4n-6 to PGG_2 via CO reaction and the reduction of PGG_2, thus forming a transient hydroxyendoperoxide (PGH_2) via the peroxidase reaction (Fig. 4.6). The PGH_2 intermediate is rapidly converted to PGI_2 by vascular endothelial cells, to TXA_2 by an isomerase in platelets, or to other prostanoids depending on the tissues involved. PGHS-2 generates prostanoids associated with mitogenesis and inflammation and is inhibited by glucocorticoids.

C20:4n-6 can be oxygenated via the 5-, 12-, and 15-LO pathways (see Fig. 4.5). The 5-LO pathway generates mainly LTB_4, LTC_4, and LTD_4 from C20:4n-6, LTs that are implicated as important mediators in proliferative and synthetic immune responses. LTB_4 in particular has been indicated as a key proinflammatory mediator in inflammatory and proliferative disorders (98). From C20:4n-6, the 12-LO pathway generates 12-L-hydroxyeicosatetraenoic acid (12-HETE) and 12-hydroperoxyeicosatetraenoic acid (12-HPETE). A proinflammatory response can be generated by 12-HETE in a variety of cell types. Products generated from C20:4n-6 metabolism by the 15-LO reaction include 15-hydroxyeicosatetraenoic acid (15-HETE), which has anti-inflammatory action and may inhibit 5- and 12-LO activities (99).

Because the major eicosanoids are synthesized from C20:4n-6, the availability of C20:4n-6 in PL pools of tissue may be a primary factor in regulating the quantities of eicosanoids synthesized by tissues in vivo. In addition, the intensity of the n-6 eicosanoid signal from the released PUFA will be stronger as C20:4n-6 becomes proportionally greater in the PUFAs. The levels of C20:4n-6 in tissue PL pools are affected by the elongation and desaturation of dietary C18:2n-6 and by the intake of C20:4n-6 (170–220 mg/day in the Western diet) (100). Although dietary concentrations of C18:2n-6 up to 2% to 3% of calories increase tissue C20:4n-6 concentrations, intakes of C18:2n-6 that are greater than 3% of calories are poorly correlated with tissue C20:4n-6 content (101). Because C18:2n-6 constitutes approximately 6% to 8% of the North American diet, moderate dietary changes in C18:2n-6 would not be expected to modulate tissue C20:4n-6 levels. Intakes of C18:2n-6 greater than 12%, however, may actually decrease tissue C20:4n-6 because of inhibition of

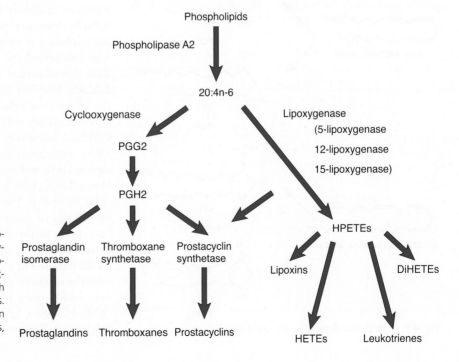

Fig. 4.6. Major pathways of synthesis of eicosanoids from arachidonic acid. *DiHETE*, dihydroxyeicosatetraenoic acid; *HETE*, hydroxyeicosatetraenoic acid; *HPETE*, hydroperoxyeicosatetraenoic acid; *PG*, prostaglandin. (Adapted with permission from Innis SM. Essential dietary lipids. In: Ziegler EE, Filer LJ, eds. Present Knowledge in Nutrition. 7th ed. Washington, DC: ILSI Press, 1996:58–66.)

Δ^6 desaturase. In contrast, dietary C20:4n-6 is much more effective in enriching C20:4n-6 in tissue PLs (101), and compared with C18:2n-6, relatively low dietary levels of C20:4n-6 may be physiologically significant in enhancing eicosanoid metabolism (100).

Diets high in n-3 FAs result in substitution of C20:4n-6 by n-3 PUFAs in membrane PLs, thus suppressing the response of C20:4n-6-derived eicosanoids by decreasing availability of the C20:4n-6 precursor and by the competitive inhibition of C20:5n-3 for eicosanoid biosynthesis (102). Although less pronounced than the effects observed with C20:5n-3 and C22:6n-3 dietary supplementation, C18:3n-3–enriched diets were observed to suppress PGE$_2$ production by peripheral blood mononuclear cells in monkeys (102). C18:3n-3 could competitively inhibit desaturation and elongation of C18:2n-6 for the conversion into C20:4n-6. The eicosanoids derived from n-3 are homologs of those derived from C20:4n-6 with which they compete (Fig. 4.7) and are associated with less active responses than n-6 eicosanoids when bound to the specific receptors.

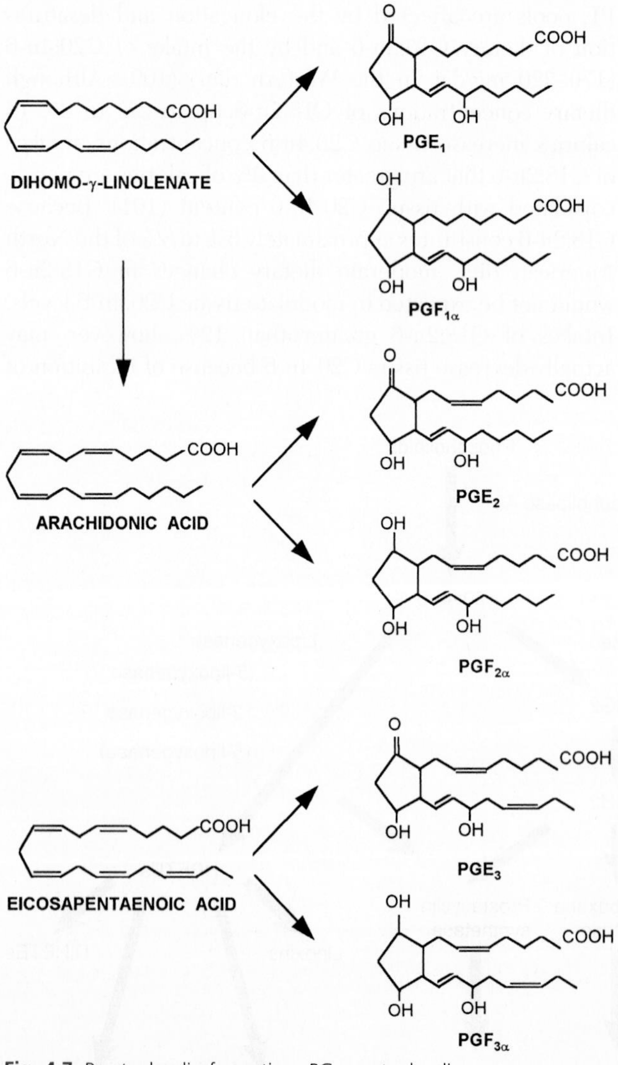

Diets rich in competing and moderating FAs (n-3 PUFAs, C18:3n-6) may produce changes in the production of eicosanoids that are more favorable with respect to inflammatory reactions. For instance, the PGE$_3$ formed from C20:5n-3 has less inflammatory effect than PGE$_2$ derived from C20:4n-6. The LTB$_5$, derived from C20:5n-3, is substantially less active in proinflammatory functions than the LTB$_4$ formed from C20:4n-6, including the aggregation and chemotaxis of neutrophils. Two 15-LO products, 15-HEPE and 17-hydroxydocosahexaenoic acid (17-HoDHE), are derived from C20:5n-3 and C22:6n-3, respectively (100). Both metabolites are potent inhibitors of LTB$_4$ formation.

Overproduction of C20:4n-6–derived eicosanoids has been implicated in many inflammatory and autoimmune disorders such as thrombosis, immune-inflammatory disease (i.e., arthritis, lupus nephritis), cancer, and psoriatic skin lesions, among others. Because typical North American diets appear to maintain n-6 PUFAs in PLs near the maximal capacity, investigators have suggested that n-6–rich diets may contribute to the incidence and severity of eicosanoid-mediated diseases including thrombosis and arthritis (103). Because platelet aggregation and activation are indicated to play a critical role in the progression toward vascular occlusion and myocardial infarction, the counterbalancing roles of TXA$_2$ and PGI$_2$ in cardiovascular functions have been emphasized. C20:4n-6 is required for platelet function as a precursor of the proaggregatory TXA$_2$. Biosynthesis of TXA$_2$ is the rate-limiting step in the aggregation of platelets, a key event in the process of thrombosis. The effects of TXA$_2$ are counteracted by PGI$_2$, a potent antiaggregatory agent that prevents adherence of platelets to blood vessel walls. Because of displacement of C20:4n-6 from membrane PLs by C18:2n-6, C18:3n-6, and C20:3n-6, stepwise increases in dietary C18:2n-6 from 3% to 40% of calories actually decreased platelet aggregation, a finding indicating inhibition of eicosanoid synthesis by these n-6 PUFAs. The antithrombotic influx C18:2n-6 is substantially less than that observed after high intakes of n-3 PUFA-rich fish oils, however (104). This finding has been related to the observations that PGI$_3$ generated from C20:5n-3 has antiaggregatory potency. Conversely, TXA$_3$ derived from C20:5n-3 has a very weak proaggregatory effect, whereas TXA$_2$ synthesis is reduced (105). Long-term ingestion of aspirin (106) and n-3 PUFA reduces the intensity of TXA$_2$ biosynthesis, which could decrease rates of cardiovascular mortality. The results of epidemiologic studies on the effects of dietary n-3 FAs on cardiovascular disease have been inconsistent, however. One prospective study demonstrated no protective effect of fish consumption on cardiovascular disease mortality and morbidity (107), whereas another showed protective effects in Japanese man and women who ate only modest amounts of fish (108). However, large clinical intervention trials involving fish oil supplementation showed a rapid onset of reduction

Fig. 4.7. Prostaglandin formation. *PG,* prostaglandin.

92. Anghel SI, Wahli W. Cell Res 2007;17:486–511.
93. Chawala A, Lee CH, Barak Y et al. Proc Nat Acad Sci U S A 2003;100:1268–73.
94. Murphy MG. J Nutr Biochem 1990;1:68–79.
95. Uauy R, Dangour AD. Nutr Rev 2006;64:S24–33;discussion S72–91.
96. Stinson AM, Wiegand RD, Anderson RE. Exp Eye Res 1991; 52:213–8.
97. Litman BJ, Mitchell DC. Lipids 1996;31(Suppl):193S–7S.
98. Cipollone F, Cicolini G, Bucci M. Pharmacol Ther 2008; 118:161–80.
99. Ziboh VA, Miller CC, Cho Y. Am J Clin Nutr 2000; 71(Suppl):361S–6S.
100. Li B, Birdwell C, Whelan J. J Lipid Res 1994;35:1869–77.
101. Whelan J, Surette ME, Hardardottir I et al. J Nutr 1993; 123:2174–85.
102. Wu D, Meydani SN, Meydani M et al. Am J Clin Nutr 1996; 63:273–80.
103. Simopoulos AP. Exp Biol Med 2008;233:674–88.
104. Hurst S, Rees S G, Randerson PF et al. Lipids 2009; 44:889–96.
105. von Schacky C, Fischer S, Weber PC. J Clin Invest 1985; 76:1626–31.
106. Anonymous. Lancet 1988;2:349–60.
107. Manger MS, Strand E, Ebbing M et al. Am J Clin Nutr 2010; 92:244–51.
108. Iso H, Kobayashi M, Ishihara J et al. Circulation 2006; 113:195–202.
109. Marchioli R, Barzi F, Bomba E et al. Circulation 2002; 105:1897–903.
110. Wall R, Ross RP, Fitzgerald GF et al. Nutr Rev 2010; 68:280–9.
111. Caughey GE, Mantzioris E, Gibson RA et al. Am J Clin Nutr 1996;63:116–22.
112. Holman RT. Essential fatty acid deficiency. Progress Chem Fats Other Lipids 1971;9:275–348.
113. Hansen HS, Artmann A. J Neuroendocrinol 2008; 20(Suppl 1):94–9.
114. Brown WR, Hansen AE, Burr GO et al. J Nutr 1938; 16:511–24.
115. Food and Nutrition Board, Institute of Medicine. Dietary Reference Intakes for Energy, Carbohydrate, Fiber, Fat, Fatty Acids, Cholesterol, Protein, and Amino Acids (Macronutrients). Washington, DC: National Academy Press, 2005.
116. Crawford MA, Golfetto I, Ghebremeskel K et al. Lipids 2004;38:303–15.
117. Crawford MA, Costeloe K, Doyle W et al. Essential fatty acids in early development. In: Bracco U, Deckelbaum RJ, eds. Polyunsaturated Fatty Acids in Human Nutrition. New York: Raven Press, 1992:93–110.
118. Koletzko B, Braun M. Ann Nutr Metab 1991;35:128–31.
119. Carlson SE, Cooke RJ, Werkman SH et al. Lipids 1992; 27:901–7.
120. Uauy R, Mena P, Wegher B et al. Pediatr Res 2000; 47:127–135.
121. Fleith M, Clandinin MT. Crit Rev Food Sci Nutr 2005; 45:205–29.
122. Koletzko B, Decsi T, Demmelmair H. Lipids 1996;31:79–83.
123. Makrides M, Neumann MA, Gibson RA. Lipids 1996; 31:115–9.
124. Russo GL. Biochem Pharmacol 2009;77:937–46.
125. Chung WL, Chen JJ, Su HM. J Nutr 2008;138:1165–71.
126. Neuringer M, Connor WE. Nutr Rev 1986;44:285–94.
127. Innis SM. Brain Res 2008 27;1237:35–43.
128. Clandinin MT, Chappell JE, Heim T. Prog Lipid Res 1981; 20:901–4.
129. Carlson SE, Rhodes PG, Ferguson MG. Am J Clin Nutr 1986; 44:798–804.
130. Makrides M, Neumann MA, Simmer K et al. Lancet 1995; 345:1463–8.
131. Brenna JT, Lapillonne A. Ann Nutr Metab 2009;55:97–122.
132. Food and Agriculture Organization/World Health Organization Expert Consultation. The Role of Fats and Oils in Human Nutrition. FAO Food and Nutrition paper 3. Rome: Food and Agriculture Organization, 1978.

SUGGESTED READINGS

Chawla, A, Repa JJ, Evans RM et al. Nuclear receptors and lipid physiology: opening the X-Files, Science 2001;294:1866–70.
Din JN, Newby DE, Flapan AD. Omega 3 fatty acids and cardiovascular disease: fishing for a natural treatment. BMJ 2004;328:30–5.
Grundy SM, Abate N, Chandalia M. Diet composition and the metabolic syndrome: what is the optimal fat intake? Am J Med 2002;113:25–9.
Jequier E, Bray GA. Low-fat diets are preferred. Am J Med 2002; 113:41–6.
Masson LF, McNeill G, Avenell A. Genetic variation and the lipid response to dietary intervention: a systematic review. Am J Clin Nutr 2003;77:1098–111.
Oh DY, Talukdar S, Bae EJ et al. GPR120 is an omega-3 fatty acid receptor mediating potent anti-inflammatory and insulin-sensitizing effects. Cell 2010;142:687–98.

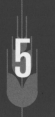

5 ENERGY NEEDS: ASSESSMENT AND REQUIREMENTS[1]

NANCY F. BUTTE AND BENJAMIN CABALLERO

ENERGETICS OF INTERMEDIATE METABOLISM

To sustain life, humans must eat. The chemical free energy of food is the only form of energy humans can use to maintain the structural and biochemical integrity of the body; to perform internal work of circulation, respiration, and muscle contraction; and to perform external work (1–3). Our ability to use the chemical free energy of food results from the development of the biochemical, structural, and physiologic apparatus that permits the transformation of chemical free energy into other energy forms essential for life. Part of the energy from food, on the order of 5%, is thermodynamically obligated for conversion to heat because the entropy of the metabolic end products is greater than the initial substances (Fig. 5.1). Conversion of food energy into high-energy biochemical compounds is an inefficient process, with approximately 50% lost as heat. Through biochemical transformations, approximately 45% of the energy of food is available to the body, primarily as adenosine triphosphate (ATP). Eventually, all the energy of food is lost from the body in the form of heat or external work.

Energy is provided in the diet by protein, carbohydrate, fat, and alcohol. The energy in foods is expressed as a unit of heat, the calorie. A calorie is defined as the amount of heat required to raise the temperature of 1 g of water by 1°C from 15°C to 16°C. The scientific international unit of energy is the joule (J), defined as the energy expended when 1 kg is moved 1 m by a force of 1 newton. In 1956, an international committee standardized the equivalency of these units as 1 cal = 4.1868 J, but the figure of 4.184 is more commonly used in nutrition studies. For practicality, a kilocalorie (kcal), which is 1000 times the energy of a calorie (cal), is commonly used in nutrition. Hence, 1 kcal = 4.184 kJ, and 1 kJ = 0.0239 kcal. Another, less frequently used unit, is the thermochemical calorie, which is the heat liberated by the combustion of 1 g of pure benzoic acid and is also equivalent to 4.184 J (1).

The potential energy contribution of food is determined experimentally by measuring the heat evolved in a bomb calorimeter when foodstuffs are completely combusted to carbon dioxide (CO_2) and water (4). The actual amount of heat evolved per gram of foodstuff varies according to its chemical composition. Average values are 4.1 kcal/g of carbohydrate, 9.3 kcal/g of fat, and 5.4 kcal/g of protein. The body cannot oxidize nitrogen, and therefore energy resulting from the oxidation of the nitrogenous component of protein is unavailable to the body. Consequently, only 4.2 kcal/g protein is potentially available to the body. The physiologic fuel value is compromised further by the apparent digestibility of various foodstuffs that vary among food sources. These factors result in physiologic fuel values of 4 kcal/g for carbohydrate, 9 kcal/g for fat, and 4 kcal/g for protein, also known as the Atwater factors. The physiologic fuel value for alcohol is 7 kcal/g (Table 5.1).

Substrate oxidation rates are a function of dietary macronutrient intake and level of energy turnover (5). Protein oxidation is largely determined by protein intake, whereas

---

[1]**Abbreviations: ATP**, adenosine triphosphate; **BAT**, brown adipose tissue; **BEE**, basal energy expenditure; **BMR**, basal metabolic rate; **CO₂**, carbon dioxide; **DLW**, doubly labeled water; **DRI**, dietary reference intake; **EE**, energy expenditure; **EER**, estimated energy requirement; **FFA**, free fatty acid; **FFM**, fat free mass; **FM**, fat mass; **HR**, heart rate; **NPRQ**, nonprotein respiratory quotient; **PAL**, physical activity level; **P:O ratio**, phosphorylation-to-oxidation ratio; **RMR**, resting metabolic rate; **RQ**, respiratory quotient; **SMR**, sleeping metabolic rate; **TEE**, total energy expenditure; **TEF**, thermic effect of food; **UCP1**, uncoupling protein-1; **VCO₂**, carbon dioxide production; **VO₂**, oxygen consumption; **VO₂max**, maximal oxygen consumption.

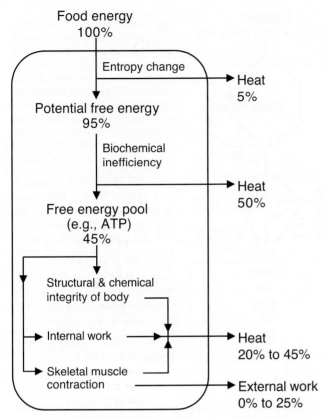

Fig. 5.1. Energy utilization within the body. The distribution of food energy within the body and its transfer to the environment as heat or external work is illustrated (see text for further details). *ATP,* adenosine triphosphate. (Reprinted with permission from Brown AC. Energy metabolism. In: Ruch TC, Patton HD, eds. Physiology and Biophysics III: Digestion, Metabolism, Endocrine Function and Reproduction. Philadelphia: WB Saunders, 1973:85–104.)

the relative contributions of glucose or free fatty acids (FFAs) to the fuel mix are more variable. Glucose oxidation is adjusted to carbohydrate intake to maintain stable glycogen stores. Fat intake, in contrast, does not promote its own oxidation, and under conditions of positive energy balance, some fat will be deposited. Most cells can use the metabolic intermediates of carbohydrates, fats, and proteins interchangeably to regenerate ATP, with a few exceptions. The brain preferentially uses glucose and is able to use ketone bodies after adaptation to starvation,

but it does not use FFAs (6). Red blood cells also depend on glucose. At rest, the brain (20%), internal organs (25% to 30%), and skeletal muscle (20%) account for the majority of energy turnover. During vigorous activity, skeletal muscle overwhelms the utilization of other tissues. In the postabsorptive state, FFAs are mainly oxidized by muscle, whereas during exertion, muscle's own glycogen reserve is used, with a subsequent shift toward use of FFAs mobilized from muscle fat stores and adipose tissue.

When alcohol is consumed, it promptly appears in the circulation and is oxidized at a rate determined largely by its concentration and by the activity of liver alcohol dehydrogenase. Oxidation of alcohol rapidly reduces the oxidation of the other substrates used for ATP regeneration. Ethanol oxidation proceeds in large part through conversion to acetate and oxidative phosphorylation. Approximately 80% of the energy liberated by ethanol oxidation is used to drive ATP regeneration, and approximately 20% is released as heat (7). Alcoholic beverages can contribute to weight gain in healthy persons consuming an otherwise adequate diet (8), in contrast to the pharmacologic effect of excessive ethanol, which can inhibit normal eating and can cause emaciation in persons with alcoholism.

Flatt and Tremblay (5) computed the ATP yield from oxidation of macronutrients based on the phosphorylation-to-oxidation (P:O) ratio and the ATP required to initiate degradation, transport, activation, and handling of the metabolic fuels (Fig. 5.2). Assuming a P:O ratio of 3:1 for the reoxidation of mitochondrial reduced nicotinamide adenine dinucleotide, the oxidation of 1 mol of glucose produces 38 mol ATP, but 2 mol is used for activation; therefore, the net ATP yield is 95%. Allowing for the costs of recycling through the Cori cycle, the glucose-alanine cycle and gluconeogenesis, the net postabsorptive ATP yield is approximately 82%. Accounting for the postprandial phase of digestion, absorption, and transport, the net ATP yield from dietary carbohydrate is 75%, such that the oxidation of 24 kcal of dietary carbohydrate is required to replace 1 mol of ATP. To calculate the ATP yield from dietary fat, the fatty acid oleate was used as an example. The oxidation of 1 mol of oleate yields 146 mol ATP but expends 5.5 mol ATP in lipolysis/reesterification and activation to oleyl-coenzyme A; therefore, the ATP yield for fat oxidation is

TABLE 5.1	**HEATS OF COMBUSTION, PHYSIOLOGIC ENERGY VALUES, HEAT EQUIVALENTS, AND CORRESPONDING VOLUMES OF OXYGEN AND CARBON DIOXIDE FOR CARBOHYDRATE, PROTEIN, FAT, AND ETHANOL OXIDATION**						

	ENERGY (kcal/g)			HEAT EQUIVALENTS			VOLUME	
FOOD	HEAT OF COMBUSTION	HUMAN OXIDATION	PHYSIOLOGIC VALUE	$\dot{V}O_2$ (kcal/L)	VCO_2 (kcal/L)	RQ	OXYGEN (L/g)	CO_2 (L/g)
Carbohydrate	4.1	4.1	4	5.05	5.05	1.00	0.81	0.81
Protein	5.4	4.2	4	4.46	5.57	0.80	0.94	0.75
Fat	9.3	9.3	9	4.74	6.67	0.71	1.96	1.39
Ethanol	7.1	7.1	7	4.86	7.25	0.67	1.46	0.98

RQ, respiratory quotient; VCO_2, carbon dioxide production; $\dot{V}O_2$, oxygen consumption.

Data from Brown AC. Energy metabolism. In: Ruch TC, Patton HD, eds. Physiology and Biophysics III: Digestion, Metabolism, Endocrine Function and Reproduction. Philadelphia: WB Saunders, 1973:85–104, with permission.

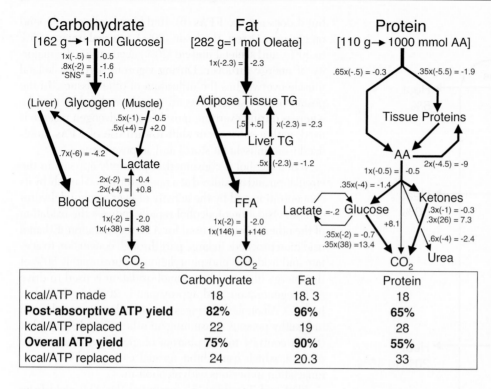

	Carbohydrate	Fat	Protein
kcal/ATP made	18	18. 3	18
Post-absorptive ATP yield	**82%**	**96%**	**65%**
kcal/ATP replaced	22	19	28
Overall ATP yield	**75%**	**90%**	**55%**
kcal/ATP replaced	24	20.3	33

Fig. 5.2. Adenosine triphosphate (ATP) yields from oxidation of carbohydrate, fat, and protein. Moles of substrate flowing through the metabolic pathways are in *brackets*, and the moles of ATP produced and expended per mole of substrate metabolized are in *parentheses*, assuming a phosphorylation-to-oxidation (P:O) ratio of 3 for the reoxidation of mitochondrial reduced nicotinamide adenine dinucleotide. For example, 38 ATPs are produced during the oxidation of 1 mole of glucose, but because of substrate handling, storage, and recycling costs, the postabsorptive ATP yield is approximately 82%, and the overall yield is 75%. *AA,* amino acid; *FFA,* free fatty acid; *SNS,* sympathetic nervous system; *TG,* triglyceride. (Reprinted with permission from Flatt JP, Tremblay A. Energy expenditure and substrate oxidation. In: Bray GA, Bouchard C, James WPT, eds. Handbook of Obesity. New York: Marcel Dekker, 1998.)

approximately 96%. Accounting for the postprandial phase, the net ATP yield from dietary fat is approximately 90%.

In the case of proteins, the oxidation of 1 mol of amino acids generates approximately 28.8 mol of ATP or 18 kcal/mol ATP. The costs of gluconeogenesis, ureagenesis, and protein resynthesis reduce the net postabsorptive ATP yield to 65%. Accounting for the postprandial phase, the overall ATP yield is 55%. Based on these estimates, the transport, storage, recycling, and activation dissipate approximately 10%, 25%, and 45% of the ATP produced in the oxidation of dietary fat, carbohydrate, and protein, respectively. Therefore, the corresponding net ATP yields are estimated to be 90%, 75%, and 55% with dietary fat, carbohydrate, and protein.

Lipogenesis from the conversion of dietary carbohydrate to fat is an inefficient process estimated at 25%. This pathway appears to be of minor importance in humans, because large amounts of dietary carbohydrate expand glycogen reserves, not body fat (9). Lipogenesis therefore does not account for the higher dissipation of dietary energy by carbohydrate compared with fat. Similarly, the energy dissipation by futile cycles or substrate cycles that dissipate ATP with no net change in the organism also appears to make only a minor contribution to overall energy economy. Futile cycles are thought to account for only a small percentage of total energy expenditure (TEE) (10).

ENERGY BALANCE

Energy balance is the accounting for the energy consumed in foods, losses in excreta, heat produced, and retention or secretion of organic compounds (4). Implicit in the delineation of energy balance is that energy is conserved. The energy balance may be expressed as follows:

$$E_{intake} - E_{feces} - E_{urine} - E_{combustible\ gas} - E_{expenditure} = E_{retention}\ or\ E_{secretion}$$

Digestible energy is the dietary energy absorbed by the gastrointestinal tract after accounting for loss in feces (11). Metabolizable energy is that energy available to the organism after accounting for losses in feces, urine, and combustible gases. Metabolizable energy is measured by meticulous energy balance techniques and was determined for human diets by Atwater in the early 1900s. The Atwater factors of 4, 9, and 4 kcal of metabolizable energy per gram of protein, fat, and carbohydrate, respectively, are widely used to express the energy content of foods in food composition tables, including those in the United States (12). The Atwater factors are applied to the protein estimated from its nitrogen content, fat determined by extraction, and carbohydrates determined by difference, after taking into account the water and ash in the food. In the United Kingdom, the metabolizable energy factors of 4, 9, and 3.75 kcal/g of protein, fat, and carbohydrate, respectively, are used in food composition tables (13). In this system, the metabolizable energy factor is applied to available carbohydrate, defined as the sum of free sugars, dextrins, starch, and glycogen, and the result is lower estimates of the caloric content of foods than in the Atwater system.

Humans can survive on foods with varying proportions of carbohydrates, fats, and proteins (14–18). The ability to shift from carbohydrate to fat as the main source of energy, coupled with substantial reserves of body fat, makes it possible to accommodate large fluctuations in energy intake and energy expenditure (EE). Energy balance is regulated by a complex set of neuroendocrine feedback mechanisms. Changes in energy intake or in EE trigger metabolic and behavioral responses aimed at restoring energy balance.

MEASUREMENT OF ENERGY INTAKE AND ENERGY EXPENDITURE

Several methods are used to assess dietary intake including weighed or observed diet records, dietary recalls and diaries, and food frequencies. It is now generally recognized that reported energy intakes tend to underestimate usual energy intake (19). Evidence of underreporting has been substantiated from measurements of TEE by the doubly labeled water (DLW) method (20, 21). Implausibly low energy intakes have been revealed when TEE was substantially greater than reported usual energy intakes in weight-stable individuals. Underreporting of food intake is pervasive, ranging from 10% to 45% depending on the age, gender, and body composition of the study subjects (22).

Methods for measuring EE include direct calorimetry, indirect calorimetry, and noncalorimetric methods (23). Direct calorimetry is the measurement of the heat emitted from the body over a given period (1, 24). A direct calorimeter chamber measures heat loss by radiation, convection, conduction, and latent heat arising from vaporization of water. Heat sink calorimeters capture the heat produced by liquid-cooled heat exchangers. Gradient layer calorimeters measure heat loss by a network of thermocouples in series surrounding the insulated chamber. Indirect calorimetry estimates heat production indirectly by measuring oxygen consumption ($\dot{V}O_2$), CO_2 production (VCO_2), and the respiratory quotient (RQ), which is equal to the ratio of the VCO_2 to $\dot{V}O_2$ (25). Indirect calorimetry arose from the observations of Lavoisier and Laplace that heat production of animals as measured by calorimetry was equal to that released when organic substances are burned, and that the same quantities of oxygen were consumed by the two processes. The RQ reflects substrate utilization. The complete oxidation of glucose results in an RQ equal to 1.0. The complete oxidation of fat and protein results in an RQ averaging about 0.71 and 0.84, respectively, depending on the chemical structure of the foodstuff. Specific RQs for FFAs range from 0.69 to 0.81. RQs of amino acids range from 0.56 to 1.00, with conventional food proteins ranging from 0.81 to 0.87. In mixed diets, the RQ is approximately 0.85. Lipogenesis, the conversion of carbohydrate to fat, can substantially increase the RQ. The conversion of fat to carbohydrate, in contrast, will lower the RQ to less than 0.70.

Substrate utilization can be determined from rates of $\dot{V}O_2$, VCO_2, and urinary nitrogen (23, 25). First, gas exchange must be corrected for the incomplete oxidation of protein. One gram of urinary nitrogen represents the combustion of an amount of protein that would require 5.92 L of oxygen and produce 4.75 L of CO_2. The $\dot{V}O_2$ and

VCO_2 associated with the protein oxidized are subtracted from the total and are used to compute a nonprotein RQ (NPRQ). The amount of protein oxidized may be calculated directly from urinary nitrogen assuming that 1 g of nitrogen represents 6.25 g of protein. The NPRQ is then used to calculate the proportions of carbohydrate and fat oxidized when the NPRQ is less than 1.00 (Table 5.2). When the NPRQ is greater than 1.00, net fat synthesis occurs, as shown in Figure 5.3. When the NPRQ is greater than 1.00, carbohydrate is used both for storage of energy and for oxidation (25).

Weir (26) demonstrated that the error in neglecting the effect of protein metabolism on the caloric equivalent of oxygen is 1% for each 12.3% of the total calories that arise from protein. The most widely used equation for the calculation of total heat output is by Weir:

$$EE \text{ (kcal)} = 3.941 \times \dot{V}O_2 \text{ (L)} + 1.106 \, VCO_2 \text{ (L)} - (2.17 \times UrN \text{ [g])}$$

or EE (kcal) $= 3.941 \times \dot{V}O_2$ (L) $+ 1 \, VCO_2$ (L)/(1 + 0.082 p)

where UrN is urinary nitrogen and p is the fraction of calories resulting from protein. Assuming approximately 12.5% of total calories will arise from protein; therefore, the foregoing equation can be reduced to the following:

$$EE \text{ (kcal)} = 3.9 \times \dot{V}O_2 \text{ (L)} + 1.1 \, VCO_2 \text{ (L)}$$

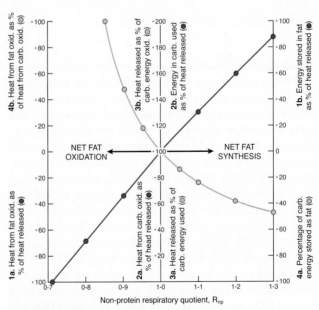

Fig. 5.3. Carbohydrate and fat utilization as a function of nonprotein respiratory quotient (NPRQ). The two curves demonstrate carbohydrate (starch, glycogen) utilization and fat (triglyceride) oxidation and synthesis with the ordinate axes displaying heat from fat oxidation as a percentage of heat released, heat from fat oxidation as a percentage of heat from carbohydrate oxidation, and the percentage of carbohydrate energy stored as fat and stored in fat as a percentage of heat released. (Reprinted with permission from Elia M, Livesey G. Theory and validity of indirect calorimetry during net lipid synthesis. Am J Clin Nutr 1988;47:591–607. Copyright American Journal of Clinical Nutrition, American Society for Clinical Nutrition.)

TABLE 5.2	NONPROTEIN RESPIRATORY QUOTIENT AND THE RELATIVE QUANTITY OF CARBOHYDRATE AND FAT OXIDIZED AND ENERGY PER LITER OF OXYGEN		
NONPROTEIN RESPIRATORY QUOTIENT	CARBOHYDRATE (g/L O_2)	FAT (g/L O_2)	ENERGY (kcal/L O_2)
0.707	0.000	0.502	4.686
0.71	0.016	0.497	4.690
0.72	0.055	0.482	4.702
0.73	0.094	0.465	4.714
0.74	0.134	0.450	4.727
0.75	0.173	0.433	4.739
0.76	0.213	0.417	4.751
0.77	0.254	0.400	4.764
0.78	0.294	0.384	4.776
0.79	0.334	0.368	4.788
0.80	0.375	0.350	4.801
0.81	0.415	0.334	4.813
0.82	0.456	0.317	4.825
0.83	0.498	0.301	4.838
0.84	0.539	0.284	4.850
0.85	0.580	0.267	4.862
0.86	0.622	0.249	4.875
0.87	0.666	0.232	4.887
0.88	0.708	0.215	4.899
0.89	0.741	0.197	4.911
0.90	0.793	0.180	4.924
0.91	0.836	0.162	4.936
0.92	0.878	0.145	4.948
0.93	0.922	0.127	4.961
0.94	0.966	0.109	4.973
0.95	1.010	0.091	4.985
0.96	1.053	0.073	4.998
0.97	1.098	0.055	5.010
0.98	1.142	0.036	5.022
0.99	1.185	0.018	5.035
1.00	1.232	0.000	5.047

Whole body respiratory calorimeters are small rooms in which the subject may reside comfortably for longer periods unencumbered by respiratory gas collection devices. In these rooms, the concentrations of oxygen (O_2) and CO_2 and airflow through the system are monitored continuously. Whole body calorimeters provide a controlled experimental environment to measure TEE and its components. Portable indirect calorimetric systems also have been devised to measure EE in field, clinical, and laboratory settings (27–29). The Douglas bag method has been used historically for many measurements of basal and resting metabolism. In this method, all expired air is collected into a nonpermeable bag with a capacity up to 150 L. After a known period, the volume of expired air at standard temperature and pressure dried, and the concentrations of O_2 and CO_2 are measured from which $\dot{V}O_2$ and $\dot{V}CO_2$ and RQ are calculated. Commercial metabolic carts in laboratory and clinical settings have largely replaced the Douglas bag method. For field measurements, several portable respirometers have been designed with oxygen analyzers as well as gas flow meters and electronics to process and store data. These systems require airtight masks, breathing valves, and nose clips to measure respiratory gas exchange quantitatively. Hood devices and canopies have been designed for more comfort, but they restrict movement.

Other methods to assess EE applicable to field conditions include heart rate (HR) monitoring and DLW. The HR monitoring method is based on the linear relationship between HR and EE (30). Because of variations resulting from age, sex, body size, fitness, and nutritional status, the relationship must be calibrated on an individual basis. Simultaneous measurements of EE and HR in subjects are performed across a range of activities to calibrate the individual. Other confounding factors such as ambient conditions, time of day, emotional state, hydration status, food and caffeine intake, and smoking may influence the EE:HR relationship. As a result, HR data on individuals are subject to error and may yield unreliable estimates of EE. When applied to groups of individuals, the HR monitoring method provides an acceptable estimate of TEE.

DLW is a stable (nonradioactive) isotope method that provides an estimate of TEE in free-living individuals. The DLW method was originally developed by Lifson et al for use in small animals (31, 32), and it was later adapted for humans (33, 34). Two stable isotopic forms of water ($H_2{}^{18}O$ and ^2H_2O) are administered to the individual, and their ^{18}O and ^2H disappearance rates from the body are monitored for 7 to 21 days, equivalent to one to three half-lives for these isotopes. The disappearance rate of ^2H_2O reflects water flux, whereas that of $H_2{}^{18}O$ reflects water flux plus VCO_2, because of the rapid equilibration of the body water and bicarbonate pools by carbonic anhydrase. The difference between the two disappearance rates is used to calculate VCO_2. Assuming an RQ, $\dot{V}O_2$ and, hence, EE are calculated. When energy balance prevails, the average RQ may be estimated from the composition of the diet by using the food quotient (35). If substantial gains or losses of body constituents are known to occur during the period of measurement, appropriate adjustments must be made in estimating the RQ. Under field conditions, this method is accurate within 5% or better. The advantage of this technique is the noninvasive, nonintrusive manner in which it measures TEE. In weight-stable individuals, the DLW method may be used to assess energy requirements. The disadvantages of the method are the high cost of ^{18}O and expensive, sophisticated mass spectrometric equipment and the expertise required to measure ^{18}O and ^2H.

HUMAN ENERGY REQUIREMENTS

Human energy requirements are composed of basal metabolism, thermogenesis, physical activity, external work, and energy costs of depositing new tissues during growth and pregnancy and secreting milk during lactation. The utilization of metabolizable energy is represented in terms of energy balance and thermal balance in Figure 5.4. Since the 1960s, a resurgence in whole body energy metabolism has led to a reexamination of the major factors contributing to TEE (2).

Basal Metabolism

The basal metabolic rate (BMR) is defined as the rate of EE in the postabsorptive state after a 12-hour overnight fast. The BMR is measured while the subject is supine, awake, and motionless in a thermoneutral environment. The BMR

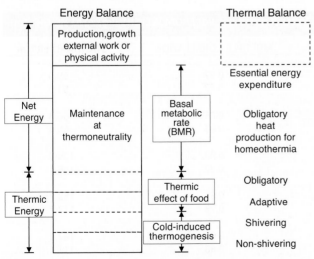

Fig. 5.4. Utilization of metabolizable energy represented in terms of energy balance and thermal balance. (Reprinted with permission from Kinney JM. Energy metabolism: heat, fuel and life. In: Kinney JM, Jeejeebhoy KN, Hill GL et al. Nutrition and Metabolism in Patient Care. Philadelphia: WB Saunders, 1988:3–34.)

represents the energy needed to sustain the metabolic activities of cells and tissues plus the energy to maintain blood circulation and respiration in the awake state. The sleeping metabolic rate (SMR) is approximately 5% to 10% lower than the BMR (36). The BMR is affected by age, gender, body composition, and nutritional and health status. For practical considerations, the resting metabolic rate (RMR) is often measured instead of the BMR. By definition, the RMR is measured under the same experimental conditions as the BMR except a 3- to 4-hour fasting period is required, and the time of day and prior physical activity are not controlled. The RMR is approximately 10% to 20% higher than the BMR. The BMR historically was normalized to body surface area, but it is now more appropriately normalized to body weight or fat free mass (FFM).

In 1932, Brody and Kleiber described the empiric relationship between BMR and body weight (1). The logarithm of metabolic rate was found to be a linear function of the logarithm of body weight, and therefore, metabolic rate could best be described as a power of body weight. When the BMR was measured across a wide range of species of varying sizes, it was estimated that

$$BMR = 70\ WT^{3/4}$$

where WT, weight, is in kg, and BMR is in kcal/kg$^{3/4}$/day

The Brody-Kleiber relationship does not hold for all species or within a species, however. Within a species, the relationship between minimal metabolism and body weight varies with a power of weight less than the 0.75 that relates to adults, because young individuals have higher metabolic rates per unit metabolic size.

In 1919, Harris and Benedict (37) published prediction equations for BMR based on sex, height, age, and weight:

$$BMR_{women}\ (kcal/day) = 665 + (9.6 \times Weight\ [kg]) + (1.8 \times Height\ [cm]) - (4.7 \times Age\ [years])$$

$$BMR_{men}\ (kcal/day) = 66 + (13.7 \times Weight\ [kg]) + (5 \times Height\ [cm]) - (6.8 \times Age\ [years])$$

Schofield et al (38) derived widely used equations for predicting BMR using data on 7549 persons. The equations predicting BMR from weight and height or from weight alone are provided in Tables 5.3 and 5.4 for separate age-sex groups. Inclusion of height and weight was shown to be advantageous for very young and elderly persons; for older children and adults, weight-alone equations performed as well as the more complex equations. Although the Schofield equations predict the BMR reasonably in some populations, they overestimated the BMR in some tropical populations by 8% to 10% (39, 40). Other studies, however, did not confirm these findings (41, 42). In addition, studies of well-nourished immigrants from tropic to temperate climates found similar BMR/kg body weight values (43–45).

FFM contains the metabolically active compartments of the body and therefore is the major predictor of basal metabolism. The contribution of FFM and fat mass (FM)

TABLE 5.3	SCHOFIELD EQUATIONS FOR ESTIMATING BASAL METABOLIC RATE (kcal/d) FROM WEIGHT (kg)			
		n	MULTIPLE CORRELATION	STANDARD ERROR
	Children: <3 y			
Males	BMR = 59.5 wt − 30.4	162	0.95	69.9
Females	BMR = 58.3 wt − 31.1	137	0.96	58.7
	3–10 y			
Males	BMR = 22.7 wt + 504.3	338	0.83	67.0
Females	BMR = 20.3 wt + 485.9	413	0.81	69.9
	10–18 y			
Males	BMR = 17.7 wt + 658.2	734	0.93	105.2
Females	BMR = 13.4 wt + 692.6	575	0.80	111.4
	Adults: 18–30 y			
Males	BMR = 15.0 wt + 692.1	2879	0.65	153.8
Females	BMR = 14.8 wt + 486.6	829	0.73	119.2
	30–60 y			
Males	BMR = 11.5 wt + 873.0	646	0.60	167.9
Females	BMR = 8.1 wt + 845.6	372	0.68	111.7
	>60 y			
Males	BMR = 11.7 wt + 587.7	50	0.71	164.8
Females	BMR = 9.1 wt + 658.4	38	0.68	108.3

BMR, basal metabolic rate; wt, weight.

Reprinted with permission from Schofield WN, Schofield C, James WPT. Basal metabolic rate. Hum Nutr Clin Nutr 1985;39C:1–96.

to the variability in RMR was examined in a metaanalysis of seven published studies (46). FFM was the single best predictor of RMR, and it accounted for 73% of the variability; FM accounted for only an additional 2%. Adjusted for FFM, the RMR did not differ between genders, but it did between lean and obese persons. In another meta-analysis, the relationship of the RMR with FFM was found to be nonlinear across a wide range of infants to adults (47). RMR/kg of weight or RMR/kg FFM falls as mass increases, because the relative contributions made by the most metabolically active tissues (brain, liver, and heart) decline as body size increases.

Basal metabolism declines with age at a rate of approximately 1% to 2% per decade in weight-constant persons (48). This decline is attributable to loss of FFM and gain of less metabolically active fat associated with aging. Endurance training may attenuate the decline in the BMR seen with aging (49). Gender differences in basal metabolism also are evident. Lower BMR in women is largely attributed to differences in body composition, although hormonal differences also may play a role. The BMR varies throughout the menstrual cycle (50, 51). The BMR is approximately 6% to 15% lower in the preovulatory (follicular) phase than in the premenstrual (luteal)

TABLE 5.4	SCHOFIELD EQUATIONS FOR ESTIMATING BASAL METABOLIC RATE (kcal/d) FROM WEIGHT (kg) AND HEIGHT (m)			
		n	MULTIPLE CORRELATION	STANDARD ERROR
	Children: <3 y			
Males	BMR = 1.67 wt + 1517 ht − 618	162	0.97	58.0
Females	BMR = 16.2 wt + 1023 ht − 413	137	0.97	51.6
	3–10 y			
Males	BMR = 19.6 wt + 130 ht + 415	338	0.83	66.8
Females	BMR = 17.0 wt + 162 ht + 371	413	0.81	69.4
	10–18 y			
Males	BMR = 16.2 wt + 137 ht + 516	734	0.93	105.0
Females	BMR = 8.4 wt + 466 ht + 200	575	0.82	108.1
	Adults: 18–30 y			
Males	BMR = 15.0 wt − 10.0 ht + 706	2879	0.65	153.2
Females	BMR = 13.6 wt + 283 ht + 98	829	0.73	117.7
	30–60 y			
Males	BMR = 11.5 wt − 2.6 ht + 877	646	0.60	167.3
Females	BMR = 8.1 wt + 1.4 ht + 844	372	0.68	111.4
	>60 y			
Males	BMR = 9.1 wt + 972 ht − 834	50	0.74	157.7
Females	BMR = 7.9 wt + 458 ht + 17.7	38	0.73	102.5

BMR, basal metabolic rate; ht, height; wt, weight.

Reprinted with permission from Schofield WN, Schofield C, James WPT. Basal metabolic rate. Hum Nutr Clin Nutr 1985;39C:1–96.

phase of the cycle. Even when BMR data are adjusted for gender differences in FFM and FM, however, differences in BMR still exist, possibly because of variations in relative contributions of organs and tissues to FFM.

The FFM compartment consists of organs and tissues with a wide range of specific metabolic rates (52). The RMRs of skeletal muscle (14.5 $kcal \cdot kg^{-1} \cdot d^{-1}$) and adipose tissue ($4.5$ $kcal \cdot kg^{-1} \cdot d^{-1}$) are low relative to the metabolic rates of brain (240 $kcal \cdot kg^{-1} \cdot d^{-1}$), liver ($200$ $kcal \cdot kg^{-1} \cdot d^{-1}$), heart, and kidneys ($440$ $kcal \cdot kg^{-1} \cdot d^{-1}$). Together, the brain, liver, heart, and kidneys account for approximately 60% to 70% of RMR in adults, but they represent less than 6% of body weight. Skeletal muscle accounts for only 20% to 30% of RMR and comprises 40% to 50% of body weight.

The contribution of organ and tissue masses to the variability in RMR has been investigated using magnetic resonance imaging and echocardiography methods to measure liver, kidney, spleen, heart, and brain masses (53–57). In a comprehensive study of 89 adults, the addition of trunk organ masses and brain explained 5% more of the variance in RMR beyond that accounted for by FFM and FM (55). Furthermore, the organ masses reduced the role of age, race, and sex in explaining the variance in RMR, in agreement with another study in elderly persons (56). The decline in RMR in growing children is attributed to both a decrease in the proportion of some metabolically active organs and tissues and changes in the metabolic rate of specific organs and tissues (54).

Ethnicity also may affect basal metabolism. Numerous studies documented lower BMR in African-American than white adults (58–61) and children (62–65). The BMR, expressed per kilogram of body weight or per kilogram of FFM, is on the order of 5% to 10% lower in African-Americans compared with whites. Differences in relative contributions of organs and tissues to FFM may explain the differences in BMR among ethnic groups. Lower RMR in African-American women compared with white women is attributed to the greater proportion of low-metabolic-rate skeletal muscle and bone in African-Americans (57).

Thermogenesis

Thermogenesis augments basal metabolism in response to stimuli unassociated with muscular activity. Stimuli include food ingestion and cold and heat exposure. Thermogenesis has two components: obligatory and facultative thermogenesis (23, 66). Obligatory thermogenesis depends on the energy cost of digesting, absorbing, and processing or storing nutrients. The magnitude of this component is determined by the metabolic fate of the ingested substrate. Obligatory thermogenesis also may be potentiated by exercise, a frequent meal pattern, and increased meal size. Facultative or regulatory thermogenesis represents the additional EE not accounted for by the known energy costs of obligatory thermogenesis. The sympathetic nervous system plays a role in modulating facultative thermogenesis.

The thermic effect of food (TEF) refers to the increase in EE elicited by food consumption (1). The increments in EE above BMR, divided by the energy content of the food consumed, vary from 5% to 10% for carbohydrate, 0% to 5% for fat, and 20% to 30% for protein. A mixed meal elicits an increase in EE equivalent to approximately 10% of the calories consumed.

Cold- and heat-induced thermogenesis refers to the increase in EE that is induced at ambient temperatures lower or higher than the zone of thermoneutrality. Studies consistently suggest that low–normal temperatures of 20°C to 22°C and high temperatures of 28°C to 30°C are associated with an increase in sedentary EE of 2% to 5% compared with temperatures of 24°C to 27°C. Because people usually adjust their clothing and environment to maintain comfort, the additional energy cost of thermoregulation has a minimal effect on TEE.

Brown adipose tissue (BAT) has long been recognized to play a unique role in facultative thermogenesis in rodents. Uncoupling protein-1 (UCP1) in the inner mitochondrial membrane of BAT is responsible for this adaptive thermogenic process. UCP1 allows brown adipocytes to dissipate the mitochondrial proton electrochemical gradient that normally drives ATP synthesis (67). Evidence of the presence of BAT in humans has prompted a reappraisal of its role in human physiology. Fluorodeoxyglucose positron emission tomography (FDG PET) used to trace tumor metastasis revealed symmetric areas of increased tracer uptake in the upper parts of the body corresponding to BAT (68). Human depots of BAT were found in the supraclavicular and the neck regions with some additional paravertebral, mediastinal, paraaortic, and suprarenal localizations. The presence of BAT-unique UCP1 demonstrated in samples of adipose tissue from the neck of 35 patients confirmed the presence of BAT (69). BAT activity is induced acutely by cold exposure and is stimulated by the sympathetic nervous system (70). BAT has the potential to be of metabolic significance in normal human physiology.

Other substances, such as caffeine, can increase the BMR by 10% to 30% for 1 to 3 hours (71). On a daily basis, normal caffeine consumption may cause a modest 3% increase in TEE (72). Drugs such as amphetamines, ephedrine, and some antidepressants stimulate the sympathetic nervous system and, in turn, increase metabolism, whereas propranolol, reserpine, or bethanidine may depress it. The effect of smoking on the BMR is unclear (73, 74), but one study showed a 10% increase in 24-hour EE in a room calorimeter associated with smoking 24 cigarettes (75).

Physical Activity

EE for physical activity represents the most variable component of TEE. Physical activity level (PAL) is defined as the ratio of daily TEE to basal energy expenditure (BEE) (TEE/BEE) and is commonly used to describe typical activity levels. PAL for sedentary individuals varied from 1.3 to 1.5, with an average value of 1.35 among nine studies (21). In whole room calorimeter studies, the TEE/BEE ratio averaged 1.32 in groups with no exercise, 1.42 in those who did 30 to 75 minutes/day of exercise, and 1.60 in those who did 100 to 180 minutes/day (76). The value of $1.4 \times$ BMR represents maintenance energy requirement and covers BMR, TEF, and minimal activity. In more active groups, the PAL ranges from 1.4 to 1.7, and it ranges from 2.0 to 2.8 in very active groups.

The energy costs of discrete physical activities have been made using indirect calorimetry (77, 78). Ainsworth et al (79) provided comprehensive tables to estimate the energy expended in discrete physical activities for adults.

The energetic efficiency for the conversion of dietary energy into physical work is remarkably constant in humans for non–weight-bearing activities (1, 3, 80–82). The metabolic cost of performing specific physical activities is highly reproducible under standardized test conditions. Under optimal conditions, the net efficiency (external work/internal energy conversion rate increase necessary to accomplish the work) of the body is approximately 25% to 27%, but under typical circumstances, the mechanical efficiency of the body is considerably less. This finding does not imply that the energy cost of activities is constant among individuals, however. Energy cost of activities among individuals varies because of differences in weight and skill. For weight-bearing physical activities, the cost is roughly proportional to body weight.

Excess postexercise $\dot{V}O_2$ refers to the small increase in EE, which occurs for some time after the exercise has been completed. Excess postexercise $\dot{V}O_2$ is estimated to be approximately 14% of the increment in expenditure that occurs during the exercise itself (83). A sustained increase in postexercise basal metabolism occurs only after intense and prolonged exercise (70% to 75% maximal $\dot{V}O_2$ [$\dot{V}O_2$max] for 80 to 90 minutes or longer), and even this increase is small relative to the energy expended in exercise. Moderate levels of exercise do not appear to increase subsequent EE markedly.

Substrate utilization during exercise depends mainly on relative intensity. Fat is the main energy source in muscle and at the whole body level during rest and mild exercise (84). As exercise intensity increases, a shift from the predominant use of fat to carbohydrate occurs. Other factors such as exercise duration, gender, training status, and dietary history play secondary roles (85). The peak rate of fat oxidation is achieved at approximately 45% of $\dot{V}O_2$max, and for exercises at greater than 50% of $\dot{V}O_2$max, the oxidation of FFAs declines in muscle, both as a percentage of total energy and on an absolute basis. The main carbohydrate energy source is muscle glycogen, supplemented by blood glucose and lactate. If exercise persists beyond 60 to 90 minutes, fat oxidation will rise as carbohydrate fuel sources become depleted. In this case, the intensity of exercise must drop because of depletion of muscle glycogen, decreased blood glucose, and fatigue (80).

Growth

In infants and children, the energy requirement includes the energy associated with the deposition of tissues. The energy requirement for growth relative to maintenance is low except for the first months of life. As a percentage of total energy requirements, the energy cost of growth decreases from 35% at 1 month to 3% at 12 months of age, and it remains low until puberty, at which time it increases to 4% (82). During childhood, girls grow slightly more slowly than boys, and girls have slightly more body fat. During adolescence, the gender differences in body composition are accentuated (86–89). Adolescence in boys is characterized by rapid acquisition of FFM, a modest increase in FM in early puberty, followed by a decline. Adolescence in girls is characterized by a modest increase in FFM and continual FM accumulation.

Pregnancy and Lactation

The additional energy requirements of pregnancy include increased basal metabolism and energy cost of physical activity and energy deposition in maternal and fetal tissues. The BMR increases as a result of the metabolic contribution of the uterus and fetus and the increased internal work of the heart and lungs (90). In late pregnancy, the fetus accounts for approximately 50% of the increment in BMR. A 3-kg fetus uses approximately 8 mL O_2/kg/minute or 56 kcal/kg/day (91). The energy cost of weight-bearing activities was increased by 19% after 25 weeks of gestation (92). The gross energy cost of non–weight-bearing activities increased on the order of 10% and the net cost on the order of 6% in late pregnancy (92). The energy cost of tissue deposition can be calculated from the amount of protein and fat deposited in the fetus, placenta, amniotic fluid, uterus, breasts, blood, extracellular fluid, and adipose tissue. Hytten and Chamberlain (90) estimated that 925 g protein and 3.8 kg fat, equivalent to 41,500 kcal, were associated with a weight gain of 12.5 kg and a birth weight of 3.4 kg.

Consistent with the additional energy cost of milk synthesis, basal metabolism of lactating women increased on the order of 4% to 5% (93–96). Although TEE may be slightly lower in the first months postpartum, TEE does not appear to differ from nonpregnant, nonlactating values thereafter (93, 94, 97, 98). Energy cost of lactation is estimated from milk production rates and the energy density of human milk. Milk production rates averaged 0.78 L/day from 0 to 6 months postpartum (99–101) and 0.6 L/day from 6 to 12 months postpartum (102). Energy density measured by bomb calorimetry or proximate macronutrient analysis averaged at 0.67 (range, 0.64 to 0.74) kcal/g (103). Energy mobilized from maternal tissue stores can subsidize the energy cost of lactation. Gradual weight loss averaging −0.8 kg/month in the first 6 months postpartum is typical in well-nourished lactating women (93).

ASSESSMENT OF ENERGY REQUIREMENTS

Energy requirements are defined as the levels of metabolizable energy intake from food that will balance EE as well as cover the needs for growth, pregnancy, and lactation. Recommendations for the nutrient intakes of individuals are generally set to provide enough to meet or exceed the requirements of almost all healthy persons in a given gender–age group, and enough to allow reasonable fast recovery of losses that may have been incurred. For most nutrients, individual requirements correspond to the population average requirement plus two standard deviations as a safety factor to ensure that the requirements provide for the needs of nearly all (~95%) the healthy persons in the population. This approach is reasonable for nutrients for which modest excess intakes present no health risks; however, excess energy intake is eventually deposited in the form of body fat, which does provide a means to maintain metabolism during periods of limited food intake, although it can result in obesity.

Desirable levels of energy intake should be commensurate with EE to achieve energy balance. Energy balance was considered inadequate as a sole criterion for setting energy requirements in the 1985 *Technical Report* published by the Food and Agriculture Organization/World Health Organization/United Nations University Expert Consultation on Energy and Protein Requirement (104), however. It stated:

> The energy requirement of an individual is a level of energy intake from food that will balance energy expenditure when the individual has a body size and composition, and level of physical activity, consistent with long-term good health; and that would allow for the maintenance of economically necessary and socially desirable physical activity. In children and pregnant or lactating women the energy requirement includes the energy needs associated with the deposition of tissues or the secretion of milk at rates consistent with good health.

This definition implies that desirable energy intakes should support healthy body weights and composition and adequate PALs. Although theoretically it is possible to maintain energy balance and to avoid excess weight gain by reducing dietary energy intake only, optimizing both energy intake *and* output has important advantages. First, some evidence suggests that the ability to control food intake may be reduced at very low PALs (105). Second, marked reductions in food intake may make it difficult to fulfill the requirements for essential nutrients such as vitamins and minerals. Implicit in this statement is that desirable energy intakes for obese persons are less than their EE, because weight loss and establishment of a lower body weight are desirable for them. For underweight persons, conversely, desirable energy intakes are greater than their EE to permit weight gain and maintenance of a higher body weight. Unlike other nutrients, body weight can be used to monitor the adequacy or inadequacy of habitual energy intake. Body weight provides a readily monitored indicator of the adequacy or inadequacy of habitual energy intake. Chronic energy deficiency or energy excess eventually will manifest as wasting or obesity. Weight-for-height indices and body mass index are used to assess the weight status of individual persons as well as population groups (106, 107).

The factorial method historically has been used to assess energy requirements (102, 108). In this approach, TEE is estimated from BEE (i.e., BMR extrapolated to 24 hours) and activity EE derived from the time devoted to different activities and the energy costs of each activity. Limitations of this approach include the accuracy of the BMR predictions, data availability of energy costs of all activities, and the difficulty in estimating random, spontaneous movement. Compared with the DLW method, the factorial method has been found to give significantly higher estimates of TEE (109, 110). Alternatively, the expansive DLW database of TEE measurements can be used to estimate energy requirements.

DIETARY REFERENCE INTAKES: ESTIMATED ENERGY REQUIREMENT

Dietary reference intakes (DRIs) are published by the Food and Nutrition Board of the Institute of Medicine and are intended for healthy persons in the United States and Canada (111). The estimated energy requirement (EER) is defined as the average dietary intake that is predicted to maintain energy balance in a healthy adult of a defined age, gender, weight, and height, and PAL consistent with health. In children and pregnant and lactating women, the EER is taken to include the needs associated with the deposition of tissues or the secretion of milk at rates consistent with health.

The EER was based on TEE measured by the DLW method (111). A normative DLW database was compiled on TEE values of 407 adults and 525 normal-weight children. Four PALs were defined to reflect sedentary, low active, active, and very active levels of EE. The sedentary PAL category (PAL = 1.0 − 1.39) reflects BEE, TEF, and activity EE. In addition to the activities that are required for independent living, the low active PAL category (PAL = 1.4 − 1.59) encompasses walking 2.5 miles/day or the equivalent EE in other activities; the active PAL category (PAL = 1.6 − 1.89) includes walking 6 miles/day or its equivalent; and the very active PAL (PAL = 1.9 − 2.5) reflects walking 12 miles/day or equivalent. Stepwise multiple linear regression was used to develop prediction equations of TEE from age, gender, weight, height, and PAL category. The general equation was as follows:

$$\text{TEE (kcal/day)} = A + B \times \text{Age (years)} + PC \times (D \times \text{Weight [kg]} + E \times \text{Height [m]})$$

where A is the constant term; B is the age coefficient; PC is the physical activity coefficient for sedentary, low active, active, and very active PAL categories; D is the

TABLE 5.5	EQUATIONS FOR ESTIMATED ENERGY REQUIREMENTS FOR GENDER-AGE GROUPINGS AND PHYSICAL ACTIVITY COEFFICIENTS FOR SEDENTARY, LOW ACTIVE, ACTIVE, AND VERY ACTIVE PHYSICAL ACTIVITY LEVELS				
GENDER, AGE CATEGORY	EQUATIONS FOR ESTIMATED ENERGY REQUIREMENTS (kcal/d)	PA PAL = SEDENTARY	PA PAL = LOW ACTIVE	PA PAL = ACTIVE	PA PAL = VERY ACTIVE
Males, Females 0–3 mo	$(89 \times$ Weight [kg] $- 100) + 175$				
Males, Females 4–6 mo	$(89 \times$ Weight [kg] $- 100) + 56$				
Males, Females 7–12 mo	$(89 \times$ Weight [kg] $- 100) + 22$				
Males, Females 13–35 mo	$(89 \times$ Weight [kg] $- 100) + 20$				
Males, 3–8 y	$88.5 - 61.9 \times$ Age [y] $+ PA \times (26.7 \times$ Weight [kg] $+ 903 \times$ Height [m]) $+ 20$	1.00	1.13	1.26	1.42
Females, 3–8 y	$135.3 - 30.8 \times$ Age [y] $+ PA \times (10.0 \times$ Weight [kg] $+ 934 \times$ Height [m]) $+ 20$	1.00	1.16	1.31	1.56
Males, 9–18 y	$88.5 - 61.9 \times$ Age [y] $+ PA \times (26.7 \times$ Weight [kg] $+ 903 \times$ Height [m]) $+ 25$	1.00	1.13	1.26	1.42
Females, 9–18 y	$135.3 - 30.8 \times$ Age [y] $+ PA \times (10.0 \times$ Weight [kg] $+ 934 \times$ Height [m]) $+ 25$	1.00	1.16	1.31	1.56
Males, >19 y	$662 - 9.53 \times$ Age [y] $+ PA \times (15.91 \times$ Weight [kg] $+ 539.6 \times$ Height [m]	1.00	1.11	1.25	1.48
Females, >19 y	$354 - 6.91 \times$ Age [y] $+ PA \times (9.36 \times$ Weight [kg] $+ 726 \times$ Height [m])	1.00	1.12	1.27	1.45

PA, physical activity coefficient; PAL, physical activity level.

Reprinted with permission from Food and Nutrition Board, Institute of Medicine. Dietary Reference Intakes for Energy, Carbohydrate, Fiber, Fat, Fatty Acids, Cholesterol, Protein, and Amino Acids. 5th ed. Washington, DC: National Academy Press, 2002.

weight coefficient; and E is the height coefficient. EER was derived from TEE, plus an allowance for growth in the case of children. The equations for predicting EER of specific gender-age groupings are shown in Table 5.5.

Infants and Children

The energy requirements of infants and young children should balance EE at PALs conducive to normal development and should allow for deposition of tissues at rates consistent with health. Because of the dominant contribution of the brain (60% to 70%), basal metabolism is highest during the first years of life (112). The BMR of term infants ranges from 43 to 60 kcal/kg/day or two to three times greater than in adults (113). The BMR and TEE are influenced by age (older greater than younger), gender (males greater than females), and feeding mode (breast-fed less than formula-fed infants) (82). The DRI for infants and young children was based on a single equation using weight alone to predict TEE, plus an allowance for growth.

Energy requirements of older children and adolescents are defined to promote normal growth and maturation and to support a desirable PAL consistent with health. Energy requirements of children and adolescents are highly variable as a result of differences in growth rate and physical activity. Mean PALs estimated by DLW, HR monitoring, time-motion/diary, and time allocation records range from 1.3 to 1.5 for children less than 5 years of age and from 1.5 to 1.9 for children 6 to 18 years who are living in urban, industrialized settings (114). Although absolute EE

increases with age, weight-specific EE decreases across adolescence, primarily because of the decrease in BMR.

Haschke (115) estimated changes in body composition during adolescence from literature values of total body water, potassium, and calcium. FFM increases in boys, with peak deposition coinciding with peak rates of height gains. The percentage of FM increases during this period in girls, and it actually declines in boys.

The energy cost of growth is more accurately estimated from the individual costs of protein and fat deposition, because the composition of weight gain varies with age. The energy cost of growth ranges from 2.4 to 6.0 kcal/g (10 to 25 kJ/g), depending on the composition of the tissues deposited (116, 117). For the DRI, the energy cost of growth is estimated to be 175 kcal/day for the age interval 0 to 3 months, 60 kcal/day for 4 to 6 months, and 20 kcal/day for 7 to 35 months. Although the composition of newly synthesized tissues varies in childhood and adolescence, these variations have a minor impact on total energy requirements, because only approximately 20 to 25 kcal/day will be required for growth.

Adults

In weight-stable adults, energy requirements are equal to their TEE. The DLW database was used to derive separate TEE predictive equations for men and women based on age, height, weight, and PAL category. The age-related decline in TEE was found to amount to approximately 10 and 7 kcal/year for men and women, respectively. Marked variation is apparent in PALs, which depend on the occupational and recreational lifestyles of adults. The DRI equations for adults were corroborated in the Observing Protein and Energy Nutrition Study (OPEN) in which TEE was measured using DLW in 450 men and women, ages 40 to 69 years (118).

Pregnancy and Lactation

Current DRIs are based on empiric longitudinal data of the changes in TEE and body composition of pregnant women. Total energy deposition during pregnancy as a result of 3.7 kg fat and 925 g protein is estimated at 39,862 kcal or 180 kcal/day. As pregnancy progresses, the increment in basal metabolism is offset partially by decreased physical activity. Longitudinal measurements of TEE throughout pregnancy indicate a median change in TEE of approximately 8 kcal/gestational week, with a range of −57 to 107 kcal/week. The DRI for the extra energy required during pregnancy (340 and 452 kcal/day during the second and third trimesters, respectively) was estimated from the sum of the median change in TEE plus the energy deposition during pregnancy. During the first trimester, no additional energy intake was recommended, because TEE changes little and weight gain is minor. Additional factors that should enter into consideration to determine individual dietary energy intake goals include prepregnancy weight, obesity, and diabetes risk, among others.

The EER during lactation is estimated from TEE, milk energy output, and energy mobilization from tissue stores. Based on milk production rates of 0.78 and 0.6 L/day from 0 to 6 months and 6 to 12 months postpartum, respectively, and an energy density of 0.67 kcal/g milk, the additional energy cost of lactation would be 523 kcal/day during the first 6 months and 402 kcal/day during the second 6 months of lactation. Based on the average weight loss (0.8 kg/month, equivalent to 170 kcal/day) of well-nourished women during 0 to 6 months postpartum, the net energy cost of lactation is 330 kcal/day from 0 to 6 months postpartum. No further weight loss is assumed; therefore, the full cost of lactation is 400 kcal/day for 6 to 12 months postpartum.

REFERENCES

1. Kleiber M. The Fire of Life: An Introduction to Animal Energetics. Huntington, NY: Robert E. Kreiger, 1975.
2. Kinney JM. Energy metabolism: heat, fuel, and life. In: Kinney JM, Jeejeebhoy KN, Hill GL et al, eds. Nutrition and Metabolism in Patient Care. Philadelphia: WB Saunders, 1988:3–34.
3. Brown AC. Energy metabolism. In: Ruch TC, Patton HD, eds. Physiology and Biophysics III: Digestion, Metabolism, Endocrine Function and Reproduction. Philadelphia: WB Saunders, 1973:85–104.
4. Blaxter K. Energy Metabolism in Animals and Man. Cambridge: Cambridge University Press, 1989:1–336.
5. Flatt JP, Tremblay A. Energy expenditure and substrate oxidation. In: Bray GA, Bouchard C, James WPT, eds. Handbook of Obesity. New York: Marcel Dekker, 1998.
6. Elia M. Fuels of the tissues. In: Garrow JS, James WPT, Ralph A, eds. Human Nutrition and Dietetics. Edinburgh: Churchill Livingstone, 2000:37–59.
7. Siler SQ, Neese RA, Hellerstein MK. Am J Clin Nutr 1999;70:928–36.
8. Suter PM, Schutz Y, Jequier E. N Engl J Med 1992;326:983–7.
9. Acheson KJ, Schutz Y, Bessard T et al. Endocrinol Metab 1984;9:E62–E70.
10. Wolfe RR. The role of triglyceride–fatty acid cycling and glucose cycling in thermogenesis and amplification of net substrate flux in human subjects. In: Muller MJ, Danforth E, Burger AG, eds. Hormones and Nutrition in Obesity and Cachexia. New York: Springer, 1990.
11. Consolazio CF, Johnson RE, Pecora LJ. The computation of metabolic balances. In: Physiological Measurements of Metabolic Functions in Man. New York: McGraw-Hill, 1963:313–25.
12. Watt BK, Merrill AL. Composition of Foods. ARS Handbook No. 8. Washington, DC: US Government Printing Office, 1963:160.
13. Paul AA, Southgate DAT. McCance & Widdowson's the Composition of Foods. 4th ed. London: Her Majesty's Stationery Office, 1978.
14. Flatt JP. Energetics of intermediary metabolism. In: Garrow JS, Halliday D, eds. Substrate and Energy Metabolism in Man. London: John Libbey, 1985:58–69.
15. Flatt JP. Rec Adv Obes Res 1978;2:211–28.
16. Flatt JP. Diabetes Metab Rev 1988;4:571–81.
17. Flatt JP. Am J Clin Nutr 1995;62:820–36.
18. Flatt JP. Am J Clin Nutr 1987;45:296–306.
19. Black AE, Prentice AM, Goldberg GR et al. J Am Diet Assoc 1993;33:572–9.
20. Schoeller D. Metabolism 1995;44:18–22.
21. Goldberg GR, Black AE, Jebb SA et al. Eur J Clin Nutr 1991;45:569–81.
22. Johnson RK, Soultanakis RP, Matthews DW. J Am Diet Assoc 1998;98:1136–40.
23. Jequier E, Acheson K, Schutz Y. Assessment of energy expenditure and fuel utilization in man. Annu Rev Nutr 1987;7:187–208.
24. Holmes FL. Lavoisier and the Chemistry of Life. Madison, WI: University of Wisconsin Press, 1985.
25. Livesey G, Elia M. Am J Clin Nutr 1988;47:608–28.
26. Weir JB. J Physiol 1949;109:1–9.
27. Webb P. Human Calorimeters. New York: Praeger, 1985.
28. McLean JA. Animal and Human Calorimetry. Cambridge: Cambridge University Press, 1987.
29. Murgatroyd PR, Shetty PS, Prentice AM. Int J Obes 1993;17:549–68.
30. Schutz Y, Weinsier RL, Hunter G. Obes Res 2001;9:368–79.
31. Lifson N, McClintock R. J Theoret Biol 1966;12:46–74.
32. Lifson N, Gordon GB, McClintock R. J Appl Physiol 1955;7:704–10.
33. Schoeller DA, Van Santen E. J Appl Physiol 1982;53:955–9.
34. Schoeller DA, Leitch CA, Brown C. Am J Physiol 1986;1:R1137–43.
35. Black AE, Prentice AM, Coward WA. Hum Nutr Clin Nutr 1986;40C:381–91.
36. Garby L, Kurzer MS, Lammert O et al. Hum Nutr Clin Nutr 1987;41:225–33.

37. Harris JA, Benedict FG. A Biometric Study of Basal Metabolism. Publication 279. Washington, DC: Carnegie Institution, 1919.

38. Schofield WN, Schofield C, James WPT. Hum Nutr Clin Nutr 1985;39C:1–96.

39. Henry CJK, Rees DG. Eur J Clin Nutr 1991;45:177–85.

40. Piers LS, Shetty PS. Eur J Clin Nutr 1993;47:586–91.

41. Henry CJK, Piggott SM, Emery B. Hum Nutr Clin Nutr 1987;41C:397–402.

42. Soares MJ, Francis DG, Shetty PS. Eur J Clin Nutr 1993; 47:389–94.

43. Ulijaszek SJ, Strickland SS. Ann Hum Biol 1991;18:245–51.

44. Geissler CA, Aldouri MS. Ann Nutr Metab 1985;29:40–7.

45. Hayter JE, Henry CJK. Eur J Clin Nutr 1993;47:724–34.

46. Nelson KM, Weinsier RL, Long CL et al. Am J Clin Nutr 1992;56:848–56.

47. Weinsier RL, Schutz Y, Bracco D. Am J Clin Nutr 1992; 55:790–4.

48. Keys A, Brozek J, Henschel A et al. The Biology of Human Starvation. Minneapolis: University of Minnesota Press, 1950.

49. Poehlman ET, Danforth E Jr. Am J Physiol 1991;261:E233–9.

50. Bisdee JT, James WP, Shaw MA. Br J Nutr 1989;61:187–99.

51. Solomon SJ, Kurzer MS, Calloway DH. Am J Clin Nutr 1982; 36:611–6.

52. Elia M. Organ and tissue contribution to metabolic rate. In: Kinney JM, Tucker HN. Energy Metabolism: Tissue Determinants and Cellular Corollaries. New York: Raven Press, 1992:61–79.

53. Gallagher D, Belmonte D, Deurenberg P et al. Am J Physiol 1998;275:E249–58.

54. Hsu A, Heshka S, Janumala I et al. Am J Clin Nutr 2003; 77:1506–11.

55. Javed F, He Q, Davidson LE et al. Am J Clin Nutr 2010; 91:907–12.

56. Wang Z, Heshka S, Heymsfield SB et al. Am J Clin Nutr 2005;81:799–806.

57. Jones A Jr, Shen W, St-Onge MP et al. Am J Clin Nutr 2004; 79:780–6.

58. Albu J, Shur M, Curi M et al. Am J Clin Nutr 1997;66:531–8.

59. Carpenter WH, Fonong T, Toth MJ et al. Am J Physiol 1998;274:E98–101.

60. Foster GD, Wadden TA, Vogt RA. Obes Res 1997;5:1–8.

61. Jakicic JM, Wing RR. Int J Obes Relat Metab Disord 1998; 22:236–42.

62. Kaplan AS, Zemel BS, Stallings VA. J Pediatr 1996;129:643–7.

63. Treuth MS, Butte NF, Wong WW. Am J Clin Nutr 2000; 71:893–900.

64. Wong WW, Butte NF, Ellis KJ et al. J Clin Endocrinol Metab 1999;84:906–11.

65. Yanovski SZ, Renolds JC, Boyle AJ et al. Obes Res 1997;5: 321–5.

66. Jequier E. Clin Endocrinol Metab 1984;13:563–80.

67. Ricquier D. Int J Obes 2010;34(Suppl 1):S3–6.

68. Nedergaard J, Bengtsson T, Cannon B. Am J Physiol Endocrinol Metab 2007;293 E444–52.

69. Zingaretti MC, Crosta F, Vitali A et al. FASEB J 2009;23: 3113–20.

70. Cannon B, Nedergaard J. Int J Obes 2010;34:S7–16.

71. Acheson KJ, Azhorska-Markiewicz B, Pittet P et al. Am J Clin Nutr 1980;33:989–97.

72. Garrow JS, Webster JD. Thermogenesis to small stimuli in human energy metabolism. In: van Es AJH, ed. Human Energy Metabolism. Wageningen, Netherlands: Agricultural University, 1985.

73. Warwick PM, Chapple RS, Thomson ES. Int J Obes 1987; 11:229–37.

74. Dallosso HM, James WPT. Int J Obes 1984;8:365–75.

75. Hofstetter A, Schutz Y, Jequier E et al. N Engl J Med 1986;314:79–82.

76. Warwick PM. Predicting food energy requirements from estimates of energy expenditure. In: Truswell AS, Dreosti IE, English RM et al, eds. Recommended Nutrient Intakes: Australian Papers. Sydney: Australian Professional Publications, 1990:295–320.

77. Durnin JVGA, Passmore R. Energy, Work and Leisure. London: Heinemann Educational Books, 1967.

78. Passmore R, Durnin JVGA. Physiol Rev 1955;35:801–40.

79. Ainsworth BE, Haskell WL, Leon AS et al. Med Sci Sports Exerc 1993;25:71–80.

80. Pahud P, Ravussin E, Jequier E. Appl Physiol 1980;48:770–5.

81. Graham TE, Adamo KB. Can J Appl Physiol 1999;24: 393–415.

82. Butte NF, Wong WW, Hopkinson JM et al. Am J Clin Nutr 2000;72:1558–69.

83. Bahr R, Ingnes I, Vaage O et al. J Appl Physiol 1987;62: 485–90.

84. Brooks GA, Mercier J. J Appl Physiol 1994;76:2253–61.

85. Brooks GA, Fahey TD, White TP et al. Exercise Physiology: Human Bioenergetics and Its Applications. 3rd ed. Mountain View, CA: Mayfield Publishing, 2000.

86. Ellis KJ. Am J Clin Nutr 1997;66:1323–31.

87. Ellis KJ, Abrams SA, Wong WW. Am J Clin Nutr 1997;65: 724–731.

88. Forbes GB. Human Body Composition: Growth, Aging, Nutrition, and Activity. New York: Springer, 1987:1–350.

89. Tanner JM. Growth at Adolescence. 2nd ed. Oxford: Blackwell Scientific Publications, 1962.

90. Hytten FE, Chamberlain G. Clinical Physiology in Obstetrics. 2nd ed. Oxford: Blackwell Scientific Publications, 1991.

91. Sparks JW. Biol Neonate 1980;38:113–9.

92. Prentice AM, Spaaij CJK, Goldberg GR et al. Eur J Clin Nutr 1996;50:S82–111.

93. Butte NF, Wong WW, Hopkinson JM. J Nutr 2001;131:53–8.

94. Forsum E, Kabir N, Sadurskis A et al. Am J Clin Nutr 1992; 56:334–42.

95. Sadurskis A, Kabir N, Wager J et al. Am J Clin Nutr 1988; 48:44–9.

96. Spaaij CJK, van Raaij JMA, de Groot LCPGM et al. Am J Clin Nutr 1994;59:42–7.

97. Goldberg GR, Prentice AM, Coward WA et al. Am J Clin Nutr 1991;54:788–98.

98. Lovelady CA, Meredith CN, McCrory MA et al. Am J Clin Nutr 1993;57:512–8.

99. Allen JC, Keller RP, Archer P et al. Am J Clin Nutr 1991; 54:69–80.

100. Butte NF, Garza C, Stuff JE et al. Am J Clin Nutr 1984;39: 296–306.

101. Heinig MJ, Nommsen LA, Peerson JM et al. Am J Clin Nutr 1993;58:152–61.

102. Dewey KG, Finley DA, Lönnerdal B. J Pediatr Gastroenterol Nutr 1984;3:713–20.

103. Neville MC. Volume and caloric density of human milk. In: Jensen RG, ed. Handbook of Milk Composition. San Diego: Academic Press, 1995:99–113.

104. Food and Agriculture Organization/World Health Organization/United Nations University. Report of a Joint Consultation: Energy and Protein Requirements. Technical Report Series 724. Geneva: World Health Organization, 1985.

105. Stubbs RJ, Highes DA, Johnstone AM et al. Am J Clin Nutr 2004;79:62–9.

106. World Health Organization. Obesity: Preventing and Managing the Global Epidemic. Report of a World Health Organization Consultation on Obesity. Geneva: World Health Organization, 1998:1–276.

107. Kuczmarski RJ, Ogden CL, Grummer-Strawn LM et al. CDC Growth Charts: United States. Advance Data from Vital and Health Statistics. 314th ed. Hyattsville, MD: US Department of Health and Human Services, 2000:1–28.

108. National Research Council, Subcommittee on the Tenth Edition of the RDAs. Recommended Dietary Allowances. 10th ed. Washington, DC: National Academy Press, 1989.

109. Haggarty P, McNeill G, Abu Manneh MK et al. Br J Nutr 1994;72:799–813.

110. Jones PJ, Martin LJ, Su W et al. Can J Public Health 1997;88:314–9.

111. Food and Nutrition Board, Institute of Medicine. Dietary Reference Intakes for Energy, Carbohydrate, Fiber, Fat, Fatty Acids, Cholesterol, Protein, and Amino Acids. 5th ed. Washington, DC: National Academy Press, 2002.

112. Holliday M, Potter D, Jarrah A et al. Pediatr Res 1967;1:185–95.

113. Schofield WN, Schofield C, James WPT. Hum Nutr Clin Nutr 1985;39C:1–96.

114. Torun B, Davies PSW, Livingstone MBE et al. Eur J Clin Nutr 1996;50:35S–81S.

115. Haschke F. Body composition during adolescence. In: Body Composition Measurements in Infants and Children. Columbus, OH: Ross Laboratories, 1989.

116. Butte NF, Wong WW, Garza C. Proc Nutr Soc 1989;48:303–12.

117. Roberts SB, Young VR. Am J Clin Nutr 1988;48:951–5.

118. Tooze JA, Schoeller DA, Subar AF et al. Am J Clin Nutr 2007;86:382–7.

SUGGESTED READINGS

Flatt JP. McCollum award lecture: diet, lifestyle and weight maintenance. Am J Clin Nutr 1995;62:820–36.

Livesey G, Elia M. Estimation of energy expenditure, net carbohydrate utilization, and net fat oxidation and synthesis by indirect calorimetry: evaluation of errors with special reference to the detailed composition of fuels. Am J Clin Nutr 1988;47:608–28.

Elia M, Livesey G. Theory and validity of indirect calorimetry during net lipid synthesis. Am J Clin Nutr 1988;47:591–607.

Nedergaard J, Bengtsson T, Cannon B. Unexpected evidence for active brown adipose tissue in adult humans. Am J Physiol Endocrinol Metab 2007;293:E444–52.

Schoeller DA, Van Santen E. Measurement of energy expenditure in humans by doubly labeled water method. J Appl Physiol 1982;53:955–9.

6

WATER, ELECTROLYTES, AND ACID–BASE METABOLISM[1]

JAMES L. BAILEY, JEFF M. SANDS, AND HAROLD A. FRANCH

WATER

Humans can survive only a few days without a source of water. This essential nutrient plays an integral role in the maintenance and regulation of normal cellular and metabolic processes. Drinking liquids accounts for most of our water intake, but humans also consume significant amounts of water from fruits and vegetables. Water is also formed in the metabolism of many foods, although the amount made is less than daily losses. Urine losses account for most excretion, but sweat, respiration, and stool losses are important contributors to daily excretion.

Water Content and Distribution

Water constitutes approximately 54% of body weight in hospitalized adults without fluid and electrolyte disorders (1). The fraction of body weight that is water is highest in infants and children and progressively decreases with aging; it also varies depending on body fat content. Women and obese persons, who have higher body fat content, tend to have less water for any given weight. As a consequence, age and body fat content, as well as other factors, must be taken into account when total body water is calculated.

Water is present in both the intracellular and extracellular fluid compartments of the body as an aqueous solution containing electrolytes. Each cell has its own separate environment, but it also communicates with other cells through the extracellular space. Because cell membranes are permeable to water, this arrangement allows the concentration of ions per liter of solution (i.e., osmolality) to be the same throughout both compartments (2). To maintain normal metabolic functions, optimal ionic strength is critically important, particularly in the intracellular fluid, because most metabolic activities occur there.

---

[1]**Abbreviations: ADH**, antidiuretic hormone; **AG**, anion gap; **ATPase**, adenosine triphosphatase; **Ca^{2+}**, calcium; **CKD**, chronic kidney disease; **Cl$^-$**, chloride; **CO$_2$**, carbon dioxide; **DASH**, Dietary Approaches to Stop Hypertension; **DI**, diabetes insipidus; **ECG**, electrocardiographic; **ENaC**, epithelial sodium channel; **FDA**, Food and Drug Administration; **FFA**, free fatty acid; **GFR**, glomerular filtration rate; **GI**, gastrointestinal; **HCl**, hydrochloric acid; **HCO$_3$$^-$**, bicarbonate; **K$^+$**, potassium; **Mg^{2+}**, magnesium; **Na$^+$**, sodium; **NaCl**, sodium chloride; **NAD + (NAD$^+$)**, nicotinamide adenine dinucleotide; **NADH**, reduced nicotinamide adenine dinucleotide; **NAE**, net acid excretion; **NaHCO$_3$**, sodium bicarbonate; **NH$_4$$^+$**, ammonium; **P**, phosphorus; **PO$_4$$^-$**, phosphate; **PRAL**, potential renal acid load; **ROMK**, renal outer medulla potassium; **RTA**, renal tubular acidosis; **SIADH**, syndrome of inappropriate antidiuretic hormone secretion; **SPS**, sodium polystyrene sulfonate.

TABLE 6.1	VOLUMES OF BODY FLUID COMPARTMENTS[a]

Intracellular volume: 24.0 L (60%)
Extracellular volume: 16.0 L (40%)
   Interstitial volume: 11.2 L (28%)
   Plasma volume: 3.2 L (8%)
   Transcellular volume: 1.6 L (4%)

[a]A physiologically normal man weighing 73 kg (160 lb) with 40 L of total body water is used as a model.

Reprinted with permission from Oh MS, Uribarri J. Electrolytes, water, and acid-base balance. In: Shils ME, Shike M, Ross AC et al, eds. Modern Nutrition in Health and Disease. 10th ed. Baltimore: Lippincott Williams & Wilkins, 2006:149–93.

The quantity of sodium (Na^+) determines the volume of the extracellular compartment. Total body water varies from 30% to 53%, depending on whether chloride (Cl^-), inulin, or sulfate is used in the determination (3). It is greater in older subjects, in women, and when Cl^- is used as a marker (1, 4). Generally, a value of 40% of total body water is considered to represent the extracellular volume. The extracellular volume can be further divided into three fractions: interstitial (space between cells) volume, plasma volume, and transcellular (sequestered) water volume, which constitute 28%, 8%, and 4%, respectively, of the total body water (5). Thus, most extracellular fluid is partitioned between the extravascular and intravascular compartments, which are in equilibrium with each other (Table 6.1). Transcellular water represents fluids that are sequestered out of osmotic equilibrium, including luminal fluid of the gastrointestinal (GI) tract, the fluids of the central nervous system, and fluid in the eye, as well as the lubricating fluids at serous surfaces (3, 6).

Composition of the Body Fluid

Clinically, we measure electrolyte concentrations in the extracellular compartment only: plasma Na^+ is 140 mEq/L, potassium (K^+) is 4 mEq/L, Cl^- is 104 mEq/L, and bicarbonate (HCO_3^-) is 24 mEq/L. Although Na^+, Cl^-, and HCO_3^- are the main solutes in the extracellular fluid, K^+, magnesium (Mg^{2+}), phosphate (PO_4^-), and proteins (with negative charges) are the dominant solutes in the cell (Table 6.2). The concentrations of individual electrolytes inside the cell cannot be measured, but in most circumstances, the osmolality is exactly the same inside and outside the cell (7–9).

Difference between Serum Sodium Concentration and Total Body Sodium

Because we measure extracellular fluid in which Na^+ is the dominant cation, we use the serum Na^+ concentration as the main determinant of the body fluid osmolality (10). Dietary intake of more or less Na^+ does not usually change the blood Na^+ concentration. An increase in dietary Na^+ is accompanied by thirst, thus leading to a nearly proportional increase in water content as the body maintains the serum osmolality, and serum Na^+ concentration remains unchanged. If dietary Na^+ decreases, the kidney ensures that a proportional amount of water is also lost, and serum osmolality is again maintained. The total body Na^+ content is reflected in the extracellular volume, which is the main determinant of the vascular volume. When the total body Na^+ content rises, an increase in the vascular volume is expected, whereas a drop in the total body Na^+ content predicts a decrease in the vascular volume. Thus, the serum Na^+ concentration

TABLE 6.2	ELECTROLYTE CONCENTRATIONS IN EXTRACELLULAR AND INTRACELLULAR FLUIDS							
	PLASMA		INTERSTITIAL FLUID		PLASMA WATER		CELL WATER (MUSCLE)	
	(mEq/L)	(mmol/L)	(mEq/L)	(mmol/L)	(mEq/L)	(mmol/L)	(mEq/L)	(mmol/L)
Na^+	140	140	145.3	145.3	149.8	149.8	13	13
K^+	4.5	4.5	4.7	4.7	4.8	4.8	140	140
Ca^{2+}	5.0	2.5	2.8	2.8	5.3	5.3	1×10^{-7}	1×10^{-7}
Mg^{2+}	1.7	0.85	1.0	0.5	1.8	0.9	7.0	3.5
Cl^-	104	104	114.7	114.7	111.4	111.4	3	3
HCO_3^-	24	24	26.5	26.5	25.7	25.7	10	10
SO_4^-	1	0.5	1.2	0.6	1.1	0.44	—	—
PO_4^-	2.1	1.2[a]	2.3	1.3	2.2	1.2[a]	107	57[b]
Protein	15	1	8	0.5	16	1	40	2.5[c]
Organic anions	5	5[d]	5.6	5.6	5.3	5.3[d]	—	—

Ca^{2+}, calcium; Cl^-, chloride; HCO_3^-, bicarbonate; K^+, potassium; Mg^{2+}, magnesium; Na^+, sodium; PO_4^-, phosphate; SO_4^-, sulfate.

[a]The calculation is based on the assumption that the pH of the extracellular fluid is 7.4 and the dissociation constant (pK_a) of dihydrogen phosphate ($H_2PO_4^-$) is 6.8.
[b]The intracellular molal concentration of phosphate is calculated from the assumption the pK_a of organic phosphate is 6.1 and the intracellular pH 7.0.
[c]The calculation is based on the assumption that each millimole of intracellular protein has on the average 15 mEq, but the nature of cell proteins is not clearly known.
[d]The assumption has been that all the organic anions are all univalent.

Reprinted with permission from Oh MS, Uribarri J. Electrolytes, water, and acid-base balance. In: Shils ME, Shike M, Ross AC et al, eds. Modern Nutrition in Health and Disease. 10th ed. Baltimore: Lippincott Williams & Wilkins, 2006:149–93.

is not a good marker of total body Na^+. Blood pressure and physical signs of volume status such as the presence or absence of edema are much better markers of total body Na^+.

Dietary Salt Intake, Edema, and Blood Pressure

As the kidney retains Na^+, total body Na^+ content increases. This results in increases in vascular volume, in cardiac output, and in arterial blood pressure. At some point, pressure natriuresis occurs and causes the kidney to lose the excess Na^+ (11). In individuals with hypertension, a long-term increase in cardiac output results in arteriolar constriction, an autoregulatory mechanism that prevents transmission of systemic blood pressures to the capillary beds. With chronic arteriolar constriction, cardiac output gradually returns to baseline; however, peripheral vascular resistance remains elevated (12). Hypertension ensues. The role of primary renal Na^+ retention as a cause of hypertension is documented in various renal diseases, primary hyperaldosteronism, and many congenital disorders that are characterized by increased renal Na^+ reabsorption. In most cases of congestive heart failure, an increase in vascular volume is not accompanied by a rise in cardiac output and arterial blood pressure. The lack of forward flow results in edema formation. Edema can also occur in conditions such as liver disease or nephrotic syndrome without an increase in vascular volume. Nevertheless, the total body Na^+ content is elevated in all these conditions.

Although renal Na^+ retention is well known to be the primary cause of secondary hypertension, the exact role of Na^+ intake in causing essential hypertension is unknown, and the degree to which dietary Na^+ should be restricted is highly debated. The National Heart, Lung, and Blood Institute of the National Institutes of Health supports the position of the National High Blood Pressure Education Program and recommends that US residents should consume no more than 2400 mg/day Na^+ (6 g salt) (13). This amount is reduced to 1500 mg/day in individuals with hypertension or with renal disease and increased in certain individuals with high Na^+ losses in sweat.

A reduction in salt intake is not accompanied initially by a reduction in renal Na^+ excretion, and so salt excretion temporarily exceeds salt intake. This imbalance leads to a reduction in extracellular volume and the effective vascular volume. Eventually, the kidney reduces salt excretion in response to a reduction in the extracellular volume, and a new balance between Na^+ intake and output is achieved. Until then, salt excretion exceeds salt intake. A reduction in the total body Na^+ content is accompanied by a reduction in the extracellular volume and a decrease in blood pressure. Those persons who have substantial salt loss before a new balance is achieved are likely to have a greater decrease in blood pressure than are those who lose little salt before a new salt balance is achieved (14, 15).

Chloride

Whereas we consider that Na^+ largely determines extracellular volume, total body Cl^- is usually regulated in exactly the same proportion as Na^+, so it is difficult to measure the effect of Cl^- on extracellular fluid volume. Thus, except in acid–base disorders, one could use the Na^+ or the Cl^- concentration to calculate changes in osmolality, and when total body Na^+ rises, total body Cl^- rises as well. The Cl^- concentration does vary in certain acid–base disorders, however, so for practical reasons the clinical standard is to use the serum or plasma Na^+ concentration for osmolality. Evidence indicates that Cl^- has effects independent of Na^+: for example, a dose of sodium chloride (NaCl) raises blood pressure to a much greater extent than does an equal dose of sodium bicarbonate ($NaHCO_3$) (16). Moreover, administration of Cl^-, but not Na^+, relieves metabolic alkalosis (see later).

Sodium and Chloride Content of Food

Despite possible differences, Na^+ and Cl^- are consumed together in most foods. Although Na^+ and Cl^- are major extracellular solutes, the amount of Na^+ contained in food is quite small because the interstitial fluid represents a small fraction of the total fluid content of foods. Moreover, although the intracellular content of Cl^- is somewhat higher than Na^+, intracellular content of both ions is still quite low (17). For these reasons, the salt content of food is low before preparation. The high intake of Na^+ and Cl^- results from salt added to food in its preparation or during cooking. On average, the Na^+ and Cl^- content in foods before processing tends to be equal; many plant-derived foods such as nuts, vegetables, fruits, and cereals contain more Cl^- than Na^+ (17), whereas meat, fish, and eggs contain more Na^+ than Cl^- (Fig. 6.1).

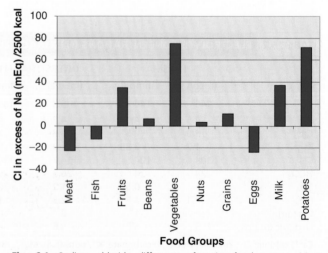

Fig. 6.1. Sodium chloride difference of major food groups. Most sodium (Na) and chloride (Cl) in food is now in the form of added salt (1:1 sodium-to-chloride ratio). In natural foods without added salt, chloride content is greater than sodium, with the exception of meat, fish, and eggs, which contain more sodium than chloride. (Reprinted with permission from Oh MS, Uribarri J. Electrolytes, water, and acid-base balance. In: Shils ME, Shike M, Ross AC et al, eds. Modern Nutrition in Health and Disease. 10th ed. Baltimore: Lippincott Williams & Wilkins, 2006:149–93.)

PATHOPHYSIOLOGY OF WATER AND OSMOLALITY

Osmolar Relations and Regulations

Measurement of Plasma Osmolality

The plasma osmolality can be measured with an osmometer or estimated as the sum of the concentration of all the solutes in the plasma. NaCl, glucose, and urea are the major constituents of the plasma that contribute to plasma osmolality. The plasma osmolality is estimated from the following formula:

$$\text{Plasma osmolality} = \text{Plasma Na}^+ \, (\text{mEq/L}) \times 2 + \text{Glucose (mg/dL)}/18 + \text{Urea (mg/dL)}/2.8$$

Na^+ always partners with its anion, Cl^-, to preserve electroneutrality, whereas the contribution of glucose and urea to the osmolality depends on fractional molecular weight. The molecular weight of glucose is 180 daltons, and that of urea is 28 daltons. Unlike NaCl or glucose, which largely remain in the plasma, urea can cross cell membranes and is not restricted to the extracellular fluid. As such, it is considered an ineffective osmol. Although urea can attain substantial concentrations in the plasma, its normal concentration is only 5 mOsm/L. Because of urea's small contribution to the total osmolality, the total osmolality is nearly equal to the effective osmolality in normal plasma.

Dangers of Changes in Osmolality

Solutes that are restricted to the extracellular fluid and that contribute to the osmolality are called effective osmols, whereas solutes that can enter the cell freely are called ineffective osmols. Examples of effective osmols include glucose and Na^+; examples of ineffective osmols are urea and alcohol. When the concentration of effective osmols increases, osmotic equilibrium is reestablished by water shifting from the cell to the extracellular fluid. Intracellular osmolality then increases to the same level as the extracellular osmolality (18–20). If ineffective osmols are added to the extracellular fluid, the osmotic equilibrium is reestablished by entry of those solutes into the cell. Because most of the solutes normally present in the extracellular fluid are effective osmols, loss of extracellular water, which can occur through insensible losses, will result in an increase in the effective osmolality and will cause a shift of water from the cells into the extracellular fluid. If extracellular osmolality is reduced, either by loss of normal extracellular solutes or by retention of water, a shift of water into the cells will occur to maintain osmolality. When the effective osmolality changes, cellular metabolism is affected, and cell swelling or shrinkage occurs as intracellular volume changes. Some of the most serious manifestations of altered osmolality are related to changes in brain cell volume because the brain is confined to a fixed space. Brain cells have the capacity to regulate their volume with time, and this explains why rapidity of alteration in osmolality is an important determinant of severity of symptoms (21).

Most of the signs and symptoms of a reduced concentration of Na^+ (hyponatremia, representing a low osmolality) are caused by brain swelling and increased intracranial pressure and include nausea or vomiting, headache, papilledema, and mental confusion (22). With increasing severity, lethargy, weakness, hyperreflexia and hyporeflexia, delirium, coma, psychosis, focal weakness, ataxia, aphasia, generalized rigidity, and seizures occur and are caused by an increase in cell volume and reduced electrolyte concentration of the brain cells. GI manifestations include abdominal cramps, a temporary loss of sense of taste and flavor, decreased appetite, nausea, vomiting, salivation, and paralytic ileus. Cardiovascular effects of hypoosmolality are usually manifested as hypotension and other signs of low effective vascular volume. Hyponatremia can also be accompanied by muscle cramps, twitching, and rigidity (23, 24).

Increased effective osmolality need not be accompanied by a high serum Na^+ concentration (hypernatremia), but hypernatremia is always accompanied by hyperosmolality. As in the hypoosmolal states, the signs and symptoms of hyperosmolality depend on the rapidity of development as well as the severity of hyperosmolality. In both human subjects and in animals, acute hyperosmolality from hypernatremia leads to subdural, cortical, and subarachnoid hemorrhages; it causes sudden shrinkage of brain cells and it creates negative pressure in the brain (25). Depression of mental status ranges from lethargy to coma. If the condition is severe, generalized seizure may also be observed but less commonly than in hypoosmolality. Muscular symptoms of hyperosmolality include muscular rigidity, tremor, myoclonus, hyperreflexia, spasticity, and rhabdomyolysis. In children with chronic hyperosmolality, spasticity, chronic seizure disorder, and mental retardation may occur (25).

Regulation of Thirst and Antidiuretic Hormone Release

If the effective osmolality rises, the hypothalamic osmoreceptor cells will shrink; this process then stimulates the thirst center in the cerebral cortex and stimulates antidiuretic hormone (ADH) production in the supraoptic and paraventricular nuclei (26, 27). If the effective osmolality declines, the osmoreceptor cells will swell; ADH production is inhibited. ADH produced in the hypothalamus is carried through long axons and is secreted from the posterior pituitary (28–30). Stimulation and inhibition of osmoreceptor cells affect production by the hypothalamus and ADH secretion by the posterior pituitary.

ADH secretion is extremely sensitive to changes in effective osmolality. A rise in the effective osmolality by just 2% to 3% stimulates ADH secretion sufficiently to result in maximally concentrated urine (25), whereas a decline in plasma osmolality of only 2% to 3% produces maximally dilute urine (<100 mOsm/L). ADH release is also regulated by nonosmotic factors such as nausea, pain, and volume (22). A low effective vascular volume (~10% decrease) provokes thirst and ADH release (31–33). These effects are mediated through baroreceptors and some humoral factors released in response to reduced blood flow. This response explains the severe thirst despite hyponatremia seen in heart or liver failure. Other factors, including β-catecholamines, angiotensin II, and physical and emotional stress, enhance ADH output. Ethanol and catecholamines inhibit the output of ADH. Lithium, certain tetracycline antibiotics (demeclocycline), foscarnet, methoxyflurane, amphotericin B, and V–2 receptor antagonists (Vaptans) inhibit the effect of ADH on the kidney (22).

To understand the effect of ADH, consider that 180 L of water are filtered through the kidney daily; 120 L are reabsorbed in the proximal tubule, and 35 L are reabsorbed in the descending limb of Henle. All this water absorption is accompanied by salt absorption (in the case of the loop of Henle in the ascending limb), however, so no net change in osmolality occurs (34). The distal convoluted and collecting tubules reabsorb salt without water, so approximately 25 L of dilute urine are delivered to the collecting duct. When ADH is totally absent, approximately 5 L of water are reabsorbed in the inner medullary collecting duct, and 20 L are excreted as the final urine. In the presence of maximal ADH, urine volume can be as low as 0.5 L/day as the urine is concentrated to as high as 1200 mOsm/L and water is reabsorbed in the cortical and medullary collecting duct (Fig. 6.2). The reabsorption of water in the collecting duct is regulated by ADH. Water is conserved as the urine is concentrated. The net effect is osmotically concentrated urine (35–44).

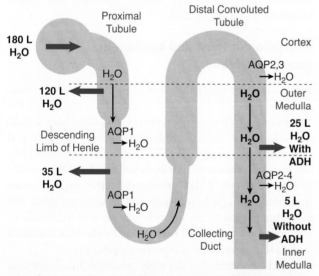

Fig. 6.2. Of the 180 L of water filtered through the kidney daily, 120 L are reabsorbed in the proximal tubule and 35 L are reabsorbed in the descending limb of Henle. Most of the remaining 25 L are reabsorbed in the collecting duct in the presence of antidiuretic hormone (ADH). When ADH is totally absent, approximately 5 L are reabsorbed in the collecting duct, and the remaining 20 L are excreted as the final urine. *AQP,* aquaporin.

Nonrenal Control of Water and Electrolyte Balance

Besides urinary losses of water, water is also lost from the skin and through normal respiration. Water is lost from the skin primarily as a means of eliminating heat, and the amount of water lost depends on the amount of heat generated in the body. In the absence of sweat or febrile illness, water loss from the skin is called insensible perspiration. Water loss from the skin depends mainly on the amount of heat generated in the body. Water loss from the skin is 30 mL/100 cal or approximately (~300 to 1000 mL/24 hours). Besides water, sweat contains Na^+ and K^+ at a concentration of approximately 50 mEq/L and 5 mEq/L, respectively, and is approximately equivalent to 0.45% normal saline. The Na^+ content of sweat varies, depending on the conditioning of the individual. An unconditioned individual placed in a hot environment (e.g., a new recruit in basic training) may have sweat that contains up to 100 mEq/L Na^+, whereas after training the Na^+ sweat content may be as low as 30 mEq/L. This difference explains why a higher dietary Na^+ intake is required for unconditioned individuals (45).

Both fats and carbohydrates serve as the major energy sources for the body. In turn, these are broken down into carbon dioxide (CO_2) and water. Both can be excreted through ventilation. Water is lost during normal ventilation because the water content of inspired air is less than that of the expired air. Ventilation is determined by the amount of CO_2 production, which is determined by the caloric expenditure. The amount of water lost during ventilation also depends on caloric expenditure:

$$\text{Respiratory water loss} = 13 \text{ mL/100 kcal at normal partial pressure of } CO_2 \text{ (P}CO_2\text{)}$$

By burning calories, water is produced that is largely lost during normal respiration. In calculating water balance, respiratory water loss may be ignored in the measurement of insensible water loss, provided metabolic water gain is also ignored. In cases of hyperventilation or fever, respiratory water loss increases disproportionately to metabolic water production (1).

The net activity of the GI tract to the level of the jejunum is secretion of water and electrolytes. The net activity from jejunum to colon is reabsorption of water and electrolytes. Most of the fluid entering the small intestine is absorbed there, and the remainder is absorbed in the colon, leaving only approximately 100 mL of water to be excreted daily in the feces. The contents of the GI tract are isotonic with plasma, and any fluid that enters the GI tract becomes isotonic. Thus, if water is ingested and vomited, solute is lost from the body.

Dehydration and Volume Depletion

In any discussion of salt and water losses, the terms *dehydration* and *volume depletion* occur. Dehydration is characterized by water loss alone or an excess loss of water to salt. Volume depletion describes the equal loss of salt and water. Salt in this case refers to NaCl, which is the main solute in the vascular space. Depending on the quantity of NaCl losses in relation to water losses, mixed forms of volume depletion and dehydration are encountered. In hypotonic dehydration, NaCl losses exceed water losses.

Volume Depletion

NaCl may be lost isotonically (i.e., at the same concentration as in the plasma) through the GI tract or directly from aspiration of the extracellular fluid from pleural effusions or ascites. With GI fluid loss, NaCl is lost with an equal or larger amount of water loss, and the osmolality of the body fluids is subsequently adjusted to isotonicity by changes in oral intake or urinary excretion of water. Isotonic fluid loss reduces only the extracellular fluid volume and can be treated with isotonic salt solution (0.9% normal saline).

Dehydration

The primary aberration in dehydration is water loss, and hypernatremia results from an increase in the concentration of Na^+ in the extracellular space. This disproportionate excess of NaCl to water in the extracellular space can occur if water intake is inadequate or water loss is excessive. Dehydration resulting from excessive water loss usually develops more rapidly than dehydration caused by reduced water intake. A lack of water intake is always caused by one of two mechanisms: (a) a defect in the thirst sensing mechanism or impaired consciousness (46, 47) or (b) a lack of available water or an inability to drink water.

Hypotonic Dehydration. Hypotonic dehydration (volume depletion with more Na^+ than water loss) occurs when the patient loses NaCl and replaces the salt with water or with water containing less NaCl than the fluid that has been lost (see the later discussion of hyponatremia). In the presence of normal renal function, NaCl loss in excess of water loss is difficult to achieve because the kidney readily excretes the excess water through the suppression of ADH. This response is blunted or absent in patients with hypotonic dehydration (48).

PRINCIPLES OF FLUID THERAPY

Goals of Salt and Water Replacement

The goal of therapy is to restore the patient to normal. Deficits in volume and water must be identified and repleted; basal requirements for electrolytes and water must be supplied daily, and ongoing salt and water losses must be quantified and provided for in the treatment plan (49, 50).

Basal Requirements

The basal requirement for water depends on sensible (urinary) and insensible losses of water (51). Fever increases both respiratory and skin water losses as a result of an increase in the basal metabolic rate. To some degree, urinary loss of water declines to compensate for these losses; however, urinary water losses do depend in part

on the total amount of solute excreted and the degree to which the kidney can concentrate the urine. Solute excretion depends mainly on salt ingestion and protein intake, but severe glycosuria causes osmotic diuresis and increases urinary water losses.

Daily Water Requirements

In the absence of fever or exercise, water loss through the skin is relatively fixed, but urinary water losses vary greatly and depend on the total amount of solute to be excreted and urinary concentrating ability. For example, for a total solute excretion of 600 mOsm/day, the urine volume will be 500 mL if urine is concentrated to 1200 mOsm/L and 6 L if urine osmolality is 100 mOsm/L. For the former individual who can maximally concentrate the urine, the minimum water requirement would be 1100 mL (500 mL for urinary water loss plus 600 mL for skin water loss at 2000 cal/day). For the latter individual who is unable to concentrate the urine, the maximal allowable water intake would be 6.6 L. In the absence of an abnormality in urinary concentrating or diluting ability, large ranges of water intake are well tolerated as the kidney adjusts and maintains fluid homeostasis (2, 52). Nevertheless, in hospitalized patients, it is best not to overestimate water requirements to avoid water intoxication. Impairment in urinary dilution, as occurs in the syndrome of inappropriate ADH secretion (SIADH), is more common than impairment in urine concentration. In a conscious patient, thirst is an effective defense mechanism, whereas patients with severe hyponatremia often lapse into coma without warning (1).

POLYURIA

Polyuria, which is arbitrarily defined as an unintentional urine volume in excess of 2.5 L/day, can be caused by either osmotic diuresis or water diuresis (1). In osmotic diuresis, urine output increases as a result of an excessive rate of solute excretion. Certain solutes such as glucose, urea, mannitol, radiopaque media, and NaCl can cause osmotic diuresis in which the solute excretion rate exceeds 60 mOsm/hour or 1440 mOsm/day in the adult (1). In water diuresis, urinary osmolality is lower than plasma osmolality because the kidney excretes dilute urine and water is not reabsorbed in the collecting duct. Major reasons for reduced water reabsorption in the collecting duct can be attributed to drinking large amounts of water, lack of ADH (53–62), or unresponsiveness to ADH (nephrogenic diabetes insipidus [DI]).

Nephrogenic DI can be either congenital or acquired. The lack of ADH can stem from a primary deficiency of ADH (central DI) or from physiologic suppression of ADH by a low serum osmolality. The latter results from the consumption or infusion of large amounts of water and is common among institutionalized patients with psychosis, particularly among those with schizophrenia (53–55, 63, 64). Various gradations of ADH deficiency can be seen. In the setting of a partial ADH deficiency, the urine osmolality is close to normal. ADH deficiency can be congenital or acquired (56–59, 60, 61). During pregnancy, ADH deficiency may be caused by excessive production of vasopressinase (gestational DI) (65, 66). Causes of polyuria are listed in Table 6.3. Note that urine outputs of more than 2.5 L may be considered desirable in patients with kidney stone formation.

Primary polydipsia is an increase in water intake in the absence of a physiologic stimulus such as hyperosmolality or volume depletion (53–55, 63, 64). It is usually psychogenic in origin, hence the term *psychogenic polydipsia*. An increase in urine output is caused by physiologic suppression of ADH secretion, and the serum Na^+ is usually at the low range of normal. Occasionally, the serum Na^+ may be low and indicates that the capacity of the GI tract to absorb water exceeds the normal capacity of the kidney to excrete water. In contrast, secondary polydipsia results from thirst stimulation in response to hyperosmolality. This condition is seen in patients with DI or patients with diabetes with severe glycosuria; the serum Na^+ usually in the high normal range.

TABLE 6.3 CAUSES OF POLYURIA

Water diuresis
  A. Lack of ADH
    1. Central diabetes insipidus
      Congenital
      Acquired (destruction of posterior pituitary)
      Tumors
      Granulomas
      Pituitary surgery
      Trauma
      Infarction
      Infection of the pituitary or hypothalamus
    2. Primary (psychogenic) polydipsia
  B. Failure of the kidney to respond to ADH
    1. Congenital nephrogenic diabetes insipidus
      Defect in the ADH receptor
      Defect in aquaporin expression
    2. Chronic renal failure
    3. Acquired nephrogenic diabetes insipidus
      Drugs
        Lithium
        Demeclocycline
        Methoxyflurane
        Heavy metals
      Interstitial kidney disease
        Amyloidosis
        Sickle cell anemia or trait
        Sarcoidosis
      Electrolyte imbalance
        Hypercalcemia
        Hypokalemia
        Obstructive uropathy
Solute diuresis
  A. Saline loading
  B. Postobstructive diuresis
  C. Hyperglycemia
  D. High-protein tube feedings
  E. Salt-wasting nephropathy

ADH, antidiuretic hormone.

Differential Diagnosis

The first step in the initial workup of polyuria should be measurement of urine osmolality (67). Osmotic diuresis can be ruled out or diagnosed solely on the basis of the rate of osmole excretion: if the excretion of osmoles exceeds a rate greater than 60 mOsm/hour or 1440 mOsm/day, this suggests osmolar diuresis. In contrast, an excretion of a large volume of maximally dilute urine at 100 mOsm/L constitutes water diuresis.

In determining the cause of water diuresis, the first step is to determine the serum Na^+ concentration. In DI, the serum Na^+ tends to be high normal, whereas in primary polydipsia, it tends to be low normal. These conditions overlap, however, and a water deprivation test (68) is needed to confirm the diagnosis. To perform this test, water is either restricted overnight or until loss of 5% of body weight occurs. If the patient has a failure to concentrate the urine maximally that subsequently improves significantly on administration of ADH, central DI is indicated. If the patient has a failure to concentrate the urine maximally and a failure to respond to ADH, nephrogenic DI should be suspected. Primary polydipsia and partial nephrogenic DI cannot be distinguished by this test. Patients with partial nephrogenic DI are frequently hypernatremic, however, whereas those with primary polydipsia are frequently hyponatremic.

Treatment

To treat osmotic diuresis, the cause of the increased solute excretion, such as poor glucose control or excessive protein intake, must be ascertained and controlled. A careful dietary history is often helpful. Administration of ADH is helpful only for central DI. Desmopressin (DDAVP), a synthetic analog of ADH, is administered intranasally, subcutaneously, or intravenously (69, 70). Nephrogenic DI cannot be treated with ADH preparations, but measures to reduce the distal delivery of salt and water (i.e., low-salt diet and thiazide diuretics) are somewhat effective (71, 72). Investigators have suggested that statin drugs may be useful to increase water channel abundance by reducing their cell surface removal in patients with nephrogenic DI (73). Reports have also noted the use of clozapine and propranolol to treat primary polydipsia in patients with schizophrenia (74), but drugs that interfere with urinary dilution, such as thiazide diuretics, will only exacerbate the problem and should be avoided.

DISORDERS OF SODIUM METABOLISM

Hyponatremia

Hyponatremia occurs when the plasma Na^+ concentration falls to less than 135 mEq/L. It is the most common electrolyte disorder and generally causes clinical concern when the concentration is less than 130 mEq/L. Pseudohyponatremia is a spurious reduction in serum

Na^+ concentration resulting from a systematic error in measurement. Changes in methodology have largely reduced this problem in most clinical centers (75); however, the presence of a nonosmotic substance (in vitro hemolysis, hyperlipidemia, hyperproteinemia, and mannitol), may still cause pseudohyponatremia (76–79).

Causes and Pathogenesis

The mechanisms responsible for a reduction in extracellular Na^+ concentration (hyponatremia) are as follows:

1. Water can shift from the cell in response to an accumulation of extracellular solutes other than Na^+ salts (78–82). Hyperglycemia causes hyponatremia by this mechanism, and the serum Na^+ decreases by 1.6 mEq/L for every 100 mg/dL rise in the serum glucose. Serum osmolality is unchanged.
2. The body can retain excess water.
3. The body can fail to retain Na^+ (83).
4. Na^+ shifts into the cells.

In examples 2, 3, and 4, hypotonicity results, and the appropriate physiologic response is suppression of ADH release, which leads to rapid excretion of excess water and correction of hyponatremia. Therefore, persistence of hyponatremia indicates the failure of this compensatory mechanism. In most instances, hyponatremia is maintained because the kidney fails to produce a water diuresis, but sometimes ingestion of water in excess of the limits of normal renal compensation is responsible. The reasons for the inability of the kidney to excrete water include renal failure, reduced delivery of glomerular filtrate to the distal nephron, and the presence of ADH. After ruling out causes of pseudohyponatremia, an assessment of extracellular fluid volume provides a useful working classification of hyponatremia (84–86).

In most cases of hyponatremia, the main reason for the fall of serum Na^+ is abnormal retention of water, which is either ingested or administered in the form of hypotonic fluids (83). Water retention can still occur despite the administration of isotonic fluid. This is seen in the setting of an increased amount of ADH, which leads to the excretion of hypertonic urine. The response is considered appropriate when ADH is released in response to hypertonicity of the body fluid or when the effective vascular volume is reduced. Hyponatremia in clinical states such as congestive heart failure and cirrhosis of the liver is associated with reduced effective vascular volume and is caused by increased secretion of ADH. Similarly, decreased perfusion may cause ADH secretion despite hyponatremia in hypothyroidism (87) and glucocorticoid deficiency states. The cerebral salt-wasting syndrome, which is defined as renal loss of salt caused by humoral substances released in response to cerebral disorders, such as acute subarachnoid hemorrhage, causes volume depletion that results in hyponatremia (88–90).

The term syndrome of inappropriate ADH (SIADH) is therefore reserved for ADH secretion that occurs despite

TABLE 6.4	CAUSES OF HYPONATREMIA

Disorders in which renal water excretion is impaired
  A. Effective circulating volume depletion
    1. Gastrointestinal losses
      Vomiting
      Diarrhea
      Tube drainage
      Intestinal obstruction
    2. Renal losses
      Diuretics
      Hypoaldosteronism
      Sodium-wasting nephropathy
    3. Skin losses
      Ultramarathon runners
      Burns
      Cystic fibrosis
    4. Edematous states
      Heart failure
      Hepatic cirrhosis
      Nephrotic syndrome
    5. Potassium depletion
  B. Thiazide diuretics
  C. Renal failure
  D. Nonhypovolemic states of ADH excess
    1. Syndrome of inappropriate ADH secretion
    2. Cortisol deficiency
    3. Hypothyroidism
  E. Decreased solute intake
Disorders in which renal water excretion is normal
  A. Primary polydipsia
  B. Reset osmostat
    1. Pregnancy
    2. Psychosis
    3. Quadriplegia
    4. Severe malnutrition

ADH, antidiuretic hormone.

hyponatremia and a normal or increased effective vascular volume. Causes of SIADH include tumors, pulmonary diseases such as tuberculosis and pneumonia, central nervous system diseases, and drugs, among others (Table 6.4) (21, 22, 91–101). Finally, mild hyponatremia may be caused by resetting of the osmostat to an osmolality lower than the usual level. In such cases, urine dilution occurs normally when the plasma osmolality is brought down to less than the reset level. Patients with chronic debilitating diseases such as pulmonary tuberculosis often manifest this phenomenon (102).

Diagnosis

The presence of a low plasma Na^+ concentration and normal osmolality suggests pseudohyponatremia (see Table 6.4). With modern analyzers, a high glucose concentration is the most common cause, and the serum Na^+ decreases by 1.6 mEq/L for every 100 mg/dL rise in the serum glucose. Hyponatremia caused by glucose is suspected from the history or by simultaneous measurements of plasma Na^+, osmolality, and glucose. Pseudohyponatremia resulting from hyperlipidemia occurs only with certain analyzers and is caused by the accumulation of chylomicrons, which consist mostly of triglycerides. This condition is obvious from the milky appearance of the serum. Substantial hyponatremia resulting from hyperlipidemia requires accumulation of more than 5 to 6 g/dL of lipids, and such a degree of hyperlipidemia does not occur with hypercholesterolemia alone.

In evaluating hyponatremia associated with hypoosmolality, the main concern is distinguishing between SIADH and hyponatremia resulting from other causes, mainly volume depletion and edematous states. The major distinction between SIADH and other causes of hyponatremia lies in the status of effective vascular volume. Effective vascular volume is normal or increased in SIADH and reduced in other disorders that cause hyponatremia. No single diagnostic test measures effective vascular volume with certainty. Physical examination is notoriously inaccurate in determining mild-to-moderate volume depletion. A more reliable method for estimating effective vascular volume is the measurement of certain laboratory parameters, all of which depend on renal responses to changes in effective vascular volume. These parameters include urinary Na^+, serum urea nitrogen, serum creatinine, and serum uric acid. Urinary Na^+ excretion of greater than 20 mEq/L, serum urea nitrogen less than 10 mg/dL, serum creatinine less than 1 mg/dL, and serum urate less than 4.0 mg/dL all suggest normal or increased effective vascular volume. The fractional excretion of urea is more reliable than the serum urea nitrogen value in determining the status of the effective vascular volume because the serum urea nitrogen also depends on protein intake. A fractional excretion of urea of less than 35% is considered an indicator of low effective vascular volume (103), whereas a fractional excretion of Na^+ less than 0.5% is thought to represent a low effective vascular volume (104). In contrast, the measurement of urine osmolality has virtually no diagnostic value and often misleads physicians.

Contrary to common belief, urine osmolality in SIADH need not be greater than plasma osmolality. Furthermore, a high urine osmolality does not necessarily support the diagnosis of SIADH because most other causes of hyponatremia are also accompanied by urine osmolality higher than plasma osmolality. The only situation in which urine osmolality may be appropriately low in the presence of hyponatremia is hyponatremia caused by primary polydipsia, and this is usually apparent when a careful history reveals polyuria and polydipsia. In all other causes of hyponatremia, urine osmolality is inappropriately increased (i.e., >100 mOsm/L) (105).

Treatment

The treatment of hyponatremia is directed at the underlying cause and may range from the addition of Na^+, the removal of water, or improvement of the organ dysfunction (cardiac, renal or hepatic). Salt is given to patients with hyponatremia resulting from salt depletion (106, 107). The speed of correction of hyponatremia is controversial but depends on the speed of development and on the patient's symptoms.

Severe symptomatic hyponatremia is a life-threatening condition and should be treated with hypertonic saline solution (108, 109), but volume overload and central pontine myelinolysis (also known as osmotic demyelinating disease) are associated with the administration of a large quantity of salt-containing solutions (110, 111). Central pontine myelinolysis, which is a demyelinating disease of the central pons and other areas of the brain, is characterized by motor nerve dysfunction. If it is severe enough, quadriplegia occurs. It is seen more often during treatment of chronic hyponatremia than of acute hyponatremia and is more frequent in malnourished and debilitated patients. Commonly accepted rates of correction of chronic hyponatremia range from 0.5 to 1.0 mEq/L/hour or less, but central pontine myelinolysis has been reported to occur when the rate of correction of hyponatremia was less than 0.5 mEq/L. A review of the literature suggested that a 4- to 6-mEq/L increase in the serum Na^+ concentration was a sufficient rise to rescue patients from complications of acute hyponatremia (109). Because the danger of central pontine myelinolysis is limited mainly to patients with asymptomatic chronic hyponatremia, rapid correction (at a rate of 1 to 2 mEq/L/hour) should be restricted to those with acute symptomatic hyponatremia (21, 112). Clinical outcomes are not improved by a rapid correction of the serum Na^+ to a level greater than 120 mEq/L (75). In cases of overcorrection, therapeutic relowering of the serum Na^+ concentration prevents brain lesions (113).

For patients admitted with volume depletion and chronic asymptomatic hyponatremia, the traditional recommendation has been administration of isotonic saline solution. With volume expansion, ADH release is suppressed. Water excretion and a rise in serum Na^+ concentration ensue. Because the rapid excretion of water following isotonic saline administration may lead to the development of central pontine myelinolysis, use of 0.45% alternating with 0.90% NaCl solution has been advocated by some clinicians. Moreover, a 4 to 6 mmol/L increase in serum Na^+ concentration is usually significant enough to improve the most severe symptoms in patients with acute hyponatremia, so a therapeutic goal of 6 mmol/day is reasonable in chronic hyponatremia even when the serum Na^+ falls to extremely low levels (114). For K^+ depletion, the appropriate treatment is with 0.45% NaCl containing 40 mEq/L K^+. Regardless, serum electrolytes should be monitored closely, with blood monitoring every 2 hours and adjustments in infusion rates made to avoid too rapid a correction.

Acute Treatment. For hyponatremia with Na^+ depletion and symptomatic hypoosmolality (e.g., confusion), intravenous administration of Na^+ as hypertonic saline solution corrects hypoosmolality effectively. The amount of Na^+ necessary to increase the Na^+ to a desired level is calculated as follows (69, 115):

$$Na^+ \text{ requirement (mEq)} = TBW \times \Delta Na$$

where TBW is total body weight and ΔNa^+ is the desired serum Na^+ 120 mEq/L minus actual serum Na^+. Na^+ is administered as a 3% NaCl solution. In emergency situations, 100 mL or 2 mL/kg bolus infusions of 3% saline can be administered rapidly over minutes in the setting of seizures and can be repeated up to two times if necessary (109, 116). Very close serial monitoring of serum Na^+ is required until blood levels are stable.

When accumulation of excess water is primarily responsible for hyponatremia, as in SIADH, water may be rapidly removed by administration of intravenous osmotic diuretics such as mannitol or urea. Loop diuretics such as furosemide alter urinary concentrating ability and hinder the kidney's ability to retain both Na^+ and water. When loop diuretics are given in conjunction with hypertonic saline, the net effect is a rise in the serum Na^+ level because Na^+ replacement exceeds water replacement. The response to furosemide cannot be accurately predicted, and frequent follow-up measurements of the serum Na^+ level must be made. Administration of hypertonic saline solution alone usually causes salt and water diuresis, but the addition of a loop diuretic makes correction of hyponatremia more predictable by preventing excretion of a concentrated urine. Besides, a diuretic prevents fluid overload. Vasopressin antagonists (vaptans) have been used to facilitate free water excretion and correct hyponatremia (117). Vasopressin mediates its biologic effects by binding to three receptor subtypes: V1A, V1B, and V2. V1A receptors are located on vascular smooth muscle, platelets, and the liver. Activation of these receptors results in vasoconstriction, platelet aggregation, and gluconeogenesis. V1B receptors are located in the anterior pituitary, and their activation stimulates adrenocorticotropic hormone (ACTH) release, whereas the V2 receptors are located in the principal cells of the renal collecting duct. Stimulation of these receptors results in water retention; conversely, antagonism of these receptors results in dilute urine and excretion of free water in the urine (118).

Intravenous conivaptan was the first vasopressin receptor antagonist to be approved by the US Food and Drug Administration (FDA) for treating euvolemic hyponatremia caused by SIADH, hypothyroidism, adrenal insufficiency, or pulmonary disorders (119). Because of its high affinity to V1A receptor, hypotension is possible. In binding to the V2 receptor, an aquaretic effect lasting for 12 hours is seen (120). Conivaptan also gained FDA approval for treating hypervolemic hyponatremia in patients with heart failure. Tolvaptan, the first oral selective V2 receptor antagonist approved for use in the United States by the FDA, was shown to increase serum Na^+ concentrations significantly compared with placebo in patients with euvolemic hyponatremia (SIADH) and hypervolemic hyponatremia (from cirrhosis, congestive heart failure), but it did not alter disease progression or mortality (118–120).

Long-Term Treatment. Chronic hyponatremia may be treated by a reduction in water intake (water restriction) or by an increase in renal water excretion. Reduction of water intake is preferable, but compliance is difficult because of the severe thirst that usually results. Hard candy and chewing gum may be helpful in keeping the mouth moist, and ice chips are more thirst quenching than an equal volume of water. If water restriction is unsuccessful, increased renal water excretion can be achieved by the use of pharmacologic agents that interfere with urine concentration. Lithium and demeclocycline increase urine output by interfering with the renal effects of ADH. Demeclocycline is more effective and has fewer side effects, but it may cause nephrotoxicity in patients with liver disease.

Administration of a loop diuretic such as furosemide in conjunction with increased salt and K^+ intake is safer than the foregoing methods. The diuretic prevents high medullary interstitial osmolality by limiting the reabsorption of salt in the loop of Henle and hence prevents a high urine concentration. Increased salt and K^+ intake increases water output by increasing the rate of solute excretion. Although vasopressin antagonists are commercially available and have been used in the acute setting, their prohibitive cost makes them difficult to use in the long-term treatment of hyponatremia (121). Nevertheless, these agents have proven useful in the treatment of heart failure, cirrhosis, and SIADH, as well as in patients with psychotic disorders (122, 123).

Hypernatremia

Hypernatremia is defined as an increased Na^+ concentration in plasma water. Whereas hyponatremia may not be accompanied by hypoosmolality, hypernatremia is always associated with an increase in the effective plasma osmolality and a reduced cell volume. An increase in the plasma osmolality should stimulate thirst. Hence, hypernatremia can occur only if the thirst mechanism is blocked, such as in the setting of altered mental status, or when an immobile patient has no access to water. Although the extracellular volume in hypernatremia may be normal, decreased, or increased, hypernatremia almost always occurs in the setting of volume depletion.

Causes and Pathogenesis

Theoretically, hypernatremia is caused by loss of water, reduced water intake, gain of Na^+, or a combination of these (Table 6.5). In gain of Na^+ in a person who has normal perception of thirst and the ability to drink water, however, the availability of water does not result in hypernatremia because a proportional amount of water is retained to maintain normal body fluid osmolality. The physiologic defense against hyponatremia is increased renal water excretion, whereas the physiologic defense against hypernatremia is an increase in water intake in response to thirst. Because thirst is such an effective and sensitive defensive mechanism against hypernatremia, it is virtually impossible to increase serum Na^+ by more than a few milliequivalents (mEq) per liter if the mechanism for drinking water is intact. Therefore, a patient with hypernatremia always has reasons for reduced water intake. Reduced water intake occurs most commonly in comatose patients, in those

TABLE 6.5   CAUSES OF HYPERNATREMIA

Water loss
  A. Insensible loss
    1. Increased sweating: fever, exercise
    2. Burns
    3. Respiratory infections
  B. Renal loss
    1. Central diabetes insipidus
    2. Nephrogenic diabetes insipidus
    3. Osmotic diuresis
        Glucose
        Mannitol
  C. Gastrointestinal loss
    1. Osmotic diarrhea
        Lactulose
        Malabsorption
        Infectious enteritides
  D. Hypothalamic disorders
    1. Primary hypodipsia
    2. Reset osmostat from volume expansion in primary
       mineralocorticoid excess
  E. Water loss into cells
    1. Seizures
    2. Severe exercise
    3. Rhabdomyolysis
Reduced water intake
  A. Defective thirst
    1. Altered mental status
    2. Thirst center defect
  B. Inability to drink water
  C. Lack of access to water
Sodium retention
  A. Administration of hypertonic sodium chloride or
     sodium bicarbonate
  B. Ingestion of sodium

patients with a defective thirst mechanism, in those patients with continuous vomiting or who lack access to water, or in those patients with mechanical obstruction resulting from a condition such as an esophageal tumor.

The excess gain of Na^+ leading to hypernatremia is usually iatrogenic. This occurs in the setting of hypertonic saline infusion, accidental entry into the maternal circulation during abortion with hypertonic saline solution, or administration of hypertonic $NaHCO_3^-$ during cardiopulmonary resuscitation or treatment of lactic acidosis. Reduced renal Na^+ excretion leading to Na^+ gain and hypernatremia usually occurs in response to dehydration caused by a primary water deficit. Water depletion resulting from DI, osmotic diuresis, or insufficient water intake leads to secondary Na^+ retention in patients who continue to ingest Na^+ or who are given Na^+ (124).

Whether hypernatremia is caused by Na^+ retention or by water loss, can be determined by examination of the patient's volume status. For example, if a patient with a serum Na^+ concentration of 170 mEq/L does not have obvious evidence of dehydration, hypernatremia is not caused entirely by water loss. To increase the serum Na^+ to 170 mEq/L through water loss alone would require a loss of more than 20% of the total body water.

Treatment

Acute Treatment. Hypernatremia is generally treated by the addition of water; when the cause is iatrogenic, Na^+ must be removed. When hypernatremia is associated with volume depletion, isotonic (0.9%) NaCl or 0.45% NaCl may be given initially to stabilize circulatory dynamics, followed by administration of hypotonic solutions to normalize the tonicity. Because rapid reduction of the plasma osmolality may result in cerebral edema, the serum Na^+ may be reduced by 6 to 8 mEq/L in the first 3 to 4 hours for acute symptomatic hypernatremia (118). As with hyponatremia, chronic hypernatremia usually does not cause central nervous system symptoms and therefore does not require rapid correction. Although investigators generally accept that a slow reduction of the serum Na^+ concentration by less than 10 mmol/L/day or 0.5 mmol/L/hour is desirable, little documented evidence exists regarding what constitutes a safe rate of rehydration.

In one study in a children's hospital in China, risk factors for cerebral edema were an initial fluid bolus, the severity of hypernatremia, and the overall hydration rate (124). Cerebral edema appeared to be mitigated if the overall hydration rate in the first 24 hours was less than 0.5 mmol/L/hour. Therefore, a safe rate of correction is 0.5 mEq/L/hour and should not exceed a 10% change in the serum Na^+ concentration during the initial 24-hour period. The amount of water needed to correct hypernatremia can be estimated using the following equation (69):

$$\text{Water deficit (L)} = TBW \times (\text{Actual } Na^+ - \text{Desired } Na^+)/\text{Desired } Na^+ = TBW \times (\Delta Na^+/\text{Desired } Na^+)$$

where ΔNa^+ is the difference between the desired and actual serum Na^+ concentration.

In the setting of hypernatremia with excess Na^+, a reduction in serum Na^+ with fluids usually initiates natriuresis. If natriuresis does not occur promptly, Na^+ may be removed with diuretics. Furosemide in combination with 5% dextrose solution may be an appropriate regimen for treatment of hypernatremia associated with excess Na^+ (69). If a hypernatremic patient with Na^+ excess has renal failure, salt can be removed by dialysis. The total water requirement must also include insensible water losses (~300 to 500 mL/24 hours) and urinary electrolyte-free water losses. The latter represents the urine water losses in excess of the volume necessary to contain urinary Na^+ in addition to K^+ at the same concentration as serum Na^+. When the urine electrolyte-free water excretion is a positive number, the serum Na^+ rises further; when it is a negative number, the effect is to decrease the serum Na^+. Urinary electrolyte-free water excretion is calculated as follows:

$$\text{Electrolyte-free water excretion} = V - (U_{Na^+} + U_{K^+})V/S_{Na^+}$$

where V is urine volume, $U_{(Na^+ + K^+)}$ is the sum of concentrations of urine Na^+ and K^+, and S_{Na^+} is serum Na^+ concentration.

Long-Term Treatment. Hypernatremic disorders that require long-term preventive therapy include DI and primary hypodipsia. Although DI is often listed as a cause of hypernatremia, it does not produce hypernatremia in the absence of a thirst defect. As such, hypernatremia can be considered a hormonal imbalance of inconvenience. Treatment is directed toward the curtailment of polydipsia and polyuria, which are the patients' main complaints. Patients with primary hypodipsia should be educated to drink water on schedule. In some instances, stimulation of the thirst center with chlorpropamide has been effective (69).

POTASSIUM METABOLISM AND ITS DISORDERS

Dietary Sources of Potassium and Handling

Because K^+ is the major intracellular cation, it is widely distributed in all foods, but the content varies greatly, depending on the type of food (Fig. 6.3). The highest K^+ content is in fruits and vegetables; the K^+ content of vegetables is particularly high when it is expressed as the content per calorie (17, 125). Among the starchy foods, the K^+ contents of polished rice and light wheat flour are particularly low, whereas the K^+ contents of potato, soybean, and buckwheat are quite high (Fig. 6.4). Although citrus fruits and bananas are often cited by health professionals as particularly rich sources of K^+, many other foods contain K^+ at higher concentration. Tomatoes, apricots, and cantaloupes contain far more K^+ than oranges and bananas when expressed as milliequivalents of K^+ per calorie (Fig. 6.5) (17). Although protein sources are not as rich in K^+ as fruits or vegetables on a per calorie basis, meats and fishes contain approximately 80 to 100 mEq/oz. Treating

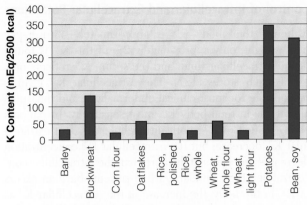

High Carbohydrate Foods

Fig. 6.4. Potassium (K) contents of major carbohydrate-containing foods. Grains, especially polished rice and light wheat flour, contain little potassium, whereas potatoes and soy beans contain large quantities of potassium. (Reprinted with permission from Oh MS, Uribarri J. Electrolytes, water, and acid-base balance. In: Shils ME, Shike M, Ross AC et al, eds. Modern Nutrition in Health and Disease. 10th ed. Baltimore: Lippincott Williams & Wilkins, 2006:149–93.)

foods with salt and then discarding the liquid (brining, boiling) induces Na^+ for K^+ exchange and reduces the K^+ content of the foods.

Dietary K^+ is almost completely absorbed in normal small intestine; approximately 10% of dietary K^+ is excreted in the stool (126). K^+ absorption in the small intestine is passive and depends on mechanisms of Na^+ and glucose absorption. Thus, it is not surprising that factors decreasing Na^+ and water adsorption also decrease K^+ adsorption. Although losses are less than that of Na^+, sweating does result in the loss of approximately 0.2 g (5 mEq)/L of K^+. This value is relatively constant with acclimation.

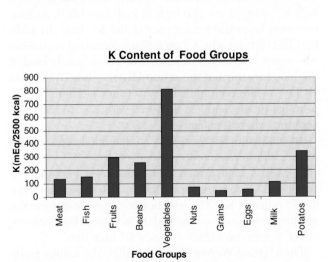

Fig. 6.3. Potassium (K) contents of major food groups. When expressed by the caloric content of food, vegetables contain the highest amounts of potassium. The potassium content of grains is quite low. (Reprinted with permission from Oh MS, Uribarri J. Electrolytes, water, and acid-base balance. In: Shils ME, Shike M, Ross AC et al, eds. Modern Nutrition in Health and Disease. 10th ed. Baltimore: Lippincott Williams & Wilkins, 2006:149–93.)

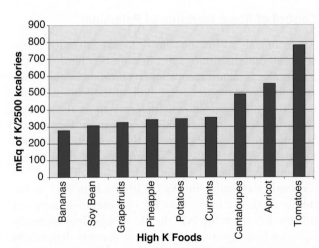

Fig. 6.5. Potassium (K) contents of major fruits. Although oranges and bananas are most often cited as fruits of high potassium content, many other fruits contain far more potassium. For example, the potassium content of apricots is more than twice that of oranges. (Reprinted with permission from Oh MS, Uribarri J. Electrolytes, water, and acid-base balance. In: Shils ME, Shike M, Ross AC et al, eds. Modern Nutrition in Health and Disease. 10th ed. Baltimore: Lippincott Williams & Wilkins, 2006:149–93.)

Control of Intracellular and Extracellular Potassium

Although total body K^+ is approximately 43 mEq/kg body weight, only approximately 2% of this K^+ is found in the extracellular fluid, and the serum K^+ reflects only extracellular stores (127). The extracellular K^+ level is responsible for most clinical abnormalities and measures alterations in total body K^+ most sensitively. In patients with a deficit of K^+, both intracellular K^+ and extracellular K^+ decrease; but the extracellular K^+ concentration decreases proportionately more than the intracellular concentration (128). Similarly, when patients have an excess of K^+ in the body, the increase in the extracellular K^+ is proportionately greater than that in the intracellular K^+.

Factors that affect the movement of K^+ into and out of cells change the levels of extracellular K^+ independently of total body stores. The rise in insulin after a meal lowers serum K^+ levels by increasing its transport into cells, thus blunting the ability of dietary K^+ to cause significantly high serum K^+ (129–132). Catecholamines (through β_2-adrenergic receptors) have a similar effect (133–135). Acidemia raises serum K^+ levels, whereas alkalemia lowers it because of shifts of hydrogen ion (H^+) into and out of the cell in exchange for K^+ (136). In general, metabolic acidosis causes greater K^+ efflux than respiratory acidosis (137). Metabolic acidosis that results from inorganic acids, such as sulfuric acid and hydrochloric acid (HCl), causes greater K^+ efflux than metabolic acidosis resulting from organic acids, such as lactic acid and ketoacids (136, 138). Significantly, meals high in net acid are generally lower in K^+, and this function protects patients from hypokalemia when such meals are consumed. In respiratory alkalosis, K^+ influx is less than that seen in metabolic alkalosis as a consequence of a drop in cellular HCO_3^- concentration (139).

Control of Renal Excretion of Potassium

Approximately 90% of the daily K^+ intake (40 to 100 mEq) is excreted in the urine (126). Because K^+ filtered at the glomerulus is almost completely reabsorbed by the proximal tubule and the ascending limb of the loop of Henle, net urinary K^+ excretion is determined at the cortical collecting duct by mechanisms shown in Figure 6.6. Secretion of K^+ occurs through the renal outer medulla K channel (ROMK) as Na^+ enters the cell through the epithelial Na channel (ENaC) (140, 141). Thus, K^+ is excreted in exchange for Na^+. Either a high Na^+ in the tubule fluid or a high blood K^+ concentration increases urinary K^+. That the Na^+ in the tubule fluid increases K^+ secretion explains the effects of thiazide diuretics in causing urinary K^+ loss. Diuretics that affect transporters in the proximal tubule (carbonic anhydrase inhibitors) and the thick ascending limb (loop diuretics) partly cause K^+ depletion by preventing K^+ absorption in these segments, but they also promote K^+ secretion by increasing Na^+ delivery to the cortical collecting duct (142–144).

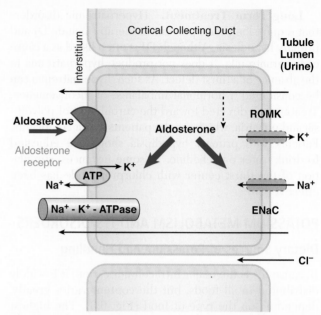

Fig. 6.6. Control of potassium (K^+) secretion at the cortical collecting duct. Sodium (Na^+) enters from the luminal fluid into the cell through the epithelial Na^+ channel (ENaC) and is transported out of the cell through Na^+/K^+-adenosine triphosphatase (ATPase) on the basolateral membrane. These processes create the luminal electrical potential that is more negative than the electrical potential of the peritubular fluid. The electrical charge imbalance created by Na^+ reabsorption is partly matched by entry of K^+ into the lumen through the renal outer medulla K^+ channel (ROMK), a K^+ channel. *ATP*, adenosine triphosphate; *Cl−*, chloride.

When anions other than Cl^- (e.g., HCO_3^-) are excreted, more Na^+ is delivered to the distal tubule, and K^+ secretion is enhanced. HCO_3^- in the tubular fluid also enhances K^+ secretion by directly stimulating ROMK activity (141). This mechanism is important because many foods with a high K^+ content are also high in base (see later), so base excretion helps the kidney excrete the K^+ load. In addition, this explains why K^+ excretion is increased in patients who vomit. The loss of stomach acid leaves base behind in the bloodstream, and the serum HCO_3^- rises. When this HCO_3^- is filtered in the kidney, it is not reclaimed in the proximal tubule, and it is delivered with Na^+ to the distal nephron, where it enhances K^+ loss.

In addition to delivery of Na^+ to the distal nephron, the plasma aldosterone concentration controls K^+ excretion (145–148). A high plasma aldosterone level increases the activity of ENaC to reabsorb Na^+ and ROMK to increase the excretion of K^+. The retention of salt and water and the resulting volume expansion leads to increased distal delivery of Na^+ which can further enhance K^+ excretion.

On a typical Western high-Na^+ diet, the kidney easily excretes K^+ because of high distal Na^+ delivery. Most of the K^+ excreted in the urine is derived from secretion at the cortical collecting duct and is determined by the amount of Na^+ delivered to that portion of the nephron. It is obvious that excretion of a large amount of K^+ requires an increased delivery of Na^+ to the cortical collecting duct (149, 150). Indeed, people may develop hypokalemia on a high-Na^+ very-low-K^+ diet, because of the obligate loss of approximately 15 mEq/L (0.6 g) of K^+ in the urine. Individuals with normal kidney function have the capacity to excrete more than 400 mEq/day (16 g/day) of K^+ without causing a clinically significant change in the serum K^+ level. In addition, an adaptation increases K^+ excretion in the stool as K^+ intake increases.

The diet of humans in preagricultural eras was much higher in K^+ intake, as a result of a higher intake of fruits, vegetables, and meat but a lower intake of grain; Na^+ intake was low because of a lack of availability. The daily dietary load of K^+ probably exceeded 300 mEq/day (~12 g/day), whereas dietary Na^+ was likely less than 90 mEq/day (~2 g/day). Based on the mechanisms discussed thus far, one would predict that the amount of Na^+ delivered to the cortical collecting duct was far less in prehistoric times than in modern times. So how do the kidneys adapt to excrete more K^+ on a low-Na^+ diet? Whereas alkali increases K secretion (even on a low-Na^+ diet) by delivering more Na^+ to the distal nephron, additional mechanisms explain K^+ excretion. High-K^+ diets decrease the amount of the thiazide-sensitive NaCl cotransporter in the distal nephron (151). The thiazide sensitive transporter is in the segment immediately before the segment expressing ENaC, so this allows more Na^+ to reach ENaC and be exchanged for K^+. It would cause more Na^+ excretion, too, if ENaC activity did not change, but ENaC is also increased by high dietary K^+. When diets are high in both K^+ and Na^+ (152), the K^+ effect on the thiazide-sensitive transporter increases Na^+ excretion to a greater extent than the effect on ENaC reduces it, thus causing a net increase in Na^+ excretion. As discussed earlier, the blood pressure rises with Na^+ intake to increase the glomerular filtration rate (GFR) and Na^+ excretion. Thus, in the setting of high Na^+, high dietary K^+ increases the amount of Na^+ excretion to lower blood pressure effectively.

The converse is also true. Low K^+ intake makes it more difficult to excrete a high Na^+ intake, and blood pressure rises as a consequence of Na^+ retention. When Na^+ intake is low, aldosterone additionally up-regulates ENaC, so that net Na^+ excretion is less influenced by K^+. A diet high in K^+ and low in Na^+ results in an increase in Na^+ reabsorption while allowing excretion of K^+. This mechanism fails only when Na^+ intake is so low that blood pressure falls and the kidney itself begins to fail.

Role of Potassium Intake on Sodium Excretion and Blood Pressure

Diets high in fruits and vegetables were shown to be beneficial in reducing blood pressure in the Dietary Approaches to Stop Hypertension (DASH) study (153, 154). Some of the blood pressure–lowering effects of these diets probably resulted from their high K^+ content. Although the combination of a low Na^+ intake and the DASH diet provided the lowest blood pressures, the DASH diet lowered the blood pressure the most when Na^+ intake was high (153, 154). The DASH investigators showed that the K^+ content of the diet enhanced Na^+ excretion for any given blood pressure. Several other studies confirmed that an increase in K^+ by 40 mEq/day reduced blood pressure more than reduction in Na^+ intake of 60 to 80 mEq/day (153–156). A high-K^+ diet likely reduces blood pressure through increased delivery of Na^+ to the distal nephron; Na^+ diuresis ensues. As discussed earlier, dietary K^+ increases Na^+ excretion to a greater extent when Na^+ intake is high, and the effect of a high-K^+ diet on blood pressure is greatest when the Na^+ intake is highest. Nevertheless, an effect is still seen at a Na^+ intake of as little as 1.6 g (an amount that is difficult to achieve on a Western diet). These data suggest that when a dietary approach is used to treat hypertension, increased K^+ intake is an effective adjunct to low Na^+ to lower blood pressure.

Hypokalemia
Causes and Pathogenesis

Because the intracellular K^+ concentration greatly exceeds the extracellular concentration, K^+ shift into the cell can cause severe hypokalemia with little change in its intracellular concentration (157–165) (Table 6.6). Alkalosis, insulin, and β_2-agonists can cause hypokalemia by shifting K^+ inside cells (158, 159). An important clinical consequence of this shift is refeeding hypokalemia. Poor intake of K^+ is rarely the sole cause of hypokalemia because poor intake of K^+ is usually accompanied by poor Na^+ intake, which decreases K^+ excretion, and low caloric intake, which causes catabolism and release of K^+ from the tissues (165). During recovery from starvation, however, insulin release causes K^+ to be transported inside the cells. Because cell mass increases during nutritional recovery, K^+, the main intracellular cation, becomes trapped inside cells, thereby leading to a drop in the extracellular level (165–167). Thus, K^+ must be watched carefully in patients with refeeding following a period of starvation or prolonged undernutrition (e.g., alcoholic patients, hospital patients with poor nutritional intake before or after admission). Phosphorus (P) and Mg^{2+} follow K^+ in many of these cases and may also become acutely decreased in the blood with refeeding of at-risk patients (165, 166).

Vomiting and diarrhea are the most common causes of hypokalemia (165). Poor intake of K^+ in patients with these conditions contributes to hypokalemia but is not the major cause. Diarrhea causes direct K^+ loss in the stool, but in vomiting, hypokalemia occurs because of direct loss in the vomitus, as well as K^+ loss in the urine. As discussed earlier, renal K^+ wasting occurs when increased aldosterone concentration is accompanied by increased distal delivery of Na^+ (168–183). Vomiting causes metabolic alkalosis, and the subsequent renal excretion of HCO_3^- leads to increased delivery of Na^+ to the distal nephron. Because of poor Na^+ intake and increased urinary losses of Na^+, aldosterone rises. Thus, vomiting increases distal

TABLE 6.6	CAUSES OF HYPOKALEMIA

Decreased net intake
  A. Low dietary intake
  B. Clay ingestion (pica)
Increased entry into cells that causes transient hypokalemia
  A. Elevation in intracellular pH
  B. Increased availability of insulin
  C. Elevated β-adrenergic activity
    1. Stress
    2. Coronary ischemia
    3. Delirium tremens
    4. Administration of β-adrenergic agonists
  D. Periodic paralysis, hypokalemic form
  E. Treatment of megaloblastic anemia
  F. Hypothermia
  G. Nutritional recovery state
Increased gastrointestinal losses
  A. Diarrhea
  B. Vomiting
  C. Intestinal drainage
  D. Laxative abuse
Increased urinary losses
  A. Diuretics
  B. Mineralocorticoid excess
    1. Primary hyperaldosteronism (adrenal adenoma or hyperplasia)
    2. Secondary hyperaldosteronism (malignant hypertension, renal artery stenosis)
  C. Increased flow to the distal nephron
    1. Salt-wasting nephropathies
    2. Diuretics
  D. Sodium reabsorption with a nonreabsorbable anion
    1. Vomiting or nasogastric suction
    2. Metabolic acidosis
    3. Penicillin derivatives
  E. Amphotericin B
  F. Hypomagnesemia
  G. Polyuria
Increased sweat losses
Dialysis

delivery of Na^+ while stimulating aldosterone production. Renal K^+ wasting ensues.

Renal loss of K^+ is common in other causes of hypokalemia. In primary aldosteronism, overactivity of the adrenal gland occurs without a secondary cause. Distal delivery of Na^+ is increased and Na^+ is retained in the distal nephron. Blood pressure rises as a consequence of volume expansion (184). In patients with secondary causes of high aldosterone, hypokalemia occurs only in conditions accompanied by increased distal Na^+ delivery. Examples include conditions in which blood pressure rises, such as renal artery stenosis and malignant hypertension. Heart failure does not lead to hypokalemia despite secondary aldosteronism unless renal Na^+ transporters are blocked. This situation occurs in the setting of loop or thiazide diuretic therapy. Defective Na^+ reabsorption, proximal to the aldosterone effective site, results in delivery of Na^+ to the cortical collecting duct. Hypokalemia follows. Bartter's and Gitelman's syndromes are genetic diseases

that lead to decreased activity of the same transporters inhibited by loop or thiazide diuretics, respectively (140, 185). Hypokalemia occurs by the same mechanisms (175–180). In chronic metabolic acidosis, hypokalemia develops because metabolic acidosis directly stimulates aldosterone secretion, reduces proximal reabsorption of NaCl, and allows increased delivery of NaCl to the distal nephron (186). With natural licorice intake, renal K^+ wasting results from the sustained mineralocorticoid activity of cortisol because licorice inhibits the enzyme 11-β-hydroxysteroid dehydrogenase and prevents the rapid metabolism of cortisol in the kidney (181–183). Artificial licorice flavor does not cause hypokalemia. Liddle's syndrome, another genetic cause of hypokalemia, is characterized by increased Na^+ channel activity. Increased K^+ secretion results (187).

Clinical Manifestations

A low serum K^+ level can be life threatening because of potentially negative changes on cardiac rate, rhythm, and conduction, as well as numerous structural and functional alterations in various organs, especially skeletal muscle (188). Hypokalemia produces abnormalities of rhythm and of rate of cardiac conduction through alteration in several physiologic states: alteration in ventricular repolarization leads to depression of the ST segment, flattening and inversion of T waves, and appearance of U waves—the most common electrocardiographic (ECG) abnormalities of hypokalemia. Combinations of altered states of polarization and conduction can produce arrhythmias, most commonly supraventricular and ventricular ectopic beats and tachycardia, atrioventricular conduction disturbances, and ventricular fibrillation. Rapidly developing hypokalemia is more likely to produce cardiac arrhythmias than is more slowly developing hypokalemia (188). Changes in organ function include cardiac and skeletal muscle cell necrosis and acute skeletal muscle rhabdomyolysis. Reduced insulin secretion and reduced intestinal motility are important nutritional effects of hypokalemia. Chronic hypokalemia may be associated with hypertension that results from decreased Na^+ excretion and kidney stone formation that results from inhibition of citrate excretion (189, 190).

Treatment

Hypokalemia is usually treated either by K^+ administration or by prevention of the renal loss of K^+. In a nonemergency setting, K^+ should be given orally in the diet or pharmacologically as KCl, K^+ phosphate, or the salt of organic acids. Administration of K^+ must take the intracellular and extracellular K^+ distribution into account. Patients who have been depleted of K^+ for prolonged periods have lower intracellular stores and require more K^+ to correct the disorder than do patients with normal K^+ stores. K^+ should be given gradually to allow time for it to shift inside cells and to prevent the extracellular concentration from rising too quickly. When K^+ is given as an oral tablet, only 40 mEq may be given safely as a single dose to allow time for K^+ to shift into the cell. The safe amount for a mixed meal has not been established (191, 192), but it is significantly greater because insulin promotes a shift of K^+ into cells. The US Institute of Medicine recommends 125 mEq (~5 g) of K^+ daily for people with normal kidney function (193). Unless ongoing losses (e.g., diarrhea, vomiting, diuretics) occur, the body's K^+ level should rise if intake is increased by as little as 40 mEq/day. In patients with prolonged hypokalemia and depleted intracellular stores, a decline in serum K^+ of 1 mEq/L generally indicates total body losses of 150 to 200 mEq of K^+, whereas a decline of 2 mEq/L indicates losses in excess of 500 mEq.

In the critical care setting, K^+ is usually given intravenously as KCl at a rate less than 10 mEq/hour. In life-threatening hypokalemia, it may be useful to estimate the number of liters of extracellular fluid as body weight in kilograms multiplied by 0.2 (194). This value multiplied by the desired increment in serum K^+ per liter provides an estimate of the amount of K^+ that can be safely given in 20 to 30 minutes without danger of hyperkalemia. A glucose-containing solution should not be used as a vehicle for KCl administration whenever serum K^+ is to be increased rapidly; glucose stimulates release of insulin, which, in turn, drives K^+ into the cells and decreases blood levels. K^+, at concentrations exceeding 40 mEq/L, may induce pain at the infusion site and may lead to sclerosis of smaller vessels. It is also advisable to avoid central venous infusion of K^+ at high concentrations, lest depolarization of the conduction tissues lead to cardiac arrest.

Renal loss of K^+ is prevented by treating its cause (e.g., removal of aldosterone-producing adenoma or by discontinuation of diuretics), by lowering distal delivery of Na^+, or by administering K^+-sparing diuretics (195). Because reduced delivery of Na^+ to the distal nephron reduces K^+ secretion, a low-salt diet helps to reduce renal K^+ loss unless a separate mechanism increases distal delivery of Na^+ (e.g., metabolic alkalosis or loop diuretics). The K^+-sparing diuretics in current use are aldosterone antagonists (e.g., spironolactone and eplerenone) and blockers of the ENaC, triamterene, and amiloride. Aldosterone antagonists are most effective in preventing renal K^+ loss if an increased mineralocorticoid concentration is responsible for hypokalemia; otherwise, the ENaC inhibitors are preferred.

Hyperkalemia

Causes and Pathogenesis
Hyperkalemia may be caused by either a shift of K^+ from the cells to the extracellular fluid (1, 19, 196, 197) or an increase in total body K^+ (Table 6.7). A shift of K^+ from inside cells can be caused by inadequate insulin (starvation type 1 diabetes) or, more commonly, by insulin resistance seen in type 2 diabetes, hyperkalemic familial periodic paralysis, administration of muscle paralytic agents (1, 19, 196, 197), administration of excess cationic amino acids such as arginine and lysine, and acute acidosis. All cause

TABLE 6.7	CAUSES OF HYPERKALEMIA

Increased intake
- A. Oral (usually with decreased excretion)
- B. Intravenous

Movement from cells into extracellular fluid
- A. Pseudohyperkalemia
  1. Mechanical puncture during venipuncture
  2. Leukocytosis (white blood cell count >100,000/mm³)
  3. Thrombocytosis (platelet count >400,000/mm³)
- B. Metabolic acidosis
- C. Insulin deficiency and hyperglycemia in uncontrolled diabetes mellitus
- D. Tissue catabolism
- E. β-Adrenergic blockade
- F. Severe exercise
- G. Digitalis overdose
- H. Periodic paralysis, hyperkalemic form
- I. Succinylcholine
- J. Arginine

Decreased urinary excretion
- A. Renal failure
- B. Effective circulating volume depletion
- C. Hypoaldosteronism
- D. Type I renal tubular acidosis, hyperkalemic form

hyperkalemia by extracellular K^+ shift. Cell death causing leakage of intracellular contents (i.e., rhabdomyolysis or hemolysis) can be associated with massive K^+ shifts. Although hyperkalemia is not as predictable in organic acidosis as in inorganic acidosis in experimental situations, hyperkalemia is common in diabetic ketoacidosis because of the lack of an insulin effect in shifting K^+ into cells (198). Hyperkalemia can also occur in severe digitalis intoxication by extracellular shift of K^+ because digitalis inhibits the Na^+/K^+-adenosine triphosphatase (ATPase) pump (199).

The kidney's ability to excrete dietary K^+ is so great that hyperkalemia rarely occurs solely on the basis of increased intake of K^+ in food. Thus, hyperkalemia is almost always the result of impaired renal excretion. The three major mechanisms of diminished renal K^+ excretion are reduced aldosterone or aldosterone responsiveness, reduced distal delivery of Na^+, and renal failure (acute or chronic). Aldosterone deficiency may be part of a generalized deficiency of adrenal hormones (e.g., Addison's disease), or it may represent a selective process (e.g., hyporeninemic hypoaldosteronism). Hyporeninemic hypoaldosteronism is the most common cause of all aldosterone deficiency states and is by far the most common cause of chronic hyperkalemia among patients who are not undergoing dialysis (19, 200). Selective hypoaldosteronism can also occur with heparin therapy, which inhibits steroid production in the zona glomerulosa (201).

In patients with reduced aldosterone secretion, any agent that limits the supply of renin or angiotensin II may provoke hyperkalemia. Examples include angiotensin-converting enzyme inhibitors, nonsteroidal anti-inflammatory agents, and β-blockers. The last category of drugs may compound the tendency to cause hyperkalemia by interfering with K^+ transport into cells. Chronic kidney disease (CKD) stage 3 or greater is often associated with decreased aldosterone levels produced by Na^+ retention and high blood pressure, but it may also cause hyperkalemia as a result of renal tubular unresponsiveness to aldosterone. This acquired aldosterone resistance may result from destruction of the distal nephron from urinary obstruction of the kidney or from interstitial nephritis. Stage 4 or greater CKD is almost always associated with an inability to excrete a K^+ load regardless of aldosterone. Genetic pseudohypoaldosteronism may also occur; this disorder may involve only K^+ secretion (pseudohypoaldosteronism type II) or Na^+ reabsorption in addition to K^+ secretion (pseudohypoaldosteronism type I) (202, 203). Severe volume depletion may cause hyperkalemia despite secondary hyperaldosteronism because of a marked reduction in delivery of Na^+ to the cortical collecting duct.

Pseudohyperkalemia, defined as a measured K^+ value higher than that present in the blood, is often caused by lysis of blood cells during the process of obtaining blood. This releases K^+ into the tube before measurement (204, 205). Repeating the blood draw is often required to verify hyperkalemia. A severe increase in platelets and leukocytes can cause pseudohyperkalemia through K^+ release during the process of coagulation (see Table 6.7).

Clinical Manifestations

K^+ helps maintain the polarization of skeletal and cardiac muscle. In severe hyperkalemia, paralysis of the skeletal muscle occurs with rapidly ascending neuromuscular weakness or paralysis. Before cardiac paralysis can develop, abnormalities of cardiac rhythm and of its rate of conduction occur. Characteristic ECG findings are used to assess the degree of cardiac involvement. The earliest, but most nonspecific, sign of hyperkalemia consists of tall, peaked T waves with shortened QT intervals. As hyperkalemia worsens, P waves flatten and QRS complexes widen progressively; then the P waves disappear entirely, and the QRS complexes merge with the T waves to stimulate a sine wave. This last rhythm is associated with a decline in cardiac output that is fatal unless rapidly treated. Other ECG findings include fascicular block and complete heart block (especially in digitalized patients), ventricular tachycardia, flutter and fibrillation, and cardiac arrest without the sine wave pattern (206, 207). Mild ECG changes have been noticed with serum K^+ levels of as low as 5.5 mEq/L. As in hypokalemia, however, the rate of development of hyperkalemia is important in the development of cardiac abnormalities. In chronic hyperkalemia, patients with K^+ levels higher than 7.0 mEq/L have had normal ECG tracings. Hyperkalemia can also cause mental confusion and paresthesias (208).

Treatment

Acute hyperkalemia may be treated by removal of K^+ from the body, by shifting extracellular K^+ into the cells, or by antagonizing K^+ action on the membrane of the cardiac

TABLE 6.8	TREATMENT OF HYPERKALEMIA

Reduction in body potassium content
  A. Reduction of intake
  B. Increased fecal secretion; potassium exchange resin and sorbitol
  C. Increased renal excretion; mineralocorticoids, increased salt intake, diuretics
  D. Peritoneal or hemodialysis
Intracellular shift of potassium
  A. Glucose and insulin
  B. Administration of alkali
  C. β-agonists: salbutamol, albuterol
Antagonism of the membrane effect of hyperkalemia
  A. Calcium salts
  B. Hypertonic sodium salts

conduction system (Table 6.8) (209–211). Antagonism of the action of K^+ on the heart with intravenous Ca^{2+} salts has the fastest effect against hyperkalemia and is used in life-threatening hyperkalemia. $CaCl_2$ and Ca gluconate are equally effective (212), but Ca gluconate is preferable because tissue damage is less when extravasation of the drug occurs during intravenous infusion. Shift of K^+ into cells can be accomplished with insulin (often given with glucose to prevent hypoglycemia), by β-adrenergic agonists (which have the advantage of the inhalation route if the patient does not have intravenous access), or by increasing the blood pH with $NaHCO_3^-$. HCO_3^- is less effective in the short term than the other approaches and partly works by diluting K^+ and increasing its excretion (211).

Removal of K^+ may be accomplished by several routes: through the GI tract with K^+ exchange resins or laxatives; through the kidney by diuretics, mineralocorticoids, and increased salt intake or saline infusion; by $NaHCO_3$ administration; and by hemodialysis or peritoneal dialysis (see Table 6.8). A K^+ exchange resin, Na polystyrene sulfonate (SPS [Kayexalate]), is more effective when it is given with agents such as sorbitol or mannitol that cause osmotic diarrhea, but no clinical trials have compared its effectiveness with other agents. Intestinal necrosis has been noted when sorbitol is given as an enema (213), so other laxatives may be preferable (214, 215). In response to reports of these complications, the FDA issued an advisory against concomitant administration of SPS with sorbitol in 2009. Because investigators thought that toxicity was related to 70% sorbitol and not 30% sorbitol, a premixed preparation of SPS in 30% sorbitol was allowed to stay on the market. More recently, reports exist showing colon necrosis following the use of premixed preparations of SPS in 30% sorbitol (216, 217). More data are needed on the benefit and harm associated with SPS and sorbitol (218). As an alternative, saline solution works by dilution and increasing distal delivery of Na^+ in patients with intact renal function. $NaHCO_3$ can also be used. When the kidney is responsive and volume overload is present, diuretics are extremely effective (219, 220). Mineralocorticoids are too slow in onset for acute use. Glycyrrhizic acid, the active ingredient of licorice, which inhibits 11-β-hydroxysteroid dehydrogenase, has been shown to decrease the serum K^+ concentration in patients undergoing dialysis. More data on pharmacokinetics and on toxicity are needed before the drug can be adopted for long-term use (221).

For chronic hyperkalemia, reduced intake of K^+ is effective in controlling high K^+. Problems with this approach include palatability, insufficient intake of fruit and vegetables (and thus fiber, antioxidants, etc.), and compliance. A thorny and unresolved problem is that despite the increased cardiac risk in patients with CKD, a low-K^+ diet restricts the very foods associated with reduction in cardiovascular disease risk. Diuretics, if needed for control of Na^+, are effective at wasting K^+ in the long term and may allow a healthier diet in some patients. Mg^{2+} wasting may be a problem when diuretics are combined with a low-K^+ diet. Some authorities advocate diuretics combined with a high-salt diet in patients without volume expansion. Renal salt retention is an important mechanism of hypertension and hypertensive cardiac damage, however, so monitoring Na^+ balance is critical. Mineralocorticoids (most often fludrocortisone (Florinef) have been used in these patients as a means of wasting K^+ (200), but mineralocorticoids have been implicated in the pathogenesis of cardiac and renal disease. $NaHCO_3$ can mildly increase K^+ excretion in patients with CKD. Because it is beneficial for its effect on acid–base balance, $NaHCO_3$ is a useful adjunct for managing these patients.

ACID–BASE BALANCE AND DISORDERS

Terminology

Changes in the proton concentration, as reflected by the pH of the blood, have a profound impact in various states with fundamental nutritional impact such as feeding, vomiting, diarrhea, and catabolism. These disorders are complex in etiology and diagnosis, however. Clinicians use numerous models (e.g., HCO_3^--anion gap [AG], base excess, strong ion difference) to classify acid–base disorders; of these, the HCO_3^--AG model is most suitable for nutrition science because it classifies disorders by the predominant species of acid or base accumulated (68, 222). In this model, acid and base come in two forms: respiratory, derived from dissolved CO_2; and metabolic, derived largely from metabolic or dietary acids and bases (19). Physiologically, a substance is an acid or a base depending on whether it will donate or accept a H^+ after metabolism in the body. CO_2 is an acid because it reacts with water to form carbonic acid. Both citric acid (in fruit sodas) and phosphoric acids (in colas) are chemically acids, but citric acid becomes a base after metabolism in the liver whereas phosphoric acid is unchanged. Thus, fruit sodas provide base and colas provide acid to the body. The term *acidosis* or *alkalosis*

refers to a pathologic process leading to acidic or alkaline pH, whereas *acidemia* and *alkalemia* refer to acidic and alkaline pH (68). This means that patients could have acidosis but actually have alkaline pH if, for example, they had combined respiratory acidosis (retaining CO_2) and metabolic alkalosis (excess consumption of base, e.g., calcium carbonate tablets).

Whole Body Acid–Base Balance

Net Acid Production

In healthy individuals, respiratory acids are derived from CO_2 from cellular respiration, whereas metabolic acids are usually derived from the diet (19, 68). On a typical Western diet, the daily production of nonvolatile acid is approximately 90 mEq/day (223). The main acid is sulfuric acid ($\sim$40 mEq/day), which originates from metabolism of the sulfur-containing amino acids methionine and cystine. Additional acid comes from organic acids that are not completely metabolized. The acid load varies greatly with the cystine and methionine content of proteins that are ingested and can be calculated from databases containing amino acid composition (223, 224). In general, when sulfur content is expressed as mEq/100 g of protein, proteins of animal sources (meat, fish, milk, and egg) contain higher amounts of sulfate for a given amount of protein than proteins of plant origin (cereal, beans, and nuts) (Fig. 6.7). The sulfur content per calorie is much greater in fruits, vegetables, and potatoes, but these food groups are not important sources of protein in the amounts usually eaten. Inorganic phosphates as food additives may also increase the acid content of food (e.g., colas).

The total amount of acid load also depends on the alkali content of food, which is present mainly as salts of organic acids (225). When both factors are considered, fruits and

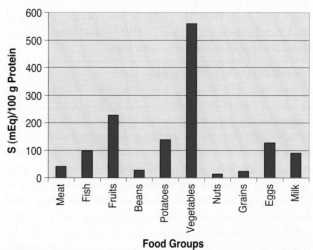

Fig. 6.7. Sulfur (S) content of food groups. (Reprinted with permission from Oh MS, Uribarri J. Electrolytes, water, and acid-base balance. In: Shils ME, Shike M, Ross AC et al, eds. Modern Nutrition in Health and Disease. 10th ed. Baltimore: Lippincott Williams & Wilkins, 2006:149–93.)

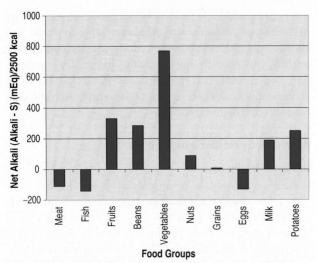

Fig. 6.8. Net alkali content of food expressed as the alkali content of food minus sulfur (S) content. Only meat, fish, and eggs have negative alkali content. Vegetables have the highest alkali content when expressed by the caloric content. (Reprinted with permission from Oh MS, Uribarri J. Electrolytes, water, and acid-base balance. In: Shils ME, Shike M, Ross AC et al, eds. Modern Nutrition in Health and Disease. 10th ed. Baltimore: Lippincott Williams & Wilkins, 2006:149–93.)

vegetables contain a large amount of net alkali; milk can be mildly acidic to alkaline, depending on the species; meat, fish, and grain have a net acid value (Fig. 6.8). Purified vegetable protein, which is devoid of organic bases, still provides a net acid load. The same is true for isolated amino acids used in parenteral nutrition and in amino acid infusions (e.g., glutamine) which are being studied in some critical care protocols. Parenteral amino acid infusions are often buffered with additional base to prevent acidosis. On typical US diets, the amount of alkali absorbed from the GI tract is approximately 30 mEq/day (225–227). If organic acids are normally metabolized to a base such as citrate and are excreted rather than metabolized, they leave their H^+ behind, thus creating a net acid load. Furthermore, stool loss of HCO_3^- and other organic bases also contributes to the acid load.

Measuring Dietary Acid or Base Load

Precise and accurate measurements of the amount of acid or base provided by the diet are difficult to obtain. As discussed earlier, measuring the acid load of the diet involves determining the number of sulfur-containing amino acids in addition to any added inorganic P. Errors arise in measuring the net alkali content of the diet, however, because these measurements are based on the metabolic fates of the components after metabolism. Ions are often used because the final metabolism of accepting an H^+ (base) involves release of cations and that of releasing an H^+ by release of anions (223). Thus, the net amount of organic base in food could be estimated from its ionic content (so-called strong ion difference) after metabolism (222). For example, the total amount of noncombustible cations (Na^+, K^+, Ca^{2+}, and Mg^{2+}) relative to the total amount

of noncombustible anions (Cl^- and P) provides a simple estimate of alkali content:

$$\text{Net alkali content} = (Na^+ + K^+ + Ca^{2+} + Mg^{2+}) - (Cl^- + 1.8\ P)$$

All units are expressed as milliequivalents per day, except P, which is expressed as millimoles per day multiplied by 1.8 and reflects the dependency of P valence on pH. Only the foregoing six ions are considered in the equation because other noncombustible ions are present in negligible amounts in the normal food. Sulfate is not included here because it is measured in the determination of the acid load.

Of course, foods induce differences in absorption, as well as stool losses of base (228). A simple method to measure net GI alkali absorption involves running the analysis on urine electrolytes instead of the diet and stool electrolytes. The method is based on the principle that noncombustible ions absorbed from the GI tract would eventually be excreted in the urine, and the individual amounts of these electrolytes excreted in the urine would equal those absorbed from the GI tract. The formula would be the same as described earlier and uses a 24-hour urine collection performed while subjects eat the diet of interest (228, 229). If the clinician has no need to know the acid or base content of a diet, but only its net acid–base effects, then renal net acid excretion (NAE) can be measured directly (see the later discussion of renal acid–base excretion) or estimated from dietary components (230, 231). Estimates of NAE have been derived from food frequency questionnaires and are based on electrolyte and protein content (230, 231). The sulfur content can be estimated from total dietary protein with a correction for dietary P. The potential base load is estimated by subtracting the effect of base using electrolytes, thus creating the so-called potential renal acid load (PRAL) (230):

$$\text{PRAL (mEq/day)} = 0.49 \times \text{Protein (g/day)} + 0.037 \times P\ (\text{mg/day}) - 0.21 \times K^+\ (\text{mg/day}) - 0.026 \times Mg^{2+}\ (\text{mg/day}) - 0.13 \times \text{Calcium } (Ca^{2+})\ (\text{mg/day})$$

PRAL correlates with renal NAE, so it is useful in epidemiologic studies, but it does not track the measured NAE in a linear fashion. An adjustment based on the metabolism or urinary loss of organic acids in the diet has been proposed. A correction factor (OA) for these organic acids on acid–base balance was measured to be OA = body surface area × 41/1.73 (232). This formula correlates with estimated intake from food frequency questionnaires and with 24-hour urine measurements (232). Thus, the best estimate of net acid load in a diet is as follows:

$$\text{NAE} = \text{PRAL} + \text{OA (232)}$$

A problem with this approach is that all ions in most foods in the diet must be known, but this is not the case for many prepackaged foods. In particular, the added P content of packaged foods is poorly known. Investigators wanted a simpler equation that used easily measurable components in the diet for use in cohort studies (231). They chose K^+, the dominant marker of organic base in the diet (and one whose content in packaged food is reported), and they performed a ratio with dietary protein, the source of dietary acid, and fit the data to measured NAE. This formula, which approximates PRAL, is useful when knowledge of the foods is more limited: NAE (mEq/day) = -10.2 + 54.5 (dietary protein [g/day]/K^+ [mEq/day]) (231). One concern with this formula is that it was verified on populations obtaining most of their protein from meat (containing ample protein and K^+). Furthermore, the usefulness of this formula in epidemiologic studies is confounded by strong dependence on components that have independent effects on health outcomes.

Buffering

Because buffering occurs, protons (H^+) added or removed from body fluids do not result in an instant change in pH (68, 233). All body buffers, including the HCO_3^--CO_2 system, are in chemical equilibrium with protons and affect the pH according to the equilibrium equation (234):

$$pH = \text{dissociation constant } (pK_a) + \log A^-/HA$$

where A is the buffer and A^- is a conjugate base of an acid HA. Because HCO_3^- and CO_2 are the major buffers of the body, pH is typically expressed as a function of their ratio, as in the Henderson–Hasselbalch equation:

$$pH = 6.1 + \log HCO_3^-/(P_{CO_2} \times 0.03)$$

where 6.1 is the pK_a of the HCO_3^- and CO_2 buffer system, and 0.03 is the solubility coefficient of CO_2.

The equation can be further simplified by combining the two constants, pK_a and the solubility coefficient of CO_2:

$$pH = 6.1 + \log HCO_3^-/(P_{CO_2} \times 0.03)$$
$$= 6.1 + \log 1/0.03 + \log HCO_3^-/P_{CO_2}$$

Hence,

$$= 7.62 + \log HCO_3^-/P_{CO_2} \quad (5)$$
$$pH = 7.62 - \log P_{CO_2}/HCO_3^-$$
$$= 7.62 + \log HCO_3^- - \log CO_2$$

When H^+ is expressed in nanomolars instead of a negative log value (pH), P_{CO_2} can be related to HCO_3^- in the following equation:

$$H(nM) = 24 \times P_{CO_2} \text{ (mm Hg)}/HCO_3^- \text{ (mM)}$$

Clinically, the Henderson–Hasselbalch equation is useful because it points out that pH depends on the HCO_3^-/P_{CO_2} ratio (74). pH increases when the ratio increases (alkalosis), and pH decreases when the ratio decreases (acidosis). The ratio may be increased by an increase in HCO_3^- (metabolic alkalosis) or by a decrease in P_{CO_2} (respiratory alkalosis). The ratio may be decreased by a decrease in HCO_3^- (metabolic acidosis) or by an increase in P_{CO_2} (respiratory acidosis).

Although the CO_2 buffer system is crucial in understanding acid–base disturbances, the complications of

acidemia and alkalemia are better explained by bone and protein buffering (235). The carbonate apatite in the bone matrix acts as a reserve of base during an acid load, which commonly occurs after a .high-protein meal. Protons interact with the carbonate to form CO_2 and water, thus liberating Ca^{2+} and P from bone. The direct effect of an acid load is bone dissolution (235). Proteins have carboxylic acid side groups that can donate or accept protons. This change in electrical charge alters protein folding or protein–protein interactions and causes cellular dysfunction; free Ca^{2+} is altered (236, 237). Acidosis increases free (ionic) Ca^{2+} by increasing the positive charges on protein and decreasing Ca^{2+} binding; alkalosis decreases free (ionic) Ca^{2+} by increasing the negative charges on protein and increasing Ca^{2+} binding.

Shifts of Protons within the Body

Protons move in a regulated fashion into cells in net exchange for K^+, but this movement is more important for K^+ than for pH regulation (137). The movement of acids and base into sequestered spaces has a far greater effect on serum pH (68, 237). For example, the movement of protons into the stomach to form stomach acid and the movement of HCO_3^- into the intestine to form bile and pancreatic secretions affect serum pH (68). The release of stomach acid causes a postprandial "alkaline tide." This effect is caused by the delay between acid secretion into the stomach before and immediately on feeding and base secretion into the intestine that occurs on gastric emptying. The urine pH rises transiently after meals as the kidney excretes some of this base and increases the net acid load associated with the meal. The urine pH then falls as alkaline bile and pancreatic secretions are replenished. This transient rise in urine pH is eliminated by drugs that block gastric acid secretion.

Renal Acid–Base Excretion

The kidney protects the body from rises in pH by simply failing to reabsorb HCO_3^- when the pH is high, but renal excretion of acid is more complex (68, 233). Acid is excreted in the form of titratable acid (free protons and buffered protons on PO_4^- and sulfate anions) and ammonium (NH_4^+). Excretion of titratable acid is usually modest because of the limited amount of buffer that produces titratable acid (i.e., P, creatinine, and urate), but it may be increased markedly in disease states (e.g., β-hydroxybutyric acid in diabetic ketoacidosis). Normally, approximately two thirds of acid excretion occurs in the form of NH_4^+, but in acidosis, NH_4^+ excretion may increase as much as 10-fold.

Nutritionally, it is critical to recognize that ammonia is required to excrete an acid load and is created from the destruction of the amino acid glutamine (238). In response to acidemia, muscle releases branched-chain amino acids that the liver converts into glutamine. The proximal tubule deaminates glutamine to form a proton, ammonia, and HCO_3^-. Thus, the mechanism for renal acid secretion relies on increased glutamine production from muscle and liver and contributes to the catabolic effects of chronic metabolic acidosis (see later) (239). High K^+ blocks ammonia production. This effect is blunted in the setting of protein malnutrition and the metabolic syndrome (233, 240).

The HCO_3^- formed from glutamine returns to the body, but the ammonia and proton are excreted into the lumen of the proximal tubule (68, 233) (Fig. 6.9). The proton is excreted in exchange for Na^+ through the Na^+ hydrogen antiporter 3. This exchange explains why altering Na^+ reabsorption affects the absorption of base in the proximal tubule, because the proton reacts with filtered HCO_3^- present in the tubule to form CO_2 and water (so-called HCO_3^- reclamation). If more HCO_3^- is filtered than the proximal tubule can reabsorb (because the blood level of HCO_3^- is high or the GFR suddenly rises), the excess is delivered to the distal nephron. Most often, this results in a loss of HCO_3^- from the body and net alkali secretion. Electroneutrality is maintained by coupling the HCO_3^- with Na^+. As discussed earlier, this HCO_3^- drag influences Na^+ and K^+ balance (138). The distal nephron contains both hydrogen pumps (primarily the vacuolar H ATPase) to add acid to the final urine and Cl^--HCO_3^- exchangers (primarily pendrin) to add base to the final urine (233). Acidemia or increased activity of the renin-angiotensin-aldosterone system increases acid secretion and decreases base secretion, whereas alkalemia or reduced activity of this physiologic system decreases acid secretion and increases base secretion.

On a Western diet, net acid secretion in the distal nephron always occurs, and the final urinary pH is acidemic (223). Potential bases in the urine such as P or uric acid buffer the pH (68, 233). The ammonia created in the proximal tubule is also excreted into the lumen and travels to the distal tubule, where it accepts protons being secreted in the distal nephron to form NH_4^+. Thus, NH_4^+ allows acid excretion without lowering the final pH of the urine.

This final urinary pH is relevant to the effects of diet on kidney stone formation (240, 241). Western diets are associated with the formation of kidney stones in an acid urine pH such as calcium oxalate and uric acid stones. Uric acid dissolves at a pH higher than 6, so uric acid stones absolutely require a persistently acidemic urine pH. As discussed earlier, protein malnutrition or metabolic syndrome lowers urinary pH during acidosis by suppressing ammonia production, and studies have shown that these conditions stimulate the formation of uric acid kidney stones (240). Thus, a stone type associated with affluent societies can be seen in developing ones as well. Consumption of excess base (e.g., calcium citrate or carbonate dietary supplements) raises the pH of the urine. At a pH higher than 6.8, PO_4^- accepts a second proton. This shift makes $CaPO_4^-$ much less soluble and leads to $CaPO_4^-$ stones, thus explaining the increased risk of kidney stones in patients taking these supplements (241).

In summary, NAE, which is equivalent to net renal production of alkali, can be determined by subtracting HCO_3^- excretion from acid excretion:

$$NAE = \text{Acid excretion} - HCO_3^- \text{ excretion} =$$
Urinary NH_4^+ + Urinary titratable acid (where titratable acid includes urinary pH + phosphates and other titratable acids − urinary HCO_3^-)

Maintenance of acid–base balance requires that net acid production equals NAE. Metabolic acidosis develops when net acid production exceeds NAE, and metabolic alkalosis develops when NAE exceeds net acid production.

Metabolic Acidosis

Metabolic acidosis is defined as an excess of protons and thus a fall in the HCO_3^- content of the body (19, 68). A reduction in HCO_3^- content may be caused by a primary increase in acid production (extrarenal acidosis) or by a primary reduction in NAE (renal acidosis) (Table 6.9). In this classification, nonrenal loss of HCO_3^- or an alkali precursor is considered part of increased acid production.

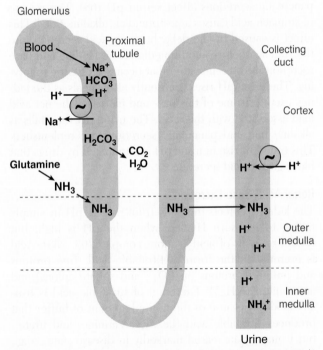

Fig. 6.9. Renal acid excretion. Bicarbonate (HCO_3^-) and sodium (Na^+) are filtered from the blood at the glomerulus. In the proximal tubule, hydrogen ions (H^+) are excreted in the urine in exchange for sodium, and the hydrogen and bicarbonate form carbonic acid, which dissolves into carbon dioxide and water. The carbon dioxide and water are reabsorbed, and the net result is that the filtered bicarbonate is not lost in the urine. The proximal tubule makes ammonia (NH_3) from glutamine, which is transported to the collecting duct. Hydrogen ions are pumped into the lumen. Some react with NH_3 to form ammonium (NH_4), which does not lower the urine pH, whereas others remain in solution to lower the urine pH. Thus, acid is excreted as hydrogen ions and ammonium, and the relative amounts of each determine the final pH of the urine.

TABLE 6.9	CAUSES OF METABOLIC ACIDOSIS
High anion gap	Anion
A. Lactic acidosis	Lactate
B. Ketoacidosis	β-Hydroxybutyric acid, acetoacetic acid
C. Renal failure	Sulfate, phosphate, urate
D. Ingestions	
1. Salicylate	Salicylate, lactate
2. Methanol	Formate
3. Ethylene glycol	Glycolate, oxalate
4. Paraldehyde	Acetate, chloroacetate
5. Toluene	Hippurate
E. Massive rhabdomyolysis	
Normal anion gap (hyperchloremic acidosis	
A. Gastrointestinal loss of bicarbonate	
1. Diarrhea	
2. Pancreatic, biliary, or intestinal fistulas	
3. Ureterosigmoidostomy	
B. Renal bicarbonate loss	
1. Type 2 (proximal) renal tubular acidosis	
C. Renal dysfunction	
1. Some cases of renal failure	
2. Hypoaldosteronism	
3. Type 1 (distal) renal tubular acidosis	
D. Ingestions	
1. Ammonium chloride	

In extrarenal acidosis, NAE is markedly increased as the kidney compensates to overcome acidosis. Conversely, NAE may be restored to normal in chronic renal acidosis because acidosis stimulates renal H^+ excretion. Normal NAE in the presence of an acidic pH suggests a defect in renal acid excretion and therefore renal acidosis. If the renal acid excretion capacity is normal, NAE should be supernormal in the presence of an acidic pH.

Complications of Acidemia

The body readily tolerates mild acute metabolic acidosis (236). This condition is seen during strenuous exercise (e.g., sprinting) when the blood pH falls to less than 7.2 without immediate adverse effects. In some ways, acute acidosis helps the body in the setting of exercise or acute illness. Principally, increased oxygen delivery to the tissues occurs through the Bohr effect as oxygen is shifted from hemoglobin to the tissues. Vasodilation and stimulation of the respiratory drive act to aid tissue respiration and minimize lactic acidosis (242). Severe metabolic acidosis (pH <7.1), however, contributes to ventricular irritability, may cause arrhythmias and resistance to the effects of catecholamines, and may lead to lower blood pressure (236, 243). Severe acidemia at a pH less than 6.8 is not well tolerated; shock, coma, respiratory failure, and death may ensue.

On a long-term basis, the body does not tolerate even small degrees of acidemia (236). Catabolism of both bone and muscle occurs with chronic acid loading even with a normal blood pH. This is because much of the catabolic response to acidemia is caused by chronic activation of the body's own mechanisms that buffer and excrete excess H^+ (236, 239). The chronic buffering of acid by bone leads to both a direct loss of bone mineral and an indirect loss related to hormonal changes (235). Elevated cortisol and parathyroid hormone levels increase bone turnover. Acidosis also induces a direct inhibition of tubular Ca^{2+} reabsorption that is independent of Ca^{2+} levels (235). In addition, acidosis causes a fall in the urinary concentration of citrate, a major urinary inhibitor of Ca^{2+} crystallization, so an increase in urinary Ca^{2+} levels is associated with an increased risk of calcium oxalate kidney stones (244). Acidosis induces both osteoporosis in adults and reduced bone growth in children, effects that are reversed by correction of the acidosis. The catabolic effects of acidosis on bone may apply to patients who merely eat a diet with a high net acid load. Adding base to the diet of middle-aged women had a positive effect on bone density (245).

Acidemia also induces negative nitrogen balance and stimulates renal ammonia excretion. As discussed earlier, muscle protein is broken down to yield amino acids that are converted to the glutamine that forms the substrate for NH_4^+ secretion (238, 239). Acid directly stimulates glutamine production by increasing muscle protein degradation and enhancing oxidation of the branched-chain amino acids to provide substrate for the liver to synthesize glutamine (240). Moreover, acidemia increases catabolic hormones such as cortisol and parathyroid hormone to increase muscle wasting further, and it induces muscle-specific resistance to the action of anabolic hormones (insulin and insulinlike growth factor-I). This catabolic effect may apply to a net acid diet: middle-aged women demonstrated marked improvement in nitrogen balance when their diets were supplemented with base (125). Base supplements are an effective ergonomic aid for sports performance (246), may be useful for muscle rehabilitation in elderly patients (247, 248), and may improve muscle mass in CKD (249). Thus, correction of acidemia has major nutritional benefits on Ca^{2+} and muscle metabolism.

High-protein diets can increase kidney damage in patients with CKD, and acidemia is one potential mediator of this effect (239). The adrenal hormone aldosterone is stimulated by acid and augments renal net acid secretion (19, 68). Aldosterone has been implicated in the progression of congestive heart failure and CKD (239, 249, 250). Although no cardiac studies have been conducted, reducing acidemia with $NaHCO_3$ has been shown to slow the loss of kidney function in patients with advanced CKD (249).

Hyperchloremic Acidosis

Metabolic acids exist in two forms: (a) they are associated with addition of HCl or the removal of equivalent amount of HCO_3^- or (b) they originate from the addition of a nonmetabolizable organic acid (19, 68, 233). When HCl is added or HCO_3^- is lost, the serum Cl^- concentration rises and the serum HCO_3^- concentration falls, thus causing so-called hyperchloremic metabolic acidosis. This condition results from the loss of HCO_3^- in the stool in the setting of diarrhea or from the retention of H^+ in CKD. When a nonmetabolized acid is added, hyperchloremic acidosis results as the organic anion is lost in the urine following release of H^+. As the HCO_3^- level falls, Cl^- shifts out of cells to maintain electroneutrality, whereas the sulfur anion is lost in the urine in the individual eating a high-protein diet. The extant proton combines with Cl^- and causes hyperchloremic acidosis. A similar effect occurs when parenteral amino acid infusions are not buffered with sufficient base.

Causes of and Therapies for Hyperchloremic Acidosis. Correct diagnosis of the cause of metabolic acidosis is important because diets and therapy vary (19, 68, 233). Diarrheal loss of HCO_3^- is the most common cause of hyperchloremic acidosis and is usually suspected from the patient's history. When diarrhea is not obvious, the culprit is often laxatives, lactose intolerance, gluten-sensitive enteropathy, hyperosmolar enteral liquid feeding products, drugs or dietary supplements that increase stool volume, or surgical drainage of HCO_3^--rich biliary or pancreatic fluid. Because urinary excretion of NH_4^+ increases as a part of renal compensatory mechanisms, indirect measurements of urine NH_4^+ can be used to confirm this diagnosis (239). Given that acidosis delays restoration of protein stores and enhances bone anabolism, the catabolic effects of chronic acidosis play a major role in the nutritional abnormalities resulting from chronic diarrhea. The use of base supplementation as K^+, Ca^{2+}, or Na^+ salts can provide significant benefit (251). In selecting feeding products, it is important to provide adequate, but not excessive, protein and to consider the osmolar load and ease of digestion to hasten recovery.

Uremic acidosis seen in acute kidney injury or CKD can be readily diagnosed by the measurement of serum creatinine and blood urea nitrogen (19, 68, 250). Because development of renal acidosis depends on acid production, it varies greatly according to the protein and vegetable content of the diet (239). Unfortunately, the low-K^+ diet that is sometimes required in advanced CKD is often deficient in organic base, and supplementary HCO_3^- tablets are required. Studies also suggest that acidosis frequently occurs at a GFR of 40 mL/minute (stage 3 CKD) when excessive protein or insufficient base is consumed or when renal tubular acidosis (RTA) is present (see later). With moderate protein restriction, uremic acidosis may develop as GFR falls to less than 20 mL/minute (stage 4 CKD) (239). Dietary protein restriction and $NaHCO_3$ are effective therapies for acidosis in CKD (239, 249, 252). Both therapies have been shown to have benefits on muscle and bone anabolism and in slowing the loss of kidney function. Protein restriction must be part of a carefully designed and monitored diet, however (see the chapter on kidney disease).

RTA occurs when the kidney cannot excrete acid and advanced CKD is absent (19, 68, 252). Three types of RTA are known. Type I RTA, also called classic RTA or distal RTA, is characterized by an inability to reduce the urine pH maximally to less than 5.5. Type I RTA can develop as a primary disorder or secondary to drug toxicity, tubulointerstitial renal diseases, autoimmune disease, or other renal diseases (252). It is associated with a low serum K^+ and kidney stones (68, 252, 253). Dietary management hinges on a K^+-rich- and base-rich diet high in fruit and vegetables and low in animal protein (see the DASH diet). K^+ base supplements are effective in treatment.

Type II RTA, also called proximal RTA, causes defective proximal HCO_3^- reabsorption (19, 68, 252). Most patients with proximal RTA have evidence of generalized proximal tubular dysfunction (i.e., Fanconi syndrome), which is manifested by bicarbonaturia, aminoaciduria, glycosuria, phosphaturia, and uricosuria. Of these conditions, renal glycosuria (glycosuria in the presence normal blood glucose) is most useful in diagnosing Fanconi syndrome. Type II RTA may be a primary disorder, secondary to genetic or acquired renal dysfunction, or induced by drugs that inhibit carbonic anhydrase. Hypokalemia is a characteristic finding of both type I and type II RTA, but it tends to be more severe in type I than in type II RTA. Because HCO_3^- losses in the urine cannot be repleted by diet alone, dietary considerations often focus on K^+ and PO_4^- repletion. High-dose therapy using K^+, Na^+, and Ca^{2+} base is required to normalize acid–base status.

Type IV RTA is caused by either aldosterone deficiency or tubular unresponsiveness to aldosterone and results in impaired renal tubular K^+ secretion and hyperkalemia (200). Although reduced H^+ secretion in the collecting duct plays a role, the major mechanism of acidosis in type IV RTA is hyperkalemia-induced impairment in ammonia production in the proximal tubule. Thus, control of K^+ is the major nutritional consideration. As discussed earlier, a diet low in K^+ is often low in base content, and $NaHCO_3$ is an effective supplement.

Anion Gap Acidosis

Massive overproduction of organic acid occurs in two life-threatening syndromes (lactic acidosis and ketoacidosis) that result from catastrophic failure in energy metabolism (19, 68, 251). Because of massive overproduction, the kidney is unable to excrete the organic acid quickly enough, and the anion is retained in the body. As the anion accumulates in the blood as a negative charge, the released H^+ causes a fall in the serum HCO_3^- concentration without any change in the serum Cl^- concentration. Because the anion is not measured on routine clinical chemistry tests, the patient's serum appears to have a missing anion (19, 68, 252). This "anion gap" is used clinically to detect acidosis secondary to nonmetabolizable organic acids that are not lost in the urine.

The term *anion gap* implies a gap between cation and anion concentrations, which obviously is not true; the concentration of total cations in the serum must be exactly equal to the concentration of total anions (19, 68). A change in serum Na^+ usually does not alter the AG because the serum Cl^- usually changes in the same direction. Given that normal serum K^+ concentration is quantitatively a minor component of serum electrolytes, the AG is estimated from the concentrations of Na^+, Cl^-, and HCO_3^- as follows:

$$AG = Na^+ - (Cl^- + HCO_3^-)$$

Because unmeasured cations outnumber unmeasured anions, the normal value is approximately 10 mEq/L (8 to 14 mEq/L). Although the total concentration of unmeasured anions (i.e., all anions other than Cl^- and HCO_3^-) is approximately 23 mEq/L, the AG is only 12 mEq/L because of the presence of approximately 11 mEq/L of unmeasured cations (i.e., all cations other than Na^+) (254). An increased AG is most often caused by accumulation of anions of acids, such as sulfate, lactate, or ketones. A decreased AG is most commonly the result of a reduction in serum albumin concentration (252, 255). Because albumin is a negatively charged protein, it is responsible for a large part of the normal AG. The AG also varies with other influences, such as severe changes in pH and hypergammaglobulinemia. Proper interpretation of a serum AG requires the knowledge of the existence of conditions that influence the AG even though they may have no direct effect on metabolic acidosis. For example, if a person with hypoalbuminemia develops lactic acidosis with renal failure, the AG could be normal because the low albumin concentration and the accumulated lactate have opposite effects on the AG. Not knowing the effect of serum albumin on AG, one could overlook the existence of lactic acidosis on the basis of a normal AG.

When the AG is increased, likely causes include organic acidosis (lactic and ketoacidosis, uremic acidosis, and acidosis resulting from certain toxins) (19, 68, 252) (see Table 6.9). Most cases of acidosis in CKD are accompanied by a normal AG, however, because the kidney still clears the sulfur from proteins adequately. Only in advanced chronic and acute renal failure is the AG increased. When the GFR falls to less than 15 mL/minute, sulfates from dietary amino acids accumulate in the blood and lead to AG acidosis.

Lactic Acidosis. In cellular metabolism, carbohydrates are first reduced to pyruvic acid (pyruvate) through glycolysis. The pyruvic acid can either enter the mitochondria to be metabolized to CO_2 and water in the presence of oxygen in the tricarboxylic acid cycle (Krebs cycle) or be recycled to lactic acid and eventually back to glucose. Thus, availability of oxygen is usually the major regulator of lactate production and explains the clinical use of lactic acidosis as a critical marker of tissue hypoxia (253). The hypoxia may arise from increased oxygen demand (e.g., exercise, seizures, cancer) or from decreased oxygen delivery (e.g., shock, severe anemia respiratory failure, carbon monoxide poisoning) (252). Lactate dehydrogenase and the cofactor reduced nicotinamide adenine dinucleotide (NADH) are required for both lactate production in the peripheral

tissue (usually muscle) and for lactate conversion back to pyruvic acid in the liver and, to a lesser extent, in the kidney. For this reason, hypoxia sometimes affects both production and metabolism of lactic acid. An elevated concentration of pyruvic acid and an increased $NADH/NAD^+$ ratio raise lactic acid production while at the same time reduce its metabolism. Decreased metabolism of lactate is largely responsible for lactic acidosis in acute alcoholism (ethanol increases the $NADH/NAD^+$ ratio), salicylate and metformin poisoning, and severe liver disease (251, 252).

Ketoacidosis. Ketoacids, acetoacetic acid, and β-hydroxybutyric acid are produced in the liver from free fatty acids (FFAs) and are metabolized by the extrahepatic tissues (19, 68, 256). Increased production of ketoacids, the main mechanism for ketoacid accumulation, requires a high concentration of FFAs and their conversion to ketoacids in the liver. Insulin deficiency is responsible for increased mobilization of FFAs from the adipose tissue, whereas glucagon excess and insulin deficiency stimulate conversion of FFAs to ketoacids in the liver. The initial step in ketoacid production from FFAs is the entry of FFAs into the mitochondria, a process that requires acylcarnitine transferase. This step is stimulated by glucagon excess. The next step is metabolism of FFAs to acetylcoenzyme A, and then finally to ketoacids. Diversion of acetyl-coenzyme A to fatty acid resynthesis requires the enzyme acetyl-coenzyme A carboxylase. Inhibition of this enzyme by insulin deficiency, glucagon excess, or an excess of stress-induced hormones further contributes to increased ketoacid synthesis.

It follows that the absence of an insulin effect, FFA availability, and increased glucagon are required for ketone formation in the liver. Although these conditions are present during prolonged starvation (starvation ketosis), full expression of life-threatening ketoacidosis occurs only in diabetic and alcoholic ketoacidosis. Only those patients with diabetes with very low insulin production (type 1 diabetes) or those patients with diabetes with the most severe insulin resistance develop severe ketoacidosis (256, 262). In patients with type 1 diabetes, the lack of insulin stimulates glucagon production to a greater extent than starvation alone and mobilizes larger amounts of FFAs. The hyperglycemia leads to Na^+ loss in the urine through osmotic diuresis, whereas nausea and vomiting lead to a decreased intake of Na^+. The lack of Na^+ compromises kidney function, traps the ketones in the body, and blocks acid excretion. Insulin, NaCl infusion, and usually additional glucose are required to treat diabetic ketoacidosis. Although ethanol is metabolized to a ketone, acetoacetate, by alcohol dehydrogenase, casual alcohol consumption does not lead to ketosis (68). Prolonged alcohol consumption in the absence of carbohydrate intake leads to a marked increase in glucagon and insulin suppression. FFA release is stimulated, whereas Na^+ depletion results from ethanol's effect as an osmotic diuretic because it is excreted in the urine. Carbohydrates and NaCl are sufficient to reverse alcoholic ketoacidosis. Because starvation is associated with relatively higher levels of insulin and lower levels of glucagon and FFAs, the amount of ketone formation is lower and does not lead to life-threatening acidemia.

The bases of the ketoacids are rapidly cleared in the urine following loss of their respective proton (19, 68, 256). The two major ketoacids, acetoacetic acid and β-hydroxybutyric acid, can be converted from one to another by β-hydroxybutyric acid dehydrogenase and the cofactor NADH. Consequently, the ratio of NADH to NAD$^+$ is the major determinant of the ratio of acetoacetic acid to β-hydroxybutyric acid. This is important because urinary testing for ketoacids detects acetoacetic acid only. When β-hydroxybutyric acid is the primary ketone, the diagnosis of ketoacidosis can be missed. This situation can occur during shock or during alcoholic ketoacidosis.

Other Types. Various different poisons can lead to AG acidosis. Salicylate (aspirin) overdose (as discussed earlier) can lead to lactic acidosis (19, 68). Like ethanol, other alcohols, including methanol (wood alcohol) and propylene glycol (antifreeze), are metabolized by alcohol and aldehyde dehydrogenase (257). Instead of the formation of acetone and subsequently acetoacetic acid with ethanol, methanol forms formaldehyde and formic acid, and ethylene glycol forms glycolic acid. Glycolic acid is eventually metabolized to oxalate. Formaldehyde causes the blindness characteristic of methanol poisoning, whereas oxalate crystallizes in the urine with Ca^{2+} at high concentrations to cause acute kidney injury. Finally, gut bacteria can create numerous organic acids that are difficult to measure when they overgrow in the GI tract.

Treatment. Correction of the underlying disorder is the best therapy for AG metabolic acidosis (258, 259). When possible, promoting metabolism of the organic acid is extremely effective. For example, when ketoacidosis is treated with insulin, the acetoacetate and β-hydroxybutyric acid are metabolized in the Krebs cycle–producing base. Thus, exogenous alkali is seldom necessary in ketoacidosis. When lactic acid results from physiologic overproduction, in exercise or during seizures, it is rapidly metabolized. Restoration of tissue oxygen delivery in hypoxia-induced lactic acid is equally effective, but it is often not possible because of the severity of the disease.

Rapid restoration of normal pH with base therapy is usually unnecessary and may be undesirable for several reasons (259). A sudden increase in extracellular pH can cause paradoxic acidosis of the cerebrospinal fluid. Rapid restoration of a normal serum HCO_3^- level in metabolic acidosis would also be undesirable because persistent hyperventilation would produce a very high blood pH. The initial aim in the treatment of severe metabolic acidosis should be to increase the blood pH to a level at which the adverse cardiovascular effects of severe acidemia can be avoided. Although the risk of acidosis varies with the age and the cardiovascular status of patients, critical care guidelines suggest acutely targeting replacement to a pH of 7.15 (243).

Respiratory Acidosis

Causes and Pathogenesis

Decreasing ventilation of the lungs causes CO_2 accumulation in the body (19, 68, 260). The causes of respiratory acidosis are usually quite apparent (Table 6.10). They include diseases of the lung (most common), respiratory muscle, respiratory nerve, thoracic cage, and airways and suppression of the respiratory center by stroke, drugs such as phenobarbital, or severe hypothyroidism. Although studies suggest subtle differences between the complications of respiratory acidosis and those of metabolic acidosis, in clinical practice, they are largely indistinguishable, except for nutritional effects on muscle. Renal compensation for respiratory acidosis involves retaining HCO_3^-, so ammonia production (and thus glutamine use) is not as severely affected (261).

TABLE 6.10	CAUSES OF ACUTE AND CHRONIC RESPIRATORY ACIDOSIS

Inhibition of the medullary respiratory center
  A. Acute
    1. Drugs: opiates, anesthetics, sedatives
    2. Central sleep apnea
    3. Cardiac arrest
  B. Chronic
    1. Extreme obesity
Disorders of the respiratory muscles and chest wall
  A. Acute
    1. Muscle weakness
        Myasthenia gravis
        Periodic paralysis
        Guillain-Barré syndrome
        Severe hypokalemia
        Severe hypophosphatemia
  B. Chronic
    1. Muscle weakness
        Poliomyelitis
        Amyotrophic lateral sclerosis
        Multiple sclerosis
        Myxedema
    2. Kyphoscoliosis
    3. Extreme obesity
Upper airway obstruction
  A. Acute
    1. Aspiration of foreign body or vomitus
    2. Obstructive sleep apnea
    3. Laryngospasm
Disorders affecting gas exchange across the pulmonary capillary
  A. Acute
    1. Exacerbation of underlying lung disease (increased carbon dioxide production with high-carbohydrate diet)
    2. Adult respiratory distress syndrome
    3. Acute cardiogenic pulmonary edema
    4. Severe asthma or pneumonia
  B. Chronic
    1. Chronic obstructive pulmonary disease
        Bronchitis
        Emphysema
        Mechanical ventilation

Treatment

All cases of respiratory acidosis are caused by alveolar hypoventilation, but in severe respiratory acidosis, efforts should be made to normalize ventilation (260). When restoration of effective ventilation is delayed and the patient is comatose or has cardiac arrhythmias, acidosis can be treated temporarily with the administration of alkali. Administration of HCO_3^- is not very effective in correcting the brain pH, however, because of the slow penetration of HCO_3^- into the central nervous system. After 24 to 96 hours, the kidneys respond to the respiratory acidosis and control the pH with renal compensation (261). As a result of the compensation, hypoxia poses a greater problem than does the chronic respiratory acidosis. Various drugs have been tried in an attempt to stimulate respiration in acute and chronic respiratory acidosis (19). The apnea of prematurity has been treated with respiratory stimulants such as doxapram and the methylxanthines, caffeine citrate, and theophylline. Caffeine occurs naturally in coffee and is a common food additive. Theophylline occurs naturally in black tea and related plants. Caffeine citrate is the consensus drug of choice for premature babies with respiratory depression. In chronic obstructive pulmonary disease, theophylline, doxapram, and progesterone derivatives including progesterone, medroxyprogesterone, and chlormadinone have been tried (262).

Metabolic Alkalosis

Causes and Pathogenesis

At a normal serum HCO_3^- concentration on a Western diet, HCO_3^- filtered at the glomerulus is virtually completely reabsorbed (68, 233, 237). As serum HCO_3^- concentration rises to more than the normal level, HCO_3^- reabsorption is incomplete, and bicarbonaturia begins. A slight increase in serum HCO_3^- to more than 24 mEq/L causes marked bicarbonaturia. Hence, when renal tubular HCO_3^- handling and GFR are normal, it is very difficult to maintain a high plasma HCO_3^- concentration unless an enormous amount of HCO_3^- is given. Therefore, maintenance of metabolic alkalosis requires two conditions: a mechanism to increase plasma HCO_3^- and a mechanism to maintain the increased concentration. HCO_3^- concentration may be increased by administration of alkali, gastric loss of HCl through vomiting or nasogastric suction, or renal generation of HCO_3^-. Plasma HCO_3^- concentration can be maintained at a high level if HCO_3^- is not filtered at the glomerulus because of advanced renal failure or if the filtered HCO_3^- is reabsorbed avidly because of an increased renal threshold for HCO_3^- (19). The two most common causes of an increased renal HCO_3^- threshold are volume depletion and K^+ depletion, but excess aldosterone may also be a cause (Table 6.11).

When metabolic alkalosis results from volume depletion, urinary excretion of Cl^- is reduced (19, 68, 237).

TABLE 6.11	CAUSES OF METABOLIC ALKALOSIS

Chloride sensitive (low urine chloride)
  A. Gastrointestinal loss of acid and chloride
    1. Vomiting, nasogastric suction
    2. Villous adenoma
  B. Renal
    1. Diuretics
    2. Posthypercapnic status
    3. Low chloride intake
    4. Hypercalcemia
    5. Anion drag (usually penicillin)
  C. Base administration
    1. Calcium base (calcium carbonate, calcium citrate) Milk alkali syndrome
    2. Sodium or potassium base (sodium bicarbonate, potassium citrate)
    3. Blood products (citrate)
    4. High acetate parenteral nutrition
With low urine chloride but no response to chloride
  A. Effective circulating volume depletion
    1. Kidney failure
    2. Heart failure
    3. Cirrhosis of liver
Chloride resistant (normal urine chloride)
  A. Increased aldosterone action
    1. Hyperaldosteronism
    2. Cushing syndrome
    3. Natural licorice
    4. Pseudohyperaldosteronism
    5. Severe hypokalemia

Measurement of urinary Na^+ is an unreliable index of volume depletion in metabolic alkalosis because excretion of HCO_3^- causes obligatory loss of Na^+ despite volume depletion. Metabolic alkalosis accompanied by low urinary Cl^- can be corrected by administration of Cl^--containing food or intravenous solution, such as NaCl or KCl, hence the term Cl^--responsive metabolic alkalosis. Patients with Cl^--responsive metabolic alkalosis are volume depleted, and the response to Cl^- alone suggests that Cl^- helps regulate extracellular volume (16). When volume depletion is caused by primary renal Na^+ loss (e.g., with diuretics), urinary loss of Cl^- is not reduced despite volume depletion. In edema-forming conditions (heart failure, cirrhosis), administration of Cl^- may not improve the metabolic alkalosis. Although the pattern of urinary excretion of Cl^- would suggest Cl^--responsive metabolic alkalosis, fluid administration usually does not restore the effective vascular volume to normal (237).

Metabolic alkalosis accompanied by normal excretion of Cl^- in urine is called Cl^--resistant metabolic alkalosis (e.g., hypokalemia-induced alkalosis); administration of Cl^- does not correct the alkalosis in such condition (237). Increased activity of aldosterone is the most common cause of Cl^--resistant alkalosis, but severe hypokalemia can also produce this condition. The renal threshold for HCO_3^- is increased in K^+ depletion because of enhanced tubular reabsorption of HCO_3^- and a decrease in GFR, which could reduce the filtered load of HCO_3^-. This condition responds rapidly to K^+ repletion.

Complications

Chronic mild alkalemia is extremely well tolerated and, as discussed earlier, may be beneficial nutritionally to counteract the negative effects of the acid Western diet (125, 245). Moderate alkalemia, however, may be a sign of volume depletion (Cl^- deficiency) from overdiuresis, chronic vomiting, heart failure, or other states (237). Ca^{2+} deposition in the kidney (stones or nephrocalcinosis) and perhaps in blood vessels may become a serious problem if the alkalemia is driven by excess base intake, especially in the form of calcium salts (237, 241).

Acutely, the major problems with metabolic alkalosis are decreased tissue oxygen delivery and a fall in Ca^{2+} (237). Just as acidemia is a vasodilator, alkalemia causes vasoconstriction. In addition, the Bohr effect reduces the release of oxygen from hemoglobin at a high pH. Thus, alkalemia is associated with decreased tissue oxygen delivery. The respiratory compensation for metabolic alkalosis is a decreased respiratory drive, so alkalosis can complicate the management of respiratory failure. Ca^{2+} (a divalent cation) binds the carboxylic acids of proteins, lowering its effective concentration. The free or ionized Ca^{2+} falls with alkalemia as proteins buffer the rise in pH by donating protons. The free negative charges bind Ca^{2+} and lower its bioavailability. Thus, the symptoms of acute severe alkalemia are largely those of hypocalcemia. At a pH higher than 7.75, sufficient free Ca^{2+} is not usually present for normal cardiac contractility, and so death rapidly ensues.

Treatment

When an increased renal HCO_3^- threshold in metabolic alkalosis is caused by a reduced effective vascular volume and hypokalemia, correction of these abnormalities leads to rapid restoration of serum HCO_3^- concentration in most patients. Correction of a low effective vascular volume is accomplished by administration of normal saline or half-normal saline solution. Sometimes, discontinuation of an offending agent (e.g., a diuretic) and restoration of normal or high salt intake are sufficient. If volume depletion is to be corrected, Cl^- must be given to replace the excreted HCO_3^-, either as NaCl or KCl (242). In certain clinical situations such as edema-forming states, treatment of reduced effective vascular volume with salt solution is not effective. In such situations, acetazolamide (Diamox), a carbonic anhydrase inhibitor, treats metabolic alkalosis as well as edema (237). Acetazolamide administration usually reduces the renal HCO_3^- threshold to a subnormal level, but the HCO_3^- threshold may remain supernormal despite the drug in patients with severe volume depletion. In renal failure, metabolic alkalosis can be treated by administration of dilute HCl or acidifying salts or by dialysis. Acidifying salts include NH_4^+Cl, arginine Cl, and lysine Cl. Metabolism of these salts results in release of HCl, which then neutralizes HCO_3^-. Direct administration of HCl into large veins has also been used. If continuous acid loss from the stomach is the cause of metabolic alkalosis, an inhibitor of acid secretion such as histamine (H_2) blockers or proton pump inhibitors may be used.

Respiratory Alkalosis

Causes and Pathogenesis

With the exception of respirator-induced alkalosis and voluntary hyperventilation, respiratory alkalosis is always the result of stimulation of the respiratory center (19, 64, 260) (Table 6.12). The two most common causes of respiratory alkalosis are hypoxic stimulation of the respiratory center and stimulation through the pulmonary receptors caused by various lung lesions, such as pneumonia, pulmonary congestion, and pulmonary embolism. Certain drugs, such as salicylate and progesterone, stimulate the respiratory center directly (263). Respiratory alkalosis is common in Gram-negative sepsis and liver disease through an unknown mechanism. Blood pH tends to be extremely high when respiratory alkalosis is caused by psychogenic stimulation of the respiratory center because the condition is usually superacute, and therefore no time exists for compensation. Complications of severe respiratory alkalemia are related to low ionized Ca^{2+} levels.

Treatment

In chronic respiratory alkalosis, treatment is usually not needed because renal compensation restores the blood pH to nearly normal values (260). The mild alkalosis may be beneficial nutritionally. In acute respiratory alkalosis resulting from psychogenic hyperventilation, PCO_2 can be increased by the use of a rebreathing bag. If this fails, then the patient may need sedation to depress the respiratory center.

TABLE 6.12	CAUSES OF RESPIRATORY ALKALOSIS

Hypoxemia
  A. Pulmonary disease
     Pulmonary edema
     Pneumonia
     Pulmonary fibrosis
     Pulmonary emboli
  B. Congestive heart failure
  C. Severe anemia
  D. High-altitude residence
Direct stimulation of the medullary respiratory center
  A. Psychogenic or voluntary hyperventilation
  B. Hepatic failure
  C. Gram-negative septicemia
  D. Salicylate intoxication
  E. Pregnancy
  F. Status after correction of metabolic acidosis
  G. Neurologic disorders: cerebrovascular accidents, pontine tumors

ACKNOWLEDGMENTS

We would like to thank Drs. Man S. Oh and Jaime Uribarri for their previous work on this chapter in the tenth edition of this textbook (19).

REFERENCES

1. Carroll HJ, Oh MS. Water, Electrolyte, and Acid-Base Metabolism. Philadelphia: JB Lippincott, 1989.
2. Berl T, Robertson GL. Pathophysiology of water metabolism. In: Brenner BM, ed. The Kidney. 6th ed. Philadelphia: WB Saunders, 2000:866–924.
3. Altman PL, Dittmer DS, eds. Blood and Other Body Fluids. Washington, DC: Federation of American Societies for Experimental Biology, 1961.
4. Gamble JL Jr, Robertson JS, Hannigan CA et al. J Clin Invest 1953;32:483–9.
5. Sterns RH, Palmer BF, eds. Nephrol Self Assess Program 2007;6:21–272.
6. Hendry EF. Clin Chem 1961;155:154–64.
7. Conway EJ. Physiol Rev 1957;37:84–132.
8. Maffly RH, Leaf A. Gen Physiol 1959;42:1257–75.
9. Conway EJ, McCormack JI. J Physiol (Lond) 1953;120:1.
10. Maffly RH, Leaf A. Nature 1958;182:60–1.
11. Selkurt EE, Womack I, Dailey WN. Am J Physiol 1965;209:95–9.
12. Mulvaney MJ. Structural changes in the resistance vessels in human hypertension. In: Laragh JH, Brenner BM, eds. Hypertension: Pathophysiology, Diagnosis, and Management, vol 1. New York: Raven Press, 1995:503–13.
13. Whelton PK, He J, Appel LJ et al. JAMA 2002;288:1882–8.
14. Oh MS, Carroll HJ. External balance of electrolytes and acids and alkali. In: Seldin DW, Giebisch G, eds. The Kidney. 3rd ed. Philadelphia: Lippincott Williams & Wilkins, 2000:33–60.
15. Guyton AC, Coleman TG, Cowley AV Jr et al. Am J Med 1972;52:584–94.
16. Papadoyannakis NJ, Stefanidis CJ, McGeowan M. Am J Clin Nutr 1984;40:623–7.
17. Lentner C. Geigy Scientific Tables, vol 1: Units of Measurement, Body Fluids, Composition of the Body, Nutrition. Basel: Ciba-Geigy, 1986:243–60.
18. Hill LL. Pediatr Clin North Am 1990;37:241–56.
19. Oh MS, Uribarri J. Electrolytes, water, and acid-base balance. In: Shils ME, Shike M, Ross AC et al, eds. Modern Nutrition in Health and Disease. 10th ed. Baltimore: Lippincott Williams & Wilkins, 2006:149–93.
20. Weisberg HF. Ann Clin Lab Sci 1978;8:155–64.
21. Mount DB. Semin Nephrol 2009;29:196–215.
22. Ellison DH, Berl T. N Engl J Med 2005;356:2064–72.
23. Arieff AI, Llack F, Massry SG. Medicine (Baltimore) 1976;55:121–9.
24. Fishman RA, Brain ED. N Engl J Med 1975;293:706–11.
25. Androgue HJ, Madias NE. N Engl J Med 2000;342:1494–9.
26. Hoffmann EK, Lambert IH, Pedersen SF. Physiol Rev 2009;89:193–277.
27. Overgaard-Steensen C, Stødkilde-Jørgensen H, Larsson A et al. Am J Physiol Regul Integr Comp Physiol 2010;299:R521–32.
28. McKinley MJ, Allen AM, Burns P et al. Clin Exp Pharmacol Physiol Suppl 1998;25:61S–7S.
29. Ibata Y, Okamura H, Tanaka M et al. Front Neuroendocrinol 1999;20:241–68.
30. Wells T. Mol Cell Endocrinol 1998;136:103–7.
31. Bourque CW, Oliet SH. Annu Rev Physiol 1997;59:601–19.
32. Olsson K. Acta Paediatr Scand Suppl 1983;305:36–9.
33. Schrier RW, Berl T, Anderson RJ. Am J Physiol 1979;236:F321–32.
34. Eaton DC, Pooler J. Vander's Renal Physiology. 7th ed. New York: McGraw-Hill, 2009.
35. Pallone TL, Turner MR, Edwards A et al. Am J Physiol Regul Integr Comp Physiol 2003;284:R1153–75.
36. Hogg RJ, Kokko JP. Urine concentrating and diluting mechanisms in mammalian kidneys. In: Brenner BM, Rector FC, eds. The Kidney. Philadelphia: WB Saunders, 1986:251–79.
37. de Rouffignac C, Jamison RL. Kidney Int 1987;31:501–672.
38. Oh MS, Halperin ML. Nephron 1997;75:84–93.
39. Sands JM, Kokko JP. Kidney Int Suppl 1996;57:93S–9S.
40. Burg MB. Am J Physiol 1995;268:F983–9.
41. Schmidt-Nielson B. Fed Proc 1977;36:2493.
42. Knepper MA. Am J Physiol 1983;245:F634–9.
43. Hogg RJ, Kokko JP. Kidney Int 1978;14:428–36.
44. Gregger R, Schlatter E, Lang F. Pflugers Arch 1983;396:308–14.
45. Shirreffs SM, Maughan RJ. Am J Physiol 1998;274:F868–75.
46. Thornton SN. Physiol Behav 2010;100:15–21.
47. Mavrakis AN, Tritos NA. Am J Kidney Dis 2008;51:851–9.
48. Elkinton JR, Winkler AW, Danowski TS. J Clin Invest 1947;26:1002–9.
49. Arieff AI. Principles of parenteral therapy. In: Maxwell MH, Kleeman CR, eds. Clinical Disorders of Fluid and Electrolyte Metabolism. 2nd ed. New York: McGraw-Hill, 1972:567–89.
50. Shoemaker WC, Walker WF. Year Book of Surgery. Chicago: Year Book Medical Publishers, 1970.
51. Adolph EF. Physiology of Man in the Desert. New York: Hafner, 1969.
52. Gaskill MB, Reilly M, Robertson GL. Clin Res 1983;31:780a.
53. Rendell M, McGrane D, Cuesta M. JAMA 1978;240:2557–9.
54. Hariprassad MK, Eisinger RP, Nadler IM et al. Arch Intern Med 1980;140:1639–42.
55. Levine S, McManus BM, Blackbourne BD et al. Am J Med 1987;82:153–5.
56. Vokes TJ, Gaskill MB, Robertson GL. Ann Intern Med 1988;108:190–5.
57. Arai K, Akimoto H, Inokami T et al. Nippon Jinzo Gakkai Shi 1999;41:804–12.
58. Leggett DA, Hill PT, Anderson RJ. Australas Radiol 1999;43;104–7.
59. Siggaard C, Rittig S, Corydon TJ et al. J Clin Endocrinol Metab 1999;84:2933–4.
60. Rutishauser J, Kopp P, Gaskill MB et al. Mol Genet Metab 1999;67:89–92.
61. Ito M, Jameson JL, Ito M. J Clin Invest 1997;99:1897–905.
62. Shibata S, Mori K, Teramoto S. No Shinkei Geka 1978;6:795–801.
63. Siegel AJ. Harv Rev Psychiatry 2008;16:13–24.
64. Dundas B, Harris M, Narasimhan M. Curr Psychiatry Rep 2007;9:236–41.
65. Nielsen S, Frokiaer J, Marples D et al. Physiol Rev 2002;82:205–44.
66. Aleksandrov N, Audibert F, Bedard MJ et al. J Obstet Gynaecol Can 2010;32:225–31.
67. Oyama H, Kida Y, Tanaka T et al. Neurol Med Chir (Tokyo) 1995;35:380–4.
68. Rose BD. Clinical Physiology of Acid-Base and Electrolyte Disorders. Chicago: R.R. Donnelley & Sons, 1989:657–60.
69. Oh MS, Carroll HJ. Crit Care Med 1992;20:94–103.
70. Loh JA, Verbalis JG. Endocrinol Metab Clin North Am 2008;37:213–34.
71. Fukuda I, Hizuka N, Takano K. Endocr J 2003;50:437–43.

72. Magaldi AJ. Nephrol Dial Transplant 2000;15:1903–5.

73. Bouley R, Hasler U, Lu HA et al. Semin Nephrol 2008;28:266–78.

74. Kirchlechner V, Koller DY, Seidl R et al. Arch Dis Child 1999;80:548–52.

75. Nguyen MK, Ornekian V, Butch AW et al. Am J Physiol 2007;292:F1652–6.

76. Oh MS, Dawood M, Carroll HJ. Proceedings of the American Society of Nephrology. Boston: American Society of Nephrology, 1993.

77. Weisberg LS. Am J Med 1989;86:315–8.

78. Nguyen MK, Rastogi A, Kurtz I. Clin Exp Nephrol 2006:10;124–6.

79. Yun JJ, Cheong I. Intern Med J 2008;38:73.

80. Milionis HJ, Liamis GL, Elisaf MS. Can Med Assoc J 2002;166:1056–62.

81. Agraharkar M, Agraharkar A. Am J Kidney Dis 1997;30:717–9.

82. Akan H, Sargin S, Turkseven F et al. Br J Urol 1996;78:224–7.

83. Agarwal R, Emmett M. Am J Kidney Dis 1994;24:108–11.

84. Berl T, Anderson RJ, McDonald KM. Kidney Int 1976;10:117–21.

85. DeFronzo RA, Their SO. Arch Intern Med 1980;140:897–902.

86. Goldberg M. Med Clin North Am 1981;65:251–69.

87. Friedmann AS, Memoli VA, North WG. Cancer Lett 1993;75:79–85.

88. Hill AR, Uribarri J, Mann J et al. Am J Med 1990;88:357–64.

89. Palmer BF. Semin Nephrol 2009;29:257–70.

90. Costa KN, Nakamura HM, Cruz LR et al. Arq Neuropsiquiatr 2009;67:1037–44.

91. Sonnenblick M, Friedlander Y, Rosin AJ. Chest 1993;103:601–60.

92. Bartter FC, Schwartz WB. Am J Med 1967;42:790–99.

93. Ajaelo I, Koenig K, Snoey E. Acad Emerg Med 1998;5:839–40.

94. Henry JA, Fallon JK, Kicman AT et al. Lancet 1998;351:1784.

95. Gold PW, Robertson GL, Ballenger JC et al. J Clin Endocrinol Metab 1983;57:952–7.

96. Hensen J, Haenelt M, Gross P. Eur J Endocrinol 1995;132:459–64.

97. North WG. Exp Physiol 2000;85:27S–40S.

98. Arlt W, Dahia PL, Callies F et al. Clin Endocrinol (Oxf) 1997;47:623–7.

99. Johnson BE, Chute JP, Rushin J et al. Am J Respir Crit Care Med 1997;156:1669–78.

100. Argani P, Erlandson RA, Rosai J. Am J Clin Pathol 1997;108:537–43.

101. Ferlito A, Rinaldo A, Devaney KO. Ann Otol Rhinol Laryngol 1997;106:878–83.

102. Koide Y, Oda K, Shimizu K et al. Endocrinol Jpn 1982;29:363–8.

103. Carvounis CP, Nisar S, Guro-Razuman S. Kidney Int 2002;62:2223–9.

104. Musch W, Thimpont J, Vandervelde D et al. Am J Med 1995;99:348–55.

105. Oh MS, Carroll HJ. Nephron 1999;82:110–4.

106. Halperin ML, Bichet DG, Oh MS. Clin Nephrol 2001;56:339–45.

107. Sterns RH. Am J Med 1990;88:557–60.

108. Sterns RH, Hix JK, Silver S. Curr Opin Nephrol Hypertens 2010;19:493–8.

109. Sterns RH, Nigwekar SU, Hix JK. Semin Nephrol 2009;29:282–99.

110. Sterns RH. Semin Nephrol 1990;10:503–14.

111. Sterns RH. Crit Care Med 1992;20:534–9.

112. Norenberg MD. Metab Brain Dis 2010;25:97–106.

113. Sterns RH, Hix JK. Kidney Int 2009;76:587–89.

114. Sterns RH, Hix JK. Am J Kidney Dis 2010;56:774–9.

115. Sterns RH. Ann Intern Med 1987;107:656–64.

116. Moritz ML, Ayus JC. Metab Brain Dis 2010;25:91–96.

117. Kumar S, Berl T. Semin Nephrol 2008;28:279–88.

118. Rozen-Zvi B, Yahav D, Gheorghiade M et al. Am J Kidney Dis 2010;56:325–37.

119. Sterns RH, Emmett M, eds. Nephrol Self Assess Program 2011;10:161–6.

120. Li-Ng M, Verbalis JG. Core Evid 2010;4:83–92.

121. Oh MS, Kim HJ. Nephron 2002;92(Suppl 1):56–9.

122. Nemerovski C, Hutchinson DJ. Clin Ther 2010;32:1015–32.

123. Josiassen RC, Curtis J, Filmyer DM et al. Expert Opin Pharmacother 2010;11:637–48.

124. Fang C, Mao J, Dai Y et al. J Paediatr Child Health 2010;46:301–3.

125. Frassetto L, Morris RC Jr, Sellmeyer DE et al. Eur J Nutr 2001;40:200–13.

126. Wingo C, Weiner ID. In: Brenner BM, ed. Brenner's and Rector's The Kidney, vol 2. Philadelphia: WB Saunders, 2000:998–1035.

127. Rastegar A, DeFronzo RA. In: Schrier RW, Gottschalk CW, eds. Diseases of the Kidney. 4th ed. Boston: Little, Brown, 1988:2921–45.

128. Shirreffs SM, Maughan RJ. Am J Physiol 1998;274:F868–75.

129. Meister B, Aperia A. Semin Nephrol 1993;13:41–9.

130. Feraille E, Carranza ML, Gonin S et al. Mol Biol Cell 1999;10:2847–59.

131. Sweeney G, Klip A. Mol Cell Biochem 1998;182:121–33.

132. Goguen JM, Halperin ML. Diabetologia 1993;36:813–6.

133. Powell WJ Jr, Skinner NS. Am J Cardiol 1966;18:73–82.

134. de la Lande IS, Manson J, Parks VJ et al. J Physiol (Lond) 1961;157:177–84.

135. Vick R, Todd E, Luedhe D. J Pharmacol Exp Ther 1972;181:139–46.

136. Adrogue HJ, Madias NE. Am J Med 1981;71:456–67.

137. Guillerm R, Radziszewski E. Undersea Biomed Res 1979;6:S91–114.

138. Perez GO, Oster JK, Vaamondi CA. Nephron 1981;27:233–43.

139. Krapf R, Caduff P, Wagdi P et al. Kidney Int 1995;47:217–24.

140. Wang WH, Giebisch G. Pflugers Arch 2009;458:157–68.

141. Welling PA, Ho K. Am J Physiol 2009;297:F849–83.

142. Giebisch GH. Kidney Int 2002;62:1498–512.

143. Halperin ML, Kamel KS. Lancet 1998;352:135–40.

144. Giebisch G. Am J Physiol 1998;274:F817–33.

145. Bock HA, Hermle M, Brunner FP et al. Kidney Int 1992;41:275–80.

146. Hollenberg NK. Hypertension 2000;35:150–4.

147. Laragh JH. J Hum Hypertens 1995;9:385–90.

148. Hall JE. Compr Ther 1991;17:8–17.

149. Stokes JB. J Clin Invest 1982;70:219–29.

150. Jamison RL. Kidney Int 1987;31:695–703.

151. Palmer B, Naderi A. J Am Soc Hypertens 2007;1:381–92.

152. Van Brummelen P, Schalekamp M, DeGraeff J. Acta Med Scand 1978;204:151–7.

153. Sacks FM, Willett WC, Smith A et al. Hypertension 1998;31:131.

154. Sacks FM, Svetkey LP, Vollmer WM et al. N Engl J Med 2001;344:3–10.

155. Geleijnse JM, Kok FJ, Grobbee DE. J Hum Hypertens 2003;17:471–80.

156. Espeland MA, Kumanyika S, Yunis C et al. Ann Epidemiol 2002;12:587–95.

157. Clemessy JL, Favier C, Borron SW et al. Lancet 1995;346:877–80.

158. Matsumura M, Nakashima A, Tofuku Y. Intern Med 2000; 39:55–7.
159. Rakhmanina NY, Kearns GL, Farrar HC 3rd. Pediatr Emerg Care 1998;14:145–7.
160. Jordan P, Brookes JG, Nikolic G et al. J Toxicol Clin Toxicol 1999;37:861–4.
161. Ogawa T, Kamikubo K. Am J Med Sci 1999;318:69–75.
162. Cannon SC. Neuromuscul Disord 2002;12:533–43.
163. Jurkat-Rott K, Mitrovic N, Hang C et al. Proc Natl Acad Sci U S A 2000;97:9549–54.
164. Bradberry SM, Vale JA. J Toxicol Clin Toxicol 1995;33:295–310.
165. Steen B. Acta Med Scand Suppl 1981;647:61–6.
166. Gariballa S. Nutr Clin Pract 2008;24:604–6.
167. Miller S. Nutr Clin Pract 2008;23:166–71.
168. Torpy DJ, Gordon RD, Lin JP et al. J Clin Endocrinol Metab 1998;83:3214–8.
169. Stowasser M, Bachmann AW, Jonsson JR et al. Clin Exp Pharmacol Physiol 1995;22:444–6.
170. Stowasser M, Bachmann AW, Jonsson JR et al. J Hypertens 1995;13:1610–3.
171. Abdelhamid S, Lewicka S, Vecsei P et al. J Clin Endocrinol Metab 1995;80:737–44.
172. Litchfield WR, New MI, Coolidge C et al. J Clin Endocrinol Metab 1997;82:3570–3.
173. Litchfield WR, Coolidge C, Silva P et al. J Clin Endocrinol Metab 1997;82:1507–10.
174. Vargas-Poussou R, Huang C, Hulin P et al. J Am Soc Nephrol 2002;13:2259–66.
175. Sakakida M, Araki E. J Clin Endocrinol Metab 2003;88:781–6.
176. Finer G, Shalev H, Birk OS et al. J Pediatr 2003;142:318–23.
177. Kunchaparty S, Palcso M, Berkman J et al. Am J Physiol 1999;277:F643–9.
178. Seyberth HW, Rascher W, Schweer H et al. J Pediatr 1985; 107:694–701.
179. Zelikovic I, Szargel R, Hawash A. Kidney Int 2003; 63:24–32.
180. Schulthesis PJ, Lorenz JN, Menton P et al. J Biol Chem 1998;273:29150–5.
181. Krozowski Z, Li KX, Koyama K et al. J Steroid Biochem Mol Biol 1999;69:391–401.
182. Heilmann P, Heide J, Hundertmark S et al. Exp Clin Endocrinol Diabetes 1999;107:370–8.
183. Song D, Lorenzo B, Reidenberg MM. J Lab Clin Med 1992;120:792–7.
184. Rossi G, Pessera A, Heagarty A. J Hypertens 2008;26: 613–21.
185. Hebert SC, Desir G, Giebisch G et al. Physiol Rev 2005; 85:319–71.
186. Nagami G. Am J Physiol 2008;294:F874–80.
187. Warnock DG. Contrib Nephrol 2001;136:1–10.
188. McKenna M, Bangsbo J Renaud J. J Appl Physiol 2008; 104:288–95.
189. Agarwal R. Hypertension 2008;52:1012–3.
190. Barri YM, Wingo CS. Am J Med Sci 1997;314:37–40.
191. Savica V, Bellinghieri G, Kopple JD. Annu Rev Nutr 2010; 30:365–401.
192. Kovesdy CP, Shinaberger CS, Kalantar-Zadeh K. Semin Dial 2010;23:353–8.
193. Sterns RH, Palmer BF, eds. Nephrol Self Assess Program 2009;8:84–6.
194. Crop M, Hoorn E, Lindemans J et al. Nephrol Dial Transplant 2007;22:3471–7.
195. Cohn JN, Kowey PR, Whelton PK et al. Arch Intern Med 2000;160:2429–36.

196. Wasserman K, Stringer WW, Casaburi R et al. J Appl Physiol 1997;83:631–43.
197. Perazella MA, Biswas P. Am J Kidney Dis 1999;33:782–5.
198. Sterns RH, Emmett M. Nephrol Self Assess Program 2011;10:129–30.
199. Reza MJ, Kovick RB, Shine KI et al. N Engl J Med 1974; 291:777–8.
200. Phelps KR, Lieberman RL, Oh MS et al. Metabolism 1980;29:186–99.
201. Phelps KR, Oh MS, Carroll HJ. Nephron 1980;25:254–8.
202. Segal A. Nat Clin Pract 2008;4:102–8.
203. Wilson FH, Kahle KT, Sabath E et al. Proc Natl Acad Sci U S A 2003;100:680–4.
204. Belot A, Ranchin B, Fichtner C et al. Nephrol Dial Transplant 2008;23:1636–41.
205. Don BR, Sebastian A, Cheitlin M et al. N Engl J Med 1990; 322:1290–2.
206. Ong YL, Deore R, El-Agnaf M. Int J Lab Hematol 2010; 32:e151–7.
207. Montague B, Ouellette J, Buller G. Clin J Am Soc Nephrol 2008;3:324–30.
208. Krishnan AV, Kiernan MC. Muscle Nerve 2007;35:273–90.
209. Greenberg A. Semin Nephrol 1998;18:46–57.
210. Mandelberg A, Krupnik Z, Houri S et al. Chest 1999;115: 617–22.
211. Wong SL, Maltz HC. Ann Pharmacother 1999;33:103–6.
212. Martin TJ, Kang Y, Robertson KM et al. Anesthesiology 1990;73:62–5.
213. McGowan CD, Saha S, Chu G et al. South Med J 2009; 102:493–7.
214. Emmett M, Hootkins RE, Fine KD et al. Gastroenterology 1995;108:752–60.
215. Gruy-Kapral C, Emmett M, Santa Ana CA et al. Am Soc Nephrol 1998;9:1924–30.
216. Thomas A, James BR, Landsberg D. Am J Med Sci 2009; 337:305–6.
217. Trottier V, Drolet S, Morcos MW. Can J Gastroenterol 2009; 23:689–90.
218. Sterns RH, Rojas M, Bernstein P et al. J Am Soc Nephrol 2010;21:733–5.
219. Palmer BF. Am J Kidney Dis 2010;56:387–93.
220. Nyirenda MJ, Tang JI, Padfield PL et al. BMJ 2009;339:b4114.
221. Farese S, Kruse A, Pasch A et al. Kidney Int 2009;75:877–84.
222. Rastegar A. Clin J Am Soc Nephrol 2009;4:1267–74.
223. Remer T, Manz F. J Am Diet Assoc 1995;95:791–7.
224. US Department of Agriculture. USDA National Nutrient Database for Standard Reference. Release 18. Washington, DC: US Department of Agriculture, 2006.
225. Lemann J Jr, Relman AS. J Clin Invest 1959;38:2215–23.
226. Oh MS. Nephron 1991;59:7–10.
227. Oh MS. Kidney Int 1989;36:915–7.
228. Oh MS, Carroll HJ. Contrib Nephrol 1992;100:89–104.
229. Lennon EJ, Lemann J Jr, Litzow JR. J Clin Invest 1966;45:1601–7.
230. Remer T, Dimitriou T, Manz F. Am J Clin Nutr 2003;77: 1255–60.
231. Frassetto LA, Todd KM, Morris RC Jr et al. Am J Clin Nutr 1998;68:576–83.
232. Berkemeyer S, Remer T. J Nutr 2006;136:1203–8.
233. Koeppen BM. Adv Physiol Educ 2009;33:275–81.
234. Soupart A, Silver S, Schrooeder B et al. J Am Soc Nephrol 2002;13:1433–41.
235. Lemann J Jr, Bushinsky DA, Hamm LL. Am J Physiol 2003;285:F811–32.

236. Franch HA, Mitch WE. J Am Soc Nephrol 1998;9:S78–81.
237. Laski ME, Sabatini S. Semin Nephrol 2006;26:404–21.
238. Welbourne TC. Am J Physiol 1987;253:F1069–76.
239. Franch HA, Mitch WE. Annu Rev Nutr 2009;29:341–64.
240. Maalouf NM, Cameron MA, Moe OW et al. Clin J Am Soc Nephrol 2010;5:1277–81.
241. Patel AM, Goldfarb S. J Am Soc Nephrol 2010;21:1440–3.
242. Hsia CC. N Engl J Med 1998;338:239–47.
243. Dellinger R, Levy M, Carlet J et al. Intensive Care Med 2008;34:17–60.
244. Taylor EN, Stampfer MJ, Curhan GC. J Am Soc Nephrol 2003;15:3225–32.
245. Sebastian A, Harris ST, Ottaway JH et al. N Engl J Med 1994;330:1776–81.
246. Webster M. Sodium bicarbonate. In: Bahrke M, Yesalis C, eds. Performance-Enhancing Substances in Sport and Exercise. Champaign, IL: Human Kinetics, 2002.
247. Mitch WE, Price SR, May RC et al. Am J Kidney Dis 1994;23:224–8.
248. Dawson-Hughes B, Castaneda-Sceppa C, Harris S et al. Osteoporos Int 2010;21:1171–9.
249. de Brito-Ashurst I, Varagunam M, Raftery MJ et al. J Am Soc Nephrol 2009;20:2075–84.
250. Kraut JA, Madias NE. Pediatr Nephrol 2011;26:19–28.
251. Morris CG, Low J. Anaesthesia 2008;63:396–411.
252. Kraut JA, Madias NE. Nat Rev Nephrol 2010;6:274–85.
253. Wagner CA. Kidney Int 2008;73:1103–5.
254. Umpierrez GE, Khajavi M, Kitabchi AE. Am J Med Sci 1996;311:225–33.
255. Chawla LS, Shih S, Davison D et al. BMC Emerg Med 2008;8:18.
256. Rewers A. Adv. Pediatr 2010;57:247–67.
257. Kraut JA, Kurtz I. Clin J Am Soc Nephrol 2008;3:208–25.
258. Oh MS, Phelps KR, Traube M et al. N Engl J Med 1979;301:249–52.
259. Sabatini S, Kurtzman NA. J Am Soc Nephrol 2009;20:692–5.
260. Oh YK. Electrolyte Blood Press 2010;8:66–71.
261. Madias NE. J Nephrol 2010;23(Suppl 16):S85–91.
262. Oh MS, Carroll HJ. Nephron 2002;91:379–82.
263. Saaresranta T, Polo-Kantola P, Irjala K et al. Chest 1999;115:1581–7.

SUGGESTED READINGS

Thornton SN. Thirst and hydration: physiology and consequences of dysfunction. Physiol Behav 2010;100:15–21.

Loh JA, Verbalis JG. Disorders of water and salt metabolism associated with pituitary disease. Endocrinol Metab Clin North Am 2008;37:213–34.

Franch HA, Mitch WE. Navigating between the Scylla and Charybdis of prescribing dietary protein for chronic kidney diseases. Annu Rev Nutr 2009;29:341–64.

7 CALCIUM[1]

CONNIE M. WEAVER AND ROBERT P. HEANEY

BIOLOGIC ROLES OF CALCIUM

In higher mammals, the most obvious role of calcium is structural or mechanical and is expressed in the mass, hardness, and strength of the bones and teeth. Calcium has another fundamental function, however: shaping key biologic proteins to activate their catalytic and mechanical

properties. A significant portion of the regulatory apparatus of the body is concerned with the protection of this second function (e.g., all the activities and roles of parathyroid hormone [PTH], calcitonin [CT], and a key activity of vitamin D). Calcium is the most tightly regulated ion in the extracellular fluid (ECF). The structural role is discussed in greater detail in the chapter on osteoporosis, whereas the cell metabolic, regulatory, and nutritional aspects of this critical element are discussed in this chapter.

Calcium and the Cell

The calcium ion (Ca^{2+}) has an ionic radius of 0.99 Å and is able to form coordination bonds with up to 12 oxygen atoms (1). The combination of these two features makes calcium nearly unique among all cations in its ability to fit neatly into the folds of the peptide chain. Cytoplasmic proteins are extremely flexible to the point of being literally floppy. They typically assume hundreds of different three-dimensional configurations each second. Some of these configurations have the capacity to bind critical ligands or to assume catalytic functions. Without calcium, these configurations are so short lived as to be of little functional significance. Calcium, when present in the cytosol in sufficient concentration, binds to, for example, aspartate and glutamate side chains on the peptide backbone and thus builds intramolecular linkages that bind together different folds of the peptide chain and "freeze" the protein into a functionally active, particular shape. Magnesium and strontium, which are chemically similar to calcium in the test tube, have different ionic radii and do not bond so well with protein. Lead and cadmium ions, by contrast, substitute quite well for calcium, and, in fact, lead binds to various calcium-binding proteins with greater avidity than does calcium itself. Fortunately, neither element is present in significant quantity in the milieu in which living organisms thrive. Nevertheless, the ability of lead to bind to the calcium-binding proteins is part of the basis for lead toxicity.

Binding of calcium to thousands of cell proteins triggers changes in protein shape that govern function (2). These proteins range from those involved with cell movement and muscle contraction to nerve transmission, glandular secretion, and even cell division. In most of these

[1]**Abbreviations: 1,25(OH)₂D**, 1,25–dihydroxyvitamin D; **AI**, adequate intake; **ATP**, adenosine triphosphate; **ATPase**, adenosine triphosphatase; **Ca²⁺**, calcium ion; **CaSR**, calcium-sensing receptor; **CT**, calcitonin; **DAG**, diacylglycerol; **ECF**, extracellular fluid; **IGF-I**, insulinlike growth factor-I; **InsP₃**, inositol-1,4,5-triphosphate; **Na⁺**, sodium ion; **NHANES**, National Health and Nutrition Examination Survey; **PTH**, parathyroid hormone; **PIP₂**, phosphatidylinositol-4,5-bisphosphate; **PTH**, parathyroid hormone; **RyR**, ryanodine receptor; **VDR**, vitamin D receptor.

situations, calcium acts both as a signal transmitter from the outside of the cell to the inside and as an activator or stabilizer of the functional proteins involved. In fact, ionized calcium is the most common signal transmitter in all of biology. It operates from bacterial cells all the way up to cells of highly specialized tissues in higher mammals.

When a cell is activated (e.g., a muscle fiber receives a nerve stimulus to contract), the first thing that happens is that calcium channels in the plasma membrane open up to admit a few calcium ions into the cytosol. These bind immediately to a wide array of intracellular activator proteins, which, in turn, release a flood of calcium from the intracellular storage vesicles (the sarcoplasmic reticulum, in the case of muscle). This second step very quickly raises cytosol calcium concentration and leads to activation of the contraction complex. Two of the many reactions involving calcium-binding proteins are of particular interest here: (a) troponin C, after it has bound calcium, initiates a series of steps that lead to the actual muscle contraction; and (b) calmodulin, a second and widely distributed calcium-binding protein, activates the enzymes that break down glycogen to release energy for contraction. In this way, calcium ions both trigger the contraction and fuel the process. When the cell has completed its assigned task, the various pumps quickly lower the cytosol calcium concentration, and the cell returns to a resting state. These processes are described in more detail later in this chapter.

If all the functional proteins of a cell were fully activated by calcium at the same time, the cell would rapidly self-destruct. For that reason, cells must keep free calcium ion concentrations in the cytosol at extremely low levels, typically on the order of 100 nmol. This is 10,000-fold lower than the concentration of calcium ion in the extracellular water outside of the cell. Cells maintain this concentration gradient by a combination of mechanisms: (a) a cell membrane with limited calcium permeability; (b) ion pumps that move calcium rapidly out of the cytosol, either to the outside of the cell or into storage vesicles within the cell; and (c) a series of specialized proteins in the storage vesicles that have no catalytic function in their own right but that serve only to bind (and hence sequester) large quantities of calcium. Low cytosolic $[Ca^{2+}]$ ensures that the various functional proteins remain dormant until the cell activates certain of them, and it does this simply by letting $[Ca^{2+}]$ rise in critical cytosolic compartments. In contrast to proteins that are activated by rising cytosolic $[Ca^{2+}]$ are enzymes such as several proteases and dehydrogenase, which are activated or stabilized by bound calcium independent of changes in $[Ca^{2+}]_i$.

OCCURRENCE AND DISTRIBUTION IN NATURE

Calcium is the fifth most abundant element in the biosphere (after iron, aluminum, silicon, and oxygen). It is the stuff of limestone and marble, coral and pearls, sea shells and egg shells, and antlers and bones. Because calcium

salts exhibit intermediate solubility, calcium is found both in solid form (rocks) and in solution. It was probably present in abundance in the watery environment in which life first appeared. Today, seawater contains approximately 10 mmol calcium per liter (approximately eight times higher than the calcium concentration in the extracellular water of higher vertebrates); and even fresh waters, if they support an abundant biota, typically contain calcium at concentrations of 1 to 2 mmol. In most soils, calcium exists as an exchangeable cation in the soil colloids. It is taken up by plants, whose parts typically contain from 0.1% to as much as 8% calcium. Generally, calcium concentrations are highest in the leaves, lower in the stems and roots, and lowest in the seeds.

In land-living mammals, calcium accounts for 2% to 4% of gross body weight. A 60-kg woman typically contains approximately 1000 to 1200 g (25 to 30 mol) of calcium in her body. More than 99% of that total is in the bones and teeth. Approximately 1 g is in the plasma and ECF bathing the cells, and 6 to 8 g are in the tissues themselves (mostly sequestered in calcium storage vesicles inside of cells, as discussed earlier).

In the circulating blood, calcium concentration is typically 2.25 to 2.5 mmol. Approximately 40% to 45% of this quantity is bound to plasma proteins, approximately 8% to 10% is complexed with ions such as citrate, and 45% to 50% is dissociated as free ions. In the ECF outside of the blood vessels, total calcium is on the order of 1.25 mmol, which differs from plasma concentration because of the absence of most plasma proteins from the ECF. It is the calcium concentration in the ECF that the cells see and that is tightly regulated by the parathyroid, CT, and vitamin D hormonal control systems.

With advancing age, humans commonly accumulate calcium deposits in various damaged tissues, such as atherosclerotic plaques in arteries, healed granulomas, other scars left by disease or injury, and often in the rib cartilages as well. These deposits are called *dystrophic calcification* and rarely amount to more than a few grams of calcium. These deposits are not caused by dietary calcium but by local injury, coupled with the widespread tendency of proteins to bind calcium. Calcification in tissues other than bones and teeth is generally a sign of tissue damage and cell death. This process is greatly exaggerated in conditions such as end stage kidney disease, when the calcium × phosphorus product of the ECF exceeds 2.5 to 3.0 $mmol^2/L^2$.

METABOLISM

Calcium metabolism and transport, as affected by age, race, and sex, on intakes approximating requirements (1000 to 1300 mg/day), are given in Table 7.1. Part of dietary calcium is absorbed into the bloodstream where it is in intimate exchange with ECF calcium. Part of the absorbed calcium is returned as endogenous secretion to the gut, where it is excreted along with unabsorbed

| TABLE 7.1 | CALCIUM (Ca) METABOLISM AS INFLUENCED BY RACE AND AGE |

LIFE STAGE (AGE [y])	mg/d[a]							
	INTAKE	ABSORBED	ENDOGENOUS SECRETION	FECAL	URINE	BONE FORMATION	BONE RESORPTION	BONE BALANCE
White pubertal girls (12–14)	1,330	494 ± 232	112 ± 35	918 ± 253	100 ± 54	1,459 ± 542	1,177 ± 436	282 ± 269
Black pubertal girls (11–14)	1,128	636 ± 188	109 ± 50	680 ± 178	46 ± 38	1,976 ± 540	1,496 ± 528	484 ± 180
Asian pubertal girls (11–15)	1,068	567 ± 27	104 ± 17	604 ± 19	87 ± 6	1,369 ± 86	992 ± 89	378 ± 22
Asian pubertal boys (11–15)	1,211	662 ± 30	154 ± 19	702 ± 20	78 ± 6	2,416 ± 95	1,986 ± 97	430 ± 24
Young white women (19–31)	1,330	283 ± 122	121 ± 39	1,138 ± 143	203 ± 79	501 ± 129	542 ± 212	−41 ± 165
Postmenopausal women (57±6)	1,083	221 ± 58	151 ± 49	1,092 ± 256	121 ± 63	307 ± 138	415 ± 192	−108 ± 110

[a]1 mg Ca = 25 μmol.

Data from Wastney ME, Ng J, Smith D et al. Am J Physiol 1996;271:R208–16; Bryant RJ, Wastney ME, Martin BR et al. Racial differences in bone turnover and calcium metabolism in adolescent females. J Endocrinol Metab 2003;88:1043–7; Spence LA, Lipscomb ER, Cadogan J et al. Differences in calcium kinetics between adolescent girls and young women. Am J Clin Nutr 2005;81:916–22; and Wu L, Martin BR, Braun MM et al. Calcium requirements and metabolism in Chinese-American boys and girls. J Bone Miner Res 2010;25:1842–9.

calcium. Part is excreted in the urine through the kidney, and part enters the slower exchange pools of soft tissue and bone. Dietary calcium influences calcium absorption and, consequently, fecal calcium and, to a lesser extent, urinary calcium excretion. An obligatory loss of calcium occurs through endogenous secretion, urine, and skin. Gender, age, and racial differences in calcium metabolism exist. Adolescents are more efficient at using calcium than are young adults, and elderly persons are the least efficient. Boys are more efficient at calcium metabolism than girls, and blacks are more efficient than whites.

Homeostatic Regulation

Plasma calcium is tightly regulated at approximately 2.5 mM (9 to 10 mg/dL). When serum calcium is more than 10% away from the population mean, one has reason to suspect disease. The regulation of serum calcium concentration involves a system of controlling factors and feedback mechanisms (Fig. 7.1).

Plasma calcium concentrations are detected by surface calcium-sensing receptors (CaSRs) found in parathyroid and the clear cells of thyroid glands, kidney, intestine, bone marrow, and other tissues. When plasma calcium concentrations are elevated, PTH release is inhibited and CT release is stimulated.

When plasma calcium concentration falls, the parathyroid gland is stimulated to release PTH. PTH increases renal phosphate clearance and renal tubular reabsorption of calcium; it activates bone resorption loci, augments osteoclast activity at existing resorption loci, and activates vitamin D to enhance intestinal calcium absorption. Activation of vitamin D occurs in two steps. An initial hydroxylation is catalyzed by vitamin D-25-hydroxylase (CYP27), a microsomal cytochrome P-450 enzyme system

in the liver. The second hydroxylation by 25-OH D-1-α-hydroxylase (CYP27B1) in the proximal convoluted tubule cells of the kidney converts the vitamin to its active potent form, 1,25-dihydroxyvitamin D [1,25(OH)$_2$D] or calcitriol. (See the chapter on vitamin D for additional details.) This

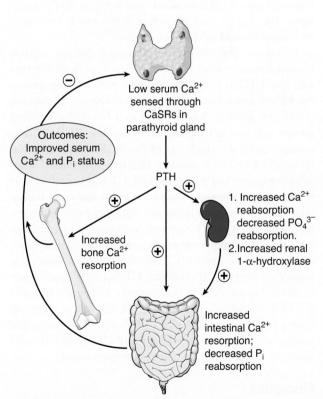

Fig. 7.1. Homeostatic regulation of calcium (Ca^{2+}) depicting the changes in vitamin D and parathyroid hormone (PTH) when plasma calcium falls to less than 2.5 mM. *CaSR,* calcium sensing receptor; *P$_i$,* inorganic phosphate; *PO$_4$$^{3-}$,* phosphate.

latter step is stimulated by PTH and is augmented by a fall in serum phosphate. PTH and $1,25(OH)_2D$ act synergistically to enhance renal tubular reabsorption of calcium and to mobilize calcium stores from bone. PTH acts in a classical negative feedback loop to raise the ECF $[Ca^{2+}]$, thereby closing the loop and reducing PTH release. Some evidence indicates that the intestine also has CYP27B1 activity that could produce $1,25(OH)_2D$ for local use; this would explain observations of increased calcium absorption with increased serum 25(OH)D levels without change in serum $1,25(OH)_2D$ levels (3).

Although the sophisticated regulatory mechanism described earlier allows a rapid response that corrects transient hypocalcemia, in the presence of a chronically calcium-deficient diet, it maintains ECF $[Ca^{2+}]$ at the cost of depleting the skeleton. The three tissues supporting serum calcium levels (i.e., gut, kidney, and bone) operate independently of one another, and altered responsiveness of any of these can increase bone fragility. For example, low fractional calcium absorption capacity was associated with increased hip fracture risk in elderly postmenopausal women (4).

When plasma calcium concentration rises in response to increased calcium absorption or increased bone resorption, extracellular Ca^{2+} binds to CaSR on the surface of parathyroid cells and thus stimulates a conformational change in the receptors leading to an inhibition of PTH secretion from the parathyroid (5). PTH augments tubular reabsorption of calcium. That reabsorption has a maximum (the T_mCa), and when that maximum is exceeded, additional filtered calcium is excreted.

In infants and children, a principal defense against hypercalcemia is release of CT by the C cells of the thyroid gland. CT is a peptide hormone with binding sites in the kidney, bone, and central nervous system. Absorption of calcium from an 8-oz feeding in a 6-month-old infant dumps 150 to 220 mg calcium into the ECF. This is enough, given the small size of the ECF compartment at that age (1.5 to 2 L), to produce fatal hypercalcemia if other adjustments are not made. Instead, CT is released, in part in response to the rise in serum calcium, but even before that, in response to gut hormones signaling coming absorption. This burst of CT slows or halts osteoclastic resorption, thus stopping bony release of calcium. Then, later, when absorption stops, CT levels also fall, and osteoclastic resorption resumes. By contrast, CT has little significance in adults because absorption is lower to begin with, and the ECF is vastly larger. As a result, absorptive calcemia from a high-calcium diet raises ECF $[Ca^{2+}]$ by only a few percentage points, and the absence of CT (as with thyroid ablation) has little impact on calcium homeostasis.

Absorption

Calcium usually is freed from complexes in the diet during digestion and is released in a soluble and typically ionized form for absorption. However, small-molecular-weight

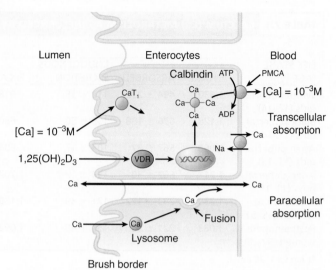

Fig. 7.2. Calcium (Ca) absorption showing active, transcellular absorption and passive, paracellular absorption. Paracellular absorption is bidirectional; transcellular absorption is unidirectional. Ca enters the cytosol down a concentration gradient. Ca enters the cell through CaT_1 and is transported across the enterocyte against an uphill gradient with the aid of vitamin D–induced calbindin, probably at least partially through endosomes and lysosomes. Finally, it is extruded at the basolateral membrane primarily by the plasma membrane calcium adenosine triphosphatase (ATPase) pump (PMCA) and secondarily by the sodium (Na^+)/Ca^{2+} exchanger or by exocytosis. *ADP*, adenosine diphosphate; *VDR*, vitamin D receptor.

complexes such as calcium oxalate and calcium carbonate can be absorbed intact (6).

Fractional calcium absorption (absorptive efficiency) generally varies approximately inversely with the logarithm of intake, but the absolute quantity of calcium absorbed increases with intake (7, 8). However, only 20% of the variation in calcium absorption can be accounted for by usual calcium intake (9). Rather, individuals seem to have preset absorptive efficiencies; approximately 60% of the variance in calcium absorption among individuals can be accounted for by their individual fractional calcium absorption (10).

Mechanisms of Absorption

Calcium absorption occurs by two pathways (Fig. 7.2):

1. Transcellular: This saturable (active) transfer involves a calcium-binding protein, calbindin.
2. Paracellular: This nonsaturable (diffusional) transfer is a linear function of calcium content of the chyme.

The relationship between calcium intake and absorbed calcium is shown in Figure 7.3. At lower calcium intakes, the active component contributes most to absorbed calcium. The Michaelis-Menten constant (K_m) for the active component in adults is calculated to be 3.2 to 5.5 mM (equivalent to a calcium load of 230 to 400 mg) (3). As calcium intakes increase and the active component becomes saturated, an increasing proportion of calcium is absorbed by passive diffusion.

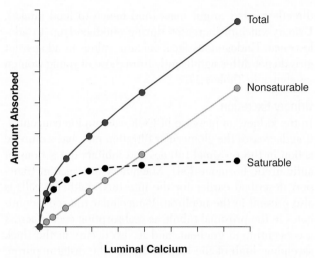

Fig. 7.3. Calcium is absorbed by both saturable and nonsaturable pathways. Total calcium transport (the sum of a saturable component [A] defined by the Michaelis-Menten equation and a concentration-dependent, nonsaturable component [B] defined by a linear equation) is described by a curvilinear function.

Active absorption is most efficient in the duodenum and next in the jejunum, but total calcium absorbed is greatest in the ileum, where residence time is the longest. In one rat study, net calcium absorption was distributed as 62% in the ileum, 23% in the jejunum, and 15% in the duodenum (11). Absorption from the colon accounts for approximately 5% to 23% (or ~1% of ingested calcium) of the total absorption in normal individuals, but it may be important in patients with small bowel resections and when colonic bacteria break down dietary complexes.

Transcellular Calcium Transport. Calcium entry into the epithelial cells occurs primarily through a calcium channel, TRPV6 (CaT$_1$) (12), although it is not a rate-limiting step (13). Calcium transfer occurs down a steep electrochemical gradient and does not require energy. The main regulator of transport across the epithelial cell against the energy gradient is 1,25(OH)$_2$D. As illustrated in Figure 7.2, 1,25(OH)$_2$D, which is responsive to serum calcium levels, regulates the synthesis of calbindin by binding with vitamin D receptor (VDR) in the cytoplasm and translocating to the nucleus, where it binds to response elements to initiate transcription of calbindin mRNA. The essentiality of VDR and 1,25(OH)$_2$D in the control of calcium absorption was established with transgenic mice (14). Intestinal calbindin, a 9-kDa protein in mammals and a 28-kDa protein in birds, is capable of binding 2 Ca^{2+} per molecule. Calbindin operates by binding Ca^{2+} on the surface of the cell and then internalizes the ions through endocytic vesicles that may fuse with lysosomes. After release of the bound calcium in the acidic lysosomal interior, the calbindin returns to the cell surface, and the Ca^{2+} ions exit the cell through the basolateral membrane (15). Using ion microscopic imaging of injected ^{44}Ca^{2+}, calcium entry into the villus was observed in vitamin D–deficient chicks, but the rapid transfer of Ca^{2+} through the cytoplasm to the basolateral pole did not occur in the absence of the ability to synthesize calbindin (16). Thus, calbindin serves both as a Ca^{2+} translocator and a cytosolic Ca^{2+} buffer to resist toxicity in chick intestine (17), but its role in mammalian intestinal epithelial cells has been questioned (3). Much remains to be understood about calcium transport across the intestine because in a double-calbindin D9k/TRPV6 knockout mouse model, calcium absorption still responded to 1,25(OH)$_2$D, although that response was reduced by 60% compared with wild-type mouse (18).

Vitamin D–induced calcium transport also involves activation of a Ca^{2+}-dependent adenosine triphosphate (ATP) pump (PMCA1b) to effect extrusion of calcium against an electrochemical gradient into the ECF (19). Relative Ca^{2+}-binding capacities across the enterocyte are brush border, 1, calbindin, 4, and the ATP-dependent Ca^{2+} pump, 10; this gradient ensures unidirectional transfer of Ca^{2+} (20). A rapid increase in calcium absorption resulting from transcaltachia, which involves 1,25(OH)$_2$D-mediated (but not transcriptional) events, also appears to be at work (3).

Paracellular Calcium Transport. In the paracellular pathway, calcium transfer occurs between the cells. Theoretically, this transfer can occur in both directions, but normally the predominant direction is from lumen into blood because much of the transfer is by solute drag, which is predominantly from lumen into ECF. The rate of transfer depends on ingested calcium load and tightness of the junctions. Calcitriol also enhances flux of ions including Ca^{2+} (21). Water probably carries calcium through the junctions by solvent drag, which is stimulated by 1,25(OH)$_2$D through induction of tight junction proteins (22).

Physiologic Factors Affecting Absorption

Various host factors affect fractional calcium absorption. Vitamin D status, intestinal transit time, and mucosal mass are the best established (23). Phosphorus deficiency, as may occur through prolonged use of aluminum-containing antacids, can cause hypophosphatemia, increased circulating levels of 1,25(OH)$_2$D, and elevated calcium absorption.

Stage of life also influences calcium absorption. In infancy, absorption is dominated by diffusion. Therefore, the vitamin D status of the mother does not affect fractional calcium absorption of young breast-fed infants. Both active and passive calcium transport is increased during pregnancy and lactation. Calbindin and plasma 1,25(OH)$_2$ and PTH levels increase during pregnancy. From midlife onward, absorption efficiency declines by approximately 0.2 absorption percentage points per year, and at menopause, an additional 2% decrease occurs (24). Decreased calcium absorption efficiency with age is related to increased intestinal resistance to 1,25(OH)$_2$D, as illustrated by a steeper slope in the relationship between fractional calcium absorption and serum 1,25(OH)$_2$D$_3$ in elderly postmenopausal women than in young premenopausal women (25). The age-related decrease in calcium absorption from intestinal resistance to $1,25(OH)_2D_3$ has been associated with decreased VDR levels (26), as well as with reduced estrogen levels (23).

Decreased stomach acid, as occurs in achlorhydria, reduces the solubility of insoluble calcium salts (e.g., carbonate, phosphate) and thus could, in theory, reduce absorption of calcium unless fed with a meal (27). Absorption of calcium supplements improves when they are taken with food irrespective of gastric acid status, perhaps by slowing gastric emptying and thereby extending the time in which the calcium-containing chyme is in contact with the absorptive surface.

VDR polymorphisms have been studied for their relationship with calcium absorption efficiency. One study showed a significant association between the VDR Fok1 polymorphism and calcium absorption in children (28).

Excretion

Loss of calcium from the body occurs in urine, feces, and sweat. Differences in losses between adult women and adolescent girls on equal and adequate calcium intakes are given in Table 7.1. This table demonstrates the conservation of calcium at the kidney for building bone during the rapid period of skeletal growth during puberty. African-American girls absorb more calcium and excrete less calcium than do white girls, and this characteristic results in greater net bone deposition (29). African-American women average 10% higher bone mineral content than do white women (30).

Turnover of the miscible calcium pool in healthy adults is approximately 16%/day, and the rapidly exchanging component (of which the ECF is a part) is approximately 40%/day. The filtered load of the kidney is determined by the glomerular filtration rate and the plasma concentration of ultrafiltrable calcium (ionized plus that bound to small-molecular-weight anions). In adults, this is approximately 175 to 250 mmol/day (7 to 10 g/day). More than 98% of this calcium is reabsorbed by the renal tubule as the filtrate passes through the nephron, but 2.5 to 5 mmol (100 to 200 mg) are excreted in the urine daily. Endogenous fecal excretory loss is similar to the amount excreted in the urine. Loss in the sweat is typically 0.4 to 0.6 mmol (16 to 24 mg)/day (31); and additional diurnal losses occur from shed skin, hair, and nails, thus bringing the total to as much as 1.5 mmol (60 mg)/day. Cutaneous losses from children average 1.3 mmol (52 mg)/day (32). Moderate exercise can increase calcium loss (33).

Endogenous Fecal Calcium

Fecal calcium includes that calcium that is unabsorbed from the diet plus calcium that enters the gut from endogenous sources, including shed mucosal cells and digestive secretions. Endogenous fecal calcium losses are approximately 2.5 to 3.0 mmol (100 to 120 mg)/day. These losses are inversely proportional to absorption efficiency and are directly related to gut mass (and hence to food intake). Urinary calcium increases during childhood up to adolescence. Endogenous fecal calcium values in adolescent girls do not differ significantly from those of young women (as shown in Table 7.1).

Urinary Excretion

In the kidney, an increase in ECF calcium ion concentration decreases the glomerular filtration rate, has a diuretic action in the proximal tubule, and inhibits the actions of antidiuretic hormone (34). Machinery for calcium transport described earlier for the intestinal epithelial cells is also present in the nephron. Paracellular transport dominates in the proximal tubule as reabsorption occurs across a concentration gradient, and it also occurs in the thick ascending limb of the loop of Henle, the distal nephron, and the collecting ducts.

Both active transport and passive transport depend on calcium load, are detected through CaSR, are stimulated by PTH and $1,25(OH)_2D$, and have a microvillar myosin I–calmodulin complex that could serve as a calcium transporter (35). PTH acts on proximal tubular cells to up-regulate CYP1α expression. Calcium enters renal epithelial cells through a calcium channel, ECaC or CaT_2 (36). Active transport occurs in the distal convoluted tubule against a concentration gradient. In the mammalian kidney, vitamin D regulation works through calbindin-$D_{28}k$, which binds 4 Ca^{2+} per molecule and shares no sequence homology with calbindin-D_9k of the intestine. This calcium-binding protein has been cloned and is regulated by both transcriptional and posttranscriptional mechanisms. Administration of $1,25(OH)_2D$ to rats induces calbindin-$D_{28}k$ mRNA and VDR mRNA in vitamin D–sufficient animals (37). However, in the absence of vitamin D, hypercalciuria is not observed, as would be predicted if mechanisms were similar to the gut. A fall in filtered load is associated with slight reductions in urine calcium. Even so, renal calcium clearance is reduced in vitamin D deficiency and is increased in PTH deficiency—findings indicating that the major effect on conservation of calcium is exerted by PTH.

During the rapid growth of adolescence, urinary calcium is little influenced by load. Absorbed calcium is diverted to bone growth at calcium intakes typically ingested, except for obligatory losses in urine, skin, and endogenous secretions. Tubular reabsorption decreases in postmenopausal women.

DIETARY CONSIDERATIONS

Dietary sources and calcium intakes have altered considerably during human evolution. Early humans derived calcium from roots, tubers, nuts, and beans in quantities believed to exceed 37.5 mmol (1500 g)/day (38) and perhaps up to twice this when they were consuming food to meet the caloric demands of a hunter-gatherer of contemporary body size. After domestication of grains, calcium intakes decreased substantially because the staple foods became grains (fruits), the plant parts that accumulate the least calcium. Pre–Iron Age milling practices were based on limestone and hence added appreciable calcium as calcium carbonate to the otherwise low-calcium flour. Consequently, the modern human on average consumes insufficient calcium to optimize bone density. The food group that supplies the bulk of the calcium in the Western diet is now the dairy food group.

Food Sources and Bioavailability

Milk and other dairy products supply more than 70% of the calcium in the US diet (39). Although corn tortillas processed with lime and dried beans provide the bulk of dietary calcium for some ethnic groups, it is difficult for most individuals to ingest sufficient quantities of calcium from foods available in a cereal-based economy without liberal consumption of dairy products. Thus, food manufacturers have developed calcium-fortified products. Many individuals have turned to dietary supplements to meet their calcium needs. However, it is prudent to remember that calcium is not the only nutrient important to health supplied by dairy products. Milk intake has been associated with intake not only of calcium but also of potassium, magnesium, zinc, riboflavin, vitamin A, folate, and vitamin D for children (40). Median intake of milk in the United States meets the recommended intake in children aged 1 to 8 years, although 25% of children do not consume the recommended 2 cups daily (41). In contrast, the median intake for older groups falls well below the recommended 3 cups daily (i.e., 1.9 cup equivalents for girls and 2.4 for boys aged 9 to 13 years, 1.5 cup for girls and 2.3 cups for boys aged 14 to 18 years, and 1.2 cup for women and 1.6 for men).

Aside from gross calcium content, potential calcium sources vary importantly in bioavailability. Fractional calcium absorption from various dairy products is similar, at approximately 30% (42). The calcium from most supplements is absorbed as well as from milk, because solubility of the salts at neutral pH has little impact on calcium absorption (43). A few calcium salts, including calcium citrate malate and calcium ascorbate, have superior absorbability. However, adjuvants added to supplements or food matrices can substantially alter bioavailability.

Several plant constituents form indigestible salts with calcium and thereby decrease absorption of their calcium. The most potent inhibitor of calcium absorption is oxalic acid, found in high concentration in spinach, rhubarb, and, to a lesser extent, sweet potatoes and dried beans (44). Calcium absorption from spinach is only 5% compared with 27% from milk ingested at a similar load (45). When these two foods of dissimilar bioavailability are coingested during the same meal, calcium fractional absorption from milk is depressed 30% of the difference between milk and spinach fed alone by the presence of spinach, and calcium fraction absorption from spinach is enhanced by 37% of the difference between milk and spinach by the presence of milk (46). The absence of complete exchange and the failure to find equal absorption from the two foods intermediate between the values for the foods fed singly suggest that calcium does not completely form a common dietary pool, as has been reported for iron and zinc.

Phytic acid, the storage form of phosphorus in seeds, is a modest inhibitor of calcium absorption. The phytic acid content of seeds, which depends on the phosphorus content of the soil where the plants are grown, influences calcium absorption (47). Fermentation, such as occurs during bread making, reduces phytic acid content by virtue of the phytase present in yeast. This process results in increased calcium absorption (48). Since the early balance studies of McCance and Widdowson, who reported negative calcium balance during consumption of whole wheat products (49), it has been assumed that fiber negatively affects calcium balance through physical entrapment or through cationic binding with uronic acid residue (50). However, it is more likely that the phytic acid associated with fiber-rich foods is the component that affects balance because purified fibers do not negatively affect calcium absorption (51). Only concentrated sources of phytate such as wheat bran ingested as extruded cereal (48) or dried beans (52) have substantially reduced calcium absorption. For other plants rich in calcium (primarily the *Brassica* genus, which includes broccoli, kale, bok choy, cabbage, and mustard and turnip greens), calcium bioavailability is as good as that from milk (53). The *Brassicas* are an anomaly in the plant kingdom in that they do not accumulate oxalate as a mechanism to detoxify excess calcium to protect against cell death.

A comparison of several foods for calcium content, bioavailability, and number of servings needed to equal the amount of calcium absorbed from one serving of milk is given in Table 7.2.

True enhancers of calcium absorption have not been well characterized. Lactose appears to enhance calcium absorption in infants. However, in adults, calcium absorption from various dairy products is equivalent regardless of the lactose content, chemical form of calcium, or presence of flavorings (54). Nondigestible carbohydrates can increase calcium absorption in the lower bowel, where they are fermented and where the resulting short-chain fatty acids produced lower pH and increase solubility of calcium (55). Some proteins can enhance calcium absorption acutely, but the effect disappears with long-term feeding when calcium absorption adapts by up-regulation of transport proteins (56).

Nutrient–Nutrient Interactions

Several nutrients and food constituents affect aspects of calcium homeostasis by means other than a simple effect on digestibility, as described earlier. Several dietary components influence urinary calcium excretion. Dietary calcium has relatively little influence on urinary calcium

TABLE 7.2	FOOD SOURCES OF BIOAVAILABLE CALCIUM					
FOOD	SERVING (g)	CALCIUM SIZE (mg)	FRACTIONAL[a] CONTENT (%)	ESTIMATED[b] ABSORBABLE ABSORPTION (mg)	SERVINGS NEEDED TO CALCIUM/ SERVING	EQUAL 1 c MILK
Milk (or 1 c yogurt or 1½ oz cheddar cheese)	260	300	32.1	96.3	1.0	
Beans, dried		177	50.0	15.6	7.8	12.3
Broccoli	71	35	61.3	21.5	4.5	
Bok choy	85	79	52.7	41.6	2.3	
Kale		65	47.0	58.8	27.6	3.5
Spinach	90	122	5.1	6.2	15.5	
Tofu, calcium set		126	258.0	31.0	80.0	1.2

C, cup.

[a]Adjusted for load; for milk, this is fractional absorption (Fx abs) = 0.889–0.0964 ln load; for low-oxalate vegetables, after adjusting by the ratio of fractional absorption determined for kale relative to milk at the same load, the equation becomes Fx abs = 0.959–0.0964 ln load.
[b]Calcium content (mg) × Fx abs.

From Weaver CM, Proulx WR, Heaney RP. Choices for achieving adequate dietary calcium with a vegetarian diet. Am J Clin Nutr 1999;70(Suppl):543S–8S, with permission.

loss, especially during growth (57). In contrast, a major determinant of urinary calcium is urinary sodium, which reflects dietary sodium (58, 59). Sodium and calcium share some of the same transport systems in the proximal tubule. In adults, each 100 mmol (2.3 g) increment of sodium excreted by the kidney pulls out approximately 0.6 to 1.0 mmol (24 to 40 mg) of accompanying calcium (60). Because urinary calcium losses account for 50% of the variability in calcium retention, dietary sodium has a tremendous potential to influence bone loss at suboptimal calcium intakes in women; each extra gram of sodium per day is projected to produce an additional rate of bone loss of 1% per year if the calcium loss in the urine comes from the skeleton (61). A longitudinal study of postmenopausal women showed a negative correlation between urinary sodium excretion and bone density of the hip (58). The investigators concluded, from the range of values available to them, that bone loss could have been prevented by either a daily dietary calcium increase of 891 mg calcium or by halving the daily sodium intake. Racial differences in the effect of dietary sodium on urinary sodium and calcium excretion are observed as early as puberty (62). White girls excrete more sodium and calcium on high-salt diets compared with black girls, a finding that may partially account for lesser vulnerability to hypertension through water retention, but greater vulnerability to osteoporosis with bone loss as they mature (62, 63).

Another dietary component that influences urinary calcium excretion is protein. Each gram of protein metabolized increases urinary calcium by approximately 1 mg; thus, doubling purified dietary proteins or amino acids in the diet increases urinary calcium by approximately 50% (64). The acid load of the sulfate produced in the metabolism of sulfur-containing amino acids that produces acid ash is mainly responsible for this increase. However, a metaanalysis concluded that little evidence exists for the acid ash effect on calcium balance (65). Increases in calcium absorption (66), decreases in endogenous

secretion (67), or the hypocalciuric effect of phosphorus in high-protein foods can offset the hypercalciuric effect of protein. At the other extreme, inadequate protein intakes compromise bone health and contribute to osteoporosis in elderly persons (68). There appear to be dietary protein–calcium interactions such that calcium absorption increases to offset the calciuric effects of high dietary protein more at low than at high calcium intakes (69). The benefits of calcium supplementation in mitigating bone loss in elderly persons are greater with higher protein intakes, however (70).

Concerns about high phosphate consumption, especially with the popular trend toward high phosphate consumption in soft drinks, has been raised for bone. A metaanalysis of calcium balance studies in response to phosphate intake showed decreased urine calcium and increased calcium retention despite increased endogenous secretion with increasing phosphate intake (71). Cola beverages have been associated with reduced bone gain in children (72), but it is more likely that the explanation is the displacement of milk than the phosphorus intake. Furthermore, cola beverages typically contain no more phosphorus per serving than orange juice and substantially less than many of the calcium-fortified orange juices now marketed.

Although caffeine in high amounts acutely increases urinary calcium (73), 24-hour urinary calcium was not altered in a double-blind, placebo-controlled trial (74). Daily consumption of caffeine equivalent to 2 to 3 cups of coffee accelerated bone loss from the spine and total body in postmenopausal women who consumed less than 744 mg calcium/day (75). The relationship between caffeine intake and bone loss in this observational study may be the result of a small decrease in calcium absorption (76) or a confounding factor such as a probable inverse association between milk intake and caffeine intake.

Fat intake has a negative impact on calcium balance only during steatorrhea. In this condition, calcium forms insoluble soaps with fatty acids in the gut.

numerous environmental factors affect bone mass (114). The main determinant of bone density in adolescent girls is calcium intake (115). During this period, urinary calcium is relatively unaffected by calcium intake (38, 57), a finding indicating an ability to use for bone accumulation all the absorbed calcium resulting from the range of intakes studied. Adequate dietary calcium influences bone size and geometry in addition to bone mass, both of which also contribute to bone strength (116).

Aside from calcium intake, other lifestyle choices that affect peak bone mass include physical activity, intake of other nutrients that affect calcium balance (covered earlier in this chapter), anorexia, and substance abuse. As may be expected, dietary calcium and exercise positively interact in forming strong skeletons (117–119). Beyond the timing of peak bone mass, lifestyle choices can affect rate of bone loss, but the window of opportunity to build bone has passed.

Adults

The mature woman has 23 to 25 mol (920 to 1000 g) body calcium, and the mature man has approximately 30 mol (1200 g) total body calcium. The population coefficient of variation around these means is approximately 15%. Total body bone mass remains relatively constant over the reproductive years, as decreases in the proximal femur and other sites after age 18 years are offset by continued growth of the forearm, total spine, and head. Then age-related bone loss occurs, which varies with the individual, but it occurs most rapidly during the first 3 years after menopause in women. The average adult loses bone at a rate of approximately 1% per year. Age-related decreases in calcium absorption and increases in urinary calcium contribute to this loss. These physiologic changes are more abrupt at menopause in women. Loss of estrogen and aging are associated with loss of intestinal VDR (3). Further, explanations for bone loss during aging include declining calcium intakes (discussed later) and physical activity and decreased levels of gonadal hormones. The calcium intake required by older adults to achieve mean maximal retention or minimal loss was determined to be 1200 mg/day by the Panel on Calcium and Related Nutrients (see Table 7.3) (117).

Pregnancy

Fetal skeletal calcium accretion is not great until the third trimester. During the third trimester, approximately 5 mmol/day (200 mg/day) of calcium are required for fetal growth. The mother's calcium absorption and renal conservation increase beginning by the second trimester to meet fetal demands and to store calcium for the subsequent lactational drain governed by PTH and IGF-I (120, 121). From before pregnancy status to the third trimester, fractional calcium absorption increases 60% to 70% (122). At low calcium intakes, the mother's skeleton is compromised to meet calcium demands of the fetus, and the fetal skeleton is protected except at exceptionally low calcium intakes (123). These changes are accompanied by a fall in biologically active PTH, increases in CT during early pregnancy, and increases in prolactin by up to 10- to 20-fold. Calcium supplementation increased bone density of neonates of malnourished women in India (124) and improved calcium balance and bone formation rates across pregnancy and lactation in women with habitual intakes of less than 500 mg/day (125). No benefits to bone mineral status of infants occurred with calcium supplementation to pregnant Gambian women whose habitual calcium intakes were 9 mmol (360 mg)/day, however (126).

Lactation

Calcium transfer to breast milk varies mainly with changes in volume; calcium concentration is relatively constant at 7 ± 0.65 mmol/L (280 ± 26 mg/L) and is independent of the calcium content of the mother's diet. Wide variability in the amount of calcium transferred to milk daily has not generally been associated with bone mineral growth or status in infancy (127). However, low dairy consumption by pregnant African-American adolescents was associated with decreased fetal femur length (128). Daily calcium transfer from maternal serum to breast milk increases from 4.2 mmol/day (168 mg/day) at 3 months following parturition to 7 mmol/day (280 mg/day) at 6 months following parturition. The increase in intestinal calcium absorption at the end of pregnancy gradually disappears after childbirth and during the lactation period. To meet the need of milk production, some renal conservation occurs, but more importantly, the maternal skeleton is depleted at a rate of approximately 1% per month; this loss is not prevented with calcium and vitamin D supplementation (129). Increased bone turnover during lactation may be under the control of PTH-related peptide (PTHrP) produced by the lactating mammary gland (130). A postlactation anabolic phase allows recovery of bone density to prelactation levels. Whether this recovery is complete in all individuals, such as older lactating women, is not known. Epidemiologic studies have found no association between pregnancy and lactation and the risk of osteoporotic fractures.

ADEQUACY OF CALCIUM INTAKE

Usual calcium intakes by age for the male and female population of the United States, as collected for the 1999 to 2004 National Health and Nutrition Examination Survey (NHANES), were compared with the 1997 AIs and tolerable upper intake levels (ULs) for calcium set by the Dietary Reference Intake Committee for the Institute of Medicine (131). Mean calcium intakes were lower than the recommended intake for calcium in persons older than 9 years. Only 21.3% of girls and women and 43.7% of boys and men in the United States had usual intakes higher than the AIs for calcium (131). Milk intake drops more than 25% from early childhood to late adolescence, and this explains the drop in calcium intake (111). As estimated from NHANES 2003 to 2006, 43% of US residents use calcium supplements (132). Calcium supplements were taken primarily by adults and substantially increased the percent of individuals meeting the AI (i.e., for men older than 71 years, 15% from food alone compared with 31% from food plus supplements; and for women older than 71 years, 39% with supplements met the AI for calcium compared with 8% from food alone).

Assessment of calcium intakes of populations is important for determining nutritional status and for drawing conclusions about the relationship between diet and health and disease. Assessing usual calcium intake of an individual is fraught with errors, however (133). Calcium intake can be assessed with food frequency questionnaires, diet recalls, diet records, or duplicate plate analysis. Duplicate plate analysis eliminates many of the errors associated with other methods but is not practical for assessing large groups of individuals. Food frequency questionnaires assess calcium better than they do some other nutrients because dairy foods are the major source of calcium, and individuals recall dairy product consumption reasonably well. Hidden calcium taken as food additives (e.g., anticaking agents), water, fortified foods, and components of pharmaceuticals can be easily overlooked, however. When calcium intakes from fortified foods were considered in assessing diets of Asian, Hispanic, and white 10- to 18-year-old children and adolescents, higher calcium intakes were observed than previously reported in national surveys, but most subgroups still fell below the recommended intakes for that age (134). The gap between calcium intakes and recommended intakes is greatest for African-Americans (135). Diet recall and diet records suffer from errors in estimating portion size, from variability in food composition, and from inadequacies of existing food composition tables. Multiple diet records can improve the estimate of an individual's average calcium intake. However, the generally large variability in calcium intake from day to day precludes confidence in estimates of usual calcium intake of an individual (136, 137).

RISKS OF EXCESS DIETARY CALCIUM

Nutritional toxicity of calcium means an elevation of blood calcium levels (hypercalcemia) by reason of overconsumption of calcium or an elevation of urine calcium excretion (hypercalciuria) to the point that either the kidneys calcify or renal stones develop. Hypercalcemia, particularly if severe, results in lax muscle tone, constipation, large urine volumes, nausea, and ultimately confusion, coma, and death. It essentially never occurs from ingestion of natural food sources. A good illustration of the safety of food calcium sources is provided by nomadic, pastoralist peoples, such as the Masai (138). Because their diets consist mostly of the milk of their herds and flocks, they have calcium intakes higher than 5000 mg/day (and often appreciably higher), roughly 5 to 10 times what people of industrialized nations ingest. Such pastoral peoples are not known to have any unusual incidence of hypercalcemia or kidney stones.

Hypercalcemia, metabolic alkalosis, and possibly renal insufficiency have been increasing, especially in postmenopausal and pregnant women with a history of excessive (typically >4 g/day) ingestion of supplemental calcium and often absorbable alkali, which raise the pH of the urine and predisposes to calcium deposits in the kidneys (139). Elderly persons are vulnerable to this "calcium alkali syndrome" because they are in a state of net bone resorption in which bone is less of a reservoir for buffering against excess calcium. Pregnant women who have enhanced calcium absorption and volume depletion may also be vulnerable.

Kidney stones are not usually caused by dietary calcium. More often, individuals with kidney stones have high urine calcium because they have a renal leak of calcium. Accordingly, they often have some degree of reduction of their skeletal calcium reserves. Lowering calcium intake in such individuals rarely affects their kidney stone problem, but it always leads to further reduction in bone mass. High calcium intakes may contribute to kidney stone formation in certain susceptible individuals. Calcium and vitamin D supplementation in the 7-year Women's Health Initiative trial was associated with a 17% increase in the risk of kidney stones (140), but the events labeled "kidney stones" were not medically confirmed. Therefore, the significance of this finding is uncertain, especially because most studies show no increase in stone risk with calcium in diet or supplements (141). In individuals with recurrent calcium oxalate stones, the stone problem is actually helped by *increasing* calcium intakes to 30 mmol (1200 mg)/day together with restricted animal protein and salt, compared with individuals on low-calcium diets of 10 mmol (400 mg) calcium/day (95). The reasons are that urinary oxalate excretion is a more important risk factor for stones, and dietary calcium binds oxalate of dietary origin in the gut, prevents oxalate absorption, and thereby reduces the urinary oxalate load.

Concerns over prolonged calcium supplementation have been raised in connection with the risk of prostate cancer (142), myocardial infarction, and vascular calcification (143). A metaanalysis reported that the use of calcium supplements was associated with almost a 30% increase in cardiovascular disease risk (144). Possible mechanisms are not established. Regarding the concern over cardiovascular end points, the beneficial effects of calcium on serum lipids and blood pressure seem inconsistent with an increased risk of disease. It is prudent not to exceed the upper level of recommended intakes from supplements while these relationships are further studied. If it turns out that a real increase in risk exists, the evidence indicates that it would apply only to supplemental sources because population studies (e.g., the Masai cited earlier and Swedish men with high dairy consumption) (145) showed, if anything, a beneficial effect on cardiovascular disease from high food calcium intakes.

CLINICAL DISORDERS INVOLVING CALCIUM

As noted earlier, low calcium intakes, coupled with low calcium absorption efficiency and high obligatory calcium losses from the body, deplete skeletal calcium reserves. In other words, low intakes cause subnormal bone mass (and strength). This is one of the contributing causes of the disorder called *osteoporosis*, which is covered in the chapter on osteoporosis. Genetic mutations can alter intracellular calcium signaling. For example, alterations in the RyR protein can lead to hypertrophy and stroke. Familial benign hypercalcemia occurs when CaSR is partially or totally inactivated. Cell injury, damage, or serious dysfunction is always associated with a rise in cytosolic calcium concentration, an association that probably reflects an impaired ability of the cell to maintain the normal 10,000-fold gradient between the interior and exterior of the cell. The rise in cytosolic calcium may worsen cell damage and hasten cell death (146).

The most common disorders of calcium metabolism (other than osteoporosis, which is multifactorial in origin), involve regulation of ECF [Ca^{2+}]. Usually, these conditions result from disorders of parathyroid gland function and are not nutritional. As noted earlier in this chapter, the skeletal calcium reserves are so vast, relative to the size of the ECF [Ca^{2+}] compartment, that simple dietary deficiency of calcium essentially never compromises ECF [Ca^{2+}] regulation. A few rare exceptions are worth noting, however, because they illustrate how the system operates.

During growth, when the demands of skeletal mineralization are highest, extremely low-calcium diets may lead to hypocalcemia, despite maximal secretory output of the parathyroid glands. One consequence of the hypersecretion of PTH is lowering of serum phosphate levels. The combination of low calcium and low phosphorus levels in the ECF results both in undermineralization of newly deposited bone matrix and in osteoblast dysfunction. The clinical result is rickets. Usually, rickets would be produced by vitamin D deficiency or hypophosphatemia from other causes or by osteoblast toxicity. As this example shows, however, rickets can sometimes be caused also by calcium deficiency alone (137).

Another example of nutritional hypocalcemia occurs as a result of magnesium deficiency, most often noted in severe alcoholism or as a result of intestinal fistula or malabsorption that causes excessive magnesium loss from the body. Magnesium, of course, is an essential cation for many cell metabolic processes (see the chapter on magnesium); and with severe magnesium depletion, many organs and systems function abnormally. The system regulating ECF [Ca^{2+}] is an example. Both PTH release from the parathyroid glands and bony response to PTH depend on magnesium, and both are defective in magnesium deficiency. Evidence that both steps are impaired is provided by the findings that PTH levels in magnesium-deficient patients fail to rise adequately in response to hypocalcemia and exogenous PTH fails to elevate bone remodeling in these patients, as it should. Magnesium repletion corrects both problems.

ACKNOWLEDGMENTS

This work was supported in part by Public Health Service (PHS) grant HD 061908.
Disclosure: CMW is a member of Pharmavite Advisory Board.

REFERENCES

1. Clapham DE. Cell 2007;131:1047–58.
2. Carafoli E, Penniston JT. Sci Am 1985;253:70–8.
3. Fleet JC, Schoch RD. In Crit Rev Clin Lab Sci 2010; 47: 181–195
4. Ensrud KE, Duong T, Cauley JA et al. Ann Intern Med 2000;132:345–53.
5. Chattopadhyay N, Brown EM. Cell Signal 2000;12:361–6.
6. Hanes D, Weaver CM, Wastney ME. FASEB J 1995;9: A283 (abstract1642).
7. Heaney RP, Saville PD, Recker RR. J Lab Clin Med 1975;85:881–90.
8. Heaney RP, Weaver CM, Fitzsimmons ML. J Bone Miner Res 1990;5:1135–8.
9. Heaney RP. Am J Clin Nutr 1991;54(Suppl):242S–57S.
10. Heaney RP, Weaver CM, Fitzsimmons ML et al. J Bone Miner Res 1990;5:1139–42.
11. Marcus CS, Lengermann FW. J Nutr 1962;77:155–60.
12. Peng JB, Cheng XZ, Berger UV et al. J Biol Chem 1999;274: 22739–46.
13. Song Y, Kato S, Fleet JC. J Nutr 2003;133:374–80.
14. Xue Y, Fleet JC. Gastroenterology 2009;136:1317–27.
15. Nemere I, Leathers V, Norman AW. J Biol Chem 1986; 261:16106–14.
16. Fulmer CA. J Nutr 1992;122:644–50.
17. Nemer I. J Nutr 1992;122:657–61.
18. Benn BS, Ajibade D, Porta A et al. Endocrinology 2008;149: 3196–3205.
19. Wasserman RH, Fullmer CS. J Nutr 1995;125(Suppl): 1971S–79S.
20. Wassermann RH, Chandler JS, Meyer SA et al. J Nutr 1992;122:662–71.
21. Chirayath MV, Gajdzik L, Hulla W et al. Am J Physiol 1998; 274:G389–96.
22. Fujita H, Sugimoto K, Inatomi S et al. Mol Biol Cell 2008;19: 1912–21.
23. Barger-Lux MJ, Heaney RP, Lanspa SJ et al. J Clin Endocrinol Metab 1995;80:406–11.
24. Heaney RP, Recker RR, Steagman MR et al. J Bone Miner Res 1989;4:469–75.
25. Pattanaungkul S, Riggs BL, Yergey AL et al. J Clin Endocrinol Metab 2000;85:4023–27.
26. Ebeling PR, Sandgren ME, Dimagno EP et al. J Clin Endocrinol Metab 1992;75:176–182.
27. Recker RR. N Engl J Med 1985;43:133–7.
28. Ames SK, Ellis KJ, Gunn SK et al. J Bone Miner Res 1999;14:740–6.

29. Bryant RJ, Wastney ME, Martin BR et al. J Endocrinol Metab 2003;88:1043–7.
30. Looker AC, Wahner HW, Dunn WL et al. Osteoporos Int 1998;8:468–89.
31. Charles P, Jenson FT, Mosekilde L et al. Clin Sci 1983;65: 415–22.
32. Palacios C, Wigertz K, Martin B et al. Nutr Res 2003;23: 401–11.
33. Martin BR, Davis S, Campbell WW et al. Med Sci Sports Exerc 2007;39:1986–6.
34. Humes HD, Ichikawa I, Troy JL et al. J Clin Invest 1978; 61:32–40.
35. Coluccio LM. Eur J Cell Biol 1991;56:286–94.
36. Hoenderop JG, van der Kemp AW, Hartog A et al. J Biol Chem 1999;274:8375–78.
37. Christakos S, Gill R, Lee S et al. J Nutr 1992;122:678–82.
38. Eaton SB, Konner M. N Engl J Med 1985;312:283–9.
39. 2005 Dietary Guidelines Advisory Committee Report. Available at: http://www.health.gov/dietaryguidelines. Accessed June 30, 2010.
40. Ballow C, Kuester S, Gillespie C. Arch Pediatr Adolesc Med 2000;154:1148–2.
41. 2010 Dietary Guidelines Advisory Committee Report. Available at: http://www.health.gov/dietaryguidelines. Accessed June 30, 2010.
42. Nickel KP, Martin BR, Smith DL et al. J Nutr 1996;126: 1406–11.
43. Heaney RP, Recker RR, Weaver CM. Calcif Tissue Int 1990;46:300–4.
44. Heaney RP, Weaver CM. Am J Clin Nutr 1989;50:830–2.
45. Heaney RP, Weaver CM, Recker RR. Am J Clin Nutr 1988;47: 707–9.
46. Weaver CM, Heaney RP. Calcif Tissue Int 1991;56:436–42.
47. Heaney RP, Weaver CM, Fitzsimmons ML. Am J Clin Nutr 1991;53:745–7.
48. Weaver CM, Heaney RP, Martin BR et al. J Nutr 1991; 121:1769–75.
49. McCance RA, Widdowson EM. J Physiol 1942;101:44–85.
50. James WPT, Branch WJ, Southgate DAT. Lancet 1978;1:638–9.
51. Heaney RP, Weaver CM. J Am Geriatr Soc 1995;43:1–3.
52. Weaver CM, Proulx WR, Heaney RP. Am J Clin Nutr 1999;70(Suppl):543S–8S.
53. Weaver CM, Heaney RP, Connor L et al. J Food Sci 2002;67:3144–7.
54. Recker RR, Bammi A, Barger-Lux MG et al. Am J Clin Nutr 1988;47:93–5.
55. Cashman KD. Br J Nutr 2002;87(Suppl):169S–77S.
56. Zhao Y, Martin BR, Wastney ME et al. Exp Biol Med 2005;230:536–42.
57. Jackman LA, Millane SS, Martin BR et al. Am J Clin Nutr 1997;66:327–33.
58. Devine A, Criddle RA, Dick IM et al. Am J Clin Nutr 1995;62:740–5.
59. Matkovic V, Ilich JZ, Andon WB et al. Am J Clin Nutr 1995;62:417–25.
60. Itoh R, Suyama Y. Am J Clin Nutr 1996;63:735–40.
61. Shortt C, Madden A, Fllynn A et al. Eur J Clin Nutr 1988;42:595–603.
62. Wigertz, K, Palacios C, Jackman LA et al. Am J Clin Nutr 2005;l81:845–50.
63. Palacios C, Wigertz K, Martin BR et al. J Clin Endocrinol Metab 2004;89:1858–63.
64. Heaney RP. J Am Diet Assoc 1993;93:1259–60.
65. Fenton TR, Lyon AW, Eliasziw M et al. J Bone Miner Res 2009;24:1835–40.
66. Kerstetter JE, O'Brien KO, Caseria DM et al. J Clin Endocrinol Metab 2005;90:26–31.
67. Spence LA, Lipscomb ER, Cadogan J et al. Am J Clin Nutr 2005;81:916–22.
68. Dawson-Hughes B. J Nutr 2003;133:852S–4S.
69. Hunt JR, Johnson LK, Roughead ZKF. Am J Clin Nutr 2009;89:1354–65.
70. Dawson-Hughes B, Harris SS. Am J Clin Nutr 2002;75:773–9.
71. Fenton TR, Lyon AW, Eliasziw M et al. Nutr J 2009;8:41–56.
72. Whiting SJ, Vatanparast H, Baxter-Jones A et al. J Nutr 2004;134(Suppl):696S–700S.
73. Hasling C, Sondergraad K, Charles P et al. J Nutr 1992; 122:1119–26.
74. Barger-Lux MJ, Heaney RP, Stegman MR. Am J Clin Nutr 1990;52:722–5.
75. Harris SS, Dawson-Hughes B. Am J Clin Nutr 1994;60: 573–8.
76. Barger-Lux MJ, Heaney RP. Osteoporos Int 1995;5:97–102.
77. Evans GH, Weaver CM, Harrington DD et al. J Hypertens 1990;8:327–37.
78. Andon MB, Ilich JZ, Tzagournio MA et al. Am J Clin Nutr 1996;63:950–3.
79. Wood RJ, Zheng JJ. Am J Clin Nutr 1997;65:1803–9.
80. Gleerup A, Rossander-Hulten L, Gramatkovski E et al. Am J Clin Nutr 1995;61:97–104.
81. Halberg L, Rossander-Hulten L, Brune M et al. Eur J Clin Nutr 1992;46:317–27.
82. Whiting SJ. Nutr Rev 1995;53:77–80.
83. Ilich-Ernst JZ, McKenna AA, Badenhop NE et al. Am J Clin Nutr 1998;68:880–7.
84. Medeiros DM, Plattner A, Jennings D et al. J Nutr 2002; 132:3135–44.
85. Berridge MJ. Nature 1993;361:315–25.
86. Brown EM. Annu Rev Nutr 2000;20:501–33.
87. Bronner F, Stein WD. J Nutr 1995;125(Suppl):1987S–95S.
88. Combs GF, Hassan N, Dellagana N et al. Biol Trace Elem Res 2008;121:193–204.
89. Barger-Lux MJ, Heaney RP. J Nutr 1994;124(Suppl):1406S–11S.
90. Weaver CM. Endocrine 2002;17:43–48.
90. Reid IR, Mason B, Horne A et al. Am J Med 2002;112: 343–47.
91. Van Vierlo LA, Arends LR, Streppel MT et al. J Hum Hypertens 2006;20:571–80.
92. Chia V, Newcomb RA. Nutr Rev 2004;62:115–20.
93. Moorman PG, Terry PD. Am J Clin Nutr 2004;80:5–14.
94. Shaukat A, Scouras N, Schunemann HJ. Am J Gastroenterol 2005;100:390–4.
95. Borghi L, Schianchi T, Meschi T et al. N Engl J Med 2002;346:77–84.
96. Heaney RP, Weaver CM. Am J Clin Nutr 1989;50:830–2.
97. Pereira MA, Jacobs DR, Van Horn L et al. JAMA 2002;287: 2081–9.
98. Chobanian AV, Bakris GL, Black HR et al. JAMA 2003;289:2560–72.
99. Heaney RP. J Am Coll Nutr 2000;19(Suppl):83S–99S.
100. Heaney RP. J Am Coll Nutr 2009;28(Suppl):82S–90S.
101. Tang BM, Eslick GD, Nowson C et al. Lancet 2007;370: 657–66.
102. Lynch MF, Griffin IJ, Hawthorne KM et al. Am J Clin Nutr 2007;85:750–4.
103. Bailey DA, McKay HA, Mirald RL et al. J Bone Miner Res 1999;14:1672–9.
104. Hill K, Braun MM, Kern M et al. J Clin Endocrind Metab 2008; 93:4743–8.
105. Wastney ME. J Clin Endocrinol Metab 2000;85:4470–5.

106. Atkinson S, McCabe GP, Weaver CM et al. J Nutr 2008; 138:1182–6.
107. Vatanparast H, Bailey DA, Baxter-Jones ADG et al. Br J Nutr 2010;103:575–80.
108. Peterson CA. J Bone Miner Res 1995;10:81–95.
109. Weaver CM, Janle E, Martin B et al. J Bone Miner Res 2009:4:1411–9.
110. Bonjour J-P. Lancet 2001;358:1208–13.
111. Teegarden D, Proulx WR, Martin BR et al. J Bone Miner Res 1995;10:711–5.
112. Lin Y-C, Lyle RM, Weaver CM et al. Bone 2003;35:546–53.
113. Heaney RP, Barger-Lux MJ, Davis KM et al. Osteoporos Int 1997;7:426–30.
114. Heaney RP, Abrams S, Dawson-Hughes B et al. Osteoporos Int 2000;11:985–1009.
115. Matkovic V, Fortana D, Tominac C et al. Am J Clin Nutr 1990;52:878–88.
116. Cheng S, Lyytikainen A, Kroger H et al. Am J Clin Nutr 2005;82:1115–26.
117. Specker B, Binkley T, Wermers J. J Bone Miner Res 2002;17(Suppl):S398.
118. Stear SJ, Prentice A, Jones SC et al. Am J Clin Nutr 2003;77:985–92.
119. Bass SL, Naughton G, Saxon L et al. J Bone Miner Res 2007;22:458–64.
120. Heaney RP, Skillman TG. J Clin Endocrinol Metab 1971; 331:661–70.
121. Zapatas CLV, Donangelo CM, Woodhouse LR et al. Am J Clin Nutr 2004;80:417–22.
122. Ritchie LD, Fung EB, Holloran BP et al. Am J Clin Nutr 1998;67:693–701.
123. Naylor KE, Igbal P, Fledeluis C et al. J Bone Miner Res 2000;15:129–37.
124. Wargovich MJ. J Am Coll Nutr 1988;7:295–300.
125. O'Brien KO, Donangelo CM, Zapato CLV et al. Am J Clin Nutr 2006;83:317–23.
126. Jarjou LMA, Prentice A, Sawo Y et al. Am J Clin Nutr 2006;83:657–66.
127. Prentice A, Laskey A, Jarjou LMA. Lactation and bone development: Implications for the calcium requirements of infants and lactating mothers. In: Bonjour J-P, Tsang RC, eds. Nutrition and Bone Development, vol 41. Philadelphia: Lippincott-Raven, 1999:127–145.
128. Chang S-C, O'Brien KO, Nathanson MS et al. Am J Clin Nutr 2003;77:1248–54.
129. Kalkwarf HJ, Specker BC, Henbi JE et al. Am J Clin Nutr 1996;63:526–31.
130. Kalkwarf HJ, Specker BL. Endocrine 2002;17:49–53.
131. Nicklas TA, O'Neil CE, Fulgoni VL. J Am Coll Nutr 2009;28(Suppl):73S–81S.
132. Bailey RL, Dodd, KW, Goldman JA, et al. J Nutr 2010;140: 817–22.
133. Boushey CJ. Clinical Approaches for Studying Calcium Metabolism and Its Relationship to Disease. In: Weaver CM, Heaney RP, eds. Calcium in Human Health. Totowa, NJ: Humana Press, 2006:65–81.
134. Novotny R, Peck L, Auld G et al. J Am Coll Nutr 2003;224: 64–70.
135. Fulgoni VL 3rd, Huth PJ, DiRienzo DB et al. J Am Coll Nutr 2004;23:651–9.
136. Weaver CM, Martin BR, Peacock M. Calcium Metabolism in Adolescent Girls. In: Burckhardt P, Heaney RP, eds. Nutritional Aspects of Osteoporosis, vol 7. New York: Raven Press, 1995:123–8.
137. Barger-Lux MJ, Heaney RP. Determinants of Calcium Absorption. In: Burckhardt P, Heaney RP, eds. Nutritional Aspects of Osteoporosis, vol 7. New York: Raven Press 1995:243–51.
138. Jackson RT, Latham MC. Am J Clin Nutr 1979;32:779–82.
139. Patel AM, Goldfarb S. J Am Soc Nephrol 2010;21:1440–3.
140. Jackson RD, La Croix AZ, Gass M et al. N Engl J Med 2006;354:669–83.
141. Heaney RP. J Am Coll Nutr 2008;27:519–27.
142. World Cancer Research Fund. Food, Nutrition, Physical Activity and the Prevention of Cancer: a Global Perspective. Am Inst Cancer Res Washington DC AICR 2007.
143. Daly RM, Ebeling PR. Nutrients 2010;2:505–22.
144. Reid IR, Bolland MJ, Grey A. Int Med J 2010;40(Suppl): S47.
145. Kaluza J, Orsini N, Levitan EB et al. Am J Epidemiol 2010;171:801–7.
146. Rasmussen H, Palmieri GMA. Altered cell calcium metabolism and human diseases. In: Rubin RP, Weiss GB, Putnsy JW Jr, eds. Calcium in Biological Systems. New York: Plenum Publishing, 1985:551–60.

SUGGESTED READINGS

Weaver CM. Osteoporosis: the early years. In: Coulston AM, Boushey CJ, eds. Nutrition: ThePrevention and Treatment of Disease. 2nd ed. New York: Academic Press, 2008:833–49.

Weaver CM, Heaney RP, eds. Calcium in Human Health. Totowa, NJ: Humana Press, 2006.

B. MINERALS

8 PHOSPHORUS[1]

KIMBERLY O. O'BRIEN, JANE E. KERSTETTER, AND KARL L. INSOGNA

---

[1]**Abbreviations: 1,25(OH)$_2$D**, 1,25-dihydroxyvitamin D; **ADHR**, autosomal dominant hypophosphatemic rickets; **AI**, adequate intake; **ARHR**, autosomal recessive hypophosphatemic rickets; **ATP**, adenosine triphosphate; **CKD**, chronic kidney disease; **DKA**, diabetic ketoacidosis; **EAR**, estimated average requirement; **FGF**, fibroblast growth factor; **GALNT3**, N-acetylgalactosaminyltransferase; **HHRH**, hereditary hypophosphatemic rickets with hypercalciuria; **NaP$_i$-2a/NaP$_i$-2b**, sodium-phosphate cotransporters; **PHEX**, phosphate-regulating gene with homologies to endopeptidases on the X-chromosome; **P$_i$**, inorganic phosphorus ion; **PTH**, parathyroid hormone; **UL**, tolerable upper intake level; **XLH**, X-linked hypophosphatemic rickets.

BRIEF HISTORICAL REVIEW

Phosphorus was discovered in 1669 by Hennig Brand, who isolated this mineral from urine. His observation that phosphorus glowed when exposed to air led to the name of this element that is based using the Greek words for light ("phos") and bearer ("phoros"). In nature, phosphorus is monoisotopic and has an atomic weight of 30.97. Two radioisotopes of phosphorus exist: ^{32}P, which has a half-life of 14.28 days; and ^{33}P, which has a half-life of 24.3 days. As early as the 1920s, George Hevesy et al used ^{32}P in plant models to elucidate the biologic roles of this mineral (1). Over the next decade, Hevesy used animal models and phosphorus radiotracers to characterize the distribution of phosphorus once absorbed into the body and to identify the integral role of phosphorus in mineralized tissues (2). Early human metabolic balance studies were undertaken in the 1940s by McCance and Widdowson (3). Their seminal studies highlighted the essential role that renal tubular phosphate handling plays in whole body homeostasis of this mineral. During this same era, Harrison and Harrison characterized the impact of parathyroid hormone (PTH) and vitamin D on phosphorus metabolism and urinary phosphorus excretion (4). Although these early studies contributed greatly to the understanding of phosphorus flux in the human body, many aspects of phosphorus metabolism remained elusive. More recently, the discoveries of the phosphatonin, fibroblast growth factor 23 (FGF23) and the FGF coreceptor Klotho gene clarified the long-term hormonal regulation of phosphorus metabolism. These advances improved our understanding of the bone-kidney axis in phosphate homeostasis and established the genetic basis for several inherited disorders of phosphorus metabolism (5–7). This enhanced understanding of the biology of phosphorus metabolism may lead to new therapies for individuals with dysregulated mineral metabolism. Better biomarkers of phosphorus homeostasis in human health and disease are still needed.

BIOCHEMISTRY AND PHYSIOLOGY

Importance

Phosphorus is a ubiquitous mineral in the human body and is integral to diverse functions ranging from the transfer of genetic information to energy utilization. Phosphorus forms the backbone of DNA and RNA and is an essential component of phospholipids that form all membrane bilayers. Many proteins, enzymes, and sugars in the body are phosphorylated, and that process often dictates the activity and function of phosphoproteins and sugars. Phosphorus is an integral component of the body's key energy source, adenosine triphosphate (ATP). Other phosphorylated proteins (e.g., creatine phosphate in muscle) serve as a rapid source of phosphate for ATP production. Phosphorus, as 2,3-diphosphoglycerate (also known as 2,3-bisphosphoglycerate), plays a vital role in the dissociation of oxygen from hemoglobin. Cellular phosphate is the main intracellular buffer and therefore is essential for pH regulation of the human body. Finally, many intracellular signaling processes depend on phosphorus-containing compounds such as cyclic adenosine monophosphate (cAMP), cyclic guanine monophosphate (cGMP) and inositol polyphosphates (e.g., inositol triphosphate or IP_3).

Distribution and Body Composition

At birth, a neonate contains roughly 20 g phosphorus (0.5 g/100 g fat free tissue), most of which is accumulated during the final 8 weeks of pregnancy (8). At maturity, total body phosphorus content increases to roughly 1.35 g/100 g fat free tissue (9) with total body phosphorus content averaging 400 g in women and 500 g in men (10).

The largest depot of phosphorus in the human body (~85%) is found in bone in the form of hydroxyapatite or $Ca_{10}(PO_4)_6(OH)_6$ (7). This compound forms the mineralized matrix of bone and contributes to the unique biomechanical properties of bone. The remaining phosphorus in the human body (~14%) is located in soft tissue, muscle, and viscera; only a small fraction (~1%) is found in the extracellular space, either as inorganic phosphorus ions (P_i), primarily in the form of phosphate (PO_4), or complexed to other cations such as calcium or magnesium (Ca^{2+} or Mg^{2+}).

Circulating Concentrations in Plasma

Eighty-five percent of plasma phosphorus is ultrafilterable whereas 15% is bound to proteins. Plasma P_i concentrations are only loosely regulated and in adults typically range from 0.8 to 1.5 mmol/L (11, 12). During infancy, childhood, and adolescence, serum P_i concentrations fall progressively from values nearly twice as high as seen in adults (e.g., 1.88 to 2.42 mmol/L) to values in the adult range. The reasons that serum phosphorus levels are high early in life are not known with certainty, but increased renal phosphate reclamation is thought to have a major role. Hypophosphatemia is defined as serum phosphate concentrations lower than 0.5 mmol/L, whereas hyperphosphatemia is considered to be present when the plasma concentration is greater than 2.2 mmol/L. Severe hypophosphatemia is associated with cardiomyopathy and skeletal myopathy. Chronic hypophosphatemia can cause rickets in children and osteomalacia in adults. Hyperphosphatemia may result in

soft tissue calcification and, when severe, can cause hypocalcemia leading to tetany and death.

A serum phosphorus concentration even slightly higher than the upper limit of normal may have some utility as a biomarker for cardiovascular disease (13–15). The mechanisms responsible for this association have not been identified, but investigators have postulated that higher serum phosphorus concentrations may reflect increased bone resorption leading to vascular calcification and osteoporosis (16). Alternatively, perhaps high plasma phosphorus concentrations may indicate an atherogenic diet (high levels of meat, butter, saturated fats, and cholesterol).

Hormones That Regulate Phosphorus Homeostasis

Three key hormones influence whole body phosphorus economy: 1,25-dihydroxyvitamin D (abbreviated 1,25[OH]₂D and also known as calcitriol), PTH, and FGF23. Calcitriol is produced in the kidney by hydroxylation of circulating 25-hydroxyvitamin D at the 1-position by the renal 1-α hydroxylase enzyme. The 1-α hydroxylase enzyme is very tightly regulated, and the result is circulating concentrations of calcitriol that are 1000-fold lower than levels of its precursor (25-hydroxyvitamin D).

PTH is produced by the four parathyroid glands, which are located adjacent to the thyroid gland. Secretion of PTH is responsive to very small changes in serum ionized calcium. A slight fall in ionized serum calcium induces a substantial rise in PTH, whereas even modest hypercalcemia causes profound suppression of PTH secretion. Serum PTH stimulates the renal 1-α hydroxylase enzyme, thus leading to an increase in calcitriol production. Calcitriol stimulates the absorption of both calcium and phosphorus from the proximal small bowel. Chronic elevations in PTH result in increased bone resorption and consequently the release of phosphorus from hydroxyapatite. Despite the actions of PTH on 1-α hydroxylase and bone, the dominant effect of PTH is to lower circulating levels of phosphorus because PTH acutely lowers the renal phosphate threshold. The renal phosphate threshold is the plasma phosphorus concentration above which phosphate begins to appear in the urine. The renal phosphate threshold is the principal determinant of the plasma serum phosphate concentration. PTH acts to reduce the renal phosphate threshold by inhibiting proximal tubular phosphate reabsorption (see later). In regulating phosphate concentrations, PTH acts through the PTHR1 receptor expressed in the proximal renal tubule and in bone. The effect of PTH to lower serum phosphate occurs within minutes of administering the hormone to humans.

Serum phosphate concentrations are also involved in the regulation of calcitropic hormones. Thus, hypophosphatemia or dietary phosphate deprivation profoundly stimulates 1-α hydroxylase (an action independent of PTH) and leads to an increase in serum 1,25(OH)₂D levels that, as noted, stimulates intestinal phosphate absorption. Conversely, elevations in serum phosphate inhibit the activity of the 1-α hydroxylase enzyme. Serum phosphate has also been shown, at least in experimental animals, to stimulate PTH secretion directly, independent of any changes in extracellular ionized calcium concentration.

Research since the mid-1990s has identified PTH-independent circulating factors, called phosphatonins, that also regulate phosphorus metabolism (17). Phosphatonins were originally isolated from individuals with oncogenic osteomalacia, a rare disease in which a mesenchymal tumor secretes a factor that lowers the renal phosphate threshold and results in hypophosphatemia. These factors also suppresses 1-α hydroxylase activity (18). To date, at least four phosphatonins have been identified, including FGF23, secreted frizzled-related protein-4 (sFRP-4), matrix extracellular phosphoglycoprotein (MEPE), and FGF7 (17). Of the phosphatonins identified, FGF23 is currently believed to be the major phosphatonin that contributes to phosphate homeostasis.

FGF23 is produced by osteocytes, specialized bone cells entombed in the mineralized matrix of the skeleton. Investigators have speculated that FGF23 serves to regulate the amount of phosphorus available for mineralization in newly formed bone matrix. Under physiologic conditions, serum phosphorus and $1,25(OH)_2D$ are major regulators of FGF23 production. Hyperphosphatemia, dietary phosphate supplementation, and $1,25(OH)_2D$ all stimulate FGF23 production whereas hypophosphatemia and dietary phosphate deprivation suppress its expression. The major effects of FGF23 are on the proximal renal tubular cell, in which FGF23 reduces the renal phosphate threshold by suppressing proximal renal tubular phosphate reabsorption. FGF23 also suppresses 1-α hydroxylase activity. The actions of FGF23 on renal tubular phosphate reabsorption occur more slowly than do those of PTH. FGF23 levels show no diurnal variation in healthy individuals, and it is currently believed that FGF23 is responsible for more long-term regulation of phosphate homeostasis.

FGF23 appears to act primarily through the FGFR1c receptor. FGF23 requires a transmembrane cofactor, α-Klotho, to activate the FGFR1c receptor. Together, the FGFR1c receptor and Klotho form a receptor complex that, when liganded by FGF23, induces a cell signaling cascade that affects phosphate homeostasis as just described. When Klotho is nonfunctional or genetically absent, FGF23 cannot act, and mice with this genetic lesion have markedly elevated serum phosphorus levels despite high circulating levels of FGF23. Working in concert, PTH, $1,25(OH)_2D$, and FGF23 ensure that serum phosphate concentrations and whole body phosphate stores remain within a normal range.

WHOLE BODY HOMEOSTASIS

Dietary Sources

Phosphorus is widely distributed in the diet and is found in milk, meat, poultry, fish, eggs, milk products, nuts, legumes, and cereal grains. Because of the large variety of foods that contain phosphorus, deficiency of this mineral is relatively uncommon in persons ingesting typical diets, which provide approximately 20 mg/kg/day or approximately 1500 mg of phosphorus daily.

Assessment of dietary phosphorus may be complicated by the fact that many food additives and common food preservatives contain phosphorus. These inorganic phosphorus salts (e.g., sodium phosphate, sodium aluminum phosphate, sodium acid pyrophosphate, monocalcium phosphate, sodium tripolyphosphate) are added during food processing because of their nonnutritive functions such as retention of moisture, smoothness, and binding. These additives may not be factored into the published phosphorus content of the food (19, 20), and the food industry is not required to include these amounts on food labels (21). Investigators have estimated that these additives may increase phosphorus intake by as much as 1000 mg/day in individuals as the relative contribution of processed food to our diets increases (22). More research on the impact of these food additives and preservatives on phosphorus homeostasis is needed because their use has been associated with higher levels of serum PTH concentrations (23).

Intestinal Phosphorus Absorption

Phosphorus reaches the absorptive surfaces of the enterocyte in the form of P_i or organic phosphorus complexes. Within the gut lumen, phosphatases help to digest and hydrolyze the organic forms into P_i. Absorption of phosphorus from the diet is highest in infants and children (in whom it ranges between 65% and 90%). Intestinal phosphorus absorption tends to decrease with aging but remains high and averages approximately 50% to 70% in adults.

Most phosphorus absorption occurs in the small intestine by load-dependent passive absorption. Active carrier-mediated absorption also occurs by a sodium-dependent process that uses the sodium-phosphorus cotransporters NaP_i-2b (NPT2B) and P_iT1. Calcitriol increases the number of NaP_i-2b cotransporters in the intestine and leads to increased efficiency of phosphorus absorption (24). Intestinal absorption can occur in the absence of calcitriol, however, as demonstrated by the relatively small difference in phosphorus absorption observed in patients with renal failure (60%) compared with that observed among healthy controls (80%) (25). In addition, humans with inactivating mutations in NaP_i-2b have normal serum phosphate concentrations, although this may simply be a result of a compensatory change in the renal phosphate threshold. An intriguing and as yet unconfirmed report (26) suggested that the duodenal mucosa secretes a novel hormone that regulates renal tubular phosphate handling. This would make teleologic sense because such a hormone would act to mitigate the hyperphosphatemia that would otherwise occur following a meal rich in phosphate.

Endogenous Phosphorus Secretion

During the process of digestion, approximately 3 mg/kg/day of phosphorus is secreted into the intestine as a component of digestive pancreatic and intestinal enzymes. Unlike endogenous fecal calcium losses, which are only minimally affected across a wide range of dietary calcium intake, endogenous fecal phosphorus excretion is responsive to alterations in dietary phosphorus intake and ranges between 0.9 and 4 mg/kg (0.03 and 1.24 mmol/kg)/day (27, 28).

Renal Phosphorus Excretion

The kidney plays the predominant role in the regulation of systemic phosphorus economy. Approximately 95% of filtered phosphate in the kidney is reabsorbed in the proximal tubule by a hormonally mediated active process. When an individual is in phosphorus equilibrium (i.e., not gaining or losing phosphorus), the amount of phosphorus lost in urine is roughly equal to the amount of phosphorus absorbed from the gastrointestinal tract. When phosphorus status is compromised, renal reclamation of phosphorus increases dramatically to maximize phosphorus retention. For example, within 24 to 48 hours of administering a zero-phosphate diet to humans, urine phosphate declines to undetectable levels.

In the kidney, phosphate enters the apical side of the proximal tubular cells by two renal sodium-phosphate cotransporters: NaP_i-2a (NPT2A) and NaP_i-2c (NPT2C) (7). Activity of these sodium-phosphate cotransporters relies on the inward sodium gradient that is generated and maintained by the sodium-potassium–ATPase pump. NaP_i-2a is electrogenic, importing three sodium atoms for each divalent P_i atom (3 Na ions: 1 phosphate), whereas NaP_i-2c is electroneutral, transporting two sodium atoms with each P_i.

The ability of the kidney to respond and modify phosphorus reabsorption in response to phosphorus status is mediated by PTH, FGF23, and circulating phosphorus concentrations. When serum phosphate concentrations are elevated (or serum ionized calcium levels fall to less than normal ranges), PTH is released from the parathyroid glands. The principal physiologic role of PTH is to respond to hypocalcemia rapidly, which it does in minutes by increasing distal renal tubular calcium absorption and reducing proximal tubular phosphate reabsorption (i.e., lowering the renal phosphate threshold). The molecular mechanism by which this occurs is through a PTH-induced internalization of the proximal renal tubular cell luminal membrane sodium-phosphate cotransporter NaP_i-2a. NaP_i-2c also plays a key role in renal phosphate reabsorption (see later) but does not appear to be as acutely regulated as NaP_i-2a.

The intracellular signaling events that mediate PTH-induced internalization of NaP_i-2a include PTH-induced activation of both protein kinase A and phospholipase C.

NaP_i-2a is stabilized at the brush-border membrane by a scaffolding protein called NHERF1 (sodium/hydrogen exchange regulatory factor 1). PTH treatment is thought to dissociate NaP_i-2a from NHERF1, with the subsequent localization of NaP_i-2a to clatherin-coated pits and then to endosomes. Internalization of the NaP_i-2a cotransporters prevents phosphorus reabsorption and increases urinary phosphorus excretion (29). The resultant fall in serum phosphorus favors a rise in serum calcium. Within hours of an increase in PTH secretion, bone resorption is increased, thus releasing both calcium and phosphorus into the circulation. The extra phosphorus does not cause a rise in plasma phosphate because of the previously noted effect on the renal phosphate threshold.

High serum phosphate concentrations, in large part by stimulating production of FGF23, suppress renal 1-α hydroxylase, which lowers circulating calcitriol levels and reduces intestinal absorption of phosphorus and calcium. Low serum phosphate concentrations have the reverse effect, in this case by lowering FGF23 levels, thereby stimulating 1-α hydroxylase enzyme activity and increasing renal production of $1,25(OH)_2D$ and ultimately intestinal absorption of phosphorus. Dietary phosphate restriction in humans causes levels of calcitriol to increase by 180%, and phosphate supplementation decreases levels by 29% (30).

FGF23 lowers the renal phosphate threshold and increases urinary phosphorus excretion by suppressing transcription of the NaP_i cotransporter genes in the proximal tubule. When the activity of these transporters is reduced, renal phosphate reabsorption is impaired, and more phosphorus is lost in the urine. FGF23 also suppresses 1-α hydroxylase activity in the proximal renal tubular cell by an as yet unknown molecular pathway. It also induces the renal 24-hydroxylase enzyme that is responsible for inactivating $1,25(OH)_2D$. These two actions lead to a fall in serum levels of $1,25(OH)_2D$. In the aggregate, FGF23 increases urine phosphorus excretion and reduces intestinal phosphorus absorption, actions that combine to reduce serum phosphorus concentrations; these effects are largely independent of changes in PTH or serum calcium. As noted, FGF23 signaling requires the transmembrane protein α-Klotho (6). Genetic deletion of Klotho in mice causes hyperphosphatemia, and these animals have a phenotype similar to mice in which FGF23 has been knocked out (31). One of the intriguing and unresolved puzzles regarding the actions of FGF23 on proximal renal tubular cell phosphate reabsorption is that a-Klotho is not expressed by this cell. Klotho is expressed by the distal renal tubular cell. Because Klotho is required for FGF23 to activate the FGFR1c receptor, it is not clear how this is accomplished. Although a soluble form of Klotho exists, it remains controversial and uncertain whether this form can effectively substitute for the transmembrane isoform.

Several human diseases that alter normal phosphorus metabolism are now known to be caused by genetic mutations in the FGF23 gene (detailed later). Of the acquired diseases in which FGF23 is thought to play a pathogenic role, renal disease is the most important. As renal function declines, the ability of the kidney to handle the dietary phosphate load is compromised, and when renal function has declined by 80%, hyperphosphatemia develops unless dietary and or medical interventions are instituted (11). Individuals with chronic kidney failure must restrict their dietary intake of phosphorus to reduce the risk of hyperphosphatemia. Without such preventive measures, the hyperphosphatemia can result in calcification of soft tissues and can lead to hypocalcemia. This condition causes a compensatory rise in PTH that is referred to as secondary hyperparathyroidism.

The rise in serum phosphorus is also accompanied by a rise in serum FGF23 in a futile attempt to correct the hyperphosphatemia. The resulting increase in serum FGF23 suppresses renal $1,25(OH)_2D$ production, thus impairing intestinal calcium absorption and exacerbating the hypocalcemia. The disturbed hormonal and mineral ion milieu seen in advanced renal diseases is thought to be responsible for the skeletal disease and accelerated vascular calcification prevalent in patients with renal failure (32). A summary of whole body phosphorus partitioning is depicted in Figure 8.1.

DIETARY PHOSPHORUS REQUIREMENTS

Traditionally, dietary phosphorus requirements were developed in close concert with dietary calcium requirements. The most recent dietary reference intake (DRI) recommendations, published in 1997, did not use this approach and instead based requirements on the phosphorus intake necessary to maintain serum phosphate

TABLE 8.1	RECOMMENDED PHOSPHORUS INTAKES[a]
LIFE STAGE GROUP	PHOSPHORUS (mg/d)
Infants	
0–6 mo	100*
7–12 mo	275*
Children	
1–3 y	460
4–8 y	500
Males	
9–13 y	**1,250**
14–18 y	**1,250**
19–30 y	**700**
31–50 y	**700**
51–70 y	**700**
>70 y	**700**
Females	
9–13 y	**1,250**
14–18 y	**1,250**
19–30 y	**700**
31–50 y	**700**
51–70 y	**700**
>70 y	**700**
Pregnancy	
14–18 y	**1,250**
19–30 y	**700**
31–50 y	**700**
Lactation	
14–18 y	**1,250**
19–30 y	**700**
31–50 y	**700**

[a]This table presents recommended dietary allowances in bold type and adequate intakes in regular type followed by an asterisk.

Data from Food and Nutrition Board, Institute of Medicine. Dietary Reference Intakes for Calcium, Phosphorus, Magnesium, Vitamin D, and Fluoride. Washington, DC: National Academy Press, 1998, with permission.

concentrations in the lower range of normal using existing serum P_i and balance data. Infant requirements were based on data available from infants fed human milk as the primary fluid milk during the first year of life.

Depending on the strength of the data available for each age group, dietary phosphorus requirements were presented as an adequate intake (AI), estimated average requirement (EAR), or recommended dietary allowance (RDA). A tolerable upper intake level (UL) was also estimated for those 1 year old and older. In infants less than 12 months of age, insufficient data on adverse events associated with phosphorus intake were available, so a UL was not established for this age group. The 1997 guidelines for dietary phosphorus intake are presented in Table 8.1.

ASSESSMENT OF PHOSPHORUS REQUIREMENTS

Dietary Assessment

Intake of phosphorus by the US population has tended to increase over the past several decades. Between 1977 and 1985, the US Department of Agriculture's national surveys suggested a slight increase (~8%) in dietary phosphorus. Food supply and disappearance data suggest an even larger

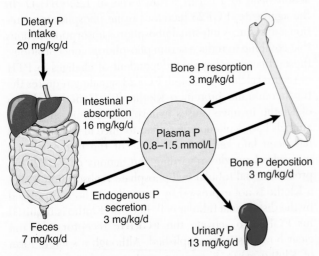

Fig. 8.1. Phosphorus economy in the human body. Overview of phosphorus economy in the human body is depicted for an adult maintaining phosphorus equilibrium. Under these conditions, urinary phosphorus losses are comparable to net phosphorus absorption, and skeletal phosphorus deposition is equal to skeletal phosphorus resorption. *P*, phosporous.

increase of approximately 13% between 1980 and 1994. Despite difficulties in estimating food intake using supply and disappearance data and the limitations of assessing phosphorus-containing food additives (as noted earlier), it appears that over the past several decades, the rise in phosphorus intake is approximately 10% to 15% (11).

A concern has been raised about phosphorus intake from sodas that contain phosphoric acid and the possible impact on bone health. The phosphorus content of soda is relatively low—50 mg/12 oz soda. The same volume of milk would contain approximately seven times the phosphorus content. The more likely culprit in soda has been postulated to be the fixed acid load imposed by the phosphoric acid and the possibility that this is buffered by bone mineral. However, epidemiologic data on this question are mixed, and short-term intervention studies do not suggest that this is likely. Perhaps the most detrimental aspect of soda consumption is the consequent displacement of nutritive-containing beverages from the diet. Phosphorus supplements are not widely used in the United States (11).

In general, foods that are high in protein are also high in phosphorus. With the possible exception of elderly persons, most US residents consume more than adequate protein and concurrently more than adequate phosphorus. Because the chance of phosphorus deficiency is so rare in free-living adults, the assessment of phosphorus status is perhaps less critical than is the assessment of other minerals or nutrients.

Assessment of Phosphorus Status

The indicators and approaches used to assess phosphorus status and to set the AI include serum phosphorus, phosphorus balance, and whole body accretion (in conditions of new tissue growth).

Studies of phosphorus partitioning in the body are limited because phosphorus is monoisotopic, and thus no minor abundance stable isotopes are available to assess in vivo partitioning and metabolism of this mineral. To monitor phosphorus status and requirements, multiple biochemical indicators have been used, including urinary phosphate concentrations, plasma phosphorus concentrations, and the phosphate content of red blood cells, leukocytes, and platelets. Urinary phosphate concentration has been used to assess dietary phosphorus intakes under normal physiologic conditions. The phosphate content of red blood cells, leukocytes, and platelets correlates well with serum phosphorus levels and has been used as an acceptable indicator of phosphorus status. Other approaches for measuring whole body phosphorus content, such as nuclear magnetic resonance and whole body neutron activation analyses, are expensive and have limited applications.

Although serum phosphorus is sometimes used as in index of whole body phosphorus status, it is not a reliable marker. As noted, the serum phosphorus concentration entirely depends on the renal phosphate threshold, which under physiologic conditions is controlled by PTH but

is also influenced by FGF23 and other hormonal factors such as growth hormone and catecholamines. Drugs that bind dietary phosphate can cause hypophosphatemia. Similarly, elevations in serum phosphorus can be a consequence of renal failure and hypoparathyroidism, as well as the ingestion of phosphate-containing laxatives such as Phospho-soda. Despite these limitations, serum phosphorus was used to establish the 1997 EAR for healthy adults. During periods of growth, serum phosphorus is not reliable indicator of phosphorus status, so the factorial approach in infants, children, and adolescents was used to establish requirements (11). Phosphorus balance studies can also be used to assess net retention of this mineral and to determine how this varies across the life cycle.

Bioavailability of Phosphorus

The ability to absorb and use phosphorus is affected by the total amount of phosphorus found in the diet and also by the type (organic versus inorganic), food origin (animal versus plant derived), and ratio of phosphorus to other dietary components. Although most food groups contain phosphorus, not all dietary sources are bioavailable. In particular, phytic acid (the storage form of phosphorus in plants) cannot be digested because humans lack the phytase enzyme. Yeast and bacteria have phytase and may allow for some degradation of phytate in the gut.

Absorption of phosphorus may be also be affected by other minerals, including magnesium, aluminum, and calcium. For example, overuse of antacids that contain aluminum hydroxide can cause phosphorus depletion particularly if the habitual diet is limiting in phosphorus. The same can be said for some calcium salts. Certain synthetic polymers such as sevelamer are used as pharmacologic binders of dietary phosphate. The impact of these compounds on the bioavailability of phosphorus has been used in human situations when reductions in dietary phosphorus absorption are desirable. For example, pharmacologic doses of calcium acetate and sevelamer are used to treat patients with kidney disease, to help prevent hyperphosphatemia.

ACQUIRED DISORDERS OF PHOSPHORUS METABOLISM

Disorders of phosphate metabolism can be characterized as either genetic or acquired. Acquired disorders are those that result from medical complications. The prevalence of acquired disorders is much higher than the prevalence of diseases associated with known genetic mutations in the identified regulators of phosphorus metabolism.

Chronic Kidney Disease

In untreated chronic kidney disease (CKD), as the glomerular filtration rate falls to less than 60 mL/minute, the frequency with which hyperphosphatemia, hypocalcemia, and secondary hyperparathyroidism are observed rises rapidly. Because of the high molecular weight of phosphate anions, they are not efficiently dialyzed. Consequently, patients undergoing hemodialysis retain approximately half of the phosphorus they consume. Because dietary phosphate can no longer be disposed of effectively, hyperphosphatemia develops. The combined effects of PTH and FGF23 may not be able to stimulate renal phosphate excretion to compensate for the falling glomerular filtration rate. Left untreated, chronic stimulation of the parathyroid glands by the combined effects of a high serum phosphorus concentration and a low serum calcium concentration, both from hyperphosphatemia and reduced renal $1,25(OH)_2D$ production, leads to parathyroid gland hyperplasia. Long-standing secondary hyperparathyroidism can eventually lead to such severe parathyroid gland hyperplasia that frank hypercalcemia develops, so-called tertiary hyperparathyroidism. The metabolic bone disease known as renal osteodystrophy is common among patients with advanced renal insufficiency as a consequence of the chronic hyperparathyroidism, vitamin D deficiency, poor calcium absorption, and accumulation of toxic moieties such as advanced glycation end products (AGEs).

In these patients, a high dietary intake of phosphorus exacerbates the hyperparathyroidism and renal osteodystrophy and may promote vascular calcification leading to potential cardiovascular events. To avoid these complications, considerable efforts are made to control the amount of phosphorus ingested and absorbed from the diet in patients with CKD while promoting the intake of calcium-rich foods. In practical terms, this is often difficult to achieve because foods that are high in calcium (e.g., dairy) are also prohibitively high in phosphorus. Similarly, restriction of dietary phosphorus may limit protein-rich foods and exacerbate protein-energy wasting in this group (33). The impracticalities of dietary phosphate restriction have led to the routine use of medications such as phosphorus binders to decrease intestinal phosphorus absorption. As noted earlier, among those agents most commonly used are calcium salts, particularly calcium acetate, and polymers such as sevelamer.

Starvation and Refeeding Syndrome

During periods of starvation, phosphate depletion occurs, yet serum phosphorus levels may remain unchanged as a consequence of increased efflux of phosphorus from muscle cells. After a period of starvation, aggressive nutritional rehabilitation (whether enteral, parenteral, or oral, particularly with carbohydrate) results in a potentially life-threatening refeeding syndrome. Refeeding syndrome was first recognized during World War II when rapid nutritional support was provided to malnourished patients. Hyperglycemia, thiamin deficiency, hypokalemia, and hypomagnesemia were all observed as part of the refeeding syndrome, but the predominant problem observed was hypophosphatemia resulting in fatal cardiac arrest. Once glucose is reintroduced to the previously malnourished patient as the primary source of energy, the rise in glucose metabolism increases the use of intracellular phosphate in the generation of ATP. This mechanism, coupled with the fact that glucose uptake into cells requires phosphate, results in a rapid fall in extracellular phosphate concentrations.

To decrease the risk of this complication, serum phosphorus concentrations (as well as potassium, magnesium, and fluid status) should be carefully monitored, and phosphorus should be supplemented as required. Other factors that may precipitate the refeeding syndrome, such as prolonged vomiting or diarrhea, prolonged fasting in the postoperative patient, cancer, gastrointestinal malabsorption diseases, and alcoholism, are also important to recognize (34).

Metabolic Bone Disease of Prematurity

Mineral deficiencies in preterm infants are common for a multitude of reasons: increased nutritional requirements for growth, delayed or inadequate enteral feedings, parenteral nutrition, unfortified human milk, malabsorption, and medication use (corticosteroids, furosemide, and methylxanthines). Impaired bone mineralization is often a consequence of these deficiencies and in this age group is referred to as the osteopenia of prematurity. This problem is thought to occur in almost one fourth of very-low-birth-weight infants who weigh less than 1500 g, and the incidence doubles for infants weighing less than 1000 g (35). Phosphorus deficiency is one of the primary nutritional causes of osteopenia of prematurity. Human milk contains approximately 150 mg/L of phosphorus. Although this amount is adequate for bone mineralization in term infants, unfortified human milk is inadequate to meet the very high calcium and phosphorus requirements of the preterm infant, particularly those weighing less than 1500 g. To avoid this complication and help meet the high phosphorus and calcium demands of the preterm infant, mineral fortifiers can be added to human milk (36).

Medical Causes of Hypophosphatemia

Many relatively common medical disorders can lead to hypophosphatemia. One such disorder is diabetic ketoacidosis (DKA). Hypophosphatemia is often observed during the treatment of DKA because the administration of insulin drives glucose and phosphate into cells and causes a rapid fall in extracellular plasma phosphate. This decline is generally self-limiting and is not associated with clinical findings, although cautious phosphorus supplementation is sometimes recommended when the serum phosphorus concentration falls to less than 2 mg/dL.

Mild hypophosphatemia can also occur as a common, generally asymptomatic consequence of hyperparathyroidism. The hypophosphatemia results from elevated circulating levels of PTH that lower the renal phosphate threshold, as discussed earlier. Fanconi syndrome can also cause hypophosphatemia. This disease can be acquired or

Cellular Homeostasis

Mg is compartmentalized within the cell, and most of it is bound to proteins and negatively charged molecules. Significant amounts of Mg are found in the nucleus, mitochondria, the endoplasmic and sarcoplasmic reticulum, and the cytoplasm (5, 6, 20). Total cell Mg concentration has been reported to range between 5 and 20 mM (15). From 90% to 95% of cytosolic Mg is bound to ligands such as ATP, adenosine diphosphate (ADP), citrate, proteins, and nucleic acids. The remainder is free Mg^{2+}, constituting 1% to 5% of the total cellular Mg (15, 21).

The concentration of free ionized Mg^{2+} in the cytoplasm of mammalian cells has ranged from 0.5 to 1.0 mM, similar to circulating ionized Mg^{2+} (6, 15). The Mg^{2+} concentration in the cell cytoplasm is maintained relatively constant even when the Mg^{2+} concentration in the extracellular fluid is experimentally varied to either high or low nonphysiologic concentrations (22). The relative constancy of the Mg^{2+} in the intracellular milieu is attributed to the limited permeability of the plasma membrane to Mg and to the operation of specific Mg transport proteins, which regulate the rates at which Mg is taken up or extruded from cells (5, 6, 15). Maintenance of a normal intracellular concentration of Mg^{2+} requires that Mg be actively transported out of the cell (15). Mg transport into or out of cells appears to require the presence of carrier-mediated transport systems. The efflux of Mg from the cell appears to be coupled to Na transport and requires extrusion of Na by Na^+/K^+-ATPase (15). Evidence also indicates a Na-independent efflux of Mg (7, 15). Mg influx appears to be linked to Na transport, but by a different mechanism than efflux (15, 23). At least seven transmembrane Mg^{2+} channels have been cloned (24). These include NIPA2 (25) and MagT1 and TUSC3 (26). Studies of human hereditary diseases (see later) have identified paracellin-1 (claudin 16), claudin 19, and two transient receptor potential channel family members, TRPM6 and TRPM7 (27–29). TRPM6 is expressed in the kidney, and TRPM7 is constitutively expressed (28). Tissues vary with respect to the rates at which Mg exchange occurs and the percentage of total Mg, which is readily exchangeable (7). The rate of Mg exchange in heart, liver, and kidney exceeds that in skeletal muscle, lymphocytes, red blood cells, brain, and testis.

The processes that maintain or modify the relationships between total and ionized internal and external Mg are incompletely understood. Changes in cytosolic Mg^{2+} regulate some channels (TRPM6 and TRPM7) (24). Mg transport in mammalian cells may be influenced by hormonal and pharmacologic factors (15). Mg^{2+} efflux was stimulated after short-term exposure of isolated perfused rat heart and liver or thymocytes to α- and β-agonists and permeant cAMP (30, 31). Activation of protein kinase C by diacylglycerol or by phorbol esters stimulates Mg^{2+} influx and does not alter efflux (32). Epidermal growth factor (EGF) has been shown to increase Mg^{2+} transport into a vascular smooth muscle cell line (33). Insulin and dextrose were found to increase ^{28}Mg uptake by several tissues, including skeletal and cardiac muscle (5, 6). The mechanism of insulin-induced Mg transport is likely the result of an effect on protein kinase C (5, 6). An insulin-induced transport of Mg into cells could be one factor responsible for the fall in the serum Mg concentration observed during insulin therapy of diabetic ketoacidosis (34). Investigators have hypothesized that this hormonally regulated Mg uptake system controls intracellular Mg^{2+} concentration in cellular subcytoplasmic compartments. The Mg^{2+} concentration in these compartments would then serve to regulate the activity of Mg-sensitive enzymes. An overall schema of cellular Mg homeostasis is shown in Figure 9.1.

Body Homeostasis

Mineral homeostasis of the individual depends on the amounts ingested, the efficiency of intestinal and renal absorption and excretion, and all other factors affecting them. A schema for human Mg balance is given in Figure 9.2.

Dietary Intake

Mg is widely distributed in plant and animal food sources, but in differing concentrations. Vegetables, fruits, grains, and animal products account for approximately 16% each; dairy products contribute 20% in adolescents and 10% beyond the third decade (35). The 1994 US Department of Agriculture Continuing Survey of Food Intakes by Individuals (CSFII) indicated that the mean daily Mg intake was 323 mg in boys and men and 228 mg in girls and women, findings similar to those of the third National Health and Nutrition Examination Survey (NHANES III). These values fall to less than the current RDA recommendation of approximately 420 mg for boys and men and 320 mg for girls and women (4). Indeed, investigators have suggested that 75% of U.S. residents have a dietary Mg intake lower than the RDA (see the later discussion of Mg requirements and http://ods.od.nih.gov/factsheets/magnesium.asp).

Intestinal Absorption

Molecular mechanisms for Mg homeostasis have been reviewed (36). In humans, the primary sites of intestinal Mg absorption are the jejunum and ileum, although absorption can occur at other sites, including the colon (37). Under normal dietary Mg intake, 30% to 40% is absorbed. Following oral ingestion, ^{28}Mg appears in the blood within 1 hour, stabilizes at the rate of 4% to 6%/hour from the second hour to the eighth hour, then decreases rapidly, and ceases at the tenth hour (38). Mg absorption has both a passive paracellular mechanism and an active transport process (Fig. 9.3). The paracellular mechanism depends on a transcellular potential difference generated by Na transport and accounts for approximately 90% of intestinal Mg absorption (37). A Mg-specific transport protein channel, TRPM6 (28), accounts for the remainder

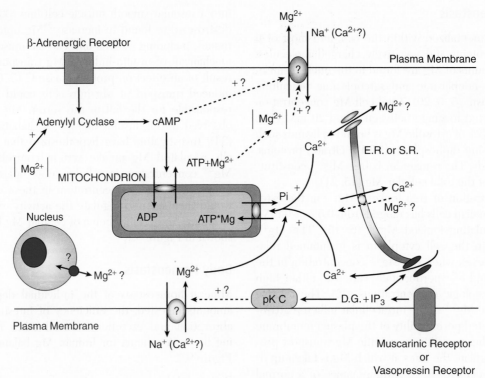

Fig. 9.1. Schema of regulation of cellular magnesium (Mg^{2+}) homeostasis in the mammalian cell. The pathways are indicated for cellular Mg^{2+} release (**upper section**) and for its uptake (**lower section**). Stimulated by β-adrenergic agonists, cyclic adenosine monophosphate (cAMP) is increased in the cytosol, which modulates mitochondrial adenine nucleotide translocase and increases the efflux of Mg^{2+} from the mitochondrion by means of an exchange of one Mg adenosine triphosphate (MgATP) for adenosine diphosphate (ADP). Activation of muscarinic receptors (in cardiac cells) or vasopressin receptors (in the liver) may stimulate an Mg^{2+} influx mechanism either by decreasing cAMP or by enhancing protein kinase C (pK C) activity by diacylglycerol (D.G.). Vasopressin receptor activation is coupled with production of inositol triphosphate (IP$_3$) from phosphatidylinositol bisphosphate, which induces release of calcium (Ca^{2+}) from the endoplasmic reticulum (E.R.) or the sarcoplasmic reticulum (S.R.). Ca^{2+} release may be associated with either Mg^{2+} influx or Mg redistribution in the nucleus or endoplasmic reticulum. *Na$^+$*, sodium. (Adapted with permission from Romani A, Marfella C, Scarpa A. Cell magnesium transport and homeostasis: role of intracellular compartments. Miner Electrolyte Metab 1993;19:282–9.)

of Mg absorption and may be influenced by certain hormones (39). Absorption of Mg as a function of intake is curvilinear (Fig. 9.3), and this pattern reflects this active saturable process and passive diffusion. Net Mg absorption increases with increasing Mg intake; however, fractional Mg absorption falls. When small amounts of Mg were fed in the form of a standard meal supplemented by varying amounts of Mg (40), fractional absorption fell progressively from approximately 65% to 70% with intake of 7 to 36 mg (0.3 to 1.5 mmol) down to 11% to 14% with intake of 960 to 1000 mg (40 mmol).

Data on absorption fractions from balance studies using differing diets have been quite variable, ranging from 35% to 70% (41). When free-living adults eating self-selected diets were evaluated periodically over the course of a year, the mean absorptive fraction averaged 21% with an average intake of 323 mg (13.4 mmol) by men and 27% with an average intake of 234 mg (9.75 mmol) by women (42).

Bioavailability

The fractional absorption of ingested Mg by healthy persons is influenced not only by its dietary concentration, but also the presence of dietary components inhibiting or promoting absorption. Long-term balance studies in healthy individuals generally indicate that increasing oral Ca intake does not significantly affect Mg absorption or retention (43). Increased amounts of Mg in the diet have been associated with either decreased Ca absorption (44) or no effect (45). Although a higher Mg intake may not affect intestinal Ca absorption, renal tubular mechanisms may increase Ca excretion (40).

Some reports showed decreased Mg absorption at high intakes of dietary phosphate, whereas others found no consistent effect (46). Increased amounts of absorbable oral Mg have been noted to decrease phosphate absorption, perhaps secondary to formation of insoluble Mg phosphate (40). Reduced absorption of Mg associated with high phosphate intake did not change Mg balance, however, because of associated decreased urinary excretion of Mg (40).

A major increase in zinc intake (from 12 to 142 mg/day) lowered Mg absorption and balance significantly (47). Vitamin B$_6$ depletion induced in young women was associated with a negative Mg balance because of increased urinary excretion (48). The presence of excessive amounts of free fatty acids and oxalate may also impair Mg absorption (49).

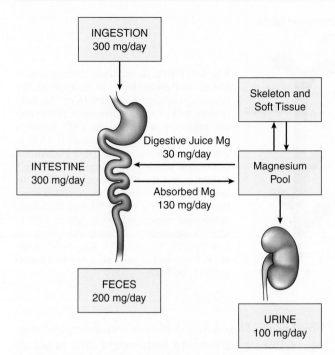

Fig. 9.2. Magnesium (Mg) homeostasis in humans. A schematic representation of its metabolic economy indicating (a) its absorption from the alimentary tract, (b) its distribution into bone, and (c) its dependence on the kidney for excretion. Homeostasis depends on the integrity of intestinal and renal absorptive processes. (Adapted with permission from Rude RK. Magnesium homeostasis. In: Bilezikian JB, Raisz L, Rodan G, eds. Principles of Bone Biology. 3rd ed. San Diego: Academic Press, 2008:487–513.)

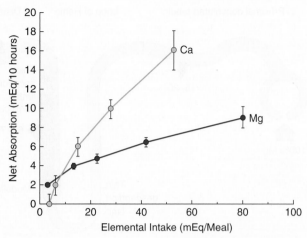

Fig. 9.3. Net magnesium (Mg) and calcium (Ca) absorption in healthy humans. The data were obtained under conditions described in reference 39 and in the text. Mean values S.E. are indicated by *vertical bars.* The absorption data for Mg represent a curved function compatible with a saturable process (at ~10 mEq/meal in this study) and a linear function reflecting passive diffusion at higher intakes. (Adapted with permission from Fine KD, Santa Ana CA, Porter JL et al. Intestinal absorption of magnesium from foods and supplements. J Clin Invest 1991;88:396–402.)

Increased intakes of dietary fiber have been reported to decrease Mg utilization in humans, presumably by reducing absorption. The introduction of uncontrolled variables, including multiple differences among dietary components in addition to fiber contents, complicates interpretation of the data, however (46). When isolated fiber was added to a basal diet, the effects of fiber itself were negative for dephytinized barley fiber (50) and positive for cellulose (51).

Absorbability of Magnesium Salts
Multiple salts of Mg are available as dietary supplements including oxide, hydroxide, citrate, chloride, gluconate, lactate, and aspartate. The fractional absorption of a salt depends on its solubility in intestinal fluids and the amounts ingested; an amount of 5 mmol (120 mg) of the acetate in gelatin capsules has been found to be an optimal dose in terms of net absorption (40). Absorption of enteric-coated Mg chloride is 67% less than that of the acetate in gelatin capsules (41). In one study, Mg citrate was found to have high solubility, even in water, whereas Mg oxide was poorly soluble, even in acid solution; better absorption of the citrate salt was demonstrated in humans (52). Little difference in absorption has been demonstrated among other salts, however (53). Mg oxide and various salts in large doses act as an osmotic laxative, with resultant diarrhea; the physician faced with a patient who

has diarrhea of uncertain origin should consider measuring fecal Mg (45).

Regulation of Intestinal Magnesium Absorption
No hormone or factor has been described that regulates intestinal Mg absorption, although several hormones may influence the TRPM6 channel, as discussed earlier. Vitamin D and its active metabolites were shown to increase intestinal Mg absorption in several studies (37). $1,25(OH)_2$-Vitamin D increases intestinal absorption in normal human subjects and in patients with chronic renal failure (54). In balance studies, vitamin D increased intestinal Mg absorption, but much less than Ca, and mean Mg balance was not affected (54). In patients with impaired Ca absorption resulting from intestinal disease who were given vitamin D, only small increases in Mg absorption were observed compared with Ca (54). Mg was absorbed by individuals with no detectable plasma $1,25(OH)_2$-vitamin D, and, in contrast to Ca absorption, no significant correlation existed between plasma $1,25(OH)_2$-vitamin D and Mg absorption (54).

Renal Regulation
Renal Filtration and Tubular Absorption. The kidney is the critical organ regulating Mg homeostasis. Mg handling is a process of filtration and reabsorption. The kidney plays a critical role in excreting the Mg that is not retained for tissue growth or turnover replacement (55). Approximately 10% (roughly 100 mmol or 2400 mg) of total body Mg is normally filtered daily through the glomeruli in the healthy adult; of this, only approximately 5% is excreted in the urine. Approximately 75% of the serum Mg is ultrafiltrable at the glomeruli. The fractional absorption of the filtered load in the various segments of

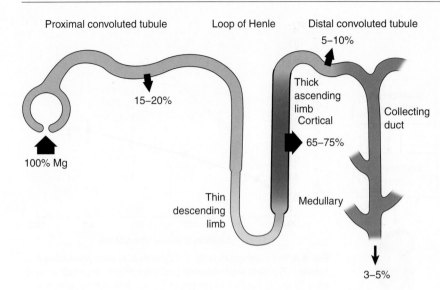

Fig. 9.4. Fractional segmental reabsorption of filtered magnesium (Mg^{2+}) in the nephron. The percentage absorption of filtered Mg^{2+} has been determined by micropuncture techniques in various laboratory animals as the Mg^{2+} proceeds through the nephron. Approximately 15% to 20% of the Mg^{2+} is reabsorbed in the proximal convoluted tubule. The major site for Mg^{2+} reabsorption is the thick ascending limb of the loop of Henle, primarily in its cortical portion. Here, 65% to 75% of Mg^{2+} leaves the lumen. In the distal convoluted tubule, 5% to 10% of Mg^{2+} is reabsorbed. (Adapted with permission from Cole DE, Quamme GA. Inherited disorders of renal magnesium handling. J Am Soc Nephrol 2000;11:1937–47).

the nephron is summarized in Figure 9.4. Paracellin-1 (claudin-16) and claudin-19 appear to mediate this transport (27, 28). The distal convoluted tubule reabsorbs 5% to 10% of filtered Mg via an active transcellular pathway. Several proteins may be involved, including the sodium chloride cotransporter (28). TRPM6 is also expressed in the distal tubule. Mutations of TRPM6 result in lower intestinal Mg absorption and renal Mg wasting (27–29).

Hormonal and Other Regulator Influences on Absorption. Experimental studies in rodents show that arginine vasopressin, glucagon, calcitonin, parathyroid hormone (PTH), and (to a lesser degree) an adrenergic agonist and insulin, when added individually to the bath of mouse segments of the cortical thick ascending limb of the loop of Henle or the distal convoluted tubule, significantly increase Mg absorption (55, 56). The physiologic significance of these observations, however, is unclear. Proof that Mg balance is normally regulated hormonally would require that certain changes in serum Mg concentration liberate one or more of these hormones into the blood and act on the tubule (56).

Although the regulatory mechanisms are unclear, certain conditions affect absorption, principally in the ascending thick limb. Inhibition occurs with hypermagnesemia and hypercalcemia (55). This is thought to occur because these cations bind to a Ca-sensitive receptor on the basolateral aspect of tubular cells; this process decreases transepithelial voltage and thereby reduces paracellular absorption of both Mg and Ca. Lowered Mg intake in experimental animals and humans rapidly decreases Mg excretion, even before serum and plasma Mg concentrations fall to less than the normal range, a finding suggesting an adaption of the kidney to Mg insufficiency (55).

Tissue Sources

Extracellular and intracellular Mg, and that in bone, fall during Mg depletion. Bone may serve as an important reservoir for Mg. Human iliac crest changes indicate a broad range of loss during depletion, with a weighted average of 18% or 1.2 mmol/kg body weight (57). In young, Mg-deficient rats and mice, the major body loss is from bone (~30% of that in bone) with much less from muscle; however, age and duration of study affect the amounts lost (58). During starvation, in a human obesity study associated with acidosis, significant amounts of Mg were lost from lean body mass and bone (59). In an experimental human study lasting approximately 3 weeks and with resulting asymptomatic hypomagnesemia, the investigators noted no significant decrease in muscle Mg; presumably, bone and other soft tissues were the sources of loss (60).

Sweat Losses

The amount of Mg lost in sweat is very small in comparison with loss of other cations. For example, in a 10-km run in 40.5 minutes with an average body weight (fluid) loss of 1.45 kg, the actual ion losses per kilogram of weight loss were as follows: Na, 800 mg; K, 200 mg; Ca, 20 mg; and Mg, 5 mg (61).

ASSESSING MAGNESIUM REQUIREMENTS

Assessment of Magnesium Intake

Table 9.2 compares the 1989 RDAs with the 1997 dietary reference intakes (DRIs) by age and gender. The DRIs are uniformly higher for children 4 years or more and for adults. Because excessive Mg intake from nonfood sources causes adverse effects, the DRI (4) established tolerable upper intake levels (UL) for such sources. The UL of supplemental Mg for adolescents and adults is 350 mg (14.6 mmol)/day. This is based on the lowest observed adverse (diarrhea) effect level (LOAEL) of 360 mg (15 mmol)/day.

According to the DRIs (Table S-3 in reference 4), infant levels are based on estimates of adequate human intake, whereas most other ages are based on balance

TABLE 9.2 COMPARISON OF 1989 AND 1997 RECOMMENDATIONS FOR DAILY INTAKES (IN MILLIGRAMS) OF MAGNESIUM

	1989[a]			1997[b]			
AGE (y)	MALE	FEMALE	AGE (y)	MALE	FEMALE		
0–0.5	40	40	0–0.5	30[c]	30[c]	AI	
0.5–1.0	60	60	0.5–1.0	74[d]	75[d]	AI	
1–3	80	80	1–3	80	80		
4–6	120	120	4–8	130	130		
7–10	170	170	9–13	240	240		
11–14	270	280	14–18	410	360		
15–18	400	300	19–30	400	310		
19–24	350	280	31–50	420	320		
25–50	350	280	51–0	420	320		
51+	350	280	>70	420	320		
Pregnant		320	≤18		400		
			19–30		350		
			31–50		360		
Lactating							
First 6 mo			≤18		400		
Second 6 mo			19–30		350		
			31–50		320		

AI, adequate intake.

[a]Food and Nutrition Board, National Research Council. Recommended Dietary Allowances. 10th ed. Washington, DC: National Academy Press, 1989.
[b]Food and Nutrition Board, Institute of Medicine. Dietary Reference Intakes for Calcium, Phosphorus, Magnesium, Vitamin D, and Fluoride. Washington, DC: National Academy Press, 1997.
[c]Intake from human milk by healthy breast-fed infants.
[d]Human milk plus solid food.

studies. The difficulties in performing balance studies with specific reference for achieving zero balance and the uncertainties presented by variability in subject energy expenditure and body build were discussed previously (62). The 1989 and 1997 US and Canadian RDAs are presented, for comparison, in Table 9.2.

Assessment of Dietary Magnesium Intake

Estimates of Mg intakes in the NHANES III (1988 to 1991) indicated that children 2 to 11 years old had median intakes much higher than their RDAs. Children aged 1 to 5 years in the lower 5th percentile took in approximately 90% of the RDA, which includes a safety factor (63). Conversely, male and female subjects from 12 to more than 60 years of age, grouped by race and ethnicity, with the exception of non-Hispanic white boys and men, had low median intakes relative to the RDAs (63).

The basis for the claims that many adolescents and adults in the United States are at risk of Mg depletion rests on the accuracy of two indices: the dietary intake data summarized in NHANES and the RDA. If either or both of these are seriously inaccurate, the extent of potential depletion will be either higher or lower. The *Third Report on Nutrition Monitoring in the United States* (1995) analyzed intake in relation to the RDA for age and gender and concluded that Mg presents a potential public health issue requiring further study (63). One reason given was that the median intakes of Mg from food were lower than the RDAs in various population groups. Assessment of Mg status at various dietary Mg intakes has not been performed. It is therefore impossible to estimate what level of intake would place one at risk for a problem associated with Mg deficiency. Serum Mg was determined by atomic absorption spectrophotometry (AAS) in 15,820 individuals in the NHANES I (1971 to 1974); 95% of adults aged 18 to 74 years had serum concentrations in the range of 0.75 to 0.96 mmol/L (1.50 to 1.92 mEq/L), with a mean of 0.85 mmol/L. Adults in the 5th percentile were at or higher than the lower limits of normal (i.e., 0.70 to 0.73 mmol/L). Although serum Mg concentration correlated with blood pressure, this parameter may not reflect true body Mg status.

ASSESSING MAGNESIUM STATUS

Analytic Procedures

Various methods have been developed to measure Mg in foods, excreta, blood, cells, and cell compartments. Because Mg is mostly within cells or in bone, assessment of Mg status is most difficult. Several laboratory techniques are used in clinical and research investigations (14). AAS has been widely used to determine total Mg in many sources and remains the reference method because it provides the greatest accuracy and precision (64), although some metallochromic indicators and dyes are commonly used in automated methods (19). Ion-selective electrodes (ISEs) can measure ionized Mg (70% of total Mg) in serum, plasma, and whole blood (22, 65). However, Ca^{2+} and lipophilic cations interfere with determination of ionized Mg. The literature indicates that ISEs from various manufacturers differ in accuracy, and from AAS, and may give misleading results in sera with low Mg concentrations (66). Moreover, in critically ill patients, the correlation between total and ionized serum Mg concentrations is poor (67).

Other techniques have been developed to assess intracellular Mg concentration, including nuclear magnetic resonance spectroscopy and fluorescent indicators (19, 21). Mg isotopes have been used as biologic tracers to follow the absorption, distribution, and excretion of the Mg ion. The radioisotope ^{28}Mg has been used in human studies (5, 68). Its value is limited by its radioactivity, its short half-life, of 21.3 hours, and its short supply.

Clinical Assessment

Total serum Mg is the only test available to clinicians for assessing Mg status (19, 69). Some reports have noted normal serum and plasma concentrations associated with a variety of illnesses but, with low values in various blood cells and other organs. Consequently, total serum and plasma Mg values in such situations may be considered unreliable indicators of depletion. The level of ionized Mg may be more relevant than that of total Mg. As discussed earlier, intermethod differences exist for ionized Mg. Therefore, reference ranges must exist for each analyzer, and they may not be comparable among different manufacturers (70).

Erythrocyte and blood mononuclear cell Mg content have been measured in experimental human Mg deficiency and in patient populations, and these measurements may be more accurate than serum Mg in assessing Mg status (19, 71, 72). These tests are not commercially available, however, and technical issues appear to limit their use in assessing Mg status in any given individual.

Assessing urinary Mg excretion may be of use. When the amount of Mg ingested is reduced, urinary Mg excretion falls fairly rapidly. Serum Mg may still be within normal limits when urine concentrations are low (73). This finding would not indicate whether the Mg deficits were acute or chronic, however. In situations in which renal Mg wasting occurs, the resulting hypomagnesemia is associated with excessive urinary Mg excretion (>1 mmol/day) (74). Such a relationship suggests renal tubular dysfunction as the cause of the hypomagnesemia.

The intravenous Mg retention test provides an estimate of the proportion of infused Mg that is retained over a given period. Persons retaining more than the percentage retained by Mg-replete individuals (e.g., 20% to 25%) are considered to have some body depletion. A suggested clinical protocol that has been tested in a relatively large number of hypomagnesemic patients, patients with chronic alcoholism, and animal controls has been published (75). This test is invasive, time consuming, nonstandardized, and expensive; and it requires hospitalization or other close supervision for the partial or full 24 hours after infusion, with careful urine collection for laboratory analysis.

RISK FACTORS AND CAUSES OF MAGNESIUM DEFICIENCY

Prevalence

The many risk factors for Mg depletion (Table 9.3) suggest that this condition is not rare in acutely or chronically ill patients. Of 2300 patients surveyed in a Veterans Administration hospital, 6.9% were hypomagnesemic; 11% of patients who had routine Mg determinations were hypomagnesemic (76). When patients were hypokalemic, hypomagnesemia occurred in 42%; 29% of those with hypophosphatemia were hypomagnesemic, 27% of those had hyponatremia, and 22% of those had hypocalcemia (76). The true prevalence of Mg depletion is unknown because this ion is not included in routine electrolyte testing in many clinics or hospitals (77). Similar high rates of depletion have been reported in studies of patients in intensive care units (78).

TABLE 9.3   CAUSES OF MAGNESIUM DEFICIENCY

Gastrointestinal disorders
  Nutritional deficiency
  Prolonged nasogastric suction/vomiting
  Acute and chronic diarrhea
  Intestinal and biliary fistulas
  Malabsorption syndromes
  Extensive bowel resection or bypass
  Acute hemorrhagic pancreatitis
  Primary intestinal hypomagnesemia (mutation of TRPM6 channel)
  Proton pump inhibitors
Renal loss
  Long-term parenteral fluid therapy
  Osmotic diuresis (glucose, urea, mannitol)
  Hypercalcemia
  Polyuric phase of acute renal failure, renal transplant, history of renal obstruction
  Non–drug-associated tubulointerstitial nephropathy
  Alcohol
  Diuretics (furosemide, hydrochlorothiazide)
  Epidermal growth factor blockers (cetuximab, panitumumab)
  Renal tubular nephrotoxins (aminoglycosides, cisplatin, amphotericin B, pentamidine)
  Calcineurin inhibitors (cyclosporin, tacrolimus)
  Genetic mutations of magnesium transport channels
  Activating mutation of the calcium-sensing receptor
Endocrine and metabolic disorders
  Diabetes mellitus (glycosuria, osmotic diuresis)
  Phosphate depletion
  Primary hyperparathyroidism
  Hypoparathyroidism
  Primary aldosteronism
  Excessive lactation
Cutaneous loss
  Sweat (athletics)
  Burns
Redistribution of magnesium to bone and soft tissues
  Hungry bone syndrome
  Parenteral nutrition/refeeding syndrome

Gastrointestinal Disorders

As discussed earlier, dietary Mg intake falls to less than the recommended intake in a large proportion of the population (4). Therefore, nutritional Mg deficiency may be observed in the presence of other conditions that impair Mg balance. Gastrointestinal disorders (Table 9.3) may lead to Mg depletion in various ways (79). The Mg content of upper intestinal tract fluids is approximately 1 mEq/L. Vomiting and nasogastric suction may therefore contribute to Mg depletion. The Mg content of diarrheal fluids and fistulous drainage is much higher (≤15 mEq/L) and, consequently, Mg depletion is common in acute and chronic diarrhea, regional enteritis, ulcerative colitis, and intestinal and biliary fistulas. Malabsorption syndromes may also result in Mg deficiency. Steatorrhea and resection or bypass of the small bowel, particularly the ileum, often results in intestinal Mg loss or malabsorption. Acute severe pancreatitis is associated with hypomagnesemia, which may result from the clinical problem causing the pancreatitis, such as alcoholism, or from saponification of Mg in necrotic parapancreatic fat (80).

Proton pump inhibitors have been reported to cause hypomagnesemia in some patients (81). The evidence implicates intestinal Mg malabsorption. A primary defect in intestinal Mg absorption, which manifests early in life with hypomagnesemia, hypocalcemia, and seizures, has been described as an autosomal recessive disorder linked to chromosome 9q22. This disorder appears to be caused by mutations in TRPM6, which expresses a protein involved with active intestinal Mg transport (38).

Renal Disorders

Excessive excretion of Mg into the urine may be the basis of Mg depletion (Table 9.3) (79, 82). Renal Mg reabsorption is proportional to tubular fluid flow, as well as to Na and Ca excretion. Therefore, long-term parenteral fluid therapy, particularly with saline solution, and volume expansion states such as primary aldosteronism and hypercalciuria, may result in Mg depletion. Hypercalcemia has been shown to decrease renal Mg reabsorption, probably mediated by Ca binding to the Ca-sensing receptor in the thick ascending limb of the loop of Henle and decreasing transepithelial voltage (83). Osmotic diuresis caused by glucosuria results in urinary Mg wasting (79).

Hypermagnesuria also occurs during the polyuric phase of recovery from acute renal failure in a native kidney, during recovery from ischemic injury in a transplanted kidney, and in postobstructive diuresis. In such cases, it is likely that residual tubule reabsorptive defects persisting from the primary renal injury play as important a role as polyuria itself in inducing renal Mg wasting (74). Renal Mg wasting has occasionally been reported in patients with acute or chronic tubulointerstitial nephritis not caused by nephrotoxic drugs, such as chronic pyelonephritis and acute renal allograft rejection (74). Alcohol ingestion may also cause renal Mg wasting and is one cause of the high prevalence of Mg deficiency in patients with chronic alcoholism (84).

Many pharmaceutical drugs may cause renal Mg wasting and Mg depletion, including diuretics such as furosemide (85), and EGF receptor blockers cetuximab and panitumumab (86)—monoclonal blocking antibodies of the EGF receptor that are used in the treatment of metastatic colorectal cancer. Renal tubular nephrotoxins (aminoglycosides, amphotericin B, cisplatin, and pentamidine) have been shown to cause renal lesions that result in hypermagnesuria and hypomagnesemia (74, 87–89). Similarly, calcineurin inhibitors (cyclosporine and tacrolimus) have been reported to result in renal Mg wasting in patients after organ transplantation that is caused by downregulation of the distal tubule Mg channel, TRPM6 (90)

Several renal Mg wasting disorders have been described that may be genetic or sporadic (91). One such disorder, which is autosomal recessive, results from mutations in the paracellin-1 gene on chromosome 3 (claudin 16). This disorder is characterized by low serum Mg, hypercalciuria, and nephrocalcinosis. Another autosomal dominant form of isolated renal Mg wasting and hypomagnesemia has been linked to chromosome 11q23 and identified as a mutation on the Na^+/K^+-ATPase γ-subunit of gene FXYD2. A mutation of the Mg channel, TRPM6, may also result in Mg wasting. Gitelman syndrome (familial hypokalemia-hypomagnesemia syndrome) is an autosomal recessive disorder caused by a genetic defect of the thiazide-sensitive Na chloride cotransporter gene on chromosome 16. Other undefined genetic defects also exist (91).

Diabetes Mellitus

Diabetes mellitus is the most common disorder associated with Mg deficiency (92). Investigators generally believe that the mechanism for Mg depletion in diabetes is renal Mg wasting secondary to osmotic diuresis generated by hyperglycosuria. Dietary Mg intake falls to less than the RDA in most patients; therefore, nutritional deprivation may also be a factor. Mg deficiency has been reported to result in impaired insulin secretion as well as in insulin resistance (93, 94), which may contribute to hypertension (95, 96). The mechanism is unclear, but it may result from abnormal glucose metabolism, given that Mg is a cofactor in several enzymes in this cycle. In addition, Mg depletion may decrease tyrosine kinase activity at the insulin receptor, and Mg may influence insulin secretion by the β cell. Mg therapy has been shown to improve diabetes control. Two studies reported that the incidence of type 2 diabetes was significantly greater in people with lower Mg intake (93, 94). Genetic variants of TRPM6 and TRPM7 have been reported to increase the risk of type 2 diabetes in women with intakes of less than 250 mg/day (97). Mg status should therefore be assessed in patients with diabetes mellitus because a vicious cycle may occur: diabetes may lead to Mg loss, and the subsequent Mg deficiency may result in impaired insulin secretion and action, with worsening diabetes control.

Other Disorders

Hypomagnesemia may accompany several other disorders (79). Phosphate depletion has been shown experimentally to result in urinary Mg wasting and hypomagnesemia. Hypomagnesemia may also accompany the "hungry bone" syndrome, a phase of rapid bone mineral accretion in subjects with hyperparathyroidism or hyperthyroidism following surgical treatment, as well as mineral accretion into soft tissue during the refeeding syndrome (98, 99). Mg loss may occur from the skin in sweat and in patients with burn injury (100, 101).

CLINICAL PRESENTATION OF MAGNESIUM DEFICIENCY

Because Mg plays an essential role in a wide range of fundamental biologic reactions, it is not surprising that Mg deficiency may lead to serious clinical symptoms. Early studies were performed in animals. Nutrient requirements of laboratory animals have been established (102).

Human subjects have been studied in the course of Mg deficiency induced by diets low in this element (79, 103), and these observations, along with those in persons who have Mg deficiency secondary to other causes, have identified the manifestations of this deficit. Symptoms and signs of deficiency are given in Table 9.4, and an algorithm of a diagnostic approach to suspected Mg deficiency is shown in Figure 9.5. Mg deficiency occurs in numerous predisposing and complicating disease states. The clinical presentation of Mg deficiency in disease states may coexist with or be masked by the signs and symptoms of the primary disorder.

Moderate-to-Severe Magnesium Deficiency

When Mg deficiency is recognized in the clinical setting, it is usually moderate to severe. Biochemical, neuromuscular, and cardiac complications are the most prevalent findings in the Mg-deficient patient.

Hypocalcemia

Ca is the major regulator of PTH secretion. Mg, however, modulates PTH secretion via the Ca^{2+}-sensing receptor in a manner similar to that of Ca (104). Although acute changes in the extracellular Mg concentrations influence PTH secretion in a manner qualitatively similar to that of Ca, Mg deficiency perturbs mineral homeostasis (104, 105). Hypocalcemia is a prominent manifestation of moderate to severe Mg deficiency. In this case, Mg therapy alone restores serum Ca concentrations to normal, whereas Ca or vitamin D therapy does not correct the hypocalcemia. One major cause for the hypocalcemia is impaired parathyroid gland function. Most patients with hypocalcemia resulting from Mg deficiency have low

TABLE 9.4	MANIFESTATIONS OF MAGNESIUM DEPLETION

Bone and mineral metabolism
  Hypocalcemia
    Impaired PTH secretion
    Renal and skeletal resistance to PTH
    Impaired formation and resistance to 1,25(OH)₂-vitamin D
  Osteoporosis
Neuromuscular manifestations
  Positive Chvostek and Trousseau sign
  Spontaneous carpo-pedal spasm
  Seizures
  Vertigo, ataxia, nystagmus, athetoid and choreiform movements
  Muscular weakness, tremor, fasciculation, and wasting
  Psychiatric: depression, psychosis
Potassium homeostasis
  Hypokalemia
    Renal potassium wasting
    Decreased intracellular potassium
Cardiovascular manifestations
  Cardiac arrhythmia
    Electrocardiographic: prolonged PR and QT intervals, U waves
    Atrial tachycardia, premature contractions, and fibrillation
    Junctional arrhythmias
    Ventricular premature contractions, tachycardia, fibrillation
    Sensitivity to digitalis intoxication
    Torsades de pointes
  Myocardial ischemia/infarction (putative)
  Hypertension
  Atherosclerotic vascular disease (putative)
Other manifestations
  Migraine
  Asthma
  Colon cancer

PTH, parathyroid hormone.

or inappropriately normal (for the prevailing serum Ca concentration) serum PTH concentrations. The administration of Mg results in an immediate rise in serum PTH. The presence of normal or even elevated serum concentrations of PTH in the presence of hypocalcemia suggests end-organ resistance to PTH action. Skeletal resistance to exogenous PTH in hypocalcemic Mg-deficient patients has been reported. Similarly, urinary excretion of cAMP or phosphate in response to PTH in such patients has been observed (104, 105).

The mechanism for impaired PTH secretion and action in Mg deficiency remains unclear. Investigators have suggested a possible defect in the second-messenger systems in Mg depletion. Adenylate cyclase has been universally found to require Mg for cAMP generation, both as a component of the substrate (MgATP) and as an obligatory activator of enzyme activity. PTH has also been shown to activate the phospholipase C second-messenger system. Mg depletion could perturb this system via several mechanisms, because a Mg^{2+}-dependent guanine nucleotide regulating protein is involved in

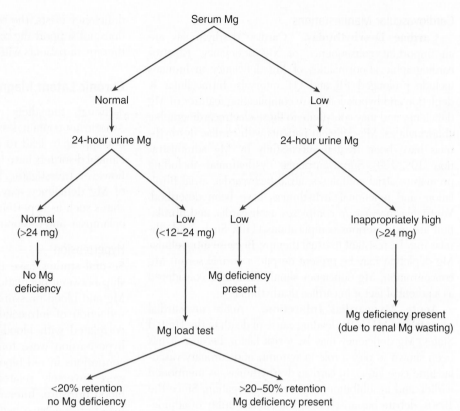

Fig. 9.5. Algorithm of a diagnostic approach to suspected magnesium (Mg) deficiency in which urine Mg levels are emphasized to distinguish the key factors leading to Mg depletion. (Adapted with permission from al Ghamdi SM, Cameron EC, Sutton RA. Magnesium deficiency: pathophysiologic and clinical overview. Am J Kidney Dis 1994;24:737–52.)

activation of phospholipase C and Mg^{2+} has been shown to be a noncompetitive inhibitor of IP_3-induced Ca^{2+} release (105).

Mg is also important in vitamin D metabolism (104, 105). Patients with hypocalcemia and Mg deficiency have also been reported to be resistant to pharmacologic doses of vitamin D, 1α-hydroxy-vitamin D and 1,25-dihydroxy-vitamin D. The exact nature of altered vitamin D metabolism in Mg deficiency is unclear. Serum concentrations of 1,25-dihydroxyvitamin D have been found to be low or low normal in most hypocalcemic Mg-deficient patients. Because PTH is a major trophic for 1,25-dihydroxyvitamin D formation, the low serum PTH concentrations could explain the low 1,25-dihydroxyvitamin D concentrations, a finding suggesting that Mg deficiency impairs the ability of the kidney to synthesize 1,25-dihydroxyvitamin D. Mg is known to support the 25-hydroxy-1α-hydroxylase in vitro (104, 105).

Hypokalemia

A common feature of Mg depletion is hypokalemia (106, 107). Experimental human Mg deficiency demonstrated negative K balance resulting from increased urinary loss. During Mg depletion, patients also lose intracellular K. Attempts to replete the K deficit with K therapy alone are not successful without simultaneous Mg therapy. The reason for this disrupted K metabolism may be related to Mg dependence of the Na^+/K^+-ATPase. During Mg depletion, intracellular Na and Ca rise, and Mg and K fall. Mg also appears to be important in regulation of K

channels in cardiac cells that are characterized by inward rectification (106, 107). This biochemical feature may be a contributing cause of the electrocardiographic findings and cardiac dysrhythmias discussed later.

Neuromuscular Manifestations

Neuromuscular hyperexcitability is a common presenting complaint of patients with Mg deficiency (79). Latent tetany, as elicited by a positive Chvostek and Trousseau sign, or spontaneous carpopedal spasm, may be present. Seizures may also occur. Although hypocalcemia contributes to the neurologic signs, Mg deficiency without hypocalcemia has been reported to result in neuromuscular hyperexcitability. Other signs may include vertigo, ataxia, nystagmus, and athetoid and choreiform movements. Muscular tremor, fasciculation, wasting, and weakness may be present. Reversible psychiatric aberrations also have been reported.

These neuromuscular problems may have several mechanisms. Mg has been shown to stabilize the nerve axon. Lowering serum Mg concentration decreases the threshold of axonal stimulation and increases nerve conduction velocity. Mg also has been shown to influence the release of neurotransmitters, such as glutamate, at the neuromuscular junction by competitively inhibiting the entry of Ca into the presynaptic nerve terminal. It is likely that a decrease in extracellular Mg would allow greater influx of Ca into the presynaptic nerves, with subsequent release of more neurotransmitters, resulting in hyperresponsive neuromuscular activity.

Cardiovascular Manifestations

Cardiac Dysrhythmias.   Cardiac dysrhythmias are an important consequence of Mg deficiency. Electrocardiographic abnormalities of Mg deficiency in humans include prolonged PR and QT intervals. Intracellular K depletion and hypokalemia are complicating features of Mg deficiency and may contribute to these electrocardiographic abnormalities. Mg-deficient patients with cardiac dysrhythmias have been treated successfully by Mg administration (108, 109). Supraventricular dysrhythmias, including premature atrial complexes, atrial tachycardia, atrial fibrillation, and junctional arrhythmias, have been described. Ventricular premature complexes, tachycardia, and fibrillation are more serious complications (110). Such dysrhythmias may be resistant to usual therapy. Because intracellular Mg depletion may be present despite a normal serum Mg concentration, Mg deficiency should always be considered as a potential factor in cardiac dysrhythmias.

Acute Myocardial Infarction.   Acute myocardial infarction (AMI) is the leading cause of death in the United States. Mg deficiency may be a risk factor, because it has been shown to play a role in systemic and coronary vascular tone (see later), in cardiac dysrhythmias, as mentioned earlier, and in inhibition of platelet aggregation. Since the 1980s, debate has arisen over the clinical utility of adjunctive Mg therapy for AMI. Although several small controlled trials suggested that adjunctive Mg therapy reduced mortality from AMI by 50%, three major trials defined our understanding regarding Mg therapy in AMI (111). The second Leicester Intravenous Magnesium Intervention Trial (LIMIT-2) was the first study with large numbers of participants. Over a 6-year period, 2316 participants with suspected AMI were randomized to receive adjunctive Mg therapy or placebo. The Mg-treated group showed an approximately 25% lower mortality rate (7.8% versus 10.3%; $p < .04$).

The fourth International Study of Infarct Survival (ISIS-4) randomized more than 58,000 participants over a 3-year period to examine the effects of captopril, nitrates, and Mg on AMI. Unlike LIMIT-2, in ISIS-4 the mortality rate in the Mg-treated group was not significantly different from that of the control group (7.64% versus 7.24%). The conclusion was that Mg therapy was not indicated in suspected AMI. Despite the null result, some investigators suggested that the ISIS-4 design masked the benefits of Mg therapy. Two major criticisms involved the timing of the Mg therapy and the severity of illness. ISIS-4 randomized participants up to 24 hours after presentation. The leading theory regarding the role of Mg therapy in AMI involves the prevention of ischemia-reperfusion injury.

The Magnesium in Coronaries (MAGIC) trial was designed to address these issues regarding ISIS-4 study design, namely, early intervention in high-risk patients (111). Over a 3-year period, 6213 participants were studied. The Mg treated group mortality at 30 days was not significantly different from the placebo group mortality (15.3% versus 15.2%). Unless a high suspicion of Mg deficiency exists, the overall evidence from clinical trials does not support the routine application of adjunctive Mg therapy in patients with AMI (112).

Chronic Latent Magnesium Deficiency

Although the diets ordinarily consumed by healthy Americans contain less Mg than the RDA (4), they do not appear to lead to symptomatic Mg depletion. Some clinical disorders have been associated with a low-Mg diet, however. Investigators have suggested that milder degrees of Mg deficiency may, over time, contribute to disease states such as hypertension, coronary artery disease, preeclampsia, and osteoporosis.

Hypertension

Several studies have demonstrated an inverse relationship between populations that have low dietary intake of Mg and blood pressure (24, 113). Hypomagnesemia and reduction of intracellular Mg have also been inversely correlated with blood pressure. Patients with essential hypertension were found to have low free Mg^{2+} concentrations in red blood cells. The Mg^{2+} concentrations were inversely related to both systolic and diastolic blood pressure. Intervention studies with Mg therapy in hypertension have had conflicting results. Several studies showed a positive blood pressure–lowering effect of Mg supplements, whereas others did not. Other dietary factors may also play a role. A diet rich in fruit and vegetables, which increased Mg intake from 176 to 423 mg/day (along with an increase in K), significantly lowered blood pressure (114). The addition of nonfat dairy products, which increased Ca intake as well, further lowered blood pressure (114). The mechanism by which Mg deficiency may affect blood pressure is not clear but may involve decreased production of prostacyclin (PGI_2), increased production of thromboxane A_2, and enhanced vasoconstrictive effect of angiotensin II and norepinephrine. Investigators have suggested that the vascular TRPM7 Mg channel may be altered in hypertension (24).

Atherosclerotic Vascular Disease

Another potential cardiovascular complication of Mg deficiency is the development of atheromatous disease (115). Lipid alterations have been reported in hypomagnesemic human subjects; however, they are often complicated by factors related to underlying lipoprotein abnormalities occurring in diabetes, coronary artery disease, myocardial infarction, and other diseases (116). Epidemiologic studies have related water hardness (Ca and Mg content) inversely to cardiovascular death rates. Platelet hyperactivity is a recognized risk factor in the development of cardiovascular diseases. Mg has been shown to inhibit platelet aggregation against certain aggregation agents. Patients with diabetes and Mg depletion have been shown to have high platelet aggregations. Mg therapy in these subjects returned the response toward normal. The antiplatelet effect of Mg may be related to the finding that Mg inhibits the synthesis of thromboxane A_2 and 12-hydroxyeicosatetraenoic acid (12-HETE), eicosanoids thought to be involved in platelet aggregation (117, 118). Mg also inhibits the thrombin-induced Ca influx in platelets and stimulates synthesis of PGI_2, a potent antiaggregatory eicosanoid.

Preeclampsia and Eclampsia

Preeclampsia complicates 1 in 2000 pregnancies in developed countries and is responsible for more than 50,000 maternal deaths per year. Mg therapy has been used for decades in both preeclampsia and eclampsia and contributes to the very low mortality rate in developed countries (119). Despite decades of use, no large randomized trial examining the efficacy of Mg therapy had been performed until the Magnesium Sulfate for Prevention of Eclampsia (MAGPIE) trial in 2002. This trial, which compared women with preeclampsia treated with either Mg sulfate ($MgSO_4$) or nimodipine, a specific cerebral arterial vasodilator, showed a lower risk (0.8% versus 2.6%) of eclampsia in the group receiving Mg therapy (119). The Mg status of women with preeclampsia has been difficult to establish. No difference was found in plasma Mg concentrations of women with preeclampsia and those of healthy pregnant women; however, women with preeclampsia had lower red blood cell Mg concentrations. Women with preeclampsia and women with preterm labor had no differences in ionized or total serum Mg. Although subtle deficits in total body Mg may contribute to hypertension during pregnancy, the role of Mg may relate more to its stabilizing neuronal and vascular effects than to correction of an electrolyte deficit. Mg therapy is clearly indicated for women with preeclampsia to decrease the incidence of eclampsia and likely to decrease overall mortality (119).

Osteoporosis

Dietary Mg restriction in animals resulted in retarded growth of the skeleton (105, 120). Osteoblastic bone formation was been shown to be reduced. An increase in the number and activity of osteoclasts in the Mg-deficient rat and mouse was reported (105, 120), even across intakes seen in the human population (121–124). Bone from Mg-deficient rats was described as brittle and fragile. Biomechanical testing directly demonstrated skeletal fragility in both rats and pigs.

In humans, epidemiologic studies demonstrated a correlation between bone mass and dietary Mg intake (105). Few studies assessed Mg status in patients with osteoporosis. Low serum and red blood cell Mg concentrations, as well as high retention of parenterally administered Mg, suggested an Mg deficit, but these results were not consistent among studies. Similarly, whereas low skeletal Mg content was observed in some studies, others found normal or even high Mg content. The effect of Mg supplements on bone mass has generally led to an increase in bone mineral density, although study design limits useful information. Larger long-term, placebo-controlled, double-blind investigations are required.

Several potential mechanisms may account for lower bone mass in Mg deficiency. Mg is mitogenic for bone cell growth, and this property may directly decrease bone formation. (105). One study suggested that the TRPM7 Mg channel is critical for osteoblast function and that Mg deficiency may thereby decrease bone formation (121). Mg also affects crystal formation; a lack of Mg results in larger, more perfect crystals, which may affect bone strength. Mg deficiency causes both serum PTH and $1,25(OH)_2D$ to fall, as discussed earlier. Given that both hormones are trophic for bone, impaired secretion or skeletal resistance may result in osteoporosis. An increased release of inflammatory cytokines was shown to result in activation of osteoclasts and increased bone resorption in rodents (105, 120, 122, 124).

Other Disorders

Mg deficiency has been associated with migraine headache, and Mg therapy has been reported to be effective in the treatment of migraine (125). Because Mg deficiency results in smooth muscle spasm, it has also been implicated in asthma; and Mg therapy has been effective in asthma in some studies (126). Finally, high dietary Mg intake has been associated with a reduced risk of colon cancer (127).

MANAGEMENT OF MAGNESIUM DEPLETION

The physician should consider all predisposing factors in patients at risk to anticipate hypomagnesemia and institute early treatments to prevent its occurrence or minimize its severity. These measures include instituting control of the underlying disease, minimizing the therapeutic insult, and initiating medical and dietary changes designed to maximize Mg retention by the intestine and kidney. When Mg depletion is evident, its cause must be determined. Before treatment is initiated, Mg, Ca, K, and Na levels in the blood and urine and the acid–base balance in blood must be determined. The amount, route, and duration of Mg administration depend on the severity of Mg depletion and its causes.

Adolescents and Adults

Seizures, acute arrhythmias, and severe generalized spasticity require immediate intravenous infusion. One to 2 g $MgSO_4 \cdot 7H_2O$ (8.2 to 16.4 mEq Mg^{2+}) is usually infused over 5 to 10 minutes, followed by continuous infusion of 6 g over 24 hours or until the condition is controlled (128). Correction of electrolytes (especially K) and acid–base imbalances should accompany Mg therapy. Additionally, serum Mg and other electrolytes should be determined at least twice daily in such patients (129, 130).

Less severe manifestations (e.g., paresthesias with latent or active tetany) are also best treated by the intravenous route, again in conjunction with appropriate therapy for the underlying condition and with correction of other electrolyte and acid–base abnormalities. When renal function is good, 6 g (48 mEq) of $MgSO_4$ may be given intravenously over 24 hours in saline or dextrose solutions, with other nutrients as required (128). This regimen may be continued for 3 to 5 days, until the signs and symptoms and electrolyte abnormalities are corrected. When the intravenous route cannot be used, intramuscular injections can be given, although these are painful. This regimen is continued for 2 or more days, and the situation is then reassessed. The dosages given must always exceed the daily losses, as indicated by serum concentrations and urinary excretion. The return to the normal or slightly higher range of serum Mg with any of these schedules is relatively rapid. Repletion of Mg lost from bone and other tissues requires more prolonged Mg therapy, however.

When intestinal absorption is normal and renal Mg wasting is present, supplements should be added to the usual diet to tolerance (onset of diarrhea) to maintain normal serum concentrations. In some instances, oral Mg may not be sufficient, and intramuscular or intravenous Mg may be required. Patients with continuing severe Mg and K losses in the urine (e.g., cisplatin nephrotoxicity or hereditary renal defects) may require long-term supplements by intravenous infusion, via an indwelling central catheter for home administration.

When depletion is modest and persistent, initial efforts should be directed to increased intake of Mg-rich foods. When necessary and feasible, supplementary oral Mg may be taken. From 300 to 600 mg may be given in divided doses three to six times per day, with a full glass of water to prevent or minimize Mg-related diarrhea and to ensure solubilization (41). For patients receiving enteral feeding, one of these salts may be dissolved in the formula. Improvement of existing steatorrhea by dietary or other medical means will decrease fecal Mg losses. Again, treatment of underlying disease and replacement of K deficits are essential.

Infants and Young Children

Symptomatic Mg depletion in infants responds well to relatively small amounts of intravenous or intramuscular Mg. When renal function is normal, parenteral administration is recommended: 3.6 to 6.0 mg (0.15 to 0.25 mmol or 0.3 to 0.5 mEq)/kg body weight as 50% $MgSO_4$ over the first several hours, followed by an equal amount, either intramuscularly or intravenously, over the remainder of the day (131). Ca may also be infused initially together with K and other electrolytes as indicated. When convulsions or arrhythmias are present in children beyond infancy, treatment may be initiated with an oral bolus of 50% $MgSO_4$ at a dose of 20 to 100 mg (1.65 to 8.25 mEq/kg) over 1 minute; this is followed by 1.0 mEq/kg given continuously thereafter (132).

In patients with chronic malabsorption (e.g., primary hypomagnesemia), 12 to 18 mg/kg (0.5 to 0.75 mmol) in multiple, divided oral doses is suggested; this dosage schedule raises serum concentrations to nearly normal without inducing diarrhea (131).

MAGNESIUM EXCESS OR TOXICITY

Mg excess or intoxication is not a common clinical problem. Mild-to-moderate elevations in the serum Mg have been observed in up to 12% of admissions in acute care hospitals, however (133). Mg intoxication is usually the result of excessive administration of Mg salts, generally in patients with impaired renal function.

Causes of Hypermagnesemia

Preeclampsia and Eclampsia

Excessive Mg administration is observed in preeclampsia and eclampsia. As discussed earlier, preeclampsia and eclampsia are the most important causes of maternal death in the United States and in many other countries (119, 134). High-dose parenteral $MgSO_4$ is the drug of choice in North America for preventing eclamptic convulsions that may occur in association with severe hypertension and other problems in late pregnancy or during labor (119, 135). A loading dose and then maintenance doses are given to maintain a high serum concentration of approximately 2 to 3 mmol/L (4–6 mEq/L) (135) or slightly higher (136). Patients with normal kidneys can excrete 40 to 60 g of $MgSO_4 \cdot 7H_2O$ per day when it is given constantly by infusion. The high doses used are rarely associated with serious side effects, because patients are closely monitored with modification of dosage as indicated.

In one report, fetuses delivered from mothers receiving high-dose Mg had hypermagnesemia of the umbilical vein and arterial blood at about the elevated levels of the mother. Serum concentrations fell progressively to normal in neonates by 48 hours, however (137).

Magnesium Overdose

Mg-containing cathartics have been given orally with activated charcoal in single or multiple doses (each of 30 g $MgSO_4 \cdot 7H_2O$ [245 mEq Mg^{2+}]) in an effort to decrease blood concentrations of drugs, as part of the treatment of patients with suspected drug overdose. Despite initially normal serum creatinine concentrations (138), 9 of 14 patients were hypermagnesemic by the third dose at 8 hours, including 4 patients with Mg concentrations of 3.0 to 5.0 mEq/L. The presence of drugs that decreased gut motility (e.g., anticholinergics or opioids) appeared related to the higher concentrations (139).

Renal Failure

In addition to the planned therapeutic hypermagnesemia noted earlier, elevated serum concentrations occur when Mg-containing drugs, usually antacids or cathartics, are ingested on a long-term basis and in relatively large amounts by individuals with advanced renal insufficiency. Because 20% or more of Mg from various salts may be absorbed, impaired renal clearance can induce significant hypermagnesemia. The common association of age- or disease-related impairment of glomerular filtration, which may be exacerbated by ingestion of potentially nephrotoxic medications (e.g., steroidal anti-inflammatory drugs for

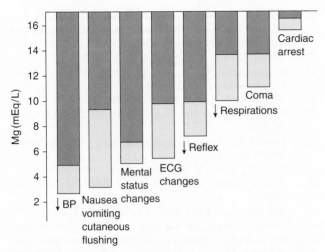

Fig. 9.6. The progression in toxic effects as hypermagnesemia becomes more severe. An early sign is a lowering of blood pressure (BP). Nausea, vomiting, and hypotension may occur in the range of 3 to 9 mEq/L; bradycardia and urinary retention also occur in this range. Electrocardiogram (ECG) changes, hyporeflexia, and secondary central nervous system depression may appear in the range of 5 to 10 mEq/L, followed at higher concentrations by life-threatening respiratory depression, coma, and asystolic cardiac arrest. (Adapted with permission from Mordes JP, Wacker EC. Excess magnesium. Pharmacol Rev 1978;29:274–300.)

arthritic pain), and the long-term use of Mg-containing antacids or laxatives contribute to the danger of significant hypermagnesemia in such individuals.

Hypermagnesemia may occur at symptomatic levels in patients with gastrointestinal disorders such as obstipation, severe constipation, ulceration, obstruction, or perforation when Mg-containing cathartics or antacids are taken, even in moderate doses, and renal insufficiency is mild or moderate (140).

Clinical Presentation of Magnesium Excess

The many potentially toxic and even lethal effects of Mg excess are summarized in Figure 9.6 (141). One of the earliest effects is a fall in blood pressure, progressing with increasing hypermagnesemia; this appears to result from inhibition of Ca^{2+} flux and the vasoconstrictive action of norepinephrine and angiotensin II (142). Mg at concentrations higher than normal relaxes vascular smooth muscle in vitro and reduces pressor responses (143). In humans, when serum Mg concentrations were roughly twice normal, the following effects were noted: systolic and diastolic blood pressures fell by an average of 10 and 8 mm Hg, respectively; renal blood flow increased significantly; and the pressor effect of angiotensin II was blunted (143). Urinary excretion of 6-keto-prostaglandin $F_{1\alpha}$ ($PGF_{1\alpha}$) increased markedly. Cyclooxygenase inhibition with indomethacin or ibuprofen completely blocked the Mg-induced fall in blood pressure, the rise in urinary 6-keto-$PGF_{1\alpha}$, and the rise in renal blood flow. The Ca channel blocker nifedipine also prevented the Mg-induced rise in 6-keto-$PGF_{1\alpha}$ and the fall in blood pressure. These findings indicate that the effect of Mg was

mediated by PGI_2 release and increased Ca^{2+} flux. With increased serum Mg, circulating PTH may drop, with associated hypocalcemia (136, 144). With maternal hypocalcemia in the treatment of eclampsia, the fetus at delivery may have a normal (137) or low serum Ca concentration (145).

Some of the effects of very high serum Mg, such as lethargy, confusion, and deterioration in renal function, may be related to the hypotension (146). Electrocardiographic changes, such as prolongation of the PR and QT intervals, occur at 5 mEq/L (2.5 mmol). Tachycardia (probably secondary to hypotension) or bradycardia may occur. At 6 mEq/L and higher, muscle weakness and hyporeflexia may occur, presumably resulting from decreased release of acetylcholine and impaired transmission at the neuromuscular junction; hypocalcemia may contribute to the progressive muscle weakness and respiratory difficulty. Complete heart block and cardiac arrest may occur at approximately 15 mEq/L (141).

Management of Hypermagnesemia

Prevention or treatment of mild-to-moderate hypermagnesemia ($\geq$1.5 mmol) requires reducing Mg intake when absorption from all sources exceeds the renal excretory capability. At higher levels, when hemodynamic instability and muscle weakness are apparent, all Mg intake should be stopped, and an acute infusion of 5 to 10 mEq of Ca over 5 to 10 minutes should be given; Ca antagonizes the toxic effects (146). Continued saline and Ca infusion will increase Mg excretion. Peritoneal dialysis or hemodialysis will remove Mg readily in the patient with poor renal function (146).

REFERENCES

1. Kruse HD, Orent ER, McCollum EV. J Biol Chem 1932;96:519–36.
2. Hirschfelder AD, Haury VG. JAMA 1934;102:1138–41.
3. Flink EB. J Am Coll Nutr 1985;4:17–31.
4. Food and Nutrition Board, Institute of Medicine. Dietary Reference Intakes for Calcium, Phosphorus, Magnesium, Vitamin D, and Fluoride. Washington, DC: National Academy Press, 1997.
5. Maguire ME, Cowan JA. Biometals 2002;15:203–10.
6. Wolf FI, Cittadini A. Mol Aspects Med 2003;24:3–9.
7. Cowan JA. Biometals 2002;15:225–35.
8. Cowan JA. Introduction to the biological chemistry of magnesium. In: Cowan JA, ed. The Biological Chemistry of Magnesium. New York: VCH Publishers, 1995:1–24.
9. Black CB, Cowan JA. Magnesium dependent enzymes in nucleic acid biochemistry; and Magnesium dependent enzymes in general metabolism. In: Cowan JA, ed. The Biological Chemistry of Magnesium. New York: VCH Publishers, 1995:137–58.
10. Knighton DR, Zheng J, Ten Eyck LF et al. Science 1991;253:407–14.
11. Litosch I. J Biol Chem 1991;266:4764–71.
12. Volpe P, Alderson-Lang BH, Nickols GA. Am J Physiol 1990;258:C1077–85.
13. Smith D. Magnesium as the catalytic center of RNA enzymes. In: Cowan JA, ed. The Biological Chemistry of Magnesium. New York: VCH Publishers, 1995:111–36.

14. Ackerman MJ, Clapham DE. N Engl J Med 1997;336:1575–86.
15. Romani A. Arch Biochem Biophys 2007;458:90–102.
16. Dorup I. Acta Physiol Scand 1994;150:7–46.
17. White RE, Hartzell HC. Biochem Pharmacol 1989;38:859–67.
18. Wallach S. Magnes Trace Elem 1990;9:1–14.
19. Endres DB, Rude RK. Disorders of bone. In: Burtis CA, Ashwood ET, Burns DE, eds. Tietz Textbook of Clinical Chemistry. 6th ed. Philadelphia: WB Saunders, 2008:711–34.
20. Romani A, Marfella C, Scarpa A. Miner Electrolyte Metab 1993;19:282–9.
21. Grubbs RD. Biometals 2002;15:251–9.
22. Quamme GA, Dai L, Rabkin SW. Am J Physiol 1993;265:H281–8.
23. Gunther T, Hollriegl V. Biochim Biophys Acta 1993;1149:49–54.
24. Touyz RM. Am J Physiol 2008;294:H1103–118.
25. Goytain A, Hines RM, Quamme GA. Am J Physiol 2008;295:C944–52.
26. Zhou H, Clapham DE. Proc Natl Acad Sci U S A 2009;106:15750–5.
27. Hou J, Renigunta A, Gomes AS et al. Proc Natl Acad Sci U S A 2009;106:15350–5.
28. Schlingmann KP, Waldegger S, Kondrad M et al. Biochim Biophys Acta 2007;1772:813–21.
29. Gunzel D, Yu AS. Eur J Physiol 2009;458:77–88.
30. Romani A, Scarpa A. FEBS Lett 1990;269:37–40.
31. Gunther T, Vormann J. Magnes Trace Elem 1990;9:279–82.
32. Romani A, Marfella C, Scarpa A. FEBS Lett 1992;296:135–40.
33. Grubbs RD. Am J Physiol 1991;260:C1158–64.
34. Kumar D, Leonard E, Rude RK. Arch Intern Med 1978;138:660.
35. Pennington JA, Young B. J Am Diet Assoc 1991;91:179–83.
36. Alexander RT, Hoenderop JG, Bindels RJ. J Am Soc Nephrol 2008;19:1451–8.
37. Kerstan D, Quamme GA. Physiology and pathophysiology of intestinal absorption of magnesium. In: Massry SG, Morii H, Nishizawa Y, eds. Calcium in Internal Medicine. Surrey, UK: Springer-Verlag, 2002:171-83.
38. Quamme GA. Curr Opin Gastroenterol 2008;24:230–5.
39. Graham LA, Ceasar JJ, Burgen AS. Metab Clin Exp 1960;9:646–59.
40. Fine KD, Santa Ana CA, Porter JL et al. J Clin Invest 1991;88:396–402.
41. Spencer H, Lesniak M, Gatza LA et al. Gastroenterology 1980;79:26–34.
42. Lakshmann FL, Rao RB, Kim WW. Am J Clin Nutr 1984;40(Suppl 6):1380–9.
43. Andon MB, Illich JZ, Tzagournis MA et al. Am J Clin Nutr 1996;63:950–3.
44. Spencer H, Osis D. Magnesium 1988;7:271–80.
45. Fine KD, Santa Ana CA, Fordtran JS. N Engl J Med 1991;324:1012–7.
46. Vormann J. Mol Aspects Med 2003;24:27–37.
47. Spencer H, Norris C, Williams D. J Am Coll Nutr 1994;13:479–84.
48. Turnlund JR, Betschart AA, Liebman M et al. Am J Clin Nutr 1992;56:905–10.
49. Franz KB. In: Itokawa Y, Durlach J, eds. Magnesium in Health and Disease. London: John Libbey, 1989:71–8.
50. Wisker E, Nagel R, Tanudjaja TK et al. Am J Clin Nutr 1991;54:553–9.
51. Slavin JL, Marlett JA. Am J Clin Nutr 1980;33:1932–9.
52. Lindberg JS, Zobitz MM, Poindexter JR et al. J Am Coll Nutr 1990;9:48–55.
53. Kuhn I, Jost V, Wieckhorst G et al. Meth Find Exp Clin Pharmacol 1992;14:269–72.

54. Rude RK, Shils ME. Magnesium. In: Shils ME, Shike M, Ross CA et al, eds. Modern Nutrition in Health and Disease. 10th ed. Philadelphia: Lippincott Williams & Wilkins, 2006:223–47.
55. Satoh J, Romero MF. Biometals 2002;15:285–95.
56. de Rouffignac C, Mandon B, Wittner M et al. Miner Electrolyte Metab 1993;19:226–31.
57. Wallach S. Magnesium 1988;7:262–70.
58. Rude RK, Gruber HE, Wei LY et al. Cacif Tissue Int 2003;72:32–41.
59. Drenick EG, Hung JF, Swendseid ME. J Clin Endocrinol l969;29:1341–8.
60. Dunn MJ, Walser M. Metabolism 1966;15:884–95.
61. Wenk C, Kuhnt M, Kunz P et al. Z Ernahrungswiss 1993;32:301–7.
62. Shils ME, Rude RK. J Nutr 1996;126:2398S–403S.
63. American Society for Experimental Biology, Life Sciences Research Office, Interagency Board for Nutrition Monitoring and Related Research. Third Report on Nutrition Monitoring in the United States. Washington, DC: US Government Printing Office, 1995.
64. Elin RJ. Magnes Trace Elem 1991–92;10:60–6.
65. Huijgen HJ, Van Ingen HE, Kok WT et al. Clin Biochem 1996;29:261–6.
66. Csako G, Rehak N, Elin RJ. Clin Chem 1996;42(Suppl):S279.
67. Escuela MP, Guerra, M, Anon, JM et al. Intensive Care Med 2005;31:151–6.
68. Haigney MC, Silver B, Tanglao E et al. Circulation 1995;92:2190–7.
69. Arnaud MJ. Br J Nutr 2008;99(Suppl 3):S24–36.
70. Cecco SA, Hristova ME, Rehak NN. Clin Chem 1997;108:564–9.
71. Rude RK, Stephen A, Nadler J. Magnes Trace Elem 1991–92;10:117–2.
72. Elin RJ, Hosseini JM, Gill JR Jr. J Am Coll Nutr 1994;13:463–6.
73. Fleming CR, George L, Stoner GL et al. Mayo Clin Proc 1996;71:21–4.
74. Rude RK. Magnesium disorders. In: Kokko JP, Tannen RL, eds. Fluids and Electrolytes. 3rd ed. Philadelphia: WB Saunders, 1996:421–45.
75. Ryzen E, Elbaum N, Singer FR, Rude RK. Magnesium 1985;4:137–47.
76. Whang R, Oei T, Aikawa JK et al. Arch Intern Med 1984;144:1794–6.
77. Whang R, Hampton EM, Whang DD. Ann Pharmacother 1994;28:220–6.
78. Ryzen E, Wagers PW, Singer FR et al. Crit Care Med 1985;13:19–21.
79. Rude RK. Magnesium homeostasis. In: Bilezikian JB, Raisz L, Rodan G, eds. Principles of Bone Biology. 3rd ed. San Diego: Academic Press, 2008:487–513.
80. Ryzen E, Rude RK. West J Med 1990;152:145–8.
81. Cundy T, Dissanayake A. Clin Endocrinol (Oxf) 2008;69:338–41.
82. Quamme GA, de Rouffignac C. Frontiers Biosci 2000;5:694–711.
83. Quamme GA. Kidney Int 1997;52:1180–95.
84. Romani AP. Magnes Res 2008;21:197–204.
85. Dyckner T, Wester PO. Acta Med Scand 1985;218:443–8.
86. Tejpar S, Piessevaux H, Claes K et al. Lancet Oncol 2007;8:387–94.
87. Lajer H, Kristensen M, Hansen HH et al. Cancer Chemother Pharmacol 2005;5:231–6.
88. Goldman RD, Koren G. J Pediatr Hematol Oncol 2004;26:421–6.
89. Wilkinson R, Lucas GL, Heath DA et al. Br Med J (Clin Res Ed) 1986;292:818–9.

90. Navaneethan SD, Sankarasubbaiyan S, Gross MD et al. Transplant Proc 2006;38:1320–2.

91. Naderi AS, Reilly RF Jr. Nat Clin Pract Nephrol 2008;4:80–9.

92. McNair P, Christensen MS, Christiansen C et al. Eur J Clin Invest 1982;12:81–5.

93. Song Y, Buring JE, Manson JE et al. Diabetes Care 2004; 27:59–65.

94. Lopez-Ridaura R, Stampfer MJ, Wiollett WC et al. Diabetes Care 2004;27:134–40.

95. Barbagallo M, Dominguez LJ, Resnick LM. Am J Ther 2007;14:375–85.

96. Gunther T. Magnes Res 2010;23:5–18.

97. Song Y, Hsu YH, Niu T et al. BMC Med Genet 2009;10:4.

98. Farese S. Ther Umsch 2007;64:277–80.

99. Ziegler TR. N Engl J Med 2009;361:1088–97.

100. Nielsen FH, Lukaski HC. Magnes Res 2006;19:180–9.

101. Berger MM, Rothen C, Cavadini C, Chiolero RL. Am J Clin Nutr 1997;65:1473–81.

102. National Research Council. Nutrient Requirements of Laboratory Animals. Washington, DC: National Academy Press, 1995. Available at: http://www.nap.edu/openbook. php?record_id=4758. Accessed June 15, 2011.

103. Shils ME. Magnesium. In: O'Dell BL, Sunde RA, eds. Handbook of Nutritionally Essential Mineral Elements. New York: Marcel Dekker, 1997:117–52.

104. Rude RK. Magnesium deficiency in parathyroid function. In: Bilezikian JP, ed. The Parathyroids. 2nd ed. New York: Raven Press, 2001:763–77.

105. Rude RK, Singer FR, Gruber HE. J Am Coll Nutr 2009; 28:131–41.

106. Whang R, Hampton EM, Whang DD. Ann Pharmacother 1994;28:220–6.

107. Huang CL, Kuo E. J Am Soc Nephrol 2007;18:2649–52.

108. Zehender M, Meinertz T, Faber T et al. J Am Coll Cardiol 1997;29:1028–34.

109. Morgan JL, Gallagher J, Peake SL et al. Crit Care Med 1995;23:1816–24.

110. Delva P. Mol Aspects Med 2003;24:53–62.

111. Antman E, Cooper H, Domanski M et al. Lancet 2002; 360:1189–96.

112. Yellon DM, Hausenloy DJ. N Engl J Med 2007;357:1121–35.

113. Sontia B, Touyz RM. Arch Biochem Biophys 2007;458:33–9.

114. Appel LJ, Moore TJ, Obarzanek E et al. N Engl J Med 1997; 336:1117–24.

115. Maier J. Mol Aspects Med 2003;24:137–46.

116. Delva P. Mol Aspects Med 2003;24:63–78.

117. Hwang D, Yen C, Nadler J. Am J Hypertens 1992;5:700–6.

118. Nadler J, Malayan S, Luong H et al. Diabetes Care 1992; 15:835–41.

119. Belfort MA, Anthony J, Saade GR et al. N Engl J Med 2003;348:302–11.

120. Rude RK, Gruber HE, Norton HJ et al. J Nutr 2004;134: 79–85.

121. Abed E, Moreau. Am J Physiol 2009;297:C360–8.

122. Rude RK, Gruber HE, Norton HJ et al. Bone 2005;37:211–9.

123. Rude RK, Gruber HE, Norton HJ et al. Osteoporosis Int 2006;17:1022–32.

124. Rude RK, Wei L, Norton HJ et al. Growth Factors 2009; 26:370–6.

125. Sun-Edelstein C, Mauskop A. Expert Rev Neurother 2009; 9:369–79.

126. Mohammed S, Goodacre S. Emerg Med J 2007;24:823–30.

127. Dai Q, Shrubsole MJ, Ness RM et al. Am J Clin Nutr 2007; 86:743–51.

128. Ryzen E. Magnesium 1989;8:201–12.

129. Ramee SR, White CJ, Savarinth JT et al. Am Heart J 1985;109:164–6.

130. Tzivoni D, Keren A. Am J Cardiol 1990;65:1397–9.

131. Stromme JH, Steen-Johnson J, Harnaes K et al. Pediatr Res 1981;15:1134–9.

132. Allen DB, Greer FR. Calcium and magnesium deficiency beyond infancy. In: Tsang RC, ed. Calcium and Magnesium Metabolism in Early Life. Boca Raton, FL: CRC Press, 1995.

133. Wong ET, Rude RK, Singer FR et al. Am Soc Clin Pathol 1983;79:348–52.

134. Roberts JM, Redman CWG. Lancet 1993;341:1447–51.

135. Cunningham FG, Lindheimer MD. N Engl J Med 1992; 326:927–32.

136. Cholst IN, Steinberg SF, Tropper PJ et al. N Engl J Med 1984;310:1221–5.

137. McGuinness GA, Weinstein MM, Cruikshank DP et al. Obstet Gynecol 1980;56:595–600.

138. Smilkstein MJ, Steedle D, Kulig KW et al. Clin Toxicol 1988; 26:51–65.

139. Nelson KB. JAMA 1996;276:1843–33.

140. Kattan M. J Pediatr 1996;129:783–5.

141. Mordes JP, Wacker EC. Pharmacol Rev 1978;29:274–300.

142. Rude RK, Mamoogian C, Ehrich P et al. Magnesium 1989; 8:266–73.

143. Altura BM, Altura BT. Magnes Bull 1986;8:338–50.

144. Eisunbud E, LoBoe CL. Arch Intern Med 1976;136:688–91.

145. Donovan EF, Tsang RC, Steichen JJ et al. J Pediatr 1980; 96:305–10.

146. Clark BA, Brown RS. Am J Nephrol 1992;12:336–43.

SUGGESTED READINGS

Cowan JA. Introduction to the biological chemistry of magnesium. In: Cowan JA, ed. The Biological Chemistry of Magnesium. New York: VCH Publishers, 1995:1–24.

Endres D, Rude RK. Disorders of bone. In: Burtis CA, Ashwood ET, Burns DE, eds. Tietz Textbook of Clinical Chemistry. 6th ed. Philadelphia: WB Saunders, 2008:711–34.

Rude RK. Magnesium deficiency and hypermagnesemia. In: Favus MJ, ed. Primer on the Metabolic Bone Diseases and Disorders of Mineral Metabolism. 7th ed. Washington, DC: American Society of Bone and Mineral Research, 2008:325–8.

Rude RK. Magnesium homeostasis. In: Bilezikian JB, Raisz L, Rodan G, eds. Principles of Bone Biology. 3rd ed. San Diego: Academic Press, 2008:487–513.

Rude RK, Shils ME. Magnesium. In: Shils ME, Shike M, Ross CA et al, eds. Modern Nutrition in Health and Disease. 10th ed. Philadelphia: Lippincott Williams & Wilkins, 2006:223–47.

(In the current edition, the text and references have been shortened at the request of the editors. Although updates have been made, the tenth edition contains some discussion and references of older literature the reader may find of interest.)

B. MINERALS

10 IRON[1]
MARIANNE WESSLING-RESNICK

HISTORICAL PERSPECTIVE

As early as the sixteenth and seventeenth centuries, chlorosis (iron deficiency anemia) was reported as a medical condition that could be treated with iron supplementation, but it was not until the turn of the twentieth century that our understanding of the essential nature of iron for heme synthesis slowly emerged (1). Since that time, the pace of discovery in the field of iron metabolism has accelerated to the current explosion in molecular information in the twenty-first century (2). This chapter highlights the most current concepts in iron homeostasis.

----

[1]**Abbreviations: 2,5-DHBA**, 2,5-dihydroxybenzoic acid; **ACD**, anemia of chronic disease; **BMP**, bone morphogenic protein; **CHr**, reticulocyte hemoglobin; **DcytB**, duodenal cytochrome B; **DMT1**, divalent metal transporter-1; **HCP1**, heme carrier protein-1; **HJV**, hemojuvelin; **HYPO**, hypochromic red blood cells; **IRE**, iron-responsive element; **IRP**, iron regulatory protein; **MCH**, mean corpuscular hemoglobin; **PCBP1**, poly(rC)-binding protein-1; **RDA**, recommended dietary allowance; **sTfR**, soluble transferrin receptor; **WHO**, World Health Organization.

CHEMISTRY AND IMPORTANCE OF IRON

Iron exists in one of two oxidation states: the ferrous form (Fe^{2+}) or the ferric form (Fe^{3+}). This chemical property results in iron's catalytic role in a multitude of redox reactions necessary to support basic metabolic functions for life. In fact, iron's central role in oxygen and energy metabolism underscores the biologic significance of this element and helps to explain why it is one of the best-studied metals in nutrition and health. These same catalytic properties of iron also confer its well-known toxicity resulting from Fenton chemistry, a reaction that generates free radicals including superoxide. Thus, iron is an essential nutrient as well as a powerful toxicant, and it is important to understand how both features are kept in balance.

Total iron body content is estimated to be 3.8 g in men and 2.3 g in women. Most body iron is found as heme iron (Fig. 10.1). Heme iron is the essential constituent for oxygen transport in hemoglobin, oxygen storage in myoglobin, and electron transport for cytochrome function in aerobic respiration, and it is even necessary for signal transduction as a cofactor for nitric oxide synthase and guanylyl cyclase. The second largest pool of iron is found in its storage form ferritin (also hemosiderin). Ferritin is a large assembly of 24 protein subunits that form a large sphere around a mineralized ferric core of several thousands of iron atoms (3). In times of demand, iron is liberated from ferritin to fulfill essential functions in oxygen transport and energy metabolism. Damage generated by reactive oxygen species arising from redox-reactive free iron is prevented by its storage in ferritin.

In similar fashion, newly absorbed iron is bound by transferrin, thereby limiting its toxic effects as it is transported in serum. Transferrin-bound iron is destined to be taken up by the transferrin receptor in peripheral tissues for storage or utilization. Transferrin has two binding sites for one iron atom each. Under normal circumstances, 30% to 40% of these iron-binding sites are filled with approximately 4 mg of total body iron. Circulating transferrin-bound iron represents a highly dynamic storage pool that can be drawn from to fulfill immediate demands. Hence the saturation state of serum transferrin plays a key role in the regulation of iron metabolism and is one of the indices used clinically to evaluate iron status.

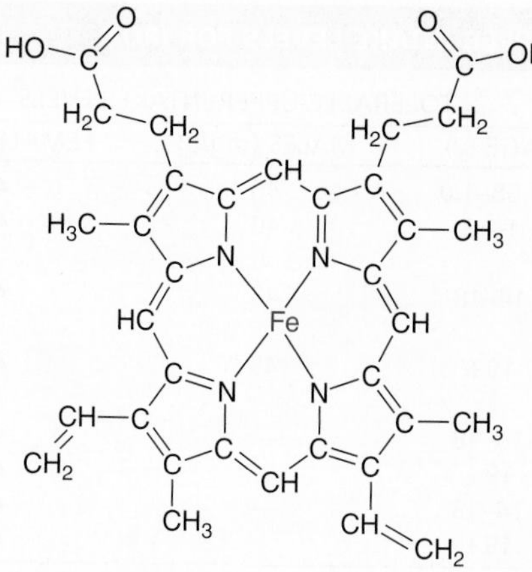

Fig. 10.1. Structure of heme.

TABLE 10.1	**FACTORS INFLUENCING IRON ABSORPTION**	
	NUTRIENTS	**ENDOGENOUS FACTORS**
Enhancers	Ascorbic acid (vitamin C)	Enhanced erythropoiesis due to
	Fructose	Hypoxia
	Citric acid	Hemorrhage
	Dietary protein	Hemolysis
	Lysine	Androgens
	Histidine	Cobalt
	Cysteine	Low iron stores
	Methionine	
Inhibitors	Oxalic acid	Infection/inflammation
	Tannins	Lack of stomach acid
	Phytate	High iron stores
	Polyphenols	
	Carbonate	
	Phosphate	
	Fiber	
	Other metal ions	

Adapted from Linder M. Nutritional Biochemistry and Metabolism with Clinical Applications. New York: Elsevier, 1985, with permission.

Iron absorption, utilization, and storage are finely tuned to maintain the metal's homeostasis. Unlike the situation with other essential elements, iron metabolism is subject to a high degree of conservation. Rather than eliminate excess iron that is not immediately required, iron is stored in ferritin for times of need, as described earlier. The nature of iron homeostasis reflects the metal's key chemical role in oxygen and energy metabolism, processes that are necessary for life and must therefore rely on a substantial reservoir of iron to support the ultimate demands of human physiology. Approximately 20 to 25 mg of iron is turned over daily with the erythrophagocytosis of senescent red blood cells, and iron that is released from heme is captured for reutilization in the production of new erythrocytes. Small amounts of iron are lost in feces (~0.6 mg/day), urine (<0.1 mg/day), and sweat (<0.3 mg/day). Menstruating women suffer an average blood loss of approximately 40 mL/cycle or 0.4 to 0.5 mg/day. Most losses are offset by the amount of iron provided in the diet, however, pathologic conditions associated with excessive blood loss such as hookworm infection or bleeding ulcers can result in greater iron demands. A key feature of iron homeostasis is that the body's iron status is maintained at the level of dietary iron absorption to prevent toxic accumulation while adequate amounts are provided to offset losses. When iron is depleted from the body, dietary iron absorption increases to meet the demand for iron, although no known regulated pathway exists for excretion of excess iron.

DIETARY SOURCES

Iron is absorbed from the diet as either heme or nonheme iron (see the following website: http://ods.od.nih.gov/factsheets/Iron-HealthProfessional). Heme iron is typically derived from hemoglobin or myoglobin and is contained in foods such as red meats, fish, and poultry. Various sources of nonheme iron, such as plant foods, are also available. This form of iron is also added to enrich and fortify foods such as cereals. Although nonheme iron is the predominant form in the diet, heme iron is more

bioavailable (4). Approximately 15% to 35% of heme iron will be assimilated, compared with 2% to 20% nonheme iron absorption. As discussed earlier, the levels of stored iron in the body influence the extent of absorption. Under low-iron conditions, dietary absorption is promoted, whereas high-iron conditions reduce absorption. Many other dietary and endogenous factors can influence iron uptake (Table 10.1). For example, ascorbate can help to reduce ferric iron to the more bioavailable form of ferrous iron (5, 6). Polyphenols and phytates can interfere with nonheme iron uptake (6). Calcium blocks uptake of both heme and nonheme iron (7), whereas other metals can inhibit nonheme iron absorption by sharing the same pathway for absorption (4). In particular, not only is lead a competitive inhibitor for uptake, but also it can disrupt steps of iron metabolism required for heme synthesis (8). Because low iron status enhances metal absorption, lead poisoning is often associated with iron deficiency in children (9).

RECOMMENDED DIETARY ALLOWANCES

The recommended dietary allowances (RDAs) set for iron by the Institute of Medicine of the National Academy of Sciences are listed in Table 10.2. Iron is considered a micronutrient: adult men require 8 mg iron/day, and during their reproductive years, girls and women require 18 mg iron/day. The typical North American diet of 12 to 18 mg iron/day should be adequate to fulfill these needs, but the requirement for iron markedly increases to 27 mg/day during pregnancy, and iron supplements are often needed to match this high demand. Infants are born with a 4- to 6-month iron supply, and an RDA has not been established for this early age. An adequate intake (AI) of 0.27 mg/day is recommended, however. Beyond this age, iron content in milk cannot entirely meet the needs of the developing child, and food sources are

TABLE 10.2	RECOMMENDED DIETARY ALLOWANCES AND TOLERABLE UPPER INTAKE LEVELS FOR IRON					
	RECOMMENDED DIETARY ALLOWANCES			TOLERABLE UPPER INTAKE LEVELS		
	AGE (y)	MALES (mg/d)	FEMALES (mg/d)	AGE (y)	MALES (mg/d)	FEMALES (mg/d)
Infants	0.58–1.0	11	11	0.58–1.0	40	40
Children	1–3	7	7	1–13	40	40
	4–8	10	10			
Adolescents	9–13	8	8	14–18	45	45
	14–18	11	15			
Adults	19–50	8	18	19+	45	45
	51+	8	8			
Pregnancy	14–18	—	27	14–18	—	45
	19–50		27	19+		45
Lactation	14–18	—	10	14–18	—	45
	19–50		9	19+		45

From Food and Nutrition Board, Institute of Medicine. Dietary Reference Intakes for Vitamin A, Vitamin K, Arsenic, Boron, Chromium, Copper, Iodine, Iron, Manganese, Molybdenum, Nickel, Silicon, Vanadium, and Zinc. Washington, DC: National Academy Press, 2001.

required to meet RDAs (7 mg/day at age 1 to 3 years and 10 mg/day at age 4 to 8 years). Iron toxicity can also pose a risk for children, and it commonly results from ingestion of excess iron supplements. Death occurs at levels of 200 to 300 mg/kg. The tolerable upper limits (UL) for iron intake are listed in Table 10.2.

IRON METABOLISM AND ITS REGULATION

The field of iron biology has made rapid advances since 2000. Many of the proteins involved in iron transport and homeostatic regulation have been identified, and their physiologic roles have been uncovered. Perhaps the most exciting breakthrough came with the discovery of iron regulatory hormone, hepcidin. Features of hepcidin regulation of iron metabolism have been compared to insulin action in glucose metabolism, thus creating a new field of iron endocrinology (10). How hepcidin regulates systemic iron homeostasis is a major focus of current investigation. At the cellular level, molecular insights into the regulation of iron-binding proteins have yielded information about regulation of iron transport, utilization, and storage that have important clinical considerations. Finally, transcriptional and posttranscriptional networks that may be activated by hepcidin-induced signaling are beginning to emerge and provide clues into the relationships between iron and inflammation.

Intestinal Iron Absorption

Because body iron status is precisely tuned by the absorption of dietary iron, it is important to understand the mechanisms involved in this process and the multiple layers that regulate the flux of iron into the system (Fig. 10.2). Because the body does not eliminate excess iron, dysregulation of intestinal iron absorption causing assimilation of too much iron will result in iron overload. Conversely, if sufficient iron is not absorbed to make up for small daily losses, the risk for iron deficiency increases. Iron is absorbed as nonheme or heme forms. Heme iron is absorbed more effectively (11), and this process does not

appear to be subject to the same regulatory mechanisms as nonheme iron uptake (12).

These findings indicate that heme and nonheme iron are taken up by independent mechanisms. A putative heme transporter called heme carrier protein-1 (HCP1)

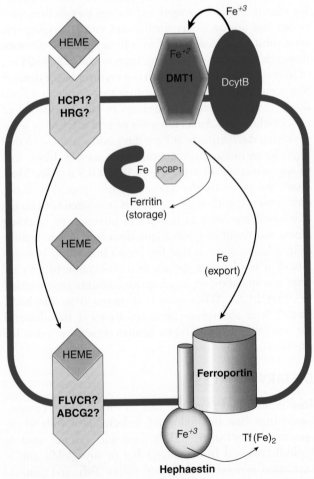

Fig. 10.2. Intestinal iron (Fe) absorption. *ABCG2*, ABC transporter; *DcytB*, duodenal cytochrome B; *DMT1*, divalent metal transporter-1; *FLVCR*, feline leukemia virus C receptor; *HCP1*, heme carrier protein-1; *HRG*, heme-responsive gene; *PCBP1*, poly(rC)-binding protein-1; *Tf(Fe)₂*, diferric transferrin.

was identified (13), but questions about its true function arose when a role in folate transport was determined for the same factor (14). HCP1 may possibly be a low-affinity transporter for heme, but its physiologic relevance remains to be better established. A different molecule, heme-responsive gene-1 or *HRG1*, has been identified as a heme transporter in *Caenorhabditis elegans* (15). Although a similar gene is present in humans, its activity has yet to be defined. Heme oxygenase may release iron from heme entering the intestinal absorptive enterocyte to join the pool of newly absorbed nonheme iron entering the cell (16). Alternatively, intact heme may be released across the basolateral surface. Feline leukemia virus C receptor (FLVCR) has been identified to function as a heme exporter in erythroid cells (17), and a second possible efflux pathway involving the ABC transporter ABCG2 (also known as breast cancer regulated protein, BCRP) has been suggested (18), but their possible roles in heme assimilation by the intestine have yet to be fully explored.

Uptake of nonheme iron by enterocytes is better understood. Although less effectively absorbed, nonheme iron is present in a greater range of foods, most typically in the ferric (Fe^{3+}) form. Reduction to Fe^{2+} is the first step in intestinal nonheme iron assimilation and is mediated by brush-border ferrireductase activity. An enzyme called duodenal cytochrome B (DcytB) has been implicated in this process (19). Although it does not appear to be an essential gene (20), DcytB is highly regulated in response to iron status in animals and humans (21–23), and a promoter polymorphism observed in the human population appears to modify serum ferritin levels in *HFE*-associated hereditary hemochromatosis (24). After reduction by DctyB or another brush-border ferrireductase, uptake of the ferrous (Fe^{2+}) form of iron is mediated by divalent metal transporter-1 (DMT1) (25–27). The low pH of the intestinal lumen is important for these initial steps because DMT1 is a proton-coupled transporter, and acidification is therefore necessary for its optimal activity (26). Like DcytB, DMT1 is also highly regulated by iron status. The small intestine expresses four transcripts of DMT1, and mRNA levels are regulated both transcriptionally and posttranscriptionally (28, 29).

Different isoforms of the protein appear to have tissue-specific function and subcellular localization (30). Iron status appears to control not only the protein and mRNA levels for DMT1 but also the distribution of the protein in various enterocyte compartments (31). Studies have shown that intestinal DMT1 is necessary for iron absorption in mice after birth, but it appears to be dispensable for other tissues—a finding suggesting that redundant activities fulfill that role (27). Human mutations in DMT1 are associated with microcytic anemia (32), consistent with its major function in dietary iron absorption. The finding that these patients also load iron is consistent with an important DMT1 function in delivering iron to erythroid cells (see the later description of the transferrin cycle).

Molecular details of the transfer of imported nonheme iron across the intestinal mucosal cell for release into

circulation have also emerged. Investigators have long speculated that a cytosolic iron chaperone directs the fate of newly absorbed intestinal iron. Only one such factor has been identified to date, however, and its function in the intestine has yet to be fully characterized. Poly(rC)-binding protein-1 (PCBP1) has been shown to deliver iron to ferritin and is ubiquitously expressed (33). When efflux from the enterocyte is impaired, intestinal iron is known to accumulate in the ferritin storage compartment (34, 35). Deletion of intestinal ferritin in mice promotes increased dietary iron absorption and dysregulated systemic iron metabolism (36). Ferritin iron stored as a result of excess dietary absorption would probably be lost from the body as enterocytes are shed from the villus tip. It seems likely that PCBP1 may function in the intestine to help load iron onto ferritin. Whether an iron chaperone function is necessary to traffic cytosolic iron across the mucosa for its entry into portal circulation is unclear, however.

An alternate model is that iron crosses the enterocyte through a vesicular trafficking pathway (37, 38), which involves intracellular transfer to a compartment with the membrane iron exporter ferroportin and the ferroxidase hephaestin, along the ultimate target iron-free apotransferrin. Each of these factors plays an important role in export of iron from the enterocyte, but whether these factors act within the lumen of intracellular vesicles or directly at the basolateral surface is not certain because they are topologically equivalent. Ferroportin is essential for iron efflux from the intestine (39). It is believed to export iron in concert with hephaestin, a membrane-bound ceruloplasmin homolog that oxidizes ferrous iron to the ferric form (35). Ceruloplasmin itself can also fulfill this function (40), and both ferroxidases provide iron to transferrin in the correct oxidation state. Transferrin binds two atoms of ferric iron and circulates in serum to deliver iron to peripheral tissues. In fact, fasting transferrin saturation is recommended as the most sensitive serum index of iron status because postprandial increases can otherwise cause false-positive indications of iron-loading (41).

The Transferrin Cycle

Circulating transferrin delivers iron by binding to cell surface receptors. Two receptors that specifically and uniquely recognize transferrin as a ligand are known. Transferrin receptor-1 has long been studied as the functional partner in iron uptake and is ubiquitously expressed (42, 43). Its closely related homolog, transferrin receptor-2, has a more restricted expression pattern and predominates in liver, where it plays an iron-sensing role in metabolism (44–46).

Uptake of iron by cells from the transferrin-receptor binding complex begins with its internalization by clathrin-mediated endocytosis (Fig. 10.3). Clathrin-coated vesicles deliver their cargo to acidic intracellular compartments called early endosomes. The low pH of this environment promotes release of iron and stabilizes the binding of apotransferrin

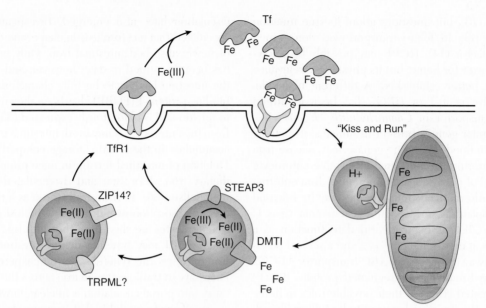

Fig. 10.3. Transferrin (Tf) cycle. *DMT1,* divalent metal transporter-1; *Fe,* iron; *STEAP3,* a ferrireductase; *TfR1,* transferrin receptor 1; *TRPML,* transient receptor potential cation channel, mucolipin subfamily (a transporter); *ZIP 14,* a zinc transporter.

to the receptor. Together, they are recycled back to the cell surface, where apotransferrin dissociates from the receptor at neutral pH (47). Reduction of ferric iron released in the lumen of the endosome is supported by the ferrireductase Steap3 (48). Subsequent transport of ferrous iron in erythroid cells is mediated by DMT1 (49). In one model, investigators proposed that reticulocyte endosomes bearing iron-bound transferrin directly deliver cargo to mitochondria for heme biosynthesis, the "kiss-and-run hypothesis" (50).

Still, other transporters may provide for iron transfer in the endosomal-lysosomal system in peripheral tissues, including Zip14 (51) and TRPML1 (52). On entering the cell cytoplasm, iron is either rapidly metabolized or stored in ferritin. A small labile iron pool exists and is in the micromolar range in most cell types. In excess, this free iron can produce reactive oxygen species that can cause cellular damage. For example, loss of iron storage as a result of tissue-specific deletion of ferritin heavy chain in mice leads to liver damage (53). Defects in transferrin's intracellular trafficking are also known to give rise to anemia in the *hbd* hemoglobin-deficit mouse model as a result of mutation of Sec15l1 of the exocyst complex (54). Emerging evidence indicates that the iron-regulated myotonic dystrophy kinase–related CDC42-binding kinase α (MRCKα) may be involved in modulating transferrin-mediated iron uptake, possibly by its association with the actin cytoskeletal network and the transferrin–transferrin receptor complex (55). Clearly, the transferrin cycle must be regulated tightly and in a coordinated manner to control the distribution of iron sufficient to meet metabolic demands but limited to avoid toxicity.

Regulation of Iron Status at the Cellular Level

A major mechanism regulating iron status at the cellular level involves posttranscriptional regulation of the

transferrin receptor, ferritin, and other key metabolic factors. Uptake of iron into cells is proportional to levels of the transferrin receptor and reflects the needs of the cell; otherwise, excess iron must be stored in ferritin to prevent oxidative damage, as described earlier. Transcripts for the transferrin receptor and ferritin are known to contain iron-responsive elements (IREs), stem-loop RNA structures that control stability and translation of the mRNAs, respectively (56, 57). IREs are bound by iron regulatory proteins (IRP1 and IRP2) to regulate expression of these and many other important factors in iron transport, utilization, and storage in a coordinated way (Table 10.3). Under low-iron conditions, IRPs confer translational control by binding to IREs present in the 5′ ends of iron storage or efflux proteins (ferritin and ferroportin) to reduce protein synthesis. At the same time, IRP binding to 3′ ends of mRNAs for iron uptake factors (transferrin receptor-1 and DMT1) increases message stability to enhance levels of transport into cells. Conversely, under high-iron conditions, IRP–IRE binding is lost, and synthesis for proteins involved in storage or efflux is increased, whereas iron uptake is reduced.

Cellular iron also exerts transcriptional effects through antioxidant elements (AREs) found in genes for ferritin heavy and light chains (58, 59). In addition, transcription of the ferritin genes is responsive to heme (iron in protoporphyrin X; see Fig. 10.1), exerted through its interactions with BACH1, a DNA-binding transcriptional repressor (60). Indirectly, ferritin levels also respond to regulation of protein levels of IRP1 and IRP2 by the iron sensing hemerythrin domain of FBXL5 (61, 62). This E3 ligase is destabilized when iron (or oxygen) is low; conversely, FBXL5 is stabilized by high iron and oxygen and is enabled to target the IRPs for degradation. To add an additional layer of complexity, IRP1 is a bifunctional

ligase parkin regulates neuronal DMT1 as well, thus providing important clues into the relationships among aging, iron, and neurodegeneration (142, 143).

Use of Iron Supplements

The frequency, severity, and global nature of the adverse effects of nutritional deficiency in iron have led to great efforts in correcting the problem. Iron fortification to prevent nutritional iron deficiency, either through the open market or government-regulated programs, has been successful in developed countries, but it has not proven as effective in less-developed countries where risk for iron deficiency is perhaps more problematic (144, 145). On an individual basis, dietary recommendations to increase food with high iron availability (e.g., meat sources), to consume foods with the ability to enhance iron absorption (e.g., vitamin C–rich sources), and to avoid foods that reduce absorption (e.g., tea) are made, and iron supplements are used to satisfy greater needs. Pregnant women, preterm or low birth weight infants, young children, and women in their reproductive years are likely to benefit from iron supplementation. People with kidney failure who are undergoing dialysis and individuals with inflammatory bowel diseases who have difficulty with iron absorption may also need iron supplements. The anemia resulting from hookworm infection and its associated blood loss is also ameliorated by iron supplementation. The use of supplements may be contraindicated in ACD, however (103).

Iron fortification policies have been criticized because they also may pose problems for people with iron overload or susceptibility for genetic or acquired iron loading. Similarly, the benefits of iron supplementation in pregnant women are controversial, given that high iron concentrations can promote oxidative stress and complications such as gestational diabetes (145, 146). As a result, weekly supplementation (as opposed to daily supplementation) and strategies focused on prevention of iron deficiency (rather than treatment of anemia) have been proposed (145, 147).

Folate is commonly provided with iron supplements in pregnant women and children and is justified not only because of the possibility that anemia stems from folic acid deficiency, but also because folate reduces the risk of neural tube defects. Nonetheless, the presence of other micronutrient deficiencies is an important concern when iron supplementation is used to treat iron deficiency anemia. Vitamin A deficiency affects iron mobilization and often coexists with iron deficiency such that providing iron alone is not as effective as supplementation with combination of these micronutrients (146). Riboflavin has similar effects. Similarly, iron deficiency can disrupt vitamin A metabolism (148), and it can limit the effectiveness of iodine supplementation (111). Thus, micronutrient supplements must be used judiciously to address metabolic problems correctly.

ASSESSMENT OF IRON STATUS

Blood loss, increased physiologic demands, and limited diet promote iron deficiency and iron deficiency anemia. ACD or inflammation is also prevalent in patients with medical illness. Important symptoms include fatigue resulting from the requirement for iron in oxidative metabolism. Clinical tests involve analysis of several indicators in blood samples (Table 10.4), with values reflecting iron depletion or iron-restricted red blood cell production (149, 150). Problems with excessive iron absorption and overload are also common, and diagnosis generally relies on the same blood tests.

Iron Deficiency and Iron Deficiency Anemia

The hallmark of frank iron deficiency anemia is low hemoglobin levels (male, <13 g/dL; and female, <12 g/dL). Transferrin saturation (<20%) and serum ferritin (<30 ng/mL) are typically low, and inflammation should be absent (see later). Mean corpuscular hemoglobin (MCH) and mean corpuscular volume (MCV) are indicators of iron deficiency in red blood cells. Vitamin B_{12} or folate deficiency can also promote anemia with or without iron deficiency, and cell size (microcytosis) is important in distinguishing iron deficiency anemia. In iron deficiency without anemia, hemoglobin levels may be normal because a large amount of iron is stored in the body. Reduced serum ferritin is the key indicator of iron depletion because this storage protein circulates in a manner dependent on iron availability. Iron deficiency is typically characterized by ferritin levels lower than 30 ng/mL. In the presence of inflammation, ferritin levels may be normal or even high because ferritin is an acute

TABLE 10.4	TESTS FOR IRON DEFICIENCY AND IRON DEFICIENCY ANEMIA	
	PARAMETERS	VALUES
Iron depletion in the body	Serum iron	50–180 mg/dL
	Transferrin	200–360 mg/dL
	Transferrin saturation	20%–50%
	Ferritin	30–300 ng/mL
	sTfR	0.76–1.76 mg/L
	Log ratio of sTfR to serum ferritin	<1
Iron deficient red cell production	Hemoglobin	12–16 g/dL (female) 13–17 g/dL (male)
	MCV	80–100 fL
	RDW	11–15
	MCH	28–35 pg
	HYPO	<5%
	CHr	28–35 pg

CHr, reticulocyte hemoglobin; HYPO, hypochromic red blood cells; MCH, mean corpuscular hemoglobin; MCV, mean corpuscular volume; RDW, red blood cell distribution width; sTFR, soluble transferrin receptor.

phase reactant protein. In this setting, iron deficiency is positively identified by low transferrin saturation (20% to 50% normal range).

Iron deficiency is also reflected in lower MCH (28 to 35 pg normal range) or higher red blood cell width (RDW, 11 to 15 normal range). Reticulocyte hemoglobin content (CHr) is an early indicator of iron deficiency that may be particularly useful for diagnosis in children because they are vulnerable to neurologic damage caused by low iron status (151). The normal adult range is 28 to 35 pg; values indicating anemia in small children are lower than 28 pg (152).

Anemia of Chronic Disease with and without Iron Deficiency

Patients with chronic or inflammatory disease are identified with a high serum C-reactive protein level greater than 0.5 mg/dL. ACD can be diagnosed by low hemoglobin concentrations (male, <13 g/dL; female, <12 g/dL) and low transferrin saturation (<20%). Serum ferritin concentrations are normal or increased (>100 ng/mL). For patients with ACD and iron deficiency, serum ferritin levels may fall into the normal range of 30 to 100 ng/mL. To determine the diagnosis of ACD with iron deficiency, a soluble form of transferrin receptor present in serum (sTfR) is useful. sTfR is proportional to the amount of surface receptors and therefore the number of progenitor erythroid cells (153). A derived value for the ratio of sTfR to log ferritin greater than 2 defines ACD with iron deficiency, whereas a ratio of sTfR to log ferritin less than 1 is typical in ACD without iron deficiency (150). Two other useful markers are CHr and hypochromic red cells (HYPO), which are less than 28 pg and less than 5% in iron deficiency, respectively. Investigators have argued that these values are the most direct indicators of functional iron deficiency whereas iron stores fail to be mobilized from the reticuloendothelial system to bone marrow in ACD (154).

Hemochromatosis

Whether genetic or acquired, hemochromatosis results from accrual of toxic levels of iron in liver, heart, and endocrine tissues. Because iron is primarily stored in liver, the determination of iron content in liver biopsies by atomic absorption spectroscopy is a definitive means of diagnosis. Transferrin saturation and serum ferritin are perhaps more useful immediate indices of the disease state, however. Both indicators reflect increased iron stores in the absence of inflammation. Transferrin saturation greater than 45% can identify most cases of *HFE*-associated hemochromatosis (155). A rise in serum ferritin usually occurs subsequent to increased transferrin saturation on iron loading, and ferritin levels higher than 1000 ng/mL are used as an indication for liver biopsy (41).

Future Prospects

Better clinical laboratory tools to assess iron status are on the horizon. Use of analyzers that provide values for CHr and HYPO (ADVIA 120 and 2120 [Bayer, now Siemens] and Sysmex XE-2100) are becoming more widespread. Advanced noninvasive and continuous monitoring devices for hemoglobin are anticipated to be of great utility for iron studies in small children (151). Serum immunoassays for hepcidin also have become available and may become routinely applied to differentiate between patients with ACD and iron deficiency and patients with ACD who do not have iron deficiency (156, 157). Magnetic resonance imaging holds great promise to determine iron content of liver in patients with iron-loading disorders (158). Hepcidin-replacement therapies are under development (10). In terms of population studies, body iron determinations based on the use of log-transformed sTfR and ferritin ratios to define iron status have been recommended by the WHO and have shown promise in monitoring the prevalence of iron deficiency in the United States (159). These and other major advances in diagnostic tools and clinical approaches are clearly keeping pace with the rapid discoveries in iron metabolism.

ACKNOWLEDGMENTS

This research is supported by the National Institutes of Health grant numbers R01 DK064750, R01 ES014638, R21 DA025573, RC1 DK086774, and R03 DA027030.

REFERENCES

1. Guggenheim KY. J Nutr 1995;125:1822–5.
2. Andrews NC. Blood 2008;112:219–30.
3. Theil EC. Annu Rev Nutr 2004;24:327–43.
4. Miret S, Simpson RJ, McKie AT. Annu Rev Nutr 2003;23: 283–301.
5. Hunt JR, Gallagher SK, Johnson LK. Am J Clin Nutr 1994; 59:1381–5.
6. Siegenberg D, Baynes RD, Bothwell TH et al. Am J Clin Nutr 1991;53:537–41.
7. Hallberg L, Brune M, Erlandsson M et al. Am J Clin Nutr 1991;53:112–9.
8. Goyer RA. Environ Health Perspect 1993;100:177–87.
9. Kwong WT, Friello P, Semba RD. Sci Total Environ 2004; 330:21–37.
10. Pietrangelo A. Gastroenterology 2010;139:393–408.
11. Hunt JR, Roughead ZK. Am J Clin Nutr 2000;71:94–102.
12. Roughead ZK, Hunt JR. Am J Clin Nutr 2000;72:982–9.
13. Shayeghi M, Latunde-Dada GO, Oakhill JS et al. Cell 2005; 122:789–801.
14. Qiu A, Jansen M, Sakaris A et al. Cell 2006;127:917–28.
15. Rajagopal A, Rao AU, Amigo J et al. Nature 2008;453: 1127–31.
16. Raffin SB, Woo CH, Roost KT et al. J Clin Invest 1974; 54:1344–52.
17. Quigley JG, Yang Z, Worthington MT et al. Cell 2004;118: 757–66.
18. Krishnamurthy P, Ross DD, Nakanishi T et al. J Biol Chem 2004;279:24218–25.
19. McKie AT, Barrow D, Latunde-Dada GO et al. Science 2001;291:1755–9.

20. Gunshin H, Starr CN, Direnzo C et al. Blood 2005;106:2879–83.
21. Latunde-Dada GO, Van der Westhuizen J, Vulpe CD et al. Blood Cells Mol Dis 2002;29:356–60.
22. Muckenthaler M, Roy CN, Custodio AO et al. Nat Genet 2003;34:102–7.
23. Nelson JE, Mugford VR, Kilcourse E et al. Am J Physiol 2010;298:G57–62.
24. Constantine CC, Anderson GJ, Vulpe CD et al. Br J Haematol 2009;147:140–9.
25. Fleming MD, Trenor CC 3rd, Su MA et al. Nat Genet 1997;16:383–6.
26. Gunshin H, Mackenzie B, Berger UV et al. Nature 1997;388:482–8.
27. Gunshin H, Fujiwara Y, Custodio AO et al. J Clin Invest 2005;115:1258–66.
28. Hubert N, Hentze MW. Proc Natl Acad Sci U S A 2002;99:12345–50.
29. Lee PL, Gelbart T, West C et al. Blood Cells Mol Dis 1998;24:199–215.
30. Lam-Yuk-Tseung S, Gros P. Biochemistry 2006;45:2294–301.
31. Ma Y, Specian RD, Yeh KY et al. Am J Physiol 2002;283:G965–74.
32. Mims MP, Guan Y, Pospisilova D et al. Blood 2005;105:1337–42.
33. Shi H, Bencze KZ, Stemmler TL et al. Science 2008;320:1207–10.
34. Edwards JA, Hoke JE, Mattioli M et al. J Lab Clin Med 1977;90:68–76.
35. Vulpe CD, Kuo YM, Murphy TL et al. Nat Genet 1999;21:195–9.
36. Vanoaica L, Darshan D, Richman L et al. Cell Metab 2010;12:273–82.
37. Alvarez-Hernandez X, Smith M, Glass J. Blood 2000;95:721–3.
38. Moriya M, Linder MC. Am J Physiol 2006;290:G301–9.
39. Donovan A, Lima CA, Pinkus JL et al. Cell Metab 2005;1:191–200.
40. Cherukuri S, Potla R, Sarkar J et al. Cell Metab 2005;2:309–19.
41. Clark P, Britton LJ, Powell LW. Clin Biochem Rev 2010;31:3–8.
42. Testa U, Pelosi E, Peschle C. Crit Rev Oncog 1993;4:241–76.
43. Enns CA, Rutledge EA, Williams AM. Biomembranes 1996;4:255–87.
44. Kawabata H, Yang R, Hirama T et al. J Biol Chem 1999;274:20826–32.
45. Robb A, Wessling-Resnick M. Blood 2004;104:4294–9.
46. Johnson MB, Enns CA. Blood 2004;104:4287–93.
47. Richardson DR, Ponka P. Biochim Biophys Acta 1997;1331:1–40.
48. Ohgami RS, Campagna DR, Greer EL et al. Nat Genet 2005;37:1264–9.
49. Fleming MD, Romano MA, Su MA et al. Proc Natl Acad Sci U S A 1998;95:1148–53.
50. Zhang AS, Sheftel AD, Ponka P. Blood 2005;105:368–75.
51. Zhao N, Gao J, Enns CA et al. J Biol Chem 2010;285:32141–50.
52. Dong XP, Cheng X, Mills E et al. Nature 2008;455:992–6.
53. Darshan D, Vanoaica L, Richman L et al. Hepatology 2009;50:852–60.
54. Lim JE, Jin O, Bennett C et al. Nat Genet 2005;37:1270–3.
55. Cmejla R, Ptackova P, Petrak J et al. Biochem Biophys Res Commun 2010;395:163–7.
56. Wallander ML, Leibold EA, Eisenstein RS. Biochim Biophys Acta 2006;1763:668–89.
57. Theil EC, Goss DJ. Chem Rev 2009;109:4568–79.
58. Wasserman WW, Fahl WE. Proc Natl Acad Sci U S A 1997;94:5361–6.
59. Torti FM, Torti SV. Blood 2002;99:3505–16.
60. Hintze KJ, Katoh Y, Igarashi K et al. J Biol Chem 2007;282:34365–71.
61. Vashisht AA, Zumbrennen KB, Huang X et al. Science 2009;326:718–21.
62. Salahudeen AA, Thompson JW, Ruiz JC et al. Science 2009;326:722–6.
63. Ye H, Rouault TA. Biochemistry 2010;49:4945–56.
64. Sheftel A, Stehling O, Lill R. Trends Endocrinol Metab 2010;21:302–14.
65. Hentze MW, Muckenthaler MU, Galy B et al. Cell 2010;142:24–38.
66. Galy B, Ferring-Appel D, Sauer SW et al. Cell Metab 2010;12:194–201.
67. Shaw GC, Cope JJ, Li L et al. Nature 2006;440:96–100.
68. Paradkar PN, Zumbrennen KB, Paw BH et al. Mol Cell Biol 2009;29:1007–16.
69. Chen W, Paradkar PN, Li L et al. Proc Natl Acad Sci U S A 2009;106:16263–8.
70. Richardson DR, Lane DJ, Becker EM et al. Proc Natl Acad Sci U S A 2010;107:10775–82.
71. Sheftel AD, Lill R. Ann Med 2009;41:82–99.
72. Devireddy LR, Hart DO, Goetz DH et al. Cell 2010;141:1006–17.
73. Levi S, Corsi B, Bosisio M et al. J Biol Chem 2001;276:24437–40.
74. Surguladze N, Patton S, Cozzi A et al. Biochem J 2005;388:731–40.
75. Li JY, Paragas N, Ned RM et al. Dev Cell 2009;16:35–46.
76. Coffman LG, Parsonage D, D'Agostino R Jr et al. Proc Natl Acad Sci U S A 2009;106:570–5.
77. Worwood M, Cragg SJ, Wagstaff M et al. Clin Sci (Lond) 1979;56:83–7.
78. Cohen LA, Gutierrez L, Weiss A et al. Blood 2010;116:1574–84.
79. De Domenico I, Vaughn MB, Paradkar PN et al. Cell Metab 2011;13:57–67.
80. Chen TT, Li L, Chung DH et al. J Exp Med 2005;202:955–65.
81. Li L, Fang CJ, Ryan JC et al. Proc Natl Acad Sci U S A 2010;107:3505–10.
82. De Domenico I, Ward DM, Kaplan J. Blood 2009;114:4546–51.
83. Asano T, Komatsu M, Yamaguchi-Iwai Y et al. Mol Cell Biol 2011.
84. Wang W, Knovich MA, Coffman LG et al. Biochim Biophys Acta 2010;1800:760–9.
85. Nicolas G, Bennoun M, Porteu A et al. Proc Natl Acad Sci U S A 2002;99:4596–601.
86. Nicolas G, Viatte L, Bennoun M et al. Blood Cells Mol Dis 2002;29:327–35.
87. Nemeth E, Tuttle MS, Powelson J et al. Science 2004;306:2090–3.
88. Verga Falzacappa MV, Vujic Spasic M, Kessler R et al. Blood 2007;109:353–8.
89. Wrighting DM, Andrews NC. Blood 2006;108:3204–9.
90. Lee P, Peng H, Gelbart T et al. Proc Natl Acad Sci U S A 2005;102:1906–10.
91. Nemeth E, Rivera S, Gabayan V et al. J Clin Invest 2004;113:1271–6.
92. Lee PL, Beutler E. Annu Rev Pathol 2009;4:489–515.
93. Babitt JL, Huang FW, Wrighting DM et al. Nat Genet 2006;38:531–9.
94. Du X, She E, Gelbart T et al. Science 2008;320:1088–92.
95. Finberg KE, Heeney MM, Campagna DR et al. Nat Genet 2008;40:569–71.
96. Silvestri L, Pagani A, Nai A et al. Cell Metab 2008;8:502–11.
97. van Dijk BA, Laarakkers CM, Klaver SM et al. Br J Haematol 2008;142:979–85.

98. Nemeth E, Roetto A, Garozzo G et al. Blood 2005;105:1803–6.
99. Schmidt PJ, Toran PT, Giannetti AM et al. Cell Metab 2008;7:205–14.
100. Gao J, Chen J, Kramer M et al. Cell Metab 2009;9:217–27.
101. Nemeth E, Valore EV, Territo M et al. Blood 2003;101:2461–3.
102. Nicolas G, Chauvet C, Viatte L et al. J Clin Invest 2002; 110:1037–44.
103. Wessling-Resnick M. Annu Rev Nutr 2010;30:105–22.
104. Shah YM, Matsubara T, Ito S et al. Cell Metab 2009;9:152–64.
105. Mastrogiannaki M, Matak P, Keith B et al. J Clin Invest 2009;119:1159–66.
106. Hahn PF, Bale WF, Ross JF et al. J Exp Med 1943;78:169–88.
107. Zimmermann MB, Hurrell RF. Lancet 2007;370:511–20.
108. World Health Organization/UNICEF/United Nations University. Iron Deficiency Anemia: Assessment, Prevention, and Control. Geneva: World Health Organization, 2001.
109. Gardner GW, Edgerton VR, Barnard RJ et al. Am J Clin Nutr 1975;28:982–8.
110. Finch CA, Gollnick PD, Hlastala MP et al. J Clin Invest 1979;64:129–37.
111. Zimmermann MB. Annu Rev Nutr 2006;26:367–89.
112. Salas RE, Gamaldo CE, Allen RP. Curr Opin Neurol 2010; 23:401–6.
113. Bhaskaram P. Br J Nutr 2001;85(Suppl 2):S75–80.
114. de Silva A, Atukorala S, Weerasinghe I et al. Am J Clin Nutr 2003;77:234–41.
115. Beard J. J Nutr 2003;133(Suppl):1468S–72S.
116. World Health Organization. The Prevalence of Anemia in Women: A Tabulation of Available Information. Geneva: World Health Organization, 1992.
117. Allen KJ, Gurrin LC, Constantine CC et al. N Engl J Med 2008;358:221–30.
118. Roncagliolo M, Garrido M, Walter T et al. Am J Clin Nutr 1998;68:683–90.
119. Lukowski AF, Koss M, Burden MJ et al. Nutr Neurosci 2010;13:54–70.
120. Shafir T, Angulo-Barroso R, Jing Y et al. Early Hum Dev 2008;84:479–85.
121. Beard JL, Connor JR. Annu Rev Nutr 2003;23:41–58.
122. Lozoff B, Beard J, Connor J et al. Nutr Rev 2006;64:S34–43.
123. Perez VP, de Lima MN, da Silva RS et al. Curr Neurovasc Res 2010;7:15–22.
124. Fredriksson A, Archer T. J Neural Transm 2007;114: 195–203.
125. Rao R, Georgieff MK. Semin Fetal Neonatal Med 2007;12: 54–63.
126. Guralnik JM, Eisenstaedt RS, Ferrucci L et al. Blood 2004; 104:2263–8.
127. Yip R, Dallman PR. Am J Clin Nutr 1988;48:1295–300.
128. Ferrucci L, Semba RD, Guralnik JM et al. Blood 2010; 115:3810–6.
129. Levenson CW, Tassabehji NM. Ageing Res Rev 2004;3: 251–63.
130. Zecca L, Youdim MB, Riederer P et al. Nat Rev Neurosci 2004;5:863–73.
131. Moalem S, Percy ME, Andrews DF et al. Am J Med Genet 2000;93:58–66.
132. Bartzokis G, Lu PH, Tishler TA et al. J Alzheimers Dis 2010; 20:333–41.
133. Lehmann DJ, Worwood M, Ellis R et al. J Med Genet 2006;43:e52.
134. Connor JR, Lee SY. J Alzheimers Dis 2006;10:267–76.
135. Crapper McLachlan DR, Dalton AJ, Kruck TP et al. Lancet 1991;337:1304–8.
136. Kaur D, Yantiri F, Rajagopalan S et al. Neuron 2003;37: 899–909.
137. Berg D. Neurochem Res 2007;32:1646–54.
138. Pezzella A, d'Ischia M, Napolitano A et al. J Med Chem 1997;40:2211–6.
139. Youdim MB, Ben-Shachar D, Yehuda S et al. Adv Neurol 1990;53:155–62.
140. Salazar J, Mena N, Hunot S et al. Proc Natl Acad Sci U S A 2008;105:18578–83.
141. Howitt J, Putz U, Lackovic J et al. Proc Natl Acad Sci U S A 2009;106:15489–94.
142. Roth JA, Singleton S, Feng J et al. J Neurochem 2010;113: 454–64.
143. Higashi Y, Asanuma M, Miyazaki I et al. J Neurochem 2004; 89:1490–7.
144. Lynch SR. Best Pract Res Clin Haematol 2005;18:333–46.
145. Pena-Rosas J, Viteri F. Cochrane Database Syst Rev 2009; (4):CD004736.
146. Allen LH. J Nutr 2002;132:813S–9S.
147. Scholl TO. Am J Clin Nutr 2005;81:1218S–22S.
148. Hodges RE, Rucker RB, Gardner RH. Ann N Y Acad Sci 1980;355:58–61.
149. Cook JD. Best Pract Res Clin Haematol 2005;18:319–32.
150. Weiss G, Goodnough LT. N Engl J Med 2005;352:1011–23.
151. Bamberg R. Clin Lab Sci 2008;21:225–31.
152. Brugnara C, Zurakowski D, DiCanzio J et al. JAMA 1999; 281:2225–30.
153. Cook JD, Flowers CH, Skikne BS. Blood 2003;101:3359–64.
154. Punnonen K, Irjala K, Rajamaki A. Blood 1997;89:1052–7.
155. McLaren CE, McLachlan GJ, Halliday JW et al. Gastroenterology 1998;114:543–9.
156. Ganz T, Olbina G, Girelli D et al. Blood 2008;112:4292–7.
157. Koliaraki V, Marinou M, Vassilakopoulos TP et al. PLoS One 2009;4:e4581.
158. Tziomalos K, Perifanis V. World J Gastroenterol 2010;16: 1587–97.
159. Cogswell ME, Looker AC, Pfeiffer CM et al. Am J Clin Nutr 2009;89:1334–42.

SUGGESTED READINGS

Pietrangelo A. Hereditary hemochromatosis: pathogenesis, diagnosis and treatment. Gastroenterology 2010;139:393–408.

Richardson DR, Ponka P. The molecular mechanisms of the metabolism and transport of iron in normal and neoplastic cells. Biochim Biophys Acta 1997;1331:1–40.

Torti FM, Torti SV. Regulation of ferritin genes and protein. Blood 2002;99:3505–16.

Hentze MW, Muckenthaler MU, Galy B et al. Two to tango: regulation of mammalian iron metabolism. Cell 2010;142:24–38.

B.   MINERALS

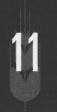

11

ZINC[1]

JANET C. KING AND ROBERT J. COUSINS

---

[1]**Abbreviations: AD**, Alzheimer disease; **AMD**, age-related macular degeneration; **EAR**, estimated average requirement; **FAO**, Food and Agriculture Organization; **GI**, gastrointestinal; **HIV**, human immunodeficiency virus; **IFN**, interferon; **K_d**, dissociation constant; **LOAEL**, lowest observed adverse effect level; **MT**, metallothionein; **NO**, nitric oxide; **RDA**, recommended dietary allowance; **UL**, tolerable upper intake level; **WHO**, World Health Organization; **ZnT**, zinc transporter.

HISTORICAL BACKGROUND

Zinc (Zn) essentiality in plants was established in 1869, in experimental animals in 1934, and in humans in 1961. The biochemical basis for essentiality has not been established, but it rests within the catalytic, structural, and regulatory roles of this micronutrient. Detailed reviews are available (1–4). A syndrome of anemia, hypogonadism, and dwarfism was reported in a 21-year-old Iranian man in 1961 who was subsisting on a diet of unrefined flat bread, potatoes, and milk. Shortly thereafter, a similar syndrome was observed in adolescent boys in Egypt who were also subsisting on a diet of flat bread and a few vegetables. Administration of a hospital diet improved growth and corrected the hypogonadism. Subsequent studies showed that the syndrome was primarily the result of a lack of zinc in the diet. Since the discovery of human zinc deficiency, interest in the biochemical and clinical aspects of zinc nutrition has increased exponentially.

CHEMISTRY

Zinc^{2+} (Zn^{2+}) is a stronger Lewis acid (electron acceptor) than iron (Fe^{3+}), but it is weaker than copper (Cu^{2+}). This property favors strong binding to thiolate and amine electron donors (5). Zinc exhibits fast ligand exchange, which is believed to be important for some biochemical functions. Zinc does not exhibit redox chemistry directly, but the release of Zn^{2+} from a Zn-thiolate cluster by an oxidant produces disulfide bonds. Zn–sulfur (S) thiolate bonds, therefore, are sensitive to cellular redox (6).

Analytical procedures focus on atomic absorption spectrophotometry and inductively coupled plasma emission. Both have working ranges suitable for biologic samples and have generated much of the literature in this chapter. Zinc reference standards are available from the National Institute of Standards and Technology (NIST). Of the zinc radioisotopes, only ^{65}Zn (half-life, 245 days) has been widely used in research. Stable isotopes of zinc and corresponding natural abundances are as follows: ^{64}Zn, 49%; ^{66}Zn, 29%; ^{67}Zn, 4%; ^{68}Zn, 19%; and ^{70}Zn, 1%. These isotopes have been effectively used in experiments with humans. Highly specific fluorescent probes for zinc, such as FluoZin-3, are coming into wide use (7). Applications include studies of zinc transport by cells and organelles and measures of labile Zn^{2+} concentrations (a putative free Zn^{2+} pool) within cells (8).

BIOCHEMICAL AND PHYSIOLOGIC FUNCTIONS

Zinc-dependent biochemical mechanisms that determine physiologic functions have received extensive study, but clear relationships with phenotype have not been defined. Zinc has a ubiquitous subcellular distribution, which hampers this situation. Consequently, zinc contrasts with iron, which exists in defined cellular components and has defined physiologic roles. Three general functional classes—catalytic, structural, and regulatory—define zinc's role in biology (9).

Catalytic Functions

Zinc serves a catalytic role in enzymes from all six enzyme classes (10). More than 300 zinc metalloenzymes have been identified. When the same enzyme identified in different species is counted only once, however, the number is much lower. How zinc is donated to apometalloenzymes has not been established. Zinc binding is a posttranslational protein modification, which likely requires a metal donor molecule or pH appropriate for zinc solubility, perhaps coordinated by events in the endoplasmic reticulum or a vesicular compartment. This process may require zinc transporter activity. An example is that a ZnT5/ZnT7 complex provides Zn^{2+} to activate tissue-nonspecific alkaline phosphatase (10).

An enzyme is generally considered a zinc metalloenzyme if the removal of zinc causes loss of activity without irreversibly altering the protein, and selective reconstitution with zinc restores the activity. Examples are the nucleotide polymerases (RNA polymerases I, II, and III), alkaline phosphatases, and the carbonic anhydrases. Unequivocal evidence of a direct link between signs of zinc deficiency or toxicity and a specific metalloenzyme has not been shown in complex organisms, and it is most likely an overt physiologic defect would occur only if the zinc-requiring enzyme was rate limiting in a critical biochemical pathway. Older literature has examples of relationships among zinc, enzyme, and disease (e.g., alcohol dehydrogenase and liver disease and RNA polymerases and growth retardation). Such enzyme changes are no longer considered as representing a critical function for zinc. Reports documenting zinc-responsive control of enzymes for intermediary metabolism, perhaps operating through effects on intracellular zinc concentrations, have been published (11, 12). Demonstrated physiologic control of some zinc transporters offers a new appreciation of the way in which coordinated Zn^{2+} fluxes in cells could influence enzyme activity (reviewed in 13).

Structural Functions

The structural function for zinc had its origin in 1985 with identification of a transcription factor having coordinating zinc-binding motifs (14). These motifs ("zinc fingers") use cysteine and histidine to form a tetrahedral Zn^{2+} coordination complex. These have the general structure $-C-X_2-C-X_n-C-X_2-C-$, where C designates cysteine or histidine and X designates other amino acids. Zinc fingers have two to four cysteines and up to two histidines. Removal of zinc from zinc finger proteins alters folding and results in loss of function and probably degradation. Classic examples of zinc finger transcription factors are the retinoic acid and calcitriol nuclear receptors. The human transcriptome has 2500 zinc finger protein genes (15). This represents approximately 8% of the genome, a finding suggesting that a significant portion of the zinc requirement is allocated to maintain occupancy of zinc finger proteins. The mouse transcriptome has a comparable number of zinc finger genes (16). Binding affinity (apparent stability constants) of the fingers varies widely (dissociation constant $[K_d] = 10^8 - 10^{11}\ M^{-1}$). By comparison, metallothionein (MT) binds zinc strongly (to a maximum $K_d = 10^{12}\ M^{-1}$) (17). Both nitrosative stress and oxidative stress can disrupt zinc finger motifs and can cause loss of function, at least for oxidative stress (18). Because zinc fingers exhibit a spectrum of binding affinities (19), some sites may be particularly facile and potentially influenced by dietary zinc through zinc transporter activity.

Zinc finger proteins have a broad cell distribution and also bind RNA molecules and facilitate protein–protein interactions. These functions broaden their biologic role to include transcriptional and translational control, modulation of those processes, and signal transduction. Interest in zinc finger motifs is considerable because of their potential as targets for therapeutic interventions, including gene therapy.

Zn/S clusters, such as those in MT, may act as low redox potential units (17). These zinc thiol clusters, when oxidized by cellular oxidants (including oxidative and nitrosative stressors), results in zinc release. The glutathione/glutathione disulfide (GSH/GSSG) redox couple and some selenium compounds influence zinc release, which potentially integrates MT into cellular redox mechanisms. Nitric oxide (NO) may also mobilize zinc from this protein's thiolate clusters (20, 21). This mobilization may be limited to the protein's beta domain (3 Zn cluster), whereas the alpha domain (4 Zn cluster) is viewed as having a detoxifying role. Increased oxidative and nitrosative stress that accompanies zinc deficiency (22, 23) may be explained in part by induction of NO synthase (24, 25).

A hybrid function between structure and regulatory is that movement of large quantities of zinc are associated with insulin secretion by pancreatic β cells, zinc metallodigestive enzyme secretion by pancreatic acinar cells, and acid secretion by parietal cells of the stomach. In the first two instances, Zn^{2+} has a stabilizing role during the secretory process, whereas Zn^{2+} may replace hydrogen ion (H^+) during gastric acid release (26, 27). The transporters

ZnT8, ZnT2, and ZIP11 are the likely major players for these functions.

Regulatory Functions

Regulation of gene expression is a biochemical role for zinc. Originally identified as an active component of the metalloregulatory mechanism for *MT* gene regulation, the metal-response element (MRE)–binding transcription factor 1 (MTF1) now is believed to provide zinc responsiveness to many genes (28, 29), including acting as a master regulatory transcription factors (30) for miRNA genes involved in gene repression. Null mutation of the *MTF1* gene produces embryonic lethality in mice, a finding indicating importance in animals. On zinc occupancy, MTF1 translocates to the nucleus, where it participates in chromatin binding through MREs of the gene promoter. Polymorphisms in the zinc finger domain of the human *MTF1* gene (31) suggest the possibility of genetic variation in the response of MTF1-regulated genes to dietary zinc intakes. A homologous transcription factor MTF2, documented to be involved in stem cell development (32), may repress genes during normal zinc status and produce activation on zinc depletion. Reciprocal expression of zinc-responsive genes, including zinc transporters, that maintain zinc homeostasis may be regulated by these and other transcription factors that provide opposite responses to zinc status.

The second regulatory role executed by zinc is as a regulator of cell signaling pathways. This places Zn^{2+} in an intracellular role that is analogous to calcium (Ca^{2+}), except at a finer level of control. A primary mode of action is through regulation of kinase and phosphorylase activity (33–35). Zn^{2+} is a powerful inhibitor of phosphatases in the low micromolar range. Such control of phosphorylation and dephosphorylation could explain many of the effects attributed to zinc on activity of phosphorylated transcription factors, cell surface receptor binding of growth factors and cytokines, and activity of key phosphorylated substrates within cells. The profound effects of zinc on the immune system may thus be traceable to effects of Zn^{2+} availability to indirectly regulate transcription factors such as the STATs, NFAT and CREBP, as well as the phosphatase, calcineurin and the cytoplasmic protein tyrosine kinase, lymphocyte-specific protein tyrosine kinase. The coordination of such activities may relate to any one or several of the 24 zinc transporters that exhibit differing specificity of expression in various cell types. Relevant examples are the influence of ZIP8 on interferon gamma (IFN-γ) production by T cells, and regulation by ZIP6 of lipopolysaccharide-induced histocompatibility complex in dendritic cells (36, 37).

Zinc is abundant in the central nervous system. A considerable portion is in the form of ionic Zn^{2+}, in concentrations referred to as $[Zn^{2+}]i$ from the picomolar up to the millimolar range in synaptic vesicles (38). Zinc affects activity of *N*-methyl-D-aspartate and γ-aminobutyric acid receptors to influence synaptic transmission. Neuronal [Zn] is tightly controlled by a brain-specific MT and members of both the ZnT and ZIP transporter families. The mechanism of zinc transport across the blood–brain barrier has not been established. Dietary zinc deficiency has been shown to alter brain zinc homeostasis (39–41). Cerebral ischemia leads to Zn^{2+} release, which participates in activation of downstream signaling cascades (particularly P13K/Akt) and oxidative and nitrosative stress that leads to necrotic, apoptotic, and autophagic death of neuronal and glial cells (38, 42).

BIOAVAILABILITY

The bioavailability of zinc is the fraction of zinc intake that is absorbed, retained, and used for physiologic functions. Zinc bioavailability in healthy individuals is determined primarily by the quantities of zinc and phytate in the diet (43). In general, the *amount* of zinc absorbed increases with the amount ingested, and the *fractional* absorption declines. However, if the diet is high in phytate, the net increase in absorbed zinc with increases in dietary intake is blunted significantly. Although changes in the quantity of bioavailable zinc directly influence the amount of zinc that is absorbed, the effect of zinc status over time on zinc absorption is questionable and, at most, plays a minor role in the maintenance of zinc homeostasis (44, 45).

Factors Affecting Bioavailability

Zinc absorption is most efficient from aqueous sources in the absence of food. With intakes lower than 5 mg, absorption is close to 100% when zinc is consumed in an aqueous solution in the fasting state (46). When zinc is ingested with food, the amount absorbed can vary from 5% to more than 50%, depending on the amount of zinc and phytate in the diet (44). Modeling studies showed that the maximal amount of zinc absorbed per day is approximately 7 mg if the diet is low in phytate and if zinc intakes are distributed throughout the day.

The efficiency of zinc absorption from plant foods is lower than that from animal source foods (43). Phytate (myoinositol hexaphosphate), which is present in plant products, especially cereals and legumes, irreversibly binds zinc in the intestinal lumen and accounts for the lower efficiency of absorption from plant foods. The negative effect on absorption is determined by the inositol hexaphosphates and pentaphosphates that bind zinc. When plant foods are fermented (leavened breads and porridges from fermented cereals), the fermenting organisms produce phytases that break down phytate and release the zinc, thus making it available for absorption (47). Because phytate is a major inhibitor of zinc absorption, the phytate–zinc molar ratio is used to estimate the likely absorption of zinc from a mixed diet. It can be calculated as follows: (phytate content of foods/660)/(zinc content of foods/65.4), where 660 and 65.4 represent the molecular or atomic weights of phytate and zinc, respectively (48). Phytate–zinc molar ratios greater than 15 are generally considered to result in relatively poor zinc bioavailability, those between 5 and 15 are considered to result in medium bioavailability, and those less than 5 are considered to result in good bioavailability. Most plant foods have phytate–zinc molar ratios greater than 15 (seeds and nuts, whole grain cereals, beans and lentils, and tubers). Zinc absorption from those plant foods generally is less than 1 mg/100 g of food, whereas approximately 2 to 2.5 mg zinc is absorbed from 100 g of meat.

A mathematical model of zinc absorption has been developed to predict the amount of zinc absorbed as a function of dietary zinc and phytate (49). This model is used to develop recommendations for the zinc fortification of flour from various cereal grains and to predict the availability of zinc from zinc-fortified cereals. Plant breeding or genetic engineering strategies that either reduce the content of inhibitors (e.g., phytate) or increase the expression of compounds that enhance zinc absorption (e.g., amino acids) have been considered to improve the bioavailability of zinc from plant foods (50).

Because calcium has the propensity to form complexes with phytate and zinc that are insoluble, investigators have proposed that the phytate–zinc molar ratio should be multiplied by the dietary calcium concentration to improve the prediction of zinc bioavailability (51). The interaction with calcium is complex, however, and the effect of calcium on the phytate–zinc interaction is not consistent. Thus, the effect of calcium is usually ignored when determining the effect of phytate on zinc absorption. Supplemental or dietary calcium without phytate has little to no effect on zinc absorption at an adequate level of intake.

Nutrient Interactions

Interactions with other divalent cations in the intestinal lumen may also influence zinc bioavailability. Isotopic tracer studies indicated that iron supplementation may interfere with zinc absorption and vice versa, but only when these supplements are provided simultaneously in aqueous solutions and in disproportionate molar doses (52). No evidence indicates interference when the supplements are delivered in nearly isosmolar amounts or with food. Some longer term studies suggested that, when iron and zinc are given together, each mineral may reduce the magnitude of the response observed with single-nutrient supplementation (53), although nutritional status is still enhanced to a considerable extent.

Less information is available regarding the interaction between zinc and copper. Shifts in the dietary zinc–copper ratios from 2:1 to 15:1 had no effect on copper absorption (54). However, some studies showed a negative effect of large-dose zinc supplements (~50 mg/day) on indicators of copper status (55). High levels of tin and cadmium inhibit zinc absorption, but the extent to which lower, physiologic levels affect absorption in humans is unknown. The relative bioavailability of nanoparticles of zinc (oxide or phosphate) is not known, but these may see use as future food additives (56).

Food Sources

The quality of dietary zinc sources is determined by the amount and bioavailability of zinc from the foods. Organs and flesh of mammals, fowl, fish, and crustaceans are the richest food sources of zinc; and because these foods do not contain phytate, they are particularly good sources of absorbable zinc. Eggs and dairy foods also are free of phytate, but they have lower zinc concentrations than organ or flesh foods. Cereals and legumes contain a modest amount of zinc, but their high phytate content reduces the amount of zinc available. Many breakfast cereals are fortified with zinc, and they are one of the major sources of zinc in the US diet. Fruits and vegetables are low in zinc.

METABOLISM

Body Zinc

Total body zinc in adult humans is between 1.5 g (females) and 2.5 g (males), making it slightly less abundant than iron. The tissue distribution of zinc is ubiquitous, however, with some tissues (e.g., the prostate) having a curiously high overall concentration. Zinc concentrations of some tissues of an adult man are shown in Table 11.1. Eighty-six percent of the total body zinc is in skeletal muscle and bone. Within organs, regional differences in zinc abundance can be striking (e.g., hippocampus of the cerebral hemispheres and β cells of the pancreas and kidney cortex). These foci of zinc concentration are believed to be functionally relevant. Approximately 95% of body zinc is intracellular, with most zinc found in the cytosol. A variable amount of cytosolic zinc may reside in vesicles. The finite amount of "free" Zn^{2+} in cells is a subject of some debate, but investigators agree that it is extremely low (8, 17). The high binding affinities of nucleic acids, protein thiols, and nitrogen ligands account for this low concentration of free Zn^{2+}.

TABLE 11.1	APPROXIMATE ZINC CONTENT OF MAJOR ORGANS AND TISSUES IN A NORMAL ADULT MAN			
	APPROXIMATE ZINC CONCENTRATION		PERCENTAGE OF BODY ZINC	
TISSUE	WET WEIGHT (μM/g)	(μg/g)	g	(%)
Skeletal muscle	0.78	51	1.53	~57
Bone	1.54	100	0.77	29
Skin	0.49	32	0.16	6
Liver	0.89	58	0.13	5
Brain	0.17	11	0.04	1.5
Kidneys	0.85	55	0.02	0.7
Heart	0.35	23	0.01	0.4
Hair	2.30	150	<0.01	~0.1
Blood plasma	0.02	1	<0.01	~0.1

Adapted from Mills CF, ed. Zinc in Human Biology. London: Springer, 1989.

Zinc Transporters

Following discovery of zinc transporters, all aspects of cellular zinc metabolism have been viewed within the context of transporter gene regulation by diet and hormones or cytokines and their genetic features, including mutations and polymorphisms in these genes that dictate phenotypic consequences. Two families of zinc transporter proteins have been defined. The ZnT family (solute carrier; SLC30A) and ZIP family (SLC39A) have numerous members (reviewed in 13). The 10 mammalian ZnTs (ZnT1 to ZnT10) are believed to facilitate zinc efflux across the cell membrane or into intracellular vesicles. In contrast, the 14 mammalian ZIP transporters (ZIP1 to ZIP14) facilitate zinc influx into cells or from vesicles. Both families exhibit tissue-specific expression. Subcellular localization does not appear uniform; rather, localization may be a function of physiologic conditions and body zinc status.

Some metal–metal interactions could be explained by specific transporters exhibiting multiple ion specificity (e.g., ZIP8 with zinc and manganese and ZIP14 with zinc and non–transferrin-bound iron). Genomic databases show that some transporter genes exhibit single nucleotide polymorphisms, which may have physiologic significance. Evidence exists that some ZnT and ZIP genes exhibit either up-regulation or down-regulation in response to zinc (13) and may contribute to the tight homeostatic control of zinc. Mechanisms responsible for regulating zinc transporters include transcription factors responsive to diet or physiologic conditions, mRNA stabilization, and intracellular proteolytic mechanisms.

Some transporters have been linked to specific genetic diseases and conditions, such as ZnT2 (low zinc in breast milk); ZIP4, (acrodermatitis enteropathica, with zinc malabsorption), and ZIP13 (Ehlers–Danlos syndrome). Other transporters have undefined associations with human disease, such as ZnT8 (type 1 and 2 diabetes), ZIP1, ZIP4, ZIP6, ZIP7, ZIP10, and ZIP14 (prostate, pancreatic, colon, or breast cancers), and ZIP14 (iron overload).

Intestinal Uptake and Absorption

The nature of absorbed zinc is not clear. As the zinc-binding macromolecules of food are liberated and degraded to smaller zinc-binding molecules during digestion, bioavailability is generally improved. Systemic factors that influence endogenous intestinal zinc secretion or result in poor hydrolysis of luminal constituents (e.g., pancreatic insufficiency; inflammatory bowel diseases) affect intestinal zinc absorption and retention.

Evidence from model systems suggests that zinc is probably transported as free solute (Zn^{2+}) or as a complex that may liberate Zn^{2+} before or after membrane transport. The way in which zinc is liberated from complexes in the neutral pH of the intestinal lumen for transport as a free solute is not known.

Absorption occurs along the entire intestinal tract (57). Perfusion studies suggested that the human jejunum exhibits the highest rate of absorption (58). Other studies with humans and animals suggested that the duodenum is quantitatively most important to the overall mass of zinc absorbed because the duodenal lumen has the highest zinc concentration after a meal (59). Endogenous secretions, including those from the pancreas, contribute to luminal zinc abundance. Overall, the extent of absorption is a function of the collective solubility of ingested zinc. Apparent absorption averages 33% and was a factor used to compute the recommended dietary allowance (RDA) (60).

Zinc absorption takes place down a concentration gradient from a relatively high luminal concentration (micromolar range) after a meal. Kinetic measurements place the Michaelis-Menten constant (K_m; affinity) for zinc uptake in the micromolar range. Maximum velocity increases during zinc-deficient conditions, a finding suggesting up-regulation of zinc transport when dietary zinc consumption is low (61, 62). Zinc uptake kinetics by the small intestine show mediated (saturable) and nonmediated (passive transport) components (61, 63). The saturable component may represent the sum of zinc transporter activity of enterocytes. The apically localized transporter ZIP4 (SLC39A4) is up-regulated in murine zinc deficiency (64, 65). A mutation of human *ZIP4* is responsible for the zinc malabsorption disorder, acrodermatitis enteropathica (66). Defective ZIP4 in this disease leads to zinc-responsive immune dysfunction and cognitive abnormalities (67).

Within enterocytes, two proteins, MT and the transporter ZnT7, influence transcellular zinc movement (68, 69) through zinc buffering and zinc trafficking into the Golgi complex to a secretory pathway, respectively. Both are dispensable, because ablation of these genes does not block zinc absorption. ZnT1 may be the major transporter that facilitates zinc efflux from enterocytes (70). Depending on dietary zinc status the transporters expressed in enterocytes undergo varying rates of synthesis, trafficking, endocytosis, and degradation. At higher luminal zinc concentrations, generated through consumption of a zinc supplement, the nonmediated (nonsaturable) component of zinc absorption may make a major contribution to total absorption. Albumin appears to be the major portal carrier for zinc after transfer across the basolateral surface of enterocytes (71).

Homeostatic Regulation

The gastrointestinal (GI) tract plays a primary role in maintaining a stable whole body zinc content, or homeostasis. At very low levels of ingested zinc, less than 1 mg/day, nearly all the zinc from a low-phytate diet is absorbed (72). Concomitantly, a reduction in zinc secretion into the intestinal lumen occurs through pancreatic secretions and from the intestine through transepithelial flux in the serosal to mucosal direction. Mechanisms regulating intestinal zinc secretion are not well understood. As the amount of ingested zinc increases, more zinc is absorbed, although the efficiency of zinc absorption declines, and endogenous losses increase accordingly to maintain zinc homeostasis. In humans, changes in zinc absorption with increasing zinc intake fit best with a saturable response model (73). Between 1 and approximately 9 mg dietary zinc/day, the efficiency of zinc absorption declines from nearly 1.0 to approximately 0.4. With intakes higher than approximately 9 mg/day, or the estimated average requirement (EAR), the fractional zinc absorption declines rapidly, a decline that helps to maintain homeostasis by minimizing the absorption of excess zinc. Up-regulation and down-regulation of zinc transporters and possibly other proteins involved in the transport of zinc underlie these adjustments in the efficiency of zinc absorption with changes in intake. Adjustments in absorption appear to occur rapidly because nearly tripling the zinc intakes reduced zinc absorption efficiency within 24 hours (46). Although zinc absorption responds rapidly to changes in intake, changes in absorption with shifts in zinc status appear to be minor by comparison. Studies in experimental animals showed that absorption increases during late pregnancy and lactation (74); it may also decline with aging (75).

Zinc Turnover and Transport

Plasma zinc comprises only 0.1% of total body zinc and, depending on species, represents 20% to 30% of the zinc in whole blood. Plasma concentrations are normally maintained within strict limits ($\sim$100 μg/dL; 15 μM), with serum concentrations slightly higher in nonhemolyzed samples. Severe human zinc depletion causes a fall in plasma zinc within approximately 2 weeks (72). With zinc intakes between 3 and 10 mg/day, plasma zinc increases and then rises very slowly until a plateau is reached with intakes between 25 and 30 mg/day (75). Plasma zinc may fluctuate by as much as 20% during a day, largely because of the effects of food ingestion. The highest values of the day occur in the morning after an overnight fast.

Plasma zinc is primarily bound to albumin (70%) (71, 76). At its normal plasma concentration of 600 μM, albumin has a molar ratio with zinc of 40:1. Zinc is easily exchanged from albumin (K_d = 7.5 M-1). α_2-Macroglobulin, a protease inhibitor and carrier of growth factors, binds zinc tightly and represents most of the remaining protein-bound zinc in plasma (3). A very small amount (i.e., $\sim$0.01%) is complexed with amino acids, especially histidine and cystine. This non–protein-bound component could be physiologically relevant and may influence urinary zinc loss. Zinc chemistry is such that virtually none circulates in a free ionized form. The flux of zinc through the plasma compartment is approximately 130 times/day (72).

A total of 70% to 80% of the blood zinc is cellular, with the concentration of leukocytes (6 mg zinc/10^6 cells) greater than that of erythrocytes (1 mg zinc/10^6 cells) (77). Erythrocyte zinc is found mostly with carbonic anhydrase (>85%), copper–zinc superoxide dismutase, and various other proteins including MT (78). In mice, membranes of erythrocytes in peripheral blood contain zinc transporter proteins, some of which are reflective of past zinc intake

(79). cDNA array analyses have shown that some leukocyte genes are very sensitive to zinc (80) and may respond to plasma zinc levels or, more likely, may reflect conditions of zinc status of progenitor cells in the bone marrow.

Kinetic data with both radioactive and stable isotopes have provided important information on zinc pool turnover in humans. Two metabolic pools (rapid [$\sim$12.5 days] and slow [$\sim$300 days]) have been identified (81, 82). Kinetically active tissues are liver more than pancreas, kidney, and spleen. Slow turnover is found in muscle and red blood cells, followed by bone and the nervous system. Using a kinetic model, cyclic adenosine monophosphate administration to rats appeared to alter the distribution and metabolism of zinc in the thymus, skin, spleen, intestine, and, especially, the bone marrow (83). Stable isotopes of zinc have been used to identify an exchangeable zinc pool (EZP) in humans (84). The pool represents the approximately 10% of whole body zinc that exchanges with the isotope in a 2-day period. Because most zinc in the body is bound to proteins, the size of the pool is influenced by the amount of lean body mass (85). A severe dietary zinc restriction causes the size of the pool to decrease by approximately one third. This may reflect the redistribution of this more rapidly turning over zinc to other tissues (72). General features of zinc metabolism are shown in Figures 11.1 and 11.2.

Dietary and Physiologic Adaptation Mechanisms

Hormonal regulation of zinc metabolism has been identified through transient fluctuations in plasma zinc. Humans experience a reproducible reduction in this level postprandially, perhaps related to metal-induced changes in insulin and other hormones (86). Plasma zinc increases during acute fasting (87) are likely caused by hormonally influenced muscle catabolism, with concomitant zinc release. Plasma zinc is transiently reduced following acute stresses (infection, trauma, surgery) (88). Hypozincemia is associated with stress and the acute phase. The underlying mechanisms are related to zinc transport into the liver and other organs, perhaps involving cytokine responsive transporters (89). Hypozincemia may be beneficial, to decrease zinc availability to microbial pathogens, provide zinc for protein synthesis, or maintain zinc signaling pathways for immune responses and generated metabolic needs. Comparable processes mediated by hepcidin occur in iron metabolism and initiate the anemia of inflammation. Stress and myocardial infarction also reduce plasma zinc in humans (90). Hemodilution, as occurs during pregnancy, oral contraceptive use, and other hormonal treatments, also lowers plasma zinc. Any condition that increases blood cell hemolysis will cause a rise in plasma zinc because intracellular zinc concentrations are higher than plasma zinc.

Storage, Recycling, and Conservation

Zinc does not have a specific storage site. However, cells have zinc in vesicles that may serve as a transient

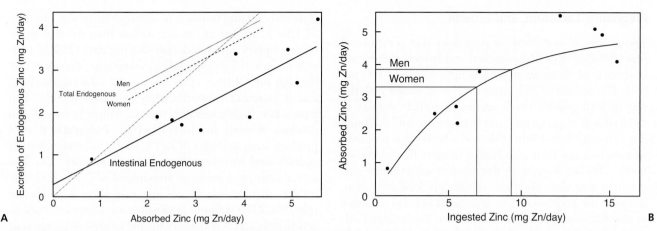

Fig. 11.1. A. The relationship between zinc losses and absorbed zinc in adult humans. The line starting at the origin (– – –) represents a hypothetical, perfect agreement between endogenous loss and absorbed zinc. The heavy line (—) represents the linear regression of actual intestinal excretion of endogenous zinc versus absorbed zinc based on data from 10 metabolic studies with isotopes. Other losses, added to intestinal endogenous losses, were used to obtain lines (- - - and – – –) for total endogenous losses for men and women. The intersect of the line of perfect agreement with that for total endogenous losses represents the amount of zinc that must be absorbed to compensate for those losses. **B.** Relationship of absorbed zinc with ingested zinc in human subjects' losses. (From Food and Nutrition Board, Institute of Medicine. Zinc. In: Dietary Reference Intakes for Vitamin A, Vitamin K, Arsenic, Boron, Chromium, Copper, Iodine, Iron, Manganese, Molybdenum, Nickel, Silicon, Vanadium, and Zinc. Washington, DC: National Academy Press, 2001, with permission.)

source of cellular zinc in times of need and as a way to protect the cell from the cytotoxicity resulting from excessive free zinc in the cytoplasm (91). For example, supplemental zinc, higher than the requirement, continued to support normal growth in chicks for 8 days after withdrawal (92). In addition, micronutrient supplements containing zinc given to Vietnamese infants either daily or weekly improved growth similarly in both groups (93).

Recycling of zinc through the erythron is analogous to that for iron. Red blood cells contain between 20 and 40 μg zinc/g hemoglobin (77), and the average circulating hemoglobin content is 750 g in adults. This represents a red blood cell zinc pool of 15 to 30 mg. The average life span of a red blood cell is 120 days; therefore, turnover for this zinc pool is between 0.12 and 0.25 mg/day (15 or 30 mg/120 days). This finding shows that a meaningful amount of zinc needs to be available to maintain erythropoiesis.

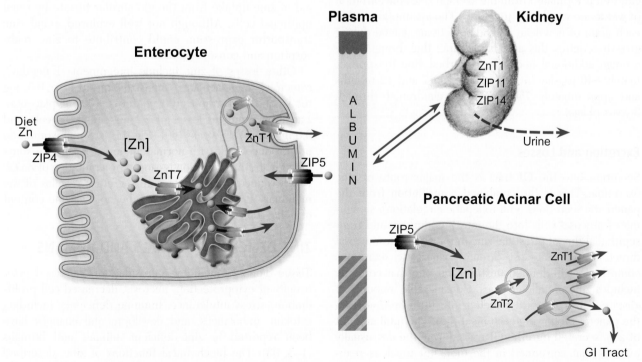

Fig. 11.2. Major transporter-mediated zinc (Zn) pathways for enteric absorption and pancreatic and renal output. *GI,* gastrointestinal; *ZnT,* zinc transporter.

Pregnancy, Lactation, and Growth

The additional zinc need for pregnancy that is estimated from the weight of tissues gained and from the zinc concentration of those tissues totals approximately 100 mg (94). The additional daily need for zinc increases with the rate of fetal growth; needs are less than 0.25 mg/day in the first half of pregnancy and between 0.5 and 0.75 mg/day in the last half. Little evidence indicates that pregnant women increase their zinc intakes to meet this additional need, a finding suggesting that modest adjustments may occur in zinc absorption or endogenous fecal excretion. Because the additional daily zinc need is small, changes in zinc homeostasis may be not evident. Severe zinc deficiency in pregnant experimental animals causes multiple teratogenic anomalies and limits fetal growth (95). Similar effects of zinc deficiency and fetal development have been observed in women with acrodermatitis enteropathica. Randomized controlled trials of zinc supplementation showed little benefit to women worldwide who were consuming typical diets with marginal to adequate zinc intakes (96).

The zinc requirement for lactation varies with changes in milk volume and zinc concentration throughout the lactation period. The need is highest in first month of lactation when the concentration is at its peak (~2.8 µg zinc/mL), and total breast milk zinc varies from 1 to 2 mg/day; it declines approximately 75% by the ninth month (97). Because of this sharp fall in milk zinc concentration, human milk alone is an inadequate source of zinc after the first 6 months (60). Milk zinc concentrations do not appear to vary with maternal zinc intake.

The additional need for zinc in growing infants and children is estimated from the average zinc concentration of wet tissue weight, 20 µg/g (60). The assumption is that each gram of new lean and adipose tissue gained during growth requires this amount of zinc, thus bringing the average additional needs for absorbed zinc to approximately 840 µg/day in infants between 7 and 12 months and approximately 750 µg/day in children 1 through 3 years of age.

Excretion and Losses

Secretion into the GI tract is the major route of zinc excretion. This is the combined contribution from the pancreatic secretions (enterohepatic circulation), sloughing of mucosal cells into the intestinal lumen, and transepithelial flux of intestinal zinc in the serosal to mucosal direction (3). Zinc lost through pancreatic secretions comprises an ill-defined mixture, but one that certainly includes zinc metalloenzymes. Considerable amounts of zinc (~3 to 5 mg) are secreted into the intestine from the pancreas following each meal (59). The total amount of zinc secreted into the GI tract during the day usually exceeds that consumed in the diet, but much is reabsorbed to maintain zinc balance (98). GI zinc excretion

is directly related function of dietary zinc intake (see Fig. 11.1B). Estimates are as low as less than 0.5 mg/day in severe dietary zinc restriction (0.3 mg/day) (72). At realistic intakes of 7 to 15 mg/day, endogenous zinc excretion through the GI tract ranges from 3.0 to 4.6 mg/day (99), and it increases proportionally at higher intakes. The pancreas is highly sensitive to zinc, which, in excess, can produce necrosis in chickens (100). Pancreatic β cells produce large amounts of ZnT8, which influences insulin stability and secretion through zinc transport (13). The acinar cells produce large amounts of MT, which closely reflects dietary zinc intake and may serve a protective role (26). ZIP5 is found in plasma membrane localized in acinar cells and is refractory to zinc intake (101), whereas ZnT2 is found with zymogen granule membranes and responds to both zinc and glucocorticoid hormone (26). ZnT1 appears to facilitate zinc secretion from acinar cells into the ductal system through the apical membrane for export to the intestinal lumen.

Urinary zinc output is low (<1 mg/day) and is refractory to change over a wide intake range (4 to 25 mg/day) (99). Starvation or trauma and other conditions that increase muscle protein catabolism increase urinary zinc as the load of amino acids filtered by the kidney increases. Some supplements that bind zinc tenaciously (e.g., zinc picolinate) may promote zinc loss in the urine (102). Glucagon has been shown to regulate zinc reabsorption by the renal tubular system (103). Some zinc transporters are expressed in kidney. Investigators have proposed that ZnT1, an efflux transporter, is oriented to the basolateral surface such that it contributes to zinc reabsorption (104). Similarly, ZIP8, ZIP11, and ZIP14 are highly expressed in kidney (13, 105) and would likely aid in zinc uptake from the glomerular filtrate by renal epithelial cells. Although not well explored, renal zinc transporter expression could contribute to zinc reabsorption and conservation.

Other losses of zinc include integument (1 mg/day), semen (1 mg/ejaculate), menstruation (0.1 to 0.5 mg total), and parturition (100 mg/fetus, 100 mg/placenta). Lactation produces losses of 2.2 mg/day at 4 weeks and 0.9 mg/day at 35 weeks (60) (Fig. 11.3). Some women do not produce milk with normal amounts of zinc. In some individuals, this condition is caused by a mutation of *ZnT2*, which reduces zinc uptake into secretory vesicles of the mammary gland and decreases the normal zinc content of milk (106).

ZINC DEFICIENCY: ANIMALS AND HUMANS

Tissue damage (including peroxidation, decreased cytotoxicity or cytoprotection, necrosis, decreased cell proliferation) stress intolerance, immune deficiency including cytokine imbalances, and developmental changes have been reported in zinc-deficient animals and humans (1–3, 93). The biochemical functions of zinc, described in the previous sections, are so basic to cellular growth,

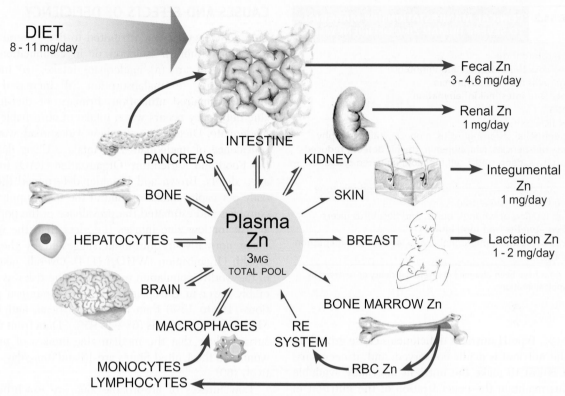

DIET
8 - 11 mg/day

INTESTINE

Fecal Zn
3 - 4.6 mg/day

PANCREAS

KIDNEY

Renal Zn
1 mg/day

BONE

SKIN

Integumental
Zn
1 mg/day

Plasma
Zn
3MG
TOTAL POOL

HEPATOCYTES

BREAST

Lactation Zn
1 - 2 mg/day

BRAIN

BONE MARROW Zn

MACROPHAGES

RE
SYSTEM

MONOCYTES
LYMPHOCYTES

RBC Zn

Fig. 11.3. Diagrammatic representation of mammalian zinc (Zn) metabolism. Tissues of high metabolic activity or particular functional significance are shown as deriving zinc from the plasma pool *(double arrows)*. Systems contributing to absorption, recycling, and loss of zinc are shown as *unidirectional arrows. RBC,* red blood cell; *RE,* reticuloendothelial.

development, and activity, however, that little wonder exists that the exact factors responsible for these effects of zinc deficiency have yet to be defined. Phenotypic outcomes of zinc functions in integrative systems can be placed in four general categories: (a) redox, peroxidation, and tissue damage; (b) apoptosis regulation; (c) cell proliferation and growth; and (d) immune regulation. These categories provide a framework to help understand the complexities of zinc deficiency.

Zinc is not a redox metal, yet tissue peroxidation and oxidative injury are occasionally observed in zinc-deficient animals. Iron accumulation leading to reactive oxygen or nitrogen radical generation could be a factor because at least one zinc transporter (ZIP14) also transports iron (107, 108). NO causes oxidative zinc release from sulfhydryl binding sites that leads to dysfunction (18, 20). Up-regulation of inducible NO synthetase in zinc deficiency may exacerbate NO-induced zinc release and cell injury (24, 65, 107). Animal-based evidence suggests that zinc protects against xenobiotic radical damage. Similarly, zinc may be a factor in regulating apoptosis through influences at various steps in the signaling cascades involved. Cells with characteristically high turnover rates (e.g., immune and epithelial cells) could be most vulnerable. Consequently, immune dysfunction and skin and intestinal disorders associated with zinc deficiency could be outcomes of altered apoptosis.

Reduced growth and cell proliferation observed in zinc deficiency could also be related to abnormal apoptosis. Further, direct effects on hormones that influence cell division or food intake (e.g., insulinlike growth factor or leptin), or the genes that produce these hormones or their receptor or alter their signal transduction pathways, could also explain the decreased growth as an outcome of zinc deficiency (109). Similarly, immune dysfunction and the susceptibility to infection in zinc deficiency could involve atypical regulation of cytokine gene function and signaling pathways that, in turn, disrupts the balance of cell-mediated versus humoral immunity (35, 110, 111). Alternatively, failure of zinc-dependent structural factors needed for antigen presentation or microbial killing could be an outcome that leads to parasitic and microbial infections secondary to zinc deficiency.

Essentiality of zinc in animals was first identified in rats (1934) and subsequently in pigs (1955). Most prominent signs of deficiency included skin lesions, a reduction in growth, and a reduction in food intake (1–3). Essentiality in humans was not shown until 1961 (2, 22). Human zinc deficiency is characterized by skin lesions, reductions in growth, delayed puberty, hypogonadism, host defense defects including infections of the epithelium, and poor appetite (Table 11.2). Zinc deficiency is characterized as a type II nutrient defi-

TABLE 11.2	CLINICAL MANIFESTATIONS OF MARGINAL TO SEVERE HUMAN ZINC DEFICIENCY[a]

Growth retardation
Delayed sexual maturation and impotence
Hypogonadism and hypospermia
Diarrhea and intestinal inflammation
Alopecia
Acroorificial skin lesions
Other epithelial lesions: glossitis, alopecia, nail dystrophy
Immune deficiencies: lymphopenia, thymic defects, reduced phagocytosis, depressed T-cell function, impaired cytokine production
Behavioral disturbances, including impaired hedonic tone
Impaired taste (hypogeusia)
Delayed healing of wounds, burns, and decubitus ulcers
Impaired appetite and food intake
Eye lesions, including photophobia and lack of dark adaptation and photic injury

[a]Some signs have been observed in severe deficiency or reversed by zinc supplementation.

ciency (3). Type II nutrient deficiencies cause growth to stop; the nutrient is avidly conserved, and, if necessary, weight is lost to make the nutrient internally available and thus maintain the concentration of the nutrient in the tissues. As such, reduced growth occurs without a concomitant reduction in zinc levels of tissues, coupled with nonspecific signs, particularly in the most metabolically active tissues.

In adult humans, depletion of zinc is a slow process because of adaptive mechanisms that involve homeostatic control of absorption and endogenous losses. Repletion of zinc deficiency appears to be rapid. Evidence from experimental animal studies suggests that some biochemical markers of zinc deficiency are normalized in a period of 24 hours. The clinical spectrum of severe zinc deficiency contrasts with what is expected with the far more prevalent condition of moderate zinc deficiency (4). Other possible signs of marginal zinc deficiency include dysfunctions in taste (hypogeusia) and smell (hyposmia). These observations have not been rigorously tested, but evidence suggests that some olfactory receptors are zinc metalloproteins.

Our current understanding of zinc deficiency in humans, much of which is marginal zinc deficiency, is based on responses to zinc supplementation. General agreement exists, from studies done in many parts of the world, that physical growth of children in some population groups benefits from zinc supplementation. In numerous studies, cognitive performance and other measures of neuropsychological performance have concomitantly improved on zinc supplementation. In other studies, impressive reductions in childhood morbidity and mortality have been produced through zinc supplementation. Most of this improvement relates to a reduction in secretory diarrhea and upper respiratory infections, including pneumonia (112).

CAUSES AND EFFECTS OF DEFICIENCY

Zinc deficiency can be attributed to five general causes, occurring either in isolation or in combination (113). These causes are (a) inadequate intake, (b) increased requirements, (c) malabsorption, (d) increased losses, and (e) impaired utilization. Primary, or diet-induced, zinc deficiency occurs when intake of absorbable zinc is inadequate. Dietary surveys show widespread, worldwide prevalence of inadequate zinc intakes. Using data from the Food and Agriculture Organization (FAO) food balance sheets, Brown and Wuehler determined the mean daily per capita intake of zinc in the food supply of 178 countries and estimated the prevalence of the population at risk for low zinc intakes (i.e., less than the weighed mean normative requirement suggested by the World Health Organization [WHO]) (114). Overall, nearly half of the world's population was at risk. The risk was considerably lower in European and North American populations (1% to 13%) than in Asian, African, and Eastern Mediterranean regions (68% to 95%). Data from national surveys show that the median zinc intakes of men and women in the United States are 13 and 9 mg/day, respectively (60).

Low intakes of absorbable zinc are exacerbated by physiologic or pathologic conditions that increase zinc requirements. Increased zinc needs for growth place infants, children, adolescents, and pregnant and lactating women at increased risk for zinc depletion. Pathologic conditions such as preterm birth, low birth weight, and diarrheal disorders reduce zinc absorption because of immaturity of the GI tract or increase intestinal losses and further raise the risk of zinc deficiency among infants and children (112).

Severe zinc deficiency is characterized by erythematous, vesiculobullous, and pustular rashes, primarily adjacent to the body orifices and at the extremities (see Table 11.2). After the onset of dermatitis, the hair may change and become hypopigmented and acquire a reddish hue. Patchy loss of hair is a common feature.

Malabsorptive Disorders

Malabsorption syndromes and inflammatory bowel diseases that alter the integrity of the mucosal cell can reduce zinc absorption and can precipitate secondary zinc deficiency states, particularly if zinc intakes are also marginal. Zinc deficiency has developed in Crohn disease, sprue, short bowel syndrome, and jejunoileal bypass. Crohn disease, or regional enteritis, is a type of inflammatory bowel disease. Low serum zinc concentrations and depressed urinary zinc excretion have been reported in patients with Crohn disease (115). Zinc depletion in Crohn disease may result from impaired absorption without appropriate reductions in excretion, hypoalbuminemia, or an internal redistribution of zinc (116, 117). Supplementation with 25 mg elemental zinc/day for 8 weeks reduced the

6. Krezel A, Hao Q, Maret W. Arch Biochem Biophys 2007; 463:188–200.

7. Gee KR, Zhou ZL, Qian WJ et al. J Am Chem Soc 2002; 124:776–8.

8. Haase H, Hebel S, Engelhardt G et al. Anal Biochem 2006; 352:222–30.

9. Cousins RJ. Zinc. In: Brown Bowman BA, Russell RM, eds. Present Knowledge in Nutrition. International Life Sciences Institute (ILSI) Nutrition Foundation. Washington, DC: ILSI Press, 2006:445–57.

10. Suzuki T, Ishihara K, Migaki H et al. J Biol Chem 2005; 280:637–43.

11. Pedrosa FO, Pontremoli S, Horecker BL. Proc Natl Acad Sci U S A 1977;74:2742–5.

12. Brand IA, Kleineke J. J Biol Chem 1996;271:1941–9.

13. Lichten LA, Cousins RJ. Annu Rev Nutr 2009;29:153–76.

14. Klug A, Schwabe JW. FASEB J 1995;9:597–604.

15. Blasie CA, Berg JM. Biochemistry 2002;41:15068–73.

16. Ravasi T, Huber T, Zavolan M et al. Genome Res 2003;13: 1430–42.

17. Krezel A, Maret W. J Am Chem Soc 2007;129:10911–21.

18. Kroncke KD, Klotz LO, Suschek CV et al. J Biol Chem 2002;277:13294–301.

19. Roesijadi G, Bogumil R, Vasak M et al. J Biol Chem 1998;273:17425–32.

20. Spahl DU, Berendji-Grun D, Suschek CV et al. Proc Natl Acad Sci U S A 2003;100:13952–7.

21. Zangger K, Oz G, Haslinger E et al. FASEB J 2001;15:1303–5.

22. Prasad AS. Curr Opin Clin Nutr Metab Care 2009;12:646–52.

23. Ho E, Ames BN. Proc Natl Acad Sci U S A 2002;99:16770–5.

24. Cui L, Blanchard RK, Cousins RJ. J Nutr 2003;133:51–6.

25. Gomez NN, Davicino RC, Biaggio VS et al. Nitric Oxide 2006;14:30–8.

26. Guo L, Lichten LA, Ryu MS et al. Proc Natl Acad Sci U S A 2010;107:2818–23.

27. Naik HB, Beshire M, Walsh BM et al. Am J Physiol 2009; 297:C979–89.

28. Lichtlen P, Wang Y, Belser T et al. Nucleic Acids Res 2001; 29:1514–23.

29. Hogstrand C, Zheng D, Feeney G et al. Biochem Soc Trans 2008;36:1252–7.

30. Lee J, Li Z, Brower-Sinning R et al. PLoS Comput Biol 2007;3:e67.

31. Otsuka F, Okugaito I, Ohsawa M et al. Biochim Biophys Acta 2000;1492:330–40.

32. Walker E, Chang WY, Hunkapiller J et al. Cell Stem Cell 2010; 6:153–66.

33. Cousins RJ, Liuzzi JP, Lichten LA. J Biol Chem 2006;281: 24085–9.

34. Yamasaki S, Sakata-Sogawa K, Hasegawa A et al. J Cell Biol 2007;177:637–45.

35. Haase H, Rink L. Annu Rev Nutr 2009;29:133–52.

36. Aydemir TB, Liuzzi JP, McClellan S et al. J Leukoc Biol 2009;86:337–48.

37. Kitamura H, Morikawa H, Kamon H et al. Nat Immunol 2006;7:971–7.

38. Sensi SL, Paoletti P, Bush AI et al. Nat Rev Neurosci 2009; 10:780–91.

39. Takeda A, Minami A, Takefuta S et al. J Neurosci Res 2001; 63:447–52.

40. Chowanadisai W, Kelleher SL, Lonnerdal B. J Nutr 2005; 135:1002–7.

41. Cote A, Chiasson M, Peralta MR, 3rd et al. J Physiol 2005; 566:821–37.

42. Kwak YD, Wang B, Pan W et al. J Biol Chem 2010;285: 9847–57.

43. Lonnerdal B. J Nutr 2000;130(Suppl):1378S–83S.

44. Hambidge KM, Miller LV, Westcott JE et al. Am J Clin Nutr 2010;91(Suppl):1478S–83S.

45. Hunt JR, Beiseigel JM, Johnson LK. Am J Clin Nutr 2008; 87:1336–45.

46. Chung CS, Stookey J, Dare D et al. Am J Clin Nutr 2008; 87:1224–9.

47. Hotz C, Gibson RS, Temple L. Int J Food Sci Nutr 2001; 52:133–42.

48. World Health Organization. Trace Elements in Human Nutrition and Health. Geneva: World Health Organization, 1996.

49. Miller LV, Krebs NF, Hambidge KM. J Nutr 2007;137:135–41.

50. Lonnerdal B. J Nutr 2003;133(Suppl):1490S–3S.

51. Fordyce EJ, Forbes RM, Robbins KR et al. J Food Sci 1987;52:440–4.

52. Sandstrom B, Davidsson L, Cederblad A et al. J Nutr 1985; 115:411–4.

53. Brown KH, Peerson JM, Baker SK et al. Food Nutr Bull 2009;30(Suppl):S12–S40.

54. August D, Janghorbani M, Young VR. Am J Clin Nutr 1989;50:1457–63.

55. Davis CD, Milne DB, Nielsen FH. Am J Clin Nutr 2000; 71:781–8.

56. Hilty FM, Arnold M, Hilbe M et al. Nat Nanotechnol 2010; 5:374–80.

57. Cousins RJ. Adv Exp Med Biol 1989;249:3–12.

58. Lee HH, Prasad AS, Brewer GJ et al. Am J Physiol 1989;256:G87–91.

59. Matseshe JW, Phillips SF, Malagelada JR et al. Am J Clin Nutr 1980;33:1946–53.

60. Food and Nutrition Board, Institute of Medicine. Zinc. In: Dietary Reference Intakes for Vitamin A, Vitamin K, Arsenic, Boron, Chromium, Copper, Iodine, Iron, Manganese, Molybdenum, Nickel, Silicon, Vanadium, and Zinc. Washington, DC: National Academy Press, 2001.

61. Hoadley JE, Leinart AS, Cousins RJ. Am J Physiol 1987; 252:G825–31.

62. Lee DY, Prasad AS, Hydrick-Adair C et al. J Lab Clin Med 1993;122:549–56.

63. Raffaniello RD, Lee SY, Teichberg S et al. J Cell Physiol 1992;152:356–61.

64. Dufner-Beattie J, Wang F, Kuo YM et al. J Biol Chem 2003;278:33474–81.

65. Liuzzi JP, Guo L, Chang SM et al. Am J Physiol 2009;296: G517–23.

66. Wang K, Zhou B, Kuo YM et al. Am J Hum Genet 2002;71:66–73.

67. Thyresson N. Acta Derm Venereol 1974;54:383–5.

68. Davis SR, McMahon RJ, Cousins RJ. J Nutr 1998;128:825–31.

69. Huang XP, Yabuki Y, Kojima M et al. Biol Chem 2007;388:129–33.

70. McMahon RJ, Cousins RJ. Proc Natl Acad Sci U S A 1998; 95:4841–6.

71. Smith KT, Failla ML, Cousins RJ. Biochem J 1979;184:627–33.

72. King JC, Shames DM, Lowe NM et al. Am J Clin Nutr 2001;74:116–24.

73. Hambidge KM, Miller LV, Westcott JE et al. Am J Clin Nutr 2010;91(Suppl):1478S–83S.

74. Davies NT, Williams RB. Br J Nutr 1977;38:417–23.

75. Fairweather-Tait SJ, Harvey LJ, Ford D. Exp Gerontol 2008;43:382–8.

76. Gibson RS, Hess SY, Hotz C et al. Br J Nutr 2008; 99(Suppl):S14–S23.

77. Milne DB, Ralston NV, Wallwork JC. Clin Chem 1985; 31:65–9.

78. Grider A, Bailey LB, Cousins RJ. Proc Natl Acad Sci U S A 1990;87:1259–62.

79. Ryu MS, Lichten LA, Liuzzi JP et al. J Nutr 2008;138:2076–83.

80. Cousins RJ, Blanchard RK, Popp MP et al. Proc Natl Acad Sci U S A 2003;100:6952–7.

81. Foster DM, Aamodt RL, Henkin RI et al. Am J Physiol 1979;237:R340–R9.

82. Wastney ME, Aamodt RL, Rumble WF et al. Am J Physiol 1986;251:R398–R408.

83. Dunn MA, Cousins RJ. Am J Physiol 1989;256:E420–30.

84. Miller LV, Hambidge KM, Naake VL et al. J Nutr 1994;124:268–76.

85. Pinna K, Woodhouse LR, Sutherland B et al. J Nutr 2001; 131:2288–94.

86. King JC, Hambidge KM, Westcott JL et al. J Nutr 1994;124:508–16.

87. Fell GS, Fleck A, Cuthbertson DP et al. Lancet 1973;1:280–2.

88. Falchuk KH. N Engl J Med 1977;296:1129–34.

89. Liuzzi JP, Lichten LA, Rivera S et al. Proc Natl Acad Sci U S A 2005;102:6843–8.

90. Prasad AS. J Am Coll Nutr 1985;4:591–8.

91. Haase H, Beyersmann D. Biometals 1999;12:247–54.

92. Emmert JL, Baker DH. Poultry Sci 1995;74:1011–21.

93. Thu BD, Schultink W, Dillon D et al. Am J Clin Nutr 1999;69:80–6.

94. Swanson CA, King JC. Am J Clin Nutr 1987;46:763–71.

95. King JC. Am J Clin Nutr 2000;71(Suppl):1334S–43S.

96. Brown KH, Hess S. Food Nutr Bull 2009;30(Suppl):S1–S188.

97. King JC, Turnlund JR. Human zinc requirements. In: Mills CF, ed. Zinc in Human Biology. London: Springer, 1989: 335–50.

98. Krebs NF. J Nutr 2000;130(Suppl):1374S–7S.

99. King JC, Shames DM, Woodhouse LR. J Nutr 2000;130 (Suppl):1360S–6S.

100. Lu J, Combs GF Jr. J Nutr 1988;118:681–9.

101. Wang F, Kim BE, Petris MJ et al. J Biol Chem 2004;279: 51433–41.

102. Seal CJ, Heaton FW. J Nutr 1985;115:986–93.

103. Victery W, Levenson R, Vander AJ. Am J Physiol 1981;240:F299–F305.

104. Cousins RJ, McMahon RJ. J Nutr 2000;130(Suppl):1384S–7S.

105. Girijashanker K, He L, Soleimani M et al. Mol Pharmacol 2008;73:1413–23.

106. Chowanadisai W, Lonnerdal B, Kelleher SL. J Biol Chem 2006;281:39699–707.

107. Mackenzie GG, Keen CL, Oteiza PI. Dev Neurosci 2002;24:125–33.

108. Liuzzi JP, Aydemir F, Nam H et al. Proc Natl Acad Sci U S A 2006;103:13612–7.

109. MacDonald RS. J Nutr 2000;130(Suppl):1500S–8S.

110. Moore JB, Blanchard RK, Cousins RJ. Proc Natl Acad Sci U S A 2003;100:3883–8.

111. Koski KG, Scott ME. Annu Rev Nutr 2001;21:297–321.

112. Walker CF, Black RE. Annu Rev Nutr 2004;24:255–75.

113. Solomons NW, Cousins RJ. Zinc. In: Solomons NW, Rosenberg IH, eds. Absorption and Malabsorption of Mineral Nutrients. New York: Alan R. Liss, 1984:125–97.

114. Brown KH, Wuehler SE. Zinc and Human Health: The Results of Recent Trials and Implications for Program Interventions and Research. Ottawa: Micronutrient Initiative, 2000.

115. McClain CJ. J Am Coll Nutr 1985;4:49–64.

116. Matsui T. J Gastroenterol 1998;33:924–5.

117. Griffin IJ, Kim SC, Hicks PD et al. Pediatr Res 2004;56:235–9.

118. Sturniolo GC, Di Leo V, Ferronato A et al. Inflamm Bowel Dis 2001;7:94–8.

119. Elmes ME, Golden MK, Love AHG. Q J Mol Med 1978;55:293–306.

120. Hogberg L, Danielsson L, Jarleman S et al. Acta Paediatr 2009;98:343–5.

121. Jones PE, Peters TJ. Gut 1981;22:194–8.

122. Andersson K-E, Bratt L, Dencker H et al. Eur J Clin Pharmacol 1976;9:423–8.

123. Madan AK, Orth WS, Tichansky DS et al. Obes Surg 2006;16:603–6.

124. Halsted CH, Keen CL. Eur J Gastroenterol Hepatol 1990;2:399–405.

125. Zhong W, McClain CJ, Cave M et al. Am J Physiol 2010;298: G625–33.

126. Szuster-Ciesielska A, Plewka K, Daniluk J et al. Toxicol Appl Pharmacol 2008;229:1–9.

127. Russell RM. Am J Clin Nutr 1980;33:2741–9.

128. McClain CJ, Su LC. Alcohol Clin Exp Res 1983;7:5–10.

129. Uriu-Hare JY, Stern JS. Diabetes 1989;38:1282–90.

130. Walter RM Jr, Uriu-Hare JY, Olin KL et al. Diabetes Care 1991;14(11):1050–6.

131. Beletate V, El Dib RP, Atallah AN. Cochrane Database Syst Rev 2007;(1):CD005525.

132. Haase H, Maret W. Biometals 2005;18:333–8.

133. Chimienti F, Devergnas S, Favier A et al. Diabetes 2004;53:2330–7.

134. Staiger H, Machicao F, Stefan N et al. PLoS One 2007;2:e832

135. Wenzlau JM, Juhl K, Yu L et al. Proc Natl Acad Sci U S A 2007;104:17040–5.

136. Brown KH, Baker SK, Committee IS. Food Nutr Bull 2009;30(Suppl):S179–S84.

137. World Health Organization, United Nations Children's Fund (UNICEF). WHO/UNICEF Joint Statement. Clinical management of acute diarrhea. Geneva: World Health Organization/UNICEF, 2004.

138. Garland ML, Hagmeyer KO. Ann Pharmacother 1998;32:63–9.

139. Kupka R, Fawzi W. Nutr Rev 2002;60:69–79.

140. Aydemir TB, Blanchard RK, Cousins RJ. Proc Natl Acad Sci U S A 2006;103:1699–704.

141. Bao S, Liu MJ, Lee B et al. Am J Physiol 2010;298:L744–54.

142. Weismann K. Dan Med Bull 1986;33:208–11.

143. Zemel BS, Kawchak DA, Fung EB et al. Am J Clin Nutr 2002;75:300–7.

144. Selimoglu MA, Ertekin V, Doneray H et al. J Clin Gastroenterol 2008;42:194–8.

145. Age-Related Eye Disease Study Research Group. Arch Ophthalmol 2001;119:1417–36.

146. Clemons TE, Kurinij N, Sperduto RD. Arch Ophthalmol 2004;122:716–26.

147. Arsenault JE, Brown KH. Am J Clin Nutr 2003;78:1011–7.

148. Lowe NM, Woodhouse LR, Sutherland B et al. J Nutr 2004;134:2178–81.

149. Lowe NM, Fekete K, Decsi T. Am J Clin Nutr 2009; 89(Suppl):2040S–51S.

150. Hess SY, Peerson JM, King JC et al. Food Nutr Bull 2007;28(Suppl):S403–29.

151. Hotz C, Peerson JM, Brown KH. Am J Clin Nutr 2003;78: 756–64.

152. Song Y, Chung CS, Bruno RS et al. Am J Clin Nutr 2009; 90:321–8.

153. Bremner I, Morrison JN, Wood AM et al. J Nutr 1987; 117:1595–602.

Physiologic Functions

The necessary presence of copper in several enzymes discussed previously gives us clues to the phenotype of copper deficiency. In many cases, symptoms of copper inadequacy can be linked with decreased activity of one or more of these copper-dependent enzymes.

Connective Tissue Formation

The copper-dependent enzyme LOX is required for normal formation of connective and bone tissue, as well as for the integrity of connective tissue in the heart and vasculature. Copper deficiency thus results in connective tissue disorders, osteoporosis, and bone defects. Skeletal perturbations have been documented in copper-deficient neonates that mirror the bone abnormalities of scurvy (vitamin C deficiency) (25). Moreover, data demonstrated that long-term copper supplementation may decrease bone loss in adult humans (26), but contradictory results have also been obtained (27).

Iron Metabolism

Copper homeostasis is intimately entwined with that of iron (28). The most obvious link is the multicopper ferroxidases, CP and HEPH; the expression and activity of both proteins is effected by dietary copper (and perhaps iron) status. During copper deficiency, CP activity is extremely low, reflecting its need for copper for proper function (29). The net effect of low copper then is that iron efflux from some tissues is impaired, including liver, to the extent of possible pathologic consequence in humans (30). Moreover, copper deficiency results in microcytic, hypochromic anemia resembling that seen in iron deficiency. This finding may be explained by decreased circulating iron levels or an inability of erythroid precursor cells to use iron for hemoglobin synthesis.

Central Nervous System

Copper plays well-known roles in the physiology of the central nervous system (CNS), including brain development. Copper is deposited in the brain late in gestational development and during the perinatal period, and as such, copper deprivation of pregnant or lactating females results in pathologic phenotypes in offspring. Many of the effects of copper deprivation can be ascribed to altered expression or activity of cuproenzymes found in the tissues of the CNS and their susceptibility to body copper levels (16). The essentiality of copper in brain development is perhaps best exemplified by the neuropathologic phenotype of infants with the genetic copper-deficiency disorder MD (31). The tremors, ataxia, perturbations in myelination of nerve fibers (hypomyelination or demyelination), and reductions seen in some neurotransmitters observed during copper deficiency likely result from decreased production of sphingolipids (as mediated by CCO) and decreased activity of dopamine β-hydroxylase and MAO.

Melanin Pigment Formation

Copper is necessary for normal pigmentation, given the copper dependency of the TYR enzyme, which is a key factor in melanin synthesis. During copper deficiency in humans and animals, depigmentation of skin and hair is commonly observed.

Cardiac Function and Cholesterol Metabolism

Several pathologic anomalies in the cardiovascular system are noted in severely copper-deficient young animals. Copper deficiency in humans may also predispose individuals to developing cardiovascular disease. Some human metabolic trials, however, showed no cardiovascular effects from the consumption of a low-copper diet, whereas other trials demonstrated the development of cardiac arrhythmias (16). Several other observational studies in humans made correlative connections between high serum copper levels and a decreased incidence of coronary heart disease; these studies were reviewed (32).

Copper deficiency is also known to lead to alterations in blood lipid profiles and blood pressure and to cause anemia. Abnormal lipid metabolism is exemplified by hypercholesterolemia and hypertriglyceridemia. It thus logically follows that because copper deficiency causes alterations in lipid metabolism and thus risk factors for atherosclerotic cardiovascular disease, it likely plays a vital role in atherogenesis (33).

Immune Function

Evidence exists that copper plays an important role in the normal functioning of the immune system; many studies have shown that systemic copper deficiency is frequently associated with an increased risk of infection (34). The reason may be that cellular and humoral factors of the immune system are altered or suppressed by copper deficiency. A commonly noted symptom in copper-deficient humans is neutropenia, and some activities of macrophages and lymphocytes are adversely affected by even marginal copper deficiency. One study in men demonstrated that in vitro stimulation of T lymphocytes was suppressed by consuming a diet with 0.36 mg copper/day for 42 days. These individuals further had decreased plasma copper levels and reduced activity of some copper-dependent enzymes, but their hematologic parameters were normal (35). These and other unmentioned findings (36) implicate copper in the ability of immune cells to respond to infectious stimuli, but definitive proof is lacking in part because of the inability to detect marginal copper deficiencies.

BIOAVAILABILITY

The relative amount of copper in the diet seems to be the major predictor of absorption levels. Several factors, including certain amino acids and proteins, iron, zinc, molybdenum, vitamin C, and carbohydrates, have been reported to exert adverse effects on the bioavailability of dietary copper, however (37). High doses of zinc induce symptoms of systemic copper deficiency, as reported in several patients who used excessive amounts of zinc-containing denture cream (38). The impact of dietary components on copper absorption may be more pronounced in neonates, because digestive function and homeostatic regulation of biliary copper excretion are immature.

Nutrient Interactions

Copper metabolism is known to be effected by iron, zinc, and vitamin C. Perturbations of dietary copper levels are also thought potentially to affect the metabolism of other nutrients, a topic not discussed here.

Iron

Copper and iron interact in numerous ways (28). Important iron–copper interactions in the gut include the regulation of HEPH by dietary copper levels and the regulation of the Menkes copper ATPase (ATP7A, a protein necessary for copper efflux) expression by iron levels (39, 40). Furthermore, liver copper levels vary inversely according to iron status for unexplained reasons (41). An unknown aspect of bone marrow iron utilization is copper dependent, because during copper deficiency, hemoglobin production is inefficient despite normal serum iron levels (28).

Zinc

High dietary zinc intake impairs copper absorption. This may in part be explained by the induction of metallothionein (MT) in enterocytes. Moreover, copper depletion has been observed in humans consuming supplements containing 50 mg of zinc daily for extended periods; this finding is, in fact, the rationale for the tolerable upper intake level (UL) for zinc of 40 mg/day for adults (42).

Ascorbic Acid

Ascorbic acid supplementation may induce copper deficiency in experimental animals and could have a similar effect in humans. In premature infants, plasma vitamin C levels were negatively correlated with serum CP and antioxidant activity (43). Other human studies also suggested that ascorbic acid supplementation may perturb serum ferroxidase activity.

Food Sources

The typical diet of an adult in the United States supplies slightly more copper than is suggested by the recommended dietary allowance (RDA; 0.9 mg/day). The richest sources of dietary copper are shellfish, seeds, nuts, organ meats, wheat bran cereal, whole grain products, and foods containing chocolate. Vegan diets contain ample copper, but absorption seems to be lower from plant foods than from other dietary sources (44). Other sources of copper include vitamin and mineral supplements, although copper is often in the Cu^{2+} oxide form, which has low bioavailability (45).

METABOLISM

Genetic Regulation

mRNA levels for many proteins involved in copper homeostasis in mammals (e.g., CTR1, ATP7A, ATP7B) do not change in response to dietary copper intake levels, a finding demonstrating a lack of control at the level of gene transcription (46). Regulation of copper intake and efflux may be controlled at a posttranscriptional level, predominantly by protein trafficking (47). In contrast, ATP7A has been shown to be induced at the transcriptional level during iron deprivation in intestinal epithelial cells (48).

Overall Body Copper Homeostasis

Copper enters the body from the diet with an average intake of approximately 1.3 mg/day (Fig. 12.1). The amount extracted from the diet daily is approximately 0.8 mg/day, which is delivered to the liver. Excretion occurs predominantly through the copper exporter ATP7B into the bile (~0.4 mg/day), and total fecal losses are approximately 1 mg/day. Copper is incorporated into CP and other cuproenzymes in the liver; CP is secreted into the blood along with atomic copper, which binds to serum proteins for copper delivery to cells of the body. Homeostatic control of body copper levels includes modulation of copper absorption in the intestine and of copper excretion in the liver.

Vectorial Transport across the Intestinal Mucosa

Dietary sources of copper and endogenous copper from various body secretions contribute to the intestinal copper pool, although biliary copper may be complexed and unavailable for absorption. Dietary copper must be reduced from the Cu^{2+} to the Cu^+ state for absorption (Fig. 12.2). At least three Cu^{2+} reductases have been identified (cytochrome b [558] ferric/Cu^{2+} reductase, STEAP 2, and CYBRD1), but the precise roles of each are not currently clear (28). Once reduced, the metal is likely transported into enterocytes by copper transporter 1 (CTR1) (49). It is also possible that divalent metal transporter 1 (DMT1) is involved in absorption of dietary copper (50). This seems plausible, particularly during dietary iron deprivation, when DMT1 mRNA and protein levels are very strongly induced in the setting of no competing iron atoms (40).

Once in cells, copper is bound by one of several chaperone proteins that deliver copper to the mitochondria (COX17; a chaperone for CCO), to the *trans*-Golgi network (ATOX1; a chaperone for the Menkes copper ATPase [ATP7A]), or to the cytosol for copper/zinc-SOD (SOD1) expression (copper chaperone for SOD1 [CCS]). Excess copper may be bound in cells by MT. Finally, copper may be transported out of enterocytes by ATP7A. Once copper exits enterocytes, the oxidizing environment of the interstitial fluids presumably converts Cu^+ copper to Cu^{2+} copper, which binds to albumin or α_2-macroglobulin for delivery in the portal blood to the liver.

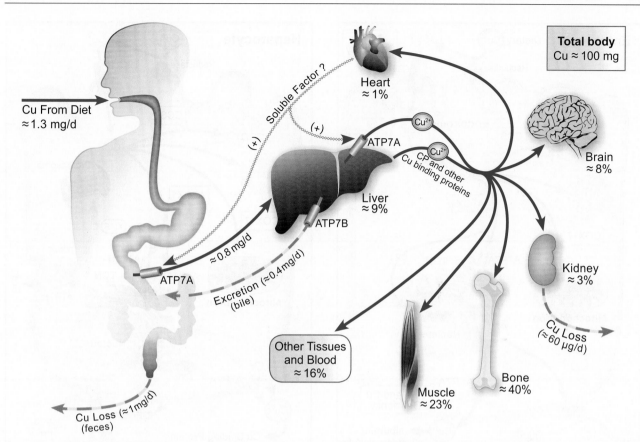

Fig. 12.1. Overall body copper (Cu) homeostasis in humans. Shown in this diagram are the major regulatory mechanisms that control body copper levels, from absorption in the diet, to distribution to various body tissues to excretory mechanisms. Two copper-exporting adenosine triphosphatases (ATPases) play critical roles in intestinal absorption (ATP7A) and biliary excretion (ATP7B). Studies have suggested that cardiac copper deficiency may signal by an unknown factor to the ATP7A copper exporter in intestine and liver to increase serum copper levels. *Numbers* under various organs indicate the approximate percentage of body copper present in that organ or tissue. Copper is predominantly in the cupric form (Cu^{2+}) in the diet and within the serum, but it must be reduced for absorption into cells lining the small intestine and other cells of the body. Once copper exits cells, the oxidizing environment of the interstitial fluids causes it to reoxidize to Cu^{2+}. Although most copper in the serum is bound to ceruloplasmin (CP), other copper-binding proteins exist because the absence of CP (in aceruloplasminemia) does not cause copper deficits in peripheral tissues.

Transport and Transfer

Absorbed copper is transported to the liver, where its first reduced and then imported by CTR1 (Fig. 12.3) (51). Inside liver cells, copper is bound to chaperones and is distributed to copper-dependent proteins. ATP7B pumps copper into the *trans*-Golgi network (TGN), where it is incorporated into CP and other cuproproteins. Excess copper stimulates the translocation of ATP7B from the TGN to the canalicular membrane of the hepatocyte and thereby facilitates excretion of copper into the bile.

Excretion

The primary excretory route for endogenous copper is through hepatocytes into bile, as mediated by ATP7B. Biliary copper and unabsorbed dietary copper are lost through the feces. Copper excretion is immature during the fetal and neonatal periods, and this explains the higher hepatic copper levels noted at these developmental stages. Cholestasis, in later life, may also lead to increased liver copper levels.

Storage

Total copper amounts in adults range from 50 to 120 mg. In general, copper is not stored in the human body; tissue copper levels thus likely reflect quantities of cuproenzymes.

Homeostatic Mechanisms

Humans have developed efficient adaptive mechanisms designed to protect against copper deficiency and toxicity. Absorption of dietary copper is regulated, with the percentage of absorption increasing when intake levels are low (52). Under conditions of high copper intake, copper may be sequestered in MT in enterocytes, and biliary excretion may also increase. Copper absorption under normal conditions is approximately 10%, a finding reflecting combined absorption and subsequent excretion of newly absorbed copper (53). These adaptive mechanisms become inefficient with chronic intake of copper lower than 0.7 mg/day; fortunately, this intake level is well below the estimated average intake in the United States of approximately 1.2 mg/day.

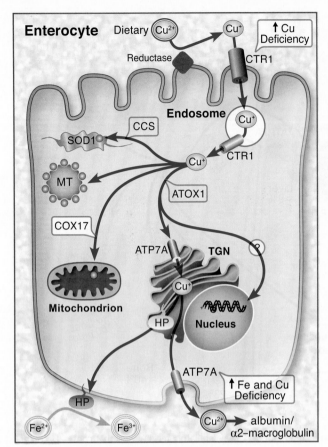

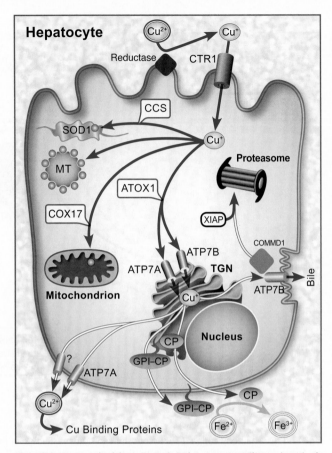

Fig. 12.2. Copper (Cu) homeostasis in enterocytes. Shown in this diagram is a single enterocyte, with the processes involved in copper absorption from the diet. Dietary copper is first reduced and then transported across the apical surface by copper transporter 1 (CTR1). Once copper enters the cytoplasmic pool, it is rapidly bound to chaperones for distribution to various cellular compartments. Copper chaperone for superoxide dismutase (CCS) delivers copper to the cytosolic copper/zinc (Cu/Zn) superoxide dismutase (SOD1); ATOX1 delivers copper to the Menkes copper-transporting adenosine triphosphatase (ATP7A) in the *trans*-Golgi network (TGN) and may also deliver copper to the nucleus where ATOX1 can act as a transcription factor to regulate genes related to cell cycle control; cytochrome c oxidase assembly homolog *(S. cerevisiae)* (COX17) delivers copper to the mitochondria. Excess copper can be bound to metallothionein (MT) under certain conditions, equating to a mucosal block to copper absorption. In the TGN, copper is incorporated into copper-containing proteins bound for the secretory pathway, including hephaestin (HP), a multicopper ferroxidase that is important to oxidize transported iron (Fe) on the basolateral surface for binding to transferrin. Under conditions of copper excess, ATP7A traffics to the basolateral membrane and functions in copper export. Once cuprous copper exits cells, it spontaneously oxidizes and is then bound by albumin and α_2-macroglobulin for transport through the portal blood to the liver. Expression of the predominant players in both the import and export processes may be up-regulated by copper deficiency (CTR1 and ATP7A), and the copper export process may also be increased during iron deficiency because ATP7A expression is strongly induced.

Fig. 12.3. Copper (Cu) homeostasis in hepatocytes. Shown is a single hepatocyte with the major proteins involved in copper homeostasis in the liver. Copper from the blood must be reduced before being transported into the cell by copper transporter 1 (CTR1). A similar host of copper chaperones bind copper (as detailed in the legend to Fig. 12.2) and facilitate movement throughout the cell; excess copper can also be stored bound to metallothionein (MT). During early life, both copper-exporting adenosine triphosphatase (ATP7A, ATP7B) are expressed in hepatocytes and may be necessary for the production of cuproproteins in the *trans*-Golgi network (TGN). After the neonatal period, ATP7A expression decreases dramatically, although studies have indicated that it may play an important role in hepatic copper export in older animals during cardiac copper deficiency (thus ATP7A is depicted on the lower membrane of the cell). A large percentage of copper in this cell type is incorporated into ceruloplasmin (CP), which is secreted into the bloodstream. A glycophosphatidylinositol (GPI)–anchored version of CP also exists in hepatocytes. Both CP proteins are ferroxidases that play critical roles in iron (Fe) release from certain tissues and cell types. Under conditions of excess body copper, ATP7B translocates to the canalicular membrane and facilitates copper excretion in the bile. ATP7B protein levels are controlled by copper metabolism (Murr1) domain containing 1 (COMMD1) and X-linked inhibitor of apoptosis (XIAP) through the proteasome pathway. Additional copper export pathways may exist in hepatocytes because a percentage of serum copper is not bound to CP and may therefore not proceed through the secretory pathway; a potential unknown copper transported is thus depicted on the lower surface of the cell. *ATOX1,* ATX1 antioxidant protein 1 homolog (yeast); *CCS,* copper chaperone for superoxide dismutase; *COX17,* cytochrome c oxidase assembly homolog *(S. cerevisiae); SOD,* superoxide dismutase.

Genetic Defects in Copper Metabolism

Copper-related diseases in humans most frequently arise because of defects in two copper export systems, resulting in MD and WD.

Menkes Disease

MD is an X-linked, recessive disorder of copper metabolism that affects multiple organ systems. As expected, most patients are male. Typical manifestations include progressive neurodegeneration, connective tissue disturbances, and unusual "kinky" hair. The disease is usually fatal by the age of 3 years; no cure exists, although copper histidine treatment (by subcutaneous injection) of affected individuals early in life has shown promise, particularly in partial amelioration of neurologic symptoms (31). The prevalence of MD varies in different regions of the world; a lower prevalence is noted in Japan and in European countries (1:300,000 to 1:360,000), but a much higher incidence is observed in Australia (1:50,000 to 100,000) (54). The underlying genetic defect is in the *ATP7A* gene, encoding a copper-translocating ATPase required for copper delivery to cuproenzymes in the secretory pathway and for cellular copper export.

Defective copper elimination from cells is the basic physiologic disturbance in MD, and most tissues (except liver and brain) accumulate excessive copper. Copper does not accumulate to toxic levels, however, at least partially because of an intestinal block to absorption of dietary copper. The lack of copper in some peripheral tissues, despite accumulation in other tissues (e.g., intestinal mucosa, muscle, spleen, and kidney), leads to signs and symptoms of systemic copper deficiency. These include low serum copper and CP activity and impaired synthesis of SOD and CCO. LOX activity is also impaired, leading to defective artery formation in the CNS and osteoporosis. Progressive nerve degeneration is noted in the brain, with consequent classic neurologic symptoms of MD (55).

Wilson Disease

WD is an autosomal recessive disease in which affected individuals exhibit abnormal copper storage (56). The underlying defect is in the *ATP7B* gene, which encodes a copper-transporting ATPase. The worldwide prevalence of WD was reported to be 1:30,000 (57). In patients with WD, systemic copper accumulation in liver, brain, and cornea (Kayser-Fleisher rings) results in multiorgan damage, particularly in brain and liver. Neurologic damage and cirrhosis may ensue if the condition is left untreated. Acute hepatitis, hemolytic crisis, and hepatic failure may also occur. Other observations include abnormally high urinary copper excretion and low CP values. Permanent organ damage can be avoided in WD by proper medical treatment, especially if initiated early in life. Typical treatment uses decoppering chelation therapy with penicillamine or trientine (58), with lifelong compliance required, or high zinc dosing (which interferes with absorption of dietary copper).

COPPER DEFICIENCY IN ANIMALS AND HUMANS

Severe copper deficiency in animals results in abnormalities in the immune, skeletal, and cardiovascular systems. Further consequences of copper deprivation are hypochromic anemia (which does not respond to iron supplementation), hypopigmentation, thrombocytopenia, and neutropenia (25). Across many species, other hallmarks of copper deficiency in addition to anemia include neutropenia and osteoporosis. More specific features are as follows: skeletal abnormalities, fractures, and spinal deformities; neonatal ataxia; depigmentation of hair and wool; abnormal keratinization of hair, wool, and fur; reproductive failure; cardiovascular abnormalities; and impaired immune function. Some of these symptoms have been observed in only one or two species, and manifestations of copper deficiency in experimental and other animals is typically more severe than observed in humans (described below).

Systemic copper deficiency in humans, which is rare, can result from ineffective absorption of dietary copper or excessive copper loss through the endogenous excretory system in the liver through bile. Several groups of individuals are however susceptible to copper deficiency including: individuals receiving total parenteral nutrition on a long-term basis and without proper copper supplementation; premature infants consuming milk-based formulas lacking adequate copper; neonates experiencing chronic diarrhea or malnutrition; hospitalized patients undergoing long-term peritoneal dialysis; patients with severe burns; patients undergoing renal dialysis; and persons consuming large doses of supplemental zinc, antacids, or copper chelators (16). Malabsorption may also result in copper deficiency. Moreover, evidence suggests an association between surgical bowel resection in the management of morbid obesity and acquired copper deficiency (59).

In humans, copper deficiency is accompanied by low serum copper levels and reduced serum ferroxidase activity. Usual pathophysiologic features include anemia, leukopenia, and neutropenia. During periods of rapid growth, osteoporosis is a common feature. Furthermore, moderate copper deficiency as a result of long-term low copper intakes in humans is a possibility. This may result in additional manifestations including arthritis, arterial disease, depigmentation, myocardial disease, and neurologic abnormalities (52). Possible additional effects of marginal copper deficiency include cardiac arrhythmias, increased serum cholesterol levels, and glucose intolerance (60). Because these observations were not duplicated in other studies, future clinical studies will be necessary before strong conclusions can be drawn.

DIETARY CONSIDERATIONS AND REQUIREMENTS

Dietary reference intakes for copper were established in 2001 (61) and are listed in Table 12.2. Based on a lack of experimental data, Adequate intake (AI) levels for copper have been established for infants 0 to 6 months of age and for those between 7 and 12 months. The RDA increases throughout childhood and adolescence and is increased from adult levels during pregnancy and lactation. ULs have also been established for copper (also listed in Table 12.2).

EVALUATION OF COPPER STATUS

Analytical Methods

The most widely used methods to quantify copper are inductively coupled plasma (ICP) emission spectroscopy and atomic absorption spectroscopy (AAS) (12). For AAS, samples are atomized with a graphite furnace (GFAA) or with an air-acetylene flame (flame AA) for electrothermal ionization. ICP is often used when more than one mineral is being quantified. Studies to determine the distribution of copper in living animals typically employ stable isotopes of copper (62) to track the absorption, utilization, excretion, and turnover of copper in biologic systems. The most common method to measure the copper isotope ratios is mass spectrometry (MS); ICP-MS and thermal ionization MS (TIMS) are the most frequently used techniques.

Assessment of Copper Status

Much effort has gone into identifying biomarkers of copper status that are sensitive to even marginal deficiency and that are noninvasive and consistently reliable (63). The most commonly used method in humans has been to quantify copper levels and the activity of various cuproenzymes in blood (16). Reductions in plasma copper and CP activity are noted in severely copper deficient-humans; intakes in experimental settings of 0.6 mg/day or less for at least a month and a half are required to see these decreases consistently. Observed reductions in serum copper and CP activity are complicated, however, by the finding that several physiologic alterations can increase copper content and CP activity of blood, including the acute phase response to infection and inflammation, pregnancy and other hormonal perturbations, and some carcinogenic phenotypes (16). Other markers in use, including SOD1 activity in erythrocytes, CCO activity in platelets and mononuclear cells, and copper content of various circulating blood cells, have shown limited usefulness in determining the copper status of humans. Recent studies have also evaluated other potential biomarkers of copper status. Studies in rats revealing alterations in serum and tissue PAM activity (64) have been correlated with similar observations in copper-deficient humans (65).

COPPER TOXICITY AND UPPER LIMITS

Copper toxicity is uncommon in humans and animals because mammals have evolved precise homeostatic control of copper in response to the propensity of the free metal to generate reactive oxygen species. Free copper in cells and in the body is extremely low; copper almost always exists in biologic systems bound to proteins. Ingestion of high copper levels may, however, override the innate checkpoints designed to regulate overall body copper levels, including, but not limited to, enhanced intestinal absorption in the absence of a physiologic demand for copper. Because of possible adverse consequences of high copper ingestion, a UL of 10 mg/day has been established for adults >19 years of age.

Copper is often included in complete nutrition and micronutrient supplements without consequence. One study supplemented adults with 10 mg Cu^{2+} gluconate daily for 12 weeks without evidence of liver damage or gastrointestinal distress (66). Despite a lack of effect of high copper intake in adults, copper toxicity risks are higher for neonates and infants, given their immature biliary excretory system and enhanced intestinal absorption apparatus. Copper loading is observed clinically today in the setting of WD and other disorders in which biliary copper excretion is impaired, such as biliary cirrhosis and biliary atresia.

TABLE 12.2	DIETARY REFERENCE INTAKE VALUES FOR COPPER[a]		
AGE	RDA (μg/d)[b]	AI (μg/d)[c]	UL (μg/d)[d]
0–6 mo	—	200	ND[e]
7–12 mo	—	220	ND
1–3 y	340	—	1,000
4–8 y	440	—	3,000
9–13 y	700	—	5,000
14–18 y	890	—	8,000
19–50 y	900	—	10,000
>51 y	900	—	10,000
Pregnancy			
14–18 y	1,000	—	8,000
19–50 y	1,000	—	10,000
Lactation			
14–18 y	1,300	—	8,000
19–50 y	1,300	—	10,000

[a]1 μg copper = 0.0157 μmol.
[b]Recommended dietary allowance. This is the intake that meets the nutrient needs of almost all (97% to 98%) of individuals in a group.
[c]Adequate intake. This is the mean intake of healthy infants receiving human milk.
[d]Tolerable upper intake levels. This is the highest level that is likely to pose no risk of adverse health effects to almost all individuals.
[e]Not determinable. The source of intake should be from food only.

ACKNOWLEDGMENTS

The writing of this chapter was supported by the National Institutes of Health grant DK074867 (to JFC).

REFERENCES

1. Bodansky M. J Biol Chem 1921;48:361.
2. Cohn EJ, Minot GR, Fulton JF et al. J Biol Chem 1927;74:1xix.
3. Wilson SAK. Brain 1912;34:295–509.
4. Mason KE. J Nutr 1979;109:1979–2066.
5. Menkes JH, Alter M, Steigleder GK et al. Pediatrics 1962; 29:764–79.
6. Danks DM, Campbell PE, Stevens BJ et al. Pediatrics 1972; 50:188–201.
7. Dyer FF, Leddicotte GW. The Radiochemistry of Copper. Washington, DC: National Academy of Sciences, National Research Council, 1961.
8. Harris ED. Copper. In: O'Dell BL, Sunde RA, eds. Clinical Nutrition in Health and Disease: Handbook of Nutritionally Essential Mineral Elements, vol 2. New York: Marcel Dekker, 1997:231–73.
9. Linder MC. Biochemistry and molecular biology of copper in mammals. In: Massaro EJ, ed. Handbook of Copper Pharmacology and Toxicology. Totowa, NJ: Humana Press, 2003:3–32.
10. McDonald A, Tipton K, O'Sullivan J et al. J Neural Transm 2007;114:783–6.
11. Dunkel P, Gelain A, Barlocco D et al. Curr Med Chem 2008;15:1827–39.
12. Turnlund JR. Copper. In: Shils ME, Shike M, Ross AC et al, eds. Modern Nutrition in Health and Disease. 10th ed. Baltimore: Lippincott Williams & Wilkins, 2006:286–99.
13. Tininello A, Pietrangeli P, De Marchi U et al. Biochim Biophys Acta 2006;1765:1–13.
14. Rodriguez C, Rodriguez-Sinovas A, Martinez-Gonzales J. Drug News Perspect 2008;21:218–24.
15. Molnar J, Fong KS, He QP et al. Biochim Biophys Acta 2003; 1647:220–24.
16. Prohaska JR. Copper. In: Bowman BA, Russell RM eds. Present Knowledge in Nutrition. 9th ed. Washington, DC: ILSI Press, 2006:458–470.
17. Czyzyk TA, Morgan DJ, Peng B et al. J Neurosci Res 2003; 74:446–55.
18. De Domenico I, Ward DM, Di Patti MC et al. EMBO J 2007; 26:2823–31.
19. Vulpe CD, Kuo YM, Murphy TL et al. Nat Genet 1999;21:195–9.
20. Hudson DM, Curtis SB, Smith VC et al. Am J Physiol 2010; 298:G425–32.
21. Chen H, Huang G, Su T et al. J Nutr 2006;136:1236–41.
22. Thomas SA, Matsumoto AM, Palmiter RD. Nature 1995; 374:643–46.
23. Fattman CL, Schaefer LM, Oury TD. Free Radic Biol Med 2003;35:236–56.
24. Oberley-Deegan RE, Regan EA, Kinnula VL et al. COPD 2009;6:307–12.
25. Uauy R, Olivares M, Gonzalez M. Am J Clin Nutr 1998; 67:952S–9S.
26. Disilvestro RA, Selsby J, Siefker K. J Trace Elem Med Biol 2010;23:165–68.
27. Baker A, Harvey L, Kajask-Newman G et al. J Nutr 1999; 53:408–12.
28. Collins JF, Prohaska JR, Knutson MD. Nutr Rev 2010;68:133–47.
29. Broderius M, Mostad E, Wendroth K et al. Comp Biochem Physiol C Toxicol Pharmacol 2010;151:473–9.
30. Thackeray EW, Sanderson SO, Fox JC et al. J Clin Gastroenterol 2011;45:153–8.
31. Kaler SG, Holmes CS, Goldstein DS et al. N Engl J Med 2008;358:605–14.
32. Easter RN, Chan Q, Lai B et al. Vas Med 2010;15:61–69.
33. Aliabadi H. Med Hypoth 2008;6:1163–66.
34. Prohaska JR, Failla ML. Copper and immunity. In: Klurfeld DM, ed. Human Nutrition: A Comprehensive Treatise. New York: Plenum Press, 1993:309–32.
35. Kelley DS, Dauda PA, Taylor PC et al. Am J Clin Nutr 1995;62:412–6.
36. White C, Lee J, Kambe T et al. J Biol Chem 2009;284: 33949–56.
37. Lonnerdal B. Am J Clin Nutr 1998;67(Suppl):1046S–53S.
38. Nations SP, Boyer PJ, Love LA et al. Neurology 2008;71: 639–43.
39. Collins JF, Franck CA, Kowdley KV et al. Am J Physiol 2005; 288:G964–71.
40. Ravia JJ, Stephen RM, Ghishan FK et al. J Biol Chem 2005; 280:36221–7.
41. Yokoi K, Kimura M, Itokawa Y. Biol Trace Elem Res 1991; 29:257–65.
42. Food and Nutrition Board, Institute of Medicine. Zinc. In: Dietary Reference Intakes for Vitamin A, Vitamin K, Arsenic, Boron, Chromium, Copper, Iodine, Manganese, Molybdenum, Nickel, Silicon, Vanadium, and Zinc. Washington, DC: National Academy Press, 2002:442–501.
43. Powers HJ, Loban A, Silvers K et al. Free Radic Res 1995; 22:57–65.
44. Hunt JR, Matthys LA, Johnson LK. Am J Clin Nutr 1998; 67:421–30.
45. Baker DH. J Nutr 1999;129:2278–79.
46. Prohaska JR, Gybina AA. J Nutr 2004;134:1003–6.
47. Van Den Berghe PV, Klomp LW. J Biol Inorg Chem 2010; 15:37–46.
48. Collins JF, Hua P, Lu Y et al. Am J Physiol 2009;297:G695–707.
49. Nose Y, Kim BE, Thiele DJ. Cell Metab 2006;4:235–44.
50. Arredondo M, Cambiazo, V, Tapia L et al. Am J Physiol 2003; 284:C1525–30.
51. Kim H, Son HY, Bailey SM et al. Am J Physiol 2009;297: G356–64.
52. Danks DM. Annu Rev Nutr 1988;8:235–57.
53. Harvey LJ, Dainty JR, Hollands WJ et al. Am J Clin Nutr 2005;81:807–13.
54. Tumer Z, Moller LB. Eur J Hum Genet 2010;18:511–8.
55. Nishihara E, Furuyama T, Yamashita S et al. Neuroreport 1998;9:3259–63.
56. Mak CM, Lam CW. Crit Rev Clin Lab Sci 2008;45:263–90.
57. Scheinberg I, Sternlieb I. Major Prob Intern Med 1984; 23:1–24.
58. Lewitt PA. Mov Disord 1999;14:555–6.
59. Griffith DP, Liff DA, Ziegler TR et al. Obesity 2009;17: 827–31.
60. Davis GK, Mertz W. Copper. In: Mertz W, ed. Trace Elements in Human and Animal Nutrition, vol 1. 5th ed. San Diego: Academic Press, 1987:301–64.
61. Trumbo P, Yates AA, Schlicker S et al. J Am Diet Assoc 2001;101:294–301.
62. Patterson KY, Veillon C. Exp Biol Med 2001;226:271–82.
63. Harvey LJ, Ashton K, Hooper L et al. Am J Clin Nutr 2009;89(Suppl):2009S–24S.

64.   Prohaska JR, Gybina AA. J Neurochem 2005;93:698–705.
65.   Prohaska JR. Neurochemical roles of copper as antioxidant or prooxidant. In: Conner JR, ed. Metals and Oxidative Damage in Neurological Disorders. New York: Plenum Press, 1997.
66.   Pratt WB, Omdahl, JL. Sorenson JR. Am J Clin Nutr 1985;42:681–82.

SUGGESTED READINGS

Harris ED. Copper. In: O'Dell BL, Sunde, RA, eds. Clinical Nutrition in Health and Disease: Handbook of Nutritionally Essential Mineral Elements, vol 2. New York: Marcel Dekker, 1997: 231–73.

La Fontaine S, Ackland ML, Mercer JF. Mammalian copper-transporting P-type ATPases, ATP7A and ATP7B: emerging roles. Int J Biochem Cell Biol 2010;42:206–9.

Lutsenko S, Bhattacharjee A, Hubbard AL. Copper handling machinery of the brain. Metallomics 2010;9:596–608.

Mason KE. A conspectus of research on copper metabolism and requirements of man. J Nutr 1979;109:1979–2066.

Prohaska JR. Copper. In: Bowman BA, Russell RM eds. Present Knowledge in Nutrition. 9th ed. Washington, DC: ILSI Press, 2006; 458–70.

Uriu-Adams JY, Scherr RE, Lanoue L et al. Influence of copper on early development: prenatal and postnatal considerations. Biofactors 2010;36:136–52.

13 IODINE[1]
PETER LAURBERG

OVERVIEW

The only established role of iodine in humans is to be a component of thyroid hormones. The hormones are essential for development and growth, and severe iodine deficiency may lead to developmental brain damage (1). Moreover, thyroid hormones participate in regulation of the daily activity of probably every single cell.

Appropriate thyroid hormone levels for the current state of every cell are obtained through several complicated systems. Iodine exerts strong autoregulatory effects on the thyroid gland to accommodate thyroid iodine utilization to daily needs for hormone production, despite large variations in iodine supply. Over time, activation of iodine autoregulatory mechanisms may lead to thyroid functional abnormalities in many individuals. Thus, the epidemiology

of thyroid disease in a population is associated with the iodine intake level, even if neither regular severe iodine deficiency nor excess is present.

HISTORICAL BACKGROUND

The history associated with iodine has been that of the iodine deficiency diseases endemic goiter and cretinism. Iodine discovery is credited to Bernard Courtois in 1811, and the first use of iodine for treatment of goiter was published in 1820 by Coindet (2, 3) in Geneva. The use of iodine in high doses for medical purposes in the early nineteenth century led to the first reports of clinical thyrotoxicosis after intake of iodine (4).

A landmark in progress was the trial performed in Ohio between 1917 and 1922 by Marine and Kimball in 4495 school children; results of this trial showed profound effects of iodine supplements on goiter frequencies (5). Voluntary iodized salt prophylaxis was introduced in Michigan in 1924.

During the same period, Hunziker, from iodine-deficient Switzerland, observed that as little as 100 µg iodine per day was effective in preventing goiter, and in 1922, voluntary iodine prophylaxis was introduced in parts of Switzerland (6).

Despite considerable knowledge on the prevention of iodine deficiency, developmental brain damage caused by iodine deficiency occurred in many parts of the world until recent decades. The formation in 1985 of the International Council for the Control of Iodine Deficiency Disorders (ICCIDD; http://www.ICCIDD.org) (7) and its subsequent activities in collaboration with the World Health Organization (WHO) and The United Nations Children's Fund (UNICEF) improved the situation, but further efforts are necessary.

DIETARY SOURCES

The dietary sources of iodine vary with the country and population sector. Data from the United States were reviewed by Pearce (8). In countries such as the United States with an extensive intake of dairy products, these foods are often the most important source. Iodine is concentrated in milk (see later), and the iodine content of dairy products is often relatively high because of

---

[1]**Abbreviations: H_2O_2,** hydrogen peroxide; **ICCIDD,** International Council for the Control of Iodine Deficiency Disorders; **KI,** potassium iodide; **MCT8,** monocarboxylate transporter 8; **NIS,** sodium iodide symporter; **T_3,** triiodothyronine; **T_4,** thyroxine; **TPO,** thyroid peroxidase; **TRH,** thyrotropin-releasing hormone; **TSH,** thyroid-stimulating hormone; **UNICEF,** United Nations Children's Fund; **WHO,** World Health Organization.

the iodine in supplements given to dairy cows. Before the Danish iodization of salt, iodine in dairy products contributed 44% of iodine intake, whereas iodine in fish products contributed 15% (9).

Countries where iodine-rich kelp products constitute a significant part of the diet (Japan, Korea) have a generally high iodine intake (10, 11), much higher than the internationally recommended levels (see later). Groundwater iodine content is low in most places. High levels may be caused by leaching of iodine-containing humic substances into aquifers, presumably from old sea bottom deposits (12, 13).

A dietary iodine source that is difficult to control is iodine from chemicals used by the food industry for other purposes. The most prominent example is the use of iodate in the baking industry in the United States, although this practice has become less common. Nonetheless, some types of bread may contain more than the recommended daily intake of iodine in a single slice, without any notification to the consumer (14). The decrease in the use of iodate by the baking industry is probably one of the main causes for the fall in median urinary iodine concentration in the US population from 320 μg/L in 1971 to 1974 (excessive; Table 13.1) to 145 μg/L in 1988 to 1994 (within recommended levels). In 2001 to 2002, it was 168 μg/L (15), and in 2003 to 2004 it was 160 μg/L (16).

The use of iodine-containing medications, radiographic contrast agents, or disinfectants may lead to very high iodine intakes in some individuals.

Multivitamins may contain iodine, often 150 μg per tablet. This is an important source of iodine intake in some populations.

A major source of iodine intake in many countries is iodized salt, to prevent iodine deficiency disorders (17). Programs differ among countries. In the United States, the iodine content of iodized salt is relatively high (45 mg of iodine/kg salt [45 ppm]), albeit with large variations among samples of salt (18), but the use of iodine is voluntary and is limited to 70% of household salt (8). Switzerland uses lower amounts of iodine in salt (20 ppm) (19), but the frequency of use is high; 95% of household salt and 70% of salt used by the food industry are iodized. In some countries, such as Denmark, the use of iodized salt is obligatory for some purposes (table salt, bread production, but not other types of food) (20), to obtain more uniform distribution of iodine intake in the population.

RECOMMENDED INTAKES

Both international and national organizations have made similar recommendations on iodine intake. Because approximately 90% of iodine in diet is excreted by the kidney, and because iodine nutrition is mostly assessed by urinary iodine measurement, recommendations are often given for urinary iodine excretion values. The recommendations given by the WHO, UNICEF, and ICCIDD (1) are outlined in Table 13.1.

TABLE 13.1	WORLD HEALTH ORGANIZATION, UNITED NATIONS CHILDREN'S FUND, AND INTERNATIONAL COUNCIL FOR THE CONTROL OF IODINE DEFICIENCY DISORDERS EPIDEMIOLOGIC CRITERIA FOR ASSESSING IODINE NUTRITION BASED ON MEDIAN URINARY IODINE CONCENTRATIONS

SCHOOL-AGE CHILDREN (≥6 y)[a]	
MEDIAN URINARY IODINE CONCENTRATION (μg/L)	**IODINE STATUS**
<20	Insufficient; severe iodine deficiency
20–49	Insufficient; moderate iodine deficiency
50–99	Insufficient; mild iodine deficiency
100–199	Adequate iodine nutrition
200–299	Above requirements
≥300	Excessive; risk of adverse health consequences (iodine-induced hyperthyroidism, autoimmune thyroid diseases)

PREGNANT WOMEN[b]	
MEDIAN URINARY IODINE CONCENTRATION (μg/L)	**IODINE STATUS**
<150	Insufficient
150–249	Adequate
250–499	Above requirements
≥500	Excessive[c]

[a]Applies to adults, but not to pregnant and lactating women. Comment: In adults, a median nonfasting urinary iodine concentration of 100 μg/L would correspond to a urinary iodine excretion of 150 μg/24 hour (71). Because small amounts of iodine are excreted in feces and sweat, intake of iodine would be 10% higher than urinary iodine excretion. The intakes recommended by the World Health Organization, United Nations Children's Fund, and International Council for the Control of Iodine Deficiency Disorders are as follows: <5 years of age, 90 μg; 6 to 12 years, 120 μg; >12 years, 150 μg; pregnancy and lactation, 250 μg/day. Iodine 1 μg/L corresponds to 7.88 nmol/L.

[b]For lactating women and for children <2 years of age, a median urinary iodine concentration of 100 μg/L can be used to define adequate iodine intake, but no other categories of iodine intake are defined. Although lactating women have the same requirement as pregnant women, the median urinary iodine is lower because part of iodine is excreted in breast milk.

[c]The term "excessive" means in excess of the amount required to prevent and control iodine deficiency. Comment: If iodine intake of the population is in general adequate with a median urinary iodine excretion of 100 to 200 μg/L in representative groups, the daily iodine intake and thyroid stores of iodine will be sufficient to cover the needs during pregnancy and lactation (23).

From World Health Organization, United Nations Children's Fund, International Council for the Control of Iodine Deficiency Disorders. Assessment of Iodine Deficiency Disorders and Monitoring Their Elimination: A Guide for Programme Managers. 3rd ed. Geneva: World Health Organization, 2007:1–99, with permission.

The iodine take recommendations of the Food and Nutrition Board of the US Institute of Medicine (21) are shown in Table 13.2. These recommendations are for iodine intakes of population groups to minimize the risk of disease and for average intakes of individuals over a period of time. The recommendations are not for evaluation

TABLE 13.2	RECOMMENDATIONS ON DIETARY INTAKES OF IODINE BY THE FOOD AND NUTRITION BOARD OF THE INSTITUTE OF MEDICINE

	RDA^a (μg/d)	AI^b (μg/d)	UL^c (μg/d)
Infants			
0–6 mo		110	
7–12 mo		130	
Children			
1–3 y	90		200
4–8 y	90		300
9–13 y	120		600
14–18 y	150		900
Women	150		1,100
Men	150		1,100
Pregnancy	220		1,100
Lactation	290		1,100

^{a}RDA, recommended dietary allowance: the average daily intake that meets the estimated iodine needs of almost all (97.5 %) individuals in the group.
^{b}AI, adequate intake: the iodine intake that appears to sustain normal thyroid structure and function in the group. Data are insufficient to establish an RDA.
^{c}UL, tolerable upper intake level: the highest level of daily iodine intake that is likely to pose no risk of adverse health effects for almost all individuals in the group.

From Food and Nutrition Board, Institute of Medicine. Dietary Reference Intakes: Iodine. Washington, DC: National Academy Press, 2001:258–89, with permission.

of individuals on a daily basis. Because of the adaptive capacities of the thyroid, most individuals adapt to days of very low or high iodine intake without incident.

The Public Health Committee of the American Thyroid Association recommends that women living in the United States and Canada receive dietary supplements that contain 150 μg iodine during pregnancy and lactation to cover the increase in need of iodine during these periods (22). Detailed recommendations on iodine intake during pregnancy and lactation have been published by WHO/UNICEF/ICCIDD (23) (see Table 13.1).

EFFECTS OF IODINE IN THE HUMAN BODY

The effects of iodine in the human body can be regarded as belonging to one of three groups:

1. Effects of deficient production of thyroid hormone caused by iodine deficiency.
2. Autoregulatory effects of iodine on the thyroid gland.
3. Extrathyroidal effects of iodine that are mostly of theoretic importance in need of final proof.

The central role of iodine is to be part of the hormones produced in the thyroid gland. Avoidance of iodine deficiency is especially important in pregnancy, to prevent developmental brain damage in the fetus.

The autoregulatory effects of iodine on the thyroid gland tend to compensate for a low iodine supply by increasing the activity of processes involved in utilization of iodine for thyroid hormone production. Other autoregulatory

processes rapidly shut down thyroid utilization of iodine after intake of excess iodine. Thus, the thyroid gland normally keeps thyroid hormone production stable despite large changes in iodine supply. The price for the complex ability to compensate for these variables is a tendency to develop thyroid disease. Because the thyroid processes activated by low and high iodine intake are different, the pattern of thyroid disease in a population depends on the level of iodine intake (24).

Extrathyroidal effects and handling of iodine have received less focus. The exception is the processes involved in transport of iodine from the mother to the breast-fed child, and to some degree also from the mother to the fetus through the placenta. This iodine is necessary for thyroid hormone production by the fetal and infant thyroid.

Investigators have suggested that iodine may function in the human body (e.g., in breast and gastrointestinal tract) to protect against reactive oxygen species (25), similar to the role of iodine in macroalgae (26). However, more evidence is necessary before a conclusion can be drawn.

Finally, very large amounts of iodine may lead to excess upper airway secretions (large iodine doses were formerly used as medication for airway problems), skin eruptions, and various other toxicities (27).

METABOLISM

Iodine in diet occurs in various forms. Most iodine-containing compounds are broken down in the gut, and the iodide is rapidly absorbed.

The absorbed iodide enters the circulating pool of inorganic iodide together with iodide released by metabolism of thyroid hormones. Most circulating iodide is either excreted by the kidney (clearance of 30 to 50 mL/minute, independent of iodine status) or concentrated in the thyroid gland (clearance from very low to more than 100 mL/minute). Thyroid uptake of iodine is low after excessive iodine intake and high in iodine deficiency, and it depends on the functional status of the thyroid (low if nonfunctional thyroid, high in stimulated thyroid). In people with a recommended iodine intake of approximately 150 μg/day, thyroid clearance of iodine is approximately half that of the kidney, and the half-life of iodide in blood is approximately 6 hours. In breast-feeding women, a considerable fraction of the circulating iodide is taken up by the mammary glands and is excreted in breast milk, as discussed later.

The iodide taken up by the thyroid is build into tyrosine groups to create monoiodotyrosines and diiodotyrosines in the 660-kDa glycoprotein thyroglobulin present in the colloid of thyroid follicles. This process is catalyzed by the membrane-bound enzyme thyroid peroxidase (TPO) in the presence of hydrogen peroxide (H_2O_2). TPO is a heme-containing protein, and interaction exists between the effects of iodine and iron deficiency (28). TPO also catalyzes the coupling of iodinated tyrosine residues in thyroglobulin to form the double-ring iodothyronines L-thyroxine (tetraiodothyronine, T_4) and L-triiodothyronine (T_3).

Thyroid hormone secretion is initiated by uptake into the follicular cells of thyroglobulin through micropinocytosis and macropinocytosis. The thyroid hormones T_4 and T_3 and iodotyrosines are liberated by hydrolysis of thyroglobulin catalyzed by lysosomal enzymes. The iodotyrosines are nearly entirely deiodinated in the follicular cells, thus preserving the iodide in the cells for hormone production. Release of T_4 and T_3 can be immediately and reversibly blocked by certain iodine-containing compounds; this finding indicates active transport of the hormones out of the follicular cells (29). Certain thyroid hormone transporters have been identified (30), but their potential role in thyroid hormone secretion has not been clarified.

The two most important regulators of thyroid activity are thyrotropin (thyroid-stimulating hormone [TSH]) and iodide by autoregulation. TSH is secreted from the anterior lobe of the pituitary, regulated by classical feedback inhibition from T_4 and T_3, and by hypothalamic signals. The most important hypothalamic factor is thyrotropin-releasing hormone (TRH), which modulates the set point of the thyroid system. Vitamin A plays a role in the activity of the pituitary-thyroidal axis (31). TSH activates all the processes involved in thyroid activities by binding to the TSH receptor.

SODIUM IODIDE SYMPORTER

Sodium iodide symporter (NIS) is central in the transport of iodine in the body (32). It is an 85-kDa membrane protein that couples the translocations of sodium (Na^+) (from high to low) and iodine (I^-) (from low to high concentration) into the cells. The most important sites of NIS are the basolateral membrane of the follicular cells of the thyroid and the lactotrophs of the lactating mammary gland, but NIS is also present in salivary glands, in the gut mucosae, in sweat glands, and in the choroid plexus of the cerebral lateral ventricles.

IODIDE AUTOREGULATION OF THE THYROID

Iodide has a strong autoregulatory function on the thyroid independent of TSH regulation of the thyroid (33). The mechanisms involved have been only partially elucidated, but they may occur through organic iodinated compounds, possibly iodolactones (34).

When iodine is scarce, practically all processes involved in iodine trapping and hormone synthesis are enhanced. Conversely, excessive iodine is rapidly followed by blocking of iodide organification (Wolff–Chaikoff effect) and of hormone secretion (an effect used therapeutically in patients with thyroid storm) and blood flow (used therapeutically before thyroid surgery to prevent bleeding). Moreover, high iodine concentrations inhibit thyroid growth and promote apoptosis of thyrocytes (35). Shortly after a load of iodine, down-regulation of NIS occurs (36),

with a reduction of thyroid iodine uptake and intrathyroid iodine content. This process tends to reestablish iodide organification (escape from the Wolff–Chaikoff effect).

IODIDE TRANSPORT INTO MILK

The lactating mammary gland concentrates iodide from blood into milk by way of NIS. A major difference between iodide transport in the mammary gland and transport in the thyroid is that iodide autoregulation and TSH stimulation have little or no effect on the mammary gland. The concentration of iodide in breast milk varies with the iodine intake of the mother.

Certain chemicals, most importantly thiocyanate and perchlorate, are competitive inhibitors of iodide transport by NIS (32), both in the thyroid gland and in the lactating mammary gland. Because of the lack of iodide autoregulation in the mammary gland, intake of such compounds affects iodide excretion into milk much more directly than such intake affects thyroid iodide uptake. Thiocyanate in rapeseed oil cakes used to feed cows may lead to low dairy milk iodine content (37). Both thiocyanate and perchlorate are important industrial waste products, and environmental pollution may worsen iodine deficiency and lead to an increase in the risk of goiter and thyroid nodules when iodine intake is low (38).

The leading cause of high levels of thiocyanate in blood is tobacco smoking, because cyanide in the tobacco smoke is detoxified in the liver to thiocyanate. Thus, tobacco smoking during the period of breast-feeding leads to a low iodine concentration in breast milk, and the neonates of smoking mothers have a low urinary iodine excretion because their iodine intake from mother's milk is low (39). Smokers also have a higher risk of goiter if their iodine intake is low (40).

ACTIONS OF THYROID HORMONES

The main actions of thyroid hormones are exerted by binding to nuclear receptors that modulate transcription of many proteins. The active hormone is T_3, which has been directly synthesized in the thyroid or derived by outer ring 5'-deiodination of T_4. In physiologically normal persons, approximately 80% of circulating T_3 has been derived from T_4 in peripheral tissues. Outer ring deiodination of T_4 to T_3 is catalyzed by type 1 or type 2 iodothyronine deiodinase, whereas type 3 iodothyronine deiodinase exclusively inactivates thyroid hormones by inner ring deiodination (41). The three deiodinases are selenoenzymes, and severe selenium deficiency interferes with normal thyroid function. Selenium may influence thyroid autoimmunity and growth by several mechanisms (42).

The iodothyronine deiodinases, as well as different types of thyroid hormone transporters and receptors, are differently distributed in tissues. The complex roles of the deiodinases in health and disease are still an area of research (43).

Investigators have shown that the Allan-Herndon-Dudley syndrome is caused by a mutation in the gene coding for the monocarboxylate transporter 8 (MCT8) transport protein (30). MCT8 is a thyroid hormone transporter, but defective transport of other substances may contribute to the clinical syndrome.

Thyroid hormone is important for brain development, as discussed later. In adult humans, the most significant effects of thyroid hormones are their overall regulation of levels of activity in many organs and tissue. Thus, excess thyroid hormone production is associated with the clinical picture of thyrotoxicosis, characterized by psychomotor hyperactivity, high pulse rate, sweating, weight loss, and tremor, whereas lack of thyroid hormone (hypothyroidism or myxedema) is associated with the opposite symptoms and signs.

EFFECTS OF DEFICIENT THYROID HORMONE PRODUCTION CAUSED BY IODINE DEFICIENCY

The most important consequences of iodine deficiency are those related to development because they may be irreversible. The importance of thyroid hormone for metamorphosis in amphibians is well characterized (44). Thyroid hormones have an equally important role in the development of the brain in mammals. For example, thyroid hormones are necessary for proper sprouting of neurons and therefore for development of neural networks (45, 46).

The clinical consequence of severe iodine deficiency in pregnancy and fetal life and during the first years is cretinism. Depending on the time and severity of thyroid hormone deficiency during development, different clinical pictures may occur. In geographic areas where cretinism caused by iodine deficiency is found, the population may have a general shift in intelligence quotient toward low values (47).

IODINE INTAKE AND THYROID DISEASE IN THE POPULATION

Investigations into the development of thyroid disease of populations, have revealed that the level of iodine intake of a population is a major determinant of the epidemiology of thyroid disease, even in areas not affected by obvious signs of iodine deficiency (24).

Figure 13.1 illustrates the principal relationship between a certain level of iodine intake and the associated risk of disease. The curve is U shaped but asymmetric, with a much steeper increase in risk with low than with high iodine intake. The diseases that may be more common at a certain level of iodine intake are indicated in Table 13.3. In addition, individual risk depends on genetics and on other environmental factors.

The diseases associated with severe iodine deficiency and, to a lesser degree, with moderate iodine deficiency (see Table 13.3) are easily understandable. Both cretinism and

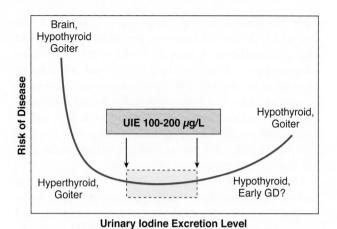

Fig. 13.1. Theoretical relationship between exposure to a certain iodine intake level over a long period and the risk of developing a thyroid disease. The *box* indicates the recommended level with a median urinary iodine excretion *(UIE)* of 100 to 200 μg/L. *GD,* Graves' disease. (Modified from Laurberg P. Prevention in endocrinology. In: Wass J, Shalet S, eds. Oxford Textbook of Endocrinology and Diabetes. Oxford: Oxford University Press, 2002:3–8, with permission.)

hypothyroidism are caused by lack of substrate for thyroid hormone production, and goiter is secondary to an increase in serum TSH and to iodide autoregulation of the thyroid.

It may seem a paradox that mild and moderate iodine deficiency will lead to a high incidence of hyperthyroidism. The type is mainly multinodular toxic goiter (48). The

TABLE 13.3	INCREASE IN RISK OF DISEASE IN THE POPULATION ASSOCIATED WITH POPULATION IODINE INTAKE OUTSIDE THE OPTIMAL LEVEL[a]	
IODINE NUTRITION	**MEDIAN URINARY IODIDE CONCENTRATION (μg/L)**	**DISEASE**
Severe iodine deficiency	<20	Cretinism Goiter Hypothyroidism Low IQ
Moderate iodine deficiency	20–49	(Hypothyroidism, low IQ) Goiter Hyperthyroidism
Mild iodine deficiency	50–99	Goiter Hyperthyroidism
Optimal	100–199	
More than adequate	200–299	Hypothyroidism Early Graves disease?
Excessive	≥300	Hypothyroidism Goiter Early Graves disease?

IQ, intelligence quotient.

[a]The exact boundaries of iodine intake associated with the different diseases depend on intake of goitrogens and other nutritional deficiencies. Subgroups of the population may have iodine intake levels that differ from those of the main population. The lower part of moderate iodine deficiency may especially be associated with risk of brain involvement in some individuals. A sudden increase from low to high iodine intake may lead to a surge of hyperthyroidism (4).

likely mechanism is that iodide autoregulation of the thyroid keeps thyroid hormone production normal, but such autoregulation is associated with a risk of multifocal mutations with multinodular growth and autonomous function of the thyroid. This development may be caused by reactive H_2O_2 that is up-regulated in iodine deficiency. Autonomous thyroid nodules do not adapt to high iodine intake, and people harboring such nodules may develop hyperthyroidism after an increase in iodine intake (the Jod-Basedow phenomenon) (4).

The pattern of disease is much different when iodine intake is higher than the recommended level (see Table 13.3). Findings include a high incidence and prevalence of thyroid hypofunction with an increase in pituitary TSH secretion. A comparative epidemiologic study showed that elderly people living in Jutland, Denmark with long-standing mild-to-moderate iodine deficiency often had low serum TSH concentrations, whereas high serum TSH was rare. In contrast, elderly persons from Iceland with long-standing high iodine intake had the opposite pattern (49). This finding has been consistent in many studies (24). For example, a study from Brazil (iodine intake evaluated as excessive by the WHO [50]) reported elevated serum TSH concentrations in 23% of white women aged 66 to 75 years (51).

With high iodine intake, indications are that Graves disease may develop at a younger age, and diffuse goiter may be more common (24).

The likely cause of low thyroid function in populations with high iodine intake is overadaptation to high iodine intake in people affected by thyroid autoimmunity. An autoimmune reaction against the thyroid is very common, especially in elderly persons, in women, and in white people. Approximately 50% of elderly white women have some degree of lymphocytic infiltration of the thyroid (52, 53). The frequency of thyroid autoimmune reaction is lower in Japanese people (53), and elevated TSH concentrations in elderly people are not that common in Japan, despite high iodine intake. Nonetheless, elevated serum TSH correlates with high iodine intake in Japan (54). Thyroid autoimmunity and elevated TSH are also less common in elderly African-Americans (52, 55) and in black Brazilians (51).

Figure 13.1 suggests that the optimal level of iodine intake corresponds to a median urinary iodide concentration of 100 to 200 µg/L, which is in accordance with WHO/UNICEF/ICCIDD recommendations (see Table 13.1). Unfortunately, the occurrence of hypothyroidism in a population becomes elevated when iodine intake increases from mildly deficient to recommended (56), but the occurrence of hyperthyroidism decreases. Thus, adjusting iodine intake of a population to minimize the risk of thyroid disease is a delicate balance.

ASSESSMENT OF IODINE NUTRITION

It is not easy to depict exact daily intake needs from iodine balance studies. Thus, recommendations are mainly based on knowledge of the association between iodine intake level and disease (57).

A landmark in the history of iodine nutrition was the report on endemic goiter in the world, by Kelly and Snedden (58), published by the WHO in 1960. In all continents and most countries, large areas were marked as endemic goiter areas. Although certain environmental agents may lead to endemic goiter because of their interaction with iodine utilization and thyroid function (59), the predominant cause of endemic goiter is iodine deficiency.

Iodine intake may be studied from a combination of diet recording and measurement of iodine contents of foods (60). The recommended primary tool to evaluate and monitor iodine nutrition of a population is measurement of urinary iodine excretion in representative groups of the population, however (1). Because the concentration of iodine in a spot urine sample generally reflects iodine intake within the last few hours, urinary concentration in an individual may vary considerably from day to day, and even within the same day, and median values from groups of samples are necessary for evaluation.

The number of spot urine samples needed to estimate the iodine level in a population with 95% confidence within a precision range of ± 10% is approximately 125, and within a precision range of ± 5%, it is approximately 500. A precision range of ± 20% in an individual would require approximately 12 urine samples (61). Thus, iodine deficiency in an individual cannot be diagnosed based on a single spot urine iodine measurement. Studies of urinary iodine excretion in populations require that several other technical details be taken into account (1, 62).

The clinical consequences of iodine deficiency may be monitored by examination of school-age children for goiter. A simple classification system is used to describe goiter, but the sensitivity and specificity for finding small goiters are low. The goiter frequency should be less than 5%. Thyroid ultrasonography gives a much more precise estimate of thyroid size. Normative values dependent on age and sex have been given (1).

Thyroglobulin is released from the thyroid in amounts that depend on thyroid size and activity. In population studies, the level of serum thyroglobulin is a sensitive indicator of iodine deficiency (63), but this value is nonspecific in individuals.

Serum TSH, measured as part of neonatal screening for congenital hypothyroidism, has been used for evaluation of iodine deficiency during pregnancy. The rationale is that low thyroid hormone production in the fetus or neonate caused by iodine deficiency would lead to a compensatory increase in fetal or neonatal pituitary TSH secretion. Careful control of the TSH measurement method is necessary. Moreover, the neonatal thyroid is very sensitive to the inhibitory effect of high iodine in the mother. Thus, a substantial percentage of elevated neonatal TSH values observed in areas of low iodine intake has been caused by vaginal application of iodine-containing sterilizers in the mother during preparation for labor (64).

NATIONAL IODINE NUTRITION PROGRAMS

Because iodine intake is so important for the risk of disease in a population and because very few populations have an adequate iodine intake from natural diet, practically all countries should have an official iodine nutrition program (1). As indicated earlier, much disease prevention can be achieved by proper regulation. The WHO regularly provides updates on iodide nutrition status worldwide, and the ICCIDD website (http://www.ICCIDD.org) is a valuable source of information.

GLOBAL IODINE NUTRITION STATUS

Although global iodine nutrition status has improved greatly since the 1980s, areas of iodine deficiency and excess remain common (47, 50). Continuous monitoring and adjustment of programs are mandatory. The recommended approach to achieve optimal iodide nutrition in most countries is the iodization of salt (1). If all salt used by households and by the food industry is iodized (universal salt iodization), this will distribute iodine quite evenly in the population.

A technical problem to consider is ensuring sufficient coverage when the use of iodized salt is voluntary. When only a fraction of the population uses iodized salt, the result is a higher than optimal intake in people using the salt and a lower than optimal intake in those not using iodized salt (65). This situation is the major reason for having mandatory iodization of salt in some countries.

Another technical detail to consider is adjustment of the iodide content of salt when salt intake is reduced to prevent cardiovascular disease (66). In principle, this is easily done, but proper adjustments require careful population-based studies of both salt intake and iodine intake.

IODIDE AS A THYROID-BLOCKING AGENT IN RADIATION EMERGENCIES

The Chernobyl reactor accident in Ukraine in 1986 resulted in massive releases of radioiodines including iodine-131 (^{131}I). With a latency of approximately 4 years, this accident was followed by a sharp increase in the incidence of thyroid cancer among children and adolescents in Belarus and the Ukraine (67). Iodine deficiency of the population with high thyroid uptake of ^{131}I may have added to the high frequency of thyroid cancer.

In Poland, where fallout from Chernobyl was fortunately only moderate, more than 10 million children received potassium iodide (KI) after the Chernobyl accident to protect against thyroid cancer. Only mild and clinically insignificant side effects of iodine were observed (68).

The March 2011 Fukushima nuclear power plant disaster in Japan caused by an earthquake and subsequent tsunami renewed focus on the distribution of iodine for the prevention of thyroid cancer. Fortunately, the iodine intake with food is high in Japan (from seaweed), and this reduces the risk of significant thyroid uptake of radioactive iodine. Current preventive measures in Japan have been to evacuate people from the area of risk and to control water and food for radioactivity to block distribution for consumption when appropriate. Shortly after the disaster, Japanese authorities distributed 230,000 doses of KI to evacuation centers from the area around the power plant as a precautionary measure. As of this writing, however, no official systematic administration of iodine to groups of the population has been initiated.

Both the WHO (69) and the US Food and Drug Administration (70) have put forward detailed recommendations on the use of KI as a thyroid-blocking agent in case of radiation emergencies. An update of the WHO recommendations is expected to be released soon.

REFERENCES

1. World Health Organization, United Nations Children's Fund, International Council for the Control of Iodine Deficiency Disorders. Assessment of Iodine Deficiency Disorders and Monitoring Their Elimination: A Guide for Programme Managers. 3rd ed. Geneva: World Health Organization, 2007:1–99.
2. Coindet JF. Ann Clin Phys 1820;15:49–59.
3. Hetzel BS. The Story of Iodine Deficiency: An International Challenge in Nutrition. Oxford: Oxford University Press, 1989:1–236.
4. Stanbury JB, Ermans AE, Bourdoux P et al. Thyroid 1998; 8:83–100.
5. Carpenter KJ. J Nutr 2005;135:675–80.
6. Bürgi H, Supersaxo Z, Selz B. Acta Endocrinol 1990;123: 577–90.
7. Stanbury JB. The Iodine Trail: Exploring Iodine Deficiency and Its Prevention around the World. Oxford: Farber Public Relations, 2008:1–202.
8. Pearce EN. Thyroid 2007;17:823–7.
9. Rasmussen LB, Ovesen L, Bülow I et al. Br J Nutr 2002;87: 61–9.
10. Nagataki S. Thyroid 2008;18:667–8.
11. Kim JY, Moon SJ, Kim KR et al. Yonsei Med J 1998;39: 355–62.
12. Laurberg P, Andersen S, Pedersen IB et al. Biofactors 2003; 19:145–53.
13. Andersen S, Guan H, Teng W et al. Biol Trace Elem Res 2009; 128:95–103.
14. Pearce EN, Pino S, He X et al. J Clin Endocrinol Metab 2004;89:3421–4.
15. Caldwell KL, Jones RL, Hollowell JG. Thyroid 2005;15: 692–9.
16. Caldwell KL, Miller GA, Wang RY et al. Thyroid 2008;18: 1207–14.
17. Andersson M, de Benoist B, Rogers L. Best Pract Res Clin Endocrinol Metab 2010;24:1–11.
18. Dasgupta PK, Liu Y, Dyke JV. Environ Sci Technol 2008; 42:1315–23.
19. Zimmermann MB, Aeberli I, Torresani T et al. Am J Clin Nutr 2005;82:388–92.

20. Laurberg P, Jørgensen T, Perrild H et al. Eur J Endocrinol 2006; 155:219–28.

21. Food and Nutrition Board, Institute of Medicine. Dietary Reference Intakes: Iodine. Washington, DC: National Academy Press, 2001:258–89.

22. Becker DV, Braverman LE, Delange F et al. Thyroid 2006; 16:949–51.

23. World Health Organization Secretariat, Andersson M, de Benoist B, et al. Public Health Nutr 2007;10:1606–11.

24. Laurberg P, Cerqueira C, Ovesen L et al. Best Pract Res Clin Endocrinol Metab 2010;24:13–27.

25. Venturi S, Venturi M. Nutr Health 2009;20:119–34.

26. Küpper FC, Carpenter LJ, McFiggans GB et al. Proc Natl Acad Sci U S A 2008;105:6954–8.

27. Pennington JA. J Am Diet Assoc 1990;90:1571–81.

28. Zimmermann MB. Annu Rev Nutr 2006;26:367–89.

29. Laurberg P. Endocrinology 1985;117:1639–44.

30. Heuer H, Visser TJ. Endocrinology 2009;150:1078–83.

31. Biebinger R, Arnold M, Koss M et al. Thyroid 2006;16:961–5.

32. Dohán O, De la Vieja A, Paroder V et al. Endocr Rev 2003; 24:48–77.

33. Ingbar SH. Mayo Clin Proc 1972;47:814–23.

34. Gärtner R, Dugrillon A, Bechtner G. Acta Med Aust 1996; 23:47–51.

35. Chen W, Man N, Shan Z et al. Exp Clin Endocrinol Diabetes 2011;119:1–8.

36. Eng PH, Cardona GR, Fang SL et al. Endocrinology 1999; 140:3404–10.

37. Laurberg P, Andersen S, Knudsen N et al. Thyroid 2002;12:897–902.

38. Brauer VF, Below H, Kramer A et al. Eur J Endocrinol 2006; 154:229–35.

39. Laurberg P, Nøhr SB, Pedersen KM et al. J Clin Endocrinol Metab 2004;89:181–7.

40. Knudsen N, Laurberg P, Perrild H et al. Thyroid 2002;12: 879–88.

41. Bianco AC, Salvatore D, Gereben B et al. Endocr Rev 2002;23:38–89.

42. Köhrle J, Gärtner R. Best Pract Res Clin Endocrinol Metab 2009;23:815–27.

43. St Germain DL, Galton VA, Hernandez A. Endocrinology 2009;150:1097–107.

44. Brown DD, Cai L. Dev Biol 2007;306:20–33.

45. Kimura-Kuroda J, Nagata I, Negishi-Kato M et al. Brain Res Dev Brain Res 2002;137:55–65.

46. Bernal J. Vitam Horm 2005;71:95–122.

47. Zimmermann, MB. Endocr Rev 2009;30:376–408.

48. Laurberg P, Pedersen KM, Vestergaard H et al. J Intern Med 1991;229:415–20.

49. Laurberg P, Pedersen KM, Hreidarsson A et al. J Clin Endocrinol Metab 1998;83:765–9.

50. Andersson M, Takkouche B, Egli I et al. Bull World Health Organ 2005;83:518–25.

51. Sichieri R, Baima J, Marante T et al. Clin Endocrinol 2007;66: 803–7.

52. Okayasu I, Hara Y, Nakamura K et al. Am J Clin Pathol 1994; 101:698–702.

53. Okayasu I, Hatakeyama S, Tanaka Y et al. J Pathol 1991; 163:257–64.

54. Konno N, Makita H, Yuri K et al. J Clin Endocrinol Metab 1994;78:393–7.

55. Hollowell JG, Staehling NW, Flanders WD et al. J Clin Endocrinol Metab 2002;87:489–99.

56. Pedersen IB, Laurberg P, Knudsen N et al. J Clin Endocrinol Metab 2007;92:3122–7.

57. Ascoli W, Arroyave G. Arch Latinoam Nutr 1970;20: 309–20.

58. Kelly FC, Snedden WW. Prevalence and distribution of endemic goitre. In: World Health Organization, ed. Endemic Goitre. WHO monograph series no. 44. Geneva: World Health Organization, 1960:27–233.

59. Gaitan E. Annu Rev Nutr 1990;10:21–39.

60. Murray CW, Egan SK, Kim H et al. J Expo Sci Environ Epidemiol 2008;18:571–80.

61. Andersen S, Karmisholt J, Pedersen KM et al. Br J Nutr 2008;99:813–8.

62. Vejbjerg P, Knudsen N, Perrild H et al. Thyroid 2009;19: 1281–6.

63. Knudsen N, Bülow I, Jørgensen T et al. J Clin Endocrinol Metab 2001;86:3599–603.

64. Chanoine JP, Boulvain M, Bourdoux P et al. Arch Dis Child 1988;63:1207–10.

65. Laurberg P, Andersen S, Pedersen IB et al. Hot Thyroidol 2007(4). Available at: http://www.hotthyroidology.com. Accessed March 18, 2011.

66. Bibbins-Domingo K, Chertow GM, Coxson PG et al. N Engl J Med 2010;362:590–9.

67. Cardis E, Howe G, Ron E et al. J Radiol Prot 2006;26: 127–40.

68. Nauman J, Wolff J. Am J Med 1993;94:524–32.

69. World Health Organization. Guidelines for Iodine Prophylaxis following Nuclear Accidents. Geneva: World Health Organization, 1999:1–30.

70. Guidance: Potassium Iodide as a Thyroid Blocking Agent in Radiation Emergencies. Rockville, MD: US Department of Health and Human Services, Food and Drug Administration, Center for Drug Evaluation and Research (CDER), 2001: 1–12. Available at: http://www.fda.gov/downloads/Drugs/ GuidanceComplianceRegulatoryInformation/Guidances/ ucm080542.pdf. Accessed March 18, 2011.

71. Laurberg P, Andersen S, Bjarnadóttir RI et al. Public Health Nutrition 2007;10:1547–52.

SUGGESTED READINGS

International Council for the Control of Iodine Deficiency Disorders. Available at: http://www.iccidd.org. Accessed March 18, 2011. (Homepage)

Preedy VC, Burrow GN, Watson RR, eds. Comprehensive Handbook on Iodine: Nutritional, Endocrine and Pathological Aspects. London: Academic Press, 2009:1–1334. (Detailed book by many specialists on various aspects of iodine)

Public Health Nutr 2007:10;1527–1611. (Special issue 12A organized by the World Health Organization and the United Nations Children's Fund on iodine intake during pregnancy and lactation)

World Health Organization, United Nations Children's Fund, International Council for the Control of Iodine Deficiency Disorders. Assessment of Iodine Deficiency Disorders and Monitoring Their Elimination: A Guide for Programme Managers. 3rd ed. Geneva: World Health Organization, 2007. (Comprehensive authoritative guidelines)

Zimmermann M, ed: Iodine efficiency. Best Pract Res Clin Endocrinol Metab 2010;24:1–158. (Special issue on iodine and disease)

14 SELENIUM[1]

ROGER A. SUNDE

[1]**Abbreviations: ApoER2**, apolipoprotein E receptor; **DRI**, dietary reference intake; **EAR**, estimated average requirement; **GPX**, glutathione peroxidase; **GSH**, glutathione; **NHANES**, third National Health and Nutrition Survey; **NOAEL**, no-observed-adverse-effect level; **RDA**, recommended dietary allowance; **Sec**, selenocysteine; **SECIS**, selenocysteine insertion sequence; **SEPN1**, selenoprotein N; **SEPP1**, selenoprotein P; **SNP**, single nucleotide polymorphism; **U**, selenocysteine (one-letter symbol); **UL**, tolerable upper intake level; **WHO**, World Health Organization.

Selenium first attracted biologic interest in the 1930s when it was found to cause poisoning of livestock that grazed in areas with high-selenium soils (1). In 1957, Schwarz and Foltz (2) reported that small amounts of selenium prevented liver necrosis in vitamin E–deficient rats, a finding indicating that selenium was an essential nutrient and not only a toxin. Soon thereafter, deficiencies of selenium and vitamin E were shown to be involved in several economically important nutritional diseases of cattle, sheep, swine, and poultry (1). The first demonstration of a biochemical function for selenium in animals came in 1973, when the element was discovered to be a constituent of the enzyme glutathione peroxidase (GPX) (3).

The importance of selenium in human nutrition was documented in 1979, when Chinese scientists reported that selenium supplementation prevented the development of a cardiomyopathy known as Keshan disease in children living in low-selenium areas (4), and New Zealand workers reported a clinical response to selenium in a selenium-depleted patient (5). Information about the role of selenium in human nutrition increased rapidly in the 1980s, and a recommended dietary allowance (RDA) for selenium was established in 1989 (6) and revised in 2000 (7). Dietary recommendations from the World Health Organization (WHO) were issued in 1996 (8). Molecular and genetic studies, in humans, animals, and other organisms, are providing extensive new information on selenoproteins and the molecular biology of selenium.

CHEMICAL FORMS

Most selenium in biologic systems is present in proteins as a constituent of amino acids. Reflecting the similarity of selenium chemistry to that of sulfur, those amino acids are usually selenocysteine and selenomethionine. Selenocysteine (Fig. 14.1) is incorporated into the peptide backbone of selenoproteins, contains selenium in the selenol form, and is often referred to as the twenty-first amino acid. The standard amino acid symbols for selenocysteine are Sec (three letters) or U (one letter). Selenol has chemical properties that are distinct from the thiol in cysteine, and selenocysteine almost always performs catalytic functions in proteins. Selenomethionine, conversely, contains selenium bound covalently to two carbon atoms

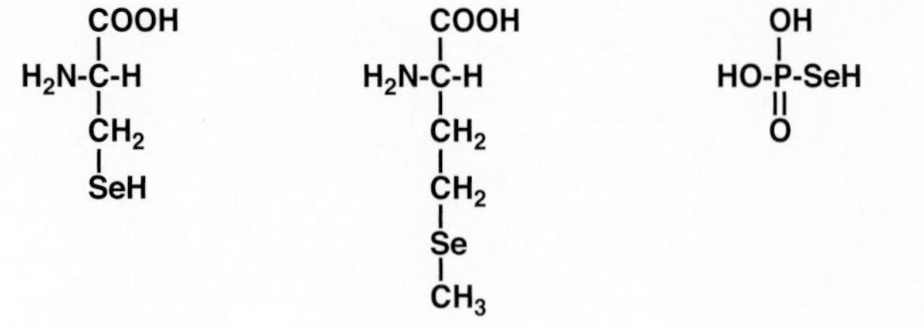

COOH
H₂N-C-H
CH₂
SeH

COOH
H₂N-C-H
CH₂
CH₂
Se
CH₃

OH
HO-P-SeH
O

Selenocysteine   *Selenomethionine*   *Selenophosphate*

Fig. 14.1. Key selenium-containing molecules found in animals. Selenocysteine is the biologically active form of the element found in selenoproteins. Its selenol is largely ionized at physiologic pH and is a stronger nucleophile than the thiol of cysteine. These chemical properties contribute to its catalytic function in selenoenzymes. Selenomethionine contains selenium covalently bound to two carbon atoms. Thus, its selenium is shielded and is not as chemically active as the selenium in selenocysteine. Selenomethionine appears to be distributed nonspecifically in the methionine pool. Selenophosphate, the product of selenophosphate kinase, is the activated form of selenium used for synthesis of selenocysteine.

and is considerably less reactive than selenocysteine. It is not known to have a biochemical function distinct from that of methionine.

A selenoprotein contains stoichiometric amounts of selenium. Selenocysteine is the form of the element in all the animal selenoproteins identified so far and in nearly all the bacterial selenoproteins. The presence of selenium in an unidentified form (not selenocysteine) that is coordinated with molybdenum in nicotinic acid hydroxylase from *Clostridium barkeri* (9) indicates that selenoproteins containing forms of the element other than selenocysteine exist in nature. In addition, some prokaryotes synthesize a modified selenouridine base found in the anticodons of a just a few tRNA species (10).

Numerous proteins contain selenium as selenomethionine in nonstoichiometric amounts and are referred to as selenium-containing proteins. This designation has low utility because virtually all proteins that contain methionine contain selenomethionine in proportion to the relative abundance of these two amino acids in the organism. This is because enzymes that attach methionine to the methionine-tRNA for incorporation into protein or that metabolize methionine cannot distinguish selenomethionine from methionine.

Selenium enters the food chain through plants that incorporate it into compounds that usually contain sulfur. The result is that plant selenium is in the form of selenomethionine and, to a lesser extent, selenocysteine and other analogs of sulfur amino acids. Fungi and higher plants do not have selenoproteins or the selenocysteine incorporation machinery necessary for synthesis of selenoproteins (11), and they do not appear to require selenium for their existence.

Some plants express an enzyme that methylates free selenocysteine, thus producing selenium-methylselenocysteine (12). This is a detoxification product, and it cannot be incorporated into protein. It accumulates to high concentrations and can be responsible for selenium poisoning in animals that eat these plants.

Selenophosphate (see Fig. 14.1) is an important intermediate compound in selenium metabolism. It is produced by selenophosphate synthetase and serves as the selenium donor for the production of selenocysteine destined for incorporation into selenoproteins (13).

Methylated forms of selenium are produced as excretory metabolites and rapidly appear in the urine and breath (14, 15). This includes a methylated selenosugar, 1β-methylseleno-N-acetyl-D-galactosamine, which is synthesized in liver and is the major selenium species in urine with usual dietary intakes of selenium (15). Additional small molecule forms of the element have been detected in blood plasma, but their identities have not been established (16).

DIETARY CONSIDERATIONS

Food Sources

The richest food sources of selenium are organ meats and seafoods (0.4 to 1.5 µg/g fresh weight)[2], followed by muscle meats (0.1 to 0.4), cereals and grains (<0.1 to >0.8), dairy products (<0.1 to 0.3), and fruits and vegetables (<0.1) (14). The wide variation in the selenium content of cereals and grains occurs because plants contain variable amounts, depending on how much soil selenium is available for uptake. For example, the selenium content of corn collected in China ranged from 0.005 to 8.1 µg/g, and the selenium content of the British diet declined from 65 to 31 µg/day after Britain switched its source of wheat from North America to Europe (14). Foods from animal sources vary somewhat in selenium content, but the degree of variation is less than in plants because of the homeostatic control of selenium metabolism in animals. The US Department of Agriculture National Nutrient Database for Standard Reference provides analytic or inferred values for the selenium content of hundreds of food items (17). Drinking water generally contributes negligible selenium to the overall intake, except in some localized highly seleniferous areas (14).

The Dietary Intake Data from the third National Health and Nutrition Survey (NHANES III) Total Diet Study found that median daily selenium intake was 149 and 98 µg for adult (19 to 50 years) men and women, respectively, between 1988 and 1994 (7). Lower daily selenium intakes, 30 µg or less, have been reported in countries with selenium-poor soils, such as New Zealand (14). Extremely low dietary selenium intakes from 3 to 22 µg/day have been reported in areas of China affected by Keshan disease. Conversely, very high dietary intakes (≤6690 µg/day) have been observed in a region of China with endemic human selenosis. The food in this area had been grown on soil contaminated with selenium leached from highly seleniferous coal fly ash (14).

---

[2]1 µg of selenium equals 0.0127 µmol of selenium

Selenoprotein W

This selenoprotein was originally identified in muscle and postulated to play a role in the development of white muscle disease, a selenium deficiency condition in sheep (51). It has since been identified in many other tissues and shown to exist in several forms. One form has GSH bound to it, a finding suggesting that selenoprotein W undergoes redox changes. Some evidence indicates that it can protect against oxidative injury. Selenoprotein W concentration decreases in selenium deficiency (51), and, at least in rodents, selenoprotein W mRNA levels in selenium deficiency decrease similarly to GPX1 (47).

Selenoprotein N

Selenoprotein N (SEPN1), one of the ER-resident proteins, is highly expressed in muscle. Human mutations in SEPN1 result in congenital muscular dystrophy initially characterized by development of a rigid spine (52). At least 30 different human mutations have been identified, all with early onset of muscle weakness, which are collectively called SEPN1-related myopathies (53). Mouse fetuses and pups lacking the SEPN1 gene develop normally, a finding suggesting a role for SEPN1 during maturation of organs or protection during stress (54).

Selenophosphate Synthetase

Two selenophosphate synthetases have been identified in animals. One contains a selenocysteine residue in its primary structure, and the other contains a cysteine residue at this position (39). Currently, however, it appears that only the selenocysteine-containing synthetase is used for selenocysteine synthesis (13).

BIOLOGIC ACTIVITY

Deficiency of selenium can lead to marked changes in many biochemical systems, but selenium deficiency alone usually does not cause disease in animals or clinical illness in free-living humans. First-generation selenium-deficient animals exhibit heightened sensitivity to certain stresses, and this is the basis of most naturally occurring conditions of selenium deficiency. One such stress is vitamin E deficiency. Simultaneous selenium and vitamin E deficiencies lead to numerous pathologic conditions in animals (1). Selenium-deficient animals are more susceptible to injury by certain chemicals such as the redox cyclers paraquat, diquat, and nitrofurantoin. These injuries are generally oxidative and may be related to decreased levels of the selenoenzymes that defend against oxidative injury (14).

When selenium deficiency or other factors result in a loss of protective selenoproteins, reactive oxygen species can increase and signal a cascade of changes. GSH S-transferase activities in rat liver, kidney, and lung rise in selenium deficiency (55), and GSH metabolism is affected by selenium deficiency (56). Certain drug-metabolizing enzymes, including the cytochrome P-450 system, are affected, some with activities increased and others with activities decreased (57). The underlying causes of these changes appear to be rises in reactive oxygen species in selenium deficiency and activation of Nrf2-responsive genes such as GSH S-transferase (58, 59).

Selenium can influence the outcome of infections. The increased virulence of Coxsackievirus B3 in selenium-deficient mice is described later.

DEFICIENCY IN HUMANS AND ANIMALS

Combined deficiency of selenium and vitamin E causes liver necrosis in rats and swine, exudative diathesis in chickens, and white muscle disease in sheep and cattle (1). In animals fed a selenium-deficient diet containing adequate levels of vitamin E, signs attributable to selenium deficiency included hair loss and growth retardation, as well as reproductive failure in rats fed a deficient diet for two generations and pancreatic degeneration in chicks fed amino acid–based diets severely deficient in selenium. Rodents fed selenium- and vitamin E–deficient diets when the essentiality of selenium was discovered grew poorly and developed necrosis and died in less than a month (2); today, with improved selenium status of the mothers, improved diets, and disease-free conditions (see Coxsackievirus later), rodents fed deficient diets no longer show reduced growth or overt disease (47), although second-generation selenium-deficient rats grow poorly compared with selenium-supplemented littermates (60).

Keshan Disease

In 1979, Chinese scientists first described in English the relationship of selenium with Keshan disease, an endemic cardiomyopathy affecting children and young women that occurs in a long belt running from northeastern to southwestern China (4). The acute form is characterized by sudden onset of insufficient heart function, whereas patients with chronic disease exhibit moderate to severe heart enlargement with varying degrees of heart insufficiency. The histopathologic features include multifocal necrosis and fibrosis of the myocardium. A series of intervention trials encompassing more than a million subjects demonstrated the protective effects of selenium supplements (61), but selenium cannot reverse the cardiac failure once it occurs. Marginal to deficient vitamin E status has also been observed in persons residing in endemic areas, and other complicating nutritional deficiencies (e.g., protein) may exacerbate the condition. Nonetheless, selenium deficiency appears to be the fundamental underlying condition predisposing persons to the development of Keshan disease. With improved economic and living conditions in China, the disease has disappeared (14).

Because certain features of Keshan disease could not be explained solely on the basis of selenium status (e.g., seasonal variation), investigators suggested that a cardiotoxic agent, such as a virus, may also be involved. Beck (62) found that a myocarditic strain of Coxsackievirus B3 *(CVB3/20)* produced more heart damage in selenium-deficient mice than in physiologically normal mice. Similarly, normal mice infected with a benign (amyocarditic) strain of Coxsackievirus B3 *(CVB3/0)* suffered no heart damage, whereas a moderate degree of heart damage was observed in infected, selenium-deficient mice. Virus isolated from the selenium-deficient mice infected with originally benign *CVB3/0* retained its cardiotoxicity when it was subsequently inoculated into physiologically normal mice, a finding indicating that the avirulent virus had converted to a virulent strain by a genotypic change. A similar phenomenon can occur with influenza virus and can develop with other nutritional imbalances, such as vitamin E deficiency and iron overload in laboratory animals or nutritional insufficiency in a human population (63). These results suggest that diet-driven mutations may be a general feature of RNA viruses and disease (62, 63).

Kashin-Beck Disease

Kashin-Beck disease is another endemic disease in China that has been associated with poor selenium status (64). This is a preadolescent or adolescent osteoarthritis, with necrotic degeneration of the chondrocytes, and with dwarfism and joint deformation resulting from these cartilage abnormalities. Aside from selenium deficiency, numerous other etiologic factors have been suggested for this condition (e.g., mycotoxins in grain, mineral imbalance, organic contaminants in drinking water). Attempts to improve the clinical condition of subjects with Kashin-Beck disease by administering selenium have not been successful. It is still possible that selenium deficiency permits the development of the illness, however (64).

Cancer

A major unresolved issue in selenium biology is whether the element has a beneficial cancer preventive effect in humans. The epidemiologic evidence linking low selenium status and an increased incidence of cancer is conflicting (65, 66), and it is often based on small differences in plasma selenium levels between controls and subjects who later developed cancer (67). Some animal experiments show that high levels of dietary selenium can protect against certain chemically or virally induced cancers (66), but examples exist in which selenium itself can stimulate tumorigenesis in rodent models (68).

Human nutritional intervention studies suggest that selenium supplements may have some beneficial effects against cancer. A study of approximately 30,000 poorly nourished rural Chinese persons found that overall cancer mortality could be reduced 13% by giving a supplement containing selenium, vitamin E, and β-carotene (69). These results may not be directly applicable to Western populations of better nutritional status, however.

In the United States, the Nutritional Prevention of Cancer Trial (NPCT) was conducted to study the effect of supplementation of 200 μg/day of selenium as selenized yeast on recurrence of nonmelanoma skin cancer (70). The study included 1312 men and women in a multicenter, double-blind, randomized, placebo-controlled trial. The outcome was that selenium supplementation provided no benefit in preventing skin cancer. Significant reductions in several secondary end points were reported, however, including a 37% reduction in total cancer incidence; 58% and 46% declines in the incidence of colorectal and lung cancers, respectively; a 50% decrease in total cancer mortality; and 63% fewer new cases of prostate cancer among men who had taken selenium for 6 ½ years than among men who took the placebo (70). This study initiated the current interest in high-selenium supplementation to prevent disease.

The original report (70) was subjected to several reanalyses, prompted by a follow-up study showing that baseline plasma selenium concentration could predict the effect of subsequent selenium supplementation on prostate cancer (71). Only the persons in the lower two tertiles of plasma selenium concentration (<1.56 μmol/L), however, had a statistically significantly lower incidence of prostate cancer resulting from selenium supplementation, whereas those in the highest tertile showed a statistically nonsignificant 20% elevation in total cancer incidence (72). Similar results were found for lung cancer (73). A report on the entire blinded period (12 years) of high-selenium yeast supplementation showed that the supplemented group had a higher incidence of squamous cell carcinoma of the skin than did the placebo group (74). Analysis of the full study also found a significantly higher diabetes incidence (hazard ratio 1.55) in selenium-supplemented subjects versus placebo subjects and a significant hazard ratio of 2.7 for selenium supplementation in subjects in the highest tertile of baseline plasma selenium level (75).

More recently, the Selenium and Vitamin E Cancer Prevention Trial (SELECT) enrolled 35,534 participants who consumed pills containing 200 μg selenium as L-selenomethionine and/or 400 mg DL-α-tocopherol acetate, or placebo pills. In 2008, however, the study was stopped because an independent monitoring committee found that selenium and vitamin E, taken alone or together for an average of 5 years, did not prevent prostate cancer, and because of suggestions of adverse effects resulting from single supplements (76). The discrepancy between these two trials is not understood, but it may involve the initial selenium status of the two populations or the form of selenium supplementation (selenized yeast versus selenomethionine).

Early studies similarly suggested an inverse link between selenium status and breast cancer, but later case-controlled, prospective studies using tissue selenium and breast cancer incidence provided no evidence for a protective effect of selenium (77). Finally, analysis of 67 intervention studies looking at low-bias risk trials also found no significant effect, either positive or negative, of selenium supplementation on all-cause mortality (78)—a finding further indicating that selenium supplementation is not a panacea. Given the foregoing, defining studies are needed showing that selenium can serve as a cancer chemopreventive agent, or can otherwise positively affect the health of US residents, before it seems prudent to recommend supernutritional selenium supplementation to the US public.

EVALUATION OF NUTRIENT STATUS

Selenium status can be evaluated by dietary and biochemical means. No known physical examination signs are associated with selenium deficiency.

Analytic Evaluation

Random urine samples are of little use in assessing selenium status because these samples are affected by dilution and by the selenium content of the previous meal (79). Blood selenium levels, which vary widely in different countries, are thought to reflect dietary intakes and selenium nutriture when they are evaluated under steady-state conditions (80). In the United States, the NHANES III reported that the 1st and 99th percentile adult (19 to 50 years) serum selenium levels were 1.23 and 2.05 μmol/L, respectively, between 1988 and 1994 (7), whereas extreme values of 0.10 and 95.0 μmol/L have been reported in areas of China affected by Keshan disease and endemic selenosis, respectively (81).

Plasma (or serum) selenium levels, which respond to selenium supplementation more rapidly than do whole blood levels, are the most commonly used index of selenium status. The NHANES III found that median serum selenium levels were 1.59 and 1.54 μmol/L for adult (19 to 50 years) men and women, respectively, between 1988 and 1994 (7). The 25th and 75th percentile values were 1.49 and 1.70 μmol/L, respectively, for men and 1.44 and 1.65 μmol/L, respectively, for women (7). Levels less than 0.63 μmol/L are often seen in healthy residents of the South Island of New Zealand (82). Serum selenium concentrations fall soon after birth and then gradually increase to adult values (79).

Determination of total selenium in blood or blood fractions provides no definitive information about the speciation of selenium in blood (18). The compartmentalization of selenium can influence the interpretation of blood selenium levels (Fig. 14.6). Intake of diets rich in selenomethionine can raise blood selenium concentrations markedly because this form of selenium is not subject to homeostatic regulation. Moreover, serum selenium does not reflect the buildup of selenium in the skeletal muscle of animals when high levels of selenomethionine are fed (83). Hair selenium was used in China to evaluate selenium status (61), but this approach may not be valid in Western countries where shampoos containing selenium are used. Toenail selenium has been suggested as a convenient noninvasive index of selenium status, but hair and nail selenium levels, at least in rats, are influenced by the form of selenium fed and the methionine content of the diet (83).

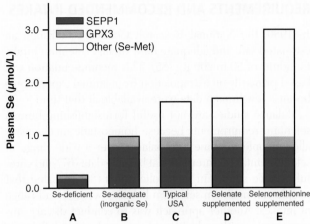

Fig. 14.6. Pools of selenium (Se) in plasma proteins. The two selenoproteins in plasma are glutathione peroxidase (GPX3) and selenoprotein P (SEPP1). Selenomethionine (Se-met) is distributed in the methionine pool and is present as such in most proteins. These three pools make up more than 95% of plasma selenium. The bar labeled *A* represents plasma from a Keshan disease–affected area in China. Bar *B* represents plasma from a selenium-adequate person who had consumed only inorganic selenium and therefore did not have any selenium in the form of selenomethionine. Bar *C* represents plasma from someone consuming more than the recommended dietary allowance of selenium, with much of it in the form of selenomethionine. Bar *D* represents plasma from the person in bar *C* after a month of supplementation with 400 μg/day selenium as selenate. Bar *E* represents plasma from the person in bar *C* after a month of supplementation with 400 μg/day selenium as selenomethionine. The selenium-deficient person has subnormal selenoproteins and selenium. All selenium-adequate samples have the same selenoprotein contents. Plasma selenium concentration in selenium-adequate persons depends on selenomethionine intake.

Assessment of selenium status by calculating the dietary intake from food composition tables is a potentially less precise procedure because of the wide variation in the selenium content of foods (14). Unless one is certain that the database used is applicable to the diet in question, the safest approach is direct chemical analysis of the diet. Nonetheless, it is possible to obtain reasonable agreement between calculated and analyzed selenium intakes if the appropriate database is available (84).

Biochemical Evaluation

Measurement of selenoproteins, such as plasma SEPP1 and GPX (see Fig. 14.5), is useful in assessing selenium nutriture. Neither value rises after the selenium requirement has been met, however. Beyond that point, values plateau and can be used only to indicate that selenium nutriture is adequate. Plasma selenium will continue to rise if increasing amounts of selenium are fed as selenomethionine (see Fig. 14.6). Thus, adequate selenium nutriture can be assumed if plasma GPX activity and SEPP1 concentration are normal or if plasma selenium concentration is 1 μmol/L or greater. Higher plasma selenium concentrations usually parallel selenomethionine intake.

REQUIREMENTS AND RECOMMENDED INTAKES

In 1980, the National Research Council established an estimated safe and adequate daily dietary selenium intake for adults of 50 to 200 μg (85). This recommendation was based primarily on extrapolation from animal experiments because few human data were available at that time.

Balance studies are not useful for establishing human selenium requirements because homeostatic mechanisms allow people to come into balance over a wide range of selenium intakes. International balance data (67) and careful balance studies in metabolic wards (86) revealed that people can maintain selenium balance over a broad range of intakes. Another approach was to conduct dietary surveys in areas with and without human selenium deficiency, that is, with and without Keshan disease. Such surveys showed that Keshan disease was not present in areas where the selenium intake was at least 19 and 13 μg/day for men and women, respectively (87). These values can be considered minimum dietary requirements for selenium.

Human selenium requirements have also been estimated by determining the dietary selenium intake needed to maximize the activity of the selenoenzyme GPX. In these studies, the diets of Chinese men of very low selenium status (residents of an area where Keshan disease is endemic) were supplemented with graded doses of selenomethionine. Plasma GPX activity tended to be greatest in those persons who received 30 μg/day or more of supplemental selenium over several months. That intake plus their habitual dietary intake (11 μg/day) yielded 41 μg/day as the lowest amount tested that caused a plateau of enzyme activity. This value, multiplied by body weight and safety factors, was the basis for the 1989 US National Research Council RDA of 70 and 55 μg selenium/day for men and women, respectively (6).

Recommended Dietary Allowances

Although North Americans should easily achieve the selenium RDA through consumption of a typical mixed US diet, persons living in countries with selenium-poor soils would have difficulty in attaining such intakes (see the earlier section on dietary considerations). For that reason, an expert consultation group of the WHO developed dietary selenium standards that were considerably lower than the US RDAs (8). The WHO, using a two-tiered system of population mean intake recommendations ("basal" and "normative"), specified the basal requirements as 21 and 16 μg selenium/day for men and women, respectively, based on the Keshan disease–based minimum dietary requirements. The WHO consultation group further specified the normative requirements as 40 and 30 μg/day for men and women, respectively, based on the Chinese plasma GPX activity data, which showed the amount of ingested selenium that was needed to achieve two thirds of the maximum attainable activity of plasma GPX. The decision to use two thirds of maximal GPX activity was

based on the observation that "abnormalities in the ability of blood cells to metabolize hydrogen peroxide became apparent only when the GPX activity in these cells declines to one-quarter or less of normal" (8).

In 2000, the US Institute of Medicine (7) established dietary reference intake (DRI) standards for selenium based on two intervention trials, one in China and the other in New Zealand. The analysis provided estimated average requirements (EARs) of 52 and 38 μg/day, respectively, based on the amount of dietary selenium needed to maximize plasma GPX activity. The average of the two EARs, 45 μg/day, was multiplied by 1.2 to account for individual variation, to yield an RDA of 55 μg/day (Table 14.2). Because women of childbearing age are prone to Keshan disease, their RDA was kept at 55 μg/day despite their smaller size. No data were available to derive an EAR for children or adolescents, so their RDAs were extrapolated downward from young adult values using an adjustment for metabolic body size and growth.

Older and younger adults seem to have similar selenium requirements, and the aging process seems to have little effect on selenium absorption or utilization, so the RDA for elderly persons was kept the same as that for young adults. For infants, because "no functional criteria of selenium status have been demonstrated that reflect response to dietary intake" (7), the adequate intake (AI) for selenium was set at 15 and 20 μg/day for the first and second 6 months of life, respectively, based on the mean selenium intake of infants fed principally with human milk. Similarly, the selenium RDA during pregnancy and lactation was calculated by adding the amount of selenium acquired by the fetus (4 μg/day) or the amount of selenium lost in the breast milk (14 μg/day), respectively, to the EAR for the nonpregnant, nonlactating woman.

TABLE 14.2	RECOMMENDED SELENIUM (Se) INTAKES AND UPPER LIMITS (μg/d)[a]		
	AGE (y)	INTAKES[b]	UL[b]
Infants	0.0–0.5	15	45
	0.5–1.0	20	60
Children	1–3	20	90
	4–8	30	150
	9–13	40	280
Adolescents	14–18	55	400
Adults	19–30	55	400
	31–50	55	400
	51+	55	400
Pregnancy		60	400
Lactation		70	400

UL, tolerable upper intake levels.

[a]1 μg Se = 0.0127 μmol.

[b]Recommended intakes and upper limits are for males and females, except for pregnancy and lactation. Intake values are recommended dietary allowances except intake values for infants. From Food and Nutrition Board. Dietary Reference Intakes for Vitamin C, Vitamin E, Selenium and Carotenoids. Washington, DC: National Academy Press, 2000, with permission.

Two more recent studies may help to refine the RDA for selenium. An initial study was conducted in China in 120 selenium-deficient subjects, with an average dietary intake of 10 μg selenium/day, who were supplemented for 20 weeks with graded levels of between 13 and 66 μg selenium/day provided in tablets as selenite or selenomethionine. Plasma GPX3 activity reached a plateau with 37 μg selenium/day as selenomethionine and 66 μg selenium/day as selenite; neither form of selenium raised SEPP1 to plateau levels (88). A second study was thus conducted using higher doses of selenium and a longer study duration; 98 selenium-deficient subjects, with an average dietary intake of 14 μg selenium/day, were supplemented for 40 weeks with graded levels of between 21 and 125 μg selenium/day provided in tablets as selenomethionine. With the longer duration, GPX3 activity was optimized by 21 μg selenium/day, and SEPP1 was optimized by 49 μg selenium/day. Including the dietary intake of 14 μg selenium/day, this results in total daily intakes of 35 and 63 μg selenium/day (89). These results indicate that plasma SEPP1 levels are a more conservative biomarker than plasma GPX3 for estimation of human selenium status and requirements. With adjustment for differences in body size between US and Chinese subjects and for uncertainty, similar to the adjustments for the current RDA (7), this finding suggests that the adult selenium RDA may be as high as 75 μg selenium/day. Studies with less deficient populations (90), however, yield lower estimated requirements, thus suggesting that values obtained in repletion studies with very selenium-deficient subjects may be an overestimate of the level required to maintain selenium status in the US population.

Finally, because mRNA levels for GPX1 and several other selenoproteins are highly regulated by selenium status at least in rodents (see Fig. 14.5), these mRNA transcripts have potential to serve as molecular biomarkers for assessment of selenium status (47, 91). Application of this approach to European subjects, however, has not been successful perhaps because the selenium status of these persons was already on the plateau region of the response curves (92, 93).

TOXICITY IN HUMANS AND ANIMALS

The level of dietary selenium needed to cause chronic selenium toxicity in animals is 4 to 5 μg/g (1). In livestock, chronic selenosis (alkali disease) is characterized by cirrhosis, lameness, hoof malformations, hair loss, and emaciation (1). Laboratory rats poisoned with selenium on a long-term basis exhibit growth depression and cirrhosis. The mechanism of selenium toxicity is not known, and the toxic effects of selenium may be modified by adaptation and certain dietary factors. No sensitive and specific biochemical test is currently available to indicate overexposure to selenium (14). The plasma selenium level can serve as an index of selenium intake when the form ingested is selenomethionine, however (see Fig. 14.6).

Public health surveys carried out in seleniferous areas of the United States failed to establish any symptom specific for selenium poisoning (14). A report from China described an outbreak of endemic selenium poisoning in humans. The most common sign of intoxication was loss of hair and nails. In high-incidence areas, lesions of the skin, nervous system, and teeth were observed. Biochemical analyses showed a change in the ratio of plasma selenium to erythrocyte selenium at selenium intakes greater than 750 μg/day. Signs of selenosis (nail changes) were seen in susceptible patients at intakes of 910 μg/day or more, corresponding to a blood selenium level of 13.3 μmol/L or higher (14). No signs or symptoms of selenium overexposure were observed among residents of seleniferous ranches in South Dakota or Wyoming whose dietary intake was as high as 724 μg/day (94).

Episodes of human selenium poisoning, however, are reported in the United States as a result of misformulation of products. In 1984, 13 persons were identified who consumed a "health food" supplement that exceeded the label declaration for selenium by 182 times (95), with the total amount of selenium consumed by these persons estimated to be between 27 and 2387 mg. Signs and symptoms of poisoning included nausea, diarrhea, irritability, fatigue, peripheral neuropathy, hair loss, and nail changes. In 2008, the US Food and Drug Administration was asked to diagnose the nature of more than 40 cases of adverse reaction to a health food supplement, with symptoms including hair loss, muscle cramps, diarrhea, joint pain, deformed fingernails, and fatigue. The product was ultimately found to contain up to more than 700 times the US RDA for selenium per serving (96).

Similarly, in 2009, 21 polo horses dropped dead because of supplement injections given just a few hours before the rapid onset of massive hemorrhaging in the lungs. The supplement, containing selenium, vitamin B_{12}, potassium, and magnesium, was presumed by those in the industry to help muscles recover from strenuous exercise. The supplement, however, was misformulated (perhaps by confusion of μg with mg), resulting in blood selenium levels 10 to 15 times higher and liver selenium levels 15 to 20 times higher than normal (97).

Tolerable Upper Intake Levels

As part of its DRIs, the Institute of Medicine established a tolerable upper intake level (UL), defined as "the highest level of daily nutrient intake that is likely to pose no risk of adverse health effects in almost all individuals" (7). For selenium, the adult UL was based on hair and nail brittleness and loss as the critical toxicologic end points. To calculate the UL, the committee used a data set provided by five Chinese persons who had recovered in 1992 from an earlier episode of selenium poisoning in 1986. During the selenosis phase, these persons were consuming 913 to 1907 μg/day of selenium (calculated from corresponding blood selenium concentrations). Six years later, during the recovery phase, the mean selenium intake of the same persons was 800 μg/day. The Chinese investigators suggested that the latter intake represented a no-observed-adverse-effect level (NOAEL), and, in fact, 800 μg/day was used to calculate the UL according to the following formula:

$$UL = NOAEL/UF$$

where UF is an uncertainty factor that encompasses all relevant uncertainties associated with extrapolating from the observed data set to the general population. To protect sensitive persons, a UF of 2 was used to calculate the UL:

$$UL = 800/2 = 400 \text{ μg/day}$$

The Institute of Medicine committee also calculated ULs for infants, children, and adolescents. An NOAEL of 7 μg/kg was identified based on the lack of adverse effects in infants consuming breast milk containing 60 μg/L. Consuming 0.78 L/day of such milk would provide an average of 47 μg/day to a 7-kg infant or 7 μg/kg/day. The 7 μg/kg/day was then used to calculate ULs for all age groups through adolescence adjusted according to body weight. Because no reports of teratogenicity or selenosis in infants born to mothers with high but not toxic intakes of selenium have been published, the ULs for pregnant and lactating women were kept the same as for nonpregnant and nonlactating women.

The current paucity of good biomarkers for high selenium status and the unresolved issue of beneficial effects of supernutritional selenium supplementation together emphasize the need for additional research to identify biomarkers for high selenium status. Yet to be identified molecular biomarkers and biochemical biomarkers have the potential to provide individualized assessment of selenium status and perhaps even to discriminate between individuals who will benefit and those adversely affected by supernutritional selenium supplementation (91).

SELENIUM-RELATED GENETICS AND HUMAN DISEASE

With the investigation of selenoproteins, the possibility exists that genetic causes of selenium deficiency will be found in humans, such as mutations in the *SEPP1* gene (26), that could be treated by feeding supernutritional amounts of selenium, similar to current studies in rodents. Inborn errors in other selenoprotein genes, such as SEPN1-related myopathies (53), or in genes important in selenium metabolism, are likely to be identified as well. In addition, research into single nucleotide polymorphisms (SNPs) of selenoprotein genes is finding that selenoprotein SNPs can elicit differences in selenoprotein biomarkers and are associated with differences in cancer risk (98–100). Similar studies in the future are likely both to expand our knowledge of the interaction of genetics and selenium status and to identify options, dietary and otherwise, for treatment of related human disease.

ACKNOWLEDGMENTS

I gratefully acknowledge the authors of the selenium chapter in the previous edition, Dr. Raymond F. Burk and Dr. Orville A. Levander, for substantial contributions to the present chapter. My work is supported by National Institutes of Health grant DK74184.

REFERENCES

1. National Research Council. Selenium in Nutrition. Washington, DC: National Academy Press, 1983.
2. Schwarz K, Foltz CM. J Am Chem Soc 1957;79:3292–3.
3. Rotruck JT, Pope AL, Ganther HE et al. Science 1973; 179:588–90.
4. Keshan Disease Research Group. Chin Med J 1979;92:471–6.
5. van Rij AM, Thomson CD, McKenzie JM et al. Am J Clin Nutr 1979;32:2076–85.
6. National Research Council. Recommended Dietary Allowances. 10th ed. Washington, DC: National Academy Press, 1989.
7. Food and Nutrition Board. Dietary Reference Intakes for Vitamin C, Vitamin E, Selenium and Carotenoids. Washington, DC: National Academy Press, 2000.
8. World Health Organization. Trace Elements in Human Nutrition and Health. Geneva: World Health Organization, 1996.
9. Gladyshev VN, Khangulov SV, Stadtman TC. Proc Natl Acad Sci U S A 1994;91:232–6.
10. Zhang Y, Gladyshev VN. Chem Rev 2009;109:4828–61.
11. Lobanov AV, Hatfield DL, Gladyshev VN. Biochim Biophys Acta 2009;1790:1424–8.
12. Neuhierl B, Bock A. Methods Enzymol 2002;347:203–7.
13. Lobanov AV, Hatfield DL, Gladyshev VN. Protein Sci 2008; 17:176–82.
14. Burk RF, Levander OA. Selenium. In: Shils ME, Shike M, Ross CA et al, eds. Modern Nutrition in Health and Disease. 10th ed. Philadelphia: Lippincott Williams & Wilkins, 2005:312–25.
15. Kobayashi Y, Ogra Y, Ishiwata K et al. Proc Natl Acad Sci U S A 2002;99:15932–6.
16. Kato T, Read R, Rozga J et al. Am J Physiol 1992;262:G854–8.
17. US Department of Agriculture. USDA National Nutrient Database for Standard Reference, release 24, 2011 (cited December 12, 2011). Available at: http://www.ars.usda.gov/ba/bhnrc/ndl. Accessed December 12, 2011.
18. Burk RF, Norsworthy BK, Hill KE et al. Cancer Epidemiol Biomarkers Prev 2006;15:804–10.
19. Yamashita Y, Yamashita M. J Biol Chem 2010;285:18134–8.
20. Hill KE, Zhou J, McMahan WJ et al. J Biol Chem 2003; 278:13640–6.
21. Schomburg L, Schweizer U, Holtmann B et al. Biochem J 2003;370:397–402.
22. Olson GE, Winfrey VP, Nagdas SK et al. Biol Reprod 2005; 73:201–11.
23. Renko K, Werner M, Renner-Muller I et al. Biochem J 2008; 409:741–9.
24. Hill KE, Zhou J, McMahan WJ et al. J Nutr 2004;134:157–61.
25. Olson GE, Winfrey VP, Nagdas SK et al. J Biol Chem 2007; 282:12290–7.
26. Burk RF, Hill KE. Biochim Biophys Acta 2009;1790:1441–7.
27. Olson GE, Winfrey VP, Hill KE et al. J Biol Chem 2008; 283:6854–60.
28. Schweizer U, Michaelis M, Köhrle J et al. Biochem J 2004; 378:21–6.
29. Sunde RA, Evenson JK. J Biol Chem 1987;262:933–7.
30. Sunde RA, Hoekstra WG. Biochem Biophys Res Commun 1980;93:1181–8.
31. Ganichkin OM, Xu XM, Carlson BA et al. J Biol Chem 2008;283:5849–65.

32. Berry MJ, Larsen PR. Endocr Rev 1992;13:207–19.
33. Böck A. Incorporation of selenium into bacterial seleno-proteins. In: Burk RF, ed. Selenium in Biology and Human Health. New York: Springer-Verlag, 1994:9–25.
34. Driscoll DM, Copeland PR. Annu Rev Nutr 2003;23:17–40.
35. Tujebajeva RM, Copeland PR, Xu XM et al. EMBO Rep 2000;1:158–63.
36. Fagegaltier D, Hubert N, Yamada K et al. EMBO J 2000;19:4796–805.
37. Chavatte L, Brown BA, Driscoll DM. Nat Struct Mol Biol 2005;12:408–16.
38. Allmang C, Wurth L, Krol A. Biochim Biophys Acta 2009;1790:1415–23.
39. Kryukov GV, Castellano S, Novoselov SV et al. Science 2003;300:1439–43.
40. Fomenko DE, Gladyshev VN. Biochemistry 2003;42:11214–25.
41. Shchedrina VA, Zhang Y, Labunskyy VM et al. Antioxid Redox Signal 2010;12:839–49.
42. Ursini F, Heim S, Kiess M et al. Science 1999;285:1393–6.
43. Spector A, Yang Y, Ho YS et al. Exp Eye Res 1996;62:521–40.
44. Olson GE, Whitin JC, Hill KE et al. Am J Physiol Renal Physiol 2010;298:F1244–53.
45. Yant LJ, Ran Q, Rao L et al. Free Radic Biol Med 2003;34:496–502.
46. Esworthy RS, Yang L, Frankel P et al. J Nutr 2005;135:740–5.
47. Barnes KM, Evenson JK, Raines AM et al. J Nutr 2009;139:199–206.
48. Kohrle J, Gartner R. Best Pract Res Clin Endocrinol Metab 2009;23:815–27.
49. Arner ES. Biochim Biophys Acta 2009;1790:495–526.
50. Hill KE, McCollum GW, Boeglin ME et al. Biochem Biophys Res Commun 1997;234:293–5.
51. Whanger PD. Biochim Biophys Acta 2009;1790:1448–52.
52. Moghadaszadeh B, Petit N, Jaillard C et al. Nat Genet 2001;29:17–8.
53. Lescure A, Rederstorff M, Krol A et al. Biochim Biophys Acta 2009;1790:1569–74.
54. Castets P, Maugenre S, Gartioux C et al. BMC Dev Biol 2009;9:46.
55. Prohaska JR, Ganther HE. Biochem Biophys Res Commun 1977;76:437–45.
56. Hill KE, Burk RF, Lane JM. J Nutr 1987;117:99–104.
57. Reiter R, Wendel A. Biochem Pharmacol 1983;32:3063–7.
58. Burk RF, Hill KE, Nakayama A et al. Free Radic Biol Med 2008;44:1617–23.
59. Suzuki T, Kelly VP, Motohashi H et al. J Biol Chem 2008;283:2021–30.
60. Thompson KM, Haibach H, Sunde RA. J Nutr 1995;125:864–73.
61. Yang G, Chen J, Wen Z et al. Adv Nutr Res 1984;6:203–31.
62. Beck MA. J Nutr 2007;137:1338–40.
63. Beck MA, Handy J, Levander OA. Trends Microbiol 2004;12:417–23.
64. Stone R. Science 2009;234:1378–81.
65. Willett WC, Stampfer MJ. BMJ 1988;297:573–4.
66. Ip C. J Nutr 1998;128:1845–54.
67. Levander OA. Annu Rev Nutr 1987;7:227–50.:227–50.
68. Birt DF, Pour PM, Pelling JC. The influence of dietary selenium on colon, pancreas, and skin tumorigenesis. In: Wendel A, ed. Selenium in Biology and Medicine. Berlin: Springer-Verlag, 1989:297–304.
69. Blot WJ, Li JY, Taylor PR et al. J Natl Cancer Inst 1993;85:1483–92.
70. Clark LC, Combs GF, Turnbull BW et al. JAMA 1996;276:1957–63.
71. Clark LC, Dalkin B, Krongrad A et al. Br J Urol 1998;81:730–4.

72. Duffield-Lillico AJ, Reid ME, Turnbull BW et al. Cancer Epidemiol Biomarkers Prev 2002;11:630–9.
73. Reid ME, Duffield-Lillico AJ, Garland L et al. Cancer Epidemiol Biomarkers Prev 2002;11:1285–91.
74. Duffield-Lillico AJ, Slate EH, Reid ME et al. J Natl Cancer Inst 2003;95:1477–81.
75. Stranges S, Marshall JR, Natarajan R et al. Ann Intern Med 2007;147:217–23.
76. Lippman SM, Klein EA, Goodman PJ et al. JAMA 2009;301:39–51.
77. Hunter DJ, Willett WC. Annu Rev Nutr 1994;14:393–418.
78. Bjelakovic G, Nikolova D, Gluud LL et al. JAMA 2007;297:842–57.
79. Thomson CD, Robinson MF. Am J Clin Nutr 1980;33:303–23.
80. Rayman MP. Lancet 2000;356:233–41.
81. Yang GQ, Wang S, Zhou R et al. Am J Clin Nutr 1983;37:872–81.
82. Robinson MF. Nutr Rev 1989;47:99–107.
83. Salbe AD, Levander OA. J Nutr 1990;120:200–6.
84. Duffield AJ, Thomson CD. Br J Nutr 1999;82:131–8.
85. National Research Council. Recommended Dietary Allowances. 9th ed. Washington, DC: National Academy of Sciences, 1980.
86. Levander OA, Sutherland B, Morris VC et al. Am J Clin Nutr 1981;34:2662–9.
87. Yang G, Ge K, Chen J et al. World Rev Nutr Diet 1988;55:98–152.
88. Xia Y, Hill KE, Byrne DW et al. Am J Clin Nutr 2005;81:829–34.
89. Xia YM, Hill KE, Li P et al. Am J Clin Nutr 2010;92:525–31.
90. Duffield AJ, Thomson CD, Hill KE et al. Am J Clin Nutr 1999;70:896–903.
91. Sunde RA. J Nutr Biochem 2010;21:665–70.
92. Sunde RA, Paterson E, Evenson JK et al. Br J Nutr 2008;99(Suppl):S37–47.
93. Pagmantidis V, Meplan C, van Schothorst EM et al. Am J Clin Nutr 2008;87:181–9.
94. Longnecker MP, Taylor PR, Levander OA et al. Am J Clin Nutr 1991;53:1288–94.
95. Helzlsouer K, Jacobs R, Morris S. Fed Proc 1985;44:1670 (abstr).
96. MacFarquhar JK, Broussard DL, Melstrom P et al. Arch Intern Med 2010;170:256–61.
97. Ballantyne C. Mystery Solved: Polo Ponies Probably Died of Selenium Overdose, 2009 (cited June 10, 2010). Available at: http://www.scientificamerican.com/blog/post.cfm?id=mystery-solved-polo-ponies-probably-2009-04-30. Accessed April 26, 2011.
98. Meplan C, Hughes DJ, Pardini B et al. Carcinogenesis 2010;31:1074–9.
99. Cooper ML, Adami HO, Gronberg H et al. Cancer Res 2008;68:10171–7.
100. Zhuo P, Goldberg M, Herman L et al. Cancer Res 2009;69:8183–90.

SUGGESTED READINGS

Food and Nutrition Board, Institute of Medicine. Selenium. In: Dietary Reference Intakes for Vitamin C, Vitamin E, Selenium, and Carotenoids. Washington, DC: National Academy Press, 2000:284–324.

Hatfield DL, Berry MJ, Gladyshev VN, eds. Selenium: Its Molecular Biology and Role in Human Health. 3rd ed. New York: Springer-Verlag, 2012:1–598.

Sunde RA. Selenium. In: Stipanuk MH, ed. Biochemical, Physiological, and Molecular Aspects of Human Nutrition. 2nd ed. Philadelphia: WB Saunders, 2006:1091–126.

B. MINERALS

15 MANGANESE[1]
ALAN L. BUCHMAN

HISTORY, CHEMISTRY, AND BIOCHEMISTRY

Manganese (Mn) was first isolated as a free metal in 1774 following the reduction of its dioxide with carbon. It was first found as a constituent of animal tissues in 1913, although a state of deficiency (in animals) was not described until 1931 (1–3). Mn is a hard, brittle metal. Its oxidation state ranges between -3 and $+7$, although the most stable valence is $+2$ and the most abundant is $4+$. Mn^{2+}, the only form absorbed by humans, is oxidized to Mn^{3+}, the oxidative state, over time in plasma. The human body contains approximately 10 to 20 mg of Mn, with 25% to 40% present in bone and 5 to 8 mg turned over on a daily basis. The biologic half-life of Mn ranges from approximately 12 to 40 days (4).

Associated Enzymes

Mn is essential as a cofactor for the metalloenzymes superoxide dismutase (SOD), xanthine oxidase, arginase, galactosyltransferase, and pyruvate carboxylase (5). It functions as a constituent of these metalloenzymes or as an enzyme activator. SOD activity is depressed in Mn-deficient animals (6). SOD protects the cell against antioxidant processes, including injury associated with radiation, chemicals, and ultraviolet light. Mn binding to arginase has significant importance in nitrogen metabolism through the ornithine cycle (7). It hydrolyzes L-arginine to urea and L-ornithine. Decreased arginase results in increased plasma ammonia in rats (8). Pyruvate carboxylase is involved in gluconeogenesis, but its activity appears minimally affected by Mn deficiency, except in newborns (6, 9). Mn also activates numerous enzymes including various decarboxylases, glutamine synthetase, hydrolases, kinases, and transferases such as glycosyltransferases, the last of which are involved in polysaccharide biosynthesis (10). Depressed galactosyltransferase activity may account for the connective tissue defects observed in Mn-deficient animals (11). Activation of these enzymes by Mn probably involves Mn binding to the protein that induces a conformational change or binding to a substrate such as adenosine triphosphate (ATP). Mn is not essential to most of these enzyme systems, which can also be activated by other metals, except for glycosyltransferases. Therefore, at least in nonprimate animals, Mn deficiency can result in defective cartilage formation in animals.

DIETARY CONSIDERATIONS

Dietary Mn is found primarily in whole grain cereals, legumes, nuts, coffee, and tea. A 1982 study of 10,000 French households found that the average daily Mn intake was 2 mg/day based on purchases of food designed to total 2000 kcal /day (8360 kJ/day) (12). Other dietary surveys in the United States, Canada, and New Zealand have shown intake to range between 2.0 and 4.7 mg/day, with vegetarians having significantly greater intake (13). Daily food intake ranges between 2 and 6 mg/day and up to 11 mg/day in vegetarian diets (13).

Orally consumed adult nutritional formulas have a range of Mn content from 0.7 to 1.2 mg/237 mL (14, 15). The actual concentration may differ from that shown on the formula label (16). In a study of 116 milk samples from 24 lactating women in Champaign-Urbana, Illinois, the concentration of Mn was found to range between 1.9 and 27.5 μg/L (0.03 and 0.50 μmol/L), with a mean value of 4.9 ± 3.9 μg/L (0.09 ± 0.07 μmol/L); infants consumed approximately 0.4 μg/kg/day (17). Bovine-based infant formula contains 30 to 75 μg/L (0.54 to 1.35 μmol/L),

[1]**Abbreviations: AI**, adequate intake; **Ca**, calcium; **Mn**, manganese; **MRI**, magnetic resonance imaging; **PN**, parenteral nutrition; **SOD**, superoxide dismutase; **UL**, tolerable upper intake level.

and soy-based formula contains approximately 100 to 300 μg/L of Mn (1.8 to 5.4 μmol/L) (18). Cow's milk has significantly more Mn than does human milk (19). For adults, most studies have shown that an intake of 2 to 5 mg/day is sufficient to remain in positive Mn balance, although individual variation is significant. For example, men absorb less Mn, but they retain it longer than do women (20).

The dietary reference intakes of the Food and Nutrition Board, Institute of Medicine for Mn are given in Table 15.1. From the criteria list, it is apparent that none of the values are based on quantitative biochemical data. Because insufficient data were available for a recommended dietary allowance to be formulated, the adequate intake (AI) value of Mn is indicated. For infants, the AI reflects the mean intake of Mn from breast milk. For adults, the AI was set based on median intakes reported in the US Food and Drug Administration Total Diet Study. Although no documented need exists for dietary Mn supplementation, absorption of Mn supplements is substantially greater in the fasting state (15). The tolerable upper intake level (UL) is described later in this chapter. Toxicity from usual dietary intake is unusual, given that only approximately 5% of dietary Mn is absorbed (16, 17).

Parenteral Nutrition

For patients who require parenteral nutrition (PN), the American Society for Parenteral and Enteral Nutrition recommended 0.06 to 0.10 mg/day in adults and 0.001 to 0.150 mg/kg for children, depending on age (18). Contamination in PN components is low (<3 to 20 μg/day); therefore, nearly all Mn in PN is derived from the addition of a multitrace metal complex (19–24). At the low end of probable requirements, however, such contamination could supply up to one third of the daily need. Data on various concentrations of Mn in patients who received long-term PN indicated that blood concentrations could be maintained at adequate levels at 60 to 120 μg/day (1.5 to 3.0 μg/kg) (25). Human deficiency, even in the absence of Mn supplementation, has not clearly been described in patients receiving PN, however, and supplementation may not be required. Mn supplementation should cease in the presence of biliary obstruction or cholestasis jaundice, because of decreased Mn excretion with subsequent accumulation in tissues (see the later discussion of toxicity).

Nutrient–Nutrient Interactions

The addition of large doses of Mn (four to eight times the AI) leads to a decrease in iron absorption by approximately one third (26). Mn supplementation leads to decreased iron absorption in iron-deficient animals, although this effect has not been demonstrated in humans (27). Investigators have also suggested that Mn absorption is enhanced in iron sufficiency and is decreased in iron deficiency (28). Therefore, Mn may possibly be recognized by the intestinal iron transport mechanism, and factors that regulate iron absorption may also then regulate Mn absorption. In no other known situations does Mn ingestion have any effect on other nutrient, metal, or medication absorption. Adding calcium (Ca) to human milk and increasing dietary phytate have been shown to reduce Mn absorption (29, 30).

Because of biliary excretion (31), balance studies are not particularly useful in the determination of daily requirements. Therefore, most estimates of absorption are based on whole body retention after 10 to 30 days of using ^{54}Mn.

		AI (mg/d)[a]	
LIFE STAGE GROUP	CRITERION	MALE	FEMALE
0–6 mo	Average manganese intake from human milk	0.003	0.003
7–12 mo	Extrapolation from adult AI	0.6	0.6
1–3 y	Median manganese intake from FDA Total Diet Study	1.2	1.2
4–8 y	Median manganese intake from FDA Total Diet Study	1.5	1.5
9–13 y	Median manganese intake from FDA Total Diet Study	1.9	1.6
14–18 y	Median manganese intake from FDA Total Diet Study	2.2	1.6
≥19 y	Median manganese intake from FDA Total Diet Study	2.3	1.8
Pregnancy			
14–18 y	Extrapolation of adolescent female AI based on body weight		2.0
19–50 y	Extrapolation of adult female AI based on body weight		2.0
Lactation			
14–18 y	Median manganese intake from FDA Total Diet Study		2.6
19–50 y	Median manganese intake from FDA Total Diet Study		2.6

TABLE 15.1 CRITERIA AND DIETARY REFERENCE INTAKE VALUES FOR MANGANESE BY LIFE STAGE GROUP

FDA, Food and Drug Administration.

[a]AI, adequate intake. The observed average or experimentally determined intake by a defined population or subgroup that appears to sustain a defined nutritional status, such as growth rate, normal circulating nutrient values, or other functional indicators of health. The AI is used if sufficient scientific evidence is not available to derive an estimated average requirement (EAR). For healthy infants receiving human milk, the AI is the mean intake. The AI is not equivalent to a recommended dietary allowance.

Reproduced with permission from Food and Nutrition Board, Institute of Medicine. Dietary Reference Intakes for Vitamin A, Vitamin K, Arsenic, Boron, Chromium, Copper, Iodine, Iron, Manganese, Molybdenum, Nickel, Silicon, Vanadium, and Zinc. Washington, DC: National Academy Press, 2001.

ABSORPTION, TRANSPORT, AND EXCRETION

Dietary Mn is absorbed by a diffusion mechanism and a transport mechanism that are rapidly saturable (32, 33). Approximately 6% to 16% of dietary Mn is absorbed (mean, 9%), with a retention half-life of 8 to 33 days (19, 34, 35). Mena (36) found that retention was 15.4% in premature infants at 10 days, but only 8.0% in term newborns and 1.0% to 3.0% in adults. The better absorption from human milk than from bovine milk or soy-based formula may be related to the decreased concentration of Mn in human milk or the increased binding of Mn in human milk to lactoferrin, the increased Ca content of bovine milk, and, for soy-based formula, the relatively large amounts of phytic acid (37, 38). No other dietary factors are known to affect Mn absorption, including ascorbic acid.

Homeostatic mechanisms control intestinal absorption; lower amounts are absorbed during periods of significant exposure (39). The cellular mechanisms that govern absorption and the mechanism that controls absorption are unknown, however. Absorption is increased in patients with hemochromatosis (34), as well as in patients with iron deficiency (36). Mn absorption is decreased in the presence of a large Ca load (40). Mn sulfate is the most soluble salt and is therefore the form found in most nutritional supplements (41). After absorption into the portal circulation, Mn may remain either free or bound preferably to transferrin (42), but also to α_2-macroglobulin (43, 44) and albumin (45) to a lesser extent, all three of which are rapidly taken up by the liver.

In serum, Mn appears to be bound primarily to transferrin (44) and an α_2-macroglobulin (46), although binding to transferrin, at least, does not appear to be essential for Mn uptake by extrahepatic tissues (47). The divalent form of Mn is firmly bound within the erythrocyte. The mechanism by which Mn is transported to and taken up by extrahepatic tissues has not yet been clearly elucidated, but it appears to involve internalization within endosomal vesicles as well as voltage-regulated Ca channels (48). Mn crosses the blood–brain barrier by carrier-mediated transport, although the specific carrier has not been elucidated (49, 50). Some evidence suggests that the primary carrier protein is divalent metal transport-1 (DMT1) (51). Conflicting data suggest otherwise, however (52). Crossgrove and Yokel (53) suggested that store-operated Ca channels are largely responsible for the transport of Mn across the blood–brain barrier. Over time, Mn^{2+} is oxidized to Mn^{3+} in plasma (54, 55) possibly by ceruloplasmin (46), which is also bound to transferrin (46). Transferrin may be the moiety that accumulates in tissues (55). When Mn is oxidized, it becomes more tightly bound to transferrin (46). Newer data suggest a possible role of the zinc transporters, ZIP8 (SLC39a8) and ZIP14 (SLC39a14) in manganese uptake (56, 57) (see also Chapter 11: Zinc). These transport processes and the potential competition of Mn ions with other divalent

and trivalent metal ions are illustrated schematically in Figure 15.1.

The trivalent form of Mn is transported and is bound to transferrin, albumin, and the $\beta(1)$-globulin transmanganin (58). It is taken up by the liver, pancreas, and kidney, although it is not clear that Mn^{3+} is stored in tissues except for bone, where 25% of the estimated 10 to 20 mg of total body Mn can be found (59). Metabolically active tissues with high numbers of mitochondria as well as pigmented structures appear to have greater Mn concentrations (6). Animal studies indicated that Mn is then secreted into bile against a concentration gradient (60).

Excretion occurs primarily through the bile, and, as such, nearly all Mn is excreted in the feces (31). Studies in the rat indicated that approximately 11% of intravenously infused Mn that is excreted into the biliary system is reabsorbed in the intestine, although some variation may exist among species. As little as 1% of an

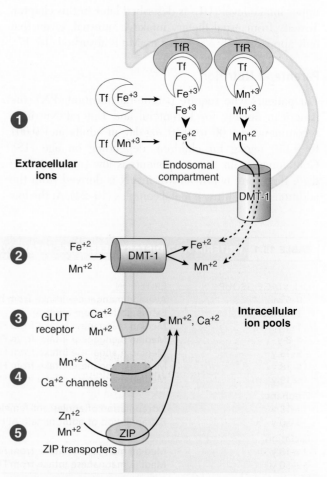

Fig. 15.1. Various transport mechanisms responsible for manganese uptake: 1, transferrin (Tf)–transferrin receptor (TfR) mediated; 2, mediated by divalent metal transporter 1 (DMT-1); 3, mediated by glutamic acid ionotropic receptor (GLUT receptor); 4, mediated by channels typically considered calcium ion channels; 5, mediated by divalent metal transporters of the zinc transporter (ZIP/SLC39) family. See references 44, 46, 48, 51 to 53, 56, 57, and 115 for related publications.

intravenously administered dose of ^{54}Mn was present in the blood 10 minutes after injection, however (61). This finding indicates enterohepatic circulation of Mn and shows that all is not eliminated necessarily by the biliary tract (62). Minimal Mn is excreted in the urine, and urinary excretion does not correlate with dietary intake (58).

ANALYTIC METHODS

Flame atomic absorption spectrophotometry is the accepted method for quantitation of Mn in biologic samples, although in the presence of low Mn concentration, graphite furnace atomic absorption is preferable (31). Inductively coupled plasma source mass spectrometry may also be used, although this technique is much more expensive (19). Whole blood concentration reflects current exposure, rather than chronic toxicity or deficiency (63). Normal whole blood concentration is 4 to 15 μg/L (73 to 274 nmol/L) when measured by atomic absorption, and it is increased in cirrhosis (64). Serum concentration of Mn is not generally useful, given that elevated intracerebral concentration may occur in the presence of normal serum concentration. In addition, serum concentrations are subject to error because the concentration may approach the limits of detection. Finally, even slight sample hemolysis may increase either plasma or serum Mn concentration dramatically.

Red blood cell Mn may also be measured because erythrocytes account for 60% to 80% of the Mn in whole blood and are a reliable indicator of tissue stores (65). When blood is obtained for analysis, the potential for contamination from Mn-containing disposable steel syringe needles must be considered; the error value may be as great as 80% (66). It is therefore appropriate to discard the initial sample obtained by syringe before obtaining blood for analysis. EDTA is the preferred anticoagulant because heparin may also be contaminated with Mn. Given that the concentration of Mn in erythrocytes is approximately 25 times greater than in serum, contamination has a less significant effect on the measurement of erythrocyte Mn as compared with serum Mn. Care must also be taken to avoid Mn-contaminated water used for dilutions during analysis (67). A three-step purification procedure including deionization, double distillation, and re-deionization is advised to achieve true blanks. In addition, because of significant contamination potential from dust, the analytic apparatus should be covered.

Mn can also be detected by magnetic resonance imaging (MRI) because the metal's atom has unpaired electrons in the level 3d orbit (68). Brain Mn content can be estimated using the Pallidal Index, a ratio of the intensity of the T1 signal in the globus pallidus to the frontal white matter signal (69). This technique may be used to help differentiate between Parkinson's disease and other neurological movement disorders.

DEFICIENCY

Human Deficiency

Human Mn deficiency has not been well documented. One patient studied in a metabolic ward who accidentally received 0.34 mg/day of Mn for 17 weeks developed delayed blood clotting, hypocholesterolemia, weight loss, slowed nail and hair growth, and reddening of his beard (70). This patient had been placed on an experimental vitamin K–free diet in an attempt to induce vitamin K deficiency. The Mn level in food was determined from food tables created before 1970, when analytic methods were not as accurate as more recent methods, and additional Mn from contamination was not considered. Unfortunately, neither blood Mn nor Mn loss was measured. Prothrombin time failed to respond to a 0.5-mg dose of vitamin K, but it responded incompletely to a 10-mg dose injected intramuscularly. Cholesterol levels fell, but only by 20 mg/dL. Whether these findings, other than the prothrombin time, improved following resumption of a normal diet was not reported. Finally, only one patient in the study developed these characteristics despite identical experimental diets. Improvement in clotting ability occurred when a standard diet was provided without any additional Mn supplementation.

Another case of purported Mn deficiency described a neonate who was dependent on total PN and who developed irregularities in bone calcification as well as bone demineralization in the presence of very low serum Mn concentration (71). These abnormalities were reportedly corrected following an unspecified amount of Mn supplementation over a 4-month period.

Finally, Friedman et al (72) described clinical and laboratory findings in a group of seven male college students who were fed a purported Mn-deficient diet in a research setting for 39 days. The serum cholesterol concentration decreased, although the subjects had been placed on a low-cholesterol diet 3 weeks before baseline evaluation, for unclear reasons. The cholesterol concentration continued to decline, however, following Mn supplementation during the repletion phase of the study. *Miliaria crystallina* dermatitis developed in five of the seven subjects during the Mn depletion period and resolved following Mn supplementation. Plasma, serum, and whole blood Mn concentration did not change during the study. Based on measured Mn losses and calculated retention (difficult to determine accurately because of the enterohepatic circulation of Mn), the investigators calculated the minimum Mn requirement to be 98.5 to 1037.0 μg/day (mean, 743 μg/day).

Experimental Animals

In various nonprimate animal species, Mn deficiency has been associated with skeletal abnormalities (10, 73), ataxia (74), decreased fertility (75), corneal degeneration (76), and abnormalities in carbohydrate and lipid metabolism, including impaired insulin production (77) and decreased serum high-density lipoprotein concentration (78–81).

TOXICITY

Toxicity affects primarily the central nervous system and was first described in 1837 in Chilean miners who were exposed to Mn-containing dust and who developed *locura manganica* (Mn madness) (82). Workers with significant occupational exposure to Mn have been observed to exhibit a manic stage initially, with insomnia, depression, and delusions, followed by anorexia, apathy, arthralgias, asthenia, headaches, irritability, lethargy, and lower extremity weakness early. Eventually, progressive alterations in gait and balance as well as tremor and Parkinson-like symptoms develop (including tremor and rigidity), consistent with Mn deposition in the basal ganglia. Symptoms may improve, but not completely resolve, and they may even continue to progress despite withdrawal from Mn exposure and improvement of MRI findings (83–85). More recently, the potential for airborne Mn toxicity was suggested in response to release of Mn^{2+} in the exhaust fumes from methylcyclopentadienyl Mn tricarbonyl, a lead-replacement additive in gasoline used to increase octane. This additive is used in parts of Europe and Canada (86).

Mn deposits primarily in the globus pallidus and subthalamic area and also in the internal capsule and white matter. Mn deposition results in an increased signal observed on T1-weighted images of a brain MRI scan. However, these lesions may also be seen in other diseases including cirrhosis and neurofibromatosis type 1, as well as in patients with basal ganglia calcification. Mn appears to alter dopaminergic neurotransmission by some unknown mechanism. Investigators have postulated that Mn binding to dopaminergic receptors leads to autooxidation of dopamine with subsequent dopamine depletion and the formation of free radicals (87), although conflicting data suggested that Mn may function as a potent antioxidant (88). This may be associated with degeneration of γ-aminobutyric acid (GABA)–minergic neurons within the globus pallidus (89, 90). Mn-induced apoptosis may also contribute to toxicity (91, 92), but it is unlikely to be the primary reason for toxicity because inhibition of apoptotic markers does not prevent cytotoxicity (93).

Several cases of possible Mn toxicity were reported in patients receiving PN at home, although not all patients were symptomatic (94–97). Whole blood concentration correlates with both MRI intensity of the globus pallidus and T1 value (98). Brain Mn deposition may occur even with a daily Mn dose of 0.1 mg (24). In some patients, the increased signal intensity in the globus pallidus dissipates following removal of supplemented Mn (although not Mn present through contamination) from the PN solutions, although the Parkinson-like symptoms often fail to improve in the absence of medical therapy (94, 95). Tremor has improved in other patients following withdrawal of Mn and a decrease in whole blood Mn concentration (99, 100). The homeostatic mechanism that controls Mn absorption becomes irrelevant when Mn is intravenously infused. Despite the lack of well-demonstrated evidence that Mn deficiency occurs in patients who require long-term PN, supplementation of PN solutions has been advised (101). This supplementation is in addition to that contained in the various PN components as a contaminant (102). Whether Mn accumulation and brain deposition of Mn are direct results of Mn toxicity or are caused by a decrease in biliary excretion mediated by PN and PN-associated liver disease is unknown, however (103).

Significantly elevated whole blood Mn concentrations have been described in patients with cholestatic jaundice (95–97). Investigators have postulated that PN-associated liver disease may, in part, be related to Mn toxicity. Given that Mn excretion is decreased in liver disease, especially cholestasis, and that bile flow is decreased during PN (104), however, the elevated Mn concentrations and brain deposition in these patients are likely the sequelae of the liver disease rather than its cause. Mn toxicity is discussed further on Chapter 84: Parenteral Nutrition.

Toxicity from increased dietary intake of Mn has not been well described in healthy humans. No adverse effects have been observed in persons ingesting an estimated 13 to 20 mg/day of Mn (105–107), although blood concentrations may increase significantly in association with lymphocyte Mn-dependent SOD activity (105). A single case report described an increased whole blood Mn concentration in a patient who received long-term cyclic enteral nutrition with concomitant substantial tea consumption (108).

Prolonged exposure to lower levels of elevated Mn intake may be associated with chronic toxicity (109). In this study, Mn sulfate (15 to 20 mg/kg per week) was administered intravenously as a weekly bolus for a period of approximately 28 weeks to cynomolgus macaque monkeys. Whole blood Mn concentrations increased significantly and were similar to those in humans with toxicity, although the administered dose was greatly in excess of what humans would receive even in PN. This Mn concentration was accompanied by mild deficits in spatial working memory and more significant deficits in nonspatial working memory, and performance was inversely associated with brain Mn concentration. Task performance improved in vehicle-treated animals. In humans, however, the level of exposure and the period of time required for the development of chronic toxicity are unclear. Toxicity, manifested by neurologic symptoms, may worsen even though toxic exposure including asymptomatic exposure ceased years earlier (110).

Yin et al (111) reported that, in mice, the cytoplasmic iron exporter ferroportin (Fpn) may function to transport Mn actively from cells in the presence of toxicity. Although the mechanism of Mn toxicity remains unknown, data suggest a role for Mn-induced oxidative stress (112). Mn is transported by a calcium (Ca^{2+}) uniporter into mitochondria, where Mn may accumulate because of slow clearance and may inhibit oxidative phosphorylation (113).

Treatment of Mn toxicity requires removal of the exposure and may require treatment with a chelating agent such as the Ca salt of ethylenediamine tetraacetic acid ($CaNa_2EDTA$) with careful clinical and biochemical monitoring (114). Controlled trials of this treatment in humans are lacking, however.

Tolerable Upper Intake Levels

The Food and Nutrition Board chose the following reasonable no-observed-adverse-effect levels of total Mn from food, water, and supplements as the UL: 2, 3, and 6 mg/day for children at ages 1 to 3 years, 4 to 8 years, and 9 to 13 years, respectively; 9 mg/day for ages 14 to 18 years and during pregnancy and lactation for adolescents; and 11 mg/day for adults more than 19 years old and for adults during pregnancy and lactation. Based on the Food and Drug Administration Total Diet Study, the highest daily dietary intake at the 95th percentile was 6.3 mg (by men aged 31 to 50 years) (12).

REFERENCES

1. Kemmerer AR, Elvehjem CA, Hart EB. J Biol Chem 1931;92:623–30.
2. Orent ER, McCollum EV. Science 1931;73:501–6.
3. Orent ER, McCollum EV. J Biol Chem 1931;92:651–78.
4. Mahoney JP, Small WJ. J Clin Invest 1968;47:643–53.
5. Schroder HA, Balassa JJ, Tipton IH. J Chronic Dis 1966;19:545–71.
6. Keen CL, Ensunsa JL, Clegg MS. Metal Ions Biol Systems 2000;37:89–121.
7. Kuhn NJ, Ward S, Piponski M et al. Arch Biochem Biophys 1995;320:24–34.
8. Brock AA, Chapman SA, Ulman EA et al. J Nutr 1994;124:340–4.
9. Baly DL, Keen CL, Hurley LS. J Nutr 1985;115:872.
10. Staley GP, Van der Lugt JJ, Axsel G et al. J S Afr Vet Assoc 1994;65:73–7.
11. Baly DL, Keen CL, Hurley LS. J Nutr 1985;115:872–9.
12. Food and Nutrition Board, Institute of Medicine. Dietary Reference Intakes for Vitamin A, Vitamin K, Arsenic, Boron, Chromium, Copper, Iodine, Iron, Manganese, Molybdenum, Nickel, Silicon, Vanadium, and Zinc. Washington, DC: National Academy Press, 2001.
13. Couzy F, Aubree E, Magnolia C et al. J Trace Elem Electrolytes Health Dis 1988;2:79–83.
14. Gibson RS. Am J Clin Nutr 1994;59:1223S–32S.
15. Sandstrom B, Davidsson L, Eriksson R et al. J Trace Elem Electrolytes Health Dis 1987;1:33–8.
16. Davidsson L, Cederblad A, Lonnerdal B et al. Am J Clin Nutr 1989;49:170–9.
17. Johnson PE, Lykken GI, Korynta ED. J Nutr 1991;121:711–7.
18. National Advisory Group on Standards and Practice Guidelines for Parenteral Nutrition. JPEN J Parenter Enteral Nutr 1998;22:49–66.
19. Stobbaerts RFJ, Ieven M, Deelstra H et al. Z Emahrungswiss 1992;31:138–46.
20. Krachler M, Rossipal E. Ann Nutr Metab 2000;44:68–74.
21. Stastny D, Vogel RS, Picciano MF. Am J Clin Nutr 1984;39:872–8.
22. Lonnerdal B. Physiol Rev 1997;77:643–9.
23. Finley JW, Johnson PE, Johnson LK. Am J Clin Nutr 1994;60:949–55.
24. Bertinet DB, Tinivella M, Balzola FA et al. JPEN J Parenter Enteral Nutr 2000;24:223–7.
25. Shike M, Ritchie ME, Shils ME. Clin Nutr 1986;34:804A.
26. Rossander-Hulten L, Brune M, Sandstrom B et al. Am J Clin Nutr 1991;54:152–6.
27. Thompson ABR, Olatunbosun P, Valberg LS. J Lab Clin Med 1971;78:642–55.
28. Finley JW. Am J Clin Nutr 1999;70:37–43.
29. Davidsson L, Cedarblad A, Lonnerdal B et al. Am J Clin Nutr 1991;54:1065–70.
30. Davidsson L, Almgren A, Jullerat MA et al. Am J Clin Nutr 1995;62:984–7.
31. Ishihara N, Matsushiro T. Arch Environ Health 1986;41:324–30.
32. Garcia-Aranda JA, Wapnir RA, Lifshitz F. J Nutr 1983;113:2601–7.
33. Bell JG, Keen CL, Lonnerdal B. J Toxicol Environ Health Res 1989;26:387–98.
34. MacDonald NS, Figueroa WG. UCLA Rep (US Atomic Energy Com) 1969;June 30:51–33.
35. Davidsson L, Cederblad A, Hagebo E et al. J Nutr 1988;118:1517–21.
36. Mena I. In: Bronner FL, Coburn JW, eds. Disorders of Mineral Metabolism. New York: Academic Press, 1981:233–70.
37. Ekmekcioglu C. Nahrung 2000;44:390–7.
38. Davidson L, Almgren A, Juillerat MA et al. Am J Clin Nutr 1995;62:984–7.
39. Mena I, Horiuchi K, Burke K et al. Neurology 1969;19:1000–6.
40. Freeland-Graves JH, Lin PH. J Am Coll Nutr 1991;10:38–43.
41. Wong-Valle J, Henry PR, Ammerman CB et al. J Anim Sci 1989;67:2409–14.
42. Rabin O, Hegedus L, Bourre JM et al. J Neurochem 1993;61:509–17.
43. Davis CD, Wolf TL, Greger JL. J Nutr 1992;122:1300–8.
44. Davidsson L, Lonnerdal B, Sandstrom B et al. J Nutr 1989;119:1461–4.
45. Davis CD, Zech L, Greger JL. Proc Soc Exp Biol Med 1993;202:103–8.
46. Harris WR, Chan Y. J Inorg Chem 1994;54:1–19.
47. Davidsson L, Lonnerdal B, Sandstrom B et al. J Nutr 1989;119:1461–4.
48. Ruth JA, Garrick MD. Biochem Pharmacol 2003;66:1–13.
49. Ascher M, Ascher JL. Neurosci Biobehav Rev 1991;15:333–40.
50. Rabin O, Hegedus L, Bourren JM et al. J Neurochem 1993;61:509–17.
51. Wu LJ, Leenders AG, Cooperman S et al. Brain Res 2004;1001:108–17.
52. Crossgrove JS, Yokel RA. Neurotoxicology 2004;25:451–60.
53. Crossgrove JS, Yokel RA. Neurotoxicology 2005;26:297–307.
54. Aisen P, Aesa R, Redfield AG. J Biol Chem 1969;244:4628–33.
55. Gibbons RA, Dixon SN, Hallis K et al. Biochem Biophys Acta 1976;444:1–10.

56. He L, Girijashanker K, Dalton TP et al. Mol Pharmacol 2006;70:171–80.

57. Girijashanker K, He L, Soleimani M et al. Mol Pharmacol 2008;73:1413–23.

58. Foradori AC, Bertinchamps A, Gulibon JM, et al. J Gen Physiol 1967;50:2255.

59. Sumino K, Hayakawa K, Shibata T et al. Arch Environ Health 1975;30:487–94.

60. Klassen C. Toxicol Appl Pharmacol 1974;29:458–68.

61. Cotzias GC, Horiuchi K, Fuenzalida S et al. Neurology 1968;18:376–82.

62. Cikrt M. Arch Toxikol 1973;31:51–9.

63. Tsalev DL, Langmyhr FJ, Gunderson N. Bull Environ Contam Toxicol 1977;17:660–6.

64. Hauser RA, Zesiewica TA, Martinez C et al. Can J Neurol Sci 1996;23:95–8.

65. Milne DB, Sims RL, Ralston NVC. Clin Chem 1990;36:450–2.

66. Versieck J. Crit Rev Clin Lab Sci 1985;22:97–184.

67. Neve J, Leclercq N. Clin Chem 1991;37:723–8.

68. Aschner M, Erikson KM, Hernandez EH et al. Neuromol Med 2009;11:252–66.

69. Krieger D, Krieger S, Jansen O et al. Lancet 1995;346:270–4.

70. Doisy EA Jr. Trace Sub Environ Health 1972;6:193–9.

71. Norose N, Terai M, Norose K. J Trace Elem Exp Med 1992;5:100–1.

72. Friedman BJ, Freeland-Graves JH, Bales CW et al. J Nutr 1987;117:133–43.

73. Smart ME. Vet Clin North Am Food Anim Pract 1985;1:13–23.

74. Erway L, Hurley LS, Fraser AS. J Nutr 1970;100:643–54.

75. Hidiroglou M. J Diary Sci 1979;62:1195–206.

76. Gong H, Amemiya T. Cornea 1999;18:472–82.

77. Baly DL, Curry DL, Keen CL et al. J Nutr 1984;114:1438–46.

78. Leach RM Jr, Lilburn MS. World Rev Nutr Diet 1978;32:123–34.

79. Everson GJ, Shrader RE. J Nutr 1968;94:89–94.

80. Amdur MO, Norris LC, Heuser GF. J Biol Chem 1946;164:783–4.

81. Kawano J, Ney DM, Keen CL et al. J Nutr 1987;117:902–6.

82. Couper J. Br Ann Med Pharm Vital Statis Gen Sci 1837;1:41–2.

83. Rodier J. Br J Ind Med 1955;12:21–35.

84. Huang CC, Lu CS, Chu NS et al. Neurology 1993;43:1479–83.

85. Huang CC, Chu NS, Lu CS et al. Neurology 1998;50:698–700.

86. Kaiser J. Science 2003;300:926–8.

87. Mergler D. Can J Neurol Sci 1996;23:93–4.

88. Sziraki I, Rauhala P, Koh KK et al. Neurotoxicology 1999;20:455–6.

89. Olanow CW, Good PF, Shinotoh H et al. Neurology 1996;46:492–8.

90. Pal KP, Samii A, Caline DB. Neurotoxicology 1999;20:227–38.

91. Desole MS, Sciola L, Delogu MR et al. Neurochem Int 1997;31:169–76.

92. Latchoumycandane C, Anantharam V, Kitazawa A et al. J Pharmacol Exp Ther 2005;313:46–55.

93. Roth JA, Walowitz J, Browne RW. J Neurosci Res 2000;61:162–71.

94. Mirowitz SA, Westrich TJ. Radiology 1992;18:535–6.

95. Ejima A, Imamura T, Nakamura S et al. Lancet 1992;339:426.

96. Taylor S, Manara AR. Anaesthesia 1994;49:1013.

97. Azaz A, Thomas A, Miller V et al. Arch Dis Child 1995;73:89.

98. Takagi Y, Okada A, Sando K et al. Am J Clin Nutr 2002;75:112–8.

99. Komaki H, Maisawa SI, Sugai K et al. Brain Dev 1999;21:122–4.

100. Nagatomo S, Umehara F, Hanada K et al. J Neurol Sci 1999;162:102–5.

101. American Society for Parenteral and Enteral Nutrition Board of Directors. JPEN J Parenter Enteral Nutr 1998;22:49–66.

102. Buchman AL, Neely M, Grossie VB Jr et al. Nutrition 2001;17:600–6.

103. Alves G, Thiebot J, Tracqui A et al. JPEN J Parenter Enteral Nutr 1997;21:41–5.

104. Messing B, Bories C, Kunstlinger F et al. Gastroenterology 1983;84:1012–9.

105. David CD, Greger JL. Am J Clin Nutr 1992;55:747–52.

106. Greger JL. Neurotoxicology 1999;20:205–12.

107. Schroeder HA, Balassa JJ, Tipton IH. J Chronic Dis 1966;19:545–71.

108. Ross C, O'Reilly DS, McKee R. Ann Clin Biochem 2006;43:226–8.

109. Schneider JS, Decamp E, Clark K et al. Brain Res 2009;1258:86–95.

110. Rosenstock HA, Simons DG, Meyer JS. JAMA 1971;217:1354–8.

111. Yin Z, Jiang H, Lee ES et al. J Neurochem 2010;112:1190–8.

112. Stredrick DL, Stokes AH, Worst TJ et al. Neurotoxicology 2004;25:543–53.

113. Gavin CE, Gunter KK, Gunter TE. Toxicol Appl Pharmacol 1992;115:1–5.

114. Herrero Hernandez E, Discalzi G, Valentini C et al. Neurotoxicology 2006;27:333–9.

115. Roth JA. Biol Res 2006;39:45–57.

SUGGESTED READINGS

Friedman BJ, Freeland-Graves JH, Bales CW et al. Manganese balance and clinical observations in young men fed a manganese-deficient diet. J Nutr 1987;117:133–43.

Girijashanker K, He L, Soleimani M et al. Slc39a14 gene encodes ZIP14, a metal/bicarbonate symporter: similarities to the ZIP8 transporter. Mol Pharmacol 2008;73:1413–23.

Roth JA. Homeostatic and toxic mechanisms regulating manganese uptake, retention, and elimination. Biol Res 2006;39:45–57.

B. MINERALS

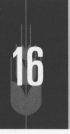

16 TRACE ELEMENTS[1]
CURTIS D. ECKHERT

[1]**Abbreviations: AI**, adequate intake; **As**, arsenic; **AsO$_2$$^-$**, arsenite; **ATPase**, adenosine triphosphatase; **B**, boron; **Ca^{2+}**, calcium; **cADPR**, cyclic adenosine diphosphate ribose; **CO$_2$**, carbon dioxide; **Cr**, chromium; **DARP**, dissimilatory arsenate-reducing prokaryote; **DRI**, dietary reference intake; **FAD**, flavin adenine dinucleotide; **FDA**, Food and Drug Administration; **GTF**, glucose tolerance factor; **Mo**, molybdenum; **NAD**, nicotinamide adenine dinucleotide; **Ni**, nickel; **PO$_3$$^-$**, phosphite; **Si**, silicon; **TPN**, total parenteral nutrition; **UL**, tolerable upper intake level; **V**, vanadium.

Elements ingested in milligrams or less per day are referred to as trace elements (1). Chemists originally used the term *trace* to indicate that concentrations were lower than the detectable limits of the analytic procedure in some of their samples. Statistical analysis cannot use words, so the practice was changed by replacing "trace" with an estimated number, often the midpoint been the lowest detectable limit and zero.

Trace elements enter the food chain from soil, water, and atmospheric particles derived from weathered geologic formations and volcanic eruptions. Two concepts are important when considering the essentiality of a trace element metals. First, evolving biologic systems were based on geochemistry and aquatic chemistry, which used metals and metalloids to perform catalytic, structural, and signaling functions. In metal-poor environments such as the ocean, organisms survive because many functions can be maintained using different metals with similar ionic radii and electronic structures. The second concept is chemical reactivity. In living systems, reactive metal atoms are not "free," but rather are stabilized by coordinate bonds to functional groups of amino acids in energetically strained (entatic) catalytic sites of proteins or are bound to ligands such as nucleotides and tetrapyrroles (2). In metalloenzymes, the strained state of metal coordination geometry stores most of the energy required to reach the critical high-energy transition state of the enzyme-substrate complex, so only small geometric changes are required to produce the activation energy needed to initiate enzymatic catalysis. One of the coordination sites on the metal atom is open for substrate binding and, in the relaxed state, binds an easily replaced ligand such as water (H_2O). The reactivity of a metal confined in this manner performs an essential biologic function, but at concentrations that exceed the capacity to coordinate or bind metal atoms, the same reactivity can damage neighboring molecules. Thus, at low levels of intake, the benefit of a trace element metal may be relative to the availability of other elements, but at high intakes, the probability of toxicity approaches certainty.

This chapter addresses several of the trace elements: arsenic (As), boron (B), chromium (Cr), molybdenum (Mo), nickel (Ni), silicon (Si), and vanadium (V). These elements are present in tissues at concentrations in the range of micrograms per kilogram and have been reported to alter some biologic process in some species. The elements Cr, Mo, Ni, and V are metals, whereas As, B, and Si are metalloids with properties of both metals and nonmetals. The term *essential* has two parts: essentiality of the biologic function and the requirement of a specific element to achieve that function. B and Mo are the only trace elements covered in this chapter that are essential for plants and whose concentration in plant foods is determined by local soil and water concentrations, as well as homeostatic mechanisms of the plant. Mo is essential for human health, and B is essential for lower vertebrates and beneficial for humans. The elements As and B are unique in that both have been proposed to have important roles in the origin of life. Evidence suggests that the other trace elements are beneficial to health under specific conditions. The benefits of these other trace elements to humans may not be unique but can be achieved using other elements or molecules.

ARSENIC

Historical Overview

As has been used as a poison for thousands of years. The ancient Syrians used inorganic salts of As as agricultural pesticides (3), and today organic arsenics such as roxarsone (4-hydroxy-3-nitrophenyl arsenic acid) are used to prevent coccidiosis in swine and improve the growth of poultry. As trioxide was such an effective human poison during the Middle Ages; it was referred to as "inheritance powder" (4). One of the curious events of European history involved the metabolism of As. William Morris (1834 to 1896) was a member of the family that owned the largest As mine in Europe. The mine polluted the ecology of Devon, England and caused pocked skin and lung disease in the local population (5). To divorce himself from the mine, William sold his share and used the proceeds to manufacture expensive wallpaper colored with the dye Scheele's green, which contained copper arsenite. Fungi in the wallpaper paste methylated the As salt into toxic trimethyl arsine. This volatile substance rose to high concentrations in the poorly ventilated rooms of the time. This is presumed to be the source of the high As levels in the hair of exiled Napoleon Bonaparte (6).

Terminology, Chemistry, Metabolic Roles, Interactions with Other Compounds, and Basic Importance in Normal Functions

As is widely distributed in nature in association with ores of metals such as copper, lead, and gold (3, 7). It is a metalloid existing in four oxidation states: As($-$III), As(0),

As(III), and As(V). The predominant form of inorganic As in aqueous and aerobic environments is arsenate (As[V] as $H_2AsO_4^-$ and $HAsO_4^{2-}$), whereas in anoxic environments, arsenite (As[III] as $H_3AsO_3^0$ and $H_2AsO_3^-$) predominates. Adsorption of arsenate on the surface of minerals such as ferrihydrite and alumina constrains its hydrologic mobility. The most common form of arsenite (AsO_2^-) is less strongly adsorbed to minerals, so its oxyanion is more mobile in environmental water (8). As has not been shown to be required for any physiologic functions in animals or humans, but deficiencies have been reported to result in myocardial damage. Its principal importance in the diet is as a toxin that can induce damage to the nervous and cardiovascular systems and increase the risk of cancer of the skin, lung, and bladder.

Dietary Sources

The total dietary intake of As from food is approximately 50 μg of As/day, of which 10 μg is inorganic. Less than 4 μg/day is derived from drinking water (9). Salt water fish contain the highest concentration of As (1662 ng/g) as arsenobetaine, a nontoxic organic form. Cereals and bakery products provide approximately 23.5 ng/g, and fats and oils contain 19 ng/g (10). The major contributors of inorganic As are rice, flour, spinach, and grape juice (11). As intakes in North America range from 0.5 to 0.81 μg/kg/day, with a median intake of 2.0 to 2.9 and 1.7 to 2.1 μg/day for men and women, respectively (12). The concentration in human milk ranges from 0.2 to 6 μg/kg wet weight. Drinking water is the primary source of inorganic As(III) and As(V).

Recommended Dietary Allowances

The Food and Nutrition Board of the Institute of Medicine has not established a dietary reference intake (DRI) or a tolerable upper intake level (UL) for dietary As (Table 16.1).

Sites of Intestinal Absorption, Blood Transport, and Intracellular Forms

Soluble forms of ingested As are readily absorbed from water (90%) and food (60% to 70%) by the human gastrointestinal tract (13, 14). Less soluble arsenosugars occur in plant products such as seaweed and are poorly absorbed (15). The proportion of inhaled As absorbed ranges from 30% to 34% (16). As bound to the skin is slowly released into the circulation (17). As is cleared from the blood in humans, although some remains bound to the cysteine residues of hemoglobin (18). It is methylated in the liver using S-adenosylmethionine as the methyl donor to methylarsonic acid and dimethylarsinic acid (19). Arsenics containing As(III) are the preferred substrates for enzymatically catalyzed methylation. Inorganic and organic As(V) is first reduced to As(III) by glutathione or other thiols and then is methylated and cycled between

TABLE 16.1	RECOMMENDED DIETARY ALLOWANCES AND UPPER LIMITS		
ELEMENT	AI	RDA	UL
Arsenic	ND		
Boron	ND		
1–3 y			3 mg/d
4–8 y			6 mg/d
9–13 y			11 mg/d
14–18 y			17 mg/d
Adults			20 mg/d
Chromium			
0–6 mo	0.2 μg/d		
7–12 mo	5.5 μg/d		
1–3 y	11 μg/d		
4–8 y	15 μg/d		
9–13 y	25 μg/d		
Adult male	35 μg/d		
Adult female	25 μg/d		
Molybdenum			
0–6 mo		2 μg/d	
7–12 mo		3 μg/d	
1–3 y		17 μg/d	300 μg/d
4–8 y		22 μg/d	600 μg/d
9–13 y		34 μg/d	1,100 μg/d
14–18 y		43 μg/d	1,700 μg/d
Adults		45 μg/d	2,000 μg/d
Pregnancy and Lactation		50 μg/d	
Nickel	ND		
1–3 y			0.2 mg/d
4–8 y			0.3 mg/d
9–13 y			0.6 mg/d
Adults			1.0 mg/d
Silicon	ND		ND
Vanadium	ND		ND

AI, adequate intake; ND, no data; RDA, recommended dietary allowance; UL, tolerable upper intake level.

the As(V) and As(III) oxidation states to form dimethylated products,

$$As^VO_4^{3-} + 2e \rightarrow As^{III}O_3^{3-} + CH_3^+ \rightarrow CH_3As^VO_3^{2-}$$
$$+ 2e \rightarrow CH_3As^{III}O_2^{2-} + CH_3^+(CH_3)_2As^VO_2^- + 2e$$
$$\rightarrow (CH_3)_2As^{III}O^- + CH_3^+$$

The mammalian enzyme responsible for catalyzing the transfer of the methyl group from S-adenosyl-L-methionine to trivalent and dimethylated arsenics is S-adenosyl-L-methionine: As(III) methyltransferase (19). Methylation efficiency in humans decreases when concentrations are high (20), and when the liver's methylating capacity is exceeded, inorganic As accumulates in soft tissues. Pretreatment of cells with small amounts of As over prolonged periods increases the methylating efficiency and thereby decreases the risk of toxicity.

Tissue accumulation is influenced by methyltransferases, and polymorphisms of these enzymes may explain the variability in individual risk for As toxicity (19). As accumulates in the liver, kidney, muscles, heart, spleen, pancreas, lungs, and brain (21). Following low-level exposure to inorganic As, its methylated metabolites are rapidly excreted in urine with small amounts of inorganic As eliminated in feces, sweat, skin desquamation, hair, and nails (22). The relative proportions of urinary As metabolites are 40% to 60% dimethylarsinic acid, 20% to 25% inorganic As, and 15% to 25% methylarsinic acid (23). One study, in which a single intravenous injection of radiolabeled trivalent inorganic As(III) was administered to human volunteers, showed that most of the As(III) was removed by urinary excretion within 2 days, and a small amount of excretion continued during the subsequent 2 weeks. The biologic half-life of As from fish is estimated to be less than 20 hours, with total clearance occurring over 48 hours. Blood concentrations may appear normal while levels in the urine remain elevated.

Functions in Metabolism and Biology

Bacteria isolated from mud taken from Mono Lake, California were able to grow using AsO_3^- in place of phosphite (PO_3^-). This finding suggests that life using AsO_3^- in place of PO_3^- was important in the origin of life on Earth and may exist on other planets (24).

A group of bacteria called dissimilatory arsenate-reducing prokaryotes (DARPs) uses As(V) as a nutrient (7). DARPs occur in anoxic environments, in the gastrointestinal tracts of animals, and in the subsurface aquifer sediments of Bangladesh (7, 25). DARPs use As in respiration by linking the oxidation of lactate to the reduction of As(V) to As(III). No unique biologic functions have been discovered for As in vertebrates.

Assessment of Nutrient Status

Methods are not available to assess nutritional status, but blood levels of As are affected by the status of folate. Methylation of ingested inorganic As to monomethylarsonic and dimethylarsinic acids requires folate-dependent one-carbon metabolism and facilitates urinary As elimination. Gamble et al (26) used folic acid supplementation (400 µg/day) to reduce total blood As concentrations from a preintervention mean ± SE of 9.86 ± 0.62 µg/L to 8.20 ± 0.50 µg/L after the intervention with folic acid ($p <$ .0001). A nonsignificant decline from 9.59 ± 0.63 µg/L to 9.14 ± 0.61 µg/L occurred in individuals receiving a placebo ($p = .10$) (26).

Specific Causes and Manifestations of Deficiency and Excess

Dabeka (10) reported symptoms associated with low dietary As intake in goats, miniature pigs, and rats. Myocardial damage was observed in lactating goats with evidence of mitochondrial membrane damage. Other manifestations include reduced growth, impaired fertility, and increased perinatal mortality. Deficiency symptoms depend on available methylating capacity (25).

The toxicity of As is based on the ability of As(III) to react with the sulfhydryl groups in proteins, thus leading to inactivation of enzymes (27). Mitochondria are the primary cellular targets of As(III), and they are where it accumulates, uncouples oxidative phosphorylation, and reduces the synthesis of adenosine triphosphate (ATP). As is also a cocarcinogen with ultraviolet radiation (20). The underlying mechanism may be inhibition of DNA repair by AsO_2^- following ultraviolet damage (28). Methylation of As competes for S-adenosylmethionine and leads to hypomethylation of DNA and potential damage (29). Acute As poisoning causes an acute paralytic syndrome characterized by cardiovascular collapse and loss of brain function resulting from necrosis of white and gray matter secondary to vasodilation (30, 31). The symptoms of As toxicity are dose dependent and include encephalopathy, gastrointestinal symptoms, skin pigmentation and dermatitis, peripheral vascular disease and neuropathy, genotoxicity, and cancer. Acute ingestion of 1 mg/kg/day of inorganic As causes anemia and hepatotoxicity. Ingestion of 10 mg/kg/day or more can result in encephalopathy and gastrointestinal disturbances. Long-term ingestion of 10 µg/kg/day in drinking water can produce arsenicism. This is an occlusive peripheral vascular disease, commonly referred to as black foot disease, in which, in extreme cases, feet turn black and develop gangrene. The US Environmental Protection Agency's maximum contaminant level (MCL) for drinking water As is 10 µg/L (16).

Long-term ingestion of low levels of inorganic As occurs over an extensive region of Southern Asia and increases the risk of cancers of the skin, bladder, and lung (32). As poisoning is a problem in Bangladesh and West Bengal, India on a scale never before encountered for a natural or synthetic toxic substance (33, 34). The problem is a consequence of attempts to meet the water demand for the large population. In the 1970s, The United Nations Children's Fund (UNICEF) and other relief international agencies drilled 6 to 10 million shallow drinking water wells to bypass sewage-tainted surface waters contaminated with cholera. The sediments in the area contained As adsorbed on the surface of iron oxides. By 1998, 61% of the shallow wells were found to be contaminated with As, thus exposing millions of people to high levels, with 200,000 reported cases of arsenicosis. The release of As from the minerals may have been initiated by the reduction of iron oxide coating on sand grains in the sediment by DARPs, inorganic carbon from peat, and methane (34).

BORON

Historical Overview

B was identified as an essential plant nutrient in 1923 (35), but it took 73 years to discover that borate esters are required to hold the cell wall scaffolding together under the enormous pressures required for cell elongation (36). B is also required for flowering and seed formation and is added to fertilizers, but deficiencies remain a major cause of crop failure throughout the world. Fungi synthesize antibiotics that contain a single B atom in their structure, and bacteria synthesize and release autoinducer AI-2, a quorum-sensing molecule with a single B atom (37).

In the search for B function, Hunt and Nielsen (38) employed a nutrient stress model. These investigators showed that B was beneficial for bone development in birds and mammals stressed with a combined deficiency of B along with calcium (Ca^{2+}), vitamin D, or magnesium. Penland (39) determined that the major change in humans subjected to 62 days of B deprivation was a deficit in executive brain function. Eckhert (40) determined that B was required even in the absence of stress by showing that the growth of embryonic rainbow trout embryos (*Oncorhynchus mykiss*) increased in a dose-dependent manner with increasing boric acid. Further evidence for its essentiality in vertebrates was obtained in a study showing that B deficiency disrupted cleavage of zebrafish zygotes. B-deficient zygotes failed to cleave properly into two cells, and from two cells to the four-cell stage, and this was reversible by repletion with boric acid (41). These observations were reinforced by studies showing B was also required for the morphogenesis of frog (*Xenopus*) embryos (42). The major symptom of B deficiency in adult zebrafish was retinal degeneration, an observation that reinforced Penland's observation that B was important for the nervous system (43).

Terminology, Chemistry, Metabolic Roles, Interactions with Other Compounds, and Basic Importance in Normal Functions

B was formed along with hydrogen, carbon, nitrogen, and oxygen during the nucleosynthesis of low-weight elements following the Big Bang (44). Borates from meteorites could stabilize glyceraldehyde, thus allowing it to combine with enediolate and stabilize ribose in the interstellar environment (45). This postulated role, in the transition between interstellar chemistry and the RNA world, has placed B center stage at the origin of life.

B, atomic number 5, has an atomic weight of 10.81 and exists as a mixture of stable isotopes ^{10}B and ^{11}B with respective abundances of 19.8% and 80.2% in the natural environment. The principal geologic forms of borate include the following: tincal (borax), $Na_2B_4O_7.10H_2O$; kernite (borax pentahydrate), $Na_2[B_4O_5(OH)_4].2H_2O$; colemanite, $Ca[B_3O_4(OH)_3].H_2O$; and ulexite, $NaCa[B_5O_6(OH)_6].5H_2O$ (44). B is a metalloid with an electronic structure of $1s^2 2s^2 p$ and oxidation state of $^{+}3$. The chemistry of B in nature is dominated by its affinity for oxygen (46). Three (trigonal) covalent bonds with oxygen form boric acid and four (tetrahedral) borates. B has a strong tendency to form a fourth bond to complete the octet of valence electrons in molecules such as halides. Soluble forms of B include boric acid $B(OH)_3$ and the monovalent anion $B(OH)_4^-$, with the predominate form

dependent on the pH of the solvent. Boric acid is a weak Lewis acid with a negative logarithm of the constant for the ionization equilibrium (pK_a) of 9.2. The structures of borate minerals contain trigonal BO_3 or tetrahedral BO_4 units forming large B-oxygen anions. Boric acid is the major form of B in physiologic fluids at concentrations with reported ranges from 2 to 100 μM B, but usually between 2 and 10 μM B. Boric acid and borate form complexes with *cis*-diol groups on the five-carbon sugars apiose in plants and ribose in animals. Physiologic concentrations of boric acid have been shown to modulate the release of endoplasmic reticular Ca^{2+} stores, one of the major processes by which cells control intracellular events in response to changes in the environment. At millimolar concentrations, boric acid inhibits serine proteases including prostate serum antigen (8).

Dietary Sources

All foods made from plants and their byproducts contain B as an essential structural component of cell walls; seeds, nuts, and vegetables contain a higher concentration than fruits and grains. Furthermore, the B content of foods reflects local soil and water conditions in which they were grown (46). The major contributors of B to the diet are those associated with the Mediterranean diet and include apples, avocados, legumes, dates, prunes, nuts, wine, whole grain breads, tomato sauces, and potatoes (47, 48).

Because diets in industrialized countries contain various plant products, the major contributors to the diet often represent less than 10% of total B intake. In developing countries, however, it is skewed to one food. For example, the top contributor in Germany is wine (15%); in Kenya, it is maize (35%); in South Korea, it is rice (6%); in Mexico, it is tortillas (56%); and in the United States, it is coffee (6%) (48, 49).

Recommended Dietary Allowances

The Food and Nutrition Board has not established a DRI for B. The ULs for different age groups are as follows: 3 mg B/day, 1 to 3 years of age; 6 mg B/day, 4 to 8 years; 11 mg B/day, 9 to 13 years, 17 mg B/day, 14 to 18 years; and 20 mg/day for pregnant and lactating women more than 19 years old and all adults (11) (see Table 16.1).

Sites of Intestinal Absorption, Blood Transport, and Intracellular Forms

Boric acid and borates are rapidly absorbed from the gastrointestinal tract with more than 90% efficiency (11). Borates are not absorbed through skin, but small amounts can be absorbed by inhalation of dust from occupational and consumer product exposures. The major form in blood and other body fluids is boric acid, which is distributed to all tissues. Human semen concentrations from physiologically normal men are four times higher than in blood in low-B regions, but the ratio is lower in men living in higher-B regions (50). This finding suggests that borate/boric acid export transporters are present in the prostate or seminal glands. More than 90% of ingested B is eliminated as boric acid in the urine of humans and rats following first-order kinetics. The half-life of renal clearance is approximately 21 hours in humans, renal reabsorption occurs when the ratio of B to creatinine is less than 1 (51). Locksley and Sweet (52) conducted a dose-response mouse toxicity study using intraperitoneal injections of borax. Tissue B concentrations increased proportionally over a range of 1.8 to 71 mg B/kg. Ku et al (53) evaluated the tissue concentrations of male rats fed a diet containing 1575 mg B/kg for 7 days. After bone, the seminal vesicles accumulated the next highest concentration and are a known target of toxic exposure in rats.

Functions in Metabolism and Biology

Unique roles have been identified for B in three different biologic processes. In vascular plants, polysaccharide chains of the most complex carbohydrate known, rhamnogalacturonan II, provide scaffolding to maintain the architecture of cells as they expand to hundreds of times their length during growth. As tremendous turgid pressure elongates the cell, borate esters link dimers of rhamnogalacturonan II together to prevent rupture (22). Several transporters have been identified in plants that move borate anions from the roots to the shoots and export B when levels become excessive (54). One transporter has been identified in animal cells, but this has not been confirmed by other laboratories (55). Myxobacteria synthesize antibiotics that contain a single B atom (56–58). Gram-positive and Gram-negative bacteria synthesize an autoinducer that contains a single B atom and coordinates gene expression among different species (59).

Hunt (60–63) proposed that B acts in animals by altering energy substrate utilization, mineral metabolism, vitamin metabolism, and enzyme activities, as well as by perturbing the immune system and more. Cui, Barranco, and Eckhert et al (64–66) used epidemiology as a tool to screen for B-responsive health effects and found that intake from food and regional groundwater was inversely associated with prostate cancer. The plausibility of this hypothesis has been confirmed in both cell culture and animal models (67). These investigators proposed that these effects were secondary to B's ability to modulate the nicotinamide adenine dinucleotide (NAD^+)/CD38/cyclic adenosine diphosphate ribose (cADPR) intercellular signaling pathway (68). Extracellular NAD^+ derived from active secretion by cells or their necrosis binds to CD38 on the plasma membrane of neighboring cells (69). CD38 is a multifunctional enzyme that converts NAD^+ to cADPR, an intracellular messenger. cADPR is released into the cytoplasm, where it binds to the ryanodine receptor, a Ca^{2+} channel that controls the release of Ca^{2+} stores in the endoplasmic reticulum into the cytoplasm. Mass spectrometry showed

boric acid bound to NAD^+ and cADPR (70, 71). Confocal Ca^{2+} imaging identified boric acid acts as a reversible competitive inhibitor of cADPR-stimulated Ca^{2+} release (72). The ability to modulate cADPR-stimulated Ca^{2+} release was within the dietary controlled blood range of healthy humans and was dose dependent. The effect occurred within seconds and led to a 30% drop in endoplasmic reticular Ca^{2+} levels. Ca^{2+} signaling and phosphorylation represent the major ways cells adapt to changes in their environment, and the relationship between Ca^{2+} and cell proliferation is well established (73).

Positive health effects of B intake have been reported in human studies and include an increase in brain executive function and prevention of cancer. Human subjects depleted of B for up to 65 days exhibited deficits in executive brain function, with minor alterations in steroid metabolism and hematologic indicators that were reversible by B supplementation (39). The risk of prostate cancer decreased with increasing B intake from either food (64) or the water supply (65, 66). The biologic plausibility of this epidemiologic association was shown in studies using human cell lines (74, 75), mice (67), and human subjects (76). Dietary boric acid inhibited the growth of xenograph human prostate cell tumors and the amount of serum antigen (prostate-specific antigen) in a murine model of cancer (67). Enlarged prostates are a major risk factor for prostate cancer. Turkish urologists used ultrasound to measure prostate volume in men who were 59 years old on average in two villages with different levels of B in the water supply. Men living in the high-B village had intakes of 6.2 mg B/day and significantly smaller prostates ($p < .0001$) than men living in the low-B village with intakes of 0.6 to 0.8 mg/day (76). One epidemiologic study did not observe a protective effect of B on the risk of prostate cancer, but this study was flawed by pooling men from low-B and high-B regions, using a database designed to compare relative amounts of elements in foods and not their absolute amounts, and estimating B concentrations of foods (77).

The protective effect of B is not limited to prostate cancer. The risk of lung cancer in women was also reported to be reduced by B in a dose-dependent manner (78) and cervical dysplasia was lower in high-B regions compared with low-B regions (79). In vitro studies have also shown boric acid reduces proliferation of breast cancer (80) and melanoma cells (81).

B was shown in numerous studies to alter bone in chicks, pigs, and rats (82). In pigs, supplementation levels of 5 mg B/kg diet increased bone bending moment in males, but not females (83). In male rats, B supplementation did not change tibia or femur resistance to bending, but dietary levels of 200 mg/kg diet increased vertebral resistance to crush force (84). In contrast, B supplementation of ovariectomized female rats did not provide protection against osteopenia or improve vertebrae strength. An epidemiologic study of Korean women who were 41 years old on average did not observe a significant relationship between B intake (0.9 mg/day) and bone density (49).

Assessment of Nutrient Status

Considerable geographic variability exists in dietary B intake (47, 85). A comparison of dietary intakes in the United States, Germany, Kenya, and Mexico showed that the United States had the lowest intake and Mexico the highest (48). The major contributors and their contribution to total B dietary intake in the United States were coffee (6.7%), milk (5.1%), apples (5.1%), beans (4.8%), and potatoes (4.8%) (86). Measuring B excretion in a 24-hour urine collection is the most objective approach to measuring B intake (87).

Specific Causes and Manifestations of Deficiency and Excess

An adequate level of B intake has not been determined. When the amount required for women's bone health is selected, the report by Kim et al (49) in Korean women suggests that 0.9 mg/day would be adequate for women. When prostate health is chosen as the end point for men, the report by Muezzinoglu et al (76) suggests 6 mg/day would be an adequate intake. No reports exist of B toxicity induced by diet in humans. Toxicity in animals requires blood concentrations greater than 1000 μM, a level 20 times higher than reported in B mine workers in the People's Republic of China who had very high intakes of 41 mg/day (50). In rats, the primary reproductive effect is degeneration of the spermatogenic epithelium of the testes leading to impaired spermatogenesis, reduced fertility, and sterility (88).

CHROMIUM

Historical Overview

Rats fed a necrogenic diet develop liver degeneration and glucose intolerance. Schwarz and Mertz (89) discovered that dietary selenium protected against the liver degeneration, and glucose intolerance could be corrected by intubating crude fractions of homogenized pig kidney or brewer's yeast. These investigators named the unknown factor in the fractions glucose tolerance factor (GTF). The fraction's activity was lost during storage, but it could be restored with wet ash of pig kidney. The researchers concluded that a trace element was required as a cofactor. They screened 43 different salts for their ability to improve the rate of glucose removal when taken orally (89) and reported the 3 most active salt preparations: a combination of Cr(II) and Cr(VI), vanadyl sulfate and Cr(VI), and Cr(III) chloride alone. From this information, the researchers concluded that Cr(III) was required for GTF activity (89). In 1998, Mertz (90) discussed the four major criticisms others had made about their conclusion and against the use of Cr(III) to treat glucose intolerance. These criticisms were as follows: (a) Cr(VI) is a carcinogen; (b) the bioavailability of Cr(III) is very low; (c) Cr(III) does not ameliorate glucose intolerance in all organisms; and (d) despite great effort, GTF had not been characterized, and different laboratories did not agree on its composition or structure (90).

Terminology, Chemistry, Metabolic Roles, Interactions with Other Compounds, and Basic Importance in Normal Functions

Cr (atomic number 24, molecular weight 59) occurs in each oxidative state from -2 to $+6$, with Cr(III) and Cr(VI) the most important in human health. Cr(III) is poorly absorbed (0.4% to 2.5%), and the remainder is excreted in feces. Cr(III) has been hypothesized to serve as a necessary cofactor for the biologic activity of Mertz's isolated factor. Mertz named the factor GTF but was unable to purify it. Vincent (91) isolated a low-molecular-weight Cr-binding substance from adipocytes called chromodulin. He proposed that activation of the insulin receptor allows Cr to enter the cell. Once absorbed, Cr binds to apochromodulin and converts it to holochromodulin, the active form. Holochromodulin binds to the insulin receptor, thus activating its receptor kinase activity and physiologic function. Wang et al (92) reported that several different Cr(III) compounds were effective at enhancing insulin receptor phosphorylation in intact cells, but they were not effective in activating a recombinant insulin receptor kinase. Anderson (93) suggested that Cr(III) increases insulin activity by both activating the insulin receptor and increasing the number of copies of the receptor.

Dietary Sources

The level of Cr in dietary plants is determined by the local soil and water conditions. Plants do not require Cr and contain less than 0.2 mg/kg, but they bioaccumulate heavy metals. When grown in soil polluted from Cr-emitting industries or when sewage sludge is used as a fertilizer, plants can accumulate high concentrations (94). Whole grains, cereals, and unrefined sugars contain the highest concentrations, with lesser amounts in fruits and vegetables, and most servings containing less than 1 to 2 μg (95). Cr also enters foods from stainless steel cooking pots and pans during cooking and in the processing of meats (96).

Recommended Dietary Allowances

The Food and Nutrition Board set an adequate intake (AI) for Cr (see Table 16.1). The infant AI was calculated from Cr levels in milk. A round adult diet is estimated to contain 13.4 μg Cr/1000 kcal. The AI for men and women has been set at 35 and 25 μg/day, respectively. A UL value for Cr has not been established.

Sites of Intestinal Absorption, Blood Transport, and Intracellular Forms

Ingested Cr(III) is poorly absorbed (0.4% to 2.5%), with the remainder excreted in feces. In rats, 80% of absorbed dietary $^{51}CrCl_3$ was reported to bind to transferrin (97).

Many different synthetic Cr(III) chelates have been synthesized in an attempt to increase its bioavailability including amino acids, vitamins, and picolinic acid. Despite years of work, the biologically active form of Cr(III) has not been identified. Urinary excretion of Cr is increased by exercise (98).

Functions in Metabolism and Biology

Cr may increase the effectiveness of insulin in controlling blood glucose, but the effect is small and inconsistent. Elucidating the function of Cr at a molecular level has proved problematic. The mode of action is proposed to involve an increase in the activity of the insulin receptor, but the specificity and target of Cr(III) remain unknown. Vincent and Anderson wrote reviews on the subject (91, 93).

Assessment of Nutrient Status

No indicator of Cr status is known at this time. Urinary Cr is related to recent Cr intake and is not a good indicator of Cr status (99).

Specific Causes and Manifestations of Deficiency and Excess

No cases of Cr deficiency in a healthy population have been reported. Three patients receiving total parenteral nutrition (TPN), including one patient for more than 3 years, exhibited symptoms of impaired glucose removal, elevated free fatty acids, peripheral neuropathy, and unexplained weight loss. The addition of 250 μg Cr to the TPN solution corrected the glucose resistance within 2 weeks (11). Anderson (93) reviewed 23 human studies designed to determine the effect of Cr(III) supplementation on blood glucose and lipids. In 5 trials, no effect was noted, but the remainder reported an improvement in glucose tolerance and an increase in high-density lipoprotein (93). The US National Institutes of Health is currently conducting a randomized double-blind study in nonobese, nondiabetic, insulin-resistant subjects. Subjects will take 500 μg Cr picolinate or placebo twice a day for 16 weeks to determine whether this supplement is effective in decreasing insulin resistance and decreasing blood lipids (100).

Cr(VI) is well established as a teratogen, genotoxin, and carcinogen, but the toxicity of Cr(III) was thought for a long time to be low because of its poor bioavailability and reactivity. Vincent (91) reviewed the toxicity of nutrient supplements containing Cr(III). Cr(III) toxicity stems from its ability to bind to nucleic acids in DNA and to the sulfhydryl groups in proteins. Cr(III) is a hapten and binds to proteins triggering immune responses that result in allergic reactions (101). Two clinical case reports of chronic interstitial nephritis attributed to the ingestion of Cr picolinate have been published (11). Cr(III), given as chromic chloride, is mildly teratogenic to the nervous system of mice (102). Cr(III) has not been considered genotoxic based on tests for mutations, DNA fragmentation, unscheduled DNA synthesis, and sister chromatid exchange assays. A test for the loss of genes (gene deletion) showed that pharmacologic concentrations of Cr(III) were more potent than Cr(VI) in causing gene deletions in both mice and yeast (103).

MOLYBDENUM

Historical Overview

Mo serves an essential role in the nitrogen cycle through its role in the molybdopterin cofactor of molybdoenzymes that are involved in nitrogen fixation and in nitrate reductase, an enzyme required for the conversion of nitrate to ammonia. Mo was recognized as essential for human xanthine oxidase activity in 1953 and for sulfite oxidase activity in 1971 (104, 105). Human essentiality is based on observations of genetic defects that cause a deficiency in the Mo cofactor that results in seizures and death of newborns within days of birth (106).

Terminology, Chemistry, Metabolic Roles, Interactions with Other Compounds, and Basic Importance in Normal Functions

The earth's crust contains approximately 1 mg/kg Mo (107). Physiologically relevant oxidations states for Mo are between $+IV$ and $+VI$ with redox potentials of -0.3 V (108). At these oxidation states, Mo has an affinity toward negatively charged O and S ligands such as oxide, sulfide, thiolates, or hydroxide and nitrogen ligands. Mo is an essential element for plants and occurs at concentrations ranging from less than 0.5 to more than 100 mg/kg in plant dry matter (109). The stable hexavalent form, molybdate(VI), MoO_4^{2-}, is very soluble at pH 7 and resembles the sulfur-transporting ion, SO_4^{2-}. Molybdate aggregates into clusters at oxidation states below $+VI$, but this action is suppressed in biologic systems by coordination of the Mo atom to dithiolene sulfurs on molybdopterin to form the molybdopterin cofactor. The molybdopterin cofactor is identical in all species and serves as the coenzyme in molybdoenzymes.

Mo accumulates as the molybdopterin cofactor in the liver, kidney, adrenal gland, and bone at concentrations that range from 0.1 to 1 mg/g wet weight (110). A pool of enzyme free metal-pterin complex, the Mo cofactor, is present in the mitochondrial outer membrane. Molybdoenzyme sulfite oxidase is located in the mitochondrial intermembrane space, and xanthine dehydrogenase and aldehyde oxidase are cytosolic enzymes (111).

Dietary Sources

The concentration of Mo in foods reflects the level of the soil and irrigation water in which they were grown. Rich sources include legumes, grains, and nuts. Low amounts are found in animals, fruits, and vegetables (112, 113).

Recommended Dietary Allowances

Data from the Total Diet Study indicated that the average Mo intake in the United States is 76 μg/day for women and 109 μg/day for men (112). The recommended AI for term infants is 0.3 μg/(kg/day) (11), but concern has been expressed that the value should be between 4 and 6 μg/(kg/day) for premature infants (114). The Food and Nutrition Board used a lowest observed adverse effect level of 0.9 mg/kg/day and uncertainty factor of 30 to determine the UL. The ULs for different age groups are as follows: 300 μg Mo/day, 1 to 3 years; 600 μg Mo/day, 4 to 8 years; 1100 μg Mo/day, 9 to 13 years, 1700 μg Mo/day, 14 to 18 years, and 2000 μg Mo/day for pregnant and lactating women more than 19 years old (11).

Sites of Intestinal Absorption, Blood Transport, and Intracellular Forms

In its most stable hexavalent form as molybdate(VI) (MoO_4^{2-}), Mo is water soluble and absorbed over a wide range of intakes. The extrinsic addition of stable isotopes of Mo to diets was used to measure absorption, retention, and excretion (115). Mo is rapidly absorbed and excreted from the kidney, with retention regulated primarily by urinary excretion. Absorption averaged 89% when daily Mo intake ranged from 25 to 122 μg/day and 93% when average intakes ranged from 466 to 1488 μg/day. Mo absorption is inhibited by high intakes of sulfate, possibly because sulfate anions compete for the same transport proteins (116, 117). Excess intake of Mo produced a copper deficiency in ruminants and nonruminants grazing on a pasture contaminated with high concentrations of Mo from industrial and mining waste (118).

Intrinsically labeled food was produced by incorporating ^{97}Mo into soybeans and kale grown in hydroponic systems (119, 120). Purees of extrinsically and intrinsically labeled soybeans and kale were then fed to 12 women. The mean 8-day absorption of Mo was 87% from extrinsic Mo, 86.1% from kale, and 56.7% from soybeans. The mean urinary excretion was 60.8% of absorbed dose for extrinsic Mo, and it was 56.6% from kale and 63.9% from soybeans.

Functions in Metabolism and Biology

The most important Mo function in mammalian systems is the transfer of oxygen to a two-electron substrate using one-electron transferring compounds such as flavin adenine dinucleotide (FAD). Coupling electron transfer and oxide exchange transfer an oxygen atom from the metal center to the substrate.

$$LMo^{VI}O_2 + X \leftrightarrow LMo^{IV}O + XO$$

where L is a ligand.

Three mammalian hydroxylases are molybdoenzymes. They include the mitochondrial enzyme sulfite oxidase, which catalyzes the oxidation of sulfite to sulfate in the metabolism of sulfur from methionine and cysteine; and two enzymes that hydroxylate heterocyclic substrates including purines and pyridines, xanthine oxidase, and aldehyde oxidase. Xanthine oxidase catalyzes the conversion of xanthine and its derivatives such as caffeine to uric acid and uric acid derivatives. Aldehyde oxidase is a metalloflavoprotein composed of FAD, Mo, and iron in a 1:1:4 ratio. It is involved in the formation of cotinine, a major metabolite of nicotine that occurs in the urine of cigarette smokers.

Assessment of Nutrient Status

Mo blood concentrations range widely in the literature (121). Isotope dilution studies reported plasma values of 5 nmol/L in subjects with an intake of 22 μg/day, 20 μmol/L at an intake of 467 μg/day, and 44 μmol/L at an intake of 1490 μg/day (122).

Specific Causes and Manifestations of Deficiency and Excess

Tungsten, the element immediately below Mo in Group 6B in the Periodic Table, has a similar ionic radius and electronic structure and forms a complex with molybdopterin that activates molybdoenzymes. Tungsten can induce Mo deficiency as measured by a decrease in molybdoenzyme activity, but it is not considered to be significant to livestock or humans because it is rarely found in the environment.

Evidence for Mo essentiality rests on clinical observations (123). The first was a case of sulfite oxidase deficiency in a child with an inborn error of metabolism. The symptoms included seizures, mental retardation, and dislocated ocular lenses, with the appearance of the unusual amino acid S-sulfocysteine in the plasma and urine, as well as high urinary levels of sulfite, thiosulfate, and taurine. A postmortem examination confirmed sulfite oxidase deficiency. Since then, nearly 50 additional cases of sulfite oxidase deficiency have been identified (123). The second observation was loss of sulfite oxidase activity in a patient with Crohn disease who was supported on TPN for 18 months (124). Symptoms developed after 1 year and included tachycardia, tachypnea, night blindness, and coma. Biochemical evaluation showed an elevation in plasma methionine, low serum uric acid, and reduced urinary levels of sulfate, thiosulfate, and uric acid. All symptoms were eliminated by the addition of 300 μg/day of ammonium molybdate to the TPN solution.

Mo deficiency has not been observed in humans, and no beneficial effects of taking supplements of the element have been documented. Observations of Mo deficiency have been limited to genetic defects that interfere with the Mo cofactor's ability to activate molybdoenzymes. Mo toxicity was induced in rats and caused renal insufficiency at levels of 80 mg/kg/day, but not at 40 mg/kg/day (96). In rabbits,

5 mg/kg/day induced weight loss and histopathologic changes in the kidney and liver (125).

NICKEL

Historical Overview

Ni was first shown to promote the growth of bacteria in 1965 (126). The biologic importance of Ni was subsequently shown in both bacteria and plants to be based on its catalytic role in four enzymes: urease, hydrogenases, CD dehydrogenase, and methyl-coenzyme M reductase. Between 1975 and 1978, diets were developed to induce deficiency symptoms in rats, chicks, pigs, and goats (127–130). The nutritional importance of Ni in humans is unknown and remains largely unstudied.

Terminology, Chemistry, Metabolic Roles, Interactions with Other Compounds, and Basic Importance in Normal Functions

Ni is in the first transition series of the Periodic Table with oxidation states of −I, 0, II, III, and IV. State II is the most important in biologic systems. Ni coordinates with the amino acids histidine, glutamic acid, and aspartate in metal centers of proteins (108), and it binds to histidine and cysteine on albumin and a macroglobulin called nickeloplasmin (131). Tissue concentrations decrease with age and are lower in 90-year-old adults than in 1-year-old children (132).

Dietary Sources

The 1984 Total Diet Study by the US Food and Drug Administration (FDA) showed that the mean Ni consumption in infants and children was 69 to 90 μg/day; and the median for adolescents, adults, and the elderly was 71 to 97 μg/day, 74 to 100 μg/day, and 80 to 97 μg/day, respectively (112). The major contributors vary in different countries. The major contributors to US diet are mixed dishes and soups (19% to 30%), grains and grain products (12% to 30%), vegetables (10% to 24%), legumes (3% to 16%), and desserts (4% to 18%). The major contributors in Canada are meat and poultry (11). Foods with the highest concentration of Ni include nuts, legumes, and chocolate (112).

Recommended Dietary Allowances

No AI or recommended dietary allowance (RDA) has been determined for Ni. The Food and Nutrition Board used a no observed adverse effect level of 5 mg/kg/day, based on decreased weight gain in rats. An uncertainty factor of 300 was derived by multiplying uncertainties of 10 each for extrapolation from rat to human, human variation, and 3 for potential toxic reproductive effects. The ULs for children 1 to 3, 4 to 8, and 9 to 13 years old were 0.2, 0.3, and 0.6 mg/day, respectively, of soluble Ni salts. The UL for adolescents and all adults was 1.0 mg/day (11).

Sites of Intestinal Absorption, Blood Transport, and Intracellular Forms

Dietary Ni is poorly absorbed, with reported values from 1% to 5% (132–135). Absorption is increased under conditions of low Ni and iron availability. A stable isotope study using ^{62}Ni reported that 29% to 40% of the metal was absorbed (109). The highest concentrations in the blood occurred 2 to 3 hours after oral intake of Ni sulfate or oxide (134, 136). The amount retained varied from 0% to 11%. Entry into brush-border epithelial cells is saturable. Movement of Ni from epithelial cells into blood is not regulated, and Ni ions move in both directions (134, 137, 138).

Functions in Metabolism and Biology

Ni has not been shown to be essential for any biochemical processes in humans. Ni is an essential component of ureases in jackbeans, ruminal bacteria, and several other plants, algae, and fungi. Ureases catalyze the degradation of urea to carbon dioxide (CO_2) and ammonia. Ni is also essential for hydrogenases in methanogenic bacteria that catalyze the conversion of hydrogen (H_2) and CO_2 to methane (CH_4). Methanogenic and acetogenic bacteria also require Ni in CD dehydrogenase, an enzyme that converts carbon monoxide to CO_2. Finally, methanogens use Ni in methylcoenzyme M reductase in the last step in the formation and liberation of methane (108, 134).

Assessment of Nutrient Status

No methods are available to assess Ni nutritional status, and urine concentrations have been reported to be higher in smokers (139). Ni blood levels in nonsmokers ranged from 0.01 to 0.26 μg/L, with a median of 0.06 μg/L, compared with a range of 0.01 to 0.42 μg/L and a median of 0.07 μg/L in smokers. Urine values in nonsmokers ranged from less than 0.01 to 4.6 μg/L, with a median of 0.5 μg/L, and values in smokers ranged from less than 0.01 to 8.2 μg/L, with a median of 1.2 μg/L ($p < .05$).

Specific Causes and Manifestations of Deficiency and Excess

Consuming dietary Ni has no known beneficial health effects in humans. Nielsen (132) reviewed the health effects of dietary Ni restriction in animals. The major observations in Ni-deprived pigs and rats were delayed sexual maturity, perinatal mortality, rough coat, and disorganization of the rough endoplasmic reticulum of the liver.

SILICON

Historical Overview

Abnormalities in bone, joints, skin, feathers, and hair in Si-deficient chickens and rats were first reported in 1972 by Carlisle (140) and by Schwarz and Milne (141). The results quickly became controversial when several other laboratories failed to observe similar changes (142). In studies in which Si supplementation of Si-deficient animals did have an effect, that effect was on the extracellular matrix and at the active site of bone formation during growth. A discussion of the controversy can be found in a review by Sripanyakorn et al (142). An epidemiologic study in 2004 observed a positive association between Si intake and bone mineral density in the hip of men and in premenopausal women, but not in postmenopausal women (143). The best evidence of biologic essentiality is in plants and diatoms. A gene family of Si transport proteins was identified in diatoms in 1997 (144).

Terminology, Chemistry, Metabolic Roles, Interactions with Other Compounds, and Basic Importance in Normal Functions

Si is the second most abundant element in the Earth's crust. The chemistry of Si in the natural world is dominated by its affinity for oxygen, to which it is tetrahedrally coordinated in minerals (145). In aqueous solution at neutral pH, Si takes the form of monosilicic acid, $Si(OH)_4$ (146). It forms stable complexes with mannitol and other polyhydroxy aliphatic hexose sugars containing two hydroxyls in the *theo* position. This results in the formation of stable polyolate complexes containing five and six coordinated Si atoms. The ease of formation and the stability of these polysilicate anions are what most likely enhance absorption and accumulation in tissue (146).

Dietary Sources

In the FDA's Total Diet Study, the major contributors of Si to the US diet were beverages (55%), primarily beer, coffee, and water, followed by grain and grain products (14%) and vegetables (8%) (147). Carrots, beetroot, and radish contain high concentrations of Si, but their bioavailability is lower than that of other vegetables (148).

Recommended Dietary Allowances

The Food and Nutrition Board has not established a DRI for Si. The mean intake of Si in adult men and women from the Total Diet Study was 40 and 19 mg/day, respectively (147). The magnitude of difference between intakes on low-fiber and high-fiber diets is approximately 21 mg/day versus 46 mg/day (149). No evidence indicates that dietary Si has any adverse effect. The use of antacids containing magnesium trisilicate has been associated with the development of urolithiasis resulting from the formation of Si-containing stones (150).

Sites of Intestinal Absorption, Blood Transport, and Intracellular Forms

The mean uptake of Si in adult men and women from the Total Diet Study was 40 and 19 mg/day, respectively (94). Si in food is broken down into the monomeric form in the gastrointestinal tract and is then absorbed. Serum Si levels reach a maximum 100 to 120 minutes following ingestion (148). Si is freely transported in the blood, possibly in a polymeric form (151). It is moved into tissue from plasma and is readily excreted. The excretion of Si in humans increases as dietary Si intake increases (152).

Urinary Si represents $41 \pm 36\%$ of total intake, a percentage suggesting that for many foods, Si content can be used as an approximate indicator of food absorption (148). This method cannot be used for the Si from root vegetables and bananas, however, because they are poorly absorbed (148).

Functions in Metabolism and Biology

Si has been reported to increase bone mineralization, but the mechanism of action remains unknown (140, 141, 153). Carlisle (154) suggested that Si is involved with phosphorus in events leading to calcification and that its primary effect is on connective tissue components, but she was never able to elucidate the biologic process. When she used an electron microprobe to determine the site of Si, however, Si was localized to the active growth areas of bone in growing mice and rats (155). The localized concentration reached a maximum during the final stages of calcification and then dissipated. Eckhert (156) suggested from this and from what is known from diatoms (157, 158) that the mechanism of the effect of Si on bone could lie in proton buffering.

Assessment of Nutrient Status

Serum Si values of 1325 healthy subjects 18 to 91 years old were measured using atomic absorption spectrometry (159). In men 18 to 59 years of age, the median was 9.5 µmol/L, and it decreased to 8.5 µmol/L at 60 to 74 years of age. The median concentration in women increased from 10.00 µmol/L at 18 to 29 years of age to 11.10 µmol/L from 30 to 44 years and decreased to 9.23 µmol/L between 45 and 59 years. In subjects 74 years old and older, the median was 7.70 µmol/L for men and 8.00 µmol/L for women.

Specific Causes and Manifestations of Deficiency and Excess

Human deficiencies of Si have not been reported. Studies in chickens, rats, and mice suggested that Si may be important for the growth of bone (148). One epidemiologic study found a positive association between Si intake and bone mineral density in men and premenopausal, but not postmenopausal, women (143). Intramuscular injections of monomethyltrisilanol and in osteoporotic patients were shown to improve trabecular bone volume and femoral bone mass density (143). Excessive intakes of Si were reported to cause urolithiasis, a deposition of calculi or uroliths containing monosilicic acid in the kidney, bladder, and urethra of grazing animals (155). In humans, adverse effects are primarily limited to silicosis, a lung disease resulting from the inhalation of silica particles. No dose-response data are available to establish a UL for Si.

VANADIUM

Historical Overview

In the 1970s, Va was reported by several laboratories to improve the growth of chickens, rats, and goats (160). The results were inconsistent, however, and Nielsen (161) suggested that the effects probably reflected poorly controlled experimental diets that provided Va at levels 10 to 100 times that found in normal diets. In 1986 and 1989, Anke (160) used better-formulated diets and compared supplemented goats (2 μg/g diet) with Va-deprived goats (10 ng/g diet). Va-deficient goats exhibited higher rates of spontaneous abortion and offspring that developed convulsions and succumbed to death at a rate of 41% during the first 3 months of life (160). Serum creatinine and β-lipoprotein concentrations were elevated and serum glucose depressed in Va-deprived goats. Rat studies showed increased thyroid weights in animals deprived of Va (162). Va is a possible carcinogen, and no evidence indicates that it is essential for humans, although pharmacologic levels promote the action of insulin and reduce blood glucose levels (162, 163).

Terminology, Chemistry, Metabolic Roles, Interactions with Other Compounds, and Basic Importance in Normal Functions

Va is a transition metal with six oxidations, of which three are biologically relevant: +III, +IV, and +V (108). Foods contain the tetravalent vanadyl [VO_2^+] and pentavalent [VO_3^-] forms. Common compounds include Va pentoxide (V_5O_5), sodium metavanadate ($NaVO_3$), sodium orthovanadate (Na_3VO_4), vanadyl sulfate ($VOSO_4$), and ammonium vanadate (NH_4VO_3). The Va ion is an enzyme cofactor and has been found to occur in certain tunicates (164). Vanadate(V) ions compete with phosphate ions and inhibit Na^+ adenosine triphosphatase (ATPase). The *ortho*vanadate ion, VO_4^{3-}, resembles the *ortho*phosphate ion, PO_4^{3-}. Unlike the phosphate ion, Va(V) is easily reduced to IV and III with biologic reductants such as glutathione (165, 166). Va-dependent enzymes include nitrogenase in bacteria and iodoperoxidase and bromoperoxidase in algae and lichens (108).

Dietary Sources

Grains and grain products contribute 13% to 30% of dietary Va. Marine organisms such as tunicates and brown algae and lichen and mushrooms are rich sources of Va (112). Eighty-eight percent of the foods evaluated in the FDA's Total Diet Study contained less than 2 μg/100 g of Va.

Recommended Dietary Allowances

Dietary intake of Va ranges from 6 to 18 μg/day (112). The Food and Nutrition Board has not assigned a DRI to Va or determined a UL.

Sites of Intestinal Absorption, Blood Transport, and Intracellular Forms

Less than 5% of ingested Va is absorbed (167, 168). Vanadyl sulfate and sodium metavanadate have been used as supplements. Va pentoxide (V_2O_3) from occupational exposures is reduced from Va(V) to (IV) in humans and other animals. Most Va is in the form of the vanadyl ion VO^{2+}(IV) in the stomach. Absorption occurs in the duodenum and upper gastrointestinal tract (169). The vanadate anion(V) is absorbed three to five times more readily than the vanadyl ion(IV). The vanadate anion(V) enters cells through nonspecific anionic channels and is reduced by glutathione (170, 171).

Va is rapidly cleared from plasma and accumulates in kidney, liver, testes, bone, and spleen. The Va anion(V) binds to the iron binding proteins, lactoferrin, transferrin, and ferritin, and tissue levels increase in rats fed Va-supplemented diets (169). Va is able to cross the placenta and is considered a reproductive toxin. Va is excreted primarily through the kidney, with a small amount through bile. Tissues with the highest concentrations include lung, teeth, thyroid, and bone (169).

Functions in Metabolism and Biology

A functional role for Va has not been identified in humans or other vertebrates. Vanadyl(IV) complexes potentiate the effect of insulin, but the underlying mechanism remains unknown (164). Oral doses of vanadyl sulfate (100 mg/day) improved both hepatic and skeletal muscle insulin sensitivity in subjects with non–insulin-dependent diabetes mellitus (NIDDM), in part by enhancing insulin's inhibitory effect on lipolysis, but they did not alter insulin sensitivity in nondiabetic subjects (172). Crystallographic analysis showed that Va as VO_4^{3-} can be incorporated into bone matrix, thus replacing PO_4^{3-} (173). Vanadate(V) anions inhibit phosphate-dependent enzymes and Na^+/ potassium (K^+)-ATPase hydrolysis. However, rats fed low dietary Va pentoxide, 1.8 to 18 mg/kg body weight, had higher alkaline phosphatase activity and DNA content in the femoral diaphysis, a finding indicating that it was beneficial, but diets containing 27 mg/kg body weight were inhibitory (174). Thus, the range between beneficial and toxic appears to be exceedingly small.

In the in vitro cell culture gilthead sea bream (*Sparus aurata* L.) model of vertebrate skeletal development, 7.5 μM vanadate increased cell proliferation, but it decreased extracellular matrix mineralization in 20% of controls (175). Va is particularly toxic to macrophages (176). Va (V) causes oxidation of thiols, including glutathione and cysteine, and introduces thiyl radicals (177). Va toxicity is mediated in part by oxygen-derived free radicals (178). Va amplifies the initial generation of singlet oxygen generated by the reduced form of NAD phosphate (NADPH) oxidase. The genotoxicity of Va pentoxide results from oxidative damage to DNA that causes DNA strand breakage.

Assessment of Nutrient Status

No methods are available to evaluate Va nutritional status.

Specific Causes and Manifestations of Deficiency and Excess

No human cases of Va deficiency have been reported. Va deficiency in goats was reported to increase rates of abortion, convulsions, bone malformations, and early death. Va as Va pentoxide is an industrial pollutant that is very toxic, but it is not present in foods. How interconvertible various forms of Va are in the stomach and when acted on by the intestinal microflora is not clear. Va toxicity symptoms include abdominal cramps, diarrhea, hemolysis, increased blood pressure, and fatigue. Va is a reproductive toxin affecting males more than females. It crosses the blood–placenta barrier, is teratogenic in rodents, and affects prepubertal animals. The International Agency for Research on Cancer (IRAC) lists Va as a possible carcinogen based on inhalation studies of Va pentoxide in animals (176). The US Environmental Protection Agency oral reference dose is 0.009 mg/kg/day (11).

REFERENCES

1. O'Dell B, Sunde R, eds. Handbook of Nutritionally Essential Mineral Elements. New York: Marcel Dekker; 1997.
2. Kaim W, Schwederski B. Some general principles. In: Bioinorganic Chemistry: Inorganic Elements in the Chemistry of Life. West Sussex, UK: John Wiley, 1994:1–38.
3. Nriagu J. Environmental Chemistry of Arsenic. New York: Marcel Dekker, 2002.
4. Megard A. Nature 2003;423:688.
5. Oremland RS, Stolz JF. Science 2003;300:939–43.
6. Jones DE, Ledingham KW. Nature 1982;299:626–7.
7. Smedley PL, Kinniburgh DG. Appl Geochem 2002;17:517.
8. Lin S, Shi Q, Nix FB et al. J Biol Chem 2002;277:10795–803.
9. Bagla P, Kaiser J. Science 1996;274:174–5.
10. Dabeka RW. Sci Total Environ 1989;89:279–89.
11. Food and Nutrition Board, Institute of Medicine. Dietary Reference Intakes for Vitamin A, Vitamin K, Arsenic, Boron, Chromium, Copper, Iodine, Iron, Manganese, Molybdenum, Nickel, Silicon, Vanadium, and Zinc. Washington, DC: National Academy Press, 2001.
12. Gunderson EL. J AOAC Int 1995;78:1352–63.
13. Hopenhayn-Rich C, Biggs M, Fuchs A, et al. Epidemiology 1996;7:117–24.
14. Yamauchi H, Kaise T, Yamamura Y. Bull Environ Contam Toxicol 1986;36:350–5.
15. Holland RH, McCall MS, Lanz HC. Cancer Res 1956;19:1154–6.
16. Wester RC, Maibach HI, Sedik L. Fundam Appl Toxicol 1993;20:336–40.
17. Benramdane L, Accominotti M, Fanton L. Clin Chem 1999;45:301–6.
18. Lu M, Wang H, Li XF et al. Chem Res Toxicol 2004;17:1733–42.
19. Agency for Toxic Substances and Disease Registry. Toxicological Profile for Arsenic. Atlanta: US Department of Health and Human Services, 2000:301–6.
20. Abernathy CO, Liu YP, Longfellow D et al. Environ Health Perspect 1999;107:593–7.
21. Abernathy CO, Thomas DJ, Calderon RL. J Nutr 2003;13:1536S–8S.
22. Marafante E, Vahter M, Norin H et al. J Appl Toxicol 1987;7:111–7.
23. Marcus WL, Rispin AS. Threshold carcinogenicity using arsenic as an example. In: Cothern C, Mehlman M, Marcus W, eds. In: Advances in Modern Environmental Toxicology, vol 15. Risk Assessment and Risk Management of Industrial and Environmental Chemicals. Princeton, NJ: Princeton Scientific, 1988:133–58.
24. Wolfe-Simon F, Blum JS, Kulp TR et al. Science 2011;332:1163–6.
25. Czarnecki DL, Baker GH. Poultry Sci 1982;61:516.
26. Gamble MV, Liu X, Slavkovich V et al. Am J Clin Nutr 2007;86:1202–9.
27. Abernathy CO, Liu YP, Longfellow D et al. Environ Health Perspect 1999;107:593–7.
28. Rossman TG, Uddin AN, Burns FJ et al. Toxicol Appl Pharmacol 2001;176:64–71.
29. Costa M. Am J Clin Nutr 1995;61(Suppl 3):666S–9S.
30. Nielsen FH. Ultratrace minerals. In: Shils ME, Olson JA, Shike M, et al, eds. Modern Nutrition in Health and Disease. 9th ed. Baltimore: Williams & Wilkins, 1999:283–303.
31. Civantos DP, Lopez RA, Aguado-Borruey JM et al. Chest 1995;108:1774–5.
32. Brouwer OF, Okenhout W, Edelbroek PM et al. Clin Neurol Neurosurg 1992;94:307–10.
33. National Research Council. Arsenic in Drinking Water. Washington, DC: National Academy Press, 1999.
34. Stokstad E. Science 2002;298:1535–6.
35. Warington K. Ann Bot 1923;37:629–72.
36. O'Neill MA, Eberhard S, Albersheim P et al. Science 2001;294:846–9.
37. Vendeville A, Winzer K, Heurlier K et al. Nat Rev Microbiol 2005;3:383–96.
38. Hunt C, Nielsen F. Interaction between boron and cholecalciferol in the chick In: Hunt C, Nielsen F, Gawthorne J, White C, eds. Trace Element Metabolism in Man and Animals. 1981:567–600.
39. Penland JG. Environ Health Perspect 1994;102(Suppl 7):65–72.
40. Eckhert CD. J Nutr 1998;128:2488–93.
41. Rowe RI, Eckhert CD. J Exp Biol 1999;37:1649–54.
42. Fort DJ, Propst TL, Stover EL et al. Biol Trace Elem Res 1998;66:237–59.
43. Eckhert CD, Rowe RI. J Trace Elem Exp Med 1999;12:213–9.
44. Copi CJ, Schramm DN, Turner ST. Science 1995;267:192–8.
45. Ricardo A, Carrigan MA, Olcott AN et al. Science 2004;303:196.
46. Loomis WD, Durst RW. BioFactors 1992;3:229–39.
47. Naghii MR, Wall L, Samman S. J Am Coll Nutr 1996;15:614–9.
48. Rainey C, Nyquist L. Biol Trace Elem Res 1998;66:79–86.
49. Kim MH, Bae YJ, Lee YS, Choi MK. Biol Trace Elem Res 2008.
50. Robbins WA, Wei F, Elashoff DA et al. J Androl 2007;29:115–21.
51. Pahl MV, Culver BD, Strong PL et al. Toxicol Sci 2001;60:252–6.
52. Locksley H, Sweet WH. Proc Soc Exp Biol Med 1954;86:56–63.
53. Ku WW, Chapin RE, Moseman RF, et al. Toxicol Appl Pharmacol 1991;111:145–51.
54. Tanaka M, Fujiwara T. Pflugers Arch 2008;456:671–7.
55. Park M, Li Q, Shcheynikov N et al. Mol Cell 2004;16:331–41.
56. Schummer D, Irschik H, Reichenbach H et al. Liebigs Ann Chem 1994;1994:283–9.
57. Dunitz JD, Hawley DM, Micklos D et al. Helv Chim Acta 1971;54:1709–13.

58. Chen TSS, Ching-Jer C, Floss HG. J Am Chem Soc 1979; 101:5826–7.

59. Chen X, Schauder S, Potier N et al. Nature 2002;415:545–9.

60. Hunt CD. J Trace Elem Exp Med 1996;9:185–213.

61. Hunt C. Environ Health Perspect 1994;102(Suppl 7):35–43.

62. Hunt CD. Biol Trace Elem Res 1998;66:205–25.

63. Hunt CD. J Trace Elem Exp Med 2003;216:291–306.

64. Cui Y, Winton M, Zhang ZF et al. Oncol Rep 2004;11: 887–92.

65. Barranco W, Hudak P, Eckhert C. Cancer Causes Control 2007;18:71–7.

66. Barranco W, Hudak P, Eckhert CD. Cancer Causes Control 2007;18:583–4.

67. Gallardo-Williams M, Chapin R, King P et al. Toxicol Pathol 2004;32:73–8.

68. Barranco WT, Eckhert CD. Cancer Lett 2004;216:21–9.

69. Lee HC. Mol Med 2006;12:317–23.

70. Kim D, Marbois B, Faull K et al. J Mass Spectrom 2003;38:632–40.

71. Kim D, Faull K, Norris AJ et al. J Mass Spectrom 2004;39: 743–51.

72. Henderson K, Salvatore L, Stella J et al. PLoS One 2009;4: 1–10.

73. Whitfield JF. Calcium in Cell Cycles and Cancer. 2nd ed. Boca Raton: CRC Press, 1995.

74. Barranco W, Eckhert C. Cancer Lett 2004;216:21–9.

75. Barranco W, Eckhert C. Br J Cancer 2006;94:884–90.

76. Muezzinoglu T, Korkmaz M, Nese N et al. Biol Trace Elem Res 2011 Mar 23 [Epub ahead of print].

77. Gonzalea A, Peters U, Lampe JW et al. Cancer Causes Control 2007;18:1131–40.

78. Mahabir S, Spitz MR, Barrera SL et al. Am J Epidemiol 2008;167:1070–80.

79. Korkmaz M, Uzgoren E, Bakirdere S et al. Environ Toxicol 2007;22:17–25.

80. Scorei R, Ciubar R, Ciofrangeanu C et al. Biol Trace Elem Res 2008;122:197–205.

81. Acerbo AS, Miller LM. Analyst 2009;134:1669–74.

82. Nielsen FH, Stoecker BJ. J Trace Elem Med Biol 2009;23: 195–203.

83. Armstrong TA, Spears JW, Crenshaw TD et al. J Nutr 2000;139:2575–81.

84. Chapin RE, Ku WW, Kenney MA et al. Fundam Appl Toxicol 1997;35:205–15.

85. Rainey C, Nyquist LA, Christensen RE et al. J Am Diet Assoc 1999;99:335–40.

86. Rainey C, Nyquist LA. Biol Trace Elem Res 1998;66:79–86.

87. Pahl MV, Culver BD, Strong PL et al. Toxicol Sci 2001;60: 252–6.

88. Fail PA, Chapin RE, Price CJ. Reprod Toxicol 1998;12:1–18.

89. Schwarz K, Mertz W. Nature 1959;85:292–5.

90. Mertz W. J Am Coll Nutr 1998;17:544–7.

91. Vincent JB. Acc Chem Res 2000;33:503–10.

92. Wang H, Kruszewski A, Brautigan DL. Biochemistry 2005; 44:8167–75.

93. Anderson RA. J Am College Nutr 2005;17:548–55.

94. Taylor FGJ, Mann LK, Dahlmann RC et al. Environmental effects of chromium and zinc in cooling-water drift. In: Cooling Tower Environment. Washington, DC: US Energy Research and Development Administration, 1975:408–26.

95. Welch RM, Carry EE. J Agric Food Chem 1975;23:479–82.

96. Anderson RA, Bryden NA, Polansky MM. Biol Trace Elem Res 1992;32:117–21.

97. Harris DC. Biochemistry 1977;16:560–4.

98. Anderson RA, Polansky MM, Bryden NA et al. J Nutr 1983; 113:276–81.

99. Anderson RA, Polansky MM, Bryden NA et al. Am J Clin Nutr 1991;54:909–16.

100. University of California, San Francisco. Chromium and Insulin Resistance. Trial identifier: NCT00846248. Available at: http://clinicaltrials.gov. Accessed November 23, 2011.

101. Polak L. Immunology of chromium. In: Burrows D, ed. Chromium: Metabolism and Toxicity. Boca Raton, FL: CRC Press, 1981:51–136.

102. Iijima S, Matsumoto N, Lu CC. Toxicology 1983;26:257–65.

103. Kirpnick-Sobol Z, Reliene R, Schiestl RH. Cancer Res 2006; 66:3480–4.

104. Richert DA, Westerfield WW. J Biol Chem 1953;203:915–23.

105. Cohen HJ, Fridovich I, Rajogopalan KV. J Biol Chem 1971; 246:374–82.

106. Johnson JL. Molybdenum. In: O'Dell BL, Sunde RA, eds. Handbook of Nutritionally Essential Mineral Elements. New York: Marcel Dekker, 1997:413–38.

107. Davis GK, Jorden R, Kubota H et al. Geochemistry and the Environment. Washington, DC: National Academy of Sciences, 1974.

108. Fraústo da Silva JJR, Williams RJP. The Biological Chemistry of the Elements: The Inorganic Chemistry of Life. New York: Oxford University Press, 2001:454.

109. Stone LR, Erdman JA, Fedder GL et al. J Range Manage 1983;36:280–5.

110. Schroeder HA, Balassa JJ, Tipton IH. J Chronic Dis 1970; 23:481–99.

111. Johnson JL, Jones HP, Rajogopalan KV. J Biol Chem 1977; 252:4995–5003.

112. Pennington JA, Jones JW. J Am Diet Assoc 1987;87:1644–50.

113. Tsongas TA, Meglen RR, Walravens PA et al. Am J Clin Nutr 1980;33:1103–7.

114. Sievers EJ. J Nutr 2003;133:236–7.

115. Turnlund JR, Keyes WR, Anderson HL et al. Am J Clin Nutr 1989;49:870–8.

116. Cardin CJ, Mason J. Biochim Biophys Acta 1975;455:937.

117. Mills CF, Bremner I. Nutritional Aspects of Molybdenum in Animals. Oxford: Pergamon Press, 1980.

118. Ladefoged O, Sturup S. Vet Hum Toxicol 1995;37:63–5.

119. Turnlund JR, Keyes WR, Peiffer GL. Am J Clin Nutr 1995; 61:1102–9.

120. Turnlund JR, Keyes WR, Peiffer GL. Am J Clin Nutr 1995; 61:790–6.

121. Allaway WH, Kubota J, Losee F et al. Arch Environ Health 1968;16:342–8.

122. Turnlund JR, Keyes WR. J Nutr Biochem 2004;25:90–5.

123. Johnson JL, Wadman SK. Molybdenum Cofactor Deficiency and Isolated Sulfite Oxidase Deficiency. 7th ed. New York: McGraw-Hill, 1995.

124. Adbumrad N, Schnieder AJ, Steel D et al. Am J Clin Nutr 1981;34:2271–83.

125. Asmangulyan TA. Gig Sanit 1965:6–11.

126. Bartha R, Ordal EJ. J Bacteriol 1965;89:1015–9.

127. Schnegg A, Kirchgessner M. Z Terphysiol Tierernahr Futtermittelkd 1975;36:63–74.

128. Nielsen FH, Myron DR, Givand SH et al. J Nutr 1975;105: 1620–30.

129. Anke M, Grun M, Dittrich D et al. Low Nickel Rations for Growth and Reproduction in Pigs. Baltimore: University Park Press, 1974.

130. Spears JW, Hatfield E, Forbes RM et al. J Nutr 1978;108: 313–20.

increased risk (16, 18). The critical indicators used to specify the UL were birth defects in women of reproductive age and liver abnormalities for all other age-sex groups. The UL is specified as 3000 μg of retinol/day for both women and men, and 600, 900, 1700, and 2800 μg retinol/day for the age ranges 0 to 3, 4 to 8, 9 to 13, and 14 to 18 years, respectively (18).

METABOLISM

A schematic of whole body vitamin A metabolism is depicted in Figure 17.2. The metabolism of retinoids is directed in part by their binding to specific proteins, as discussed next, and by various enzymes that convert retinol to its storage form, mobilize REs, and oxidize retinol and retinal to RA, as subsequently discussed. Several processes in vitamin A metabolism are regulated by vitamin A metabolites, resulting in a certain level of autoregulation.

Chaperone Proteins That Facilitate Vitamin A Metabolism

Chaperones belonging to the families of retinoid-binding proteins and retinoid receptors are critical for the normal metabolism of vitamin A. Retinoid-binding proteins confer aqueous solubility to lipophilic molecules and serve as guides for the transport and metabolism of specific retinoids, whereas the nuclear receptors mediate the functions of RA.

Plasma Transport Proteins: Retinol-Binding Protein and Transthyretin

Approximately 95% of the vitamin A present in plasma is in the form of all-*trans*-retinol, and nearly all of it is bound to retinol-binding protein (RBP), which is sometimes referred to by its gene designation *RBP4*. RBP is described as holo-RBP when retinol is bound to it and as apo-RBP

in the absence of retinol. RBP is a 21-kDa protein belonging to the lipocalin family that has the overall structure of a "β-barrel." Each protein molecule binds one molecule of retinol within a hydrophobic cavity, with the hydroxyl group of retinol oriented toward the surface of RBP (21). RBP circulates bound to the protein transthyretin (TTR, previously known as prealbumin), which is one of the plasma transport proteins for thyroxine. The association between a molecule of RBP and a tetramer of TTR is noncovalent; this association serves to stabilize holo-RBP, as shown in vitro and in vivo (22–24). Some other retinoids bind to RBP but in a less stable manner. For example, the retinol analog 4-HPR binds to RBP, but the complex interacts relatively weakly with TTR. As a result, RBP is more readily lost in urine, and plasma retinol concentrations are reduced (23, 25). α-Retinol, apparently because of its more planar overall structure than retinol (formally β-retinol), does not bind effectively to RBP (26).

Although the rate of synthesis of RBP is normally high, the plasma concentration is relatively low, approximately 1 to 3 μM, at least as compared with other plasma proteins (27). This is related to the rapid turnover of RBP, with a half-life of approximately 0.5 days for the holoprotein and 4 hours for apo-RBP (24). Because the formation of the holo-RBP-TTR complex (23) increases its molecular weight, to approximately 75 kDa, complex formation slows the rate of loss of RBP in the kidneys.

The gene *RBP4* encoding RBP covers approximately 1000 base pair of cDNA, and its mRNA is one of the most highly expressed in the liver (27), with mRNA expression localized to hepatocytes (28). *RBP4* mRNA is also expressed in adipose tissue and kidney at approximately 3% to 10% of the level present in liver (27), a finding suggesting that these organs may also synthesize

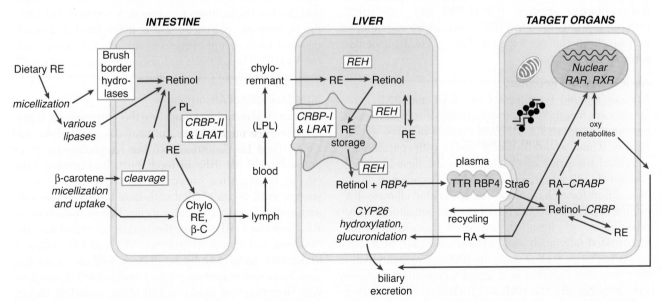

Fig. 17.2. Major reactions in retinoid metabolism. *CRABP*, cellular retinoic acid–binding protein; *CRBP*, cellular retinol-binding protein; *LPL*, lipoprotein lipase; *LRAT*, lecithin: retinol acyltransferase; *PL*, phospholipid; *RA*, retinoic acid; *RAR*, retinoic acid receptor; *RBP*, retinol-binding protein; *RE*, retinyl ester; *REH*, retinyl ester hydrolase; *RXR*, retinoid X receptor; *Stra6*, stimulated by RA gene 6; *TTR*, transthyretin.

RBP protein. Adipose-derived RBP may function as an adipokine and play a role in glucose homeostasis (29), and numerous studies have correlated its levels with various metabolic parameters. Whether it is a causative factor or a correlative biomarker is still unclear, however.

The liver is the main, but not the only, site of synthesis of TTR (22). The molar concentration of TTR in plasma is higher than that of RBP, and thus most TTR circulates as the free tetramer. Numerous TTR polymorphisms are known, and although some of them affect thyroxine or RBP binding, most are associated with familial amyloidotic polyneuropathies (22).

Cellular Retinoid-Binding Proteins

Several cellular retinoid-binding proteins act as intracellular chaperones for retinol, retinal or RA (30, 31). The cellular RBPs (CRBPs) CRBP-I, II, and III belong to the fatty acid binding protein/CRBP family, are of similar size, approximately 14.6 kDa, and have a β-clam structure with a hydrophobic binding site that binds a single molecule of retinol with its hydroxyl group inward (30). CRBP-I, the most abundant form expressed in liver, kidney, testes, and other tissues, binds all-*trans*-retinol, whereas CRBP-II binds both all-*trans*-retinol and retinal and is abundant in enterocytes (32). Neither appreciably binds 9-*cis*-retinoids. CRBP-III and CRBP-IV are present in heart, skeletal muscle, kidney, and some other tissues, but they are less well studied (31).

The cellular RA-binding proteins (CRABP) CRABP-I and CRABP-II, which are structurally similar to the CRBP proteins, bind all-*trans*-RA (33). They are also expressed in tissue-specific patterns, generally at lower concentrations than CRBPs (31). Both are expressed in the developing embryo but usually not in the same cells, a finding suggesting that they perform different functions.

Two other cellular retinoid-binding proteins, cellular retinal-binding protein (CRALBP) and interstitial retinoid-binding protein (IRBP) are expressed almost exclusively in the eye (see the later section on ocular retinoid metabolism).

Nuclear Retinoid Receptors

Nuclear retinoid receptors of the RAR and RXR gene families are members of the superfamily of steroid/thyroid hormone receptors (3, 4). Each consists of three genes: *RAR*-α, β, and γ, and *RXR*-α, β, and γ, with considerable structural similarity, especially within the ligand-binding domain of each subgroup (34, 35). Tissue expression, however, differs for each receptor. The RARs bind all-*trans*-RA exclusively. The RARs can bind 9-*cis*-RA, but, alternatively, other physiologic ligands have been suggested, including unsaturated fatty acids and phytanic acid (36). Synthetic "rexinoids" selectively activate the RXRs (37). Additionally, they may also function in a ligand-independent manner (38). Functionally, the RXR and RAR bind to each other as heterodimers, which, in turn, bind to specific DNA sequences in retinoid-responsive genes, as described

later. The binding of ligand, for example, of all-*trans*-RA to RAR, induces a conformational change in the receptor that facilitates its interaction other proteins, including coactivator or corepressor proteins, enzymes that modify chromatin-bound histones, basal transcription factors, and RNA polymerases (3, 35). The amount of retinoid receptor protein available for ligand binding can be regulated by transcription, posttranscriptional modification, proteolysis, and protein trafficking (35). The RXRs also form heterodimers with other nuclear receptors, including the vitamin D receptor, peroxisome proliferator-activated receptor (PPAR), farnesoid X receptor (FXR), liver X receptor (LXR), and receptors for certain drugs and xenobiotics (34), thus participating in various regulatory networks.

The retinoid-response elements to which RAR-RXR heterodimers bind are typically a direct repeat (DR) of the hexanucleotide sequence (A/G)/(G/T)GTCA, with either five or two intervening nucleotides, referred to as a DR-5 or DR-2, respectively, which are most often located in the 5′-regulatory region of retinoid-responsive genes. Some, however, lie in introns or outside of genes (39). CRABP-II, RAR-β, and CYP26A1 (discussed in the section on metabolism) contain one or more retinoic acid response element (RARE), which provides a means for RA to self-regulate certain aspects of its own metabolism and functions. For many genes, despite evidence of their physiologic regulation by RA, no RARE has been identified, and they could be regulated indirectly (39).

Intestinal and Hepatic Retinoid Metabolism

Metabolism is characterized by extensive interorgan trafficking of retinol, cycles of retinol esterification to form RE and of the hydrolysis of RE to regenerate retinol, and stepwise oxidative metabolism. Approximately 70% of dietary vitamin A is absorbed, even when intake is high, and this has implications for vitamin A overload and toxicity. In contrast, plasma retinol is maintained at a nearly constant level, except in states of vitamin A deficiency and excess (19). Thus, tissues are normally exposed to a well-regulated supply of plasma retinol.

Intestinal Retinol Absorption

Vitamin A absorption comprises the processes of digestion, emulsification, uptake, intracellular metabolism, and export from the intestine into the lymphatic system or portal blood (40). REs in foods must be liberated from chyme by digestive enzymes, and REs, regardless of source, must be emulsified with fatty acids and bile salts and incorporated into lipid micelles before hydrolysis by RE hydrolases (REH) and the uptake of retinol into the duodenal and jejunal enterocytes. REHs include colipase-dependent pancreatic lipase (41), as well as microvillus membrane-associated enzymes. Conditions that interfere with digestion and lipid emulsification, including dietary fat less than approximately 5%, may reduce the efficiency of vitamin A absorption (18).

After uptake of free retinol by enterocytes (42), approximately 95% is esterified as REs (43). Retinol for esterification is carried by CRBP-II to the membrane-bound enzyme lecithin: retinol acyltransferase (LRAT), which transfers the fatty acid in the stereospecific nomenclature (sn)-1 position of membrane-associated phosphatidyl choline (lecithin) to retinol, thus forming RE. The composition of sn-1 fatty acids in lecithin dictates that LRAT will form a mixture of retinyl palmitate in quantities greater than stearate, oleate, and linoleate in most tissues. LRAT is an obligatory enzyme, as shown by studies in mice that lack LRAT and accumulate little RE in their tissues (44). The newly formed REs, along with triglycerides and cholesteryl esters, are packaged into the lipid core of the nascent chylomicron (41). The quantity of RE formed in the enterocyte and the amount of RE per chylomicron particle vary in direct proportion to the amount of vitamin A being absorbed and esterified at the time (45), which can vary from nil after a meal free of vitamin A up to several milligrams per gram of lipid after ingestion of a high–vitamin A meal or vitamin A supplement (45).

The trafficking of chylomicron RE is mainly determined by the metabolism of the chylomicron itself. Chylomicrons enter the lymphatic system and then the venous circulation, and they peak in concentration in plasma approximately 2 to 6 hours after meals. Whereas chylomicron triglycerides are rapidly metabolized in tissues containing lipoprotein lipase (LPL), the chylomicron remnant contains nearly all the original RE, except for a small fraction that may transfer into tissues during the LPL reaction or exchange with plasma lipoproteins. Because of the very rapid hepatic uptake of chylomicron remnants, dietary REs have a short half-life, less than 20 minutes, in the plasma of normal subjects (46). If chylomicron clearance is impaired or the absorption of RE is extremely high, then REs may be found in plasma at more than a few percent of total retinol concentration. Some tissue uptake of RE may take place through lipoprotein receptors (47), or during lipolysis by LPL (48, 49). Approximately 60% to 80% of dietary RE is taken up by the liver during the process of chylomicron remnant clearance, however.

Chylomicrons also contain a minor portion of unesterified retinol (5% to 10% of total vitamin A), which may more readily exchange with tissues and lipoproteins. Additionally, some small fraction of newly absorbed vitamin A is oxidized to polar retinoids in the intestinal mucosal cells. RA is absorbed bound to albumin (27). Portal venous blood RA increases after a dose of β-carotene (50), and most likely after vitamin A.

In isotope kinetic studies, approximately 70% to 90% of a physiologic dose of vitamin A was absorbed (51). The process of retinol absorption is relatively unregulated, and absorption is high even when the dose is very large (18), a situation that may contribute to the development of hypervitaminosis A (see later section). Chylomicrons in humans contain a minor proportion of intact β-carotene (52), but mostly RE. In rodents, nearly all carotene is cleaved and absorbed as RE.

Hepatic Metabolism

The liver plays a central role in whole body retinoid homeostasis. The RE molecules in chylomicron remnants are hydrolyzed soon after uptake by the liver (53, 54). Whereas this process appears insensitive to vitamin A status, what happens after this initial hydrolysis depends greatly on vitamin A status. In a study that traced the metabolism of chylomicron ^{3}H-RE, in vitamin A–adequate rats most of the ^{3}H was initially taken up by hepatocytes, but it was then transferred within 2 hours into hepatic stellate cells (HSCs) (54), which contain the CRBP-I and lecithin retinol acyltransferase (LRAT) necessary to synthesize RE and to store REs within their cytoplasmic lipid droplets (55). These REs make up approximately 50% to 85% of total body vitamin A, more than 90% as RE, in the well-nourished state (56). In contrast, in vitamin A–deficient rats, very little retinol was transferred to HSCs (54); instead, retinol rapidly appeared in the plasma compartment. That liver LRAT expression and activity decline progressively as vitamin A deficiency develops is known (45). Therefore, the reduction in hepatic LRAT is likely part of a regulatory mechanism that spares the little remaining retinol for other uses, such as secretion as holo-RBP or conversion to RA.

The proportion of CRBP as apo-CRBP also increases as vitamin A status declines, and apo-CRBP stimulates the hydrolysis of RE by REH (57). The result is that essentially all vitamin A in the liver can be mobilized and used. Conversely, when vitamin A is administered to deficient animals, holo-RBP is very rapidly secreted, and then hepatic LRAT expression increases (58), resulting in restoration of normal plasma retinol and the appearance of stored REs within a few hours. Although most studies have been conducted in mice and rats, human retinol metabolism is likely to be similar, based on a similar range of vitamin A levels in human liver specimens (59), as well as observations of a similar rapid rise in the plasma of vitamin A–deficient persons after vitamin supplementation.

Hepatic Synthesis and Secretion of Retinol-Binding Protein

Hepatocytes synthesize RBP as a 24-kDa preprotein that is cleaved during translation to form the mature 21-kDa protein (27). The movement of RBP through the secretory pathway depends on its combining with retinol to form holo-RBP (60). In vitamin A deficiency, RBP mRNA stays relatively constant, but RBP protein accumulates within the hepatocytes as apo-RBP, to be released as holo-RBP on vitamin A repletion. In vitamin A–deficient rats, the concentrations of plasma retinol and RBP rose from nearly undetectable to a level higher than normal in approximately 5 hours after vitamin A repletion and then stabilized at a normal level (61). These findings provide the rationale for the relative dose response (RDR) test, described later, which is used clinically.

Retinoids in Plasma

Retinol

In healthy humans in the fasting state, plasma vitamin A is mainly in the form of retinol (>95%). Plasma REs are elevated transiently after vitamin A–containing meals as a result of the REs in chylomicrons and their remnants. If RE constitutes 5% to 10% of the total retinol in fasting plasma, however, then this suggests an abnormal situation, such as impaired chylomicron clearance or an excessive intake of dietary vitamin A (hypervitaminosis A; see later). Considerable variation exists among animal species in retinol transport in plasma: whereas most rodents used in laboratory research resemble humans and transport mostly of their plasma vitamin A as retinol, most of the plasma vitamin A in great apes and several species of carnivores is found as RE bound to lipoproteins (62). In dogs, plasma REs were present in the fasted state, and, surprisingly, even after weeks on a vitamin A–deficient diet (63).

Plasma retinol concentrations in adults normally range from approximately 1 to 3 μmol/L (equivalent to 28 to 86 μg/dL). Day-to-day variation is low. The molar ratio of plasma retinol to RBP is approximately 0.82, indicating that some apo-RBP is normally present in plasma (64). The median plasma retinol concentration measured in the National Health and Nutrition Examination Survey (NHANES) is age related, lower in young children than in adolescents and higher in adult men than in premenopausal women (65). After 50 years of age, values are similar in men and women. In women using oral contraceptives, the retinol concentration is 15% to 35% higher. In newborns, values are lower for premature infants than for full-term infants (66).

Plasma retinol values of less than 0.35, less than 0.70, and less than 1.05 μmol/L are often interpreted as indicating states of severe deficiency, marginal deficiency, and subclinical low vitamin A status, respectively. Based on analysis of serum retinol in NHANES from 1988 to 1994, the prevalence of low serum retinol lower than 0.70 μmol/L in all strata of the US population was very low (67). The prevalence of serum retinol lower than 1.05 μmol/L was 16.7% to 33.9% in children aged 4 to 8 years and 3.6% to 14.2% in children aged 9 to 13 years, depending on sex and racial or ethnic group, but it was higher in non-Hispanic black and Mexican American children than in non-Hispanic white children even after controlling for covariates. As reviewed in the literature (68), the WHO and other organizations use plasma retinol as one criterion for determining whether low vitamin A status is a public health problem in regions or countries.

Because of the relatively short half-life of plasma RBP and TTR, approximately 0.5 day and 2 to 3 days,

respectively (24), their replacement requires a high rate of protein synthesis. Plasma RBP levels are sensitive to changes nutritional and physiologic conditions and are significantly reduced in protein and energy malnutrition (69), infection and inflammation (70, 71), and trauma (72, 73). Conversely, the synthesis of RBP and the concentration of plasma holo-RBP generally respond rapidly during the recovery phase, and thus RBP is considered a useful clinical indicator of visceral protein status and the response to nutritional support (74, 75).

Plasma retinol and RBP levels are usually reduced in diseases of the liver, kidney, and thyroid gland (76), as well as during inflammation. Low levels were reported in patients with primary biliary cirrhosis and primary sclerosing cholangitis (77). Several aspects of retinol storage and transport are perturbed during inflammation, including a loss of RE from HSCs, which develop a myofibroblastic phenotype (78), and reduced synthesis of both RBP and TTR in the liver (70). Patients with inflammation had lower concentrations of plasma RBP, retinol, all-*trans*- and 13-*cis*-RA, which were all negatively correlated with the level of C-reactive protein (CRP), a biomarker of inflammation (79). Fex et al (79) speculated that "the decrease in serum retinol and RA concentration, which occurs in inflammation, may create an 'acute vitamin A deficiency,' which may be a factor contributing to the excess mortality associated with measles in children with marginal vitamin A deficiency and in patients with AIDS."

Genetic deficiencies of RBP are rare, but low RBP was described in a detailed study of two teenage sisters in Germany who presented at clinic with impaired vision (night blindness) (80). These siblings were shown to carry two mutated alleles of the RBP gene that resulted in two different single amino acid substitutions in the RBP protein. Although their plasma retinol and RBP concentrations were 0.19 μmol/L and less than 0.60 μmol/L, respectively, their growth and development appeared normal. Interestingly, their plasma RA levels were also normal. Because their diet was adequate in vitamin A, it was considered most likely that most of their tissues, except their eyes, received adequate vitamin A from chylomicrons and that sufficient RA was produced from this precursor. A similar picture was observed in *RBP4*-null mice, with low plasma retinol and abnormal electroretinograms, which improved after several months on a vitamin A–adequate diet (81). These studies suggest that the eyes are relatively more sensitive to a deficiency of circulating holo-RBP than are other tissues for which enough vitamin A can be obtained through metabolism of dietary vitamin A or uptake of RA from plasma. Mutations in the TTR gene affecting the binding of TTR with holo-RBP also are associated with low plasma RBP levels (82). The finding of Stra6 (stimulated by RA gene 6), a receptor for RBP, as relatively abundant on the surface of retinal pigment epithelium (RPE) cells (see the section on uptake of vitamin

A from plasma into cells) also suggests that the retina depends on holo-RBP as a source of retinol.

Relationship of Plasma Vitamin A with Liver Vitamin A Storage

Data compiled by Olson (19) first showed that plasma retinol is held at a nearly constant level across a wide range of liver vitamin A concentrations, from a low of approximately 20 μg/g liver to a high of approximately 300 to 500 μg/g liver. Plasma retinol begins to fall only when the liver is nearly depleted of vitamin A. The value of less than 20 μg retinol/g liver is often considered a cutoff point for inadequate liver vitamin A reserves. At elevated levels of liver vitamin A, approximately 300 to 500 μg retinol/g, plasma vitamin A rises, but even then little rise in holo-RBP occurs, and nearly the entire increase in plasma *total* retinol results from the presence of REs in lipoproteins (19, 64).

Uptake of Vitamin A from Plasma into Cells

The transmembrane protein Stra6 functions as a receptor for RBP (83), and the uptake of RBP-bound retinol by Stra6 is aided by coupling to the LRAT reaction, which esterifies retinol intracellularly (83, 84). The intracellular retinoid concentration often exceeds the concentration in plasma (14, 85). Stra6 is relatively abundant in the RPE, where LRAT is also high. In the lungs of neonatal rats, vitamin A alone and combined with RA increased Stra6 and LRAT expression, thus resulting in significantly high RE formation (86). The genetic disorder Matthew-Wood syndrome has been attributed to mutations in Stra6 (84), and deletion of the Stra6 gene disrupted vitamin A homeostasis in developing zebrafish (84).

Many types of cells store RE, although the levels are usually much lower than in the liver. Extrahepatic stellate cells are present in lung, intestine, kidney, pancreas, and probably many other tissues, where they are thought to store vitamin A as RE that can be later released and used locally for the formation of RA or released back to plasma as retinol (87). Humans and laboratory rodents are similar in storing most vitamin A in the liver, but among other species considerable differences exist, with some carnivores having much higher RE levels in kidney than liver (88).

In the kidney, apo-RBP is readily filtered, as is any holo-RBP that has dissociated from TTR. The multiligand receptor megalin (gp330), which can bind both TTR and RBP, as well as several other nutrient-related transport proteins, has been shown to aid in the reuptake of RBP and retinol. Megalin is present on the apical surface of renal proximal tubule cells (89). Whereas a portion of the RBP that is taken up is degraded intracellularly, some fraction undergoes transcytosis across the renal tubule cells, with consequent the recycling of retinol back to plasma (89). In mice null for the megalin gene, the uptake of RBP into the renal proximal tubules was defective, and the loss of retinol and RBP in urine was significantly elevated (90).

Tissues containing low-density lipoprotein receptors or scavenger receptors are probably involved in the uptake of RE contained in plasma lipoproteins, as demonstrated in cell culture studies (47).

Retinol Recycling

An important feature of retinol physiology is the recycling of retinol from the plasma to tissues and back again to the plasma compartment. Recycling is believed to help regulate plasma retinol levels at the relatively steady levels that are typical for this nutrient. Based on studies using computer-based compartmental modeling in rats, each molecule of retinol recycles an average of 9 to 11 times among the liver, plasma, kidneys, and other tissues before it is irreversibly degraded (51, 91). One study found that the recycling number remained fairly constant even though the total body vitamin A pool size of individual rats varied some 40-fold (51). A compartmental analysis of data from a healthy young man who had consumed 105 μmol of ^{13}C-labeled retinyl palmitate showed that 50 μmol of retinol passed through plasma each day, whereas only 4 μmol/day was degraded (91). In contrast to retinol, the RBP molecule does not appear to be recycled (24), and this finding suggests that RBP must be resynthesized de novo in various tissues for retinol to be recycled. Consistent with this suggestion, RBP mRNA is found in numerous tissues, although relatively little is known about the rates of RBP synthesis therein. Compartmental analysis has also revealed that retinol turnover changes, apparently as a means to conserve vitamin A, when dietary intake is low and the liver is nearly depleted of retinol. Other conditions that have been shown to affect whole body retinol turnover include retinoid treatment, inflammation, and exposure to hepatotoxic agents (51).

Other Retinoids in Plasma and Tissues

The concentration of plasma RA and related metabolites is typically in the low nanomolar range and RA is bound to serum albumin (14, 31), whereas the more polar metabolites may be loosely protein bound or have sufficient aqueous solubility to be partly in the free state. Metabolites including 13-*cis*-RA and 13-*cis*-4-oxo-RA are present in human plasma, and their concentrations increased two- to fourfold in healthy human subjects who ingested retinyl palmitate at levels in excess of normal intakes (92), as well as after consumption of liver high in vitamin A (93). The more polar products of retinoid oxidation are increasingly more aqueous soluble, and the glucuronide conjugates are considered water soluble.

RA is sufficiently lipophilic to be taken into cells by simple diffusion, but the possibility that membrane channels or transporters are involved has not been eliminated. The concentration of RA in tissues is usually higher than in plasma, perhaps because of sequestration of RA by cytoplasmic CRABPs. Plasma uptake versus production intracellularly contributes different proportions to the RA content of various tissues. In the rat, approximately 80% of RA in the liver was derived by uptake from plasma, whereas most of the RA in testis was produced locally, presumably by the oxidation of retinol (85).

Cellular Retinoic Acid Metabolism

RA concentrations are regulated by both biosynthesis and oxidation. Several different enzymes have been shown to be capable of producing and degrading RA. Many questions remain about their specific functions in different tissues in vivo, however. The oxidation of retinol to retinal has been attributed to several retinol dehydrogenases (RDHs) that are members of the short-chain dehydrogenase/reductase superfamily. These enzymes have relatively broad substrate specificities, including for certain steroids (94, 95). In vitro, some RDHs preferentially oxidize all-*trans*-retinol and others the *cis* isomers of retinol. Additionally, some alcohol dehydrogenases oxidize retinol to retinal (96). The oxidation of retinol to retinal is generally considered rate limiting for RA production, and the concentration of retinal within most tissues is very low, for example, less than 2% as compared with unesterified retinol in a study of mouse liver (13).

The oxidation of retinal to RA is an irreversible process. Multiple enzymes have been implicated in forming RA, including members of the retinal dehydrogenase (RALDH) family and the cytochrome P-450 gene family. *RALDH2* is the gene most firmly established as being critical for RA production, especially during embryogenesis, when deletion of the gene is lethal. In mice null for the *RALDH2* gene, the administration of RA to the dam rescued the phenotype, a finding providing strong evidence for the importance of *RALDH2* and for its role in RA production (97).

The biologic significance of 13-*cis*-RA and 9-*cis*-RA is not clear (98). 13-*cis*-RA is a natural metabolite of vitamin A in human plasma. 13-*cis*-RA possesses bioactivity similar to that of all-*trans*-RA in some assays, and it is useful clinically (see the later section on other uses of retinoids), but it has not been shown to bind significantly to RARs or RXRs, and thus its mechanism of action is unclear. Possibly, 13-*cis*-RA functions as a "prodrug" that undergoes slow isomerization to all-*trans*-RA. The physiologic role of 9-*cis*-RA, which has been widely employed in research studies especially as a ligand for the RXRs, is also controversial. No enzymatic mechanism has been described for conversion of all-*trans*-RA to either *cis* isomer (98). In vitro, however, some conversion occurs nonenzymatically (14). Because CRABP-I and CRABP-II preferentially bind the all-*trans*-RA isomer of RA, this form could preferentially be stabilized and targeted within cells (30). CRABP-I also may facilitate the oxidation of all-*trans*-RA to more polar products (30, 99), whereas for CRABP-II it has been proposed to shuttle RA to the nucleus, interact with RAR-α, and participate in the regulation of target gene transcription (100, 101).

Numerous microsomal cytochrome P-450 enzymes, especially of the CYP26 family, have been described that are capable of the oxidative hydroxylation of RA, at least in biochemical studies. Based on in vivo studies, the CYP26 family of cytochrome P-450 enzymes is of particular interest because of its inducibility by RA in several tissues and cell types (102). CYP26A1 mRNA is most abundant in liver, intestine, and reproductive organs (102). The promoter region of the *CYP26A1* gene contains multiple RAREs, which function in a cooperative manner to induce a high level of expression, especially in RA-treated liver and liver cells in culture (103, 104). The mRNA for CYP26B1 is most highly expressed in cephalic tissue (105, 106), and it is readily induced in the lung by treatment of animals RA (86). The gene for CYP26C1 is expressed in embryonic brain, and this form of CYP26 appears to be the only one capable of oxidizing both *cis* and *trans* isomers of RA (107). After oxidation, the retinoid structure often undergoes glucuronidation (see Figs. 17.1 and 17.2), resulting in water-soluble metabolites (9), which have a short in vivo half-life.

Retinoid Excretion

The renal clearance of RBP is estimated to be equivalent to approximately 7/8 L/day of plasma in a 70-kg human (24). As discussed earlier, the protein megalin is implicated as a type of receptor for RBP in the proximal tubules that facilitates the recovery and reuptake of retinol and RBP (90). Polar retinoids such as the glucuronides described earlier are directly secreted from the liver and excreted in bile.

Kidney diseases that affect filtration rate are typically associated with higher plasma levels of retinol and RBP (76), as well as TTR (108). Apo-RBP, which normally is rapidly filtered from plasma in the glomerulus because of its poor binding to TTR, may provide a signal to the liver to stimulate the output of holo-RBP, to maintain plasma retinol homeostasis (109). Retinol is lost from the kidneys in conditions of diarrhea (110) and severe infections with proteinuria (111).

FUNCTIONS

Ocular Retinoid Metabolism

In 1913, Ishihara suggested that a "fatty substance" in the plasma is necessary both for the synthesis of rhodopsin in the retina and for the maintenance of the cornea, and this investigator proposed that night blindness and keratomalacia develop when this substance is deficient (112). It is now well understood that vitamin A plays two distinct roles: as 11-*cis*-retinal in the processes of photoisomerization and signal transduction in the retina (113); and as RA in the conjunctival membranes and the cornea, where it promotes cell differentiation, normal morphology, and the barrier function of these membranes.

The rod photoreceptor cells, specialized for vision in dim light and sensing motion, contain abundant rhodopsin, each molecule of which contains a molecule of 11-*cis*-retinal bound to a specific lysine reside in Schiff base linkage. As Figure 17.3 depicts, the absorption of a photon of light by rhodopsin's 11-*cis*-retinal triggers its

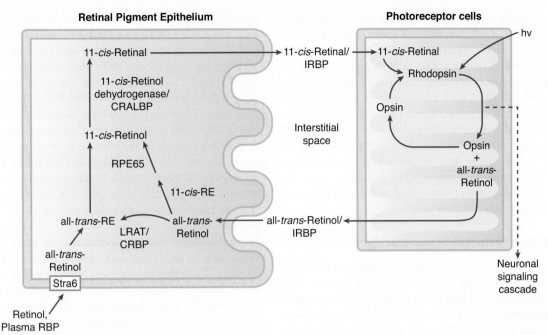

Fig. 17.3. Retinoid metabolism in vision. *CRALBP,* cellular retinal-binding protein; *CRBP,* cellular retinol-binding protein; *IRBP,* interstitial retinoid-binding protein; *LRAT,* lecithin: retinol acyltransferase; *RBP,* retinol-binding protein; *RE,* retinyl ester; *RPE,* retinal pigment epithelium; *Stra6,* stimulated by retinoic acid.

photoisomerization. This process results in a complex signal transduction cascade and in the production of all-*trans*-retinal, which is released from the opsin molecule. The photoisomerization process (photobleaching) occurs in fractions of a second. Signals generated simultaneously by multiple rod cells are integrated by nearby ganglion cells and are communicated by the optic nerve to the brain's visual cortex (114).

For vision to continue after photobleaching, 11-*cis*-retinal must be regenerated. Most of the enzymatic reactions that form 11-*cis*-retinal take place in the RPE, a layer of epithelial cells separated from the photoreceptor cells by the interphotoreceptor space. In brief, all-*trans*-retinal is first reduced enzymatically to all-*trans*-retinol in the photoreceptor cell outer segments, and then it is transported by IRBP through the interphotoreceptor space to the RPE (115). In the RPE, most of the retinol is esterified by LRAT and a palmitoylated, membrane-bound form of the protein RPE65 that form a local pool of RE (114, 116). Plasma retinol also enters this pool after uptake by Stra6. The cycle continues when REs are hydrolyzed and isomerized by the RPE-specific protein RPE65 to regenerate 11-*cis*-retinol (117), followed by oxidation resulting in the regeneration of 11-*cis*-retinal. The latter reaction is facilitated by CRALBP in the RPE cells (118). After 11-*cis*-retinal is transported back to the photoreceptor cells, it can react again with opsin to regenerate rhodopsin (113). When the contents of the RE pool becomes depleted, as in the case of vitamin A deficiency, then the regeneration of 11-*cis*-retinal and the reformation of rhodopsin occur

much more slowly. The clinical consequence is night blindness (poor dark adaptation after exposure to bright light) (1), which is further discussed later.

A similar cycle occurs in the color-sensitive cone cells located mainly in the foveal region. Each cone cell expresses a red-, green-, or blue-specific opsin that is responsive to part of the visible light spectrum (113). The cone visual cycle rapidly regenerates 11-*cis*-retinal for binding to cone opsins. Some of the cone cycle reactions take place within the cone cells, and some occur in the nearby Müller cells, with IRBP likely functioning between them (119).

Most night blindness is the result of a lack of dietary vitamin A and is reversed after adequate vitamin A is provided. At least one other form of night blindness, Sorsby fundus dystrophy, has a genetic origin causing retinal degeneration in an autosomal dominant manner. In patients with early-stage disease, the condition was reported to improve within a week after intake of 50,000 IU (~15,000 μg) of vitamin A (120, 121).

Investigators have described several mutations and deletions of vitamin A–metabolizing proteins that affect visual function (122, 123). Mutations in LRAT, RDHs, and RPE65 are associated with retinal dystrophy and mutations of the RDH5 with fundus albipunctatus. The RDH12 has been associated with cone-rod degeneration (124), and it was reported to be the most frequently mutated gene in young subjects with retinitis pigmentosa in a Spanish genotyping study (125).

In the cornea and conjunctiva, vitamin A is essential for cell differentiation and the structural integrity of these tissues. Although the cornea is avascular, it receives vitamin A in tear fluid, because the lacrimal gland synthesizes and secretes RBP (126). As vitamin A deficiency develops, mucus production by the goblet cells of the conjunctival membranes becomes reduced, and the cornea becomes dry (xerosis) (1). Bitot spots (desquamated cellular debris and bacteria) may develop. These changes are reversible by vitamin A if it is administered in time. If vitamin A deficiency continues, however, the condition is likely to progress to irreparable damage, including keratomalacia, corneal ulceration, and irreversible blindness (see the chapter on clinical manifestations of nutritional deficiencies and toxicities for illustrations).

Prenatal and Postnatal Development

The role of vitamin A compounds in development has been studied since the 1930s. Early work in rat, mouse, and chick embryos showed that the presence of either vitamin A deficiency or vitamin A excess at critical periods of development caused severe malformations, involving especially craniofacial structures, limbs, and visceral organs (127). It is now understood that retinoid signaling begins soon after gastrulation. Moreover, an appropriate level of RA is critical for the normal formation of structures derived from neural crest cells and somites, and later on in the period of organogenesis for the correct development of the heart, lungs, eyes, gonads, urogenital tract, and other organs (127–129). When RA is administered by oral gavage to pregnant mice at embryonic day 9.5, limb development is abnormal, with limb shortening and an abnormal number of digits (fingers or toes). Studies in which RA-soaked beads were implanted in specific regions of chick and mouse embryonic tissues further demonstrated that an excess of RA alters the development of nearby structures.

The embryo is thought to be able to produce its own RA from maternally derived retinol because several genes involved in RA production, signaling, and catabolism are expressed when the embryonic body pattern is forming. These include the RALDH2 (referred to as Aldh1a2 in mice), RARβ, and CYPA1, which are expressed in temporally and spatially regulated patterns, often in adjacent cells or layers, but seldom within the same cells. Based on such observations, investigators believe that the local production of RA results in the diffusion of RA, forming a gradient of RA concentrations, to which nearby cells are exposed. The expression of genes within these cells is sensitive to the concentration of RA, and other regulatory signals, to which the cells are exposed (127). Based on regional patterns of gene expression, it appears that RA production is turned on, evidenced by RALDH2, and then extinguished in specific patterns in different regions of the embryo, as evidenced by expression of CYP26 genes. Investigators have extensively debated whether RA itself is an endogenous morphogen that controls vertebrate development or whether it acts as an inducer of other primary morphogenetic signals (130). Retinoid signaling is part of a complex network that involves proteins of the *Hox*, *Hedgehog*, fibroblast growth factor (*Fgf*), and *Wnt* signaling pathways that also regulate the timing and development of various body structures (131).

CYP26B1 plays a role in the sex specification of the gonads, which are still undifferentiated at the midembryonic stage. Whereas RA, which is known to stimulate meiosis (132), is produced in the mesonephros adjacent to the developing gonads of both sexes, by embryonic day 13.5 in the mouse only the male gonad expresses CYP26B1, apparently in Sertoli cells. Concomitantly, the relative amount of RA in the male gonad is reduced to 25% of that in the female gonad. In other studies, CYP26B1, together with an unknown secreted meiosis inhibitory factor, inhibited meiosis specifically in male germ cells (133). Bowles et al (134, 135) concluded that CYP26B1 in Sertoli cells, acting as a meiosis inhibiting factor in males, holds the key to the appropriate timing of male germ cell maturation by retarding meiosis in the male fetal testis.

In late gestation, at approximately embryonic day 16, RBP can be detected in rat liver (136). Organ-specific gene expression patterns in the perinatal period have also been described for other retinoid-binding proteins, as well as nuclear retinoid receptors, and RE deposition in the liver, lungs, small intestine, and other tissues (86, 137). Early in the postnatal period, the lungs are of special interest because they undergo extensive alveolarization, and vitamin A is implicated in accelerating this maturation process (138). In mouse and rat models, RA promotes alveolarization even in the presence of hyperoxia or dexamethasone, which is known to slow the process (138). Providing vitamin A either alone or combined with RA significantly increases the content of lung RE in the postnatal period while at the same time regulating the expression of retinoid homeostatic genes, including *LRAT, CYP26B1*, and *Stra6* (86). A Cochrane Database Review of clinical studies conducted in very-low-birthweight infants concluded that supplementation of infants who weighed less than 1500 g with vitamin A (5000 IU, or 2.5 mg three times weekly) is associated with reductions in the mortality rate and in the requirement for oxygen at 1 month of age (139).

Tissue Repair

A large body of research has shown that RA is one of the principal regulators of cell differentiation and tissue repair. In 1925, Wolbach and Howe (140) discovered that the epithelial lining of many tissues become flattened (squamous), dry, and keratinized in vitamin A deficiency. Research continuing to the present has shown that RA is a key player in the regulation of many different genes that regulate cell cycle progression or that function as transcription factors, receptors, enzymes, soluble signaling molecules, or structural proteins (4, 39). These findings provide the rationale for investigating retinoids as therapeutic agents in numerous conditions.

As two out of many examples, RA improved lung alveolar repair (141), including in some models of emphysema (142). In vitamin A–deficient rats subjected to partial small bowel resection, the adaptive response was inhibited, whereas the administration of RA improved the intestinal adaptive response, as shown by crypt cell proliferation, reduced apoptosis, extracellular matrix synthesis, and increased enterocyte migration rate (143).

Immunity

Poor resistance to infection was one of the earliest recognized pathologic features of vitamin A deficiency. It is now well established that vitamin A–deficient animals and humans are more susceptible to natural infections or respond poorly to immunologic challenges (144) (see the chapter on nutrition and infectious disease). Vitamin A and its metabolite, RA, are recognized as important regulators of several types of immune cells with roles in T-cell differentiation. Vitamin A and RA are especially influential in regulating the balance of Th1 to Th2 T-helper cells, in which vitamin A favors Th2 development (144). Vitamin A and RA also regulate the balance of FoxP3-positive T-regulatory cells and Th17 cells, in which RA and transforming growth factor-β promote the T-regulatory cell phenotype (145) associated with intestinal homeostasis and prevention of autoimmune disorders (146) while suppressing the development of Th17 cells, which are generally proinflammatory. Vitamin A deficiency results in impaired T-cell and B-cell trafficking in the intestine, associated with impaired expression of adhesion molecules and other lymphocyte homing factors (147, 148). It is currently understood that dendritic cells in intestinal mucosal lymph nodes produce or respond to RA in a way that favors their induction of T-regulatory over Th17 cells (146). RA also regulates B-cell maturation (149), the magnitude of the antibody response (150), and various aspects of innate and mucosal immunity (151, 152).

ASSESSMENT OF VITAMIN A STATUS

Vitamin A status exists as a continuum of states for which deficient, marginal, adequate, excessive, and toxic represent convenient descriptors (45, 153). Some of the plasma and liver changes indicative of these conditions are listed in Table 17.2. Investigators have been especially interested in ways to assess vitamin A deficiency and marginal vitamin A status in noninvasive or minimally invasive ways (68, 154).

Indicators and Tests

Biochemical

A low concentration of vitamin A or RBP in plasma, breast milk, or tear fluid may indicate vitamin A deficiency. Despite the limitations of plasma retinol for assessing the vitamin A status of individuals, it is still useful for characterizing the status of large populations (68). Plasma RBP is a good surrogate for serum retinol in vitamin A deficiency (155), but values of both are likely to be low during when protein or energy is inadequate to maintain RBP synthesis, as well as during inflammation. An analysis of NHANES data showed that low plasma retinol is inversely related to the level of CRP, a positive acute phase protein considered a marker of inflammation. This finding suggests

			VULNERABLE GROUPS/
RANGE	PLASMA RETINOL	CLINICAL SIGNS	MOST COMMON SITUATIONS
Deficient	<0.35 µmol/L[a]	Night blindness; other ocular manifestations common	Preschool-age children and pregnant or lactating women with low vitamin A intakes; inflammation and poor nutritional status
Marginal	0.35–0.70[b] µmol/L	None or minimal (positive plasma response to vitamin A)[c]	Children, pregnant women in vulnerable populations, often with high rates of infection[d]
Adequate	>1.05–3.00 µmol/L	None	Typical of a well-nourished general population
Excessive	Upper normal to >3 µmol/L[e]	Not apparent or mild; may have elevated liver enzymes in plasma indicative of liver damage	Long-term supplement use; frequent intake of foods (e.g., liver) high in preformed vitamin A
Toxic	Similar to above, with circulating retinyl esters in fasting plasma	Headache; bone or joint pain; elevated liver enzymes and clinical signs of liver disease; very high vitamin A in liver and increased levels in extrahepatic tissues	Food faddists and users of high-dose vitamin A supplements; patients treated with retinoids[f]

TABLE 17.2   TYPICAL FINDINGS ASSOCIATED WITH CATEGORIES OF VITAMIN A STATUS

[a]Very rarely, plasma retinol may be low because of hereditary familial low retinol-binding protein (see text); 0.35 µmol/L = 10 µg retinol/dL.
[b]The range 1.05 to 0.70 µmol/L is sometimes used to indicate marginal status, and <0.70 µmol/L is used to indicate vitamin A deficiency. These ranges may be more appropriate for adults, in whom median plasma retinol levels are higher than those in children (see text).
[c]Positive relative dose response (RDR) or modified (MRDR) test.
[d]Low plasma retinol in inflammation may indicate an acute phase response associated with reduced RBP production, rather than deficient vitamin A storage (see text).
[e]Retinol and RBP are normal, whereas total retinol is elevated as a result of retinyl esters, and liver total retinol exceeds approximately 300 µg/g.
[f]Retinoid administration typically reduces, not increases, plasma retinol levels.

that persons with adequate vitamin A status and mild inflammation, as may exist in the generally healthy US population sampled by NHANES, could be misclassified as having low (inadequate) vitamin A based on their lower serum retinol values, when the reduction is the result of inflammation (156).

Liver total retinol is considered the "gold standard," but it is rarely obtainable in human studies. Indirect assays of liver vitamin A reserves have been developed. In the RDR test, a small dose of retinol (1.6 to 3.5 μmol [450 to 1000 μg]) is given orally in oil, and plasma is sampled at baseline and again approximately 5 hours later—the time of the peak plasma retinol response. An increase in plasma retinol of more than 20% compared with the baseline concentration generally is interpreted as an indication that hepatic vitamin A reserves are inadequate for maintaining a normal rate of secretion of holo-RBP. Subsequently, a modified RDR (MRDR) test that is similar in principle but uses a dose of vitamin A_2 (3,4-didehydroretinol) was developed. These tests have proved useful as indicators of low vitamin A reserves in clinical research settings, and they have been adapted for limited use in population-based studies (68).

Tracer methods using stable isotopes of retinol have been used as research tools to quantify total body retinol, as reviewed by Furr et al (157).

Eye Signs

Conjunctival xerosis with Bitot spots in young children (WHO classification X1B) is strongly associated with vitamin A deficiency (1, 68). A prevalence of more than 0.5% XIB classification in young children is one of the criteria used by the WHO to identify significant rates of vitamin A deficiency. Tests of night blindness have been developed to be suitable for field use in young children; night blindness is also significant in pregnant women in regions of low vitamin A intake (158). The histologic evaluation of the conjunctiva by conjunctival impression cytology (CIC) has been used as a field operative test for low vitamin A status (154). Further characteristics are described later in the section "Who Is at Risk?"

Dietary Assessment

Dietary data are of greatest value in assessing the food habits of populations. Vitamin A is concentrated in relatively few foods, which may be consumed infrequently. Comparisons of dietary histories and food frequency questionnaire methods have been reported (159). It is important to take vitamin A–containing supplements into account.

CAUSES AND MANIFESTATIONS OF DEFICIENCY AND OF EXCESS

Vitamin A Deficiency

By WHO criteria, vitamin A deficiency is considered a public health problem based on the regional prevalence of traditional eye signs of severe deficiency (e.g., corneal xerosis, Bitot spots), as well as population-based cutoff levels for subclinical indicators (e.g., low serum retinol <0.7 μmol/L in 15% or more of a defined population or low breast milk retinol) (68). The prevalence of vitamin A deficiency in young children increases after weaning, most likely a reflection of a combination of maternal vitamin A deficiency, resulting in a limited transfer of maternal vitamin A to the fetus and low breast milk vitamin A, and inadequate vitamin A in the postweaning diet of the child (160). Vitamin A deficiency has also been described as worsening low iron status, resulting in a condition known as vitamin A deficiency anemia (161).

According to WHO estimates, providing adequate vitamin A to children in parts of the world where vitamin A deficiency is still prevalent will reduce young child mortality by 23% to 34% (1, 160, 162). The effect on infant mortality is now unclear because some studies reported reductions in mortality by vitamin A supplementation during the first 2 days of life (163), whereas others reported sex-dependent differences in mortality, with a reduction in boys but an increase in girls given vitamin A as neonates (164). Currently, vitamin A supplementation is promoted by WHO/UNICEF to reduce child mortality in regions where vitamin A deficiency is still a public health problem (5). Typical doses in capsule form contain 15 to 60 mg (50,000 to 200,000 IU) of retinol, depending on age, which are administered at 3- to 6-month intervals (165). Providing vitamin A in high-dose form does not seem essential because a study that supplied vitamin A weekly at an RDA-level dose reported a 50% reduction in mortality (166, 167). In pregnant Nepali women, a weekly low dose of vitamin A or β-carotene reduced pregnancy-related mortality (158). Because of the potential teratogenicity of a high intake of vitamin A in early gestation, supplementation with vitamin A in women of reproductive age is limited to the first 6 weeks postpartum (see further in the later section on clinical signs of toxicity and hypervitaminosis A).

Who Is at Risk?

Diseases that involve poor absorption of lipids including impaired pancreatic or biliary secretion, Crohn disease, celiac disease, radiation enteritis, ileal resection or damage, and various infections increase the risk of deficiency of vitamin A, as well as other nutrients.

The symptoms and signs of vitamin A deficiency have been studied in greater detail than have those of any other nutritional deficiency disorder. The eye is primarily involved, and xerophthalmia predominantly affects young children. Impaired dark adaptation or night blindness is an early symptom and can be elicited by a careful history and some simple tests in a poorly illuminated room. Photopic and color vision, mediated by the retinal cones, is usually unaffected.

Dryness (xerosis) and unwettability of the bulbar conjunctiva follow. CIC, as described in the section on assessment of vitamin A status, is abnormal at this stage. Bitot spots, an accumulation of desquamated cells most commonly seen in the interpalpebral fissure on the temporal aspect of the conjunctiva, is another sign (see the chapter on manifestations of nutrient deficiencies and toxicities). In older children and adults, Bitot spots may be stigmata of past deficiency, or they may be entirely unrelated to vitamin A deficiency when local trauma is responsible. Corneal involvement, starting as a superficial punctate keratopathy and proceeding to xerosis and varying degrees of "ulceration" and liquefaction (keratomalacia), frequently results in blindness. Punctate degenerative changes in the retina (xerophthalmic fundus) are rare signs of chronic deficiency usually seen in older children. Corneal scars may have many causes, but those that are bilateral in the lower and outer part of the cornea of a person with a history of past malnutrition or measles often signal earlier vitamin A deficiency.

Extraocular manifestations include perifollicular hyperkeratosis, an accumulation of hyperkeratinized skin epithelium around hair follicles most commonly seen on the lateral aspects of the upper arms and the thighs. This finding is also seen in starvation and has been attributed to a deficiency of B-complex vitamins or essential fatty acids. Other changes associated with vitamin A deficiency may include impaired taste, anorexia, vestibular disturbance, bone changes with pressure on cranial nerves, increased intracranial pressure, infertility, and congenital malformations (168).

Hypervitaminosis A and Adverse Effects

Hypervitaminosis A can be induced acutely by a very high intake of vitamin A, but it is most often the result of long-term intake of lower, but still excessive, amounts of vitamin A, particularly excessive use of vitamin A–containing supplements, food faddism such as an excessive consumption of liver, or self-medication with vitamin A preparations (16). The severity of adverse effects depends on the dosage and includes severe headache, nausea, skin irritation, pain in bones and joints, coma, and death. The side effects of prescription retinoids (retinoid toxicity) are similar. Side effects vary with both dosage and the structure of the retinoid analog (169).

Clinical Signs of Toxicity (Hypervitaminosis A)

Most of the features of hypervitaminosis A are related to a rise in intracranial pressure: nausea, vomiting, headache, vertigo, irritability, stupor, fontanel bulging (in infants), papilledema, and pseudotumor cerebri (mimicking brain tumor) (170). Pyrexia and peeling of the skin also occur.

Chronic poisoning produces a bizarre clinical picture that is often misdiagnosed because of failure to consider excessive vitamin A intake (170). It is characterized by anorexia, weight loss, headache, blurred vision, diplopia, dry and scaling pruritic skin, alopecia, coarsening of the hair, hepatomegaly, splenomegaly, anemia, subperiosteal new bone growth, cortical thickening (especially bones of

hands and feet and long bones of the legs), and gingival discoloration. The x-ray appearance may assist in making a correct diagnosis. Cranial sutures are widened in the young child.

Birth Defects (Teratogenesis)

Vitamin A and other retinoids are powerful teratogens in both pregnant experimental animals and women (170, 171). These agents cause fetal malformations (exencephaly, craniofacial malformations, eye defects, and cardiac abnormalities) that are quite similar across animal species and in humans (127, 172). The Teratology Society reviewed the literature in 1987 and concluded that at least seven case reports of adverse pregnancy outcome associated with a daily intake of vitamin A of 25,000 IU or more had been published (173). In a study of the relationship between dietary vitamin A intake and birth defects in more than 22,000 pregnant US women (174), the investigators concluded that the risk of birth defects was significantly higher in women who consumed more than 10,000 IU/day (3000 μg/day) of retinol during the periconceptual period. This study was in part the basis for setting the UL at 3000 μg retinol/day (18). Concerns have been raised about the frequent consumption of foods very high in vitamin A such as liver (>100,000 IU [~33,000 μg retinol] per 100 g) by pregnant or potentially pregnant women (93).

Acidic retinoids approved by the US Food and Drug Administration (FDA) that are marketed in the United States mainly for the therapy of skin disorders (see later) are now used under very strict FDA regulations that have been put in place to prevent exposure to retinoids during pregnancy and resulting birth defects (175). The risk of teratogenesis may, however, persist for many months after discontinuation of the drug (172). Adverse effects of depression and other psychiatric effects have also been claimed (176).

Liver Abnormalities

The IOM committee reviewed case reports of liver abnormalities associated with elevated long-term intakes of vitamin A (18). Human data are potentially confounded by other factors related to liver damage such as the following: alcohol intake; hepatitis A, B, and C; hepatotoxic medication; or preexisting liver disease. Consistency and specificity were found for the following liver disorders associated with prolonged high intakes of vitamin A: evidence of excessive vitamin A in perisinusoidal stellate cells, perisinusoidal fibrosis, hyperplasia, and hypertrophy of HSCs. The level of intake reported for these cases ranged from 1500 to more than 14,000 μg/day over periods of ranging from 1 to 30 years.

Bone Mineral Loss

Animal, human, and laboratory research generally supports an association between a high intake of vitamin A and a loss of bone mineral density, a risk factor for osteoporosis. A study of lifelong vitamin A supplementation in the rat did not find evidence for adverse effects on bone, however (177). Significant evidence indicates that long-term intake of larger dose supplements of retinol (intakes of retinol >300 μg/day) is associated with an increased risk of bone fractures in older Swedish men and women, as well as in women in the United States (178).

RETINOIDS AS THERAPEUTIC AGENTS

Dermatology

All-*trans*-RA, 13-*cis*-RA (isotretinoin [Accutane]) and etretinate (Tegison, Tigason) are used therapeutically for conditions including severe cystic acne and psoriasis, both as systemic drugs and as topical treatments (179). Topically applied retinoids are used for reversal of photodamaged skin (180). The effects of retinoids on the skin are likely to involve several mechanisms, including reduced cell proliferation, improved epidermal differentiation, modulation of dermal growth factors and their receptors, inhibition of sebaceous gland activity (180), and suppression of androgen formation (181). These actions may account for the comedolytic and anticomedogenic activity of systemic and topically applied retinoids (182). Topical retinoids result in greatly reduced systemic exposure. A pharmacokinetic model assessed the internal exposure to all-*trans*-RA applied topically to skin as four to six orders of magnitude lower than that from a minimally teratogenic oral dose (183).

Cancer Prevention and Treatment

In many epidemiologic studies, lower intakes of vitamin A have been associated with a higher risk of certain cancers, especially those of epithelial origin (184, 185). In experimental animals, vitamin A deficiency increased tumor incidence and susceptibility to chemical carcinogens. Investigators have hypothesized that aberrant changes in tissue retinoid metabolism and retinoid signaling through nuclear receptors may contribute to tumor growth and cancer progression (186). Evidence does not, however, support any benefit of consuming dietary vitamin A at intakes greater than the RDA (185).

All-*trans*-RA has been shown to be a highly successful drug for the treatment of acute promyelocytic leukemia (APL). This form of leukemia is characterized by a specific chromosomal translocation t(15,17) that interrupts a copy of the *RARα* gene, which is located at 17q21, and thus results in aberrant retinoid signaling. Researchers in Shanghai first reported in 1986 that a high dose of all-*trans*-RA induced a complete remission in a substantial proportion of patients with APL. This study and larger follow-up trials in the United States and Europe led to the widespread adoption of all-*trans*-RA in the treatment of APL (187, 188).

Unexpectedly, the use of RA in patients with APL also revealed a new high-risk syndrome, which occurs in some patients. Referred to as RA syndrome (188), this disorder includes fever, respiratory distress, hypotension, and renal failure and is fatal in a significant percentage of patients. To minimize this complication, all-*trans*-RA is now given for a shorter time, followed by conventional chemotherapy to eliminate the leukemogenic cells. Patients treated with all-*trans*-RA gradually become refractory to its differentiating activity, and those who have a relapse of APL after chemotherapy are often resistant to further treatment with all-*trans*-RA. The reason appears to be increased retinoid catabolism, at least in part.

ACKNOWLEDGMENTS

Support for my research was provided by the National Institutes of Health grants DK-41479, CA-90214, and HD-66982, and the Dorothy Foehr Huck endowment to the Pennsylvania State University. I thank Douglas Heimburger and Maurice E. Shils for material on clinical manifestations of vitamin A deficiency and toxicity.

REFERENCES

1. Sommer A. J Nutr 2008;138:1835–9.
2. Wald G. Science 1968;162:230–9.
3. Germain P, Chambon, Eichele G et al. Pharmacol Rev 2006; 58:712–25.
4. Balmer JE, Blomhoff R. J Lipid Res 2002;43:1773–808.
5. World Health Organization. Prevention and Control of Vitamin A Deficiency, Xerophthalmia and Nutritional Blindness: Proposal for a Ten-Year Programme of Support to Countries. Document NUT/84.5 Rev 1. Geneva: World Health Organization, 1985.
6. United Nations Children's Fund. Reduce child mortality. In: Millennium Development Goals. 2011. Available at: http://www.unicef.org/mdg/childmortality.html. Accessed November 29, 2011.
7. Tanumihardjo SA, Howe JA. J Nutr 2005;135:2622–6.
8. Tamura K, Kagechika H, Hashimoto Y et al. Cell Diff Dev 1990;32:17–26.
9. Formelli F, Barua AB, Olson JA. FASEB J 1996;10:1014–24.
10. Pilkington T, Grogden RN. Drugs 1992;43:597–627.
11. Gundersen TE, Blomhoff R. J Chromatogr A 2001;935:13–43.
12. Furr HC. J Nutr 2004;134(Suppl):281S–5S.
13. Kane M, Folias AE, Napoli JL. Anal Biochem 2008;378:71–9.
14. Kane MA, Folias AE, Wang C et al. Anal Chem 2008;80: 1702–8.
15. Ross AC. Methods Enzymol 1990;189:81–4.
16. Office of Dietary Supplements, National Institutes of Health. Vitamin A. Available at: http://ods.od.nih.gov/factsheets/list-all/VitaminA. Accessed November 30, 2011.
17. Food and Agriculture Organization/World Health Organization. Requirements of Vitamin A, Thiamine, Riboflavin, and Niacin. Report of a Joint Food and Agriculture Organization/World Health Organization Expert Committee. FAO nutrition meetings report series no. 41. WHO technical report series no. 362. Geneva: World Health Organization, 1967.
18. Food and Nutrition Board, Institute of Medicine. Dietary Reference Intakes for Vitamin A, Vitamin K, Arsenic, Boron, Chromium, Copper, Iodine, Iron, Manganese, Molybdenum, Nickel, Silicon, Vanadium, and Zinc. Washington, DC: National Academy Press, 2001.
19. Olson JA. J Natl Cancer Inst 1984;73:1439–44.
20. Food and Agriculture Organization/World Health Organization. Vitamin A. In: Human Vitamin and Mineral Requirements. Report of a joint FAO/WHO expert consultation. Geneva: World Health Organization, 2001.

Terminology and Glossary of Terms

The terminology used in the vitamin D field is confusing to many experts and nonexperts alike. A glossary of relevant terms is provided here to help the reader:

Vitamin D: Nutritional term coined in the 1920s to mean a substance that possesses the full antirachitic activity of the parent molecule vitamin D_3. The term is now often employed as a short form for the class of compounds with the biologic activity of $1\alpha,25$-dihydroxyvitamin D, abbreviated as $1\alpha,25$-$(OH)_2D$ and also known as calcitriol. It is also occasionally used to mean a summation of both vitamin D_2 and vitamin D_3 forms (14), especially in the reporting of clinical assay results where serum 25-hydroxyvitamin D (25-OH-D) is used to mean the sum of 25-hydroxyvitamin D_2 (25-OH-D_2) and 25-hydroxyvitamin D_3 (25-OH-D_3) forms.

Vitamin D_3: This natural derivative of 7-dehydrocholesterol is made in the skin (see Fig. 18.1 for structure).

Vitamin D_2: Artificial or plant-derived form of vitamin D often used in food fortification, in daily dietary supplements, and in high-potency pharmaceutical preparations. It is metabolized to an active form, $1\alpha,25$-$(OH)_2D_2$, in a manner similar to the natural vitamin D_3. Vitamins D_2 and D_3 are considered biologically equivalent in terms of their ability to cure rickets.

Renal 1α-hydroxylase: Proximal tubular form of the enzyme responsible for the final 1α-hydroxylation step of vitamin D activation, comprising three proteins, the key one being the cytochrome P-450 (CYP) protein CYP27B1. Renal 1α-hydroxylase is regulated by calcium (Ca^{2+}) and phosphate (PO_4^{3-}) ions through the hormones parathyroid hormone (PTH) and fibroblast growth factor 23 (FGF-23).

Extrarenal 1α-hydroxylase: 1α-Hydroxylase, as evidenced by CYP27B1 protein, expressed in nonrenal tissues, especially where it locally produces $1\alpha,25$-$(OH)_2D_3$ that is believed to act in an autocrine or paracrine manner. It is regulated by cytokines and not by PTH and FGF-23.

Vitamin D receptor (VDR): Target cell protein that binds $1\alpha,25$-$(OH)_2D_3$, as well as specific sequences (vitamin D–responsive elements [VDREs]) in the genome to regulate gene expression of vitamin D–dependent genes at the transcriptional level. VDR does not bind any other metabolite with strong affinity, thus making it unlikely that vitamin D and 25-OH-D have any direct effect on gene expression under normal circumstances.

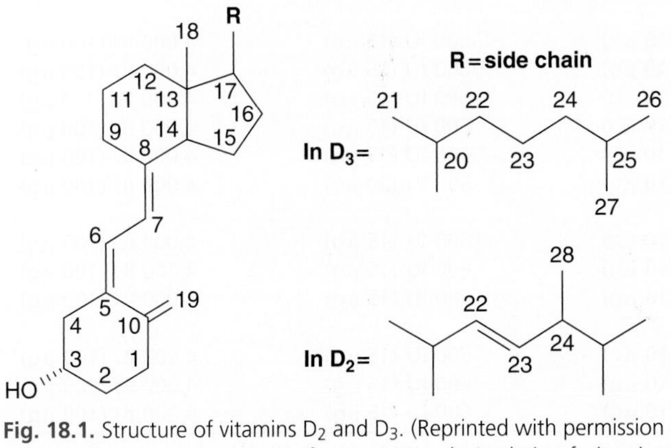

DIETARY SOURCES OF VITAMIN D

As already pointed out, vitamin D can be derived from either endogenous synthesis in the skin or from the diet. In the strictest use of the term, vitamin D is therefore not a vitamin, at least during the summer months. Consequently, it should be referred to as a prohormone. Dietary sources become critical during the winter months (above 43 degrees north between October and April) when the zenith angle of the sun is such that UVB light does not penetrate the atmosphere and synthesis of vitamin D_3 in the skin is insignificant. Unfortunately, dietary sources of vitamin D are few, and most foodstuffs are devoid of vitamin D. The only significant sources of vitamin D (D_2 or D_3) are animal liver, fatty fish (e.g., salmon, halibut, cod), egg yolks, and fish oils. Unfortified cow's milk is not a rich source. Because human milk is an extremely poor source of vitamin D, breast-fed infants require a vitamin D supplement. Most grains, lean meat, vegetables, and fruits are virtually devoid of measurable amounts of vitamin D. Although vitamin D_2 can be derived from the plant sterol ergosterol, the likelihood that this provitamin D_2 will be UV irradiated naturally seems low, even though some cultures sun-dry vegetables. The artificial irradiation of shitake mushrooms, a rich source of ergosterol, has increased the possibility of finding vitamin D_2 in the diet.

Food fortification with either synthetic vitamin D_2 or, later, vitamin D_3 was pioneered and patented in the United States in the 1930s by Steenbock. His concept was to fortify staples such as breakfast cereals, milk, and margarine with vitamin D, initially in the form of irradiated ergosterol, to ensure delivery of this scarce nutrient and also to overcome the seasonal variability in potency found in natural sources (e.g., fish oils). This public health initiative to fortify certain foods with vitamin D eradicated rickets in the United States and virtually everywhere else in the world where it was introduced. In Quebec, Canada, which was the last province or state in North America to introduce vitamin D fortification, statistics showed a dramatic decline in the annual incidence of rickets cases at a downtown Montreal hospital (Ste Justine pour les Enfants) from 130 per 1000 to

Fig. 18.1. Structure of vitamins D_2 and D_3. (Reprinted with permission from Makin HLJ, Jones G, Kaufmann M et al. Analysis of vitamins D, their metabolites and analogues. In: Makin HLJ, Gower DB, eds. Steroid Analysis. New York: Springer, 2010:967–1096.)

virtually 0 per 1000 over an 8-year span between 1968 and 1976; this period coincided with provincial legislation making it mandatory for dairies to fortify milk (15). A few countries resisted vitamin D fortification programs, not because they believed that they would be unsuccessful in the eradication of rickets but because of financial questions about whether government or industry would pay for the programs or out of concern about vitamin D intoxication in the neonatal period—fears that were proved largely unfounded.

RECOMMENDED DIETARY ALLOWANCES OF VITAMIN D

The dietary reference intakes (DRIs) were reviewed in a report published by a panel of the Institute of Medicine (IOM) at the National Academy of Sciences in Washington, DC (16). The chosen parameters for reporting optimal vitamin D intakes are currently adequate intake (AI) for the newborn to 1-year life stage and recommended dietary allowance (RDA) for all other life stages. Excessive intake is defined as tolerable upper intake level (UL) for all age groups; and the DRI values for the various life stage groups are provided in Table 18.1.

CURRENT UNDERSTANDING ABOUT VITAMIN D ACTIVATION AND INACTIVATION

Vitamin D_3 is synthesized from the sterol 7-dehydrocholesterol by a process involving UVB light in the wavelengths 290 to 315 nm (17) (Fig. 18.2). UV irradiation opens the 9,10-bond of the provitamin to give a previtamin D_3 intermediate in the upper layers of the skin before it is isomerized nonenzymatically by heat to give vitamin D_3 in the lower layers. Transport of vitamin D_3 is carried by a specific plasma protein, vitamin D–binding protein (DBP), from skin to storage tissues or to the liver for the first step of activation. The D vitamins can also be derived from the diet, both as vitamin D_3 and vitamin D_2. Transport to storage depots or liver in the dietary case is on chylomicrons, although some evidence indicates that transfer from chylomicrons to DBP may also occur during transit. Vitamin D from skin or dietary sources does not circulate for long in the bloodstream, but instead is immediately taken up within hours by adipose tissue or liver for storage or activation (18).

Ultimately, vitamin D_3 undergoes its first step of activation (Fig. 18.3), namely, 25-hydroxylation in the liver. Over the years, some controversy has existed over whether 25-hydroxylation of vitamin D_3 is carried out by one enzyme

TABLE 18.1	VITAMIN D DIETARY REFERENCE INTAKES BY LIFE STAGE (AMOUNT/DAY)			
LIFE STAGE GROUP	AI	EAR	RDA	UL
Infants				
0–6 mo	400 IU (10 μg)	—	—	1,000 (25 μg)
7–12 mo	400 IU (10 μg)	—	—	1,500 (38 μg)
Children				
1–3 y	—	400 IU (10 μg)	600 IU (15 μg)	2,500 IU (63 μg)
4–8 y	—	400 IU (10 μg)	600 IU (15 μg)	3,000 IU (75 μg)
Males				
9–13 y	—	400 IU (10 μg)	600 IU (15 μg)	4,000 IU (100 μg)
14–18 y	—	400 IU (10 μg)	600 IU (15 μg)	4,000 IU (100 μg)
19–30 y	—	400 IU (10 μg)	600 IU (15 μg)	4,000 IU (100 μg)
31–50 y	—	400 IU (10 μg)	600 IU (15 μg)	4,000 IU (100 μg)
51–70 y	—	400 IU (10 μg)	600 IU (15 μg)	4,000 IU (100 μg)
>71 y	—	400 IU (10 μg)	800 IU (20 μg)	4,000 IU (100 μg)
Females				
9–13 y	—	400 IU (10 μg)	600 IU (15 μg)	4,000 IU (100 μg)
14–18 y	—	400 IU (10 μg)	600 IU (15 μg)	4,000 IU (100 μg)
19–30 y	—	400 IU (10 μg)	600 IU (15 μg)	4,000 IU (100 μg)
31–50 y	—	400 IU (10 μg)	600 IU (15 μg)	4,000 IU (100 μg)
51–70 y	—	400 IU (10 μg)	600 IU (15 μg)	4,000 IU (100 μg)
>71 y	—	400 IU (10 μg)	800 IU (20 μg)	4,000 IU (100 μg)
Pregnancy				
14–18 y	—	400 IU (10 μg)	600 IU (15 μg)	4,000 IU (100 μg)
19–31 y	—	400 IU (10 μg)	600 IU (15 μg)	4,000 IU (100 μg)
31–50 y	—	400 IU (10 μg)	600 IU (15 μg)	4,000 IU (100 μg)
Lactation				
14–18 y	—	400 IU (10 μg)	600 IU (15 μg)	4,000 IU (100 μg)
19–31 y	—	400 IU (10 μg)	600 IU (15 μg)	4,000 IU (100 μg)
31–50 y	—	400 IU (10 μg)	600 IU (15 μg)	4,000 IU (100 μg)

AI, adequate intake; EAR, estimated average requirement; IU, international unit; RDA, recommended dietary allowance; UL, tolerable upper intake level.

Reproduced with permission from Food and Nutrition Board, Institute of Medicine. Dietary Reference Intakes for Calcium and Vitamin D. Washington, DC: National Academy Press, 2011.

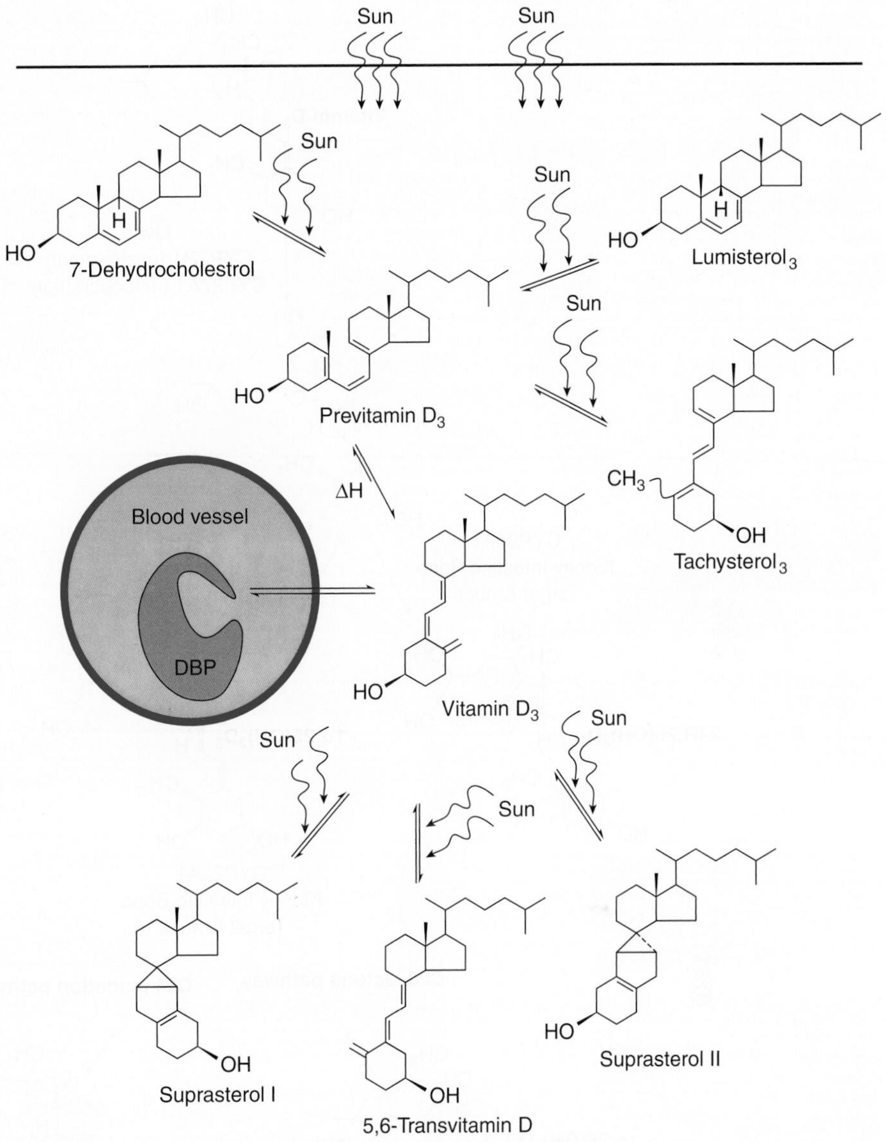

Fig. 18.2. Photochemical events that lead to the production and regulation of vitamin D_3 in the skin. *DBP,* vitamin D–binding protein; *Sun,* ultraviolet B rays as a component of sunshine. (Reprinted with permission from Holick MF. Photobiology of vitamin D. In: Feldman D, Pike JW, Glorieux FH, eds. Vitamin D, 2nd ed. New York: Elsevier, 2005:37–46).

or two and whether this cytochrome P-450–based enzyme is found in mitochondrial or microsomal fractions of liver (18). Biochemical research has established that one human mitochondrial enzyme (CYP27A1) and several microsomal cytochrome P-450 enzymes (including CYP2R1, CYP3A4 and CYP2J3) are able to carry out the 25-hydroxylation of vitamin D_2 or vitamin D_3, or both (see Fig. 18.3) (reviewed in 19). The physiologic relevance of one of these enzymes, CYP2R1, is particularly pertinent because of a single report of a human mutation at Leu99Pro within the CYP2R1 gene in an individual with rickets (20); the enzyme is a 1α-OH-D_2-25-hydroxylase with a high affinity for its vitamin D_2 substrate (21). Investigations have provided a crystal structure of CYP2R1 with several of the known vitamin D substrates bound in the active site (22). Furthermore, a genome-wide association study of the genetic determinants of serum 25-hydroxyvitamin D concentrations (23) concluded that the chromosomal locus for CYP2R1 (11p15) showed the second strongest association of only a

handful of sites in the whole genome; the others were DBP (or Gc), CYP24A1, and 7-dehydrocholesterol reductase (DHR7). Notably, variants of the other 25-hydroxylases, such as CYP27A1 or CYP3A4, were not identified as associated with serum 25-OH-D concentrations. This finding suggests that CYP2R1 is the most physiologically-relevant 25-hydroxylase.

The product of the 25-hydroxylation step, 25-OH-D_3, is the major circulating form of vitamin D_3 and in humans is present in plasma at concentrations in the range 10 to 80 ng/mL (25 to 200 nmol/L) (24). The main reason for the extended plasma half-life of 25-OH-D_3 is its strong affinity for DBP, and the DBP-XO mouse shows accelerated rates of clearance and low 25-OH-D_3 levels (25). Serum levels of 25-OH-D_3 therefore represent a measure of the vitamin D status of the animal in vivo.

The circulating metabolite, 25-OH-D_3, is converted to the active form of vitamin D known as calcitriol or $1\alpha,25$-(OH)$_2$D$_3$. The second step of activation, 1α-hydroxylation,

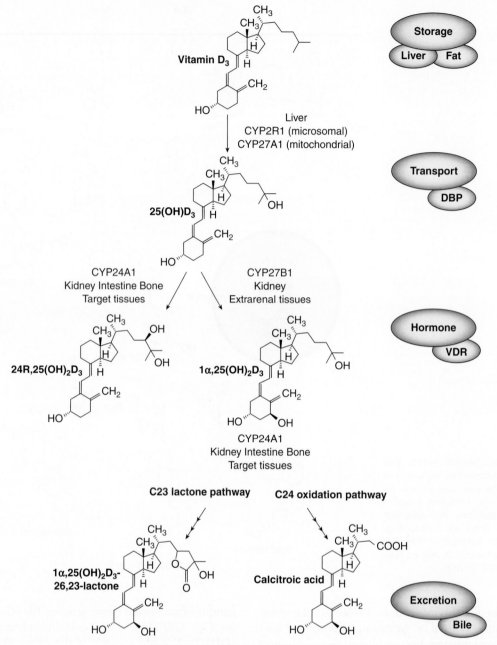

Fig. 18.3. Metabolism of vitamin D_3. Current knowledge of the key metabolites in vitamin D metabolism in conjunction with the enzymes (all cytochrome P-450s) involved in their production. The hormonal form, $1\alpha,25\text{-}(OH)_2D_3$, is the sole "active" form through a transcriptional mechanism involving target cell machinery, in particular the vitamin D receptor (VDR). The regulation of the enzyme system involves induction of CYP27B1 by parathyroid hormone and fibroblast growth factor 23 during a shortage of $1\alpha,25\text{-}(OH)_2D_3$ and induction of the CYP24A1 by the hormone itself during excess. Calcitroic acid is the biliary excretory product of $1\alpha,25\text{-}(OH)_2D_3$ generated by CYP24A1. A similar pathway exists for vitamin D_2. *DBP,* vitamin D–binding protein.

occurs primarily in the kidney (18). The synthesis of *circulating* $1\alpha,25\text{-}(OH)_2D_3$ in the normal, nonpregnant mammal appears to be the exclusive domain of the kidney. A specific mechanism appears to involve the cell surface receptors megalin and cubilin to provide uptake of the substrate, in the form of the 25-OH-D/DBP complex, by renal proximal cells (see Fig. 18.3) (26). Megalin knockout mice show reduced vitamin D metabolite levels and vitamin D deficiency. Additional evidence for renal synthesis of circu-

lating calcitriol stems from clinical medicine. Patients with chronic kidney disease exhibit reduced $1\alpha,25\text{-}(OH)_2D_3$ levels and frank rickets or osteomalacia resulting from a deficiency of $1\alpha,25\text{-}(OH)_2D_3$ that is caused by lack of renal-1α-hydroxylase, a situation that can be reversed by $1\alpha,25\text{-}(OH)_2D_3$ hormone replacement therapy (27). The cytochrome P-450 enzyme, CYP27B1, representing the 1α-hydroxylase enzyme, was cloned virtually simultaneously from several species including rat, human, and mouse

(28–31). Investigators had known for some time that the kidney mitochondrial 1α-hydroxylase enzyme comprises three proteins—a cytochrome P-450, a ferredoxin, and a ferredoxin reductase for activity—and is strongly down-regulated by 1α,25-$(OH)_2D_3$ and up-regulated by PTH as part of the calcium homeostatic loop (32). Investigators showed that a similar phosphate homeostatic loop also exists involving FGF-23, seemingly the long-postulated "phosphatonin" hormone that down-regulates CYP27B1 enzyme activity presumably at the transcriptional level (33). The promoter for the CYP27B1 gene appears to contain the necessary regulatory elements (cyclic AMP response elements [CREs] and negative VDREs) necessary to explain the observed physiologic regulations of PTH and 1α,25-$(OH)_2D_3$, respectively, at the transcriptional level. Whether additional elements exist to explain the action of FGF-23 through the klotho receptor remains to be addressed (33). Human CYP27B1 gene mutations result in vitamin D dependency rickets type 1 (VDDR-I) (34), a disease state first proposed, in 1973, to result from a genetic defect of the 1α-hydroxylase enzyme (35). Two independent groups generated the analogous mouse CYP27B1 knockout model by deletion of the cyp27B1 gene, and the 1α,25-$(OH)_2D_3$–deficient model revealed further insights into the regulation of the gene by different stimuli and subtleties in the roles of 1α,25-$(OH)_2D_3$ (36, 37).

The final piece of the vitamin D metabolic machinery has been elucidation of the catabolism of 25-OH-D_3 and 1,25-$(OH)_2D_3$ in the body. This involves another cytochrome P-450 enzyme named CYP24A1, originally known as the 25-OH-D-24-hydroxylase. CYP24A1 inactivates both 25-OH-D_3 and 1α,25-$(OH)_2D_3$ by subjecting these metabolites to 24-hydroxylation and thus giving rise initially to 24R,25-$(OH)_2D_3$ and 1α,24,25-$(OH)_3D_3$, respectively (38, 39) (see Fig. 18.3).

Currently, some speculation exists that 24-hydroxylated metabolites may play a unique biologic role in bone fracture repair, but most of the evidence favors the concept that 24-hydroxylation is primarily an inactivating step. The enzyme 24-hydroxylates both 25-OH-D_3 and 1α,25-$(OH)_2D_3$, the latter with a 10-fold higher efficiency (40, 41). In the complete absence of DBP, however, this substrate discrimination is less evident. Because the circulating level of 25-OH-D_3 is approximately 1000 times higher than that of 1α,25-$(OH)_2D_3$, the clearance of products of 25-OH-D_3 by CYP24A1 (e.g., 24R,25-$(OH)_2D_3$) is readily evident in the bloodstream. The enzyme, particularly the renal form, appears to be expressed at high constitutive levels in the normal animal and may be involved in the inactivation and clearance of excess 25-OH-D_3 from the circulation.

Conversely, the extrarenal 24-hydroxylase appears to be primarily involved in target cell destruction of 1α,25-$(OH)_2D_3$ (42). Indeed, CYP24A1 has now been shown to be expressed fairly ubiquitously, in particular wherever the VDR is expressed. CYP24A1 enzyme activity has been demonstrated in various cell lines representing specific vitamin D target organs (intestine, CaCo2 cells; osteosarcoma, UMR-106 cells; kidney, LLC-PK1 cells; keratinocyte, HPK1A and HPK1A-ras). Researchers have shown that 24-hydroxylation is the first step in the C-24 oxidation pathway, a five-step, vitamin D–inducible, ketoconazole-sensitive pathway that changes the hydroxylated vitamins D molecules to water-soluble truncated products such as the biliary form, calcitroic acid (43, 44).

Although with human, rat, and mouse CYP24A1, the formation of calcitroic acid is the main pathway, other CYP24A1 isoforms, in particular the guinea pig and opossum analogs, predominantly carry out a 23-hydroxylation pathway to a 26,23-lactone product (45). The biologic value for the synthesis of the 26,23-lactone remains unknown, but the switch to the 23-hydroxylation pathway can be effected by a single Ala326Gly mutation in human CYP24A1 (45). In most biologic assays, the intermediates and truncated products of these 23- and 24-hydroxylation pathways possess lower or negligible biologic activity. Furthermore, many of these compounds have little or no affinity for DBP, thus making their survival in plasma tenuous at best. Polymerase chain reaction (PCR) studies of CYP24A1 led to the detection of CYP24A1 mRNA in a wide range of tissues, thereby corroborating the earlier studies reporting widespread 24-hydroxylase enzyme activity in most, if not all, calcitriol target cells.

Additional studies showed that mRNA transcripts for CYP24A1 are virtually undetectable in naive target cells, not exposed to 1α,25-$(OH)_2D_3$, but are dramatically induced by a VDR-mediated mechanism within hours of exposure to 1α,25-$(OH)_2D_3$ (46). In fact, the promoters of both human and rat CYP24A1 genes possess a double VDRE that has been shown to mediate the calcitriol-dependent induction of CYP24 enzyme in both species. It is therefore attractive to propose that not only is 24-hydroxylation an important step in the inactivation of excess 25-OH-D_3 in the circulation but also it is involved in the inactivation of 1α,25-$(OH)_2D_3$ inside target cells. As such, one can hypothesize that C-24 oxidation is a target cell attenuation or desensitization process that constitutes a molecular switch to turn off calcitriol responses inside target cells (47).

Loss-of-function mutations of human CYP24A1 result in the condition known as idiopathic infantile hypercalcemia (IIH) (48) characterized by hypercalcemia, hypercalciuria, nephrolithiasis and nephrocalcinosis which supports a counterregulatory role for CYP24A1 in vitamin D metabolism. The CYP24A1-knockout mouse exhibits a similar hypercalcemic phenotype and in 50% of animals is severe enough to cause death at around weaning. Conversely, surviving animals have unexplained changes in bone morphology involving excess unmineralized osteoid that could suggest an alternative role for 24-hydroxylase in bone mineralization, although double knockouts lacking both CYP24A1 and VDR do not exhibit this bone phenotype (49). Surviving CYP24A1 null animals have been shown to possess a much reduced ability to clear a bolus dose of

$[1\beta\text{-}^3H]1\alpha,25\text{-}(OH)_2D_3$ from their circulation as compared with normal, wild-type littermates (50). Thus, not much evidence exists for efficient non–CYP24A1-mediated backup excretory systems for calcitriol catabolism.

Calcitroic acid, the final water-soluble biliary product of $1\alpha,25\text{-}(OH)_2D_3$ catabolism, is probably not synthesized in liver because C-24 oxidation does not occur in hepatoma cells and presumably must therefore be transferred from target cells to liver by some plasma carrier. Although calcitroic acid has been found in various tissues in vivo (51), details of its transfer to bile have not been elucidated. Some emerging evidence indicates that high concentrations of vitamin D compounds can be metabolized by the general purpose liver cytochrome P-450 enzyme, CYP3A4, which is induced in intestine by calcitriol (52–54).

ROLE OF CALCITRIOL IN THE REGULATION OF VITAMIN D–DEPENDENT GENE EXPRESSION

Current dogma holds that vitamin D, through its hormonal form $1\alpha,25\text{-}(OH)_2D_3$ (calcitriol), is a central regulator of calcium and phosphate homeostasis and also promotes cellular differentiation and limits cell division of selected cell types (18). Calcitriol achieves these functions through a VDR-mediated mechanism in which the hormone directly regulates gene expression at the transcriptional level of many different vitamin D–dependent genes in vitamin D target cells (55), coding for proteins that, in turn, regulate cellular events such as intestinal calcium transport and cell division (18) (Fig. 18.4). As in the classical steroid hormone model, $1\alpha,25\text{-}(OH)_2D_3$ enters the cell by traversing the plasma membrane in a free form and binds strongly to the VDR inside the nucleus (dissociation constant $[K_d] = 2 \times 10^{-10}$ M). The liganded or occupied VDR specifically targets only vitamin D–dependent genes by interacting with a specific sequence found upstream of the vitamin D–dependent gene. The sequence, known as a VDRE, is a tandem repeating oligonucleotide of six base pairs containing a 3-nucleotide spacer that is situated normally upstream of the 5' end of the vitamin D–responsive gene. A consensus VDRE (AGGTCAnnnAGGTCA) is found in the rat and human osteocalcin genes, the rat calbindin-9K

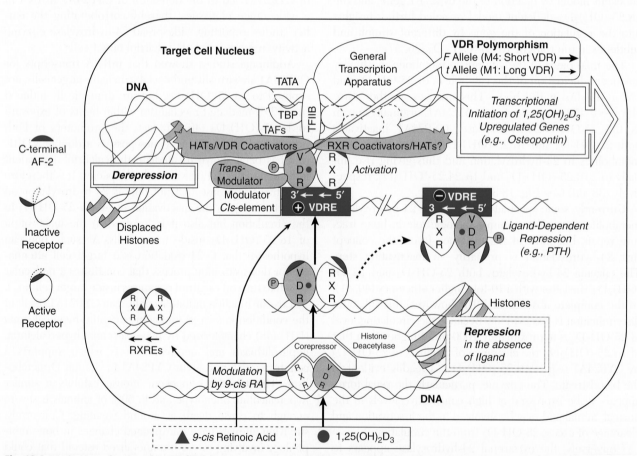

Fig. 18.4. Mechanism of action of $1\alpha,25\text{-}(OH)_2D_3$ in gene expression at the transcriptional level. The simple target cell takes up $1\alpha,25\text{-}(OH)_2D_3$ as the free ligand originally ferried to the target cell bound to vitamin D–binding protein. The illustration shows the key elements of the transcriptional machinery including the vitamin D receptor (VDR), retinoid X receptor (RXR), and various coactivators in regulation of this machinery. *HAT,* histone acetyl transferase; *PTH,* parathyroid hormone; *RA,* retinoic acid; *RXRE,* retinoid X receptor response element; *TAF, TBP,* and *TFIIB,* transcription factors; *VDRE,* vitamin D–responsive element. (Reprinted with permission from Haussler MR, Whitfield GK, Haussler CA et al. The nuclear vitamin D receptor: biological and molecular regulatory properties revealed. J Bone Miner Res 1998;13:325–49.)

gene, and the mouse osteopontin gene, whereas more complex elements are found in the collagen type I gene and the pre-pro-PTH gene, where these elements play a negative or suppressive role. Further research showed that VDR requires a heterodimeric partner called the *retinoid X receptor* (RXR) and a plethora of other transactivators, termed a *DRIP complex,* to transactivate genes (56).

The current model suggests that occupation of the ligand-binding domain of the VDR component triggers a protein conformational change in the AF-2 domain of the C-terminus of the VDR (56) that allows recruitment of positive transcription factors and shedding of transcriptional inhibitory factors that lead to increased formation of a transcription initiation complex and an increased rate of gene transcription. The complexity of this mechanism and the number of specific and general transcription factors involved are impressive.

CALCEMIC AND NONCALCEMIC FUNCTIONS FOR VITAMIN D

From autoradiographic studies using radiolabeled calcitriol (57), VDR protein distribution studies (58), gene chip arrays (59), and data from various gene knockout mice (36, 37, 50, 60), investigators now recognize that vitamin D, in the form of calcitriol, acts on many different cells around the body. The spectrum of vitamin D–dependent genes is not limited to a handful of specific calcium and phosphate transport–related genes but is broad and is probably in the hundreds (61). The vitamin D–dependent genes point to several physiologic functions of $1\alpha,25\text{-}(OH)_2D_3$ (18), which are usually divided into calcemic and noncalcemic roles. *Calcemic roles* include the regulation of blood calcium and phosphate concentrations by actions at intestine, bone, parathyroid, and kidney. *Noncalcemic roles* include cell differentiation and antiproliferative actions in various cell types, such as bone marrow (osteoclast precursors and lymphocytes), immune system, skin, breast and prostate epithelial cells, muscle, and intestine.

Although most of the calcemic actions of calcitriol have been known since the early twentieth century, when dietary vitamin D deficiency was first demonstrated, the noncalcemic roles have emerged only from more subtle studies involving experiments probing the mechanism of action of calcitriol at the molecular level and from studies of the VDR knockout mouse (62).

The calcemic roles of calcitriol are mediated through regulation of a series a calcium-related genes such as the calcium channel proteins (TRPV5 and 6), the cellular calcium-binding proteins (calbindins 9K and 28K), and the calcium pumps (e.g., calcium-dependent adenosine triphosphatases: $PMCA_{1b}$ and the sodium/Ca^{2+} exchanger, NCX1), which together would explain the movement of Ca^{2+} across membranes of intestinal and kidney cells (62). Although various VDR knockout mouse models showed a 60% decrease in intestinal calcium

absorption and a reduced expression of all these proteins (62), in the process demonstrating their vitamin D dependence, somewhat paradoxically TRPV6 knockout mice (63, 64) and calbindin-9K knockout mice (65, 66) provided mainly negative or inconclusive data that these proteins are involved in calcium absorption. Obvious explanations for these observations are that TRPV6 and calbindin-9k knockout mice have unknown compensatory vitamin D–dependent calcium transport mechanisms and that the calcium pumps are the key vitamin D–dependent components (62). Given the known effects of calcitriol on phosphate transport in intestine, a similar set of genes including the type 2b sodium–phosphate cotransporter must also exist for phosphate (33, 67).

The noncalcemic actions of calcitriol, especially on cell division and differentiation, are the result of effects on the cell cycle at the G_0 to G_1 transition. $1\alpha,25\text{-}(OH)_2D_3$ has been shown to have the following actions: it up-regulates p21 and p27 cyclin-dependent kinase inhibitors, a process that results in the dephosphorylation of the retinoblastoma protein, which inhibits the transcription of the mammalian transcription factors E2F required for cell cycle progression (68, 69); it up-regulates the transcription factor homeobox gene HOXA10 (70); and it regulates the dephosphorylation of p70S6 kinase, implicated in the cell cycle arrest in the G_1 to S phase transition in breast and colon cancer cells, respectively (71). Alteration to growth factor signaling is another route by which $1\alpha,25\text{-}(OH)_2D_3$ and analogs have been observed to inhibit cell growth (72). Several mechanisms whereby $1\alpha,25\text{-}(OH)_2D_3$ can induce apoptosis in cancer cells have been identified and include the following: (a) modulation of the relative amounts of antiapoptotic Bcl-2 and proapoptotic Bax (73, 74); (b) activation of proapoptotic μ-calpain by increasing cellular calcium concentration (75); and (c) interaction with other signaling pathways that may lead to apoptosis, including through insulinlike growth factor and tumor necrosis factor (76, 77). Results obtained from the VDR knockout mouse suggest that $1\alpha,25\text{-}(OH)_2D_3$ could play a role in the differentiation of specialized cell types. For example, keratinocytes from VDR knockout animals exhibited uncontrolled hyperplasia as well as a reduction in the expression of the keratinocyte differentiation markers including involucrin and loricrin, and these animals were more prone to carcinogen-induced tumorigenesis when compared with the wild-type animals (78–80). Markers of terminal keratinocyte differentiation were also reduced in the CYP27B1 knockout animals, a finding implying a role for $1\alpha,25\text{-}(OH)_2D_3$ in keratinocyte differentiation.

These discoveries in the basic science of vitamin D formed a basis to search for new functions or applications for vitamin D and, in some cases, are further supported by fairly convincing epidemiologic data (81). The actions of calcitriol in the immune system, skin, muscle, pancreas, kidney, and brain led to claims that vitamin D deficiency is associated with the pathogenesis of psoriasis, certain

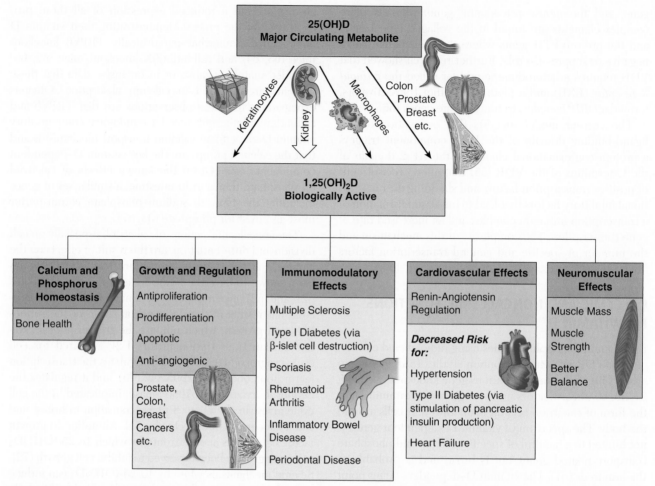

Fig. 18.5. Calcemic and noncalcemic actions of calcitriol. The figure provides the range of biologic effects of calcitriol around the body through renally produced hormone by the local synthesis by the extrarenal 1α-hydroxylase (CYP27B1). Disease states associated with vitamin D deficiency are also indicated. (Reprinted with permission from Holick MF. High prevalence of vitamin D inadequacy and implications for health. Mayo Clin Proc 2006;81:353–73.)

types of cancer, and autoimmune diseases such as multiple sclerosis and diabetes. These actions also point to roles for calcitriol in the synthesis of antimicrobial peptides, blood pressure regulation, and muscle cell differentiation. Consequently, these noncalcemic applications of vitamin D can now be potentially added to the calcemic roles in calcium- and phosphate-related diseases such as rickets and osteomalacia, hyperparathyroidism, and osteoporosis (18, 81) (Fig. 18.5).

EMERGENCE OF EXTRARENAL CYP27B1 AND THE IMPORTANCE OF SERUM 25-HYDROXYVITAMIN D LEVELS

Epidemiologic data (82, 83) placed increased emphasis on monitoring serum levels of 25-OH-D, the circulating precursor to 1α,25-(OH)$_2$D, because serum 25-OH-D values correlate well, and better than do serum 1α,25-(OH)$_2$D values, with certain clinical parameters (e.g., bone mineral density). Why may serum 25-OH-D levels be a better

health indicator than serum 1α,25-(OH)$_2$D levels? This is best addressed in a newly emerging concept of an extrarenal 1α-hydroxylase that is expressed in many sites outside the kidney and that augments the kidney-produced serum "endocrine" 1α,25-(OH)$_2$D with locally produced "autocrine" or "paracrine" 1α,25-(OH)$_2$D to promote additional roles for vitamin D outside the classical functions in calcium and phosphate homeostasis. This hypothesis had its roots in ideas developed in prostate disease (84), but it has been broadened to explain the wide distribution of the 1α-hydroxylase and VDR in skin, immune system, and intestine (85–87). In fact, the original concept of the extrarenal 1α-hydroxylase enzyme activity is already 2 decades old. Investigators suggested that an *extrarenal* 1α-hydroxylase may manifest in several physiologic or pharmacologic situations. A placental 1α-hydroxylase was reported in the late 1970s and proved to be difficult to purify. Since cloning of the renal enzyme, however, its presence in placental tissue has been confirmed by real-time PCR of CYP27B1 mRNA and by specific antibody studies of the immunodetectable protein of CYP27B1 (88, 89).

Before the use of calcitriol and its analogs in clinical medicine, occasional reports surfaced of anephric individuals who had been given large doses of vitamin D or 25-OH-D$_3$ and who had measurable blood levels of a metabolite. This metabolite displaced $1\alpha,25$-(OH)$_2$D$_3$ in receptor binding assays (90, 91), a finding suggesting the existence of a significant extrarenal source of the 1α-hydroxylase. The concept was given additional momentum with work demonstrating the existence of loosely regulated 25-OH-D$_3$–1α-hydroxylase activity in sarcoid tissue that can cause elevated plasma $1\alpha,25$-(OH)$_2$D$_3$ levels and, in turn, hypercalciuria and hypercalcemia in patients with sarcoidosis (92). The induction of extrarenal 1α-hydroxylase in macrophages by cytokines (e.g., interferon-γ) and growth factors as part of the inflammatory response was confirmed using molecular probes (93, 94), and even its role in antimicrobial peptide cathelicidin synthesis has been elucidated.

CYP27B1 mRNA and protein have been detected in many other extrarenal locations (95). This knowledge has given rise to the concept that extrarenal CYP27B1 augments circulating $1\alpha,25$-(OH)$_2$D$_3$ with local production of $1\alpha,25$-(OH)$_2$D$_3$ (96, 97). The locally high concentrations of $1\alpha,25$-(OH)$_2$D$_3$ in certain sites such as skin, prostate, and breast are believed to give tissue-specific patterns of gene expression that, in turn, limit cell growth and lead to tissue-specific differentiation of specific cell types. Occasionally, as in sarcoidosis, locally high extrarenally synthesized calcitriol leaves the tissue and leaks out into the main circulation (92).

An important physiologic role for extrarenal 1α-hydroxylase is also associated with the importance of circulating 25-OH-D levels that provide the substrate for this extrarenal enzyme, as well as for the renal enzyme. Support has grown for the idea that the serum 25-OH-D concentration is an excellent predictor or biomarker of the noncalcemic actions of the D vitamins in the health of the immune system, skin, bone, certain epithelial cells, and muscle (81) and is superior even to the serum $1\alpha,25$-(OH)$_2$D concentration.

ASSESSMENT OF NUTRIENT STATUS: SERUM 25-HYDROXYVITAMIN D AS A POTENTIAL BIOMARKER FOR HEALTH

Because serum 25-OH-D serves as a substrate not only for the kidney but also wherever 1α-hydroxylase is found, the new theory has suggested wider use of the serum 25-OH-D parameter for monitoring vitamin D nutritional status. This theory has also led to a reevaluation of the optimal circulating 25-OH-D level. The IOM report defined the different nutritional categories (16) as follows: (a) vitamin D deficiency remains defined as a 25-OH-D level lower than 20 ng/mL; (b) vitamin D sufficiency is

defined as a 25-OH-D level between 20 and 50 ng/mL; and (c) vitamin D toxicity is defined as a 25-OH-D level higher than 50 ng/mL.

Other investigators defined another category between deficiency and sufficiency that is known as *insufficiency* (24). These investigators used a higher threshold of more than 30 ng/mL between inadequacy and adequacy. Some clinical chemists also use a much higher toxicity threshold of more than 80 ng/mL. Observed serum 25-OH-D values in US residents from 2003 to 2006 National Health and Nutrition Examination Survey (NHANES) data ranged from 5 to 50 ng/mL, however.

Central to controversies over the optimal ranges for serum 25-OH-D is that different health agencies (98) embrace different values for the important threshold between deficiency and sufficiency. Some vitamin D experts, like the IOM, set this value lower, at approximately 20 ng/mL, based on the blood level that results in normalization of bone health in 97.5% of the population (RDA), and these experts suggested that higher values constitute normalcy (99). Other experts endorsed the concept of an insufficiency range and suggested that the normal range starts somewhere between 20 and 60 ng/mL. Within this group, some experts emphasized the 25-OH-D threshold as the inflection point (at ~32 ng/mL) in a serum PTH/25-OH-D plot above which PTH values are normalized. Yet another group of bone experts used data emerging from NHANES studies of bone density or muscle strength parameters in broad populations of physiologically normal US women (100, 101) or in large epidemiologic correlations of serum 25-OH-D with breast, colon, and prostate cancer incidence to suggest that the sufficiency threshold may be set at 40 ng/mL or even higher.

The IOM report (16) evaluated two Agency for Healthcare Research and Quality (AHRQ) reports and more than 1000 studies in reaching the conclusion that vitamin D status could be based only on bone health, because data from nonskeletal health outcomes were inconclusive, contradictory, or negative. Time will tell whether investigators will need to reevaluate this perspective and set a higher normal range and thus new thresholds for vitamin D supplementation. Meanwhile, the 2011 IOM recommendations should be used as an appropriate guide for all North Americans because these guidelines are based on a thorough analysis of the best data currently available.

Serum 25-OH-D methodology uses both antibody-based and liquid chromatography tandem mass spectrometry–based approaches and provides reasonably reliable values for the physiologically relevant parameter, which is total 25-OH-D (sum of 25-OH-D$_2$ and 25-OH-D$_3$). Current controversies surrounding vitamin D methodology were reviewed (102), and most vitamin D analysts voluntarily subscribed to a global vitamin D external quality assessment scheme (DEQAS) that oversees assay and analyst performance four times each year.

If serum 25-OH-D is found to be lower than 20 ng/mL, clear justification exists for supplementation with appropriate doses of vitamin D for periods of approximately 6 weeks. Because of the time delay between vitamin D ingestion and a rise in the serum 25-OH-D levels and because 25-OH-D has a half-life of 15 to 20 days in the blood, no reason exists to measure serum 25-OH-D until 4 months after treatment begins. Most clinicians recommend monitoring serum 25-OH-D annually.

In evaluation of serum 25-OH-D levels, many otherwise normal individuals living at northern latitudes (>42 degrees), where skin synthesis is compromised for 6 months of the year, show 25-OH-D levels in the range of 10 to 40 ng/mL and are thus classified by some experts as insufficient, as least for part of the year (24).

BIOEQUIVALENCE OF VITAMIN D_2 VERSUS VITAMIN D_3

Qualitatively, vitamins D_2 and D_3 exhibit identical sets of biologic responses around the body, primarily through the VDR-mediated regulation of gene expression described earlier for calcitriol (18, 56). Physiologic responses to vitamin D_2 and D_3 hormones include regulation of calcium and phosphate homeostasis and regulation of cell proliferation and cell differentiation of specific cell types (18). Quantitatively, considerable biochemical evidence indicates that most of the individual steps involved in the metabolism and actions of vitamin D_2 and D_3 are identical (18). With the discovery of the critical importance of metabolism in vitamin D action, a series of vitamin D_3 metabolites was isolated and identified in the late 1960s and early 1970s; these metabolites included 25-OH-D_3, 1α,25-$(OH)_2D_3$, and 24R,25-$(OH)_2D_3$ (18). This discovery was followed by the identification of their vitamin D_2 counterparts: 25-OH-D_2, 1α,25-$(OH)_2D_2$, and 24R,25-$(OH)_2D_2$ (18). Noteworthy here was that the structural features unique to the vitamin D_2 side chain did not preclude either the 25-hydroxylation or 1α-hydroxylation steps in activation of the molecule or the first step of inactivation, namely, 24-hydroxylation.

Studies relating to the biochemistry of vitamin D since the late 1970s also documented that none of the steps in the specific vitamin D signal transduction cascade appeared to discriminate discernibly between the two vitamin D homologs at the molecular level. These steps include the following: transport of vitamin D by DBP; 25-hydroxylation by CYP2R1; 1α-hydroxylation by CYP27B1; binding of 25-OH-D to the transport protein DBP; binding of 1,25-$(OH)_2D$ to the VDR; 24-hydroxylation of 25-OH-D or 1,25-$(OH)_2D$ by CYP24A1; and metabolic clearance of 1,25-$(OH)_2D_3$, all of which are similar for both vitamins D_2 and D_3 (18). The implication is that specific signal transduction systems designed to respond to vitamin D_3 also respond to physiologic doses of vitamin D_2 equally well.

Although reports suggested that certain species (e.g., avian species and New World monkeys) (103, 104) discriminate against vitamin D_2, in humans, investigators have long assumed that the two vitamins are essentially equipotent. In 1940, Park (105) reviewed biopotency comparisons of viosterol (vitamin D_2) and cod liver oil (vitamin D_3) from more than 40 rickets treatment studies, and although he suggested that many of the studies were of "poor quality" he concluded, "For practical purposes the vitamin D in viosterol may be regarded as being equal to the vitamin D of cod liver oil. If viosterol is inferior to cod liver oil, rat unit for rat unit, the differences cannot be great" (105). Thus, the historical viewpoint in the medical literature that vitamin D_2 and vitamin D_3 are equipotent in treating rickets seems to have been reinforced by subsequent comparisons in rodents (106, 107) and by frequent reports assuming that the two vitamins have similar effects in humans (108).

Since 2000, the dogma that vitamins D_2 and D_3 are bioequivalent has been challenged (109), and this has led to numerous efforts to reexamine the biopotency of the two forms in humans. Most, if not all, of these studies have been based on a surrogate, nonfunctional marker for biologic activity, namely, comparison of the plasma 25-OH-D levels achieved after equivalent dosing of vitamin D_2 and vitamin D_3.

Multiple studies have provided evidence to suggest that vitamin D_2 is severalfold less effective in raising or maintaining 25-OH-D levels compared with vitamin D_3 (110–113), whereas other studies have not been able to demonstrate a discrimination against vitamin D_2 and have argued that similar rises in 25-OH-D levels can be achieved with both forms (114–116). Part of the apparent conflict between these different studies is almost certainly the result of the significant variation in study designs, with differences in the size, frequency, and duration of dosing (that ranges from daily 1000 IU/day doses for several months or years to 50,000 IU in a single dose), formulation, mode of administration, and baseline serum 25-OH-D (i.e., degree of deficiency). Whereas the study of Armas et al (111) used single doses of 50,000 IU and found markedly accelerated clearance of 25-OH-D_2 as compared with 25-OH-D_3, the study of Holick et al (115) used daily doses of 1000 IU for 11 weeks and found the same rises in 25-OH-D and similar absolute 25-OH-D levels at the end of the dosing period. Nevertheless, the complexity of the factors affecting the rise in serum vitamin D_3 and serum 25-OH-D_3 following various orally administered doses of vitamin D_3 cannot be overstated and were highlighted in the pharmacokinetic work of Heaney et al (117).

This continuing debate about the relative biopotency of vitamin D_2 and vitamin D_3 can also be put into the context of frequent claims that vitamin D_2 compounds are less toxic than their vitamin D_3 counterparts in numerous mammalian species from rodents to primates (101–102, 113). The implication of these diverse studies is that vitamin D_2 compounds may show differences in pharmacokinetics, particularly using pharmacologic doses (e.g., 50,000 IU/dose) (111), that are reflected in terms of the lower toxicity of vitamin D_2 but not necessarily a lower potency to cure rickets using physiologic doses (e.g., 1000 IU/day) (115).

The challenge of the observed findings in dietary studies is to explain the in vivo discrimination against vitamin D_2 at higher doses (110–113), discrimination consistent with the reports of lower toxicity (106–107, 118), whereas at lower doses relative equipotency exists between the two vitamin forms. Among the possible explanations for this concentration-dependent phenomenon are the reports that vitamin D_2 and vitamin D_3 could be differentially susceptible to nonspecific inactivating modifications such as those occurring to various drugs in the liver. These enzymes could include any of the liver CYPs that are known to metabolize vitamin D compounds differently, such as CYP27A1, which 25-hydroxylates vitamin D_3 and 24-hydroxylates vitamin D_2 (18); and CYP3A4, which 24- and 25-hydroxylates vitamin D_2 substrates more efficiently than vitamin D_3 substrates (119, 120) and 23R- and 24S-hydroxylates $1\alpha,25\text{-}(OH)_2D_3$ (52). CYP3A4 has been shown to be selectively induced by $1\alpha,25\text{-}(OH)_2D$ in the intestine (52, 53).

Both CYP27A1 and CYP3A4 are known to have significantly lower Michaelis-Menten constant (K_m) values for vitamin D compounds (18) in the micromolar range, a property that questions their physiologic but not their pharmacologic relevance. Investigators (121) have shown that both human intestinal microsomes and recombinant CYP3A4 break down $1\alpha,25\text{-}(OH)_2D_2$ at a significantly faster rate than $1\alpha,25\text{-}(OH)_2D_3$. This finding suggests that this nonspecific cytochrome P-450 enzyme may limit vitamin D_2 action preferentially in target cells where it is expressed (53, 121), especially in the pharmacologic dose range. Thus, one explanation for the discrimination against vitamin D_2 could be the selective catabolism of vitamin D_2 by nonspecific cytochrome P-450 enzymes (e.g., CYP3A4) in liver and intestine. The same type of mechanism involving differential induction of nonspecific CYPs may also underlie the long-standing reports that coadministered drug classes, such as anticonvulsants (122, 123), cause accelerated degradation of vitamin D_2.

POPULATIONS AT RISK FOR VITAMIN D DEFICIENCY

Because human breast milk is such a poor source of vitamin D, breast-fed infants constitute an important group to target for vitamin D supplementation. At particular risk are breast-fed, dark-skinned children of African or Asian descent, especially those living in northern climates, such as Canada. Over the past few decades, sporadic reports have noted persistent vitamin D deficiency rickets almost always in breast-fed, dark-skinned Canadians of African or Asian descent, but the total number of cases,

even in a major metropolitan center such as Toronto, is small (17 over a 5-year period from 1988 to 1993) (124). Nevertheless, both Canadian and US pediatric societies have emphasized vitamin D supplementation programs and have recommended that daily intakes of vitamin D be doubled to 400 IU or 10 μg in this life stage.

Other life stages or groups at risk of vitamin D deficiency include individuals living at high latitude (Inuit), especially those who have forsaken their traditional high vitamin D–rich seafood diets and individuals with dark skin including those of African, Indian, Pakistani, or Sri Lankan descent who are living at northerly latitudes (125). These individuals have limited exposure to UV light or require longer exposure to UV light to make adequate amounts of vitamin D. Reports suggest that these groups have lower serum 25-OH-D than their lighter-skinned neighbors, a characteristic that may make them more susceptible to vitamin D deficiency during at least part of the year.

Another group at risk of vitamin D deficiency identified consists of individuals with high body mass index (BMI). With the increase in obesity to epidemic proportions in the United States and Western countries, much interest has been shown in the association of increasing BMI and vitamin D deficiency (126, 127). The widely held belief is that the vitamin D deficiency is the result of the sequestration of dietary vitamin D by adipose tissue. Because vitamin D is lipophilic, when it is absorbed from the gut, it enters the circulation, first on chylomicrons, and then is only partially transferred to DBP and at a very slow rate (5). Vitamin D has a relatively low affinity for DBP; reviews estimate this at between $10^{-5}M$ and $10^{-7}M$ (128). Transport of dietary vitamin D contrasts significantly with that of vitamin D_3 made during skin synthesis, which is mainly DBP bound (129). The consequences of chylomicron transport of dietary vitamin D include the possibility of uptake by peripheral tissues, such as adipose tissue and muscle, as a result of the action of lipoprotein lipase (128) and a short plasma half-life of 4 to 6 hours (128). In contrast, the half-life of vitamin D stores is 2 months. The nutritional outcome of the sequestration of dietary vitamin D by adipose tissues is increased variability in the rise of serum 25-OH-D in response to vitamin D supplementation with increasing BMI. In contrast, weight loss studies show that even modest weight losses result in rises in serum 25-OH-D, presumably because of mobilization of adipose tissue stores that parallels adipose tissue depletion.

One group at particular risk of vitamin D deficiency is that of patients with chronic kidney disease, 80% to 100% of whom have extremely low 25-OH-D levels (130). This situation is further complicated by high levels of FGF-23 secondary to phosphate retention, which results in CYP27B1 down-regulation as well as increased 25-OH-D catabolism caused by CYP24A1 up-regulation (131). Correction of serum 25-OH-D into the sufficient range results in some improvement in most vitamin D–related outcomes in patients with chronic kidney disease, and in patients undergoing dialysis, vitamin D supplementation even improves their survival (131, 132). Whether vitamin D supplementation also leads to benefits for various vitamin D–related health outcomes for the physiologically normal population is still to be proved in appropriate randomized controlled trials.

ACUTE TOXICITY CAUSED BY VITAMIN D

Numerous animal studies involving systematic vitamin D intoxication have been conducted since the late 1970s in various species, including rats, cows, pigs, rabbits, dogs, and horses (128). Vitamin D_3 intoxication results in elevation of the blood levels of several metabolites, including vitamin D_3, 25(OH)D_3, 24,25(OH)$_2D_3$, 25,26(OH)$_2D_3$, and 25(OH)D_3-26,23-lactone, although it rarely raises plasma $1\alpha,25(OH)_2D_3$ levels. Results of studies by Horst et al (reviewed in 128) in pigs and dairy cows were quite definitive in suggesting that renal CYP27B1 is effectively turned off.

Focus therefore shifted to the levels of other vitamin D metabolites correlated with toxicity, especially the plasma threshold of 25-OH-D that must be exceeded to cause hypercalcemia. Shephard and DeLuca (133) acutely intoxicated rats with graded oral doses of vitamin D_3 (0.65 to 6500 ng/day for 14 days) or 25-OH-D_3 (0.46 to 4600 ng/day for 14 days) and used high-performance liquid chromatography and competitive binding assays to measure vitamin D metabolites post-mortem. The findings showed that serum vitamin D_3 and 25(OH)D_3 levels rose to micromolar levels in plasma of rats given the highest intakes of vitamin D_3 and resulted in marked hypercalcemia. Dihydroxylated metabolites, including 24,25-(OH)$_2D_3$, 25,26-(OH)$_2D_3$, and 25(OH)D_3-26,23-lactone, also rose to levels higher than 40 ng/mL, but the level of plasma $1\alpha,25(OH)_2D_3$ remained within the normal range. A dose of 460 ng/day of 25-OH-D_3 resulted in serum 25(OH)D_3 levels of 436 ± 53 ng/mL with normocalcemia, but such animals had no vitamin D burden. Based on this finding and on various studies in several animal species, it appears that the serum 25-OH-D levels associated with acute toxicity are always in excess of 200 ng/mL.

For ethical reasons, no systematic studies of vitamin intoxication have been conducted in humans. Numerous anecdotal reports collected over the years have described accidental vitamin D intoxication with either vitamin D_3 or vitamin D_2, however (reviewed in 128, 134). Because many of these studies involved measuring 25-OH-D and sometimes $1\alpha,25$-(OH)$_2$D, it is worth reviewing the vitamin D metabolite values that correlate with overt toxicity symptoms. Although an occasional report did find evidence of modest elevation of $1\alpha,25$-(OH)$_2$D levels (128), all reported that 25-OH-D levels were well above the normal range at between 284 and 635 ng/mL. In a study of 35 hypervitaminotic patients with hypercalcemia resulting from chronic ingestion of overfortified milk (135), the average 25-OH-D level was 224 ng/mL (range, 56 to 596 ng/mL). In an extended family group accidentally intoxicated with a veterinary vitamin D concentrate (peanut oil solution containing

2×10^6 IU cholecalciferol), Pettifor et al (136) showed that 25-OH-D levels ranged from 339 to 661 ng/mL in intoxicated family members, whereas plasma $1\alpha,25$-(OH)$_2$D values were within the normal range in 8 of 11 patients.

A perusal of these data and the anecdotal reports led reviewers in this field to the same conclusion (128, 134), namely, that hypercalcemia results only when 25-OH-D_3 levels have been consistently higher than 200 ng/mL. The mechanism of vitamin D toxicity is unknown but is thought to involve vitamin D metabolites exceeding the vitamin D–carrying capacity of the DBP of the plasma. Displacement of one of the elevated metabolites, $1\alpha,25(OH)_2D$ or 25-OH-D, into the target cell results in increases in unregulated biologic effects. Recent studies with the CYP27B1-knockout mouse which is unable to make $1\alpha,25$-(OH)$_2D_3$ from 25-OH-D_3 suggests that 25-OH-D_3 and not $1\alpha,25$-(OH)$_2D_3$ is the toxic form (137). Both knockout animals and their normal wild-type littermates are intoxicated at the same dietary vitamin D intakes.

With the increasingly popular call in the scientific literature (96, 99) and even in the lay press for higher vitamin D supplementation, the question of vitamin D toxicity has switched to this: What are the long-term risks of moderately high doses of vitamin D? An honest answer to this important question is that we do not know whether vitamin D supplementation that produces serum 25-OH-D levels of 50 to 100 ng/mL is safe or whether it causes any long-term side effects. Individuals with serum 25-OH-D levels in this range (e.g., lifeguards, outdoor workers) do not have acute toxicity (e.g., hypercalcemia), but whether they suffer more subtle side effects (e.g., more renal stones, higher cancer rates, higher mortality rates) has yet to be determined. Cancer epidemiologic data suggest that certain cancers show a U-shaped curve in response to vitamin D supplementation: low levels of serum 25-OH-D are strongly associated with an increased cancer risk, and moderately high levels of serum 25-OH-D greater than 50 ng/mL also show a risk, albeit at a lower risk level than in deficiency (138). Concern has been expressed that long-term ingestion of moderately high vitamin D intakes may cause changes in vascular calcification.

Experimentation using the hypercholesterolemic, low-density lipoprotein receptor knockout mouse model rendered uremic by partial nephrectomy with low endogenous 1,25-(OH)$_2$D production exhibited accelerated vascular calcification, but this was reversed by graded doses of various vitamin D analogs (139). This model suggests that, contrary to popular belief, vitamin D compounds protect the vasculature from calcification, and only at very high doses do they trigger adverse effects through increasing serum Ca^{2+} and PO_4^{3-}. Results of epidemiologic studies are consistent with these animal data (140). Consequently, vitamin D supplementation that does not result in changes in calcium and phosphate homeostasis may be safe, and the serum 25-OH-D threshold for acute vitamin D toxicity (>200 ng/mL) may also turn out to be predictive for long-term risk. Currently, the normal range for serum 25-OH-D currently used by clinical chemistry laboratories is between 20 and 80 ng/mL, or even between 20 and 100 ng/mL (24), although NHANES data suggest that most US residents have values between 5 and 50 ng/mL (16). This range may change significantly because the IOM Committee recommendations include using a narrower normal range of 20 to 50 ng/mL in view of concerns about long-term effects of chronic vitamin D dosing (16). North Americans should be reassured that the ULs selected for different age groups (4000 IU for 9 to more than 71 years) still include a large safety margin, at least based on acute toxicity symptoms (hypercalcemia).

REFERENCES

1. Whistler D. De morbo puerili Anglorum, quem patrio idiomate indigenae vocant. The rickets MD thesis, University of Leiden, Leiden, Netherlands, 1645.
2. Glisson F. De Rachitide sive morbo puerili qui vulgo. The rickets dicitur. London, 1650.
3. Sniadecki J. 1840. Cited by Mozolowski W. Nature 1939;143:121.
4. Palm TA. Practitioner 1890;45:270–9.
5. Percival T. Essays Medical, Philosophical and Experimental on the Medical Use of Cod-Liver Oil, vol 2. London, 1789.
6. Raczynski J. C R Assoc Int Pediatr 1913;308.
7. Huldschinsky K. Dtsch Med Wochenschr 1919;45,712–3.
8. Hess AF, Unger JF Pappenheimer AM. J Exp Med 1922;36:427–46.
9. Mellanby E. Lancet 1919;1:407–12.
10. McCollum EV, Simmonds N, Becker JE et al. J Biol Chem 1922;53:293–312.
11. Hess AF, Weinstock M. J Biol Chem 1924;62:301–13.
12. Steenbock H, Black A. J Biol Chem 1924;61:408–22.
13. Windaus A, Schenck F, van Werder F. Hoppe Seylers Z Physiol Chem 1936;241:100–3.
14. Makin HLJ, Jones G, Kaufmann M et al. Analysis of vitamins D, their metabolites and analogues. In: Makin HLJ, Gower DB, eds. Steroid Analysis. New York: Springer, 2010:967–1096.
15. Delvin EE, Glorieux FH, Dussault M et al. Med Biol 1978;57:165–70.
16. Food and Nutrition Board, Institute of Medicine. Dietary Reference Intakes for Calcium and Vitamin D. Washington, DC: National Academy Press, 2011.
17. Holick MF. Photobiology of vitamin D. In: Feldman D, Pike JW, Glorieux FH, eds. Vitamin D. 2nd ed. New York: Elsevier, 2005:37–46.
18. Jones G, Strugnell SA, DeLuca HF. Physiol Rev 1998;78:1193–231.
19. Prosser DE, Jones G. Trends Biochem Sci 2004;29:664–73.
20. Cheng JB, Levine MA, Bell NH et al. Proc Natl Acad Sci U S A 2004;101:7711–5.
21. Jones G, Byford V, West S et al. Anticancer Res 2006;26:2589–96.
22. Strushkevich N, Usanov SA, Plotnikov AN et al. J Mol Biol 2008;380:95–106.
23. Wang TJ, Zhang F, Richards JB et al. Lancet 2010;376:180–8.
24. Hollis BW: Detection of vitamin D and its major metabolites. In: Feldman D, Pike JW, Glorieux FH, eds. Vitamin D. 2nd ed. New York: Elsevier, 2005:931–50.
25. Safadi FF, Thornton P, Magiera H et al. J Clin Invest 1999;103:239–51.
26. Willnow TE, Nykjaer A. Endocytic pathways for 25-hydroxyvitamin D₃. In: Feldman D, Pike JW, Glorieux FH, eds. Vitamin D. 2nd ed. New York: Elsevier, 2005:153–63.
27. Martinez I, Saracho R, Montenegro J et al. Nephrol Dial Transplant 1996;11:22–8.
28. St-Arnaud RH, Messerlian SH, Moir JM et al. J Bone Miner Res 1997;12:1552–9.
29. Takeyama K, Kitanaka S, Sato T et al. Science 1997;277:1827–30.
30. Monkawa T, Yoshida T, Wakino S et al. Biochem Biophys Res Commun 1997;239:527–33.
31. Fu GK, Lin D, Zhang MYH et al. Mol Endocrinol 1997;11:1961–70.
32. Armbrecht HJ, Hodam TL, Boltz MA. Arch Biochem Biophys 2003;409:298–304.
33. Quarles LD. Am J Physiol 2003;285:E1–9.
34. Yamamoto K, Uchida E, Urushino N et al. J Biol Chem 2005;280:30511–6.
35. Fraser D, Kooh SW, Kind P et al. N Engl J Med 1973;289:817–22.
36. Dardenne O, Prud'homme J, Arabian A et al. Endocrinology 2001;142:3135–41.
37. Panda DK, Miao D, Bolivar I et al. J Biol Chem 2004;279:16754–66.
38. Holick MF, Schnoes HK, DeLuca HF et al. Biochemistry 1972;11:4251–5.
39. Holick MF, Kleiner-Bossaller A, Schnoes HK et al. J Biol Chem 1973;248:6691–6.
40. Ohyama Y, Okuda K. J Biol Chem 1991;266:8690–5.
41. Tenenhouse HS, Yip A, Jones G. J Clin Invest 1988;81:461–5.
42. Jones G, Vriezen D, Lohnes D et al. Steroids 1987;49:29–53.
43. Makin G, Lohnes D, Byford V et al. Biochem J 1989;262:173–80.
44. Reddy GS, Tserng KY. Biochemistry 1989;28:1763–9.
45. Prosser D, Kaufmann M, O'Leary B et al. Proc Natl Acad Sci U S A 2007;104:12673–8.
46. Shinki T, Jin CH, Nishimura A et al. J Biol Chem 1992;267:13757–62.
47. Lohnes D, Jones, G. J Nutr Sci Vitaminol (Tokyo) 1992;Spec No:75–8.
48. Schlingmann KP, Kaufmann M, Weber S et al. New Engl J Med 2011;365:410–21.
49. St-Arnaud R, Arabian A, Travers R et al. Endocrinology 2000;141:2658–66.
50. Masuda S, Byford V, Arabian A et al. Endocrinology 2005;146:825–34.
51. Esvelt RP, Schnoes HK, DeLuca HF. Biochemistry 1979;18:3977–83.
52. Xue Y, Hashizume T, Shuhart MC et al. Mol Pharmacol 2006;69:56–65.
53. Thummel KE, Brimer C, Yasuda K et al. Mol Pharmacol 2001;60:1399–406.
54. Thompson PD, Jurutka PW, Whitfield GK et al. Biochem Biophys Res Commun 2002;299:730–8.
55. Haussler MR, Whitfield GK, Haussler CA et al. J Bone Miner Res 1998;13:325–49.
56. Whitfield GK, Jurutka PW, Haussler C et al. Nuclear receptor: structure-function, molecular control of gene transcription and novel bioactions. In: Feldman D, Pike JW, Glorieux FH, eds. Vitamin D. 2nd ed. New York: Elsevier, 2005:219–62.
57. Stumpf WE. Histochem Cell Biol 1995;104:417–27.
58. Pike JW. Annu Rev Nutr 1991;11:189–216.
59. White JH. J Steroid Biochem Mol Biol 2004;89–90:239–44.
60. Yoshizawa T, Handa Y, Uematsu Y et al. Nat Genet 1997;16:391–6.
61. Pike JW, Zella LA, Meyer MB et al. J Bone Miner Res 2007;22(Suppl 2):V16–9.
62. Bouillon R, Carmeliet G, Verlinden L et al. Endocr Rev 2008;29:726–76.

63. Benn BS, Ajibade D, Porta A et al. Endocrinology 2008;149: 3196–205.
64. Bianco SD, Peng JB, Takanaga H et al. J Bone Miner Res 2007;22:274–85.
65. Kutuzova GD, Akhter S, Christakos S et al. Proc Natl Acad Sci U S A 2006;103:12377–81.
66. Lee GS, Lee KY, Choi KC et al. J Bone Miner Res 2007;22: 1968–78.
67. Xu H, Bai L, Collins JF et al. Am J Physiol 2002;282:C487–93.
68. Liu M, Lee MH, Cohen M et al. Genes Dev 1996;10:142–53.
69. Wang Q, Jones JB, Studzinski GP. Cancer Res 1996;56:264–7.
70. Rots NY, Liu M, Anderson EC et al. Mol Cell Biol 1998;18:1918.
71. Bettoun DJ, Buck DW, Lu JF et al. J Biol Chem 2002;277:24847–50.
72. Masuda S, Jones G. Mol Cancer Ther 2006;5:797–808.
73. Wagner N, Wagner KD, Schley G et al. Exp Eye Res 2003;77:1–9.
74. James SY, Mackay AG, Colston KW et al. J Steroid Biochem Mol Biol 1996;58:395–401.
75. Mathiasen IS, Sergev IN, Bastholm L et al. J Biol Chem 2002;277:30738–45.
76. Xie SP, James SY, Colston KW. J Endocrinol 1997;154:495–504.
77. McGuire TF, Trump DL, Johnson CS. J Biol Chem 276:26365–73.
78. Xie ZJ, Komuves L, Yu QC et al. J Invest Dermatol 2002;118:11–6.
79. Sakai Y, Demay MB. Endocrinology 2000;141:2043–9.
80. Zinser GM, Sundberg JP, Welsh J. Carcinogenesis 2002;23:2103–9.
81. Holick MF. Am J Clin Nutr 2004;80(Suppl):1678S–88S.
82. Grant WB, Garland CF. Nutr Cancer 2004;48:115–23.
83. Grant WB, Garland CF. J Intern Med 2002;252:178–9.
84. Schwartz GG, Hulka BS. Anticancer Res 1990;10:1307–11.
85. Bikle DD, Chang S, Crumrine D et al. J Invest Dermatol 2004;122:984–92.
86. Bises G, Kallay E, Weiland T et al. J Histochem Cytochem 2004;52:985–9.
87. Jones G, Ramshaw H, Zhang A et al. Endocrinology 1999; 140:3303–10.
88. Zeohnder D, Bland R, Williams MC et al. J Clin Endocrinol Metab 2001;86:888–94.
89. Somjen D, Katzburg S, Stern N et al. J Steroid Biochem Mol Biol 2007;107:238–44.
90. Barbour GL, Coburn JW, Slatopolsky E et al. N Engl J Med 1981;305:440–3.
91. Dusso AS, Finch J, Brown A et al. J Clin Endocrinol Metab 1991;72:157–64.
92. Adams JS, Gacad MA, Singer FR et al. Ann N Y Acad Sci 1986,465:587–94.
93. Dusso AS, Kamimura S, Gallieni M et al. J Clin Endocrinol Metab 1997;82:2222–32.
94. Stoffels K, Overbergh L, Giulietti A et al. J Bone Miner Res 2006;21:37–47.
95. Hewison M, Adams JS. Extra-renal 1α-hydroxylase activity and human disease. In: Feldman D, Pike JW, Glorieux FH, eds. Vitamin D. 2nd ed. New York: Elsevier, 2005:1379–402.
96. Holick MF. N Engl J Med 2007;357:266–81.
97. Jones G. Semin Dial 2007;20:316–24.
98. Kidney Disease Outcomes Quality Initiative of the National Kidney Foundation. Am J Kidney Dis 2003;42(Suppl 3):S1–202.
99. Hollis BW. J Nutr 2005;135:317–22.
100. Bischoff-Ferrari HA, Dietrich T, Orav EJ et al. Am J Med 2004;116:634–9.
101. Bischoff-Ferrari HA, Dietrich T, Orav EJ et al. Am J Clin Nutr 2004;80:752–8.
102. Jones G, Horst RL, Carter G et al. J Bone Miner Res 2007;22(Suppl 2):V11–5.
103. Chen PS, Bosmann HB. J Nutr 1964;83:133–9.
104. Marx SJ, Jones G, Weinstein RS et al. J Clin Endocrinol Metab 1989;69:1282–90.
105. Park EA. JAMA 1940;115:370–9.
106. Roborgh JR, de Man T. Biochem Pharmacol 1960;2:1–6.
107. Roborgh JR, de Man T. Biochem Pharmacol 1960;3:277–82.
108. Whyte MP, Haddad JG, Walters DD et al. J Clin Endocrinol Metab 1979;48:906–11.
109. Houghton LA, Vieth R. Am J Clin Nutr 2006;84:694–7.
110. Trang HM, Cole DE, Rubin LA et al. Am J Clin Nutr 1998;68:854–8.
111. Armas LA, Hollis BW, Heaney RP. J Clin Endocrinol Metab 2004;89:5387–91.
112. Romagnoli E, Mascia ML, Cipriani C et al. J Clin Endocrinol Metab 93:3015–20.
113. Leventis P, Kiely PD. Scand J Rheumatol 2009;38:149–53.
114. Rapuri PB, Gallagher JC, Haynatzki G. Calcif Tissue Int 2004;74:150–6.
115. Holick MF, Biancuzzo RM, Chen TC et al. J Clin Endocrinol Metab 2008;93:677–81.
116. Thacher TD, Obadofin MO, O'Brien KO et al. J Clin Endocrinol Metab 2009;94:3314–21.
117. Heaney RP, Armas LA, Shary JR et al. Am J Clin Nutr 2008;87:1738–42.
118. Hunt RD, Garcia FG, Walsh RJ. J Nutr 1972;102:975–86.
119. Gupta RP, Hollis BW, Patel SB et al. J Bone Miner Res 2004;19:680–8.
120. Gupta RP, He YA, Patrick KS et al. J Clin Endocrinol Metab 2005;90:1210–9.
121. Jones G, Byford V, Helvig C et al. Abstract presented at the 14th International Vitamin D Workshop, Brugge, Belgium, October 4–8, 2009.
122. Tjellesen L, Gotfredsen A, Christiansen C. Calcif Tissue Int 1985;37:218–22.
123. Hosseinpour F, Ellfolk M, Norlin M et al. Biochem Biophys Res Commun 2007;357:603–7.
124. Binet A, Kooh SW. Can J Public Health 1996;87:227–30.
125. Wu H, Gozdzik A, Barta JL et al. Nutr Res 2009;29:255–61.
126. Wortsman J, Matsuoka LY, Chen TC et al. Am J Clin Nutr 2000;72:690–3.
127. Reinehr T, de Sousa G, Alexy U et al. Eur J Endocrinol 2007;157:225–32.
128. Jones G. Am J Clin Nutr 2008;88(Suppl):582S–6S.
129. Haddad JG, Matsuoka LY, Hollis BW et al. J Clin Invest 1993;91:2552–5.
130. Gonzalez EA, Sachdeva A, Oliver DA et al. Am J Nephrol 2004;24:503–10.
131. Judd SE, Tangpricha V. Am J Med Sci 2009;338:40–4.
132. Drechsler C, Pilz S, Obermayer-Pietsch B et al. Eur Heart J 2010;31:2253–61.
133. Shephard RM, DeLuca HF. Arch Biochem Biophys 1980;202:43–53.
134. Vieth R. Bone Miner 1990;11:267–72.
135. Blank S, Scanlon KS, Sinks T et al. Am J Public Health 1995;85:656–9.
136. Pettifor JM, Bikle DD, Cavaleros M et al. Ann Intern Med 1995;122:511–3.
137. DeLuca HF, Prahl JM, Plum LA. Arch Biochem Biophys. 2011;505:226-30.
138. Grant WG. Dermatoendocrinology 2009;1:289–93.
139. Mathew S, Lund RJ, Chaudhary LR et al. J Am Soc Nephrol 2008;19:1509–19.
140. Giovannucci E. Curr Atheroscler Rep 2009;11:456–61.

19 VITAMIN E[1]

MARET G. TRABER

[1]**Abbreviations: α-CEHC**, 2,5,7,8-tetramethyl-2-(2_-carboxyethyl)-6-hydroxychroman; **α-TTP**, α-tocopherol transfer protein; **γ-CEHC**, 2,7,8-trimethyl-2-(2_carboxyethyl)-6-hydroxychroman; **ABC**, ATP-binding cassette; apo, apolipoprotein; **AVED**, ataxia with vitamin E deficiency; **CRALBP**, cellular retinaldehyde-binding protein; **DRI**, dietary reference intake; **EAR**, estimated average requirement; **HDL**, high-density lipoprotein; **HOPE**, Heart Outcomes Prevention Evaluation; **IOM**, Institute of Medicine; **IU**, international unit; **LDL**, low-density lipoprotein; **MDR**, multidrug resistance gene or p-glycoprotein; **NGT**, 2,7,8-trimethyl-2-(4,8,12-trimethyldecyl)-5-nitro-6-chromanol; **NPC1L1**, Niemann-Pick C1 -like 1; **PLTP**, phospholipid transfer protein; **PUFA**, polyunsaturated fatty acid; **RDA**, recommended dietary allowance; **ROO·**, peroxyl radical; **TPN**, total parenteral nutrition; **UL**, tolerable upper intake level; **VLDL**, very-low-density lipoprotein.

HISTORICAL OVERVIEW

In 1922, Evans and Bishop (1), during their investigations of infertility, first described fetal resorption as a symptom of vitamin E deficiency in rats fed "rancid lard." In 1936, Evans et al (2) isolated a factor from wheat germ and named it "α-tocopherol," a name derived from the Greek "tokos" (offspring) and "pherein" (to bear), with an "ol" to indicate that it was an alcohol. Two other tocopherols, β- and γ-, with lower biologic activities, were isolated from vegetable oils (3). These early observations formed the foundation for defining the "biologic activity" of vitamin E, which is based on its ability to prevent or reverse specific vitamin E deficiency symptoms (4). Now it is recognized that the various forms are not interconvertible, and only α-tocopherol meets human requirements (5).

Vitamin E deficiency symptoms in various animal species were reviewed by Machlin (4). Necrotizing myopathy, fetal death and resorption, anemia, and accumulation of lipofuscin (a fluorescent pigment of "aging") in tissues have been observed in vitamin E–deficient animals. Progressive, peripheral, sensory neuropathy is the first sign of vitamin E deficiency in humans (6).

Horwitt et al (7, 8) attempted to induce vitamin E deficiency in men by feeding a diet low in vitamin E for 6 years to volunteers at the Elgin (Illinois) State Hospital in the 1950s. These data were used in 2000 to set the recommended dietary allowance (RDA) for vitamin E (5), discussed later.

It was not until the mid-1960s that vitamin E deficiency was described in children with fat malabsorption syndromes, as reviewed (9). Subsequently, vitamin E–deficient patients with peripheral neuropathies but without fat malabsorption were described (10). Studies in such patients opened new avenues in vitamin E investigations because these patients were found to have a genetic defect in the hepatic α-tocopherol transfer protein (α-TTP) (11, 12).

TERMINOLOGY

The Institute of Medicine (IOM), Food and Nutrition Board, defined that only α-tocopherol meets human vitamin E requirements (5). Molecules with α-tocopherol antioxidant activity include four tocopherols and four tocotrienols (Fig. 19.1), however. These molecules have similar chromanol structures: trimethyl (α-), dimethyl (β- or γ-), and monomethyl (δ-); tocopherols have a phytyl side chain, whereas tocotrienols have an unsaturated side chain. α-Tocopherol synthesized by condensation of trimethyl hydroquinone with racemic isophytol (13) contains eight stereoisomers (arising from the three chiral centers: 2′, 4′, and 8′, specifically: *RRR, RSR, RSS, RRS, SRR, SSR, SRS,* and *SSS*) and is designated *all-rac-*α-tocopherol (incorrectly called *dl-*α-tocopherol) (see Fig. 19.1). The naturally occurring *RRR-*α-tocopherol (formerly called *d-*α-tocopherol) is only one of the eight stereoisomers present in *all-rac-*α-tocopherol. The IOM (5) defined that human vitamin E requirements are met only by *2R-*α-tocopherols, that is, half of the stereoisomers in *all-rac-*α-tocopherol. Previously, γ-tocopherol and other vitamin E forms were included as sources of vitamin E; these forms no longer are included because of a lack of evidence showing they have health benefits in humans (5).

The IOM definition of vitamin E has led to confusion about vitamin E units. The definition of the unit used on supplement labels derives from units set by the US Pharmacopoeia (14). These supplements often contain esters of α-tocopherol, such as α-tocopheryl acetate, succinate, or nicotinate. Previously, the vitamin E international

unit (IU) was defined as 1 IU = 1 mg *all-rac-*α-tocopheryl acetate or 0.67 mg *RRR-*α-tocopherol, or 0.74 mg *RRR-*α-tocopheryl acetate. The IOM (see Table 6.1 in reference 5), however, defined the vitamin E requirement in milligrams of *2R-*α-tocopherol and provided conversion factors, such that 1 mg *all-rac-*α-tocopherol is equal to 0.5 mg *RRR-*α-tocopherol.

Vitamin E as defined by IOM (5):

$$\text{IU } \textit{all-rac-}\alpha\text{-tocopherol or its esters}$$
$$= 0.45 \text{ mg } 2R\text{-}\alpha\text{-tocopherol}$$

$$\text{IU } \textit{RRR-}\alpha\text{-tocopherol or its esters}$$
$$= 0.67 \text{ mg } 2R\text{-}\alpha\text{-tocopherol}$$

Thus, a 400-IU pill of *d-*α-tocopherol contains 268 mg *2R-*α-tocopherol (400 IU × 0.67 mg/IU), whereas a 400 IU pill of *dl-*α-tocopherol contains 180 mg *2R-*α-tocopherol (400 IU × 0.91 mg/IU ÷ 2).

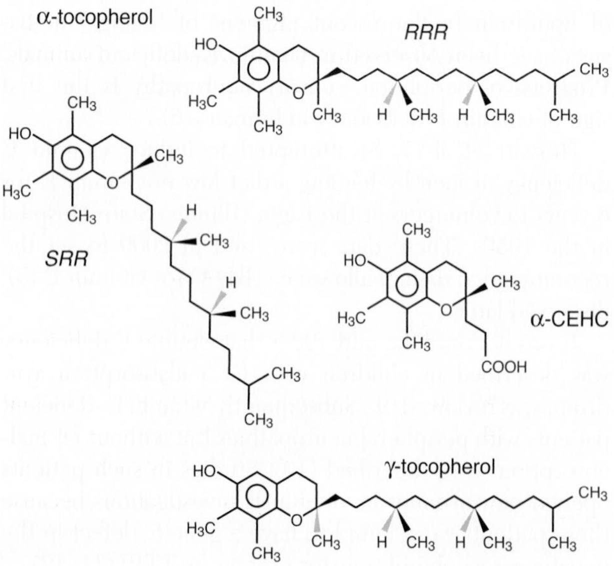

CHEMISTRY

Antioxidant Activity

Vitamin E functions in vivo as a chain-breaking antioxidant, as reviewed (15). It is a potent peroxyl radical scavenger and especially protects polyunsaturated fatty acids (PUFAs). When peroxyl radicals (ROO·) are formed, these react 1000 times faster with vitamin E (Vit E-OH) than with PUFA (RH) and form the tocopheroxyl radical (Vit E–O·):

In the presence of vitamin E: ROO· + Vit E-OH → ROOH + Vit E–O·

In the absence of vitamin E: ROO· + RH → ROOH + R·

R· + O$_2$ → ROO·

In this way, vitamin E prevents further lipid autooxidation.

The two-electron oxidation product of α-tocopherol is α-tocopheryl quinone. Other α-tocopherol oxidation products that may be formed include 4a,5-epoxy- and 7,8-epoxy-8a (hydroperoxy) tocopherones and their respective hydrolysis products, 2,3-epoxy-α-tocopherol quinone and 5,6-epoxy-α-tocopherol quinone (16, 17). These products are formed during in vitro oxidation; however, their importance in vivo is unknown. Further oxidation products, including dimers, trimers, and other adducts, have also been described (18).

Vitamin E Antioxidant Network

The tocopheroxyl radical (Vit E–O·) formed in membranes emerges from the lipid bilayer into the aqueous domain, as reviewed (19). It is here that the tocopheroxyl radical reacts with vitamin C (or other reductants serving as hydrogen donors, AH), thereby oxidizes the latter, and returns, vitamin E to its reduced state.

Vit E–O· + AH → Vit E–OH + A·

Fig. 19.1. Structures of α- and γ-tocopherols and α-2,5,7,8-tetramethyl-2-(2′-carboxyethyl)-6-hydroxychroman (α-CEHC). Eight naturally occurring forms of vitamin E are recognized. Shown is *RRR-*α-tocopherol with naturally occurring stereochemistry; the three chiral centers can give rise to eight different stereoisomers in synthetic vitamin E (*all-rac-*α-tocopherol). These are *RRR-, RRS-, RSR-, RSS-, SRR-, SSR-, SRS-,* and *SSS-*. Shown is *SRR-*α-tocopherol; its dramatic structural difference is readily apparent and explains why only *2R-*α-tocopherols meet the human vitamin E requirement. Also shown is *RRR-*γ-tocopherol and the α-tocopherol metabolite, CEHC. Note that it has opposite stereochemistry from the parent compound.

Biologically important hydrogen donors include ascorbate (vitamin C) and thiols, especially glutathione. This phenomenon led to the idea of vitamin E recycling in which the antioxidant function of the vitamin E radical is continuously restored by other antioxidants and by the metabolic activity of cells (20). Regeneration of tocopherol from its radical by vitamin C appears to be a physiologically relevant mechanism, based on studies in humans (see next section), as well as in guinea pigs (21–23) and other rodents (24).

Increased Utilization of Vitamin E by Humans under Oxidative Stress

Oxidative stress caused by ultramarathon running was shown to increase rates of plasma vitamin E disappearance in humans (25). Moreover, prior vitamin E and C supplementation decreased markers of lipid peroxidation in runners (26). Chronic oxidative stress and inflammation caused by cigarette smoking also increased α-tocopherol fractional disappearance rates in cigarette smokers compared with nonsmokers (27). Moreover, the smokers with the lowest plasma ascorbic acid concentrations had the fastest α-tocopherol disappearance rates, presumably because vitamin C regenerates vitamin E (28). In a subsequent study, Bruno et al (29) showed that not only was marginal vitamin C status in smokers associated with increased rates of vitamin E disappearance from plasma but also these rates could be normalized by prior vitamin C supplementation. Importantly, both α- and γ-tocopherols were similarly affected by vitamin C status, a finding suggesting that oxidation of the tocopherols is the mechanism for the faster vitamin E disappearance in the presence of low vitamin C status (29).

Structure-Function Relationships of Vitamin E Forms

Numerous reports have noted health benefits of non–α-tocopherols as anti-inflammatory agents, antioxidants, and antiangiogenic compounds both in atherosclerosis and in cancer protection, as reviewed (30, 31). One mechanism in which α-tocopherol cannot participate is scavenging reactive nitrogen species. In vitro, γ-, β- or δ-tocopherols can be nitrated (32–34). Hoglen et al (35) demonstrated that 5-nitro-γ-tocopherol (2,7,8-trimethyl-2-[4,8,12-trimethyldecyl]-5-nitro-6-chromanol [NGT]) is the major reactive product between peroxynitrite and γ-tocopherol. NGT has been detected in the plasma of zymosan-treated rats (36), in the plasma of patients with coronary artery disease (37) and of cigarette smokers (38), and in brains collected post-mortem from patients with Alzheimer disease (39).

DIETARY SOURCES

The richest food sources of vitamin E are almonds, sunflower seeds, and edible vegetable oils (40), which contain varying proportions of the eight homologs: α-, β -, γ-, and δ-tocopherols or tocotrienols. *RRR*-α-tocopherol is especially high in wheat germ oil, safflower oil, and sunflower oil, whereas soybean and corn oils contain predominantly γ-tocopherol, as well as some tocotrienols. Foods that have been fortified with *all-rac*-α-tocopheryl acetate include some breakfast cereals, tomato juice, orange juice, and milk.

DIETARY REFERENCE INTAKES

The dietary reference intakes (DRIs) for vitamin C, vitamin E, selenium, and carotenoids were published in 2000 (5). The DRIs distinguish between *RRR*- and *all-rac*-α-tocopherol because these structures are physically different and have different fates with respect to transport and metabolism (5).

The estimated average requirement (EAR) was based on the amount of 2R-α-tocopherol intake that reversed in vitro peroxide-induced erythrocyte hemolysis in men who were vitamin E deficient as a result of consuming a vitamin E–deficient diet for 5 years, as reviewed (5). The RDA values for α-tocopherol by life stage are given in Table 19.1. The EAR of 12 mg 2R-α-tocopherol was chosen because intakes at this level and above resulted in plasma α-tocopherol concentrations that prevented in vitro hydrogen peroxide–induced erythrocyte hemolysis. The assumption was made that men and women would have similar requirements because women, despite their

TABLE 19.1	DIETARY REFERENCE INTAKE VALUES FOR VITAMIN E BY LIFE STAGE GROUP[a]	
LIFE STAGE GROUP	RDA[b] (mg/d)	AI[c] (mg/d)
0–6 mo		4
7–12 mo		5
1–3 y	6	
4–8 y	7	
9–13 y	11	
14–18 y	15	
>18 y	15	
Pregnancy		
≤18 y	15	
19–50 y	15	
Lactation		
≤18 y	19	
19–50 y	19	

[a]In units of mg 2R-α-tocopherol.
[b]RDA, recommended dietary allowance. The intake that meets the nutrient needs of almost all (97% to 98%) of individuals in a group.
[c]AI, adequate intake. The observed average or experimentally determined intake by a defined population or subgroup that appears to sustain a defined nutritional status, such as growth rate, normal circulating nutrient values, or other functional indicators of health. The AI is used if sufficient scientific evidence is not available to derive an estimated average requirement. For healthy infants receiving human milk, the AI is the mean intake. The AI is not equivalent to an RDA.

Reproduced with permission from Food and Nutrition Board, Institute of Medicine. Dietary Reference Intakes for Vitamin C, Vitamin E, Selenium, and Carotenoids. Washington, DC: National Academy Press, 2000.

lower body weight, have a larger percentage body fat needing antioxidant protection. The RDA for adults (both men and women ≥19 years old), defined as $2R$-α-tocopherol, is 15 mg/day.

The tolerable upper intake level (UL) was set at 1000 mg/day for vitamin E (any form of supplemental α-tocopherol) (5). This was one of the few UL that was set using data from rats because sufficient and appropriate quantitative data assessing long-term adverse effects of vitamin E supplements in humans were not available.

The amount of α-tocopherol consumed by most US adults is sufficient to prevent overt symptoms of deficiency (41). The actual quantities consumed by US adults are closer to 8 mg, however, as assessed by various surveys (42–44). Thus, 93% of men and 96% of women in the United States do not consume 12 mg vitamin E daily (45). The report from the 2010 Dietary Guidelines Committee acknowledged this discrepancy between intake and recommendations but did not promote consumption of most foods containing high amounts of α-tocopherol because these are generally high-fat foods (45a).

Most people do not consume 15 mg α-tocopherol daily, and therefore they may be at increased risk for various chronic diseases. Previously, the Alpha-Tocopherol Beta-Carotene cancer prevention trial found that daily supplements (vitamin E [50 mg dl-α-tocopheryl acetate] or β-carotene [20 mg]) for 5 years did not decrease cancer incidence (46). A subsequent report assessing baseline vitamin E status and dietary intakes described the 29,092 men who had been followed for 19 years since the study's initiation, during which time 13,380 deaths ensued. The men at baseline in the highest compared with the lowest serum α-tocopherol quintiles had significantly lower risks of total and cause-specific mortality, including cardiovascular disease and cancer (47). The optimum relative reductions in mortality occurred at serum α-tocopherol concentrations of 13 to 14 mg/L (30 to 32 μmol/L) or higher and were associated with an estimated dietary vitamin E intake of 12 mg α-tocopherol (47), a dietary value not different from the EAR (12 mg) proposed by the IOM (5). This finding suggests a health benefit of obtaining the RDA amount of vitamin E from the diet.

PHYSIOLOGIC FACTORS INFLUENCING UTILIZATION

Digestion and Intestinal Absorption

The efficiency of vitamin E absorption is low (<50%) and depends on processes necessary for fat digestion and uptake into enterocytes (41). The bioavailability of vitamin E increases with increasing fat content of foods eaten with vitamin E supplements or food fortificants (48–50).

The trafficking of vitamin E through the absorptive cells is not well understood; no intestinal tocopherol transfer proteins have been described (41). Discrimination among

forms of vitamin E does not occur during their absorption and secretion in chylomicrons. The intestinal cells package chylomicrons containing triglycerides, free and esterified cholesterol, phospholipids, and apolipoproteins (especially apolipoprotein [apo] B48). In addition, fat-soluble vitamins, carotenoids, and other fat-soluble dietary components are incorporated into chylomicrons (41). Anwar et al (51) demonstrated that the primary pathway for vitamin E absorption is through chylomicrons, but in the absence of a functional microsomal triglyceride transfer protein necessary for chylomicron formation, high-density lipoproteins (HDLs) participate in vitamin E absorption. The critical role of bile acids for vitamin E absorption also suggests that the key steps in vitamin E absorption are, first, entry into the enterocyte, followed by packaging into chylomicrons (41).

Vitamin E absorption appears to be mediated similarly to cholesterol absorption. Niemann-Pick C1-like 1 (NPC1L1), a sterol transport protein, is critical for cholesterol uptake into the enterocyte (52, 53). Similarly, vitamin E absorption is facilitated by NPC1L1 (54), a finding leading to the suggestion that people who have a defect in the NPC1L1 gene may have defective vitamin E absorption (55). The prevalence of NPC1L1 defects relative to defects in vitamin E absorption in humans has not been extensively elucidated.

Plasma Transport

Unlike other fat-soluble vitamins, which have their own specific plasma transport proteins, vitamin E is transported nonspecifically in lipoproteins in the plasma. During chylomicron catabolism in the circulation and delipidation by lipoprotein lipase, some of the newly absorbed vitamin E is transferred to circulating lipoproteins and is delivered to the liver (Fig. 19.2) (41). During this process, vitamin E is also transferred to HDLs, which readily transfer vitamin E to other circulating lipoproteins. Kostner et al (56) demonstrated that the phospholipid transfer protein (PLTP) catalyzed vitamin E exchange between lipoproteins at a rate that represents transfer of approximately 10% of the plasma vitamin E per hour.

The liver, not the small intestine, discriminates among various vitamin E forms. Following partial delipidation of chylomicrons and their uptake by the liver, fats are repackaged in very-low-density lipoproteins (VLDLs), as reviewed (41), and $2R$-α-tocopherol is selectively secreted into plasma. During the VLDL delipidation cascade, low-density lipoproteins (LDLs) are formed. Some α-tocopherol remains with LDLs and some is transferred to HDLs. Thus, the major plasma lipoproteins, LDLs and HDLs, become enriched with α-tocopherol (Fig. 19.3).

A pharmacokinetic model of vitamin E transport in plasma has been developed using data from studies with deuterium-labeled stereoisomers of α-tocopherol (RRR- and SRR-) (57). In control subjects, the fractional

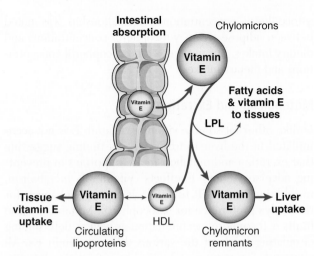

Fig. 19.2. Pathways for absorption of vitamin E and its delivery to tissues during chylomicron catabolism. Vitamin E absorption requires bile acids (secreted from the liver) and fatty acids and monoglycerides (released from dietary fat by pancreatic enzymes) for micelle formation. Following uptake into enterocytes of the intestine, all forms of dietary vitamin E are incorporated into chylomicrons (41). These triglyceride-rich lipoproteins are secreted into the circulation, where lipolysis by lipoprotein lipase (LPL) bound to the endothelial lining of capillary walls takes place. The resultant chylomicron remnants are mainly taken up by the liver. During lipolysis, various forms of vitamin E can be transferred to tissues or to high-density lipoproteins (HDLs). Vitamin E can exchange between HDL and other circulating lipoproteins, which can also deliver vitamin E to peripheral tissues.

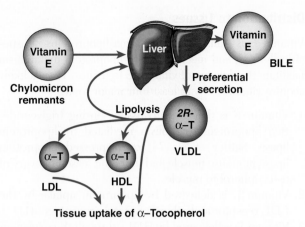

Fig. 19.3. Pathways for the preferential delivery of α-tocopherol to peripheral tissues. Chylomicron remnants containing various forms of vitamin E are taken up by the liver. In the liver, the α-tocopherol transfer protein seems preferentially to incorporate α-tocopherol into nascent very-low-density lipoproteins (VLDLs) (41). Following VLDL secretion into plasma, lipolysis of VLDL by lipoprotein lipase and hepatic triglyceride lipase results in the preferential enrichment of circulating lipoproteins with *RRR*-α-tocopherol. The metabolism of these lipoproteins results in the delivery of *RRR*-α-tocopherol to peripheral tissues. *HDL*, high-density lipoprotein; *LDL*, low-density lipoprotein.

disappearance rates of deuterium-labeled *RRR*-α-tocopherol (0.4 ± 0.1 pools per day) were significantly ($p < .01$) slower than for *SRR*- (1.2 ± 0.6). The apparent half-life of *RRR*-α-tocopherol in normal subjects was approximately 48 hours, consistent with the "slow" disappearance of plasma *RRR*-α-tocopherol (57). Because *RRR*-α-tocopherol is returned to the plasma, its apparent turnover is slow. This hepatic recirculation of *RRR*-α-tocopherol results in the daily replacement of nearly all the circulating *RRR*-α-tocopherol.

Hepatic α-Tocopherol Transfer Protein

α-TTP (30–35 kDa) has been isolated from humans and a variety of animals. The human protein has 94% homology to the rat protein, as well as some homology both to the cellular retinaldehyde-binding protein (CRALBP) in the retina and to sec14, a PLTP (58). The gene has been localized to the 8q13.1–13.3 region of human chromosome 8 (58, 59). The crystal structure has also been described (60, 61). Various human mutations have also been described (62).

α-TTP belongs to a family of hydrophobic ligand-binding proteins that have a *cis*-retinal binding motif sequence (CRAL_TRIO). This motif is also shared with CRALBP and yeast phosphatidylinositol transfer protein (Sec14p). Panagabko et al (63) showed that all of the CRAL_TRIO members bind α-tocopherol to some extent, but only α-TTP appears to have sufficient

affinity to serve as a physiologic α-tocopherol transfer mediator.

α-TTP is expressed by hepatocytes (64), and α-TTP mRNA has also been detected at low levels in rat brain, spleen, lung, and kidney (65). α-TTP is a critical factor during pregnancy; it is increased at the site of implantation (66, 67), expressed in the syncytiotrophoblast and trophoblast cells of the human placenta (67–69), and is additionally expressed by the human yolk sac (70). Early failure of pregnancy is associated with lipid peroxidation, with resultant damage to the syncytiotrophoblast (71). Jauniaux et al (70) suggested that during very early human fetal development, the human embryo obtains α-tocopherol from the yolk sac. Thus, it is likely that α-tocopherol is needed both by the fetus and by the mother to protect her from the oxidative stress of the rapidly growing fetus.

In vitro, α-TTP preferentially transfers α-tocopherol, compared with other dietary vitamin E forms, between liposomes and microsomes (72). Hypothetically, this selective transfer of α-tocopherol is responsible for the in vivo α-TTP action enriching nascent VLDLs secreted with *RRR*-α-tocopherol (73). When this hypothesis was tested in an α-TTP–expressing hepatic cell line (McARH7777 cells), however, α-TTP–mediated α-tocopherol secretion was not directly coupled with VLDL secretion (74). Thus, the *mechanism* by which α-TTP facilitates α-tocopherol secretion into plasma is unknown. Progress in this area is highlighted by studies demonstrating the ability of the purified α-TTP in vitro to fold properly, bind, and transfer vitamin E (75), as well as the use of fluorescent α-tocopherol analogs to follow trafficking and oxidation (76, 77).

Distribution to Tissues

Vitamin E is transported in plasma lipoproteins nonspecifically (41), and mechanisms of lipoprotein metabolism facilitate the delivery of vitamin E to tissues. Tissues likely acquire vitamin E by at least four major routes:

1. Vitamin E is delivered to tissues during triglyceride-rich lipoprotein catabolism mediated by lipoprotein lipase. Sattler et al (78) overexpressed lipoprotein lipase in mouse muscle and found increased delivery of α-tocopherol to muscle.
2. Vitamin E is delivered by lipoprotein uptake by the LDL receptor and other lipoprotein receptors (41).
3. Vitamin E is delivered by HDLs through the scavenger receptor-BI (SR-BI) (79), which delivers lipoprotein contents to cells.
4. Vitamin E rapidly exchanges among lipoproteins, as well as between lipoproteins and membranes. Therefore, exchange mechanisms may enrich membranes with vitamin E, as reviewed (41).

ABCA1 is an ATP-binding cassette (ABC) transporter that transports cellular cholesterol and phospholipids from cells to lipid-poor HDL. Oram et al (80) identified that ABCA1 facilitates uptake of α-tocopherol by HDLs. ABCA1 also facilitates α-tocopherol secretion mediated by α-TTP from hepatocytes in vitro, when apoAI is used as an acceptor (81). Mice lacking ABCA1 have severe deficiency of fat-soluble vitamins, including α-tocopherol (82). Clearly, ABCA1 is important in α-tocopherol trafficking; its physiologic role with regard to vitamin E appears to involve cellular α-tocopherol efflux.

Deuterated α-tocopherol has been used to assess the kinetics and distribution of α-tocopherol into various tissues in rats (83), guinea pigs (84), and humans (85). From these studies, it is apparent that groups of tissues, such as erythrocytes, liver, and spleen, are in rapid equilibrium with the plasma α-tocopherol pool and readily replace "old" with "new" α-tocopherol (86). Other tissues such as heart, muscle, and spinal cord have slower α-tocopherol turnover rates. Brain shows the slowest α-tocopherol turnover rate, perhaps because it expresses α-TTP (65, 87). In humans, the peripheral nerves (6) are the most susceptible tissues to α-tocopherol deficiency (88).

The mechanisms of tocopherol release from tissues are not well characterized. More than 90% of the human body pool of α-tocopherol is located in the adipose tissue, with more than 90% of adipose tissue α-tocopherol in fat droplets. In α-tocopherol–deficient humans, adipose tissue α-tocopherol content is lower than in physiologically normal subjects, although it is not clear whether this is the result of decreased delivery, increased export, or increased utilization (89). Thus, the analysis of adipose tissue α-tocopherol content provides a useful estimate of long-term vitamin E intakes. El-Sohemy et al (90) reported, in nearly 500 Costa Rican subjects, that adipose tissue α-tocopherol concentrations were higher than

γ-tocopherol concentrations. A relationship was noted between adipose tissue γ-tocopherol concentrations and dietary intakes, but not between α-tocopherol concentrations and dietary intakes.

Metabolism and Excretion

Unlike other fat-soluble vitamins, vitamin E is not accumulated in the liver to toxic levels, a finding suggesting that excretion and metabolism are important in preventing adverse vitamin E effects. Vitamin E metabolism, in addition to α-TTP function, is a key mechanism for the body's preference for α-tocopherol. Metabolism also limits α-tocopherol accumulation as well as determining circulating levels of the various dietary vitamin Es. All vitamin E forms are metabolized by ω-oxidation by cytochrome P-450s (CYPs), followed by β-oxidation, conjugation, and excretion in urine (91) or bile (92). Most ingested vitamin E, because of its relatively low intestinal absorption, is excreted in the feces.

Hepatic Metabolism

The liver is one site of vitamin E metabolism (93–95). It is unknown whether other tissues can also metabolize vitamin E, although a lung cancer cell line, A549, has also been successfully used to study metabolism (96, 97).

Vitamin E metabolites, for example α-CEHC (2,5,7,8-tetramethyl-2-[2′-carboxyethyl]-6-hydroxychroman; see Fig. 19.1) and γ-CEHC (2,7,8-trimethyl-2 [2′carboxyethyl]-6-hydroxychroman) are derived from α-tocopherols and α-tocotrienols and from γ-tocopherols and γ-tocotrienols, respectively (93, 98). In addition to α-CEHC, 13′OH-α-tocopherol and α-CMBHC (carboxymethyl butyl hydroxychroman) have been reported (95). Metabolism of γ-tocopherol or γ-tocotrienols generates 9′-, 11′-, and 13′-γ-carboxychromanols (97, 99). The process of β-oxidation by the liver appears to take place primarily in the mitochondria, with some activity in the peroxisomes (100).

High α-tocopherol intakes (e.g., most vitamin E supplements) lead to increases of plasma α-tocopherol, decreases of γ-tocopherol (101) and increases in both α-CEHC (102) and γ-CEHC excretion (98, 103). γ-CEHC excretion increases because γ-tocopherol is more actively metabolized to CEHCs than is α-tocopherol (98, 104, 105).

Hepatic CYP4F2 is involved in ω-oxidation of α- and γ-tocopherols (106). Sontag and Parker (107), however, also showed that CYP4F2 activity toward α-tocopherol was limited and that α-tocopherol stimulated the ω-hydroxylation of non–α-tocopherol forms of vitamin E. Although CYP4F2 most likely initiates vitamin E metabolism, it is not specific for vitamin E, because it is necessary in eicosanoid metabolism to regulate inflammation (108).

CYP3A has also been proposed to be involved in vitamin E metabolism based on the observation that CYP3A inhibitors and stimulators altered CEHC production (93,

37. Morton LW, Ward NC, Croft KD et al. Biochem J 2002; 364:625–8.

38. Leonard SW, Bruno RS, Paterson E et al. Free Radic Biol Med 2003;38:813–9.

39. Williamson KS, Gabbita SP, Mou S et al. Nitric Oxide 2002;6:221–7.

40. Sheppard AJ, Pennington JAT, Weihrauch JL. Analysis and distribution of vitamin E in vegetable oils and foods. In: Packer L, Fuchs J, eds. Vitamin E in Health and Disease. New York: Marcel Dekker, 1993:9–31.

41. Traber MG. Vitamin E. In: Shils ME, Olson JA, Shike M et al, eds. Modern Nutrition in Health and Disease. 9th ed. Baltimore: Williams & Wilkins, 1999:347–62.

42. Ma J, Hampl JS, Betts NM. Am J Clin Nutr 2000;71:774–80.

43. Ford ES, Sowell A. Am J Epidemiol 1999;150:290–300.

44. Kushi LH, Fee RM, Sellers TA et al. Am J Epidemiol 1996;144:165–74.

45. Maras JE, Bermudez OI, Qiao N et al. J Am Diet Assoc 2004;104:567–75.

45a. 2010 Dietary Guidelines Committee, US Department of Agriculture. Dietary Guidelines for Americans, June 23, 2010. Available at: http://www.cnpp.usda.gov/dietaryguidelines.htm. Accessed July 21, 2010.

46. Albanes D, Heinonen OP, Taylor PR et al. J Natl Cancer Inst 1996;88:1560–70.

47. Wright ME, Lawson KA, Weinstein SJ et al. Am J Clin Nutr 2006;84:1200–7.

48. Hayes KC, Pronczuk A, Perlman D. Am J Clin Nutr 2001;74: 211–8.

49. Bruno RS, Leonard SW, Park S-I et al. Am J Clin Nutr 2006;83: 299–304.

50. Leonard SW, Good CK, Gugger ET et al. Am J Clin Nutr 2004;79:86–92.

51. Anwar K, Iqbal J, Hussain MM. J Lipid Res 2007;48:2028–38.

52. Altmann SW, Davis HR Jr, Zhu LJ et al. Science 2004;303: 1201–4.

53. Davis HR Jr, Altmann SW. Biochim Biophys Acta 2009;1791: 679–83.

54. Narushima K, Takada T, Yamanashi Y et al. Mol Pharmacol 2008;74:42–9.

55. Yamanashi Y, Takada T, Suzuki H. Pharmacogenet Genomics 2009;19:884–92.

56. Kostner GM, Oettl K, Jauhiainen M et al. Biochem J 1995;305:659–67.

57. Traber MG, Ramakrishnan R, Kayden HJ. Proc Natl Acad Sci U S A 1994;91:10005–8.

58. Arita M, Sato Y, Miyata A et al. Biochem J 1995;306:437–43.

59. Doerflinger N, Linder C, Ouahchi K et al. Am J Hum Genet 1995;56:1116–24.

60. Meier R, Tomizaki T, Schulze-Briese C et al. J Mol Biol 2003;331:725–34.

61. Min KC, Kovall RA, Hendrickson WA. Proc Natl Acad Sci U S A 2003;100:14713–8.

62. Schuelke M. Ataxia with vitamin E deficiency. In: Pagon RA, Bird TC, Dolan CR et al, eds. GeneReviews [serial online] May 20, 2005 [updated September 4, 2007]. Available at: http://www.ncbi.nlm.nih.gov/bookshelf/br.fcgi?book=gene&part=aved. Accessed July 14, 2010.

63. Panagabko C, Morley S, Hernandez M et al. Biochemistry 2003;42:6467–74.

64. Yoshida H, Yusin M, Ren I et al. J Lipid Res 1992;33: 343–50.

65. Hosomi A, Goto K, Kondo H et al. Neurosci Lett 1998;256: 159–62.

66. Jishage K, Arita M, Igarashi K et al. J Biol Chem 2001; 273:1669–72.

67. Kaempf-Rotzoll DE, Igarashi K, Aoki J et al. Biol Reprod 2002;67:599–604.

68. Kaempf-Rotzoll DE, Horiguchi M, Hashiguchi K et al. Placenta 2003;24:439–44.

69. Rotzoll DE, Scherling R, Etzl R et al. Eur J Obstet Gynecol Reprod Biol 2008;140:183–91.

70. Jauniaux E, Cindrova-Davies T, Johns J et al. J Clin Endocrinol Metab 2004;89:1452–8.

71. Hempstock J, Jauniaux E, Greenwold N et al. Hum Pathol 2003;34:1265–75.

72. Sato Y, Hagiwara K, Arai H et al. FEBS Lett 1991;288:41–5.

73. Traber MG, Rudel LL, Burton GW et al. J Lipid Res 1990; 31:687–94.

74. Arita M, Nomura K, Arai H et al. Proc Natl Acad Sci U S A 1997;94:12437–41.

75. Panagabko C, Morley S, Neely S et al. Protein Express Purif 2002;24:395–403.

76. Wang Y, Panagabko C, Atkinson J. Bioorg Med Chem 2010;18:777–86.

77. West R, Panagabko C, Atkinson J. J Org Chem 2010;75: 2883–92.

78. Sattler W, Levak-Frank S, Radner H et al. Biochem J 1996; 318:15–9.

79. Mardones P, Strobel P, Miranda S et al. J Nutr 2002;132:443–9.

80. Oram JF, Vaughan AM, Stocker R. J Biol Chem 2001;276: 39898–902.

81. Shichiri M, Takanezawa Y, Rotzoll DE et al. J Nutr Biochem 2010;21:451–6.

82. Orso E, Broccardo C, Kaminski WE et al. Nat Genet 2000;24:192–6.

83. Ingold KU, Burton GW, Foster DO et al. Lipids 1987;22: 163–72.

84. Burton GW, Wronska U, Stone L et al. Lipids 1990;25:199–210.

85. Burton GW, Traber MG, Acuff RV et al. Am J Clin Nutr 1998;67:669–84.

86. Burton GW, Traber MG. Annu Rev Nutr 1990;10:357–82.

87. Copp RP, Wisniewski T, Hentati F et al. Brain Res 1999; 822:80–7.

88. Traber MG, Sokol RJ, Ringel SP et al. N Engl J Med 1987;317:262–5.

89. Steephen AC, Traber MG, Ito Y et al. JPEN J Parenter Enteral Nutr 1991;15:642–52.

90. El-Sohemy A, Baylin A, Ascherio A et al. Am J Clin Nutr 2001;74:356–63.

91. Brigelius-Flohé R, Traber MG. FASEB J 1999;13:1145–55.

92. Kiyose C, Saito H, Kaneko K et al. Lipids 2001;36:467–72.

93. Birringer M, Pfluger P, Kluth D et al. J Nutr 2002;132:3113–8.

94. Parker RS, Swanson JE. Biochem Biophys Res Commun 2000;269:580–3.

95. Mustacich DJ, Leonard SW, Devereaux MW et al. Free Radic Biol Med 2006;41:1069–78.

96. Yang WC, Regnier FE, Jiang Q et al. J Chromatogr A 2010;1217:667–75.

97. Freiser H, Jiang Q. J Nutr 2009;139:884–9.

98. Lodge JK, Ridlington J, Vaule H et al. Lipids 2001;36:43–8.

99. Freiser H, Jiang Q. Anal Biochem 2009;388:260–5.

100. Mustacich DJ, Leonard SW, Patel NK et al. Free Radic Biol Med 2010;48:73–81.

101. Handelman GJ, Machlin LJ, Fitch K et al. J Nutr 1985;115: 807–13.

102. Schultz M, Leist M, Elsner A et al. Methods Enzymol 1997;282:297–310.

103. Smith KS, Lee C-L, Ridlington JW et al. Lipids 2003;38: 813–9.
104. Traber MG, Elsner A, Brigelius-Flohe R. FEBS Lett 1998; 437:145–8.
105. Swanson JE, Ben RN, Burton GW et al. J Lipid Res 1999;40:665–71.
106. Sontag TJ, Parker RS. J Biol Chem 2002;277:25290–6.
107. Sontag TJ, Parker RS. J Lipid Res 2007;48:1090–8.
108. Kalsotra A, Strobel HW. Pharmacol Ther 2006;112:589–611.
109. Birringer M, Drogan D, Brigelius-Flohe R. Free Radic Biol Med 2001;31:226–32.
110. Parker RS, Sontag TJ, Swanson JE. Biochem Biophys Res Commun 2000;277:531–4.
111. Ikeda S, Tohyama T, Yamashita K. J Nutr 2002;132:961–6.
112. Kluth D, Landes N, Pfluger P et al. Free Radic Biol Med 2005;38:507–14.
113. Ohnmacht S, Nava P, West R et al. Bioorg Med Chem 2008;16:7631–8.
114. Stahl W, Graf P, Brigelius-Flohe R et al. Anal Biochem 1999;275:254–9.
115. Pope SA, Burtin GE, Clayton PT et al. Free Radic Biol Med 2002;33:807–17.
116. Cho JY, Kang DW, Ma X et al. J Lipid Res 2009;50:924–37.
117. Jiang Q, Freiser H, Wood KV et al. J Lipid Res 2007;48: 1221–30.
118. Christians U. Ther Drug Monit 2004;26:104–6.
119. Mustacich DJ, Gohil K, Bruno RS et al. J Nutr Biochem 2009;20:469–76.
120. Mustacich DJ, Shields J, Horton RA et al. Arch Biochem Biophys 1998;350:183–92.
121. Mustacich DJ, Vo AT, Elias VD et al. Free Radic Biol Med 2007;43:610–8.
122. Shearer MJ, Bach A, Kohlmeier M. J Nutr 1996;126: 1181S–6S.
123. Harrington DJ, Booth SL, Card DJ et al. J Nutr 2007;137: 1763–8.
124. McDonald MG, Rieder MJ, Nakano M et al. Mol Pharmacol 2009;75:1337–46.
125. Lee IM, Cook NR, Gaziano JM et al. JAMA 2005;294:56–65.
126. Glynn RJ, Ridker PM, Goldhaber SZ et al. Circulation 2007;116:1497–503.
127. Traber MG. Nutr Rev 2008;66:624–9.
128. Tovar A, Ameho CK, Blumberg JB et al. Nutr Metab (Lond) 2006;3:29.
129. Booth SL, Golly I, Sacheck JM et al. Am J Clin Nutr 2004;80:143–8.
130. Barella L, Muller PY, Schlachter M et al. Biochim Biophys Acta 2004;1689:66–74.
131. Helson L. Thromb Res 1984;35:11–8.
132. Sokol RJ, Heubi JE, Iannaccone ST et al. N Engl J Med 1984;310:1209–12.
133. Traber MG, Jialal I. Lancet 2000;355:2013–4.
134. Morley S, Cross V, Cecchini M et al. Biochemistry 2006;45:1075–81.
135. Qian J, Atkinson J, Manor D. Biochemistry 2006;45:8236–42.
136. Morley S, Cecchini M, Zhang W et al. J Biol Chem 2008;283:17797–804.
137. Zhang WX, Frahm G, Morley S et al. Lipids 2009;44:631–41.
138. Yokota T, Shiojiri T, Gotoda T et al. Ann Neurol 1997;41: 826–32.
139. van Soest S, Westerveld A, de Jong PT et al. Surv Ophthalmol 1999;43:321–34.
140. Berson EL, Rosner B, Sandberg MA et al. Arch Ophthalmol 1993;111:761–72.
141. Lemoyne M, Van Gossum A, Kurian R et al. Am J Clin Nutr 1987;46:267–72.
142. Di Donato I, Bianchi S, Federico A. Neurol Sci 2010;31: 511–5.
143. Stephens NG, Parsons A, Schofield PM et al. Lancet 1996;347:781–6.
144. Boaz M, Smetana S, Weinstein T et al. Lancet 2000;356:1213–8.
145. Salonen RM, Nyyssonen K, Kaikkonen J et al. Circulation 2003;107:947–53.
146. Gruppo Italiano per lo Studio della Streptochinasi nell'Infarcto Miocardico. Lancet 1999;354:447–55.
147. Yusuf S, Dagenais G, Pogue J et al. N Engl J Med 2000;342:154–60.
148. Cheung MC, Zhao XQ, Chait A et al. Arterioscler Thromb Vasc Biol 2001;21:1320–6.
149. Brown BG, Zhao XQ, Chait A et al. N Engl J Med 2001;345:1583–92.
150. Waters DD, Alderman EL, Hsia J et al. JAMA 2002;288: 2432–40.
151. Vivekananthan DP, Penn MS, Sapp SK et al. Lancet 2003;361:2017–23.
152. Berry D, Wathen JK, Newell M. Clin Trials 2009;6:28–41.
153. Miller ER, 3rd, Paston-Barriuso R, Dalal D et al. Ann Intern Med 2005;142:37–46.
154. Bjelakovic G, Nikolova D, Gluud LL et al. JAMA 2007;297:842–57.
155. Levy AP, Gerstein HC, Miller-Lotan R et al. Diabetes Care 2004;27:2767.
156. Milman U, Blum S, Shapira C et al. Arterioscler Thromb Vasc Biol 2008;28:1–7.
157. Sesso HD, Buring JE, Christen WG et al. JAMA 2008; 300:2123–33.
158. Gaziano JM, Glynn RJ, Christen WG et al. JAMA 2009;301: 52–62.
159. Lippman SM, Klein EA, Goodman PJ et al. JAMA 2009; 301:39–51.
160. Pinsky PF, Miller A, Kramer BS et al. Am J Epidemiol 2007; 165:874–81.
161. Steiner M, Glantz M, Lekos A. Am J Clin Nutr 1995;62: 1381S–4S.

SUGGESTED READINGS

Di Donato I, Bianchi S, Federico A. Ataxia with vitamin E deficiency: update of molecular diagnosis. Neurol Sci 2010;31:511–5.
Food and Nutrition Board, Institute of Medicine. Dietary Reference Intakes for Vitamin C, Vitamin E, Selenium, and Carotenoids. Washington, DC: National Academy Press, 2000.
Morley S, Cecchini M, Zhang W et al. Mechanisms of ligand transfer by the hepatic tocopherol transfer protein. J Biol Chem 2008;283:17797.
Schuelke M. Ataxia with vitamin E deficiency. In: Pagon RA, Bird TC, Dolan CR et al, eds. GeneReviews [serial online] May 20, 2005 [updated September 4, 2007]. Available at: http://www.ncbi.nlm.nih.gov/bookshelf/br.fcgi?book=gene&part=aved. Accessed July 14, 2010.
Traber MG, Atkinson J. Vitamin E, antioxidant and nothing more. Free Radic Biol Med 2007;43:4.

C. VITAMINS

VITAMIN K[1]

JOHN W. SUTTIE

Vitamin K was discovered in 1929 by Henrik Dam (1), when he noted that chicks ingesting diets that had been extracted with nonpolar solvents to remove cholesterol developed subdural or muscular hemorrhages and that blood taken from these animals clotted slowly. Other investigators conducting studies of diet-related hemorrhage in animals (2), and by 1935, Dam (3) proposed the existence of a new fat-soluble factor, vitamin K. During the late 1930s, investigators established that menadione, 2-methyl-1,4-naphthoquinone, had vitamin K activity, and the vitamin was isolated from alfalfa as a yellow oil.

---

[1]**Abbreviations: AI**, adequate intake; **ApoE**, apolipoprotein E; **DRI**, dietary reference intake; **EAR**, estimated average requirement; **Gla**, γ-carboxyglutamic acid; **GRP**, Gla-rich protein; **HCO_3^-**, bicarbonate; **INR**, international normalized ratio; **K_m**, Michaelis-Menten constant; **MGP**, matrix Gla protein; **MK**, menaquinone; **OC**, osteocalcin; **PT**, prothrombin time; **RDA**, recommended dietary allowance; **ucOC**, undercarboxylated osteocalcin; **VKDB**, vitamin K deficiency bleeding; **VKORC1**, vitamin K epoxide reductase complex subunit 1.

This form, vitamin K_1, was characterized as 2-methyl-3-phytyl-1,4-naphthoquinone (4), and it was synthesized by Doisy's group at St. Louis University. The Doisy group also isolated a form of the vitamin from putrefied fish meal that was called vitamin K_2 and contained an unsaturated polyprenyl side chain at the 3-position of the naphthoquinone ring. Early investigators recognized that the vitamin K activity of some sources of the vitamin, such as putrefied fish meal, was the result of bacterial synthesis, and they also realized that several different vitamers of the K_2 series had differing chain length polyprenyl groups at the 3-position.

At the time that vitamin K was isolated and characterized, the only plasma proteins known to be involved in blood coagulation were prothrombin and fibrinogen. Dam et al (5) isolated a crude prothrombin fraction from chick plasma and demonstrated that the activity of this fraction was decreased when it was obtained from a vitamin K–deficient chick. The hemorrhagic condition resulting from obstructive jaundice or biliary problems was also shown to be caused by poor utilization of vitamin K, and these bleeding episodes were initially specifically attributed to a lack of prothrombin. A real understanding of thrombus formation and of the various soluble and cellular factors involved in regulating the generation of thrombin from prothrombin did not begin until the mid-1950s. As factors VII, IX, and X were discovered through the study of patients with clotting disorders, these factors were shown to depend on vitamin K for synthesis. For a considerable time, these three factors and prothrombin were the only proteins known to require vitamin K for their synthesis.

CHEMICAL STRUCTURE AND NOMENCLATURE

The term *vitamin K* is used as a generic descriptor of 2-methyl-1,4-naphthoquinone (menadione or vitamin K_3) and all derivatives of this compound that exhibit an antihemorrhagic activity in animals fed a vitamin K–deficient diet (Fig. 20.1). The major dietary source of vitamin K is green plants and is generally called vitamin K_1, but it is preferably called phylloquinone (USP phytonadione). The compound, 2-methyl-3-farnesylgeranyl-1,4-naphthoquinone), first isolated from putrefied fish meal, is one of a series of vitamin K compounds with unsaturated side chains called multiprenylmenaquinones that

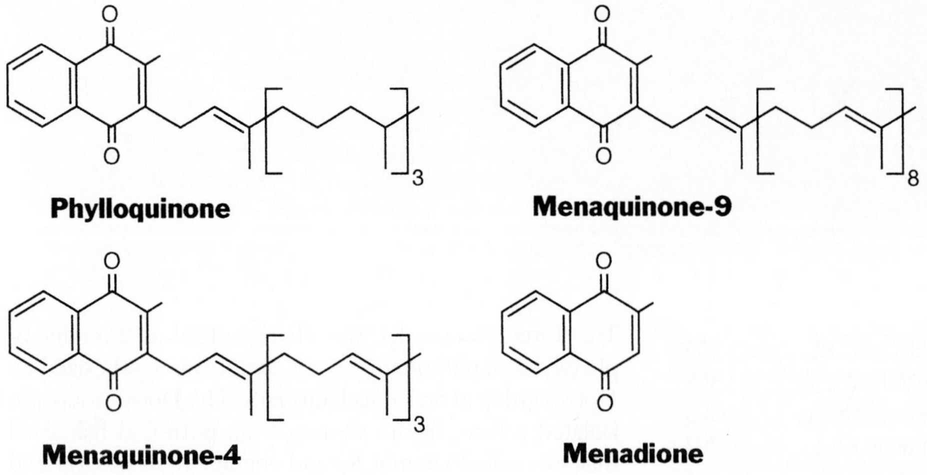

Phylloquinone

Menaquinone-9

Menaquinone-4

Menadione

Fig. 20.1. Structures of vitamin K active compounds. Phylloquinone (vitamin K_1) synthesized in plants is the main dietary form of vitamin K. Menaquinone-9 is a prominent member of a series of menaquinones (vitamin K_2) produced by intestinal bacteria, and menadione, vitamin K_3, is a synthetic compound that can be converted to menaquinone-4 by animal tissues.

are produced by a limited number of anaerobic bacteria and are present in large quantities in the lower bowel. This particular menaquinone (MK) has 7 isoprenoid units, or 35 carbons, in the side chain; it was once called vitamin K_2, but that term is currently used to describe any of the vitamers with an unsaturated side chain, and this compound would be identified as MK-7. Vitamins of the MK series with up to 13 prenyl groups have been identified, but the predominant forms found in the gut are MK-7 through MK-9. MK-4 (2-methyl-3-geranylgeranyl-1,4-naphthoquinone) can be formed in animal tissues by alkylation of menadione (6) and is the biologically active tissue form of the vitamin used when menadione is taken as a dietary supplement.

SOURCES AND UTILIZATION OF VITAMIN K

Analysis, Food Content, and Bioavailability

Standardized procedures suitable for the assay of the vitamin K content of foods are available, and sufficient values have been obtained (7) to provide a reasonable estimate of dietary intake of the vitamin (Table 20.1). Green, leafy vegetables are the foods with the highest phylloquinone content in most diets. Foods providing substantial amounts of the vitamin to most of the population are spinach (380 µg/100 g), broccoli (180 µg/100 g), and iceberg lettuce (35 µg/100 g). Fats and oils also contribute to the daily vitamin K intake of many individuals.

The phylloquinone content of oils varies considerably; soybean oil (190 µg/100 g) and canola oil (130 µg/100 g) have a high content, and corn oil (3 µg/100 g) is a poor source. The source of fat or oil has a major influence on the vitamin K content of margarine and prepared foods with a high fat content. The process of hydrogenation to convert plant oils to solid margarines or shortening converts some of the phylloquinone to 2′,3′-dihydrophylloquinone with a completely saturated side chain. The biologic activity of this form of the vitamin is lower than that of phylloquinone but has not been accurately determined. Investigators have found that the intake of this form of

the vitamin by the US population is 20% to 25% that of phylloquinone (8).

The bioavailability of phylloquinone from various foods in human subjects has been difficult to assess. Initial studies compared the increase in plasma phylloquinone from the consumption of green vegetables with that of pure phylloquinone. These limited studies suggested that the bioavailability of phylloquinone from various vegetable

TABLE 20.1	PHYLLOQUINONE CONCENTRATION OF COMMON FOODS[a]		
FOOD ITEM	µg/100 g	FOOD ITEM	µg/100 g
Vegetables		Fats and Oils	
Collards	440	Soybean oil	193
Spinach	380	Canola oil	127
Salad greens	315	Cottonseed oil	60
Broccoli	180	Olive oil	55
Brussels sprouts	177	Margarine	42
Cabbage	145	Butter	7
Bib lettuce	122	Corn oil	3
Asparagus	60		
Okra	40	Prepared foods	
Iceberg lettuce	35	Salad dressings	100
Green beans	33	Coleslaw	80
Green peas	24	Mayonnaise	41
Cucumbers	20	Beef chow mein	31
Cauliflower	20	Muffins	25
Carrots	10	Doughnuts	10
Tomatoes	6	Potato chips	15
Potatoes	1	Apple pie	11
		French fries	5
Protein sources		Macaroni/cheese	5
Dry soybeans	47	Lasagna	5
Dry lentils	22	Pizza	4
Liver	5	Hamburger/bun	4
Eggs	2	Hot dog/bun	3
Fresh meats	<1	Baked beans	3
Fresh fish	<1	Bread	3
Whole milk	<1		

[a]Median values.

Modified from Food and Nutrition Board, Institute of Medicine. Dietary Reference Intakes for Vitamin A, Vitamin K, Arsenic, Boron, Chromium, Copper, Iodine, Iron, Manganese, Molybdenum, Nickel, Silicon, Vanadium, and Zinc. Washington DC: National Academy Press, 2001.

sources should not be considered more than 15% to 20% as available as phylloquinone consumed as a supplement. The availability of phylloquinone from vegetable oil added to corn oil was found to be about twice that from broccoli. The use of stable isotopes labeled phylloquinone should result in more accurate measurements of bioavailability (9–11). These findings demonstrate that meal composition is an important factor (12).

A limited number of foods, mainly cheeses, do contain a significant (50 to 70 μg/100 g) amount of long-chain MKs, and a fermented soybean product, natto, that is consumed mainly in the Japanese market contains nearly 1000 μg/100 g of MK-7. Limited data indicate that the absorption of long-chain MKs may be substantially higher than the absorption of phylloquinone from green vegetables (13).

Absorption and Transport of Vitamin K

Phylloquinone, the predominant dietary form of the vitamin, is absorbed from the intestine through the lymphatic system (14), and absorption is decreased in patients with biliary insufficiency or various malabsorption syndromes. Phylloquinone in plasma is predominantly carried by the triglyceride-rich lipoprotein fraction containing very-low-density lipoproteins and chylomicron remnants, although some is located in the low-density lipoprotein and high-density lipoprotein fractions (15). Plasma phylloquinone concentrations in a physiologically normal population have been shown to have a mean of approximately 1.0 nmol/L (~0.45 ng/mL), with a wide range in values from 0.3 to 2.6 nmol/L (16). As expected from this route of transport, plasma phylloquinone concentrations are strongly correlated with plasma lipid levels (17).

The major route of entry of phylloquinone into tissues appears to be through clearance of chylomicron remnants by apolipoprotein E (ApoE) receptors. The polymorphism of ApoE influences fasting plasma phylloquinone concentrations. This response is correlated with the hepatic clearance of chylomicron remnants from the circulation, with ApoE2 having the slowest rate of removal (18). The secretion of phylloquinone from the liver and the process by which the vitamin moves among organs are not yet understood.

The total human body pool of phylloquinone is very small, and turnover is rapid. A peak of circulating phylloquinone concentration following absorption has been shown to be rapidly decreased (half-life ~15 minutes), followed by a slower decrease (half-life ~2.5 hours) (10). Although the total amount of vitamin K is relatively high, long-chain MKs, rather than phylloquinone, are the major source of the vitamin in liver (2). Data based on liver biopsies of patients fed diets very low in vitamin K before surgery indicate that approximately two thirds of hepatic phylloquinone was lost in 3 days (19). These findings are consistent with a small pool size of phylloquinone that turns over very rapidly. The large amount of MKs in the liver, however, turns over at a much lower rate.

The major route of ingested phylloquinone excretion is through the feces, and very little unmetabolized vitamin is excreted. Many details of the metabolic transformation of the vitamin are currently lacking, but investigators have shown that the side chains of phylloquinone and MK-4 are shortened to seven or five carbon atoms yielding a carboxylic acid group at the end (14, 20). These [5]C and [7]C-aglycones, which are the major metabolites of phylloquinone, are excreted in the urine at concentrations that are related to the intake of the vitamin (21). Studies have also shown that glucuronides of menadione are excreted in urine at an amount that is positively related to phylloquinone (22). The mechanism by which menadione is cleaved from various sources of vitamin K or its metabolites is not known. Evidence indicates the existence of numerous other unidentified metabolites, and it also shows that treatment of patients with warfarin, which results in a substantial conversion of the body pool of phylloquinone to phylloquinone-2,3-epoxide, leads to the generation of new metabolites.

Utilization of Menaquinones from the Large Bowel

Substantial amounts of vitamin K in the form of long-chain MKs are known to be present in the human gut. Relatively few of the bacteria that comprise the normal intestinal flora are major producers of MKs. Obligate anaerobes of the *Bacteroides (B. fragilis), Eubacterium, Propionibacterium,* and *Arachnia* genera are major producers, however, as are facultatively anaerobic organisms such as *Escherichia coli.* The amount of vitamin K in the gut can be quite large, and the amounts found in total intestinal tract contents from five patients who underwent colonoscopy ranged from 0.3 to 5.1 mg (23), with MK-9 and MK-10 the major contributors. These amounts are considerably larger than the daily dietary requirement for the vitamin, which is less than 100 μg/day. Long-chain MKs, mainly MK-6, MK-7, MK-10, and MK-11, are present at very low levels in plasma, but they have been found in human liver at levels that greatly exceed the phylloquinone concentration (24).

A major question remaining is how these very lipophilic compounds that are present as constituents of bacterial membranes are absorbed from the lower bowel. Little evidence on the route of absorption and transport of these vitamins to the liver is available.

Vitamin K deficiency in the adult human that is characterized by vitamin K–responsive hypoprothrombinemia is a very rare condition, and numerous case reports of antibiotic-induced hypoprothrombinemia are often cited as evidence of the importance of bacterial MKs. These antibiotic-induced hypoprothrombinemias have historically been presumed to result from a decrease in the synthesis of MKs by gut organisms (25), with the underlying assumption that MKs are important in satisfying at least a portion of the normal human requirement for vitamin K. In nearly all these case reports, however, evidence of decreased MK synthesis in the presence of antibiotic treatment is lacking, and the drugs themselves may have influenced hemostatic control. The difficulty in producing a clinically significant deficiency in human subjects, such as an increased prothrombin time (PT) by dietary restriction, and the known rapid turnover of the body phylloquinone pool strongly suggest that MKs do contribute to maintaining adequate vitamin K status (24), but the magnitude of the contribution cannot be determined with the available data.

VITAMIN K–DEPENDENT PROTEINS

Hemostasis-Related Plasma Proteins

Prothrombin, the circulating zymogen of the procoagulant thrombin, was the first protein shown to depend on vitamin K for its synthesis. Prothrombin was also the first protein demonstrated to contain γ-carboxyglutamic acid (Gla) residues. Plasma clotting factors VII, IX, and X were all initially identified because their activity was decreased in the plasma of a patient with a hereditary bleeding disorder (26), and these factors were subsequently shown to depend on vitamin K$_I$ for their synthesis. Until the mid-1970s, these four vitamin K–dependent clotting factors were the only proteins known to require this vitamin for their synthesis.

A complex series of events (Fig. 20.2), which lead to the generation of thrombin by proteolytic activation of protease zymogens (27, 28), is essential for hemostasis. The vitamin K–dependent clotting factors are involved in these activation and propagation events through membrane-associated complexes with each other and with accessory proteins. All these proteins contain a number of Gla residues, and their amino terminal Gla domain is very homologous, with 10 to 13 Gla residues in each, in essentially the same position as in prothrombin.

In addition to the classic vitamin K–dependent proteins, three more Gla-containing plasma proteins with similar homology have been discovered. Protein C and protein S participate in thrombin-initiated inactivation of factor V and therefore play an anticoagulant rather than a procoagulant role in normal hemostasis (29). In addition to the Gla domain, with approximately 40 residues, the vitamin K–dependent proteins have other common features. The Gla domain of prothrombin is followed by two kringle domains, which are also found in plasminogen, and a serine protease domain. Factors VII, IX, and X and protein C contain two epidermal growth factor domains and a serine protease domain, whereas protein S contains four epidermal growth factor domains but is not a serine protease. The function of the seventh Gla-containing plasma protein (protein Z), which is not a protease zymogen, has been shown to have an anticoagulant function under some conditions (30). Because these proteins play a critical role in hemostasis, they have been extensively studied; the cDNA and genomic organization of each of them is well documented,

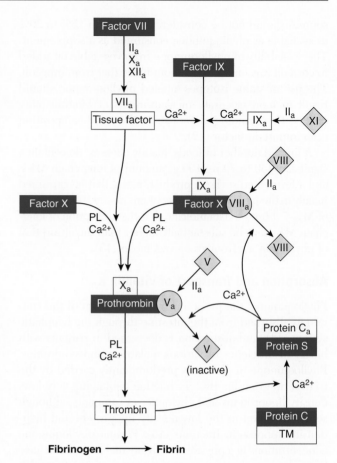

Fig. 20.2. Vitamin K–dependent clotting factors involved in blood coagulation. The vitamin K–dependent procoagulants (prothrombin and factors VII, IX, and X) circulate as zymogens of serine proteases until converted to their active (subscript a) forms. Initiation of this process occurs when vascular injury exposes tissue factor to blood (extrinsic pathway). The product of the activation of one factor can activate a second zymogen, and this cascade effect results in the rapid activation of prothrombin to thrombin and the subsequent conversion of soluble fibrinogen to the insoluble fibrin clot. Some of the steps in this activation involve an active protease, a second vitamin K–dependent protein substrate, and an additional plasma protein cofactor *(circles)* to form a calcium (Ca^{2+})-mediated association with a phospholipid (PL) surface. The formation of activated factor X can also occur through thrombin activation of factor XI and subsequently factor IX (intrinsic pathway). The other two vitamin K–dependent proteins participate in hemostatic control as anticoagulants, not procoagulants. Protein C is activated by thrombin (factor II$_a$) in the presence of an endothelial cell protein called thrombomodulin (TM). Activated protein C functions in a complex with protein S to inactivate factors V$_a$ and VIII$_a$ and to limit clot formation.

and many genetic variants of these proteins have been identified as risk factors in coagulation disorders (31).

Proteins Found in Calcified Tissue

The first vitamin K–dependent Gla-containing protein discovered that was not located in plasma was isolated from bone (32, 33). This 49-residue protein containing 3 Gla residues was called osteocalcin (OC) or bone Gla protein (BGP), and it had little structural homology with the vitamin K–dependent plasma proteins. Although OC is the second most abundant protein in bone, its function is not yet clearly defined. Rats maintained on a protocol of anticoagulant treatment and vitamin K administration to prevent bleeding problems developed fusion of the proximal tibia growth plate (34). This finding suggests that OC is involved in some manner in the control of tissue mineralization or skeletal turnover, but OC gene knockout mice have been shown to produce more dense bone rather than a defect in bone formation (35).

OC produced in bone appears in plasma at concentrations that are high in young children and approach adult levels at puberty, and its concentrations are increased in Paget disease and other conditions of rapid bone turnover. Bone also contains a second low-molecular-weight (79 residue) protein with 5 Gla residues isolated from bone and is called matrix Gla protein (MGP). This protein has a structural relationship with OC but is also present in other tissues and is synthesized in cartilage and many other soft tissues (37). The protein has been difficult to study because of its hydrophobic nature, relative insolubility, and tendency to aggregate. As with OC, details of its physiologic role are unclear, but in studies with MGP knockout mice, death ensued from spontaneous calcification of arteries and cartilage (38). Arterial calcification was also demonstrated in a warfarin-treated rat model (39).

More recently, additional vitamin K–dependent proteins associated with calcified tissue have been identified. Although evidence to support a specific function in calcified tissues is lacking, the plasma protein, protein S, which is produced in the liver, is also synthesized by bone cells. Gla-rich protein (GRP), the most extensively carboxylated protein known (40), was initially found in sturgeon cartilage and was subsequently demonstrated to be expressed and accumulated in the soft tissue of rats and humans. Although the metabolic role of this protein has not been established, it appears to play a role in connective tissue calcification (41). A protein expressed by mesenchymal stroma cells, periostin, has been demonstrated to contain four Gla-rich fascilin-like domains (42). Its role is not known, and periostin null mice are grossly normal at birth, but severely growth retarded (43).

Other Proteins

Limited numbers of other mammalian proteins have been found to contain Gla residues and therefore depend on vitamin K for their synthesis. One such protein is Gas 6, a ligand for the tyrosine kinase Axl (44), which appears to be a growth factor for mesangial and epithelial cells. Two proline-rich Gla proteins (PRGP-1 and PRGP-2) were discovered) as integral membrane proteins with an extracellular amino terminal domain that is rich in Gla residues (45). Subsequently, two other members of this transmembrane Gla protein family (TMG-3 and TMG-4) were cloned (46). The specifics of the role of these cell surface receptors are not yet known. Vitamin K–dependent proteins are not confined to vertebrates, and many toxic venom peptides secreted by marine *Conus* snails are rich in Gla

residues (47). Vitamin K–dependent proteins have also been found in snake venom (48), and the carboxylase has been cloned from certain vertebrates, the *Conus* snail, a tunicate, and drosophila (49). The strong sequence homology of the carboxylase enzyme from these phylogenetic systems suggests that this posttranslational modification of glutamic acid is of ancient evolutionary origin, and that numerous vitamin K–dependent proteins are yet to be discovered.

BIOCHEMICAL ROLE OF VITAMIN K

A period of approximately 40 years elapsed between the discovery of vitamin K and the determination, beginning in the 1960s, of its metabolic role. Early theories that vitamin K controlled the production of specific proteins at a transcriptional level could not be proven. Abnormalities of clotting times in anticoagulated patients suggested that a circulating inactive but immunochemically similar form of prothrombin, referred to as "abnormal prothrombin," was present in increased concentrations in the plasma of these patients.

Characterization of the abnormal prothrombin isolated from the plasma of cows fed the anticoagulant dicumarol led directly to an understanding of the metabolic role of vitamin K. This protein lacked the specific calcium-binding sites present in normal prothrombin and did not demonstrate the calcium-dependent association with negatively charged phospholipid surfaces that was known to be essential for prothrombin activation. Acidic peptides were obtained by proteolytic enzyme digestion of prothrombin and were shown to contain Gla, a previously unrecognized acidic amino acid (50, 51). Gla residues could not be obtained by proteolysis of the abnormal prothrombin. All 10 of the glutamic acid residues in the first 42 residues of bovine prothrombin were subsequently shown to be posttranslationally γ-carboxylated to form these effective calcium-binding groups.

Vitamin K–Dependent Carboxylase

The discovery of Gla residues in prothrombin led to the demonstration that crude rat liver microsomal preparations contained an enzymatic activity (the vitamin K–dependent carboxylase) that promoted a vitamin K–dependent incorporation of ^{14}C bicarbonate ($H^{14}CO_3^-$) into endogenous precursors of vitamin K–dependent proteins present in these preparations (52). Small peptides containing adjacent Glu-Glu sequences such as Phe-Leu-Glu-Glu-Val were substrates for the enzyme, and they were used to study the properties of this unique carboxylase. The rough microsomal fraction of liver was highly enriched in carboxylase activity, and the carboxylation event was located to the luminal side of the rough endoplasmic reticulum. The vitamin K–dependent carboxylation reaction does not require adenosine triphosphate, and the energy to drive this carboxylation reaction is derived from the oxidation of the reduced, hydronaphthoquinone, form of vitamin K (vitamin KH_2) by O_2 to form vitamin K-2,3-epoxide (Fig. 20.3).

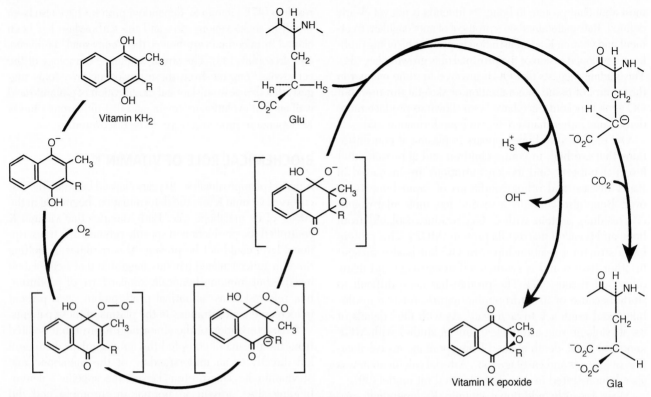

Fig. 20.3. The vitamin K–dependent γ-glutamyl carboxylase. The available data support an interaction of oxygen (O_2) with vitamin KH_2, the reduced (hydronaphthoquinone) form of vitamin K, to form an oxygenated intermediate that is sufficiently basic to abstract the γ-hydrogen of the glutamyl residue. The products of this reaction are vitamin K-2,3-epoxide and a glutamyl carbanion. Attack of CO_2 on the carbanion leads to the formation of a γ-carboxyglutamyl residue (Gla). The bracketed peroxy, dioxetane, and alkoxide intermediates have not been identified in the enzyme catalyzed reaction but are postulated based on model organic reactions, and the available data are consistent with their presence.

The lack of a requirement for biotin and studies of the carbon dioxide/bicarbonate (CO_2/HCO_3^-) requirement indicate that CO_2 rather than HCO_3^- is the active species in the carboxylation reaction. Studies of substrate specificity at the vitamin K–binding site of the enzyme have shown that although some differences in biologic activity can be measured, phylloquinone, MK-4, and the predominant intestinal forms of the vitamin, MK-6 and MK-8, are all effective substrates. Synthesis and assay of large numbers of high (Michaelis-Menten constant (K_m)) low-molecular-weight peptide substrates of the enzyme failed to reveal any unique sequences surrounding the Glu residue that are needed as a signal for carboxylation.

Very few of the proteins secreted by the liver to the plasma are vitamin K dependent, so an efficient mechanism for recognizing the precursors of the vitamin K–dependent proteins is an essential prerequisite for efficient carboxylation. Cloning of the vitamin K–dependent proteins revealed that their primary gene products contain a very homologous domain between the amino terminus of the mature protein and the signal sequence that targets the polypeptide for the secretory pathway. This propeptide region appears to be both a docking or recognition site for the enzyme (53) and a modulator of the activity of the enzyme by decreasing the apparent K_m of the Glu site substrate (54). All vitamin K–dependent proteins contain

this approximately 18-residue sequence, which is cleaved before secretion of the protein.

Although the carboxylase-binding affinities of the propeptides for different proteins differ significantly (55), propeptides are required for efficient carboxylation. The role of vitamin K in the overall reaction catalyzed by the enzyme is to abstract the hydrogen on the γ-carbon of the glutamyl residue to allow attack of CO_2 at this position. The association between epoxide formation, Gla formation, and γ-C-H bond cleavage has been studied, and the reaction efficiency, defined as the ratio of Gla residues formed to gg-C-H- bonds cleaved, has been shown to be independent of Glu substrate concentrations and to approach unity at high CO_2 concentrations (56).

Identification of an intermediate chemical form of vitamin K that could be sufficiently basic to abstract the γ-hydrogen of the glutamyl residue was first proposed by Dowd et al (57). These investigators suggested that an initial attack of O_2 at the naphthoquinone carbonyl carbon adjacent to the methyl group results in the formation of a dioxetane ring, which generates an alkoxide intermediate. This intermediate is hypothesized to be the strong base that abstracts the γ-methylene hydrogen and leaves a carbanion that can interact with CO_2. This pathway leads to the incorporation of one atom of molecular oxygen into vitamin K epoxide and the second to water (58, 59).

Although the general scheme shown in Figure 20.3 is consistent with all the available data, the details of this mechanism are not yet clear.

Although progress in purifying the enzyme was slow, the enzyme was eventually purified to near homogeneity (60) and cloned (61). The carboxylase is a unique 758-amino acid residue protein with a sequence suggestive of an integral membrane protein, with some membrane spanning domains in the N-terminus and a C-terminal domain located in the lumen of the endoplasmic reticulum. Investigators demonstrated that the multiple Glu sites on the substrate for this enzyme are carboxylated processively as they are bound to the enzyme by their propeptide (62), whereas the Gla domain undergoes intramolecular movement to reposition each Glu for catalysis, and release of the carboxylated substrate is the rate limiting step in the reaction (63). Further details of the morphology of the enzyme within the membrane, location and identification of key active site residues, and the wide distribution of the enzyme within the animal kingdom are available in published reviews (2, 49, 64, 65).

Vitamin K Epoxide Reductase

As vitamin K–dependent proteins are degraded, the Gla residues released are not used to form new proteins or metabolized but are excreted in the urine (66).

The amount of Gla excreted by an adult human is in the range of 50 μmol/day, so a similar amount must be formed each day. The dietary requirement of vitamin K is only approximately 0.2 μmol/day, and tissue stores are very low. A mole of vitamin is oxidized for each mole of Gla formed, and the vitamin K-2,3-epoxide generated by the carboxylase is actively recycled by an enzyme called the vitamin K epoxide reductase.

The hepatic ratio of the epoxide relative to that of the vitamin was increased in animals administered the 4-hydroxycoumarin anticoagulant warfarin (67). This finding led to the theory that warfarin inhibition of vitamin K action is indirect, through inhibition of the 2,3-epoxide reductase. Blocking of this enzyme prevents the reduction of the epoxide to both the quinone form of the vitamin and the carboxylase substrate, vitamin KH$_2$. The study of the activity of the epoxide reductase in livers of warfarin-resistant rats (68) was key to understanding (69, 70) the details of the vitamin K cycle (Fig. 20.4).

Three forms of vitamin K—the quinone (K), the hydronaphthoquinone (KH$_2$), and the 2,3-epoxide (KO)—can feed into this liver vitamin K cycle. In normal liver, the ratio of vitamin K-2,3-epoxide to the less oxidized forms of the vitamin is approximately 1:10, but it can increase to a majority of epoxide in an anticoagulated animal. The epoxide reductase is now known (71, 72) to be a small, 163-amino acid, single-chain integral membrane

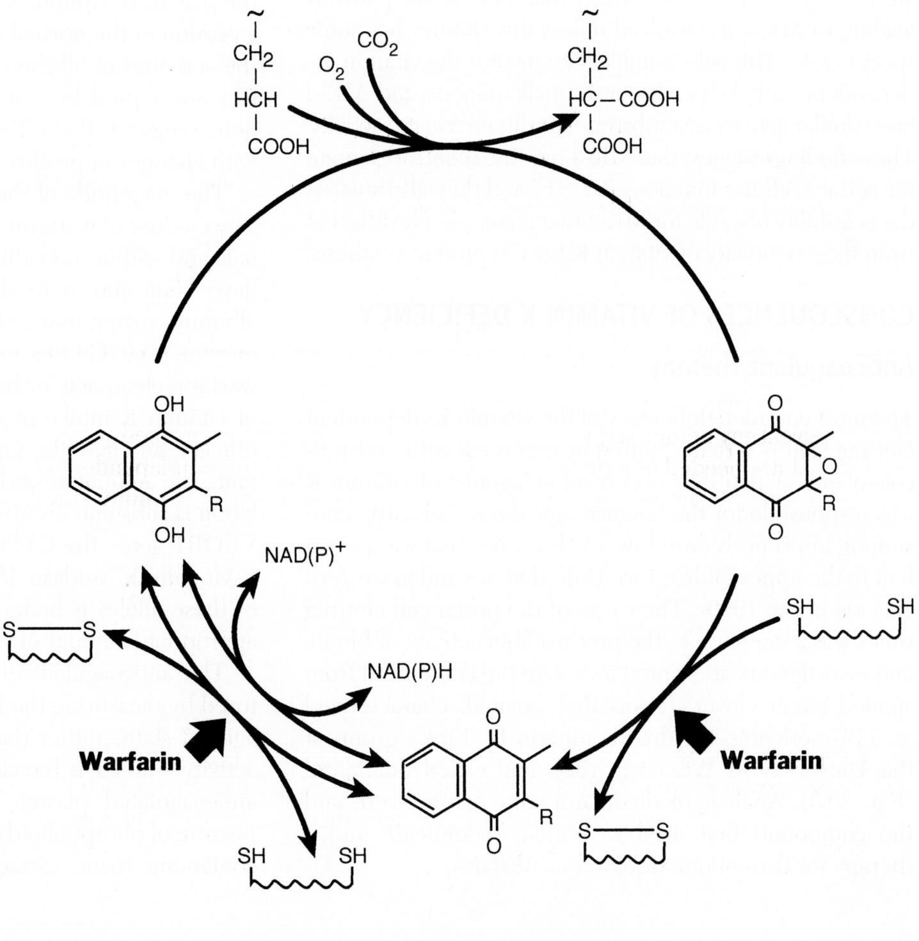

Fig. 20.4. Tissue metabolism of vitamin K. Vitamin K epoxide formed in the carboxylation reaction is reduced to the quinone form of the vitamin by a warfarin-sensitive pathway, vitamin K epoxide reductase (VKORC1), which is driven by a reduced dithiol. The naphthoquinone form of the vitamin can be reduced to the hydronaphthoquinone form either by the same warfarin-sensitive dithiol-driven reductase or by one or more of the hepatic reduced nicotinamide adenine dinucleotide (NADH) or NADH phosphate (NADPH)–linked quinone reductases, which are less sensitive to warfarin.

protein vitamin K epoxide reductase complex subunit 1 (VKORC1). Although other cellular reductases can reduce the quinone form of vitamin K (73), investigators have shown that VKORC1 knockout mice die soon after birth of a blood clotting factor deficiency (74). The enzyme contains a cysteine-based redox center, but regeneration of VKORC1 following vitamin K epoxide reduction requires a redox protein that has not yet been identified.

Synthesis and Function of Menaquinone-4

MK-4 is not a major product of bacterial synthesis of vitamin K within the large bowel, and investigators have known for some time that animals have the ability to convert menadione to MK-4. Studies of vitamin K metabolism in poultry in the early 1990s found that the liver of chicks fed phylloquinone as a source of vitamin K also contained a large amount of MK-4. High liver concentrations of MK-4 are apparently limited to chicks, but certain extrahepatic tissues such as brain, salivary gland, and pancreas of rats and humans fed phylloquinone also contain a much higher concentration of MK-4 than of phylloquinone (75, 76).

Tissue formation of MK-4 from phylloquinone fed to gnotobiotic rats (77, 78) and the demonstration that cultured cells can convert phylloquinone to MK-4 (78, 79) showed that bacterial action is not involved in the conversion. During the conversion, the phytol side chain of phylloquinone is removed and is replaced by a geranylgeranyl side chain. Details of the mechanism of this conversion are lacking, but it seems unlikely that a metabolic pathway leading to MK-4 has evolved unless this vitamer has some specific role. This role is unlikely to involve the vitamin K–dependent carboxylase, because phylloquinone and MK-4 have similar activity as a substrate for this enzymatic activity. These findings suggest that MK-4 may be a control element for certain cellular functions (80, 81), and they also suggest the possibility of a role for MK-4 that is completely different from the essentiality of vitamin K for Gla protein synthesis.

CONSEQUENCES OF VITAMIN K DEFICIENCY

Anticoagulant Therapy

The most common deficiency of the vitamin K–dependent clotting factors is that acquired by treatment with oral anticoagulants. A naturally occurring antagonist of vitamin K was responsible for the hemorrhagic disease of cattle consuming improperly cured sweet clover hay that was prevalent in the upper midwestern United States and in western Canada in the 1920s. The cause of the prolonged clotting times was a decrease in the prothrombin activity of blood, and investigators attempted to isolate the compound from spoiled sweet clover. It was first isolated, characterized as 3-3′-methylbis-4-hydroxycoumarin by Link's group at the University of Wisconsin (82), and called dicumarol (Fig. 20.5). Analogs of dicumarol were synthesized, and the compound first used as both a rodenticide and a therapy for thrombotic disease was warfarin.

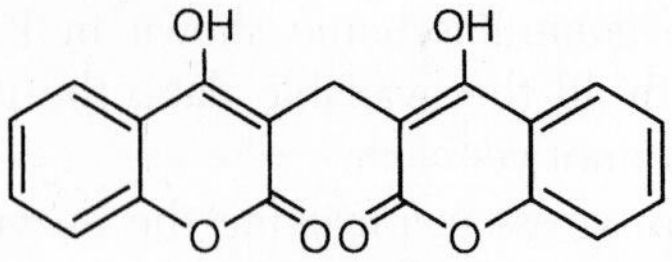

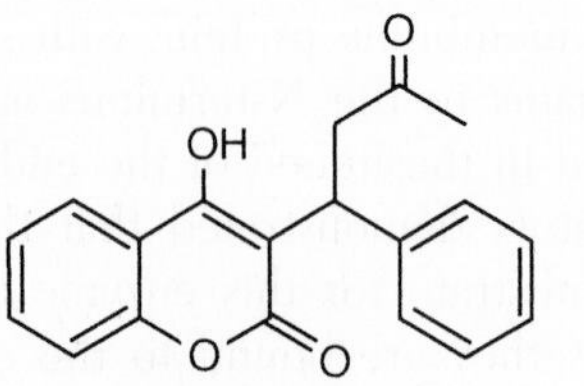

Fig. 20.5. Structure of dicumarol and warfarin. Dicumarol was the compound isolated from sweet clover as a toxic hemorrhagic factor, and warfarin is the most commonly used of several 4-hydroxycoumarin anticoagulants.

Although warfarin has a very favorable pharmacologic profile and is essentially the only coumarin derivative prescribed in North America, structurally related compounds such as acenocoumarol, phenprocoumon, and ticlomarol are widely used in Europe. The pharmacology and clinical uses of these drugs are similar to those of warfarin.

Warfarin acts as an inhibitor of the vitamin K epoxide reductase. The results of this action are an acquired deficiency of vitamin K at the tissue level and the secretion to the plasma of vitamin K–dependent proteins lacking all or a portion of the normal number of Gla residues. Although the activities of all the vitamin K–dependent clotting factors are altered by warfarin treatment, the available evidence suggests that efficacy of treatment is best correlated with changes in prothrombin activity.

The magnitude of the anticoagulant effect produced by a given dose of warfarin varies substantially among individuals and within individual patients over time. Some drugs have been shown to displace warfarin from its plasma albumin carrier, induce the hepatic cytochrome P-450 isoenzyme CYP2C9 that metabolizes warfarin, interfere with warfarin clearance, or bind warfarin in the gut. Alterations of vitamin K intake or absorption can also alter warfarin efficacy, and genetic variability is also undoubtedly important. The amount of warfarin needed to stabilize anticoagulation is substantially affected by polymorphism within the VKOR1 gene, the CYP2C9 gene, and the CYP4F2 gene, a vitamin K oxidase (83, 84). Pharmacogenetic testing of these alleles is being used to assist in determining the appropriate amount of warfarin needed for patients (85).

The anticoagulant effect of warfarin therapy is monitored by measuring the PT, a measure of combined procoagulant status rather than a true measure of prothrombin activity. The PT is the clotting time of a mixture of citrate-anticoagulated plasma, calcium, and thromboplastin, a mixture of phospholipid and tissue factor, or a tissue factor–containing tissue extract. Thromboplastin reagents vary widely in their composition, and because some reagents are much more sensitive than others, plasma from a warfarin-treated patient may yield very different PTs when tested with different thromboplastins. To overcome this problem, the international normalized ratio (INR) is used as a standardized method for reporting PT results. The INR allows interconversion of PT ratios (patient PT/mean normal PT) by use of an international sensitivity index that corrects for differences in thromboplastin sensitivities.

The goal of anticoagulant therapy is the achievement of steady-state levels of vitamin K–dependent procoagulants in the range of 10% to 30% of normal (INR of 2 to 3). The most common complication of anticoagulant therapy, bleeding, is directly related to the INR; few episodes of bleeding occur at a stable INR of less than 4.0, and a relatively high incidence occurs with INRs greater than 7.0. Excessive anticoagulation can be brought back to the desired level by lowering the warfarin dose or, if levels are severely out of range, by subcutaneous or even slow intravenous infusion of phylloquinone.

Hemorrhagic Disease of the Newborn

Hemorrhagic disease of the newborn or early vitamin K deficiency bleeding (VKDB) occurring during the first week of life in healthy-appearing neonates is the classic example of a human vitamin K deficiency (86). Low placental transfer of phylloquinone, low clotting factor levels, a sterile gut, and the low vitamin K content of breast milk all contribute to this disease. Although the incidence is low, the mortality rate from intracranial bleeding is high, and prevention by oral or parenteral administration of vitamin K immediately following birth is the standard cure. Late VKDB is a syndrome occurring between 2 and 12 weeks of age, predominantly in exclusively breast-fed infants (87) or in infants with severe intestinal malabsorption problems. Although oral administration of vitamin appears to be as effective as parenteral administration to prevent early VKDB, it may not be as effective for preventing late VKDB.

A report in the early 1990s (88) suggested that intramuscular injection of vitamin K to infants was associated with an increased incidence of certain childhood cancers. This suggestion led to a switch to oral administration of vitamin K in some countries and an increase in the incidence of late VKDB. Subsequent studies failed to show a correlation between the use of intramuscular vitamin K and the incidence of childhood leukemia or other cancers (89, 90). The current recommendations of the American Academy of Pediatrics (91) are that "vitamin K (phylloquinone) should be given to all newborns as a single, intramuscular dose of 0.5 to 1 mg."

Adult Deficiencies

Reports of uncomplicated adult deficiencies of vitamin K are rare, and most diets contain an adequate amount of vitamin K. The historical indication of a vitamin K deficiency, hypoprothrombinemia that responded to vitamin K administration, depended on the relatively insensitive PTs to assess adequacy of the vitamin K–dependent clotting factors.

Vitamin K deficiency has been reported in patients subjected to long-term total parenteral nutrition, and supplementation of the vitamin is advised under these circumstances. Low lipid intake or impaired lipid absorption resulting from the lack of bile salts adversely affects vitamin K absorption, as will malabsorption syndromes and other gastrointestinal disorders (e.g., cystic fibrosis, sprue, celiac disease, ulcerative colitis, regional ileitis, *Ascaris* infection, and short bowel syndrome).

These reports and numerous cases of a vitamin K–responsive hemorrhagic event in patients receiving antibiotics have been extensively reviewed (25). Most of these cases are assumed to result from decreased gut MK utilization by these patients, but many cases may represent low dietary intake alone. The second- and third-generation cephalosporins have been implicated in many hypoprothrombinemic episodes (92), and it is likely that these drugs exert weak carboxylase inhibition or a coumarin-like response that may be more important than an influence on the gut bacterial population.

Experimentally induced vitamin K deficiencies that are sufficiently severe to reduce PT measurements are rare. An often cited study (93) investigated the vitamin K requirement of starved, intravenously fed debilitated patients who were given antibiotics to decrease intestinal vitamin K synthesis. A significant degree of vitamin K–responsive hypoprothrombinemia was clearly established in these subjects. More recently, controlled studies using diets containing approximately 10 μg/day or less of phylloquinone demonstrated alterations using more sensitive markers of vitamin K status (94, 95), but a clinically significant decrease in PT was not seen.

ROLE IN SKELETAL HEALTH

Although MGPs, protein S, and GRPs are also synthesized or are located in bone or cartilage, the large amount of OC in bone has attracted attention as a possible factor in bone health. Small amounts of this protein circulate in plasma. Concentrations are four to fivefold higher in young children than in adults and reach adult levels at puberty. A fraction of the circulating OC in individuals within the physiologically normal population is not completely γ-carboxylated and can be influenced by vitamin K status (96–98). Most studies have defined undercarboxylated OC (ucOC) as the fraction that does not adsorb to hydroxyapatite under standard conditions. Depending on assay conditions and specific epitopes detected by the assay kits used, the fraction of ucOC reported in normal populations has ranged from 30% to 40% to less than 10%.

Clearly, the normal dietary intake of vitamin K is not sufficient to maximally γ-carboxylate OC. Supplementation with 1 mg phylloquinone per day (~10 × the current dietary reference intake [DRI]) is required to achieve maximal γ-carboxylation (99). Early reports linking this apparent marker of vitamin K insufficiency with bone health included epidemiologic observations that a low vitamin K intake is associated with increased hip fracture risk (100) and reports that ucOC is correlated with low bone mass (101). These associations do not necessarily imply causation, and they may simply be surrogate markers of general nutrient deficiencies. Patients receiving oral anticoagulant therapy have very high ucOC levels, and attempts to correlate this treatment with alterations in bone mineral density have not yielded consistent outcomes (102). The demonstration that transgenic mice lacking the OC gene showed increased rather than decreased bone mineral also suggests that the impact of OC status on bone mineralization is not yet understood (35).

Vitamin K supplementation in the form of MK-4 has been common therapy for osteoporosis in Japan and other Asian countries for several years. The standard prescription is for 45 mg of MK-4/day, a pharmacologic rather than a nutritional approach. Many rather small trials assessing bone mineral density or fracture rates of postmenopausal osteoporotic women have been conducted (103, 104), with varying responses. A postmarketing research study with 2000 subjects found decreases in new fractures in only a small subpopulation (105). Supplementation with this large amount of MK-4 has not been widely used outside of Asia, but some more recent placebo-controlled randomized clinical trials assessing the impact of supplementation of 200 μg to 5 mg of phylloquinone on skeletal health were conducted (106–110). These studies were directed toward changes in bone mineral density or bone turnover markers and did not support the view that vitamin K supplementation will have a positive role in decreasing bone fracture rate (111, 112).

MATRIX GLA PROTEIN AND VASCULAR CALCIFICATION

Early studies of MGP knockout mice found that these animals died of massive calcification of large arteries within 8 weeks of birth (38, 39), and other efforts to block MGP carboxylation in rats led to rapid calcification of the elastic lamellae of arteries and heart valves. These findings led to human studies relating low MGP activity to various aspects of soft tissue and blood vessel calcification. Reports of an association between low vitamin K intake and aortic calcification have been published (113), and a clinical trial indicated that supplementation with 500 μg of phylloquinone for 3 years slightly diminished the progression of coronary artery calcification in older men and women (114).

If vitamin K status does have an influence on vascular calcification, patients who have been treated with warfarin for years should be particularly susceptible to coronary calcification. Studies have had mixed results (115–117),

and more data will be needed to define more clearly the risk of vascular calcification that may be related to warfarin therapy. A genetic disorder, pseudoxanthoma elasticum, is also linked to the control of ectopic calcification by MGP (118, 119), given that undercarboxylated MGP is increased in patients with this disease. Although the involvement of MGP in regulating vascular calcification appears established, the clinical value of supplemental vitamin K has not yet been determined (120, 121).

DIETARY REQUIREMENTS

Reference values for vitamin K intake, established by the Dietary Reference Intakes Project of the Food and Nutrition Board of the Institute of Medicine, have been published (7). Ample data have established that essentially all individuals do not consume sufficient vitamin K to γ-carboxylate their circulating OC maximally and that supplementation with approximately 1 mg/day of phylloquinone is needed to achieve this response. Because the clinical significance of this apparent deficiency has not been established, these indices of adequacy were not used to set a reference value. The only clinically significant indicator of vitamin K status is PT, and alterations in the PT by changes in dietary intake alone are uncommon to nonexistent. Because circulating phylloquinone concentration depends highly on the previous day's intake, it is also not a satisfactory indicator of an adequate intake.

Intakes of vitamin K that are in the range of 10% of normal under controlled conditions have been demonstrated to result in decreases in urinary Gla excretion and increases in under-γ-carboxylated prothrombin, which can be measured by a commercially available immunoassay. No studies using a range of intakes that would allow the calculation of an estimated average requirement (EAR) are available, however.

The recommended dietary allowance (RDA), the historical term that is used to indicate requirements, is defined as the intake sufficient for nearly all (97% to 98%) individuals and can be calculated from the EAR. Because data are insufficient data to determine an EAR, the DRI used was the adequate intake (AI). The value is defined as "the recommended average daily intake level based on observed or experimentally determined approximations or estimates of nutrient intake by a group (or groups) of apparently healthy people that are assumed to be adequate."

AIs of infants are based on the phylloquinone content of human milk and assume that infants also receive prophylactic vitamin K at birth (Table 20.2). AIs for children, adolescents, and adults are based on the highest median intake for each age group reported by the third National Health and Nutrition Examination Survey (NHANES III). Based on those data, the intakes of pregnant or lactating women do not differ from those of the general population.

TABLE 20.2	ADEQUATE INTAKES OF VITAMIN K[a]
POPULATION	**µg/d OF VITAMIN K**
0–6-mo-old infants	2.0
7–12-mo-old infants	2.5
1–3-y-old children	30.0
4–8-y-old children	55.0
9–13-y-old boys and girls	60.0
14–18-y-old boys and girls[b]	75.0
19–>70-y-old men	120.0
19–>70-y-old women[b]	90.0

[a]Dietary reference intakes.
[b]No alteration of intake for pregnancy or lactation.

Reproduced with permission from Food and Nutrition Board, Institute of Medicine. Dietary Reference Intakes for Vitamin A, Vitamin K, Arsenic, Boron, Chromium, Copper, Iodine, Iron, Manganese, Molybdenum, Nickel, Silicon, Vanadium, and Zinc. Washington DC: National Academy Press, 2001.

Because indications of toxicity following the ingestion of large amounts of vitamin K are not available, the DRI process was unable to define a tolerable upper intake limit (UL) for vitamin K.

REFERENCES

1. Dam H. Biochem Z 1929;215:475–92.
2. Suttie JW. Vitamin K in Health and Disease. Boca Raton, FL: CRC Press Taylor & Francis Group, 2009.
3. Dam H. Nature 1935;135:652–3.
4. MacCorquodale DW, Cheney LC, Binkley SB et al. J Biol Chem 1939;131:357–70.
5. Dam H, Schonheyder F, Tage-Hansen E. Biochem J 1936; 30:1075–9.
6. Dialameh GH, Yekundi KG, Olson RE. Biochim Biophys Acta 1970;223:332–8.
7. Food and Nutrition Board, Institute of Medicine. Dietary Reference Intakes for Vitamin A, Vitamin K, Arsenic, Boron, Chromium, Copper, Iodine, Iron, Manganese, Molybdenum, Nickel, Silicon, Vanadium, and Zinc. Washington DC: National Academy Press, 2001.
8. Booth SL, Webb DR, Peters JC. J Am Diet Assoc 1999; 99:1072–6.
9. Kurilich AC, Britz SJ, Clevidence BA et al. J Agric Food Chem 2003;51:4877–83.
10. Jones KS, Bluck LJC, Wang LY et al. Eur J Clin Nutr 2008; 62:1273–81.
11. Fu X, Peterson JW, Hdeib M. Anal Chem 2009;81:5421–5.
12. Jones KS, Gluck LJC, Wang LY et al. Br J Nutr 2009;102: 1195–1202.
13. Schurgers LJ, Vermeer C. Haemostasis 2000;30:298–307.
14. Shearer MJ, Newman P. Thromb Haemost 2008;100:530–47.
15. Lamon-Fava S, Sadowski JA, Davidson KW et al. Am J Clin Nutr 1998;67:1226–31.
16. Sadowski JA, Hood SJ, Dallal GE et al. Am J Clin Nutr 1989; 50:100–8.
17. Saupe J, Shearer MJ, Kohlmeier M. Am J Clin Nutr 1993; 58:204–8
18. Kohlmeier M, Saupe J, Drossel HJ et al. Thromb Haemost 1995;74:1252–4.
19. Usui Y, Tanimura H, Nishimura N et al. Am J Clin Nutr 1990;51:846–52.
20. Wiss O, Gloor H. Vitam Horm 1966;24:575–86.
21. Harrington DJ, Booth SL, Card DJ et al. J Nutr 2007;137: 1763–8.
22. Thijssen HHW, Vervoort LMT, Schurgers LJ et al. Br J Nutr 2006;95:260–6.
23. Conly JM, Stein K. Am J Gastroenterol 1992;87:311–6.
24. Suttie JW. Annu Rev Nutr 1995;15:399–417.
25. Savage D, Lindenbaum J. Clinical and experimental human vitamin K deficiency. In: Lindenbaum J, ed. Nutrition in Hematology. New York: Churchill Livingstone, 1983:271–320.
26. Giangrande PLF. Br J Haematol 2003;121:703–12.
27. Dahlback B. Lancet 2000;355:1627–32.
28. Mann KG. Chest 2003;124(Suppl):4S–10S.
29. Esmon CT. Chest 2003;124(Suppl):26S–32S.
30. Yin ZF, Huang ZF, Cui J, et al. Proc Natl Acad Sci U S A 2000;97:6734–8.
31. Endler G, Mannhalter C. Clin Chim Acta 2003;330:31–55.
32. Hauschka PV, Lian JB, Gallop PM. Proc Natl Acad Sci U S A 1975;72:3925–9.
33. Price PA, Otsuka AS, Poser JW et al. Proc Natl Acad Sci U S A 1976;73:1447–51.
34. Price PA, Williamson MK, Haba T et al. Proc Natl Acad Sci U S A 1982;79:7734–8.
35. Ducy P, Desbois C, Boyce B et al. Nature 1996;382:448–52.
36. Price PA, Williamson MK. J Biol Chem 1985;260:14971–5.
37. Fraser JD, Price PA. J Biol Chem 1988;263:11033–6.
38. Luo G, Ducy P, McKee MD et al. Nature 1997;386:78–81.
39. Price PA, Faus SA, Williamson MK. Arterioscler Thromb Vasc Biol 1998;18:1400–7.
40. Viegas CSB, Simes DC, Laize V. J Biol Chem 2008;283: 36655–64.
41. Viegas CSB, Cavaco S, Neves PL. Am J Pathol 2009;175: 2288–98.
42. Coutu DL, Wu JH, Monette A. J Biol Chem 2008;238: 17991–18001.
43. Rios H, Koushik SV, Wang H. Mol Cell Biol 2005;25:11131–44.
44. Manfioletti G, Brancolini C, Avanzi G et al. Mol Cell Biol 1993;13:4976–85.
45. Kulman JD, Harris JE, Haldeman BA et al. Proc Natl Acad Sci U S A 1997;94:9058–62.
46. Kulman JD, Harris JE, Xie L et al. Proc Natl Acad Sci U S A 2001;98:1370–5.
47. McIntosh JM, Olivera BM, Cruz LJ et al. J Biol Chem 1984; 259:14343–6.
48. Brown MA, Hambe B, Furie B et al. Toxicon 2002;40:447–53.
49. Bandyopadhyay PK. Vitamin K–dependent gamma-glutamylcarboxylation: an ancient posttranslational modification. In: Litwack G, ed. Vitamin K. New York: Academic Press, 2008:157–85.
50. Stenflo J, Ferlund P, Egan W et al. Proc Natl Acad Sci U S A 1974;71:2730–3.
51. Nelsestuen GL, Zytkovicz TH, Howard JB. J Biol Chem 1974;249:6347–50.
52. Esmon CT, Sadowski JA, Suttie JW. J Biol Chem 1975; 250:4744–8.
53. Furie B, Furie BC. N Engl J Med 1992;326:800–6.
54. Knobloch JE, Suttie JW. J Biol Chem 1987;262:15334–7.
55. Presnell SR, Stafford DW. Thromb Haemost 2002;87:937–46.
56. Suttie JW. Vitamin K. In: Zempleni J, Rucker RB, McCormick DB et al, eds. Handbook of Vitamins. Boca Raton, FL: CRC Press Taylor & Francis Group, 2007:111–52.
57. Dowd P, Ham SW, Geib SJ. J Am Chem Soc 1991;113:7734–43.
58. Dowd P, Ham SW, Naganathan S et al. Annu Rev Nutr 1995;15:419–40.

59. Berkner KL. Annu Rev Nutr 2005;25:127–49.
60. Wu SM, Morris DP, Stafford DW. Proc Natl Acad Sci U S A 1991;88:2236–40.
61. Wu SM, Cheung WF, Frazier D et al. Science 1991;254:1634–6.
62. Stenina O, Pudota BN, McNally BA et al. Biochemistry 2001;40:10301–9.
63. Hallgren KW, Hommema EL, McNally BA et al. Biochemistry 2002;41:15045–55.
64. Presnell SR, Stafford DW. Thromb Haemost 2002;87:937–46.
65. Berkner KL. Vitamin K–dependent carboxylation. In: Litwack G, ed. Vitamin K. New York: Academic Press, 2008;78:131–56.
66. Shah DV, Tews JK, Harper AE et al. Biochim Biophys Acta 1978;539:209–17.
67. Bell RG, Matschiner JT. Nature 1972;237:32–3.
68. Lund M. Nature 1964;203:778.
69. Zimmermann A, Matschiner JT. Biochem Pharmacol 1974;23:1033–40.
70. Hildebrandt EF, Suttie JW. Biochemistry 1982;21:2406–11.
71. Rost S, Fregin A, Ivaskevicius V et al. Nature 2004;427:537–41.
72. Li T, Chang CY, Jim DY et al. Nature 2004;427:541–4.
73. Tie JK, Stafford DW. Structure and function of vitamin K epoxide reductase. In: Litwack G, ed. Vitamin K. New York: Academic Press, 2008;78:103–30.
74. Spohn G, Kleinridders A, Wunderlich FT et al. Thromb Haemost 2009;101:1044–50.
75. Thijssen HHW, Drittij-Reijnders MJ. Br J Nutr 1994;72:415–25.
76. Thijssen HHW, Drittij-Reijnders MJ. Br J Nutr 1996;75:121–7.
77. Ronden JE, Drittij-Reijnders MJ, Vermeer C et al. Biochim Biophys Acta 1998;1379:69–75.
78. Davidson RT, Foley AL, Engelke JA et al. J Nutr 1998;128:220–3.
79. Okano T, Shimomura Y, Yamane M et al. J Biol Chem 2008;283:11270–9.
80. Yoshida T, Miyazawa K, Kasuga I. Int J Oncol 2003;23:627–32.
81. Tabb MM, Sun A, Zhou C. J Biol Chem 2003;278:43919–27.
82. Link KP. Circulation 1959;19:97–107.
83. Flockhart DA, O'Kane D, Williams MS et al. Genet Med 2008;10:139–50.
84. McDonald MG, Rieder MJ, Nakano M et al. Mol Pharmacol 2009;75:1337–46.
85. Gage BF, Eby C, Johnson J et al. Clin Pharmacol Ther 2008;84:326–31.
86. Lane PA, Hathaway WE. J Pediatr 1985;106:351–9.
87. Greer FR. Nutr Res 1995;15:289–310.
88. Golding J, Greenwood R, Birmingham K et al. BMJ 1992;305:341–6.
89. Roman E, Fear NT, Ansell P et al. Br J Cancer 2002;86:63–9.
90. Fear NT, Roman E, Ansell P et al. Br J Cancer 2003;89:1228–31.
91. American Academy of Pediatrics Committee on Fetus and Newborn. Pediatrics 2003;112:191–2.
92. Weitekamp MR, Aber RC. JAMA 1983;249:69–71.
93. Frick PG, Riedler G, Brogli H. J Appl Physiol 1967;23:387–9.
94. Allison, PM, Mummah-Schendel LL, Kindberg CG et al. J Lab Clin Med 1987;110:180–8.
95. Booth SL, O'Brien-Morse ME, Dallal GE et al. Am J Clin Nutr 1999;70:368–77.
96. Sokoll, IJ, Booth SL, O'Brien ME et al. Am J Clin Nutr 1997;65:779–84.
97. Sokoll, IJ, Sadowski JA. Am J Clin Nutr 1996;63:566–73.
98. Binkley NC, Krueger DC, Engelke JA et al. Am J Clin Nur 2000;72:1523–8.
99. Binkley NC, Krueger DC, Kawahara TN et al. Am J Clin Nutr 2002;76:1055–60.
100. Booth SL, Tucker KI, Chen H et al. Am J Clin Nutr 2000;71:1201–8.
101. Vergnaud P, Garnero P, Meunier PJ et al. J Clin Endocrinol Metab 1997;82:719–24.
102. Caraballo PJ, Gabriel SE, Castro MR et al. Osteoporosis Int 1999;9:441–8.
103. Iwamoto J, Sato Y, Takeda T et al. Nutr Res 2009;29:221–8.
104. Cockayne S, Adamson J, Lanham-New S et al. Arch Intern Med 2006;166:1256–61.
105. Tamura T, Morgan SL, Takimoto H. Arch Intern Med 2007;167:94.
106. Braam LAJ, Knapen MHJ, Geusens P et al. Calcif Tissue Int 2003;73:21–6.
107. Bolton-Smith C, McMurdo MET, Paterson CR et al. J Bone Miner Res 2007;22:509–12.
108. Booth SL, Dallal G, Shea MK et al. J Clin Endocrinol Metab 2008;93:1217–23.
109. Binkley N, Harke JM, Krueger D et al. J Bone Miner Res 2009;24:983–91.
110. Cheung AM, Tile L, Lee Y et al. PLoS Med 2008;5:1461–72.
111. Gundberg C. J Bone Miner Res 2009;24:980–2.
112. Shea MK, Booth SL. Nutr Rev 2008;66:549–57.
113. Jie KS, Bots ML, Vermeer C et al. Atherosclerosis 1995;116:117–23.
114. Shea MK, O'Donnell CJ, Hoffmann U et al. Am J Clin Nutr 2009;89:1799–1807.
115. Donovan JL, Whittaker P. Circulation 2006;114(Suppl II):30.
116. Rennenberg RJ, van Varik BJ, Schurgers LJ et al. Blood 2010;115:5121–3.
117. Villines TC, O'Malley PG, Feuerstein IM et al. Calcif Tissue Int 2009;85:494–500.
118. Gheduzzi D, Boraldi F, Annovi G et al. Lab Invest 2007;87:998–1008.
119. Hendig D, Zarbock R, Szliska C et al. Clin Biochem 2008;41:407–12.
120. Wallin R, Schurgers LJ, Wajih N. Thromb Res 2008;122:411–7.
121. Schurgers LJ, Cranenburg ECM, Vermeer C. Thromb Haemost 2008;100:593–603.

21 | THIAMIN[1]

CHANTAL BÉMEUR AND ROGER F. BUTTERWORTH

HISTORICAL OVERVIEW

Chinese medical texts referred to the condition known as beriberi as early as 2700 BC, but it was not until 1884 AD that Takaki, a surgeon general in the Japanese navy, showed that the disease was the consequence of a dietary inadequacy. Many years later, Eijkman, a military doctor in the Dutch East Indies, discovered that fowl fed a diet of cooked, polished rice developed paralysis that he attributed to a nerve poison in the endosperm of the grain.

A colleague, Grijns, later correctly interpreted the connection between excessive consumption of polished rice and beriberi. Indeed, he concluded that rice contained an essential nutrient in the outer layers of the grain that was removed in polishing (1). In 1911, Funk isolated an antineuritic substance from rice bran that he called a "vitamine" because it contained an amino group. Dutch chemists went on to isolate and crystallize the active agent whose structure (Fig. 21.1) was determined in 1934 by Williams, a US chemist. Thiamin was synthesized in 1936.

CHEMISTRY AND METABOLISM

Thiamin, a water-soluble vitamin also known as vitamin B or aneurin, is chemically defined as 3-(4-amino-2-methyl-pyrimidyl-5-methyl)-5(2-hydroyethyl)-4-methylthiazolium (see Fig. 21.1) and has a molecular weight (as the hydrochloride salt) of 337.3 (2). Aqueous solutions of thiamin are stable at acid pH but are unstable in alkaline solutions or when exposed to ultraviolet light. Both the pyrimidine and thiazole moieties (see Fig. 21.1) are required for biologic activity (3). Thiamin is readily cleaved at the methylene bridge by sulfite treatment at pH 6.0.

DIETARY SOURCES AND RECOMMENDED DIETARY ALLOWANCES

Thiamin concentrations are highest in yeast and in the pericarp and germ of cereals (3, 4). Table 21.1 summarizes major dietary sources of thiamin. Nowadays, most cereals and breads are fortified with thiamin. Conversely, milk and dairy products, seafood, and most fruits are poor sources of thiamin. Thiamin is also absent from refined sugars. Thiamin is sensitive to high temperatures, and prolonged cooking of foods may result in a loss of thiamin content. Baking of bread, for example, leads to a 20% to 30% reduction in thiamin content, and pasteurization of milk may also result in thiamin losses of up to 20%. In contrast, freezing of foods does not result in significant reductions of thiamin content. Because thiamin is a water-soluble vitamin, significant amounts are lost in discarded cooking water. Thiamin is also destroyed by rays and by ultraviolet irradiation of food stuffs (3, 4). Dietary reference intake values for thiamin by life stage group (4) are shown in Table 21.2.

---

[1]**Abbreviations: α-KTG**, α-ketoglutarate dehydrogenase; **BBB**, blood-brain barrier; **eNOS**, endothelial nitric oxide synthase; **HPLC**, high-performance liquid chromatography; **IgG**, immunoglobulin G; **KP**, korsakoff psychosis; **NMDA**, N-methyl-D-aspartate; **TDP**, thiamine diphosphate; **TTP**, thiamine triphosphate; **WE**, Wernicke encepalopathy.

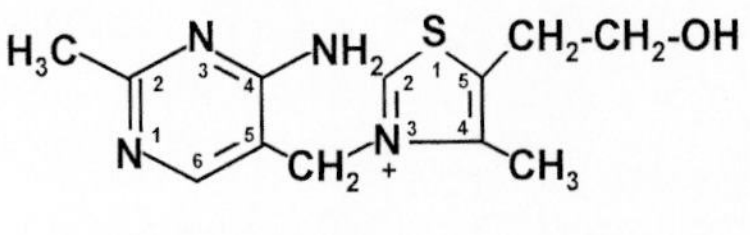

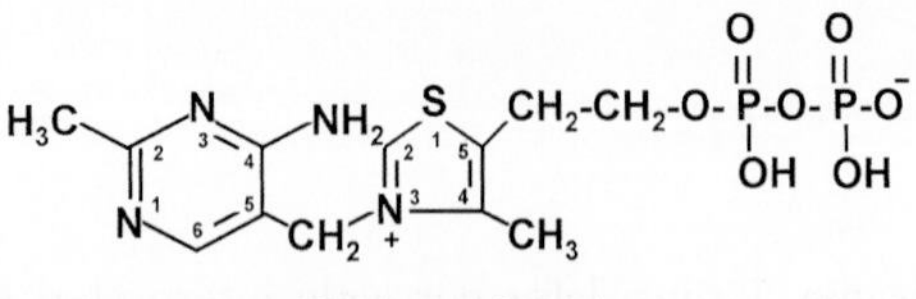

Fig. 21.1. The thiamin molecule consists of a pyrimidine ring and a thiazole moiety, which are linked by a methylene (CH_2) bridge. Thiamin is a water-soluble white crystalline solid.

TABLE 21.1	THIAMIN CONTENT OF COMMON FOOD
FOOD TYPE	THIAMIN CONTENT (mg/100 g)
Wheat flour (whole meal)	0.4–0.5
Rice	
Whole rice	0.50
Polished rice	0.03
Rice bran	2.30
Vegetables	
Peas	0.36
Other legumes	0.4–0.6
Potatoes	0.10
Cow's milk	0.04
Meats	
Beef	0.3
Lamb	0.2
Pork	≤1.0
Poultry	0.1
Refined sugars	Nil

THIAMINASES AND ANTITHIAMIN COMPOUNDS IN FOODS

Certain foods contain thiaminases—thermolabile enzymes that rapidly degrade thiamin (3). Thiaminase I is encountered in some raw fish, shellfish, and ferns, as well as in microorganisms such as *Clostridium thiaminolyticus*. Thiaminase II, which has an action distinct from that of thiaminase I, is found in other organisms such as *Candida aneurinolytica*. Thiaminases act during food storage or during passage through the gastrointestinal tract. Consequently, regular consumption of raw fish (with or without fermentation), raw shellfish, and ferns is a risk factor for the development of thiamin deficiency.

Antithiamin compounds are thermostable and have been identified in some ferns, teas, and betel nut, in which the toxic agents were found to be analogs of polyphenolic compounds such as tannic acid (tannin).

ABSORPTION, TRANSPORT, AND EXCRETION

Thiamin is absorbed by the small intestine by two distinct mechanisms, namely, active transport (at concentrations <2 μmol/L) and passive diffusion (at higher concentrations) (3). Active thiamin transport is greatest in jejunum

TABLE 21.2	CRITERIA AND DIETARY REFERENCE INTAKE VALUES FOR THIAMIN BY LIFE STAGE GROUP					
		EAR[a] (mg/d)		RDA[b] (mg/d)		
LIFE STAGE GROUP	CRITERION	MALE	FEMALE	MALE	FEMALE	AI[c] (mg/d)
0–6 mo	Average thiamin intake from human milk					0.2
7–12 mo	Extrapolation from adult requirements					0.3
1–3 y	Extrapolation from adult EAR	0.4	0.4	0.5	0.5	
4–8 y	Extrapolation from adult EAR	0.5	0.5	0.6	0.6	
9–13 y	Extrapolation from adult EAR	0.7	0.7	0.9	0.9	
14–18 y	Extrapolation from adult EAR	1.0	0.9	1.2	1.0	
18–>70 y	Depletion/repletion studies; erythrocyte transketolase activity	1.0	0.8	1.2	1.1	
Pregnancy						
14–50 y	Adult female EAR plus estimated daily thiamin accumulation by fetus		1.2		1.4	
Lactation						
14–50 y	Adolescent female EAR plus average amount of thiamin secreted in human milk		1.2		1.4	

[a]EAR, estimated average requirement, the intake that meets the estimated nutrient needs of half the individuals in a group.
[b]RDA, recommended dietary allowance, the intake that meets the estimated nutrient needs of almost all (97% to 98%) individuals in a group.
[c]AI, adequate intake, the observed average of experimentally determined intake by a defined population or subgroup that appears to sustain a defined nutritional status, such as growth rate, normal circulating nutrient values, or other functional indicators of health. The AI is used if sufficient scientific evidence is not available to derive an EAR. For healthy infants receiving human milk, the AI is the mean intake. The AI is not equivalent to an RDA.

Reproduced with permission from Food and Nutrition Board, Institute of Medicine. Dietary Reference Intakes for Thiamin, Riboflavin, Niacin, Vitamin B_6, Folate, Vitamin B_{12}, Biotin, and Choline. Washington, DC: National Academy Press, 1998:58–86.

TABLE 21.3	THIAMIN TURNOVER RATES IN PERIPHERAL NERVE, SPINAL CORD, AND BRAIN REGIONS

THIAMIN TURNOVER RATE (μg/g tissue/h)	
Peripheral nerve	0.58
Spinal cord	0.39
Brain	
Cerebellum	0.55
Medulla oblongata	0.54
Pons	0.45
Hypothalamus	0.36
Midbrain	0.29
Striatum	0.27
Cerebral cortex	0.16

Adapted from Rindi G, Patrini C, Comincioli V et al. Thiamine content and turnover rates of some rat nervous regions, using labeled thiamine as a tracer. Brain Res 1980;181:369–80, with permission.

and ileum. Intestinal transport of thiamin is rate limiting in humans. Following uptake from the gastrointestinal tract, thiamin is transported by the portal blood to the liver.

In the normal adult human body, total thiamin concentrations have been estimated to be of the order of 25 to 30 mg. Skeletal muscle, heart, liver, kidney, and brain contain relatively high thiamin concentrations. Thiamin turnover rates in brain are region dependent (Table 21.3), with highest turnover rates evident in more caudal brain structures such as striatum and cerebral cortex (5). Given these relatively fast turnover rates and because thiamin is not stored to any large extent in tissue, a continuous dietary supply is necessary. Thiamin and its acid metabolites (2-methyl-4-amino-5-pyrimidine carboxylic acid, 4-methylthiazole-5-acetic acid, and thiamin acetic acid) are excreted principally in the urine (3).

ASSESSMENT OF THIAMIN STATUS

Measurements of blood thiamin levels and urinary thiamin excretion are not reliable indicators of thiamin status. Consequently, these measurements have been replaced by indirect assays of thiamin status based on measurement and activation of the thiamin diphosphate (TDP)-dependent enzyme transketolase in red blood cell hemolysates (6) or direct measurement of TDP in these hemolysates using high-performance liquid chromatography (HPLC) (7).

Erythrocyte Transketolase Activation Assay

The widely used erythrocyte transketolase activation assay is based on measurement of transketolase activity in hemolysates of red blood cells in the absence of (and in the presence of) added excess cofactor (TDP). The enzymatic reaction catalyzed by transketolase is as follows:

$$\Leftrightarrow$$

Xylulose-5-phosphate + ribose-5-phosphate D sedo-heptulose-7-phosphate + glyceraldehyde-3-phosphate

Samples of hemolyzed whole blood are incubated at 37°C with the enzyme substrate (ribose-5-phosphate) in a buffer at pH 7.4, with or without added TDP (10 mM). The product, sedoheptulose-7-phosphate, produced per milliliter of blood per hour, is a measure of transketolase activity. The difference in enzymatic activity between the sample to which excess TDP has been added and the sample without added excess cofactor is then defined as the *TDP effect*.

In physiologically normal human volunteers, hemolysate transketolase activities are in the range of 90 to 160 μg sedoheptulose formed/mL per hour, and the TDP effect values range from 0% to 15%, depending on the levels of circulating TDP in normal subjects. Patients with marginal thiamin deficiency have TDP effect values in the 15% to 25% range, and those with values in excess of 25% are generally considered thiamin deficient. Following parenteral thiamin administration to thiamin-deficient patients, TDP effect values generally return to normal ranges within 24 hours (6).

High-Performance Liquid Chromatography

The advent of HPLC led to the publication of several procedures to measure thiamin and its phosphate esters in blood directly. One of the most reliable of these methods makes use of HPLC and precolumn derivatization. Blood samples are hemolyzed and deproteinized with perchloric acid, and supernatants are then oxidized to their thiochrome derivatives following the addition of potassium ferricyanide and sodium hydroxide and subsequent neutralization. When this technique is used, analysis times are short and recovery is excellent. The reference value for TDP in healthy volunteers is 120 ± 17.5 nmol/L (8). The HPLC method is precise and yields results similar to those of the erythrocyte activation assay (9).

FUNCTIONS OF THIAMIN IN METABOLISM

Enzyme Cofactor

After uptake into the cell, thiamin is rapidly phosphorylated to its diphosphate ester (TDP), previously referred to as thiamin pyrophosphate. TDP is an essential cofactor for enzymes involved in glucose and amino acid metabolism (10–12). Such enzymes include the following: transketolase, a key component of the pentose shunt pathway; pyruvate dehydrogenase complex, an enzyme complex situated at the point of entry of pyruvate carbon into the tricarboxylic acid cycle; α-ketoglutarate dehydrogenase (α-KGDH), a rate-limiting enzyme and constituent of the tricarboxylic acid cycle; and branched-chain keto acid dehydrogenases. The first three of these TDP-dependent enzymes are implicated in glucose and energy metabolism by the cell, as shown in simplified schematic form in Figure 21.2.

Not surprisingly, given the mitochondrial localization of the dehydrogenases and the importance of the pentose

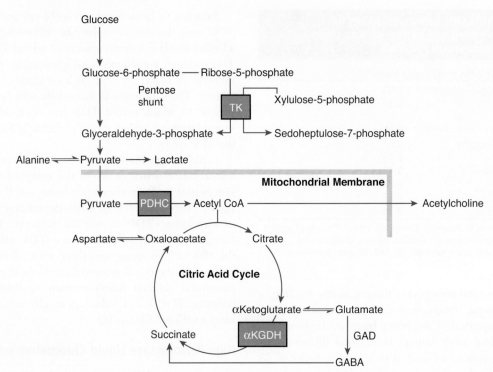

Fig. 21.2. Thiamin diphosphate–dependent enzymes. *CoA,* coenzyme A; *GABA,* γ-aminobutyric acid; *GAD,* glutamic acid decarboxylase; *αKGDH,* α-ketoglutarate dehydrogenase; *PDHC,* pyruvate dehydrogenase complex; *TK,* transketolase.

shunt pathway in cellular glucose metabolism, thiamin deficiency has a plethora of metabolic consequences, including a reduction of tricarboxylic acid intermediates, reduced synthesis of high-energy phosphates (13), and the accumulation of alanine (12) and lactate (14). Alterations of brain pH resulting from focal lactic acidosis could contribute to the pathogenesis of thalamic neuronal damage and consequent cerebral dysfunction in thiamin deficiency (15). In the brain, where the tricarboxylic acid cycle is essential for the synthesis of neurotransmitters such as acetylcholine and γ-aminobutyric acid, thiamin deficiency also results in a decrease in their synthesis (12, 16) (see Fig. 21.2). Addition of thiamin to thiamin-deprived cellular preparations in vitro (17) or to intact thiamin-deficient animals (12) results in rapid normalization in activities of TDP-dependent enzymes and their associated metabolites and neurotransmitters (12). This reversible metabolic phenomenon has been referred to as *the biochemical lesion* in thiamin deficiency.

Component of Neuronal Membranes

Electrical stimulation of nerve preparations results in the release of thiamin, a finding that led to the proposal that thiamin has a cellular function distinct from its role in the form of TDP as enzyme cofactor. The enzyme TDP phosphoryltransferase, which is expressed in brain, liver, kidney, and heart, may further phosphorylate TDP to thiamin triphosphate (TTP). Although the precise role of TTP has not yet been identified, investigators have suggested that

it activates high-conductance chloride channels (18). TTP also has regulatory properties on certain proteins involved in the clustering of acetylcholine receptors, properties suggestive of a direct role in the regulation of cholinergic neurotransmission (19).

TTP is rapidly hydrolyzed to TDP (by the action of TTPase), then to thiamin monophosphate (by the action of TDPase), and finally to free thiamin (by the action of thiamin monophosphatase). Studies suggest that thiamin phosphorylation-dephosphorylation reactions represent a compartmentalized series of processes in brain involving both neurons and surrounding glial cells (20). Genes coding for the enzymes involved in thiamin phosphorylation and dephosphorylation are being cloned and characterized, and this information is expected to assist greatly in our understanding of the role of these processes in cellular function.

CAUSES OF THIAMIN DEFICIENCY

Thiamin deficiency may result from inadequate dietary intake of the vitamin as well as from decreased absorption, defective transport, increased requirements, and enhanced losses (4). Populations at particularly high risk for the development of thiamin deficiency include those with alcoholism, human immunodeficiency virus and acquired immunodeficiency syndrome (HIV/AIDS) (21), gastrointestinal and liver diseases, and persistent vomiting (hyperemesis gravidarum) (22), as well as those receiving parenteral nutrition (16) when thiamin is omitted from the formula in error or when the thiamin is destroyed by prolonged contact with the amino acid solution. Certain drugs such as the antihyperglycemic agent tolazamide may also cause thiamin deficiency (23). Thiamin deficiency is also seen in hunger strikers and in patients with anorexia nervosa.

HUMAN THIAMIN DEFICIENCY DISORDERS

Human disorders resulting from thiamin deficiency include several forms of beriberi and Wernicke encephalopathy (WE). Furthermore, abnormalities of TDP-dependent enzymes have been reported in many different neurodegenerative and inherited metabolic disorders.

Beriberi

Clinical manifestations of beriberi vary with age (see also the chapter on manifestations of nutrient deficiency and excess). The three major forms of the disorder are dry beriberi, wet beriberi, and infantile beriberi (3). *Dry beriberi* is characterized principally by peripheral neuropathy consisting of symmetric impairment of sensory, motor, and reflex functions that affects distal more than proximal limb segments and causes calf muscle tenderness. *Wet beriberi* is associated with edema, tachycardia, cardiomegaly, and congestive heart failure in addition to peripheral neuropathy. Hemodynamic changes in wet beriberi include high cardiac output and low peripheral resistance. Rarely, patients have fulminant or "shoshin" beriberi, the major features of which are tachycardia and circulatory collapse.

Developing brain is more sensitive than adult brain to the deleterious effects of thiamin deficiency (24, 25). For example, it is well established that infantile beriberi occurs in infants breast-fed by mothers who themselves may be asymptomatic. Reports from many world populations continue to describe a high prevalence of thiamin deficiency and its complications in pregnant and lactating women, a population known to have increased thiamin requirements. Victims of trade embargoes as well as displaced persons in refugee camps are populations at particular high risk for the development of maternal thiamin deficiency (26). Increased sequestration of thiamin by the fetus and placenta during the third semester of pregnancy is thought to result in increased thiamin requirements. Thiamin concentrations are higher in umbilical cord blood compared with maternal blood, a finding consistent with preferential delivery of thiamin to the developing infant.

Eating a staple diet of polished rice and concurrently ingesting foods containing thiaminases or antithiamin compounds continue to be the major causes of maternal thiamin deficiency in many parts of the world. For example, white rice often lacks nutrient enrichment, including thiamin (27). Other causes of maternal thiamin deficiency include alcohol abuse, gastrointestinal disease, hyperemesis gravidarum, and HIV/AIDS. Investigators have shown that maternal thiamin deficiency contributes

to intrauterine growth retardation (24), a condition that results in delayed myelination of the brain that may be related to reduced activity of TDP-dependent enzymes. Maternal thiamin deficiency may also contribute to the pathogenesis of the fetal alcohol syndrome.

Infantile beriberi commonly manifests between the ages of 2 and 6 months. Infants may have cardiac, aphonic, or pseudomeningitic forms of the disorder. Infants with cardiac beriberi frequently have a loud piercing cry, vomiting, and tachycardia (3). Convulsions are common, and death may ensue if thiamin is not administered promptly.

Wernicke Encephalopathy (Wernicke–Korsakoff Syndrome)

WE is a common neuropsychiatric complication of chronic alcoholism (10). It is also encountered in patients with severe gastrointestinal disease, those with HIV/AIDS (21), and patients who receive injudicious administration of parenteral glucose or hyperalimentation without adequate B-vitamin supplementation (21). In brain tissue obtained at autopsy from patients with WE, activities of all three TDP-dependent enzymes are reduced (28).

In patients with alcoholism, thiamin deficiency results from inadequate dietary intake of the vitamin, reduced absorption resulting from gastrointestinal disease, and reduced liver thiamin stores caused by hepatic steatosis or fibrosis (10). In addition, ethanol itself inhibits thiamin transport in the gastrointestinal system and blocks brain phosphorylation of thiamin to its cofactor form (TDP) (29).

The diagnosis of WE is based generally on the acute appearance of ocular palsies, nystagmus, and gait ataxia as well as disorders of mentation (1). In addition, more than 80% of patients with WE show signs of peripheral neuropathy. However, these diagnostic criteria are nonspecific, and the diagnosis of WE is missed in many patients with alcoholism (30) as well as in those with HIV/AIDS (21). The reason for the high degree of underdiagnosis rests with the overzealous use of the classic triad of symptoms (ophthalmoplegia, ataxia, confusion) espoused by many textbooks. In practice, many cases of WE confirmed at autopsy do not manifest this triad of symptoms, and patients may show only psychomotor slowing or apathy (21). A rewriting of this textbook definition of WE is long overdue. In the meantime, thiamin deficiency should be suspected in all patients with grossly impaired nutritional status associated with chronic diseases, with particular attention paid to patients with chronic alcoholism, gastrointestinal diseases, HIV/AIDS, and persistent vomiting. Thiamin should be administered parenterally in a timely manner. It is essential to administer thiamin to all patients before infusions of glucose or parenteral nutrition are given.

Korsakoff psychosis (KP) is generally considered to occur with deterioration of brain function in patients initially diagnosed with WE (1). However, KP may be present at the time of diagnosis of WE or even, in a few cases, present without WE symptoms. KP is an amnestic-confabulatory syndrome characterized by retrograde and anterograde amnesia, impairment of conceptual functions, and decreased spontaneity and initiative.

Neuropathology

Hemorrhagic lesions of mammillary bodies and periventricular regions of the thalamus are observed in the acute stages of WE (31). Multiple acute insults eventually give rise to a chronic lesion, characterized by loosening of the neuropil (the region between neuronal cell bodies in the gray matter of the brain and spinal cord) and cell loss that manifests as mammillary body atrophy and ventricular dilatation. Also observed in WE is a significant loss of neurons in the cerebellar vermis, a phenomenon referred to as *alcoholic cerebellar degeneration*.

Magnetic resonance imaging may be used to confirm the diagnosis and to assess the extent of brain lesions. This imaging method allows the assessment of neurodegeneration and neuronal recovery (32). Mammillary body atrophy and loss of thalamic tissue leading to ventricular enlargement, as well as cerebellar atrophy, are clearly discernible (33).

Genetics

Although thiamin deficiency is very common in patients with alcoholism, only relatively few patients (10% to 12%) go on to develop WE. This observation led to the proposal of a genetic predisposition to the disorder. Much attention in this regard has been paid to the TDP-dependent enzyme transketolase. Initially, investigators proposed that a reduction in affinity of transketolase for its cofactor (TDP) could represent one such genetic abnormality. Reports of both biochemical and chromatographic variants of transketolase in cells from patients with WE have appeared in the literature (34, 35). The coding sequences of the transketolase gene were compared between cells from physiologically normal individuals and cells from patients with WE, however, and no significant differences were observed (36). This finding suggests that transketolase alterations are posttranslational.

Thiamin Diphosphate–Dependent Enzymes in Brain in Neurodegenerative Diseases

Reduced activities of TDP-dependent enzymes are found in brain tissue obtained at autopsy from patients with Alzheimer disease (37, 38). Activities of α-KGDH in particular, are significantly reduced in both genetic and sporadic forms of the disease. Decreased activities of α-KGDH have also been described in the brains of patients with other neurodegenerative diseases including Parkinson disease and progressive subnuclear palsy (11). The most plausible explanation for the selective loss of α-KGDH activity in these diseases may relate to the deleterious effects of oxidative stress resulting from the cell death cascade mechanisms in these disorders (11).

Other Thiamin Deficiency–Related Disorders

Other disorders in which a putative role for thiamin deficiency has been implicated include subacute necrotizing encephalomyelopathy, opsoclonic cerebellopathy (a paraneoplastic syndrome), and Nigerian seasonal ataxia. In addition, several inherited disorders of TDP-dependent enzymes have been reported (39). Some of these inherited disorders may respond to thiamin treatment. End stage chronic liver failure results in thiamin deficiency caused principally by depletion of liver thiamin stores. Consequently, brain dysfunction secondary to thiamin deficiency in chronic liver failure may occur (40).

Clinical Response to Thiamin Administration

Parenteral thiamin should be administered promptly to patients suspected of having beriberi or WE. Doses in the 50- to 100-mg range are initially administered intravenously or intramuscularly to replenish cellular thiamin stores (particularly liver) (3). Parenteral rather than oral thiamin administration is particularly important in patients with gastrointestinal disease or alcoholism, in whom thiamin absorption is likely to be impaired.

In wet beriberi, rapid improvement consisting of reduction in heart rate, respiratory rate, and clearing of pulmonary congestion occurs generally within 24 hours (3). Rapid improvements are also seen in infants with dry beriberi. Recovery of impaired sensation and motor weakness, in contrast, may take several weeks or months.

Response to thiamin administration in patients with WE is variable, depending on the symptoms and the degree of neuronal cell loss. Ophthalmoplegia (nystagmus, ptosis) generally improves rapidly (within 24 hours), a finding suggesting that these symptoms are the result of biochemical (metabolic) lesions in oculomotor and vestibular nuclei. Gait ataxia, conversely, responds more sluggishly to thiamin administration because, in most cases, loss of cerebellar neurons is significant (41). Similarly, the amnestic deficit that is generally thought to result from lesions in the medial-dorsal nucleus of the thalamus shows variable response to thiamin administration, and most patients have some residual memory deficit. Improvements of peripheral neuropathy in both beriberi and WE syndrome may require several months of thiamin treatment (41). In addition, complete recovery from WE has been demonstrated following aggressive thiamin treatment (42).

Selective Neuronal Cell Death Resulting from Thiamin Deficiency

Investigators have proposed that thiamin deficiency leads to two distinct types of neuropathologic lesions. The first type, characterized by neuronal disintegration, mild endothelial swelling, and sparing of the neuropil, is generally confined to the thalamus and inferior olives. Conversely, destruction of the neuropil, endothelial swelling, and neuronal sparing occur in mammillary bodies and periventricular brainstem nuclei (43). Several mechanisms have been proposed to explain the phenomenon of selective neuronal cell damage and death resulting from thiamin deficiency. These mechanisms include cellular energy failure, oxidative and nitrosative stress, N-methyl-D-aspartate (NMDA) receptor–mediated excitotoxicity, and blood–brain barrier (BBB) breakdown.

Cellular Energy Failure

As discussed earlier, thiamin deficiency is characterized by decreased brain concentrations of TDP and reduced activity of TDP-dependent enzymes (12). Attention has been focused particularly on the role of decreased α-KGDH in the pathogenesis of neuronal cell death resulting from thiamin deficiency because it is well established that α-KGDH is a rate-limiting enzyme in the tricarboxylic acid cycle responsible for cellular energy production.

Prolonged reductions in activity of α-KGDH resulting from thiamin deficiency lead to decreased glucose (pyruvate) oxidation and increased brain concentrations of alanine and lactate. Studies of oxidative metabolism in mitochondria isolated from the brains of thiamin-deficient animals revealed decreased respiration using α-ketoglutarate as substrate but no such changes in respiration using succinate (8), a finding consistent with decreased activities of α-KGDH (see Fig. 21.2). High-energy phosphates in thiamin deficiency are decreased in brainstem (13). Decreased activity of α-KGDH resulting from thiamin deficiency also reduces synthesis of amino acid neurotransmitters such as glutamate and γ-aminobutyric acid (12). Focal accumulation of lactate leading to reduced pH has been described (14), and disintegration of mitochondria has also been reported in degenerating diencephalic neurons of thiamin-deficient animals (11). Furthermore, investigators have suggested that impaired branched-chain ketoacid metabolism could contribute to the neuronal dysfunction and ultimate thalamic neuronal cell death observed in thiamin deficiency (44).

Oxidative and Nitrosative Stress

Accumulation of reactive oxygen species has been reported in brain in thiamin deficiency (45). Other indicators consistent with oxidative and nitrosative stress in brain as a result of thiamin deficiency include reports of early activation of microglia (11, 46) and increased expression of inducible nitric oxide synthase leading to increased nitrotyrosine immunoreactivity in vulnerable brain regions (47), as well as reports of increased expression of heme oxygenase-1, intercellular adhesion molecule-1, S-nitrosocysteine and cyclo-oxygenase-2 (11, 48, 49). Evidence suggests that vascular factors also contribute to thiamin deficiency–related brain damage. Such factors include increases of endothelial nitric oxide synthase (eNOS) (50). Moreover, targeted disruption (knockdown) of the eNOS gene attenuates the neuronal cell death in thiamin-deficient mice (11, 48). eNOS knockdown, but not knockdown of inducible NOS or neuronal NOS, leads to a reduction in protein tyrosine nitration.

This finding suggests a major role of eNOS as the source of nitric oxide–related nitrosative stress in thiamin deficiency. Furthermore, treatment of thiamin-deficient rats with the antioxidant N-acetylcysteine prevents the down-regulation of astrocytic glutamate transporter or excitatory amino acid transporter (EAAT-2) and increases neuronal survival (51). Reactive oxygen species production results in decreased expression of astrocytic glutamate transporters and reduced activities of α-KGDH, with the potential to result in an amplification of cell death mechanisms in thiamin deficiency (52) (see also the chapter on oxidant defenses).

NMDA Receptor–Mediated Excitotoxicity

The nature of the neuropathologic damage resulting from thiamin deficiency is similar to some degree to that encountered in excitotoxic brain injury (i.e., brain injury resulting from excessive stimulation of NMDA receptors by glutamate, a process known as *excitotoxicity* and shown to result in excessive accumulation of intracellular calcium leading to the activation of cell death mechanisms). Evidence consistent with a role of excitotoxicity in the pathogenesis of thiamin deficiency–related brain damage includes the finding of increased extracellular glutamate in brain regions that are particularly vulnerable to thiamin deficiency (53) and the report that pretreatment with the NMDA receptor antagonist MK801 leads to significant neuroprotection (54). One possible explanation for the increased extracellular brain concentrations of glutamate in thiamin deficiency is the reported loss in expression of high-affinity glutamate transporters in vulnerable brain regions (55, 51).

Blood–Brain Barrier Breakdown

The hemorrhagic lesions characteristic of experimental thiamin deficiency and of WE in humans are indicative of a breakdown of the BBB. Studies using immunoglobulin G (IgG) as an indicator of BBB integrity in thiamin-deficient animals revealed increased IgG immunoreactivity in inferior colliculus and inferior olive before the onset of cell death in these regions as well as in the medial thalamus (56–58). Microglial activation leading to the release of reactive oxygen species and cytokines is an early cellular event responsible for BBB breakdown resulting from thiamin deficiency (46). Investigators have also demonstrated that thiamin deficiency is associated with alterations in tight junction proteins (occludin, zona occludens-1, and zona occludens-2) and matrix metalloproteinase-9 (58). These alterations could be responsible for the initiation of changes to BBB integrity in thiamin deficiency (58).

REFERENCES

1. McCollum EV. A History of Nutrition. Cambridge, MA: Riverside Press, Houghton Mifflin, 1957.
2. International Union of Nutritional Sciences Committee on Nomenclature. J Nutr 1990;120:7–14.
3. Tanphaichitr V. Thiamin. In: Shils ME, Olsen JA, Shike M et al., eds. Modern Nutrition in Health and Disease. 9th ed. Baltimore: Lippincott Williams & Wilkins, 1999.

4. Food and Nutrition Board, Institute of Medicine. Dietary Reference Intakes for Thiamin, Riboflavin, Niacin, Vitamin B6, Folate, Vitamin B12, Biotin, and Choline. Washington, DC: National Academy Press, 1998:58–86.

5. Rindi G, Patrini C, Comincioli V et al. Brain Res 1980;181: 369–80.

6. Dreyfus PM. N Engl J Med 1962;267:596–8.

7. Mojzisova G, Kuchta M. Physiol Res 2001;50:529–35.

8. Parker WD Jr, Haas R, Stumpf DA et al. Neurology 1984;34: 1477–81.

9. Talwar D, Davidson H, Cooney J et al. Clin Chem 2000;46: 704–10.

10. Butterworth RF. Drug Alcohol Rev 1993;12:315–22.

11. Gibson GE, Zhang H. Neurochem Int 2002;40:493–504.

12. Butterworth RF, Héroux M. J Neurochem 1989;52:1079–84.

13. Aikawa H, Watanabe IS, Furuse T et al. J Neuropathol Exp Neurol 1984;43:276–87.

14. Hakim AM. Ann Neurol 1984;16:673–9.

15. Navarro D, Zwingmann C, Chatauret N et al. Metab Brain Dis 2008;23:115–22.

16. Harper CG. Aust N Z J Med 1980;10:230–5.

17. Pannunzio P, Hazell AS, Pannunzio M et al. J Neurosci Res 2000;62:286–92.

18. Cooper JR, Pincus JH. Neurochem Res 1979;4:223–39.

19. Bettendorff L. Metab Brain Dis 1994;9:183–209.

20. Butterworth RF. Nutr Res Rev 2003;16:277–84.

21. Butterworth RF, Gaudreau C, Vincelette J et al. Metab Brain Dis 1991;6:207–12.

22. Nightingale S, Bates D, Heath PD et al. Postgrad Med J 1982;58:558–9.

23. Kwee IL, Nakada T. N Engl J Med 1983;309:599–600.

24. Butterworth RF. Am J Clin Nutr 2001;74:712–3.

25. Fournier H, Butterworth RF. Metab Brain Dis 1990;5:77–84.

26. McGready R, Simpson JA, Cho T et al. Am J Clin Nutr 2001;74:808–13.

27. Leon Guerrero RT, Gebhardt SE, Holden J et al. J Am Diet Assoc 2009;109:1738–43.

28. Butterworth RF, Kril JJ, Harper CG. Alcohol Clin Exp Res 1993;17:1084–8.

29. Rindi G, Imarisio L, Patrini C. Biochem Pharmacol 1986;35:3903–8.

30. Harper C. J Neurol Neurosurg Psychiatry 1979;42:226–31.

31. Kril JJ. Metab Brain Dis 1996;11:9–17.

32. Dror V, Eliash S, Rehavi M et al. Brain Res 2010;1308: 176–84.

33. Charness ME, DeLaPaz RL. Ann Neurol 1987;22:595–600.

34. Blass JP, Gibson GE. N Engl J Med 1977;297:1367–70.

35. Mukherjee AB, Svoronos S, Ghzanfari A et al. J Clin Invest 1987;79:1039–43.

36. McCool BA, Plonk SG, Martin PR et al. J Biol Chem 1993;268:1397–04.

37. Gibson GE, Sheu KF, Blass JP et al. Arch Neurol 1988;45: 836–40.

38. Butterworth RF, Besnard AM. Metab Brain Dis 1990;5: 179–84.

39. Blass JP. Inborn errors of pyruvate metabolism. In: Stanbury JB, Wyngaarden JB, Frederckson DS et al., eds. Metabolic Basis of Inherited Disease. 5th ed. New York: McGraw-Hill, 1983.

40. Butterworth RF. Metab Brain Dis 2009;24:189–96.

41. Maurice V, Adams RD, Collins GH. The Wernicke-Korsakoff Syndrome and Related Neurologic Disorders Due to Alcoholism and Malnutrition. Philadelphia: FA Davis, 1989.

42. Paparrigopoulos T, Tzavellas E, Karaiskos D et al. In Vivo 2010;24:231–3.

43. Trovik A. Science 1985;11:179–90.

44. Navarro D, Zwingmann C, Butterworth RF. Metab Brain Dis 2008;23:445–55.

45. Langlais PJ, Anderson G, Guo SX et al. Metab Brain Dis 1997;12:137–43.

46. Todd KG, Butterworth RF. Glia 1999;25:190–8.

47. Calingasan NY, Park LC, Calo LL et al. Am J Pathol 1998;153:599–610.

48. Beauchesne E, Desjardins P, Hazell AS et al. J Neurochem 2009;111:452–9.

49. Gu B, Desjardins P, Butterworth RF. Metab Brain Dis 2008;23:175–87.

50. Kruse M, Navarro D, Desjardins P et al. Neurochem Int 2004;45:49–56.

51. Hazell AS, Sheedy D, Oanea R et al. Glia 2010;58:148–56.

52. Desjardins P, Butterworth RF. Mol Neurobiol 2005;31:17–25.

53. Hazell AS, Butterworth RF, Hakim AM. J Neurochem 1993;61:1155–8.

54. Langlais PJ, Mair RG. J Neurosci 1990;10:1664–74.

55. Hazell AS, Rao KV, Danbolt NC et al. J Neurochem 2001;78:560–8.

56. Calingasan NY, Baker H, Sheu KF et al. Exp Neurol 1995;134:64–72.

57. Harata N, Iwasaki Y. Metab Brain Dis 1995;10:159–74.

58. Beauchesne E, Desjardins P, Hazell AS et al. Neurochem Int 2009;55:275–281.

SUGGESTED READINGS

Beauchesne E, Desjardins P, Hazell AS et al. Altered expression of tight junction proteins and matrix metalloproteinases in thiamine-deficient mouse brain. Neurochem Int 2009;55:275–81.

Butterworth RF. Maternal thiamine deficiency: still a problem in some world communities. Am J Clin Nutr 2001;74:712–3.

Food and Nutrition Board, Institute of Medicine. Dietary Reference Intakes for Thiamin, Riboflavin, Niacin, Vitamin B6, Folate, Vitamin B12, Biotin, and Choline. Washington, DC: National Academy Press, 1998:58–86.

Maurice V, Adams RD, Collins GH. The Wernicke-Korsakoff Syndrome and Related Neurologic Disorders Due to Alcoholism and Malnutrition. Philadelphia: FA Davis, 1989.

22 RIBOFLAVIN[1]

HAMID M. SAID AND A. CATHARINE ROSS

Riboflavin (vitamin B_2) was initially isolated from milk whey in a nonpure form in 1879 (1), followed by determination of its structure and identification of its major coenzymes, flavin mononucleotide (FMN) and flavin adenine dinucleotide (FAD) (2–5). Although free riboflavin has little biologic activity, its coenzymes FMN and FAD play essential roles in normal cellular functions, growth, and development. Specifically, FMN and FAD act as cofactors for certain enzymes (flavoproteins) involved in electron transfer reactions (e.g., energy production reactions, metabolic conversion of essential micronutrients such as that of folate, vitamin B_6, niacin), drug metabolism, toxin detoxifying, and electron scavenging pathways. Riboflavin deficiency, also called ariboflavinosis, leads to degenerative changes in the nervous system, endocrine dysfunction, anemia, and skin disorders as well as inflammation of the lining of the mouth, tongue, and throat; cracks at the corners of the mouth (angular cheilitis); and red and itchy eyes (from vascularization of the cornea). Riboflavin deficiency and suboptimal levels occur in persons with alcoholism and in patients with inflammatory bowel syndrome and diabetes, as well as in elderly persons.

---

[1]**Abbreviations: EGRAC**, erythrocyte glutathione reductase activity coefficient; **FAD**, flavin adenine dinucleotide; **FMN**, flavin mononucleotide; **G6PD**, glucose-6-phosphate dehydrogenase; **Na$^+$**, sodium; **RDA**, recommended dietary allowance; **RFT**, riboflavin transporter.

CHEMISTRY, BIOCHEMISTRY, AND FUNCTION OF RIBOFLAVIN AND DERIVATIVES

The riboflavin molecule (7,8-dimethyl-10-(1′-D-ribityl)-isoalloxazine) is composed of an isoalloxazine planar ring to which a ribitol side chain is bound (Fig. 22.1). Free riboflavin has a molecular weight of 376.4, acts as a weak base in aqueous solutions, and is fluorescent. The vitamin has modest water solubility, which limits its use in parenteral and oral aqueous preparations. The riboflavin molecule is photosensitive and degrades to lumiflavin (7,8,10-trimethyl-isoalloxazine; Fig. 22.2) and lumichrome (7,8-dimethyl-alloxazine; see Fig. 22.2) at alkaline and neutral–acidic solutions, respectively. Both lumiflavin and lumichrome are biologically inactive compounds, yet they compete with riboflavin for uptake by different cells. Thus, prolonged phototherapy in neonates with jaundice and in patients with certain skin disorders may negatively affect normal body and cellular riboflavin homeostasis.

In the diet, riboflavin exists mostly in the form of FAD and FMN, with little in the free form. FMN is produced enzymatically by phosphorylation of the 5′-hydroxymethyl terminus of the ribityl side chain of the riboflavin molecule. This reaction is catalyzed by the enzyme flavokinase (Fig. 22.3). When FMN is further modified by the addition of a pyrophosphate-bridged adenyl moiety, a reaction that is catalyzed by FAD synthetase (also known as FAD pyrophosphorylase), the more abundant FAD form of the vitamin is produced (see Fig. 22.3). Conversion of free riboflavin to its coenzyme forms takes places mainly in the cytoplasm, although some conversion has also been reported to take place in the mitochondria (6–9). Riboflavin conversion to FMN and FAD appears to be affected by thyroid hormones, an effect that appears to be mediated by flavokinase activation (10–12). Riboflavin can be regenerated from FMN and FAD in reactions that involve several phosphatases (see Fig. 22.3).

FAD is used more than FMN as a coenzyme by most cellular flavoproteins in the different metabolic pathways. In addition to generating a more biologically active form of the vitamin, cellular conversion of riboflavin to FMN and FAD also serves as a trapping and retaining mechanism for this essential micronutrient in the cell. Most of the intracellular flavoproteins are located in the mitochondria;

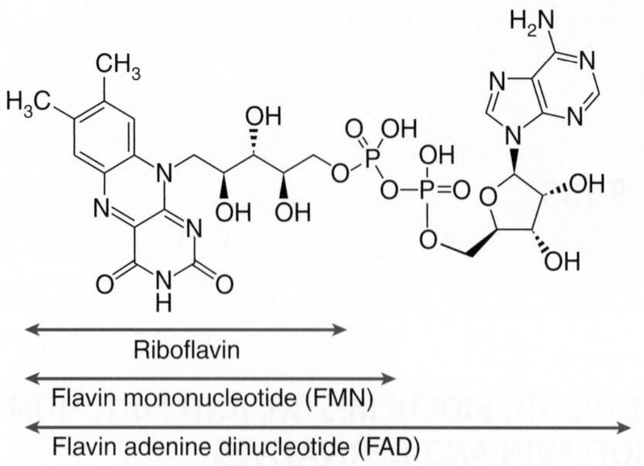

Riboflavin

Flavin mononucleotide (FMN)

Flavin adenine dinucleotide (FAD)

Fig. 22.1. Structure of riboflavin and its coenzymes flavin mononucleotide (FMN) and flavin adenine dinucleotide (FAD).

FAD (or riboflavin) is imported into this organelle by a mechanism that is different from that involved in the mitochondrial uptake of flavoproteins (9, 12–15). Transport of FAD and riboflavin into the mitochondria appears to be occurred by a specific carrier-mediated system in the mitochondrial membrane (14). Little is known about how this system is regulated at the cellular and molecular levels and about the factors that affect its function.

ASSESSMENT OF RIBOFLAVIN STATUS

Most flavins in the plasma exist in the form of free riboflavin, although some FMN and FAD are also present. All plasma flavins are associated with plasma proteins, and mostly with albumin. Two main methods are commonly used to assess riboflavin nutritional status. The first method is based on the determination of activity known as the erythrocyte glutathione reductase activity coefficient, abbreviated as EGRAC (16, 17), and the second is based on fluorometric measurement of urinary excretion of riboflavin over a period of 24 hours (expressed as total amount of riboflavin excreted or in relation to creatinine excretion). A newer method involving estimation of the activity of erythrocyte pyridoxine phosphate oxidase has been described (18). This method appears to be especially suited for use in populations with a high prevalence of glucose-6-phosphate dehydrogenase (G6PD)

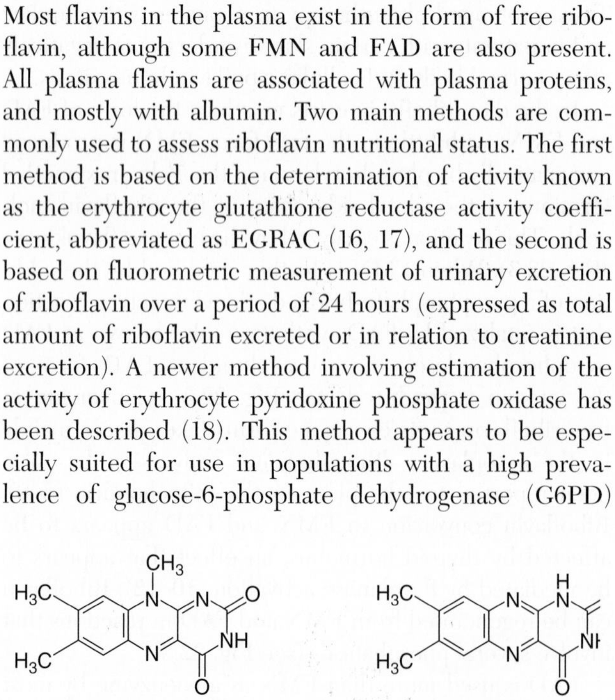

Lumiflavin

Lumichrome

Chlorpromazine

Fig. 22.2. Structure of riboflavin and related compounds.

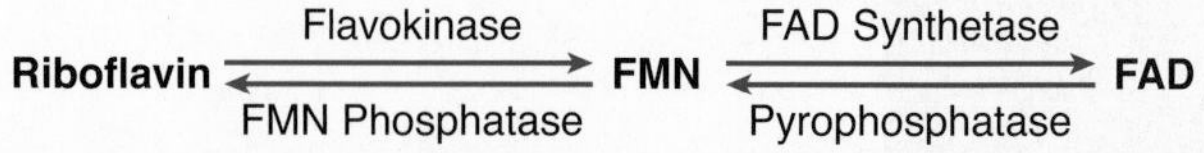

Fig. 22.3. Interconversion of riboflavin to its coenzymes flavin mononucleotide (FMN) and flavin adenine dinucleotide (FAD).

deficiency (18). Estimation of riboflavin status in patients with G6PD deficiency by means of the erythrocyte glutathione reductase activity method may mask riboflavin deficiency because G6PD deficiency is known to be associated with enhanced binding of FAD to erythrocyte glutathione reductase (19). Other methods available to measure the levels of riboflavin and its derivatives in biologic samples include high-performance liquid chromatography and binding of riboflavin and its derivative to specific flavoproteins (20).

PHYSIOLOGY OF RIBOFLAVIN

Intestinal Absorption

Humans and all other mammals cannot synthesize riboflavin, and thus they must obtain the vitamin from exogenous sources through intestinal absorption. The intestine therefore plays a central role in regulating and maintaining normal riboflavin body homeostasis. The intestine is exposed to two sources of riboflavin: a dietary source, which is processed and absorbed in the small intestine; and a bacterial source in which riboflavin is generated by the normal microflora in the large intestine and absorbed in that region of the gut (21). Riboflavin in the diet exists mainly in the form of FMN and FAD, which are noncovalently bound to proteins; free riboflavin exists only in small amounts in the diet. The first step in the processing of dietary FMN and FAD is their release from proteins by the combined action of gastric acid and intestine-associated hydrolases. The released FMN and FAD molecules are then hydrolyzed to free riboflavin in the intestinal lumen and surface through the action of alkaline phosphatases before absorption (22).

The mechanism of intestinal absorption of free riboflavin in the small intestine has been the subject of extensive investigations using various human and animal intestinal preparations. These preparations have ranged from intact intestinal tissue to purified vesicles isolated from the individual membrane domains of the polarized intestinal absorptive cells (i.e., from the apical brush-border membrane and from the basolateral membrane) (22–30). Collectively, these investigations have shown that absorption of free riboflavin occurs mainly in the proximal part of the small intestine and involves a specific sodium (Na^+)-independent, carrier-mediated system. This system is inhibited in a competitive manner by riboflavin structural analogs, such as lumiflavin and lumichrome, and by amiloride (a Na^+/hydrogen [H^+] exchange inhibitor) (24). The intestinal riboflavin uptake process is also inhibited by chlorpromazine (a tricyclic phenothiazine drug), a compound that shares structural similarities with riboflavin (25). Although some of the internalized riboflavin is phosphorylated inside the absorptive cells (31), only free riboflavin exits across the basolateral membrane. The latter process again involves a specific electroneutral, carrier-mediated mechanism (25).

The amount of riboflavin generated by the normal microflora of the large intestine depends on the type of the ingested diet. Higher amounts of riboflavin are produced following ingestion of a vegetable-based diet compared with a meat-based diet (32). In addition, considerable amounts of the bacterially produced riboflavin exist in the large intestinal lumen in the form of free riboflavin (32, 33), and thus are available for absorption. Indeed, studies have shown that the large intestine is capable of absorbing luminally introduced free riboflavin (34, 35). The mechanism involved in riboflavin uptake by colonocytes has been characterized and involves an efficient and specific carrier-mediated mechanism that is similar to the one described in the small intestine (36, 37). Considering the time that the luminal content resides in the large intestine, it is reasonable to assume that this source of riboflavin contributes to the host's overall riboflavin nutrition, especially the cellular nutrition of the localized colonocytes. These colonocytes are known to depend on luminal content for other nutrients (e.g., short-chain fatty acids produced by bacteria are used by the colonocytes for energy production). Further studies, however, are needed to determine the exact level of contribution of this source of riboflavin to whole body riboflavin nutrition and the way in which environmental factors may affect such contribution.

Newer insights have been gained into the molecular identity of the systems involved in the intestinal riboflavin uptake process (38, 39). Two potential transport systems have been identified: riboflavin transporter-1 (RFT-1) and riboflavin transporter-2 (RFT-2) (38, 39). RFT-2 appears to be a more promising candidate than RFT-1 because it transports riboflavin with much greater efficiency. Both systems, however, are expressed in the intestine (38, 39). Further studies are needed to determine which of these uptake system contributes mostly to riboflavin absorption in the native intestine in vivo.

Fluctuation in the dietary level of riboflavin plays a role in regulating the intestinal riboflavin uptake process. Investigators showed that riboflavin deficiency was associated with a significant and specific up-regulation in intestinal riboflavin uptake, whereas oversupplementation with pharmacologic concentrations of riboflavin resulted in a significant and specific down-regulation in riboflavin uptake (24, 36, 40). These adaptive changes in the intestinal riboflavin uptake process appeared to be mediated by transcriptional mechanisms (24, 36, 40). The intestinal riboflavin uptake process was also found to be under the regulation of pathways mediated by intracellular protein kinase A and calcium/calmodulin (28, 36). Further, the intestinal riboflavin absorption process has been shown to undergo ontogenic regulation, with higher uptake during the suckling period compared with adulthood (41).

Excretion and Reabsorption in the Kidney

The kidney also plays an important role in regulating and maintaining normal body homeostasis of riboflavin by controlling the level of the vitamin that is lost in the urine. Under the normal condition of sufficient riboflavin intake, the amount of riboflavin that appears in the urine per day is approximately 120 μg, with free riboflavin representing between 60% and 70% of the total urinary flavin. Other flavin metabolites that have been identified in the urine include 7- and 8-hydroxymethylflavins, lumichrome, 10-formylmethylflavin, 10-(2′-hydroxyethyl) flavin, 8α-flavin peptides, and 5′ riboflavinyl peptide ester (17, 41–47).

In the kidney, physiologic levels of riboflavin are filtered through the glomeruli and are then reabsorbed in the proximal tubule through an efficient and specific carrier-mediated process (48–53). This process is again adaptively up-regulated in riboflavin deficiency and is under the regulation of specific intracellular protein kinase–mediated pathways (48–53). When the plasma level of riboflavin is high (following ingestion of high doses of riboflavin), tubular secretion of riboflavin also occurs to enhance excretion of the vitamin from the body (48–53).

Transport in Other Epithelia

With regard to riboflavin transport in the placenta, studies of cell culture models and membrane vesicles isolated from the apical (maternal-facing) and basal (fetal-facing) membranes of the syncytiotrophoblast from full-term human placentas have shown the involvement of a specific and regulated carrier-mediated process (7, 54–56).

Studies have also characterized riboflavin transport in the liver, which plays an important role in normal riboflavin metabolism and is the site of maximal utilization of the vitamin. The results again have shown the involvement of a carrier-mediated process that is regulated by extracellular riboflavin levels and by a specific intracellular regulatory pathway (57–59).

Uptake of riboflavin by human retinal pigment epithelium, which provides riboflavin to the metabolically active retina, has also been examined. The results have shown the involvement of a specific carrier-mediated mechanism that is up-regulated in riboflavin deficiency and is under the control of specific intracellular regulatory pathways (60).

Secretion in Milk

Both riboflavin and FAD are found in human and cow's milk; concentrations in human milk are higher than in cow's milk (61, 62). The level of flavin in milk depends on maternal dietary intake of the vitamin (63, 64). Secretion of free riboflavin and FAD into milk appears to involve two separate mechanisms, with transport of riboflavin in the mammary gland mediated by the multidrug transport breast cancer resistance protein (BCRP/ABCG2), an ABC transporter (65). Other flavin metabolites found in the milk include

10-(2'-hydroxyethyl)flavin, 7- and 8-hydroxymethylribo-flavin, 10-formylmethylflavin, and lumichrome (59, 61, 62).

RIBOFLAVIN DEFICIENCY

Deficiency of riboflavin, ariboflavinosis, is often accompanied by other nutrient deficits. Clinical signs and symptoms include lesions on the outside of lips (cheilosis) and corners of the mouth (angular stomatitis), inflammation of the tongue (glossitis), redness or bloody (hyperemia) and swollen (edema) mouth or oral cavity, the inflammatory skin condition seborrheic dermatitis, anemia, and peripheral nerve dysfunction (neuropathy), among other signs (see the chapter on manifestations of nutrient deficiency and toxicity). People at risk for deficiency include those with congenital heart disease, some cancers, and excessive alcohol intake. The conversion of riboflavin into FAD and FMN is impaired in hypothyroidism and adrenal insufficiency (11, 43, 66).

Excretion of riboflavin is enhanced by diabetes mellitus, trauma, stress, and oral contraceptive use. When riboflavin intake is very high, excess riboflavin is excreted in urine. Because of the participation of FAD in intermediary metabolism, fatty acid oxidation is impaired. Riboflavin acts in concert with thiamin, niacin, and pantothenic acid, in reactions that include pyruvate dehydrogenase and α-ketoglutarate dehydrogenase, and in the metabolism of vitamin B_6 (conversion of pyridoxine or pyridoxamine phosphates to pyridoxal phosphate is catalyzed by a flavoprotein). Marginal riboflavin status may be associated with increased plasma homocysteine levels as a result of the requirement for riboflavin for 5,10-methylene tetrahydrofolate reductase, a key enzyme of folate metabolism. A hierarchy of cellular metabolic changes during the onset of riboflavin deficiency has been proposed: the core electron transfer chain required for adenosine triphosphate synthesis is preserved, whereas the enzymes required for the first step of fatty acid β-oxidation are diminished (67).

Riboflavin deficiency ranges from mild to severe. Mild deficiency is detectable only by biochemical assays (elevated EGRAC or reduced erythrocyte glutathione reductase activity). Riboflavin supplementation also results in changes that are detectable biochemically. In a systematic review of numerous riboflavin supplementation studies that used EGRAC or basal glutathione reductase activity to determine riboflavin status, EGRAC (14 studies) and glutathione reductase activity (5 studies) showed a highly significant association with riboflavin intake, although substantial study-to-study heterogeneity was noted (68). Changes in EGRAC or glutathione reductase appear to be suitable biomarkers for changes in riboflavin intake in populations with severe to normal baseline intakes (68).

Investigators have known or assumed for some time that riboflavin deficiency is relatively prevalent in parts of the developing world with limited intakes of foods of animal origin, principally milk, eggs, and meats, which contain higher concentrations of the vitamin. Children and

pregnant women are most likely to be affected. A 24-hour dietary recall study conducted in urban women of reproductive age living in Mali identified riboflavin as one of the four micronutrients for which the probability of adequacy was lowest (69). Other studies evaluated multiple micronutrient supplementation as a means to improve diet quality and various health-related biomarkers, but riboflavin itself was not specifically tested. A study conducted in Poland that used EGRAC to assess riboflavin status in 20- to 25-year-old men and women found biochemical evidence of riboflavin deficiency in 33.7% of women and 25% of men (70). The investigators associated these findings with lower intakes of riboflavin during a 7-day period in which dietary intake was recorded (70).

Investigators have also shown interest in whether mild-to-moderate riboflavin deficiency is prevalent in affluent countries, and whether it may be part of a syndrome of suboptimal health or may affect the utilization of other micronutrients. Powers et al (71) reported results of a randomized clinical trial of riboflavin supplementation in women in the United Kingdom who were 19 to 25 years old and were low milk consumers; improvements in hematologic status served as the primary end point. The study group had elevated EGRAC values of more than 1.4 at baseline and was randomized to receive 2 or 4 mg of riboflavin or a placebo for 8 weeks. Riboflavin status, assessed by reduction in EGRAC values, improved dose dependently. Hemoglobin status improved significantly and was greatest for the tertile of riboflavin-supplemented women with the highest baseline EGRAC values of greater than 1.65. The investigators suggested that consideration should be given to raising the currently accepted EGRAC threshold for deficiency.

SOURCES AND RECOMMENDED DIETARY ALLOWANCES

Riboflavin, which occurs largely as a component of digestible coenzymes, is present in most plant and animal tissues. Especially good sources are eggs, organ meats (liver and kidney), lean meats, and milk. The US Department of Agriculture Continuing Survey of Food Intakes by Individuals found that food groups that supply more than 5% of total riboflavin intake are milk and milk drinks, bread and bread products, mixed foods (including sandwiches with meat, poultry, or fish as main ingredients), ready-to-eat cereals, and mixed foods with grain as the main ingredient (72). Among vegetables, Brussels sprouts and broccoli contain more riboflavin per weight and calorie than most other vegetables or fruits. Whole grains contain more riboflavin than milled, refined grains. Vitamin B–enriched breads and cereals are significant sources of riboflavin in the United States and other countries with similar nutrient fortification policies. Losses occur during cooking as a result of leaching of the heat-stable, light-sensitive flavins into water. Bioavailability is estimated at approximately 95% of food flavin, up to approximately 27 mg per single meal or dose (72).

TABLE 22.1	DIETARY REFERENCE INTAKE VALUES FOR RIBOFLAVIN BY LIFE STAGE GROUP		
LIFE STAGE GROUP	**RDA (mg/d)**[a]		**AI**[b] **(mg/d)**
	MALE	**FEMALE**	
0–6 mo			0.3
7–12 mo			0.4
1–3 y	0.5	0.5	
4–8 y	0.6	0.6	
9–13 y	0.9	0.9	
14–18 y	1.3	1.0	
19–>70 y	1.3	1.1	
Pregnancy	1.4		
Lactation	1.6		

[a]RDA, recommended dietary allowance, is the intake that meets the nutrient need of almost all (97% to 98%) individuals in a group.
[b]AI is adequate intake. For healthy infants receiving human milk, the AI is the mean intake.

Reprinted with permission from Food and Nutrition Board, Institute of Medicine. Riboflavin. In: Dietary Reference Intakes: Thiamin, Riboflavin, Niacin, Vitamin B₆, Vitamin B₁₂, Pantothenic Acid, Biotin, and Choline. Washington, DC: National Academy Press, 1998:87–122.

The requirement for riboflavin, in contrast to that for thiamin, does not increase when energy use is increased (72). Recommended dietary allowances (RDAs) (Table 22.1) for riboflavin are given in milligrams/day. For conversion, 1 μmol riboflavin equals 0.376 mg, or inversely, 1 mg riboflavin equals 2.66 μmol. Clinical signs of deficiency in adults can be prevented with intakes of riboflavin greater than 0.4 mg/1000 kcal, but more than 0.5 mg/1000 kcal may be required to maintain tissue reserves in adults and children, as reflected in urinary excretion, red cell riboflavin, and erythrocyte glutathione reductase.

For infants, an adequate intake, based on the content of riboflavin in human milk (0.35 mg/L) and the volume that is consumed, is now suggested as 0.3 mg/day for those 0 to 6 months of age and 0.4 mg/day for those 7 to 12 months of age (see Table 22.1). The RDA values for riboflavin (72) for children progressively increase on the basis of body weight from 0.5 to 1.3 mg/day for the age ranges of 1 to 3 years, up to 18 years, with slightly greater amounts recommended for boys than for girls. Pregnancy and lactation impose extra demands, and an additional 0.3 mg/day and 0.5 mg/day, respectively, are deemed appropriate, added to the RDA for adult women.

Safety and Adverse Effects

When supplementation or therapy with riboflavin is warranted, oral administration of 5 to 10 times the RDA usually is satisfactory.

Toxicity from ingestion of excess riboflavin is doubtful. No toxic or adverse effects of high riboflavin intake in humans are known. A research study that administered 60 mg of supplemental riboflavin and 11.6 mg of riboflavin

as a bolus intravenous dose reported no adverse effects (73). The Food and Nutrition Board of the Institute of Medicine did not establish a tolerable upper intake level when the RDAs were revised in 1998 (72).

ACKNOWLEDGMENTS

We would like to thank the US Department of Veterans Affairs (HMS) and the National Institutes of Health (DK56061, DK58057 to HMS and DK41479, CA90214 and HD66982 to ACR) for their kind support of our work.

REFERENCES

1. McCollum EV, Kennedy C. J Biol Chem 1916;24:491.
2. Stern KG, Holiday ER. Ber Dtsch Chem Ges 1934;67:1104.
3. Theorell H. Biochem Z 1934;272:155.
4. Theorell H. Biochem Z 1937;290:293.
5. Warburg O, Christian V. Biochem Z 1938;295:261.
6. Merrill AH Jr, Lambeth JD, Edmondson DE et al. Annu Rev Nutr 1981;1:281–317.
7. Huang SN, Swaan PW. J Pharmacol Exp Ther 2001;298:264–71.
8. McCormick DB. Riboflavin. In: Brown ML, ed. Present Knowledge in Nutrition. 6th ed. Washington, DC: International Life Sciences Institute Press, 1990:146–54.
9. Barile M, Brizio C, Valenti D et al. Eur J Biochem 2000;267:4888–4900.
10. Rivlin RS. Riboflavin. In: Bowman BA, Russel RN, eds. Present Knowledge in Nutrition. 8th ed. Washington, DC: International Life Sciences Institute Press, 2001:191–8.
11. Lees SS, McCormick DB. Arch Biochem Biophys 1985;237:197–201.
12. Cimino JA, Jhangiani S, Schwartz E et al. Proc Soc Exp Biol Med 1987;184:151–3.
13. Spaan AN, Ijlst L, van Roermund CWT et al. Mol Genet Metab 2005;86:441–7.
14. Nagao M, Tanaka K. J Biol Chem 1992;267:17925–32.
15. Barile M, Passarella S, Bertoldi A et al. Arch Biochem Biophys 1993;305:442–7.
16. Sauberlich HE, Judd WH. Am J Clin Nutr 1972;25:756–62.
17. Briggs M, ed. Vitamins in Human Biology and Medicine. Boca Raton, FL: CRC Press, 1981.
18. Mushtaq S, Su H, Hill MH et al. Am J Clin Nutr 2009;90:1151–9.
19. Flatz G. Nature 1970;226:755.
20. Kodentsova VM, Vrzhesinskaya OA, Spirichev VB. Ann Nutr Metab 1995;39:455–60.
21. Wrong OM, Edmonds CJ, Chadwich WS. Vitamins. In: The Large Intestine: Its Role in Mammalian Nutrition and Homeostasis. New York: Wiley, 1981:157–66.
22. Daniel H, Binninger E, Rehner G. Int J Vitam Nutr Res 1983;53:109–14.
23. Daniel H, Wille U, Rehner G. J Nutr 1983;113:636–43.
24. Said HM, Ma TY. Am J Physiol 1994;266:G15–21.
25. Said HM, Hollander D, Khani R. Biochim Biophys Acta 1993;1148:263–8.
26. Tomei S, Yuasa H, Inoue K. Drug Deliv 2001;8:119–24.
27. Said HM, Khani R, McCloud E. Proc Soc Exp Biol Med 1993;202:428–34.
28. Said HM, Ma TY, Grant K. Am J Physiol 1994;267:G955–9.
29. Hegazy E, Schwnk M. J Nutr 1983;113:1702–7.
30. Middleton HM. J Nutr 1985;120:588–93.
31. Gastaldi G, Ferrari G, Verri A et al. J Nutr 2000;130:2556–61.

32. Iinuma S. J Vitam 1955;2:6–13.

33. Ocese O, Pearson PB, Schwiegert BS. J Nutr 1948;35:577–90.

34. Sorrell MP, Frank O, Thomson AD et al. Am J Clin Nutr 1971;24:924–9.

35. Kasper H. Am J Protocol 1970;21:341–5.

36. Said HM, Ortiz A, Moyer MP et al. Am J Physiol 2000;278: C270–6.

37. Yuasa H, Hirobe M, Tomei SA et al. Biopharm Drug Dispos 2000;21:77–82.

38. Yonezawa A, Masuda S, Katsura T et al. Am J Physiol 2008; 295:C632–41.

39. Yamamoto S, Inoue K, Ohta KY et al. J Biochem 2009; 145:437–43.

40. Said HM, Khani R. Gastroenterology 1993;105:1294–8.

41. Said HM, Ghishan FK, Greene HL et al. Pediatr Res 1985; 19:1175–8.

42. Ohkawa H, Ohishi N, Yagi K. J Biol Chem 1983;258:5623–8.

43. McCormick DB. Riboflavin. In: Shils ME, Shike M, Olson JA et al, eds. Modern Nutrition in Health and Disease. 9th ed. Baltimore: Williams & Wilkins, 1999:391–9.

44. Chastain JL, McCormick DB. J Nutr 1987;117:468–75.

45. Chia CP, Addison R, McCormick DB. J Nutr 1978;108: 373–81.

46. Chastain JL, McCormick DB. Biochim Biophys Acta 1988; 967:131–4.

47. Chastain JL, McCormick DB. Am J Clin Nutr 1987;46:830–4.

48. Yanagawa N, Shih RN, Jo OD et al. Am J Physiol 2000; 279:C1782–6.

49. Yanagawa N, Jo OD, Said HM. Biochim Biophys Acta 1998;1415:56–62.

50. Kumar CK, Yanagawa N, Ortiz A et al. Am J Physiol 1998; 274:F104–10.

51. Yanagawa N, Jo OD, Said HM. Biochim Biophys Acta 1997; 1330:172–8.

52. Lowy RJ, Spring KR. J Membr Biol 1990;117:91–9.

53. Spector R. J Pharmacol Exp Ther 1982;221:394–8.

54. Moe AJ, Plas DR, Powell KA et al. Placenta 1994;15:137–46.

55. Zempleni J, Link G, Kubler W. Int J Vitam Nutr Res 1992; 62:165–72.

56. Dancis J, Lehanka J, Levitz M. Pediatr Res 1985;19:1143–6.

57. Said HM, McCloud E, Yanagawa N. Biochim Biophys Acta 1995;1236:244–8.

58. Said HM, Ortiz A, Ma TY et al. J Cell Physiol 1998;176: 588–94.

59. Aw YT, Jones DP, McCormick DB. J Nutr 1983;113:1249–54.

60. Said HM, Wang S, Ma TY. J Physiol 2005;566:369–77.

61. Roughead ZK, McCormick DB. J Nutr 1990;120:382–8.

62. Roughead ZK, McCormick DB. Am J Clin Nutr 1990;52: 854–7.

63. Ortega RM, Quintas ME, Martinez RM et al. J m Coll Nutr 1999;18:324–9.

64. Allen LH. J Nutr 2003;133:3000S–7S.

65. van Herwaarden AE, Wagenaar E, Merino G et al. Mol Cell Biol 2007;27:1247–53.

66. Powers HJ. Proc Nutr Soc 1999;58:435–40.

67. Ross NS, Hansen TP. Biofactors 1992;3:185–90.

68. Hoey L, McNulty H, Strain JJ. Am J Clin Nutr 2009;89: 1960S–80S.

69. Kennedy G, Fanou-Fogny N, Seghieri C et al. J Nutr 2010; 140:2070S–8S.

70. Szczuko M, Seidler T, Mierzwa M et al. Int J Food Sci Nutr 2011;62:431–8.

71. Powers HJ, Hill MH, Mushtag S et al. Am J Clin Nutr 2011; 93:1274–84.

72. Food and Nutrition Board, Institute of Medicine. Riboflavin. In: Dietary Reference Intakes: Thiamin, Riboflavin, Niacin, Vitamin B_6, Vitamin B_{12}, Pantothenic Acid, Biotin, and Choline. Washington, DC: National Academy Press, 1998:87–122.

73. Zempleni J, Galloway JR, McCormick DB. Am J Clin Nutr 1996;63:54–66.

SUGGESTED READINGS

Fujimura M, Yamamoto S, Murata T et al. Functional characteristics of the human ortholog of riboflavin transporter 2 and riboflavin-responsive expression of its rat ortholog in the small intestine indicate its involvement in riboflavin absorption. J Nutr 2010; 140:1722–7.

Powers HJ, Hill MH, Mushtag S et al. Correcting a marginal riboflavin deficiency improves hematologic status in young women in the United Kingdom (RIBOFEM). Am J Clin Nutr 2011;93:1274–84.

Zempleni J, Galloway JR, McCormick DB. Pharmacokinetics of orally and intravenously administered riboflavin in healthy humans. Am J Clin Nutr 1996;63:54–66.

23 | NIACIN[1]

JAMES B. KIRKLAND

HISTORICAL OVERVIEW

Pellagra is the clinical disease of niacin deficiency in humans. It is mainly caused by dependence on corn as a staple food. Although pellagra likely occurred at a low incidence throughout history, it reached epidemic proportions in the southern United States and Europe as corn-based agriculture spread (1). The term *pellagra* was derived from the Italian name for the condition, meaning "rough skin." Corn does contain niacin, but in tightly

bound structures; this binding is heat stable, although it is sensitive to alkaline treatment (2). Native Americans had developed various alkaline processing techniques to release the existing niacin, and the importance of this processing was not recognized when Columbus brought corn back to Europe (1).

Pellagra is characterized by the three "Ds" of dermatitis (sun sensitive), dementia, and diarrhea. Diarrhea is the least unique of these, but it leads to a vicious cycle of worsening status of niacin and other nutrients. Anorexia also tends to set in as the deficiency progresses, usually leading up to the death of the patient. The development of the more unique signs of dermatitis and dementia can be unpredictable from patient to patient, thus making diagnosis of pellagra difficult in many cases. The epidemic in the southern United States occurred largely in people working outdoors, and sun-induced skin lesions were a clinical focus (3). Similar outbreaks occurred in Spain, Italy, and Egypt during the 1700s and 1800s. The reported incidence in northern Europe was much lower (3), but cooler weather and indoor work environments may have caused pellagra to manifest as poorly diagnosed dementia, for which unfortunate patients were often confined to an asylum and fed a disease-perpetuating corn-based diet. Even in the southern United States in the 1900s, outbreaks of pellagra were described in asylum populations (3). Women were much more likely to develop pellagra than men, possibly because of an unequal division of food resources (1).

Remarkably, it took several hundred years for the dietary reliance on corn to be accepted as the cause of pellagra, although corn consumption was originally proposed to carry a disease or toxin. Starting in 1915, Dr. Joseph Goldberger conducted clinical trials in which pellagra was induced in prison populations and was cured or prevented by balanced diets or yeast supplements (4). Although nicotinic acid was first isolated in 1867, its role as the active vitamin was not identified until 1937, when black tongue in dogs was used as an animal model of pellagra (5). A host of publications in 1937 to 1938 demonstrated that nicotinic acid cured pellagra in humans (3), and Drs. Douglas Spies, Marion Arthur Blankenhorn, and Clark Niel Cooper were named by *Time* magazine as Men of the Year for their contributions.

---

[1]**Abbreviations: ACMS**, 2-amino-3-carboxymuconic-6-semialdehyde; **ACMSD**, 2-amino-3-carboxymuconic-6-semialdehyde decarboxylase; **ADP**, adenosine diphosphate; **ART**, mono-ADP-ribosyltransferase; **ATP**, adenosine triphosphate; **BER**, base excision repair; **CICR**, calcium-induced calcium release; **DRI**, dietary reference intake; **GI**, gastrointestinal; **GRP**, glucose-regulated-protein; **IP3**, inositol triphosphate; **NAADP**, nicotinic acid adenine dinucleotide phosphate; **NAD**, nicotinamide adenine dinucleotide; **NADH**, reduced nicotinamide adenine dinucleotide; **NADP**, nicotinamide adenine dinucleotide phosphate; **NADPH**, reduced nicotinamide adenine dinucleotide phosphate; **NER**, nucleotide excision repair; **NFκB**, nuclear factor κB; **PARP**, poly(ADP-ribose) polymerase; **RDA**, recommended dietary allowance; **TCA**, tricarboxylic acid; **UL**, tolerable upper intake level.

Nicotinamide adenine dinucleotide (NAD$^+$) was first identified in yeast extracts in 1906 (6), but its redox capabilities were not described until 1936 (7), followed by the connection of reduced NAD (NADH) formation with adenosine triphosphate (ATP) production in 1949 (8). For several decades, research focused on the extensive redox roles of NAD and NAD phosphate (NADP) in animal, plant, and microbial metabolism. An important advance was made in 1966, with the first publication on adenosine diphosphate (ADP)-ribose formation (9). This advance led up to our current knowledge of poly- and mono-ADP-ribosylation of proteins (10) as well as the formation of cyclic ADP-ribose (11) and of O-acetyl-ADP-ribose by sirtuins (12). These discoveries allowed a much better understanding of the unique metabolic origin of pellagra.

TERMINOLOGY AND CHEMISTRY

The term *niacin* can have broad or narrow meaning. In the broader sense, as in the "niacin content of a diet," it could refer to the combination of nicotinic acid and free and nucleotide-bound nicotinamide, all of which would directly contribute to niacin status. In its narrow meaning, niacin refers to nicotinic acid, and the term niacin is used in this manner in the extensive literature on the pharmacologic use of nicotinic acid in the treatment of dyslipidemias and other conditions.

From an ecologic perspective, niacin is introduced into the food chain, predominantly by plants, as nicotinic acid, nicotinamide, and the amino acid tryptophan (Fig. 23.1). Plants often synthesize provitamin metabolites for purposes quite distinct from those of human cells. Plants do use nicotinic acid to form pyridine nucleotides, but plants also use nicotinic acid to form large amounts of alkaloids, such as nicotine (13) and trigonelline (14), for purposes such as pest resistance and growth regulation. Some nicotinamide is formed in plants from nicotinic acid during pyridine nucleotide synthesis and may be released during plant cellular metabolism or during the digestion of plant matter in the human gastrointestinal (GI) tract.

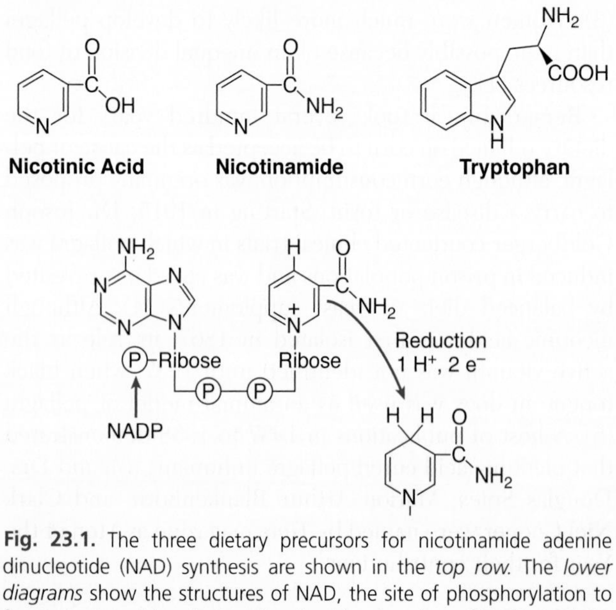

Nicotinic acid and nicotinamide (niacinamide) are position 3 derivatives of the pyridine ring structure (carboxylic acid in the former, carboximide in the latter structure) (see Fig. 23.1). Tryptophan is an essential amino acid in animals, synthesized in plants as a derivative of an indole structure. Despite the differences in ring structure, tryptophan is used to form niacin in many plants (15), and it is used to form NAD$^+$ in the liver of animals, with variable efficiency and poor control with respect to niacin status (16, 17).

The biologically active forms of niacin compounds are the NAD and NADP coenzymes (see Fig. 23.1). The C-4 position on the pyridine ring of the nicotinamide moiety participates in oxidation and reduction reactions. Because of the electronegativity of the amide group and the nitrogen at position 1 on this ring, hydride ions can readily reduce the oxidized C-4 position. This is the basis for the enzymatic hydrogen transfer reactions that are ubiquitous among organisms. With respect to the nonredox functions of NAD, the glycosidic linkage between nicotinamide and ribose is a high-energy bond, and cleavage of this bond drives all types of ADP-ribose transfer reactions in the forward direction.

The oxidized and reduced forms of the coenzymes are designated NAD$^+$ or NADP$^+$ and NADH or NADPH, respectively. The designations NAD and NADP are used to describe the total pools. This is often necessary if the method of quantification does not distinguish between oxidized and reduced forms or if a general statement about the nucleotide pool is made. The total pool of all four forms may be referred to as NAD(P). NAD and NADP have strong ultraviolet absorption at 340 nm in their reduced forms, and this is often used to monitor the oxidation or reduction of these cofactors in enzyme assays.

DIETARY SOURCES

Several categories of foods are good sources of niacin by different mechanisms. Starting with plant-based foods, nuts, legumes, and grains have approximately 2 to 5 mg per average serving, and they are important sources, given the consumption level of these staple foods. Niacin in these foods is largely in the form of nicotinic acid, in some cases bound in poorly available structures as seen in corn. Muscle-based foods, such as poultry, beef, and fish, provide approximately 5 to 10 mg per average serving, mainly in the form of preformed nucleotides, which release nicotinamide during digestion. A third category of niacin-rich foods is created through fortification, usually of flour and cereal products. In Canada and the United States, these products are fortified with approximately 5 mg/100 g flour. The eventual niacin content of ready-to-eat breakfast cereals can range up to 60 mg/100 g of

Nicotinic Acid   **Nicotinamide**   **Tryptophan**

Fig. 23.1. The three dietary precursors for nicotinamide adenine dinucleotide (NAD) synthesis are shown in the *top row.* The *lower diagrams* show the structures of NAD, the site of phosphorylation to form nicotinamide adenine dinucleotide phosphate (NADP), and the change in ring structure during reduction.

dry cereal, however, according to the US Department of Agriculture National Nutrient Database (18).

The last category of niacin-rich foods consists of high-protein foods that provide tryptophan, converted at low efficiency in the liver to NAD. The contribution of tryptophan is not generally included in the niacin content of a food, but it is included in a calculation of niacin equivalents (1 NE = 1 mg niacin = 60 mg tryptophan, or milligrams niacin + milligrams tryptophan/60). The efficiency of tryptophan conversion is not easily predictable because it will be less efficient with low tryptophan intakes (16, 17).

Niacin in plant products is present mainly in the form of nicotinic acid, although much of it exists in poorly understood bound forms. These bound forms have been studied in wheat bran, corn, and other grains, and they are heterogeneous mixtures of polysaccharides and glycopeptides to which nicotinic acid is esterified (2). In corn, most nicotinic acid is bound, and the tryptophan content is low, thus making pellagra a likely outcome when corn is consumed as a staple grain without alkaline processing. These conditions still occur in developing countries, and outbreaks of pellagra are periodically described (19). Conversely, in the United States, the average daily intake of niacin climbed from approximately 16 mg in the 1930s to approximately 32 mg in 2004 (20) as a result of fortification and increased intake of cereal products. Thus, the incidence of clinically obvious pellagra in developed countries is extremely low. Some evidence still points to subclinical deficiencies in developed countries, however, based on low blood NAD/NADP ratios (21). Niacin deficiency and clinical signs of pellagra may appear in combination with other conditions including anorexia nervosa (22), alcoholism (23), acquired immunodeficiency syndrome (24), cancer (25), and chemotherapy (26).

RECOMMENDED DIETARY ALLOWANCES AND TOLERABLE UPPER INTAKE LIMITS

The Dietary Reference Intake (DRI) values adopted by the United States and Canada include recommended dietary allowances (RDAs), which range from 2 to 8 mg/day in infants and children to 14 mg/day in women and 16 mg/day in men (Table 23.1). The tolerable upper intake levels (ULs) range from 10 to 20 mg/day in children up to 35 mg/day in adults. The UL values only apply to niacin

supplements plus niacin fortification, and they are based on the nicotinic acid–induced skin flush response. The skin flush is uncomfortable, but it is not directly related to any real health problems. Very few people have persistent skin flush responses to this level of niacin, and most niacin supplements as well as all B-50, B-75, and B-100 complex formulations greatly exceed the stated UL. Niacin supplements up to 500 mg are freely available for purchase.

Physicians prescribe nicotinic acid up to 3000 mg/day to treat dyslipidemias. This treatment can be effective in decreasing low-density lipoprotein cholesterol and increasing high-density lipoprotein cholesterol (27). The strong skin flush responses decrease over time and can be modulated with cyclooxygenase inhibitors, but patients do struggle with compliance. These higher intakes of niacin also cause some side effects other than skin flush including nausea and, in rare cases, liver injury. The doubling in niacin intake between 1930 and 2005 in the United States preceded the increase in obesity and diabetes in children, and intervention trials showed that very large doses of nicotinamide can impair glucose tolerance (20). The relevance of these results to normal variation in dietary niacin status is uncertain.

The pharmacologic effects of high doses of nicotinic acid and nicotinamide occur by some common and some distinct mechanisms (28), and their deleterious effects need to be researched and assessed separately. Even single effects, such as inhibition of poly(ADP-ribose) polymerases, may have both beneficial and harmful effects on health (29). Very high levels of niacin intake can stress methyl donor status (30) and increase blood homocysteine levels (31). At this point, it is clear that the current UL values are not being enforced, and the potential exists for toxicity of higher doses of nicotinic acid or nicotinamide supplements. Further work should be done to define more valid upper limits, which can then be applied in the marketplace.

SITES OF INTESTINAL ABSORPTION, BLOOD TRANSPORT, AND INTRACELLULAR FORMS

Preformed nicotinamide and nicotinic acid can be absorbed slowly through the stomach lining, but absorption in the small intestine is more rapid. Intact nucleotides are degraded in the upper small intestine to form free nicotinamide. The mechanisms of intestinal absorption

TABLE 23.1	RECOMMENDED DIETARY ALLOWANCES FOR NIACIN[a]							
AGE (y)	0–0.5	0.5–1	1–3	4–8	9–13	≥14	PREGNANCY	LACTATION
RDA(mg)	2	4	6	8	12	Female: 14 Male: 16	18	17

RDA, recommended dietary allowance.

[a]Values are niacin equivalents (NEs), except for values in infants younger than 6 months, which are expressed as preformed niacin.

Data from Food and Nutrition Board, Institute of Medicine. http://www.iom.edu/~/media/Files/Activity%20Files/Nutrition/DRIs/DRI_Vitamins.pdf. Accessed July 27, 2012.

are not fully clear in the current literature. Low concentrations of nicotinic acid and nicotinamide may be transported by sodium-dependent facilitated diffusion (32) or by proton cotransporters (33) or anion antiporters (34). Higher concentrations of both forms appear to be absorbed by passive diffusion, which will come into play with supplement use.

Once absorbed from the lumen into the intestinal mucosa, nicotinamide may be converted to NAD (Fig. 23.2, reactions 4 and 5) or released into the portal circulation. Conversely, physiologic levels of nicotinic acid are largely converted through the Preiss-Handler pathway to NAD (32) (see Fig. 23.2, reactions 1, 2, and 3). NAD glycohydrolases release nicotinamide into the portal circulation (see Fig. 23.2, reaction 7). The liver then takes up and converts

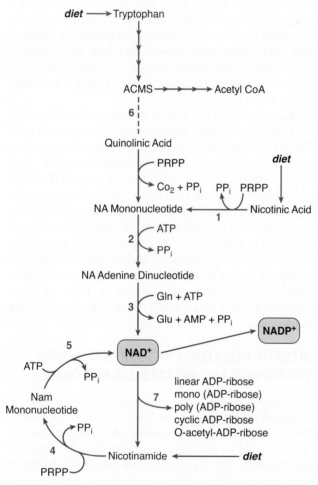

Fig. 23.2. The synthesis and nonredox reactions of pyridine nucleotides. Reactions 1 to 3 constitute the Preiss-Handler pathway for de novo synthesis of nicotinamide adenine dinucleotide (NAD$^+$). Reactions 4 and 5 are used to convert dietary or endogenous nicotinamide into NAD$^+$. Reaction 6 is a spontaneous chemical reaction required for the formation of NAD$^+$ from tryptophan. At position 7 are a large family of varied adenosine diphosphate (ADP)-ribosylation and NAD glycohydrolase reactions. *ACMS*, 2-amino-3-carboxymuconic-6-semialdehyde; *AMP*, adenosine monophosphate; *ATP*, adenosine triphosphate; *CoA*, coenzyme; *Gln*, glutamine; *NA*, nicotinic acid *Nam*, nicotinamide; *PP$_i$*, pyrophosphate *PRPP*, phosphoribosyl pyrophosphate.

most of the remaining nicotinic acid in the portal blood to NAD, which it cleaves to release nicotinamide as needed into the systemic circulation. Red blood cells also take up nicotinic acid and nicotinamide, thus forming a circulating reserve pool of pyridine nucleotides (35, 36).

The liver is a central player in niacin metabolism. The liver receives nicotinamide and some nicotinic acid through the portal circulation as well as nicotinamide released from other extrahepatic tissues. In the liver, nicotinic acid and nicotinamide are metabolized to NAD or to yield compounds for urinary excretion, depending on niacin status. The liver is also the site of tryptophan conversion to NAD. The liver has very high basal levels of NAD, which are further increased by extra dietary niacin and create a medium-term storage pool that can be used to maintain blood nicotinamide levels (32). The liver also produces various methylated and hydroxylated products of both nicotinic acid and nicotinamide for urinary excretion. In humans, nicotinamide is primarily methylated to produce N^1-methylnicotinamide, whereas nicotinic acid is conjugated with glycine to form nicotinuric acid. Unmodified nicotinic acid and nicotinamide can be found in the urine as a consequence of high dietary intake (32) because methyl donor capacity may become limiting (30).

Plants and microorganisms form nicotinic acid, nicotinamide, and tryptophan, which act as the dietary sources for the pyridine ring structure in mammals. Preiss and Handler (37) initially described the pathway for conversion of nicotinic acid to NAD in animal cells (Fig. 23.2, reactions 1, 2, and 3). Dietrich et al (38) showed that nicotinamide is salvaged by combining with phosphoribosyl pyrophosphate and then ATP to produce NAD directly (Fig. 23.2, reactions 4 and 5). Nicotinamide is not demethylated to form nicotinic acid in humans, except by bacteria in the GI tract, which can occur at high levels of nicotinamide intake (28).

A small proportion of tryptophan catabolized in the liver results in NAD formation, thus supporting niacin status. Most tryptophan is fully catabolized through 2-amino-3-carboxymuconic-6-semialdehyde (ACMS) to acetyl coenzyme. ACMS is catabolized by ACMS decarboxylase (ACMSD). If ACMS accumulates, some of it degrades spontaneously to quinolinic acid (see Fig. 23.2, reaction 6), to allow formation of NAD. Thus, the production of NAD from tryptophan is favored by high activity of tryptophan or indoleamine 2,3-dioxygenase, low activity of ACMSD, and high activity of quinolinate phosphoribosyltransferase, all of which lead to a wide range in the efficiency of tryptophan to niacin conversion among species and individuals (39–41). This pathway appears to be regulated, in part, to minimize quinolinate neurotoxicity during high protein intake (42), starvation, and ketosis (43).

The traditional estimate of efficiency for tryptophan to NAD conversion is 1/60. This leads to the concept of niacin equivalents (1 NE = 1 mg niacin = 60 mg tryptophan). Significant individual variation exists, however (44).

More importantly, a lack of tryptophan conversion is noted at low levels of tryptophan intake (16). In studies, young men consuming a diet containing 6 NE/day (RDA = 16 NE) for 5 weeks started receiving an additional 240 mg/day of tryptophan. This addition of 4 NE/day had no effect on blood NAD, and it appears that protein turnover takes precedence over niacin synthesis when tryptophan levels are low. This finding was also reported in animal models (17). At the same time, high-protein diets and tryptophan supplements cure pellagra, and a genetic defect in tryptophan absorption, known as Hartnup disease, can cause pellagra in persons with marginal diets.

ASSESSMENT OF NUTRIENT STATUS

At normal-to-low niacin intakes, most urinary excretion is of nicotinamide metabolites because nicotinic acid is efficiently converted into metabolically active nucleotides. As an individual becomes niacin deficient, the urinary excretion of N-methyl-2-pyridone-5-carboxamide decreases to a greater extent than does that of N-methylnicotinamide, with a ratio of less than 1 suggesting niacin deficiency (45). Human studies by Fu et al (16) subsequently showed that red blood cell NAD decreases during niacin deficiency, although the NADPH pool is very stable. These findings led to the use of (NAD/NAD + NADP) × 100, referred to as the niacin number, as an easily obtained index of human niacin deficiency (21, 25, 46). This result was reproduced in other cell types in culture (47) and animal models (48) and showed a specific loss of the NAD$^+$ pool during niacin deficiency. This topic is considered later in the discussion of the mechanisms of cellular disruption during niacin deficiency.

FUNCTIONS IN METABOLISM

Redox Reactions

The most critical function of the pyridine nucleotides likely is support of the oxidation and reduction reactions that are found throughout metabolism in all organisms. The oxidized nicotinamide ring in NAD$^+$ or NADP$^+$ can accept one electron at the positively charged nitrogen and a second electron (with associated proton) at the C-4 carbon (see Fig. 23.1). The formation of a separate NADP pool is critical to the support of both oxidative and reductive processes, and the NAD kinase responsible for this is highly conserved among all levels of organisms (49). The phosphorylation itself does not affect the redox properties of the cofactor, but it allows for enzyme specificity between the NAD and NADP pools. Consequently, the NAD pool is maintained in a largely oxidized state (as NAD$^+$), primarily by components of the electron transport chain.

Conversely, the NADP pool is maintained largely in a reduced state (as NADPH), primarily by the hexose monophosphate shunt (pentose phosphate pathway). The oxidizing NAD$^+$/NADH redox couple can then be linked to enzymes that oxidize substrates (e.g., glycolytic reactions, oxidative decarboxylation of pyruvate, oxidation of acetate in the tricarboxylic acid [TCA] cycle, oxidation of alcohol, β-oxidation of fatty acids) and drive them forward by mass action. The reducing NADPH/NADP$^+$ redox couple can be linked to enzymes that reduce substrates (e.g., fatty acid and cholesterol synthesis, manufacture of deoxyribonucleotides, detoxification of hydrogen peroxide). The critical nature of these reactions can be seen from the central pathways that depend completely on their function including glycolysis, the TCA cycle, the electron transport chain, fatty acid synthesis, and β-oxidation.

Poly(ADP-Ribose) Formation

Poly(ADP-ribose) was discovered in 1966 by Paul Mandel's group (9). Poly(ADP-ribose) polymerase-1 (PARP-1) was the first synthetic enzyme identified, because it is an abundant protein that represents the majority of cellular PARP activity. Eventually, PARP-1 knockout mice were found to synthesize 5% to 10% of control levels of poly(ADP-ribose), and a search for related enzymes led to the discovery of PARP-2, PARP-3, vault-PARP, tankyrase and tankyrase 2, PARP-7 (dioxin-inducible), and PARP-10 (50, 51).

PARP-1 contains 2 zinc fingers that allow the enzyme to bind specifically to strand breaks in DNA and signal the catalytic portion of the protein to initiate poly(ADP-ribose) synthesis (52). More than 30 nuclear proteins may act as acceptors, but most of the poly(ADP-ribose) is synthesized on PARP-1 itself. This "automodification" of PARP-1 is critical to its function in DNA repair. Automodification of PARP-1 occurs by homodimerization of PARP-1 or heterodimerization of PARP-1 and PARP-2 (53). As PARP becomes more poly(ADP-ribosyl)ated, it takes on a negative charge, which eventually causes it to be repelled from DNA and lose catalytic activity (54).

PARP-2 is similar to PARP-1, with an abbreviated DNA-binding domain. PARP-1 and PARP-2 both interact with XRCC1 in the regulation of base excision repair (BER) (55). Both PARP-1 and PARP-2 null mice survive and reproduce, although they display genomic instability; double knockouts die in utero, thus demonstrating a redundancy of activity between these two enzymes (56).

PARP-3 lacks nick-sensing ability, but it can heterodimerize with PARP-1 and tends to localize to the centrosome (51). PARP-4, or VPARP, is found in association with vault particles, which are massive ribonucleoprotein particles present in the cytosol of mammalian cells (51). The role of PARP-4, and vault particles in general, is not well understood. Tankyrase and tankyrase 2 are found around telomeres, the repetitive sequences at the end of mammalian chromosomes (51). Their PARP activity causes relaxation of the folded telomere tips that allows telomerase access to the DNA terminus, which it elongates. Telomerase is required by dividing cells to prevent erosion and instability at the ends of the chromosome. PARP-7 and PARP-10 can poly(ADP-ribosyl)ate histones and may regulate gene expression (51).

It is beyond the scope of this chapter to describe the function of this superfamily of PARP enzymes in detail. Mechanistically, poly(ADP-ribose) has a strong negative charge similar to DNA. Proteins that are covalently modified with polymer are then repelled from DNA or other negatively charged binding partners. Additionally, the covalent modification can directly alter the activity of a protein (57). Clouds of negatively charged polymer around sites of DNA damage can repel other strands of DNA and can help to prevent deleterious translocation events. Finally, many proteins have specific, noncovalent, high-affinity binding sites for poly(ADP-ribose) and are thereby drawn to sites of polymer formation. These varied mechanisms have been most thoroughly studied in relation to the functions of PARP-1 and PARP-2 (PARP-1/2) in DNA repair. Briefly, activation of PARP-1/2 in response to DNA damage leads to a cascade of events. Activated PARP-1/2, bound to a DNA strand break, will covalently modify nearby histones, thus causing them to be repelled from DNA and leading to local chromatin relaxation.

Additionally, histones have high-affinity polymer-binding sites and are drawn out of nearby chromatin to bind to the cloud of poly(ADP-ribose) attached to PARP-1/2. This chromatin relaxation allows assembly of a complex of repair enzymes that is further aided by attraction of specific proteins with high-affinity polymer-binding motifs such as XRCC1, p53, XPA, ATM, DEC, topoisomerase, DNA ligase, and DNA polymerase (58). After the repair complex has been fully assembled, the automodified PARP-1/2 can be repelled from the DNA to allow the repair process to be completed. Inhibition of PARP-1 activity, or very low cellular NAD levels, can cause PARP-1 to remain stuck to the site of DNA damage and can prevent repair from proceeding (28).

Another area of interest is the role of PARP enzymes in controlling gene expression, likely using physical properties similar to those described earlier. PARP-1 does bind to DNA in the absence of strand breaks and can be catalytically activated by certain secondary structures in DNA (59). Thus, PARP-1 can regulate chromatin structure and cause assembly of transcription factors in the absence of DNA damage. For example, PARP-1 has been shown to be required for neural plasticity and learning (60), processes thought to be driven more by regulation of gene expression than by DNA strand breaks. Similarly, interest has grown in the role of PARP-1 in the regulation of nuclear factor κB (NFκB) signaling and inflammation (61). Although this pathway likely has positive effects in responding to infection, these signals worsens tissue injury in many acute models such as heart attack and stroke, organ transplantation, and septic shock as well as in chronic models such as diabetes and cardiovascular disease (29). Many investigators have demonstrated that PARP-1 inhibition can greatly diminish the severity of these disease processes. This finding has caused quite a controversy in the literature on PARP-1 and health. Many publications show the need for PARP activity to maintain genomic stability and long-term health, whereas many others demonstrate the negative impact of PARP-1 activity on the progression of numerous important human health issues (29). To make the most effective clinical use of PARP modifiers, including catalytic inhibitors and niacin supplementation, the positive and negative roles of PARP enzymes in each stage of each disease process must be defined.

Mono ADP-Ribosylation Reactions

In this class of reactions, a single ADP-ribose unit is moved from NAD^+ to an amino acid residue on an acceptor protein (10, 62). The bacterial toxins of the cholera, pertussis, and diphtheria pathogens and *Pseudomonas* ADP-ribosylate host G-proteins that disrupt host cellular function. Mammalian cells are now known to contain numerous endogenous mono-ADP-ribosyltransferases (ARTs) (10), which act on various amino acid side chains as ADP-ribose acceptors. Ecto-ARTs are secreted or expressed on the outside of cells, whereas endo-ARTs work inside cells. Some ecto-ARTs include ART1 (ADP-ribosylates integrins and controls myogenesis) and ART2 (induces apoptosis through ADP-ribosylation of an ATP-gated ion channel) (63). Normally, extracellular NAD^+ levels are very low, and the source of substrate for ecto-ARTs may involve NAD channels in the plasma membrane or NAD released from injured cells. These ideas suggest that NAD itself may be used as a signal of the metabolic state of a cell or as a signal for the death of nearby cells, thus leading to signaling events that may be paracrine or autocrine in nature.

Endo-ARTs act inside the cell. G-proteins are important components of cell signaling and have been shown to be substrates for arginine-specific ADP-ribosylation (10). This process could control various pathways, depending on what the G-protein is controlling. Elongation factor 2 is another G-protein that is a substrate for an endo-ART (64). Another substrate of endo-ART activity is the 78-kDa glucose-regulated protein (GRP78), a molecular chaperone that aids in the correct folding of secreted proteins in the lumen of the endoplasmic reticulum. During metabolic or environmental stress, GRP78 is mono(ADP-ribosyl)ated, and this process may decrease the rate of protein secretion during times of nutritional stress while at the same time preventing a total shutdown that would eventually kill the cell (10).

Cyclic ADP-ribose, Linear ADP-ribose, *O*-Acetyl-ADP-ribose, Nicotinic Acid Adenine Dinucleotide Phosphate, and Calcium Signaling

In 1993, a metabolite of NAD^+ known to cause intracellular calcium mobilization was identified as cyclic ADP-ribose (65). Calcium concentrations are approximately

10,000-fold higher outside cells relative to the cytosol. Transient increases in intracellular calcium, arriving through the plasma membrane or released from intracellular stores (e.g., endoplasmic reticulum, mitochondria, lysosomes), regulate processes from neurotransmission to insulin release by β cells, muscle cell contraction, and T-lymphocyte activation, among others (66). Cyclic ADP-ribose participates in the process of calcium-induced calcium release (CICR). For example, an impulse traveling along a nerve axon arrives at a synapse in which voltage-gated channels allow a certain amount of calcium to cross the plasma membrane. This calcium causes the formation of inositol triphosphate (IP3) and cyclic ADP-ribose, which bind to ryanodine and IP3 receptors, respectively, thus causing more calcium release from intracellular stores. If intracellular calcium reaches a certain threshold, signals for the release of neurotransmitters will be sufficient to cause the impulse to be propagated across the synapse. Similar calcium release events occur in both the presynaptic and postsynaptic boutons, which enhance or dampen the strength of synapses and are involved in essentially all aspects of nervous system function.

More recently, a contaminant of commercial $NADP^+$ was found to mobilize calcium and was identified as nicotinic acid adenine dinucleotide phosphate ($NAADP^+$). $NAADP^+$ has been found in cultured cells and whole tissues and has been shown to respond to physiologic events (67). Although the mechanism of formation of $NAADP^+$ from $NADP^+$ remains uncertain, $NAADP^+$ is, surprisingly, made by the same enzymes that make cyclic ADP-ribose under in vitro conditions (11). The enzymes responsible for $NAADP^+$ formation in vivo have not been identified. $NAADP^+$ causes calcium release through two-pore channels, which may initiate or amplify CICR (68). Finally, this same class of enzymes forms linear ADP-ribose, either directly from NAD^+ or by hydrolyzing cyclic ADP-ribose (11). Linear ADP-ribose is also formed through the formation and turnover of poly ADP-ribose. Linear ADP-ribose also causes calcium release, through TRPM2 channels (69). TRPM2 channels can also release calcium in response to another NAD^+ metabolite, O-acetyl-ADP-ribose, which results from sirtuin activity. The emerging picture is that control of intracellular calcium release is a result of overlapping signals from IP3, cyclic ADP-ribose, linear ADP-ribose, O-acetyl-ADP-ribose, and $NAADP^+$. Clearly, calcium signaling is heavily integrated with pyridine nucleotide metabolism and the energy status of the cell.

Sirtuin Function

Another role for NAD^+ is as a substrate for the sirtuins, a family of NAD-dependent protein deacetylases. The acetyl group is transferred from various proteins onto ADP-ribose, with the release of nicotinamide. The mammalian sirtuin family has seven members, the most

thoroughly researched of which is SIRT1(mammals)/Sir2(yeast, worms, flies) (12). Excitement grew as Sir2 was found to mediate the life extension effects of caloric restriction in yeast, worm, and fly models. Resveratrol, a polyphenol found in grape products, was found to activate Sir2 and extend lifespan in the absence of caloric restriction (70), thereby boosting interest in red wine and health. Many questions remain about the exact mechanism of life span extension and whether SIRT1 in mammals functions in all the same ways as Sir2 in simpler animal models.

SIRT1 functions as a protein deacetylase, whereas SIRT2 through SIRT7 have a mixture of deacetylase and ADP-ribosyl transferase activities (12). Early work established that SIRT1 acted to deacetylate histones and p53. Deacetylation of histones leads to a more compact chromatin structure and gene silencing. In theory, niacin deficiency could lead to a more open DNA structure, with more active gene expression and greater sensitivity to damage and translocation events. SIRT1 appears to link control of chromatin structure to cellular energy status. SIRT1 may control the chromatin microenvironment around sites of DNA damage. Activation of PARP-1/2 at strand breaks creates a localized depression in NAD^+ and an increase in nicotinamide. This inhibits SIRT1 activity, thus allowing acetylation of histones and leading to chromatin relaxation (71), which aids access of repair enzymes (Fig. 23.3).

Other substrates that are deacetylated by SIRT1 include p53, FOXO, Ku70, p300, Rb, NFκB, and PGC-1α (72)—findings suggesting that the metabolic impact of sirtuin activation is complex. p53 controls cell cycle checkpoints, DNA repair, and apoptosis, and acetylation appears to enhance p53 stability and accumulation by inhibiting ubiquitination. Thus, SIRT1 action appears to hinder p53 function and act as a tumor promoter (72). Many other substrates will have to be studied to determine the balance of SIRT1 actions with respect to apoptosis, genomic stability, and cancer.

SIRT1 has the potential to extend longevity through chromatin structure and genomic stability, but it also appears to be extensively involved in the regulation of gene expression related to control of energy metabolism in

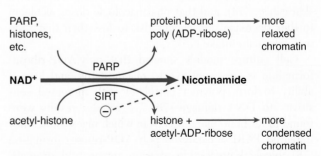

Fig. 23.3. Potential interactions between poly(ADP-ribose) polymerases (PARP) and sirtuins (SIRT) in the control of chromatin structure. *ADP,* adenosine monophosphate; *NAD,* nicotinamide adenine dinucleotide.

critical tissues such as liver, skeletal muscle, adipose tissue, and pancreas (12). SIRT1 activation, on balance, appears to maintain insulin sensitivity and decrease the risk of type 2 diabetes (12, 70). Much remains to learn about sirtuins and human health and life span extension.

SPECIFIC CAUSES AND MANIFESTATIONS OF DEFICIENCY AND EXCESS STATES

Early researchers probably attributed the pathologic features associated with niacin deficiency to disruptions in redox cycling because this was the only metabolic role known for niacin at that time. However, the distinctive clinical signs of pellagra (dementia, sun-sensitive dermatitis) are better explained in relation to the ADP-ribosylation functions of NAD. The redox functions of pyridine nucleotides are too critical to lose and may be preserved as long as possible during niacin deficiency through high enzyme affinities and subcellular compartmentalization (1). During niacin deficiency, it is mainly the NAD^+ pool that declines, whereas NADH, $NADP^+$, and NADPH are maintained, and the GSH/GSSG (reduced and oxidized glutathione) couple is not impaired (48). NAD is known to be concentrated in the mitochondria, where it can serve multiple redox functions while being protected from use by most ADP-ribosyltransferases in the cell (see later) (1). The powerful techniques of metabolomics should soon be brought to bear on the analysis of intermediary metabolism at different levels of niacin status and give us a better idea of the responsiveness of redox reactions to niacin status in different tissues in whole animal models.

The sun sensitivity of pellagra is dramatic and is not found with deficiencies of related redox nutrients such as riboflavin or iron. From experience with familial sun sensitivity disorders, such as xeroderma pigmentosum, sun sensitivity is generally recognized to reflect problems in DNA repair pathways such as nucleotide excision repair (NER). No major genetic deficiencies occur in base excision repair (BER) genes, likely because they are critical for survival. Low niacin status and decreased PARP activity could impair NER, BER, and other pathways for DNA repair, given the broad participation of PARP enzymes in these processes (73). Mouse models showed that niacin deficiency increases the incidence of ultraviolet-induced skin cancer (74), and that pharmacologic doses of niacin further decrease skin cancer risk to less than that seen with adequate intake (75).

Cell culture models showed that poly(ADP-ribose) formation is very sensitive to niacin status, and loss of ability to form polymer correlates with increased sensitivity to DNA damage (76, 77). Similar results were found in rat bone marrow cells in which niacin deficiency impaired PARP-1 catalyzed poly(ADP-ribose) formation (78), blocked nucleotide excision repair, and dramatically increased genomic instability (79), thus increasing the development of nitrosourea-induced leukemias (80).

These findings raise the question of niacin status and cancer risk in humans. Data do not appear to be available on long-term skin cancer risk in niacin-deficient human populations. The native population of the Transkei region in South Africa has a high risk of esophageal cancer (81). A maize-based, low-protein diet is the staple for these people, and pellagra is common. Esophageal ulcerations and esophagitis, frequent in patients with pellagra, have been associated with development of carcinoma of the esophagus. Studies of other populations have linked corn consumption with esophageal cancer risk (82–85). In summary, the sun sensitivity of pellagra and other forms of genomic instability are probably related to low levels of poly(ADP-ribose) synthesis, definitely by PARP-1, and possibly by other members of the PARP family.

The other unique response to niacin deficiency is pellagrous dementia, which can progress from general depression to profound disruption of neural function similar to schizophrenia. Patients may have auditory and visual hallucinations and display paranoid, suicidal, and aggressive behaviors (86). Throughout the history of pellagrous epidemics, many patients in asylums for the insane were probably merely niacin deficient, even when skin lesions were not present. This situation is illustrated by a report of 11 cases admitted to the Georgia State Sanitarium in the early 1900s (87). Most of these patients with dementia showed no skin lesions initially and were not immediately diagnosed with pellagra. Dr. Little successfully treated 10 of the 11 patients with a nutrient-rich diet, starting with a combination of raw eggs in sweet milk.

Starting in 1937, numerous clinical reports of the response of patients with pellagra to nicotinic acid therapy were published. Clinicians reported that the most rapid and dramatic improvements were in the area of neural function. The signs of pellagrous dementia often disappeared virtually overnight. Patients were able to recall their mental disturbances and marvel at their disappearance. This shows that niacin deficiency is disrupting a short-term process, such as cell signaling and neural transmission, as opposed to causing a degeneration of brain structure. Like sun sensitivity, dementia is not observed with deficiencies of other redox active nutrients such as riboflavin and iron. Pellagra generally involves deficiencies of protein, energy, and micronutrients in addition to niacin, such as riboflavin and thiamin. Following niacin therapy, riboflavin supplementation may be needed to resolve the oral lesions, and thiamin may be needed to treat peripheral nerve problems. Some researchers have focused on decreased tryptophan metabolites, including quinolinic acid and serotonin (88), to explain pellagrous dementia, but the rapid improvement in central nervous system function following niacin supplementation is more supportive of the role of NAD metabolites.

It is now apparent that neural function can be altered by changes in various ADP-ribosylation reactions. PARP-1 activity is required for long-term potentiation of synapses in

of stroke (81, 82). Concurrent folate and vitamin B$_{12}$ supplementation complicated assessment of the effects of vitamin B$_6$ alone. Nevertheless, large-scale randomized trials that attempted to examine the effect of vitamin B$_6$ supplementation on secondary prevention have yielded largely negative results (83).

Several hypotheses may explain how vitamin B$_6$ deficiency affects VD. In addition to effects on multiple pathways of homocysteine metabolism (75), vitamin B$_6$ status may affect VD through effects on lipid metabolism (84), endothelial function (85), thrombogenesis (84), and inflammation (74). Low plasma PLP or low vitamin B$_6$ intake has been associated with elevated levels of plasma CRP, an indicator of inflammation (74, 86, 87). When comparing the association of plasma PLP levels and circulating CRP in healthy patients and patients with coronary artery disease, the association was observed only in the healthy patients (69). In addition, controlled dietary vitamin B$_6$ restriction did not affect plasma CRP in healthy young subjects (57). Investigators have suggested that the requirement for vitamin B$_6$ increases in inflammation (86). The mechanism relating plasma PLP and CRP or other inflammatory markers warrants further examination. The inhibitory role proposed for vitamin B$_6$ in platelet aggregation in vivo is unlikely (88), and all other hypotheses remain unproven.

The importance of adequate vitamin B$_6$ status for proper immune function, particularly cell-mediated and to a lesser degree humoral immunity, has been known for many years. Lymphoid tissue atrophy, reduced lymphocyte content of lymph tissues, extended allograft survival, and depressed antibody production, as well as reductions in lymphocyte proliferation, phagocytic activity of macrophages, and T-cell–mediated cytotoxicity in vitro, are all characteristic of vitamin B$_6$–deficient animals (89). In human studies, lymphocytes isolated from vitamin B$_6$–deficient subjects display reduced proliferation and reduced interleukin-2 production in response to mitogens (60, 90), in addition to reduced antibody production in response to immunization (89). Supplementation of vitamin B$_6$ has been reported to ameliorate immune responses in inflammatory conditions. In apparent contrast, proinflammatory cytokines were suppressed in patients with rheumatoid arthritis who were given 100 mg/day of vitamin B$_6$ (91). Critically ill patients supplemented with high doses of vitamin B$_6$ showed improved cell-mediated immune responses after 14 days (92). Depressed lymphocyte proliferation in vitamin B$_6$ deficiency may stem from impaired DNA synthesis resulting from reduced activity of SHMT, a key enzyme in de novo synthesis of purines and thymidine (see Fig. 24.3, reaction 1). The immune systems of elderly persons appear particularly sensitive to inadequate vitamin B$_6$ status (90), and this population may benefit from vitamin B$_6$ supplementation (93). Vitamin B$_6$ depletion-repletion studies in young and old subjects suggest that intake of vitamin B$_6$ equal to the current RDA may be insufficient to maximize immunocompetence (60, 90).

A role for vitamin B$_6$ in cancer was suggested by perturbations of vitamin B$_6$ metabolism observed in patients with breast cancer and within tumors (94). The level of exposure to vitamin B$_6$ is inversely proportional to cell proliferation in experimental models of cancer, as reviewed in Komatsu et al (94). Several epidemiologic studies reported an inverse relationship between vitamin B$_6$ intake or plasma PLP and colorectal cancer risk (95). This protective effect was suggested to be independent of effects of vitamin B$_6$ status on one-carbon metabolites and inflammatory biomarkers (96). Higher levels of plasma PLP have also been associated with a lower risk of lung cancer (97). This association has been suggested in other cancers as well, but the results are inconsistent (98–100). Few clinical trial data are available to assess causality for low vitamin B$_6$ status in cancer. Potential protective effects of vitamin B$_6$ include modulation of steroid hormone action (101), maintenance of one-carbon metabolism, and maintenance of immune function (102).

The nervous system relies on certain PLP-dependent enzymes for neurotransmitter synthesis, as explained earlier. Serotonin production and γ-aminobutyric acid production are particularly sensitive to vitamin B$_6$ status in rats, and this sensitivity may account for changes in thyroid hormone levels and seizure activity observed in vitamin B$_6$–deficient animals (33). In addition, these studies suggest a strong role for vitamin B$_6$ in cognitive development. PN-dependent seizure is a rare inherited condition in humans that begins before or within days of birth, ceases immediately on intravenous PN administration, and is controllable through daily PN supplementation (~0.2 to 3 mg/kg body weight) (103). The disease is now known to be caused by mutations in the gene encoding for α-aminoadipic semialdehyde dehydrogenase (104). Loss of activity of the dehydrogenase results in accumulation of piperideine-6-carboxylate, which condenses with and inactivates PLP (104). The resulting reduction in PLP-dependent glutamate decarboxylase activity is presumed to cause the seizures (105). As discussed earlier, seizures also occurred in infants consuming infant formula deficient in vitamin B$_6$ (51). Abnormal brain wave activity was observed in these infants, as well in some adult subjects examined in vitamin B$_6$ deficiency studies (106). Attempts to correct suspected neurotransmitter abnormalities with PN treatment in conditions such as headache, chronic pain, behavioral disorders, depression, autism, Down syndrome, schizophrenia, and various neuropathies have met with limited success (107). Although the positive association between plasma total homocysteine and cognitive decline, dementia, and Alzheimer disease in elderly persons implies a potential link between vitamin B$_6$ status and these conditions, few studies have found any association between vitamin B$_6$ status and cognitive function (108–110). Both low plasma PLP and low dietary vitamin B_6 intake have been associated with higher likelihood of depressive symptoms (111, 112).

Multiple links exist between vitamin B_6 status and diabetes (113). The roles of vitamin B_6 in gluconeogenesis and glycogenolysis are described in the earlier section on vitamin B_6 function. Low concentrations of plasma B_6 vitamers observed in type 1 or type 2 diabetes may be related to increased plasma alkaline phosphatase activity or the acute suppressive effect of an oral glucose load on plasma PLP concentration. Supraphysiologic concentrations of PLP inhibit advanced glycation reactions in vitro (114). Similarly, high-dose vitamin B_6 administration markedly inhibited accumulation of advanced glycation end products in streptozotocin-induced diabetic rats (115) and improved diabetic neuropathy (116). Claims regarding PM treatment have not been fully evaluated clinically. Biochemical and functional indices indicate that declining vitamin B_6 status occurs with aging in both animals and humans (117, 118). Although the cause of these observations is uncertain, reduced dietary intake, impaired renal function, and effects of inflammation and the acute phase response on vitamin B_6 metabolism are possible contributors (118). These indices, as well as immune function, are improved by PN supplementation (93, 119). In controlled nutritional studies, vitamin B_6 intakes needed to restore biochemical, functional, and immunologic indices of B_6 status in elderly persons to levels considered normal for younger populations were greater than the current RDA for this age group (90, 120).

Vitamin B_6 status also is perturbed in individuals with impaired renal function (121, 122). Low vitamin B_6 status is associated with elevated post–methionine load homocysteine concentrations in renal transplant recipients, which can be ameliorated with supplemental vitamin B_6 (123). Hemodialysis-induced peripheral neuropathy and sensory abnormalities also respond to supplemental PN (124). Vitamin B_6 deficiency and hyperhomocysteinemia, which are independent risk factors for VD (72), are prevalent in patients with renal disease and are coincident with elevated VD risk in this population (122). Patients with renal disease who were supplemented with B vitamins had lower plasma homocysteine concentration than were patients treated with a placebo, but the treatment did not improve survival or reduce the incidence of cardiovascular events (125).

Vitamin B_6 metabolism is perturbed in patients with rheumatoid arthritis (126). Patients have significantly lower plasma PLP concentrations (127), even at similar vitamin B_6 intakes (128). Depletion of vitamin B_6 was shown to be tissue specific in a rodent model of arthritis, a finding that implies redistribution of PLP to tissues that may have a higher demand for the coenzyme (129). Supplementation with 100 mg PN/day, but not at 50 mg PN/day, suppressed production of proinflammatory cytokines in patients with rheumatoid arthritis (91, 130).

PHARMACOLOGIC PYRIDOXINE THERAPY AND PYRIDOXINE TOXICITY

In addition to the uses of supplemental PN mentioned earlier, congenital homocystinuria has been successfully treated with 250 to 500 mg PN/day (131). PN also improves hematopoiesis in patients with specific forms of sideroblastic anemia (132). Pharmacologic doses of vitamin B_6 also have been used, with little proof of efficacy, to alleviate the symptoms of dysmenorrhea, morning sickness, asthma, carpal tunnel syndrome, and hyperoxaluria, among other conditions (133). Those studies that showed benefit of supplemental PN often were small and poorly controlled. Trials of PN therapy for premenstrual syndrome, the treatment that may represent the most frequent use of large PN doses, yielded equivocal results (134).

Although efficacy is questionable in many cases, PN treatment at pharmacologic doses continues to be used, either prescribed or self-administered, as stand-alone or adjunct therapy for many of the conditions mentioned earlier. Persistent PN use is the result, in part, of low perceived toxicity of PN supplementation compared with traditional medical approaches. However, long-term intake of pharmacologic doses of PN (>500 mg/day) is associated with a risk of sensory neuropathies, which are reversed on withdrawal of the PN supplements (53). The Food and Nutrition Board of the Institute of Medicine established a tolerable upper intake level of vitamin B_6 at 100 mg/day, to prevent neuropathy (53). This quantity of vitamin B_6 intake is not approachable by dietary means other than supplementation.

VITAMIN B_6–DRUG INTERACTIONS

Certain drugs, including cycloserine, hydralazine, phenelzine, gentamycin, penicillamine, isoniazid, and L-dopa, antagonize vitamin B_6 status by covalently binding to the carbonyl group of PLP or PL; this process reduces the availability of the PLP coenzyme (135). The asthma drug theophylline interferes with PLP production by inhibition of PL kinase (136). Vitamin B_6 status usually is recovered through PN supplementation without reducing drug efficacy (135). PN supplementation was previously contraindicated in patients treated with L-dopa for Parkinson disease because PN enhances peripheral metabolism of the drug (133). Concurrent treatment with a peripheral decarboxylase inhibitor can be used to preserve the effectiveness of L-dopa during PN supplementation, however. Alcohol intake antagonizes vitamin B_6 status through production of acetaldehyde, which competes with PLP for binding sites of PLP-dependent enzymes (137). Because chronic alcoholism likely increases vitamin B_6 catabolism through this mechanism, PN supplementation may be advisable for patients affected by this disease.

Tryptophan metabolism was reported to be perturbed in users of oral contraceptives (138). The pattern of excreted tryptophan metabolites was similar to that seen in vitamin B$_6$ deficiency, a finding suggesting that oral contraceptives affect vitamin B$_6$ status. Studies have confirmed lower plasma PLP levels in oral contraceptive users (61, 139), but the mechanism to account for this association has not been elucidated.

REFERENCES

1. Mackey AD, Davis SR, Gregory JF. Vitamin B$_6$. In: Shils ME, Shike M, Ross AC, et al, eds. Modern Nutrition in Health and Disease. 10th ed. Baltimore: Lippincott Williams & Wilkins, 2005:452–461.
2. Gyorgy P. Nature 1934;133:448–9.
3. Lepkovsky S. Science 1938;87:169–70.
4. Keresztesy JC, Stevens JR. Proc Soc Exp Biol Med 1938;38:64–5.
5. Gyorgy P. J Am Chem Soc 1938;60:983–4.
6. Kuhn R, Wendt G. Ber Dtsch Chem Ges 1938;71B:780–2.
7. Ichiba A, Michi K. Sci Papers Inst Phys Chem Res 1938;34:623–6.
8. Snell EE. Annu Rev Nutr 1989;9:1–19.
9. Gunsalus IC, Bellamy WD, Umbreit WW. J Biol Chem 1944;155:685–6.
10. American Institute of Nutrition. J Nutr 1990;120:12–9.
11. Leklem JE, Machlin LJ.Vitamin B-6. New York: Marcel Dekker, 1991:341.
12. Said HM. Annu Rev Physiol 2004;66:419–46.
13. Tarr JB, Tamura T, Stokstad ELR. Am J Clin Nutr 1981;34:1328–37.
14. Roth-Maier DA, Kettler SI, Kirchgessner M. Int J Food Sci Nutr 2002;53:171–9.
15. Gregory JF III. Eur J Clin Nutr 1997;51(Suppl 1):S43–8.
16. Andon MB, Reynolds RD, Moser-Veillon PB et al. Am J Clin Nutr 1989;50:1050–8.
17. Ink SL, Gregory JF III, Sartain DB. J Agric Food Chem 1986;34:857–62.
18. Trumbo PR, Gregory JF III, Sartain DB. J Nutr 1988;118:170–5.
19. Nakano H, McMahon LG, Gregory JF III. J Nutr 1997;127:1508–13.
20. Gregory JF III, Trumbo PR, Bailey LB et al. J Nutr 1991;121:177–86.
21. McMahon LG, Nakano H, Levy MD et al. J Biol Chem 1997;272:320–25.
22. Mackey AD, Henderson GN, Gregory JF III. J Biol Chem 2002;277:26858–64.
23. Ink SL, Mehansho H, Henderson LM. J Biol Chem 1982;257:4753–7.
24. Coburn SP, Mahuren JD, Kennedy MS et al. Biofactors 1988;1:307–12.
25. Mehansho H, Henderson LM. J Biol Chem 1980;255:11901–7.
26. McCormick DB, Chen H. J Nutr 1999;129:325–7.
27. Merrill AH, Henderson JM. Ann N Y Acad Sci 1990;585:110–7.
28. Van Hoof VO, De Broe ME. Crit Rev Clin Lab Sci 1994;31:197–293.
29. Fonda ML. J Biol Chem 1992;267:159–78.
30. Coburn SP. Ann N Y Acad Sci 1990;585:76–85.
31. Coburn SP, Lewis DL, Fink WJ et al. Am J Clin Nutr 1988;48:291–4.
32. Zhang Z, Gregory JF III, McCormick, DB. J Nutr 1993;123:85–9.
33. Dakshinamurti K, Paulose CS, Viswanathan M et al. Ann N Y Acad Sci 1990;585:128–44.
34. Davis SR, Stacpoole PW, Williamson J et al. Am J Physiol 2004;286:E272–9.
35. Lamers Y, Williamson J, Gilbert LR et al. J Nutr 2007;137:2647–52.
36. Lima CP, Davis SR, Mackey AD et al. J Nutr 2006;136:2141–7.
37. Scheer JB, Mackey AD, Gregory JF. J Nutr 2005;135:233–8.
38. Davis SR, Quinlivan EP, Shelnutt KP et al. J Nutr 2005;135:1045–50.
39. Davis SR, Scheer JB, Quinlivan EP et al. Am J Clin Nutr 2005;81:648–55.
40. Lamers Y, O'Rourke B, Gilbert LR et al. Am J Clin Nutr 2009;90:336–43.
41. Lamers Y, Williamson J, Theriaque DW et al. J Nutr 2009;139:666–71.
42. Bergami R, Maranesi M, Marchetti M et al. Int J Vitam Nutr Res 1999;69:315–21.
43. Cho YO, Leklem JE. J Nutr 1990;120:258–65.
44. Black AL, Guirard BM, Snell EE. J Nutr 1978;108:670–7.
45. Coburn SP, Ziegler PJ, Costill DL et al. Am J Clin Nutr 1991;53:1436–42.
46. Hurford MT, Marshall-Taylor C, Vicki SL et al. Clin Chim Acta 2002;321:49–53.
47. Gregory JF. J Food Comp Anal 1988;1:105–23.
48. Gregory JF, Sartain DB. J Agric Food Chem 1991;39:899–905.
49. Kabir H, Leklem JE, Miller LT. J Food Sci 1983;48:422–5.
50. Gregory JF, Fennema OR. Vitamins. New York: Marcel Dekker, 2007:429–521.
51. Coursin DB. JAMA 1954;154:406–8.
52. Gregory JF III, Carmel R, Jacobsen DW.Vitamin B$_6$ Deficiency. New York: Cambridge University Press, 2001:307.
53. Food and Nutrition Board, Institute of Medicine. Dietary Reference Intakes for Thiamin, Riboflavin, Niacin, Vitamin B$_6$, Folate, Vitamin B$_{12}$, Pantothenic Acid, Biotin, and Choline. Washington, DC: National Academy Press, 1998:150.
54. Leklem JE. J Nutr 1990;120(Suppl):S1503–7.
55. Lumeng L, Ryan MP, Li TK. J Nutr 1978;108:545–53.
56. Ubbink JB, van der Merwe A, Delport R et al. J Clin Invest 1996;98:177–84.
57. Davis SR, Quinlivan EP, Stacpoole PW et al. J Nutr 2006;136:373–8.
58. Lamers Y, Williamson J, Ralat M et al. J Nutr 2009;139:452–60.
59. Hansen CM, Shultz TD, Kwak HK et al. J Nutr 2001;131:1777–86.
60. Kwak HK, Hansen CM, Leklem JE et al. J Nutr 2002;132:330–8.
61. Morris MS, Picciano MF, Jacques PF et al. Am J Clin Nutr 2008;87:1446–54.
62. West KD, Kirksey A. Am J Clin Nutr 1976;29:961–9.
63. Reynolds RD, Polansky M, Moser PB. J Am Diet Assoc 1984;84:1339–44.
64. Ulvik A, Ebbing M, Hustad S et al. Clin Chem 2010;56:755–63.
65. Rhinehart JF, Greenberg LD. Am J Pathol 1949;25:481–91.
66. Smolin LA, Crenshaw TD, Kurtycz D et al. J Nutr 1983;113:2122–33.
67. Clarke R, Smulders Y, Fowler B et al. Semin Vasc Med 2005;5:75–6.
68. Selhub J, Jacques PF, Wilson PWF et al. JAMA 1993;270:2693–8.

69. Cheng CH, Lin PT, Liaw YP et al. Nutrition 2008;2:239–44.
70. Hron G, Lombardi R, Eichinger S et al. Haematologica 2007;92:1250–3.
71. Page JH, Ma J, Chiuve SE et al. Circulation 2009;120:649–55.
72. Kelly PJ, Shih VE, Kistler JP et al. Stroke 2003;34:e51–4.
73. Vanuzzo D, Pilotto L, Lornbardi R et al. Eur Heart J 2007; 28:484–91.
74. Friso S, Jacques PF, Wilson PW et al. Circulation 2001;103: 2788–91.
75. McKinley MC. Proc Nutr Soc 2000;59:221–37.
76. Albert CM, Cook NR, Gaziano JM et al. JAMA 2008;299: 2027–36.
77. Galan P, Kesse-Guyot E, Czernichow S et al. BMJ 2010;341:36.
78. Hankey GJ, Eikelboom JW, Baker RI et al. Lancet Neurol 2010;9:855–65.
79. Lonn E, Yusuf S, Arnold MJ et al. N Engl J Med 2006;354:1567–77.
80. Toole JF, Malinow MR, Chambless LE et al. JAMA 2004; 291:565–75.
81. Saposnik G, Ray JG, Sheridan P et al. Stroke 2009;40: 1365–72.
82. Spence JD, Bang H, Chambless LE et al. Stroke 2005;36: 2404–9.
83. Ebbing M, Bonaa KH, Arnesen E et al. J Intern Med 2010;268:367–82.
84. Brattstrom L, Stavenow L, Galvard H. Scand J Clin Lab Invest 1990;50:873–7.
85. Miner SE, Cole DE, Evrovski J et al. J Heart Lung Transplant 2001;20:964–9.
86. Morris MS, Sakakeeny L, Jacques PF et al. J Nutr 2010;140:103–10.
87. Shen J, Lai CQ, Mattei J et al. Am J Clin Nutr 2010;91: 337–42.
88. Schoene NW, Chanmugam P, Reynolds RD. Am J Clin Nutr 1986;43:825–30.
89. Chandra RK, Sudhakaran L. Ann N Y Acad Sci 1990;585: 404–23.
90. Meydani SN, Ribaya-Mercado JD, Russel RM et al. Am J Clin Nutr 1991;53:1275–80.
91. Huang SC, Wei JC, Wu, DJ et al. Eur J Clin Nutr 2010; 64:1007–13.
92. Cheng CH, Chang SJ, Lee BJ et al. Eur J Clin Nutr 2006; 60:1207–13.
93. Talbott MC, Miller LT, Kerkvliet NI. Am J Clin Nutr 1987; 46:659–64.
94. Komatsu S, Yanaka N, Matsubara K et al. Biochim Biophys Acta 2003;1647:127–30.
95. Larsson SC, Orsini N, Wolk A. JAMA 2010;303:1077–83.
96. Lee JE, Li HJ, Giovannucci E et al. Cancer Epidemiol Biomarkers Prev 2009;18:1197–1202.
97. Johansson M, Relton C, Ueland PM et al. JAMA 2010; 303:2377–85.
98. Ames BN, Wakimoto P. Nat Rev Cancer 2002;2:694–704.
99. Gibson TM, Weinstein SJ, Mayne ST et al. Cancer Cause Control 2010;21:1061–9.
100. Stevens VL, McCullough ML, Sun J et al. Am J Clin Nutr 2010;91:1708–15.
101. Allgood AE, Cidlowski JA. J Biol Chem 1992;267:3819–24.
102. Brown RR. Possible role for vitamin B-6 in cancer prevention and treatment. In: Leklem JE, Reynolds, RD, eds. Clinical and Physiological Applications of Vitamin B-6. New York: Alan R. Liss, 1988:279–301.
103. Gupta VK, Mishra D, Mathur I et al. J Paediatr Child Health 2001;37:592–6.
104. Mills PB, Struys E, Jakobs C et al. Nat Med 2006;12:307–9.
105. Baxter P. Biochim Biophys Acta 2003;1647:36–41.
106. Kretsch MJ, Sauberlich HE, Newburn E. Am J Clin Nutr 1991;53:1266–74.
107. Pfeiffer SI, Norton J, Nelson L et al. J Autism Dev Disord 1995;25:481–93.
108. Balk EM, Raman G, Tatsioni A et al. Arch Intern Med 2007;167:21–30.
109. Brady CB, Gaziano JM, Cxypoliski RA et al. Am J Kidney Dis 2009;54:440–9.
110. Ford AH, Flicker L, Alfonso H et al. Neurology 2010;75: 1540–7.
111. Merete C, Falcon LM, Tucker KL. J Am Coll Nutr 2008;27: 421–7.
112. Skarupski KA, Tangney C, Li H et al. Am J Clin Nutr 2010;92: 330–5.
113. Leklem JE. Ann N Y Acad Sci 1992;669:34–43.
114. Bender DA. Br J Nutr 1999;81:7–20.
115. Nakamura S, Li H, Adijiang A et al. Nephrol Dial Transplant 2007;22:2165–74.
116. Jolivalt CG, Mizisin LM, Nelson A et al. Eur J Pharmacol 2009;612:41–7.
117. van den Berg H, Bode W, Mocking JA et al. Ann N Y Acad Sci 1990;585:96–104.
118. Bates CJ, Pentieva KD, Prentice A et al. Br J Nutr 1999;81: 191–201.
119. Schrijver J, Westermarck T, Tolonen M et al. Vitamin B-6 status and the effect of supplementation in Finnish and Dutch elderly. In: Leklem J, Reynolds, RD, eds. Clinical and Physiological Applications of Vitamin B-6. New York: Alan R. Liss, 1988:127.
120. Ribaya-Mercado JD, Russel RM, Sahyoun N et al. J Nutr 1991;121:1062–71.
121. Lindner A, Bankson DD, Stehman-Breen C et al. Am J Kidney Dis 2002;39:134–45.
122. Robinson K, Gupta A, Dennis V et al. Circulation 1996;94:2743–8.
123. Bostom AG, Gohh RY, Beaulieu AJ et al. Ann Intern Med 1997;127:1089–92.
124. Okada H, Moriwaki, K, Kanno Y et al. Nephrol Dial Transplant 2000;15:1410–3.
125. Jamison RL, Hartigan P, Kaufman JS et al. JAMA 2007;298: 1163–70.
126. Roubenoff R, Roubenoff RA, Selhub J et al. Arthritis Rheum 1995;38:105–9.
127. Chiang EP, Bagley PJ, Roubenoff R et al. J Nutr 2003;133: 1056–9.
128. Woolf K, Manore MM. J Am Diet Assoc 2008;108:443–53.
129. Chiang EP, Smith DE, Selhub J et al. Arthritis Res Ther 2005;7:R1254–62.
130. Chiang EPI, Selhub J, Bagley PJ et al. Arthritis Res Ther 2005;7:R1404–R11.
131. Barber GW, Spaeth GL. J Pediatr 1969;75:463–78.
132. Mason DY, Emerson PM. Br Med J 1973;1:389–90.
133. Bernstein AL. Ann N Y Acad Sci 1990;585:250–60.
134. Wyatt KM, Dimmock PW, Jones PW et al. BMJ 1999;318: 1375–81.
135. Bhagavan BM. Curr Concepts Nutr 1983;12:1–12.
136. Ubbink JB, Delport R, Becker PJ et al. J Lab Clin Med 1989;113:15–22.
137. Lumeng L. J Clin Invest 1978;62:286–93.
138. Rose DP. Nature 1966;210:196–7.
139. Lussana F, Zighetti ML, Bucciarelli P et al. Thromb Res 2003;112:37–41.

C. VITAMINS

25 PANTOTHENIC ACID[1]

PAULA R. TRUMBO

HISTORICAL OVERVIEW

Pantothenic acid belongs to the group of B vitamins. The name is a Greek derivation meaning "from everywhere." Earlier names used for pantothenic acid include vitamin B_5, chick antidermatitis factor, antidermatosis vitamin, and chick antipellagra factor. Pantothenic acid was isolated by R. J. Williams et al in 1931 (1), and this isolate was shown to be a single acidic substance essential for the growth of yeast in 1933 (2). The structure of pantothenic acid was later determined in 1939 (3). In 1940, Williams et al successfully synthesized pantothenic acid (4), thus showing its relationship with inositol, thiamin, biotin, and vitamin B_6 as to the growth of yeast (5). These researchers also developed assays for the isolation and measurement of pantothenic acid (6). In 1947, Lipmann et al identified pantothenic acid as one of the components of coenzyme A (CoA). The accepted biochemical structure of CoA was published in 1953 (7). It was not until 1954 that Bean and

Hodges (8) reported that pantothenic acid is essential in human nutrition. Pantothenic acid–containing CoA has since been shown to be essential to the respiratory tricarboxylic acid (TCA) cycle, fatty acid synthesis and degradation, and many other metabolic and regulatory processes.

TERMINOLOGY, CHEMISTRY, AND BIOCHEMISTRY

Pantothenic acid is water soluble, exists as a yellow viscous oil, and is unstable to acids, bases, and heat. Pantothenic acid, $d(+)-\alpha$-(-dihydroxy-β,β-dimethylbutyryl-β-alanine), is synthesized by microorganisms through an amide linkage of β-alanine and pantoic acid (Fig. 25.1). Pantetheine consists of a β-mercaptoethylamine group added to pantothenate in humans. CoA is composed of 4'-phosphopantetheine linked by an anhydride bond to adenosine 5'-monophosphate, modified by a 3'-hydroxyl phosphate. In addition to serving as a component of CoA, 4'-phosphopantetheine is linked to certain proteins. 4'-Phosphopantetheine has been shown to be an essential cofactor in the biosynthesis of fatty acids (e.g., fatty acid synthetase), peptides (e.g., antibiotics), and polyketides (9).

Pantothenate, in the form of CoA, performs multiple roles in cellular metabolism. CoA facilitates the transfer of acetyl or acyl groups. β-Oxidation of fatty acids and the oxidative degradation of amino acids depend on CoA and thereby make the catabolic products available to the TCA cycle. Furthermore, acetyl CoA provides acetyl groups to oxaloacetic acid for the formation of citrate in the TCA cycle. The condensation of three acetyl CoA molecules yields 3-hydroxy-3-methylglutaryl-CoA (HMG CoA), an intermediate in cholesterol synthesis.

DIETARY SOURCES

Free and conjugated pantothenic acid is found in various plants and animals foods. Approximately 85% of dietary pantothenic acid exists as CoA or phosphopantetheine (10). Major sources of pantothenic acid include beef, chicken, liver, eggs, tomato products, broccoli, potatoes, and whole grains (11, 12) (Table 25.1). Pantothenic acid is added to various foods, such as breakfast cereals, beverages, and baby foods. Fruit products and corn-based

[1]**Abbreviations: AI**, adequate intake; **ATP**, adenosine triphosphate; **CoA**, coenzyme A; **NBIA**, neurodegeneration with brain iron accumulation; **PKAN**, pantothenate kinase–associated neurodegeneration; **TCA**, tricarboxylic acid.

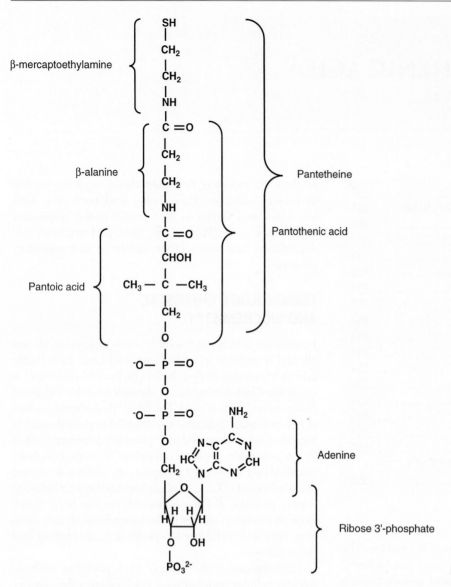

Fig. 25.1. Coenzyme A and intermediaries.

and presweetened cereals are among the poorest sources of pantothenic acid.

A review of studies in North America and the United Kingdom reported that the average pantothenic acid concentration in mature breast milk ranges from 2.2 to 2.5 mg/L (13). The pantothenic acid concentration in human milk has been reported to be 6.7 mg/L, with no change occurring from 1 to 6 months postpartum (14). The pantothenic acid content in human milk correlates with maternal intake of the vitamin (15). In one report, the concentration of pantothenic acid in breast milk increased from 0.48 to 2.45 mg/L within 4 days after parturition (16).

RECOMMENDED DIETARY ALLOWANCES

In 1989, an estimated safe and adequate daily intake (ESADDI) of 4 to 7 mg/day of pantothenic acid was set because subjects were shown to excrete this level through the urine and feces (17). Based on a scientific review of the data for setting dietary reference intakes (DRIs), the determination was that the information for setting an estimated average requirement (EAR) was insufficient, and, therefore, a recommended dietary allowance (RDA) could not be set. An adequate intake (AI) value was set for pantothenic acid for all life stage and gender groups, however (Table 25.2) (18). The AI for infants 0 to 6 months old

	PANTOTHENIC ACID
TABLE 25.1	**PANTOTHENIC ACID CONTENT OF FOODS**
FOOD	PANTOTHENIC ACID (mg/100g EDIBLE PORTION)
Beef, ground, cooked	0.33
Bran, 100%	1.73
Broccoli, raw	0.53
Cashew nuts	1.22
Chicken, fried	1.00
Eggs, hard-boiled	1.40
Liver, fried	5.92
Milk, canned	0.76
Mushrooms, cooked	2.16
Potato, baked	0.86
Rice, white	1.13
Tomato products	0.75

TABLE 25.2	ADEQUATE INTAKE FOR PANTOTHENIC ACID
AGE (MALE AND FEMALE)	ADEQUATE INTAKE (mg/d)[a]
0–6 mo[b]	1.7
7–12 mo	1.8
1–3 y	2
4–8 y	3
9–13 y	4
14–18 y	5
≥19 y	5
Pregnant women	6
Lactating women	7

[a]Based on usual intakes for groups 1 year old and older (see text).
[b]Based on the average contents of pantothenic acid in human milk consumed by infants (see text).

represents the average daily intake of pantothenic acid for infants exclusively fed human milk. The AI for men and for nonpregnant and pregnant women is based on usual pantothenic acid intakes by adults in the United States. The AI for children 1 to 18 years old was set by extrapolating from the adult AI, based on body weight and growth factors. The AI during lactation is 7 mg/day because approximately 2 mg of pantothenic acid is secreted in human milk daily (18).

United States nutrition surveys do not estimate intakes of pantothenic acid. The mean pantothenic acid intake of men and women of different ages in Quebec in 1990 fell from approximately 6 to 3 mg/day with advancing age (18). The average intake of pantothenic acid was 5.5 and 4.0 g/day for the male and female population, respectively, of New Brunswick, Canada (19). Usual intakes of approximately 4 to 7 mg/day have been reported for adolescents and adults of various ages (18). The average dietary intake estimated for pregnant and lactating women has been reported at 2.8 mg/1000 kcal (20) or 7.6 mg/day for lactating women (14); for pregnant women living in Boston, the estimated intake was 6.6 mg/day (21); and for elderly persons, it was 5.9 mg/day (22). The average daily intake of pantothenic acid from multivitamin/mineral supplements has been estimated at 10 mg/day (23).

PHYSIOLOGIC ASPECTS

Digestion, Absorption, and Excretion

Dietary CoA is hydrolyzed in the intestinal lumen to dephospho-CoA, pantetheine, and phosphopantetheine. Pantetheine is further hydrolyzed by pantetheinase to pantothenic acid. Although pantothenic acid may be absorbed by passive diffusion, it is absorbed into the bloodstream of animals by a saturable, sodium-dependent active transport mechanism (24). Studies in mice indicated that the kinetics for this active transport system is not affected by variation in dietary intake levels of the vitamin (25). Although animal studies demonstrated that intestinal microflora synthesize pantothenic acid (25), the contribution to absorbed pantothenic acid in humans is unknown.

Absorbed pantothenic acid is transported by the red blood cells throughout the body (26). The vitamin is also transported in the free acid form in the plasma at a concentration of approximately 1 μg/mL (27). (The molecular weight of pantothenic acid is 219.24 g/mol; 1 mg equals 4.56 μmol; 1 μg/mL equals 4.56 μmolar [μM]). Concentrations in red blood cells are higher than in plasma. Maximum pantothenate concentrations occurred 3 minutes following intravenous injection and subsequently decreased, a finding suggesting that the vitamin is rapidly taken up by red blood cells and other tissues (28). A large increase in red blood cell pantothenate concentration was observed in men following the injection of a multivitamin mixture that included 45 mg D-panthenol (29).

Animal studies showed that, following the intraluminal administration of radiolabeled pantothenate or CoA, approximately 40% was located in muscle, 10% in the liver, and 10% in the intestine (30). Because pantothenic acid is an essential component for the biosynthesis of CoA, most tissues transport the vitamin through an active sodium cotransport mechanism (31, 32). Most of the pantothenic acid in tissues is present as CoA, with lesser amounts present as acyl carrier protein and free pantothenic acid.

Before urinary excretion, CoA is hydrolyzed to pantothenate in a multistep reaction. Pantothenic acid is excreted in urine and is typically measured by microbiologic assay. When subjects were given 100 mg/day of pantothenic acid, urinary excretion was only 60 mg/day. This finding suggests that the vitamin can be stored when intake levels are high or the fractional bioavailability is relatively low.

Bioavailability

Data on the bioavailability of dietary pantothenic acid are limited. One study reported that dietary pantothenic acid was, on average, 50% (40% to 61%) bioavailable compared with the pure form of the vitamin (calcium pantothenate) given in a formula diet (33). Approximately 60% of ingested pantothenic acid was excreted in urine when subjects were fed three different experimental diets (34).

Genetic Factors

Pantothenate kinase–associated neurodegeneration (PKAN) is a major cause of neurodegeneration with brain iron accumulation (NBIA). NBIA is a rare, inherited neurologic movement disorder in which a mutation of the PANK2 gene results in a deficiency of pantothenate kinase and therefore inadequate synthesis of CoA. NBIA is characterized by dystonia, parkinsonism, and iron accumulation in the brain (35). Approximately 25% of affected individuals have atypical presentations (e.g., prominent speech defects and psychiatric disturbances) with late onset (age greater than

10 years) (36). *PANK2* is one of four known pantothenate kinases and is the only known gene to be associated with PKAN (36). Acanthocytosis and a defect in plasma lipoproteins have also been noted in association with the *PANK2* mutations (37). The efficacy of pantothenate supplementation in mitigating the symptoms of PKAN is unknown; however, some anecdotal reports have suggested improvement with supplementation (36).

FUNCTIONS IN METABOLISM

Synthesis of Coenzyme A

The first step in the synthesis of CoA is phosphorylation of pantothenic acid, which is catalyzed by pantothenate kinase. Following this, an adenosine triphosphate (ATP)–dependent condensation of 4'-phosphopantothenic acid with cysteine yields 4'-phosphopantothenoylcysteine, which is decarboxylated to 4'-phosphopantetheine (38). CoA is formed by a series of transfers of adenosine monophosphate and phosphate from ATP to 4'-phosphopantetheine. Approximately 95% of CoA is located in the mitochondria. Because CoA does not cross the mitochondrial membrane, the final site of CoA synthesis is thought to be within the mitochondria (39).

Cellular Metabolism

Pantothenate, usually in the form of CoA, performs multiple roles in cellular metabolism (40). Acetyl-CoA is central to the energy-yielding oxidation of glycolytic products and other metabolites through the mitochondrial TCA cycle. The first step of the TCA cycle involves the condensation of acetyl-CoA with oxaloacetate to yield citrate and subsequently succinyl-CoA, which provides energy for guanosine diphosphate phosphorylation. The β-oxidation of fatty acids and the oxidative degradation of amino acids are also CoA-dependent processes; the catabolic products of these processes become available to the respiratory TCA cycle for further degradation and energy production.

Pantothenic acid is required for the synthesis, by biosynthetically competent species, of several essential molecules including sphingolipids, leucine, arginine, and methionine. CoA is also required for the synthesis of isoprenoid derivatives, such as farnesol, cholesterol, steroid hormones, vitamin A, vitamin D, and heme A. Some of the isoprenoids are further bound to certain proteins, such as viral Ras proteins. Succinyl-CoA is required for the synthesis of δ-amino-levulinic acid, which is the precursor of the porphyrin rings in hemoglobin and the cytochromes and the corrin ring of vitamin B_{12}. CoA provides the essential acetyl group to the neurotransmitter acetylcholine, to serotonin in its conversion to melatonin, and to the acetylated sugars present in glycoproteins and glycolipids (*N*-acetylglucosamine, *N*-acetylgalactosamine, and *N*-acetylneuramic acid).

Protein Acetylation

Most soluble proteins are *N*-terminally acetylated by CoA. *N*-Acetylation appears to alter the structure of certain proteins, thereby altering function or metabolism. Peptide hormones are acetylated, a process that alters their hormone activity. For example, acetylation results in the activation of α-melanocyte–stimulating hormone and the inactivation of β-endorphin. Acetylation of histones alters the conformation of chromatin and changes its sensitivity to nucleases. Two classes of proteins are internally acetylated: histones and α-tubulin. Acetylation of histones neutralizes the charge of acetylated lysine residues and thereby weakens interactions between the nucleosomes that depend on histone *N*-terminal tails. Histones that are highly acetylated tend to be associated with newly synthesized DNA or DNA that is transcriptionally active. Acetylated chromatin has a more unfolded conformation, as indicated by its increased sensitivity to nucleases (41). Hyperacetylation of histones H3 and H4 has been shown to decrease the supercoiling within the nucleosome (42).

Acetylation and deacetylation regulate the assembly and disassembly of microtubules. Microtubules, which are essential components of the cellular cytoskeleton, are assembled from α- and β-tubulin dimers that polymerize and depolymerize continuously. Acetylation of α-tubulin occurs in the assembled microtubule and appears to stabilize microtubules (43). Deacetylation appears to be associated with depolymerization of microtubules (44).

Protein Acylation

Many different cellular proteins are covalently modified with long-chain fatty acids donated by fatty acyl CoA. The fatty acids, myristic acid and palmitic acid, are commonly added to proteins by acylation. This modification affects the location and activity of many proteins, including those involved with signal transduction. Myristolated proteins are located in the cytoplasm, plasma membrane, endoplasmic reticulum, and nuclear membrane. Myristolation of proteins is irreversible and often combines with other protein modifications for regulation of the protein's activity or localization. Because of the reversibility of palmitoylation, this process has a regulatory function. Guanosine triphosphate–binding proteins, Src and Src-related tyrosine kinases, and most viral and cellular Ras proteins comprise an extensive group of proteins that become modified by addition of myristate or palmitate. Palmitoylation is required for oncogenic viral Ras proteins to bind to the plasma membrane and transform cells and for vesicular transport through the Golgi stacks (45). Transmembrane receptors that are palmitoylated include the insulin receptor and the iron-transferrin receptor. Palmitate is acylated to certain membrane proteins involved with the cytoskeleton, including fibronectin and gap junction proteins (46). Several neuronal proteins are modified with palmitate. Acetylcholinesterase, which degrades the neurotransmitter acetylcholine, is bound to the cell membrane by palmitoylation (47). The reversible palmitoylation of proteins is involved with neural development by influencing neural motility and outgrowth in the developing brain (48).

ASSESSMENT OF STATUS

Analytical Methods

Blood, urine, and tissue pantothenic acid concentrations are often measured by microbiologic growth assays, animal bioassay, or radioimmunoassay. Microbiologic assays for measuring pantothenic acid are highly sensitive and specific, but they are slow and tedious to perform. Results of radioimmunoassay compare favorably with those obtained by microbiologic methods. Samples containing bound vitamin (biologic sources excluding urine) must be hydrolyzed with enzymes or chemicals to release the pantothenate component of CoA before being assayed. Enzymes used to release pantothenic acid include papain, mylase-P, diastase, and clarase. High-performance liquid chromatography methods, coupled with mass spectrometry or fluorometric detection, have also been shown to be sufficiently sensitive for measuring pantothenic acid in urine (49, 50). Quantification of pantothenic acid in biologic samples has been developed using stable isotope dilution assay (51) and enzyme-linked immunosorbent assay (52).

Blood Concentrations

Blood concentrations of pantothenic acid that are lower than 100 μg/dL have been suggested to indicate inadequate intake (53). Whole blood pantothenic acid concentrations have been reported to be significantly correlated with intake (54). Whole blood concentrations fell from 8.9 to 6.4 μmol/L when men were fed a diet devoid of pantothenic acid for up to 9 weeks (55). When the men were supplemented with 10 mg/day of pantothenic acid for 9 weeks, no difference in whole blood concentration was noted, compared with baseline. Dietary pantothenic acid intake did not correlate with blood concentration in a group of elderly subjects; however, when a supplement containing pantothenic acid was taken, blood concentration increased markedly (56).

Pantothenic acid intake and serum concentration were reported to correlate in adolescents, whereas no correlation was observed in adults (57). Plasma concentrations did not reflect changes in intake or status of pantothenic acid (29). The correlation between dietary and erythrocyte pantothenic acid in a group of well-nourished adolescents was 0.4, and average erythrocyte concentration was 1.5 μmol/L (334 ng/L) (54). At parturition, the pantothenic acid concentration was five times lower in the mother's serum compared with the infant's (16).

Urinary Excretion

A dose-response relationship between dietary intake and urinary excretion of pantothenic acid was shown in women (58, 59). This correlation was also confirmed in adolescents (57). Urinary pantothenic acid concentrations in women fed a diet low in pantothenic acid (2.8 mg/day) exceeded the intake level; suggesting that body stores were being lost or that synthesis was occurring (58). The body has been shown to conserve pantothenic acid (60).

CAUSES AND MANIFESTATIONS OF DEFICIENCY AND EXCESS

Information on the causes of deficiency or overexposure of pantothenic acid in humans is limited. Because pantothenic acid is present, to some extent, in all foods, a deficiency in humans is rare except in severe malnutrition, and it most likely occurs in conjunction with other nutrient deficiencies. During World War II, prisoners of war in Japan, the Philippines, and Burma experienced numbness in their toes and painful burning sensations in their feet. These symptoms were relieved with pantothenic acid supplementation, but not when other B-complex vitamins were given (61). When given a diet completely devoid of pantothenic acid (57) or when given an antagonist of pantothenic acid metabolism (62, 63), subjects experienced irritability, restlessness, sleep disturbances, numbness, and gastrointestinal disturbances.

Pantothenic acid has been suggested to aid in wound healing (64, 65) by increasing the number of migrating dermal fibroblasts (66) through modulation of gene expression (67). Low blood concentrations of pantothenic acid have been reported in patients with rheumatoid arthritis (68). One randomized double-blind study showed that daily supplementation with 1 g calcium pantothenate resulted in a significant reduction in pain in patients with rheumatoid arthritis (69) (see also the chapter on rheumatic and arthritis diseases). Evidence demonstrated that a class of pantothenic acid analogs represses the proliferation of the human malaria parasite, *Plasmodium falciparum* (70). Prospective observational studies have reported a significant positive association between pantothenic acid intake and birth weight (71) and birth length (21).

Administration of pantothenate analogs to humans has occurred with unintentionally deleterious side effects. Hopantenate is an analog of pantothenic acid, in which γ-amino butyric acid (GABA) replaces β-alanine. Hopantenate was used in Japan in individuals with emotional disturbance secondary to cerebrovascular disease and to alleviate tardive dyskinesia symptoms induced by tranquilizers. As a result, the patients exhibited severe side effects, including lactic acidosis, hypoglycemia, hyperammonemia, and eventually acute encephalopathy (72). These effects were also demonstrated in dogs and were shown to be caused by pantothenic acid deficiency. Dogs given an equivalent amount of pantothenic acid and calcium hopantenate did not develop the disorder (73).

No adverse effects of overconsumption of pantothenic acid in humans have been reported. For this reason, the Institute of Medicine did not set a tolerable upper intake level (UL) for pantothenic acid (18). When patients were treated with up to 15 g/day of pantothenic acid, however, symptoms of lupus erythematosus, nausea, and gastrointestinal distress were reported (74, 75). The toxic oral dose (LD$_{50}$) for mice was determined to be 10 g/kg, which led to death by respiratory failure (15). A study in which rats were provided up to 3% of their diet as calcium pantothenate for 29 days demonstrated that adverse effects (enlargement of testis, diarrhea, and hair damage) were observed at 3% but not at 1% (76). The investigators suggested that the lowest-observed-adverse-effect level (LOAEL) and no-observed-adverse-effect level (NOAEL) for pantothenic acid should be 3% and 1%, respectively. This information, along with an uncertainty factor that takes into consideration the use of animal data, can be used for setting a UL.

REFERENCES

1. Williams RJ, Bradway EM. J Am Chem Soc 1931;53:783.
2. Williams RJ, Lyman CM, Goodyear GH et al. J Am Chem Soc 1933;55:2912–27.
3. Williams RJ, Weinstock HH, Rohrmann E et al. J Am Chem Soc 1939:89:199–206.
4. William RJ, Mitchell HK, Weinstock HH et al. J Am Chem Soc 1940;62:1784–5.
5. Williams RJ, Eakin RE, Snell EE. J Am Chem Soc 1940; 62:1204–7.
6. Pennington D, Snell EE, William RJ. J Biol Chem 1940;135: 213–22.
7. Baddiley J, Thain EM, Novelli GD et al. Nature 1953;171:76–9.
8. Bean WB, Hodges RE. Proc Soc Exp Biol Med 1954;86:693–9.
9. Plesofsky-Vig N, Brambl R. Annu Rev Nutr 1988;8:461–82.
10. Bender DA, Bender AE, eds. Nutrition: A Reference Handbook. Oxford: Oxford University Press, 1997.
11. Walsh JH, Wyse BW, Hansen RG. J Am Diet Assoc 1981; 78:140–4.
12. US Department of Agriculture, Agricultural Research Service. USDA National Nutrient Database for Standard Reference. Release 16. Nutrient Data Laboratory. 2003. Available at: http://www.ars.usda.gov/ba/bhnrc/ndl. Accessed December 5, 2011.
13. Picciano MF. Water-soluble vitamins in milk. In: Jensen RG, ed. Handbook of Milk Composition. San Diego: Academic Press, 1995.
14. Johnston L, Vaughan L, Fox HM. Am J Clin Nutr 1981;34: 2205–9.
15. Song WO, Chan GM, Wyse BW et al. Am J Clin Nutr 1984; 40:317–24.
16. Robinson AF, Folkers K, eds. Vitamins and Coenzymes. New York: John Wiley, 1964.
17. National Research Council. Recommended Dietary Allowances. Washington, DC: National Academy Press, 1989:169–73.
18. Food and Nutrition Board, Institute of Medicine. Dietary Reference Intakes for Thiamin, Riboflavin, Niacin, Vitamin B$_6$, Folate, Pantothenic Acid, Biotin, and Choline. Washington, DC: National Academy Press, 1998;357–73.
19. New Brunswick Department of Health and Wellness. Appendix E. In: New Brunswick Nutrition Survey. Fredericton, New Brunswick, Canada: New Brunswick Department of Health and Wellness, 1997.
20. Song WO, Wyse BW, Hansen RG. J Am Diet Assoc 1985;85: 192–8.
21. Lagiou P, Mucci L, Tamimi R et al. Eur J Nutr 2005;44:52–9.
22. Srinivasan V, Christensen N, Wyse BW et al. Am J Clin Nutr 1981;34:1736–42.
23. Park SY, Murphy SP, Martin CL et al. J Am Diet Assoc 2008;108:529–33.
24. Fenstermacher DK, Rose DC. Am J Physiol 1986;250: G155–60.
25. Stein ED, Diamond JM. J Nutr 1989;119:1973–83.
26. Eissenstat BR, Wyse BW, Hansen RG. Am J Clin Nutr 1986; 44:931–37.
27. Fox HM. Pantothenic acid. In: Machlin LJ, ed. Handbook of Vitamins. New York: Marcel Dekker, 1984:437.
28. Tahiliani AB, Beinlich CH. Vitam Horm 1991;46:165–28.
29. Baker H, Frank O, Thomson AD et al. Am J Clin Nutr 1969;22:1469–75.
30. Shibata K, Gross CJ, Henderson LM. J Nutr 1983;113:2107–15.
31. Barbarat B, Podevin RA. J Biol Chem 1986;261:14455–60.
32. Prasad PD, Ramamoorthy S, Leibach FH et al. Placenta 1997;18:527–33.
33. Tarr JB, Tamura T, Stocksatd EL. Am J Clin Nutr 1981;34: 1328–37.
34. Yu BH, Kies C. Plant Foods Hum Nutr 1993;43:87–95.
35. Hayflick SJ, Westaway SK, Levinson B et al. N Engl J Med 2003;348:33–40.
36. Gregory A, Hayflick SJ. Pantothenate kinase-associated neurodegeneration. In: Pagon RA, Bird TD, Dolan CR, Stephens K, eds. GeneReviews. Seattle: University of Washington, 2008.
37. Ching KH, Westaway SK, Levinson B et al. Neurology 2002; 58:1673–4.
38. Brown G. J Biol Chem 1959;234:370–8.
39. Robishaw JD, Berkick D, Neely JR. J Biol Chem 1982;257: 10967–72.
40. Combs GF. The Vitamins: Fundamental Aspects in Nutrition and Health. New York: Academic Press, 1992:352.
41. Ridsdale JA, Hendzel MJ, Delcuve GP et al. J Biol Chem 1990;265:5150–6.
42. Norton VG, Marvin KW, Yau P et al. J Biol Chem 1990; 265:19848–52.
43. Plesofsky-Vig N, Brambl R. Annu Rev Nutr 1988;8:461–82.
44. Lim SS, Sammak PJ, Borisy GG. J Cell Biol 1989;109:253–63.
45. Pfanner N, Orci L, Glick BS et al. Cell 1989;59:95–102.
46. Maneti S, Dunia I, Benedetti EL. FEBS Lett 1990;262:356–8.
47. Randall WR. J Biol Chem 1994;269:12367–74.
48. Hess DT, Patterson SI, Smith DS et al. Nature 1993;366: 562–5.
49. Heudi O, Fontannaz P. J Sep Sci 2005;28:669–72.
50. Takahashi K, Fukuwatari T, Shibata K. J Chrom B 2009; 877:2168–72.
51. Rychlik M J Agr Food Chem 2000;48:1175–81.
52. Gonthier A, Boullanger P, Fayol V et al. J Immunoassay 1998; 19:167–94.
53. Sauberlich HE, Skala, JH. Laboratory Tests for the Assessment of Nutritional Status. Cleveland: CRC Press, 1974:88.
54. Eissenstat BR, Wyse BW, Hansen RG. Am J Clin Nutr 1986; 44:931–7.
55. Fry PC, Fox HM, Tao HG. J Nutr Sci Vitaminol (Tokyo) 1976; 22:399–46.
56. Wyse BW, Hansen RG. Fed Proc 1977;36:1169.
57. Kathman JV, Kies C. Nutr Res 1984;4:245–50.
58. Fox HM, Linkswiler H. J Nutr 1961;75:451–4.
59. Tsuiji T, Fukuwatari T, Sasaki S et al. Nutr Res 2010;30: 171–8.

60. Karnitz LM, Gross CJ, Henderson LM. Biochim Biophys Acta 1984;769:486–92.

61. Glusman M. Am J Med 1947;3:211–23.

62. Hodges RE, Ohlson MA, Bean WB. J Clin Invest 1958;37: 1642–57.

63. Hodges RE, Bean WB, Ohlson MA et al. J Clin Invest 1959; 38:1421–25.

64. Aprahamian M, Dentiger A, Stock-Damage C et al. Am J Clin Nutr 1985;41:578–89.

65. Lacroix B, Didier E, Grenier JF. Int J Vit Nutr Res 1988; 58:407–13.

66. Weimann BI, Hermann D. Int J Vit Nutr Res 1999;69:113–9.

67. Widerholt T, Heise R, Skazik C et al. Exp Dermatol 2009; 18:969–78.

68. Barton-Wright EC, Elliot WA. Lancet 1963;26:862–3.

69. Einstein P, Scheiner SA, eds. Overcoming the Pain of Inflammatory Arthritis: The Pain-Free Promise of Pantothenic Acid. Garden City, NY: Avery, 1999.

70. Lehane SM, Marchetti RV, Spry C et al. J Biol Chem 2007; 282:25395–405.

71. Haggarty P, Campbell DM, Duthie S et al. Br J Nutr 2009; 102:1487–97.

72. Otsuka M, Akiba T, Okita Y et al. Jpn J Med 1990;29:324–8.

73. Noda S, Haratake J, Sasaki A et al. Liver 1991;11:134–42.

74. Welsh AL. Arch Dermatol 1952;65:137–48.

75. Welsh AL. Arch Dermatol 1954;70:181–98.

76. Shibata K, Takahashi C, Fukuwatari T et al. J Nutr Sci Vitaminol (Tokyo) 2005;51:385–91.

SUGGESTED READINGS

Expert Group on Vitamins and Minerals. Review of Pantothenic Acid. London: Food Standards Agency, 2002.

Gregory A, Hayflick SJ. Pantothenate kinase-associated neurodegeneration. In: Pagon RA, Bird TD, Dolan CR et al., eds. GeneReviews. Seattle: University of Washington, 2008.

US Department of Agriculture, Agricultural Research Service. USDA National Nutrient Database for Standard Reference, Release 22. Nutrient Data Laboratory Home Page. 2008. Available at: http://www.ars.usda.gov/ba/bhnrc/ndl. Accessed December 5, 2011.

26 FOLIC ACID[1]

PATRICK J. STOVER

HISTORICAL BACKGROUND

Also known as vitamin B_9, vitamin B_c, vitamin M, *Lactobacillus casei* factor, folacin, and pteroyl-L-glutamic acid, folic acid was first discovered by Wills and Mehta in 1931 as a factor in yeast ("Wills' factor") that corrected the macrocytic anemia of pregnant Hindu women in India (1). The factor was later isolated from spinach leaves and was given the name folic acid (Latin *folium,* "leaf") by Mitchell et al in 1941, who demonstrated that it was required for growth of *Streptococcus lactis*

R (*Streptococcus faecalis*) (2). In 1945, the chemical synthesis of pure crystalline folic acid was reported in the journal *Science* (3). Synthetic folic acid was effective in reversing megaloblastic anemia that was refractory to treatment with liver extracts, but this agent was not able to prevent or improve neurologic damage that progressed from anemia that is now known to be caused by vitamin B_{12} deficiency.

Shortly after the discovery of folic acid as a growth-promoting factor, the development of folate antagonists as chemotherapeutics was undertaken by the Nobel Laureates Hitchings and Elion. In 1948, the folate antagonists aminopterin and, shortly thereafter, methotrexate were developed and administered to patients with childhood acute lymphoblastic leukemia and found to be effective treatments (4). This success led to the development of numerous anticancer and antimicrobial agents over the following 50 years that targeted folate-requiring enzymes. Beginning in the 1950s to the present time, folate-dependent enzymes were purified to homogeneity, biochemical pathways were elucidated, and later, their genes were cloned and structures determined. Beginning in the 1980s, the importance of folic acid in prevention of chronic diseases, certain cancers, and birth defects gained appreciation. This knowledge led to fortification of the food supply with folic acid in the United States, Canada, and other countries to prevent a class of common birth defects known as neural tube defects (NTDs). An excellent review of the history of folic acid was published in 2001 by Hoffbrand and Weir (1).

OVERVIEW OF FOLATE AND FOLIC ACID

Folate is a generic term that refers to a family of water-soluble B vitamins that are found in natural food and in biologic organisms (Fig. 26.1). Folates function as a family of enzyme cofactors that carry and chemically activate single carbons (referred to as one-carbons) for biosynthetic reactions. Folate is required for the biosynthesis of ribonucleotides and deoxyribonucleotide precursors for DNA synthesis. It is also required for amino acid metabolism, including the remethylation of homocysteine to methionine, and therefore functions in the regulation of gene expression by methylation. Hence, folate cofactors are

---

[1]**Abbreviations: AdoHcy**, S-adenosylhomocysteine; **AdoMet**, S-adenosylmethionine; **AICARFT**, phosphoribosylaminoimidazole-carboxamide formyltransferase; **DFE**, dietary folate equivalent; **DHF**, dihydrofolate; **DHFR**, dihydrofolate reductase; **DNMT**, DNA methyltransferase; **GARFT**, phosphoribosylglycinamide formyltransferase; **GNMT**, glycine *N*-methyltransferase; **LINE-1**, long interspersed nuclear element-1; **MTHFD**, methylenetetrahydrofolate dehydrogenase; **MTHFR**, methylenetetrahydrofolate reductase; **MTR**, methionine synthase; **NADPH**, reduced nicotinamide adenine dinucleotide phosphate; **NTD**, neural tube defect; **PCFT**, proton-coupled folate transporter; **RDA**, recommended dietary allowance; **SHMT**, serine hydroxymethyltransferase; **THF**, tetrahydrofolate; **TYMS**, thymidylate synthase.

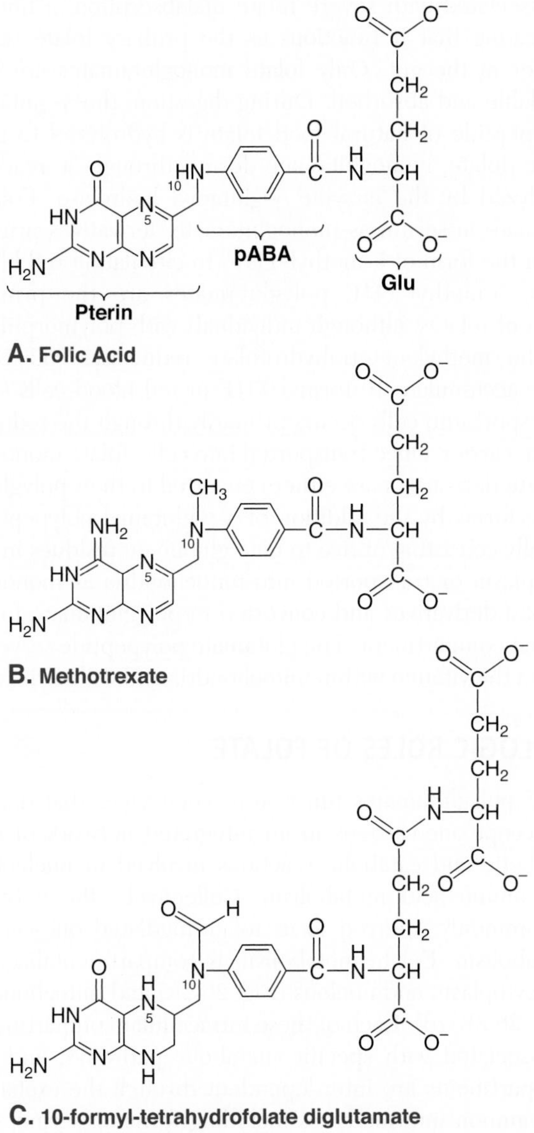

A. Folic Acid

B. Methotrexate

C. 10-formyl-tetrahydrofolate diglutamate

Fig. 26.1. The chemical structure of folic acid **(A)**, methotrexate **(B)**, and 10-formyl-tetrahydrofolate diglutamate **(C)**. Folic acid contains a pterin ring that is bridged to *para*-aminobenzoic acid (PABA) through a methylene group to form pteroic acid. The addition of the glutamate residue (Glu) through a peptide linkage results in the formation of folic acid. Methotrexate (4-amino-10-methylpteroylglutamic acid) **(B)** is a folate analog, antagonist, and pharmaceutical agent that inhibits the activity of DHFR. Once transported into the cell, folic acid is reduced to tetrahydrofolate and is modified by the addition of a glutamate polypeptide containing up to nine glutamate residues linked by unusual γ-peptide linkages. THF is also modified by the addition of single carbons at the N5 or N10 position or that bridge the N5 and N10 positions. The carbon moieties are carried at the oxidation states of formate, formaldehyde, or methanol. The structure of 10-formyl-tetrahydrofolate diglutamate is shown in **C**.

found in virtually all forms of life. Tetrahydrofolate (THF), which is the fully reduced form of the vitamin, carries one-carbons at one of three different oxidation levels ranging from methanol to formate (5, 6). The one-carbons are covalently bound to the N5 or N10 position of THF. In the cell, five different one-carbon substituted forms of THF are present: 10-formyl-THF; 5-formyl-THF;

5,10-methenyl-THF; 5,10-methylene-THF; and 5-methyl-THF, and each of these forms is interconverted in the cell through enzyme-mediated catalysis. Folates are also modified through the addition of a glutamate polypeptide that is polymerized through unusual γ-linked peptide bonds (7). The polyglutamate polypeptide increases the affinity of folate cofactors for folate-dependent enzymes and is required to retain folates within the cell and subcellular organelles. Folic acid (see Fig. 26.1) is not a biologically active form of folate, but it can serve as a provitamin because it is converted to the reduced, natural form of folate once transported into cells. It is an oxidized form of folate generated during the oxidative degradation of folate and normally does not accumulate in cells, although most degradation of THF is irreversible with degradation products that include oxidized pterin and *para*-aminobenzoylglutamate (8). Folic acid is also a synthetic form of folate present in fortified foods and in dietary supplements.

DIETARY SOURCES

Folate is a vitamin and therefore must be acquired from the diet. Folate nutritional status is supported by the intake of the vitamin found in natural foods as well as dietary supplements and fortified foods (9). The best dietary sources of natural folate include fresh fruits, leafy green vegetables, yeast, liver, and legumes (10). Natural folates found in food are chemically labile and readily undergo irreversible oxidative degradation during food preparation and cooking. 5-Methyl-THF and formyl-substituted THF are the primary forms of folate present in natural foods, and they are also among the more stable forms of the vitamin. Folic acid, the synthetic, fully oxidized, and stable provitamin, is present in dietary supplements and fortified food (see Fig. 26.1). Folic acid has greater bioavailability than natural food folate because of its chemical stability and lack of a polyglutamate moiety, which impairs absorption across the intestinal epithelium (11). Once transported into the cell, folic acid is reduced to dihydrofolate (DHF) and subsequently THF by the enzyme DHF reductase (DHFR), and once fully reduced, folic acid is indistinguishable from natural food folate. Low levels of DHFR expression may result in the appearance of folic acid in the serum of individuals with high levels of folic acid intake (9). Evidence indicates that the total DHFR activity is highly variable among individuals—a finding that may indicate a variable capacity to metabolize folic acid among individuals (12).

RECOMMENDED DIETARY ALLOWANCES AND FOLIC ACID FORTIFICATION

The recommended intakes of folate established by the Food and Nutrition Board of the Institute of Medicine are shown in Table 26.1 (13). Dietary folate requirements are expressed as dietary folate equivalents (DFEs) because

TABLE 26.1	DIETARY REFERENCE INTAKES FOR FOLATE[a]
GROUP	INTAKE (µg OF DFE/d)
Infants (mo)	Adequate intake
0–5	65
6–11	80
Children and adolescents (y)	Recommended dietary allowance
1–3	150
4–8	200
9–13	300
14–18	400
Adults (y)	Recommended dietary allowance
≥19	400
Pregnant women	600
Lactating women	500

DFE, dietary folate equivalent.

[a]Requirements are expressed as dietary folate equivalents, to account for the increased bioavailability of folic acid compared with natural food folate.

Data from Food and Nutrition Board, Institute of Medicine. Folate. In: Dietary Reference Intakes for Thiamin, Riboflavin, Niacin, Vitamin B6, Folate, Vitamin B12, Pantothenic Acid, Biotin, and Choline. Washington, DC: National Academy Press, 1998:196–305; and Bailey LB, Gregory JF III. Folate metabolism and requirements. J Nutr 1999;129:779–82.

of the need to adjust for the increased bioavailability of folic acid compared with natural food folate (11). Folic acid is estimated to be 1.7 times more bioavailable than natural food folate. The recommended dietary allowance (RDA) for both men and women is 400 µg/day DFEs. The requirement for women of childbearing age is 400 µg of folic acid from fortified foods and supplements, in addition to food folate consumption from a varied diet (13). The tolerable upper intake level for adults was set at 1000 µg/day of folic acid exclusive of food folate, based on concerns that elevated intake of folic acid would exacerbate neurologic consequences of vitamin B12 deficiency.

The United States and Canada mandated the addition of folic acid at a level of 140 µg/100 g of product to enriched flour in 1998 to achieve a predicted intake of 100 µg/day folic acid to reduce the incidence of NTDs (14). Before folic acid fortification, the median folate intake from food was estimated to be 250 µg/day. Population intake levels increased by 529 µg DFE/day between the interval 1998 to 1994 (before fortification) and 1999 to 2000 (after fortification) and then decreased by 135 mg between 1999 to 2000 and 2003 to 2004 (14). Folic acid fortification increased serum and red blood cell folate concentrations in the United States and decreased total plasma homocysteine levels by 6% to 13% (15, 16).

SITES OF INTESTINAL ABSORPTION

Folate absorption across the intestinal epithelium occurs in the acidic environment of the upper small intestine through the proton-coupled folate transporter (PCFT) (17), which was originally and probably incorrectly discovered as a heme transporter. Loss of PCFT function is associated with severe folate malabsorption, a finding indicating that it functions as the primary folate transporter in the gut. Only folate monoglutamates are bioavailable and absorbed. During digestion, the γ-glutamyl polypeptide of natural food folate is hydrolyzed to generate folate monoglutamate forms through a reaction catalyzed by the enzyme γ-glutamyl hydrolase. Folates circulate in serum as monoglutamate derivatives primarily in the form of 5-methyl-THF. In circulating red blood cells, 5-methyl-THF polyglutamates are the primary form of folates, although individuals with polymorphisms in the methylenetetrahydrofolate reductase (MTHFR) gene accumulate 10-formyl-THF in red blood cells (18). Transport into cells occurs primarily through the reduced folate carrier. Once transported into cells, folate monoglutamate derivatives are either converted to their polyglutamate forms by the addition of a γ-glutamyl polypeptide, usually consisting of five to nine glutamate residues in the cytoplasm or transported into mitochondria as monoglutamate derivatives and converted to polyglutamate forms in that compartment. The glutamate polypeptide serves to retain the vitamin within mitochondria and within the cell.

BIOLOGIC ROLES OF FOLATE

THF polyglutamates function as coenzymes that donate or accept one-carbons in an integrated network of biosynthetic and catabolic reactions involved in nucleotide and amino acid metabolism. Collectively, the network is commonly referred to as folate-mediated one-carbon metabolism. Folate metabolism is compartmentalized in the cytoplasm and nucleus (Fig. 26.2A) and mitochondria (Fig. 26.2B) (6). Each of these intracellular compartments is associated with specific metabolic pathways, and the compartments are interdependent through the exchange of common intermediates including formate, serine, and glycine (see Fig. 26.2B) (5, 19). Folate-mediated one-carbon metabolism also requires the water-soluble vitamins riboflavin (vitamin B2), niacin (vitamin B3), choline, pantothenic acid (vitamin B5), pyridoxal phosphate (vitamin B6), and cobalamin (vitamin B12) for its function (6) (see Fig. 26.2).

Cytoplasm

The de novo biosynthesis of purine and thymidylate nucleotides and the remethylation of homocysteine to methionine occur in the cytoplasm. The cytoplasm is the only compartment in the network that involves all the one-carbon substituted forms of THF (6). Formate serves as the primary source of one-carbon units for cytoplasmic one-carbon transfer reactions and is derived from amino acid catabolism in mitochondria (5, 20). In an adenosine triphosphate–dependent reaction, formate condenses with THF to form 10-formyl-THF, catalyzed by the 10-formyl-THF synthetase activity of the multifunctional enzyme methylenetetrahydrofolate dehydrogenase 1 (MTHFD1).

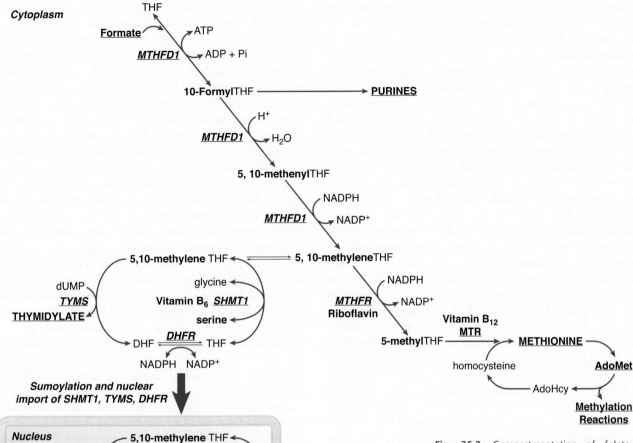

A

B

Fig. 26.2. Compartmentation of folate-mediated one-carbon metabolism in the cytoplasm, mitochondria, and nucleus. **A.** One-carbon metabolism in the cytoplasm is required for the de novo synthesis of purines and thymidylate and for the remethylation of homocysteine to methionine. One-carbon metabolism in the nucleus synthesizes thymidylate from uridylate and serine, and it occurs during the S phase of the cell cycle. **B.** One-carbon metabolism in the mitochondria is required to generate formate for one-carbon metabolism in the cytoplasm. The folate and amino acid carriers of the one-carbon unit are indicated by **bold type**. *AdoHcy*, S-adenosylhomocysteine; *AdoMet*, S-adenosylmethionine; *ADP*, adenosine diphosphate; *ATP*, adenosine triphosphate; *DHF*, dihydrofolate; *DHFR*, dihydrofolate reductase; *DMGD*, dimethylglycine dehydrogenase; *dUMP*, deoxyuridine monophosphate; *GCS*, glycine cleavage system; *mFTHFS*, mitochondrial formyltetrahydrofolate synthetase; *mMTHFC*, mitochondrial methenyltetrahydrofolate cyclohydrolase; *mMTHFD*, mitochondrial methylenetetrahydrofolate dehydrogenase; *MTHFR*, methylenetetrahydrofolate reductase; *MTR*, methionine synthase; *M-tRNA-FT*, methionyl-tRNA formyltransferase; *NAD*, nicotinamide adenine dinucleotide; *NADP*, nicotinamide adenine dinucleotide phosphate; *NADPH*, reduced nicotinamide adenine dinucleotide phosphate; *Pi*, inorganic phosphate; *SD*, sarcosine dehydrogenase; *SHMT1*, cytoplasmic serine hydroxymethyltransferase; *THF*, tetrahydrofolate; *TYMS*, thymidylate synthase.

Therefore, MTHFD1 is the primary entry point of one-carbons into the one-carbon metabolic network in the cytoplasm. The folate-dependent de novo synthesis of purine nucleotides involves 10 reactions and occurs through the formation of a multiple-enzyme complex termed a *purineosome*, which assembles when exogenous sources of purines are not available (21). The activated formyl moiety of 10-formyl-THF is incorporated into the number 2 and number 8 positions of the purine ring. In the third reaction of de novo purine biosynthesis, phosphoribosylglycinamide formyltransferase (GARFT) catalyzes the 10-formyl-THF–dependent conversion of glycinamide ribotide (GAR) to form formylglycinamide ribonucleotide (FGAR) and THF (see Fig. 26.2). In the ninth reaction, phospho-ribosylaminoimidazolecarboxamide formyltransferase (AICARFT) catalyzes the 10-formyl-THF–dependent conversion of aminoimidazolecarboxamide ribotide (AICAR) to formylaminoimidazolecarboxamide ribonucleotide (FAICAR) and THF. Transformed cells are dependent on de novo purine biosynthesis, which accounts for the effectiveness of chemotherapeutic antifolates that target GARFT or AICARFT, including 6-R-dideazatetrahydrofolate (DDATHF; lometrexol that specifically targets GARFT) (22–24). Methotrexate (4-amino-10-methylpteroylglutamic acid) inhibits several folate-dependent enzymes, including both GARFT and AICARFT, by depleting 10-formyl-THF.

Alternatively, the one-carbon of 10-formyl-THF can be enzymatically reduced to 5,10-methylene-THF through the cyclohydrolase and reduced nicotinamide adenine dinucleotide phosphate (NADPH)–dependent dehydrogenase activities of MTHFD1. The de novo synthesis of thymidylate requires 5,10-methylene-THF as the one-carbon donating cofactor. 5,10-methylene-THF and uridylate are converted to thymidylate and DHF in a reaction catalyzed by the enzyme thymidylate synthase (TYMS). For this reaction, 5,10-methylene-THF serves both as a one-carbon donor and also as a source of two electrons through the oxidation of THF to DHF. THF is regenerated from DHF in a reaction catalyzed by the NADPH-dependent enzyme DHFR. To complete the de novo thymidylate synthesis cycle, THF is concerted to 5,10-methylene-THF by the three catalytic activities of MTHFD1, as described earlier, or alternatively by the vitamin B$_6$–dependent enzyme serine hydroxymethyltransferase (SHMT1 and SHMT2α). The SHMT isozymes catalyze the conversion of serine to glycine to generate 5,10-methylene-THF from THF (see Fig. 26.2) (25). Several chemotherapeutic agents that target TYMS have been developed, including the fluoropyrimidines 5-fluorouracil (5-FU) and 5-fluoro-2-deoxyuridine (FdUrd), and the antifolates raltitrexed, pemetrexed, and methotrexate. These agents have been proven effective in the treatment of head, neck, breast, stomach, and colon cancers (26). These agents decrease TYMS catalytic function while also increasing cellular TYMS concentrations (27, 28) by preventing TYMS from binding to its mRNA or by decreasing the rate of ubiquitin-independent enzyme degradation (29, 30).

The remethylation of homocysteine to methionine occurs through folate-dependent and folate-independent pathways. For the folate-dependent pathway, 5,10-methylene-THF is reduced to 5-methyl-THF in a reaction catalyzed by the NADPH- and flavin adenine dinucleotide (FAD)–dependent enzyme MTHFR. 5-Methyl-THF is a cofactor for homocysteine remethylation to methionine, which is catalyzed by methionine synthase (MTR) in a vitamin B$_{12}$–dependent reaction that converts 5-methyl-THF and homocysteine to methionine and THF. Homocysteine can be converted to methionine in a folate-independent reaction catalyzed by the enzyme betaine homocysteine methyltransferase, a reaction in which betaine serves as the one-carbon donor. Once formed, methionine can be adenosylated to form S-adenosylmethionine (AdoMet), which is a cofactor and one-carbon donor for numerous other methylation reactions (31). S-Adenosylhomocysteine (AdoHcy) is a product of AdoMet-dependent transmethylation reactions and is cleaved to form adenosine and homocysteine, which completes the homocysteine remethylation pathway.

These three metabolic pathways in the cytoplasm are highly interconnected and interdependent. Folate-dependent enzymes bind folate polyglutamate cofactors tightly with binding constants in the low micromolar or nanomolar range. The cellular concentration of folate-binding proteins exceeds that of folate derivatives (which are present at 25 to 35 μM), and therefore, the concentration of free folate in the cell is negligible (8, 32, 33). Consequently, independent of their origin, metabolic impairments of one-carbon metabolism rarely affect a single pathway, but rather they influence the entire network. This primarily occurs because the folate-dependent pathways compete for a limiting pool of folate cofactors in the cytoplasm (8, 34).

Mitochondria

Mitochondria contain as much as 40% of total cellular folate, and folate polyglutamates in mitochondria are a distinct pool that does not exchange with folate polyglutamates in the cytoplasm (35). In this compartment, one-carbon metabolism is required to formylate Met-tRNA to form fMet-tRNA, which is used for the initiation of mitochondrial protein synthesis. A primary role of one-carbon metabolism in mitochondria is to generate formate for one-carbon metabolism in the cytoplasm, however. Both pathways require 10-formyl-THF (see Fig. 26.2B). Formate can be generated from the THF-dependent catabolism of the amino acids glycine, serine, dimethylglycine, and sarcosine, although serine and glycine are the primary sources of formate (36, 37). These amino acids donate a one-carbon to THF, thus generating 5,10-methylene-THF, which is subsequently oxidized to form 10-formyl-THF through the activities of MTHFD2 and MTHFD1L (20). Formate derived in mitochondria traverses to the cytoplasm for use in cytoplasmic one-carbon metabolism (5).

Nucleus

Approximately 10% of total liver folates reside in the nuclear compartment (38). Nuclear one-carbon metabolism functions to generate thymidylate from uridylate (25) during the S phase of the cell cycle and during ultraviolet radiation-induced DNA damage (39). The enzymes that constitute the entire thymidylate synthesis pathway, including the enzymes SHMT1, SHMT2α, TYMS, and DHFR, are modified by the small ubiquitin-like modifier (SUMO), which facilitates the nuclear translocation of the entire pathway (25). SHMT is the only source of one-carbons for nuclear thymidylate synthesis; mice lacking SHMT1 exhibit impaired thymidylate synthesis and elevated uracil in nuclear DNA (40). The necessity for redundancy in the compartmentation of de novo thymidylate synthesis in the cytoplasm and nucleus is not known.

REGULATION OF THE CELLULAR METHYLATION POTENTIAL AND IMPACT OF VITAMIN B_{12} DEFICIENCY

The cellular methylation potential is highly regulated, primarily through the control of AdoMet synthesis and use. AdoMet synthesis occurs only when cellular AdoMet concentrations are depleted, and excess AdoMet is consumed when its levels are elevated. Both regulatory processes occur through a single mechanism that involves interactions among the metabolites AdoMet, 5-methyl-THF, MTHFR, and glycine N-methyltransferase (GNMT), an enzyme that catalyzes the AdoMet-dependent methylation of glycine to sarcosine for the purpose of disposing excess cellular AdoMet (41). Because AdoMet is an allosteric inhibitor of MTHFR, 5-methyl-THF, which is the cofactor for the folate-dependent remethylation of homocysteine to methionine, is synthesized only when AdoMet levels are depleted. This feedback inhibition of MTHFR by AdoMet ensures that folate cofactors are available for nucleotide synthesis when the methylation potential is adequate to support cellular methylation reactions.

AdoMet levels are also maintained through the allosteric inhibition of GNMT by 5-methyl-THF (42). The depletion of 5-methyl-THF levels that results from the AdoMet inhibition of MTHFR activates GNMT, which, in turn, lowers AdoMet levels through the conversion of glycine to sarcosine. GNMT prevents the cellular accumulation of AdoMet. Mice lacking GNMT exhibit a 36-fold elevation in AdoMet concentrations and a 100-fold increase in the AdoMet/AdoHcy ratio. They also exhibit fatty liver (43). Humans with mutations in GNMT have been identified with similar metabolic disruptions seen in the *Gnmt* null mice (43). GNMT expression is regulated by vitamin A (44) and glucocorticoids (45), thus providing a mechanism whereby signals and nutrients unrelated to one-carbon metabolism can influence cellular methylation reactions and potentially epigenetic processes (41).

Vitamin B_{12} deficiency has a major impact on the folate-mediated one-carbon network and disrupts both homocysteine remethylation and nucleotide biosynthesis. This disruption is the metabolic origin of megaloblastic anemia. Vitamin B_{12} deficiency, whether from nutritional deficiency or excessive exposure to nitrous oxide, impairs MTR activity. Lack of MTR activity disrupts the homocysteine remethylation pathway and depletes AdoMet concentrations, thereby activating MTHFR. MTHFR activation causes cellular folate to accumulate as 5-methyl-THF, a condition often referred to as the folate "methyl trap." Because the MTHFR-catalyzed generation of 5-methyl-THF is essentially irreversible in vivo, accumulation of 5-methyl-THF can impair purine and thymidylate de novo biosynthesis, as occurs in severe vitamin B_{12} deficiency (46).

ANALYTIC METHODS AND BIOMARKERS OF IMPAIRED ONE-CARBON METABOLISM

Certain clinically useful biomarkers are responsive to dietary folate intake and can be used to assess folate status and disruptions in folate-mediated one-carbon metabolism. Most of the functional metabolic biomarkers that report on folate status lack specificity, however, because they are also responsive to nutritional status for other B vitamins as well as for common variants in genes that encode folate-dependent enzymes (47, 48). Impairments in the folate metabolic network can result from primary dietary folate deficiency and from deficiencies of other nutrients that function in one-carbon metabolism, including vitamin B_6, vitamin B_{12}, and riboflavin, from excessive alcohol intake, or from genetic variation that influences the activity or expression of folate-dependent enzymes (see Fig. 26.2) (19).

Folate levels are measured in serum or red blood cells to assess folate status in individuals as well as in epidemiologic and population status (13). Red blood cell folate concentrations are the preferred indicators of long-term folate status (47). The reason is that folate enters the red blood cells only during their development in the bone marrow, and therefore, these values reflect the average folate status over the life span of the adult red blood cell, which is 120 days. A value of 140 ng/mL of red blood cell folate is considered the lower limit of folate sufficiency. Serum folate levels report on both long-term status and recent folate intake and thus should be measured repeatedly when folate status is assessed. Plasma levels lower than 7 nM indicate negative folate balance. The persistence of this condition usually progresses to megaloblastic anemia.

Measuring folate levels is particularly challenging because of the multiple chemical forms of the vitamin and its chemical liability (8). Microbiologic assay has been the method of choice until fairly recently, in part because it measures growth of *Lactobacillus casei* when exposed to all forms of folate monoglutamates and can tolerate high quantities of ascorbate that are required to prevent folate oxidation during sample preparation and assay. Radioisotope and chemiluminescent, and high-performance chromatography methods have also been widely used (48). The high-performance chromatography methods have the advantage of distinguishing among folate one-carbon and polyglutamate forms (49). Similarly, newer mass spectrometry methods are capable of resolving and quantifying the one-carbon forms of folate (50). The distribution of the one-carbon forms of folate in serum or erythrocytes may serve as a more robust biomarker of folate status or functional indicator of impaired one-carbon metabolism. All the existing methods are prone to errors of accuracy and precision, as discussed elsewhere (48).

Two sensitive biomarkers of impaired folate metabolism are uracil content in nuclear DNA (51, 52) and elevations in homocysteine concentrations in plasma and tissue (47). Decreased rates of deoxythymidine triphosphate (dTTP) synthesis result in the incorporation of deoxyuridine triphosphate (dUTP) into DNA, because DNA polymerases do not discriminate between dUTP and dTTP (51, 53). Uracil content in white blood cell DNA may not be a robust surrogate for uracil content in tissue, however, so its utility for clinical and population assessment of folate status remains uncertain (54). As mentioned earlier, total plasma homocysteine is responsive to folate status and has been used to assess folate status in the clinic and in population studies because decreased rates of folate-dependent homocysteine remethylation result in elevations in cellular and plasma homocysteine (31). Total plasma homocysteine is also responsive to vitamin B_6 and vitamin B_{12} status as well as genetic variation in the *MTHFR* gene (47, 48, 55). Elevated homocysteine also results in elevated AdoHcy concentrations because the equilibrium for the hydrolysis AdoHcy to adenosine and homocysteine favors AdoHcy synthesis (56). AdoHcy is a potent inhibitor of AdoMet-dependent methylases including DNA and protein methyltransferases (57), and AdoHcy accumulation causes hypomethylated DNA in white blood cells (18, 58–60). AdoMet, AdoHcy, and the AdoMet/AdoHcy ratio have also been explored as functional indicators of folate status (61). Other biomarkers of whole body folate deficiency include DNA hypomethylation, elevated formiminoglutamate in urine (an intermediate in folate-dependent histidine catabolism), and neutrophil hypersegmentation (62, 63).

The biomarkers that were used to determine the RDA for dietary folate intake by the Institute of Medicine include erythrocyte folate concentrations and plasma homocysteine and folate concentrations (47). Both are responsive to inadequate dietary intake of folate. As stated earlier, however, secondary nutrient deficiencies including vitamin B_6 and B_{12}, genetics, and gender can influence metabolic biomarkers such as homocysteine that are used to assess whole body folate status (64). Men tend to exhibit higher levels than women (47). The reference interval for total plasma homocysteine varies among research laboratories. A value of 10 μM total plasma homocysteine has been suggested to be a cutoff to assess folate status in populations. Erythrocyte folate concentrations less than 140 ng/mL indicate folate deficiency, but these concentrations are also influenced by genetic variation, including the common 677 C$\rightarrow$ T polymorphism in the *MTHFR* gene (18). Increasing evidence indicates that dietary folate requirements may differ by *MTHFR* genotype (65).

FOLATE AND EPIGENETICS

Epigenetics commonly refers to the inheritance of traits independent of DNA primary sequence, and this term is often used to describe the transmission of DNA methylation patterns and potentially other covalent chromatin modifications that may be heritable (66). The term is often associated with various biologic phenomena including X chromosome inactivation and metabolic and nutritional imprinting. The influence of maternal nutrition during gestation and the suckling period on fetal and neonatal traits is referred to as *metabolic imprinting* (67). Experimental animal models support the concept that maternal nutrition can influence the developing fetus and neonate by altering DNA methylation patterns and altering gene expression patterns. These genomic changes persist throughout the lifetime of the animal and result in risk phenotypes such as obesity and metabolic syndrome that increase the risk of adult-onset disease including cardiovascular disease and certain cancers (68). Dietary exposures that are associated with metabolic programming phenomena include caloric undernutrition and overnutrition, as well as intake levels of specific dietary components including protein, fatty acids, folate, choline, methionine, and combinations of these B vitamins and methyl donors (69–74).

Dietary folate and intake of other B vitamins and metabolites of one-carbon metabolism can induce alterations in DNA methylation patterns that are potentially heritable (75). The only established mechanism whereby folate influences epigenetic processes is through the homocysteine remethylation pathway. Cellular AdoMet and AdoHcy levels influence the activity of AdoMet-dependent methyltransferases, albeit by distinct mechanisms. AdoMet is the substrate for transmethylation reactions catalyzed by methyltransferases including DNA and histone methyltransferases. AdoHcy, the product of AdoMet-dependent methyltransferase reactions, binds tightly and inhibits many AdoMet-dependent enzymes through product inhibition and therefore is a physiologically relevant inhibitor of chromatin methylation. The ratio of cellular AdoMet to AdoHcy concentrations has often been referred to as the *cellular methylation potential* (56). AdoHcy, which accumulates when homocysteine accumulates (see Fig. 26.1), is the more important determinant of cellular methylation capacity and global DNA methylation compared with AdoMet concentrations in human lymphocytes (76). In cystathionine β-synthase–deficient mice, which exhibit elevated homocysteine and AdoHcy, AdoHcy, but not AdoMet, predicts global DNA hypomethylation (77). Similarly, vitamin B_{12} deficiency causes elevated homocysteine and DNA hypomethylation in rodents (78).

Many examples of the impact of folate and other B-vitamin dietary deficiencies on global DNA CpG methylation have been reported. Mice fed a folate-deficient diet for 32 weeks exhibited 60% elevations in serum homocysteine and global DNA hypomethylation in splenocytes (reduced 9.1%) and colonic epithelial cells (reduced 7.2%), without changes in allelic-specific methylation at the mouse B1 element or the genetically imprinted genes *H19* or *Oct4* (52). These effects may be mediated through elevations in homocysteine. In an endothelial cell culture model, exposure to homocysteine (to 50 μm) was sufficient to reduce by 30% DNA methyltransferase 1 (DNMT1) activity without affecting DNMT1 protein levels. Homocysteine exposure diminished DNA CpG methylation within the repressive cyclin-dependent element of the cyclin A promoter, thus leading to depressed *cyclin A* transcription. These results are consistent with a role for homocysteine-induced elevations in AdoHcy ratio in the regulation of DNMT1 activity (79). In human studies, genetic impairments that elevate homocysteine are also associated with global DNA hypomethylation. A common polymorphism in the *MTHFR* gene, C677T, is associated with reduced MTHFR enzyme activity and elevated homocysteine levels (80) as well as reduced methylation potential and DNA hypomethylation in lymphocytes (18). Folate nutritional status and global DNA CpG methylation do not exhibit a linear dose-response relationship, however. Folic acid supplementation in humans at 1 mg/day was shown not to alter long interspersed nuclear element-1 (LINE-1) methylation density, a proxy for DNA global methylation, in normal colonic mucosa cells (81).

More severe elevations in plasma homocysteine, at levels shown in patients with homocystinuria (plasma levels higher than 50 μM), exhibited DNA CpG hypomethylation and biallelic expression of both sex-linked and imprinted genes. The magnitude of the shift from monoallelic expression to biallelic expression depended on homocysteine concentrations. Supplemental folic acid corrected the DNA hypomethylation and restored imprinted patterns of gene expression (82). However, in the absence of severe genetic disruptions, as seen in patients with homocystinuria, or severe dietary deficiencies, no evidence indicates that one-carbon metabolism influences gene silencing associated with classical parent-of-origin-specific genetic imprinting.

In transformed tissue, folate deficiency or genetic impairment in one-carbon metabolism affects both global and allelic-specific CpG methylation differently from that observed in nontransformed cells. Folate nutritional status and LINE-1 methylation do not correlate in normal colonic mucosa, but some evidence indicates that folate status does affect LINE-1 methylation once neoplasia develops (83). Similarly, the common C677T polymorphism in *MTHFR* is associated with increased promoter methylation in colon cancer (84). A study by de Vogel et al (85) showed that the variants of MTR (A2756) and MTR reductase (A66G) genes may reduce mutL homolog 1 (*MLH1*) promoter hypermethylation in colorectal cancer. In non–small cell lung cancers, folate levels in tumors correlate with global methylation, using LINE-1 methylation as a surrogate and allelic-specific methylation at the promoters of CDH13, RUNX3, but not MYOD1, RASSF1P16, APC, RARB. This study supports the concept that folate levels influence both global and some allelic-specific methylation in transformed cells (86).

Although alterations in one-carbon metabolism and the cellular methylation potential can alter DNA methylation patterns and affect gene expression, the ability of maternal dietary folate and other metabolites of one-carbon metabolism to establish and then memorize specific changes in chromatin methylation appears to be possible only within specific developmental windows (87). Harnessing the diet-epigenetic relationship will require further advances in our understanding of methylation targeting and limits of epigenetic plasticity in embryonic and adult stem cells as well as more differentiated cell lineages.

FOLATE AND NEURAL TUBE DEFECTS

NTDs are neurodevelopmental anomalies that result from a failure of the neural tube to close during early embryonic development (88). They are among the most common congenital birth defects in humans, with a worldwide prevalence ranging from 0.5 to 60/10,000 births (89). The most common and severe NTDs include spina bifida, which results from a failure of posterior neural tube to close and results in exposure of the spinal cord and life-long paralysis, and anencephaly, which is lethal and defined by absence of the cranial vault and brain secondary to failure of the anterior neural tube to close. Maternal folic acid supplementation is the most effective intervention that is known to prevent NTDs, and it may prevent up to 70% of NTDs (90). In the United States and Canada, folic acid fortification of enriched flour was initiated in 1998 to lower the incidence of NTDs, and this public health intervention has been successful (91). Human genetic variation that contributes to a woman's risk of having an NTD-affected pregnancy includes genes that encode the folate-dependent enzymes MTHFR (92–94) and MTHFD1 (95). Both maternal and fetal *MTHFR* variants contribute to risk, whereas *MTHFD1* risk is exclusively maternal.

The impaired metabolic pathway responsible for NTDs has not been established. Homocysteine is cytotoxic at high levels and induces oxidative stress, but mouse models of inborn errors of metabolism that exhibit severe hyperhomocysteinemia, including MTHFR deletion, do not develop NTDs. Similarly, elevated homocysteine in fetal culture medium does not induce NTDs in developing embryos (96). Impairments in AdoMet-dependent methylation reactions, including genomic methylation, have also been proposed to underlie the origin of NTD.

Decreased chromatin methylation may affect neural tube closure by affecting cellular differentiation (97) or cellular migration processes (98, 99), both of which are critical for neural tube formation. In support of this notion, mice with targeted deletion of the de novo DNMT enzyme Dnmt3b exhibit altered differentiation capacity in ES cells (100), and embryos have NTDs. These findings confirm the essentiality of de novo methylation and cell differentiation in neural tube closure. Targeted deletion of genes that mediate DNA methylation-mediated suppression of gene expression also result in NTDs (101). The relevance of these mouse models to human NTDs, if any, is not known, however, nor is it known whether these NTDs can be prevented with folic acid.

Human embryos with NTDs have been shown to exhibit impaired de novo thymidylate synthesis (102), a finding indicating a potential causal correlation between impaired thymidylate biosynthesis and NTDs. The rapid proliferation of the neuroepithelium during neural tube formation requires robust de novo nucleotide biosynthesis to maintain rates of cell division and limit uracil accumulation in DNA. Impairments in thymidylate biosynthesis during DNA replication and repair decrease rates of cell division during the critical period of neural tube closure (103). Mouse models of genomic instability also exhibit NTDs, although genomic instability resulting from increased uracil accumulation in DNA has not been investigated (104–106). Disruption of the murine Pax3 gene, which encodes a homeobox transcription factor, causes 100% penetrant spina bifida and impaired de novo thymidylate biosynthesis (107, 108). Maternal in utero folic acid supplementation or supplementation of culture media with either thymidine or folic acid prevented NTDs in homozygous Pax3 null embryos, whereas methionine supplementation exacerbated the NTD phenotype. Collectively, the literature indicates that thymidylate biosynthesis is a strong candidate for the causal biosynthetic pathway involved in folate-responsive NTD pathogenesis. However, human epidemiologic and murine fetal culture models have also identified choline as a modifier of NTD risk (109).

Choline interacts with folate-mediated one-carbon metabolism by two distinct mechanisms. Choline degradation is a source of one-carbon units for one-carbon metabolism in the cytoplasm. Choline biosynthesis from glycine is folate dependent, requiring three equivalents of AdoMet. The developing embryo may also be at risk for developmental anomalies resulting from vitamin B_{12} deficiency. Increasing evidence from cross-sectional studies indicates that NTD-affected pregnancies that are not prevented by maternal folic acid supplementation or wheat flour folic acid fortification may result from vitamin B_{12} deficiency, although no randomized control trials have been conducted (110). Additional research is required to demonstrate conclusively which disruptions in one-carbon metabolism are causal and which are bystanders in the etiology of folate-responsive developmental anomalies.

The potential role of other nutrients in the origin of NTD should be considered.

FOLATE IN CANCER AND CHRONIC DISEASE

Impairments in one-carbon metabolism, as indicated primarily by elevated plasma homocysteine or low circulating folate concentrations, have been shown to be associated with cardiovascular disease (111, 112), cancers (113), and cognitive decline (114). Gene–diet interactions are thought to be fundamental to the origins of virtually all folate-associated chronic disease. Genetic variation in the one-carbon metabolic network has been shown to be associated with cancer risk; the MTHFR 677C → T polymorphism is associated with an increased risk of NTDs but a decreased risk of colon cancer (115). Although mechanisms have yet to be established, proposed mechanisms underlying these disorders include the modification of cellular proteins by homocysteine that leads to loss of function (116, 117), alterations in genome methylation and gene expression profiles, uracil accumulation in DNA, and subsequent genome instability (118). Proposed roles of low folate status in carcinogenesis have been the subject of several excellent reviews (113, 119). Low folate status increases uracil content in DNA (52), which can lead to double strand breaks and altered DNA methylation patterns, all of which contribute to carcinogenesis. Folate has also been proposed to be a two-edged sword in relation to cancer risk. Whereas folate deficiency may increase the risk of cancer initiation, it has also been proposed to accelerate the growth of established cancers.

Randomized placebo-controlled clinical trials have not conclusively validated observational studies indicating a preventive role for folate in cardiovascular disease and cancer. Secondary prevention trials have failed to demonstrate an effect of homocysteine lowering on cardiovascular disease outcomes (120). Similarly, randomized clinical trials do not support a role for folic acid supplementation in the prevention of colon cancer (121, 122). This last finding indicates that cancer risk may be associated only with overt folate deficiency. Given the role of folate in nucleotide biosynthesis, investigators have suggested that elevated folate status may accelerate cellular transformation or tumor growth in colon cancer, but definitive evidence from randomized controlled trials has not fully supported this hypothesis to date (122, 123).

Folate-mediated one-carbon metabolism remains an attractive target for nutritional intervention to prevent or manage chronic disease, but a more comprehensive understanding of the causal pathways, their regulation, and mechanism of pathogenesis is required. Genome wide association studies are indicating a role for one-carbon metabolism in mitochondria in vascular disease (124), but virtually nothing is known about the regulation of one-carbon metabolism in this compartment, including whether formate production is limiting in the one-carbon network. A more comprehensive understanding of folate metabolism and its regulation should provide a better mechanistic appreciation of the role of folate in human disease and should lead to the design of more effective therapies and preventive strategies.

REFERENCES

1. Hoffbrand AV, Weir DG. Br J Haematol 2001;113:579–89.
2. Mitchell HK, Snell EE, Williams RJ. J Am Chem Soc 1941; 63:2284.
3. Angier RB, Boothe JH, Hutchings BL et al. Science 1945; 102:227–8.
4. Farber S, Diamond LK. N Engl J Med 1948;238:787–93.
5. Appling DR. FASEB J 1991;5:2645–51.
6. Fox JT, Stover PJ. Vitam Horm 2008;79:1–44.
7. Moran RG. Semin Oncol 1999;26(Suppl 6):24–32.
8. Suh JR, Herbig AK, Stover PJ. Annu Rev Nutr 2001;21:255–82.
9. Yang Q, Cogswell ME, Hamner HC et al. Am J Clin Nutr 2010;91:64–72.
10. Allen LH. Food Nutr Bull 2008;29(2 Suppl):S20–34; discussion S35–7.
11. Bailey LB. Nutr Rev 1998;56:294–9.
12. Bailey SW, Ayling JE. Proc Natl Acad Sci U S A 2009;106: 15424–9.
13. Food and Nutrition Board, Institute of Medicine. Folate. In: Dietary Reference Intakes for Thiamin, Riboflavin, Niacin, Vitamin B_6, Folate, Vitamin B_{12}, Pantothenic Acid, Biotin, and Choline. Washington, DC: National Academy Press, 1998: 196–305.
14. Quinlivan EP, Gregory JF III. Am J Clin Nutr 2007;86:1773–9.
15. Ganji V, Kafai MR. J Nutr 2009;139:345–52.
16. Pfeiffer CM, Osterloh JD, Kennedy-Stephenson J et al. Clin Chem 2008;54:801–13.
17. Zhao R, Matherly LH, Goldman ID. Expert Rev Mol Med 2009;11:e4.
18. Friso S, Choi SW, Girelli D et al. Proc Natl Acad Sci U S A 2002;99:5606–11.
19. Stover PJ. Nutr Rev 2004;62:S3–12; discussion S13.
20. Christensen KE, MacKenzie RE. Bioessays 2006;28:595–605.
21. An S, Kumar R, Sheets ED et al. Science 2008;320:103–6.
22. Beardsley GP, Moroson BA, Taylor EC et al. J Biol Chem 1989;264:328–33.
23. Erba E, Sen S, Sessa C et al. Br J Cancer 1994;69:205–11.
24. Zhao R, Goldman ID. Oncogene 2003;22:7431–57.
25. Anderson DD, Stover PJ. PLoS One 2009;4:e5839.
26. Takemura Y, Jackman AL. Anticancer Drugs 1997;8:3–16.
27. Gorlick R, Metzger R, Danenberg KD et al. J Clin Oncol 1998;16:1465–9.
28. Van der Wilt CL, Pinedo HM, Smid K et al. Cancer Res 1992;52:4922–8.
29. Forsthoefel AM, Pena MM, Xing YY et al. Biochemistry 2004;43:1972–9.
30. Kitchens ME, Forsthoefel AM, Rafique Z et al. J Biol Chem 1999;274:12544–7.
31. Finkelstein JD. Semin Thromb Hemost 2000;26:219–25.
32. Schirch V, Strong WB. Arch Biochem Biophys 1989;269:371–80.
33. Strong WB, Tendler SJ, Seither RL et al. J Biol Chem 1990; 265:12149–55.
34. Scott JM, Dinn JJ, Wilson P et al. Lancet 1981;2:334–7.
35. Lin BF, Huang RF, Shane B. J Biol Chem 1993;268:21674–9.
36. Davis SR, Stacpoole PW, Williamson J et al. Am J Physiol 2004;286:E272–9.
37. Lamers Y, Williamson J, Theriaque DW et al. J Nutr 2009; 139:666–71.
38. Shin YS, Chan C, Vidal AJ et al. Biochim Biophys Acta 1976;444:794–801.
39. Fox JT, Shin WK, Caudill MA et al. J Biol Chem 2009; 284:31097–108.
40. MacFarlane AJ, Liu X, Perry CA et al. J Biol Chem 2008; 283:25846–53.
41. Luka Z, Mudd SH, Wagner C. J Biol Chem 2009;284:22507–11.
42. Luka Z, Loukachevitch LV, Wagner C. Biochim Biophys Acta 2008;1784:1342–6.
43. Luka Z, Capdevila A, Mato JM et al. Transgenic Res 2006; 15:393–7.
44. Nieman KM, Rowling MJ, Garrow TA et al. J Biol Chem 2004;279:45708–12.
45. Rowling MJ, Schalinske LK. J Nutr 2003;133:3392–8.
46. Scott JM. Proc Nutr Soc 1999;58:441–8.
47. Selhub J, Jacques PF, Dallal G et al. Food Nutr Bull 2008; 29(Suppl):S67–73.
48. Green R. Food Nutr Bull 2008;29(Suppl):S52–63; discussion S64–6.
49. Bagley PJ, Selhub J. Clin Chem 2000;46:404–11.
50. Hannisdal R, Gislefoss RE, Grimsrud TK et al. J Nutr 2010; 140:522–6.
51. Blount BC, Mack MM, Wehr CM et al. Proc Natl Acad Sci U S A 1997;94:3290–5.
52. Linhart HG, Troen A, Bell GW et al. Gastroenterology 2009; 136:227–35.
53. Ames BN. Ann N Y Acad Sci 1999;889:87–106.
54. Hazra A, Selhub J, Chao WH et al. Am J Clin Nutr 2010; 91:160–5.
55. Barbosa PR, Stabler SP, Machado AL et al. Eur J Clin Nutr 2008;62:1010–21.
56. Finkelstein JD. Clin Chem Lab Med 2007;45:1694–9.
57. Clarke S, Banfield K. S-Adenosylmethionine–dependent methyltransferases. In: Carmel R, Jacobson DW, eds. Homocysteine in Health and Disease. Cambridge: Cambridge University Press, 2001.
58. Friso S, Choi SW, Dolnikowski GG et al. Anal Chem 2002; 74:4526–31.
59. Jaenisch R, Bird A. Nat Genet 2003;33(Suppl):245–54.
60. Huang C, Sloan EA, Boerkoel CF. Curr Opin Genet Dev 2003;13:246–52.
61. Obeid R, Kostopoulos P, Knapp JP et al. Clin Chem 2007; 53:326–33.
62. Lindenbaum J, Allen RH. Clinical spectrum and diagnosis of folate deficiency. In: Bailey LB, ed. Folate in Health and Disease. New York: Marcel Dekker, 1995.
63. O'Connor DL. Prog Food Nutr Sci 1991;15231–54.
64. Bailey LB, Gregory JF III. J Nutr 1999;129:779–82.
65. Solis C, Veenema K, Ivanov AA et al. J Nutr 2008;138:67–72.
66. Ptashne M. Curr Biol 2007;17:R233–6.
67. Waterland RA, Garza C. Am J Clin Nutr 1999;69:179–97.
68. Stover PJ, Harlan WR, Hammond JA et al. Curr Opin Lipidol 2010;21:136–40.
69. Plagemann A, Harder T, Brunn M et al. J Physiol 2009; 587:4963–76.
70. Sinclair KD, Allegrucci C, Singh R et al. Proc Natl Acad Sci U S A 2007;104:19351–6.
71. Zeisel SH. Am J Clin Nutr 2009;89:673S–7S.
72. Suter MA, Aagaard-Tillery KM. Semin Reprod Med 2009; 27:380–90.
73. Lillycrop KA, Slater-Jefferies JL, Hanson MA et al. Br J Nutr 2007;97:1064–73.
74. Burdge GC, Slater-Jefferies J, Torrens C et al. Br J Nutr 2007;97:435–9.

75. Waterland RA, Jirtle RL. Mol Cell Biol 2003;23:5293–300.
76. Yi P, Melnyk S, Pogribna M et al. J Biol Chem 2000;275: 29318–23.
77. Caudill MA, Wang JC, Melnyk S et al. J Nutr 2001;131:2811–8.
78. Brunaud L, Alberto JM, Ayav A et al. Digestion 2003;68:133–40.
79. Jamaluddin MD, Chen I, Yang F et al. Blood 2007;110:3648–55.
80. Frosst P, Blom HJ, Milos R et al. Nat Genet 1995;10:111–3.
81. Figueiredo JC, Grau MV, Wallace K et al. Cancer Epidemiol Biomarkers Prev 2009;18:1041–9.
82. Ingrosso D, Cimmino A, Perna AF et al. Lancet 2003; 361:1693–9.
83. Schernhammer ES, Giovannucci E, Kawasaki T et al. Gut 2010;59:794–9.
84. Oyama K, Kawakami K, Maeda K et al. Anticancer Res 2004; 24:649–54.
85. de Vogel S, Wouters KA, Gottschalk RW et al. Cancer Epidemiol Biomarkers Prev 2009;18:3086–96.
86. Jin M, Kawakami K, Fukui Y et al. Cancer Sci 2009;100: 2325–30.
87. Waterland RA. Epigenetics 2009;4:523–5.
88. Beaudin AE, Stover PJ. Birth Defects Res A Clin Mol Teratol 2009;85:274–84.
89. International Centre for Birth Defects. Birth Defects Annual Report. Rome: International Center for Birth Defects, 2000.
90. Blencowe H, Cousens S, Modell B et al. Int J Epidemiol 2010;39(Suppl 1):i110–21.
91. Ray JG. Food Nutr Bull 2008;29(Suppl):S225–30.
92. Botto LD, Yang Q. Am J Epidemiol 2000;151:862–77.
93. Blom HJ, Shaw GM, den Heijer H et al. Nat Rev Neurosci 2006;7:724–31.
94. van der Put NM, Blom HJ. Eur J Obstet Gynecol Reprod Biol 2000;92:57–61.
95. Brody LC, Conley M, Cox C et al. Am J Hum Genet 2002; 71:1207–15.
96. Watanabe M, Osada J, Aratani Y et al. Proc Natl Acad Sci U S A 1995;92:1585–9.
97. Kobayakawa S, Miike K, Nakao M et al. Genes Cells 2007; 12:447–60.
98. Issaeva I, Zonis Y, Rozovskaia T et al. Mol Cell Biol 2007; 27:1889–903.
99. Rahnama F, Shafiei F, Gluckman PD et al. Endocrinology 2006;147:5275–83.
100. Jackson M, Krassowska A, Gilbert N et al. Mol Cell Biol 2004;24:8862–71.
101. Kim JK, Huh SO, Choi H et al. Mol Cell Biol 2001;21:7787–95.
102. Dunlevy LP, Chitty LS, Burren KA et al. Brain 2007;130:1043–9.
103. Keller-Peck CR, Mullen RJ. Brain Res Dev Brain Res 1997;102:177–88.
104. Herrera E, Samper E, Blasco MA. Embo J 1999;18:1172–81.
105. Hollander MC, Sheikh MS, Bulavin DV et al. Nat Genet 1999;23:176–84.
106. Wang X, Wang RH, Li W et al. J Biol Chem 2004;279:29606–14.
107. Fleming A, Copp AJ. Science 1998;280:2107–9.
108. Wlodarczyk BJ, Tang LS, Triplett A et al. Toxicol Appl Pharmacol 2006;213:55–63.
109. Zeisel SH. Annu Rev Nutr 2006;26:229–50.
110. Thompson MD, Cole DE, Ray JG. Am J Clin Nutr 2009; 89:697S–701S.
111. McNulty H, Pentieva K, Hoey L et al. Proc Nutr Soc 2008; 67:232–7.
112. Bazzano LA. Am J Med Sci 2009;338:48–9.
113. Martinez ME, Marshall JR, Giovannucci E. Nat Rev Cancer 2008;8:694–703.
114. Vogel T, Dali-Youcef N, Kaltenbach G et al. Int J Clin Pract 2009;63:1061–7.
115. Ma J, Stampfer MJ, Giovannucci E et al. Cancer Res 1997; 57:1098–102.
116. Hubmacher D, Cirulis JT, Miao M et al. J Biol Chem 2010; 285:1188–98.
117. Perla-Kajan J, Jakubowski H. FASEB J 2010;24:931–6.
118. Mason JB. Nutr Rev 2009;67:206–12.
119. Hubner RA, Houlston RS. Br J Cancer 2009;100:233–9.
120. Smulders YM, Blom HJ. J Inherit Metab Dis 2011;34:93–9.
121. Cole BF, Baron JA, Sandler RS et al. JAMA 2007;297:2351–9.
122. Wu K, Platz EA, Willett WC et al. Am J Clin Nutr 2009; 90:1623–31.
123. Ebbing M, Bonaa KH, Nygard O et al. JAMA 2009;302:2119–26.
124. Samani NJ, Erdmann J, Hall AS et al. N Engl J Med 2007; 357:443–53.

SUGGESTED READING

Hoffbrand AV, Wier DG. The history of folic acid. Br J Haematol 2001;113:579–89.

C. VITAMINS

27 COBALAMIN (VITAMIN B$_{12}$)[1,2]

RALPH CARMEL

---

[1]**Abbreviations: CoA**, coenzyme A; **FBCM**, food-bound cobalamin malabsorption; **holo-TC II**, holotranscobalamin II; **IF**, intrinsic factor; **MCV**, mean corpuscular volume; **MMA**, methylmalonic acid; **PA**, pernicious anemia; **SCCD**, subclinical cobalamin deficiency; **TC**, transcobalamin; **THF**, tetrahydrofolic acid.
[2]Système Internationale units: 1 ng cobalamin = 0.738 pmol.

HISTORICAL BACKGROUND

The history of cobalamin is inextricably bound to the disease that provides the most common setting for its clinical deficiency, even though cobalamin deficiency can arise from many other causes. The reader is referred to excellent reviews of the dramatic scientific and clinical story (1, 2). In 1849, Addison reported several patients with a "remarkable form of anemia" that was accompanied by languor and restlessness, among other signs and symptoms. Although Addison mistakenly attributed the anemia to adrenal disease, his report is considered to be the first of the disease whose often fatal course later led Biermer to name it "pernicious anemia" (PA). That name is less apt now because the easily treated disease is no longer pernicious and because the disease is defined by its underlying gastric defect and not its anemic manifestation, which is sometimes minimal or even absent. Indeed, the strikingly megaloblastic anemia, although characteristic, is not specific to PA or even to cobalamin deficiency.

The classical experiments by Minot and Murphy (3) transformed the lethal course of PA by feeding affected patients large amounts of liver and documenting their hematologic improvement. For this work, they shared a Nobel Prize. The second important contribution was Castle's discovery that patients with PA responded effectively to an "extrinsic factor" in the ingested liver or meat when it was combined with an "intrinsic factor" (IF) in gastric juice (4). This demonstration sealed the long-suspected connection of PA with achylia gastrica. The third critical achievement was the identification of cobalamin as the extrinsic factor. The synthesis of cobalamin (5, 6) was accompanied by elucidation of its structure by Hodgkin (7), who was also awarded a Nobel Prize for her crystallographic work.

As biosynthetic fermentation made cyanocobalamin readily available, PA became easy to treat. The vitamin also became one of the most frequently given injections in the United States and acquired the dubious status of a frequently misused placebo and "energizer." Having lost its grim implications, cobalamin deficiency began to be viewed with complacency by some health professionals, at times to their patients' disadvantage.

The past several decades have extended methodologic advances in accurate and sensitive metabolic assays that allow identification of cobalamin deficiency at even earlier stages of development. As a result, asymptomatic subclinical cobalamin deficiency (SCCD) (8, 9) is now understood to be far more prevalent than the relatively rare state of clinical deficiency (10). This subclinical expansion has had major epidemiologic ramifications. Molecular understanding of cobalamin transport and metabolism and of their varied disorders has also advanced, with exploration of genetic influences and interactions with the environment and with acquired disorders.

BIOCHEMISTRY

Cobalamin contains a planar tetrapyrrole (corrin), at whose center sits a cobalt atom, and has critically attached moieties (Fig. 27.1). The cobalt fluctuates among monovalent, divalent, and trivalent states, with the reduced, monovalent cob(I)alamin being the active form. Linked to cobalt in the α position below the corrin plane is the 5,6-dimethylbenzimidazole nucleotide. Also linked to the cobalt atom but extending above the plane (β position) is any one of several interchangeable prosthetic moieties that lend their names to the cobalamin. The most important cobalamins are methylcobalamin, in which methyl is the prosthetic moiety, and deoxyadenosylcobalamin, in which 5'-deoxyadenosine is the β-linked moiety. Methylcobalamin predominates in cytoplasm and serves as a cofactor with 5-methyltetrahydrofolic acid (methylTHF) in the methylation of homocysteine to methionine (Fig. 27.2). Deoxyadenosylcobalamin predominates in mitochondria, where it serves as a cofactor in the intramolecular rearrangement of L-methylmalonyl-coenzyme A (CoA) to succinyl-CoA in propionate metabolism (Fig. 27.3). These two are the only known roles for cobalamin in humans.

Other cobalamins include hydroxocobalamin, which is very stable and occurs widely; aquocobalamin; and sulfitocobalamin. Cyanocobalamin is a stable biosynthetic pharmaceutical that requires conversion to other cobalamins to become metabolically active; the term *vitamin*

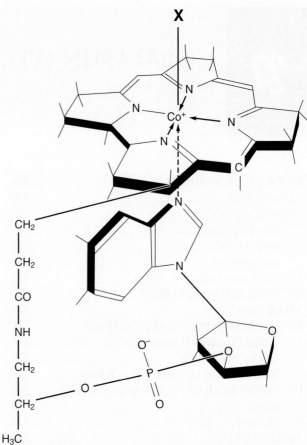

Fig. 27.1. The structure of cobalamin. Attached to the central cobalt atom of the corrin tetrapyrrole and to one of the pyrrole rings is the α-ligand, the 5,6-dimethylbenzimidazole nucleotide, extending below the corrin plane. The β-ligand (marked as *X* in the figure) above the plane can be any of several moieties such as methyl, 5'-deoxyadenosyl, hydroxyl, or cyanide. (Reprinted with permission from Carmel R. Megaloblastic anemias: disorders of impaired DNA synthesis. In: Greer JP, Foerster J, Lukens JL et al, eds. Wintrobe's Clinical Hematology. 11th ed. Philadelphia: Lippincott Williams & Wilkins, 2004.)

B$_{12}$ refers specifically to cyanocobalamin (5), but it often serves as a catch-all name for cobalamins as a whole. Altered corrinoids with structural deletions are nonfunctional in humans but can find their way into tissues (11), even though cobalamin carriers, other than transcobalamin (TC) I, bind them poorly compared with functional cobalamins (12–14).

Many confusing terminologies have been applied to the cobalamin-binding proteins. This chapter uses TC I and TC II for the two plasma carriers, terms with the longest usage and in conformity with the genetic nomenclature of *TCN1* and *TCN2*, respectively. Others introduced the names haptocorrin and transcobalamin, respectively. An older, common name for TC I in the literature was R binder.

ANALYTIC METHODS

Analytic methods to diagnose cobalamin deficiency fall into two categories: measures of cobalamin amount, such

the neurologic nuances and distinctions continue to be debated (103). The frequency of neurologic dysfunction has varied in part because it is less quantifiable than hematologic changes and its diagnosis, especially when changes are subtle, depends on the observers' expertise. Estimates suggest that more than half of patients with PA display neurologic findings (103, 104). Neurologic deficits can be the earliest and, in up to 27% of cases, even the sole clinical expression of cobalamin deficiency (26, 104, 105). For unknown reasons, the severities of hematologic and neurologic manifestations tend to be inversely related in patients (104, 106), and the same expression tends to recur at relapse (100, 104, 107). Just as many patients with PA present with only anemia as present with only neurologic changes. Genetic polymorphism of methylene THF reductase, which diverts methylene THF away from generating methylTHF and toward thymidylate synthesis (see Fig. 27.2), seems not to be a factor (108).

The distribution and characteristics of the neuropathy and myelopathy tend to be stereotypical but not specific to cobalamin deficiency. Histologically, myelin loss is followed by axonal degeneration and gliosis, and the larger, more myelinated fibers are preferentially affected (107). The myelopathy affects the posterior and lateral columns, thus giving rise to "subacute combined degeneration" of the spinal cord. Symptoms tend to be symmetric and begin in the feet and later ascend to affect the legs, hands, and trunk (17, 104). The early clinical manifestations are diminished vibratory and position sense and paresthesias, but ataxia often follows, as can spasticity, incontinence, and other disabling manifestations. Motor function is largely spared, although gait disturbances and spasticity may become incapacitating. Cerebral manifestations can range from memory, mood, or personality changes to psychosis and occasionally delirium (103–105). Autonomic dysfunction, optic neuritis, and visual changes occur sometimes.

Magnetic resonance imaging may demonstrate surprisingly large patches of demyelination throughout the brain, in addition to classical upper spinal cord involvement. Electroencephalographic and other electrophysiologic abnormalities are common (109, 110), and they may occur even in asymptomatic patients (9, 111, 112).

Neurologic abnormalities usually respond within a few weeks to months to cobalamin therapy, with complete response in 47% of cases and partial response in most of the rest (104). Complete irreversibility occurs in only 6%, unlike the universal correction of the anemia (unless complicated by coexisting anemias). The irreversibility is unpredictable but appears tied to the initial extent of the neurologic involvement and often to undue therapeutic delay in patients with a relentless cause of deficiency such as PA (103, 104, 113, 114). High folate intake or therapy has also been a suspected contributor; neurologically affected patients tend to have higher serum folate levels than unaffected patients (106, 115), but it is unclear

if cobalamin-related metabolism or high folate intake explains the higher levels. The partial response of cobalamin-deficiency anemia to folate sometimes delays recognition of the cobalamin deficiency (17, 103). Whether folate therapy simply delays recognition of cobalamin deficiency or can sometimes directly accelerate neurologic worsening remains unsettled. Our continued ignorance about the basic mechanisms whereby cobalamin deficiency produces neurologic changes has stymied progress to date.

Other Clinical Manifestations

Nonhematologic and nonneurologic abnormalities also occur in clinical deficiency and reverse with cobalamin therapy (17, 31). These include the following: occasional glossitis, sometimes severe enough to be the dominant symptom; unexplained weight loss; transient intestinal malabsorption; skin darkening, reddish hair, and nail pigment changes, especially in darker skinned patients; and biochemical evidence of impaired bone formation.

Metabolic Explanations for the Clinical Manifestations

The megaloblastic anemia of cobalamin deficiency arises from cobalamin's biochemical intersection with folate metabolism and is identical to folate deficiency anemia. The "methylTHF trap" hypothesis (116, 117) provides a compelling focus on the methylation of homocysteine by methionine synthase, which requires both methylTHF and methylcobalamin (see Fig. 27.2). This irreversible reaction is impaired in cobalamin deficiency, and methylTHF, the most abundant folate but one unable to flow through the folate cycle via any other reaction, accumulates as other critical folates diminish. The reduced production of methionine, and therefore also of S-adenosylmethionine, which fuels many critical methylations, stimulates conversion of methyleneTHF to methylTHF in an attempt to generate more S-adenosylmethionine, but that only augments the trapping of folates as methylTHF. The trap also reduces methyleneTHF availability for deoxyuridylate conversion to thymidylate. Excess uracil replaces thymidine incorporation into DNA, and active excision repair leads to strand breaks and ultimately to interphase arrest. This process appears to be a major contributor to megaloblastic conversion, but it may not be the entire explanation (31).

The mechanism for the neurologic manifestations of cobalamin deficiency is unknown. Hypotheses have included abnormal myelinization resulting from impaired propionic acid metabolism, MMA toxicity to neural cells, the accumulation of nonfunctional cobalamin analogs, and possible effects of cytokines. Many observations, including the limitation of classical neurologic deficits to genetic cobalamin disorders involving hyperhomocysteinemia alone and not those involving methylmalonic aciduria alone, favor the methionine synthase block as a linchpin, but the details are elusive. Cerebrospinal fluid studies in indirect models suggested that *S*-adenosylmethionine depletion may cause the neurologic dysfunction in cobalamin deficiency (118). However, this would not explain the neurologic differences between cobalamin and folate deficiencies. Moreover, low plasma *S*-adenosylmethionine was reported to be a better predictor of anemia than of neurologic manifestations in patients with PA (106); plasma cysteine and folate levels were the most significant biochemical predictors of neurologic dysfunction.

Subclinical Cobalamin Deficiency and the Public Health

SCCD was first described in 1985 (8, 9, 111), and its defining characteristics are shown in Table 27.4. A low cobalamin value by itself is insufficient evidence of SCCD and requires metabolic support. The early, preclinical phases of PA satisfy the definition of SCCD (119) before they progress to the clinical stage, but most cases of SCCD are unrelated to PA or IF-related malabsorption (9, 10, 85). Most causes of SCCD are unknown, and only 30%

TABLE 27.4	CRITERIA FOR SUBCLINICAL COBALAMIN DEFICIENCY

The diagnosis requires all four of the following criteria to be met:
1. Any two or more of the following test abnormalities must be present[a]:
   - Elevated methylmalonic acid[b]
   - Elevated plasma homocysteine[b]
   - Low serum cobalamin[c]
   - Low serum holotranscobalamin II
   - Abnormal deoxyuridine suppression test
2. The abnormal methylmalonic acid and homocysteine results must respond to cobalamin therapy.[d,e]
3. Clinical signs of cobalamin deficiency must be absent.[f]
4. Pernicious anemia must be ruled out.[g]

[a]A lone abnormality is not reliable because each biomarker has limited sensitivity and specificity and because clinical confirmation, by definition, is unavailable in subclinical deficiency.

[b]The serum creatinine level must also be normal. Elevated creatinine suggests the likelihood of spuriously high metabolite values.

[c]The subject must not be pregnant or have transcobalamin I deficiency, conditions that feature spuriously low cobalamin levels. These conditions nevertheless coexist with subclinical deficiency on occasion.

[d]The therapy must provide sufficient cobalamin: either a single injection of 100 to 1000 μg or oral 1000 μg doses daily for a week.

[e]Any rise in cobalamin and holotranscobalamin II levels after cobalamin therapy simply reflects the influx of vitamin and has no diagnostic or metabolic implications or specificity.

[f]Subclinical deficiency is often encountered in persons undergoing evaluation for unrelated clinical findings that initially mimic cobalamin deficiency, such as anemia. The temptation to link subclinical deficiency to coexisting but nonspecific clinical findings such as nonmacrocytic anemia must be avoided (subclinical deficiency causes no anemia and the anemia of cobalamin deficiency is macrocytic).

[g]Anti–intrinsic factor antibody should be measured in every cobalamin-deficient patient to rule out pernicious anemia, which is the most common cause of clinical deficiency but is occasionally encountered at a preclinical stage before it inevitably and irreversibly progresses to a clinical stage.

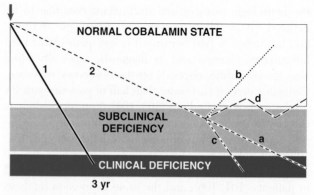

Fig. 27.6. Schematic illustration of the diverse courses that cobalamin deficiency states may follow, depending on their underlying causes. The fields represent, from **top** to **bottom**, the normal cobalamin state, subclinical deficiency (mild metabolic abnormalities without clinical signs or symptoms), and clinical deficiency (mild and then progressively more severe hematologic or neurologic [or both] manifestations). The *arrow* **(upper left)** marks the onset of gradual cobalamin depletion whose progressions are arbitrarily represented as linear: *line 1*, the depletion produced by severe, permanent malabsorption typified by pernicious anemia; *line 2*, a less complete, less inexorable disruption of cobalamin balance (e.g., dietary insufficiency or a malabsorption limited to food-bound cobalamin). Based on published direct and indirect (but nonsystematic) observations, the diagram posits a slower course of unknown duration that increases the time spent transiting through subclinical deficiency, which may explain why subclinical deficiency is seen more often than clinical deficiency. At some point, this course may *(line a)* eventually progress sufficiently to produce clinical, symptomatic deficiency; *(line b)* remit completely for reasons that may or may not be known (e.g., remission of food-bound cobalamin malabsorption following unrelated antibiotic therapy); *(line c)* accelerate and reach clinical deficiency more quickly (e.g., chronic gastritis transforms into pernicious anemia as intrinsic factor secretion disappears); or *(line d)* fluctuate indefinitely between normal and mildly subclinical deficiency states. (Reprinted with permission from Carmel R. Biomarkers of cobalamin [vitamin B-12] status in the epidemiologic setting: a critical overview of context, applications, and performance characteristics of cobalamin, methylmalonic acid, and holotranscobalamin II. Am J Clin Nutr 2011;94[Suppl1]:348S–58S.)

to 50% of cases are associated with FBCM (10, 85, 88). SCCD progression to clinical deficiency is not guaranteed, unlike the inevitable progression of PA. SCCD and its causes may be static, progress glacially, fluctuate, remit spontaneously, or occasionally accelerate, such as when chronic gastritis transforms into PA and cobalamin absorption plummets (Fig. 27.6). As a result, prognosis in SCCD and PA differs, and so must management.

SCCD accounts for more than 80% of the cobalamin deficiency detected in population surveys (28, 30). The often static or even transient course of SCCD (16, 53, 85) indicates that epidemiologic and clinical data are not interchangeable (16, 69, 120); the IF-related malabsorption in clinical deficiency usually predicts inevitable progression if left untreated.

Like clinical deficiency, SCCD is more common in the aged population (85, 86). Low cobalamin levels occur in 5% to 15% of elderly persons, almost all of whom absorb free cobalamin adequately as shown with the Schilling test and appear to have adequate cobalamin intake (10, 85, 90). Cobalamin-related metabolic abnormalities accompany only 60% to 70% of those low cobalamin levels (30, 121), which suggests that one third of such persons may not have SCCD or be cobalamin deficient at all. Moreover, isolated metabolic abnormalities often appear to be spurious. Longitudinal study (1 to 4 years) reported that 84% of isolated MMA elevations reversed spontaneously or remained stationary (53)—a finding supporting older, limited observations that many persons with SCCD remain asymptomatic for many years (122).

The known neurologic consequences of clinical cobalamin deficiency explain the persisting disquiet about similar risks in SCCD. When tested, some patients with SCCD have demonstrated subtle cobalamin-responsive neurologic and electrophysiologic changes without apparent impact on health (111, 112). Nevertheless, the extensive literature on cognitive risks in SCCD is controversial. Observational studies cannot prove causation, and disentangling the influence of cobalamin status from influences of folate, other B vitamins, and most especially homocysteine has been difficult (123–125). Initial clinical trials were equally inconclusive and often negative (126–130).

Two more recent clinical trials now provide evidence that high daily doses of B vitamins may delay cognitive decline and reduce brain atrophy progression (130a, 130b), but important aspects need attention (125). The justifiable use of a combination of cobalamin, folic acid, and pyridoxine leaves the effective vitamin or vitamins unidentified; indeed, an earlier trial reported cognitive improvement with folic acid alone (130c). Responders to the three-vitamin regimen tended to have high baseline homocysteine levels (130a)—a finding suggesting that response may not occur when homocysteine is normal. Yet, baseline MMA, which is more specific to cobalamin status, tended to be normal in responders; this fact casts uncertainty on the role of SCCD, especially because of recurrent observations in these and other studies that cobalamin-related data were only slightly "less normal" than in control subjects (125), and despite a proposal that cobalamin status may be abnormal despite normal metabolic data (130d). Moreover, the subjects had mild cognitive dysfunction at baseline, and this leaves unknown whether normal elderly persons or those with advanced dysfunction will benefit. Finally, the need for high doses will preclude food fortification (130e).

Other unresolved statistical associations with low or low-normal cobalamin levels are protean: insulin resistance in children of mothers with marginal cobalamin status, depression, osteopenia, infertility, tinnitus, and some cancers. To lend some perspective to this partial list, the data are often statistical exercises in which, for example, comparisons of the highest quartile to the lowest lend undue influence to outliers, which are rarely investigated in detail. Indeed, higher cobalamin levels are sometimes similarly associated with adverse outcomes (131), yet may reflect TC I changes more than cobalamin status (42, 131).

Randomized clinical trials alone can determine whether cobalamin therapy modifies any of the many proposed risk associations with SCCD, which affects several million people in the United States. Studies must also confirm and clarify the effect of combined B vitamin therapy on cognitive decline. Adverse effects of chronically high intake of the B vitamins are currently unknown.

CAUSES OF DEFICIENCY

Identifying what caused a cobalamin deficiency is essential in patient care and also has important public health and research implications. It determines how the deficiency is best managed, what its course and prognosis are likely to be, and what associations and complications are probable. The causes are grouped in Table 27.5 by categories of mechanisms, arranged in the sequence of events from cobalamin intake through cellular use shown in Figure 27.4.

Dietary Causes

For reasons already discussed, adult vegetarians and even vegans take many years to develop cobalamin deficiency. The consequences tend to be mild (e.g., borderline macrocytosis without anemia) or, most often, purely biochemical (132, 133); notable clinical deficiency is

TABLE 27.5	CAUSES OF COBALAMIN DEFICIENCY[a]

Inadequate dietary intake
  Veganism
  Infants of vegan mothers (especially if also breast-fed by them)
  Long-term, highly restricted diets (e.g., phenylketonuria diet)
Gastrointestinal malabsorption
  Malabsorption of all cobalamin (free and food-bound)
    Pernicious anemia: acquired or hereditary
    Total gastrectomy
    Partial gastrectomy (~30% of cases)
    Ileal disease or damage (e.g., tropical sprue, ileal surgery)
    Hereditary cobalamin malabsorption (Imerslund-Gräsbeck syndrome)
    Bacterial overgrowth of the small bowel
    Parasitic infestation (e.g., *Diphyllobothrium latum*)
  Malabsorption limited to food-bound cobalamin
    Atrophic gastritis
    Partial gastrectomy (affects >50% of cases)
    Other gastric surgery (e.g., gastric stapling, vagotomy)
    Inhibitors of gastric acid secretion (e.g., omeprazole)
Metabolic disorders
  Acquired
    Nitrous oxide toxicity
  Hereditary
    Transcobalamin II deficiency
    cbl mutations

[a]Claims for some unproven causes of cobalamin deficiency dot the literature. Examples are entities associated with cobalamin malabsorption but not yet convincingly linked to deficiency (e.g., pancreatic insufficiency, gastric acid-suppressing drugs), drugs associated with occasionally low cobalamin levels without proof of malabsorption or deficiency (e.g., metformin), and automatic equation of *Helicobacter pylori* infection with cobalamin deficiency.

uncommon. Dietary cobalamin insufficiency is particularly common among Hindus and other lifelong vegetarians, but chronic dietary limitations may occur in other settings also (134). Contributing gastrointestinal factors have not always been excluded in geographic studies.

Consequences may be greater when restricted intake begins in childhood, perhaps because of smaller body stores, the requirements of growth, and the greater vulnerability of the developing brain. Children may display cognitive problems, and metabolic abnormalities sometimes persist despite dietary relaxation (135).

An often catastrophic syndrome affects infants born to vegan mothers or mothers with mild, undiagnosed PA with subnormal breast milk cobalamin content who rely heavily on breast-feeding their babies (136–139). These children often develop severe neurologic complications including seizures and developmental problems, whereas the mothers have only asymptomatic SCCD. The frequency is unknown, but it may be the most common cause of clinical cobalamin deficiency in babies.

Pernicious Anemia and Other Causes of Malabsorption of All Cobalamin

Severe malabsorption of all cobalamin, which was diagnosable with the now unavailable Schilling test (17, 31), was shown to cause 94% of clinically expressed cases of deficiency (46). PA, in which IF secretion is lost irretrievably, accounted for 76% of the cases. Its frequency varies; a survey of elderly community dwellers in Los Angeles discovered that 1.9% had PA in a mild, early, and often subclinical state of deficiency (119).

In the slow evolution of classic acquired PA, atrophic gastritis, typically autoimmune and usually sparing the antrum, begins in late middle age. PA supervenes when parietal cell damage progresses to cause loss of IF (87). However, most chronic gastritis with achlorhydria may cause FBCM without progressing to PA. Once IF secretion fails, cobalamin depletion begins (or accelerates), leading to clinical deficiency several years later, typically in old age. PA sometimes affects young adults and even children (17), especially among black women and, to a lesser degree, Latin Americans (140). The immune features of PA include two autoantibodies: the more prevalent one is directed against the hydrogen, potassium-adenosine triphosphatase pump of parietal cells but is not specific for PA; the less frequent but diagnostically more specific antibody is directed against IF (31). Various autoimmune disorders coexist with PA, the most common being thyroid disorders (141); other immune disorders include vitiligo, myasthenia gravis, immune cytopenias, and agammaglobulinemia (17, 31). Iron deficiency, often (but not always) attributable to the iron malabsorption of achlorhydric gastritis, coexists in half of cases (142). The most worrisome complication in PA is an increased risk of gastric cancer and carcinoid tumors (31, 87, 143, 144).

A rarer form of PA results from the isolated loss of gastric IF secretion caused by mutations in the *GIF* gene (145, 146). Clinical cobalamin deficiency usually appears in the first few years of life (147).

Partial gastric resection sometimes causes malabsorption of free as well as food-bound cobalamin. Loss of IF or significant cobalamin parasitization by increased bacteria colonizing the upper small bowel can be responsible, and clinical deficiency occurs in 15% to 30% of patients (31, 148). Most often, however, postgastrectomy malabsorption limits itself to food-bound cobalamin, which is mild and causes SCCD only (149).

Bacterial overgrowth in the small bowel, resulting from blind loops, impaired gut motility, or giant diverticula, can parasitize ingested cobalamin and produce a malabsorptive picture and clinical deficiency. The fish tapeworm, *Diphyllobothrium latum*, can do the same but is infrequently seen today.

Intestinal causes of severe, IF-related malabsorption are disorders of the ileum, the major site for IF-mediated absorption. Acquired causes include tropical sprue, damage to the ileum by surgical bypass, resection, or radiation, and ileal bladder reserve pouches (17, 31, 46). Other nutrients are often absorbed poorly as well. Hereditary malabsorption of cobalamin (Imerslund-Gräsbeck syndrome) causes isolated cobalamin malabsorption early in life (147). It arises from mutations of the gene for cubilin (150, 151) or of the gene for amnionless (73). The children usually also have minor proteinuria, which reflects defective cubilin in the renal tubule.

Malabsorption Limited to Food-Bound Cobalamin

Mild malabsorption limited to inadequate release of cobalamin from food, and thus its decreased transfer to IF, was discovered in 1973 in cobalamin-deficient patients with normal Schilling test results (149). The FBCM was tied to gastric surgery or to chronic gastritis, usually with diminished acid and pepsin secretion (88); IF secretion was intact. Other causes include bariatric gastric procedures (152, 153) and manipulations to suppress acid secretion, most often, drugs such as proton-pump inhibitors. FBCM affects 30% to 50% of persons with SCCD, but it also occurs in 10% to 15% of persons without deficiency and in rare patients with severe deficiency (88).

Helicobacter pylori infection occurred in 78% of patients with FBCM and in 44% of those without FBCM (154). Histologic and functional gastric studies suggested that infected patients with FBCM had mild gastritis and hypochlorhydria, whereas uninfected patients had severe atrophic gastritis and achlorhydria (155); study in a small subset showed that antibiotics reversed the FBCM in *H. pylori*–infected patients but not in uninfected ones. The role of *H. pylori* remains unsettled (69, 156), despite provocative but problematic reports of improved cobalamin status after antibiotic therapy.

The FBCM data from the active period of investigation has been reviewed in detail (88), but many studies after the late 1990s became unreliable as absorption testing disappeared (157). As discussed elsewhere (157), some investigators substituted unproven diagnostic criteria whose misdiagnosis of FBCM cast doubt on data and conclusions, such as claims that persons with presumed FBCM respond to small oral cobalamin doses. Other assumptions and lack of absorption data cloud intriguing reports suggesting that clinical improvement of cobalamin deficiency in *H. pylori*–infected subjects are treated with antibiotics alone (69).

Drugs

Unlike drugs that affect cobalamin metabolism directly (e.g., nitrous oxide), drugs with other actions, such as inhibitors of absorption, are likely to produce cobalamin deficiency only when they are taken uninterruptedly for many years. Thus, many drugs such as colchicine, omeprazole, and alcohol can induce cobalamin malabsorption but rarely lead to cobalamin deficiency. Metformin, which is taken on a long-term basis, has been associated with low cobalamin levels, but the mechanism and whether cobalamin deficiency exists are poorly documented.

Metabolic Disorders

Clinical cobalamin deficiency develops much more quickly in disorders that disrupt cellular uptake and use of cobalamin than in malabsorptive conditions. Serum cobalamin levels often remain normal or even rise in cellular disorders. The most common acquired metabolic disorder is long-term, recurrent exposure to nitrous oxide, which oxidatively destroys cobalamin and the methionine synthase to which it is attached (158). Inhalant abuse of nitrous oxide is particularly widespread among young people (159), and it can produce severe neurologic and mental changes. Although surgery provides too transient an exposure to produce clinical consequences, severe postoperative neurologic dysfunction can occur if a patient with unrecognized clinical cobalamin deficiency, such as PA, receives the nitrous oxide (160, 161).

Hereditary metabolic disorders are rare. These disorders include TC II deficiency in which failure of cellular uptake of cobalamin causes megaloblastic anemia and, occasionally, neurologic complications and immune dysfunction. Various *cbl* mutations affect methionine synthase or methionine synthase reductase activity, whose manifestations range from very mild and delayed to severe developmental, neurologic, and hematologic consequences that can be lethal in infancy, as often happens with *cblC*, the most common mutation. Other sources can be consulted for details of this complex, rapidly developing area (147, 162).

Cobalamin-Related Disorders that Do Not Cause Cobalamin Deficiency

Chronic pancreatic insufficiency can produce abnormal Schilling test results because pancreatic secretion is inadequate to degrade TC I/haptocorrin and release its cobalamin to IF in the gut (see Fig. 27.4). The disorder is sometimes claimed to cause cobalamin deficiency despite the absence of clinically convincing reports. Patients with hyperthyroidism and some malignant diseases may have increased cobalamin requirements, yet clinical consequences appear negligible.

Hereditary deficiency of TC I produces spuriously low serum cobalamin levels (see the earlier section on serum cobalamin). Because cellular cobalamin metabolism is unaffected, the low cobalamin levels are typically discovered incidentally in adults (27, 163). The role of TC I, which limits access of corrinoid analogs to cells and may withhold cobalamin from bacteria, is uncertain. Homozygous or compound heterozygous *TCN1* mutations cause virtually undetectable TC I with cobalamin levels lower than 100 ng/L, whereas simple heterozygosity causes modest TC I and cobalamin reductions (32, 33, 163). Originally thought rare, mild TC I deficiency may explain 15% of all low cobalamin levels (27), and it is typically mistaken for and treated as cobalamin deficiency.

Diagnostic Tests for Causes of Cobalamin Deficiency

Serum cobalamin and metabolite assays identify cobalamin deficiency but not its cause. Identifying the cause has great clinical and scientific importance, not just for diagnostic accuracy but also for its prognostic implications and management guidance on duration of therapy and disease complications (15, 157). Tests of cobalamin absorption have long been mainstays (17, 31) because clinical deficiency is malabsorptive in 94% of cases (46). The disappearance of the classic Schilling test to measure the absorption of oral, radiolabeled cobalamin and to differentiate between gastric and intestinal defects created a major diagnostic vacuum (157). Modified versions to assess FBCM (88, 149) are also unavailable. A newer absorption test, based on holo-TC II response to oral cobalamin (164), has not yet undergone adequate assessment of its performance characteristics and clinical sensitivity and specificity.

Surrogate tests for cobalamin malabsorption have limited value. Measuring serum antibody to IF is helpful because it is highly specific for diagnosing PA, unlike the parietal cell antibody (165, 166). However, only 50% to 70% of patients with PA have the anti-IF antibody, and the test provides no diagnostic information about other disorders. Serum gastrin is elevated and pepsinogen I is decreased in 80% to 90% of patients with PA, but both tests lack specificity (167). Combining either test with IF antibody seems the best approach today in diagnosing PA.

No reliable surrogate markers exist for the no longer available absorption tests for FBCM. Unproven indirect diagnostic criteria (168) predispose to misdiagnoses (157).

The diagnostic approach in children must consider genetic disorders, as well as the entities that also affect adults. MMA and homocysteine testing should always be included in children because cobalamin levels may be normal in genetic disorders of cellular uptake and metabolism and because the two tests help narrow down the genetic possibilities and diagnostic focus. The complex approach is discussed elsewhere (147). Low cobalamin levels in very early infancy suggest maternal cobalamin deficiency as their cause; the mother should also be tested.

TREATMENT OF DEFICIENCY

Even a 1-μg injection of cobalamin suffices to reverse the megaloblastic anemia of cobalamin deficiency temporarily, but the goals of treatment include repletion of stores and preventing relapse, not just reversal of manifestations. Management requires ascertainment of the cause of the deficiency. Only knowing the cause can allow informed decisions about duration (ranging from a brief course to lifelong treatment), doses, and routes of cobalamin therapy (15).

Vegetarians and Other Patients with Normal Absorption

The normal cobalamin absorption in vegetarians allows use of small oral supplements (e.g., 5 μg). Larger doses exceed the capacity of the IF system, and only 1% to 2% of the excess can be assimilated (see Table 27.2). It is prudent for vegetarians to take preventive cobalamin supplements, especially during pregnancy and while breast-feeding, and to avoid nitrous oxide anesthesia.

Patients Who Cannot Absorb Any Cobalamin

This category includes patients with PA, which is irreversible, and intestinal diseases with impaired IF-cobalamin absorption. Together, these disorders comprise more than 90% of clinically apparent cases of cobalamin deficiency. The optimal goal is to replete cobalamin stores. Larger parenteral doses produce greater absolute retention despite greater excretory losses (17, 31, 68). After a short course of daily to weekly injections, monthly 100- or 1000-μg doses of cyanocobalamin provide average retentions of 55 or 100 μg, respectively (Table 27.6). Patients can be taught to self-inject. For unknown reasons, perhaps related to clearance variations, occasional patients may require more frequent injections (15, 68).

Patients with PA also respond to oral cobalamin, provided the dose is taken daily and is large enough (e.g., 1000 μg) so that the average 1.2% bioavailability provides enough absorbed vitamin (68, 169). Oral therapy avoids the discomfort, inconvenience, and cost of monthly injections, but it is not trouble-free in PA (15). Clinical responses are sometimes suboptimal (170), equivalent efficacy for severe neurologic symptoms is not fully proven, compliance with the usually lifelong requirement may wane, and relapse occurs sooner after discontinuance of oral therapy than discontinuance of parenteral therapy (171). Noncompliance and relapse complicate all modes of cobalamin treatment (100), and they can be traced to poor understanding by patients and sometimes to physicians' complacency about cobalamin therapy.

Patients with Malabsorption Limited to Food-Bound Cobalamin

Patients with FBCM absorb free, unbound cobalamin and theoretically should absorb cobalamin from supplements normally. However, that assumption may be premature (69). Patients often respond incompletely to oral doses as high as 50 μg after gastric surgery, a known cause of FBCM (152, 153), and some elderly persons with SCCD (but unknown absorption status) had incomplete metabolic responses until doses reached 500 μg (95–97). The optimal oral doses and the effect of meals on their bioavailability, which can be significant in patients with PA (68), await formal study in elderly patients with and without documented FBCM.

TABLE 27.6   RETENTION OF INTRAMUSCULAR INJECTION DOSES OF COBALAMIN, WITH COMPARISON OF CYANOCOBALAMIN AND HYDROXOCOBALAMIN[a]

INTRAMUSCULAR INJECTION DOSE	CYANOCOBALAMIN		HYDROXOCOBALAMIN	
	AMOUNT RETAINED	% RETAINED	AMOUNT RETAINED	% RETAINED
10 μg	9.7 μg	97%	—	—
100 μg	55 μg	55%	92 μg	92%
500 μg	150 μg	30%	375 μg	75%
1,000 μg	150 μg	15%	710 μg	71%

[a]The amounts retained may be overestimated because they are based on losses by urinary excretion only. For example, losses by other routes (e.g., biliary) may conceivably differ between the two forms of cobalamin.

Data from Chanarin I. The Megaloblastic Anaemias. 2nd ed. Oxford: Blackwell Scientific, 1979:311.

Patients with Subclinical Cobalamin Deficiency

SCCD is severalfold more common than clinical deficiency in the population, but the need to treat it is not yet proven. The specific clinical role of SCCD and the benefit of treating with cobalamin was not addressed in the recent demonstration of cognitive prophylaxis (130a, 130b) because the response occurred with high doses of folic acid, cobalamin, and pyridoxine in subjects without proven SCCD.

As discussed in the previous section, the cobalamin doses needed to simply improve metabolic status in SCCD itself can be surprisingly, and unpredictably, high (95–97, 152, 153). Many surveys of supplementation have suggested that small oral doses are effective in the whole study population, often without identifying the small SCCD subset at risk of nonresponsiveness hidden by the normal, responsive, majority. If supplementation is deemed necessary for SCCD, the metabolic response must be monitored and doses adjusted accordingly (15). The duration of intervention, whether brief or lifelong, is also unclear in most persons with SCCD because the causes of deficiency are often unknown.

Patients with Metabolic Disorders

Treatment of nitrous oxide toxicity must be started early and should be parenteral because reversal can be incomplete. The optimal cobalamin form and the possible value of adding folic acid are uncertain. Prevention is important whenever possible, and cobalamin levels and blood counts should be tested preoperatively if nitrous oxide use is anticipated.

Most patients with hereditary disorders of metabolism require parenteral therapy and sometimes auxiliary measures as well. Other sources can be consulted for therapeutic details and rationales (147).

Monitoring and Response to Cobalamin Therapy

Monitoring response has many virtues; it provides ultimate confirmation that the diagnosis was correct and allows early identification of nonresponsiveness or complications (15). In clinically overt deficiency, reticulocyte counts show rises within 2 to 3 days and peak at 7 to 10 days (15, 17, 31). Failure of full hematologic normalization by 8 weeks suggests that the diagnosis was incorrect or another form of anemia, usually iron deficiency, coexists. Neurologic response, both clinical and electrophysiologic, also begins within the first few weeks, but its course and rate vary, and response can evolve over many months (104); approximately 6% of patients have irreversible damage.

Biochemical improvement, which is the only measurable response in asymptomatic SCCD, begins within a week. MMA and homocysteine levels reach normality after 1 to 2 weeks (22, 23), but they do not respond to folic acid given instead. Monitoring metabolites is preferable to vitamin levels (cobalamin or holo-TC II), which rise whether therapy is effective or not. Maintenance therapy must continue for as long as the causative disorder persists.

Food Fortification

The conceptual and practical requirements for cobalamin fortification have been reviewed (172). The case for fortification arises from a confluence of considerations: the potential to augment prevention of neural tube and perhaps other birth defects (173); the high frequency of SCCD in elderly persons; and the possibility of mitigating neurologic risks that high folic acid intake may pose in persons with unsuspected clinical cobalamin deficiency.

Those are important goals, but the brief for them must overcome the many information gaps (172). Although folic acid fortification has been successful, it does not predict success for cobalamin fortification (130e). Two important differences exist between the two fortifications. One is that bioavailability in the chief targeted subpopulation was never at issue with folic acid but is problematic with cobalamin. Cobalamin bioavailability now appears surprisingly poor, not just in PA but in many elderly persons with SCCD or FBCM (69, 95–97, 152, 153), a shortcoming suggesting that small fortification doses may not suffice in an important target subpopulation. Moreover, bioavailability may be compromised when cobalamin is taken with meals (68), which is the setting for fortification. Population studies of metabolic response to cobalamin supplements have generally provided limited information on the response of subsets at special risk. The first controlled study of fortified food (bread that provided a high daily amount of 9.6 μg) showed overall improvement in a small cohort (174). However, elevated MMA became normal in only 7 of the 15 subjects, and details about the nonresponders or about absorption status were unavailable.

Other issues that need resolution are whether SCCD indeed causes the neurocognitive abnormalities possibly associated with it and whether giving cobalamin in smaller doses can reverse or prevent them. Potential adverse effects of fortification also need consideration, guided by the experience from combined folic acid and high-dose cobalamin supplementation that detected increased risks of cancer (175) and reduction of renal function in diabetic patients (176). Should adverse effects emerge, cobalamin accumulation may not be quickly dissipated because cobalamin turnover is very slow (172). Opinions differ, but all can agree that prospective clinical trials must address these important questions, including the crucial question of dose.

Characteristics of Cobalamin Preparations

Hydroxocobalamin is a suitable alternative to cyanocobalamin; its superior retention allows less frequent maintenance injections. Documentation of advantages for methylcobalamin is limited. Nasal and sublingual preparations have not been studied systematically.

Cobalamin has little toxicity even at high doses. However, the nonphysiologic injected form, cyanocobalamin, accumulates in red blood cells when doses reach 1000 μg or more (177). Allergic reactions can occur during routine therapy, and they can be severe (178). Autoantibody to TC II sometimes appears following injection of high-retention cobalamin preparations and produces very high serum cobalamin levels (38), but harmful effects have not been noted.

INTERACTIONS

Folate

Cobalamin and folate are linked by close metabolic, clinical, and therapeutic connections (see also the chapter on folic acid). Cobalamin's narrow dietary sources, slow rate of depletion, and highly specific, yet occasionally vulnerable, IF-dependent absorption processes explain why cobalamin deficiency, unlike folate deficiency, tends to be a drawn out malabsorptive deficiency state limited chiefly to cobalamin. As cobalamin deficiency progresses, it usually raises methylTHF levels (and thus serum folate) as predicted by the methylTHF trap hypothesis, whereas the poor cellular retention of methylTHF lowers red blood cell folate levels. Folate deficiency lowers plasma cobalamin levels by unknown mechanisms; the levels rebound after folate therapy. Both vitamin deficiencies induce homocysteine elevation.

The anemia of cobalamin deficiency often responds to folate therapy, although the response can be partial and transient, but neurologic manifestations do so much less often (17, 113, 114). Data are insufficient to determine whether the sharply increased folate intake in the United States since 1997 has compromised the early hematologic diagnosis of cobalamin deficiency or worsened its neurologic complications. Cognitive findings related to the high folate status–low cobalamin status combination have conflicted in three epidemiologic studies (179–181), perhaps because the subsets at risk were all small and neurocognitive testing was too limited (120). An unexpected, incidental finding was that the combination of low cobalamin and high folate levels was associated with greater MMA abnormalities than when folate status was normal (181, 182). The nature of those metabolic associations is unclear. However, indirect evidence (183) supports the likelihood that the subjects with that unusual metabolic combination had severe cobalamin deficiency (such as PA), which elevates serum folate, and did not have SCCD with unusually high folate intake (120). No evidence emerged to link the metabolic patterns to cognitive status.

Folate intake and cobalamin status interactions raise other issues in specialized medical settings. For example, patients with sickle cell diseases are routinely given folic acid because their chronic hemolytic anemia raises their folate requirements. However, reports now suggest that patients with sickle cell disease can develop PA despite

their young age (163, 184). It seems prudent to screen such patients for clinical cobalamin deficiency periodically if they continue to take folic acid supplements.

Iron

More than half of patients with PA develop iron deficiency (142), often because the atrophic gastritis underlying PA also compromises iron absorption. However, the increased risk of gastric cancer in patients with PA mandates a search for blood loss. When iron and cobalamin deficiency anemias coexist, the expected hematologic characteristics of either clinical entity may be blurred by the other (31, 101); MCV may be high, normal, or low, and markers of iron status can be masked by severe, untreated cobalamin deficiency sometimes (17). The mixed anemia may fail to respond if only one of the two required hematinics is given.

REFERENCES

1. Kass L. Pernicious Anemia. Philadelphia: WB Saunders, 1976.
2. Wintrobe MM. Blood, Pure and Eloquent: A Story of Discovery, of People, and of Ideas. New York: McGraw-Hill, 1980.
3. Minot GR, Murphy WP. JAMA 1926;87:470–6.
4. Castle WB. Am J Med Sci 1929;178:748–64.
5. Rickes EL, Brink NG, Koniuszy FR et al. Science 1948; 107:396–7.
6. Smith EL, Parker LFJ. Biochem J 1948;43:viii–ix.
7. Hodgkin DC, Kamper J, Mackay M et al. Nature 1956;178:64–6.
8. Carmel R, Karnaze DS. JAMA 1985;253:1284–7.
9. Carmel R, Sinow RM, Karnaze DS. J Lab Clin Med 1987;109:454–63.
10. Carmel R. Annu Rev Med 2000;51:357–75.
11. Kondo H, Kolhouse JF, Allen RH. Proc Natl Acad Sci U S A 1980;77:817–21.
12. Kolhouse JF, Kondo H, Allen NC et al. N Engl J Med 1978;299:785–92.
13. el Kholty S, Guéant JL, Bressler L et al. Gastroenterology 1991;101:1399–408.
14. Hardlei RF, Nexo E. Clin Chem 2009;55:1002–10.
15. Carmel R. Blood 2008;112:2214–21.
16. Carmel R. Am J Clin Nutr 2011;94(Suppl 1):348S–58S.
17. Chanarin I. The Megaloblastic Anaemias. 2nd ed. Oxford: Blackwell Scientific, 1979.
18. Carmel R, Brar S, Agrawal A et al. Clin Chem 2000;46:2017–8.
19. Vlasveld LT, van't Wout JKW, Meuwissen P et al. Clin Chem 2006;52:17–8.
20. Carmel R. Blood 2005;106:1136–7.
21. Stabler SP, Marcell PD, Podell ER et al. J Clin Invest 1986; 77:1606–12.
22. Allen RH, Stabler SP, Savage DG et al. Am J Hematol 1990; 34:90–8.
23. Lindenbaum J, Savage DG, Stabler SP et al. Am J Hematol 1990;34:99–107.
24. Adams J, Boddy K, Douglas A. Br J Haematol 1972;23:297–305.
25. Mollin DL, Anderson BB, Burman JF. Clin Haematol 1976; 5:521–46.
26. Carmel R. Arch Intern Med 1988;148:1712–4.
27. Carmel R. Clin Chem 2003;49:1367–74.
28. Lindenbaum J, Rosenberg IH, Wilson PWF et al. Am J Clin Nutr 1994;60:2–11.
29. van Asselt DZB, de Groot LCPGM, van Staveren WA et al. Am J Clin Nutr 1998;68:328–34.

30. Carmel R, Green R, Jacobsen DW et al. Am J Clin Nutr 1999;70:904–10.

31. Carmel R. Megaloblastic anemias: disorders of impaired DNA synthesis. In: Greer JP, Foerster J, Rodgers GM et al, eds. Wintrobe's Clinical Hematology. 12th ed. Philadelphia: Lippincott Williams & Wilkins, 2009:1143–72.

32. Carmel R, Parker J, Kelman Z. Br J Haematol 2009;147:386–91.

33. Carmel R, Parker J, Kelman Z. Blood 2009;114(Suppl):abstract 1989.

34. Hazra A, Kraft P, Lazarus R et al. Hum Mol Genet 2009;18:4677–87.

35. Tanaka T, Scheet P, Giusti B et al. Am J Hum Genet 2009;84:477–82.

36. Carmel R. Semin Hematol 1999;36:88–100.

37. Carmel R, Vasireddy H, Aurangzeb I et al. Clin Lab Haematol 2001;23:365–71.

38. Skouby AP, Hippe E, Olesen H. Blood 1971;38:769–74.

39. Carmel R, Tatsis B, Baril L. Blood 1977;49:987–1000.

40. Carmel R. Large vitamin B$_{12}$–binding proteins and complexes in human serum. In: Zagalak B, Friedrich W, eds. Vitamin B$_{12}$: Proceedings of the Third European Symposium on Vitamin B$_{12}$ and Intrinsic Factor. Berlin: Walter de Gruyter, 1979:777–90.

41. Jeffery J, Millar H, MacKenzie P et al. Clin Biochem 2010;43:82–8.

42. Carmel R. Cobalamin-binding proteins in man. In: Silber R, Gordon AS, LoBue J et al, eds. Contemporary Hematology-Oncology, vol 2. New York: Plenum, 1981:79–129.

43. Bolann BJ, Soll JD, Schneede J et al. Clin Chem 2000;46:1744–50.

44. Rasmussen K, Moller J, Lyngbak M et al. Clin Chem 1996;42:630–6.

45. Vogiatzoglou A, Oulhaj A, Smith AD et al. Clin Chem 2009;55:2198–206.

46. Savage DG, Lindenbaum J, Stabler SP et al. Am J Med 1994;96:239–46.

47. Carmel R, Rasmussen K, Jacobsen DW et al. Br J Haematol 1996;93:311–8.

48. Lewerin C, Ljungman S, Nilsson-Ehle H. J Intern Med 2007;261:65–73.

49. Monsen ALB, Refsum H, Markestad T et al. Clin Chem 2003;49:2067–75.

50. Bjorke-Monsen AL, Torvik I, Saetran H et al. Pediatrics 2008;122:83–91.

51. Hvas AM, Ellegaard J, Nexo E. Clin Chem 2001;47:1396–404.

52. Bailey R, Carmel R, Green R et al. Am J Clin Nutr 2011;94:552–61.

53. Hvas AM, Ellegaard J, Nexo E. Arch Intern Med 2001;161:1534–41.

54. Sentongo TA, Azzam R, Charrao J. J Pediatr Gastroenterol Nutr 2009;48:495–7.

55. Carmel R, Jacobsen DW. Homocysteine in Health and Disease. Cambridge: Cambridge University Press, 2001.

56. Refsum H, Smith AD, Ueland PM et al. Clin Chem 2004;50:3–32.

57. Lindemans J, Schoester M, van Kapel J. Clin Chim Acta 1983;132:53–61.

58. Brady J, McGregor L, Valente E et al. Clin Chem 2008;54:567–73.

59. Morkbak AL, Hvas AM, Milman N et al. Haematologica 2007;92:1171–2.

60. Goringe A, Ellis R, McDowell I et al. Haematologica 2006;91:231–4.

61. Carmel R. Clin Chem 2002;48:407–9.

62. Chen X, Remacha AF, Sardà MP et al. Am J Clin Nutr 2005;81:110–4.

63. Martens AF, Barg H, Warren MJ. Appl Microbiol Biotechnol 2002;58:275–85.

64. Food and Nutrition Board, Institute of Medicine. Dietary Reference Intakes: Thiamin, Riboflavin, Niacin, Vitamin B$_6$, Folate, Vitamin B$_{12}$, Pantothenic Acid, Biotin, and Choline. Washington, DC: National Academy Press, 1998:306–56.

65. Watanabe F. Exp Biol Med 2007;232:1266–74.

66. Tucker KL, Rich S, Rosenberg I et al. Am J Clin Nutr 2000;71:514–22.

67. Vogiatzoglou A, Smith AD, Nurk E et al. Am J Clin Nutr 2009;89:1078–87.

68. Berlin H, Berlin R, Brante G. Acta Med Scand 1968;184:247–58.

69. Carmel R, Sarrai M. Curr Hematol Rep 2006;5:23–33.

70. del Corral A, Carmel R. Gastroenterology 1990;98:1460–6.

71. Allen RH, Seetharam B, Podell E et al. J Clin Invest 1978;61:47–54.

72. Moestrup SK, Verroust PJ. Annu Rev Nutr 2001;21:407–28.

73. Fyfe JC, Madsen M, Hojrup P et al. Blood 2004;103:1573–9.

74. Pedersen GA, Chakraborty S, Steinhauser AL et al. Traffic 2010;11:706–20.

75. Quadros EV, Regec AL, Khan KM et al. Am J Physiol 1999;277:G161–6.

76. Waters HM, Dawson DW. Clin Lab Haematol 1999;21:169–72.

77. Kalra S, Li N, Yammani RR et al. Arch Biochem Biophys 2004;431:189–96.

78. Namour F, Olivier JL, Abdelmoutalleb I et al. Blood 2001;97:1092–8.

79. Quadros EV, Nakayama Y, Sequeira JM. Blood 2009;113:186–92.

80. Jiang W, Sequeira JM. Nakayama Y et al. Gene 2010;466:49–55.

81. Birn H. Am J Physiol Renal Physiol 2006;291:F22–36.

82. Cowland JB, Borregaard N. J Leukoc Biol 1999;66:989–95.

83. Hall CA. Clin Sci Mol Med 1977;53:453–7.

84. Burger RL, Schneider RJ, Mehlman CS et al. J Biol Chem 1975;250:7707–13.

85. Carmel R. Am J Clin Nutr 1997;66:750–9.

86. Nilsson-Ehle H. Drugs Aging 1998;12:277–92.

87. Carmel R. Pernicious anemia: definitions, expressions, and the long-term consequences of atrophic gastritis. In: Holt PR, Russell RM, eds. Chronic Gastritis and Hypochlorhydria in the Elderly. Boca Raton, FL: CRC Press, 1993:99–114.

88. Carmel R. Baillieres Clin Haematol 1995;8:639–55.

89. Selhub J, Jacques PF, Wilson PWF et al. JAMA 1993;270:2693–8.

90. Howard JM, Azen C, Jacobsen DW et al. Eur J Clin Nutr 1998; 52:582–7.

91. Ervin RB, Wright JD, Wang CY et al. Advance Data from Vital and Health Statistics. No. 339. Hyattsville, MD: National Center for Health Statistics, 2004.

92. Bor MV, Lydeking-Olsen E, Moller J et al. Am J Clin Nutr 2006;83:52–8.

93. Bor MV, von Castel-Roberts KM, Kauwell GPA et al. Am J Clin Nutr 2010;91:571–7.

94. Kaufman DW, Kelly JP, Rosenberg I et al. JAMA 2002;287:337–44.

95. Seal EC, Metz J, Flicker L et al. J Am Geriatr Soc 2002;50:146–51.

96. Garcia A, Paris-Pombo A, Evans L et al. J Am Geriatr Soc 2002;50:1401–4.

97. Rajan S, Wallace JI, Brodkin KI et al. J Am Geriatr Soc 2002;50:1789–95.

98. Herbert V. Trans Assoc Am Physicians 1962;75:307–20.

99. Carmel R. Arch Intern Med 1979;139:47–50.

100. Savage D, Lindenbaum J. Am J Med 1983;74:765–72.
101. Chan CW, Liu SY, Kho CS et al. Int J Lab Haematol 2007;29:163–71.
102. Carmel R. Sem Hematol 2008;45:224–34.
103. Reynolds EH. Lancet Neurol 2006;5:949–60.
104. Healton EB, Savage DG, Brust JC et al. Medicine (Baltimore) 1991;70:229–45.
105. Lindenbaum J, Healton EB, Savage DG et al. N Engl J Med 1988;318:1720–8.
106. Carmel R, Melnyk S, James SJ. Blood 2003;101:3302–8.
107. Pant SS, Asbury AK, Richardson EP Jr. Acta Neurol Scand Suppl 1968;44:1–36.
108. Carmel R, Pullarkat V. Br J Haematol 2003;120:907–9.
109. Fine EJ, Soria E, Paroski MW et al. Muscle Nerve 1990;13:158–64.
110. Hemmer B, Glocker FX, Schumacher M et al. J Neurol Neurosurg Psychiatry 1998;65:822–7.
111. Karnaze DS, Carmel R. Arch Neurol 1990;47:1008–12.
112. Carmel R, Gott PS, Waters CH et al. Eur J Haematol 1995;54:245–53.
113. Rundles RW. Blood 1946;1:209–19.
114. Ungley CC. Brain 1949;72:382–427.
115. Magnus EM. Eur J Haematol 1987;39:39–43.
116. Noronha JM, Silverman M. On folic acid, vitamin B$_{12}$, methionine and formiminoglutamic acid metabolism. In: Heinrich HC, ed. Vitamin B$_{12}$ und Intrinsic Factor 2. Europäisches Symposion. Stuttgart: Enke, 1962:728–36.
117. Herbert V, Zalusky R. J Clin Invest 1962;41:1263–76.
118. Bottiglieri T, Hyland K, Reynolds EH. Drugs 1994;48:137–52.
119. Carmel R. Arch Intern Med 1996;156:1097–100.
120. Carmel R. Am J Clin Nutr 2009;90:1449–50.
121. Metz J, Bell AH, Flicker L et al. J Am Geriatr Soc 1996;44:1355–61.
122. Waters WE, Withey JL, Kilpatrick GS et al. Br J Haematol 1971;20:521–6.
123. Smith AD. Food Nutr Bull 2008;29:S143–72.
124. Ho RCM, Cheung MWL, Fu E et al. Am J Geriatr Psychiatry 2011;19:607–17.
125. Carmel R. Curr Opin Gastroenterol 2012;28:151–8.
126. Malouf R, Areosa Sastre A. Cochrane Database of Syst Rev 2003:CD004394. .
127. McMahon JA, Green TJ, Skeaff CM et al. N Engl J Med 2006;354:2564–72.
128. Balk EM, Raman G, Tatsioni A et al. Arch Intern Med 2007;167:21–30.
129. Aisen PS, Schneider LS, Sano M et al. JAMA 2008;300:1774–83.
130. Wald DS, Kasturiratne A, Simmonds M. Am J Med 2010; 123:522–7.
130a. Smith AD, Smith SM, de Jager CA et al. PLoS One 2010;5:e12244.
130b. de Jager CA, Oulhaj A, Jacoby R et al. Int J Geriatr Psychiatry 2012;27:592–600.
130c. Durga J, van Boxtel MPJ, Schouten EG et al. Lancet 2007;369:208–16.
130d. Smith AD, Refsum H. Am J Clin Nutr 2009;89(Suppl):707S–11S.
130e. Carmel R. J Inher Metab Dis 2011;34:67–73.
131. Collin SM, Metcalfe C, Refsum H et al. Cancer Epidemiol Biomarkers Prev 2010;19:1632–42.
132. Refsum H, Yajnik CS, Gadkari M et al. Am J Clin Nutr 2001; 74:233–41.
133. Carmel R, Mallidi PV, Vinarskiy S et al. Am J Hematol 2002;70:107–14.
134. Stabler SP, Allen RH. Annu Rev Nutr 2004;24:299–326.
135. Louwman MWJ, van Dusseldorp M, van den Vijver FJR et al. Am J Clin Nutr 2000;72:762–9.
136. Higginbottom MC, Sweetman L, Nyhan WL. N Engl J Med 1978;299:317–23.
137. Graham SM, Arvela OM, Wise GA. J Pediatr 1992;121:710–4.
138. Grattan-Smith PJ, Wilcken B, Procopis PG et al. Mov Disord 1997;12:39–46.
139. Centers for Disease Control and Prevention. MMWR Morb Mortal Wkly Rep 2003;52:61–4.
140. Carmel R, Johnson CS, Weiner JM. Arch Intern Med 1987;147:1995–6.
141. Carmel R, Spencer CA. Arch Intern Med 1982;142:1465–9.
142. Carmel R, Weiner JM, Johnson CS. JAMA 1987;257:1081–3.
143. Borch K. Scand J Gastroenterol 1986;21:21–30.
144. Sjoblom SM, Sipponen P, Miettinen M et al. Endoscopy 1988;20:52–6.
145. Yassin F, Rothenberg SP, Rao S et al. Blood 2004;103:1515–7.
146. Tanner SM, Li Z, Perko JD et al. Proc Natl Acad Sci U S A 2005;102:4130–3.
147. Watkins D, Rosenblatt DS. Inherited disorders of folate and cobalamin transport and metabolism. In: Valle D, Beaudet AL, Vogelstein B et al, eds. The Online Metabolic and Molecular Bases of Inherited Disease. New York: McGraw-Hill, 2011: part 17, chap 155. Available at: http://www.ommbid.comract/part17/ch155.
148. Sumner AE, Chin MM, Abraham JL et al. Ann Intern Med 1996;124:469–76.
149. Doscherholmen A, Swaim WR. Gastroenterology 1973;64:913–9.
150. Aminoff M, Carter JE, Chadwick RB et al. Nature Genet 1999;21:309–13.
151. Kristiansen M, Aminoff M, Jacobsen C et al. Blood 2000;96: 405–9.
152. Provenzale D, Reinhold RB, Golner B et al. J Am Coll Nutr 1992;11:29–35.
153. Rhode BM, Arseneau P, Cooper BA et al. Am J Clin Nutr 1996;63:103–9.
154. Carmel R, Aurangzeb I, Qian D. Am J Gastroenterol 2001; 96:63–70.
155. Cohen H, Weinstein WM, Carmel R. Gut 2000;47:638–45.
156. Dierkes J, Ebert M, Malfertheiner P, et al. Dig Dis 2003;21: 237–44.
157. Carmel R. J Nutr 2007;137:2481–4.
158. Guttormsen AB, Refsum H, Ueland PM. Acta Anaesthesiol Scand 1994;38:753–6.
159. Ng J, Frith R. Lancet 2002;360:384.
160. Schilling RF. JAMA 1986;255:1605–6.
161. Kinsella LJ, Green R. Neurology 1995;45:1608–10.
162. Quadros EV. Br J Haematol 2009;148:195–204.
163. Carmel R, Bellevue R, Kelman Z. Am J Hematol 2010;85:436–9.
164. Hardlei TF, Morkbak AL, Bor MV et al. Clin Chem 2010;56:432–6.
165. Carmel R. Clin Exp Immunol 1992;89:74–7.
166. Waters HM, Dawson DW, Howarth JE et al. J Clin Pathol 1993;46:45–7.
167. Carmel R. Am J Clin Pathol 1988;90:442–6.
168. Andres E, Kurtz JE, Perrin AE et al. Am J Med 2001;111:126–9.
169. Kuzminski AM, Del Giacco EJ, Allen RH et al. Blood 1998;92:1191–8.
170. Kondo H. Acta Haematol 1998;99:200–5.
171. Magnus EM. Scand J Haematol 1986;36:457–65.
172. Carmel R. Food Nutr Bull 2008;29:S177–87.
173. Li F, Watkins D, Rosenblatt DS. Mol Genet Metab 2009;98:166–72.
174. Winkels RM, Brouwer IA, Clarke R et al. Am J Clin Nutr 2008;88:348–55.
175. Ebbing M, Bonaa KH, Nygard O et al. JAMA 2009;302:2119–26.
176. House AA, Eliasziw M, Cattran D et al. JAMA 2010;303:1603–9.

177. Gimsing P, Hippe E, Helleberg-Rasmussen I et al. Scand J Haematol 1982;29:311–8.

178. Tordjman R, Genereau T, Guinnepain T et al. Eur J Haematol 1998;60:269–70.

179. Morris MS, Jacques PF, Rosenberg IH et al. Am J Clin Nutr 2007;85:193–200.

180. Clarke R, Sherliker P, Hin H et al. Br J Nutr 2008;100:1054–9.

181. Miller JW, Garrod MG, Allen LH et al. Am J Clin Nutr 2009;90:1586–92.

182. Selhub J, Morris MS, Jacques PF. Proc Natl Acad Sci U S A 2007;104:19995–20000.

183. Mills JL, Carter TC, Scott JM et al. Am J Clin Nutr 2011; 94:495–500.

184. Dhar M, Bellevue R, Carmel R. N Engl J Med 2003;348: 2204–7.

SUGGESTED READINGS

Banerjee R. B$_{12}$ trafficking in mammals: a case for coenzyme escort service. ACS Chem Biol 2006;1:149–59.

Carmel R. How I treat cobalamin (vitamin B$_{12}$) deficiency. Blood 2008;112:2214–21.

Carmel R, Sarrai M. Diagnosis and management of clinical and subclinical cobalamin deficiency: advances and controversies. Curr Hematol Rep 2006;5:23–33.

Healton EB, Savage DG, Brust JC et al. Neurologic aspects of cobalamin deficiency. Medicine (Baltimore) 1991;70:229–45.

Stabler SP, Allen RH. Vitamin B$_{12}$ deficiency as a worldwide problem. Annu Rev Nutr 2004;24:299–326.

Watanabe F. Vitamin B$_{12}$ souces and bioavailability. Exp Biol Med 2007;232:1266–74.

28 BIOTIN[1]

DONALD M. MOCK

HISTORY OF DISCOVERY

Although a growth requirement for the "bios" fraction had been demonstrated in yeast, Boas first demonstrated the mammalian requirement for a factor—biotin—in rats fed egg-white protein. The severe dermatitis, hair loss, and neuromuscular dysfunction were termed "egg-white injury" and were cured by a factor present in liver. The critical event in this egg-white injury of both humans and rats is the highly specific and very tight binding (dissociation constant = 10^{-15}M) of biotin by avidin, a glycoprotein found in egg white. From an evolutionary standpoint, avidin probably serves as a bacteriostat in egg white; consistent with this hypothesis is the observation that avidin is resistant to a broad range of bacterial proteases. Because avidin is also resistant to pancreatic proteases, dietary avidin binds dietary biotin and biotin synthesized by intestinal microbes and thus prevents absorption. Cooking denatures avidin and renders it susceptible to digestion and unable to interfere with absorption of biotin.

STRUCTURE, CHEMISTRY, AND BIOCHEMISTRY

Structure

Biotin is a bicyclic compound (Fig. 28.1). One ring contains a ureido group; the other contains sulfur and has a valeric acid side chain. The structure of biotin was elucidated independently by Kogl and by du Vigneaud in the early 1940s (1). Eight stereoisomers exist, but only one (designated d-[+]-biotin or, simply, biotin) is found in nature and is enzymatically active.

Regulation

In mammals, biotin serves as an essential cofactor for five carboxylases, each of which catalyzes a critical step in intermediary metabolism. Biotin exists in free and bound pools within the cell that are responsive to changes in biotin status (2). The pool size is likely determined by a balance among cellular uptake, cellular release, incorporation into apocarboxylases and histones, release from these biotinylated proteins during turnover, and catabolism to inactive metabolites.

Attachment of biotin to the apocarboxylase (see Fig. 28.1) is a condensation reaction catalyzed by holocarboxylase synthetase (HCS). An amide bond is formed between the carboxyl group of the valeric acid side chain of biotin and the ε-amino group of a specific lysyl residue in the apocarboxylase; these apocarboxylase regions contain sequences of amino acids that tend to be highly

---

[1]**Abbreviations: ACC**, acetyl-CoA carboxylase; **AMP**, adenosine monophosphate; **CoA**, coenzyme A; **HCS**, holocarboxylase synthetase; **MCC**, methylcrotonyl-CoA carboxylase; **Na+**, sodium; **PC**, pyruvate carboxylase; **PCC**, propionyl-CoA carboxylase; **SMVT**, sodium-dependent multivitamin transporter.

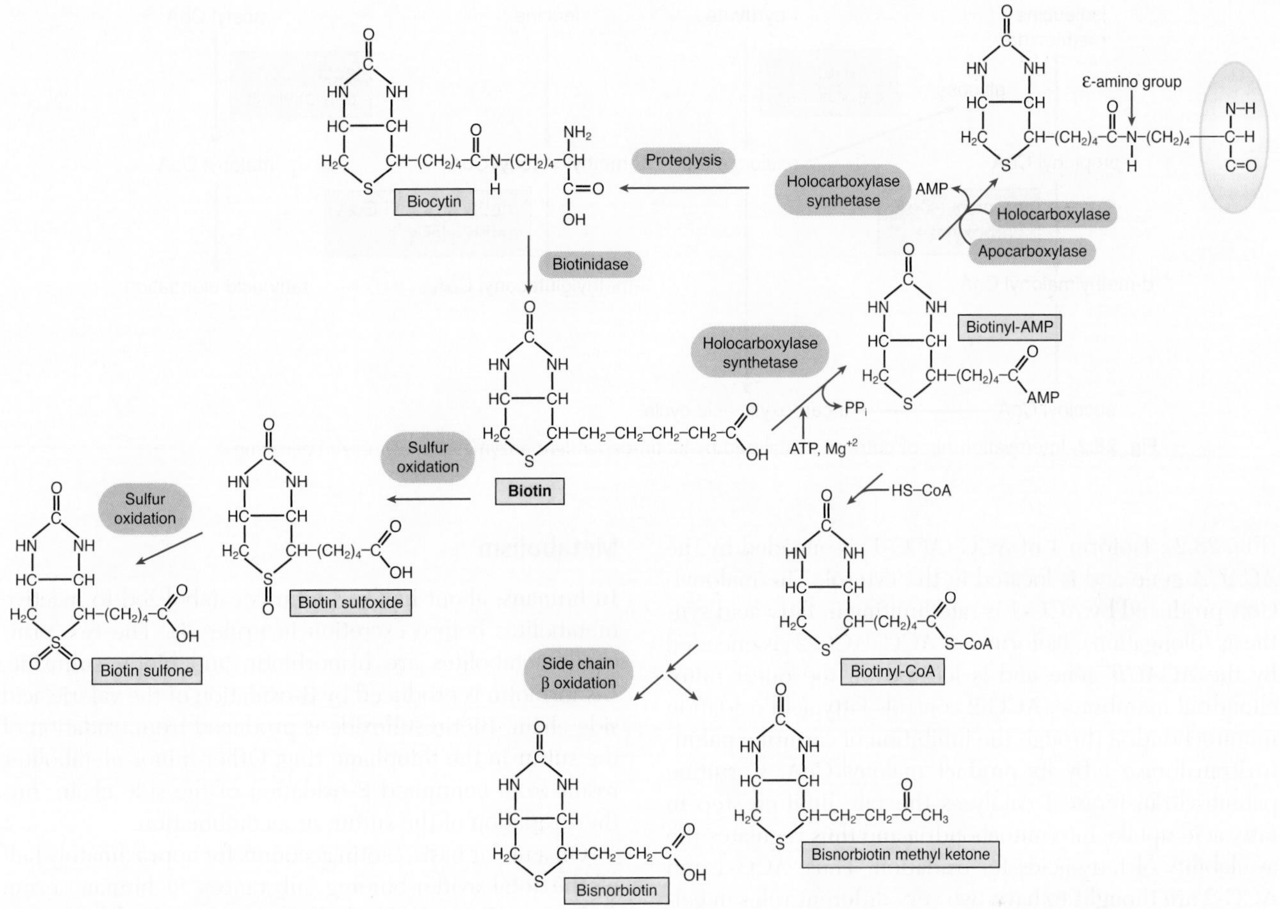

Fig. 28.1. Biotin metabolism and degradation. *Ovals* denote enzymes or enzyme systems; *rectangles* denote biotin, intermediates, and metabolites. *AMP*, adenosine monophosphate; *ATP*, adenosine triphosphate; *CoA*, coenzyme A; *Pp_i*, pyrophosphate; *asterisk*, site of attachment of carboxyl moiety.

conserved within and among species for the individual carboxylases.

Regulation of intracellular mammalian carboxylase activity by biotin remains to be elucidated. However, the interaction of biotin synthesis and production of holoacetyl–coenzyme A (CoA) carboxylase in *Escherichia coli* has been extensively studied. In the bacterial system, the availability of the apocarboxylase protein and of biotin (as the intermediate biotinyl–adenosine monophosphate [AMP]) act together to control the rate of biotin synthesis by direct interaction with promoter regions of the biotin operon, which, in turn, controls a cluster of genes that encode enzymes that catalyze the synthesis of biotin.

In the normal turnover of cellular proteins, holocarboxylases are degraded to biocytin (ε-N-biotinyl-L-lysine) or biotin linked to an oligopeptide containing at most a few amino acid residues (see Fig. 28.1). Biotinidase (biotin amide hydrolase, EC 3.5.1.12) releases biotin for recycling. The clinical manifestations of biotinidase deficiency appear to result largely from a secondary biotin deficiency. The genes for HCS and human biotinidase have been cloned, sequenced, and characterized (3).

Chemistry

All five of the mammalian carboxylases catalyze the incorporation of bicarbonate as a carboxyl group into a substrate and employ a similar catalytic mechanism. In the carboxylase reaction, the carboxyl moiety is first attached to biotin at the ureido nitrogen opposite the side chain; then the carboxyl group is transferred to the substrate. The reaction is driven by the hydrolysis of adenosine triphosphate. Subsequent reactions in the pathways release carbon dioxide. Thus, these reaction sequences rearrange the substrates into more useful intermediates, but they do not violate the classic observation that mammalian metabolism does not result in the *net* fixation of carbon dioxide (4).

Biotin-Dependent Carboxylases

The five biotin-dependent mammalian carboxylases are acetyl-CoA carboxylase (ACC; EC 6.4.1.2) isoforms I and II, pyruvate carboxylase (PC: EC 6.4.1.1), methylcrotonyl-CoA carboxylase (MCC; EC 6.4.1.4), and propionyl-CoA carboxylase (PCC; EC 6.4.1.3).

Both acetyl-CoA carboxylases catalyze the incorporation of bicarbonate into acetyl-CoA to form malonyl-CoA

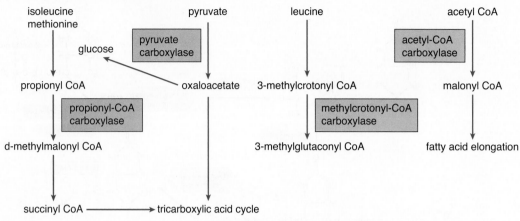

Fig. 28.2. Interrelationship of pathways catalyzed by biotin-dependent enzymes *(boxes)*. *CoA*, coenzyme A.

(Fig. 28.2). Isoform 1 of ACC (ACC-1) is encoded by the *ACACA* gene and is located in the cytosol. The malonyl-CoA produced by ACC-1 is rate limiting in fatty acid synthesis (elongation). Isoform 2 of ACC (ACC-2) is encoded by the *ACACB* gene and is located on the outer mitochondrial membrane. ACC-2 controls fatty acid oxidation in mitochondria through the inhibition of carnitine palmitoyltransferase I by its product malonyl-CoA. Carnitine palmitoyltransferase I catalyzes the rate limiting step in fatty acid uptake into mitochondria and thus regulates the availability of fatty acids for oxidation. Thus, ACC-1 and ACC-2 are thought to have two very different roles in cellular metabolism; one controls fatty acid synthesis, and the other controls fatty acid oxidation. An inactive mitochondrial form of ACC may also serve as storage for biotin (5).

The three remaining carboxylases are mitochondrial. PC catalyzes the incorporation of bicarbonate into pyruvate to form oxaloacetate, an intermediate in the Krebs tricarboxylic acid cycle (see Fig. 28.2). In gluconeogenic tissues (i.e., liver and kidney), the oxaloacetate can be converted to glucose. Deficiency of PC is probably the cause of lactic acidemia, central nervous system lactic acidosis, and abnormalities in glucose regulation observed in biotin deficiency and biotinidase deficiency (see later).

MCC catalyzes an essential step in the degradation of the branched-chain amino acid leucine (see Fig. 28.2). Deficient activity of MCC leads to metabolism of 3-methylcrotonyl-CoA to 3-hydroxyisovaleryl-CoA, 3-hydroxyisovaleryl-carnitine, and 3-hydroxyisovaleric acid by an alternate pathway (1). Increased urinary excretions of 3-hydroxyisovaleryl-carnitine and 3-hydroxyisovaleric acid reflect deficient activity of MCC and are biomarkers of biotin deficiency (1, 6).

PCC catalyzes the incorporation of bicarbonate into propionyl-CoA to form methylmalonyl-CoA; methylmalonyl-CoA undergoes isomerization to succinyl-CoA and enters the tricarboxylic acid cycle (see Fig. 28.2). In a fashion analogous to MCC deficiency, deficiency of PCC leads to increased urinary excretion of 3-hydroxypropionic acid and 3-methylcitric acid.

Metabolism

In humans, about half of biotin is catabolized to inactive metabolites before excretion in urine (4). The two principal metabolites are bisnorbiotin and biotin sulfoxide. Bisnorbiotin is produced by β-oxidation of the valeric acid side chain. Biotin sulfoxide is produced from oxidation of the sulfur in the thiophane ring. Other minor metabolites result from continued β-oxidation of the side chain, further oxidation of the sulfur, or a combination.

On a molar basis, biotin accounts for approximately half of the total avidin-binding substances in human serum and urine (Table 28.1). During pregnancy and long-term anticonvulsant treatment, accelerated biotin catabolism is thought to contribute to biotin deficiency.

Measurement of Biotin and Metabolites

For measuring biotin at physiologic concentrations (i.e., 100 pmol/L to 100 nmol/L), various assays have been proposed, and a few have been used to study biotin nutriture. For a more detailed review, please refer to the study by Mock (7). Most published studies of biotin nutriture have used one of two basic types of biotin assays: bioassays or avidin-binding assays.

Bioassays generally have adequate sensitivity to measure biotin in blood and urine, especially with modifications using injected agar plates or metabolic radiometry. However, the bacterial bioassays (and perhaps the eukaryotic bioassays

TABLE 28.1	NORMAL RANGE FOR BIOTIN AND METABOLITES IN HUMAN SERUM AND URINE[a]	
COMPOUND	SERUM (pmol/L)	URINE (nmol/24 h)
Biotin	133–329	18–127
Bisnorbiotin	21–563	6–39
Biotin sulfoxide	0–120	5–19

[a]Normal ranges (minimum–maximum) are reported (*n* = 15 for serum; *n* = 16 for urine).

approximately 70 µg/day (300 nmol/d) for the Swiss population. This result is in reasonable agreement with the estimated dietary intake in Canada of 60 µg/day (71) and in Britain of 35 µg/day (72, 73).

TOXICITY

Daily doses up to 200 mg orally and up to 20 mg intravenously have been given to treat biotin-responsive inborn errors of metabolism and acquired biotin deficiency. Toxicity has not been reported.

ACKNOWLEDGMENTS

Nell Matthews and Marie Tippett provided assistance in preparation of this chapter.

REFERENCES

1. Mock DM. Biotin. In: Ziegler EE, Filer LJ Jr, eds. Present Knowledge in Nutrition. 7th ed. Washington, DC: International Life Sciences Institutes, Nutrition Foundation, 1996:220–35.
2. Lewis B, Rathman S, McMahon R. J Nutr 2001;131:2310–5.
3. Wolf B. Disorders of biotin metabolism. In: Scriver CR, Beaudet AL, Sly WS et al., eds. The Metabolic and Molecular Basis of Inherited Disease. 8th ed. New York: McGraw-Hill, 2001:3151–77.
4. Mock DM. Biotin. In: Shils ME, Olson JA, Shike M et al., eds. Modern Nutrition in Health and Disease. 9th ed. Baltimore: Lippincott Williams & Wilkins, 1999:459–66.
5. Shriver BJ, Roman-Shriver C, Allred JB. J Nutr 1993;123:1140–9.
6. Stratton SL, Horvath TD, Bogusiewicz A et al. Am J Clin Nutr 2010;92:1399–405.
7. Mock DM. Biotin. In: Brown M, ed. Present Knowledge in Nutrition. 6th ed. Blacksburg, VA: International Life Sciences Institute, Nutrition Foundation, 1990:189–207.
8. Mock DM, Nyalala JO, Raguseo RM. J Nutr 2001;131:2208–14.
9. Said H. J Nutr 2008;139:158–62.
10. Balamurugan K, Ortiz A, Said HM. Am J Physiol Gastrointest Liver Physiol 2003;285:G73–7.
11. Mardach R, Zempleni J, Wolf B et al. J Clin Invest 2002;109:1617–23.
12. Subramanya SB, Subramanian VS, Kumar JS et al. Am J Physiol Gastrointest Liver Physiol 2011;300:G494–501.
13. Spector R, Mock DM. J Neurochem 1987;48:400–4.
14. Spector R, Mock DM. Neurochem Res 1988;13:213–9.
15. Ozand PT, Gascon GG, Al Essa M et al. Brain 1999;121:1267–79.
16. Zeng WQ, Al-Yamani E, Acierno JS Jr et al. Am J Hum Genet 2005;77:16–26.
17. Subramanian VS, Marchant JS, Said HM. Am J Physiol Cell Physiol 2006;291:C851–9.
18. Mantagos S, Malamitsi-Puchner A, Antsaklis A et al. Biol Neonate 1998;74:72–4.
19. Mock DM. J Nutr 2009;139:154–7.
20. Mock DM, Mock NI, Langbehn SE. J Nutr 1992;122:535–45.
21. Mock DM, Mock NI, Dankle JA. J Nutr 1992;122:546–52.
22. Mock DM, Stratton SL, Mock NI. J Pediatr 1997;131:456–8.
23. Daberkow RL, White BR, Cederberg RA et al. J Nutr 2003;133:2703–6.
24. Grafe F, Wohlrab W, Neubert RH et al. J Invest Dermatol 2003;120:428–33.
25. Fujimoto W, Inaoki M, Fukui T et al. J Dermatol 2005;32:256–61.
26. Velazquez A, Martin-del-Campo C, Baez A et al. Eur J Clin Nutr 1988;43:169–73.
27. Krause KH, Berlit P, Bonjour JP. Ann Neurol 1982;12:485–6.
28. Krause KH, Berlit P, Bonjour JP. Int J Vitam Nutr Res 1982;52:375–85.
29. Mock DM, Dyken ME. Neurology 1997;49:1444–7.
30. Wang KS, Mock NI, Mock DM. J Nutr 1997;127:2212–6.
31. Mock DM, Mock NI, Lombard KA et al. J Pediatr Gastroenterol Nutr 1998;26:245–50.
32. Said HM, Redha R, Nylander W. Am J Clin Nutr 1989;49:127–31.
33. Takechi R, Taniguchi A, Ebara S et al. J Nutr 2008;138:680–4.
34. Czeizel AE, Dudás I. N Engl J Med 1992;327:1832–5.
35. Zempleni J, Mock D. Proc Soc Exp Biol Med 2000;223:14–21.
36. Said HM, Sharifian A, Bagherzadeh A et al. Am J Clin Nutr 1990;52:1083–6.
37. Nisenson A. J Pediatr 1957;51:537–48.
38. Nisenson A. Pediatrics 1969;44:1014–5.
39. Erlichman M, Goldstein R, Levi E et al. Arch Dis Child 1981;567:560–2.
40. Livaniou E, Evangelatos GP, Ithakissios DS et al. Nephron 1987;46:331–2.
41. Yatzidis H, Koutisicos D, Agroyannis B et al. Nephron 1984;36:183–6.
42. Koutsikos D, Fourtounas C, Kapetanaki A et al. Ren Fail 1996;18:131–7.
43. Descombes E, Hanck AB, Fellay G. Kidney Int 1993;43:1319–28.
44. Mock NI, Malik MI, Stumbo PJ et al. Am J Clin Nutr 1997;65:951–8.
45. Mock DM, Henrich-Shell CL, Carnell N et al. J Nutr 2004;134:317–20.
46. Mock DM, Henrich CL, Carnell N et al. Am J Clin Nutr 2002;76:1061–8.
47. Mock DM, Henrich CL, Carnell N et al. J Nutr Biochem 2002;13:462–70.
48. Horvath TD, Stratton SL, Bogusiewicz A et al. Anal Chem 2010;82:4140–4.
49. Horvath TD, Stratton SL, Bogusiewicz A et al. Anal Chem 2010;82:9543–8.
50. Stratton SL, Horvath TD, Bogusiewicz A et al. J Nutr 2011;141:353–8.
51. Sander JE, Packman S, Townsend JJ. Neurology 1982;32:878–80.
52. Suchy SF, Rizzo WB, Wolf B. Am J Clin Nutr 1986;44:475–80.
53. Suchy SF, Wolf B. Am J Clin Nutr 1986;43:831–8.
54. Mock DM. J Pediatr Gastroenterol Nutr 1990;10:222–9.
55. Stanley JS, Mock DM, Griffin JB, Zempleni J. J Nutr 2002;132:1854–9.
56. Hymes J, Fleischhauer K, Wolf B. Clin Chim Acta 1995;233:39–45.
57. Gralla M, Camporeale G, Zempleni J. J Nutr Biochem 2008;19:400–8.
58. Chew YC, West JT, Kratzer SJ et al. J Nutr 2008;138:2316–22.
59. Kobza K, Sarath G, Zempleni J. BMB Rep 2008;41:310–5.
60. Camporeale G, Oommen AM, Griffin JB et al. J Nutr Biochem 2007;18:760–8.
61. Wijeratne SS, Camporeale G, Zempleni J. J Nutr Biochem 2010;21:310–6.

62. Healy S, Perez-Cadahia B, Jia D et al. Biochem Biophys Acta 2009;1789:719–33.

63. Healy S, Heightman TD, Hohmann L et al. Protein Sci 2008;18:314–28.

64. Chauhan J, Dakshinamurti K. J Biol Chem 1991;266: 10035–8.

65. Dakshinamurti K, Desjardins PR. Can J Biochem 1968;46: 1261–7.

66. Collins JC, Paietta E, Green R et al. J Biol Chem 1988;263:11280–3.

67. Greene HL, Hambridge KM, Schanler R et al. Am J Clin Nutr 1988;48:1324–42.

68. Hardinge MG, Crooks H. J Am Diet Assoc 1961;38:240–5.

69. Guilarte TR. Nutr Rep Int 1985;32:837–45.

70. Staggs CG, Sealey WM, McCabe BJ et al. J Food Compost Anal 2004;17:767–76.

71. Hoppner K, Lampi B, Smith DC. Can Inst Food Sci Technol J 1978;11:71–4.

72. Bull NL, Buss DH. Hum Nutr Appl Nutr 1982;36A:125–9.

73. Lewis J, Buss DH. Br J Nutr 1988;60:413–24.

SUGGESTED READINGS

Gralla M, Camporeale G, Zempleni J. Holocarboxylase synthetase regulates expression of biotin transporters by chromatin remodeling events at the SMVT locus. J Nutr Biochem 2008;19:400–8.

Mock DM, Said H. Introduction to advances in understanding of the biological role of biotin at the clinical, biochemical, and molecular level. J Nutr 2009;139:152–3.

Zeng WQ, Al-Yamani E, Acierno JS Jr et al. Biotin-responsive basal ganglia disease maps to 2q36.3 and is due to mutations in SLC19A3. Am J Hum Genet 2005;77:16–26.

29 VITAMIN C[1]

MARK LEVINE AND SEBASTIAN J. PADAYATTY

[1]**Abbreviations: DRI**, dietary reference intake; **EAR**, estimated average requirement; **G6PD**, Glucose-6-phosphate dehydrogenase; **HPLC**, high-performance liquid chromatography; K_m, Michaelis-Menten constant; **NHANES**, National Health and Nutrition Examination Survey; **NIH**, National Institutes of Health; **RDA**, recommended dietary allowance; **UL**, tolerable upper intake level; $\dot{V}_{max}$, maximal velocity.

HISTORY

Scurvy, which we now know is caused by vitamin C deficiency, was described by Egyptians circa 3000 BC and by Hippocrates circa 500 BC (1). Although sixteenth- and seventeenth-century sailor-explorers knew of scurvy, its fatal outcome, and its cure with fruits, lime, or plant products, the disease persisted among sailors and in northern latitudes whenever and wherever fruits and vegetables were scarce.

In 1753, James Lind published *A Treatise of the Scurvy*, a landmark controlled study showing that scurvy was easily treated (2). In clinical experiments at sea, Lind divided 12 patients with severe scurvy into 6 groups. Each group received a different treatment, including cider, vinegar, seawater, or citrus fruit. The results unequivocally demonstrated that citrus fruit cured scurvy. Unfortunately, Lind included cold climate, dampness, lack of fresh air, and foggy weather as causative agents, thereby obscuring the clear outcome of his clinical trial. Only in 1795 did the British Royal Navy make it mandatory to issue an ounce of citrus juice (lemon, and later lime) daily to every sailor after 2 weeks at sea, but this rule was not enforced until 1804. Sailors in merchant navies continued to develop scurvy until the citrus fruit provision became mandatory following the Merchant Shipping Act in 1854.

Scurvy remained widespread during the American Civil War and World War I. After World War I, research intensified to identify the antiscorbutic principle. Using ox adrenal glands, oranges, and cabbages, Albert Szent-Gyorgyi in 1928 isolated a six-carbon reducing substance. In 1932, the laboratories of Szent-Gyorgyi and C.G. King independently confirmed that this substance was the antiscorbutic principle (3, 4). Szent-Gyorgyi named it ascorbic acid, and he was awarded the Nobel Prize for this research in 1937.

TERMINOLOGY, CHEMISTRY, METABOLIC ROLES, INTERACTIONS WITH OTHER COMPOUNDS, AND BASIC IMPORTANCE IN NORMAL FUNCTIONS

Terminology and Chemical Properties: Formation, Oxidation-Reduction, and Degradation

Vitamin C (L-ascorbic acid, ascorbate), a water-soluble micronutrient essential for humans, is a six-carbon α-ketolactone weak acid with a pH of 4.2 and a molecular weight of 176 (Fig. 29.1). Plants use glucose and fructose to synthesize vitamin C. Vitamin C is abundant in plant leaves and in chloroplasts, and it may have a role in photosynthesis, stress resistance, plant growth, and development. Most mammals synthesize vitamin C from glucose in the liver, whereas some birds, reptiles, and amphibians synthesize the vitamin in the kidney (5). Vitamin C is not synthesized by humans and nonhuman primates because of their lack of gulonolactone oxidase, the terminal enzyme in the biosynthetic pathway of vitamin C from glucose. The gulonolactose oxidase gene became nonfunctional in a common primate ancestor (5). Guinea pigs, capybaras, bats, and some fish also do not synthesize ascorbate (6). For all species unable to synthesize ascorbate, it is a vitamin by definition and must be obtained exogenously. Animals unable to synthesize vitamin C usually obtain sufficient amounts from plant diets, but they develop scurvy in captivity without adequate dietary supplementation (7).

Vitamin C is an electron donor, or reducing agent (see Fig. 29.1), and all its known functions are attributable to this property. Vitamin C sequentially donates two electrons from the double bond between carbons two and three. When these electrons are lost, vitamin C is oxidized, and another compound is reduced, thereby forestalling oxidation of the reduced compound. Vitamin C is therefore commonly known as an antioxidant.

With loss of the first electron, vitamin C oxidizes to the ascorbate free radical (semidehydroascorbic acid). In comparison with other free radicals, the ascorbate radical is relatively stable and unreactive. Reactive free radicals are reduced by vitamin C, and the less reactive ascorbate radical is formed in their place. This is the basis for characterizing vitamin C as a good free radical scavenger, or antioxidant (8). Because of the short half-lives (i.e., $<10^{-3}$ seconds) of most free radicals, they cannot be measured directly and instead are measured indirectly by

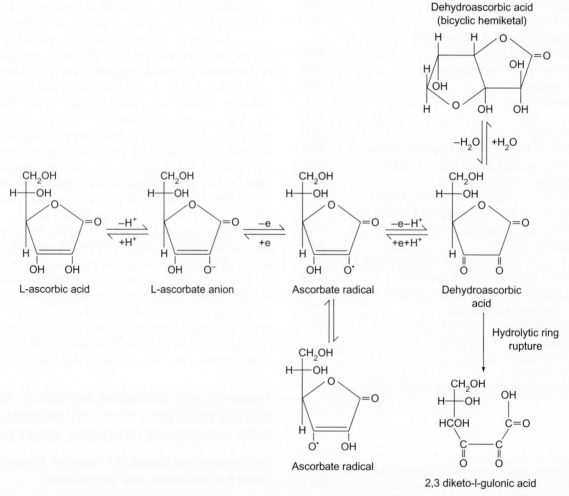

Fig. 29.1. Ascorbic acid metabolism. Ascorbic acid and many of its metabolites exist in several resonant forms. These are not shown for simplicity, but two resonant forms of ascorbate radical are shown. Dehydroascorbic acid may exist in many structural forms. The nondehydrated form of dehydroascorbic acid and its hydrated bicyclic hemiketal forms are shown. 2,3 Diketo-l-gulonic acid undergoes further metabolism resulting in several metabolites including the clinically significant product oxalate. (From Washko PW, Welch RW, Dhariwal KR et al. Ascorbic acid and dehydroascorbic acid analyses in biological samples. Anal Biochem 1992;204:1–14. Modified and reproduced with permission of *Analytical Biochemistry*.)

using other agents that form radical species with longer half-lives. The half-life of the ascorbate radical is long enough to be measured directly by electron paramagnetic resonance, however. Ascorbate radical half-life depends on concentration, the presence of trace metals, and oxygen, and it can vary from 10^{-3} seconds to minutes.

After formation, the ascorbate radical is either reversibly reduced to vitamin C or loses a second electron and is thereby oxidized to dehydroascorbic acid (8). Although this substance is more stable than the ascorbate radical, the stability of dehydroascorbic acid depends on its concentration, temperature, and pH, and it is often stable for only minutes (9). Dehydroascorbic acid may exist in one of several different structural forms (see Fig. 29.1). Its dominant form in vivo is uncertain, but a good candidate is the hydrated hemiketal (10). Because dehydroascorbic acid is probably not an acid in vivo, the designation "dehydroascorbate" is incorrect. Formation of both the ascorbate radical and dehydroascorbic acid from vitamin C in biologic systems is mediated by oxidants such as molecular oxygen with or without trace metals (iron and copper), superoxide, hydroxyl radical, hypochlorous acid, and reactive nitrogen species.

In biologic systems, dehydroascorbic acid has two fates. One is to become hydrolyzed, with irreversible rupture of the ring to yield 2,3-diketogulonic acid. Although 2,3-diketogulonic acid metabolism is not well characterized, its metabolic products probably include oxalate, threonate, xylose, xylonic acid, and lynxonic acid (9). Carbons from vitamin C were reported to be expired as carbon dioxide in animals, but this probably does not occur in humans (11). Of vitamin C metabolites formed by dehydroascorbic acid hydrolysis, oxalate is an end product with clinical significance (see the section "Manifestations of Vitamin C Deficiency and Excess").

The second fate of dehydroascorbic acid is to become reduced, either to the ascorbate radical by addition of one electron, or to vitamin C by addition of two electrons. Dehydroascorbic acid reduction in biologic tissues occurs chemically or is protein dependent (5). Chemical reduction of dehydroascorbic acid is mediated in vivo by glutathione, with formation of glutathione disulfide. Enzymatic reduction of dehydroascorbic acid in vivo, with an electron donor, is often faster than by chemical reduction alone. Reduced nicotinamide adenine dinucleotide phosphate–dependent regenerating enzymes include 3-α-hydroxysteroid dehydrogenase and thioredoxin reductase. Glutathione-dependent regenerating enzymes include glutaredoxin (thioltransferase), protein disulfide isomerase, and dehydroascorbate (sic) reductase, with Michaelis-Menten constants (K_ms) for dehydroascorbic acid of 250 μM to several millimolars. Protein (enzyme)-mediated reduction results in ascorbate formation without ascorbate radical as an intermediate, as described for glutaredoxin.

Ascorbate radical can also be reduced to vitamin C. Although the reducing activities responsible have not been purified, several reducing activities have been reported in membranes of mitochondria, microsomes, and erythrocytes. The cytosolic enzyme thioredoxin reductase also reduces the ascorbate radical (5).

In humans, ascorbate radical and dehydroascorbic acid reduction efficiency is incomplete. When vitamin C is removed from diets of healthy humans, deficiency occurs by 30 days, even if the subjects were initially saturated with vitamin C (12, 13) (see the discussion about pharmacokinetics under the section "Physiology"). These data are a summed measure of both oxidation and reduction rates. The overall direction is vitamin C utilization, in which ascorbic acid is oxidized to dehydroascorbic acid, and dehydroascorbic acid undergoes irreversible hydrolysis.

Metabolic Roles, Biochemistry, and Importance in Normal Functions

General Principles of Vitamin C as an Electron Donor

Vitamin C is considered an outstanding antioxidant because of its reduction (redox) potential as an electron donor, taking into account anticipated concentrations in vivo. Under standard chemical conditions, the reduction potential of the couple dehydroascorbic acid/vitamin C is approximately +0.06 volts (9). Reduction potentials are based on the Nernst equation:

$$E = E° + \frac{RT}{nF} \quad \ln \frac{[\text{electron acceptor}]}{[\text{electron donor}]}$$

Because vitamin C loses electrons sequentially, with ascorbate radical as an intermediate, the reduction potential for the dehydroascorbic acid/ascorbic acid couple is the sum of the dehydroascorbic acid/ascorbate radical and ascorbate radical/ascorbic acid couples. The redox potential of the couple ascorbate radical/ascorbic acid is approximately +0.3 volts under standard conditions (8, 9). Based on only this redox potential, ascorbic acid would not appear to be a good reducing agent. Standard reduction potentials assume each member of the redox pair is at 1 M concentration, pH 7, at 25°C, however. Varying concentrations of each species are taken into account by the Nernst equation for calculating reduction potentials, and these can change when concentrations of electron donor and acceptor are different. Under physiologic conditions, predicted concentrations are ascorbic acid >> dehydroascorbic acid >> ascorbate radical, so that the summed redox potentials become favorable for reduction of many oxidizers (8, 9).

In addition to its redox potential, other properties of ascorbic acid make it an excellent biochemical electron donor. After one electron loss, the product ascorbate radical under physiologic conditions is relatively harmless and nonreactive, and it produces little superoxide because of poor reactivity with oxygen (8). As noted earlier, some dehydroascorbic acid is reduced by cells to ascorbic acid, for reuse (14).

Reductive Functions

Enzymatic Functions.   Vitamin C is an electron donor for 17 enzymes (15–17), 3 of which are in fungi and are involved in reutilization pathways for pyrimidines or deoxynucleosides. In mammals, vitamin C is a cofactor for 14 different enzymes that are either monooxygenases or dioxygenases (Table 29.1). The monooxygenases dopamine β-monooxygenase and peptidyl glycine α-monooxygenase incorporate a single oxygen molecule into a substrate, either dopamine for norepinephrine synthesis or a peptide with a terminal glycine for peptide amidation. The remaining 12 mammalian enzymes are dioxygenases, which incorporate molecular oxygen (O_2), but with each oxygen atom incorporated in a different way (15, 16). Nine dioxygenases add hydroxyl groups to proline or lysine. Of these, three prolyl 4-hydroxylase isoenzymes add hydroxyl groups to the amino acid proline in the collagen molecule, to stabilize its triple helix structure (18). Four prolyl 4-hydroxylases add hydroxyl groups to proline in hypoxia-inducible factor (HIF) (17). Two additional dioxygenases, prolyl-3-hydroxylase and lysyl hydroxylase, also modify collagen (18). Of the remaining three mammalian dioxygenase enzymes, two participate in different steps of biosynthesis of carnitine, necessary for fatty acid transport into mitochondria for adenosine triphosphate synthesis

(19), and the remaining dioxygenase participates in tyrosine metabolism. Scurvy possibly is the result of impaired function of ascorbate-dependent enzymes.

Nonenzymatic Reductive Functions: Vitamin C as an Antioxidant In Vitro.   Vitamin C may have nonenzymatic functions resulting from its redox potential or free radical intermediate. In vitro evidence suggests that vitamin C has a role as a chemical reducing agent both intracellularly and extracellularly (see Table 29.1). Intracellular vitamin C may prevent intracellular protein oxidation in tissues with millimolar ascorbate concentrations and high oxidant production or oxygen concentration, such as neutrophils, monocytes, macrophages, lung, and tissues of the eye that are exposed to light (20).

In vitro, extracellular vitamin C may protect against oxidants and oxidant-mediated damage. Aqueous peroxyl radicals and lipid peroxidation products in isolated plasma are quenched by vitamin C (21, 22), which is preferentially oxidized before the plasma antioxidants uric acid, tocopherol, and bilirubin. In vitro, extracellular vitamin C affects several pathways involved in atherogenesis, including protection of low-density lipoprotein (LDL) from metal-catalyzed oxidation and regeneration of oxidized α-tocopherol (vitamin E) as a lipid-soluble antioxidant (21–23) (see also the chapter on vitamin E).

TABLE 29.1	PUTATIVE ENZYMATIC AND NONENZYMATIC EFFECTS OF VITAMIN C IN HUMANS
COFACTOR FOR ENZYMES	
ENZYME	FUNCTION OF ENZYME
Dopamine β-monooxygenase	Norepinephrine biosynthesis (57)
Peptidyl-glycine α-amidating monooxygenase	Amidation of peptide hormones (114)
Prolyl 4-hydroxylase (Three collagen isoenzymes)	Collagen hydroxylation (18)
Four HIF isoenzymes	HIF hydroxylation (17)
Prolyl 3-hydroxylase	
Lysyl hydroxylase	
Trimethyllysine hydroxylase	Carnitine biosynthesis (19)
γ-Butyrobetaine hydroxylase	
4-Hydroxyphenylpyruvate dioxygenase	Tyrosine metabolism (115)
REDUCING AGENT	
SITE	ACTION
Small intestine	Promote iron absorption (106)
ANTIOXIDANT	
SITE	ACTION
Cells	Regulate gene expression and mRNA translation, prevent oxidant damage to DNA and intracellular proteins (20, 116, 117)
Plasma	Increase endothelium-dependent vasodilatation, reduce extracellular oxidants from neutrophils, reduce low-density lipoprotein oxidation, quench aqueous peroxyl radicals and lipid peroxidation products (22)
Stomach	Prevent formation of N-nitroso compounds (118)
PROOXIDANT	
TARGET	EFFECT
DNA	DNA damage (37)
Lipid hydroperoxidase	Decomposition of lipid peroxidase leading to DNA damage (36)
Ascorbate radical targets	Damage to some cancer cells (39, 45)

HIF, hypoxia-inducible factor.

Adapted from Padayatty SJ, Daruwala R, Wang Y et al. Vitamin C: molecular actions to optimum intake. In: Cadenas E, Packer L, eds. Handbook of Antioxidants. 2nd ed. New York: Marcel Dekker, 2002:117–145, with permission of Marcel Dekker Inc, New York.

Because α-tocopherol also prevents oxidation of LDL in vitro (23), recycling of oxidized α-tocopherol by vitamin C was hypothesized to decrease atherosclerosis, as part of the oxidation modification hypothesis (24). Unfortunately, vitamin C has minimal effects on markers of oxidation and endothelial activation in humans (25), the oxidative modification hypothesis has not been supported by most clinical trials (26), and the evidence is limited that α-tocopherol recycling occurs in vivo (27, 28).

Caution is necessary in extrapolating conclusions from in vitro experiments to in vivo conditions (20). Reactions in vitro may not have a specific requirement for vitamin C as an antioxidant in vivo, and the type or concentration of the oxidant used in vitro may not be relevant in vivo. Oxidation in vitro is often induced by copper or iron, either added exogenously or as unintended trace contaminants in culture media. In vitro, metal-catalyzed LDL oxidation requires free copper or iron and relatively long lag periods for induction of oxidation. In vivo, both metals are tightly bound to proteins and may not be available to oxidize physiologic concentrations of vitamin C.

Extracellular vitamin C could have other effects as an antioxidant. For example, extracellular vitamin C may reduce oxidants from activated neutrophils (14) or macrophages that otherwise could damage collagen or fibroblasts (29). Extracellular vitamin C in the intestinal lumen may keep iron reduced, facilitate iron absorption, and quench reactive oxidants in the stomach and duodenum (see the section "Functional Consequences in Humans").

Other Cell Functions. In vitro, vitamin C may have other nonenzymatic intracellular functions. Vitamin C has been reported to regulate gene transcription, mRNA stabilization, and signal transduction for certain genes. Examples include the following genes: collagen types I and III, elastin, acetylcholine receptor, fos-related antigen-1 (fra-1), activator protein-1 (AP-1), nuclear factor-κB (NF-κB), some forms of cytochrome P-450, tyrosine hydroxylase, collagen integrins, some ubiquitins, some osteoblastic marker proteins, and phosphatidylinositol transfer protein (30–32). Vitamin C may regulate mRNA translation (33) and also may stabilize intracellular tetrahydrobiopterin, thus perhaps enhancing endothelial nitric oxide synthesis (34).

Effects of vitamin C on many of these pathways should be interpreted cautiously. Often, control cells have no vitamin C. No corresponding in vivo condition exists, other than severe scurvy. Sometimes added ascorbate concentrations are high enough to generate oxidants inadvertently, oxidants that are responsible for observed effects (30, 35).

Prooxidant Functions

Some investigators proposed that vitamin C, under physiologic conditions and acting as an electron donor, could initiate prooxidant reactions, such as increasing 8-oxo-adenine in DNA or decomposition of lipid hydroperoxides (36, 37). The physiologic relevance of these systems is unclear, whether because vitamin C concentrations were not truly physiologic, in vitro conditions were not representative of in vivo physiology, or experimental artifacts may have complicated interpretation of the measurements. In vivo data do not support a prooxidant effect of physiologic concentrations of vitamin C (13). Potential functions as a prooxidant when vitamin C is at pharmacologic concentrations (38, 39) are discussed in the sections "Physiology" (discussion on pharmacokinetics) and "Functional Consequences in Humans."

DIETARY SOURCES AND INTAKE

Food Sources of Vitamin C

The fruits and seeds of plants act as sink organs for synthesized ascorbate (Table 29.2). Because vitamin C is labile, its content in plant foods may vary depending on season, transportation, shelf time, storage, and cooking practices. Generally, 200 to 300 mg daily of vitamin C can be obtained from five servings of fruits and vegetables if a wide variety is consumed, whereas fruit and vegetable consumption restricted to a narrow selection may provide less vitamin C (40). Vitamin C is also available as a supplement in tablet and powder form, alone or in combination with other vitamins (20).

Intake in The United States

In the third National Health and Nutrition Examination Survey (NHANES III) (1988–1991), median dietary intake of vitamin C in 20- to 59-year-old subjects was 85 mg/day in men and 67 mg/day in women, with some variation based on race and ethnicity (41). Mean intake was somewhat higher, perhaps because of skewing by users of high-dose supplements (42). Approximately 37% of men and 24% of women consumed less than 2.5 servings of fruits and vegetables daily (41). Some intake data did not take into account vitamin C from supplements, but whether supplements changed total vitamin C consumption substantially is unclear. Despite a small increase in vitamin C ingestion compared with earlier NHANES II data, 10% to 25% of the US population had mean vitamin C intakes at or below dietary reference intake (DRI) values (20, 42).

Since NHANES III, newer vitamin C data from NHANES, now conducted as a continuous survey (see the chapter on national surveys on nutritional status and nutrient intake), were obtained in 2003 and 2004 from 7277 noninstitutionalized civilians (43). Mean plasma vitamin C concentrations (in subjects ≥6 years old) were 48 μM in male subjects and 54.8 μM in female subjects. Vitamin C intake and fruit and vegetable consumption remained largely unchanged between the two surveys (pharmacokinetics data discussed later in the section "Physiology" can be used to convert plasma values to estimated intake). Vitamin C deficiency, defined as plasma vitamin C concentrations lower than 11.4 μM, was present in 8.2% of male subjects and 6% of female subjects

TABLE 29.2	FOOD SOURCES OF VITAMIN C		
SOURCE (PORTION SIZE)	**VITAMIN C (mg)**	**SOURCE (PORTION SIZE)**	**VITAMIN C (mg)**
Fruit		**Vegetables**	
Cantaloupe (1/4 medium)	60	Asparagus, cooked (1/2 cup)	10
Fresh grapefruit (1/2 fruit)	40	Broccoli, cooked (1/2 cup)	60
Honeydew melon (1/8 medium)	40	Brussels sprouts, cooked (1/2 cup)	50
Kiwi (1 medium)	75	Cabbage	
Mango (1 cup, sliced)	45	Red raw, chopped (1/2 Cup)	20
Orange (1 medium)	70	Red, cooked (1/2 cup)	25
Papaya (1 cup, cubes)	85	Raw, chopped (1/2 cup)	10
Strawberries (1 cup, sliced)	95	Cooked (1/2 cup)	15
Tangerines or tangelos (1 medium)	25	Cauliflower, raw or cooked (1/2 cup)	25
Watermelon (1 cup)	15	Kale, cooked (1/2 cup)	55
Juice		Mustard greens, cooked (1 cup)	35
Grapefruit (1/2 cup)	35	Pepper, red or green	
Orange (1/2 cup)	50	Raw (1/2 cup)	65
Fortified Juice		Cooked (1/2 cup)	50
Apple (1/2 cup)	50	Plantain, sliced, cooked (1/2 cup)	15
Cranberry juice cocktail (1/2 cup)	45	Potato, baked (1 medium)	25
Grape (1/2 cup)	120	Snow peas	
		Fresh, cooked (1/2 cup)	40
		Frozen, cooked (1/2/ cup)	20
		Sweet potato	
		Baked (1 medium)	30
		Vacuum can (1 cup)	50
		Canned, syrup-pack (1 cup)	20
		Tomato	
		Raw (1/2 cup)	15
		Canned (1/2 cup)	35
		Juice (6 fluid oz)	35

From Levine M, Rumsey SC, Daruwala R et al. Criteria and recommendations for vitamin C intake. JAMA 1999;281:1415–23, with permission of the American Medical Association.

(see the section "Assessment of Vitamin C Status"). Vitamin C deficiency was more common in some population subgroups, including low-income subjects and smokers. In men at least 20 years old, 18% of smokers were vitamin C deficient, in contrast to 5.3% of nonsmokers. For women, corresponding values were 15.3% and 4.2%, respectively.

DIETARY REFERENCE INTAKES

General Strategies for Deriving Recommendations

Ideally, recommendations for optimum intake of vitamin C should be based on intakes that produce good health and on clinical outcomes in relation to different intakes (doses) of vitamin C from foods. Without such data, other measures in combination can be used: dietary availability, steady-state concentrations in plasma or tissues in relation to doses, bioavailability, urinary excretion, adverse effects, biochemical and molecular functions in relation to concentrations, beneficial effects in relation to doses, and prevention of deficiency (15, 42). Although data are available for some parameters (12, 13), clinical outcome data that describe the optimal intake of vitamin C in health and to prevent disease are lacking (38) (see the section "Functional Consequences in Humans").

Dietary Reference Intake Values

DRI values for vitamin C were set by the Institute of Medicine (42). Calculations of the estimated average requirement (EAR) were based on neutrophil vitamin C concentrations in men, putative vitamin C antioxidant action in neutrophils, and urinary vitamin C excretion in men, an approach reviewed elsewhere (38). The EAR for men 19 years old and older was determined as 75 mg/day. Based on body weight differences between genders, requirements for women were extrapolated, and the EAR for women 19 years old and older was set at 60 mg/day. EAR values were then used to calculate recommended dietary allowances (RDAs) for vitamin C in the United States and Canada, and thus RDAs were set at 90 mg/day for men and 75 mg/day for women (Table 29.3). Actual rather than extrapolated data for women became available only after the release of the foregoing DRI values (13), and they have not been incorporated into these guidelines. Based on these newer pharmacokinetics data, other countries have set vitamin C intake recommendations at 100 to 110 mg daily (13).

Pregnancy

Plasma vitamin C concentrations decrease during pregnancy, perhaps secondary to hemodilution, active transfer to the fetus, or increased renal loss. Vitamin C deficiency

TABLE 29.3   DIETARY REFERENCE INTAKE VALUES FOR VITAMIN C[a]

LIFE STAGE	GENDER	AGE	EAR	RDA	AI	UL
Infants (mo)		0–6			40	[b]
		7–12			50	
Children (y)	Boys and	1–3	13	15		400
	girls	4–8	22	25		650
	Boys	9–13	39	45		1,200
		14–18	63	75		1,800
	Girls	9–13	39	45		1,200
		14–18	56	65		1,800
Adults (y)	Men	19–30	75	90		2,000
		31–50	75	90		
		51–70	75	90		
		>70	75	90		
	Women	19–30	60	75		
		31–50	60	75		
		51–70	60	75		
		>70	60	75		
Pregnancy (y)		14–18	66	80		1,800
		19–30	70	85		2,000
		31–50	70	85		
Lactation (y)		14–18	96	115		1,800
		19–30	100	120		2,000
		31–50	100	120		
Smokers (y)	Men	>19	110	130[c]		
	Women	>19	95	115[c]		

AI, adequate intake; EAR, estimated average requirement; RDA, recommended dietary allowance; UL, tolerable upper intake level.

[a]Dietary reference intake values for vitamin C in milligrams, by life stage and gender.
[b]It is not possible to establish UL values for infants and children, for whom the source of vitamin C intake should be infant formula and food only.
[c]Whereas EARs were stated for smokers, RDAs for smokers were not explicitly documented. RDAs for smokers are calculated based on stated EAR × 1.2.

Adapted from the Food and Nutrition Board, Institute of Medicine. Dietary Reference Intakes for Vitamin C, Vitamin E, Selenium, and Carotenoids. Washington, DC: National Academy Press, 2000. From Levine M, Padayatty SJ, Katz A et al. Dietary allowances for vitamin C: recommended dietary allowances and optimal nutrient ingestion. In: Asard H, May JM, Smirnoff N, eds. Vitamin C Function and Biochemistry in Animals and Plants. London: BIOS Scientific Publishers, 2004:291–316, with permission of BIOS Scientific Publishers, London.

during pregnancy is associated with increased risk of infection, premature rupture of membranes, premature delivery, and eclampsia. It is unknown whether vitamin C deficiency contributes to these conditions or simply indicates poor general nutrition. An increased in intake from 75 mg daily in nonpregnant women to 85 mg/day during pregnancy was recommended, based on data that 7 mg/day of vitamin C prevents scurvy in infants (42).

Use in Disease

Data were insufficient to recommend additional vitamin C other than in pregnant women, lactating women, and smokers (42).

Upper Level

The tolerable upper intake level (UL) for vitamin C was set at 2 g/day, based on adverse gastrointestinal effects at higher doses (42).

PHYSIOLOGY

General Physiology and Tissue Distribution

Absorbed vitamin C reaches the liver through the hepatic portal venous system. Beyond the hepatic vein, vitamin C appears in the general circulation and is not protein bound. In blood, ascorbic acid is either the dominant chemical species or the only one (44). In the kidney, vitamin C is freely filtered through glomeruli and is reabsorbed in proximal collecting tubules. When reabsorption becomes saturated, the remaining vitamin C is excreted unchanged in urine.

Vitamin C distributes freely in the extracellular space as a water-soluble micronutrient (45), and it is accumulated by almost all human tissues (Table 29.4). As an approximate conversion, 1 g of tissue equals 1 mL of internal volume. Concentration gradients range from a minimum of approximately 2-fold to 5-fold, to a maximum of approximately 100-fold for the pituitary and adrenal glands. Red blood cells are the only cells in which internal concentrations of vitamin C are less than plasma concentrations (46). Because many measurements were performed on postmortem specimens and before the advent of accurate high-performance liquid chromatography (HPLC) assays, literature values may be underestimates.

It is uncertain why vitamin C is accumulated in millimolar concentration in many cells. For some types of cells, ascorbate may function as an enzyme cofactor. In the adrenal medulla, vitamin C is a cofactor for norepinephrine biosynthesis from dopamine. In the

TABLE 29.4	VITAMIN C CONTENT OF HUMAN TISSUES[a]		
ORGAN/TISSUE	VITAMIN C CONCENTRATION	ORGAN/TISSUE	VITAMIN C CONCENTRATION
Pituitary gland	40–50	Lungs	7
Adrenal gland	30–40	Skeletal muscle	3–4
Eye lens	25–31	Testes	3
Liver	10–16	Thyroid	2
Brain	13–15	Cerebrospinal fluid	3.8
Pancreas	10–15	Plasma	0.4–1.0
Spleen	10–15	Saliva	0.07–0.09
Kidneys	5–15		

[a]Ascorbic acid content of human tissues (mg/100 g of wet tissue, mg/100 mL for fluids) (119, 120). Values given are approximate and may vary with ascorbic acid intake, age, and possibly disease states.

Adapted from Hornig D. Distribution of ascorbic acid, metabolites and analogues in man and animals. Ann N Y Acad Sci 1975;258:103–18, with permission of the New York Academy of Sciences, New York.

pituitary and perhaps the pancreas, vitamin C may be a cofactor for amidation of peptide hormones. In fibroblasts, osteoblasts, and chondrocytes, vitamin C is a cofactor for proline and lysine hydroxylation, and it perhaps regulates collagen or elastin gene transcription. Vitamin C has several postulated roles that are incompletely characterized, often involving antioxidant action, in neutrophils, monocytes, lens, retina, cornea, peripheral and central neurons, liver, pancreas, skeletal muscle, and endothelial cells. The purpose of accumulated vitamin C is uncertain in lymphocytes, platelets, adrenal cortex, testis, and ovary.

Transport and Accumulation Principles

Ascorbate is accumulated intracellularly by two distinct pathways: active transport as ascorbate and facilitated transport as dehydroascorbic acid through ascorbate recycling. In the former pathway, ascorbic acid itself is transported by one of two known sodium-dependent transporters, SLC23A1 and SLC23A2, which are also termed SVCT1 and SVCT2 (sodium-dependent vitamin C transporter) (47, 48). The SVCTs are members of the nucleobase transporter superfamily and are dissimilar to other sodium-dependent transporters. SVCT1 (SLC23A1) is localized to intestine, liver, and kidney and is an epithelial cell transporter; it has a Michaelis-Menten constant (K_m) of approximately 100 to 200 μM and a maximal velocity ($\dot{V}_{max}$) of approximately 1 mM. These values are consistent with predicted vitamin C concentrations in the intestinal lumen after oral ingestion, in the portal venous system, and in the proximal renal tubule. SVCT2 (SLC23A2) is more widely distributed among tissues; it has a K_m of approximately 5 to 10 μM and $\dot{V}_{max}$ of approximately 60 to 100 μM. These values are within the range of vitamin C concentrations found in human tissues, as described later. Both these transporters are sodium and energy dependent and do not transport dehydroascorbic acid (10).

The second mechanism for ascorbate accumulation in cells is ascorbate recycling. In this pathway, external ascorbic acid is oxidized to dehydroascorbic acid, which is then transported by facilitated glucose transporters 1 to 4 and is immediately reduced to ascorbic acid intracellularly (10, 14). The affinity of dehydroascorbic acid for at least some facilitated glucose transporters is greater than that of glucose. Intracellular dehydroascorbic acid reduction is mediated by glutathione or reducing proteins, as discussed earlier.

Vitamin C accumulation in vivo is probably driven by sodium-dependent vitamin C transport, although specific tissues may use the dehydroascorbic acid–ascorbate recycling pathway. Mice lacking SVCT2 have a severe vitamin C deficiency in many tissues and die at birth, a finding indicating that sodium-dependent vitamin C transport is the dominant mechanism (49). It is difficult to reconcile these findings with proposals that dehydroascorbic acid transport is the primary pathway for ascorbate accumulation (50). Dehydroascorbic acid–ascorbate recycling likely depends on dehydroascorbic acid availability. Using HPLC assays, only trace amounts of dehydroascorbic acid are found in blood and plasma (44). Dehydroascorbic acid would have to be formed locally for ascorbate recycling to occur. This mechanism may be relevant for cells such as neutrophils that generate diffusible oxidants, so that the extracellular ascorbic acid will be oxidized to dehydroascorbic acid, or for the one cell type that does not express SVCTs, the red blood cell. Ascorbate analogs that are accumulated by only one transport mechanism may advance the understanding of the dominant mechanism of vitamin C accumulation in vivo (10).

Other vitamin C transporters probably exist, but they have not been identified. SVCT1 knockout mice absorb vitamin C, a finding suggesting that another absorptive transporter exists or is induced (51). Because vitamin C is a charged molecule at physiologic pH and is not diffusible, transporters should mediate efflux as well as influx. Once transported into the intestinal epithelial cells, vitamin C must exit to reach the mesenteric vein; the process is similar for renal tubule cells, for the reabsorption of vitamin C into the circulation. In animals that synthesize ascorbate, it must exit hepatocytes. In addition, vitamin C is released by the adrenal, ovary, testes, stomach, and brain (52–56). Identification of vitamin C efflux transporters awaits future work.

Pharmacokinetics

Background

A key means to determine vitamin recommendations, for any vitamin, is from concentration–function relationships. Graphically, these are x axis/y axis relationships, with the x axis representing vitamin intake (or concentration) and the y axis representing function. Before the establishment of DRIs, y axis measures for vitamin C and other vitamins were based on prevention of deficiency, with added safety margins. For DRIs, vitamin concentration–function relationships are based not only on prevention of deficiency, but also on prevention of chronic disease (42). Although such data are difficult to obtain, they are essential for making ideal nutrient intake recommendations (7, 57).

Concentration (x axis) data are provided by pharmacokinetics, which describe how vitamin doses affect vitamin concentrations. For vitamin C, depletion–repletion studies in humans are the pharmacokinetics study design of choice. Plasma vitamin C is measured because samples are readily available, measurements reflect extracellular concentrations (45), vitamin C is not protein bound, and dehydroascorbic acid is either not present or is present in amounts too small to detect (44).

Depletion–Repletion Studies: Vitamin C Concentrations Are Tightly Controlled as a Function of Dose

Depletion–repletion studies for vitamin C have been conducted with both outpatients and inpatients. Most outpatient depletion–repletion studies are limited by uncertainty about true vitamin C consumption, a problem solved by using inpatients. In early inpatient depletion–repletion studies that were conducted in prisoners, body stores of vitamin C prevented the development of moderate to advanced scurvy for less than 6 weeks, and physical signs of scurvy were prevented by 10 mg/day of vitamin C (58–60). Before the establishment of DRIs, these data were the basis of vitamin C RDAs. These data are limited by an imprecise vitamin C assay, a diet that probably was deficient in other nutrients, a small number of subjects, and a narrow dose range.

Inpatient depletion–repletion studies that addressed these concerns were conducted at the National Institutes of Health (NIH) with healthy men and women (12, 13). These studies provided comprehensive dose concentration data using HPLC assays for analysis, and some results were used to calculate vitamin C DRIs. In these studies, 7 healthy men and 15 women, maintained as inpatients for 5 to 7 months, received diets with a dietary intake of less than 5 mg/day of vitamin C and supplements to prevent other nutrient deficiencies. Vitamin C depletion was induced by the fourth week in all subjects, with plasma vitamin C concentrations falling to less than 7 to 8 μM. Repletion followed, in which subjects were given a fixed daily dose of vitamin C, at escalating doses, until a fasting steady-state plasma vitamin C level was achieved. The fasting steady-state level was defined as 5 or more consecutive measurements, obtained over at least 7 days, for which the mean plasma vitamin C values had a mean (SD) of less than 10%. At steady state for each dose, bioavailability studies were performed (see later), circulating blood cells were isolated for vitamin C measurements, and 24-hour urine samples were collected for vitamin C and metabolites. When sample collections were completed, subjects were advanced to the next higher dose of vitamin C, a new steady state was reached, and the sampling sequence was repeated. Vitamin C doses were 30, 60, 100, 200, 400, 1000, and 2500 mg, administered in water as divided doses twice daily in the fasting state.

From these studies, extensive pharmacokinetics data for vitamin C were obtained. All plasma values from 15 women, and the depletion–repletion design, are shown (Fig. 29.2). Every steady-state calculation for every subject is displayed as a function of dose for men and women (Fig. 29.3). At plasma concentrations of up to 100 mg/day, a steep sigmoidal relationship was seen between vitamin C intake dose and vitamin C plasma concentration, and small changes in dose produced large changes in plasma concentration. At doses of up to 100 mg/day, women achieved a higher fasting steady-state plasma vitamin C concentration than men. At doses of 400 mg/day or higher, fasting steady-state plasma concentrations equaled 70 to 80 μM and increased little with higher doses. These data show that vitamin C plasma concentrations are tightly controlled as a function of oral dose in both sexes. Underlying mechanisms, described next, include intake and intestinal absorption, tissue accumulation, utilization, and renal reabsorption and excretion.

Mechanisms of Tight Control

Absorption. The efficiency of intestinal absorption of vitamin C is assessed by bioavailability, with absolute bioavailability the most accurate measurement. Data describing absolute bioavailability of vitamin C from foods are not available. Absolute bioavailability of pure vitamin C, however, as determined in the NIH study of healthy men at steady state, was calculated using standard area-under-curve pharmacokinetics and a multicompartment model (12, 61). Based on convention, bioavailability is expressed as a percentage, with 100% indicating complete absorption. Vitamin C bioavailability was 80% or greater for doses of 15 to 100 mg/day and decreased to less than 50% for 1250 mg/day (Table 29.5), findings indicating that intestinal absorption contributes to tight control of vitamin C concentrations.

Ascorbate is absorbed in the small intestine (14). It is unclear whether ascorbate, dehydroascorbic acid, or both, is or are the species transported across the brush-border epithelium. Although SVCT1 is localized to the small intestine, SVCT1 knockout mice absorb an ascorbate analog that, when oxidized, is not transported by glucose transporters (10, 51). These data suggest that another sodium-dependent ascorbate transporter exits in small intestine.

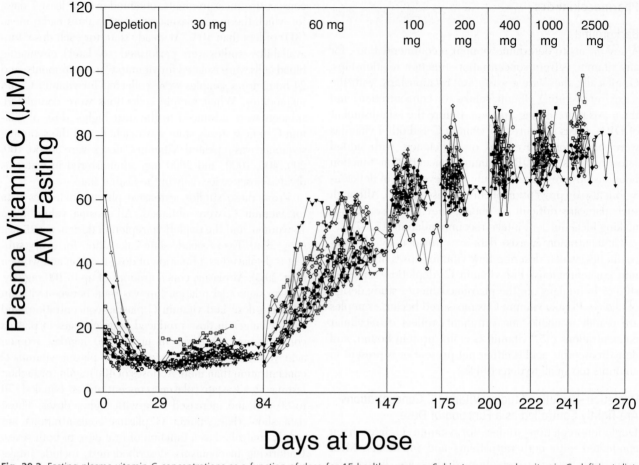

Fig. 29.2. Fasting plasma vitamin C concentrations as a function of dose for 15 healthy women. Subjects consumed a vitamin C–deficient diet, resulting in plasma and tissue vitamin C depletion. Vitamin C in solution was then administered by mouth at the doses shown until steady state was reached for each dose. (From Levine M, Wang Y, Padayatty SJ et al. A new recommended dietary allowance of vitamin C for healthy young women. Proc Natl Acad Sci U S A 2001;98:9842–6, with permission of the National Academy of Sciences, Washington, DC.)

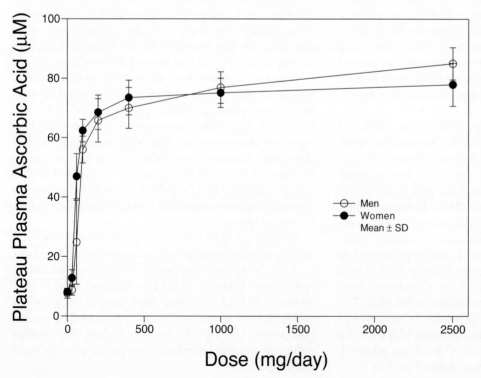

Fig. 29.3. The relationship between oral doses of vitamin C and the mean fasting steady-state plasma ascorbic acid concentration in 7 healthy men (12) and 15 healthy women (13). The daily doses of vitamin C were 30, 60, 100, 200, 400, 1000 and 2500 mg. The dose-concentration curve is sigmoidal, with its steep portion between 30 and 100 mg of vitamin C daily. The figure shown is a composite of previously published dose concentration curves for men and women (12, 13). (Data from Levine M, Conry-Cantilena C, Wang Y et al. Vitamin C pharmacokinetics in healthy volunteers: evidence for a recommended dietary allowance. Proc Natl Acad Sci U S A 1996;93:3704–9; and Levine M, Wang Y, Padayatty SJ et al. A new recommended dietary allowance of vitamin C for healthy young women. Proc Natl Acad Sci U S A 2001;98:9842–6, with permission.)

TABLE 29.5	BIOAVAILABILITY OF VITAMIN C[a]	
	BIOAVAILABILITY OF ASCORBIC ACID	
	METHOD USING AREA UNDER CURVE ANALYSES	METHOD USING MULTICOMPARTMENT MATHEMATICAL MODEL
DOSE (mg)	MEAN (%) (SD)	MEDIAN (%)
15	—	89
30	—	87.3
50	—	58
100	—	80
200	112 (25)	72
500	73 (27)	63
1,250	49 (25)	46

[a]Bioavailability of vitamin C in healthy men at steady state for each dose. Vitamin C bioavailability for three doses was calculated using area under curve analyses (12). This method could not be used for doses lower than 200 mg, when vitamin C did not have a constant volume of distribution or a constant rate of clearance (61).

Data from Levine M, Conry-Cantilena C, Wang Y et al. Vitamin C pharmacokinetics in healthy volunteers: evidence for a recommended dietary allowance. Proc Natl Acad Sci U S A 1996;93:3704–9; and Graumlich JF, Ludden TM, Conry-Cantilena C et al. Pharmacokinetic model of ascorbic acid in healthy male volunteers during depletion and repletion. Pharm Res 1997;14:1133–9, with permission.

Accumulation. Tight control of plasma vitamin C concentrations results, in part, from concentration-dependent cell and tissue accumulation. In healthy humans, only limited tissue samples can be obtained, including the following: neutrophils, monocytes, lymphocytes, and platelets, all blood components; semen and seminal fluid from men; and urine (62). Because of their ready availability, circulating cells were used as a proxy for other tissues to determine vitamin C concentration in relation to dose over an 83-fold range (Fig. 29.4). Intracellular vitamin C concentrations, always higher than plasma concentrations, increased as the dose of vitamin C increased from 30 to 100 mg/day. As doses increased further, intracellular concentrations remained constant. Cells achieved plateau concentrations before plasma (see Figs. 29.3 and 29.4), a finding consistent with SVCT2 transporter kinetics and the contribution of tissue accumulation to tight control.

Utilization. Vitamin C concentrations may be affected by utilization rates, which can change steady-state values. Utilization rates may be affected by differences in transporter activity, recycling, enzyme efficiency, or conditions that accelerate utilization, such as oxidative stress. Although alternative explanations exist, increased utilization may account for low vitamin C concentrations in smokers and in patients with critical illness, acute myocardial infarction, diabetes, and pancreatitis (15, 63–67). Utilization rates also differ even among healthy humans (see Fig. 29.2) (7, 13, 59).

Renal Reabsorption and Excretion. With normal renal function, small molecules (i.e., glucose, amino acids) are filtered through glomeruli and are reabsorbed in the renal tubules. Based on tubular reabsorptive transport, individual nephrons have a maximal capacity to absorb specific substances, termed the *tubular maximum.* When the tubular maximum is within the range of plasma concentrations, the kidney has a central role in homeostasis.

Specific characteristics and mechanisms of vitamin C handling by the kidney are emerging. Although earlier data described a low but constant amount of vitamin C in

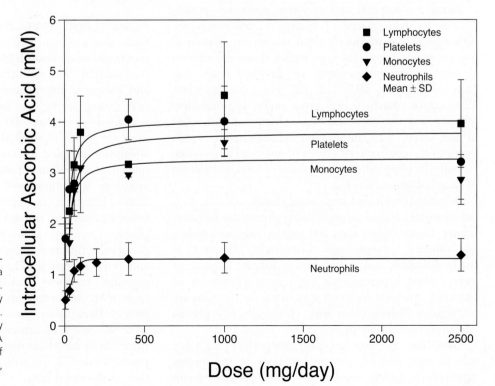

Fig. 29.4. Intracellular vitamin C concentrations in circulating cells as a function of dose in healthy women. Cells were isolated when steady state was achieved for each dose. (From Levine M, Wang Y, Padayatty SJ et al. Proc Natl Acad Sci U S A 2001;98:9842–6, with permission of the National Academy of Sciences, Washington, DC.)

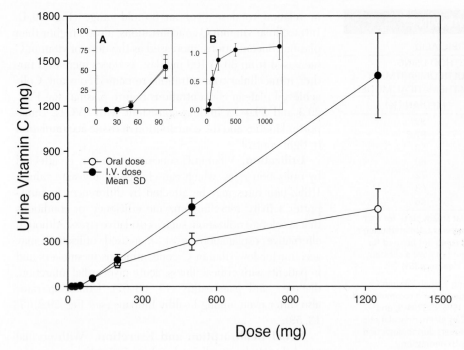

Fig. 29.5. Urinary vitamin C excretion as a function of single vitamin C doses at steady state. Vitamin C excretion over 24 hours was determined after administration of single doses given either orally or intravenously. *Inset* **A,** Vitamin C excretion for single oral or intravenous doses of 15 to 100 mg. The *x* axis indicates dose, and the *y* axis indicates the amount (mg) excreted in urine. *Inset* **B,** Fractional excretion (the fraction of the dose excreted) after intravenous administration of single doses of vitamin C. The *x* axis indicates dose, and the *y* axis indicates fractional excretion (vitamin C excreted in urine in milligrams divided by the vitamin C dose in milligrams). (From Levine M, Wang Y, Padayatty SJ et al. Proc Natl Acad Sci U S A 2001;98:9842–6, with permission of the National Academy of Sciences, Washington, DC.)

urine (68), with improved measurements no ascorbic acid was detected in urine at steady state when doses were less than 100 mg/day in men and 60 mg/day in women (12, 13) (Fig. 29.5). It is likely that vitamin C is freely filtered by the glomeruli and reabsorbed in proximal tubules by SVCT1 (51), and that a tubular maximum for vitamin C is within the range of plasma concentrations (12, 13). An exact tubular maximum, although not yet available, would be valuable for determining intake recommendations.

Renal reabsorption and excretion make key contributions to tight control of vitamin C concentrations. Although in the previously cited studies no vitamin C was excreted at low doses, at higher doses, all vitamin C administered intravenously or absorbed orally was excreted (see Fig. 29.5) (12, 13). For example, when 1250 mg of vitamin C was given orally, approximately 600 mg was absorbed and was subsequently excreted in the urine. With intravenous administration, which bypasses the confounding effects of intestinal absorption, virtually the entire administered doses of 500 and 1250 mg of vitamin C were excreted.

In patients with end stage renal disease, vitamin C is not excreted because no appreciable glomerular filtration occurs. Doses higher than 200 mg/day may accumulate and produce hyperoxalemia. Conversely, vitamin C is freely dialyzable and is lost during dialysis. Because of worry about hyperoxalemia from overreplacement of vitamin C, patients with end stage renal disease who are undergoing dialysis often have chronically low plasma vitamin C concentrations (69).

Genetics. Because ascorbate transporters play a key role in tight control, genetic variations in transporter expression or activity could modify tight control of vitamin

C concentrations in healthy humans. For both known vitamin C transporters, single nucleotide polymorphisms occur in the respective genes, including those shown to decrease SVCT1 (SLC23A1) transport activity (51). Decreased SVCT1 transport would decrease vitamin C renal reabsorption, thus leading to lower plasma vitamin C concentrations (51). Supportive data from a population study (70) suggest that genetic variations in vitamin C transporters affect tight control.

Bypassing Tight Control: Pharmacology
Gram doses of ascorbate can be ingested as oral supplements, although doses higher than 3 g produce diarrhea (see section "Manifestations of Vitamin C Deficiency and Excess"). Investigators reported that with maximal oral dosing every few hours, plasma concentrations remained lower than 300 μM (71). Plasma concentrations are tightly controlled because of limited intestinal absorption coupled to renal excretion, in turn a consequence of saturation of renal tubular reabsorption. When ascorbate is administered intravenously (parenterally), limited intestinal absorption is bypassed, and millimolar concentrations of vitamin C occur within minutes in plasma. Over several hours, homeostasis is restored by glomerular filtration, saturation of tubular reabsorption, and renal excretion (71, 72). In humans, intravenous ascorbate produces peak plasma concentrations of 25 to 30 mM, concentrations that are several hundred-fold greater than those from food ingestion. Intravenous ascorbate use is pharmacologic use, not nutritional use. Intravenous ascorbate use, as a drug, appears to be surprisingly safe (72, 73), with potential therapeutic application, as discussed later.

FUNCTIONAL CONSEQUENCES IN HUMANS

Benefits of Vitamin C Consumption from Fruits and Vegetables

The National Cancer Institute recommendation that healthy people consume at least 5 fruit and vegetable servings daily is based on more than 200 studies that describe inverse associations between cancer occurrence and increased fruit and vegetable intake or intake of antioxidant nutrients, including vitamin C (74, 75). In retrospect, many of these studies were flawed, because they were case-control studies, because health-conscious persons were overrepresented, or because of differences in subject recall (76). Newer prospective data indicate that the association is weak, at best, between cancer prevention and ingestion of fruits and vegetables (76–78).

Based primarily on observational epidemiology, an association exists between fruit and vegetable intake and protection against cardiovascular disease (76, 78–80). Fruit and vegetable intake under controlled conditions was associated with a decrease in blood pressure (81), a risk factor for cardiovascular disease. However, nutrition prevention or clinical intervention trials confirming that fruits and vegetables themselves are protective are lacking (80).

For prevention of both cancer and cardiovascular disease, it is unknown whether associated benefits of fruit and vegetable intake result from vitamin C itself, from vitamin C in addition to other components of fruits and vegetables, or from fruit and vegetable components independent of vitamin C (15). Vitamin C may simply be a surrogate marker for fruit and vegetable consumption or other healthy lifestyle practices. Fruit and vegetable consumption provides micronutrients, bulk, roughage, and satiety.

Outcome Studies

Vitamin C from foods and supplements has been investigated for prevention of cancer, cardiovascular disease, stroke, and age-related eye diseases, with conflicting and often disappointing results (20, 82–86). In some observational studies, vitamin C consumption from both food and supplements correlated with reduced mortality (87) and a lower risk of ischemic heart disease, (82) particularly when subjects had low intakes of vitamin C (83). In an intervention study, vitamins C and E slowed the progression of carotid atherosclerosis (88), but a protective effect for atherosclerosis was not observed by other investigators (20, 89). In large-scale interventional studies, when vitamin C was partially obtained from foods but was also consumed in combination with other antioxidant vitamins as a supplement, no benefit in preventing cancer or reducing vascular disease was observed (86).

Consistent with mouse studies (51), vitamins C and E decreased preeclampsia or hypertension in pregnant women with low vitamin concentrations at study entry (90). These findings were not confirmed in healthier populations, probably because subjects were near saturation with ascorbate at study entry (91, 92).

Observational data have indicated that vitamin C supplementation may prevent cataract, (84), but a large prospective study showed no effect, when vitamin C supplements were combined with vitamin E and β-carotene (93). In a large placebo-controlled study, combined supplements of vitamin C, vitamin E, β-carotene, and zinc reduced the odds of developing advanced age-related macular degeneration once the disease was present (94), but evidence is lacking that antioxidant vitamins, including vitamin C, prevent macular degeneration (95). No large-scale interventional studies of disease prevention have been reported with vitamin C as the sole supplement.

Vitamin C supplementation was also tested for potential effects on outcome for hypertension, endothelial dysfunction, and respiratory diseases. Investigators noted a modest effect on lowering blood pressure in some but not all subjects, and no large-scale studies are available (96). Many studies showed that vitamin C diminishes endothelial vasomotor dysfunction and induces vasodilation when administered arterially. However, intra-arterial (parenteral) administration bypasses tight control, and resulting plasma ascorbate concentrations are far higher than those that are achievable orally. Vitamin C supplements for 3 days potentiated nitroglycerin-induced vasodilatation, but it is unknown whether this effect would persist long term (97). Vitamin C supplements probably do not prevent acute respiratory infections in healthy populations (98), nor do they provide benefit in asthma treatment (99).

Although vitamin C supplements were effective in treating pressure sores in a small study, the findings were not confirmed (100). The original findings may have simply indicated that the control subjects were deficient in vitamin C, and supplementation corrected the deficiency. Despite scant data, vitamin C supplements are sometimes still used in elderly persons for healing pressure sores because of the low risk of this treatment approach, the possibility that the treatment population has an ascorbate deficiency, and difficulty in treating the condition.

Effects of Vitamin C in the Gastrointestinal Tract

Vitamin C is secreted in gastric juice, and it achieves concentrations severalfold higher than plasma values (55). Vitamin C content is low in the gastric juice of patients with atrophic gastritis and *Helicobacter pylori* infection, and eradication of the bacterium increases gastric vitamin C secretion (101). Vitamin C can potentially quench reactive oxygen metabolites in the stomach and duodenum and can prevent formation of mutagenic N-nitroso compounds. Whether clinical benefit ensues is controversial. Intake of foods high in vitamin C usually correlates with a reduced risk of gastric cancer (75, 102), but whether vitamin C itself or other substances in vitamin C–rich plant-derived foods are responsible is unknown. In a population at high risk for gastric cancer, vitamin C supplementation, with and without anti-*H. pylori* treatment, was associated with regression of precancerous lesions (103). In one large prospective case-control study, an inverse association was noted between plasma ascorbate concentration and gastric cancer risk, but another large study found no association between long-term vitamin C supplementation and reduced mortality from stomach cancer (102, 104). A metaanalysis of antioxidant supplements for prevention of gastrointestinal cancers, including ascorbate, indicated that supplement use did not correlate with decreased mortality and perhaps correlated with increased mortality (105).

In the small intestine, vitamin C reduces iron and thereby promotes iron absorption (see also the chapter on iron). A dose of 20 to 60 mg/day of vitamin C, found in vitamin C–rich foods, enhanced small intestinal iron absorption 1.5-fold to 10-fold, depending on iron status, vitamin C dose, and test meal type (106). The effect of vitamin C on raising hemoglobin concentration was modest (107). Clinically, vitamin C is administered with iron to increase its absorption, especially in pregnancy.

Effects of Pharmacologic Ascorbate

Pharmacologic ascorbate concentrations, achieved only by parenteral administration, produce hydrogen peroxide in the extracellular fluid but not in blood through reduction of molecular oxygen to form superoxide (39, 45). Hydrogen peroxide and pharmacologic ascorbate and trace metals produce reactive oxygen species that are selectively toxic to cancer cells in vitro and in animal models of cancer (39, 45). Pharmacologic ascorbate, by the same mechanism, has shown promise in treating infections (39). Clinical trials are necessary to learn whether pharmacologic ascorbate has efficacy in treating specific cancers in humans as an adjunct to chemotherapy.

Functions in Relation to Concentration In Vivo: Limitations and Summary

The definitive function of vitamin C in humans in vivo, except to prevent scurvy, remains a mystery. Nearly all tissues concentrate vitamin C, including many that lack enzymes known to require it, a finding implying that this vitamin has other unrecognized functions in vivo. Current in vivo understanding of the 14 vitamin C–dependent enzymes and other nonenzymatic functions, as discussed earlier, remains incomplete. It is attractive to think of vitamin C as a critical antioxidant or electron donor in vivo, but conclusive evidence is lacking (20).

Currently, investigators lack definitive evidence that a particular vitamin C concentration or intake amount produces a clinically beneficial outcome, other than preventing deficiency (20). Consuming five to nine servings of fruits and vegetables per day provides 200 to 400 mg of vitamin C and results in steady-state fasting plasma concentrations of 70 to 80 μM. Whether such vitamin C concentrations in vivo optimize biochemical functions or improve clinical outcomes is unclear.

Whereas vitamin C pharmacokinetics provide fundamental knowledge about concentrations (the x axis), a paucity of data exists on the effect of these concentrations on function (the y axis) in vivo. Even without definitive y axis data, x axis data provide key insight to human outcome studies, which ideally should recognize tight control and the steep relationship between oral vitamin C doses and concentrations. To determine whether vitamin C affects a given outcome, subjects with different vitamin C concentrations must be compared (15, 92). Unfortunately, many outcome studies have compared subjects with different vitamin C intakes rather than different vitamin C concentrations. This common design flaw, unfortunately, remains a key limitation of vitamin C outcome studies. If subjects with the lowest intake are already beyond the steep portion of the pharmacokinetics curve (see Fig. 29.3), increasing intake will not increase concentrations, and outcomes should not differ. Future outcome studies should compare subjects with a range of vitamin C concentrations rather than intake. The same x-y axis approach for physiology can reveal the possible benefit of pharmacologic ascorbate, when tight control is transiently bypassed with parenteral ascorbate administration.

ASSESSMENT OF VITAMIN C STATUS

In the absence of clinical scurvy, vitamin C status is based on white cell (leukocyte) or plasma ascorbate measurements; plasma ascorbate is used more often because of technical ease. Vitamin C deficiency is considered present when plasma concentrations are less than 11.4 μM (0.2 mg/dL) (43, 108). Marginal vitamin C status, with a moderate risk of developing deficiency, is indicated by plasma concentrations between 11.4 and 28.4 μM (0.2 to 0.5 mg/dL) (43, 108). Saturation occurs at plasma concentrations of approximately 70 μM and higher (12, 13).

Because no functional measure of vitamin C status exists other than clinical scurvy, values for deficiency and marginal status are arbitrary. For deficiency, values were obtained with an assay that overestimated vitamin C concentrations at low values (58–60). In scurvy, the clinical findings of hemorrhage and hyperkeratosis do not occur until plasma concentrations are less than 5 μM (12, 13). The first symptom of scurvy is fatigue, which unfortunately, is perhaps the most common general symptom in medicine. Fatigue occurs under controlled conditions when plasma vitamin C concentrations are less than approximately 20 μM (12, 20). Marginal vitamin C status is based on the risk of developing frank deficiency and can be thought of as representing reserve stores of vitamin C. If vitamin C ingestion were to cease, a plasma vitamin C concentration of 28 μM represents an approximate 2- to

3-week reserve to prevent clinical scurvy. With intake at the RDA level for vitamin C for both men and women, plasma values are approximately 45 μM (12, 13).

MANIFESTATIONS OF VITAMIN C DEFICIENCY AND EXCESS

Deficiency

Scurvy

Frank scurvy is now rare in industrialized countries. It occurs mainly in the following groups: malnourished populations; patients with cancer cachexia and malabsorption; persons with alcoholism, drug addicts, and poor or elderly persons with inadequate diets; institutionalized individuals; and those consuming idiosyncratic diets (109). Scurvy occurs in war-torn areas and refugee camps. Subclinical vitamin C deficiency may be more common, but symptoms are nonspecific and therefore are not easily attributed to lack of vitamin C. Historically, Lind noted that the earliest symptoms of scurvy are weakness and lassitude (2). Signs and symptoms of scurvy are further described in the chapter on manifestations of nutrient deficiencies and toxicities. Diagnosis of scurvy is based on clinical findings and is confirmed by low plasma vitamin C concentrations. If untreated, scurvy is fatal, and treatment should not be delayed for laboratory confirmation.

Treatment and Prevention. Treatment should be initiated with vitamin C 100 mg three times daily. An initial intravenous dose of 60 to 100 mg of vitamin C may be given. Children may be given 100 to 200 mg/day either orally or parenterally. With prompt diagnosis and treatment, permanent damage can be prevented. Steady-state plasma concentrations from vitamin C doses of 100 mg/day will forestall deficiency for approximately 1 month (12, 15).

Adverse Effects of Vitamin C Excess

Gastrointestinal Tract

Vitamin C is generally safe and well tolerated, with few dose-related side effects (15, 42). Because ingestion of 3 g or more at once causes osmotic diarrhea and bloating, the UL has been set at 2 g daily. Vitamin C enhances iron absorption from the small intestine. Long-term vitamin C use may increase the risk of iron overload in susceptible patients, including those with hemochromatosis, thalassemia major, sickle cell disease, sideroblastic anemia, and those who need multiple, frequent red blood cell transfusions (110). Such patients should avoid large doses of vitamin C, but not fruits and vegetables (111). In healthy individuals, vitamin C in doses as high as 2 g daily over 18 months did not induce iron overabsorption (112).

Blood

Glucose-6-phosphate dehydrogenase (G6PD) deficiency is an X-linked inherited disease that may cause hemolytic crises, most often on exposure to oxidant stress. In people with G6PD deficiency, hemolysis was precipitated by vitamin C given intravenously and by single oral doses of at least 6 g (73).

Kidney

Vitamin C doses of 3 g may cause transient hyperuricosuria, but this does not occur at doses lower than 1 g/day. Doses higher than 1 g/day may increase oxalate excretion in persons with known or occult hyperoxaluria and may precipitate oxalate kidney stone formation (15). Whether gram doses of vitamin C contribute to hyperoxaluria remains unclear (42, 69). In large-scale studies of healthy people who had no prior history of kidney stones, increased vitamin C consumption from food and supplements did not increase kidney stone formation (113). In patients with renal failure who were undergoing long-term hemodialysis, hyperoxalemia was induced by repeated intravenous vitamin C doses higher than 500 mg (69). To prevent oxalosis, vitamin C intake in these patients should probably not exceed 200 mg/day (15).

Miscellaneous

Vitamin C, at doses of 250 mg and higher, may cause false-negative results for stool occult blood with guaiac-based tests. Vitamin C intake should be reduced to less than 250 mg for several days before such testing. Several harmful effects have been erroneously attributed to vitamin C, including hypoglycemia, rebound scurvy, infertility, mutagenesis, and destruction of vitamin B_{12} (15).

REFERENCES

1. Clemeston CAB. Classical scurvy: a historical review. In: Vitamin C. Boca Raton, FL: CRC Press, 1989:1–10.
2. Lind J. Lind's Treatise on Scurvy. In: Stewart CP, Guthrie D, eds. Bicentenary volume. Edinburgh: Edinburgh University Press, 1953:1–440.
3. Svirbely J, Szent-Gyorgyi A. Biochem J 1932;26:865–70.
4. King CG, Waugh WA. Science 1932;75:357.
5. Linster CL, Van Schaftingen E. FEBS J 2007;274:1–22.
6. Cueto GR, Allekotte R, Kravetz FO. J Wildl Dis 2000;36:97–101.
7. Levine M. N Engl J Med 1986;314:892–902.
8. Buettner GR. Arch Biochem Biophys 1993;300:535–43.
9. Lewin S. Vitamin C: Its Molecular Biology and Medical Potential. London: Academic Press, 1976:5–39.
10. Corpe CP, Lee JH, Kwon O et al. J Biol Chem 2005;280:5211–20.
11. Baker EM, Halver JE, Johnsen DO et al. Ann N Y Acad Sci 1975;258:72–80.
12. Levine M, Conry-Cantilena C, Wang Y et al. Proc Natl Acad Sci U S A 1996;93:3704–9.
13. Levine M, Wang Y, Padayatty SJ et al. Proc Natl Acad Sci U S A 2001;98:9842–6.
14. Rumsey SC, Levine M. J Nutr Biochem 1998;9:116–30.
15. Levine M, Rumsey SC, Daruwala R et al. JAMA 1999;281:1415–23.
16. Levine M, Rumsey SC, Wang Y et al. Vitamin C. In: Stipanuk MH, ed. Biochemical and Physiological Aspects of Human Nutrition. Philadelphia: WB Saunders, 2000:541–67.
17. Myllyharju J. Ann Med 2008;40:402–17.
18. Prockop DJ, Kivirikko KI. Annu Rev Biochem 1995;64:403–34.

19. Rebouche CJ. Am J Clin Nutr 1991;54(Suppl):1147S–52S.
20. Padayatty SJ, Katz A, Wang Y et al. J Am Coll Nutr 2003;22:18–35.
21. Carr AC, Frei B. Am J Clin Nutr 1999;69:1086–1107.
22. Polidori MC, Mecocci P, Levine M et al. Arch Biochem Biophys 2004;423:109–15.
23. Jialal I, Fuller CJ. Can J Cardiol 1995;11:97G–103G.
24. Steinberg D. Nat Med 2002;8:1211–7.
25. Van Hoydonck PGA, Schouten EG, Manuel-Y-Keenoy B et al. Eur J Clin Nutr 2004;58:1587–93.
26. Kris-Etherton PM, Lichtenstein AH, Howard BV et al. Circulation 2004;110:637–41.
27. Jacob RA, Kutnink MA, Csallany AS et al. J Nutr 1996;126:2268–77.
28. Bruno RS, Leonard SW, Atkinson J et al. Free Radic Biol Med 2006;40:689–97.
29. Nualart FJ, Rivas CI, Montecinos VP et al. J Biol Chem 2003;278:10128–33.
30. Duarte TL, Lunec J. Free Radic Res 2005;39:671–86.
31. Li Y, Schellhorn HE. J Nutr 2007;137:2171–84.
32. Griffiths HR, Willetts RS, Grant MM et al. Br J Nutr 2008;101:1432–9.
33. Toth I, Bridges KR. J Biol Chem 1995;270:19540–4.
34. Heller R, Unbehaun A, Schellenberg B et al. J Biol Chem 2001;276:40–7.
35. Houglum KP, Brenner DA, Chojkier M. Am J Clin Nutr 1991;54(Suppl):1141S–3S.
36. Lee SH, Oe, T, Blair IA. Science 2001;292:2083–6.
37. Podmore ID, Griffiths HR, Herbert KE et al. Nature 1998;392:559.
38. Levine M, Padayatty SJ, Katz A et al. Dietary allowances for vitamin C: recommended dietary allowances and optimal nutrient ingestion. In: Asard H, May JM, Smirnoff N, eds. Vitamin C Function and Biochemistry in Animals and Plants. London: BIOS Scientific Publishers, 2004:291–316.
39. Chen Q, Espey MG, Sun AY et al. Proc Natl Acad Sci U S A 2008;105:11105–9.
40. Johnston CS. JAMA 1999;282:2118.
41. Life Sciences Research Office, Federation of American Societies for Experimental Biology, Interagency Board for Nutrition Monitoring and Related Research. Third Report on Nutrition Monitoring in the United States. Report no. 2. Washington, DC: US Government Printing Office, 1995.
42. Food and Nutrition Board, Institute of Medicine. Dietary Reference Intakes for Vitamin C, Vitamin E, Selenium, and Carotenoids. Washington, DC: National Academy Press, 2000.
43. Schleicher RL, Carroll MD, Ford ES et al. Am J Clin Nutr 2009;90:1252–63.
44. Dhariwal KR, Hartzell WO, Levine M. Am J Clin Nutr 1991;54:712–6.
45. Chen Q, Espey MG, Sun AY et al. Proc Natl Acad Sci U S A 2007;104:8749–54.
46. Evans RM, Currie L, Campbell A. Br J Nutr 1982;47:473–82.
47. Tsukaguchi H, Tokui T, Mackenzie B et al. Nature 1999;399:70–5.
48. Daruwala R, Song J, Koh WS et al. FEBS Lett 1999;460:480–4.
49. Sotiriou S, Gispert S, Cheng J et al. Nat Med 2002;8:514–7.
50. Huang J, Agus DB, Winfree CJ et al. Proc Natl Acad Sci U S A 2001;98:11720–4.
51. Corpe CP, Tu H, Eck P et al. J Clin Invest 2010;120:1069–83.
52. Koba H, Kawao K, Yamashita K. Tohoku J Exp Med 1971;104:65–71.
53. Musicki B, Kodaman PH, Aten RF et al. Biol Reprod 1996;54:399–406.
54. Rebec GV, Wang Z. J Neurosci 2001;21:668–75.
55. Schorah CJ, Sobala GM, Sanderson M et al. Am J Clin Nutr 1991;53(Suppl):287S–93S.
56. Padayatty SJ, Doppman JL, Chang R et al. Am J Clin Nutr 2007;86:145–9.
57. Levine M, Dhariwal KR, Washko PW et al. Am J Clin Nutr 1991;54(Suppl):1157S–62S.
58. Baker EM, Hodges RE, Hood J et al. Am J Clin Nutr 1969;22:549–58.
59. Baker EM, Hodges RE, Hood J et al. Am J Clin Nutr 1971;24:444–54.
60. Hodges RE, Hood J, Canham JE et al. Am J Clin Nutr 1971;24:432–43.
61. Graumlich JF, Ludden TM, Conry-Cantilena C et al. Pharm Res 1997;14:1133–9.
62. Fraga CG, Motchnik PA, Shigenaga MK et al. Proc Natl Acad Sci U S A 1991;88:11003–6.
63. Padayatty SJ, Levine M. Am J Clin Nutr 2000;71:1027–8.
64. Alberg A. Toxicology 2002;180:121–37.
65. Bonham MJ, Abu-Zidan FM, Simovic MO et al. Br J Surg 1999;86:1296–1301.
66. Long CL, Maull KI, Krishnan RS et al. J Surg Res 2003;109:144–8.
67. Cunningham JJ. J Am Coll Nutr 1998;17:105–8.
68. Kallner A, Hartmann D, Hornig D. Am J Clin Nutr 1979;32:530–9.
69. Handelman GJ. Nephrol Dial Transplant 2007;22:328–1.
70. Timpson NJ, Forouhi NG, Brion MJ et al. Am J Clin Nutr 2010;92:375–82.
71. Padayatty SJ, Sun H, Wang Y et al. Ann Intern Med 2004;140:533–7.
72. Hoffer LJ, Levine M, Assouline S et al. Ann Oncol 2008;19:1969–74.
73. Padayatty SJ, Sun AY, Chen Q et al. PloS One 2010;5: e11414.
74. Ames B, Gold L, Willett W. Proc Natl Acad Sci U S A 1995;92:5258–65.
75. Byers T, Guerrero N. Am J Clin Nutr 1995;62(Suppl):1385S–92S.
76. Willett WC. J Natl Cancer Inst. 2010;102:510–1.
77. Boffetta P, Couto E, Wichmann J et al. J Natl Cancer Inst 2010;102:529–37.
78. Hung HC, Joshipura KJ, Jiang R et al. J Natl Cancer Inst 2004;96:1577–84.
79. Khaw KT, Bingham S, Welch A et al. Lancet 2001;357:657–63.
80. Dauchet L, Montaye M, Ruidavets JB et al. Eur J Clin Nutr 2010;64:578–86.
81. Sacks FM, Svetkey LP, Vollmer WM et al. N Engl J Med 2001;344:3.
82. Osganian SK, Stampfer MJ, Rimm E et al. J Am Coll Cardiol 2003;42:246–52.
83. Nyyssonen K, Parviainen MT, Salonen R et al. BMJ 1997;314:634–8.
84. Jacques PF, Chylack LT Jr, Hankinson SE et al. Arch Ophthalmol 2001;119:1009–19.
85. Jacobs EJ, Henion AK, Briggs PJ et al. Am J Epidemiol 2002;156:1002–10.
86. Heart Protection Study Collaborative Group. Lancet 2002;360:23–33.
87. Enstrom JE, Kanim LE, Klein MA. Epidemiology 1992;3:194–202.
88. Salonen RM, Nyyssonen K, Kaikkonen J et al. Circulation 2003;107:947–53.
89. Sesso HD, Buring JE, Christen WG et al. JAMA 2008;300:2123.
90. Chappell LC, Seed PT, Briley AL et al. Lancet 1999;354:810–16.
91. Roberts JM, Myat, L, Spong CY et al. N Engl J Med 2010;362:1282.

92. Padayatty SJ, Levine M. N Engl J Med 2006;355:1065.
93. Age-Related Eye Disease Study Research Group. Arch Ophthalmol 2001;119:1439–52.
94. Age-Related Eye Disease Study Research Group. Arch Ophthalmol 2001;119:1417–36.
95. Evans J. Eye 2008;22:751–60.
96. Harrison DG, Gongora MC. Med Clin North Am 2009;93:621–35.
97. Bassenge E, Fink N, Skatchkov M et al. J Clin Invest 1998;102:67–71.
98. Douglas RM, Hemila H, D'Souza R et al. PLoS Med 2005;2:503.
99. Kaur B, Rowe BH, Arnold E. Cochrane Database Syst Rev 2009;(1):CD000993.
100. ter Riet G, Kessels AG, Knipschild PG. J Clin Epidemiol 1995;48:1453–60.
101. Sobala GM, Schorah CJ, Shires S et al. Gut 1993;34:1038–41.
102. Jenab M, Riboli E, Ferrari P et al. Br J Cancer 2006;95:406–15.
103. Correa P, Fontham ET, Bravo JC et al. J Natl Cancer Inst 2000;92:1881–8.
104. Jacobs EJ, Connell CJ, McCullough ML et al. Cancer Epidemiol Biomarkers Prev 2002;11:35–41.
105. Bjelakovic G, Nikolova D, Simonetti RG et al. Lancet 2004;364:1219–28.
106. Hallberg L, Brune M, Rossander-Hulthen L. Ann N Y Acad Sci 1987;498:324–32.
107. Cook JD, Reddy MB. Am J Clin Nutr 2001;73:93–8.
108. Jacob RA, Skala JH, Omaye ST. Am J Clin Nutr 1987;46:818–26.
109. Anonymous. N Engl J Med 1995;333:1695–1702.
110. Nienhuis AW. N Engl J Med 1981;304:170–1.
111. Barton JC, McDonnell SM, Adams PC et al. Ann Intern Med 1998;129:932–9.
112. Cook JD, Watson SS, Simpson KM et al. Blood 1984;64:721–6.
113. Gerster H. Ann Nutr Metab 1997;41:269–82.
114. Prigge ST, Kolhekar AS, Eipper BA et al. Nat Struct Biol 1999;6:976–83.
115. Lindblad B, Lindstedt G, Lindstedt S. J Am Chem Soc 1970;92:7446–9.
116. Hitomi K, Tsukagoshi N. Subcell Biochem 1996;25:41–56.
117. Toth I, Rogers JT, McPhee JA et al. J Biol Chem 1995;270:2846–52.
118. Helser MA, Hotchkiss JH, Roe DA. Carcinogenesis 1992;13:2277–80.
119. Hornig D. Ann N Y Acad Sci 1975;258:103–18.
120. Voigt K, Kontush A, Stuerenburg HJ et al. Free Radic Res 2002;36:735–9.

SUGGESTED READINGS

Asard H, May JM, Smirnoff N, eds. Vitamin C Function and Biochemistry in Animals and Plants. London: BIOS Scientific Publishers, 2004.
Corti A, Casini AF, Pompella A. Cellular pathways for transport and efflux of ascorbate and dehydroascorbate. Arch Biochem Biophys 2010;500:107–15.
Food and Nutrition Board, Institute of Medicine. Dietary Reference Intakes for Vitamin C, Vitamin E, Selenium, and Carotenoids. Washington, DC: National Academy Press, 2000.
Li Y, Schellhorn HE. New developments and novel therapeutic perspectives for vitamin C. J Nutr 2007;137:2171–84.
Lykkesfeldt J, Poulsen HE. Is vitamin C supplementation beneficial? Lessons learned from randomised controlled trials. Br J Nutr 2010;103:1251–9.
Padayatty SJ, Katz A, Wang Y et al. Vitamin C as an antioxidant: evaluation of its role in disease prevention. J Am Coll Nutr 2003;22: 18–35.

30 CHOLINE[1]

STEVEN H. ZEISEL

Choline was discovered in 1862 and was chemically synthesized in 1866 (1), but it was not recognized as one of the nutrients required by humans until 1998 (2). The importance of choline as a nutrient in animals was first appreciated more than 50 years earlier, during the pioneering work on insulin (3). Depancreatized dogs, maintained on insulin, developed fatty infiltration of the liver and died. Administration of raw pancreas prevented fatty liver and hepatic damage; the active component was the choline moiety of pancreatic phosphatidylcholine (4). The recognition that choline was needed by humans took so long because, like vitamin D, the choline moiety can be produced endogenously (when phosphatidylcholine is formed from phosphatidylethanolamine, mainly in the liver). Investigators assumed that this biosynthesis could meet human needs, but this is not true in most men and postmenopausal women (5). The gene for the enzyme catalyzing this biosynthesis is induced by estrogen (6), and some young women may not need to eat choline (5).

As discussed in more detail later, genetic variation also contributes to a wide variation in the dietary requirement for choline.

In 1998, the US Institute of Medicine's Food and Nutrition Board established an adequate intake (AI) and tolerable upper intake limit (UL) for choline (Table 30.1) (2). The AI is approximately 550 mg/70 kg body weight, with more recommended during pregnancy and lactation. The AI for infants is estimated from the calculated intake from human breast milk. The UL for choline (see Table 30.1) was derived from the lowest-observed-adverse-effect level (hypotension) in humans and is 3 g/day for an adult (2). Human studies of choline requirements in children or infants have not been conducted. As discussed later, women need less dietary choline because of enhanced endogenous biosynthesis (5, 6), but pregnancy and lactation require large amounts of choline and likely increase the requirement for this nutrient (7).

Choline has several important functions: it is a source of methyl groups needed to make S-adenosylmethionine, it is a part of the neurotransmitter acetylcholine, and it is a part of the predominant phospholipids in membranes (phosphatidylcholine and sphingomyelin) (8). Betaine, formed from choline, is an important osmolyte in the kidney glomerulus and helps with the reabsorption of water from the kidney tubule (9). Although they represent a smaller proportion of the total choline pool, important metabolites of choline include platelet-activating factor, choline plasmalogens, lysophosphatidylcholine, phosphocholine, and glycerophosphocholine (8).

DIETARY SOURCES

Many foods eaten by humans contain significant amounts of choline and esters of choline (10, 11). Eggs and liver are excellent sources of choline; one egg contains approximately 33% of the daily requirement (see the US Department of Agriculture's website for a list of dietary sources of choline and betaine: http://www.nal.usda.gov/fnic/foodcomp/Data/Choline/Choline.html). Humans on an ad libitum diet ingest between 150 and 600 mg choline/day (as free choline and choline esters) (12–17). In the 2005 National Health and Nutrition Examination Survey, only a few participants in all age groups in the United States ate diets achieving the recommended intake for choline (~550 mg/day/70 kg body

---

[1]**Abbreviations: AI**, adequate intake; **CDP-choline**, cytidine diphosphocholine; **CHDH**, choline dehydrogenase; **ERE**, estrogen-response elements; **LTP**, long-term potentiation; **MTHFR**, methylenetetrahydrofolate reductase; **PEMT**, phosphatidylethanolamine N-methyltransferase; **SNP**, single nucleotide polymorphisms; SRE, sterol-responsive element; **TPN**, total parenteral nutrition; **UL**, tolerable upper intake level; **VLDL**, very-low-density lipoprotein.

TABLE 30.1	DIETARY REFERENCE INTAKE VALUES FOR CHOLINE		
POPULATION	AGE	AI	UL
Infants	0–6 mo	125 mg/d, 18 mg/kg	Not possible to establish[a]
	6–12 mo	150 mg/d	
Children	1–3 y	200 mg/d	1,000 mg/d
	4–8 y	250 mg/d	1,000 mg/d
	9–13 y	375 mg/d	2,000 mg/d
Males	14–18 y	550 mg/d	3,000 mg/d
	≥19 y	550 mg/d	3,500 mg/d
Females	14–18 y	400 mg/d	3,000 mg/d
	≥19 y	425 mg/d	3,500 mg/d
Pregnancy	All ages	450 mg/d	Age-appropriate UL
Lactation	All ages	550 mg/d	Age-appropriate UL

[a]Source of intake should be food and formula only

From Food and Nutrition Board, Institute of Medicine. Dietary Reference Intakes for Folate, Thiamin, Riboflavin, Niacin, Vitamin B$_{12}$, Pantothenic Acid, Biotin, and Choline. Washington DC: National Academy Press, 1998:390–422, with permission.

weight) (18). Foods also contain the choline metabolite betaine (10), which cannot be converted to choline but can be used as a methyl donor, thereby sparing some choline requirements (19). Plant-derived food sources can be a rich source of betaine (named after beets), but only membrane-rich plant components (e.g., wheat germ) contain significant amounts of choline.

Human breast milk is rich in choline compounds (20). The bioavailability of choline may differ between human milk and infant formulas (20, 21), because they contain different amounts of the various choline compounds. In 2007, most commercial infant formulas were modified to "humanize" their choline content to approximate the amount present in mature human breast milk. Where does all this choline in human milk come from? Mammary epithelial cells are capable of concentrative uptake of choline from maternal blood (22) and of the biosynthesis of choline de novo (23) through phosphatidylethanolamine N-methyltransferase (PEMT) activity; this is the only pathway for endogenous biosynthesis of the choline moiety. The free choline content of human milk is very high at the start of lactation and diminishes by 30 days postpartum (24). Breast milk phosphatidylcholine and plasma choline concentrations are influenced by dietary choline intake, and a dietary supplement of phosphatidylcholine can further increase breast milk choline, betaine, and phosphocholine concentrations (25).

DIGESTION AND ABSORPTION

The extent to which dietary choline is bioavailable depends on the efficiency of its absorption from the intestine. In adults, some ingested choline is metabolized before it can be absorbed from the gut. Gut bacteria degrade choline to form betaine and to make methylamines (26) and may destroy enough diet-derived choline to influence the human dietary requirement (27, 28). Some of the variation in human requirements may be caused by differences in the intestinal microbiome. The free choline surviving

these fates is absorbed by the intestine by carrier-mediated transport (29, 30). At this time, no other component of the diet has been identified as competing with choline for transport by intestinal carriers. Both pancreatic secretions and intestinal mucosal cells contain enzymes (phospholipases A$_1$, A$_2$, and B) capable of hydrolyzing phosphatidylcholine in the diet. The free choline that is formed enters the portal circulation of the liver (31).

Large amounts of choline are delivered to the fetus across the placenta, where choline transport systems pump it against a concentration gradient (32). The placenta is one of the few nonnervous tissues to store large amounts of choline as acetylcholine (33). Perhaps this is a special reserve storage pool that ensures delivery of choline to the fetus. In utero, the fetus is exposed to very high choline concentrations, with a progressive decline in blood choline concentration thereafter until adult levels are achieved after the first weeks of life (34). In fact, plasma or serum choline concentrations are six to sevenfold higher in the fetus and newborn than they are in the adult (35, 36). High levels of choline circulating in the neonate presumably ensure enhanced availability of choline to tissues. Neonatal rat brain efficiently extracts choline from blood (37), and increased serum choline in the neonatal rat is associated with twofold higher choline concentration in neonatal brain than is present later in life. Supplementing choline during the perinatal period further increases choline metabolite concentrations in blood and brain (38).

All tissues accumulate choline by diffusion and mediated transport, but uptake by liver, kidney, mammary gland, placenta, and brain is especially important (30, 39). A specific carrier mechanism transports free choline across the blood–brain barrier at a rate that is proportional to serum choline concentration, and, in the neonate, this choline transporter has especially high capacity (37, 40). Hepatectomy increases the half-life of choline and results in an increase in blood choline concentration. The rate at which liver takes up choline is sufficient to explain the rapid disappearance of choline injected systemically.

The kidney also accumulates choline (41). Some of this choline appears in the urine unchanged, but most is oxidized within the kidney to form betaine (42–45) and glycerophosphocholine (46). Both substances are important intracellular osmoprotectants within kidney. Mean free choline concentrations in the plasma of azotemic humans are several times greater than in normal controls (47). Hemodialysis rapidly removes choline from the plasma (48, 49). Renal transplantation in humans lowers plasma choline from 30 μM in the azotemic patient to 15 μM within 1 day (50).

METABOLISM

Only a small fraction of dietary choline is acetylated (Fig. 30.1), catalyzed by the activity of choline acetyltransferase (51). This enzyme is highly concentrated in the terminals of cholinergic neurons, but it is also present in such nonnervous tissues as the placenta. The availability of choline and acetyl-coenzyme A (CoA) influences choline acetyltransferase activity. In brain, it is unlikely that choline acetyltransferase is saturated with either of its substrates, so choline (and possibly acetyl-CoA) availability determines the rate of acetylcholine synthesis (51). Increased brain acetylcholine synthesis is associated with an augmented release into the synapse of this neurotransmitter (52–54). Choline taken up by brain may first enter a storage pool (perhaps the phosphatidylcholine in membranes) before it is converted to acetylcholine (55). The choline phospholipids in cholinergic neurons comprise a large precursor pool of choline available for use in acetylcholine synthesis (56). This feature may be especially important in neurons with increased demands for choline to sustain acetylcholine release (e.g., when particular cholinergic neurons fire frequently or when the supply of choline from the extracellular fluid is inadequate).

The methyl groups of choline can be made available from one-carbon metabolism, on conversion to betaine (8) (see Fig. 30.1). Formation of betaine involves oxidation to betaine aldehyde in the inner mitochondrial membrane (57, 58), followed by oxidation of betaine aldehyde (catalyzed by betaine aldehyde dehydrogenase or by a nonspecific aldehyde dehydrogenase in the mitochondria and in the cytosol) to form betaine. Liver and kidney are the major sites of choline oxidation. Betaine cannot be reduced back to choline. Thus, the oxidation pathway acts to diminish the availability of choline to tissues while at the same time scavenging some methyl groups. This pathway is also important for mitochondrial adenosine triphosphate (ATP) generation, because mice with the choline dehydrogenase (*Chdh*) gene knocked out have defective mitochondrial ATP production (58).

The demand for choline as a methyl-group donor is probably the major factor that determines how rapidly a diet deficient in choline will induce pathologic features. The metabolisms of choline, methionine, and methylfolate are closely interrelated (see Fig. 30.1). The pathways intersect at the formation of methionine from homocysteine. Betaine:homocysteine methyltransferase, a zinc metalloenzyme (59), catalyzes the methylation of homocysteine using the choline metabolite betaine as the methyl donor (59, 60). In an alternative pathway, 5-methyltetrahydrofolate:homocysteine methyltransferase regenerates methionine by using a methyl group derived de novo from the one-carbon pool (61). Perturbing the metabolism of one of the methyl donors results in compensatory changes in the other methyl donors because of the intermingling of these metabolic pathways (62–68).

Rats ingesting a choline-deficient diet showed diminished tissue concentrations of methionine and S-adenosylmethionine (66) and of total folate (63). Methotrexate, which is widely used in the treatment of cancer, psoriasis, and rheumatoid arthritis, limits the availability of methyl groups by competitively inhibiting dihydrofolate reductase, a key enzyme in intracellular folate metabolism. Rats treated with methotrexate have diminished pools of all choline metabolites in liver (69). Choline supplementation reverses the fatty liver caused by methotrexate administration (70–73).

Genetically modified mice with defective methylene tetrahydrofolate reductase (MTHFR) activity become choline deficient (74). This observation is important because many humans have genetic polymorphisms that alter the activity of this enzyme (75, 76), and choline intake exceeding current dietary recommendations preserves markers of cellular methylation and attenuates DNA damage in men with the MTHFR C677T genotype (67).

The interrelationship between choline and folate is especially interesting because multiple studies in humans have demonstrated that individuals with diminished folate status are much more likely to have babies with neural tube defects (2, 77). In humans, women in the lowest quartile for dietary choline intake had an increased risk for having a baby with a neural tube defect or a cleft palate (15, 78). In mice, depletion of choline was associated with development of neural tube defects (79, 80). In addition, the intermingling of choline and homocysteine metabolism is important because increased plasma homocysteine concentration is an independent risk factor for cardiovascular disease (81). Homocysteine concentrations are lower when people eat diets higher in choline content (16, 82).

Elegant regulatory mechanisms control phosphatidylcholine biosynthesis and hydrolysis (83, 84). Synthesis occurs by two pathways (see Fig. 30.1). In the first pathway, choline is phosphorylated and then converted to cytidine diphosphocholine (CDP-choline). This high-energy intermediate, in combination with diacylglycerol, forms phosphatidylcholine and cytidine monophosphate. In the alternative pathway, phosphatidylethanolamine is sequentially methylated to form phosphatidylcholine, by using S-adenosylmethionine as the methyl donor.

an authentic sample should be demonstrated; and (c) if possible, a mass spectrum should be obtained that allows for at least one confirmation of the molecular mass. For quantitative analysis by HPLC, an internal control, such as echinenone, is needed to assess the efficiency of extraction procedures. Full elucidation of the structure requires a fully assigned NMR spectrum and, for chiral compounds, comparison of a circular dichroism spectrum with that of an authentic reference sample.

Carotenoids are unstable and are vulnerable when exposed to oxygen, heat, light, and acid. Precautions and special procedures must be used to minimize the risk of degradation and the formation of artifacts. All analytic procedures should be carried out in an inert atmosphere (nitrogen or argon), at room temperature (~20°C), in the dark or in diffused light, under acid-free conditions, and with freshly purified, peroxide-free solvents. Geometric (cis-trans) isomerization occurs readily when carotenoids are exposed to factors such as light or heat and slowly occurs even in isolated or purified samples. Plasma or tissue samples should be stored at −80°C to minimize degradative reactions and isomerization.

Noninvasive resonance Raman spectroscopic techniques show promise for measuring carotenoids in situ in the skin and the retina (30, 31). Carotenoids in the skin of the palm of the hand can be measured using a portable Raman device. Emission of light of 488 nm is used to estimate total carotenoids, and emission of light of 514 nm is used to estimate lycopene. The lack of power to separate individual carotenoids, except lycopene, is a limit to research, but great potential exists for monitoring carotenoid status from fruit and vegetable intake or the effect of carotenoid supplementation in human trials. Lutein and zeaxanthin, major macular pigments of the human retina, can also be measured using resonance Raman spectroscopic techniques (30). This noninvasive detection technique can be a screening method for macular pigment levels in the general population.

Stable isotope techniques that use intrinsically labeled carotenoids have proven useful in determining carotenoid bioavailability, bioconversion, and bioefficacy from different human food sources (27). Although these methods are costly and complex, they can distinguish between dosed and endogenous carotenoids and can determine the vitamin A equivalency of provitamin A carotenoids.

ABSORPTION, BIOAVAILABILITY, AND TRANSPORT

Much of the research on carotenoids to date has concentrated on β-carotene. The efficiency of absorption of a moderate dose of β-carotene in oil is approximately 9% to 22%. Humans (along with monkeys, ferrets, and gerbils, but excluding rats, mice, and rabbits unless they are given very high doses) absorb a significant portion of intact carotenoids directly and circulate or accumulate them in their plasma, liver, and peripheral tissues. The median

concentrations of carotenoids were reported in NHANES III (see Table 31.1). The half-life of plasma carotenoids ranges from up to 12 days for β-carotene, α-carotene, and cryptoxanthin, to 12 to 33 days for lycopene, and 33 to 61 days for zeaxanthin and lutein (32).

The bioavailability of β-carotene from vegetables is generally low (33). The mnemonic acronym SLAMENGHI lists the major contributors that affect carotenoid bioavailability. SLAMENGHI stands for species of carotenoids, linkages molecular level, amount of carotenoid, matrix effectors, nutrient status, genetics, host-related factors, and interactions among these variables (33). These factors are discussed in detailed in the literature (34, 35).

Carotenoids embedded in their food matrix cannot be absorbed efficiently. Food processing and cooking that cause the mechanical breakdown of the food matrix and the release of carotenoids can improve intestinal absorption. After release from the food matrix, ingested carotenoids must be emulsified and solubilized into micelles before they are absorbed into the intestinal mucosa (Fig. 31.3).

Previous research assumed that the process of carotenoid absorption occurred by passive diffusion. More recent studies, however, indicated the involvement of an active process for the uptake of carotenoids through the scavenger receptor class B type 1 protein transporter (SR-B1) (36). SR-B1 is found in the human small intestine, as well as the liver, adrenals, ovaries, placenta, kidneys, prostate, and brain. Therefore, SR-B1 may be partially responsible for the transport of carotenoids from lipoprotein to tissues and from tissues to lipoproteins (37). A diet-responsive regulatory network involving the intestine-specific homeobox (ISX) transcription factor was shown to regulate intestinal β-carotene uptake and vitamin A production by a negative feedback regulatory mechanism (36). ISX repressed both expression of intestinal BCO1 (38) and SR-B1 (39), which facilitates the absorption of dietary lipids and carotenoids (34). Because ISX is under the control of retinoic acid and retinoic acid receptor (RAR) receptor–dependent mechanisms, during vitamin A insufficiency, both BCO1 expression and SR-B1 expression are induced to increase absorption and conversion of β-carotene to vitamin A (see Fig. 31.3). Cleavage of β-carotene by BCO1 produces retinal, which can be oxidized to retinoic acid. Retinoic acid induces the expression of the ISX transcription factor and then represses expression of both BCO1 and SR-B1, to complete the dietary feedback mechanism (see Fig. 31.3).

Another protein, CD36, a surface membrane glycoprotein in the duodenum and jejunum involved in the uptake of long-chain fatty acids and oxidized low-density lipoproteins (LDLs), may also play a role in movement of carotenoids into cells. Although the same factors that influence the absorption of β-carotene may affect other carotenoids similarly, more investigation of the absorption of individual carotenoids and their cis isomers is needed.

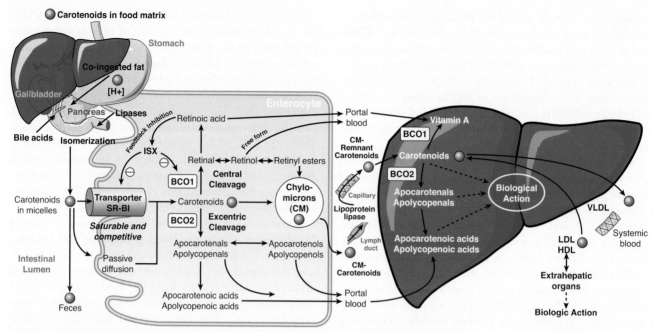

Fig. 31.3. Simplified schematic illustration of absorption, metabolism, and transport of carotenoids. *BCO1,* β-carotene-15,15′-oxygenase; *BCO2,* β-carotene-9′,10′-oxygenase; *HDL,* high-density lipoprotein; *LDL,* low-density lipoprotein; *VLDL,* very-low-density lipoprotein. (See text for detailed information).

After β-carotene is taken up by the mucosa of the small intestine, it is either cleaved by BCO1 or BCO2 into vitamin A and other metabolites or packaged into chylomicrons and secreted into the lymphatic system for transport to the liver and other peripheral tissues (see Fig. 31.3). Some polar metabolites can be directly transported into the liver through the portal blood system (40). β-Carotene, retinyl esters, retinol, and the less polar metabolites are absorbed into the lymph, whereas the more polar metabolites, which include β-apocarotenals, retinoyl-β-glucuronide, retinyl-β-glucuronide, and retinoic acid, are taken up directly into the portal blood (40). The differential absorption of β-carotene and its metabolites into lymph or portal blood seems to depend on the polarity of the metabolites involved.

Chylomicrons in the bloodstream are partially degraded by lipoprotein lipase, a process that leaves chylomicron remnants that are quickly taken up by the liver (see Fig. 31.3, and see also the chapter on lipids, sterols, and their metabolites). Some carotenoids may be released from these lipoproteins and taken up directly by extrahepatic tissues. In the fed state, the liver stores or secretes the carotenoids in very-low-density lipoproteins (VLDLs) and (LDLs). In the fasting state, plasma carotenes are found mainly in LDL. Xanthophylls (lutein, zeaxanthin, and β-cryptoxanthin) are located mainly in both LDL and high-density lipoproteins (HDLs), and small proportions are located in VLDLs. LDL transport accounts for approximately 55%, HDL transport for 31%, and VLDL transport for 14% of total blood carotenoids. Specific factors that regulate tissue uptake,

recycling of carotenoids back to the liver, and excretion are not yet understood (35).

METABOLISM

Central Cleavage Pathway

For provitamin A carotenoids, central cleavage is the main pathway leading to the formation of vitamin A. Carotenoids such as β-carotene, α-carotene, and β-cryptoxanthin are cleaved symmetrically at their central double bond by BCO1 (5, 6, 41), and they are present in several mouse and human tissues (e.g., liver, kidney, intestinal tract, and testis) (7, 42). Purified recombinant human BCO1 enzyme cleaves β-carotene in vitro with a Michaelis-Menten constant (K_m) and maximal velocity ($\dot{V}_{max}$) of 7 μM and 10 nmol retinal/mg/minute, respectively (43). Retinal formed from β-carotene can be subsequently reduced to retinol or oxidized further to form retinoic acid (see Fig. 31.1; see also the chapter on vitamin A for details). Nonprovitamin A carotenoids, such as lycopene, were cleaved by purified recombinant murine BCO1 with much lower (7) or no activity (9, 44).

Four conserved histidines and one conserved glutamate residue are essential for the catalytic mechanism of BCO1, presumably for the coordination of the iron cofactor required for catalytic activity (10). Chicken BCO1 showed substrate specificity toward a broad array of carotenoid substrates including α-carotene, β-carotene, γ-carotene, β-cryptoxanthin, apo-4′-carotenal, and apo-8′-carotenal (44). In light of this evidence, it appears that the presence of at least one unsubstituted β-ionone ring is sufficient for catalytic cleavage of the central carbon 15,15′ double bond.

Eccentric Cleavage Pathway

Building on evidence that the eccentric cleavage of β-carotene leads to a series of homologous carbonyl cleavage products (15, 45), the existence of this pathway was confirmed by the molecular identification of BCO2 in mice, humans, zebra fish, and ferrets (17, 18). BCO2 shares overall sequence homology with BCO1, as well as the same conserved pattern of histidine residues and glutamate residues presumably involved in binding the iron cofactor in both proteins (10, 17). BCO2 is highly expressed in the liver and testis and at lower levels in the kidney, lung, heart, spleen, prostate, intestine, stomach, colon, and brain (17, 18).

Recombinant ferret BCO2 cleaved all-*trans*-β-carotene to form β-apo-10′-carotenal in a pH-dependent and time-dependent linear manner with a pH optimum between 8.0 and 8.5. The reaction exhibited Michaelis-Menten kinetics, with an estimated K_m of 3.5 ± 1.1 μM for β-carotene and a V_{max} of 32.2 ± 2.9 pmol β-apo-10′-carotenal/mg/hour. β-Apocarotenals can be cleaved further by BCO1 to produce retinol and retinoic acid (46, 47), or they can be oxidized to their corresponding apo-β-carotenoic acids (see Fig. 31.1). Apo-β-carotenoic acids may then undergo a process similar to β-oxidation of fatty acids, until further oxidation is blocked by the methyl group at the C13 position (48). This shortening produces retinoic acid from β-carotene (48). β-Apo-12′-carotenal and β-apo-10′-carotenal were isolated from ferret intestinal mucosa after perfusion of β-carotene in vivo (49, 50), and β-apo-8′-carotenal was detected in humans given an oral dose of all-*trans* [10,10′,11,11′-^{14}C]-β-carotene (51).

Although the exact contribution of BCO2 to vitamin A biosynthesis remains unknown (52), kinetic results suggest that β-apocarotenals may be intermediate compounds in the production of retinoids from β-carotene. Indeed, the perfusion of β-apo-14′-carotenal in ferrets increased the formation of retinoic acid and retinol in vivo (47), and the feeding apo-8′-carotenal restored the retinol serum levels in vitamin A–depleted rats (53). Data show that the mutation in the bovine *BCO2* gene results in increased adipose, serum, and milk β-carotene concentrations and decreased liver retinol (54, 55).

Although BCO1 catalyzes the cleavage of provitamin A carotenoids with much greater activity than nonprovitamin A carotenoids, the activity of BCO2 is higher toward nonprovitamin A carotenoids, such as *cis*-lycopene isomers, lutein, and zeaxanthin, than toward β-carotene as a substrate (18, 19). These observations highlight the emerging role of central and eccentric cleavage of β-carotene and other carotenoids (both provitamin A and nonprovitamin A) in vertebrate metabolism and health. The almost ubiquitous expression of carotenoid oxygenases indicates that many tissues may contribute to their own metabolic homeostasis. However, whether the formation of other β-apocarotenals found in vitro and in vivo is the result of further metabolism of the β-apocarotenoid cleavage product or whether these substances are the primary cleavage products of additional carotene oxygenases remains to be discovered.

Genetic Factors

Variability in β-carotene absorption and metabolism is well documented in humans (56). Although regulation of BCO1 (53) and SR-B1 (36) may partially explain this variability, several genetic alterations identified in humans also affect β-carotene absorption and metabolism. SNPs within components of lipoprotein metabolism, such as apolipoprotein B, lipoprotein lipase, and SR-B1, are associated with altered plasma carotenoid in humans (37). These genes have a profound effect not only on carotenoid absorption but also on the tissue distribution. An SNP within the *SRB1* gene has been identified as a risk factor for age-related macular degeneration (57). An elevation in plasma β-carotene and a decrease in plasma retinol were demonstrated in an individual possessing a heterozygous mutation in the *BCO1* gene (58). Biochemical analysis of the mutant BCO1 protein identified the replacement of a highly conserved threonine residue by a methionine residue. Kinetic characterization demonstrated an approximately 90% decrease in activity compared with wild-type BCO1.

Certain SNPs are also identified in the protein-coding region of the human *BCO1* gene, thus resulting in several different protein variants (29, 58, 59). Women carrying either the 267S+379S or 379V variant in *BCO1* displayed decreased intestinal β-carotene conversion efficiency (59). In a separate study, an SNP located upstream of the *BCO1* gene was associated with increased β-carotene and α-carotene blood levels (29). Lycopene, lutein, and zeaxanthin levels were lower in SNP carriers. Nonetheless, the presence of SNPs within the *SRB1* and *BCO1* genes may partially explain low-absorber or low-converter phenotypes.

Although no reports exist of genetic alterations in the human *BCO2* gene, animal genetic reports have provided evidence of broad substrate specificity of BCO2. The bovine *BCO2* gene was shown to contain an SNP that resulted in a truncated and presumably nonfunctional BCO2 protein (54, 55). In Norwegian white sheep (*Ovis aries*), a nonsense mutation in the *BCO2* gene was significantly associated with a yellow adipose phenotype (60). In chickens, a yellow skin phenotype is associated with an SNP in the *BCO2* gene (61). The decrease in skin β-carotene 9′,10′-monooxygenase leads to the yellow skin pigmentation of domestic chickens, a finding suggesting a decreased ability to cleave the xanthophylls lutein and zeaxanthin, which are the major accumulated carotenoids in chicken skin (62).

Regulation

Knowledge of the molecular and regulatory framework of carotenoid metabolism is far from complete. Molecular studies of the mouse and human BCO1 promoter demonstrate the presence of a peroxisome proliferator-response element (PPRE) (63, 64). Peroxisome proliferator-activated receptor γ (PPARγ) and retinoid X receptor α (RXRα) agonists can transactivate the BCO1 promoter-reporter when they are cotransfected with the corresponding nuclear receptor (63). The human BCO1 promoter contains an additional enhancer element in the form of a myocyte enhancer factor-2 (MEF2) binding site (64). In rats supplemented with lycopene, BCO1 expression was significantly decreased in adrenal gland and kidney (65). Fatty acid binding protein-3, a PPARγ target gene, was down-regulated in parallel with BCO1. In BCO1-knockout mice, a gross impairment in lipid metabolism was observed (52). Investigators have suggested that cleavage products of β-carotene may refine the crosstalk among the nuclear receptors that regulate lipid metabolism (66). The relationship between carotenoid and lipid metabolism deserves further inquiry.

Unlike with BCO1, little evidence is available regarding regulation of BCO2. A molecular analysis failed to identify a PPRE within the mouse BCO2 promoter (65). Some insight into BCO2 regulation is gained from studying BCO1-knockout mice, which, compared with wild-type mice, have significantly elevated hepatic BCO2 expression (52, 67). This finding suggests the presence of concerted mechanisms governing the expression of BCO1 and BCO2.

Much of the evidence produced thus far indicates that supplementation with various carotenoids, especially non-provitamin A carotenoids, may affect BCO2 expression. In male adult ferret, a significant fourfold increase in lung BCO2 expression was observed after 9 weeks of lycopene supplementation (18). A separate study in rats showed that lycopene supplementation for various times resulted in subtle yet significant down-regulation of BCO2 expression in several tissues (65). Chronic alcohol consumption increased BCO1 mRNA expression as well as both PPARγ and PPARα protein and mRNA expression (68). As expected, BCO1 expression was highly and positively correlated with PPARγ expression (63, 69). A small but significant increase in BCO2 protein and mRNA expression also occurred, positively correlated with both PPARγ and PPARα expression. Taken together, these results indicate that dietary factors, especially carotenoid supplementation, may influence BCO2 expression.

BIOLOGIC FUNCTIONS OF CAROTENOIDS AND THEIR METABOLITES

Early studies focused on the provitamin A carotenoids, in particular β-carotene, but research since 1980 has provided a framework for understanding other carotenoids and how their functions may benefit human health. β-Carotene, β-cryptoxanthin, lutein, zeaxanthin, and lycopene may have unique biologic roles in protecting against the development of several chronic and degenerative diseases, including vitamin A deficiency and its related health problems (e.g., anemia, growth retardation, immune competence impairment, infections, and xerophthalmia) (70), age-related macular degeneration (71), cardiovascular disease (72), certain cancers (73), and skin lesions (74), including erythropoietic protoporphyria (75). Investigators have proposed that carotenoids have a role in metabolic syndrome (76), bone health (77), and cognitive function (78). Whether carotenoids are important food components with health benefits remains to be confirmed, however.

Although both cell culture and animal model studies provide strong evidence that carotenoids and their metabolites are active in several biologic activities (see later; Fig. 31.4), demonstrating these molecular effects in human systems, a process that involves multiple genetic and epigenetic events, is challenging. Specifically, the plasma values of carotenoids are biomarkers for consumption of diets rich in fruits and vegetables that contain other potentially bioactive nutrients, so association does not necessarily prove that carotenoids are the active compounds. As our understanding of carotenoid metabolism, molecular biologic properties, and their interactions with genetic and epigenetic factors improves, greater insight will be achieved into the role and application of carotenoids and their metabolites in human health and disease.

Retinoid-Dependent Activity

The most clearly defined human biologic function of carotenoids is their vitamin A activity. Provitamin A carotenoids, through central cleavage, serve as precursors to vitamin A and represent the major dietary sources of vitamin A for much of the world's population. Through vitamin A action, provitamin A carotenoids exert effects on several critical life processes, including vision, reproduction, metabolism, differentiation, hematopoiesis, bone development, pattern formation during embryogenesis, and tumorigenesis (see the chapter on vitamin A).

Provitamin A carotenoids can serve as direct precursors for all-*trans*- and 9-*cis*-retinoic acid (79, 80), which are ligands for RAR and RXR. In one study, β-carotene was able to maintain normal tissue levels of retinoic acid and inhibit the activation of mitogen-activated protein kinase pathways, cell proliferation, and phosphorylation of p53 (81). Certain eccentric cleavage metabolites, such as β-apocarotenoic acid, can also induce RARβ expression and transactivate the RARβ2 promoter by metabolism to the potent RAR ligand, all-*trans*-retinoic acid (82). Therefore, the molecular mode of the action of provitamin A carotenoids is likely to be mediated by retinoic acid through transcriptional activation of a series of genes (20).

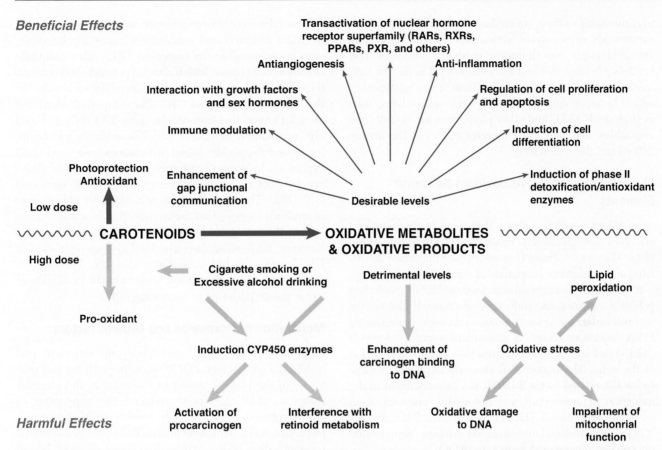

Fig. 31.4. Schematic illustration of potential biologic effects, both beneficial and harmful, attributed to carotenoids and their metabolites to human health. Although small quantities of carotenoid metabolites may offer protection against chronic diseases and certain cancers, larger amounts may be harmful, especially when coupled with a highly oxidative environment (e.g., the lungs of cigarette smokers or liver of excessive alcohol drinkers). *CYP450*, cytochrome P-450; *PPAR*, peroxisome proliferator-activated receptor; *PXR*, pregnane X receptor; *RAR*, retinoic acid receptor; *RXR*, retinoid X receptor.

Retinoid-Independent Activity

The discovery of the eccentric cleavage of carotenoids heightened interest in carotenoid cleavage products and their possible biologic role in humans. The production of apocarotenoids and apolycopenals was demonstrated in several studies (19, 51, 67, 83). Without being converted into retinoids, the nonvolatile apocarotenoids and apolycopenoids can inhibit cell growth (84–87), stimulate differentiation (88), transactivate nuclear receptors (84), or antagonize nuclear receptor activation (83, 89). The volatile apocarotenoid β-ionone has also been shown to inhibit cell proliferation and induce apoptosis both in vitro (90–92) and in vivo (93). β-Cryptoxanthin dose dependently increases RARE-dependent promoter activity in cells cotransfected with an RAR expression vector (94) is shown to bind and activate RAR receptors without its conversion into retinoids (95). Beyond participating in known retinoid signaling pathways, carotenoids may possibly be able to interact directly with transcription factors without their conversion into retinoids.

Antioxidant Activity

Free radicals can cause cellular damage by reacting with proteins, lipids, carbohydrates, and DNA, and they may be involved in the etiology of human diseases such as cancer, cardiovascular disease, and age-related diseases. Much of the biologic activity ascribed to carotenoids is attributed to their antioxidant capabilities (e.g., functioning as free radical scavengers and, in the case of lutein and zeaxanthin, as blue light filters that possibly prevent photo damage of the retina) (72). Indeed, the antioxidant properties of many carotenoids are well documented in the in vitro systems where they are believed to play critical roles in protecting against chronic disease (72). Accurate data regarding the antioxidant effects of carotenoids alone in in vivo biologic systems are limited, however.

Because most in vivo studies use fruit and vegetable products that contain various micronutrients and phytochemicals, including other carotenoids, polyphenols, vitamin C, and vitamin E, caution must be used when attributing the beneficial effects of vegetables and fruits to carotenoids or their antioxidant activity. Thus, although carotenoids demonstrate antioxidant activity in certain animal models, no definitive evidence indicates that carotenoids from diet and food sources act as in vivo antioxidants in human studies. In addition, a synergistic interaction between carotenoids and other antioxidants, such as vitamins E and C and other phytonutrients in fruits and vegetables, may play more important roles in the human antioxidant defense system.

Phase II Enzymes and Antioxidant-Response Elements

Accumulating evidence shows that some of the beneficial effects of carotenoids may result from the induction of the phase II enzymes. Phase II enzymes have important detoxifying and antioxidant properties in combating reactive oxygen species and foreign substances (xenobiotics), including potential carcinogens. Induction of phase II detoxifying and antioxidant enzymes is mediated through *cis*-regulatory DNA sequences known as antioxidant-response elements (AREs) that are located in the promoter or enhancer region of the gene. The major ARE transcription factor nuclear factor E2–related factor 2 (Nrf2) is a primary agent in the induction of antioxidant and detoxifying enzymes, such as heme oxygenase-1 (HO-1), glutathione S-transferases (GSTs), and reduced nicotinamide adenine dinucleotide phosphate:quinone oxidoreductase (NQO1).

Under normal conditions, most of the Nrf2 is sequestered in the cytoplasm by Kelch-like erythroid Cap'n'Collar homolog-associated protein 1' (Keap 1), and only residual nuclear Nrf2 binds to the ARE to drive basal activities. Exposure to certain carotenoids leads to the dissociation of the Nrf2-Keap1 complex in the cytoplasm and the translocation of Nrf2 into the nucleus (21, 84, 96). The nuclear accumulation of Nrf2 subsequently activates target genes of phase II antioxidant enzymes. Not only β-carotene, but also some nonprovitamin A carotenoids including lycopene, lutein, canthaxanthin, and astaxanthin, can induce several phase II enzymes both in vivo and in vitro (97, 98).

Gap Junction Communication

Gap junction communications (GJCs) are cell-to-cell channels that enable connected cells to exchange nutrients, waste products, and information. GJCs are implicated in the control of cell growth through adaptive responses of differentiation, proliferation, and apoptosis. Each gap junction is derived from 6 connexin proteins from each adjacent cell for a total of 12 connexin proteins. The connexin family includes more than 20 connexins; however, connexin 43 (Cx43) is the most widely expressed and is the form most often induced by retinoids and carotenoids (99). Both provitamin A and nonprovitamin A carotenoids can inhibit carcinogen-induced neoplastic transformation (100) and up-regulate Cx43 mRNA expression.

Several lines of in vitro evidence indicate that carotenoid oxidative products and metabolites, especially lycopene, may be responsible for increased GJC. After complete oxidation of lycopene with hydrogen peroxide and osmium tetroxide, Aust et al (101) isolated an oxidative metabolite that effectively increased GJC. The compound, identified as 2,7,11-trimethyl-tetradecahexaene-1,14-dial, induced GJC comparably to retinoic acid. The oxidative metabolite lycopene-5,6-epoxide, found in tomatoes, increased Cx43 expression in human keratinocytes, and the central cleavage product of lycopene, acycloretinoic acid, increased GJC (102). That the effect was achieved only at high concentrations suggests that the contribution of acycloretinoic acid to the activity of lycopene on GJC may be minimal, however. RAR antagonists also inhibited up-regulation of GJC by retinoids but not carotenoids (103). This finding, which warrants further study, suggested the possibility of two separate pathways of increasing GJC.

Modulation of Hormones and Growth Factors

Steroid hormones (e.g., androgens and estrogen) and insulinlike growth factor (IGF) signaling systems may play a role in the biologic action of carotenoids, in particular lycopene (104). Lycopene reduced the expression of 5α-reductase-1 in rat prostate tumors (105). Lycopene, phytoene, and phytofluene inhibited the estrogen-induced transactivation of the estrogen-response element bound by the nuclear estrogen receptors ERα and ERβ (106). The IGF signaling system may also play a role in the biologic action of lycopene (107).

Consistent with previous in vitro findings, epidemiologic studies demonstrated that a higher dietary intake of lycopene is associated with lower circulating levels of IGF-I (108) and higher levels of IGF-binding proteins (IGFBPs) (109, 110). The IGFBP-3 level was increased by lycopene supplementation and decreased by smoke exposure. Lycopene supplementation increased plasma IGFBP-3 levels and was associated with inhibition of cigarette smoke–induced lung squamous metaplasia, decreased proliferating cell nuclear antigen, and induction of apoptosis (111). These results, along with others, suggest that interference of IGF-I signaling may be an important mechanism by which lycopene could exert anti-cancer activity.

EFFECTS RELATED TO HIGH DOSAGE

In the early 1980s, two key publications, (112, 113), revealed that β-carotene could be an antioxidant and anti-cancer agent. This finding greatly stimulated the field of carotenoid research, and several intervention trials using pharmacologic doses of β-carotene (some 10 to 15 times more than the average dietary consumption) as a chemo-preventive agent were performed. Unfortunately, in 1994 to 1996, the human trials concluded without evidence of a beneficial effect and actually showed an increased risk

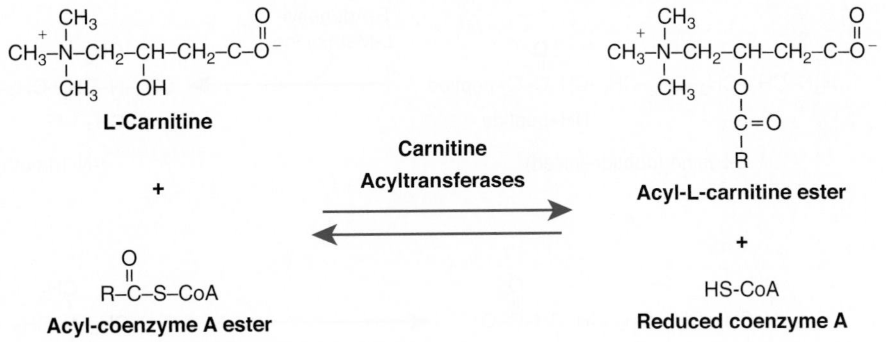

Fig. 32.1. Carnitine structure and metabolic interconversions. *CoA*, coenzyme A; *HS-CoA*, coenzyme A.

medium-chain dicarboxylic acids) were different, compared with infants consuming the same formulas but supplemented with carnitine (10). An expert panel commissioned by the US Food and Drug Administration's Center for Food Safety and Applied Nutrition recommended a minimum carnitine content in infant formulas of 7.5 μmol/100 kcal, and a maximum level of 12.4 μmol/100 kcal, a value similar to the upper limit reported for human milk (11). These recommendations were made on the basis of reported biochemical differences when infants were fed carnitine-free diets, compared with similar diets with carnitine, and despite the lack of evidence that carnitine is essential for the term infant.

HOMEOSTATIC MECHANISMS

Carnitine homeostasis in humans is maintained by the dynamic interactions of endogenous synthesis, acquisition from dietary sources, maintenance of concentration gradients across cell membranes, and regulation of renal reabsorption and excretion of carnitine.

Absorption and Bioavailability

Absorption of carnitine likely involves a combination of active transport and passive diffusion across the intestinal mucosal barrier. Evidence has accumulated from in vivo and in vitro studies, using several experimental preparations, to demonstrate that active transport of carnitine occurs across the apical brush-border membrane of enterocytes, but not across the basal membrane (9). A passive component, at least at the serosal surface, is strongly suggested by experimental studies in rats (12, 13) and Caco–2 cells (14) that demonstrated relatively rapid entry of carnitine into enterocytes from the luminal medium, but very slow appearance in the serosal perfusate or medium.

Approximately 63% to 75% of carnitine is absorbed from the normal omnivorous diet (15). The remainder is almost entirely degraded by bacteria in the large intestine. Primary organic degradation products of carnitine are trimethylamine (excreted in urine as trimethylamine oxide) and γ-butyrobetaine (excreted primarily in feces). Carnitine is not degraded by enzymes of animal origin (16).

Biosynthesis

Humans are able to synthesize carnitine from the essential amino acids lysine and methionine (Fig. 32.2). Lysine provides the carbon chain and nitrogen atom, and three methionine molecules (as S-adenosyl-L-methionine) provide the methyl groups for one molecule of carnitine (17). Methylation of the epsilon (ε) amino group of lysine is catalyzed by one or more protein:lysine methyltransferases. Lysine residues destined for carnitine synthesis must be peptide linked; no evidence indicates that free lysine is enzymatically methylated in mammals. ε-N-Trimethyllysine is released for carnitine synthesis through normal mechanisms of protein hydrolysis.

ε-N-Trimethyllysine undergoes four sequential enzymatic reactions (17): hydroxylation at position two of the carbon chain, catalyzed by ε-N-trimethyllysine hydroxylase (EC 1.14.11.8); aldol cleavage between carbons two and three of the carbon chain, catalyzed by serine hydroxymethyltransferase (EC 2.1.2.1); oxidation of the resulting aldehyde by any of several oxidized nicotinamide adenine dinucleotide (NAD1)–requiring aldehyde dehydrogenases (including one with high specificity for γ-N-trimethylaminobutyraldehyde); and a second hydroxylation, catalyzed by γ-butyrobetaine hydroxylase (EC 1.14.11.1). cDNAs coding for each of these four enzymes have been cloned and sequenced (18). All enzymes in the pathway except γ-butyrobetaine hydroxylase are ubiquitous in mammalian tissues. The last enzyme in the pathway is not found in cardiac or skeletal muscle (17). γ-Butyrobetaine hydroxylase activity is highest in liver and testes. In some species, including humans, it is abundant in kidney.

The normal rate of carnitine synthesis in humans is approximately 1.2 μmol/kg body weight/day (7). This estimate was obtained from normal rates of urinary carnitine excretion by strict vegetarians, who acquire very little carnitine (~0.1 μmol/kg body weight/day) from dietary sources. Direct measurement of the rate of carnitine synthesis technically is not feasible (7). The problems of isotope dilution (only a very small percentage of the body lysine pool is used for carnitine synthesis) and uniform mixing within the body pool are overwhelming and preclude direct measurement of rates of carnitine synthesis from lysine. Direct determination of rates of carnitine synthesis

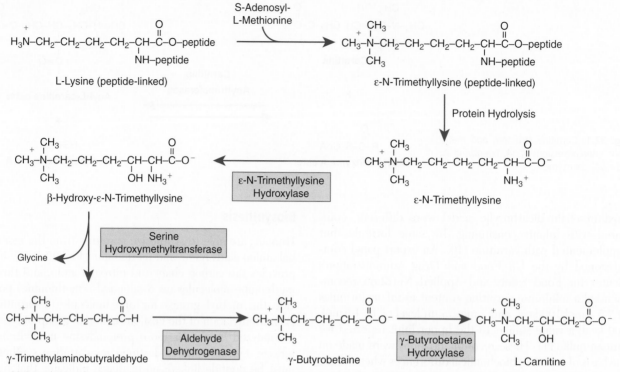

Fig. 32.2. Pathway of carnitine biosynthesis in mammals. (Adapted with permission from Rebouche CJ. Ascorbic acid and carnitine biosynthesis. Am J Clin Nutr 1991;54(Suppl):1147S–52S.)

from ε-N-trimethyllysine by isotopic conversion is also impractical because this precursor does not readily cross cell membranes, and thus pools of intracellular free ε-N-trimethyllysine cannot be labeled uniformly.

The rate of carnitine synthesis in mammals is regulated by the availability of ε-N-trimethyllysine, which, in turn, is determined by the extent of peptide-linked lysine methylation and by the rate of protein turnover (7). ε-N-Trimethyllysine destined for carnitine synthesis probably is derived from the general protein pool and not from any single or small group of proteins. Provision of excess lysine in the diet may increase carnitine synthesis modestly (19), but the evidence is indirect, and the mechanism (e.g., increased flux through protein synthesis, methylation and turnover, or stimulation of a putative vestigial capability to methylate free lysine) has not been identified. The rate of carnitine biosynthesis does not appear to be affected by the magnitude of dietary carnitine intake or by changes in renal handling of carnitine.

Transport and Excretion

Carnitine is concentrated in most tissues of the body. In humans, the intracellular concentrations of carnitine in skeletal muscle and liver are approximately 76 and 50 times higher, respectively, than that in extracellular fluid (~50 μmol/L). Approximately 97% of all carnitine in the body is in skeletal muscle. Six carnitine transporters have been identified: three organic cation transporters

OCTN1, OCTN2, and OCTN3; a carnitine transporter, CT2; an organic anion transporter, Oat9S; and an amino acid transporter, $ATB^{0,+}$.

OCTN1 is expressed in many tissues (although not in human adult liver) (20), but it has relatively low affinity (translocation rate constant, K_t = 412 μM) and specificity for carnitine (21). This pH-dependent, 63–kDa transporter may be responsible for secretion of carnitine and its short-chain esters across the renal epithelial brush-border membrane (22, 23). Carnitine is transported into most tissues by a high-affinity (K_t = 3 to 5 μM), sodium (Na^+) gradient–dependent organic cation transporter, OCTN2 (24, 25). This 63–kDa transporter is highly expressed in the heart, placenta, skeletal muscle, kidney, pancreas, testis, and epididymis (20, 25) and weakly expressed in brain, lung, and liver (26). OCTN2 binds carnitine, acetylcarnitine, and propionylcarnitine with comparable affinity (27). It is likely to be quantitatively the most important carnitine transporter in all tissues except testis.

OCTN3 is expressed primarily and at a high level in the testes, and it has higher specificity for carnitine than OCTN1 or OCTN2 (20). Unlike with OCTN2, carnitine transport by OCTN3 is not driven by an inwardly directed Na^+ gradient. A murine Octn3–green fluorescent protein construct was expressed in HepG2 cells, where it localized in peroxisomes (28). CT2 was found only in the luminal membrane of human epididymis and has high specificity for L-carnitine (29). This protein may serve to secrete L-carnitine from epididymal epithelium

33 CYSTEINE, TAURINE, AND HOMOCYSTEINE[1,2]

MARTHA H. STIPANUK

---

[1]**Abbreviations: Cys**, cysteine (any form), with thiol and disulfide forms indicated as CySH, CySSCy, and CySSR; **cyst(e)ine**, Cys or cystine; **EAR**, estimated average requirement; **Glu**, glutamate; **Gly**, glycine; **GSH**, glutathione; **Hcy**, homocysteine (any form), with thiol and disulfide forms indicated as HcySH, HcySSHcy, and HcySSR; **homocyst(e)ine**, Hcy or homocystine; **H$_2$S**, hydrogen sulfide; **K$_m$**, Michaelis-Menten constant; **Met**, methionine; **NHANES III**, Third National Health and Nutrition Examination Survey; **RDA**, recommended dietary allowance; **SAA**, sulfur amino acid; **SAH**, S-adenosylhomocysteine; **SAM**, S-adenosylmethionine; **TauT**, taurine transporter; **tCys**, sum of all forms of plasma Cys including those present as thiol, half-disulfide, mixed disulfide, and protein-bound disulfide; **tHcy**, sum of all forms of Hcy; **THF**, tetrahydrofolate; **TPN**, total parenteral nutrition; **UL**, tolerable upper intake level.
[2]**List of compounds:** cysteine, 121.2 g/mol; glutathione (reduced form), 307.3 g/mol; homocysteine, 135.2 g/mol; methionine, 149.2 g/mol; taurine, 125.1 g/mol

HISTORICAL INTRODUCTION

Cysteine (Cys) is a sulfur-containing amino acid, whereas taurine is a product of Cys oxidation, and homocysteine (Hcy) is a metabolite of methionine (Met), which also serves as a precursor of Cys sulfur. The importance of sulfur amino acids (SAAs) for growth or protein synthesis was first recognized in 1915, when Osborne and Mendel (1) demonstrated that the addition of cystine to a low-casein diet resulted in restoration of rapid growth of rats. Womack et al. (2) demonstrated that cyst(e)ine was not essential for rats when dietary Met was adequate and that the effect of cyst(e)ine resulted from its ability to replace part, but not all, of the Met in the diet. Rose and Wixom (3) demonstrated the same relationship between Met and cyst(e)ine requirements in their studies of amino acid requirements of men. Thus, only Met is considered an essential amino acid, but in practice the Met or total SAA requirement is usually met by a combination of Met and cyst(e)ine. N-Acetylcysteine, which is readily deacetylated to Cys, is used clinically in the treatment of acetaminophen overdose and for prevention of radiocontrast-induced nephropathy.

During the last decades of the twentieth century, the nutritional importance of taurine and the clinical significance of Hcy were recognized. Taurine is an end product of Cys catabolism. It was first isolated from the bile of the ox (*Box taurus*) in 1827 (4). Interest in taurine surged following the discovery in 1975 that cats fed diets containing little or no taurine suffered retinal degeneration accompanied by low retinal and plasma taurine concentrations (5). This finding was soon followed by the observation that infants fed purified formulas lacking taurine had lower plasma and urine taurine levels than did infants fed pooled human milk (6, 7). As a consequence of increasing evidence of a possible role of taurine in development, taurine has been added to most human infant formulas since the mid-1980s. Numerous possible therapeutic applications of taurine have been suggested, including treatment of patients with hypertension, cardiovascular disease, diabetes, hepatic disorders, chronic renal failure, sepsis, and inflammatory disorders.

Hcy, a metabolite of Met and precursor of the sulfur atom in Cys biosynthesis, was discovered by du Vigneaud in 1932 (8) as the product of Met demethylation. The role of homocyst(e)ine in the conversion of Met sulfur to Cys (the transsulfuration pathway by which the sulfhydryl group of Hcy replaces the hydroxyl group of serine to form Cys) was studied in the years to follow, and investigators showed that homocyst(e)ine could support the growth of animals fed diets deficient in Cys, Met, or choline. Homocystinuria, an inborn error of metabolism, was identified in 1962 when individuals with mental retardation were screened for abnormal urinary amino acid patterns (9). Subsequently, investigators recognized that small increases in plasma Hcy concentrations were associated with folate, vitamin B_{12}, or vitamin B_6 deficiency and with increased risk of cardiovascular disease, neural tube defects, and various other diseases found in the general population (10–13).

CHEMISTRY, NOMENCLATURE, AND CELLULAR/EXTRACELLULAR FORMS

The structures of Cys, Hcy, and taurine and their relations with precursor amino acids (Met and serine) are shown in Figure 33.1. As in other amino acids with an asymmetric carbon atom, the L-isomers of Met, Hcy, and Cys are the biologically active forms. Both Hcy and Cys have a free sulfhydryl group. The carbon skeleton of Hcy, which is derived from Met, has one more carbon than does the carbon chain of Cys, which is derived from serine. Taurine, 2-aminoethane sulfonate, is formed from Cys by removal of the carboxyl group and oxidation of the sulfur to form a sulfonic acid group. The carboxyl (pK_a ~1.7), sulfonic (pK_a ~1.5), sulfhydryl (pK_a ~8.3), and amino (pK_a ~9 to 11) groups all undergo ionization; the zwitterionic forms shown in Figure 33.1 are the dominant species at physiologic pH.

DIETARY CONSIDERATIONS, TYPICAL INTAKES, AND RECOMMENDED INTAKES

The body's need for Cys must be met by the diet and may be supplied either as preformed cyst(e)ine or as its

sulfur precursor Met. The carbon skeleton for cyst(e)ine biosynthesis is provided by serine, which can be synthesized in the body. Under most circumstances, sufficient taurine can apparently be synthesized from the SAAs, but taurine may be classified as conditionally essential under some conditions. Little Hcy is present in the diet, but it is formed in the process of Met metabolism in the body. No dietary requirement exists for Hcy intake.

Methionine and Cyst(e)ine

The SAAs, Met and Cys, are normally consumed as components of dietary proteins. Normal Western diets provide approximately 2 to 4 g/day of SAAs for adults (14). Based on the Third National Health and Nutrition Examination Survey (NHANES III; 1988 to 1994), the mean Met intake of 31- to 50-year-old men and women was 2.3 ± 0.04 and 1.6 ± 0.2 (standard error [SE]) g/day, or 15.4 and 10.7 mmol/day, respectively. Mean Cys intake for the same age group was 1.3 ± 0.02 and 0.89 ± 0.01 g/day, or 10.7 and 7.4 mmol/day, respectively. Thus, mean total SAA intake was 26.1 and 18.1 mmol/day, respectively, for men and women. SAAs tend to be more abundant in animal and cereal proteins than in legume proteins, and the ratio of Met to Cys tends to be higher in animal proteins than in plant proteins (Table 33.1).

For adults, the current estimated average requirement (EAR) for Met plus Cys intake is 15 mg · kg^{-1} · day, and the recommended dietary allowance (RDA) is 19 mg · kg^{-1} · day (14). Considering that approximately one third of the SAA requirement on a weight basis is taken in as Cys rather than Met, the current RDA is consistent with the estimated safe intake of Met (21 mg · kg^{-1} · day^{-1}) reported by Di Buono et al (15) but less than the estimated safe intakes (25 mg · kg^{-1} · day^{-1}) determined by Young et al (16) and Storch et al (17). The current EAR for protein intake is 0.66 g · kg^{-1} · day, and the RDA is 0.8 g · kg^{-1} · day^{-1}. Thus, a desirable amino acid pattern for adults includes at least 24 mg Met plus Cys per gram of protein (i.e., 19 mg/0.8 g = 24 mg/g). Mixtures of proteins consumed in the United States actually contain a higher proportion of SAAs, approximately 35 mg Met plus Cys per gram of protein. The RDA for SAAs (1.3 g/day for a 70-kg adult) is easily met in diets commonly consumed in the United States. Even the lowest Met plus Cys intakes reported in NHANES III (1st percentile; 1.87 for men and 1.4 g for women in the 31- to 50-year age bracket) exceeded the current RDA (14).

The current RDA for SAAs for pregnant and lactating women is 25 and 26 mg · kg^{-1} · day^{-1}. For infants and children, the SAA RDA is 43 mg · kg^{-1} · day^{-1} for 7- to 12-month-old infants, 28 mg · kg^{-1} · day^{-1} for 1- to 3-year-old children, 22 mg · kg^{-1} · day^{-1} for 4- to 8-year-old children, 22 and 21 mg · kg^{-1} · day^{-1} for 9- to 13-year-old boys and girls, and 21 and 19 mg · kg^{-1} · day^{-1} for 14- to 18-year-old boys and girls (14). The Institute of Medicine did not establish a tolerable upper intake level

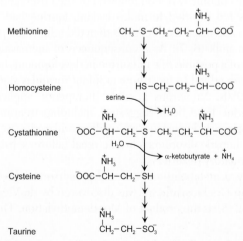

Fig. 33.1. Structures and metabolic relations of sulfur amino acids.

TABLE 33.1	METHIONINE AND CYSTEINE CONTENT OF SELECTED FOODS			
	AMOUNT		PATTERN	
	METHIONINE	CYSTEINE	METHIONINE	CYSTEINE
FOOD	(mg/100 g Edible Portion)		(mg/g Protein)	
Cheese, cheddar	652	125	26	5
Milk, whole	83	30	25	9
Egg, whole, chicken	392	289	32	24
Chicken, flesh only, cooked roasted	800	370	28	13
Beef, round, separable lean only	557	224	26	11
Wheat flour, whole meal	186	278	14	21
Corn grits, regular, dry	196	237	22	22
Oats, regular, dry	266	398	17	25
Peanut butter	292	365	10	13
Soybean, green, cooked	150	113	12	9
Brown rice, dry	142	152	19	21

(UL) for Cys or Met intake because data were insufficient for dose-response assessment and derivation of a UL for healthy adults.

Despite the availability of food proteins that provide ample amounts of SAAs, it is likely that some individuals have inadequate intakes, either because of inadequate intake of total protein or because of selection of a restricted variety of proteins that provide inadequate SAAs. Analysis of diets of long-term vegans living in California indicated an average protein intake of 64 g/day and an SAA intake of 1.04 g (7.6 mmol)/day (18); this is equivalent to an intake of approximately 15 mg · kg^{-1} · day^{-1} of SAAs and an amino acid pattern of 16 mg Met plus cyst(e)ine per gram of protein. This level of intake would meet the EAR, but not the RDA, for SAAs. Adults with higher-than-average requirements would be at risk of inadequate intake. Careful selection of plant proteins to ensure an adequate intake of SAAs may be important for individuals consuming strict vegan diets.

Mixtures of proteins typically consumed in the United States supply approximately 40% of the total SAAs as Cys and 60% as Met on a molar basis. This distribution would seem to allow optimal use of SAAs based on estimates of approximately 50% for the ability of Cys to replace Met in the diet. In cases of limited ability to convert Met to Cys (whether from hepatic dysfunction, inborn errors of Met metabolism to Cys, or prematurity), the total amount of SAAs in the diet, the balance of Cys and Met, and the adequacy of taurine should be considered.

Taurine

Taurine is not considered to be an essential nutrient because it is an end product of SAA metabolism. Nevertheless, a considerable amount of taurine may be obtained from the diet. Food taurine content has not been widely determined, but data from several reports (19–22) are summarized in Table 33.2. Taurine is present in most animal foods and is either absent or present in very low

levels in most plant foods. Relatively high concentrations of taurine have been reported for some lower plants such as seaweeds (22).

Consistent with the large range of taurine content of foods, the taurine content of typical diets varies widely. Analysis of the diets of strict vegans living in England yielded no detectable taurine, whereas the diets of omnivores contained 463 ± 156 (SE) μmol/day (23). The analyzed taurine intake of adults fed omnivorous diets in a clinical study center in the United States was 1000 to 1200 μmol/day (19). In a cross-sectional study involving 24 populations in 16 countries (24), the highest median urinary taurine levels were found in adults in Beppu, Japan (2181 and 1590 μmol/day for men and women, respectively), whereas the lowest median urinary excretions of taurine

TABLE 33.2	TAURINE CONTENT OF SELECTED FOODS
FOOD	TAURINE CONTENT
Animal foods	
Poultry	89–2,245 μmol/100 g wet weight
Beef and Pork	307–489 μmol/100 g wet weight
Processed meats	251–981 μmol/100 g wet weight
Seafood	84–6,614 μmol/100 g wet weight
Cow's milk	18–20 μmol/100 mL
Yogurt, ice cream	15–62 μmol/100 mL
Cheese	Not detected
Plant foods	
Most fruits, vegetables, seeds, cereals, grains, beans, peanuts	Not detected
Soybeans, chickpeas, black beans, pumpkin seeds, some nuts[a]	≤1–4 μmol/100 g wet weight
Seaweeds (marine algae)	1.5–100 μmol/100 g wet weight

[a]Low reported values should be regarded as upper limits because contamination of food or methodologic interference by compounds that coelute with taurine could account for these low concentrations of taurine.

Values from Laidlaw et al. (19), Pasantes-Morales et al. (20), Roe and Weston (21), and Kataoka and Ohnishi (22).

were observed in men in St. John, Canada (192 μmol/day) and women in Moscow, Russia (128 μmol/day). The large variation in taurine excretion largely reflects the range of dietary intake of animal foods, especially of seafood.

Taurine-supplemented beverages have been popular for decades in Japan, where Taisho Pharmaceutical's Lipovitan is a favored drink. Since the 1990s, these taurine-supplemented beverages have become increasingly popular in many other countries, including the United States. Examples of taurine-supplemented energy drinks include Red Bull, Dark Dog, Monster, and Rockstar, which contain 1000 mg (8000 μmol) per 240- or 250-mL can. Clearly, consumption of taurine-supplemented beverages dramatically increases taurine intake to eight or more times the typical intakes in a population. Nevertheless, little reason exists to conclude that the amounts of taurine in these beverages have either therapeutic benefits or adverse effects.

Breast-fed infants receive taurine from their mother's milk. The taurine content of milk from lactating women was reported to be 413 ± 71 (SE) μmol/L for early milk (1 to 7 days) and 337 ± 28 μmol/L for later milk (>7 days) (25, 26). The mean taurine concentration of milk from lactating lacto-ovo vegetarian women is only slightly lower than that of omnivores (26). The mean taurine content of milk of lactating vegan women is lower than that of lactating omnivores, but values between the two groups overlap considerably, and the taurine concentration in milk of vegan mothers is approximately 30 times the level in the cow's milk–based infant formulas used before the mid-1980s (23).

Because strict vegan diets tend to be lower in total SAA content and virtually free of taurine, individuals consuming vegan diets are at somewhat greater risk of inadequate SAA status. Adult humans who consume a strict vegetarian diet have been reported to have lower plasma taurine concentrations and greatly reduced urinary taurine excretion compared with omnivores. Vegans consuming little or no preformed taurine are healthy, however, and the children born to and nursed by vegan mothers appear to have normal growth and development (23).

Nevertheless, by general consensus, taurine is considered to be conditionally essential during infant development and probably for adults in some special circumstances. Because the brain and retina of human infants are not fully developed at birth and may be vulnerable to the effects of taurine deprivation, it has been judged prudent to supplement human infant formulas and pediatric feeding solutions with taurine (7, 27). During the 1980s, manufacturers of infant formulas began adding taurine to their products, and currently taurine is added to virtually all human infant formulas and pediatric parenteral solutions throughout the world (28). Taurine is added to infant formulas at levels comparable to those in human milk or at somewhat higher levels in formulas for premature infants (19).

ABSORPTION, TRANSPORT, AND EXCRETION

Intestinal Absorption

Absorption of the products of protein digestion across the intestinal epithelium is highly efficient (~95% to 99%). Dietary Met, a precursor of Cys, is transported by neutral amino acid transport systems $B^{0,+}$ (SLC6A14) and L (SLC7A8 + SLC3A2), and as Met-containing peptides by the peptide transport system (PEPT1), across the luminal (brush-border) membrane of enterocytes. Met can exit enterocytes into the interstitial fluid through the alanine, serine, and Cys (asc) preferring system (SLC7A10 + SLC3A2). Dietary Cys is absorbed as CySH, CySSCy, and as Cys-containing peptides by a variety of L-amino acid and peptide transport systems in the small intestinal mucosa. Transport of Cys (CySH) is accomplished by the sodium (Na^+)–dependent neutral amino acid transporter system B (SLC6A19) in the apical membrane and by the Na^+-independent system asc (SLC7A10 + SLC3A2) in the basolateral membrane of the intestinal mucosa cells. Cystine (CySSCy) is transported by system $B^{0,+}$ (SLC7A9 + SLC3A1) and x_c^- (SLC7A11 + SLC3A2), both Na^+-independent systems that are present in the apical membranes of the intestinal mucosa (29, 30).

Efficient absorption of taurine is facilitated by two apical membrane transporters: the β-amino acid or taurine transporter (TauT; SLC6A6), which is a Na^+ and chloride (Cl^-)–dependent carrier that serves taurine, β-alanine, and γ-aminobutyric acid; and the hydrogen ion (H^+)–coupled transporter PAT1 (SLC36A1) that may be important only when taurine intakes are very high (31). Efflux of taurine from the enterocyte across the basolateral membrane may also be mediated by TauT (32). The intestinal uptake of taurine and the expression of the TauT in the intestine do not respond to the level of dietary SAAs or taurine (33).

The reabsorption of the taurine-conjugated bile acids secreted into the lumen of the bile occurs in the ileum, and this enterohepatic reabsorption plays an important role in taurine conservation. Apical uptake of luminal bile acids is mediated by the Na^+-dependent bile acid transporter ASBT (SLC10A2) in the distal ileum, whereas efflux across the basolateral membrane may result from the heterodimeric organic solute transporter Ostα-Ostβ (34).

Blood Transport and Intracellular Forms

The small intestinal cells use dietary SAAs for protein and glutathione (GSH) synthesis and also have the capacity for SAA catabolism (35). Amino acids enter the plasma and circulate as free amino acids until they are removed by tissues. The disulfide forms of Cys (protein-bound Cys, PSSCy, and cystine, CySSCy) dominate in the more oxidized extracellular environment. The plasma membranes of cells in tissues have various amino acids transporters, similar to those in the small intestine, that take up Cys from the plasma. System x_c^- is up-regulated in response to oxidative stress or amino acid deficiency and allows uptake of more cystine to facilitate GSH and protein synthesis (36–38).

The liver removes a substantial proportion of the SAAs from the portal circulation and uses them for synthesis of protein and GSH or for catabolism to taurine and sulfate. GSH is exported into plasma, and this Cys-containing tripeptide as well as its metabolites, CysGly and γ-GluCys, can be a source of Cys to tissues. Most of the Cys in cells exists in peptide (GSH) or polypeptide/protein forms. For free Cys, the thiol form of Cys (CySH) dominates intracellularly.

Plasma Hcy levels are normally low because Hcy is not normally present in the diet and only very small amounts are normally released from tissues into the plasma. Intracellularly, low concentrations of Hcy are present in free (HcySH) and protein-bound (PSSHcy) forms. Extracellularly, Hcy is present predominantly as mixed disulfides of Hcy with protein (PSSHcy) or Cys (HcySSCy).

Physiologic and Genetic Factors Influencing Use or Production of Cysteine, Homocysteine, and Taurine

Cyst(e)ine Transport

Cys uptake can be diminished and its loss from the plasma increased by defects in cystine transport. Cystinuria is an inherited disorder of cystine and dibasic amino acid transport by the system $b^{0,+}$ transporter that is expressed by the kidney and small intestine (39–41). Because other intestinal amino acid and peptide transporters are not affected, these amino acids are generally absorbed from the intestine in sufficient amounts. The defect in the renal transporter results in elevated levels of lysine, ornithine, arginine, and cystine in the urine, however, because of the lack of reabsorption of these amino acids by the proximal tubular cells of the kidney (42). The major complication of cystinuria is the formation of cystine kidney stones because cystine is a highly insoluble amino acid with an aqueous solubility limit of 250 mg/L (1 mmol/L).

In another genetic disorder of cystine transport, cystinosis, cystine reutilization is prevented, and this leads to the accumulation of cystine in lysosomes. In cystinosis, mutations in the gene for cystinosin give rise to the lack of a functional lysosomal cystine transporter (43). This situation causes cystine from degraded proteins to accumulate inside the lysosomes of cells and leads to tissue damage. Malfunctioning kidneys and corneal crystals are the main initial features of the disorder. Patients with cystinosis are usually treated by administration of the thiol cysteamine to reduce intracellular cystine. Cysteamine enters the lysosome and reacts with cystine to form Cys and a Cys-cysteamine disulfide, which are both able to leave the lysosome through other transport systems.

Methionine Metabolism to Homocysteine and Cysteine

Because Cys can be synthesized in the body from Met (Hcy) sulfur and serine, Cys levels can be affected by Met intake and by various factors that influence Met metabolism, including the pathways for Met transmethylation, Hcy remethylation, and Hcy transsulfuration, which are summarized in Figure 33.2. Met is metabolized

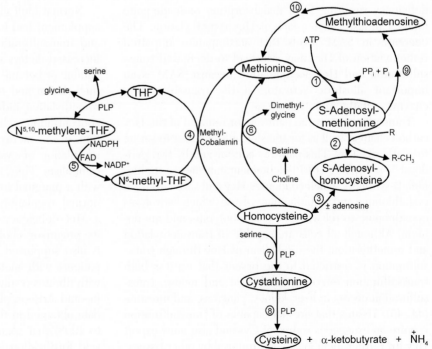

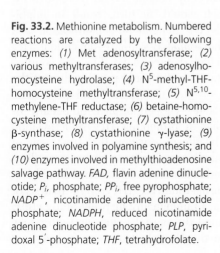

Fig. 33.2. Methionine metabolism. Numbered reactions are catalyzed by the following enzymes: *(1)* Met adenosyltransferase; *(2)* various methyltransferases; *(3)* adenosylhomocysteine hydrolase; *(4)* N^5-methyl-THF-homocysteine methyltransferase; *(5)* $N^{5,10}$-methylene-THF reductase; *(6)* betaine-homocysteine methyltransferase; *(7)* cystathionine β-synthase; *(8)* cystathionine γ-lyase; *(9)* enzymes involved in polyamine synthesis; and *(10)* enzymes involved in methylthioadenosine salvage pathway. *FAD,* flavin adenine dinucleotide; P_i, phosphate; PP_i, free pyrophosphate; $NADP^+$, nicotinamide adenine dinucleotide phosphate; *NADPH,* reduced nicotinamide adenine dinucleotide phosphate; *PLP,* pyridoxal 5′-phosphate; *THF,* tetrahydrofolate.

by formation of S-adenosylmethionine (SAM), transfer of the methyl group to various substrates forming S-adenosylhomocysteine (SAH), and the hydrolysis of SAH to form Hcy. Thus, Hcy formation depends on Met intake and on the regulation and function of the Met transmethylation pathway that leads to Hcy formation. The liver is uniquely able to respond to elevated intake or plasma concentration of Met with increased SAM formation because hepatocytes express a liver-specific high Michaelis-Menten constant (K_m) isozyme of Met adenosyltransferase that is encoded by the gene *MAT1A*. Other tissues, as well as the liver, express the low-K_m isozyme encoded by the gene *MAT2*. Although the equilibrium of SAH hydrolase actually favors formation of SAH, the reaction is normally driven forward by rapid removal of the products Hcy and adenosine. Accumulation of SAH can impair transmethylation reactions by allosteric inhibition of methyltransferases.

The Hcy generated by hydrolysis of SAH has two likely metabolic fates, remethylation and transsulfuration. In remethylation, Hcy acquires a methyl group from N^5-methyltetrahydrofolate (N^5-methyl-THF) or from betaine to form Met. In transsulfuration, the sulfur is transferred to serine to form Cys, and the remainder of the Hcy molecule is catabolized to α-ketobutyrate and ammonium. Disorders of Hcy remethylation to Met result in Hcy accumulation and reduced regeneration of Met (and hence SAM) by using methyl groups donated directly by N^5-methyl-THF or betaine. Remethylation disorders may result from genetic mutations causing a lack of functional Met synthase, a lack of functional coenzyme (methylcobalamin), or a lack of synthesis of the cosubstrate (N^5-methyl-THF). Alternatively, a lack of vitamin B_{12} or folate coenzymes secondary to vitamin deficiency resulting from malabsorption or inadequate intake can also cause a lack of Hcy remethylation. The decrease in SAM levels that accompanies impaired remethylation of Hcy may also lead to decreased transsulfuration and Hcy accumulation because SAM is an important allosteric activator of the transsulfuration enzyme cystathionine β-synthase.

Transsulfuration is the pathway for removal of the Hcy carbon chain as well as for transfer of Met sulfur to serine to synthesize Cys. This pathway is catalyzed by two pyridoxal 5′-phosphate-(PLP)–dependent enzymes: cystathionine β-synthase, which condenses Hcy and serine to form cystathionine; and cystathionine γ-lyase, which hydrolyzes cystathionine to release Cys, α-ketobutyrate, and ammonium. Although all cells are capable of transmethylation and remethylation, the catabolism of Hcy through transsulfuration is restricted to the tissues that express both transsulfuration enzymes. In the rat and mouse, transsulfuration occurs in liver, kidney, pancreas, and intestine (44, 45). Tissues that are not capable of transsulfuration require an exogenous source of Cys and also must export Hcy for further metabolism and removal by other tissues.

As may be predicted, the overexpression of cystathionine β-synthase (on chromosome 21) in children with Down syndrome results in significantly reduced plasma levels of Hcy, Met, SAH, and SAM and in significant increases in plasma cystathionine and Cys (46). In contrast, inborn errors of metabolism that lead to a lack of functional cystathionine β-synthase result in dramatic elevation of tissue and plasma levels of Hcy. Lack of the second enzyme in the transsulfuration pathway, cystathionine γ-lyase, results in accumulation of cystathionine in tissues and the loss of cystathionine in the urine, but no apparent disorder. Nevertheless, a lack of either enzyme impairs the synthesis of Cys from Met (Hcy) sulfur and decreases the supply of Cys to the body.

Met intake provides the substrate for Hcy formation. At typical intakes of SAAs, Hcy formation in men was approximately 19 mmol/day, and Cys formation by transsulfuration of part of this Hcy was approximately 12 mmol/day. In men fed an SAA-free diet, Hcy formation was reduced to 6 mmol/day, and Cys formation was reduced to 2 mmol/day (17, 47). The balance of the Hcy was remethylated back to Met. A major mechanism for regulation of Hcy remethylation versus transsulfuration in response to Met or methyl group availability is the allosteric effects of SAM (48). SAM is both an inhibitor of $N^{5,10}$-methylene-THF reductase and an activator of cystathionine β-synthase (see also the chapter on folic acid). Hence, when the cellular SAM concentration is low, the synthesis of N^5-methyl-THF proceeds uninhibited, and cystathionine synthesis is suppressed, thus favoring Hcy remethylation or Met synthesis. Conversely, when the SAM concentration is high, inhibition of N^5-methyl-THF synthesis and stimulation of transsulfuration favor Hcy catabolism and Cys biosynthesis.

Normal adult subjects given a control diet with a betaine supplement had increased rates of Met transmethylation and transsulfuration (49). This finding suggests that an increased dietary supply of methyl groups in the form of choline or betaine may increase Met catabolism by transmethylation and transsulfuration. Presumably, increased remethylation induced by betaine would increase SAM concentration, which would, in turn, result in inhibition of N^5-methyl-THF–dependent remethylation and stimulation of cystathionine β-synthase–dependent Hcy catabolism. Thus, a high dietary intake of betaine coupled with a marginal intake of Met could possibly disrupt the normal regulation of Met metabolism and precipitate a Met deficiency state. The importance of betaine or its precursor choline in promoting Hcy remethylation is also supported by the observation that treatment of patients with metabolic syndrome or diabetes mellitus with fibrates resulted in abnormal renal excretion of betaine and a rise in plasma total Hcy (tHcy) (50). Analysis of data obtained in the Framingham Offspring Study (1995 to 1998) that spanned the period before and after folic acid fortification in the United States was analyzed for the association of choline plus betaine intake and plasma tHcy. During the period before supplementation, a higher intake of choline plus betaine was associated with lower concentrations of both fasting tHcy and post–Met-load tHcy, but this association was no longer present in the period after fortification (51).

Cyst(e)ine is said to have a Met-sparing effect by reducing Met catabolism through the transsulfuration pathway, and this process appears to occur with intakes of typical food proteins in which the Met-to-Cys ratio ranges from approximately 1:1 to 2:1 (52). Maximal sparing of Met is approximately 64%, as judged by observations on subjects consuming excess cyst(e)ine and minimal Met (53). The action of supplemental cyst(e)ine when it is added to an SAA-free diet or to a low-Met diet may be explained at least partially by promotion of the incorporation of Met into protein such that less Met is catabolized (54, 55). The action of cyst(e)ine, when it is used to replace part of the dietary Met, thus keeping the total SAA level the same, may be explained by a reduction in the hepatic concentrations of Met and SAM and, hence, less activation and reduced activity of hepatic cystathionine β-synthase. When the Met-to-cyst(e)ine ratio of the diet was increased from 1:0 to 1:1 to 1:3, the ratio of metabolism of Hcy by remethylation versus transsulfuration increased from 0.75 to 1.3 to 1.9 (53). Less catabolism of Hcy by transsulfuration would result in an increase in the recycling of Hcy to Met by using methyl groups generated by the folate coenzyme system (see the chapter on folic acid).

Other mechanisms of regulation of transsulfuration may also play a role in the conversion of Hcy to Cys. Redox regulation of cystathionine β-synthase may provide a means to promote transsulfuration at the expense of remethylation, independently of methylation status, when the body has an increased need for Cys for GSH synthesis. Flux of Hcy through transsulfuration appears to be increased under oxidizing conditions, and this up-regulation of transsulfuration has been associated with oxidation of the heme moiety in the N-terminal domain or targeted proteolysis of the C-terminal domain of cystathionine β-synthase (56, 57). In addition, hepatic cystathionine β-synthase gene expression is increased by glucagon and glucocorticoids and decreased by insulin (58, 59). Hormonal regulation of hepatic cystathionine β-synthase expression may serve to conserve Met for protein synthesis in the fed state and to promote catabolism of the Met/Hcy carbon chain to α-ketobutyrate, a gluconeogenic substrate, in the starved state.

Hyperhomocysteinemia

An increase in plasma tHCy could result from an increased production rate (i.e., transmethylation), a decreased rate of removal by transsulfuration, a decreased rate of remethylation to Met, or a decrease in the uptake and metabolism or excretion of homocyst(e)ine by the kidney. The last three mechanisms have been well established.

Severe forms of elevated tissue and plasma Hcy levels that also result in excretion of Hcy, homocystine, and mixed disulfides of Hcy in the urine are caused by inborn errors of metabolism that are typically referred to as *homocystinuria*. The most common cause of homocystinuria (urinary Hcy >10 μmol/24 hours) is a lack of cystathionine β-synthase activity, which is commonly associated with plasma tHcy concentrations higher than 200 μmol/L in untreated patients and has a worldwide incidence of 1 in 335,000 births (60). A second inborn error of metabolism that causes homocystinuria is a lack of $N^{5,10}$-methylene-THF reductase activity (see also the chapter on folic acid). This second condition is the major known inborn error affecting folate metabolism and the second leading known cause of homocystinuria. A third group of inborn errors giving rise to homocystinuria are those affecting various steps in synthesis of methylcobalamin, an essential cofactor for methionine synthase (see also the chapter on cobalamin). Homocystinuria results in profound disorders (including ocular abnormalities, cardiovascular thromboembolic episodes, and mental retardation) if the condition is not detected and treated soon after birth with vitamin B_6 or folate and vitamin B_{12} supplementation, betaine supplementation, or a Met-restricted, Cys-supplemented diet (61).

Much milder forms of elevated tHcy levels result in plasma tHcy values that are only mildly or moderately elevated (e.g., >14 to 16 μmol/L) (62, 63). The exact overall prevalence of mild or moderate hyperhomocysteinemia in the general population is not known, but it has been measured for various cohorts, and the disorder is relatively common. Heterozygosity for the mutations giving rise to homocystinuria cannot account for a substantial proportion of the observed cases of mild-to-moderate hyperhomocysteinemia, because of the low frequency of these mutations (<0.2%). In contrast, mutations that result in expression of functional enzymes with impaired activity account for a substantial proportion of observed cases, particularly in individuals with low folate or vitamin B_{12} intake. The most common genetic cause of hyperhomocysteinemia is the C677T (Ala222Val) variant of $N^{5,10}$-methylene-THF reductase, which gives rise to a reduction in enzyme activity (64, 65). The frequency of the C677T polymorphism varies among racial and ethnic groups (see also the chapter on polymorphisms). Up to approximately 12% of white and Asian populations are homozygous for this mutation, and approximately 30% to 40% are heterozygous (66). African Americans exhibit much lower prevalence of the C677T mutation; less than 1.5% of this population is homozygous for this polymorphism. In populations who routinely consume food supplemented with folic acid, the C677T polymorphism of $N^{5,10}$-methylene-THF reductase has less effect on the tHcy level, although a significant effect can still be detected (67, 68).

Nutritional disorders that potentially lead to mild-to-moderate hyperhomocysteinemia, particularly in individuals with underlying genetic predispositions, are deficiencies of folate, vitamin B_{12}, and vitamin B_6 (69, 70). As noted earlier, the de novo synthesis of Met methyl groups requires both vitamin B_{12} and folate coenzymes, whereas transsulfuration requires the vitamin B_6 coenzyme PLP.

Mild-to-moderate hyperhomocysteinemia (i.e., tHcy between 15 and 100 μmol/L) has also been observed in patients with renal disease. Plasma Hcy is significantly increased in patients with moderate renal failure and rises steeply in terminal uremia (71, 72). The rise in plasma Hcy in patients with renal failure is thought to result from the loss of renal parenchymal uptake and metabolism of plasma Hcy rather than from the decreased urinary excretion of Hcy.

Certain drugs interfere with normal Hcy metabolism by causing secondary functional vitamin deficiencies. For example, theophylline is a vitamin B_6 antagonist, and valproate and carbamazepine have antifolate activity. Treatment of patients with metabolic syndrome or diabetes mellitus with fibrates resulted in abnormal renal excretion of betaine and a rise in plasma tHcy (50). These drugs can cause elevated plasma tHcy levels as a result of decreased remethylation of Hcy.

Cysteine Metabolism to Taurine and Inorganic Sulfur

Metabolic pathways for Cys are shown in Figure 33.3. To some extent, Cys levels may be influenced by the demand for Cys as substrate for reversible incorporation into proteins and GSH and by the demand for producing coenzyme A, taurine, and inorganic forms of sulfur from Cys. In general, however, Cys levels in tissues and plasma appear to be tightly controlled at the level of Cys catabolism to taurine and sulfate, which is regulated by changes in the concentration and activity of cysteine dioxygenase

in direct response to changes in tissue Cys level (45, 73). Cys concentrations are generally maintained at a level that permits adequate rates of both protein and GSH synthesis. When SAA intake is marginal, preservation of Cys levels occurs at the expense of taurine and sulfate production. GSH acts as a reservoir of Cys. When SAA intake is insufficient, net hydrolysis of GSH helps to preserve plasma Cys concentrations and protect protein synthesis. Thus, the synthesis of GSH, taurine, and inorganic forms of sulfur is strongly influenced by the availability of Cys as substrate.

Taurine synthesis requires the presence of both cysteine dioxygenase and cysteinesulfinate decarboxylase, and cysteine dioxygenase activity is normally the rate-limiting factor in taurine production. Significant expression of the cysteine dioxygenase gene is indicated by the presence of mRNA for cysteine dioxygenase in human liver, kidney, and lung (74); rodents have high levels of both cysteine dioxygenase and cysteinesulfinate decarboxylase in liver, kidney, lung, pancreas, and adipose tissue (45). Implications of polymorphisms in cysteine dioxygenase have not been extensively explored, but a high incidence of clinical and biochemical features consistent with low cysteine dioxygenase activity have been reported in individuals with liver diseases and rheumatoid arthritis (75, 76).

The human liver has been reported to have a low activity of cysteinesulfinate decarboxylase (77). Nevertheless, adult humans seem to have a significant ability to synthesize taurine. In vivo assessment of the ability of adults to synthesize taurine, based on incorporation of ^{18}O (from inhaled $^{18}O_2$) into taurine, resulted in conservative estimates of synthesis in the range of 200 to 400 μmol/day (78). These estimates are equivalent to 1% to 3% of the total SAA intake and compare favorably with the mean taurine excretion of approximately 250 μmol/day observed in strict vegans

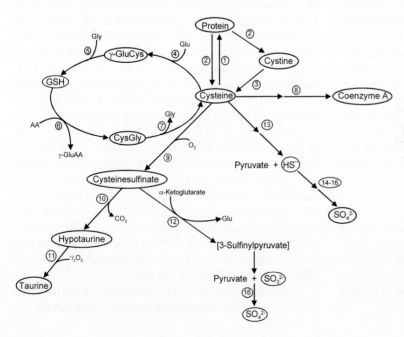

Fig. 33.3. Pathways of cysteine metabolism. Numbered reactions are catalyzed by the following enzymes or pathways: *(1)* protein synthesis; *(2)* protein degradation; *(3)* GSH-thioltransferase or nonenzymatic thiol-disulfide exchange of cystine with GSH; *(4)* γ-glutamylcysteine synthetase; *(5)* GSH synthetase; *(6)* GSH transpeptidase; *(7)* dipeptidase; *(8)* pathway of coenzyme A synthesis; *(9)* cysteine dioxygenase; *(10)* cysteinesulfinate decarboxylase; *(11)* enzymatic or nonenzymatic oxidation of hypotaurine; *(12)* aspartate (cysteinesulfinate) aminotransferase; *(13)* cysteinesulfinate-independent or desulfhydration pathways of cyst(e)ine catabolism; *(14)* sulfide oxidation by sulfide quinone oxidoreductase, sulfur dioxygenase, and thiosulfate sulfurtransferase (rhodanese); *(15)* GSH-dependent thiosulfate reductase; and *(16)* sulfite oxidase. *GSH,* glutathione; *GLU,* glutamate; *HS,* hydrogen sulfide; *CYS,* cysteine.

consuming an essentially taurine-free diet (18, 23). Thus, the percentage of the SAA intake or total urinary sulfur excretion that is represented by urinary taurine in humans fed taurine-free diets is similar to that observed in rats fed taurine-free diets (2% to 6%) (79). The similar pattern of metabolism between rats and humans seems to dispute the common statement that the rat has a high capacity for taurine synthesis whereas humans have a low capacity. It seems possible that a relatively high hepatic cysteine dioxygenase activity in humans may permit high rates of Cys catabolism to cysteinesulfinate, and that relatively high concentrations of cysteinesulfinate may allow adequate rates of taurine synthesis despite relatively low cysteinesulfinate decarboxylase activity.

Cysteinesulfinate produced by cysteine dioxygenase is also substrate for aspartate (cysteinesulfinate) amino-transferase, which transaminates cysteinesulfinate to its unstable keto acid that decomposes to yield pyruvate and sulfite. In addition, Cys is catabolized by desulfhydration reactions catalyzed by cystathionine β-synthase and cystathione γ-lyase. These desulfhydration pathways are thought to be important for the production of hydrogen sulfide (H_2S), which is thought to be an important regulatory or signaling molecule. For Cys metabolism in intact animals, both Cys concentration and cysteine dioxygenase activity change in the same direction: cysteine dioxygenase activity is low when Cys concentration is low, and the limited catabolism of Cys under these conditions is mainly the result of the desulfhydration pathways. In contrast, cysteine dioxygenase activity is high when Cys concentration is high, and Cys is readily catabolized by cysteine dioxygenase–mediated pathways to taurine and sulfite/sulfate, thus bypassing production of H_2S. The estimated percentage flux of Cys through cysteine dioxygenase–mediated pathways was 8.0% for rats fed an SAA-deficient diet and 70.6% for rats fed an SAA-adequate diet (45).

Excretion

The reabsorptive epithelium of the kidney proximal tubule has transport systems similar to those of the absorptive epithelium of the intestine, and the kidney efficiently reabsorbs amino acids from the filtrate. Renal reabsorption of Cys and Met is normally very high (>94%), and the loss of amino acids in the urine is normally negligible (80). Urinary Met excretion has been reported to be 22 to 41 μmol/day, and urinary cyst(e)ine excretion by adults has been reported as 63 to 285 μmol/day (23, 81). Thus, typical urinary excretion of these amino acids accounts for 0.2% to 2% of average daily intake.

Urinary excretion of extracellular Hcy is limited, even in individuals with defective Hcy metabolism, because of the extensive binding of plasma Hcy to proteins that limits its filtration and because of the normally active renal reabsorption of free Hcy. Of the plasma Hcy filtered by the kidney, only approximately 1% to 2% is excreted in the urine (82). Normal urinary Hcy excretion ranges from

3.5 to 9.8 μmol/day (82). Very high levels of Hcy in urine indicate an inborn error of metabolism that also causes a severe elevation in plasma tHcy concentration. For example, Hcy excretion in urine of patients with $N^{5,10}$-methylene-THF reductase deficiency ranged from 15 to 667 μmol/day (83).

In contrast to Cys and Hcy, taurine is not usually completely reabsorbed, and fractional excretion may vary over a wide range. Normally, the kidneys regulate the body pool size of taurine and adapt to changes in dietary taurine intake by regulation of TauT transporter expression in the proximal tubule brush-border membrane. During periods of inadequate dietary intake of taurine or of its SAA precursors, more taurine is reabsorbed from the filtrate as a result of enhanced TauT activity, less taurine is excreted in the urine, and more of the tissue taurine stores are maintained. The renal taurine concentration seems to be the signal for changes in renal taurine transporter activity, which are brought about by changes in TauT expression, activity, and subcellular localization (84–86).

Consistent with variation in taurine intake, and with adaptive regulation of taurine reabsorption, urinary taurine levels vary widely. Urinary taurine levels of 250 μmol/day have been reported for adult vegans consuming diets with no preformed taurine, whereas excretion of taurine by adult omnivores is usually greater than 600 μmol/day, and values greater than 1000 μmol/day are common (18, 23, 81). Daily taurine excretion of less than 90 μmol/day has been reported for individuals in Finland and Canada, and excretion of more than 2000 μmol/day has been reported for individuals in Taiwan and Japan (24).

FUNCTIONS OF CYSTEINE AND TAURINE

Cys, whether formed from Met and serine by transsulfuration or supplied preformed in the diet, serves as a precursor for synthesis of proteins and of the tripeptide GSH (γ-glutamylcysteinylglycine) and several other essential molecules, as shown in Figure 33.3. At intakes near the requirement, a large proportion of available Cys is used for synthesis of proteins and of GSH. Protein turnover and GSH hydrolysis by γ-glutamyl transpeptidase and dipeptidase result in release of Cys back into the amino acid pool. Cys is also precursor for synthesis of coenzyme A and for production of taurine and inorganic sulfur, all of which involve loss of the Cys moiety as such. The functions of GSH, taurine, and inorganic sulfur are discussed briefly here. The functions of coenzyme A are discussed in the chapter on pantothenic acid.

Both the reactive sulfhydryl group of cysteine residues in proteins and the ability of these residues to form disulfide linkages play important roles in protein structure and function. GSH is the major intracellular thiol, and the intracellular ratio of oxidized (GSSG) to reduced (GSH) is greater than 500 (87, 88). GSH serves as a supply of reducing equivalents or electrons and is involved in protection of cells from oxidative damage (see also the chapter on oxidant defenses) through reduction of hydrogen peroxide and organic peroxides by GSH peroxidases and nonenzymatic inactivation of free radicals by donation of hydrogen to the radical. GSH is an important source of reducing equivalents for the intracellular reduction of cystine to CySH. This process can occur by thiol-disulfide exchange or enzymatically by thioltransferase, with GSH providing the reducing equivalents. All these processes result in oxidation of GSH to GSSG. Because GSSG can be reduced back to GSH through the GSH reductase reaction, which uses oxidized nicotinamide adenine dinucleotide phosphate/reduced nicotinamide adenine dinucleotide phosphate ($NADP^+$/NADPH) as the oxidant/reductant, GSH plays a role in maintenance of the cellular redox state.

GSH may participate in the transport of amino acids through the membrane-bound enzyme γ-glutamyl transpeptidase. γ-Glutamyl transpeptidase, the same enzyme responsible for extracellular hydrolysis of GSH, catalyzes the transfer of the γ-glutamyl group of GSH to the α-amino group of an acceptor amino acid such as cystine or glutamine. The γ-glutamyl amino acid is transported into the cell, where the amino acid is released, and the glutamyl moiety cyclizes to 5-oxoproline, which is then hydrolyzed to regenerate glutamate (Glu). The CysGly dipeptide that is the byproduct of γ-glutamyl-transpeptidation can by hydrolyzed to Cys and glycine either extracellularly or intracellularly by dipeptidases; hence, no net consumption of amino acids occurs as a result of this transport cycle.

GSH also serves as a cosubstrate for several reactions including certain steps in leukotriene synthesis and melanin polymer synthesis. GSH is the substrate for a group of enzymes, GSH S-transferases, that form GSH conjugates from various acceptor compounds including various xenobiotics (89). These conjugates are normally degraded by the enzymes of the γ-glutamyl cycle to yield the cysteinyl derivatives, which may be acetylated using acetyl coenzyme A to become mercapturic acids, which are excreted in the urine. This process is usually a detoxification and excretion process.

Taurine has multiple functions and plays an important role in several physiologic processes, but many of these are poorly understood (90). The best understood function of taurine is its role in bile acid conjugation (27). Taurine conjugates are the major metabolites of taurine formed in vertebrates. Taurocholate is a very efficient bile acid because of the low pK_a of the sulfonic acid group, which facilitates taurocholate's ionization and, hence, detergent action, solubility, slower reabsorption, and higher intraluminal concentration. In adults, the ratio of taurocholate and glycocholate is approximately 3:1, but this ratio varies from individual to individual and with changes in the hepatic concentration of taurine. In men consuming a high-fat and high-cholesterol diet, oral supplementation with taurine (6 g/day) for 3 weeks resulted in a decrease in low-density lipoprotein cholesterol and total cholesterol (91).

Taurine also serves as a conjugation substrate for certain other compounds, such as all-*trans*-retinoic acid, and increases polarity, aqueous solubility, and, in most cases, clearance from the body. In addition, taurine is essential for two novel modifications of uridines in several mammalian mitochondrial (mt) tRNAs (5-taurinomethyl-2-thiouridine in mt tRNAs for lysine, glutamine and Glu, and 5-taurinomethyl-uridine in mt tRNAs for tryptophan and leucine) (92). These modified uridines are found at the anticodon wobble position in the tRNAs, and mutations causing a lack of these taurine modifications are found in patients with the mitochondrial encephalomyopathies mitochondrial myopathy, encephalopathy, lactic acidosis, and stroke (MELAS) and myoclonic epilepsy with ragged red fibers (MERRF) (93).

Taurine is present in high concentrations in many human tissues (~25 μmol/g wet weight in retina and leukocytes), and several physiologic actions of taurine in various tissues have been studied (27, 85). Unfortunately, these actions are not well understood despite several decades of intensive work (7, 21, 40). Taurine is involved in osmoregulation and is an important organic osmolyte (94). The movement of taurine, as well as electrolytes, into or out of the cell is a major contributor to the volume regulation that accompanies an osmotic insult. Some of the actions of taurine may be caused by activation of osmotic-linked signaling pathways, such as enhanced gene expression, changes in the phosphorylation status of proteins, or cytoskeletal changes (95, 96).

Taurine has an antioxidant effect, as judged by its ability to decrease the accumulation of oxidative markers (protein carbonyls or thiobarbituric acid reactive substances such as malondialdehyde that form during lipid peroxidation) and by the decrease in taurine in tissues of aged or diabetic animals (97, 98). The mechanism of this antioxidant effect of taurine is not clear. Taurine may minimize lipid peroxidation through its membrane-stabilizing activity or through its modulation of intracellular calcium (Ca^{2+}) homeostasis and involvement in phospholipid-Ca^{2+} interactions. Taurine directly acts as an antioxidant in the removal of hypochlorite (HOCl), a strong oxidant generated from peroxide and chloride by myeloperoxidase in activated neutrophils. The taurine chloramine thus formed is released from the neutrophils. Taurine chloramine acts as a potent anti-inflammatory agent.

Taurine is clearly involved in development. Substantial evidence supports a crucial role of taurine during the prenatal and postnatal development of the central nervous and visual systems. The specific manner in which taurine participates in these events is not clear, although taurine can act as an agonist at receptors of the inhibitory γ-aminobutyric acid–ergic (GABAergic) and glycinergic neurotransmitter systems (99). In primates deprived of taurine, retinal changes, impaired visual acuity, and degenerative ultrastructural changes in photoreceptor outer segments have been observed, and changes are more severe in younger animals (27, 85, 100). Some human infants and children whose only nutrition was taurine-free parenteral infusion or taurine-devoid formulas have exhibited ophthalmoscopically and electrophysiologically detectable retinal abnormalities and immature brainstem auditory evoked responses (27, 85).

Sulfur from both Met and Cys is ultimately released as inorganic sulfur if the Cys is not converted to taurine. In the desulfhydration pathways of Cys catabolism (pathways catalyzed by the two transsulfuration enzymes, cystathionine β-synthase and cystathionine γ-lyase), the thiol group is cleaved from the carbon chain before sulfur oxidation, thus giving rise to H_2S (mainly hydrogen sulfide anion [HS^-]). These reactions may be critical for provision of reduced sulfur because mammals do not have the ability to reduce sulfate or sulfite to thiosulfate or sulfide. Reduced sulfur can be stored as bound sulfane sulfur (e.g., $R-[S]_n-SH$) is tissues and released when needed (101). H_2S appears to be a major physiologic endothelial-derived relaxing factor, which may signal by S-sulfhydration of proteins (i.e., formation of CyS-SH persulfide residues) and lead to the opening of potassium adenosine triphosphate (K_{ATP}) channels (102, 103). H_2S also appears to serve a regulatory signaling role in the nervous system (104) and the body's defense systems (105). The sulfur of Cys is also essential as a source of unoxidized sulfur for synthesis of iron-sulfur clusters for iron-sulfur proteins, for modification of specific uridine residues in tRNAs (thiouridine), and for molybdopterin coenzyme biosynthesis (106, 107). For these processes, the mitochondrial cysteine desulfurase (iron-sulfur cluster synthetase, NFS1) removes the sulfur from cysteine and presents it as an enzyme-bound persulfide for delivery to sulfur-accepting proteins that commit the sulfur to various synthetic pathways.

Sulfide is oxidized to thiosulfate (inner sulfur), sulfite, and finally sulfate by a series of reactions, whereas sulfite is oxidized to sulfate by sulfite oxidase. Most of the inorganic sulfur is eventually oxidized to sulfate, and most of the sulfur from SAA intake is eventually excreted in the urine as sulfate. In the cell, an activated form of sulfate, 3′-phospho-5′-phosphosulfate (PAPS), serves as the substrate for a variety of sulfotransferase reactions. Many structural compounds are sulfated; in particular, the oligosaccharide chains of proteoglycans contain many sulfated sugar residues. Tyrosine residues in certain secreted and integral membrane proteins undergo sulfation as a posttranslational modification. In addition, many compounds of both endogenous and exogenous origin are excreted as sulfoesters; sulfoesters of steroid hormones and of the drug acetaminophen are examples. Inorganic sulfur is largely obtained from the metabolism of Cys in the body, and sulfur as such is not considered as an essential inorganic nutrient in the diet. Nevertheless, animal studies suggested that dietary inorganic sulfate may improve growth, feed efficiency, and sulfation of cartilage proteoglycans when SAA intake is insufficient (108).

ASSESSMENT OF SULFUR AMINO ACID STATUS

SAA adequacy has generally been assessed by measures of nitrogen balance or growth. Although growth and nitrogen balance have been used to define the nutritional requirements for amino acids, they are not necessarily good indicators of whether SAA intake is sufficient for optimal rates of production of GSH, inorganic sulfur, or taurine.

Adult human subjects remain in sulfur balance with approximately 14 to 28 mmol of sulfur equivalents excreted per day, primarily as inorganic sulfate. In studies of children and adults, free sulfate accounted for approximately 77% to 92%, ester sulfate for approximately 7% to 9%, taurine for approximately 2% to 6%, and cyst(e)ine for approximately 0.6% to 0.7% of the total urinary sulfur excretion. Because dietary taurine intake can be quite variable, taurine excretion can vary greatly. Other sulfur-containing compounds found in urine in trace amounts (<0.2% of total sulfur) include Met, Hcy, cystathionine, N-acetylcysteine, mercaptolactate, mercaptoacetate, thiosulfate, and thiocyanate (81, 109). Nakamura et al (110), in a study of young Japanese women, found that free sulfate, but not ester sulfate or taurine, was significantly correlated with urea excretion. This finding suggests that free sulfate excretion is a good index of SAA intake.

Normal Plasma Levels of Cysteine, Homocysteine, and Taurine

Normal values for plasma total Cys (tCys), GSH, and related aminothiols are shown in Figure 33.4. Cys is the major plasma thiol; tHcy is present at 10% or less of the concentration for tCys, and total GSH (tGSH) is present at less than 1% of the tCys concentration. Both Cys and Hcy are predominantly present as protein-bound disulfides, with intermediate concentrations of disulfides (predominantly CySSCy and HcySSCy) and with very low concentrations of free thiols. More than half of the plasma tGSH is present in the free thiol form. The Cys-containing peptides derived from GSH turnover, cysteinylglycine (CysGly) and γ-glutamylcysteine (γGluCys), are also present in plasma and tissues.

Mean plasma tCys concentrations in healthy adults range from approximately 220 to 320 μmol/L (111–114). Mean plasma tHcy was 11.9 μmol/L (median, 11.6), with a range of 3.5 to 66.8 μmol/L in 1160 subjects 67 to 95 years old (69). This assessment was done in Framingham Heart Study cohort survivors in 1988 and 1989 before folic acid fortification in the United States (69). Mean plasma tHcy is slightly less for younger than for older adults and for women than for men (62, 115–117).

The diagnosis of hyperhomocysteinemia is based on acceptance of a cutoff value, but no specific established cutoff points have been established for normal plasma Hcy. Use of 90th percentile values as cutoffs resulted in use of plasma tHcy values higher than 14 to 16 μmol/L as indicators of hyperhomocysteinemia before folic acid fortification (62, 63). A lower cutoff for the normal range

	Reduced		Oxidized			Total	Reduced/Total Ratio
			Free		Protein-Bound		
Cysteine	CySH	14	RSSCy	88	PSSCy	196	250	0.056
Cysteinylglycine	HSCyGly	4	RSSCyGly	5	PSSCyGly	18	29	0.14
Homocysteine	HcySH	0.05	RSSHcy	1	PSSHcy	10	11	0.0045
Glutathione	GSH	4	RSSG	1.5	PSSG	1.6	6	0.67
γ-Glutamylcysteine	γ-GluCySH	0.6	RSSCyGlu	2	PSCyGlu	1	3	0.20

Fig. 33.4. Concentrations of various forms of the major aminothiols in human plasma. The designation RSH is used to represent the reduced thiol form, RSSR or RSSR' is used to represent the disulfide of the thiol with itself or another thiol, and PSSR is used to represent protein-bound disulfides. *PS*, sulfhydryl group of cysteinyl residue in protein; *RS*, unspecified thiol, usually CySH in plasma. Mean values for plasma aminothiols are based on the data of Mansoor et al. (111, 113) and Andersson et al. (112).

may be appropriate, however, because the frequency distribution of plasma tHcy concentrations is positively skewed, and improved vitamin status can decrease the 90% cutoff value by 20% to 25% (117, 118). For folate-supplemented populations (food or supplements), Refsum et al (117) suggested upper reference limits of 12 μmol/L for adults (15 to 65 years of age), with a lower cutoff for children (8 μmol/L) and a higher cutoff for elderly persons (16 μmol/L). Homocysteinemia has been classified according to plasma tHcy levels as moderate (15 to 30 μmol/L), intermediate (>30 to 100 μmol/L), or severe (>100 μmol/L) (117), and such a classification should be helpful in determining appropriate treatment.

A wide range of plasma taurine concentrations has been reported for human subjects. Trautwein and Hayes (119) reviewed values reported in the literature and found that the reported mean plasma concentration of taurine in human subjects ranged from 39 to 116 μmol/L. Whole blood taurine ranged between 160 and 320 μmol/L, with a mean of 225 μmol/L in a small sample of adults (119). Plasma taurine concentrations change more rapidly in response to changes in taurine intake than do whole blood concentrations, and whole blood taurine concentrations are not correlated with plasma taurine concentrations, except during periods of depletion or excess intake. Plasma taurine concentrations are somewhat lower in vegans than in omnivores and somewhat lower in girls and women than in boys and men (18, 23). The urinary taurine level can be used as an indicator of adequate taurine status because taurine excretion increases as plasma taurine concentration or taurine intake or biosynthesis increases.

Measurement of Aminothiols and Taurine

The protein binding and redox status of different plasma aminothiols are interactive as a result of presumed ongoing redox cycling and disulfide exchange reactions.

For example, Hcy displaces protein-bound Cys or CysGly (113). After ingestion of a Met load or of a protein-containing meal, protein-bound Cys tends to decrease, probably because of displacement of protein-bound Cys by Hcy (111, 114). Such redistributions make it difficult to measure specific forms of Cys or Hcy accurately, so measures of tHcy or tCys are generally used in clinical studies. Food intake can affect the total levels of aminothiols and taurine in plasma, particularly if protein-rich meals or taurine-rich foods are consumed.

Careful handling of blood samples is essential for measurement of plasma concentrations of aminothiols and taurine. Blood should be rapidly cooled and centrifuged in a refrigerated centrifuge to prevent alteration of aminothiol and taurine levels resulting from transport in or out of blood cells or SAA metabolism within blood cells to alter the concentrations of these compounds (120). Hemolysis or contamination of the plasma fraction with platelets or white cells interferes with accurate analysis of plasma taurine or plasma GSH because the concentrations of both taurine and GSH are higher in the cellular fraction of blood (119). Once plasma has been obtained, tHcy, tCys, and taurine levels will be stable, and the plasma can be stored for several years at −20° C.

CAUSES AND MANIFESTATIONS OF DEFICIENCY OR EXCESS

Possible Causes of Deficiency of Cysteine or Taurine

Immaturity

Immaturity may be associated with a conditional requirement for both Cys and taurine (see also the chapter on nutrition in infancy and childhood). Preterm infants (<32 weeks' gestation) have a low capacity for transsulfuration (low cystathionine γ-lyase activity), low plasma Cys concentrations, elevated plasma cystathionine concentrations, and a low rate of GSH synthesis from Met in erythrocytes (121, 122). These observations all suggest that transsulfuration may be insufficient to meet the Cys requirements of the very premature infant. Full-term, formula-fed infants have also been observed to have high cystathionine and low taurine levels in urine, a finding that suggests a limited capacity for transsulfuration even in term infants (123).

In addition to a limited capacity to convert Met to Cys and hence to taurine (low synthetic rate), several other characteristics of premature infants contribute to the conditional requirement of these children for taurine or Cys (7, 85). First, the premature infant may have a greater requirement for Cys because of more rapid growth and for taurine because of a likely role of taurine in development of the nervous and visual systems. The brain and retina of developing animals have high taurine concentrations, and morphologic and functional impairments have been observed in animals deprived of taurine during development. Second, premature infants are born with lower stores of taurine than are mature infants. Third, the β-amino acid transport system (TauT) in the immature kidney does not adapt to poor taurine status by increasing reabsorption of taurine. The urinary taurine content of premature neonates is markedly elevated, with a fractional excretion ranging from 38% to 60% compared with a fractional excretion lower than 10% in term infants. Premature infants who received parenteral nutrition solutions devoid of taurine had high urinary taurine excretion rates despite very low plasma taurine values (84, 124, 125). By contrast, term neonates given a taurine-deficient parenteral nutrition solution can maintain plasma taurine concentrations by increased renal reabsorption of taurine, with as little as 1% of the filtered taurine load being excreted.

Hepatic Dysfunction

Because liver is the major site for transsulfuration and taurine synthesis, hepatic dysfunction can have adverse effects on SAA status. Investigators found that patients with advanced forms of liver dysfunction or cirrhosis had low plasma taurine, Cys, and GSH concentrations; an elevated plasma cystathionine concentration; decreased urinary taurine excretion; and an increased urinary excretion of Cys and cystathionine (126, 127). These patients appeared to have a decreased ability to metabolize Met to Cys, with cystathionine accumulation; and a decreased ability to metabolize Cys to taurine and inorganic sulfate, with thiosulfate, Cys, and N-acetylcysteine accumulation.

Total Parenteral or Enteral Nutrition

Patients receiving long-term total parenteral nutrition (TPN) have experienced adverse effects on their SAA status, as a result of both the route of administration and the composition of the TPN solutions (see also the chapter on parenteral nutrition). The amino acid mixtures used for TPN solutions usually contain little if any Cys, because Cys is rapidly converted to its disulfide, cystine, which is very insoluble in aqueous solution. Taurine is not routinely added to adult TPN solutions. Hence, patients receiving TPN must synthesize both Cys and taurine from the Met provided by TPN. The synthesis of Cys and taurine from Met is restricted when first-pass metabolism by the liver is bypassed by parenteral alimentation, however. In adult subjects who were given parenteral alimentation solutions free of Cys by different routes, plasma Cys concentration dropped markedly when feeding was by the parenteral route, whereas the Cys concentration rose when feeding was switched to the oral route (128). The liver apparently removes much of the Met on the first pass when solutions are administered by the oral route such that Cys and taurine synthesis from Met is facilitated.

Even enteral feeding including taurine may be marginal for ill patients, however. In a group of hospitalized male patients receiving long-term enteral nutrition, Cho et al (129) found that, despite an average intake of 337 μmol taurine/day, fasting serum and urinary taurine levels were much lower in patients receiving enteral nutrition for 48 months than in patients receiving enteral nutrition for only 6 months. Boelens et al (130) reported that patients with multiple trauma had low plasma taurine concentrations that were increased by glutamine supplementation, a finding suggesting that supplementation of enteral formulas with both taurine and glutamine would enhance taurine status.

Drug Metabolism

Various drugs and toxins are partially metabolized and excreted by conjugation with sulfate, GSH (mercapturic acid synthesis), or even taurine. Acetaminophen, a widely used analgesic and antipyretic drug, is excreted mainly as glucuronide and sulfate conjugates; a much smaller amount is excreted as the mercapturic acid. Rats fed up to 1 g (6.6 mmol) of acetaminophen per 100 g diet experienced dose-dependent inhibition of growth that was independent of hepatotoxicity and that could be overcome by addition of Met or Cys to the diet (131, 132). Lauterburg and Mitchell (131) found that therapeutic doses of acetaminophen (600 and 1200 mg, or 4 and 8 mmol) administered to healthy adult subjects markedly stimulated the rate of turnover of the pool of Cys available for the synthesis of GSH. Patients and volunteers with prolonged ingestion of acetaminophen in doses of 2 to 4 g (13 to 26 mmol) produced a maximum of 0.6 mmol/hour of acetaminophen sulfate, compared with a total sulfur excretion rate of 0.3 to 1.1 mmol/hour (133). A marginal SAA intake accompanied by prolonged ingestion of high doses of drugs or toxins that are metabolized by sulfate or GSH conjugation could have adverse effects on both SAA status and drug metabolism.

Possible Toxicity of Cysteine or Taurine

Large doses of Cys or cystine have been shown to be neuroexcitotoxic in several species. Single injections of

Cys (0.6 to 1.5 g/kg body weight) into 4-day old rat pups resulted in massive damage to cortical neurons, permanent retinal dystrophy, atrophy of the brain, and hyperactivity (134–136). Subcutaneous injection of Cys at doses higher than 1.2 g/kg into 4- to 5-day-old mice resulted in hypoglycemia and dose-dependent neurotoxicity (137, 138). Long-term survivors showed evidence of hippocampal brain damage and impaired hippocampal-related behavior; morphologic changes in brain histology were prevented when animals were given glucose after the Cys injection (137). The mechanism by which Cys induces brain damage and whether it results from its enhanced neuroexcitatory potential or its potent hypoglycemic effect are controversial. These observations have given rise to concerns about administration of excess cyst(e)ine to humans, especially to infants. The doses used to produce toxicity in the animal studies were 33 to 83 times the mean daily intake of Cys in the United States (or 12 to 31 times the mean intake of total SAAs), however, so toxicity seems very unlikely when food is the sole source of amino acids.

Studies in rodents have also demonstrated the influences of dietary SAAs on lipid metabolism; 2% to 5% (by weight) L-cystine resulted in elevated plasma cholesterol concentration, increased hepatic cholesterol biosynthesis, and depressed plasma ceruloplasmin activity (139). Excess L-Cys (0.8 or 2% of diet by weight) did not result in an elevation in plasma cholesterol, whereas the addition of 0.8% L-Met did (122, 133). Rodent diets typically contain about 6 g total SAAs per kilogram (0.6% by weight), so the levels of cystine that negatively affect blood lipids was three to eight times the typical level of total SAAs in rodent diets.

Sturman and Messing (140) found no evidence of adverse effects of prolonged feeding of high-taurine diets ($\leq$1 g or 8 mmol taurine/100 g diet) on adult female cats or their offspring. In fact, taurine may protect against toxic effects of some other compounds. Taurine addition to cat diets provided some protection against the adverse effects of the high level of cystine, a finding supporting a neuroprotective role of taurine against the excitotoxic damages in the mammalian nervous system (141). Experience with human consumption of taurine-supplemented energy drinks supports a low toxicity level for taurine.

Possible Adverse Effects of Hyperhomocysteinemia

Although Hcy is not provided in any substantial amount by typical foods, certain types of diets (e.g., high Met and low folate and vitamin B_{12}) can promote elevated Hcy levels, especially in individuals with genetic predispositions for hyperhomocysteinemia (51, 142). Because many studies have shown an apparent association of mild-to-moderate hyperhomocysteinemia with cardiovascular diseases such as atherosclerotic and ischemic cardiovascular diseases, stroke, and venous thromboses, hyperhomocysteinemia is considered a risk factor for vascular disease of the coronary, cerebral, and peripheral arteries (10, 11, 72, 115, 118). Additionally, epidemiologic studies have shown

associations between hyperhomocysteinemia and neuropsychiatric disorders such as Alzheimer disease (see the chapter on nutritional influences on the nervous system), developmental disorders such as neural tube defects, and complications of pregnancy such as placental abruption or infarction and unexplained pregnancy loss (12, 13, 143, 144). In populations of individuals with atherosclerotic disease, mild hyperhomocysteinemia is observed about as frequently as hypercholesterolemia or hypertension. A metaanalysis of 12 prospective and 18 retrospective studies, published in 2002, indicated that a 25% lower tHcy (i.e., 3 μmol/L lower in populations with mean tHcy of 11 to 12 μmol/L) was associated with an 11% lower risk of coronary artery disease and a 19% lower risk of stroke (145). Similarly, a metaanalysis of 92 studies with at least 1 of 3 end point measures indicated that a 5-μmol/L increase in the plasma tHcy concentration was associated with a 33% increase in risk of coronary artery disease, a 60% increase in risk of stroke, and a 59% increase in risk of deep vein thrombosis (146).

In a multicenter study of patients with severe hyperhomocysteinemia caused by inborn errors resulting in a deficiency of cystathionine β-synthase activity, long-term therapy to lower Hcy (Met restriction, B-vitamin supplementation, and betaine supplementation over a mean patient treatment time of 17.9 years) lowered plasma tHcy of most patients from well in excess of 150 μmol/L to the intermediate range (30 to 100 μmol/L) (147). This change was associated with approximately a 90% reduction in number of vascular events as calculated by comparison with the predicted number of vascular events for patients if left untreated (147). The number of vascular events predicted for untreated patients was calculated based on the historical documentation of disease progression in untreated patients before their diagnosis (61). This documentation was based on data obtained from 629 individuals in response to an international questionnaire survey of patients with cystathionine β-synthase deficiency (61). The history of success of treatment of patients with homocystinuria resulting from cystathionine β-synthase deficiency and other inborn errors of metabolism has clearly established the marked benefit of nutritional therapy to lower tHcy levels in reducing the incidence of vascular events in patients with severe hyperhomocysteinemia.

Several mechanisms by which Hcy itself may promote cardiovascular disease have been studied, but the precise role of Hcy is uncertain. Indeed, it seems likely that Hcy could act by multiple mechanisms. Some mechanisms may depend on direct effects of Hcy, such as oxidation of Hcy to homocystine or mixed disulfides accompanied by generation of reactive oxygen species, homocysteinylation of proteins resulting from reactivity of Hcy with thiol groups, or formation of homocysteine thiolactone, which reacts with the amino group of lysine residues in proteins to form N-homocysteinylated protein. Other mechanisms could be indirect. For example, a high Hcy level could lead to an elevation of SAH compared with SAM, and this change could lead to altered methylation of DNA and other compounds.

In contrast to the clear causal relationship of severe hyperhomocysteinemia and cardiovascular disease, the relationship between mild-to-moderate hyperhomocysteinemia and the risk of cardiovascular disease is uncertain (148, 149). Although early short-term studies showed an association of mild or moderate hyperhomocysteinemia and risk of cardiovascular disease, and although early short-term trials to lower tHcy levels showed some apparent benefit, several subsequent long-term trials did not show any benefit of lowering plasma tHcy levels by B-vitamin therapy in individuals with mild hyperhomocysteinemia (149, 150). Most of these large, randomized controlled trials were conducted in subjects with prior cardiovascular incidents (e.g., nondisabling cerebral infarction or recent myocardial infarction) or in subjects with increased risk of cardiovascular disease (subjects with diabetes mellitus or chronic kidney disease), and all studies involved treatment with folic acid, vitamin B_{12}, and vitamin B_6 for periods ranging from 2 to 7.3 years (151–160). In these trials, B-vitamin therapy was successful in generating a 20% to 30% decrease in plasma tHcy levels, but no significant effect of treatment on cardiovascular endpoints was observed. In fact, in several studies, groups given the B-vitamin therapy actually had worse outcome than the placebo groups (154, 156, 157). Collectively, these studies suggest that treatment of patients with established vascular disease with vitamin therapy is not an effective strategy.

The failure of the long-term randomized controlled trial of B-vitamin therapy leaves us with unanswered questions. Is elevated tHcy is a marker but not the actual cause of vascular pathogenesis? Perhaps some common undefined factor causes elevation of tHcy and increased risk of vascular events. Several studies looking at biochemical markers other than tHcy found that lowering tHcy by B-vitamin supplementation had no effect on plasma levels of SAH and SAM, plasma levels of inflammatory markers, endothelial dysfunction, or hypercoagulability (161–164). Alternatively, is high-dose B-vitamin therapy beneficial in individuals with severely elevated tHcy levels but not in those with mildly elevated tHcy levels? Perhaps high-dose B-vitamin therapy has adverse effects that offset the benefit of lowering plasma tHcy levels when tHcy is severely elevated but not when it is only mildly elevated.

Some data suggest that lowering plasma tHcy levels may do more to prevent cardiovascular disease than to reverse the progression of established dysfunction. Stroke mortality rates in the United States and Canada declined from the period before folate fortification (1990 to 1997) to the years after fortification (1998 to 2002), whereas this trend was not observed in England and Wales, where folate fortification was not mandatory (165). In a 3-year, double-blind clinical trial of high-dose B-vitamin supplementation in healthy subjects with no signs or symptoms of cardiovascular disease, supplemented subjects with a baseline tHcy concentration greater than 9.1 μmol/L had a lower rate of carotid artery intima media thickness progression compared with the placebo group, although no difference was noted between treated and placebo groups for the progression of aortic or coronary artery calcification (166). More research will be needed to answer questions about whether lowering plasma tHcy is the appropriate therapeutic target, whether high-dose B-vitamin therapy is the correct therapy, and whether reducing tHcy levels would have more value as a preventive than a therapeutic treatment.

REFERENCES

1. Osborne TB, Mendel LR. J Biol Chem 1915;20:351–78.
2. Womack M, Kemmerer KS, Rose WC. J Biol Chem 1937; 121:403–10.
3. Rose WC, Wixom RL. J Biol Chem 1955;216:763–73.
4. Tiedemann F, Gmelin L. Ann Physik Chem 1827;9:326–37.
5. Hayes KC, Carey RE, Schmidt SY. Science 1975;188:949–51.
6. Sturman JA, Rassin DK, Gaull GE. Life Sci 1977;21:1–22.
7. Sturman JA. Physiol Rev 1993;73:119–47.
8. du Vigneaud VE. Trail of Research in Sulfur Chemistry and Metabolism and Related Fields. Ithaca, NY: Cornell University Press, 1952.
9. Carson NAJ, Neill DW. Arch Dis Child 1962;37:505–13.
10. Clarke R, Daly L, Robinson K et al. N Engl J Med 1991; 324:1149–55.
11. Robinson K, Mayer E, Jacobsen DW. Cleve Clin J Med 1994; 61:438–50.
12. Steegers-Theunissen RPM, Boers GHJ, Trijbels FJM et al. Metabolism 1994;43:1475–80.
13. Wouters MCAJ, Boers GHJ, Blom HJ et al. Fertil Steril 1993; 60:820–5.
14. Food and Nutrition Board, Institute of Medicine. Dietary Reference Intakes for Energy, Carbohydrate, Fiber, Fat, Fatty Acids, Cholesterol, Protein, and Amino Acids. Washington, DC: National Academy Press, 2000.
15. Di Buono M, Wykes LJ, Ball RO et al. Am J Clin Nutr 2001;74:756–60.
16. Young VR, Wagner DA, Burini R et al. Am J Clin Nutr 1991; 54:377–85.
17. Storch KJ, Wagner DA, Burke JF et al. Am J Physiol 1988;255: E322–31.
18. Laidlaw SA, Shultz TD, Cecchino JT et al. Am J Clin Nutr 1988;47:660–3.
19. Laidlaw SA, Grosvenor M, Kopple JD. J Parenter Enteral Nutr 1990;14:183–8.
20. Pasantes-Morales H, Quesada O, Alcocer L et al. Nutr Rep Int 1989;40:793–801.
21. Roe DA, Weston MO. Nature 1965;203:287–8.
22. Kataoka H, Ohnishi N. Agric Biol Chem 1986;50:1887–8.
23. Rana SK, Sanders TAB. Br J Nutr 1986;56:17–27.
24. Yamori Y, Liu L, Ikeda K et al. Hypertens Res 2001;24: 453–7.
25. Rassin DK, Sturman JA, Gaull GE. Early Hum Dev 1978; 2:1–13.
26. Kim ES, Cho KH, Park MA et al. Adv Exp Med Biol 1996; 403:571–7.
27. Huxtable RJ. Physiol Rev 1992;72:101–63.
28. Agostoni C, Carratu B, Boniglia C et al. J Am Coll Nutr 2000;19:434–8.
29. Burdo J, Dargusch R, Schubert D. J Histochem Cytochem 2006;54:549–57.
30. Dave MH, Schulz N, Zecevic M et al. J Physiol 2004;558: 597–610.

31. Anderson CM, Howard A, Walters JR et al. J Physiol 2009; 587:731–44.

32. Roig-Pérez S, Ferrer C, Rafecas M et al. J Membr Biol 2009; 228:141–50.

33. Satsu H, Kobayashi Y, Yokoyama T et al. Amino Acids 2002; 23:447–52.

34. Dawson PA, Lan T, Rao A. J Lipid Res 2009;50:2340–57.

35. Bauchart-Thevret C, Stoll B, Chacko S et al. Am J Physiol 2009;296:E1239–50.

36. Lee JI, Dominy JE Jr, Sikalidis AK et al. Physiol Genomics 2008;33:218–29.

37. Sikalidis AK, Stipanuk MH. J Nutr 2010;140:1080–5.

38. Sato H, Nomura S, Maebara K et al. Biochem Biophys Res Commun 2004;325:109–16.

39. Palacin M, Chillaron J, Mora C. Biochem Soc Trans 1996;24: 856–63.

40. Mora C, Chillaron J, Calonge MJ et al. J Biol Chem 1996; 271:10569–76.

41. Chillaron J, Estevez R, Mora C et al. J Biol Chem 1996; 271:17761–70.

42. Sakhaee K. Miner Electrolyte Metab 1994;20:414–23.

43. Kalatzis V, Antignac C. Pediatr Nephrol 2003;18:207–15.

44. Finkelstein JD. Am J Clin Nutr 2003;77:1094–5.

45. Stipanuk MH, Ueki I. J Inherit Metab Dis 2011;34:17–32.

46. Finkelstein JD. Am J Clin Nutr 1998;68:224–5.

47. Storch KJ, Wagner DA, Burke JF et al. Am J Physiol 1990; 258:E790–8.

48. Selhub J, Miller J. Am J Clin Nutr 1992;55:131–8.

49. Storch KJ, Wagner DA, Young VR. Am J Clin Nutr 1991; 54:386–94.

50. Lever M, George PM, Slow S et al. Cardiovasc Drugs Ther 2009;23:395–401.

51. Lee JE, Jacques PF, Dougherty L et al. Am J Clin Nutr 2010;91:1303–10.

52. Di Buono M, Wykes LJ, Ball RO et al. Am J Clin Nutr 2001; 74:761–6.

53. Di Buono M, Wykes LJ, Cole DEC et al. J Nutr 2003; 133:733–9.

54. Stipanuk MH, Benevenga NJ. J Nutr 1977;107:1455–67.

55. Stipanuk MH. Annu Rev Nutr 2004;24:539–77.

56. Taoka S, Lepore BW, Kabil O et al. Biochemistry 2002;41: 10454–61.

57. Zou CG, Banerjee R. J Biol Chem 2003;278:16802–8.

58. Jacobs RL, Stead LM, Brosnan ME et al. J Biol Chem 2001;276:43740–47.

59. Ratnam S, Maclean KN, Jacobs RL et al. J Biol Chem 2002; 277:42912–8.

60. Yap S. J Inherit Metab Dis 2003;26:259–65.

61. Mudd SH, Skovby F, Levy HL et al. Am J Hum Genet 1985; 37:1–31.

62. Dalery K, Lussier-Cacan S, Selhub J et al. Am J Cardiol 1995;75:1107–11.

63. Bostom AG, Jacques PF, Nadeau MR et al. Atherosclerosis 1995;116:147–51.

64, Rozen, R. Semin Thromb Hemost 2000;26:255–61.

65. Jacques PF, Bostom AG, Williams RR et al. Circulation 1996;93:7–9.

66. Bailey LB, Gregory JF 3rd. J Nutr 1999;129:919–22.

67. Tsai MY, Loria CM, Cao J et al. Mol Genet Metab 2009; 98:181–6.

68. Tsai MY, Loria CM, Cao J et al. J Nutr 2009;139:33–7.

69. Selhub J, Jacques PF, Wilson PWF et al. JAMA 1993;270: 2693–8.

70. Ubbink JB, van der Merwe A, Delport R et al. J Clin Invest 1996;98:177–84.

71. Arnadotti M, Hultberg B, Nilsson-Ehle P et al. Scand J Clin Invest 1996;56:41–6.

72. Chauveau P, Chadefaux B, Conde M et al. Miner Electrolyte Metab 1996;22:106–9.

73. Stipanuk MH, Ueki I, Dominy JE Jr et al. Amino Acids 2009;37:55–63.

74. Shimada M, Koide T, Kuroda E et al. Amino Acids 1998; 15:143–50.

75. Davies MH, Ngong JM, Pean A et al. J Hepatol 1995;22: 551–60.

76. Bradley H, Gough A, Sokhi RS et al. J Rheumatol 1994; 21:1192–6.

77. Gaull GE, Rassin DK, Raiha NCR et al. J Pediatr 1977;90: 348–55.

78. Irving CS, Marks L, Klein PD et al. Life Sci 1986;38:491–5.

79. Bella DL, Stipanuk MH. Am J Physiol 1995;269:E910–7.

80. Paauw JD, Davis AT. Am J Clin Nutr 1994;60:203–6.

81. Martensson J, Hermansson G. Metabolism 1984;33:425–8.

82. Refsum H, Helland S, Ueland PM. Clin Chem 1985;31:624–8.

83. Erbe RW. Inborn errors of folate metabolism. In: Blakley RL Whitehead VM, eds. Folates and Pterins, vol 3. New York: Wiley, 1986:413–65.

84. Jensen H. Biochim Biophys Acta 1994;1194:44–52.

85. Sturman JA, Chesney RW. Pediatr Nutr 1995;42:879–97.

86. Voss JW, Pedersen SF, Christensen ST et al. Eur J Biochem 2004;271:4646–58.

87. DeLeve LD, Kaplowitz N. Pharmacol Ther 1991;52:287–305.

88. Meister A. Pharmacol Ther 1991;51:155–94.

89. Hinchman CA, Ballatori N. J Toxicol Environ Health 1994; 41:387–409.

90. Bouckenooghe T, Remacle C, Reusens B. Curr Opin Clin Nutr Metab Care 2006;9:728–33.

91. Mizushima S, Nara Y, Sawamura M et al. Adv Exp Med Biol 1996;403:615–22.

92 Suzuki T, Suzuki T, Wada T et al. Nucleic Acids Res Suppl 2001;1:257–8.

93. Yasukawa T, Kirino Y, Ishii N et al. FEBS Lett 2005;579: 2948–52.

94. Chiarla D, Giovannini I, Siegel JH. Amino Acids 2003;24: 89–93.

95. Schaeffer S, Takahashi K, Azuma J. Amino Acids 2000;19:527–46.

96. Schaeffer SW, Pastukh V, Solodushko V et al. Amino Acids 2002;23:395–400.

97. Eppler B, Dawson R Jr. Biochem Pharmacol 2001;62:29–39.

98. DiLeo MAS, Santini SA, Cercone S et al. Amino Acids 2002;23:401–6.

99. Albrecht J, Schousboe A. Neurochem Res 2005;30:1615–21.

100. Militante JD, Lombardini JB. Nutr Neurosci 2002;5:75–90.

101. Ishigami M, Hiraki K, Umemura K et al. Antioxid Redox Signal 2009;11:205–14.

102. Gadalla MM, Snyder SH. J Neurochem 2010;113:14–26.

103. Yang G, Wu L, Jiang B et al. Science 2008;322:587–90.

104. Tan BH, Wong PT, Bian JS. Neurochem Int 2010;56:3–10.

105. Mancardi D, Penna C, Merlino A et al. Biochim Biophys Acta 2009;1787:864–72.

106. Shi R, Proteau A, Villarroya M et al. PLoS Biol 2010;8: e1000354.

107. Noma A, Sakaguchi Y, Suzuki T. Nucleic Acids Res 2009;37: 1335–52.

108. Anderson JO, Warnick RE, Dalai RK. Poult Sci 1975;54:1122–8.

109. Martensson J. Metabolism 1982;31:487–92.

110. Nakamura H, Kajikawa R, Ubuka T. Amino Acids 2002; 23:427–31.

111. Mansoor MA, Bergmark C, Svardal AM et al. Arterioscler Thromb Vasc Biol 1995;15:232–40.

112. Andersson A, Isaksson A Brattstrom L et al. Clin Chem 1993;39:1590–7.

113. Mansoor MA, Ueland PM, Svardal AM. Am J Clin Nutr 1994;59:631–5.

114. Guttormsen AB, Schneede J, Fiskerstrand R et al. J Nutr 1994;124:1934–41.

115. Nygård O, Vollset SE, Refsum H et al. JAMA 1995;274:1526–33.

116. Rasmussen K, Moller J, Lyngbak M et al. Clin Chem 1996;42:630–6.

117. Refsum H, Smith AD, Ueland PM et al. Clin Chem 2004;50:3–32.

118. Ubbink JH, Becker PJ, Vermaak WJH et al. Clin Chem 1995;41:1033–7.

119. Trautwein EA, Hayes KC. Am J Clin Nutr 1990;52:758–64.

120. Malinow MR, Axthelm MK, Meredith MJ et al. J Lab Clin Med 1994;123:421–9.

121. Miller RG, Jahoor F, Jaksic T. J Pediatr Surg 1995;30:953–8.

122. Vina J, Vento M, Garcia-Sala F et al. Am J Clin Nutr 1995;61:1067–9.

123. Martensson J, Finnstrom O. Early Hum Dev 1985;11:333–9.

124. Zelikovic I, Chesney RW, Friedman AL et al. J Pediatr 1990;116:301–6.

125. Helms RA, Christensen ML, Storm MC et al. J Nutr Biochem 1995;6:462–6.

126. Chawla RK, Berry CJ, Kutner MH et al. Am J Clin Nutr 1985;42:577–84.

127. Martensson J, Foberg U, Fryden A et al. Scand J Gastroenterol 1992;27:405–11.

128. Steglink LD, den Besten L. Science 1972;178:514–6.

129. Cho KH, Kim ES, Chen JD. Adv Exp Med Biol 2000;483:605–12.

130. Boelens PG, Houdijk APJ, de Thouars HN et al. Am J Clin Nutr 2003;77:250–6.

131. Lauterburg BH, Mitchell JR. J Hepatol 1987;4:206–11.

132. McLean AEM, Armstrong GR, Beales D. Biochem Pharmacol 1989;38:347–52.

133. Sugiyama K, Akai H, Muramatsu K. J Nutr Sci Vitaminol 1986;32:537–49.

134. Sandberg M, Orwar O, Hehmann A. J Neurochem 1991;57:S152.

135. Pedersen OO, Lund-Karlsen R. Invest Ophthalmol Vis Sci 1980;19:886–92.

136. Lund-Karlsen R, Grofova I, Malthe-Sorenssen D et al. Brain Res 1981;208:167–80.

137. Gazit V, Ben-Abraham R, Pick CG et al. Pharmacol Biochem Behav 2003;75:795–9.

138. Gazit V, Ben-Abraham R, Coleman R et al. Amino Acids 2004;26:163–8.

139. Yang B-S, Wan Q, Kato N. Biosci Biotechnol Biochem 1994;58:1177–8.

140. Sturman JA, Messing JM. J Nutr 1992;122:82–8.

141. Imaki H, Sturman JA. Nutr Res 1990;10:1385–400.

142. Jakubowski H, Zhang L, Bardeguez A et al. Circ Res 2000;87:45–51.

143. Mills JL, Scott JM, Kirke PN et al. J Nutr 1996;126(Suppl):756S–60S.

144. Selhub J, Jacques PF, Bostom AG et al. N Engl J Med 1995;332:286–91.

145. Homocysteine Studies Collaboration. JAMA 2002;288:2015–22.

146. Wald DS, Law M, Morris JK. BMJ 2002;325:1202.

147. Yap S, Boers GH, Wilcken B et al. Arterioscler Thromb Vasc Biol 2001;21:2080–5.

148. Antoniades C, Antonopoulos AS, Tousoulis D et al. Eur Heart J 2009;30:6–15.

149. Joseph J, Handy DE, Loscalzo J. Cardiovasc Toxicol 2009;9:53–63.

150. Heinz J, Kropf S, Domröse U et al. Circulation 2010;121:1432–8.

151. Hankey GJ, Green DJ, Eikelboom J et al. BMC Cardiovasc Disord 2008;8:24.

152. Jamison RL, Hartigan P, Kaufman JS et al. JAMA 2007;298:1163–70.

153. Albert CM, Cook NR, Gaziano JM et al. JAMA 2008;299:2027–36.

154. Lonn E, Yusuf S, Arnold MJ et al. N Engl J Med 2006;354:1567–77.

155. Saposnik G, Ray JG, Sheridan P et al. Stroke 2009;40:1365–72.

156. Toole JF, Malinow MR, Chambless LE et al. JAMA 2004;291:565–75.

157. Løland KH, Bleie O, Blix AJ et al. Am J Cardiol 2010;105:1577–84.

158. Ebbing M, Bleie Ø, Ueland PM et al. JAMA 2008;300:795–804.

159. Bønaa KH, Njølstad I, Ueland PM et al. N Engl J Med 2006;354:1578–88.

160. den Heijer M, Willems HP, Blom HJ et al. Blood 2007;109:139–44.

161. Green TJ, Skeaff CM, McMahon JA et al. Br J Nutr 2010;103:1629–34.

162. Khandanpour N, Armon MP, Jennings B et al. Br J Surg 2009;96:990–8.

163. Bleie O, Semb AG, Grundt H et al. J Intern Med 2007;262:244–53.

164. Dusitanond P, Eikelboom JW, Hankey GJ et al. Stroke 2005;36:144–6.

165. Yang Q, Botto LD, Erickson JD et al. Circulation 2006;113:1335–43.

166. Hodis HN, Mack WJ, Dustin L et al. Stroke 2009;40:730–6.

SUGGESTED READINGS

Bauchart-Thevret C, Stoll B, Burrin DG. Intestinal metabolism of sulfur amino acids. Nutr Res Rev 2009;22:175–87.

Joseph J, Handy DE, Loscalzo J. Quo vadis: whither homocysteine research? Cardiovasc Toxicol 2009;9:53–63.

Refsum H, Smith AD, Ueland PM et al. Facts and recommendations about total homocysteine determinations: an expert opinion. Clin Chem 2004;50:3–32.

Sikalidis AK, Stipanuk MH. Growing rats respond to a sulfur amino acid–deficient diet by phosphorylation of the alpha subunit of eukaryotic initiation factor 2 heterotrimeric complex and induction of adaptive components of the integrated stress response. J Nutr 2010;140:1080–5.

Stipanuk MH, Ueki I. Dealing with methionine/homocysteine sulfur: cysteine metabolism to taurine and inorganic sulfur. J Inherit Metab Dis 2011;34:17–32.

34 GLUTAMINE[1]
THOMAS R. ZIEGLER

The amino acid glutamine, classically categorized as a nonessential amino acid, has become one of the most intensively studied nutrients in nutrition support research (1–9). Numerous studies in animal models of catabolic stress or intestinal mucosal injury support beneficial effects of parenteral or enteral glutamine supplementation (10–12). In addition, most, but not all, of the clinical outcome studies to date indicate that enteral and parenteral feedings supplemented with L-glutamine or glutamine dipeptides exert beneficial metabolic or clinical effects in various clinical conditions (3–9).

Glutamine is the most abundant amino acid in human blood and skeletal muscle as well as in the body's total free amino acid pool (1, 2, 11, 13). Glutamine exhibits dynamic interorgan metabolism and is physiologically important in several central metabolic processes, including use as a preferential fuel (energy source) for intestinal mucosal and immune cells (10, 13–16).

Several aspects of glutamine metabolism have direct relevance to nutrition support in clinical medicine, including strong evidence that glutamine becomes conditionally essential during certain catabolic states, when glutamine requirements in certain tissues exceed endogenous glutamine production and delivery to glutamine-using tissues (1, 6–9, 11, 13–21). During illness, skeletal muscle exports large amounts of glutamine into the blood (>35% of all amino acid nitrogen) (17–20). Concomitantly, glutamine-using tissues (e.g., the gut, kidney, and immune cells) markedly increase glutamine uptake and metabolism (1, 9, 11, 13–16). When tissue glutamine use exceeds endogenous production, muscle glutamine levels fall, followed by a decrease in plasma levels, typically as a function of illness severity (1, 2, 20).

Provision of conventional parenteral nutrition (PN) or enteral nutrition (EN) by tube feedings or oral supplements does not adequately meet glutamine requirements in some patients during severe illness (see the later chapters on EN and PN for information on methods of specialized EN and PN support). However, exogenous glutamine, particularly when given intravenously, markedly affects protein anabolism in surgical and other types of catabolic patients (1–4). In addition, in clinical randomized controlled trials (RCTs), primarily those comparing administration of glutamine-supplemented PN and EN with glutamine-free PN and low-glutamine EN, glutamine-supplemented PN has shown the greatest potential benefit in a wide range of catabolic clinical conditions (5–9).

BIOCHEMISTRY

As a classic nonessential amino acid, glutamine (Fig. 34.1) is synthesized endogenously in the cell cytoplasm from other amino acids, predominately branched-chain amino acids and glutamate (Glu) (16). Glutamine has two amine moieties, an α-amino group and a terminal amide group (1). Glutamine synthesis via Glu involves incorporation of ammonium ion, catalyzed by glutamine synthetase and driven by the hydrolysis of one adenosine triphosphate (ATP). Glutamine synthetase is particularly active in perivenous

---

[1]**Abbreviations: ASPEN**, American Society for Parenteral and Enteral Nutrition; **ATP**, adenosine triphosphate; **BMT**, bone marrow transplantation; **EN**, enteral nutrition; **ESPEN**, European Society for Enteral and Parenteral Nutrition; **GH**, growth hormone; **GI**, gastrointestinal; **Glu**, glutamate; **GSH**, glutathione; **HE**, hepatic encephalopathy; **ICU**, intensive care unit; **ORS**, oral rehydration solution; **PN**, parenteral nutrition; **RCT**, randomized controlled trial; **SBS**, short bowel syndrome; **SCCM**, Society of Critical Care Medicine; **TCA**, tricarboxylic acid

RANDOMIZED CONTROLLED CLINICAL TRIALS OF GLUTAMINE SUPPLEMENTATION

Since the 1980s, hundreds of published clinical studies in various adult and pediatric patient groups have explored the efficacy of various regimens of enteral glutamine and use of intravenous L-glutamine or glutamine dipeptides as a component of PN or given intravenously as a single agent. This chapter focuses primarily on results of metaanalysis and clinical practice guidelines that have evaluated this large amount of clinical research data, particularly rigorous, double-blind RCTs in intensive care unit (ICU) and surgical patients and in individuals with cancer and short bowel syndrome (SBS) or diarrheal diseases, respectively.

Enteral Glutamine Supplementation

Based on available clinical RCTs in adults with burns, trauma, and other critical illnesses requiring intensive care, the 2006 European Society for Enteral and Parenteral Nutrition (ESPEN) clinical practice guidelines concluded that enteral glutamine should be supplemented in EN in patients suffering from burns or trauma (dose not specified), but that data were insufficient to support glutamine supplementation in surgical or heterogeneous critically ill patients (97). The 2009 American Society for Parenteral and Enteral Nutrition (ASPEN)/Society of Critical Care Medicine (SCCM) clinical practice guidelines for adult ICU patients concluded that the addition of enteral glutamine to EN regimens should be considered in burn, trauma, and mixed ICU patients, at doses providing 0.3 to 0.5 g/kg/day (98).

Also in 2009, the Canadian Critical Care Clinical Practice Guidelines Committee concluded that enteral glutamine (0.3 to 0.5 g/kg/day) should be considered in adult burn and trauma patients, but that data were insufficient to support the routine use of enteral glutamine in other critically ill patients (99). The Canadian metaanalysis of data noted modest treatment effects with wide confidence intervals and heterogeneity across studies (99). Although this report noted no safety issues, it found a large treatment effect with respect to reduced length in hospital stay, but with highly skewed data, and stated that the available studies were all single-center trials with a low likelihood of reproducibility in other settings (99).

In an RCT of 41 adult burn patients, 19 received enteral L-glutamine (26 g/day) by feeding tube and 22 received an isonitrogenous mixture of aspartic acid, asparagine, and glycine with EN (100). Positive blood cultures were significantly more frequent in controls than in glutamine-treated patients (threefold), and the mortality rate was significantly lower in the glutamine versus the control group (100). A large multicenter trial is under way to confirm these findings. Zhou et al (101) studied enteral alanyl-glutamine (0.35 g glutamine/kg/day)

versus placebo in 40 adult burn patients given isonitrogenous, isocaloric tube feedings and found that glutamine decreased intestinal permeability to sugar markers (an index of gut barrier function), improved wound healing, and decreased hospital costs. Similar positive results were reported in another Chinese trial of 47 severely burned patients given enteral glutamine (0.5 g/kg/day) for 14 days versus placebo (102).

Houdijk et al (103) performed an RCT in 72 adult trauma patients who received isonitrogenous, isocaloric tube feeds containing 3.5 g glutamine/100 g protein (isonitrogenous control) versus 30.5 g glutamine/100 g protein. Five of 29 (17%) of the glutamine-supplemented patients had pneumonia compared with 14 of 31 (45%) of the control patients ($p < .02$). Bacteremia occurred in 2 (7%) patients in the glutamine group and in 13 (42%) in the control group ($p < .005$). One patient in the glutamine group developed clinical sepsis compared with 8 (26%) control patients ($p < .02$) (103).

In an RCT of medical ICU patients provided enteral tube feeding with L-glutamine (12 to 18 g/day) versus isonitrogenous glycine (control group, 2 to 3 g glutamine/day), Jones et al (104) reported no differences between groups in morbidity or mortality, but hospital costs were lower in the glutamine group. In a large ($N = 363$) RCT of critically ill patients requiring mechanical ventilation, Hall et al (105) found no differences in infection rates, hospital mortality, or 6-month mortality in patients receiving a median L-glutamine dose of 19 g/day versus those receiving isonitrogenous glycine as the control, primarily by tube feedings. It is possible that differences in clinical outcome between these studies are related to the dose of enteral glutamine used or clinical characteristics of the patients. In a small unblinded study of adult ICU patients with severe trauma requiring resuscitation for shock, enteral L-glutamine (0.5 g/kg/day) added to tube feedings was found to be safe and was associated with improved EN tolerance as compared with controls given isonitrogenous unsupplemented tube feedings (106).

In mechanically ventilated adult patients with clinical evidence of hypoperfusion or sepsis, Heyland et al (107) conducted a pilot dose-finding, 2 × 2 RCT of enteral L-glutamine (30 g/day) combined with parenteral L-alanyl-L-glutamine dipeptide (0.35 g/kg/day), the glutamine regimen combined with antioxidants (parenteral selenium and enteral selenium, β-carotene, vitamin E, and vitamin C), the antioxidant regimen alone, or placebo (107). The glutamine-supplemented and other treatments were given independently of the EN or PN prescribed by the primary physicians and were found to be safe; these data have informed a large ($N = 1200$) well-powered multicenter trial with study sites in Canada, the United States, and Europe that is nearing completion (107). This study will define the utility of enteral plus parenteral glutamine supplementation in adult critical illness.

Several double-blind RCTs of enteral glutamine have been conducted in critically ill neonates and infants, and the results of these have been summarized in comprehensive reviews (108, 109). In a single-center study by Neu et al (110), in 68 very low birth weight neonates, L-glutamine supplementation of infant formula from day 3 to 30 of life (≤0.31 g/kg/day) decreased hospital-acquired sepsis without a change in length of stay, growth parameters, or morbidity as compared with control infants who received unsupplemented formula. However, in a larger 20-center RCT of 649 infants with birth weight between 500 and 1250 g who were given L-glutamine (0.3 g/kg/day) versus water placebo in enteral feedings, no differences were noted in infectious complications, retinopathy of prematurity, growth, length of hospital stay, or mortality, although the glutamine-treated infants showed improved indexes of GI tract function and less severe neurologic sequelae than controls (111).

In another RCT of very low birth weight neonates, van den Berg et al (112) found that L-glutamine supplementation to a goal of 0.3 g/kg/day, versus isonitrogenous alanine, did not improve feeding tolerance or short-term outcome in these infants, but it did significantly reduce infectious morbidity (e.g., one or more serious infections). In a 2012 Cochrane report, Moe-Byrne et al (113) concluded that the available data from good-quality RCTs indicate that enteral (or parenteral) glutamine supplementation is safe, but it does not confer clinical outcome benefits for preterm infants. Several other small metabolic and clinical studies of enteral glutamine in children with various other acute and chronic illnesses, including critical illness, GI diseases, and sickle cell disease, have been performed and were comprehensively reviewed by Mok and Hankard (109). The authors concluded that, although glutamine is promising in some conditions and is clinically safe, further rigorous trials of enteral glutamine supplementation are needed in pediatric patients in general (109).

Enteral glutamine has been studied in numerous RCTs in adult and pediatric patients with cancer (82, 109, 114). The results of these studies are mixed. Some studies showed improvements with various regimens of oral L-glutamine in oral mucositis, some GI functions, and nutritional and immunologic parameters following chemotherapy or irradiation (82, 109, 114). In a systematic review and metaanalyses using Cochrane methodology to evaluate the use of glutamine after BMT, Crowther et al (115) concluded that oral glutamine may reduce mucositis and opioid requirements; however, most of the studies performed have been small, have used poor methodology, and were heterogenous in terms of glutamine routes of administration, dosing schedules, chemotherapy regimens, and diseases (115). The ASPEN clinical practice guidelines on nutrition support in cancer patients do not make recommendations regarding oral or enteral glutamine (116).

Given glutamine's positive effect on various GI functions in animal models (see Table 34.3), several studies have examined the efficacy of enteral glutamine in patients with SBS. Only two double-blind RCTs have examined the efficacy of oral or enteral glutamine alone in SBS. Scolapio et al (117), in a small crossover study of eight adults with SBS who were given a high–complex carbohydrate and low-fat diet without L-glutamine (0.45 g/kg/day) during an 8-week active period and an 8-week control period, found that glutamine did not significantly improve intestinal morphology, GI transit, D-xylose absorption, or stool output.

Duggan et al (118), in a pilot unblinded trial of 20 infants with GI disease (primarily SBS) who required PN, found that enteral glutamine supplementation (goal dose of 0.4 g/kg/day; n = 9) was well tolerated. However, glutamine supplementation had no effect on the duration of PN, tolerance of enteral feedings, or intestinal absorptive or barrier functions versus controls who received an isonitrogenous mixture of nonessential amino acids in EN (n = 11).

Several clinical trials have explored enteral L-glutamine combined with a modified, individualized SBS diet and recombinant human growth hormone (GH) as a method to enhance intestinal adaptation and decrease malabsorption and thus PN requirements in adult SBS (119–124). In pilot unblinded studies of Byrne et al (119, 120), in which adult patients with SBS served as their own controls, the combination of a modified individualized oral diet designed to decrease malabsorption (e.g., small frequent feedings, use of oral rehydration solutions [ORSs], elimination of simple sugars), GH, and oral L-glutamine (30 g/day) increased sodium, water, and energy absorption and decreased fecal weight while also facilitating weaning from PN.

Two subsequent small double-blind RCTs, with somewhat different methodologies, were unable to confirm these results in adults with SBS. Scolapio et al (121) gave oral L-glutamine (0.63 mg/kg/day), recombinant GH, and a high–complex carbohydrate, low-fat diet versus modified diet alone for 21 days each in a crossover study in eight patients. No improvement in macronutrient absorption, stool volume, or small intestinal morphology was observed with the active therapy, although body weight, lean body mass, and sodium absorption each improved. Szkudlarek et al (122) provided GH and glutamine (both oral and parenteral) or placebo for 28 days to patients who remained on their usual diet. No improvement in energy, fat, carbohydrate, or nitrogen absorption or in fecal volume loss was observed, although body weight, lean body mass, and sodium absorption improved, as in the previously mentioned study.

A later double-blind RCT in 41 adults with PN-dependent SBS was performed by Byrne et al (123). After a period of clinical stabilization and dietary optimization with individualized SBS diets in all subjects, patients were randomized to oral glutamine (30 g/day) and GH placebo (control group; $n = 9$), glutamine placebo and GH (0.1 mg/kg/day; $n = 16$), or glutamine and GH ($n = 16$) for 4 weeks. Patients receiving GH showed significantly greater reductions in PN volume needs than corresponding reductions in the glutamine-alone group; however, patients who received GH and glutamine showed the greatest reductions in PN needs (123). At the 3-month follow-up, only patients who had received GH with glutamine maintained significant reductions in PN needs compared with the patients treated with oral glutamine alone (123).

Several double-blind RCTs of enteral L-glutamine mixed in ORSs or in breast milk have been performed in children with diarrheal diseases or malnutrition, or both, in developing countries; safety has been established, but efficacy has been mixed in these trials (109, 124–129). Ribeiro et al (124) studied the addition of L-glutamine (90 mmol/L) to standard World Health Organization ORSs in infants with acute noncholera diarrhea and found no differences in stool output, duration of diarrhea, growth, or other parameters as compared with standard ORSs. Yalçin et al (125) found that oral L-glutamine (0.3 g/kg/day for 7 days) decreased the duration of diarrhea but did not alter weight gain or infection frequency in children aged 6 to 24 months who had acute diarrhea. Gutiérrez et al (126), in a study of 147 children with acute noncholera diarrhea, found no differences in stool output or hydration status in those randomized to L-glutamine–supplemented (20 g/L) ORSs versus those randomized to standard glutamine-free ORSs.

In 80 malnourished hospitalized children with or without diarrhea, Lima et al (127) found that ORSs supplemented with L-glutamine (16.2 g/day for 10 days) improved intestinal barrier function (sugar permeability) compared with controls receiving ORSs with isomolar glycine, but without differences between groups in duration of diarrhea or growth. In a separate Brazilian study of 107 malnourished children, Lima et al (128) found that children randomized to oral alanyl-glutamine dipeptide (24 g/day) mixed with whole milk for 10 days demonstrated improved growth indexes over 120 days compared with control children receiving isonitrogenous glycine in whole milk.

In a study by Williams et al (129) of 93 growth-faltering Gambian infants, oral L-glutamine (added to expressed breast milk for 5 to 6 months) did not improve intestinal permeability, growth parameters, or plasma immunoglobulins compared with control infants receiving an isonitrogenous mix of other nonessential amino acids. Table 34.4 shows major clinical findings from RCTs of enteral glutamine supplementation.

Parenteral Glutamine Supplementation

Many RCTs comparing intravenous L-glutamine or glutamine dipeptides as a component of PN compared with

TABLE 34.4	MAJOR CLINICAL FINDINGS FROM RANDOMIZED CONTROLLED CLINICAL TRIALS ON ENTERAL GLUTAMINE SUPPLEMENTATION[a]

Safety of glutamine administration established in adult and pediatric studies

Apparent efficacy in adult burn patients to decrease hospital-acquired infections, length of stay

Possible efficacy in adult trauma patients to decrease hospital-acquired infections

Possible efficacy in critically ill infants to reduce hospital-acquired infections

Mixed results on efficacy of oral glutamine to decrease mucositis in patients with cancer who are receiving chemotherapy and/or irradiation

Efficacy not established as a single gut trophic agent in adult patients with short bowel syndrome (possible efficacy when combined with recombinant human growth hormone)

Mixed results on efficacy of glutamine added to oral rehydration solutions or to diet to improve intestinal functions or growth in infants with noncholera diarrhea and/or malnutrition

[a]See text for references and discussion.

glutamine-free PN have been performed (2, 4–9). The first clinical outcome RCT was published in 1992, and it showed that glutamine-supplemented PN (0.57 g/kg/day) improved nitrogen balance and decreased total hospital infections and length of stay in critically ill adults after allogeneic BMT for hematologic malignant disease compared with glutamine-free PN (50). A subsequent RCT with similar PN glutamine doses in a mixed group of BMT recipients confirmed the reduction in length of hospital stay and bacteremia, but not overall infection rates (130). Subsequent RCTs by Griffiths et al (131, 132) showed the efficacy of L-glutamine-supplemented PN (25 g/day) in medical ICU patients to improve 6-month survival and decrease hospital infections. Goeters et al (133), in a mixed group of ICU patients, found that PN supplemented with alanyl-glutamine dipeptide (0.3 g/kg/day) also resulted in improved 6-month survival rates versus control subjects.

In a double-blind RCT in 168 patients requiring PN, Powell-Tuck et al (134) compared standard PN with isonitrogenous PN containing 20 g L-glutamine/day. No differences in septic complications, PN duration, length of stay, quality of life scores, overall mortality, 6-month mortality, ICU mortality, or cause of death were observed between groups, although subgroup analysis showed that glutamine was associated with a significant reduction in length of stay in surgical patients (134).

Wischmeyer et al (135) gave intravenous L-glutamine (0.57 g/kg/day) versus an isonitrogenous mixture of glutamine-free amino acids to adult burn patients in a small RCT and found that glutamine treatment reduced bacteremia. In 2002, Novak et al (136) concluded in a systematic review that parenteral glutamine supplementation may be associated with a reduction in infectious complication rates and shorter hospital stay, whereas in critically ill patients, glutamine supplementation may be associated with a reduction in complication and mortality rates, with the greatest benefit in patients receiving high-dose parenteral glutamine.

Subsequent double-blind RCTs in surgical ICU patients in France and the United States, respectively, demonstrated that PN supplemented with L-alanyl-L-glutamine dipeptide (0.5 g/kg/day) significantly decreased hospital-acquired infections (137, 138). Based on available data from RCTs, the 2009 ESPEN clinical practice guidelines for PN in the ICU concluded that when PN is indicated in ICU patients, the amino acid solution should contain 0.2 to 0.4 g/kg/day of L-glutamine (e.g., 0.3 to 0.6 g/kg/day alanyl-glutamine dipeptide) (139).

In contrast, after evaluating the same data, the 2009 ASPEN/SCCM clinical practice guidelines for adult ICU patients concluded that addition of glutamine, if available, should be considered in PN regimens; no dose recommendations were given (98). Also in 2009, the Canadian Critical Care Clinical Practice Guidelines Committee concluded that when PN is prescribed to critically ill patients, parenteral glutamine supplementation is strongly recommended, but that data are insufficient to generate recommendations for intravenous glutamine in critically ill patients receiving EN (99).

In the metaanalysis, the authors noted that, in patients receiving PN, a decrease in mortality, a shorter length of hospital stay, and a moderate reduction in infectious complications were associated with the use of glutamine (99). Given the similar pattern of reduced mortality and infections from the majority of the studies, the likelihood that the results will be replicated in other settings was deemed to be good, and a dosing range of glutamine of 0.2 to 0.57 g/kg/day was considered reasonable (99). A more recent metaanalysis of 14 RCTS in postoperative surgical patients, with a total of 587 patients randomized, concluded that glutamine-supplemented PN was beneficial by shortening the length of hospital stay and reducing the morbidity of postoperative infectious complications (140).

Many RCTs on the efficacy of glutamine-supplemented PN have been performed in preterm and critically ill infants (84–87, 109, 113). However, a 2012 Cochrane report on the efficacy of glutamine supplementation to prevent morbidity and mortality within 6 RCTs concluded that, despite generally good methodologic quality, metaanalysis did not detect a statistically significant effect of glutamine supplementation on mortality or major neonatal morbidities, including infection (87). The largest RCT, a multicenter trial on 1433 critically ill premature infants, used a glutamine-supplemented PN that substituted 20% of total essential and nonessential amino acids with glutamine in the experimental group (86). Thus, the essential

amino acid intake in the glutamine supplemented group was lower than that controls (by 20%); this, coupled with the fact that the targeted goal of 3.0 g/kg/day amino acids until day 10 of age was not achieved, could have limited comparability of nutrient intake between the study groups (109).

In 2011, ASPEN published a position paper on the utility of glutamine-supplemented PN based on current data from RCTs incorporated in seven published metaanalyses and three Cochrane reviews, with a focus on patients with critical illness, following surgery, after BMT, in acute pancreatitis, and in other miscellaneous conditions (5). The report also summarized the recommendations on glutamine-supplemented PN in published clinical practice guidelines from ASPEN and the Canadian guidelines for ICU patients (98), ASPEN guidelines for patients with cancer (116), and 2009 ESPEN clinical practice guidelines for patients with critical illness (139), cancer (141), pancreatitis (142), liver disease (143), and GI disease (144), as well as following surgical procedures (145). ICU guidelines are summarized earlier.

To summarize the guidelines outlined in the ASPEN report (5), ASPEN and ESPEN guidelines note that parenteral glutamine *may* benefit patients undergoing hematopoietic cell transplantation (116, 141); and ESPEN guidelines note that data are insufficient to recommend parenteral glutamine in inflammatory bowel disease, hepatic disease, or intestinal failure (143, 144); that parenteral glutamine supplementation (>0.30 g/kg alanyl-glutamine dipeptide) should be considered in acute pancreatitis (142); and that glutamine-supplemented PN may be of benefit in surgical patients (145). The summary and recommendations of the 2011 ASPEN position paper, based on a comprehensive and critical evaluation of the scientific literature, are outlined in Table 34.5.

Three large RCTs on the efficacy of parenteral glutamine supplementation in ICU patients have been published since the 2011 ASPEN position paper was completed. Wernerman et al (146) gave 413 clinically similar adult ICU patients receiving conventional EN with or without PN at 11 Scandinavian ICU centers parenteral alanyl-glutamine as a separate infusion (0.28 g glutamine/kg/day; n = 205) versus saline placebo infusion (n = 208). Patients were analyzed as intent to treat and per protocol (those given supplementation for >3 days). Significantly lower ICU mortality was reported in the per protocol group given parenteral glutamine versus controls, but no change in organ dysfunction scores or 6-month mortality between groups was noted (146).

Andrews et al (147) performed a 2 × 2 factorial RCT in 502 adult ICU patients from 10 Scottish ICU centers randomized to receive PN containing L-glutamine (20.2 g/day), supplemental selenium (500 μg/day), both glutamine and selenium, or neither (control). The investigators found no effect of glutamine supplementation (intent to treat or ≥5 days of glutamine-containing PN) on

TABLE 34.5	GUIDANCE FROM THE 2011 AMERICAN SOCIETY FOR ENTERAL AND PARENTERAL NUTRITION POSITION PAPER ON PARENTERAL GLUTAMINE SUPPLEMENTATION

Parenteral glutamine administration is associated with decreased infectious complications, hospital length of stay, and possibly decreased mortality in critically ill postoperative or ventilator-dependent patients requiring parenteral nutrition.

Parenteral glutamine may be beneficial in other adult surgical patients (e.g., patients undergoing major abdominal surgery) or critically ill nonventilated patients requiring PN; however, because of heterogeneity in patient populations studied, more research is needed on specific subgroups of patients who may benefit from glutamine-supplemented PN.

The trend is toward fewer positive blood cultures with use of parenteral glutamine in adult hematopoietic stem cell transplant recipients receiving PN. The full potential benefit of PN glutamine supplementation remains unclear in this patient population because results vary in data derived from allogeneic versus autologous transplants.

Parenteral glutamine may be beneficial in adult burn patients or patients with acute pancreatitis who require PN.

Because of available data in pediatric and neonatal patients, no recommendations on use of PN glutamine supplementation can be made in these patients.

PN glutamine supplementation should probably be given early and in doses larger than 0.2 g/kg/day to be effective.

To date, no evidence indicates that parenteral glutamine is harmful. No absolute contraindications to the use of parenteral glutamine exist, but liver function tests should be monitored in all patients, and parenteral glutamine should be used with caution in patients with end stage hepatic failure or hepatic insufficiency.

Further research is needed on glutamine-supplemented PN in the following areas: specific adult patient populations, pediatric patients, use of glutamine supplementation in combination with parenteral and enteral nutrition or enteral or oral nutrition alone, efficacy of dipeptide versus free L-glutamine, timing and dosing, cost-to-benefit analysis, and further elucidation of parenteral glutamine's mechanisms of action.

Parenteral free L-glutamine is available on an individual prescription, pharmacy-compounded basis in the United States. However, the practicality of compounding free L-glutamine for use in or with PN should be weighed with the benefits that may be gained with its use.

ASPEN recommends that an FDA-approved parenteral glutamine dipeptide solution be made available for use in the United States based on the professional judgment of prescribers.

ASPEN, American Society for Parenteral and Enteral Nutrition; FDA, Food and Drug Administration; PN, parenteral nutrition.

Adapted from Vanek VW, Matarese LE, Robinson M et al. A.S.P.E.N. position paper: parenteral nutrition glutamine supplementation. Nutr Clin Pract 2011;26:479–94, with permission.

infectious complications, morbidity, or mortality, although the median duration of glutamine-supplemented PN therapy was only 5 days (147).

Grau et al (148) studied 127 adult ICU patients at 12 Spanish hospitals who were deemed to require PN for 5 to 9 days. Clinically similar patients were randomized to glutamine-free PN ($n = 68$), and the others were randomized to receive isonitrogenous, isocaloric PN containing 0.5 g/kg/day alanyl-glutamine. Intent-to-treat analysis showed no statistically significant differences between the 2 study groups, with the exception of lower urinary tract infections with glutamine. However, per protocol analysis (those who received study PN for ≥ 5 days; $n = 53$ in the glutamine group and $n = 64$ in the control glutamine-free group), showed that glutamine supplementation of PN was associated with significantly decreased rates of hospital-acquired pneumonia and urinary tract infections, without a change between groups in hospital or 6-month mortality (148). Blood glucose and insulin requirements were significantly lower in the glutamine group, a finding suggesting improved insulin sensitivity (148). In late 2011, the methodology of a large Australian prospective triple-blind controlled clinical trial was reported in which trauma patients receiving and tolerating EN will be randomized to receive either 0.5 g/kg/day of intravenous alanyl-glutamine or intravenous placebo by continuous infusion, and clinical outcomes will be monitored (149).

CONCLUSIONS AND FUTURE RESEARCH DIRECTIONS

Glutamine is a dynamic nutrient with key roles in metabolism. Numerous in vitro and animal studies have demonstrated the anabolic, trophic, and cytoprotective effects of supplementation with this classically nonessential amino acid. Glutamine depletion in muscle occurs in skeletal muscle; plasma glutamine concentrations decrease during severe catabolic illness in humans (e.g., infection or sepsis, trauma, burns), and requirements for glutamine appear to exceed endogenous production (1, 2). Taken together, existing data strongly suggest that glutamine becomes a conditionally essential nutrient under these conditions (1).

Glutamine supplementation of EN or PN support is a safe and promising approach that appears to improve the metabolic and clinical efficacy of nutrition support therapy in some patients. RCTs with parenteral administration of glutamine (>0.2 g/kg/day) have often shown superior clinical efficacy compared with RCTs with enteral glutamine supplementation (3–7). However, despite extensive clinical investigation since the 1980s on the efficacy of glutamine supplementation as a component of nutritional support, additional data are still needed to define optimal glutamine dosing and the patient subgroups who may benefit most from this amino acid (8). This information should become available in the coming years with the completion of several rigorous ongoing RCTs.

ACKNOWLEDGMENTS

I would like to thank Dr. Alan C. Buchman for his previous work on this chapter in the tenth edition of this textbook.

REFERENCES

1. Lacey JM, Wilmore DW. Nutr Rev 1990;48:297–309.
2. Ziegler TR, Smith RJ, Byrne TA et al. Clin Nutr 1993; 12(Suppl 1):S82–90.
3. Heyland DK, Dhaliwalm R, Day AG et al. JPEN J Parenter Enteral Nutr 2007;31:109–18.
4. Wischmeyer PE. Curr Opin Gastroenterol 2008;24:190–7.
5. Vanek VW, Matarese LE, Robinson M et al. Nutr Clin Pract 2011;26:479–94.
6. Wernerman J. Ann Intensive Care 2011;1:25.
7. Griffiths RD. Acta Anaesthesiol Scand 2011;55:769–71.
8. Yarandi SS, Zhao VM, Hebbar G et al. Curr Opin Clin Nutr Metab Care 2011;14:75–82.
9. Soeters PB, Grecu I. Ann Nutr Metab 2011;60:17–26.
10. Souba WW, Smith RJ, Wilmore DW. JPEN J Parenter Enteral Nutr 1985;9:608–17.
11. Souba WW. Annu Rev Nutr 1991;11: 285–308.
12. Ziegler TR, Bazargan N, Leader LM et al. Curr Opin Clin Nutr Metab Care 2000;3:355–62.
13. Wilmore DW. J Nutr 2001;131(Suppl):2543S–9S.
14. Windmueller HG, Spaeth AE. J Biol Chem 1978;253:69–76.
15. Newsholme EA, Crabtree B, Ardawi MS. Q J Exp Physiol 1985;70:473–89.
16. Souba WW, Austgen TR. JPEN J Parenter Enteral Nutr 1990;14(Suppl):90S–3S.
17. Marliss EB, Aoki TT, Pozefsky T et al. J Clin Invest 1971; 50:814–7.
18. Askanazi J, Furst P, Michelsen CB et al. Ann Surg 1980; 191:465–72.
19. Vinnars E, Furst P, Liljedahl SO et al. JPEN J Parenter Enteral Nutr 1980;4:184–7.
20. Roth E, Funovics J, Mühlbacher F et al. Clin Nutr 1982; 1:25–41.
21. Roth E. J Nutr 2008;138:2025S–31S.
22. Deutz NE. Clin Nutr 2008;27:321–7.
23. Ligthart-Melis GC, Deutz NE. Am J Physiol Endocrinol Metab 2011;301:E264–6.
24. Watford M, Vincent N, Zhan Z et al. J Nutr 1994;124:493–9.
25. Curthoys NP, Lowry OH. J Biol Chem 1973;248:162–8.
26. Lenders CM, Liu S, Wilmore DW et al. Eur J Clin Nutr 2009;63:1433–9.
27. Kuhn KS, Schuhmann K, Stehle P et al. Am J Clin Nutr 1999; 70:484–9.
28. Ganapathy V, Ganapathy ME, Leibach FH. Protein digestion and assimilation. In: Yamada T, Alpers DH, Kalloo AN et al, eds. Text Book of Gastroenterology. 5th ed. Oxford: Wiley-Blackwell; 2009:464–77.
29. Fei YJ, Sugawara M, Nakanishi T et al. J Biol Chem 2000; 275:23707–17.
30. Bode BP. J Nutr 2001;131(Suppl):2475S–85S.
31. Baird FE, Beattie KJ, Hyde AR et al. J Physiol 2004;559:367–81.
32. Leibach FH, Ganapathy V. Annu Rev Nutr 1996;16:99–119.
33. Franch HA, Mitch WE. J Am Soc Nephrol 1998;9(Suppl): S78–81.
34. Ziegler TR, Benfell K, Smith RJ et al. JPEN J Parenter Enteral Nutr 1990;14:137S–46S.
35. Déchelotte P, Darmaun D, Rongier M et al. Am J Physiol 1991;260:G677–82.
36. van de Poll MC, Ligthart-Melis GC, Boelens PG et al. J Physiol 2007;581:819–27.
37. Darmaun D, Messing B, Just B et al. Metabolism 1991;40: 42–4.
38. Smith RJ. JPEN J Parenter Enteral Nutr 1990;14:40S–44S.
39. Windmueller HG, Spaeth AE. Arch Biochem Biophys 1976; 175:670–6.
40. Evans ME, Jones DP, Ziegler TR. J Nutr 2003;133:3065–71.
41. Evans ME, Jones DP, Ziegler TR. Am J Physiol 2005;289: G388–96.
42. Häussinger D, Graf D, Weiergräber OH. J Nutr 2001; 131(Suppl):2509S–14S.
43. Iwashita S, Williams P, Jabbour K et al. J Appl Physiol 2005;99:1858–65.
44. Bakalar B, Duska F, Pachl J et al. Crit Care Med 2006;34: 381–6.
45. Thibault R, Welsh S, Mauras N et al. Am J Physiol 2008; 294:G548–53.
46. Bergstrom J, Furst P, Noree LO et al. J Appl Physiol 1974; 36:693–7.
47. Rodas PC, Rooyackers O, Hebert C et al. Clin Sci (Lond) 2012;122:591–7.
48. Stehle P, Mertes N, Puchstein C et al. Lancet 1989;1:231–3.
49. Furst P, Albers S, Stehle P. JPEN J Parenter Enteral Nutr 1990;14:118S–24S.
50. Ziegler TR, Young LS, Benfell K et al. Ann Intern Med 1992;116:821–8.
51. Hammarqvist F, Strömberg C, von der Decken A et al. Ann Surg 1992;216:184–91.
52. Morlion BJ, Stehle P, Wachtler P et al. Ann Surg 1998;227: 302–8.
53. Klimberg VS, Souba WW, Salloum RM et al. J Surg Res 1990; 48:319–23.
54. Fläring UB, Rooyackers OE, Wernerman J et al. Clin Sci (Lond) 2003;104:275–82.
55. Luo M, Fernandez-Estivariz C, Jones DP et al. Nutrition 2008;24:37–44.
56. Xue H, Sawyer MB, Field CJ et al. J Nutr 2008;138:740–6.
57. Alves WF, Aguiar EE, Guimarães SB et al. Ann Vasc Surg 2010;24:461–7.
58. Xue H, Sufit AJ, Wischmeyer PE. JPEN J Parenter Enteral Nutr 2011;35:188–97.
59. Jonas CR, Gu LH, Nkabyo YS et al. Am J Physiol 2003;285: R1421–9.
60. Singleton KD, Wischmeyer PE. Am J Physiol Regul 2007; 292:R1839–45.
61. Ziegler TR, Ogden LG, Singleton KD et al. Intensive Care Med 2005;31:1079–86.
62. Hamiel CR, Pinto S, Hau A et al. Am J Physiol 2009;297: C1509–19.
63. Weitzel LR, Wischmeyer PE. Crit Care Clin 2010;26:515–25.
64. Rao RK, Samak G. J Epith Biol Pharmacol 2012;5 (Suppl 1-M7):47–54.
65. Li N, Neu J. J Nutr 2009;139:710–4.
66. Van der Hulst RRWJ, von Meyenfeldt MF, van Kreel BK et al. Lancet 1993;341:1363–5.
67. Tian J, Hao L, Chandra P et al. Am J Physiol 2009;296: G348–55.
68. Hou YC, Chiu WC, Yeh CL et al. Am J Physiol 2012;302: L174–83.
69. Sakiyama T, Musch MW, Ropeleski MJ et al. Gastroenterology 2009;136:924–32.
70. Boukhettala N, Claeyssens S, Bensifi M et al. Amino Acids 2012;42:375–83.

71. O'Dwyer ST, Smith RJ, Hwang TL et al. JPEN J Parenter Enteral Nutr 1989;13:579–85.
72. Ziegler TR, Evans ME, Fernandez-Estívariz C et al. Annu Rev Nutr 2003;23:229–61.
73. Ban K, Kozar RA. J Leukoc Biol 2008;84:595–9.
74. Ko HM, Oh SH, Bang HS et al. J Immunol 2009;182:7957–62.
75. Fan J, Meng Q, Guo G et al. Burns 2010;36:409–17.
76. Bartlett DL, Charland S, Torosian MH. Ann Surg Oncol 1995;2:71–6.
77. Xue H, Le Roy S, Sawyer MB. Br J Nutr 2009;102:434–42.
78. Todorova VK, Kaufmann Y, Hennings L et al. J Nutr 2010;140:44–8.
79. Lim V, Korourian S, Todorova VK et al. Oral Oncol 2009;45:148–55.
80. Shewchuk LD, Baracos VE, Field CJ. J Nutr 1997;127:158–66.
81. Klimberg VS, McClellan JL. Am J Surg 1996;172:418–24.
82. Kuhn KS, Muscaritoli M, Wischmeyer P et al. Eur J Nutr 2010;49:197–210.
83. Lowe DK, Benfell K, Smith RJ et al. Am J Clin Nutr 1990;52:1101–6.
84. Lacey JM, Crouch JB, Benfell K et al. JPEN J Parenter Enteral Nutr 1996;20:74–80.
85. Vaughn P, Thomas P, Clark R et al. J Pediatr 2003;142:662–8.
86. Poindexter BB, Ehrenkranz RA, Stoll BJ et al. Pediatrics 2004;113:1209–15.
87. Mohamad Ikram I, Quah BS, Noraida R et al. Singapore Med J 2011;52:356–60.
88. Berg A, Bellander BM, Wanecek M et al. Intensive Care Med 2006;32:1741–6.
89. Berg A, Bellander BM, Wanecek M et al. Clin Nutr 2008;27:816–21.
90. Masini A, Efrati C, Merli M. Metab Brain Dis 2003;18:27–35.
91. Ditisheim S, Giostra E, Burkhard PR. BMC Gastroenterol 2011;11:134.
92. Lemberg A, Fernández MA. Ann Hepatol 2009;8:95–102.
93. Kuhn KS, Stehle P, Fürst P. JPEN J Parenter Enteral Nutr 1996;20:292–5.
94. Griffiths RD, Jones C, Palmer TE. Nutrition 1997;13:295–302.
95. Albers S, Wernerman J, Stehle P et al. Clin Sci (Lond) 1988;75:463–8.
96. Steininger R, Karner J, Roth E et al. Metabolism 1989;38S:78–81.
97. Kreymann KG, Berger MM, Deutz NE et al. Clin Nutr 2006;25:210–23.
98. McClave SA, Martindale RG, Vanek VW et al. JPEN J Parenter Enteral Nutr 2009;33:277–316.
99. Heyland DK, Dhaliwal R, Drover JW et al. JPEN J Parenter Enteral Nutr 2003;27:355–73.
100. Garrel D, Patenaude J, Nedelec B et al. Crit Care Med 2003;31:2444–9.
101. Zhou YP, Jiang ZM, Sun YH et al. JPEN J Parenter Enteral Nutr. 2003;27:241–5.
102. Peng X, Yan H, You Z et al. Burns 2004;30:135–9.
103. Houdijk AP, Rijnsburger ER, Jansen J et al. Lancet 1998;352:772–6.
104. Jones C, Palmer TE, Griffiths RD. Nutrition 1999;15:108–15.
105. Hall JC, Dobb G, Hall J et al. Intensive Care Med 2003;29:1710–6.
106. McQuiggan M, Kozar R, Sailors RM et al. JPEN J Parenter Enteral Nutr 2008;32:28–35.
107. Heyland DK, Dhaliwalm R, Day A et al. JPEN J Parenter Enteral Nutr 2007;31:109–18.
108. van Zwol A, Neu J, van Elburg RM. Nutr Rev 2011;69:2–8.
109. Mok E, Hankard R. J Nutr Metab 2011;2011:617597.
110. Neu J, Roig JC, Meetze WH et al. J Pediatr 1997;13:691–9.
111. Vaughn P, Thomas P, Clark R et al. J Pediatr 2003;142:662–8.
112. van den Berg A, van Elburg RM, Westerbeek EA. Am J Clin Nutr 2005;81:1397–404.
113. Moe-Byrne T, Wagner JV, McGuire W. Cochrane Database Syst Rev 2012;(3):CD001457.
114. Ziegler TR. J Nutr 2001;131(Suppl):2578S–84.
115. Crowther M, Avenell A, Culligan DJ. Bone Marrow Transplant 2009;44:413–25.
116. August DA, Huhmann MB, ASPEN Board of Directors. JPEN J Parenter Enteral Nutr 2009;33:472–500.
117. Scolapio JS, McGreevy K, Tennyson GS et al. Clin Nutr 2001;20:319–23.
118. Duggan C, Stark AR, Auestad N et al. Nutrition 2004;20:752–6.
118. Byrne TA, Morrissey TB, Nattakom TV et al. JPEN J Parenter Enteral Nutr 1995;19:296–302.
120. Byrne TA, Persinger RL, Young LS et al. Ann Surg 1995;222:243–54.
121. Scolapio JS, Camilleri M, Fleming CR et al. Gastroenterology 1997;113:1074–81.
122. Szkudlarek J, Jeppsen PB, Mortensen PB. Gut 2000;47:199–205.
123. Byrne TA, Wilmore DW, Iyer K et al. Ann Surg 2005;242:655–61.
124. Ribeiro Júnior H, Ribeiro T, Mattos A et al. J Am Coll Nutr 1994;13:251–5.
125. Yalçin SS, Yurdakök K, Tezcan I et al. J Pediatr Gastroenterol Nutr 2004;38:494–501.
126. Gutiérrez C, Villa S, Mota FR et al. J Health Popul Nutr 2007;25:278–284.
127. Lima AA, Brito LF, Ribeiro HB et al. J Pediatr Gastroenterol Nutr 2005;40:28–35.
128. Lima NL, Soares AM, Mota RM et al. J Pediatr Gastroenterol Nutr 2007;44:365–74.
129. Williams EA, Elia M, Lunn PG. Am J Clin Nutr 2007;86:421–7.
130. Schloerb PR, Amare M. JPEN J Parenter Enteral Nutr 1993;17:407–13.
131. Griffiths RD, Jones C, Palmer TE. Nutrition 1997;13:295–302.
132. Griffiths RD, Allen KD, Andrews FJ et al. Nutrition 2002;18:546–52.
133. Goeters C, Wenn A, Mertes N et al. Crit Care Med 2002;30:2032–37.
134. Powell-Tuck J, Jamieson CP, Bettany GE et al. Gut 1999;45:82–8.
135. Wischmeyer PE, Lynch J, Liedel J et al. Crit Care Med 2001;29:2075–80.
136. Novak F, Heyland DK, Avenell A et al. Crit Care Med 2002;30:2022–9.
137. Déchelotte P, Hasselmann M, Cynober L et al. Crit Care Med 2006;34:598–604.
138. Estivariz CF, Griffith DP, Luo M et al. JPEN J Parenter Enteral Nutr 2008;32:389–402.
139. Singer P, Berger MM, Van den Berghe G et al. Clin Nutr 2009;28:387–400.
140. Wang Y, Jiang ZM, Nolan MT et al. JPEN J Parenter Enteral Nutr 2010;34:521–9.
141. Bozzetti F, Arends J, Lundholm K et al. Clin Nutr 2009;28:445–54.
142. Gianotti L, Meier R, Lobo DN et al. Clin Nutr 2009;28:428–35.

143. Plauth M, Cabré E, Campillo B et al. Clin Nutr 2009;28: 436–44.

144. Van Gossum A, Cabre E, Hébuterne X et al. Clin Nutr 2009; 28:415–27.

145. Braga M, Ljungqvist O, Soeters P et al. Clin Nutr 2009;28: 378–86.

146. Wernerman J, Kirketeig T, Andersson B et al. Acta Anaesthesiol Scand 2011;55:812–8.

147. Andrews PJ, Avenell A, Noble DW et al. BMJ 2011;342:d1542.

148. Grau T, Bonet A, Miñambres E et al. Crit Care Med 2011;39: 1263–8.

149. Al Balushi RM, Paratz JD, Cohen J et al. BMJ Open 2011; 1:e000334.

SUGGESTED READINGS

Griffiths RD. Can the case for glutamine be proved? Acta Anaesthesiol Scand 2011;55:769–71.

Moe-Byrne T, Wagner JV, McGuire W. Glutamine supplementation to prevent morbidity and mortality in preterm infants. Cochrane Database Syst Rev 2012;(3):CD001457.

Soeters PB, Grecu I. Have we enough glutamine and how does it work? A clinician's view. Ann Nutr Metab 2012;60:17–26.

Vanek VW, Matarese LE, Robinson M et al. A.S.P.E.N. position paper: parenteral nutrition glutamine supplementation. Nutr Clin Pract 2011;26:479–94.

Wernerman J. Glutamine supplementation. Ann Intensive Care 2011;1:25.

35

ARGININE, CITRULLINE, AND NITRIC OXIDE[1]

YVETTE C. LUIKING, LETICIA CASTILLO, AND NICOLAAS E.P. DEUTZ

HISTORICAL INTRODUCTION

Arginine is a semiconditional or conditional essential amino acid, which implies that healthy adults have no specific nutritional need for arginine. In neonates, in infants, and in certain conditions, however, endogenous arginine synthesis is not sufficient to meet the requirements; this deficiency can be related to insufficient synthesis of arginine precursors such as citrulline. Beyond protein synthesis, arginine is a metabolite in the urea cycle and is a well-known substrate for ureagenesis in the liver. In the 1980s, an endothelium-derived relaxing factor (EDRF) was found in endothelial cells (1). EDRF was subsequently identified as nitric oxide (NO) with L-arginine as its precursor (2), thus enhancing the functional relevance of arginine. Investigators also became increasingly aware that NO is a ubiquitous molecule, present in cardiovascular and nervous system cells as well as in inflammatory cells, with many physiologic functions and pathophysiologic implications (3–5).

Citrulline is a nonprotein amino acid, a characterization implying that it is not used in protein synthesis. Its name is derived from the Latin *Citrullus vulgaris*, which means watermelon, from which it was first isolated in 1930s. The relevance of citrulline was long neglected because citrulline was largely seen as an intermediary of the urea cycle. This perception changed, however, as a result of work on the interorgan exchange of citrulline and the identification of citrulline as a precursor for de novo arginine synthesis (6). More recently, the identification of plasma citrulline as a biomarker of intestinal functional mass (7) and evidence of the direct action of citrulline as a promoter of muscle protein synthesis (8) have added to our understanding of citrulline's biologic relevance. Citrulline is now suggested as a conditional essential amino acid, at least in persons with disorders characterized by compromised intestinal function (9–11).

METABOLISM AND FUNCTION IN HEALTH

L-Arginine is a basic amino acid. Its structure is illustrated in Figure 35.1. L-Arginine has a molar mass of 174.2 g/mol and is characterized by a guanidino group. Citrulline is an α-amino acid. Its structure is illustrated in Figure 35.2. Citrulline has a molar mass of 175.19 g/mol and is characterized by a ureido group (10).

The metabolism of arginine and citrulline can roughly be divided into a synthesis pathway and a utilization or catabolic pathway, with interorgan exchange of metabolites (Figs. 35.3 and 35.4). Pharmacokinetic studies indicate that citrulline is relatively better absorbed and has higher systemic bioavailability than arginine (12).

Arginine

Arginine Synthesis Pathway

Arginine is mainly available from protein breakdown in the body and from food intake. The jejunum is the major site for intestinal absorption of dietary arginine. Only approximately 20% of protein synthesis is derived directly from dietary

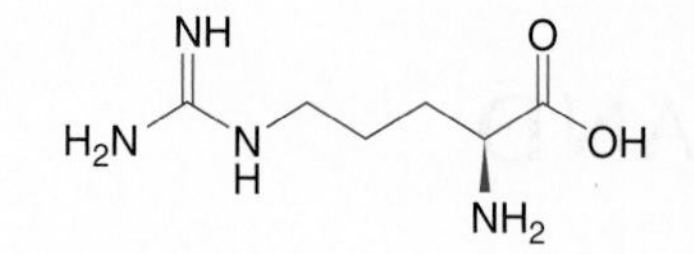

Fig. 35.1. Chemical structure of L-arginine.

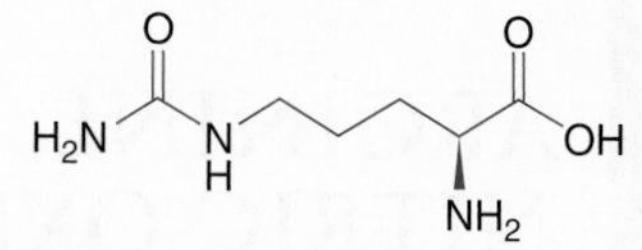

Fig. 35.2. Chemical structure of citrulline.

amino acid intake. This finding implies that approximately 80% of protein synthesis involves recycling of amino acids from protein breakdown. Moreover, arginine is synthesized endogenously or de novo in the proximal renal tubule by conversion of citrulline to arginine through a partial urea cycle by the enzymes argininosuccinate synthase (ASS) and argininosuccinate lyase (ASL) (13–16). This conversion is part of the intestinal-renal axis, as demonstrated in animal and human studies (6, 17–19). Under normal conditions, this pathway contributes approximately 10% to 15% to whole body arginine production (20, 21), in which citrulline availability is the limiting factor for renal arginine synthesis (15). In contrast to adults, the conversion to arginine in neonates is limited to intestinal arginine synthesis from dietary proline and the conversion of citrulline to arginine by the enzymes ASS and ASL (22). This first-pass de novo synthesis provides 50% of the arginine needed by neonates (23). In the postabsorptive state, whole body arginine flux in healthy adults is approximately 70 to 90 μmol/kg/hour (24).

Arginine Catabolic Pathway

Apart from being an essential component of body proteins, arginine plays a key role in several other metabolic pathways that involve various enzyme systems (3, 4, 12, 25–27), as follows:

1. The arginase pathway is quantitatively the most important. Fifteen percent of arginine flux will enter this pathway (20). This finding implies the degradation of arginine to ornithine and urea by the enzyme arginase, of which two isoforms are known (arginase type I and type II). Type I cytosolic arginase is expressed in the liver, as part of the urea cycle. A full urea cycle is present only in the liver and implies detoxification of ammonia and urea synthesis through five reaction steps to excrete excess nitrogen from the body. Type II mitochondrial arginase is expressed at low levels in extrahepatic tissues and cells (e.g., brain, kidney, small intestine, red blood cells, and immune cells) and is involved in the synthesis of ornithine, proline, and glutamate (28, 29). Through ornithine and derived polyamines (putrescine, spermine, and spermidine), arginine is important for cell growth and differentiation (30). By means of proline, which is hydroxylated to form hydroxyproline, arginine is involved in collagen formation, tissue repair, and wound healing (31). Approximately 40% of arginine that is absorbed from the intestinal lumen is degraded in the first pass (32) because of relatively high arginase activity in the intestinal mucosa.

2. Arginine is converted to NO by three isoforms of the enzyme NO synthase (NOS), with concomitant formation of citrulline (33, 34). Approximately 1.5% of arginine flux enters this pathway (20). NOS-1 (neuronal NOS) and NOS-3 (endothelial NOS) enzymes produce NO that acts as a neurotransmitter and as a vasodilator, respectively (34). NO synthesized by NOS-2 (inducible NOS) at high levels has immune regulatory functions, such as control or killing of infectious pathogens, modulation of cytokine production, and T-helper cell

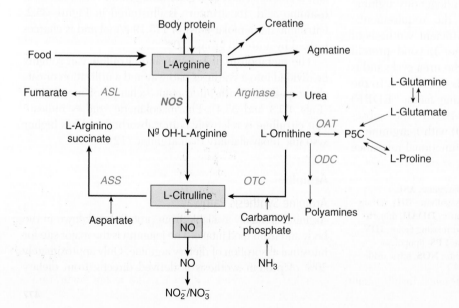

Fig. 35.3. Metabolic pathway of arginine, citrulline, and nitric oxide (NO). In this schematic overview of arginine, citrulline, and NO metabolism, arginine is derived from food, body protein, and de novo synthesis from citrulline. Arginine is the substrate for synthesis of body proteins, NO and citrulline, urea and ornithine, creatine, and agmatine. Citrulline is derived from food (minor amount) and from endogenous synthesis from glutamine and arginine. *ASL*, argininosuccinate lyase; *ASS*, argininosuccinate synthase; *NO*, nitric oxide, *NOS*, nitric oxide synthase; *OAT*, ornithine aminotransferase; *ODC*, ornithine decarboxylase; *OTC*, ornithine transcarbamoylase; *P5C*, pyrolline-5-carboxylate. (Data with permission from references 24, 27, and 86.)

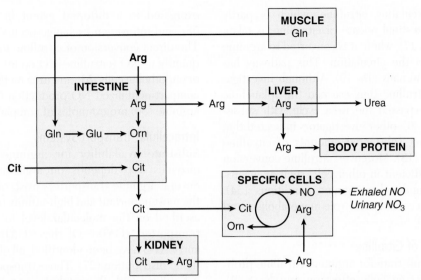

Fig. 35.4. Interorgan arginine and citrulline metabolism. Dietary arginine (Arg) is taken up by the intestine and is released through the portal circulation to the liver where a large part is converted to urea. A complete urea cycle is present only in the liver, whereas part of the cycle occurs in various organs, with interorgan exchange of metabolites. Citrulline (Cit), largely derived from intestinal conversion of glutamine (Gln), bypasses the liver and is converted back to arginine in the kidneys. In specific cells (e.g., immune cells or endothelial cells), arginine and citrulline can be converted to nitric oxide (NO) or ornithine (Orn) and polyamines. NO is exhaled in air or excreted as urinary nitrate (NO3) after conversion in blood to nitrite and nitrate. The metabolic state (fasted or fed), pathophysiologic condition, and drive for homeostasis are determinants of the pathways followed. (Data with permission from Cynober L, Moinard C, De Bandt JP. The 2009 ESPEN Sir David Cuthbertson. Citrulline: a new major signaling molecule or just another player in the pharmaconutrition game? Clin Nutr 2010;29:545–51; and Deutz NE. The 2007 ESPEN Sir David Cuthbertson Lecture: amino acids between and within organs. The glutamate-glutamine-citrulline-arginine pathway. Clin Nutr 2008;27:321–7.)

development. Moreover, this NO derived from NOS-2 acts cytoprotective as a free radical scavenger (35) when it is induced by elevated circulating cytokine concentrations (mainly tumor necrosis factor-α, and interleukin [IL]-1, IL-6, and IL-8) or microbial products (e.g., lipopolysaccharide [LPS]) during inflammatory processes (33, 34, 36–38). This property has led to the suggestion that arginine could have a great potential as an immune modulator (39, 40), and it may prove useful in enhancing the immune response in various models of immunologic challenges (41).

3. A large amount of arginine (~10% of arginine flux, equal to ~2.3 g arginine/day in humans) is used for the biosynthesis of creatine through the interorgan cooperation of kidneys, pancreas, liver, and skeletal muscle (27). Creatine is an important constituent of skeletal muscle and neurons and acts as an energy source for these tissues. Creatine is excreted in urine as creatinine (27).

4. Finally, agmatine is a decarboxylation product of arginine and acts as a cell signaling molecule (3).

Other Direct Actions of Arginine

In addition to its role as an intermediary in the synthesis of functional products, arginine also acts as a secretagogue because it stimulates release of several hormones such as insulin, glucagon, somatostatin, prolactin, growth hormone, and its peripheral mediator, insulinlike growth factor-I (30, 42). Arginine has the strongest insulinogenic effect of all the amino acids (27).

Citrulline

Citrulline Synthesis Pathway

Citrulline is synthesized by enterocytes in the small intestine that convert glutamine and proline through the glutamate-to-ornithine pathway (43). The final step in this synthesis pathway is the conversion of ornithine to citrulline, catalyzed by the enzyme ornithine transcarbamoylase (OTC) or ornithine carbamoyltransferase. Aside from the liver, where OTC is an enzyme in the urea cycle, OTC is present only in enterocytes (27). Glutamine is considered the main precursor for citrulline synthesis, as demonstrated by the close relationship between glutamine uptake and citrulline release by the intestine (44), which provides 60% to 80% of citrulline (19, 45–48). Moreover, arginine has been suggested as a source of citrulline through arginase and OTC metabolic pathways (49), and interorgan exchange of ornithine may also contribute to citrulline synthesis in the intestine (50). An additional amount of citrulline comes from nonintestinal sources. The intracellular arginine-citrulline cycle related to NO production in endothelial cells seems a likely candidate, as suggested in mice, humans, and endothelial cell studies (18, 46, 51). In the postabsorptive state, whole body citrulline flux in healthy adults is approximately 10 to 15 μmol/kg/hour (52, 53).

Citrulline Catabolic Pathway

Unlike most amino acids, citrulline is not incorporated into protein, but it can be converted to only arginine.

A large part of circulating citrulline, which is partly derived from the intestinal release of citrulline, is taken up by the kidneys (6, 17), where it is converted to arginine that is released into the circulation. This pathway has been confirmed in humans (18, 19). Although investigators thought that citrulline thus escaped the splanchnic sequestration and bypassed the urea cycle with subsequent nitrogen loss (30), other investigators indicated that the liver does extract substantial amounts of citrulline from the portal vein (18). Moreover, citrulline conversion to arginine is also efficient in other cells such as macrophages, especially under low-arginine conditions (54). This gives citrulline a considerable role in metabolism and regulation of NO (10).

Other Direct Actions of Citrulline

Besides acting as a substrate for arginine, citrulline probably also has a direct anabolic effect on muscle (8, 9). Moreover, citrulline is a major hydroxyl radical scavenger, which, in watermelon, is protective in environments inducing oxidative stress, such as drought (55).

DIETARY SOURCES AND NUTRITIONAL NEEDS

The major nutritional sources of arginine are dietary proteins. The amount of arginine is relatively high in seafood, nuts, seeds, algae, meats, rice protein concentrate, and soy protein isolate. The milk of most mammals (including cows, humans, and pigs) is relatively low in arginine (4). Daily dietary arginine intake in healthy individuals is approximately 4 to 6 g (42, 56), but 25% of the US adult population consumes less than 2.6 g/day (57). This dietary arginine intake seems minor, however, compared with the whole body arginine flux of approximately 15 to 20 g/day (20, 53).

Apart from watermelon, in which citrulline can be found in small quantities (1 g of citrulline in 780 g of watermelon), citrulline intake through food is nearly absent (10). No recommended dietary allowances are available for either arginine or citrulline.

FACTORS THAT INFLUENCE UTILIZATION AND METABOLISM

Several factors can modulate arginine, citrulline, and NO metabolism. These factors can be either endogenous (intrinsic) or exogenous (extrinsic).

Endogenous Influencing Factors

Endogenous factors that modulate arginine, citrulline, and NO metabolism are compartmentalization of metabolism, intracellular transport systems, coupling among enzymes, competition among enzymes that convert arginine to its metabolites, and endogenous NOS inhibitors.

Compartmentalization of Metabolism

The reason for compartmentalization of metabolism is that the enzymes in arginine-citrulline metabolism are expressed to a different extent in various organs (27, 58), and interorgan exchange occurs (see Fig. 35.4) (44). The direct conversion of citrulline to arginine and subsequently to NO (citrulline-NO cycle) in macrophages (59) or endothelial cells (51) and urea metabolism in the liver or compartmentalized NO production from protein-derived arginine (50) are examples of compartmentalization.

Intracellular Transport Systems

Substrate availability for arginine-requiring catabolic enzymes also depends on arginine transport systems. Several arginine transporters exist, of which system y^+ is the most important and high-affinity transport mechanism, ascribed on the molecular level to cationic amino acid transporters (CATs). Of these CATs, CAT-1, CAT-2(B), and CAT-3 have been identified, all of which differ in their tissue distribution (27). These transport systems are often colocalized with the catabolic enzymes and as such can modulate cellular arginine metabolism (27). For example, CAT-1 arginine transporter and endothelial NO synthase enzyme are colocalized in plasma membrane caveolae (60), which facilitate specific channelling of arginine to NO production without mixing with the total intracellular pool (58). Lysine, ornithine, and certain endogenous NOS inhibitors use the same transporter as arginine and may thereby compete for transporter capacity in conditions of low arginine (58, 61). For citrulline, no evidence indicates the presence of a specific transporter in any cell type, and transport by the usual generic amino acid transporters is demonstrated (10).

Coupling among Enzymes

The close coupling between, for example, de novo arginine synthesis from citrulline and NO production is supported by colocalization in endothelial cells of NOS3, ASS, and ASL (51). This could make ASS and ASL therapeutic targets for modulating endothelial NO production (51). This concept also applies to immune cells, especially under conditions of low arginine (54). Citrulline can thus be a precursor for NO, with resulting citrulline "recycling."

Competition among Enzymes That Convert Arginine to Its Metabolites

For instance, arginase reciprocally regulates NO levels in endothelial cells by competing with NOS for the arginine substrate (27, 62, 63). Inhibition of ASS by NO limits the risk of uncontrolled excessive NO production (10).

Endogenous Nitric Oxide Synthase Inhibitors

Asymmetric dimethylarginine (ADMA) is the most powerful endogenous and competitive nonspecific NOS inhibitor because it competes with L-arginine for the active site of NOS and for y^+ mediated uptake into cells (64). ADMA is derived from the catabolism of posttranslational modified proteins that contain methylated arginine residues. ADMA is metabolized by dimethylaminohydrolase (DDAH) to citrulline and methylamines and is excreted in urine (65). Increased protein catabolism and impaired renal function could therefore contribute to elevated ADMA levels. High expression of DDAH makes the liver important in the metabolism of ADMA, and hepatic dysfunction is a prominent determinant of ADMA concentration (65–68).

Exogenous Influencing Factors

Exogenous factors that modulate arginine, citrulline and NO metabolism are dietary factors, bacterial products, and pharmacologic manipulation of NO production and signaling.

Dietary Factors

Dietary Arginine. Following intestinal absorption, portal flux of arginine controls ureagenesis not only because arginine is a substrate for ureagenesis but also because it is an allosteric activator of ureagenesis key enzyme N-acetylglutamate synthetase (69). Thus, dietary arginine favors its own catabolism as well as that of other amino acids through ureagenesis. This is confirmed in healthy adults on a low-arginine diet, who have reduced arginine catabolism (arginine oxidation with conversion to ornithine) with maintained de novo arginine and reduced plasma arginine (52, 70, 71). Reduced arginine availability may limit NO synthesis because provision of the arginine pool for NO synthesis largely depends on extracellular sources of arginine (20, 72–76). Direct postprandial utilization of meal arginine for NO is considered low, however (77). L-Arginine supplementation, conversely, can increase the competitive advantage over ADMA for NO production (78) and over lysine for intracellular transport (61).

Dietary Protein Intake. When protein intake is low and ureagenesis must be slowed down to spare nitrogen, an alternative controlling pathway is activated. Intestinal arginase and OTC are activated, resulting in the conversion of arginine into citrulline. The newly formed citrulline is released into the portal vein, but it is not taken up by the liver, to facilitate low arginine influx into the liver. Citrulline is subsequently converted back to arginine in the kidney. By limiting ureagenesis, arginine and other amino acids are spared and become available in the periphery for muscle protein synthesis (8, 9, 30).

Dietary Glutamine or Its Dipeptide. This is an effective source of arginine through the glutamine-citrulline-arginine pathway, and it is more effective when given enterally than parenterally (47, 79).

Diet-Induced Insulin. Diet-induced insulin secretion stimulates NO production in endothelial cells by increasing the production of reduced nicotinamide adenine dinucleotide phosphate (NADPH) and tetrahydrobiopterin (BH_4) in endothelial cells, a process that may modulate tissue blood flow (80).

Bacterial Products

Bacterial products such as bacterial endotoxins can influence the arginine transporter and subsequently affect NOS activity (81, 82). Inflammatory cytokines can up-regulate CAT-2 arginine transporters (81, 82), and down-regulate CAT-1 arginine transporters (82). As a result, transport of arginine to NOS-2 is increased, whereas transport to NOS-3 is decreased. Because both macrophages and bacteria express arginase, this may be a mechanism whereby infectious pathogens shut down an important effector arm of the immune response locally and prolong their own survival (83). The arginase-dependent depletion of arginine in interferon-γ/LPS-stimulated macrophages causes an anti-inflammatory cytokine IL-13–mediated downregulation of NOS-2 protein, which can subsequently be restored by L-arginine administration (83).

Pharmacologic Manipulation of Nitric Oxide Production and Signaling

NO donors, such as nitroglycerin, are well known and are used as vasodilators to treat heart conditions such as angina and chronic heart failure. NOS inhibitors have also been developed, but none of these agents are currently used in clinical practice for any disorder. The main reason is that NOS inhibitors such as L-nitro-monomethylarginine (L-NMMA) or L-nitro-arginine-methylesther (L-NAME) are not NOS-isoform specific, and this limits their therapeutic applicability. More specific inhibitors, especially of NOS-2, are still in the clinical trial phase with potential application for inflammatory diseases. Other new treatment options under development are targeted at cyclic guanylate phosphate or the rate-limiting cofactor BH_4 (84).

ASSESSMENT OF NUTRIENT STATUS AND METABOLISM

Metabolic pathways can be measured either by using surrogate or indirect markers or by using direct markers of actual metabolic fluxes.

Surrogate or Indirect Markers

Surrogate metabolic markers can include plasma concentrations and levels of enzymes involved in the metabolic pathways or their metabolites. Because these markers do not directly measure synthesis or utilization, they can be considered indirect indicators.

Plasma Concentrations of Arginine and Citrulline

Plasma concentration of arginine is normally in the range of 80 to 100 μM in postabsorptive state (85). For citrulline, the normal postabsorptive concentration is in the range of 25 to 40 μM (10, 85). In the fed state, plasma levels of arginine increase, also depending on the dietary arginine content, whereas plasma citrulline levels vary less between postabsorptive and fed states. High-performance liquid chromatography is the most commonly applied analytic method for amino acid analyses, using either ion exchange or reversed phase column chromatography (10).

Arginine Metabolic Enzymes

Gene expression for specific enzymes or enzyme activity in cells of various organs indicates the maximal capacity of enzymes to convert substrate into product. However, this does not give the actual conversion rate of substrate into product. Although the relevance of specific enzyme isoforms (e.g., for NOS) can be explored, only measurement of the actual conversion rate at relevant concentrations gives full insight. Conversely, inhibiting the activity of enzymes or using knockout animals with a specific enzyme deficiency can provide an alternative way to gain metabolic insight into the role of specific enzymes.

Metabolites (Nitric Oxide, Nitrate, and Nitrite)

The half-life of NO in blood is very short (<1 second) because of rapid oxidation by oxyhemoglobin to nitrate and nitrite (cumulatively indicated as NOx), binding of NO to several cell structures, or NO scavenging. Therefore, NO in vivo is often measured as the concentration of its metabolites (NOx) as a surrogate indicator of NO production (86). NOx can be measured in plasma or within cells, such as polymorphonuclear neutrophils (87), or in saliva, where it is partly derived from bacterial NO production in the oral cavity (88). NOx analysis is widely available and relatively easy, but it can be biased by dietary nitrate intake, renal clearance rate, or (gut) bacterial production. For a review of NOx analysis, see Bryan and Grisham (89). Measurement of NO in exhaled air is also relatively easy and is used as a marker for pulmonary inflammation. However, the shape of the exhaled NO profile is affected by variability in ventilation and NO production, which may affect the physiologic interpretation (90).

Direct Measurement by Isotope Techniques

A more sophisticated and more direct method is the measurement of production and disappearance rates by using isotopes of arginine and citrulline labeled with stable carbon, hydrogen, or nitrogen and sampling of arterial or arterialized blood for measurement of isotope enrichments. The mixture of isotope-labeled amino acids needs to be composed carefully, especially when several metabolic pathways are measured simultaneously. However, this approach also requires more advanced analytic techniques, such as the combination of gas or liquid chromatography and mass spectrometry to measure isotopic enrichments (91, 92). The details given here are limited to arginine, citrulline, and NO production directly and do not describe other metabolic routes such as protein metabolism (92).

Arginine and Citrulline Production

Arginine and citrulline production can be measured as the whole body rate of appearance (R_a) of arginine and citrulline, respectively. By using a constant intravenous infusion of labeled arginine or citrulline and assuming a single-pool model, R_a can be calculated during isotope steady state when plasma isotope enrichment is stable (92).

De Novo Production of Arginine from Citrulline. This can be measured as the conversion of stable isotope–labeled citrulline to arginine (e.g., L-[ureido-^{13}C-^{2}H$_2$]-citrulline to L-[^{13}C-guanidino-^{2}H$_2$]-arginine). Simultaneous infusion of (a differently) labeled arginine enables the calculation of the absolute de novo production of arginine from citrulline (5, 24).

Arginine Utilization

Nitric Oxide Production. NO production can be measured as the conversion of intravenous or orally administered stable isotope–labeled arginine (e.g., L-[guanidino-^{15}N$_2$-^{2}H$_2$]- or L-[guanidino-^{15}N$_2$]-arginine) to labeled NO metabolites (^{15}NOx). ^{15}NOx can be measured in urine by sampling over a certain time, with correction for creatinine excretion after bolus tracer infusion (77, 93, 94). Alternatively, the fractional or absolute synthetic rate can be measured in plasma or whole blood during steady-state arginine tracer infusion (95, 96). Another approach is measurement of the conversion of labeled arginine to citrulline (e.g., L-[ureido-^{15}N-^{2}H$_2$]- or L-[ureido-^{15}N]-citrulline), which is produced stoichiometrically with NO. Simultaneous infusion of labeled citrulline (e.g., L-[ureido-^{13}C]- or L-[ureido-^{13}C-^{2}H$_2$]-citrulline) and arterial (or arterialized) blood sampling enables the calculation of the absolute rate of whole body NO production (20). Other combinations of labels are possible. In addition to measurements in healthy humans, this method can be applied in various clinical conditions, including in both neonates (97) and adult patients (98, 99) and in animal models (50, 100). Discrepancies exist between NO production as measured by NOx and stable isotopes, however, and they question the validity of the techniques. An increase in NOx with no concomitant increase in (stable isotope–measured) NO production (98, 99) may result from altered renal function, extracellular volume changes, or delayed conversion of NO to nitrate. Conversely, NO production as measured by stable isotopes may not account for possible intracellular or organ compartmentalization and thus may underestimate NO production (24). Therefore, the stable isotope–measured NO production probably represents minimal NO production, and production rates reported vary between 0.15 and 2.2 μmol/kg/hour in healthy subjects, between 0.14 and 0.25 μmol/kg/hour in pregnant women, and between 0.20 and 0.80 μmol/kg/hour in patients with sepsis (24, 98, 99, 101). Differences in isotopes, equations, and analytic techniques may underlie this variation, but they make it difficult to compare absolute values of NO production among studies.

Urea Synthesis. Urea synthesis from arginine can be measured as the conversion of labeled arginine to urea (e.g., L-[guanidono-^{15}N$_2$-^{2}H$_2$]- or L-[guanidino-^{15}N$_2$]-arginine to ^{15}N$_2$-urea). This conversion can be further quantified by simultaneous infusion of a differently labeled urea isotope (e.g., ^{13}C-urea) (99).

METABOLISM AND FUNCTION IN DISEASE

Arginine and Nitric Oxide

In various disease states, arginine metabolism is altered with regard to both synthesis and catabolism. This change can result in an imbalance between metabolic pathways and alteration of the fasting blood arginine level, which in healthy conditions is kept at homeostasis. Moreover, this altered metabolism has functional consequences. Endothelial dysfunction resulting in hemodynamic alterations (e.g., blood pressure changes, especially hypertension, and microcirculation) and immune alterations are well known.

Compared with healthy individuals, plasma levels of arginine are decreased in stressed patients (102), and the decrease is more marked in patients with sepsis (103–105). However, levels of other amino acids besides arginine may also decrease (104, 106, 107). In sepsis, the lower plasma arginine concentration was related to worse survival (103). In healthy adults ingesting a low-arginine diet, plasma arginine levels are reduced, but this is associated with reduced arginine catabolism whereas de novo arginine production is maintained (52, 70, 71). In disease states, however, this intestinal-renal pathway resulting in de novo arginine synthesis from citrulline may be impaired (99), such as due to for example, by intestinal or renal failure (15, 105, 108), thus contributing to reduced plasma arginine (16, 21, 109, 110). In the synthesis pathways of arginine, an increase of protein breakdown may mask the decline in arginine from de novo synthesis, with subsequent maintenance of total arginine production, as observed in septic patients, for example (105, 111).

In the catabolic pathways of arginine, increased protein synthesis (e.g., for acute phase proteins) and altered enzyme activation can occur, as noted in sepsis. For enzymes, these changes may be isoform specific, demonstrated by increased NOS-2 activity with down-regulation of other NOS isoforms during sepsis (112–116). This process may reduce NO production enzyme specifically, with lowered overall NO production (98, 99). ADMA levels are elevated in critically ill patients and are considered a causative factor in the development of multiple organ failure with impaired blood flow (65, 68). Elevation of ADMA levels is also a strong and independent risk factor for mortality in the intensive care unit (66). Increased plasma arginine clearance (98) can also result from enhanced arginase activity and may subsequently reduce arginine availability for other catabolic pathways. Moreover, increased arginine oxidation is observed during sepsis in pediatric patients (111), and it indicates increased use of arginine as an energy source in these children.

Citrulline

Citrulline metabolism, which includes both its endogenous production and its conversion to arginine, can be altered in disease, with a change in plasma citrulline. Related to its metabolic origin, the plasma citrulline concentration also reflects intestinal metabolic function and is therefore a potential marker for enterocyte mass and function (117). This is based on the lowered citrulline levels, first observed in patients with short bowel syndrome (7) and celiac disease with villous atrophy (118) and later reported in patients undergoing abdominal radiation therapy as potential markers for treatment-related gut damage and epithelial cell loss (119–121). Moreover, reduced plasma citrulline is observed in urea cycle disorders (e.g., OTC deficiency) (10), sepsis (99), and human immunodeficiency virus (HIV) infection (122). In HIV infection, a low citrulline level (<22 µmol/L) has been suggested as an indicator of the need for parenteral nutrition in patients with concomitant intestinal infections or HIV enteropathy (122). An elevated plasma citrulline concentration, conversely, can be caused by renal failure (123).

Reduced citrulline production and availability compromise de novo arginine production and subsequent NO production, as shown in genetically modified mice expressing only 5% to 10% of OTC activity (50, 100). OTC deficiency is characterized by elevated plasma glutamine and ammonia and reduced citrulline and arginine plasma levels (124, 125). Moreover, overt signs of disease in these mice under normal conditions are limited to growth retardation, abnormal skin and hair, hyperammonemia, and impaired cognition (125, 126). In humans, OTC deficiency is relatively uncommon (1 in 80,000 births), more pronounced in male patients, and dominant or recessive, depending on the involved mutation (10).

DEFICIENCY AND SUPPLEMENTATION

Reduced intake in disease or undernutrition can result in deficiency and can increase the nutritional need. In disease, impaired intestinal absorption (127) and impaired organ function, such as intestinal (10) or renal dysfunction (123), may further compromise citrulline and arginine metabolism and availability.

Arginine

Based on its pluripotent functions, arginine has been used in supplemental nutrition for surgical patients, burned patients, and patients with sepsis and cancer to benefit regulation of blood pressure, wound healing, immunomodulation, or as an anabolic stimulus. However, the benefits of arginine in these conditions are not uniformly proven or accepted. Arginine intake varying between 3 g/day and more than 100 g/day has been used in clinical studies. Single doses of 3 to 8 g appear to be safe and rarely provoke adverse events (78), but single doses higher than 9 g, especially when they are part of a daily dosing regimen of more than 30 g, can be associated with gastrointestinal discomfort, nausea, and (osmotic) diarrhea (128). These effects result from L-arginine-induced water and electrolyte secretion that is mediated by NO, which acts as an absorbagogue at low levels and as a secretagogue at high levels (128).

In human sepsis arginine is always supplemented in a mixture of amino acids and other nutrients but never as a single amino acid. In patients with sepsis, this approach is referred to as immunonutrition (129–132). Several review and opinion papers on its use have been published (133–140), but conclusions on the benefits and potential use in sepsis vary. Beneficial effects of arginine supplementation were observed in patients with sickle cell disease and pulmonary hypertension in the prevention of age-related glomerular injury, in reversing impaired vasodilation in clinically asymptomatic hypercholesterolemic adults, and in improving wound healing (141–145). A growing body of evidence indicates that arginine supplementation is beneficial in growth, health, and disease and may provide novel and effective therapies for obesity, diabetes, and metabolic syndrome (4).

Citrulline: An Alternative Source for Arginine or an "Independent Amino Acid"?

In healthy adults who received a single oral dose of 2, 5, 10, or 15 g of citrulline, investigators showed that short-term administration of citrulline was safe and well tolerated, that citrulline is a very potent precursor for arginine and ornithine, that plasma levels of insulin and growth hormone were not affected by citrulline administration, and that urinary excretion of citrulline remained low (<5%) even at high doses (146). At the highest doses, citrulline accumulated in the plasma, whereas arginine levels increased less than expected, thus suggesting possible saturation of renal conversion of citrulline to arginine (146). Another source of citrulline that is used in some applications is citrulline malate, which is also administered as an antiasthenia treatment in hyperammonemia to lower ammonia levels quickly (10).

As a substrate for de novo arginine production, citrulline supplementation may restore the arginine balance and metabolism, including NO production and related functions. Citrulline was demonstrated to be a potential substitute to restore NO production in an arginine-deprived in vitro model of macrophages, whereas glutamine interfered with citrulline-mediated NO production (54). Therefore, in conditions of acute or chronic inflammation with arginine deficiency, citrulline supplementation may be a powerful way to restore NO production (8). In sickle cell disease, oral citrulline supplementation may maintain elevated higher arginine levels and nearly normal total leukocyte and neutrophil counts, and therefore it may be a useful palliative therapy (147).

Citrulline supplementation is able to restore nitrogen balance, generate large amounts of arginine in rats with short bowel syndrome, and increase muscle protein content (+20%), as well as muscle protein synthesis

(+90%), in elderly malnourished rats (148, 149). These findings suggest that citrulline could play a pivotal role in maintaining protein homeostasis. The determination of the underlying mechanisms involved in citrulline's action is important for the development of new nutritional strategies in malnourished patients with compromised intestinal functions (8, 9) and in elderly people with sarcopenia (10).

ACKNOWLEDGMENTS

The project described was supported by award number R01GM084447 from the National Institute of General Medical Sciences to Nicolaas Deutz and Robert Wolfe and by award number DK- 62363 to Leticia Castillo. The content is solely our responsibility and does not necessarily represent the official views of the National Institute of General Medical Sciences or the National Institutes of Health.

We have no disclosures to report. Y.C. Luiking is an employee of Danone Research in The Netherlands.

REFERENCES

1. Moncada S, Radomski MW, Palmer RM. Biochem Pharmacol 1988;37:2495–501.
2. Palmer RM, Ashton DS, Moncada S. Nature 1988;333:664–6.
3. Morris SM Jr. J Nutr 2007;137:1602S–9S.
4. Wu G, Bazer FW, Davis TA et al. Amino Acids 2009;37: 153–68.
5. Luiking YC, Engelen MPKJ, Deutz NEP. Curr Opin Clin Nutr Metab Care 2010;13:97–104.
6. Windmueller HG, Spaeth AE. Am J Physiol 1981;241: E473–80.
7. Crenn P, Coudray-Lucas C, Thuillier F et al. Gastroenterology 2000;119:1496–505.
8. Cynober L, Moinard C, De Bandt JP. Clin Nutr 2010;29: 545–51.
9. Moinard C, Cynober L. J Nutr 2007;137:1621S–5S.
10. Curis E, Nicolis I, Moinard C et al. Amino Acids 2005;29: 177–205.
11. Curis E, Crenn P, Cynober L. Curr Opin Clin Nutr Metab Care 2007;10:620–6.
12. Cynober L. J Nutr 2007;137:1646S–9S.
13. Tizianello A, De Ferrari G, Garibotto G et al. J Clin Invest 1980;65:1162–73.
14. Featherston WR, Rogers QR, Freedland RA. Am J Physiol 1973;224:127–9.
15. Dhanakoti SN, Brosnan JT, Herzberg GR et al. Am J Physiol 1990;259:E437–42.
16. van de Poll MCG, Soeters PB, Deutz NEP et al. Am J Clin Nutr 2004;79:185–97.
17. Yu YM, Burke JF, Tompkins RG et al. Am J Physiol 1996;271:E1098–109.
18. van de Poll MC, Siroen MP, van Leeuwen PA et al. Am J Clin Nutr 2007;85:167–72.
19. Ligthart-Melis GC, van de Poll MC, Boelens PG et al. Am J Clin Nutr 2008;87:1282–9.
20. Castillo L, Beaumier L, Ajami AM et al. Proc Natl Acad Sci U S A 1996;93:11460–5.
21. Dejong CH, Welters CF, Deutz NE et al. Clin Sci (Colch) 1998;95:409–18.
22. Urschel KL, Shoveller AK, Uwiera RR et al. J Nutr 2006; 136:1806–13.
23. Bertolo RF, Burrin DG. J Nutr 2008;138:2032S–9S.
24. Luiking YC, Deutz NE. Curr Opin Clin Nutr Metab Care 2003;6:103–8.

25. Morris SM Jr. J Nutr 2004;134:2743S–7S; discussion 65S–67S.
26. Flynn NE, Meininger CJ, Haynes TE et al. Biomed Pharmacother 2002;56:427–38.
27. Wu G, Morris SM Jr. Biochem J 1998;336:1–17.
28. Jenkinson CP, Grody WW, Cederbaum SD. Comp Biochem Physiol B Biochem Mol Biol 1996;114:107–32.
29. Morris SM Jr. Br J Pharmacol 2009;157:922–30.
30. Cynober L. Gut 1994;35:S42–5.
31. Schaffer MR, Tantry U, Thornton FJ et al. Eur J Surg 1999;165:262–7.
32. Castillo L, Chapman TE, Yu YM et al. Am J Physiol 1993;265:E532–9.
33. Knowles RG, Moncada S. Biochem J 1994;298:249–58.
34. Moncada S, Higgs A. N Engl J Med 1993;329:2002–12.
35. Titheradge MA. Biochim Biophys Acta 1999;1411:437–55.
36. Groeneveld AB, Hartemink KJ, de Groot MC et al. Shock 1999;11:160–6.
37. Nakae H, Endo S, Kikuchi M et al. Surg Today 2000;30:683–8.
38. Groeneveld PH, Kwappenberg KM, Langermans JA et al. Cytokine 1997;9:138–42.
39. Reynolds JV, Daly JM, Zhang S et al. Surgery 1988;104:142–51.
40. Daly JM, Reynolds J, Sigal RK et al. Crit Care Med 1990;18:S86–93.
41. Li P, Yin YL, Li D et al. Br J Nutr 2007;98:237–52.
42. Visek WJ. J Nutr 1986;116:36–46.
43. Windmueller HG, Spaeth AE. J Biol Chem 1974;249:5070–9.
44. Deutz NE. Clin Nutr 2008;27:321–7.
45. Boelens PG, Melis GC, van Leeuwen PA et al. Am J Physiol Endocrinol Metab 2006;291:E683–90.
46. Boelens PG, van Leeuwen PA, Dejong CH et al. Am J Physiol Gastrointest Liver Physiol 2005;289:G679–85.
47. Ligthart-Melis GC, van de Poll MC, Dejong CH et al. JPEN J Parenter Enteral Nutr 2007;31:343–48; discussion 9–50.
48. van de Poll MC, Ligthart-Melis GC, Boelens PG et al. J Physiol 2007;581:819–27.
49. Marini JC, Didelija IC, Castillo L et al. Am J Physiol Endocrinol Metab 2010;299:E69–79.
50. Marini JC, Erez A, Castillo L et al. Am J Physiol Endocrinol Metab 2007;293:E1764–71.
51. Flam BR, Eichler DC, Solomonson LP. Nitric Oxide 2007;17:115–21.
52. Castillo L, Chapman TE, Sanchez M et al. Proc Natl Acad Sci U S A 1993;90:7749–53.
53. Castillo L, Sanchez M, Vogt J et al. Am J Physiol 1995;268:E360–7.
54. Bryk J, Ochoa JB, Correia MI et al. JPEN J Parenter Enteral Nutr 2008;32:377–83.
55. Akashi K, Miyake C, Yokota A. FEBS Lett 2001;508:438–42.
56. Heys SD, Gardner E. J R Coll Surg Edinb 1999;44:283–93.
57. King DE, Mainous AG 3rd, Geesey ME. Nutr Res 2008;28:21–4.
58. Cynober LA. Nutrition 2002;18:761–6.
59. Wu GY, Brosnan JT. Biochem J 1992;281:45–8.
60. McDonald KK, Zharikov S, Block ER et al. J Biol Chem 1997;272:31213–6.
61. Luiking YC, Deutz NE. J Nutr 2007;137:1662S–8S.
62. Bansal V, Ochoa JB. Curr Opin Clin Nutr Metab Care 2003;6:223–8.
63. Li H, Meininger CJ, Hawker JR Jr et al. Am J Physiol Endocrinol Metab 2001;280:E75–82.
64. Leiper J, Vallance P. Cardiovasc Res 1999;43:542–8.
65. Cooke JP. Arterioscler Thromb Vasc Biol 2000;20:2032–7.
66. Nijveldt RJ, Teerlink T, Van Der Hoven B et al. Clin Nutr 2003;22:23–30.
67. Nijveldt RJ, Teerlink T, Siroen MP et al. Clin Nutr 2003;22:17–22.
68. Nijveldt RJ, Teerlink T, van Leeuwen PA. Clin Nutr 2003;22:99–104.
69. Cynober L, Le Boucher J, Vasson MP. Nutritional Biochemistry 1995;6:402–13.
70. Castillo L, Sanchez M, Chapman TE et al. Proc Natl Acad Sci U S A 1994;91:6393–7.
71. Tharakan JF, Yu YM, Zurakowski D et al. Clin Nutr 2008;27:513–22.
72. Hallemeesch MM, Cobben DC, Soeters PB et al. Clin Nutr 2002;21:111–7.
73. Hallemeesch MM, Soeters PB, Deutz NE. Am J Physiol Renal Physiol 2002;282:F316–23.
74. Mitchell JA, Gray P, Anning PD et al. Eur J Pharmacol 2000;389:209–15.
75. Morris SM Jr, Billiar TR. Am J Physiol 1994;266:E829–39.
76. Bune AJ, Shergill JK, Cammack R et al. FEBS Lett 1995;366:127–30.
77. Mariotti F, Huneau JF, Szezepanski I et al. J Nutr 2007;137:1383–9.
78. Boger RH. J Nutr 2007;137:1650S–5S.
79. Ligthart-Melis GC, van de Poll MC, Vermeulen MA et al. Am J Clin Nutr 2009;90:95–105.
80. Wu G, Meininger CJ. Biofactors 2009;35:21–7.
81. Reade MC, Clark MF, Young JD et al. Clin Sci (Lond) 2002;102:645–50.
82. Schwartz D, Schwartz IF, Gnessin E et al. Am J Physiol Renal Physiol 2003;284:F788–95.
83. El-Gayar S, Thuring-Nahler H, Pfeilschifter J et al. J Immunol 2003;171:4561–8.
84. Domenico R. Curr Pharm Des 2004;10:1667–76.
85. Van Eijk HM, Dejong CH, Deutz NE et al. Clin Nutr 1994;13:374–80.
86. Kelm M. Biochim Biophys Acta 1999;1411:273–89.
87. Sureda A, Cordova A, Ferrer MD et al. Free Radic Res 2009;43:828–35.
88. Sato EF, Choudhury T, Nishikawa T et al. J Clin Biochem Nutr 2008;42:8–13.
89. Bryan NS, Grisham MB. Free Radic Biol Med 2007;43:645–57.
90. Suresh V, Shelley DA, Shin HW et al. J Appl Physiol 2008;104:1743–52.
91. van Eijk HM, Luiking YC, Deutz NE. J Chromatogr B Analyt Technol Biomed Life Sci 2007;851:172–85.
92. Wolfe RR, Chinkes DL. Isotope Tracers in Metabolic Research: Principles and Practice of Kinetic Analysis. 2nd ed. Hoboken, NJ: John Wiley, 2004.
93. Blouet C, Mariotti F, Mathe V et al. Exp Biol Med (Maywood) 2007;232:1458–64.
94. Magne J, Huneau JF, Delemasure S et al. Nitric Oxide 2009;21:37–43.
95. Jahoor F, Badaloo A, Villalpando S et al. Am J Clin Nutr 2007;86:1024–31.
96. Tessari P, Coracina A, Puricelli L et al. Am J Physiol Endocrinol Metab 2007;293:E776–82.
97. Urschel KL, Rafii M, Pencharz PB et al. Am J Physiol Endocrinol Metab 2007;293:E811–8.
98. Kao CC, Bandi V, Guntupalli KK et al. Clin Sci (Lond) 2009;117:23–30.
99. Luiking YC, Poeze M, Ramsay G et al. Am J Clin Nutr 2009;89:142–52.

100. Luiking YC, Hallemeesch MM, van de Poll MC et al. Am J Physiol Endocrinol Metab 2008;295:E1315–22.
101. Kurpad AV, Kao C, Dwarkanath P et al. Eur J Clin Nutr 2009;63:1091–7.
102. Vente JP, von Meyenfeldt MF, van Eijk HM et al. Ann Surg 1989;209:57–62.
103. Freund H, Atamian S, Holroyde J et al. Ann Surg 1979; 190:571–6.
104. Milewski PJ, Threlfall CJ, Heath DF et al. Clin Sci (Lond) 1982;62:83–91.
105. Luiking YC, Steens L, Poeze M et al. Clin Nutr 2003;22 (Suppl 1):S26.
106. Garcia-Martinez C, Llovera M, Lopez-Soriano FJ et al. Cell Mol Biol (Noisy-le-grand) 1993;39:537–42.
107. Bruins MJ, Lamers WH, Meijer AJ et al. Br J Pharmacol 2002;137:1225–36.
108. Prins HA, Nijveldt RJ, Gasselt DV et al. Kidney Int 2002;62:86–93.
109. Evoy D, Lieberman MD, Fahey TJ 3rd et al. Nutrition 1998;14:611–7.
110. Wakabayashi Y, Yamada E, Yoshida T et al. J Biol Chem 1994;269:32667–71.
111. Argaman Z, Young VR, Noviski N et al. Crit Care Med 2003;31:591–7.
112. Kirkeboen KA, Strand OA. Acta Anaesthesiol 1999;43: 275–88.
113. Beach PK, Spain DA, Kawabe T et al. J Surg Res 2001;96: 17–22.
114. Hallemeesch MM, Janssen BJA, De Jonge WJ et al. Am J Physiol Endocrinol Metab 2003;285:E871–5.
115. Malmstrom RE, Bjorne H, Oldner A et al. Shock 2002;18: 456–60.
116. Helmer KS, West SD, Shipley GL et al. Gastroenterology 2002;123:173–86.
117. Crenn P, Messing B, Cynober L. Clin Nutr 2008;27:328–39.
118. Crenn P, Vahedi K, Lavergne-Slove A et al. Gastroenterology 2003;124:1210–9.
119. Lutgens LC, Deutz N, Granzier-Peeters M et al. Int J Radiat Oncol Biol Phys 2004;60:275–85.
120. Lutgens LC, Blijlevens NM, Deutz NE et al. Cancer 2005; 103:191–9.
121. Lutgens L, Lambin P. World J Gastroenterol 2007;13: 3033–42.
122. Crenn P, De Truchis P, Neveux N et al. Am J Clin Nutr 2009; 90:587–94.
123. Ceballos I, Chauveau P, Guerin V et al. Clin Chim Acta 1990; 188:101–8.
124. Yudkoff M, Daikhin Y, Nissim I et al. J Clin Invest 1996; 98:2167–73.
125. Batshaw ML, Yudkoff M, McLaughlin BA et al. Gene Ther 1995;2:743–9.
126. Marini JC, Lee B, Garlick PJ. J Nutr 2006;136:1017–20.
127. Gardiner KR, Gardiner RE, Barbul A. Crit Care Med 1995;23:1227–32.
128. Grimble GK. J Nutr 2007;137:1693S–701S.
129. Bower RH, Cerra FB, Bershadsky B et al. Crit Care Med 1995;23:436–49.
130. Atkinson S, Sieffert E, Bihari D. Crit Care Med 1998;26: 1164–72.
131. Galban C, Montejo JC, Mesejo A et al. Crit Care Med 2000;28:643–8.
132. Bertolini G, Iapichino G, Radrizzani D et al. Intensive Care Med 2003;29:834–40.
133. McCowen KC, Bistrian BR. Am J Clin Nutr 2003;77:764–70.
134. Heyland DK, Novak F, Drover JW et al. JAMA 2001;286: 944–53.
135. Suchner U, Heyland DK, Peter K. Br J Nutr 2002;87 (Suppl 1):S121–32.
136. Koretz RL. Gastroenterology 1995;109:1713–4.
137. Heyland DK, Samis A. Intensive Care Med 2003;29:669–71.
138. Weimann A, Bastian L, Bischoff WE et al. Nutrition 1998; 14:165–72.
139. Georgieff M, Tugtekin IF. Kidney Int Suppl 1998;64:S80–3.
140. Heyland DK, Dhaliwal R, Drover JW et al. JPEN J Parenter Enteral Nutr 2003;27:355–73.
141. Reckelhoff JF, Kellum JA Jr, Racusen LC et al. Am J Physiol 1997;272:R1768–74.
142. Morris CR, Morris SM Jr, Hagar W et al. Am J Respir Crit Care Med 2003;168:63–9.
143. Boger RH, Bode-Boger SM, Szuba A et al. Circulation 1998;98:1842–7.
144. Gurbuz AT, Kunzelman J, Ratzer EE. J Surg Res 1998;74: 149–54.
145. Barbul A, Lazarou SA, Efron DT et al. Surgery 1990;108:331–6; discussion 6–7.
146. Moinard C, Nicolis I, Neveux N et al. Br J Nutr 2008;99: 855–62.
147. Waugh WH, Daeschner CW 3rd, Files BA et al. J Natl Med Assoc 2001;93:363–71.
148. Osowska S, Duchemann T, Walrand S et al. Am J Physiol Endocrinol Metab 2006;291:E582–6.
149. Osowska S, Moinard C, Neveux N et al. Gut 2004;53:1781–6.

SUGGESTED READINGS

Curis E, Nicolis I, Moinard C et al. Almost all about citrulline in mammals. Amino Acids 2005;29:177–205.

Cynober L, Moinard C, De Bandt JP. The 2009 ESPEN Sir David Cuthbertson. Citrulline: a new major signaling molecule or just another player in the pharmaconutrition game? Clin Nutr 2010;29:545–51.

Deutz NE. The 2007 ESPEN Sir David Cuthbertson Lecture: amino acids between and within organs. The glutamate-glutamine-citrulline-arginine pathway. Clin Nutr 2008;27:321–7.

Luiking YC, Engelen MP, Deutz NE. Regulation of nitric oxide production in health and disease. Curr Opin Clin Nutr Metab Care 2010;13: 97–104.

Wu G, Bazer FW, Davis TA et al. Arginine metabolism and nutrition in growth, health and disease. Amino Acids 2009;37:153–68.

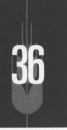

36 FUNCTIONAL FOODS AND NUTRACEUTICALS IN HEALTH PROMOTION[1]

JOHN MILNER, CHERYL TONER, AND CINDY D. DAVIS

Belief in the medicinal attributes of foods has directed attention to foods that may have health benefits over and beyond their supply of essential nutrients. The links between several so-called functional foods and health continue to mount. However, a clear understanding of the impacts of dietary exposure on the health of individuals is still evolving. What is evident is that truly miracle foods or food components do not exist. Functional foods must be considered in the context of the other constituents of the diet as well as the consumer's genetics and environmental exposures. Insults such as excess or insufficient calories, viruses, bacteria, and environmental toxins can influence the biologic response. Nevertheless, evidence from clinical trials, epidemiologic observations, preclinical models, and cell culture systems provide clues to the biologic consequences of individual foods and their components as a function of amount and duration of exposure. To take advantage of factors in eukaryotic cells that influence growth, development, and disease prevention, one must understand genetic and epigenetic events, transcription regulation, protein

targets, and the formation of small-molecular-weight signals more clearly. Although all food and beverages can influence these key cellular processes, the circumstances under which maximum benefits occur remain to be determined. Deciphering who will benefit most or be placed at risk from specific functional foods is exceedingly complex, but it holds promise to influence human health and disease risk.

DEFINITION OF FUNCTIONAL FOODS

Functional foods are foods and food components that provide health benefits beyond basic nutrition. They do more than simply provide nutrients because they assist in maintaining health and thereby reducing the risk of disease. Collectively, these foods represent a continuum of items that contain ingredients or natural constituents in conventional, fortified, enriched, and enhanced foods. The term first surfaced in Japan in the 1980s, when government approval was granted for functional foods called Foods for Specified Health Use (FOSHU) (1). In Japan, a manufacturer who wishes to apply to the government for approval under FOSHU must tabulate and summarize all available publications as well as internal reports that deal with the effectiveness of the product and its ingredients. The summary must include in vitro metabolic and biochemical studies, in vivo investigations, and randomized controlled trials in Japanese people (2). Since the 1980s, this concept has been embraced by many in the scientific and lay communities to promote healthy eating throughout the world.

Belief in functional foods by consumers is driven by multiple factors, including "natural is good," a plethora of health and structure function claims and other communications, the perception that prevention through food is less costly than the use of drug or other medical treatments, belief in diminished side effects of foods versus drugs, and the increasing acceptance that a healthy diet promotes general well-being and curbs the risk of disease (3–5). This concept is not new. Almost 2500 years ago, Hippocrates, considered by some to be the father of Western medicine, proclaimed "Let food be thy medicine, and medicine be thy food."

Although consumers appear to identify with foods having health benefits (6), the positive and negative actions of specific bioactive foods constituents continue to captivate the scientific community (7–9). The study of bioactive food constituents is becoming more common in the

---

[1]**Abbreviations: DSHEA**, Dietary Supplement Health and Education Act; **FDA**, Food and Drug Administration; **FDAMA**, Food and Drug Administration Modernization Act; **FOSHU**, Foods for Specified Health Use; **FTC**, Federal Trade Commission; **NCD**, noncommunicable disease; **NLEA**, Nutrition Labeling and Education Act; **SNP**, single nucleotide polymorphism.

TABLE 36.1	FUNCTIONAL FOODS WITH POTENTIAL HEALTH BENEFITS[a]
SUSPECTED HEALTH-PROMOTING FUNCTIONAL FOOD	**POTENTIAL BIOACTIVE INGREDIENT**
Soy	Genistein, daidzein, equol
Tomatoes	Lycopene
Spinach	Folate
Mushrooms	β-Glucans
Broccoli	Sulforaphane
Garlic	Allyl sulfur
Nuts	Flavonoids
Fish	n-3 fatty acids
Oats and other grains	Fiber, β-glucan, flavonoids
Blueberries	Polyphenols
Green tea	Catechins

[a]While considerable evidence indicates that each of these foods provides health benefits, all do not appear to provide the same benefits, and thus significant variability exists in the scientific literature. Controlled intervention studies that adequately evaluate changes in key biomarkers associated with health as a function of exposure (concentration and time) are needed.

scientific literature. Approximately 3000 publications listed in PubMed in 2011 were captured by the term "functional foods." Evidence of the ability of some functional foods to affect health is building, yet the response varies, depending on the study design and a host of factors discussed in more detail later. Functional foods with the strongest evidence of a biologic response are depicted in Table 36.1.

The earliest functional foods in the United States arose from the addition of poorly consumed nutrients to broadly consumed foods or ingredients. Examples include iodized salt to prevent goiter and vitamin D–fortified milk to prevent rickets. Today, products such as calcium-fortified orange juice, spreads with n-3 fatty acids, folate-enriched flour, and green tea extract–fortified drinks are just some examples of items that fall under the functional foods umbrella. Not all are new items, given that fermented foods such as kimchee and yogurts with live bacteria are also considered functional. Unfortunately, the definition of a functional food is so inclusive that nothing is excluded, and thus a truly "nonfunctional food" appears not to exist.

The functional food industry, consisting of food, beverage, and supplement sectors, continues to experience incredible growth. BCC Research, a resource of high-quality market research, estimated that the global market of functional foods may reach $176.7 billion in 2013. Although foods and supplements are projected to do much better than average, the best growth may occur in the beverage sector (10). This kind of growth is propelled not only by innovation and new products that satisfy the demand by consumers for more healthy food choices but also by health claims covering a gamut of issues.

DEFINITION OF NUTRACEUTICALS

Nutraceuticals are also receiving increased recognition because of their link with health. The term itself is a portmanteau of the words nutrition and pharmaceutical and congers images of a nutrient with a druglike action. The term was coined by Dr. Stephen L. DeFelice, founder and chairman of the Foundation for Innovation in Medicine in Mountainside, New Jersey. Typically, such products range from isolated nutrients, dietary supplements, and specific diets to genetically engineered foods, herbal products, and processed foods. Nutraceuticals are typically considered components of alternative medicine. As research has progressed, however, nutraceuticals have become more widely accepted (11).

In the United States, the Food and Drug Administration (FDA) is responsible for regulations and oversight of claims that manufacturers propose to make about the nutrient content and biologic response to functional foods in terms of health or body function. The FDA does not officially recognize the term "functional food." Nevertheless, the FDA does regulate these foods according to whether it is considered a conventional food, a food additive, a dietary supplement, a medical food, or a food for special dietary use (12).

DIETARY SUPPLEMENTS

Dietary supplements are products that contain nutrients derived from food products. They are typically provided in concentrated form as a liquid or a capsule and are intended to supplement the diet. The Dietary Supplement Health and Education Act of 1994 (DSHEA) provided clarification on the constituents of dietary supplements. Ingredients may include vitamins, minerals, herbs or other botanical products (excluding tobacco products), amino acids, and substances such as enzymes, organ tissues, glandular material, and metabolites. A dietary supplement may also include extracts or concentrates, provided in the form of powders, tablets, capsules, soft gels, or liquids. Concerns about the adequacy of the food supply and health care costs are surely factors that have fostered interest in the use of dietary supplements. Unfortunately, evidence to support the health benefits of these supplements is scant, and concern is increasing that the overzealous intake of these supplements may be harmful (13). The terms *nutraceuticals*, *functional foods*, *bioactive food components*, and *dietary supplements* are often used interchangeably, and thus these compounds are difficult to separate in terms of definition and biologic consequences.

DRIVERS FOR FUNCTIONAL FOODS AND NUTRACEUTICALS

Noncommunicable diseases (NCDs), including cancer, cardiovascular disease, diabetes, and the metabolic syndrome, account for 60% of all deaths globally (14). In low- to middle-income countries, the prevalence of NCD is increasing as these countries undergo socioeconomic improvement (15). The United Nations General Assembly agreed

Overall, the response to anthocyanin exposure on vision does not appear to be consistent, based on the studies presented (125, 126). Dose and length of feeding are clearly factors affecting outcomes. Positive effects have been observed at intakes in the range of 300 to 600 mg/day over a period of several months. However, consumption of these levels of anthocyanins from foods is difficult unless one consistently consumes foods containing high anthocyanin levels.

Other Effects

Although published data are limited, fruits and berries may be protective through antioxidant mechanisms in preventing DNA damage, and they may also affect cell division, apoptosis, and angiogenesis (127). Hou (128) summarized some of the molecular mechanisms whereby anthocyanins may have cancer chemoprevention properties, including those related to antioxidants and induction of apoptosis in tumor cells. In a preliminary human trial, subjects with early memory changes were given blueberry juice. After 12 weeks, improved paired associate learning and word list recall were observed (129). A study in rats indicated that anthocyanins improve learning and memory of rats with estrogen deficit caused by ovariectomy (130).

Purified anthocyanins from varying sources have been shown to decrease lipid deposition in rodent models of obesity (131). In the few studies in which anthocyanins were consumed as a part of the whole food or berry, antiobesity effects were not generally observed (132, 133). However, effects were observed with whole blueberries that protected against some of the disorders associated with obesity, including inflammation (134). Anthocyanins have been shown to regulate adipocytokine gene expression and to ameliorate adipocyte dysfunction related to obesity and diabetes. Alterations in lipogenesis and lipolysis in adipose tissue, as well as in numerous adipokine and cytokine signaling pathways, have been suggested to explain the effects of anthocyanins on the development of obesity (135, 136).

DIETARY SOURCES AND INTAKES OF FLAVONOIDS

Data on the flavonoid content of selected foods come primarily from US Department of Agriculture flavonoid database unless indicated otherwise (http://www.nal.usda.gov/fnic/foodcomp/Data/Flav/flav.html) (Table 37.1). Data on the quercetin content of foodstuffs are limited, but available data suggest a range of 2 to 250 mg quercetin/kg wet weight in fruits, 0 to 100 mg/kg in vegetables (with onions being especially high), 4 to 16 mg/L in red wine, 10 to 25 mg/L in tea, and 2 to 23 mg/L in fruit juices (137, 138). The daily consumption of flavonols is difficult to estimate because values depend on accurate assessment of feeding habits and flavonol content in foods. The average dietary intake of quercetin in the Netherlands was estimated to be 16 mg/day (137). The overall flavonoid (flavonols and flavones) intake in a population of women in the United States was estimated to be 24.6 ± 18.5 mg/day, of which quercetin was the major contributor (70.2%) (139). The mean intake of flavonoids (including flavonols, flavones, and flavanones) was estimated to be 24.2 ± 26.7 mg/day, 28.6 ± 12.3 mg/day, and 25.9 mg/day in the populations of Finland, Denmark, and the Netherlands, respectively (16, 140, 141). However, these investigators did not include monomeric, oligomeric, or polymeric flavan-3-ols in their estimation.

The major flavan-3-ols are catechin, epicatechin, epicatechin-3-gallate, epigallocatechin, and epigallocatechin-3-gallate (see Fig. 37.1). Fruits, teas, and chocolate are common sources of the catechins. Arts et al (142) estimated that the mean intake of flavan-3-ol monomers in the Netherlands was 50 mg/day, with tea being the major contributor (65.2% to 87.3%), followed by chocolate and apple. The daily intake of flavan-3-ol monomers from tea was estimated to be in the range of 12.7 to 34.2 mg/day/person for adults in the United States, based on the data of Lakenbrink et al (143). The total intake of flavan-3-ol monomers was estimated to be 17.1 to 38.6 mg/day/person for adults in the United States after the contribution of flavan-3-ols from other foods are included (144).

PAs are most prevalent in fruits and berries, but they are also found in chocolate (145), a few cereals and beans, nuts, and cinnamon (144). The foods that lack PAs and those containing PAs have been surveyed (71). The initial calculation of average daily intake of oligomeric and polymeric PAs by Gu et al (144), of 53.6 mg/day/person, is higher than that of monomeric flavan-3-ols and is twice as high as the combined overall intake of other flavonoids, including flavonols, flavones, and flavanones. PAs are likely among the major flavonoids ingested in the Western diet. Variations in PA intake among individuals are expected to be large because of different eating habits. People who eat a medium-sized apple every day can easily ingest 100 mg of PAs daily. People who take dietary supplements, such as Pycnogenol or grape seed extract, can ingest several hundred milligrams of PAs. The average daily intake of PA for infants of 6 to 10 months old is estimated to be 3.1 mg/day/kg body weight, which is four times higher than the average intake in adults of 20 or more years of age (0.77 mg/day/kg body weight) (144). Intake of PAs in 6- to 10-month-old infants increases markedly with the addition of fruits to the complementary foods.

The total dietary flavonoid intake by a Mediterranean population of Spanish adults was estimated to be 269 (median) and 313 (mean) mg/day. The most abundant flavonoid subgroup was PAs (60.1%), followed by flavanones (16.9%), flavan-3-ols (10.3%), flavonols (5.9%), anthocyanidins (5.8%), flavones (1.1%), and isoflavones (<0.01%). The main sources of total flavonoid intake were apples (23%), red wine (21%), unspecified fruit (12.8%), and oranges (9.3%) (146).

TABLE 37.1	FLAVONOID CLASSES AND CONCENTRATIONS[a] OF MAJOR COMPOUNDS IN EACH CLASS IN SELECTED FOODS AND POSSIBLE HEALTH EFFECTS	

CLASS (MAJOR COMPOUNDS)	CONCENTRATION	SITE OF ACTION/HEALTH EFFECTS (REFERENCES)
Flavones (Apigenin, Luteolin)		
Celery	5.9	Anticancer effects (22, 147, 148)
Celery hearts	22.6	
Peppers	1–7	
Spinach, raw	1.1	
Tea, green, brewed	0.3	
Flavonols (Quercetin, Kaempferol, Myricetin, Isorhamnetin)		
Onions	15.4–38.7	Antioxidants in vivo (33, 37, 38, 41)
Kale	22.9–34.4	Anti-inflammatory effects (42)
Cocoa	20.1	
Broccoli	9.4	
Blueberries	3.9	
Spinach	4.9	
Blackberries	1.1	
Tea	3.8	
Celery	3.5	
Beans	3.1–3.4	
Lettuce	2.6	
Grapefruit	0.9	
Tomatoes	0.6	
Flavanones (Hesperetin, Naringenin, Eriodictyol)		
Lemons	49.8	Anti-inflammatory effects (149)
Lemon juice	18.4	Anticancer effects (149)
Oranges	43.9	Drug interactions (51, 52)
Grapefruit	54.5	
Flavan-3-ols (e.g., Catechin, Epicatechin, Gallocatechin, Epigallocatechin)[b]		
Tea, black	114	Antioxidants in vivo
Tea, green	133	Anticancer effects in the gastrointestinal tract
Chocolate	13.4–53.5	(14, 63, 65, 70, 150)
Blackberries	18.7	Cardiovascular protection (56)
Apples	9.1	
Proanthocyanidins[c]		
Blueberries, cultivated	180	Prevention of low-density lipoprotein
Blueberries, lowbush	332	oxidation (86, 87)
Cranberries	419	Urinary tract infection factor: A-type (93)
Apple	70–126	Antidiabetic effects (95–97, 151)
Peaches	67	
Plums	215–257	
Sorghum, high tannin	788	
Pinto beans, raw	796	
Pinto beans, simmered	26	
Red beans	457	
Kidney beans	564	
Hazelnuts	501	
Pecans	494	
Pistachios	237	
Almonds	184	
Anthocyanins (Cyanidin, Delphinidin, Peonidin, Petunidin, Malvidin, Pelargonidin)[d]		
Elderberry	1,550	Vascular permeability (118)
Chokeberry	1,486	Vision effects (120–124, 126)
Blueberry	415	Anticancer effects (128)
Blackberry	317	Angiogenesis (127)
Cranberry	148	Obesity (131, 132, 152, 153)
Cherry	124	
Raspberry	96	
Strawberry	22	
Plum	20	
Nectarine	6	
Peach	5	
Red leaf lettuce	2	
Apple	1	

[a]Expressed as mg/100g fresh weight. Data from the US Department of Agriculture flavonoid database (http://www.ars.usda.gov/SP2UserFiles/Place/12354500/Data/Flav/Flav02-1.pdf) unless indicated otherwise. This table is not intended to be complete, and numbers presented are averages or ranges. Concentrations can vary considerably depending on environmental growing conditions, processing, and other conditions. Readers are encouraged to refer to the original database for more complete information.
[b]Most foods containing proanthocyanidins contain monomeric flavan-3-ols.
[c]From data of Gu et al (144) expressed as the total of all oligomers plus polymers (see the original publication for a breakdown of the individual components).
[d]From data of Wu et al (154) expressed as total of all anthocyanins in various glycosylated forms.

REFERENCES

1. Harborne JB. The Flavonoids: Advances in Research Since 1980. London: Chapman & Hall, 1988.
2. Harborne JB. The Flavonoids: Advances in Research Since 1986. London: Chapman & Hall, 1994.
3. Harborne JB. Phytochemistry 2000;55:481–504.
4. Bidlack WR, Omaye ST, Meskin MS et al. Phytochemicals: A New Paradigm. Lancaster, PA: Technomic Publishing, 1998.
5. Meskin M. Phytochemicals as Bioactive Agents. Boca Raton, FL: CRC Press, 2000.
6. Meskin M, Bidlack WR, Davies AJ et al. Phytochemicals in Nutrition and Health. Boca Raton, FL: CRC Press, 2002.
7. Meskin M, Bidlack WR Davies, AJ et al. Phytochemicals: Mechanisms of Action. Boca Raton, FL: CRC Press, 2003.
8. Middleton E Jr, Kandaswami C, Theoharides TC. Pharmacol Rev 2000;52:673–751.
9. Middleton E Jr, Kandaswami C. The impact of plant flavonoids on mammalian biology: implications for immunity, inflammation and cancer. In: Harborne JB, ed. The Flavonoids: Advances in Research Since 1986. London: Chapman & Hall, 1994:619–52.
10. Middleton E Jr, Kandaswami C. Biochem Pharm 1992;43:1167–79.
11. Beecher GR. J Nutr 2003;133:3248S–54S.
12. Havsteen BH. Pharmacol Ther 2002;96:67–202.
13. Lambert JD, Yang CS. Mutat Res 2003;523–524:201–8.
14. Yang CS, Landau JM, Huang MT et al. Annu Rev Nutr 2001;21:381–406.
15. Nijveldt RJ, van Nood E, van Hoorn DE et al. Am J Clin Nutr 2001;74:418–25.
16. Hertog MG, Hollman PC, Katan MB et al. Nutr Cancer 1993;20:21–9.
17. Hollman PC, Hertog MG, Katan MB. Biochem Soc Trans 1996;24:785–9.
18. Hertog MG, Feskens EJ, Hollman PC et al. Lancet 1993;342:1007–11.
19. Keli SO, Hertog MG, Feskens EJ et al. Arch Intern Med 1996;156:637–42.
20. Aherne SA, O'Brien NM. Nutrition 2002;18:75–81.
21. Prior RL. Phytochemicals. In: Shils ME, Shike M, Ross AC et al, eds. Modern Nutrition in Health and Disease. 10th ed. Baltimore: Lippincott Williams & Wilkins, 2006:582–94.
22. Engelmann C, Blot E, Panis Y et al. Phytomedicine 2002;9:489–95.
23. Fotsis T, Pepper MS, Montesano R et al. Baillieres Clin Endocrinol Metab 1998;12:649–66.
24. Walle T. Semin Cancer Biol 2007;17:254–362.
25. Griffiths LA, Smith GE. Biochem J 1972;130:141–51.
26. Hollman PC, De Vries JH, Van Leeuwen SD et al. Am J Clin Nutr 1995;62:1276–82.
27. Rasmussen SE, Breinholt VM. Int J Vitam Nutr Res 2003;73:101–11.
28. Murota K, Terao J. Arch Biochem Biophys 2003;417:12–17.
29. Crespy V, Morand C, Besson C et al. J Agric Food Chem 2002;50:618–21.
30. Walgren RA, Karnaky KJ Jr, Lindenmayer GE et al. J Pharmacol Exp Ther 2000;294:830–6.
31. Walgren RA, Lin JT, Kinne RK et al. J Pharmacol Exp Ther 2000;294:837–43.
32. Walle T, Otake Y, Walle UK et al. J Nutr 2000;130:2658–61.
33. Morand C, Crespy V, Manach C et al. Am J Physiol 1998;275:R212–9.
34. Hollman PC, van Trijp JM, Mengelers MJ et al. Cancer Lett 1997;114:139–40.
35. Prior RL. Am J Clin Nutr 2003;78:570S–78S.
36. Aura AM, O'Leary KA, Williamson G et al. J Agric Food Chem 2002;50:1725–30.
37. da Silva EL, Piskula MK, Yamamoto N et al. FEBS Letters 1998;430:405–8.
38. Shirai M, Moon JH, Tsushida T et al. J Agric Food Chem 2001;49:5602–8.
39. Graefe EU, Derendorf H, Veit M. Int J Clin Pharm Ther 1999;37:219–33.
40. Suri S, Liu XH, Rayment S et al. Br J Pharmacol 2009;159:566–75.
41. Liu S, Hou W, Yao P et al. Toxicol In Vitro 2009;24:516–22.
42. Harasstani OA, Moin S, Tham CL et al. Inflamm Res 2010;59:711–21.
43. Shanely RA, Knab AM, Nieman DC et al. Free Radic Res 2010;44:224–31.
44. Tsuji M, Yamamoto H, Sato T et al. J Bone Miner Metab 2009;27:673–81.
45. Davis JM, Murphy EA, Carmichael MD et al. Am J Physiol Regul Integr Comp Physiol 2009;296:11.
46. Quindry JC, McAnulty SR, Hudson MB et al. Int J Sport Nutr Exerc Metab 2008;18:601–16.
47. Dumke CL, Nieman DC, Utter AC et al. Appl Physiol Nutr Metab 2009;34:993–1000.
48. Utter AC, Nieman DC, Kang J et al. Res Sports Med 2009;17:71–83.
49. Nielsen IL, Dragsted LO, Ravn-Haren G et al. J Agric Food Chem 2003;51:2813–20.
50. Manthey JA, Grohmann K, Guthrie N. Curr Med Chem 2001;8:135–53.
51. Lohezic-Le Devehat F, Marigny K, Doucet M et al. Therapie 2002;57:432–45.
52. Ameer B, Weintraub RA. Clin Pharmacokinet 1997;33:103–21.
53. Rietveld A, Wiseman S. J Nutr 2003;133:3285S–92S.
54. Manach C, Williamson G, Morand C et al. Am J Clin Nutr 2005;81:230S–42.
55. Khanal RC, Howard LR, Wilkes SE et al. J Agric Food Chem 2010;58:11257–64.
56. de Pascual-Teresa S, Moreno DA, Garcia-Viguera C. Int J Mol Sci 2010;11:1679–703.
57. Natsume M, Osakabe N, Oyama M et al. Free Radic Biol Med 2003;34:840–9.
58. Stalmach A, Troufflard S, Serafini M et al. Mol Nutr Food Res 2009;53:S44–S53.
59. Stalmach A, Mullen W, Steiling H et al. Mol Nutr Food Res 2010;54:323–34.
60. Higdon JV, Frei B. Crit Rev Food Sci Nutr 2003;43:89–143.
61. Frei B, Higdon JV. J Nutr 2003;133:3275S–84S.
62. Arts IC, Jacobs DR Jr, Gross M et al. Cancer Causes Control 2002;13:373–82.
63. Katiyar SK, Mukhtar H. J Cell Biochem 1997;64:59–67.
64. Yang CS, Chung JY, Yang G et al. J Nutr 2000;130:472S–78S.
65. Chung FL, Schwartz J, Herzog CR et al. J Nutr 2003;133:3268S–74S.
66. Kuo YC, Yu CL, Liu CY et al. Cancer Causes Control 2009;20:57–65.
67. Khan N, Mukhtar H. Cancer Lett 2008;269:269–80.
68. Inoue M, Robien K, Wang R et al. Carcinogenesis 2008;29:1967–72.
69. Chen D, Milacic V, Chen MS et al. Histol Histopathol 2008;23:487–96.
70. Arab L, Il'yasova D. J Nutr 2003;133:3310S–18S.
71. Gu L, Kelm MA, Hammerstone JF et al. J Agric Food Chem 2003;51:7513–21.

72. Deprez S, Mila I, Huneau JF et al. Antioxid Redox Signal 2001;3:957–67.

73. Donovan JL, Manach C, Rios L et al. Br J Nutr 2002;87: 299–306.

74. Spencer JP, Chaudry F, Pannala AS et al. Biochem Biophys Res Commun 2000;272:236–41.

75. Rios LY, Bennett RN, Lazarus SA et al. Am J Clin Nutr 2002;76:1106–10.

76. Gu L, House SE, Rooney L et al. J Agric Food Chem 2007;55:5326–34.

77. Déprez S, Brezillon C, Rabot S et al. J Nutr 2000;130:2733–8.

78. Rios LY, Gonthier MP, Remesy C et al. Am J Clin Nutr 2003;77:912–8.

79. Holt RR, Lazarus SA, Sullards MC et al. Am J Clin Nutr 2002;76:798–804.

80. Urpi-Sarda M, Monagas M, Khan N et al. Anal Bioanal Chem 2009;394:1545–56.

81. Serra A, Macia A, Romero MP et al. Br J Nutr 2010;103:944–52.

82. Appeldoorn MM, Vincken JP, Gruppen H et al. J Nutr 2009;139:1469–73.

83. Stoupi S, Williamson G, Viton F et al. Drug Metab Dispos 2010;38:287–91.

84. Stoupi S, Williamson G, Drynan JW et al. Arch Biochem Biophys2010;501:73–8.

85. Schewe T, Kuhn H, Sies H. J Nutr 2002;132:1825–9.

86. Wan Y, Vinson JA, Etherton TD et al. Am J Clin Nutr 2001;74:596–602.

87. Murphy KJ, Chronopoulos AK, Singh I et al. Am J Clin Nutr 2003;77:1466–73.

88. Mao TK, Van De Water J, Keen CL et al. Exp Biol Med 2003;228:93–9.

89. Tyagi A, Agarwal R, Agarwal C. Oncogene 2003;22:1302–16.

90. Ye X, Krohn RL, Liu W et al. Mol Cell Biochem 1999;196: 99–108.

91. Mao TK, Powell JJ, Water JVD et al. Int J Immunother 1999;15:8.

92. Tebib K, Besancon P, Rouanet JM. J Nutr 1994;124:2451–57.

93. Foo LY, Lu Y, Howell AB et al. J Nat Prod 2000;63:1225–8.

94. Anderson RA, Broadhurst CL, Polansky MM et al. J Agric Food Chem 2004;52:65–70.

95. Khan A, Safdar M, Khan MH et al. Diabetes Care 2003; 26:3215–18.

96. Montagut G, Onnockx S, Vaque M et al. J Nutr Biochem 2010;21:476–81.

97. Montagut G, Blade C, Blay M et al. J Nutr Biochem 2010; 21:961–7.

98. Prior RL. Absorption and metabolism of anthocyanins: potential health effects. In: Meskin M, Bidlack WR, Davies AJ et al, eds. Phytochemicals: Mechanisms of Action. Boca Raton, FL: CRC Press, 2004:1–19.

99. Clifford MN. J Sci Food Agric 2000;80:1063–72.

100. Strack D, Wray V. The Anthocyanins. In: Harborne JB, ed. The Flavonoids: Advances in Research Since 1986. London: Chapman & Hall, 1993.

101. Wang H, Cao G, Prior RL. J Agric Food Chem 1997;45:304–09.

102. Macheix J, Fleuriet A, Billot J. Fruit Phenolics. Boca Raton, FL: CRC Press, 1990.

103. Passamonti S, Vrhovsek U, Mattivi F. Biochem Biophys Res Commun 2002;296:631–6.

104. Mulleder U, Murkovic M, Pfannhauser W. J Biochem Biophys Methods 2002;53:61–66.

105. Wu X, Cao G, Prior RL. J Nutr 2002;132:1865–71.

106. Matsumoto H, Inaba H, Kishi M et al. J Agric Food Chem 2001;49:1546–51.

107. Miyazawa T, Nakagawa K, Kudo M et al. J Agric Food Chem 1999;47:1083–91.

108. Cao G, Muccitelli HU, Sanchez-Moreno C et al. Am J Clin Nutr 2001;73:920–6.

109. McGhie TK, Walton MC. Mol Nutr Food Res 2007;51:702–13.

110. Bub A, Watzl B, Heeb D et al. Eur J Nutr 2001;40:113–20.

111. Tsuda T, Horio F, Osawa T. FEBS Lett 1999;449:179–82.

112. Wu X, Pittman HE, Prior RL. J Agric Food Chem 2006; 54:583–9.

113. Mazza G, Kay CD, Cottrell T et al. J Agric Food Chem 2002;50:7731–37.

114. Felgines C, Texier O, Besson C et al. J Nutr 2002;132:1249–53.

115. Selma MV, Espin JC, Tomas-Barberan FA. J Agric Food Chem 2009;57:6485–501.

116. Kay CD, Kroon PA, Cassidy A. Mol Nutr Food Res 2009; 53(Suppl 1):S92–101.

117. Woodward G, Kroon P, Cassidy A et al. J Agric Food Chem 2009;57:5271–8.

118. Boniface R, Robert AM. Klin Monatsbl Augenheilkd 1996; 209:368–72.

119. Xia M, Ling W, Zhu H et al. Atherosclerosis 2009;202:41–7.

120. Zadok D, Levy Y, Glovinsky Y. Eye 1999;13:734–6.

121. Nakaishi H, Matsumoto H, Tominaga S et al. Altern Med Rev 2000;5:553–62.

122. Perossini M, Guidi G, Chiellini S et al. Ottal Clin Ocul 1987;113:1173–90.

123. Orsucci PN, Rossi M, Sabbatini G et al. Clin Ocul 1983;5: 377–81.

124. Muth ER, Laurent JM, Jasper P. Altern Med Rev 2000;5: 164–73.

125. Kalt W, Hanneken A, Milbury P et al. J Agric Food Chem 2010;58:4001–07.

126. Upton R. Bilberry Fruit *Vaccinium myrtillus* L. Santa Cruz, CA: American Herbal Pharmacopoeia, 2001.

127. Prior RL, Joseph J. Berries and fruits in cancer chemoprevention. In: Bagchi D, Preuss HG, eds. Phytopharmaceuticals in Cancer Chemoprevention. Boca Raton, FL: CRC Press, 2004: 465–79.

128. Hou DX. Curr Mol Med 2003;3:149–59.

129. Krikorian R, Shidler MD, Nash TA et al. J Agric Food Chem 2010;58:3996–4000.

130. Varadinova MG, Docheva-Drenska DI, Boyadjieva NI. Menopause 2009;16:345–9.

131. Prior RL. CAB Rev Perspect Agric Vet Sci Nutr Nat Resources 2010;5:1–9.

132. Prior RL, Wilkes S, Rogers T et al. J Agric Food Chem 2010;58:3970–6.

133. Prior RL, Wu X, Gu L et al. J Agric Food Chem 2008;56: 647–53.

134. DeFuria J, Bennett G, Strissel KJ et al. J Nutr 2009;139:1510–6.

135. Tsuda T, Matsumoto H. New therapeutic effects of anthocyanins: antiobesity effect, antidiabetes effect, and vision improvement. In: Mine Y, Shahidi F, Miyashita K, eds. Nutrigenomics and Proteomics in Health and Disease: Food Factors in Gene Interactions. New York: John Wiley and Sons, 2009:273–90.

136. Tsuda T, Ueno Y, Yoshikawa T et al. Biochem Pharmacol 2006;71:1184–97.

137. Hertog MG, Hollman PC, Katan MB. J Agric Food Chem 1992;40:2379–83.

138. Hertog MG, Hollman PC, Putte B. J Agric Food Chem 1993;41:1242–46.

139. Sesso HD, Gaziano JM, Liu S et al. Am J Clin Nutr 2003;77: 1400–8.

140. Knekt P, Kumpulainen J, Jarvinen R et al. Am J Clin Nutr 2002;76:560–8.

141. Geleijnse JM, Launer LJ, Van der Kuip DA et al. Am J Clin Nutr 2002;75:880–6.

142. Arts IC, Hollman PC, Feskens EJ et al. Eur J Clin Nutr 2001;55:76–81.

143. Lakenbrink C, Engelhardt UH, Wray V. J Agric Food Chem 1999;47:4621–4.

144. Gu L, Kelm MA, Hammerstone JF et al. J Nutr 2004;134:613–7.

145. Keen CL. J Am Coll Nutr 2001;20:436S–39S.

146. Zamora-Ros R, Andres-Lacueva C, Lamuela-Raventos RM et al. J Am Diet Assoc 2010;110:390–8.

147. Fotsis T, Pepper MS, Aktas E et al. Cancer Res 1997;57:2916–21.

148. Lin SY, Chang HP. Methods Find Exp Clin Pharmacol 1997;19:367–71.

149. Manthey JA, Grohmann K, Montanari A et al. J Nat Prod 1999;62:441–44.

150. Yang CS, Landau JM. J Nutr 2000;130:2409–12.

151. Anderson OM, Jordheim M. Anthocyanins. In: Andersen OM, Markham KR, eds. Flavonoids: Chemistry, Biochemistry and Applications. Boca Raton, FL: CRC Press, 2004.

152. Prior RL, Wu X, Gu L et al. Mol Nutr Food Res 2009;53:1406–18.

153. Prior RL, Wilkes S, Rogers T et al. FASEB J 2009;23:350.2.

154. Wu X, Beecher GR, Holden JM et al. J Agric Food Chem 2006;54:4069–75.

SUGGESTED READINGS

de Pascual-Teresa S, Moreno DA, Garcia-Viguera C. Flavanols and anthocyanins in cardiovascular health: a review of current evidence. Int J Mol Sci 2010;11:1679–703.

Galvano F, La Fauci L, Vitaglione P et al. Bioavailability, antioxidant and biological properties of the natural free-radical scavengers cyanidin and related glycosides. Ann 1st Super Sanita 2007;43:382–93.

Rasmussen SE, Frederiksen H, Struntze Krogholm K et al. Dietary proanthocyanidins: occurrence, dietary intake, bioavailability, and protection against cardiovascular disease. Mol Nutr Food Res 2005;49:159–74.

Romier B, Schneider Y, Larondelle Y et al. Dietary polyphenols can modulate the intestinal inflammatory response. Nutr Rev 2009;67:363–78.

38 PROBIOTICS AND PREBIOTICS AS MODULATORS OF THE GUT MICROBIOTA[1]

SANDRA TEJERO, IAN R. ROWLAND, ROBERT RASTALL, AND GLENN R. GIBSON

Driven by the increasing burden of gastrointestinal disease, the functional foods market has moved heavily toward gut-derived events. Specifically, these foods target the human gut to stimulate beneficial microbial genera either directly, by providing growth substrates to promote the growth of an individual's autochthonous "healthy flora" selectively (prebiotics), or by using live microbial additions (probiotics). Bifidobacteria and lactobacilli are the most common targets for in vivo within the large intestine for such fortification. The use of probiotics and prebiotics carries little to no risk for consumers, but it holds much promise for improved health and well-being. This chapter discusses the main types of probiotics and prebiotics and briefly describes some of the clinical applications of each approach (Table 38.1).

PROBIOTICS

The first widely accepted definition of probiotics was made by Fuller (1): "a live microbial feed supplement which beneficially affects the host by improving its intestinal microbial balance." A more recent formal definition of probiotics was proposed by the World Health Organization (FAO/WHO): "live microorganisms which, when administered in adequate amounts, confer a health benefit to the host" (2). Both definitions, as well as others that have been touted, rely on viability of the strains during ingestion and within the product. This requirement is key for probiotic efficacy.

Any health claims associated with a probiotic food product, including claims about disease risk reduction, are strictly regulated by the European Food Safety Authority (EFSA) in the European Union and the Food and Drug Administration (FDA) in the United States. Probiotics must be safe and devoid of any toxic potential and belong to the category of "generally regarded as safe" (GRAS) substances. Current issues are becoming protracted in the legislative arena, driven largely by disagreements on what constitutes a health claim when foods such as probiotics and prebiotics are considered.

Numerous studies have been published on the benefits of oral supplementation with certain probiotics on human health. These studies provide evidence of the important roles of probiotics to prevent, ameliorate, and possibly treat some disorders and diseases (3–5). It is difficult for legislators to ignore this scientific literature (>7000 PubMed articles on probiotics alone) in their deliberations on claim efficacy. Given the track record of success with probiotics and prebiotics as well as their history of safety, robust claims based on sound scientific evidence are overdue.

Probiotics are usually strains of lactic acid–producing bacteria, in particular members of the *Lactobacillus* and *Bifidobacterium* genera. This use is not least the result of the long and safe history of these bacteria in the manufacture of dairy products. Other microorganisms have also been developed as potential probiotics, including *Bacillus coagulans*, *Escherichia coli*, and *Saccharomyces*.

Probiotic Products

The most common delivery system for live microbes is dairy products such as milk, yogurt, and cheese. This use may have historical reasons because the Russian immunologist Elie Metchnikoff proposed in 1907 that lactobacilli present in yogurt played an important role in the prolongation of human life by promoting health (6). This proposal is generally seen as the birth of the probiotic concept. Technologic advances are making it possible to market a novel range of products, such as capsules and tablets, with advantages

---

[1] **Abbreviations: ADD**, antibiotic-associated diarrhea; **CDI**, *Clostridium difficile* infection; **CFU**, colony-forming units; **DP**, degree of polymerization; **FISH**, fluorescence in situ hybridization; **FOS**, fructooligosaccharide; **GOS**, galactooligosaccharide; **IBD**, inflammatory bowel disease; **IBS**, irritable bowel syndrome; **IMO**, isomaltooligosaccharide; **LGG**, *Lactobacillus rhamnosus* GG; **MOS**, mannooligosaccharide; **SOS**, soy oligosaccharide; **TD**, traveler's diarrhea; **XOS**, xylooligosaccharide.

TABLE 38.1	DESIRED CHARACTERISTICS OF PROBIOTICS AND PREBIOTICS
Probiotics	Beneficial effect when consumed
	Lack of pathogenicity and toxicity
	Large numbers of viable cells
	Ability to survive and metabolize in the gut
	Retained viability during storage and use
	If incorporated into a food, good sensory qualities
Prebiotics	Resistance to gastric acidity and hydrolysis by mammalian enzymes and gastrointestinal absorption
	Ability to be fermented by intestinal microflora
	Selective stimulation of growth and/or activity of intestinal bacteria associated with health and well-being

of longer shelf life, easier administration, straightforward distribution requirements, and storage at ambient temperatures. These products are based on spray or freeze drying technology, which preserves bacteria for extended periods.

Saarela et al (7) investigated the stability of *Bifidobacterium animalis* spp. *lactis* VTT E-D12010 during freeze drying, storage, and acid and bile exposure by using a milk-free culture medium and cryoprotectants to produce cells for non–milk-based applications. These investigators concluded that it was feasible to develop non–milk-based production technologies for probiotic cultures. This would give an advantage for the use of probiotics in individuals with lactose intolerance or in strict vegetarians.

Some other investigators have supported this technology by conducted in vitro studies (8, 9) and double-blind, placebo-controlled trials (10, 11).

Selection Criteria

Investigators generally agree that, to be effective, probiotics have to survive passage through the upper gastrointestinal tract by exhibiting resistance to the low pH, bile salts, and pancreatic enzymes (12–14). This is a challenge that some probiotics may not meet. However, given the level of evidence in human studies for positive health outcomes, it is apparent that many strains are able to compensate for the harsh physicochemical conditions of the gastrointestinal tract.

Another important aspect of probiotics is safety, and many investigators have reviewed the different requirements for a probiotic to be regarded as "safe" (15–17). Furthermore, probiotics need certain technologic properties to be cultured on large scale, in addition to an acceptable shelf life (15).

Probiotics and the Gut

Probiotic bacteria exert their activity mainly in the human gastrointestinal tract. Most health-related studies of probiotics have focused on this activity. This discussion is divided into noninfectious and infectious disorders. Some studies that are important for gauging probiotic success are summarized here. However, probiotics also act prophylactically by reducing the risk of disease. This use should be considered when considering the frequent question on when to use probiotics: Should healthy persons take these products? The answer is "yes" if the consumer wishes to help avoid gut difficulties such as gastroenteritis. The caveat is that the strains should be recognized probiotics and able to meet the various selection criteria that are required. Different strains are almost certain to exert different effects, as noted in the examples given in this discussion.

Noninfectious Disorders

Probiotics are claimed to be effective in a wide range of gastrointestinal disorders, particularly in diarrhea, irritable bowel syndrome (IBS), and inflammatory bowel disease (IBD). The potential of probiotics to alleviate IBS symptoms was shown in several studies carried out since 2000. IBS is a significant challenge because of its ubiquity, difficulty in diagnosis, and lack of therapeutic strategies. Trials have also shown a placebo effect, and this chapter cites studies in which the investigators controlled for this effect.

Evidence for efficacy in IBS has been generated from several studies.

O'Mahony et al (18) reported that further than improvement in symptoms, the consumption of *Bifidobacterium infantis* was associated with the normalization of the basal ratio of interleukin-10 to interleukin-12 (anti-inflammatory/proinflammatory cytokine). This ratio was lower in patients with IBS than in matched healthy controls, a finding suggesting an immune-modulating ability for this intervention. In a 4-week double-blind study by Whorwell et al (19), 362 adult patients were randomized to receive 1 of 3 different doses of freeze-dried encapsulated *B. infantis* 35624 or placebo. A dose of 10^8 colony-forming units (CFU)/mL showed the best scores in relation to abdominal pain, bloating, bowel dysfunction, incomplete evacuation, straining, and the passage of gas (19).

In a more recent double-blind, placebo-controlled study, 298 adults diagnosed with IBS were randomized to receive an *E. coli* preparation or placebo. Significant improvements in pain relief and typical symptoms were observed in the treatment group (20).

IBDs such as Crohn disease, ulcerative colitis, and pouchitis are recurrent inflammatory disorders of the colon and small intestine with a complex, undefined origin. Microbial involvement has been suggested, and if this is the case, then the potential for probiotic interventions against the culprit microorganisms is feasible.

In relation to maintain remission in Crohn disease, a study of 32 adults that compared the effect of treatment with mesalamine or the yeast *Saccharomyces boulardii* in combination with mesalamine demonstrated significantly fewer relapses in the second group, a finding supporting the beneficial effect of S. *boulardii* (21). In a more recent study of 34 patients with Crohn disease, the group receiving S. *boulardii* showed an improvement in intestinal permeability compared with a placebo group (22).

In active Crohn disease, further research is required because some studies (23, 24) could not show definite conclusions on the efficacy of probiotic therapy. Clinical efficacy of the probiotic mixture VSL #3 (a mixture of 4 species of lactobacilli, 3 species of bifidobacteria, and *Streptococcus thermophilus*) was assessed in a study of 34 ambulatory patients with active ulcerative colitis. Probiotic organisms were detected in 3 of 11 patients following microbiologic analysis of mucosal biopsies, and an induction of remission or response rate of 77% was observed (25). Another study (26) demonstrated that VSL #3 treatment of patients with ulcerative colitis produced an increase in fecal concentrations of VSL #3 bacteria and helped to maintain remission, because only 4 of 20 patients experienced relapse. Given that VSL #3 is a complex mixture of probiotic strains, it is currently unclear which of the individual constituents was responsible for the effects seen.

In relation to pouchitis, Gionchetti et al (27) assessed a reduction in the incidence of pouchitis in the treated group (10%) compared with the placebo group (40%) in 40 patients after ileal pouch-anal anastomosis for ulcerative colitis. Moreover, Mimura et al (28) later confirmed the effectiveness of this probiotic mixture in antibiotic-introduced remission in 36 patients with recurrent or chronic pouchitis who were randomized to receive either a daily dose of VSL #3 or placebo. Gosselink et al (29) reported a lower rate in episodes of pouchitis after pouch formation in patients receiving *Lactobacillus rhamnosus* GG (LGG), than in patients not treated with this probiotic.

Infectious Disorders

Probiotics have been shown to be promising for the management of infectious disorders. This approach holds much promise and shows how probiotics may be useful in disease prevention. Frequent travelers, hospitalized persons, and older persons are examples of high-risk populations that may benefit from using effective probiotics.

Increasing evidence shows that probiotic treatment can alleviate acute infectious diarrhea, mainly in infants and children. Several metaanalyses (30–33) reported some moderate effects in relation to the duration of diarrhea observed after therapeutic treatment with probiotics. The probiotic that has shown the best efficacy, in this regard, to date is LGG. Some of the controlled trials using LGG are discussed here.

In a double-blind, placebo-controlled trial developed by Shornikova et al (34), 123 children aged between 1 and 36 months who had acute diarrhea received oral rehydration and 5×10^9 CFU of LGG or placebo orally. LGG significantly shortened the duration of rotavirus diarrhea, but not of diarrhea with a confirmed bacterial cause. In another study involving 39 children, the group consuming LGG showed a significantly shorter duration in episodes of diarrhea and enhanced immunoglobulin A secretion, considered a parameter of local immune defense (35). Guandalini et al (3) carried out a controlled trial in which 287 children 1 month to 3 years old were randomized to receive either a live preparation of LGG or placebo; a reduction in almost 1 day in the course of the diarrhea was observed in the treatment group.

Probably the most extensively investigated use of probiotics related to infectious disorders is as adjunctive treatment to reduce antibiotic-associated diarrhea (AAD) in patients receiving antibiotic therapy. A metaanalysis by Szajewska et al (36) of data from five randomized-controlled trials showed that S. *boulardii* significantly reduced the risk of diarrhea in patients (adults and children) treated with antibiotics for any reason (mainly respiratory tract infections). Another metaanalysis also suggested that although S. *boulardii* and *Lactobacillus* spp. had the potential to prevent AAD, their efficacy remained to be proven (37).

McFarland (38) conducted a metaanalysis to compare the efficacy of probiotics for the prevention of AAD and treatment of *Clostridium difficile* infections (CDIs). Thirty-one randomized, controlled, blinded efficacy trials in humans involving 3164 subjects were included. The conclusions were that S. *boulardii*, LGG and some probiotic mixtures were the most effective, and in 25 of these controlled trials, the risk of developing AAD was significantly reduced.

Of further interest is the role of probiotics as an adjunct to metronidazole or vancomycin, antibiotics most commonly used to treat CDIs. Colonic CDI, a common complication of antibiotic therapy, can lead to colitis or pseudomembranous colitis. So far, only a few randomized, controlled trials can be found in the literature on the use of probiotics for the prevention of CDI, but the number is even more limited for treatment of CDI.

In a double-blind, placebo-controlled study (39), 135 hospital patients were randomized to receive a probiotic drink containing *Lactobacillus casei* DN-114 001 (*L. casei Imunitass*) $(1 \times 10^8$ CFU/mL), S. *thermophilus* $(1 \times 10^8$ CFU/mL), and *Lactobacillus bulgaricus* $(1 \times 10^7$ CFU/mL) or a placebo drink twice a day. Patients started intake of the drinks within 48 hours of antibiotic therapy and continued for 1 week after they stopped taking antibiotics. The results observed that only 12% of the patients in the probiotic group developed diarrhea associated with antibiotic use compared with 34% in the placebo group, and no subject in the probiotic group had diarrhea caused by C. *difficile* compared with 17% of patients in the placebo group. These promising results suggest that probiotics are useful to help manage CDI-associated diarrhea.

Administration of probiotics has also been studied as a promising strategy for reducing episodes of traveler's diarrhea (TD). In a metaanalysis of probiotics for the prevention of TD, McFarland (40) described 12 of 940 screened studies that met the inclusion and exclusion criteria (40). The pooled relative risk indicated that probiotics significantly prevent TD (relative risk = 0.85; 95% confidence interval, 0.79, 0.91; $p < .001$); several probiotics (*S. boulardii* and a mixture of *Lactobacillus acidophilus* and *Bifidobacterium bifidum*) had significant efficacy. No serious adverse reactions were reported (40).

Other Disorders

A relationship between probiotic consumption and colon cancer development was shown in studies with animal models (41, 42). For a long time, the main focus for probiotics was to treat gastrointestinal tract disorders and diseases (43). However, probiotics have also been suggested to have some effects for the prevention of allergic diseases such as atopic eczema (44–46).

PREBIOTICS

Another approach to increase the number of beneficial bacteria in the human intestinal microbiota is through the introduction of prebiotics into the diet. Investigators increasingly recognize that the species composition of the microbiota can be modified by relatively small changes in the diet such as the introduction of certain nondigestible carbohydrates. A prebiotic is defined as "a nondigestible food ingredient that beneficially affects the host by selectively stimulating the growth and/or activity of one or limited number of bacteria in the colon that confer benefits upon host well-being and health" (47). The concept was updated by Gibson et al (48), and the evidence for established and emerging prebiotics was reviewed. Most of the interest in the development of new prebiotics aims at nondigestible oligosaccharides—short-chain polysaccharides that consist of 2 to 20 saccharide units. Examples of these include inulin-type fructans, galactooligosaccharides (GOSs), isomaltooligosaccharides (IMOs), xylooligosaccharides (XOSs), soy oligosaccharides (SOSs), glucooligosaccharides, and lactosucrose (49, 50). Prebiotics owe their derivation to the probiotic concept and were first developed to influence gut microbiota but without survival issues in the intervention used. They are a far more recent development than probiotics, and fewer studies exist. Prebiotics alter the indigenous flora components in a selective manner. The health outcomes are more or less similar to those of probiotics, and this aspect of prebiotic science is therefore not discussed here.

Several studies demonstrated the important contribution of prebiotic substrates to the human gastrointestinal microbiota. The traditional targets for prebiotics are *Bifidobacterium* spp. and *Lactobacillus* spp. (47). Reports from in vitro studies revealed that prebiotics can modify the gastrointestinal tract microbial community by increasing bifidobacteria or lactobacilli numbers and thus can improve the health of the human gut and also enhance nonspecific immune responses (51, 52).

Furthermore, intervention studies supported the positive role of prebiotics on the microbial ecology of the human gut

(53–58). A review summarized the health aspects associated with prebiotics that stimulate bifidobacteria (59).

Types of Prebiotics

Fructooligosaccharides

Fructooligosaccharides (FOS) comprise a major class of bifidogenic oligosaccharides in terms of both production volume and use. FOSs are polymers of D-fructose joined by β-(2-1) bonds. Molecules with degree of polymerization (DP) between 3 and 5 are referred to as oligofructose, and those with a DP between 2 and 60 are referred to as inulin (60). FOS occurs naturally in a range of plants such as chicory, onion, garlic, tomato, and banana. FOSs are resistant to gastric acidity and hydrolysis by human digestive enzymes (sucrase, maltase, isomaltase, or lactase) and α-amylase of pancreatic excretions (61).

Chicory-derived FOS are among the most studied and well-established prebiotics. Wang and Gibson (51) determined the prebiotic effects of FOS in an in vitro study during comparison with a range of reference carbohydrates. Bacterial growth showed preferential fermentation by bifidobacteria, whereas populations of *E. coli* and *Clostridium perfringens* remained at relatively low levels. A later study by Gibson and Wang (62) determined the bifidogenic effect of oligofructose in single-stage continuous culture systems inoculated with human fecal bacteria. FOS preferentially enriched for bifidobacteria, compared with both inulin and sucrose.

A volunteer trial of healthy adults consuming 15 g/day of FOS showed significantly stimulated bifidobacterial levels (which became the predominant bacterial group enumerated) (63). Subsequent studies similarly demonstrated a major shift in the intestinal bacterial composition after ingestion of FOS, with bifidobacteria increasing significantly (64, 65). Harmsen et al (66) conducted an in vivo study in which 14 adult volunteers received 9 g/day of inulin for a period of 2 weeks. Quantification of bacterial groups by fluorescence in situ hybridization (FISH) showed a significant increase in bifidobacteria and a significant decrease in the *Eubacterium rectale–Clostridium coccoides* group. It therefore appears that inulin and FOS could be classified as prebiotic because they fulfil all the criteria that were stated. This latter study was important because it used molecular-based characterization of the microbiota.

Galactooligosaccharides

GOSs consist of β-(1-6) linked and β-(1-4) galactopyranosyl units linked to a terminal glucopyranosyl residue through an α-(1-4) glycosidic bond. GOSs have been reported in fermented milk as a result of β-galactosidase activity of starter cultures (67). These oligosaccharides are synthesized from lactose by a β-galactosidase transfer reaction resulting in the formation of a family of disaccharides to hexasaccharides, with end products depending on the source of the enzyme. The enzyme transfers the galactose moiety of a β-galactoside to an acceptor containing a hydroxyl group. In vitro studies demonstrated that GOS supports the growth of bifidobacteria in mixed culture and decreases the number of pathogenic bacteria.

In vivo studies have shown fecal bifidobacterial levels are stimulated, in healthy human adults, by consumption of different amounts of GOSs. One such study, involving 12 human volunteers who had abnormally low numbers of fecal bifidobacteria, demonstrated that consumption of GOSs resulted in a significant degree of bifidogenesis (68). However, once GOS intake ceased, the bifidobacterial numbers returned to initial levels. In some cases, this increased bifidobacterial population was accompanied by a decrease in *Bacteroides*.

Lactulose

Lactulose (4-*O*-β-D-galactopyranosyl-D-fructose) is also considered to be prebiotic (at sublaxative doses) and is manufactured by the isomerization of lactose. A double-blind, placebo-controlled parallel study demonstrated that lactulose increased the number of bifidobacteria and lactobacilli in feces, whereas *Bacteroides* and clostridia decreased (69). Another more recent study demonstrated a statistically significant and selective increase in bifidobacteria after administration of lactulose (70).

Emerging Prebiotics

Currently in Europe and the United States, two major prebiotics are used in food manufacturing (FOSs and GOSs). However, several emerging forms have not been tested as rigorously as FOSs or GOSs. Some of these ingredients are listed and further discussed here.

Isomaltooligosaccharides

IMOs are manufactured from starch by a two-stage enzymatic process (using α-amylase, pullulanase, and α-glucosidase) and are mixtures of α-1-6-glucosides such as isomaltose, isomaltotriose, panose, and isomaltotetraose (71). Pure culture studies showed that bifidobacteria metabolized IMOs faster than other intestinal bacteria (72). Other studies suggested that IMOs could reduce numbers of *C. perfringens* and Enterobacteriaceae in vivo, but they did not increase bifidobacterial numbers (71). The minimum effective dose of IMO to induce a significant increase in fecal bifidobacteria numbers of healthy men was 8 to 10 g/day (73).

Soy Oligosaccharides

SOSs are α-galactosyl sucrose derivatives isolated from soy bean whey during soy protein manufacture. The predominant oligosaccharides are the trisaccharide raffinose and the tetrasaccharide stachyose, which are nondigestible oligosaccharides and can therefore reach the colon (74). In vitro studies suggested that SOSs stimulate the growth of bifidobacteria to a far greater degree than any other organisms tested (75). Feeding SOSs to healthy human volunteers elicited a higher fecal recovery of bifidobacteria than the control diet (76).

Xylooligosaccharides

XOSs are chains of xylose molecules linked by β-1-4 bonds and mainly consist of xylobiose, xylotriose, and xylotetraose (77). XOSs are produced from xylan extracted mainly from corncobs. Xylan is hydrolyzed to XOS by the controlled activity of the enzyme 1,4-xylanase (78). Pure culture studies showed that XOS was metabolized by bifidobacteria (*B. bifidum, B. infantis,* and *Bifidobacterium longum*), but not by lactobacilli (79). An in vivo study of male rats suggested that XOSs were preferentially fermented by bifidobacteria and produced higher short-chain fatty acid levels when XOSs formed 6% of the diet (80).

Polydextrose

Polydextrose is a carbohydrate manufactured from glucose, which is partially metabolized in the body. In an in vitro gut simulator system, polydextrose was added, and the effect on colonic microbiota was evaluated by both FISH and percentage of guanine and cytosine (%G + C) profiling. Polydextrose appeared to have a stimulatory effect on colonic bifidobacteria throughout the system at both concentrations of 1% and 2% (seen by both FISH and %G + C analysis). Increased butyrate production after the administration of polydextrose was also observed compared with FOS (81). An in vivo study of rats showed that when polydextrose was combined with lactitol, the microbial composition was altered in a favorable way by significantly decreasing production of amines and branched-chain fatty acids and increasing butyrate production (82). Human studies are currently sparse.

Mannooligosaccharides

Mannan is a byproduct of the coffee industry. Its conversion to mannooligosaccharides (MOSs) is by thermal hydrolysis (83). A double-blind, placebo-controlled, crossover human intervention study showed that MOSs in a coffee product could selectively stimulate lactobacilli at both 3 and 5 g/day MOS intake (84).

Recent Research

Since 2000, Gibson et al have researched and developed a prebiotic GOS. BiMuno is a synthetic lactose-based oligosaccharide that, following ingestion, passes unchanged to the colon, where it serves as an energy source for saccharolytic colonic bacteria. BiMuno specifically increases populations of beneficial colonic bifidobacteria. It therefore is a recognized prebiotic. The following summarizes current progress:

- The GOS is synthesized from enzymes in *B. bifidum* 41171. Traditionally, GOS is made from yeasts or bacilli. However, use of a known probiotic is relevant because the bifidobacteria are the target genera for GOS metabolism. This strain has now been fully genome sequenced (http://www.broad. mit.edu/annotation/genome/Bifidobacterium_group/ MultiHome.html).

- BiMuno has been tested in vitro, in pigs, and in humans for its prebiotic effect (85, 86).
- Human studies in IBS (56), elderly persons (54), and TD (55) are complete and show initial efficacy.
- The synbiotic effects are now being researched with appropriate probiotics.
- The prebiotic is currently being tested in high-level athletes. This approach is driven by the hypothesis that intake will reduce the risk of gastroenteritis and concomitant effects upon performance.
- Research has shown that the gut microflora of both obese humans and mouse models of obesity is altered compared with lean counterparts. This finding raises the possibility of modulating the gut microflora as a novel strategy in tackling the epidemic of obesity and diabetes sweeping the developed world. A human study in markers of metabolic syndrome and dietary-based microbiota modulation by BiMuno is ongoing.

CONCLUSION

Functional foods have always been a popular area of nutrition, but they have also attracted some skepticism. These agents appear to be a simple way to improve health management in some conditions in selected patients, particularly when functional foods are directed toward gastrointestinal outcomes. The mode of operation of probiotics versus prebiotics differs in that probiotics are living microbes in the diet, whereas prebiotics fortify certain indigenous genera and species (see Table 38.1). What can be said with confidence is that the scientific basis for either approach has improved markedly since 2000 with the application of the latest technologies. These range from high-throughput molecular-based technologies for monitoring the gut microbiota (87) to metabonomic and proteomic outcomes that assess functionality. Probiotic and prebiotic applications can now be backed up by accurate determinations of mechanism of effect). This information has improved the scientific quality of the small trials undertaken to date and also may potentially increase consumer confidence in developed products. The types of legislative claims that can be made remain a gray, area but clinical and translational research is increasingly producing reliable information. Given the low risk associated with the intake of functional foods and their ready availability to consumers, investigators must study the potential clinical efficacy of these agents further in rigorous, randomized controlled trials.

REFERENCES

1. Fuller R. J Appl Bacteriol 1989;66:365–78.
2. Food and Agriculture Organization, World Health Organization. Joint FAO/WHO Working Group Report on Drafting Guidelines for the Evaluation of Probiotics in Food, London, Ontario, Canada, April 30 and May 1, 2002:1-11.
3. Guandalini S, Pensabene L, Zikri MA et al. J Pediatr Gastroenterol Nutr 2000;30:54–60.
4. Chapman CM, Gibson GR, Rowland I. Eur J Nutr 2011;50:1–17
5. de Vrese M, Winkler P, Rautenberg P et al. Clin Nutr 2005;24:481–91.
6. Metchnikoff E. The Prolongation of Life. London: Heinemann, 1907.
7. Saarela M, Virkajarvi I, Alakomi HL et al J Appl Microbiol 2005;99:1330–9.
8. Miyamoto-Shinohara Y, Imaizumi T, Sukenobe J et al. Cryobiology 2000;41:251–5.
9. Klayraung S, Viernstein H, Okonogi S. Int J Pharm 2009;370:54–60.
10. Francavilla R, Lionetti E, Castellaneta SP et al. Helicobacter 2008;13:127–34.
11. Kotowska M, Albrecht P, Szajewska H. Aliment Pharmacol Ther 2005;21:583–90.
12. Nemcová R. Vet Med 1997;42:19–27.
13. Mattila-Sandholm T, Mättö J, Saarela M. Int Dairy J 1999;9:25–35.
14. Dunne C, O'Mahony L, Murphy L et al. Am J Clin Nutr 2001;73:386–92.
15. Salminen S, von Wright A, Morelli L et al. Int J Food Microbiol 1998;44:93–106.
16. Saarela M, Mogensen G, Fonden R et al. J Biotechnol 2000;84:197–215.
17. Snydman DR. Clin Infect Dis 2008;46:104–11.
18. O'Mahony L, McCarthy J, Kelly P et al. Gastroenterology 2005;128:541–551.
19. Whorwell PJ, Altringer L, Morel J et al. Am J Gastroenterol 2006;101:1581–90.
20. Enck P, Zimmermann K, Menke G et al. Gastroenterol 2009;47:209–14.
21. Guslandi M, Mezzi G, Sorghi M et al. Dig Dis Sci 2000;45:1462–64.
22. Garcia Vilela E, De Lourdes De Abreu Ferrari M, Oswaldo Da Gama Torres H et al. Scand J Gastroenterol 2008;43:842–48.
23. Malchow HA. J Clin Gastroenterol 1997;25:653–8.
24. Gupta P, Andrew H, Kirschner BS et al. J Pediatr Gastroenterol Nutr 2000;31:453–7.
25. Bibiloni R, Fedorak RN, Tannock GW et al. Am J Gastroenterol 2005;100:1539–46.
26. Venturi A, Gionchetti P, Rizzello F et al. Aliment Pharmacol Ther 1999;13:1103–8.
27. Gionchetti P, Rizzello F, Helwig U et al. Gastroenterology 2003;124:1202–9.
28. Mimura T, Rizzello F, Helwig U et al. Gut 2004;53:108–14.
29. Gosselink MP, Schouten WR, van Lieshout LM et al. Dis Colon Rectum 2004;47:876–84.
30. Szajewska H, Mrukowicz JZ. J Pediatr Gastroenterol Nutr 2001;33:17–25.
31. Van Niel CW, Feudtner C, Garrison MM et al. Pediatrics 2002;109:678–84.
32. Huang JS, Bousvaros A, Lee JW et al. Dig Dis Sci 2002;47:2625–34.
33. Allen SJ, Okoko B, Martinez E et al. Cochrane Database Syst Rev 2004;(2):CD003048.
34. Shornikova AV, Isolauri E, Burkanova L et al. Acta Paediatr 1997;86:460–5.
35. Kaila M, Isolauri E, Soppi E et al. Pediatr Res 1992;32:141–4.
36. Szajewska H, Dziechciarz P, Mrukowicz J. Aliment Pharmacol Ther 2006;23:217–27.
37. D'Souza AL, Rajkumar C, Cooke J et al. BMJ 2002;324:1361.
38. McFarland LV. Am J Gastroenterol 2006;101:812–22.

39. Hickson M, D'Souza AL, Muthu N et al. BMJ 2007; 335:80–4.

40. McFarland LV. Travel Med Infect Dis 2007;5:97–105.

41. Rowland IR, Rumney CJ, Coutts JT et al. Carcinogenesis 1998;19:281–85.

42. Yamazaki K, Tsunoda A, Sibusawa M et al. Oncol Rep 2000; 7:977–82.

43. Collado MC, Meriluoto J, Salminen S. Lett Appl Microbiol 2007;45:454–60.

44. Kalliomäki M, Salminen S, Poussa T et al. J Allergy Clin Immunol 2007;119:1019–21.

45. Kuitunen M, Kukkonen K, Juntunen-Backman K et al. J Allergy Clin Immunol 2009;123:335–41.

46. Abrahamsson TR, Jakobsson T, Bottcher MF et al. J Allergy Clin Immunol 2007;119:1174–80.

47. Gibson GR, Roberfroid MB. J Nutr 1995;125:1401–12.

48. Gibson GR, Probert HM, Loo JV et al. Nutr Res Rev 2004;17:259–75.

49. Rastall RA, Maitin V. Curr Opin Biotechnol 2002;13:490–6.

50. Gibson GR, Berry Ottaway P, Rastall RA. Prebiotics: New Developments in Functional Foods. Oxford: Chandos, 2000.

51. Wang X, Gibson GR. J Appl Bacteriol 1993;75:373–80.

52. Rhoades J, Manderson K, Wells A et al. J Food Protect 2008;71:2272–7.

53. Costabile A, Klinder A, Fava F et al. Br J Nutr 2008;99: 110–20.

54. Vulevic J, Drakoularakou A, Yaqoob P et al. Am J Clin Nutr 2008;88:1438–46.

55. Drakoularakou A, Tzortzis G, Rastall RA et al. Eur J Clin Nutr 2010;64:146–52.

56. Silk DB, Davis A, Vulevic J et al. Aliment Pharmacol Ther 2009;29:508–18.

57. Rowland IR, Tanaka R. J Appl Bacteriol 1993;74:667–74.

58. Kleessen B, Schwarz S, Boehm A et al. Br J Nutr 2007;98: 540–9.

59. Roberfroid M, Gibson GR, Hoyles L et al. Br J Nutr 2010; 104(Suppl 2):S1–63.

60. Conway P. Asia Pac J Clin Nutr 1996;5:10–4.

61. Roberfroid MB. J Nutr 2007;137(Suppl):2493S–502S.

62. Gibson GR, Wang X. FEMS Microbiol Lett 1994;118: 121–8.

63. Gibson GR, Beatty ER, Wang X et al. Gastroenterology 1995;108:975–82.

64. Menne E, Guggenbuhl N, Roberfroid M. J Nutr 2000;130: 1197–9.

65. Tuohy KM, Kolida S, Lustenberger A et al. Br J Nutr 2001;86:341–8.

66. Harmsen HMJ, Raangs GC, He T et al. Appl Environ Microbiol 2002;68:2982–90.

67. Tzortzis G, Goulas AK, Gibson GR. Appl Microbiol Biotechnol 2005;68:412–6.

68. Ballongue J, Schumann C, Quignon, P. Scand J Gastroenterol 1997;32:41–4.

69. Tuohy KM, Ziemer CJ, Kinder A et al. Microb Ecol Health Dis 2002;14 165–73.

70. Pham TT, Shah NP. J Agric Food Chem 2008; 56: 4703-9.

71. Kohmoto T, Fukui F, Takaku H et al. Agric Biol Chem 1991;55:2157–9.

72. Kohmoto T, Fukui F, Takaku H et al. Bifid Microflora 1988;7:61–9.

73. Cummings JH, Macfarlane GT, Englyst HN. Am J Clin Nutr 2001;73:415S–20S.

74. Saito Y, Takano T, Rowland I. Microb Ecol Health Dis 1992;5:105–10.

75. Wada K, Watabe J, Mizutani J et al. J Agric Chem Soc Japan 1992;66:127–35.

76. Hopkins MJ, Cummings JH, Macfarlane GT et al. J Appl Microbiol 1998;85:381–6.

77. Playne MJ, Crittenden R. Bull Int Dairy Found 1996;313:10–22.

78. Campbell JM, Fahey GC, Wolf BW. J Nutr 1997;127:130–36.

79. Jaskari J, Kontula P, Siitonen A et al. Appl Microbiol Biotechnol 1998;49:175-81.

80. Probert HM, Apajalahti JH, Rautonen N et al. Appl Environ Microbiol 2004;70:4505–11.

81. Peuranen S, Tiihonen K, Apajalahti JH et al. Br J Nutr 2004;91:905–14.

82. Asano I, Nakamura Y, Hoshino H et al. Nippon Nogeikagaku Kaishi 2001;75:1077–83.

83. Janardhana V, Broadway MM, Bruce MP et al. J Nutr 2009;139:1404–9.

84. Tzortzis G, Goulas AK, Gee JM et al. J Nutr 2005;135: 1726–31.

85. Depeint F, Tzortzis G, Vulevic J et al. Am J Clin Nutr 2008;87:785–91.

86. Walton GE, van den Heuvel EG, Kosters MH et al. Br J Nutr 2012;107:1466–74.

87. Chapman CM, Gibson GR, Rowland I. Eur J Nutr 2011; 50:1–17.

SUGGESTED READINGS

Chapman CM, Gibson GR, Rowland I. Health benefits of probiotics: are mixtures more effective than single strains? Eur J Nutr 2011;50:1–17.

Charalampopoulos D, Rastall RA, eds. Prebiotics and Probiotics: Science and Technology. New York: Springer, 2010

Gibson GR, Roberfroid MB, eds. A Handbook of Prebiotics. Boca Raton, FL: Taylor & Francis, 2008.

Gibson GR, Scott KP, Rastall RA et al. Dietary prebiotics: current status and new definition. IFIS Functional Foods Bull 2010;7:1–19.

Saulnier DM, Kolida S, Gibson GR. Microbiology of the human intestinal tract and approaches for its dietary modulation. Curr Pharm Des 2009; 15: 1403–14.

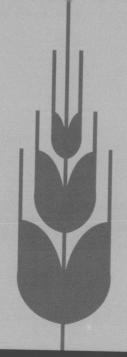

PART II

NUTRITIONAL ROLES IN INTEGRATED BIOLOGIC SYSTEMS

39 NUTRITIONAL REGULATION OF GENE EXPRESSION AND NUTRITIONAL GENOMICS[1]

ROBERT J. COUSINS AND LOUIS A. LICHTEN

Gene expression is a term that has different interpretations. These interpretations are dictated by the context in which the term is used. For example, phenotypes of health or disease are manifestations of gene expression. Similarly, the mechanics and control factors for gene transcription and mRNA translation that influence which proteins are produced also constitute gene expression. From the standpoint of nutritional influences on gene expression, processes are envisioned in which dietary conditions, either through direct interaction of specific nutrients with transcription factors (TFs) or mRNA–binding proteins or, more commonly, through indirect or exocrine means, produce changes that define phenotypic expression. The technical approaches described in this tutorial chapter are central to all research in contemporary biologic science and are actively applied in the nutritional sciences.

HISTORICAL PERSPECTIVE

Although the classic experiments of Nobel laureates François Jacob and Jacques Monod in 1961 were conducted in bacteria, they demonstrated that genes, under nutrient control through an operon, influence synthesis of enzymes involved in the metabolism of that nutrient (1).

Experiments with mammalian systems with specific nutrients followed after the operon model was proposed. Classic experiments of particular note were those demonstrating that polyribosome formation depended on the presence of essential amino acids in the diet, and the interaction of metabolites of vitamin A and vitamin D with nuclear receptors to produce physiologic effects.

GENE REGULATION BY NUTRIENTS

Nutrient regulation of gene expression is a well-recognized research emphasis in contemporary nutritional science. It is difficult to separate direct effects of individual nutrients on gene expression from those produced indirectly through physiologically controlled mediators and modulating molecules that are responsive to the diet. Consequently, experiments at the level of individual cells are essential to identify effects of nutrients that are clearly direct. However, interpretation of cell-level findings must be kept within an integrative context of the multicellular organ system to appreciate fully how dietary components and patterns influence the expression of genes in various tissues. The way in which the diet—in concert with hormones, cytokines, and growth factors—interacts to influence the differential expression of specific genes has reached a level of awareness that a new term, nutritional genomics (or nutrigenomics/nutrigenetics), has evolved to describe such relationships (2). Nutritional genomics includes all genetic factors, including epigenetic events, as they modulate individual genes and gene networks. It is one of a growing number of terms in general use in the nutritional sciences literature (Table 39.1), and it tends to replace the former term *nutrient–gene interactions*. The latter is a narrow term that implies a direct interaction of a nutrient with a gene. The closest examples of a nutrient–gene interaction may include nutrient binding to a TF for subsequent interaction with a response element of a gene, the methylation of specific genes, nutrient influenced acylation of TFs, or nutrient inhibition and activation of pathways that influence gene activation.

A generalized cell showing different modes of gene regulation by nutrients is illustrated in Figure 39.1. A "direct" effect of some nutrients (active metabolites of vitamins A and D; zinc; n-3 fatty acids and sterols) on gene transcription is shown in which, subsequent to ligand binding to

[1]**Abbreviations: ATP**, adenosine triphosphate; **ChIP**, chromatin immunoprecipitation; **CoA**, coenzyme A; **ES**, embryonic stem; **FAS**, fatty acid synthase; **HIF**, hypoxia-inducible factor; **miRNA**, micro RNA; **PCR**, polymerase chain reaction; **siRNA**, small interfering RNA; **TF**, transcription factor; **USF1**, upstream transcription factor-1.

TABLE 39.1	TERMS FREQUENTLY USED IN STUDIES ON NUTRITIONAL REGULATION OF GENE EXPRESSION

Term	Definition	Term	Definition
Acetylome	Reversible acetylation at the whole proteome level	Nuclear receptor	A transcription factor protein that requires a ligand (e.g., calcitriol for nuclear translocation and DNA binding)
Chromatin immunoprecipitation (ChIP)	Transcription factor antibodies precipitate DNA fragments to identify genes regulated by a specific transcription factor	Nutritional genomics	Genomic studies that relate nutritional factors in regulation of genes that influence cellular processes genome wide
cis-Acting	DNA elements on the same strand as a structural gene, to which transcription factors bind to and initiate transcription	Ortholog	A gene with similar function to a gene in evolutionarily related to species; ortholog comparisons help predict gene function
DNA array	Immobilized sequences of single-stranded DNA (probe) on a matrix that allows hybridization of mRNAs for quantitation of transcript abundance (also called gene chips or DNA chips)	PAGE	Polyacrylamide gel electrophoresis
Epigenetic	Nonmutational modification of a gene (e.g., by methylation and histone changes that influence expression of a specific gene)	PCR	Polymerase chain reaction
Exon-intron junction	A junction between a block of coding sequence (exon) and an adjacent block of noncoding sequence (intron) present in DNA and in precursor messenger RNA (pre-mRNA)	Polygenic	Disease or phenotypic characteristic caused by more than one gene
Functional genomics	Relationship of genes, proteins, and regulatory networks with physiologic function	Protein array	Antibodies or other proteins immobilized to a matrix allowing abundance of specific proteins to be qualitatively detected or interacting proteins to be identified
Genomics	Study of the singular or collective roles that genes play in cellular processes as influenced by external factors; prefixes such as chemo-, epi-, pharmaco-, or toxico- can define specialization in genomics	Proteomics	Proteome-wide analysis of protein structure, posttranslational modification, interactions, and function
Haplotype	A set of DNA variations, or polymorphisms, usually inherited together; haplotype can refer to a combination of alleles or to a set of single nucleotide polymorphisms found on the same chromosome	qPCR	Quantitative PCR in which the relative abundance of a sequence (mRNA derived cDNA) is compared to a normalizing sequence
Homolog	Gene that has the same evolutionary origin and function in two or more species	Response element	Portion of a gene sequence that must be present for that gene to respond to a stimulus; response elements are binding sites for transcription factors
In silico	In or by means of computer simulation of complex biologic systems; term frequently used in microarray research in which extensive computational algorithms or comparisons are executed	RNA interference (RNAi or siRNA)	Use of short RNA molecules, frequently derived from double-stranded RNA, that, on introduction into cells and complementary hybridization to specific mRNA, decrease gene expression
Metabolomics	Global analysis of all metabolites in a complex system	Single nucleotide polymorphism (SNP)	Single base substitution in coding sequence of a gene; frequently determines phenotypic differences in a population (human genome has ~10 million SNPs)
Micro RNA (miRNA)	Short regulatory form of RNA that binds to a target RNA molecule and generally suppresses its translation	Systems biology	Study of complex interactions of organ systems down to molecules
Monogenic	Disease or phenotypic characteristic produced by a single gene	trans-Acting factors	DNA-binding proteins (transcription factor) are trans because they are products of genes from other chromosomes that bind to regulatory elements; transcription factors that bind some nutrients are trans-acting factors
Noncoding RNAs	Segments of RNA that are not translated into amino acid sequences but may be involved in the regulation of gene expression	Transcription factor (TF)	Proteins that bind regulatory regions of a gene and influence the transcription rate of the gene. Some bind to nutrients vitamins and minerals for activity
		Transcriptome	All transcribed mRNAs within a cell or tissue at a particular time

a specific TF, cytoplasmic to nuclear translocation of the complex occurs, and interaction through a specific domain of the factor with a response element sequence (specific nucleotide sequence) of the regulatory region produces a change in transcription rate of the gene. In most situations involve a complex of multiple TFs and modifying proteins. Amino acid deprivation at the cellular level may activate transcription from specific defense genes through *cis*-acting nutrient-sensing response elements (see also Chapter 47: Mechanisms of Nutrient Sensing). The control of translation of specific mRNAs by iron is another example of a "direct" nutrient effect on gene expression, in this case at the level of mRNA stability and translation efficiency, to increase the abundance of a protein. Repression of mRNA by micro RNA leading to mRNA degradation is also shown in Figure 39.1.

Frequently, gene regulation by nutrients is complex. Multiple and interconnected factors, including nutrient effects on signal transduction pathways, epigenetic effects on specific genes, gene polymorphisms, alternative mRNA splicing and translation, and posttranslational modifications, converge to define indirect effects on expression of a specific gene. Studies have shown that nutritionally responsive TFs (e.g., sterol regulatory element–binding protein [SREBP]) are able to influence activity of numerous promoters through TF isoforms and coregulatory nuclear proteins that regulate lipid metabolic genes (3). Hypoxia-inducible factor (HIF) induced by iron deficiency similarly regulates multiple genes of iron metabolism (4). Metal-response element binding transcription factor-1 (MTF1)–activated nuclear translocation and DNA binding by interacting with zinc induces multiple zinc-regulatory and zinc-transporter proteins (5). Moving further clockwise around the nuclear envelope, Figure 39.1 shows the influence of TF phosphorylation, which can be either activating or deactivating. Zinc-repressing phosphatase activity, with sustained TF activation, is given as an example (6). Citrate, a product of intermediary metabolism, can diffuse into the nucleus, and adenosine triphosphate (ATP)–citrate lyase activity produces acetyl-coenzyme A (CoA). Nuclear acetyl-CoA leads to histone acetylation and activation of hexokinase 2 and other glucose-metabolizing enzymes and possibly to global changes in acetylation and gene expression (7). An example of the complexity in nutrient gene regulation is the fatty acid synthase (FAS) gene (8). During fasting, FAS is held in check by upstream transcription factors-1 and 2 (USF1 and USF2), TFs that are deacetylated by histone deacetylases (HDACs), thus leading to FAS promoter inactivation. On feeding, USF1 is phosphorylated; this process generates interactions with numerous other interacting TFs (>7) to produce increased USF1 acetylation and FAS promoter activation.

Numerous dietary constituents, most notably folic acid and one-carbon donors, influence DNA methylation (9). This process leads to a conversion of cytosine to thymidine through a methylation reaction. When the CpG sequences of gene promoters are methylated, the affinity

of the TF for the target gene is altered. As a result of this DNA methylation, the transcription rate for the gene can be substantially altered. These concepts and their effects on genetic variation are described in detail in Chapter 40: Genetic Variation: Effect on Nutrient Utilization and Metabolism, and Chapter 41: Epigenetics.

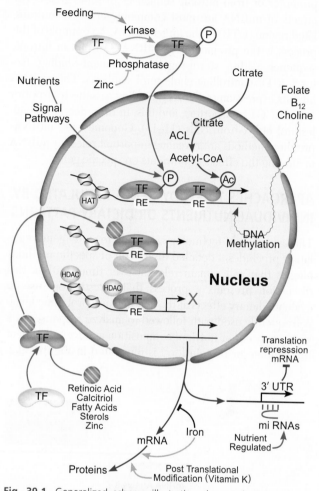

Fig. 39.1. Generalized scheme illustrating the regulation of gene expression by nutrients. Metabolites of some fat-soluble vitamins (retinoic acid and calcitrol), fatty acids, sterols, and zinc bind to specific transcription factor (TF) and produce nuclear translocation and binding to specific DNA sequences (response elements) of target genes. TFs binding retinoic acid, calcitrol, and fatty acids are called nuclear receptors and bind DNA as heterodimers or homodimers. Histone deacetylases (HDAC) and histone acetyltransferases (HAT) regulate histone activity by acetylation and are components of larger DNA-binding complexes. Some nutrients activate transmembrane receptors, which activate intracellular signaling pathways to initiate or modify gene expression. Some nutrients influence TF phosphorylation and thus influence gene expression. Intranuclear ATP-citrate lyase can convert citrate to acetyl-coenzyme A (CoA) and through TF acetylation influences gene expression. Some nutrients including folate and vitamin B₁₂ influence gene expression through DNA methylation. Some nutrients regulate genes that produce micro RNAs (miRNAs) that repress gene expression primarily through repressing translation of target mRNAs. Iron and some other nutrients influence gene expression at the posttranscriptional level through control of degradation of some specific mRNAs and stabilization of other specific mRNAs. Posttranslational modification of proteins can be produced by specific nutrients (e.g., vitamin K). *Ac,* acetyl; *ACL,* acyl-CoAlyase; *P,* phosphoryl (group); *RE,* response element.

Small RNA sequences are known to hybridize to mRNAs and result in translational repression or mRNA destabilization and degradation (10). It is now clear that such RNAs, as double-stranded RNA of approximately 22 nucleotides called micro RNAs (miRNAs), regulate many physiologic responses in animals. miRNAs are transcribed by their own promoter or from intronic sequences of some genes. The targets of miRNA are most commonly in the 3′ untranslated region (UTR) of the target mRNA. An example of this process is the production of miRNA-33 from an intronic sequence within sterol-regulatory element-binding factor-2, a TF controlling cholesterol synthesis. This miRNA inhibits expression of the ATP-binding cassette transporter G1 (ABCG1 transporter), and this, in turn, decreases cholesterol efflux from cells (11–13). Genome-wide miRNA-profiling methods are revealing important roles for miRNA in altering the effects of nutrients on specific genes.

APPROACHES TO STUDY GENES REGULATED BY INDIVIDUAL NUTRIENTS OR DIETARY PATTERNS

The explosion of technology available to study gene regulation precludes a detailed discussion of specific methodologies that will remain relevant over time. Rather, this discussion presents a process that investigators use to evaluate dietary effects at the genome and proteome level. A frequently used path followed to analyze responses of a single nutrient or nutrient composition and formulation at the genome or protein level is illustrated in Figure 39.2.

Vendors are increasingly targeting products that facilitate sample acquisition and preservation. An example is the ability to obtain blood cells by methods that allow stabilization of RNA. This is particularly important in clinical and field (intervention) protocols in which analyses are usually delayed. Protein analyses have similar limitations; nevertheless, methods extending to mass spectral identification of proteins and metabolites regulated by specific genes are now available. Websites of commercial vendors can provide excellent tutorials on applicable methods.

The approach outlined in Figure 39.2 shows how the abundance of a known transcript can be evaluated by quantitative real-time polymerase chain reaction (qPCR). This technology has become the frontline method of choice for most research involving gene expression. Northern analysis has the advantage of an estimate of transcript size, but it is hindered by requiring a labeled DNA probe (usually with phosphorus-32 [^{32}P]); only limited replicates can be processed, and the method is not quantitative. In situ hybridization can identify a site of mRNA abundance within a cell and could establish a nutrient response within a given cell type or tissue. The method is not considered quantitative. Analysis at the genome-wide level most frequently uses DNA microarrays to obtain profiles of transcripts that increase or decrease in response to feeding a particular diet or specific nutrient. This approach detects potential associations and can identify previously unknown nutrient-responsive targets. PCR arrays are narrower in scope and are used to identify genes within a given process

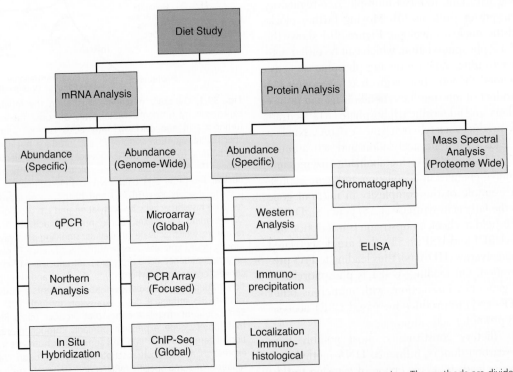

Fig. 39.2. Flow diagram of some analytic approaches used to identify nutrient effects on gene expression. The methods are divided into those at the transcript and protein levels. *ChIP-seq,* chromatin immunoprecipitation with sequencing; *ELISA,* enzyme-linked immunosorbent assay; *PCR,* polymerase chain reaction; *qPCR,* quantitative real-time polymerase chain reaction.

(e.g., oxidative stress, apoptosis, or a given cell signaling pathway). Chromatin immunoprecipitation with sequencing (ChIP-seq) takes advantage of ChIP to immunoprecipitate a TF associated with DNA, followed by massively parallel DNA sequencing to identify genes occupied by the specific TF. Specificity and selectivity of the identification rest with the selected antibody. The method enables researchers to identify novel loci for specific nutrition-related diseases and traits. An early example of this technology is the identification of vitamin D receptor–binding targets and the increased DNA-binding targets produced by calcitriol stimulation (14).

The flow chart in Figure 39.2 also provides an overview of techniques to answer questions related to nutritionally responsive processes at the proteome level. The abundance of a specific protein is most typically estimated by a blotting procedure. The proteins are separated by size by polyacrylamide gel electrophoresis (PAGE), and then the protein of interest is detected immunologically with a specific antibody. Sensitivity is increased through secondary antibodies linked to a reagent that produces luminescence before detection by x-ray film exposure. The latter process is frequently referred to as immunoblotting or Western blotting. Immunoprecipitation is a much less frequently used technique, but it can be a valuable aid for sample enrichment before a further analytic procedure to detect a target protein. Antibodies are also used to detect specific proteins in histologic specimens. The method can

accurately identify the location of a protein within a cell and if the protein is subject to trafficking within the cell. For example, the endosomal recycling of nutrient transporters in response to nutrient availability can be visualized through these methods. Enzyme-linked immunosorbent assay (ELISA) methods are widely used in nutrition research and in clinically related studies to measure specific proteins of interest. Most frequently, these are small proteins and peptides, such as cytokines, found in serum samples. Chromatography is less widely used as a method that leads to the identification of a specific protein with a nutritionally related process, but it can be an important first step in a protein purification assay (e.g., ion-exchange chromatography) before detection of the abundance of the protein by a method with greater specificity.

The field of proteomics is relatively new to nutrition-related studies, but it has exceptional promise as an analytic and research aid (15). The identification of specific proteins in an analytic sample most typically uses matrix-assisted laser desorption/ionization mass spectrometry (MALDI-MS). This approach is extremely useful because of the extensive protein and peptide databases that are available (see Fig. 39.2). These methods are gaining popularity to identify and measure nutritionally responsive biomarkers (16–18).

Figures 39.3 and 39.4 model the way in which most studies related to nutritional processes can be conducted. At the gene level, an initial aim is to establish whether

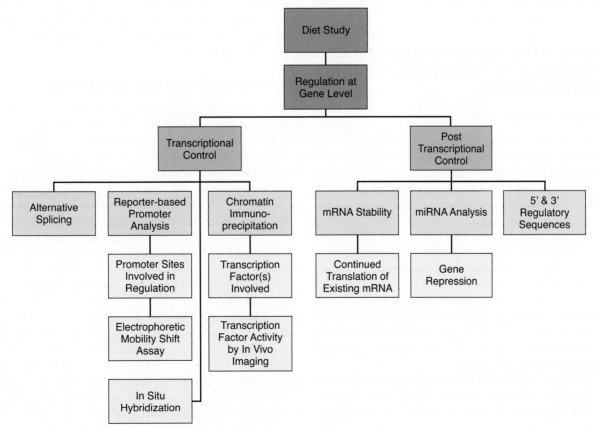

Fig. 39.3. Flow diagram of research approaches to define nutrient effects on gene regulation. *miRNA,* micro RNA.

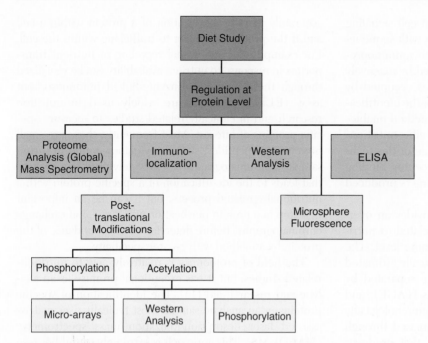

Fig. 39.4. Flow diagram of research approaches to define nutrient effects on regulation at the protein level. *ELISA,* enzyme-linked immunosorbent assay.

the mode of nutritional regulation is transcriptional or posttranscriptional, or both. Subsequent analyses are then directed at promoter activity, mRNA stability, and repression by miRNA. At the protein level, the studies are more analytically focused, based on abundance and cellular localization. Nevertheless, important mechanistic studies aimed at nutritionally responsive acetylation and phosphorylation processes are important in evaluating posttranslational modifications.

APPROACHES TO IDENTIFY AND MANIPULATE GENES REGULATED BY INDIVIDUAL NUTRIENTS OR DIETARY PATTERNS

Transgenic Animals

The term *transgenic* refers to both overexpression and deletion of expression of a specific gene. However, transgenesis most frequently is used to describe the technique that results in overexpression of a structural gene. The transgenic overexpression technique involves production of a construct consisting of a promoter and structural gene. The promoter can be the gene's normal promoter (homologous) or a different promoter (heterologous). A purified sample of the construct is injected into fertilized eggs (usually murine or porcine). If the construct DNA becomes appropriately integrated into the genome, transgenic animals will be produced from those eggs after the eggs are returned to foster mothers for the full gestation period. Selective breeding can produce homozygous lines of animals carrying transgenes.

Transgenic animals have been used to address questions of nutritional interest. A notable example is overexpression of the glucose transporter (GLUT4) in mice using the aP2 fatty acid–binding protein promoter and a genomic

DNA fragment containing the entire human *GLUT4* gene (19). Overexpression resulted in higher glucose transport rates, lower glucose tolerance curves, and greater body fat. Unfortunately, most transgenic mice strains do not exhibit such dramatic changes in phenotype or give unanticipated outcomes. The number of nutritionally relevant genes that have been overexpressed in transgenic mice is now extensive. Many strains of transgenic mice are available through distributors of laboratory animals and through mutant mouse research centers supported by the National Institutes of Health.

Gene Knockout (Null Mutation) Animals

Gene-knockout technology provides the opportunity to eliminate expression of a specific gene (null mutation). As a result, the normal gene product is not produced. Null mutations produce phenotypes that run the gamut from embryonic lethality to no apparent effect. Consequently, the technology is not exactly the genetically engineered counterpart to spontaneous mutations that occur in the laboratory animals and are propagated by selective breeding techniques. These mutations usually result in altered function of the gene product. The *ob* gene mutation of mice is an example of a spontaneous mutation (20).

The technique of creating a knockout animal model or null mutation is more correctly called gene targeting by homologous recombination. The targeted gene is disrupted in one allele (producing heterozygotes with the null mutation). Two approaches to developing knockout mice are used (21). The original approach is to isolate the murine gene under investigation, identify the exons by mapping, delete part of an exon, and replace it with the gene encoding neomycin resistance (which produces a marker for selection). An entire exon can also be deleted. This construct is the gene-targeting vector. The targeting vector is linearized and is transfected into embryonic stem (ES) cells by microinjection or electroporation. The transfected cells are then injected into blastocysts that have been removed from pregnant mice, and the transfected cells are introduced into pseudopregnant mice. The second, and more recent, approach can provide cell type–specific targeting of a gene deletion. The gene is engineered to have *loxP* sites on either side, and by ES cell technology, a transgenic line is created that carries the target gene.

Extensions of these methods have been employed to create conditional-knockout mutations (22). In this approach, Cre recombinase is expressed with a tissue-specific promoter. This allows production of mice whose genes are inactivated in a tissue-specific mode or during a specific period of development. Alternatively, a library of mutant ES cells covering much of the mouse genome is available through the International Gene Trap Consortium (http://www.genetrap.org). Gene trapping is a high-throughput method that uses vectors that produce *lacZ* fusion sequences with native endogenous gene transcripts and disrupt normal transcription of that gene (23, 24). A method for posttranslational modification of specific gene trap vectors, flanked *lox* site insertion (Floxin), is applicable to generation of conditional loss-of-function modifications of gene trap ES cells (25). Other technologies such as the use of proprietary zinc-finger nuclease technology to produce targeted gene ablation are applicable to mutant mouse development.

Numerous nutritionally relevant knockout models have addressed important questions about nutrient metabolism and function. Examples are the intestinal targets of hormonal form of vitamin D (calcitrol) that control calcium absorption (26, 27). Frequently, complete ablation of a gene leads to embryonic lethality because of loss of gene function, whereas in other cases the standard knockout of a gene may have no major phenotypic effect. To prevent these phenotypic outcomes an alternative is to produce conditional-knockout mice. The adaptive induction of iron absorption through HIF and the role of heart-specific knockout of the Ctr1 copper transporter revealing a systemic signaling mechanism in copper metabolism are examples (4, 28). An interesting extension of knockout technology is to cross-breed transgenic mice and knockout mice. When this technique is skillfully applied, valuable insights into metabolic pathways and phenotypes can be produced. For example, breeding transgenic mice overexpressing apolipoprotein A-I to apolipoprotein E null mice produced an increased high-density lipoprotein concentration and increased atherosclerotic lesions (29). Cross-breeding of such models has generated interest.

Inhibition of Gene Expression by RNA Interference

Antisense RNA technology has been used as a research tool for a limited number of genes of nutritional interest. The principle is that a small RNA sequence complementary (antisense) to a target mRNA can inhibit its translation or stimulate its degradation. Early use of antisense RNA sequences for gene silencing employed short synthetic oligonucleotides to inhibit the translation of specific mRNAs transiently by hybridization. These oligonucleotides appear to be taken up by some tissues. In these cases, antisense DNA sequences are introduced into specific areas of the brain.

The use of small interfering RNA (siRNA) has become widely accepted as an approach to gene silencing at the cell level (30, 31). Animals have retained an ancestral defense system that degrades double-stranded RNA by using an RNase (i.e., Dicer) to RNA sequences of 21 to 23 base pair (bp) in length, called siRNA. These RNA strands bind to target mRNA and promote its degradation. A synthetic oligonucleotide can replace the siRNA. In practice, double-stranded RNAs (200 to 1000 bp) or short RNAs (20 to 25 bp) produced with commercially available reagents, expression vectors, and enzymes are available to accomplish gene silencing. A disadvantage of the siRNA approach to gene suppression is that suppression is leaky; that is, inhibition of a specific gene is not 100%, as is the case with a knockout. Furthermore, the gene silencing achieved is frequently transient rather than stable. The development of small hairpin RNA (shRNA) vectors has circumvented the approach of transient siRNA transfection of cells to inhibit genes of interest. The technology has gained use for silencing genes of nutritional interest. An advantage of siRNA for gene silencing is that it allows knockdown of genes that would be otherwise lethal if knocked out in the embryo.

CONCLUSIONS

The area of nutrition and gene expression has developed rapidly and is now a recognized research discipline (nutritional genomics) in nutritional sciences. Because our knowledge of animal and human genomes is now complete, the technologies described here and new approaches still waiting to be developed will continue to have a profound impact on nutrition as a field and on our understanding of how diet and genetics influence phenotypic expression.

ACKNOWLEDGMENTS

Appreciation is expressed to the National Institute of Diabetes and Digestive and Kidney Diseases and the Boston Family Endowment from the University of Florida for long-term research support.

REFERENCES

1. Jacob F, Monod J. J Mol Biol 1961;3:318–56.
2. Muller M, Kersten S. Nat Rev Genet 2003;4:315–22.
3. Bennett MK, Seo YK, Datta S et al. J Biol Chem 2008;283: 15628–37.
4. Shah YM, Matsubara T, Ito S et al. Cell Metab 2009;9:152–64.
5. Wang Y, Lorenzi I, Georgiev O et al. Biol Chem 2004;385: 623–32.

6. Aydemir TB, Liuzzi JP, McClellan S et al. J Leukoc Biol 2009;86:337–48.
7. Wellen KE, Hatzivassiliou G, Sachdeva UM et al. Science 2009;324:1076–80.
8. Wong RH, Chang I, Hudak CS et al. Cell 2009;136:1056–72.
9. Tibbetts AS, Appling DR. Annu Rev Nutr 2010;30:57–81.
10. Bartel DP. Cell 2009;136:215–33.
11. Rayner KJ, Suarez Y, Davalos A et al. Science 2010;328:1570–3.
12. Najafi-Shoushtari SH, Kristo F, Li Y et al. Science 2010; 328:1566–9.
13. Marquart TJ, Allen RM, Ory DS et al. Proc Natl Acad Sci U S A 2010;107:12228–32.
14. Ramagopalan SV, Heger A, Berlanga AJ et al. Genome Res 2010;20:1352–60.
15. Bantscheff M, Schirle M, Sweetman G et al. Anal Bioanal Chem 2007;389:1017–31.
16. Moresco JJ, Dong MQ, Yates JR 3rd. Am J Clin Nutr 2008; 88:597–604.
17. Kussmann M, Panchaud A, Affolter M. J Proteome Res 2010; 9:4876–87.
18. Linke T, Ross AC, Harrison EH. J Chromatogr A 2004; 1043:65–71.
19. Shepherd PR, Gnudi L, Tozzo E et al. J Biol Chem 1993; 268:22243–6.
20. Ingalls AM, Dickie MM, Snell GD. J Hered 1950;41:317–8.
21. Leiter EH. Diabetologia 2002;45:296–308.
22. Liu P, Jenkins NA, Copeland NG. Genome Res 2003;13: 476–84.
23. Yamamura K, Araki K. Cancer Sci 2008;99:1–6.
24. Lee T, Shah C, Xu EY. Mol Hum Reprod 2007;13:771–9.
25. Singla V, Hunkapiller J, Santos N et al. Nat Methods 2010; 7:50–2.
26. Kutuzova GD, Akhter S, Christakos S et al. Proc Natl Acad Sci U S A 2006;103:12377–81.
27. Benn BS, Ajibade D, Porta A et al. Endocrinology 2008; 149:3196–205.
28. Kim BE, Turski ML, Nose Y et al. Cell Metab 2010;11: 353–63.
29. Plump AS, Scott CJ, Breslow JL. Proc Natl Acad Sci U S A 1994;91:9607–11.
30. Morris KV, Chan SWL, Jacobsen SE et al. Science 2004; 27:1289–92.
31. Rondinone CM. Biotechniques 2006;40:S31–6.

SUGGESTED READINGS

Bartel DP. MicroRNAs: target recognition and regulatory functions. Cell 2009;136:215–33.

Ramagopalan SV, Heger A, Berlanga AJ et al. A ChIP-seq defined genome-wide map of vitamin D receptor binding: associations with disease and evolution. Genome Res 2010;20:1352–60.

Wong RH, Chang I, Hudak CS et al. A role of DNA-PK for the metabolic gene regulation in response to insulin. Cell 2009;136: 1056–72.

Tibbetts AS, Appling DR. Compartmentalization of mammalian folate-mediated one-carbon metabolism. Annu Rev Nutr 2010;30:57–81.

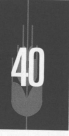

40 | GENETIC VARIATION: EFFECT ON NUTRIENT UTILIZATION AND METABOLISM[1]

PATRICK J. STOVER AND ZHENGLONG GU

HUMAN GENETIC VARIATION

Genetic variation contributes to individual phenotypic differences within and among human populations, including metabolic traits and differential susceptibility to common chronic and metabolic diseases. Metabolic impairments are integral components of chronic diseases, developmental anomalies, cancers, neurologic disorders, and most other pathologic processes. Often they precede anatomic and other signs of disease. Clinical investigations of inborn errors of metabolism provided some of the earliest and conclusive evidence that (a) metabolic impairments are heritable, (b) genes can modify nutrient use and metabolism, (c) metabolic impairments cause disease, and (d) the functional consequences of genetic mutations can be attenuated significantly by targeted nutritional therapies that compensate for and, less often, avoid genetically induced metabolic impairments.

Phenylketonuria provides a classic paradigm that demonstrates the potential effectiveness of diet in modifying deleterious phenotypes that result from genetic mutations that alter metabolism. Phenylalanine-restricted diets lessen and may even prevent severe cognitive deficits in children who carry mutations in the phenylalanine hydroxylase gene (1). Inborn errors of metabolism are generally recessive and are relatively rare in most populations, and the initiation or progression of the associated disorders can be managed by diet or nutrition in some, but not all, cases.

Inborn errors of metabolism are typically monogenic disorders that follow Mendelian modes of inheritance and therefore are well characterized with respect to their molecular and genetic bases. However, the most prevalent human metabolic disorders are complex polygenic diseases with contributions from multiple low-penetrant susceptibility alleles, and the risks associated with these alleles are modifiable by both lifestyle and environmental factors, including one or more dietary components.

The genetic and biochemical causes of many cancers and chronic diseases, including cardiovascular disease and type 2 diabetes mellitus, remain unidentified. These disorders do not conform to classic Mendelian inheritance patterns, and therefore genetic approaches based on "simple" linkage analyses are not always possible. Genomic approaches, enabled by the availability of complete genome sequences from several mammalian species and generation of a comprehensive catalog of human genetic variation, have been successful in identifying susceptibility genotypes that modify metabolism, change nutritional requirements, and contribute to metabolic disease. Furthermore, through evolutionary genomics, the origins and consequences of human

---

[1]**Abbreviations: ADH**, alcohol dehydrogenase; **ALDH**, aldehyde dehydrogenase; **AMY1**, salivary amylase gene; **ApoE**, apolipoprotein E; **CEU**, Utah residents with Northern and Western European ancestry from the CEPH (Centre d'Etude du Polymorphisme Humain) collection; **CNV**, copy number variation, **GWAS**, genome-wide association study; **HapMap**, Human Haplotype Map Project; $\mathbf{k_{cat}}$, maximal rate of product formation at infinite substrate concentration; $\mathbf{K_m}$, Michaelis-Menten constant; **LCT**, lactase gene; **LD**, linkage disequilibrium; **LDL**, low-density lipoprotein; **LP**, lactase persistence; **MAF**, minor allele frequency; **meC**, methylcytosine; **MTHFR**, methylenetetrahydrofolate reductase gene; **PCSK9**, proprotein convertase subtilisin-like kexin type 9; **SNP**, single nucleotide polymorphism; **YRI**, Yoruba in Ibadan, Nigeria (West Africa).

genetic variation are decipherable, and allelic variants and interacting environmental risk factors that impair metabolic pathways or modify optimal dietary requirements can be inferred.

Origin of Human Genetic Variation

The pattern of human genetic variation is determined by interactions among different evolutionary forces. The generation of primary sequence differences in DNA is a function of the DNA mutation rate; the expansion of the mutation within a population is a function of recombination, demographic history (e.g., fluctuations in effective population size, substructure, and migration), selection (the effect of the mutation on an organism's fitness), and random process (genetic drift) (2, 3). Not all sequence variation has phenotypic consequences (2). DNA sequence that does not affect function can mutate freely without consequences; whereas changes in DNA sequences that encode information or function may alter physiologic process, and therefore the propagation and expansion of such sequences will be more constrained.

Most human genetic variations present in noncoding regions, including those found in intronic and intergenic regions, are assumed to be selectively neutral and therefore a function of the DNA mutation rate (2), which is estimated to be approximately 2.5×10^{-8} mutations per nucleotide per generation. However, this rate is not uniformly distributed across the whole genome (4). The highest mutation rates for a human gene are approximately 1×10^{-5} per generation (5).

Many factors contribute to DNA mutation rates. DNA replication and recombination do not occur with complete fidelity and thereby account for a significant portion of observable mutation rates. Polymerase error rates and DNA mutations are affected by nutrients including iron, B vitamins, and antioxidants. For example, inhibition of folate-dependent deoxythymidine monophosphate synthesis results in the misincorporation of deoxyuridine triphosphate into DNA (6). Purine and pyrimidine bases within DNA also undergo spontaneous chemical mutation; cytosine spontaneously deaminates to uracil with a frequency of 100 mutations/genome/day, and purine nucleotides undergo depurination mutations at a rate of 3000 mutations/genome/day. DNA repair systems are effective in detecting and correcting most of these mutations (7).

Genotoxic xenobiotics, both natural products and synthetic chemicals, are present in the food supply and can modify DNA chemically and increase mutation rates. One class of natural compounds, aflatoxins, can dramatically increase DNA mutation rates, trigger cancers in somatic cells, and lead to localized cancer epidemics (8). DNA mutation rates are affected by dietary antioxidants (9) as well as by excesses in pro-oxidant nutrients including iron (10). However, only mutations that occur in the germ line contribute to a species' heritable genetic variation.

DNA mutation rates and polymorphism frequency vary throughout the human genome. Such region-specific differences within the genome have been attributed to the frequency of DNA recombination and to the mutagenic potential of specific nucleotide sequences. The most common genetic mutation within the human genome is the C to T transition (11). The sequence CpG is enriched in the promoter regions of mammalian genes and is recognized by DNA methylases, which convert the cytosine base (C) to methylcytosine (meC). meC density within the genome is modifiable by dietary folate and one-carbon donors, and fetal methylation patterns established in utero can be metastable and can influence gene expression into adulthood (12).

Cytosine methylation influences the transcription rates of genes by altering the affinity of DNA binding transcription factors or by enabling the recruitment of meC binding proteins that serve to silence gene transcription, or both. DNA methylation usually is associated with gene silencing and is critical for the inactivation of imprinted genes and X chromosome inactivation. Mutations at CpG dinucleotides occur approximately 10 times more frequently than at other loci, presumably because meC deaminates spontaneously to thymidine (T), whereas C deaminates to uracil. Uracil is recognized as foreign to DNA and is excised by the DNA repair enzymes, whereas T is not recognized as foreign. The sequence CpG is underrepresented in the human genome, and its frequency has decreased throughout evolution, consistent with that inherent instability (11).

DNA recombination rates also vary throughout the human genome. Recombination creates genetic variation by reshuffling existing genetic variation. The recombination rate was estimated to be 1 cM/Mb to approximately 1.33 cM/Mb; however, it is also very heterogeneous across the human genome: approximately 33,000 "recombination hotspots" account for approximately 50% to 60% of the crossover events, but they occupy only approximately 6% of the human genome sequence (3, 13–16). Investigators have observed that genes that interact with the environment (e.g., immunity, cell adhesion, signaling) tend to locate at genomic regions with high recombination rates whereas those genes that do not experience low recombination (17). Recombination is also correlated with levels of genetic variation, a finding indicating that recombination itself may be mutagenic (18).

Mutations that expand within a population contribute to genetic variation as polymorphisms, and this process is the basis for the molecular evolution of genomes. The expansion of mutations within a population occurs through the process of genetic drift or natural selection. Drift is a stochastic process that results from chance assortment of chromosomes at meiosis. Only a few of all possible zygotes are generated or survive to reproduce (19); therefore, mutations can expand in the absence of selection through random fluctuations in the transmission of alleles from one generation to the next, resulting from the random sampling of gametes. Because drift generally has a greater impact on allele frequencies in smaller populations, human demographic history has been a major force in shaping human genetic variation. Severe reductions in population size (bottleneck) can lead to a reduction in genetic variability, whereas rapid expansions can increase genetic variation (3).

Migration and population admixture also affect allele frequency. Modern humans originated in Africa, and small subpopulations migrated to the rest of the world within the past 100,000 years (2). As a consequence, African populations have more genetic variations than other populations (20–22). Investigators have shown that significantly more deleterious variations exist in the European populations than in the African populations, a finding indicating that genetic variation caused by demographic history has significant health consequences (23). Specific diseases, such as breast cancer, Tay-Sachs disease, Gaucher disease, Niemann-Pick disease, and familial hypercholesterolemia within the Old Order Amish and Hutterite populations may be accounted for by demographic history (19).

Selection is another important evolutionary force that shapes human genetic variation. Most substitutions in the genome are functionally neutral and do not have fitness consequences on their carriers. However, more and more genetic loci have been found to deviate from the neutral null model under various statistical tests, and the results suggest adaptive evolution. When a new mutation arises that affects the fitness in specific environmental contexts, (i.e., the capability to reproduce and propagate the genotype of its carriers), it will be subject to natural selection, which is defined as the differential contribution of genetic variants to future generations. The three general types of selection are positive, purifying, and balancing selection.

When a new mutation increases the fitness of its carriers, positive selection (adaptive evolution) drives the allele to high frequency in a population. Lactase tolerance provides a good example of positive selection (2). Purifying selection, also called negative selection, drives deleterious alleles to low frequency or extinction.

Balancing selection occurs when an allele has heterozygote advantage or it is selected only when it reaches a specific frequency (frequency-dependent selection) (24). One of the best examples of balancing selection is illustrated by the variation in the hemoglobin gene, in which heterozygosity of a variant gene confers resistance against malaria infection, whereas homozygosity results in sickle cell anemia.

Because selection changes rates of molecular evolution at defined loci within the genome, not all genes are expected to evolve at the same rate. Comparison of mammalian genome sequences has permitted the identification of genes that have undergone accelerated evolution (25). These rapidly evolving genes are assumed to enable adaptation and thus to have been positively selected because adaptive mutations expand within populations at accelerated rates relative to neutral mutations. The proportion of

amino acid substitutions that result from positive selection is estimated to be 35% to 45% (26). Specific examples of adaptive evolution include glucose-6-phosphate dehydrogenase (G6PD) in malaria (27), the lactase gene (LCT) in lactase persistence (20), amylase in starch digestion (28), and C-C chemokine receptor 5 (CCR5) in immune defense (29).

Comparison of mammalian genome sequences provides evidence that environmental exposures, including pathogens and dietary components, have been selective forces throughout evolution. These selective forces have influenced the generation of polymorphic alleles that alter the use and metabolism of dietary components and may be responsible for the generation of metabolic disease alleles across ethnically diverse human populations (27, 30). Variations that result from positive selection are expected to arise from region-specific selective factors. Therefore, the prevalence of specific functional polymorphisms may be associated with specific geographic or ethnic human populations to the degree that different selective pressures are operative across populations.

Specific allelic variants may be adaptive only in certain environments and neutral or less favored in others (24, 31). For example, the relatively high prevalence of the E6V polymorphism in the β-globin gene is likely the result of an adaptation to the region-specific environmental challenge of the malaria parasite in African populations. This disease allele has high frequency in the population because it enhanced fitness toward the region-specific environmental challenge of malaria in heterozygotes. Identifying and understanding the mechanism for the adaptive evolution of gene variants facilitate the discovery of human disease alleles. For example, a "thrifty gene" hypothesis was proposed to explain the epidemic of obesity and type 2 diabetes (5). The putatively advantageous mutations may have resulted in more efficient adaptations to fasting conditions (e.g., more rapid decreases in basal metabolism) or physiologic responses that facilitate excessive intakes in times of plenty. Adaptive alleles may be recessive disease alleles, or they may become disease alleles even in heterozygote individuals when the environmental conditions change profoundly, such as those brought about by the advent of civilization and agriculture, including alterations in the nature and abundance of the food supply (5).

CLASSIFYING HUMAN GENETIC VARIATION

The primary sequence of the human genome contains approximately 3.2 billion nucleotide base pairs that are organized into chromosomes that range in size from 50 million to 250 million base pairs. The first human genome sequence was obtained from 5 to 10 persons of diverse ethnic and geographic backgrounds or ancestry (2). The human genome, including both nuclear and mitochondrial DNA, contains an estimated 23,000 genes that serve as templates for 35,000 transcripts that encode information required for the synthesis of all cellular proteins, although a biologic function has not yet been determined for all human genes (32). Other genes encode functional RNA molecules, including tRNAs, small nuclear RNAs, ribosomal RNA, and microRNA (33), which serve various roles in protein synthesis, mRNA processing, or gene expression regulation (34, 35).

Genes account for approximately 2% of the total human DNA primary sequence; the remaining DNA is termed *noncoding* and serves structural and/or regulatory or no known roles. The number of genes encoded within the genome does not limit the biologic complexity of the mammalian cell. A single gene can encode more than one RNA or protein product through posttranscriptional and posttranslational processing reactions, including RNA editing, alternative splicing, protein splicing, and other modifications (e.g., differential phosphorylation) (36, 37). As a result of such RNA and protein processing, and modification reactions, more than 100,000 proteins with distinct primary sequences can be derived from the human genome.

Human genetic variation is a product of complex and reciprocal interactions among the genome and environmental exposures and is manifested through the formation and propagation of primary sequence alterations in DNA (38). Primary sequence variation among humans is referred to as polymorphism and constitutes one of the molecular bases for human phenotypic variation, including variations in human behavior, morphology, and susceptibility to disease (38).

Polymorphisms arise in populations through the independent and sequential processes of genetic mutation followed by expansion of the mutant allele within the population, and environment can modify both these processes. Human genetic variation was originally estimated to be approximately 0.1% (39). However, with improvements in technology that enabled the identification of structural rearrangements, investigators now estimate a 1% to 3% difference between any two sets of human chromosomes (40, 41). Human genetic variations are usually categorized into common and rare, according to the minor allele frequency (MAF, the frequency of the less common allele) in human populations. Common variations, also called polymorphisms, have an MAF of at least 1% in human populations (38). Genetic variants meeting the MAF threshold include single nucleotide changes and structural alterations, and they can result from mutations ranging from a single nucleotide base change to alterations of several hundred bases through deletions, insertions, translocations, inversions, and duplications (17).

Single Nucleotide Polymorphisms

Single nucleotide polymorphisms (SNPs) are the simplest and most common type of polymorphism and are estimated to represent approximately 90% of all human DNA polymorphisms. SNPs differ from somatic mutations in

that they are present in the germ line and therefore are heritable. SNPs are defined as nucleotide base pair differences in the primary sequence of DNA and can be single base pair insertions, deletions, or substitutions of one base pair for another. Nucleotide substitutions are the most common polymorphism; insertion or deletion mutations occur at one tenth the frequency (4).

The density of SNPs in the human genome varies within and among human chromosomes, and it ranges from 1 in 1000 bases to 1 in 100 to 300 bases. Investigators have estimated that approximately 10 to 15 million SNPs exist in human genomes (39, 42). Nucleotide substitutions within protein coding regions of a gene can be classified as either nonsynonymous substitutions, which result in an amino acid replacement substitution within a protein, or synonymous (silent) substitutions, which do not change amino acid sequence resulting from degeneracy in the genetic code. Nonsynonymous SNPs in coding regions are more functionally relevant because they change the amino acid sequence of the encoded proteins, and they subsequently have the potential to affect virtually every aspect of protein function, including protein folding and stability, enzymatic functions, allosteric regulation, and posttranslational modification. However, synonymous substitution can also have important functional consequences by altering mRNA splicing and protein translation efficiency. SNPs in introns, promoters, and intergenic regions may also be involved in regulating gene expression.

SNPs contribute to susceptibility for common diseases and developmental anomalies, and polymorphic alleles have been identified that increase the risk of common disorders including neural tube defects, cardiovascular disease, cancers, hypertension, and obesity (39). SNPs also influence physiologic responses to environmental exposures including diet (43), pharmaceuticals (44), pathogens, and toxins (25), and therefore many SNPs have diagnostic value. High-density human SNP maps facilitate the identification of disease risk alleles through gene mapping studies of complex disease, including low-penetrant alleles that make relatively small contributions to the initiation and or progression of the disorder.

Haplotypes

Genetic variants across the human genome are not always independent of each other. SNPs that are physically close with respect to primary DNA sequence usually do not segregate. As a result of meiotic recombination, DNA sequence and the variation within this sequence are inherited in "blocks." SNPs that are captured within these blocks are said to be in linkage disequilibrium (LD), which is defined as the nonrandom association of alleles at a nearby locus. Inherited blocks of genetic variation are referred to as haplotypes. The size of the haplotype block depends on the number of meiotic recombination events that have occurred historically within a population. Therefore, the average haplotype block length varies among populations as a result of human evolutionary history: approximately 22 kb for European and Asian populations and approximately 11 kb for African populations (39, 45). However, the pattern of LD is not evenly distributed across the genome. Because genetic variants in the same haplotype tend to be redundant in defining unique genetic variation, investigators have estimated that approximately 1 million SNPs can capture most human genetic variation (39).

The Human Haplotype Map Project (HapMap) was proposed to generate a list of common SNPs that can characterize human genetic variation (46). Phase I of the project started in 2003. Approximately 1 million SNPs in 270 individuals from 4 populations, including 30 family trios from the Yoruba in Ibadan, Nigeria (YRI), 30 trios from the Centre d'Etude du Polymorphisme Humain collection of Utah residents (CEU), 45 unrelated Han Chinese in Beijing (CHB), and 45 unrelated Japanese in Tokyo (JPT), were genotyped, and the data were released in 2005 (13). The generation of this SNP panel provided a detailed picture of the distribution of recombination and LD across the human genome in different populations. In 2007, phase II of the project released more than 3 million SNPs for the same 270 individuals (14). Phase III of the project revealed another approximately 1.6 million SNPs from 1115 individuals in 11 human populations (46, 47). Encouraged by the success of the HapMap project, the Human 1000 Genomes Project, initiated in 2008, will determine whole genome sequences for more than 1000 individuals. Successful completion of the project will provide a very deep catalog of all human genetic variation.

Structural Change and Copy Number Variation

Structural variations are broadly defined as all genomic alterations that are not single nucleotide substitutions, such as insertions, deletions, inversions, block substitutions, duplications, translocations, and copy number variations (CNVs) (17, 42). Retrotransposons are the most abundant transposable elements. Retrotransposons are classified by their sizes into long interspersed nuclear elements *(LINE)*, which encode all necessary genetic components for movement within the genome and to integrate within DNA, and short interspersed nuclear elements *(SINE)*, which require other transposable elements for mobility. The most abundant *SINE* is 280 base pair *Alu* element. An estimated 1.4 million copies are present in the human genome, and they occupy approximately 10% of the human genomic sequence. More than 1200 *Alu* elements in the human genome integrated after early human migrations; a new *Alu* insertion occurs every 200 births (48). Therefore, current human populations are polymorphic for the presence or absence of these insertions (38).

Insertion of transposable elements can have significant functional consequences by disrupting genes, altering gene regulation, and contributing to the coding region of nearby genes. New *Alu* insertions directly cause approximately

0.1% of human genetic disorders including Apert syndrome, cholinesterase deficiency, and breast cancer. Approximately 0.3% of human genetic disease results from *Alu*-mediated unequal homologous recombination events resulting in other inherited disorders including type 2 insulin-resistant diabetes and familial hypercholesterolemia (48). *Alu*-mediated unequal homologous recombination events are inhibited by CpG methylation of the element.

CNV represents a copy number change involving a DNA segment that is approximately 1 kb or larger (49, 50), excluding those arising from insertion or deletion of transposable elements (50). CNV represents another major source of genetic variation, and it affects more nucleotides per genome than SNPs, with different estimates ranging from 12% to 30% of the genome (41, 49). The estimated genome-wide mutation rate of CNV ranges from 1.7×10^{-6} to 1.0×10^{-4} per locus per generation, which is 100 to 10,000 times higher than nucleotide substitution rates (41). CNVs may exert their functional impacts through several mechanisms, such as modifying gene dosage, disrupting coding region, interfering with proper splicing, and altering regulation of a nearby gene. Therefore, CNVs are subject to selection (42, 49). CNVs resulting from duplication are more tolerated by the genome than are those resulting from deletion (50).

When different functional categories are observed, exonic CNVs are subject to the strongest purifying selection, followed by intronic CNVs, and finally intergenic CNVs (49). CNVs can be subject to positive selection by contributing to regional adaptation, and they are enriched in genes that function in the immune system and muscle development (49). Association studies have identified hundreds of CNVs contributing to phenotypic diversity, disease, and drug sensitivity; and CNVs are involved in starch digestion (28), steroid hormone and xenobiotic metabolism, prostate cancer (51), nicotine metabolism, regulation of food intake and body weight, neurodevelopment and neurologic disorders, colonic Crohn disease, toxin resistance, coronary heart disease risk, Alzheimer disease, human immunodeficiency virus infection, and progression of acquired immunodeficiency syndrome (50, 52–54).

FUNCTIONAL CONSEQUENCES OF GENETIC VARIATION

The metabolism of individual dietary components is affected by the activity, expression, and stability of protein transporters and enzymes. Polymorphisms affect gene expression as well as the physical and kinetic properties of cellular proteins, and thereby influence the flux through metabolic pathways and the steady-state concentration of reaction intermediates.

Gene Expression

High-throughput gene expression profiling (e.g., microarray, RNAseq) approaches have identified a large number of eQTLs (expression quantitative trait loci) (55–61). Both *cis*- and *trans*-regulatory polymorphisms influence gene expression differences within or among human populations. Which mechanism is more prevalent, however, is still controversial (55, 57, 59, 62, 63). Both SNPs and CNVs have dramatic influences on gene expression. To compare their relative importance, a study investigated the association between expression of 14,925 genes and genome-wide SNPs and CNVs in HapMap individuals. The results indicate that SNPs and CNVs contributed 83.6% and 17.7% to gene expression variations among these individuals, respectively (64).

Polymorphisms in the insulin 5' promoter decrease insulin expression and increase the risk of type 1 diabetes mellitus; the risk of type 2 diabetes mellitus is associated with polymorphisms in the calpain-10 gene promoter (65). Polymorphisms have been identified that affect the transcription of many metabolic and nutrient transport proteins including alcohol dehydrogenase (ADH), apolipoproteins, catalase, cytochrome P-450 family members, glucokinase, lipase, and the vitamin D receptor (66). Retroviral polymorphisms have been identified that influence gene expression by altering promoter methylation status in mice, and the degree of silencing depends on dietary folate and other one-carbon donors (12).

Global differential gene expression patterns among human populations have also been investigated (67–70). Genes in the inflammatory pathway and antimicrobial hormonal response are more likely to change expression from population to population; this finding indicates that gene expression differences among human populations could have resulted from local adaptation during human evolution (71). Another study identified 356 transcript clusters that have differential expression between the CEU and YRI samples (70). Twenty-seven genes show signal for adaptive evolution in at least 1 population. Among these 27 genes, certain metabolism-related molecular functions (e.g., lipid binding, metal ion binding, and transcription factor activity) are enriched, thus supporting the idea that differential gene expression among populations could have played important roles in adaptation to regionally specific dietary intake (71).

Protein Function

The rate of enzyme-catalyzed reactions is determined by the concentration of both enzyme (E) and substrate (S), and by the intrinsic Michaelis-Menten kinetic properties (Michaelis-Menten constant [K_m] and catalytic constant [k_{cat}]) of the enzyme (or transport protein).

$$E + S \rightarrow ES \rightarrow E + P$$

The Michaelis-Menten constant, K_m, refers to the affinity of E for S and is defined as the substrate concentration required for the enzyme to achieve half-maximal velocity. Formation of the ES complex requires productive collisions between the enzyme and substrate and is governed by the law of mass action. Therefore, the rate of an enzyme-catalyzed reaction is usually directly proportional to the molecular concentrations of the reacting substances (both E and S). Breakdown of the ES complex to product (P) is determined by k_{cat}, which refers to the maximal rate of product formation at infinite substrate concentration (all enzyme is present as an ES complex).

Genetic variation influences both the formation of the ES complex and the rate of P generation. Polymorphisms affect the formation of the ES complex by influencing the concentration of E or the affinity of E for S (K_m). SNPs influence the concentration of E by altering its rate of synthesis (gene expression or mRNA stability) or rate of degradation (protein stability and turnover). Nonsynonymous substitutions that affect the K_m alter the concentration of substrate required to drive the formation of ES.

Therefore, SNPs that increase K_m result in the accumulation of metabolic intermediates in cells. SNPs also can influence k_{cat}, which is the rate of formation of P, by affecting the maximum rate of catalysis (conversion of S to P at infinite S concentration). Alterations in k_{cat} can influence rates of nutrient uptake or clearance of metabolic intermediates and overall net flux through a metabolic pathway in a substrate-independent manner.

Similarly, genetic variation can affect the expression level and function of nutrient transporters and receptors. Functional effects include alterations in the affinity of transporters and receptors for nutrients, which can influence intracellular and plasma nutrient levels. Changes in transporter or receptor activity or abundance of these proteins in the membrane can affect rates of nutrient uptake and clearance. Genetic variation can also influence nutrient uptake and use indirectly by altering the expression and function of signaling peptides and hormones that regulate metabolic pathways.

IDENTIFICATION OF GENETIC VARIATION THAT AFFECTS NUTRIENT METABOLISM AND USE

Genomes that confer either nutrient requirements that cannot be met by the mother, or severe metabolic disruptions that impair basic physiologic processes, will be selected against in large part because of fetal loss or the failure to survive to reproduce. Some common SNPs in genes that encode metabolic enzymes are not in Hardy–Weinberg equilibrium (alleles are not inherited at the expected frequency) because the homozygous state reduces fetal viability (30). Nearly 62% of all human conceptuses are not viable and do not survive to the twelfth week of gestation (72, 73). Genomes that survive gestation but confer atypical nutrient requirements or inefficient metabolism may encode one or more disease-causing alleles, and the penetrance of the disease allele may be modifiable by diet. High-dose vitamin therapy can rescue impaired metabolic reactions that result from genetic mutations and polymorphisms that decrease the affinity of substrates and cofactors for the encoded enzyme (K_m). Polymorphic risk alleles that affect nutrient metabolism and use have been identified with candidate gene approaches, and more recently they have been inferred from nonbiased comparative genomic analyses.

Locating Genes of Interest

Linkage Analysis and Genome-Wide Association Study

Linkage analyses and association studies are two commonly used approaches to map causal alleles underlying human traits and diseases. Linkage analysis investigates candidate regions underlying the trait of interest in normal and affected individuals from the same family and determines whether genetic markers across the genome are inherited together with the trait. The tool has its limited power for research in complex diseases because sample sizes are usually small. The resolution can be so low that it is difficult to narrow candidate regions (74, 75).

Association studies investigate the coinheritance of genetic markers and the trait of interest in large population studies (38, 74, 76). The candidate gene approach, which is frequently used in epidemiologic studies, is a type of direct association study that tests correlations between each candidate causal variant with the trait of interest. This methodology has better resolution than linkage analysis, but it can be greatly limited by the knowledge on the trait of interest. Candidate genes are selected based on knowledge of metabolic pathways and predictions that their impairment results in metabolic phenotypes that either mirror a particular disease state or affect the concentration of a biomarker associated with chronic disease. The candidate gene approach has been successful in identifying many disease susceptibility alleles (43), but it is limited by incomplete knowledge of transcriptional and metabolic networks and by inconsistent findings among studies. Furthermore, because many SNPs are in LD, it is not always possible to determine with certainty whether an individual SNP or allele is functional and disease causing or is linked to a causal polymorphism through genetic hitchhiking.

Genome-wide association study (GWAS) is an indirect approach that does not require prior knowledge of candidate genes underlying the trait of interests. The method uses a set of genetic markers, currently more than 1 million SNPs across the whole human genome, to detect associations between a particular genomic region and the trait of interest by using thousands of or even tens of thousands of normal and affected individuals (46). Facilitated by SNPs identified through the HapMap project and the development of large-scale genotyping platforms, GWAS has been widely used and has generated candidate loci that may be causal for various complex diseases (77–85). The list of traits examined by GWAS is currently growing almost on a daily basis, and the new candidate genes generated from these studies provide novel hypotheses for disease initiation and progression.

Adaptive Evolution and Genome-Wide Selection Scans

Adaptive evolution may have played important roles in determining human specific traits that are different from other closely related primate species and human population specific traits, such as appearance, disease susceptibility, and dietary response. Detecting positively selected alleles provides another approach to facilitate identifications of genes that play important roles in determining these traits (86, 87). Genetic adaptation during evolution can lead to unique features in a genome that are different from neutral expectation.

Statistical methods have been developed to identify these adaptive signals. The methods to detect adaptive evolution can be grouped into species comparison using divergence data and population comparison using polymorphism data (87, 88). Methods for interspecies comparison include the following: the dN/dS or Ka/Ks test, (89, 90) which searches for a significantly elevated ratio of nonsynonymous to synonymous changes in gene coding regions; and the Hudson, Kreitman, and Agaude (HKA) (91) and McDonald–Kreitman (MK) (92) tests, which identify significantly different distributions of genetic polymorphism within species in comparison to divergence among species.

Population-based methods can also be grouped into two categories: "frequency-spectrum based" and "haplotype based." Both positive selection and negative selection reduce genetic variation in selected regions: positive selection increases the frequency of advantageous alleles, and negative selection removes deleterious mutations. Different selection tests, such as Tajima's D test (93), Fu and Li's test (94), and Fay and Wu's H test (95), have been developed to detect such reduction in genetic variation that differs from neutral expectation. As human ancestors migrated out of Africa and colonized different locations, human populations evolved in isolation, and allele frequencies became uniquely distributed in different populations either from random drift or from local adaptation. The F_{st} test, designed to detect such population differences, provides potential target loci that were subject to regional adaptation (96). Furthermore, the previously mentioned MK test for species comparison can also be modified to compare polymorphism data among populations.

The haplotype-based approaches to detect positive selection were made possible by the success of HapMap project and further development of large-scale genotyping capability. Adaptive evolution increases the frequency of alleles faster than the neutral expectation. Therefore, the genetic variants that are in the same haplotype with the selected alleles will also increase in frequency. During this process, recombination does not have sufficient time to break down the haplotype as efficiently as it does under neutral expectation. As a result, adaptive evolution can lead to a significantly longer haplotypes than the neutral expectation in the genome with high frequency in a population. Different haplotype-based methods, such as extended haplotype homozygosity (EHH) and relative EHH (REHH) (97), integrated haplotype score (iHS) (24), Cross Population EHH (XP-EHH) (98), and LD decay (LDD) test (99) were developed. These methods successfully identified hundreds of genes that may have gone through adaptive evolution in different human populations (24, 88, 97, 99–102), with many involved in nutrient metabolism.

GENETIC VARIATION AND NUTRIENT METABOLISM

One-Carbon Metabolism (Folate Metabolism)

Folate-mediated one-carbon metabolism is essential for the de novo biosynthesis of purines and thymidylate and the remethylation of homocysteine to methionine. The pathway is important for DNA synthesis and genome methylation (103). Genetic variants of enzymes in folate metabolic pathway, including the methylenetetrahydrofolate reductase gene *(MTHFR)* (104) and the methylenetetrahydrofolate dehydrogenase gene *(MTHFD1)* (105), are associated with altered metabolism and an increased risk of birth defects in folate-deficient individuals. These deleterious variants may also be beneficial under certain environments. For example, individuals with C677T in *MTHFR* show a decreased risk of developing colon cancer (106). Both deleterious and beneficial effects of C677T in *MTHFR* are influenced by dietary intake of folate and alcohol, a finding indicating that interactions between genetics and environment are critical for defining disease status of the genetic variants. This example illustrates the role that dietary interventions can play in modifying risks associated with potentially deleterious gene variants. The evolutionary mechanisms leading to distribution of genetic variants in one-carbon metabolism in different human populations remain to be illustrated.

Starch Digestion

CNVs can modify gene dosage and change levels of gene expression. A study of the salivary amylase gene *(AMY1)* illustrated that CNV may have played an important role in dietary adaptation (28). The gene has extensive variation in copy number, which was found to be positively correlated with AMY1 protein level, both among individuals and among human populations. Populations that consume high-starch diets exhibited a higher copy number of *AMY1* genes than populations that consumed low levels of starch. Comparison with other closely related primate species indicates that the increase in *AMY1* gene copy number occurred in the human lineage. Indeed, the low level of nucleotide divergence among different *AMY1* gene copies indicates a very recent origin of *AMY1* gene duplication (~200,000 years ago). Taken together, these results indicate that adaptation to a regional food system may have played an important role in modulating the human genome and causing genetic variation among human populations.

Alcohol Metabolism

The metabolism of ethanol varies widely among human ethnic populations. Ethanol is oxidized to acetaldehyde by the enzyme ADH; acetaldehyde is subsequently oxidized to acetic acid by aldehyde dehydrogenase (ALDH). Three genes encode the class I ADH (ADH1) isozymes. The active enzyme is a homodimer or heterodimer composed of subunits encoded by ADH1A, ADH1B, and ADH1C. ADH1B and ADH1C are highly polymorphic, and variations in ADH1B show the greatest functional effects with respect to catalytic activity, affinity of the protein for ethanol, and rates of alcohol clearance from tissues. The ADH1B°1 variant predominates in whites and African-Americans, whereas the ADH1B°2 variant predominates in Japanese and Chinese populations. The origin and spread of this protective allele in East Asia were shown to coincide with the emergence and expansion of rice domestication and alcohol production, a finding indicating the role of Neolithic dietary shift in shaping the human genome (107). The ADH1B°3 variant is mostly restricted to persons of African descent.

The second enzyme in the pathway, ALDH, is also polymorphic. Populations of Asian descent carry a common dominant null allelic variant (E487K) and develop a "flush" reaction when they consume alcohol that results from accumulation of the metabolic intermediate acetaldehyde. Individuals with high-activity ADH or low-activity ALDH2 are at lower risk of alcoholism than are other individuals (108–110).

Lactose Tolerance

Lactase hydrolyzes lactose, the main carbohydrate in milk, into glucose and galactose. After weaning, most mammals, including humans, lose the ability to digest lactose as a result of reduced lactase expression. However, northern European and African pastoralist populations maintain the ability to digest milk lactose into adulthood (lactase persistence [LP]) (20, 111). Two SNPs (C/T-13910 and G/A-22018) identified in the *cis*-regulatory elements of the lactase gene *(LCT)* were shown to be important for the LP phenotype in European populations (112).

Three other SNPs (G/C-14010, T/G-13915, and C/G-13907) in the regulatory region of the *LCT* gene were identified to be significantly associated with LP phenotype in African populations, a finding indicating that the LP trait evolved independently during human evolution (20). Haplotype-based natural selection tests show that the adaptive sweep of different lactase variants in European and African populations occurred approximately within the past 7000 years, consistent with the time when humans established cattle domestication. This classic example of dietary adaptation indicates that human cultural elements, in this case cattle domestication and adult milk consumption, played an important role in shaping the modern human genome.

Iron Metabolism

Hereditary hemochromatosis is a recessive iron storage disease common in populations of European descent, with an incidence of 1 in 300 persons. A common polymorphism in the *HFE* gene (C282Y), which encodes a protein that regulates iron levels, is associated with the disease phenotype in 60% to 100% of Europeans, although mutations in other genes are also associated with the phenotype. Iron storage diseases exist in Asia and Africa, where the *HFE* C282Y allele is essentially absent. The penetrance of the C282Y *HFE* allele for the iron overload phenotype varies widely among homozygotes, with some persons being asymptomatic. The *HFE* C282Y polymorphism expanded in human populations relatively recently and may have conferred unidentified selective advantages (113).

Lipid Metabolism

Apolipoprotein E (Apo-E) functions in lipid metabolism and cholesterol transport. The frequencies of three major Apo-E isoforms (E2, E3, and E4) vary in different human populations. These protein isoforms differ in their affinity both for lipoprotein particles and for low-density lipoprotein (LDL) receptors. Investigators estimated that Apo-E allelic variation could account for approximately 7% of variation in cholesterol concentrations in human populations (114). In controlled dietary studies of low-fat and high-cholesterol diets, serum cholesterol levels increased in E4/E4 individuals but not in those with E3/E2 and E2/E2 genotypes. In human population studies, carriers of the E2 allele tend to display lower levels of plasma cholesterol than do E4 carriers. Furthermore, the E4 allele is associated with hypercholesterolemia and an increased risk of late-onset Alzheimer disease.

Proprotein convertase subtilisin-like kexin type 9 (PCSK9) is a serine protease that regulates the plasma level of LDL (115). Loss of function mutations lower plasma LDL levels and are associated with a reduced risk of cardiovascular diseases (116). Loss of function mutations, including two nonsense (Y142X, C679X) (117) and two missense (L253F, A443T) (115) mutations, inactivate PCSK9 in some African-American individuals and are associated with an approximately 35% reduction in plasma LDL levels. Another missense mutation, R46L, which also inactivates PCSK9, is common in European-Americans.

CONCLUSION

The comprehensive identification of human genetic variation will enable an understanding of the molecular basis of phenotypic differences among individuals at the highest possible resolution. More than 1000 human genomes will be sequenced through the 1000 Genomes Project Consortium (118). The information will empower prediction of disease risk and guide dietary approaches to disease prevention and management. The understanding of human genetic variations and their impact on metabolism will lead to an era of personalized nutrition, when dietary recommendations can be tailored to optimize their interactions with individual genetic makeup.

ACKNOWLEDGMENTS

We thank Mr. Ye Kaixiong for his help during the writing of this chapter.

REFERENCES

1. van Spronsen FJ. Mol Genet Metab 2010;100:107–10.
2. Campbell MC, Tishkoff SA. Annu Rev Genomics Hum Genet 2008;9:403–33.
3. Nielsen R, Hubisz MJ, Hellmann I et al. Genome Res 2009; 19:838–49.
4. Nachman MW, Crowell SL. Genetics 2000;156:297–304.
5. Diamond J. Nature 2003;423:599–602.
6. Blount BC, Mack MM, Wehr CM et al. Proc Natl Acad Sci U S A 1997;94:3290–5.
7. Linhart HG, Troen A, Bell GW et al. Gastroenterology 2009; 136:227–235 e3.
8. Chen T, Heflich RH, Moore MM et al. Environ Mol Mutagen 2010;51:156–63.
9. Moore SR, Hill KA, Heinmoller PW et al. Environ Mol Mutagen 1999;34:195–200.
10. Shigenaga MK, Ames BN. Basic Life Sci 1993;61:419–36.
11. Walser JC, Furano AV. Genome Res 2010;20:875–82.
12. Waterland RA, Jirtle RL. Mol Cell Biol 2003;23:5293–300.
13. International HapMap Consortium. Nature 2005;437:1299–320.
14. Frazer KA, Ballinger DG, Cox DR et al. Nature 2007;449: 851–61.
15. Coop G, Wen X, Ober C et al. Science 2008;319:1395–8.
16. Myers S, Bottolo L, Freeman C et al. Science 2005;310: 321–4.
17. Frazer KA, Murray SS, Schork NJ et al. Nat Rev Genet 2009;10:241–51.
18. Lercher MJ, Hurst LD. Trends Genet 2002;18:337–40.
19. Tishkoff SA, Verrelli BC. Annu Rev Genomics Hum Genet 2003;4:293–340.
20. Tishkoff SA, Reed FA, Ranciaro A et al. Nat Genet 2007;39: 31–40.
21. Hinds DA, Stuve LL, Nilsen GB et al. Science 2005;307: 1072–9.
22. Stajich JE, Hahn MW. Mol Biol Evol 2005;22:63–73.
23. Lohmueller KE, Indap AR, Schmidt S et al. Nature 2008; 451:994–7.
24. Voight BF, Kudaravalli S, Wen X et al. PLoS Biol 2006;4:e72.
25. Clark AG, Glanowski S, Nielsen R et al. Science 2003;302: 1960–3.
26. Wolfe KH, Li WH. Nat Genet 2003;33(Suppl):255–65.
27. Tishkoff SA, Varkonyi R, Cahinhinan N et al. Science 2001; 293:455–62.
28. Perry GH, Dominy NJ, Claw KG et al. Nat Genet 2007; 39:1256–60.
29. Smith MW, Dean M, Carrington M et al. Science 1997; 277:959–65.
30. Stover PJ. Food Nutr Bull 2007;28(Suppl Int):S101–15.
31. Penyalver R, Oger PM, Su S et al. Mol Plant Microbe Interact 2009;22:713–24.
32. International Human Genome Sequencing Consortium. Nature 2004;431:931–45.
33. Washietl S. Methods Mol Biol 2010;609:285–306.

34. Fabian MR, Sonenberg N, Filipowicz W. Annu Rev Biochem 2010;79:351–79.

35. Wittmann J, Jack HM. ScientificWorldJournal 2010;10: 1239–43.

36. Keren H, Lev-Maor G, Ast G. Nat Rev Genet 2010;11: 345–55.

37. Nilsen TW, Graveley BR. Nature 2010;463:457–63.

38. Feero WG, Guttmacher AE, Collins FS. N Engl J Med 2010;362:2001–11.

39. Manolio TA, Brooks LD, Collins FS. J Clin Invest 2008;118: 1590–605.

40. Venter JC. Nature 2010;464:676–7.

41. Zhang F, Gu W, Hurles ME et al. Annu Rev Genomics Hum Genet 2009;10:451–81.

42. Eichler EE, Nickerson DA, Altshuler D et al. Nature 2007;447:161–5.

43. Stover PJ, Caudill MA. J Am Diet Assoc 2008;108:1480–7.

44. McCarthy JJ, Hilfiker R. Nat Biotechnol 2000;18:505–8.

45. Gabriel SB, Schaffner SF, Nguyen H et al. Science 2002;296:2225–9.

46. International HapMap Consortium. 2010 Nature 467:52–58.

47. Duan S, Huang RS, Zhang W et al. Pharmacogenomics 2009;10549–63.

48. Batzer MA, Deininger PL. Nat Rev Genet 2002;3:370–9.

49. Conrad DF, Pinto D, Redon R et al. Nature 2010;464:704–712.

50. Freeman JL, Perry GH, Feuk L et al. Genome Res 2006;16: 949–61.

51. Xue Y, Sun D, Daly A et al. Am J Hum Genet 2008;83: 337–46.

52. Redon R, Ishikawa S, Fitch KR et al. Nature 2006;444: 444–54.

53. Tuzun E, Sharp AJ, Bailey JA et al. Nat Genet 2005;37: 727–32.

54. Sebat J, Lakshmi B, Troge J et al. Science 2004;305:525–8.

55. Morley M, Molony CM, Weber TM et al. Nature 2004; 430:743–7.

56. Cheung VG, Spielman RS, Ewens KG et al. Nature 2005;437:1365–9.

57. Stranger BE, Forrest MS, Dunning M et al. Science 2007; 315:848–53.

58. Montgomery SB, Sammeth M, Gutierrez-Arcelus M et al. Nature 2010;464:773–7.

59. Hull J, Campino S, Rowlands K et al. PLoS Genet 2007;3:e99.

60. Kwan T, Benovoy D, Dias C et al. Genome Res 2007;17: 1210–8.

61. Kwan T, Benovoy D, Dias C et al. Nat Genet 2008;40: 225–31.

62. Pickrell JK, Marioni JC, Pai AA et al. Nature 2010;464; 768–72.

63. Wittkopp PJ, Haerum BK, Clark AG. Nature 2004; 430:85–8.

64. Stranger BE, Forrest MS, Clark AG et al. PLoS Genet 2005;1:e78.

65. Guttmacher AE, Collins FS. N Engl J Med 2002;347: 1512–20.

66. Rockman MV, Wray GA. Mol Biol Evol 2002;19:1991–2004.

67. Storey JD, Madeoy J, Strout JL et al. Am J Hum Genet 2007;80:502–9.

68. Spielman RS, Bastone LA, Burdick JT et al. Nat Genet 2007;39:226–31.

69. Huang RS, Duan S, Kistner EO et al. Pharmacogenet Genomics 2008;18:545–9.

70. Zhang W, Duan S, Kistner EO et al. Am J Hum Genet 2008;82:631–40.

71. Zhang W, Dolan ME. Evol Bioinform Online 2008;4:171–9.

72. Edmonds DK, Lindsay KS, Miller JF et al. Fertil Steril 1982;38:447–53.

73. Edwards RG. Int J Dev Biol 1997;41:255–62.

74. Witte JS. Annu Rev Public Health 2010;31:9–20.

75. Risch N Merikangas K. Science 1996;273:1516–7.

76. Borecki IB, Province MA. Adv Genet 2008;60:51–74.

77. Sladek R, Rocheleau G, Rung J et al. Nature 2007;445: 881–5.

78. Samani NJ, Erdmann J, Hall AS et al. N Engl J Med 2007;357:443–53.

79. McPherson R, Pertsemlidis A, Kavaslar N et al. Science 2007;316:1488–91.

80. Weedon MN, Lango H, Lindgren CM et al. Nat Genet 2008;40:575–83.

81. Scuteri A, Sanna S, Chen WM et al. PLoS Genet 2007;3:e115.

82. Amundadottir LT, Sulem P, Gudmundsson J et al. Nat Genet 2006;38:652–8.

83. Graham RR, Kozyrev SV, Baechler EC et al. Nat Genet 2006;38:550–5.

84. Klein RJ, Zeiss C, Chew EY et al. Science 2005;308:385–9.

85. Zhang HF, Qiu LX, Chen Y et al. Hum Genet 2009;125: 627–31.

86. Oleksyk TK, Smith MW, O'Brien SJ. Philos Trans R Soc Lond B Biol Sci 2010;365:185–205.

87. Kelley JL, Swanson WJ. Annu Rev Genomics Hum Genet 2008;9:143–60.

88. Oleksyk TK, Zhao K, De La Vega FM et al. PLoS One 2008;3:e1712.

89. Nielsen R, Yang Z. Genetics 1998;148:929–36.

90. Yang Z, Nielsen R. J Mol Evol 1998;46:409–18.

91. Hudson RR, Kreitman M, Aguade M. Genetics 1987;116: 153–9.

92. McDonald JH, Kreitman M. Nature 1991;351:652–4.

93. Tajima F. Genetics 1989;123:585–95.

94. Fu YX. Genetics 1997;147:915–25.

95. Fay JC, Wu CI. Genetics 2000;155:1405–13.

96. Weir BS, Hill WG. Annu Rev Genet 2002;36:721–50.

97. Sabeti PC, Reich DE, Higgins JM et al. Nature 2002;419: 832–7.

98. Sabeti PC, Varilly P, Fry B et al. Nature 2007;449:913–8.

99. Wang ET, Kodama G, Baldi P et al. Proc Natl Acad Sci U S A 2006;103:135–40.

100. Bustamante CD, Fledel-Alon A, Williamson S et al. Nature 2005;437:1153–7.

101. Carlson CS, Thomas DJ, Eberle MA et al. Genome Res 2005;15:1553–65.

102. Nielsen R, Williamson S, Kim Y et al. Genome Res 2005; 15:1566–75.

103. Fox JT, Stover PJ. Vitam Horm 2008;79:1–44.

104. Christensen KE, Rohlicek CV, Andelfinger GU et al. Hum Mutat 2009;30:212–20.

105. Brody LC, Conley M, Cox C et al. Am J Hum Genet 2002; 71:1207–15.

106. Ma J, Stampfer MJ, Giovannucci E et al. Cancer Res 1997; 57:1098–102.

107. Peng Y, Shi H, Qi XB et al. BMC Evol Biol 2010;10:15.

108. Bosron WF, Li TK. Hepatology 1986;6:502–10.

109. Loew M, Boeing H, Sturmer T et al. Alcohol 2003;29:131–5.

110. Crabb DW, Matsumoto M, Chang D et al. Proc Nutr Soc 2004;63:49–63.

111. Itan Y, Powell A, Beaumont MA et al. PLoS Comput Biol 2009;5:e1000491.

112. Enattah NS, Sahi T, Savilahti E et al. Nat Genet 2002;30: 233–7.

113. Toomajian C, Kreitman M. Genetics 2002;161:1609–23.

114. Inoue K, Lupski JR. Annu Rev Genomics Hum Genet 2002;3: 199–242.

115. Kotowski IK, Pertsemlidis A, Luke A et al. Am J Hum Genet 2006;78:410–22.

116. Horton JD, Cohen JC, Hobbs HH. Trends Biochem Sci 2007;32:71–7.

117. Cohen JC, Boerwinkle E, Mosley TH Jr et al. N Engl J Med 2006;354:1264–72.

118. The 1000 Genomes Project Consortium Nature 2010 467:1061–1073.

SUGGESTED READING

Feero WG, Guttmacher AE, Collins FS. Genomic medicine: an updated primer. N Engl J Med 2010;362:2001–11.

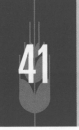

EPIGENETICS[1]

PAUL HAGGARTY

OVERVIEW

The human genome contains information that is not fully described by the DNA sequence alone. This so-called epigenetic information (from the Greek έπί, meaning "on" or "over") is laid over the genetic information in the genome. It fundamentally affects the way in which the sequence information in DNA is used, and it is essential to the identity and the healthy functioning of cells. Epigenetic processes have been implicated in a wide range of health outcomes including cancer, cognition, cardiovascular disease, diabetes, and reproductive function; and our understanding of the effect of environmental factors, such as diet and lifestyle on epigenetic status, is growing rapidly.

Epigenetics encompasses a collection of mechanisms that define the phenotype of a cell without affecting the genotype (1). In molecular terms, it represents a range of mechanisms including DNA methylation, histone modification, remodeling of nucleosomes and higher order chromatin reorganization, and regulation by noncoding RNAs (1). A key characteristic of the epigenetic signal is that it is heritable and can be passed from somatic cell to daughter cell during mitosis and even across the generations during meiosis (1–6). Understanding of the epigenetic regulation of individual genes has increased greatly, but coordinated epigenetic control of the genome on a much larger scale may be even more important. The human genome is made up of accessible regions of euchromatin and poorly accessible regions of heterochromatin, and these regions

determine the ability of the transcriptional machinery of the cell to access genetic information (5, 6). These regions may span many genes, and epigenetic regulation is critical to the transition between these states (7).

DNA methylation is probably the most widely studied epigenetic mechanism in relation to nutrition. Methylation in mammalian cells takes place at a cytosine located 5' to a guanosine (CpG site). A significant component of the global methylation signature (average level of methylation across the entire genome) is accounted for by the transposable elements that make up approximately 45% of the entire genome and are usually heavily methylated (~90%). The transposons include the long interspersed nuclear elements (*LINE1*), the intracisternal A particle (*IAP*), short interspersed nuclear elements (*SINE*), and the *Alu* family of human *SINE* elements characterized by the action of the Alu restriction endonuclease (8, 9). Some classes of transposon are able to move around the genome and can cause abnormal function and disease if they are inserted into an important conserved sequence (5, 8, 9). Within the genes that code for proteins, the most striking epigenetic distinction is between the imprinted and the nonimprinted genes. Most autosomal genes are expressed equally from both parental alleles, but imprinted genes are an exception.

Genomic imprinting refers to the epigenetic marking of genes in a manner specific to the parent of origin within the germ cells such that the subsequent expression pattern depends on the parent from whom the allele was derived (1, 4–6). Imprinted genes are particularly important in prenatal growth, placental function, and brain function and behavior (10–12). Imprinted genes are unusually found downstream of regions of DNA that have a high density of CpG sites (5). Approximately 80% of imprinted genes are found in clusters with other imprinted genes, and this arrangement is thought to reflect coordinated regulation of the genes within a chromosomal domain (5). Regions rich in CpG sites, known as CpG islands, are found in gene bodies, endogenous repeats, and transposable elements and are thought to be important in transcriptional repression (3). The process of demethylation is in many ways as important to epigenetic regulation as is methylation. Demethylation occurs in the mismatch repair pathway, but it is not known whether this is the primary mechanism by which removal of methyl groups is achieved

---

[1]**Abbreviations: *IGF-2*,** insulinlike growth factor-II gene; **SINE,** short interspersed nuclear element; **LINE1,** long interspersed nuclear elements; **IAP,** the intracisternal A particle; **BRCA1,** breast cancer 1 early onset gene.

in epigenetic remodeling (13). Epigenetic status varies among individuals (14–16) and even between genetically identical monozygotic twins (17). Much research has been carried out to determine whether this variation is important to health and whether it is influenced by nutrition.

HEALTH AND DISEASE

Investigators are currently interested in the importance of epigenetic factors in the origin of human disease (4, 18). Epigenetic change has been implicated in all the major chronic diseases affecting humans. Historically, cancer is the disease in which epigenetics has been studied most extensively. A common observation in human tumors is epigenetic change, including altered methylation of DNA (19–21) and the histones associated with DNA (22). Hypomethylation in tumor cells is thought to be an early trigger that predisposes cells to genomic instability and hypermethylation of specific genes thought to be involved in carcinogenesis and disease progression (23). Certain imprinted genes are known tumor suppressors involved in cell proliferation (24). Loss of imprinting (gain or loss of DNA methylation or loss of allele-specific gene expression) is also a common characteristic of many cancer types, including breast, lung, colon, liver, and ovary (24). Imprinting syndromes, in which the imprint is disrupted or absent, are associated with diabetes (25) and cancer risk (26), in addition to impairment of normal function that leads to obesity and impaired cognitive development (2). Although only approximately 1% of all human genes are imprinted, our understanding that imprinting status may be important for several health outcomes is growing (4).

Patients with vascular disease have significantly altered DNA methylation compared with healthy controls (27). Altered global DNA methylation has also been observed in mouse and rabbit atherosclerotic lesions (28), and studies in an atherogenic mouse model have shown that altered DNA methylation precedes the development of atherosclerosis (29). Altered methylation of the estrogen receptor-α gene has also been demonstrated in coronary atherosclerotic plaques compared with normal proximal aorta; the methylation status changes with aging (30). Epigenetic mechanisms have been implicated in Alzheimer disease (31), mental impairment, and normal cognitive function (12, 32–34).

NUTRITIONAL EFFECTS

Nutrition can influence epigenetic status by the following means:

- The availability of substrate used to mark DNA and histones epigenetically
- Direct effects on the cellular machinery involved in setting and interpreting the epigenetic mark
- Direct effects on the structure and function of the genome

The ultimate methyl donor for epigenetic methylation reactions is the folate-methylation cycle, and specifically the metabolite S-adenosylmethionine (SAM). Nutritional and genetic factors that affect the activity of this cycle also influence epigenetic marking. Poor folate status and elevated homocysteine have been linked to human DNA lymphocyte hypomethylation (35, 36). Mutation in the methylenetetrahydrofolate gene, which is involved in the provision of methyl groups, interacts with folate status to influence DNA methylation (37, 38). Direct effects of folate on the structure and function of the genome related to epigenetics are also possible. The human genome has more than 20 folate-sensitive fragile sites, which are regions of chromatin that fail to compact normally during mitosis in the presence of folate and thymidine deficiency (23).

Other B vitamins have also been implicated in epigenetic regulation. Examples include niacin and chromatin structure and function (39), as well as biotin binding to histones and its effect on retrotransposons (40). Acetylation of histones, another important epigenetic mechanism, is under the control of histone deacetylase, which is inhibited by sulforaphane, a compound found in cruciferous vegetables (41). Alcohol is also known to interact with methyl group metabolism. Animal models of chronic alcohol exposure result in altered DNA methylation (42, 43), and DNA methylation has been shown to vary with alcohol exposure in humans (44, 45). Polyphenols in green tea, coffee, and soybeans are thought to influence epigenetic status by a direct effect on the DNA methyltransferases that add the methyl group to DNA (46–48).

WINDOWS OF SENSITIVITY

Many epigenetic events are restricted to specific phases of development, cellular differentiation, and cell division. Epigenetic regulation is central to the coordinated development of human gametes, the early embryo, and the fetus, and the entire period before birth is marked by intense epigenetic activity (6). The transgenerational nature of imprinting raises the possibility that epigenetic risk accumulated by one generation may be passed on to the next. Extensive research in the field of nutritional epigenetics has focused on the long-term health consequences of nutritional exposure before birth.

Numerous studies in pregnant rodents demonstrated that epigenetic regulation of specific genes in the offspring was influenced by the maternal intake of methyl donors such as folic acid, choline, betaine (40, 41), folic acid and low protein (49), and phytoestrogens (4, 50) during pregnancy. In human pregnancy, higher levels of methylation of the insulin-like growth factor-II gene (*IGF-2*) have been observed in the umbilical cord blood DNA in babies of mothers who took folic acid supplements during pregnancy (51). *IGF-2* methylation in children has also been reported to be related to birth weight (51), which is itself related to the risk of cardiovascular disease, diabetes, obesity, and cancer in later life (52). Altered *IGF-2* methylation was also observed in women 60 years after prenatal exposure to famine during the Dutch Hunger Winter of 1944 and 1945, and these changes appeared to be associated with increased breast cancer risk (53).

Windows of epigenetic sensitivity to nutrition are not restricted to the period before birth, but they may occur throughout the life span (54). The nutritionally programmed epigenome could become fixed and propagated during mitosis or meiosis in several ways (Fig. 41.1).

EPIDEMIOLOGY

Given the fundamental nature of epigenetic control of gene expression, it is perhaps not surprising that epigenetic status varies with disease or that nutrition, which is known to influence gene expression, also influences epigenetic status. More important are whether epigenetic change is on the causal pathway to the development of disease and whether this process is influenced by nutrition. This relationship is relatively easy to establish in animal models, but species differences in epigenetic regulation and the origin of disease limit the usefulness of such models when investigating the determinants of human health. On the other hand, establishing causality in human nutritional studies presents its own challenges.

Humans have multiple epigenomes, depending on the tissue type and stage of development (7). Indeed, epigenetic change is a key event in the differentiation of tissues. In most nutritional studies, investigators often can sample only peripheral blood or buccal cell DNA. The critical tissues and organs that regulate and determine health and disease (liver, pancreas, heart, vasculature, brain) can be sampled only in the most invasive of protocols or in very specific study designs (e.g., detection of the epigenetic signature within minute traces of tumor tissue DNA

released into the peripheral blood in cancer studies [55]). The rationale for blood and buccal cell sampling is that epigenetic status within these cells either is indicative of key epigenetic events in the tissues and organs of interest or is simply a useful predictive biomarker of disease.

The logic of nutritional biomarker discovery is that the measurement is responsive to nutrition and that it predicts future health and disease risk. It is preferable if the biologic basis for the biomarker response to nutrition and the mechanism linking this biomarker to health are known, but this knowledge is not essential: For some of the most useful nutritional biomarkers the precise link to the development of disease is still a matter of controversy. Examples include plasma homocysteine (54) and the increasing use of multidimensional information (proteomics, metabolomics, genomics) produced using peripheral blood cells. Epigenetic signals within blood and buccal cells may be useful biomarkers if they can be shown to predict disease or detect covert disease, irrespective of whether the mechanism has been established. However, an understanding of mechanism offers up many more possibilities.

Epigenetic Tide

A growing body of evidence indicates that, for some genes at least, the epigenetic signal in peripheral blood and buccal cells reflects epigenetic status in the tissues. A metaphor for this would be the ebb and flow of the tide, which causes all boats rise and fall together (Fig. 41.2); whatever the particular epigenome of each cell type in the body, the level of methylation within particular genes or regions of chromatin may rise and fall together in response to environmental exposures. However, the validity and utility of this approach are likely to depend on the epigenetic parameter being measured.

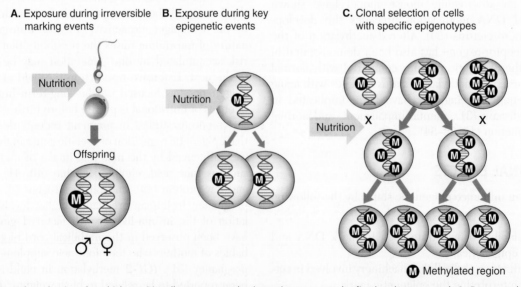

Fig. 41.1. Potential mechanisms by which nutritionally programmed epigenetic status may be fixed and propagated. **A.** Exposure during irreversible marking events (e.g. imprinting). **B.** Exposure during transcriptional activity or key epigenetic processes (e.g. mitosis). **C.** Clonal selection following the generation of a range of cellular epigenotypes in response to nutritional exposure (e.g., [24]).

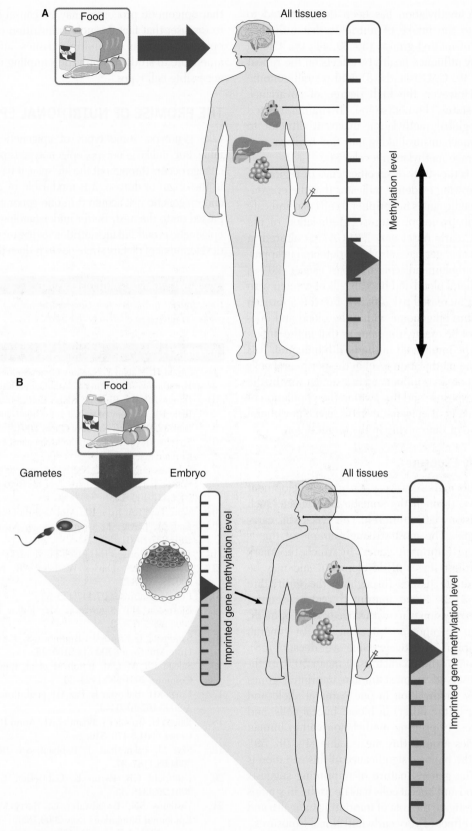

Fig. 41.2. Ways in which the population distribution of general epigenetic status, or epigenotype within specific genomic locations, within tissues may be inferred from blood and buccal cell sampling. **A.** Epigenetic tide. **B.** Echoes of early development.

Global DNA methylation has been demonstrated to be responsive to the intake of nutrients that influence the availability of methyl groups (35–39, 44, 45). Global methylation may influence health by effects on the repeat elements (5, 8, 9), CpG islands (3), and overall genome stability (23). However, the high degree of covariance among folate status, homocysteine, B-vitamin–related genotype, and global methylation makes it difficult to identify causal mechanisms linking nutrition to disease on the basis of average methylation levels (54).

More useful is the study of specific genes or regions of the genome. Growing evidence indicates that the epigenetic status of specific genes in peripheral cells may indicate status within the tissues of interest. Methylation of the breast cancer 1, early onset gene *(BRCA1)* is altered in tumor cells, but changes have also been detected in apparently normal epithelium adjacent to breast cancer (20), as well as in peripheral blood and buccal cells of women with the disease or at increased risk (56, 57). For this approach to work, the entire epigenome within the blood and buccal cells need not be exactly the same as that in the organ, tissue, or cell type implicated in the health outcome. It is sufficient that the methylation level in the peripheral cells and in the target organ is influenced in a similar way by the environmental exposure and that, within the population of interest, the ranking of epigenetic status in the peripheral cells is indicative of the ranking in the target organ.

Echoes of Early Exposure

Some epigenetic marks set very early in development are passed down through the somatic cell lineage such that, many divisions later, different cell types still carry the original signal. The most striking example of this is found within the imprinted genes, in which the mark is set at the earliest stages of development and may be retained in multiple tissues throughout the entire life span (see Fig 41.2). Some imprinted regions acquire tissue-specific expression, vary with stage of development, or may undergo epigenotype spreading (5). In general, however, the imprint is relatively stable over decades (58). This can be seen in the characteristic mean 50% methylation level observed in most human imprinted genes (reflecting 100% methylation in one parental allele and 0% methylation in the other) in blood, buccal cells, and numerous tissues. Imprinting methylation within human populations varies around this mean value (16, 58, 59), and interest in the biologic significance of this variation is considerable. The general nature of imprinting suggests that human blood and buccal cells may be useful in studies designed to investigate the role of imprinting in health and disease and the effect of very early nutritional exposures.

Whether resulting from early life events or nutrient exposures in adulthood, epigenetic status in tissues remote from those in which disease is manifested has been shown both to predict disease and to reflect key epigenetic changes in the target tissue. These observations suggest that epigenetic processes may be causal in the transition to disease, that factors such as nutrition can have general epigenetic effects on multiple tissues, and that these are amenable to study through the sampling of DNA in easily accessible cell types.

THE PROMISE OF NUTRITIONAL EPIGENETICS

Like genotype, some types of epigenetic mark are heritable, but, unlike genotype, epigenotype is plastic. Epigenetic change occurs throughout the life span, it has been implicated in the origin of disease, it is modifiable by diet and lifestyle, and epigenetic risk acquired in one generation may even be passed on to the next. Better understanding of the biology of epigenetic events linking nutrition to disease would help in the development of dietary strategies to reduce the risk of disease.

ACKNOWLEDGMENTS AND DISCLOSURE

I am grateful to the Scottish Government for support and declare no conflict of interest in relation to this work.

REFERENCES

1. Sasaki H, Matsui Y. Nat Rev Genet 2008;9:129–40.
2. Horsthemke B, Buiting K. Adv Genet 2008;61:225–46.
3. Illingworth RS, Bird AP. FEBS Lett 2009;583:1713–20.
4. Jirtle RL, Skinner MK. Nat Rev Genet 2007;8:253–62.
5. Reik W, Walter J. Nat Rev Genet 2001;2:21–32.
6. Strachan T, Read AP. Human Molecular Genetics 4. New York: Garland Science, 2010.
7. Schones DE, Zhao K. Nat Rev Genet 2008;9:179–91.
8. Walter J, Hutter B, Khare T et al. Cytogenet Genome Res 2006;113:109–15.
9. Waterland RA, Jirtle RL. Mol Cell Biol 2003;23:5293–5300.
10. Reik W, Davies K, Dean W et al. Novartis Found Symp 2001;237:19–31.
11. Tycko B, Morison IM. J Cell Physiol 2002;192:245–58.
12. Wilkinson LS, Davies W, Isles AR. Nat Rev Neurosci 2007;8:832–843.
13. Reik W. Nature 2007;447:425–32.
14. Bjornsson HT, Sigurdsson MI, Fallin MD et al. JAMA 2008;299:2877–83.
15. Sandovici I, Kassovska-Bratinova S, Loredo-Osti JC et al. Hum Mol Genet 2005;14:2135–43.
16. Sakatani T, Wei M, Katoh M et al. Biochem Biophys Res Commun 2001;283:1124–30.
17. Fraga MF, Ballestar E, Paz MF et al. Proc Natl Acad Sci U S A 2005;102:10604–9.
18. Jiang YH, Bressler J, Beaudet AL. Annu Rev Genomics Hum Genet 2004;5:479–510.
19. Szyf M, Pakneshan, P, Rabbani, SA. Biochem Pharmacol 2004;68:1187–97.
20. Umbricht CB, Evron E, Gabrielson E et al. Oncogene 2001;20:3348–53.
21. Vasilatos SN, Broadwater G, Barry WT et al. Cancer Epidemiol Biomarkers Prev 2009;18:901–14.
22. Fraga MF, Ballestar E, Villar-Garea A et al. Nat Genet 2005;37:391–400.
23. Robertson KD. Nat Rev Genet 2005;6:597–610.
24. Feinberg AP, Ohlsson R, Henikoff S. Nat Rev Genet 2006;7:21–33.
25. Temple IK, Shield JP. J Med Genet 2002;39:872–5.

26. Rump P, Zeegers MP, van Essen AJ. Am J Med Genet Assoc 2005;136:95–104.

27. Castro R, Rivera I, Struys EA et al. Clin Chem 2003;49:1292–6.

28. Hiltunen MO, Turunen MP, Hakkinen TP et al. Vasc Med 2002;7:5–11.

29. Lund G, Andersson L, Lauria M et al. J Biol Chem 2004;279:29147–54.

30. Post WS, Goldschmidt-Clermont PJ, Wilhide CC et al. Cardiovasc Res 1999;43:985–91.

31. Mattson MP. Ageing Res Rev 2003;2:329–42.

32. Levenson JM, Sweatt JD. Nat Rev Neurosci 2005;6:108–18.

33. Tsankova N, Renthal W, Kumar A et al. Nat. Rev Neurosci 2007;8:355–67.

34. Haggarty P, Hoad G, Harris SE et al. PLoS One 2010;5:e11329.

35. Jacob RA, Gretz DM, Taylor PC et al. J Nutr 1998;128:1204–12.

36. Yi P, Melnyk S, Pogribna M et al. J Biol Chem 2000;275:29318–23.

37. Friso S, Choi SW, Girelli D et al. Proc Natl Acad Sci U S A 2002;99:5606–11.

38. Stern LL, Mason JB, Selhub J et al. Cancer Epidemiol Biomarkers Prev 2000;9:849–53.

39. Kirkland JB. J Nutr 2009;139:2397–2401.

40. Zempleni J, Chew YC, Bao B et al. J Nutr 2009;139:2389–92.

41. Ho E, Clarke JD, Dashwood RH. J Nutr 2009;139:2393–6.

42. Choi SW, Stickel F, Baik HW et al. J Nutr 1999;129:1945–50.

43. Garro AJ, McBeth DL, Lima V et al. Alcohol Clin Exp Res 1991;15:395–8.

44. Bonsch D, Lenz B, Reulbach U et al. J Neural Transm 2004;111:1611–6.

45. Bonsch D, Lenz B, Kornhuber J et al. Neuroreport 2005;16:167–70.

46. Fang M, Chen D, Yang CS. J Nutr 2007;137:223S–8S.

47. Lee WJ, Zhu BT. Carcinogenesis 2006;27:269–77.

48. Fang MZ, Wang Y, Ai N et al. Cancer Res 2003;63:7563–70.

49. Lillycrop KA, Phillips ES, Jackson AA et al. J Nutr 2005;135:1382–6.

50. Dolinoy DC, Weidman JR, Waterland RA et al. Environ Health Perspect 2006;114:567–72.

51. Steegers-Theunissen RP, Obermann-Borst SA, Kremer D et al. PLoS One 2009;4:e7845.

52. UK Scientific Advisory Committee on Nutrition. The influence of maternal, fetal and child nutrition on the development of chronic disease in later life. London TSO 2011.

53. Heijmans BT, Tobi EW, Stein AD et al. Proc Natl Acad Sci U S A 2008;105:17046–9.

54. Haggarty P. Proc Nutr Soc 2007;66:539–47.

55. Laird PW. Nat Rev Cancer 2003;3:253–66.

56. Snell C, Krypuy M, Wong EM et al. Breast Cancer Res 2008;10:R12.

57. Widschwendter M, Apostolidou S, Raum E, et al. PLoS One 2008;3:e2656.

58. Sandovici I, Leppert M, Hawk PR et al. Hum Mol Genet 2003;12:1569–78.

59. Waterland RA, Jirtle RL. Nutrition 2004;20:63–8.

SUGGESTED READINGS

Feinberg AP. Phenotypic plasticity and the epigenetics of human disease. Nature 2007;447:433–40.

Feinberg AP, Ohlsson R, Henikoff S. The epigenetic progenitor origin of human cancer. Nat Rev Genet 2006;7:21–33.

Jirtle RL, Skinner MK. Environmental epigenomics and disease susceptibility. Nat Rev Genet 2007;8:253–62.

Margueron R, Reinberg D. Chromatin structure and the inheritance of epigenetic information. Nat Rev Genet 2010;11:285–96.

Reik W, Walter J. Genomic imprinting: parental influence on the genome. Nat Rev Genet 2001;2:21–32.

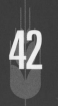

42 NUTRITIONAL PHYSIOLOGY OF THE ALIMENTARY TRACT

SHELBY SULLIVAN, DAVID ALPERS, AND SAMUEL KLEIN

---

[1]**Abbreviations: AgRP**, Agouti-related peptide; **α-MSH**, α-melanocyte-stimulating hormone; **ATPase**, adenosine triphosphatase; **CART**, cocaine and amphetamine-regulated transcript; **CCqaK**, cholecystokinin; **Cl**, chloride; **CNS**, central nervous system; **EC**, enterochromaffin cells; **ECL**, enterochromaffinlike; **ENS**, enteric nervous system; **GALT**, gut-associated lymphoid tissue; **GI**, gastrointestinal; **GIP**, glucose-dependent insulinotropic peptide; **GLP**, glucagon-like peptide; **GLUT**, glucose transporter; **GRP**, gastrin-releasing peptide; **H⁺**, hydrogen; **HCO₃⁻**, bicarbon; **Ig**, immunoglobulin; **IGF-I**, insulinlike growth factor-I; **ILF**, isolated lymphoid follicle; **K**, potassium; **LCT**, long-chain triglyceride; **MC4R**, melanocortin-4 receptor; **MCT**, medium-chain triglyceride; **MMC**, migrating motor complex; **Na**, sodium; **NO**, nitric oxide; **NPY**, neuropeptide Y; **OXM**, oxyntomodulin; **POMC**, proopiomelanocortin; **PP**, pancreatic polypeptide; **PRR**, pattern recognition receptor; **PYY**, peptide YY; **SCFA**, short-chain fatty acid; **SGLT1**, sodium-glucose cotransporter-1; **VIP**, vasoacintestinal polypeptide.

The alimentary tract is a tubular structure that extends from the posterior oropharynx to the anus. Its primary function is to digest and absorb ingested nutrients. The purpose of this chapter is to review the structural and functional components of the alimentary tract and describe the interactions of these components in response to a meal. The gastrointestinal (GI) tract flora and GI immune system are also reviewed briefly because of their importance in overall gut function.

GASTROINTESTINAL TRACT STRUCTURE

Substructures and Cells

The structure of the GI tract is reviewed briefly, with a consideration of the localization of numerous cells and substructures that are critical for its function. The GI tract consists of four contiguous segments: the esophagus, stomach, small intestine, and colon (Fig. 42.1). The wall of each segment contains four distinctive layers: the mucosa, submucosa, muscularis propria, and serosa or adventitia (Fig. 42.2). The mucosa is composed of three distinct layers: the epithelium, lamina propria, and muscularis mucosae. The epithelial layer forms a barrier between the lumen and the underlying tissues. Many of the different region-specific secretory, absorptive, and barrier functions of the alimentary tract are accounted for by differences in the type and distribution of various differentiated epithelial cell populations along the length of the gut. Thus, the epithelium shows the greatest degree of variability among different regions of the GI tract. The lamina propria is a connective tissue space between the epithelium and the thin layer of muscle fibers, the muscularis mucosae, which forms the lower boundary of the mucosa. The lamina propria contains many cells involved in immunologic functions, including immunoglobulin (Ig)-secreting plasma cells, macrophages, and lymphocytes. In addition, abundant lymphoid nodules are present, often extending through the muscularis mucosae into the underlying submucosa. Subepithelial fibroblasts produce collagen and many other extracellular matrix components that underlie the basal lamina of the epithelium. These fibroblasts and the extracellular matrix that they secrete have an important role in regulating cell proliferation and differentiation events within the overlying epithelium.

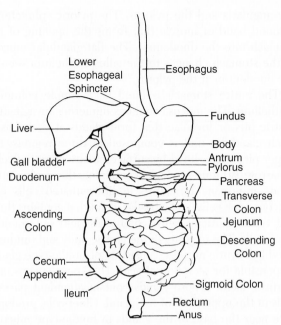

Fig. 42.1. Anatomy of the stomach, small intestine, and large intestine. The duodenum is located in the retroperitoneal space and bends around the head of the pancreas. The jejunum lies within the peritoneal cavity and begins at the ligament of Trietz. Jejunal bowel loops are predominantly located in the left and middle upper abdomen. The proximal ileum lies in the middle abdominal region. The distal ileum lies in the right lower quadrant and joins the colon at the ileal cecal valve. The *cutout* reveals the duodenum and the ligament of Trietz that lie behind the transverse colon.

The mucosal epithelium contains numerous enteroendocrine cells, in addition to cells that serve secretory, absorptive, and barrier functions. The enteroendocrine cells, found in gastric, intestinal, and colonic epithelium, are characterized by their polygonal shape, broad base, and numerous basilar membrane–bound secretory granules. Enteroendocrine cells are joined to other adjacent cells in the epithelium via junctional complexes located near the apical pole. The regulatory peptides or bioamine products stored in the basally located secretory granules are secreted through the basolateral membrane and act through paracrine or endocrine mechanisms as mediators of GI secretion, absorptive function, and motility in response to luminally and/or basolaterally derived signals.

The submucosa extends from the mucosa to the muscularis externa and contains numerous small to moderate-sized veins, arteries, and lymphatic channels surrounded by connective tissue. Ganglion cells and autonomic nerve fibers of the Meissner plexus are also found in the submucosa. Fibers of this submucosal plexus together with the myenteric plexus form the enteric nervous system (ENS), which regulates and coordinates numerous intestinal functions, including motility. Additionally, scattered lymphoid aggregates or nodules may be found in this layer of the gut wall.

The muscularis propria is organized into two layers of muscle: an inner circular layer, in which muscle cells circle the intestine, and an outer longitudinal layer, in which muscle cells run parallel with the long axis of the intestine. In the upper esophagus, skeletal muscle fibers interdigitate with smooth muscle fibers, whereas the muscularis of the remaining alimentary tract is composed entirely of smooth muscle.

Esophagus

The adult esophagus is approximately 25 cm long and extends from the posterior oropharynx at the level of

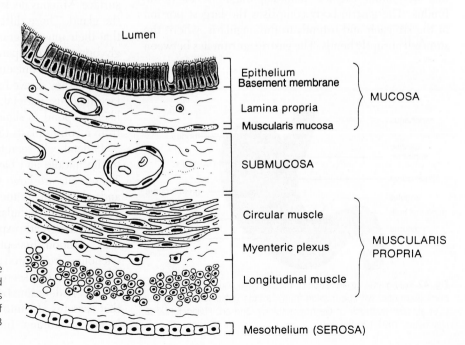

Fig. 42.2. Schematic organization of the wall of the gastrointestinal tract. (Reprinted with permission from Yamada T, Alpers DH, Owyang C et al, eds. Textbook of Gastroenterology. 2nd ed. Philadelphia: JB Lippincott, 1991:142.)

the cricoid cartilage to just below the diaphragmatic hiatus, where it enters the stomach at the esophagogastric junction. The esophageal mucosa is lined with a thick incompletely keratinized stratified squamous epithelium that provides protection against abrasion during passage of a swallowed food bolus and against refluxed stomach acid. The lamina propria contains occasional lymphoid aggregates and mucosal glands that secrete neutral mucus. Submucosal glands that secrete acidic mucus extend through the lamina propria and muscularis mucosae and are most abundant in the upper half of the esophagus.

In the upper esophagus, skeletal muscle fibers blend with the smooth muscle fibers found throughout the rest of the esophagus. The upper esophageal sphincter consists of a thickened band of oblique muscle. These skeletal muscle fibers are under voluntary control and are involved in regulating the initial passage of a swallowed bolus into the upper esophagus. The remaining smooth muscle of the muscularis is innervated by parasympathetic fibers originating from the vagus nerve. A thickened band of circular smooth muscle adjacent to the esophagogastric junction forms the lower esophageal sphincter. Contraction of this specialized region of smooth muscle, coupled with the abrupt angulation of the esophagus as it passes through the diaphragmatic hiatus, where it joins the gastric cardia, provides a mechanism for preventing reflux of the acid contents of the stomach into the esophagus.

Stomach

The stomach is an asymmetric organ that extends from the gastroesophageal junction in the cardia to the duodenum (Fig. 42.3). The upper portion of the stomach that lies under the left hemidiaphragm is called the fundus. The gastric body comprises the largest portion of the stomach and extends to the angularis, where the stomach abruptly bends. The gastric antrum lies between

the angularis and the pylorus. The pyloric sphincter is a round band of muscle that forms the opening of the stomach into the duodenum. The flat glandular mucosa of the stomach changes to the villus epithelium seen in the duodenum at the pylorus.

The entire stomach is lined by a simple columnar epithelium. The mucosa contains numerous invaginating gastric pits or foveolae that form glands at their bases. Each glandular unit is composed of three regions: the upper pit region, lined by surface mucus-secreting cells; a narrow isthmus or neck, containing the proliferative zone, and many immature undifferentiated cells and mucous neck cells; and a basilar gland that contains three cell types—parietal cells, chief cells, and enteroendocrine cells. The majority of the gastric body and fundus is lined by oxyntic mucosa, consisting of fundic-type glands responsible for secretion of acid (H^+), pepsinogens, and intrinsic factor. These glands contain abundant parietal cells in the upper half of the gland. Chief cells predominate near the base of the glands in fundic-type mucosa. The cardiac glands, found in the first 3 to 4 cm adjacent to the esophagogastric junction, are primarily mucus-secreting glands with few parietal or chief cells. Pyloric glands in the prepyloric antrum are coiled and are remarkable for their fairly long foveolae and increased population of enteroendocrine cells.

Surface mucous cells form a uniform population of columnar epithelial cells lining the surface mucosa and gastric pits. These cells secrete a glycoprotein-rich neutral mucous layer that protects the epithelium from the acid environment of the stomach (1). Surface mucous cells are constantly shed into the gastric lumen and are replaced by replication of undifferentiated cells within the neck or isthmus region of each gastric gland that differentiate during migration up the foveola and onto the gastric mucosal surface. Mucous neck cells are also present in the neck of the gland. These differ from the surface mucous cells in that their mucous granules are larger, they contain acidic glycoproteins compared with the neutral glycoproteins of the surface mucous cells, and although they secrete mucous, they derive from the stem cell precursors for surface mucous, parietal, chief, and endocrine cells (2) and likely respond to signals from the mesenchyme, possibly from myofibroblasts (3).

Parietal cells secrete hydrochloric acid and are located in the middle and basilar portions of the gastric glands. These cells are large with clear or acidophilic cytoplasm and abundant mitochondria. These cells have well-developed intracellular canaliculi containing a microvillus border that greatly expands the apical surface available for acid secretion. Receptors for histamine, gastrin, and acetylcholine are located at the basolateral surface and regulate parietal cell secretory function. Hydrogen/potassium (H^+/K^+)-adenosine triphosphatase (ATPase), the enzyme that secretes H^+ into the lumen, is located on the canalicular membrane. Intrinsic factor, a binding protein for

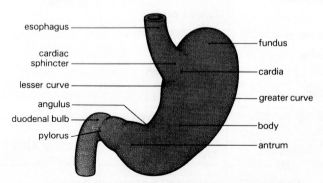

Fig. 42.3. Regional organization of the stomach and proximal duodenum. (Reprinted with permission from Yamada T, Alpers DH, Owyang C et al, eds. Textbook of Gastroenterology. 2nd ed. Philadelphia: JB Lippincott, 1991:1304.)

esophagus — fundus
cardiac sphincter — cardia
lesser curve — greater curve
angulus — body
duodenal bulb — antrum
pylorus

vitamin B_{12}, is secreted by parietal cells. In addition, parietal cells play a role in the regulation of gastric mucosa cell lineage differentiation. The growth factors transforming growth factor (TGF)-α, heparin-binding epidermal growth factor-like growth factor, and amphiregulin as well as the morphogen sonic hedgehog (a peptide involved in gastric cellular growth an differentiation) are produced by parietal cells (2, 4).

Chief cells or zymogenic cells are found near the base of the gastric glands. These cells contain an extensive basilar rough endoplasmic reticulum and supranuclear zymogen granules, reflecting their role in the production of pepsinogens and other proteases. Pepsinogens are synthesized and secreted by these cells into the gastric lumen. Hydrochloric acid in the lumen catalyzes the conversion of the proenzyme pepsinogen to the active pepsins that begin digestion of proteins to lower-molecular-weight polypeptides.

Enteroendocrine cells are most abundant in the prepyloric antrum and secrete many different neuropeptides and regulatory molecules that are discussed later. These cells are classified as open or closed cells. Open cells have apical membranes that are in contact with the lumen, whereas closed cells are not in contact with the lumen. Gastrin-secreting G cells predominate in the antrum (an example of open endocrine cell), enterochromaffin cells (ECs) are found throughout the gastric mucosa and secrete serotonin and either substance P or motilin, glucagon-secreting A cells are found in the proximal third of the stomach, and somatostatin-secreting D cells (an example of a closed endocrine cell) can be found in both the upper third of the stomach and the antrum but not in the midstomach. This complex web of enteroendocrine signals is important in integrating responses to both luminal conditions and basolateral signals.

Layers

The stomach has four tissue layers. The first of the layers is the mucosa, which is lined by the epithelial cells outlined in the preceding and also contains lamina propria and a thin muscular layer called the muscularis mucosae. The layer beneath the mucosa is the submucosa. This is a connective tissue layer that contains blood vessels, lymphatics, and nerves. The next layer is the muscularis propria, which is comprised of three muscle layers: the oblique muscle, the circular muscle layer (which becomes the pyloric sphincter), and an outer longitudinal muscle. The final layer is the serosa.

Small Intestine

The small intestine extends from the gastric pylorus to the ileocecal valve and is divided into three regions: the duodenum, the jejunum, and the ileum (5).

Duodenum

The duodenum is approximately 30 cm in length and is fixed in place, molded around the head of the pancreas.

Histologically, the duodenum is characterized by the presence of abundant submucosal Brunner glands that secrete alkaline mucus. The first portion of the duodenum, known as the bulb, is attached to a mesentery that is folded onto the posterior wall of the peritoneal cavity. The second (descending), third (transverse), and fourth (ascending) portions of the duodenum are retroperitoneal in location. Bile and pancreatic secretions enter the second portion of the duodenum from the common bile duct at the ampulla (papilla) of Vater. The junction of the duodenum and the jejunum is defined by the position of the ligament of Treitz, where the duodenum reenters the peritoneal cavity. No change occurs in the histologic appearance of the small intestine at this transition.

Jejunum and Ileum

The jejunum and ileum are mobile because of their attachment to an extensive mesentery. The proximal two fifths of the small intestine beyond the ligament of Treitz are defined as jejunum, whereas the distal three fifths are ileum. The jejunum has a larger diameter, more prominent folds, and longer villi than the ileum. The ileum is characterized by the presence of abundant lymphoid follicles (Peyer patches) in the submucosa.

The length of the jejunum and ileum in adults ranges from 320 to 846 cm. Several structural features of the small intestine amplify the mucosal surface area available for nutrient absorption to more than 200 m^2, which is larger than a doubles tennis court (Fig. 42.4). Magnification of the surface area is achieved by a series of folds and invaginations. First, the cylinder of the intestine is heaped up into circular folds (plicae circulares) involving both submucosa and mucosa. These folds are particularly prominent in the jejunum. Second, the mucosal surface is further expanded by the presence of numerous villi, long fingerlike projections of mucosa containing an arteriole, vein, and central draining lacteal. Third, the apical surface of each small intestinal epithelial cell along the villi is covered by microvilli, providing thousands of hills and valleys for surface expansion. The presence of folds, villi, and microvilli increase the surface area to 600 times that of the surface area present in a simple cylinder.

Epithelium

The simple columnar epithelium that lines the small intestine is composed of four principal differentiated cell types—absorptive enterocytes, goblet cells, Paneth cells, and enteroendocrine cells. Cells are joined to adjacent cells by junctional complexes that regulate the paracellular movement of fluid and macromolecules (see fluid and electrolytes section). Absorptive enterocytes are responsible for digestion of dipeptides, tripeptides, and disaccharides, and for nutrient absorption. The microvilli of absorptive enterocytes are supported by a central core of actin filaments that join with a dense terminal web of actin and myosin filaments oriented parallel to the apical surface of the enterocyte. The apical surface is covered by

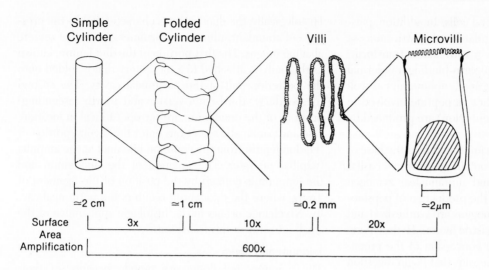

Fig. 42.4. The intestinal surface area is expanded by the presence of intestinal folds (plicae conniventes) and villi. Microvilli further expand the surface area of epithelial cells in contact with luminal contents. These structural features taken together expand the surface area of the small intestine by approximately 600-fold. (Reprinted with permission from Yamada T, Alpers DH, Owyang C et al, eds. Textbook of Gastroenterology. 2nd ed. Philadelphia: JB Lippincott, 1991:327.)

a glycoprotein-rich glycocalyx. Many enterocyte-encoded proteins important for digestive function are present at the apical surface, including dipeptidases, disaccharidases, enterokinase, and intestinal alkaline phosphatase. Goblet cells are flask-shaped cells with large apical vesicles that store and secrete mucus. Mucus secreted by the goblet cell forms a viscous gel that functions both as a lubricant and to protect the surface epithelium against adherence of invading pathogens. Goblet cells also secrete small cysteine-rich proteins (trefoil factors) that participate in host defense. Paneth cells reside at the base of the intestinal crypts and produce proteins involved in antibacterial defenses, including lysozyme and a variety of defensins.

Most enteroendocrine cells contain a large number of neuroendocrine mediators (see the section on GI hormones) (Table 42.1). The distribution of individual enteroendocrine cell subpopulations within the epithelium differs along the length of the small intestine. Although enteroendocrine cells arise from the same stem cell as the other differentiated cell types found in the small intestine, they have a much longer half-life than enterocytes or goblet cells. Thus, their migration onto and along the intestinal villi is uncoupled from the migration of the other epithelial cell types in the intestine. A small population of enteroendocrine cells do exist that differ from other enteroendocrine cells in that they do not contain secretory granules. An example is the brush cell in mice, which produces endogenous opioids as well as uroguanylin (a trypsin-resistant hormone that may act to increase bicarbonate [HCO_3^-] secretion) and express Trpm5, a molecule required for signal transduction in taste cells. It is unclear how these cells regulate digestion in humans (6).

Renewal

Under normal physiologic circumstances, cells within the intestinal epithelium are continuously and rapidly replaced by migration of cells onto the villus from several adjacent crypts of Lieberkühn or intestinal glands (Fig. 42.5). The four principal differentiated cell types of the small intestinal epithelium are all derived from multipotent stem cell(s) located near the base of each intestinal crypt (7). These crypt stem cells divide rarely to produce a daughter stem cell (self-renewal) as well as a more rapidly replicating transit cell (8). Transit cells, in turn, undergo four to six rapid cell divisions in the proliferative zone located in the lower half of each crypt, and their progeny subsequently differentiate during a bipolar migration away from this zone. Goblet cells and enterocytes undergo terminal differentiation as they are rapidly translocated upward from the zone of proliferation to the apical extrusion zone (a process lasting 48 to 72 hours) located adjacent to the villus tip, where they undergo apoptosis and are sloughed into the lumen. Paneth cells arise during downward migration to the crypt base, and enteroendocrine cells differentiate during migration from the zone of proliferation in either direction. Cell renewal, migration, and differentiation are interrelated processes that are regulated at multiple levels.

Layers

The small intestine is similar to the stomach in that it has four layers: mucosa, submucosa, muscularis propria, and serosa. However, some differences exist. The serosal lining is thinner than the stomach and as it transitions to the small bowel, it becomes continuous with the mesentery. The muscularis propria only contains two muscle layers (the outer longitudinal layer and the inner circular layer) compared with three in the stomach. Between these two layers is the myenteric nerve plexus. The submucosa is similar, but with more prominent vascular structures for absorption. The mucosa is also similar with epithelial cell layer, lamina propria, and a thin layer of muscle called the muscularis mucosae.

TABLE 42.1	GASTROINTESTINAL HORMONES		
PEPTIDE	ACTION	SITE OF RELEASE	STIMULANT
Endocrine			
Gastrin	Stimulates: 　Gastric acid secretion 　Histamine release 　Growth of gastric oxyntic gland 　mucosa 　Inhibits apoptosis 　Inhibits somatostatin	Antrum (duodenum)	Peptides Amino acids Distention Vagal stimulation GRP, PACAP, NPY
CCK	Stimulates: 　Gallbladder contraction 　Pancreatic enzyme secretion 　Somatostatin secretion 　Pancreatic bicarbonate secretion 　Growth of exocrine pancreas Inhibits gastric emptying Inhibits gastric acid production Appetite suppressant	Duodenum Jejunum	Peptides Amino acids Fatty acids >8 C in length, monitor peptide, diazepam-binding inhibitor, CCK-releasing peptide
Secretin	Stimulates: 　Pancreatic bicarbonate secretion 　Biliary bicarbonate secretion 　Somatostatin secretion 　Growth of exocrine pancreas 　Pepsin secretion Inhibits: 　Gastric acid secretion 　Trophic effect of gastrin	Duodenum	Acid Pancreatic phospholipase A_2 Possibly bile and fatty acids
GIP	Stimulates insulin release Inhibits gastric acid secretion Inhibits gastric acid secretion	Duodenum Jejunum	Glucose Amino acids Fatty acids
Peptide YY	Ileal brake Appetite suppressant May inhibit pancreatic secretion	Ileum Colon	Fatty acids Glucose
Motilin	Stimulates gastric and duodenal motility	Duodenum Jejunum	Ach, 5-HT_3
Oxyntomodulin	Inhibit gastric emptying Inhibit exocrine pancreatic secretions Appetite suppressant	Ileum Colon	Carbohydrate, protein, fat
Pancreatic polypeptide[a]	Inhibits: 　Pancreatic bicarbonate secretion 　Pancreatic enzyme secretion 　Gastric motility Appetite suppressant	Pancreas Colon	Protein Vagal stimulation
Enteroglucagon[a]	Inhibits gastric emptying	Ileum	Glucose Fat
Amylin (islet amyloid polypeptide)	Inhibit gastric emptying Inhibit glucagon secretion Appetite suppressant	Pancreas	Nutrient ingestion
Neurocrine			
VIP	Relaxes sphincters Relaxes gut circular muscle Stimulates intestinal secretion Stimulates pancreatic secretion Stimulate somatostatin release	Mucosa and smooth muscle of GI tract	Released from neurons and immune cells
GRP (bombesin)	Stimulates gastrin release Stimulates somatostatin release May stimulate exocrine pancreatic secretions	Gastric mucosa	Nutrient ingestion
Substance P	Mediates pain reflexes	Spinal afferent neurons	Afferent nerve input
Enkephalins, endomorphins, dynorphins	Stimulates smooth muscle contraction Inhibits intestinal secretion	Mucosa and smooth muscle of GI tract	Unknown,? Trpm5 cation channel

(Continued)

TABLE 42.1	GASTROINTESTINAL HORMONES *(Continued)*		
PEPTIDE	ACTION	SITE OF RELEASE	STIMULANT

Paracrine
Somatostatin
	Inhibits:
	  Gastrin release
	  Other peptide hormone release
	  Gastric acid secretion
	  Exocrine pancreatic secretions
		Gastric antrum and fundus
		Pancreatic islets
			Acid
			Gastrin, GRP, VIP, PACAP,
			secretin, ANP, β_2/β_3–adrenergic
			agonists adrenomedullin,
			amylin, adenosine, CGRP
			Vagus, histamine, and
			interferon-γ inhibits release,

GLP-1, GLP-2	Stimulates insulin secretion, Increase proliferation, Inhibits apoptosis Inhibits motility (ileal brake) Appetite suppressant	Small bowel	Nutrient ingestion
Insulinlike growth factor-I	Increase proliferation	Gut mucosal cells, liver	Nutrient ingestion
Histamine[b]	Stimulates gastric acid secretion	Oxyntic gland mucosa ECL cell	gastrin
Epidermal growth factor	Stimulates proliferation Stimulates pepsinogen secretion Decrease gastric acid, increase gland cells	Salivary gland	Possible damage to the mucosa (ulceration or resection)
Leptin	Regulates food intake at hypothalamus, decreases NPY release	Adipose tissue, chief cells	CCK, gastric volume, glucose, cytokines
Ghrelin	Stimulates food intake, GH release	Gastric endocrine cells in the fundus	Fasting

Ach, acetylcholine; ANP, atrial natriuretic peptide; CCK, cholecystokinin; ECL, enterochromaffinlike; CGRP, calcitonin gene-related peptide; GH, growth hormone; GI, gastrointestinal; GIP; glucose-dependent insulinotropic peptide; GLP, glucagon-like peptide; GRP, gastrin-releasing peptide; 5-HT$_3$, 5-hydroxytryptamine; NPY, neuropeptide Y; PACAP, pituitary adenylate–cyclase activation peptide; VIP, vasoactive intestinal polypeptide.

[a]Unknown physiologic function.
[b]Histamine is an amine, not a peptide.

Data from Furness JB, Clerc N, Vogalis F et al. The enteric nervous system and its extrinsic connections. In: Yamada T, Alpers DH, Kaplowitz N et al, eds. Textbook of Gastroenterology. 5th ed. Philadelphia: Lippincott Williams & Wilkins, 2009:15–39; and from Hasler WL. Motility of the small intestine and colon. In: Yamada T, Alpers DH, Kaplowitz N et al, eds. Textbook of Gastroenterology. 5th ed. Philadelphia: Lippincott Williams & Wilkins, 2009:207–30.

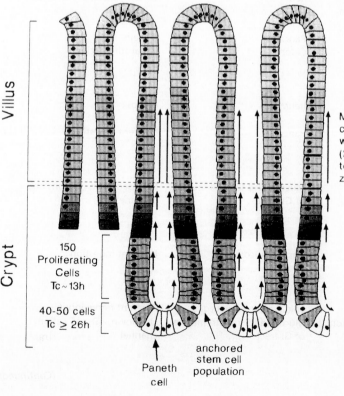

Fig. 42.5. Schematic organization of the epithelium in the adult mouse small intestine. The small intestinal crypt contains approximately 250 cells. The lower 5 cell positions contain 40 to 50 cells that have an average cycle time (Tc) of 26 hours or longer. This region includes Paneth cells and is postulated to include undifferentiated, anchored stem cells at the fifth cell position above the base. The undifferentiated cells divide asymmetrically to give rise to proliferating transit cells (Tc ~13 hours) that migrate upward toward the villus and subsequently differentiate into enterocytes, goblet cells, and enteroendocrine cells. Paneth cells differentiate during downward translocation to the crypt base. Senescent cells are extruded near the villus tips. (Reprinted with permission from Yamada T, Alpers DH, Owyang C et al, eds. Textbook of Gastroenterology. 2nd ed. Philadelphia: JB Lippincott, 1991:1561.)

Colon

Structure

The colon is approximately 100 to 150 cm in length, extending from the ileocecal valve to the proximal rectum (see Fig. 42.1) (9). The colon consists of the cecum, ascending colon, hepatic flexure, transverse colon, splenic flexure, descending colon, and sigmoid colon. The terminal ileum enters the cecum on its posteromedial border at the ileocecal valve. The cecum is a large blind pouch approximately 7.5 to 8.5 cm in diameter that projects from the antimesenteric side of the ascending colon. The appendix extends from a narrow opening in the base of the cecum. The diameter of the colon diminishes progressively; the sigmoid colon is approximately 2.5 cm in diameter and is the narrowest portion of the colon. The omentum is attached to the transverse colon on its anterior superior edge. The ascending colon, descending colon, rectum, and posterior surface of the hepatic and splenic flexures are fixed retroperitoneal structures and therefore lack a complete serosal layer. The cecum, transverse, and sigmoid colon are intraperitoneal and are covered by a complete serosal layer.

Three principal differentiated epithelial cell types are present in the adult colonic epithelium: absorptive colonocytes, goblet cells, and enteroendocrine cells. As found in the small intestine, all these cell lineages appear to be derived from a common epithelial stem cell precursor. Undifferentiated cells, replicating cells, and enteroendocrine cells predominate near the base of each colonic gland (crypt). Cells belonging to each of the principal cell lineages differentiate as they migrate away from the zone of proliferation toward the surface epithelium. The average life span of goblet cells and absorptive cells, from their birth deep in the crypt to the point at which they are sloughed into the lumen, is approximately 6 days. As in the small intestine, some enteroendocrine cell subtypes appear to have a much longer life span than goblet cells or absorptive colonocytes.

As absorptive colonocytes differentiate during their migration up the crypt, they develop short microvilli and clear apically oriented vesicles containing a fibrillar glycoprotein-rich secretory product that may contribute to a glycocalyx. These apical vesicles are lost, and microvilli elongate and increase in number as the maturing absorptive cells emerge onto the surface epithelium. At this point, alkaline phosphatase activity appears on the brush border and the basolateral membranes have acquired a considerable amount of sodium $(Na^+)/K^+$-ATPase activity, reflecting their function in water and electrolyte transport.

Many different enteroendocrine cell types are found within the colonic epithelium, including L cells, which contain both enteroglucagon and peptide YY (PYY); cells that secrete only PYY; EC_1 cells, which secrete serotonin, substance P, and leu-enkephalin; pancreatic polypeptide (PP)-secreting cells; and rare somatostatin-secreting cells. Enteroendocrine cells are more numerous in the appendix and the rectum than in the rest of the colon.

Layers

The inner circular muscle fibers form a continuous layer around the colon. The outer longitudinal smooth muscle fibers are condensed into three bands (taeniae coli) equidistant around the circumference of the colon. Haustra are the bulging sacculations that form between adjacent taeniae coli. The serosa is a mesothelially derived cell layer that covers the peritoneal aspects of the colonic wall. Therefore, regions of the ascending colon, the descending colon, and the rectum that do not lie within the peritoneal cavity have no outer serosal layer.

Appendix

The appendix is similar in histologic organization to the rest of the colon. The mucosa of the appendix consists of deep folds lined with a columnar epithelium forming simple tubular or forked glands. This epithelium contains abundant goblet cells and enteroendocrine cells. Numerous lymphoid nodules are found in the lamina propria. The normal histologic architecture of the adult appendix is often replaced by fibrous scar tissue as a result of subclinical bouts of appendicitis.

Rectum

The rectum is approximately 12 to 15 cm in length and extends from the sigmoid colon to the anal canal following the curve of the sacrum (see Fig. 42.1). The rectal wall consists of mucosal, submucosal, inner circular, and outer longitudinal muscular layers. No serosal layer exists in the rectum. The anal canal is approximately 3 cm long. The anal verge is the junction between anal and perianal skin. Anal epithelium (anoderm) lacks hair follicles, sebaceous glands, and sweat glands. The dentate line is the true mucocutaneous junction located just above the anal verge. A 6- to 12-mm transitional zone exists above the dentate line, where the squamous epithelium of the anoderm becomes cuboidal and then columnar epithelium.

VASCULATURE

Blood and lymphatic vessels provide the transportation system for delivering absorbed nutrients to other body tissues (10). In addition, the arterial blood supply provides nutrients to the alimentary tract itself. In the small intestine, each villus contains a single arteriole that breaks into a capillary network at the villus tip before anastomosing with a draining venule. Each villus contains a lymphatic vessel (lacteal) that drains into a submucosal plexus connected to larger lymphatics. In the colon, arterioles pass between crypts to the epithelial cell surface and form a network of capillaries around the crypts. Lymphatic vessels in the colon do not extend higher than the base of the crypts.

Blood from the small intestine and colon drain into the portal vein that delivers absorbed water-soluble nutrients directly to the liver, where these nutrients can be metabolized or released directly into the hepatic veins and ultimately into the systemic circulation (11). Bile salts absorbed in the terminal ileum travel through the portal vein to the liver, where they can be secreted back into the small intestine, providing an enterohepatic circulation for bile salt recycling, which is critical for normal bile salt homeostasis and fat absorption. Intestinal lymphatic vessels, which are closely associated with arteries supplying the alimentary tract, carry absorbed fat-soluble nutrients to the thoracic duct, which drains into the left subclavian vein and the systemic circulation.

Adequate intestinal blood flow is critical because it provides the oxygen necessary for intestinal cell survival. Therefore, GI tract blood flow is carefully regulated by metabolic, vascular, and hormonal factors to ensure adequate tissue oxygenation (12). Food ingestion increases intestinal blood flow and oxygen requirements (13).

ENTERIC NERVOUS SYSTEM AND MOTILITY

The ENS is able to regulate such complex and diffuse motility functions by its vast network throughout the GI tract. The ENS consists of approximately 100 million nerve cell bodies (neurons) and their processes that are embedded in the wall of the GI tract (Fig. 42.6). These neurons lie in clusters (ganglia) and are segregated largely into two layers: (a) the myenteric ganglia, which form a continuous plexus between the circular and longitudinal muscle layers of the muscularis propria and extend from the upper esophagus to the internal anal sphincter; and (b) the submucous plexus, which is located in the submucosa and is especially prominent in the small and large intestines. The processes from these ganglia form dense networks and innervate the muscularis propria, muscularis

mucosae, epithelium, and other structures. Also, nonganglionated plexuses supply all of the layers of the tubular GI tract accompanying the arteries that supply the gut wall.

The ENS has many different types of neurons (Table 42.2). Moreover, these neurons may differ in function in different regions of the digestive tract. Excitatory motor neurons innervate the longitudinal and circular smooth muscle and muscularis mucosae. In addition, they innervate enteric endocrine cells and Peyer patches. Secretomotor neurons in the small and large intestine and gallbladder regulate water and electrolyte secretion. In the stomach, they stimulate acid secretion. Interneurons are present in all regions of the gut, but their characteristics vary more than those of other neuron types. They are present as a chain within the myenteric plexus that runs from mouth to anus. Intrinsic reflex pathways that control gut movement, blood flow, and secretion are activated by sensory neurons that respond to mechanical and chemical stimuli and to distention. These neurons are now known as intrinsic primary afferent neurons. Intrinsic primary afferent neurons are multiaxonal and connect to other intrinsic primary afferent neurons, motor neurons, and interneurons. They differ from extrinsic sensory neurons because their responses can be modified by synapses at the cell body.

The ENS is connected to the central nervous system (CNS) by transmission along axons in both directions, from GI tract to brain and from brain to ENS. The connections are largely through the vagus nerve and pathways leaving the spinal cord. Most vagal fibers (75% to 90%) are afferent fibers that interact with neurons in the nucleus tractus solitarius in the midbrain. Because relatively few efferent vagal fibers exist compared with the large number

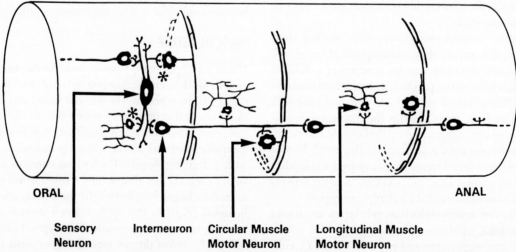

ORAL **ANAL**

Sensory **Interneuron** **Circular Muscle** **Longitudinal Muscle**
Neuron **Motor Neuron** **Motor Neuron**

Fig. 42.6. The pathways for propulsive reflexes in the intestine. A short segment of intestine is represented, on which the descending inhibitory reflex pathway and the first connections of the ascending pathway are depicted. They provide outputs to ascending and descending interneurons and monosynaptic connections to motor neurons *(asterisk)*. The interneurons form descending and ascending chains and provide outputs to motor neurons. In the descending pathway, some neurons excite the longitudinal muscle, and some neurons inhibit the circular muscle. Ascending reflex pathways supply inputs to excitatory longitudinal muscle motor neurons and excitatory circular muscle motor neurons. (Reprinted with permission from Yamada T, Alpers DH, Owyang C et al, eds. Textbook of Gastroenterology. 2nd ed. Philadelphia: JB Lippincott, 1991:15.)

TABLE 42.2	TYPES OF NEURONS IN THE ENTERIC NERVOUS SYSTEM	
LOCATION	**FUNCTION**	**CHEMICAL TRANSMITTER**
Circular muscle	Excitatory motor neurons	Ach, tachykinins
	Inhibitor motor neurons	NO, ATP, VIP, PACAP
Longitudinal muscle	Excitatory motor neurons	Ach, tachykinins
	Inhibitory motor neurons	GABA, VIP, ATP, PACAP
Muscle layers	Primary sensory neurons	Ach, CGRP, tachykinins
	Interneurons (sensorimotor reflex, MMC)	ChAT, 5-HT, somatostatin
	Secretomotor (gut endocrine cells, gastric glands)	Varies, GRP for nerves innervating G cells
Submucosa	Secretomotor/vasodilator	Ach, VIP/GAL (type 2)
	Secretomotor (not vasodilator)	Ach
	Intrinsic primary afferent neurons	Tachykinins (presumed)

Ach, acetylcholine; ATP, adenosine triphosphate; CGRP, calcitonin gene-related peptide; GABA, γ-aminobutyric acid; GAL, galanin; GRP, gastrin-releasing peptide; 5-HT, 5-hydroxytryptamine; MMC, migrating motor complex; NO, nitric oxide; PACAP, pituitary adenylate cyclase–activating peptide; VIP, vasoactive intestinal polypeptide.

Adapted from Furness JB, Clerc N, Vogalis F et al. The enteric nervous system and its extrinsic connections. In: Yamada T, Alpers DH, Kaplowitz N et al, eds. Textbook of Gastroenterology. 5th ed. Philadelphia: Lippincott Williams & Wilkins, 2009:15–39, with permission.

of ENS neurons, the vagus functions more to initiate activity of the integrated circuits in the ENS rather than to coordinate gut function by direct signaling. Efferent centers in the spinal cord can receive efferent signals from the CNS, which are relayed to the ENS. In addition, the spinal centers can process afferent signals from the gut (14).

The vagal and spinal components comprise the extrinsic branches of the autonomic nervous system, including the parasympathetic and sympathetic systems (Fig. 42.7). The striated muscles in the upper esophagus and external anal sphincter are directly innervated by cholinergic

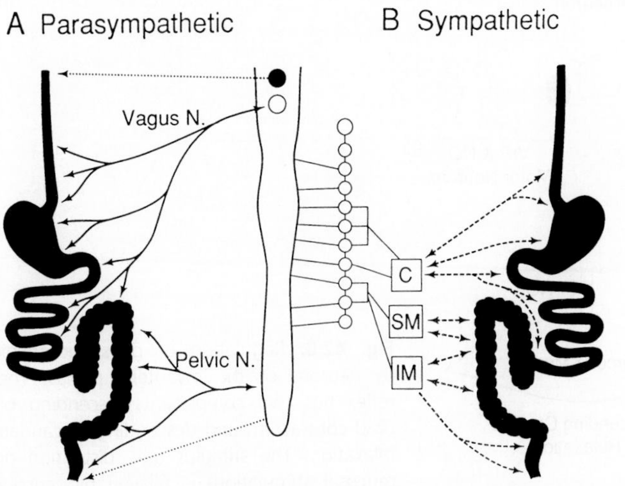

Fig. 42.7. The extrinsic branches of the autonomic nervous system. **A.** Parasympathetic. *Dashed lines* indicate cholinergic innervation of the striated muscle in the esophagus and external anal sphincter. *Solid lines* indicate afferent and preganglionic innervation of the remaining gastrointestinal tract. **B.** Sympathetic. *Solid lines* denote the afferent and preganglionic efferent pathways between the spinal cord and the prevertebral ganglia. *Dotted lines* indicate the afferent and postganglionic efferent innervation. *C,* celiac; *IM,* inferior mesenteric; *SM,* superior mesenteric. (Reprinted with permission from Johnson LR, Alpers DH, Jacobson ED et al, eds. Physiology of the Gastrointestinal Tract, vol 1. 3rd ed. New York: Raven Press, 1994:451.)

fibers, whereas the remaining gut is innervated by a variety of neural mediators, including acetylcholine, gut peptides, and nitric oxide (NO). These preganglionic fibers form synapses with the enteric plexuses, which in turn are connected with smooth muscle, secretory, and endocrine cells. The sympathetic nervous system contains preganglionic connections between prevertebral ganglia and the spinal cord, but the gut itself is innervated by postganglionic connections, mediated largely by epinephrine and norepinephrine. These postganglionic fibers innervate the plexuses of the ENS, as do the parasympathetic fibers, but the sympathetic fibers also directly innervate blood vessels, smooth muscle layers, and mucosal cells.

The sympathetic nervous system affects intestinal secretion, blood flow, and motility. The sensory fibers that accompany the sympathetic nerves (intestinofugal neurons) are primary sensory neurons that are not part of the autonomic nervous system, and are not really "sympathetic" sensory nerves. Sympathetic efferent neurons inhibit motility by decreasing contractile activity and constricting sphincters. These various effects can be relayed along the gut to other regions before returning to the region of the initial stimulus by means of prevertebral ganglia connections. Examples of these inhibitory reflexes include slowing of gastric emptying by acidity or hypertonicity in the upper small intestine.

Intestinal smooth muscle is of the unitary type and is characterized by spontaneous activity, including active tension to stretching, and activity that is not initiated by nerves, but modulated by them. The circular muscle is innervated by both excitatory and inhibitory motor neurons and forms a thick syncytium surrounding the submucosa. Contraction shortens the radius but increases the length of each fiber, and in turn, of the syncytium. In contrast, the longitudinal muscle layer surrounding the circular muscle is thin, is shortened by contraction (with enlarged radius), and is only innervated by excitatory neurons. Electrical slow waves derive from the muscle itself and trigger action potentials, which lead to contractile activity. Action potentials in intestinal smooth muscle are propagated through gap junctions from cell to cell, creating an electrical syncytium.

The regulation of peristalsis, the smallest unit of the propulsive reflex, is one of the simplest of the programmed motor activities of the ENS but is still quite complex (Fig. 42.8). Two components of the reflex, orad contraction and caudad relaxation, combine to move intestinal contents in a caudad direction. The propulsive movement is the end result of contractions and relaxations of the longitudinal and circular external muscles and the muscularis mucosae. The circular muscle has the major role in mixing and propulsion by ring contractions that decrease the diameter of the intestine, whereas the longitudinal muscle creates shortening of the segment by sleeve contractions with little alteration in luminal diameter. Excitatory and inhibitory motor neurons supply the muscle, and inhibitory reflexes modulate these activities by monitoring luminal contents. Multiple chemical mediators are involved in this reflex (see Fig. 42.8 and Table 42.1).

Many GI tract motor patterns have been described and involve complicated interactions between a series of stimulatory and inhibitory impulses from the ENS to GI smooth muscle. Intestinal smooth muscle consists of circular and longitudinal muscle layers, so the interaction of

muscular contraction between layers determines the pattern of motility. The two most important motility patterns are the migrating motor complex (MMC) and peristalsis, which are programmed by the ENS (15).

The MMC, the major complex fasting motility pattern in mammals, is cyclic and passes from the stomach to the terminal ileum (16). The migrating myoelectric complex consists of coordinated activity that empties the stomach and sweeps down the intestine, lasts for 84 to 112 minutes, and is separated into three phases. During phase I, very little motor activity occurs, with only a small amount of forward propulsion. In phase II, irregular contractions occur, and duodenal cross-sectional diameter also increases. This may be to accommodate biliary secretions, which also occurs during this phase. Propulsion occurs during this phase, with rapid propulsion in the transition from phase II to phase III. Phase III lasts only for 5 to 10 minutes of the MMC cycle, but propagates contractions over much longer distances than in phase II, with contractions starting in the gastric body. In addition, a few of the contractions in phase III are retrograde, which reflux duodenal contents and HCO_3^- into the antrum of the stomach. This increases the pH in this region of the stomach and may act to protect the mucosa in the fasting state. The maximal frequency of contractions is determined by the slow wave frequency (myocyte cell membrane potential

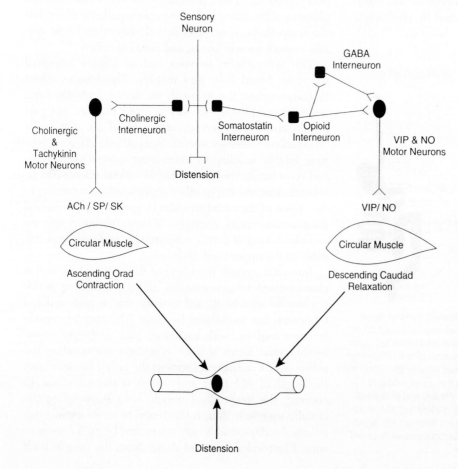

Fig. 42.8. Regulation of peristaltic reflex by neurons of the myenteric plexus. The reflex has two components: ascending or orad contraction and descending or caudad relaxation. The stimulus (i.e., distention or mucosal stimulation) is relayed by sensory neurons to cholinergic interneurons coupled to vasoactive intestinal peptide (VIP) and nitric oxide synthase (NOS) neurons caudad and acetylcholine (Ach) and tachykinin (SP, SK) neurons orad. Somatostatin, opioid, and γ-aminobutyric acid (GABA) neurons exert a modulatory influence on VIP and NOS neurons. (Reprinted with permission from Yamada T, Alpers DH, Owyang C et al, eds. Textbook of Gastroenterology. 2nd ed. Philadelphia: JB Lippincott, 1991:105.)

fluctuations which occur with a certain frequency and along the length of the bowel), which is 11 to 12 contractions per minute in the duodenum and 7 to 8 contractions per minute in the ileum. The functional role of these interdigestive movements is to clear the gut for the next meal. During fasting, the fundus of the stomach is in a state of partial contraction. The pressure created by this partial contraction decreases with a food bolus in response to receptive relaxation (stimulated swallowing) and gastric accommodation (stimulated by gastric distention) (17).

In the fed pattern, the contractions in the stomach mimic those of phase II of the MMC. This lasts until the stomach is empty and starts 5 to 10 minutes after eating commences. These contractions propel the food distally and proximally in the stomach, ultimately mixing and grinding the food. The amount of time food is in the stomach depends on the number of calories consumed and the amount of fat consumed (17). In the small intestine and colon, the MMC is replaced by a fed pattern of contraction. This is characterized by intermittent phasic contractions throughout the small intestine. Again, increased fat content increases the amount of time spent in this fed motor pattern. The return of the MMC after feeding is not well understood, but the first MMC contractions may start more distally in the small bowel. It is unclear what signals are involved (16).

The presence of luminal nutrients can increase absorption by feedback regulation of intestinal motility, called the ileal brake. Fat or carbohydrate in the ileum stimulate the release of PYY, glucagon-like peptide-1 (GLP-1), and possibly oxyntomodulin (OXM) from ileal endocrine cells (18). These hormones then enter the systemic circulation and inhibit gastric emptying, thereby slowing down small intestinal transit. Thus, this ileal brake

mechanism enhances absorption by increasing the contact time between luminal nutrients and intestinal mucosa. Although luminal nutrients in the colon also have some effect on PYY and GLP-1 secretion, they have not been shown to affect small bowel transit times in humans at doses able to alter small bowel transit times when infused in the ileum (18).

GASTROINTESTINAL HORMONES

The largest endocrine organ in the human body is the GI tract, and the first hormone ever discovered was secretin, a peptide hormone produced in the GI tract. The GI tract hormones are briefly reviewed in this section. The mucosa of the GI tract differs from other endocrine organs in that the endocrine and peptidergic neurons are found diffusely throughout the GI tract (19). These endocrine and peptidergic neurons produce regulatory substances that are critical for the precise coordination of activities necessary to handle a meal. These substances are mostly peptides that communicate by endocrine, neurocrine, and paracrine pathways (Fig. 42.9; see Table 42.1), and some of the GI tract hormones can act via more than one communication route. Endocrine peptides are hormones released from sensory cells in the intestine in response to a mechanical or chemical stimuli and enter the bloodstream to act on a distant target organ. Gut neurocrine peptides are produced within the ENS and are located in nerves within the gut itself. Most of these peptides (and their receptors) are also produced by the brain and represent a gut–brain axis. Paracrine peptides (and histamine, an amine) are produced by intestinal cells and act on adjacent or nearby cells. This can occur either by direct cellular extension to other cells, or release of the

Fig. 42.9. Three mechanisms of communication mediate responses in the gastrointestinal (GI) tract. The three mechanisms of communication that mediate responses are endocrine, neurocrine, and paracrine. For the endocrine mechanism, sensory cells respond to stimuli by releasing transmitters that travel by way of the blood to their target cells or tissues. Many examples of endocrine sensory cells through the GI tract respond to either mechanical or chemical stimuli to release their hormones. Some types of endocrine cells respond to changes in pH or osmolality, whereas others respond to changes in specific nutrients. For the neurocrine mechanisms, the sensing and transmissions to the target tissue are completely mediated by nerves and neurotransmitters. Nerves sense stimuli such as nutrients, pH, and osmolality in the luminal contents, as well as movement of the contents and distention of the gut lumen. (Reprinted with permission from Raybould H, Pandol SJ. Integrated Response to a Meal. Undergraduate Teaching Project, Unit 29. Bethesda, MD: American Gastroenterological Association, 1995.)

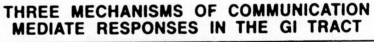

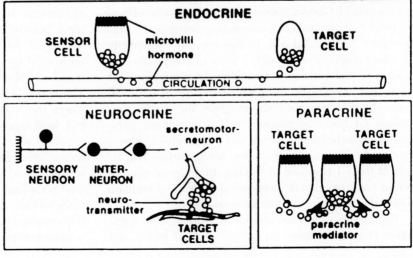

peptide (or histamine) into the mucosa (e.g., somatostatin, histamine) or into the intestinal lumen (e.g., monitor peptide, cholecystokinin [CCK]-releasing peptide, trefoil peptides).

The GI tract hormones have multiple effects, both short term in response to a meal, and more delayed on the growth and differentiation of enteric cells. Table 42.1 lists the better-characterized GI tract hormones. Many of the GI tract hormones that are important in response to a meal are produced by cells in the upper GI tract and act on the components of the upper GI tract (e.g., gastrin, CCK, secretin, motilin, glucose-dependent insulinotropic peptide [GIP], somatostatin, neuropeptide Y [NPY], leptin, ghrelin). All three major macronutrients (protein, carbohydrate, fat) are responsible for the release of these substances. Because the coordination of function in the upper intestinal tract is so crucial, involving the stomach, duodenum, pancreas, and gallbladder, it is not surprising that these sites are most important in the release of GI hormones.

The specificity and coordination of action of GI hormones depend on three major factors: the multiple functions of each hormone, the paracrine actions between neuroendocrine and mucosal cells, and the regulatory functions of the ENS. Most GI hormones have multiple actions and mediate both stimulatory and inhibitory functions (e.g., gastrin, CCK, secretin, GIP, vasoactive intestinal polypeptide [VIP], enkephalins) (see Table 42.1). Other GI hormones or amines are solely stimulatory (e.g., histamine, motilin, gastrin-releasing peptide [GRP], monitor peptide, CCK-releasing peptide), or inhibitory (e.g., somatostatin, PP). Thus, release of these hormones has the potential to create multiple effects on GI organs coordinated in time. The presence of multiple cells in the mucosa, each possessing receptors to many of the GI hormones, also helps to create specificity of response. For example, in isolated cell systems, CCK stimulates acid production. However, CCK injected into the intact animal does not stimulate acid production because of the greater effect of CCK on the D cell–producing somatostatin, an inhibitor of acid secretion, than on the parietal cell that produces acid. Gastrin, conversely, has the reverse effects on those two mucosal cells, stimulating gastric acid secretion from the parietal cell. In this way, the multiplicity of mucosal-specific cells adds a layer of complexity and control to the presence of multiple hormones present in the mucosa. Finally, the ENS, with its many neuronal connections to mucosal cells, integrates the stimuli controlling GI hormone release. Both preganglionic parasympathetic cholinergic nerves and postganglionic fibers, mediated by neurocrine peptides, are important regulators of the GI response to feeding. In addition, chemosensory neurons detect intraluminal events and regulate mucosal function by intrinsic mucosal reflexes.

Peptide hormones are also involved in appetite regulation (see the chapter on control of food intake and appetite). Hormones such as GLP-1, CCK, PYY, PP, OXM, amylin, insulin, glucagon, and ghrelin interact with the brain in both the hypothalamus and in the brainstem (area postrema) by passage through the blood–brain barrier, acting via vagal-brainstem-hypothalamic pathways, or both. All of these hormones listed, with the exception of ghrelin, result in decreased caloric intake and are considered appetite suppressing. Ghrelin is produced by the endocrine cells in the gastric fundus, and intravenous infusions of ghrelin in lean persons stimulate appetite and consumption of food (20).

Some peptide hormones are important mitogens for the cells of the intestinal tract. Gastrin stimulates the growth of gastric oxyntic gland mucosa. GLP-1 and GLP-2 are produced in gut endocrine cells. These peptides are released by nutrient ingestion, and regulate cell proliferation and differentiation in the intestine in addition to their role in energy disposal. Insulinlike growth factor-I (IGF-I) is also produced by gut mucosal cells and is a potent trophic factor for intestinal mucosa, principally targeting epithelial cells, endothelial cells, and fibroblast (21). GLP-1 and GLP-2 also have antiapoptotic activity, thereby enhancing their effect on mucosal growth (22).

INTEGRATED RESPONSE TO A MEAL

The integrated response of the GI tract to a meal represents a coordinated series of events that includes the regulation of food intake, stimuli-evoked responses in anticipation of the meal, ingestion and transfer of the meal to the stomach, digestion and absorption of the meal, and the elimination of waste products of the meal, bringing into play all of the individual regulatory controls reviewed earlier.

Regulation of Food Intake

The GI tract is involved in the earliest part of feeding, beginning with the control of nutrient ingestion. Peptide hormones and other neurotransmitters in the gut have been implicated in the short-term regulation of energy intake, although reasons for intake of food by humans is very complex and includes both short-term "satiety signals" and long-term regulatory factors or "signals of adiposity" (23). Intake of food is also influenced by olfactory and visual signals, taste of food, mood, social situations, and degree of physical activity. The hypothalamic and brainstem centers are main sites where these signals converge and are integrated to control food intake. Leptin is the best-studied peripheral regulator of energy intake, and is produced in adipose tissue; although adiponectin, resistin, and interleukin-6 also produced by adipose tissue also likely play a role in modifying food intake. Neurotransmitters involved in the CNS include dopamine, serotonin, opiates (enkephalin, β-endorphin, and dynorphins), endocannabinoids and γ-aminobutyric acid (24) as well as the neuropeptides

NPY, Agouti-related peptide (AgRP), pro-opiomelano-cortin (POMC) and cocaine and amphetamine-regulated transcript (CART), α-melanocyte-stimulating hormone (α-MSH), and melanocortin-4 receptor (MC4R). Gut hormones that have been suggested as regulators of food intake include GLP-1, CCK, PYY, PP, OXM, amylin, insulin, glucagon, orexin, bestatin, and ghrelin; however, this section focuses on GLP-1, PYY, CCK, insulin, and ghrelin and their effects on neurotransmitters and neuropeptides.

In the CNS, both the hypothalamus and the brainstem integrate signals from the periphery to regulate food intake. Multiple nuclei in the hypothalamus are involved in the regulation of food intake. The lateral hypothalamus, the ventromedial hypothalamic areas, the paraventricular nucleus, and the arcuate nucleus are likely the most involved. Signals come from the periphery through neural pathways as well as endocrine mechanisms (possibly through a leaky blood–brain barrier near the median eminence of the hypothalamus or the area postrema of the brainstem) (25).

GLP-1, PYY, and CCK, act as satiety factors through neural pathways. Receptors for these hormones are found on vagal afferent nerve fibers in the splanchnic region (26, 27). Peripheral infusions of GLP-1 and PYY have led to decreases in food intake at meals, although oral administration has led to mixed results because of their short half-lives. CCK also reduces meal size; however, long-term administration leads to an increase in meal frequency, compensating for the decrease in meal size. Leptin and insulin are thought to act similarly through endocrine mechanisms. Both leptin and insulin stimulate neurons in the hypothalamus that produce POMC and CART. POMC/CART stimulate α-MSH production, which binds to MC4R in the paraventricular nucleus to suppress food intake. They also inhibit neurons that produce NPY and AgRP, which are potent stimulators of food intake (23, 25). The phenotype of leptin deficiency in *ob/ob* mice and in human congenital leptin deficiency is very similar, including early-onset obesity, increased food intake, hypometabolism, hyperinsulinemia, and defective function of the hypothalamopituitary-thyroidal axis. Replacement of leptin in deficient humans has dramatic effects on intake of food, but none on the basal metabolic rate, even in the face of weight loss. Deletion of the NPY gene partially reverses the phenotype in *ob/ob* mice, confirming the balance between the actions of leptin and NPY. Although no monogenic disorders of NPY overexpression have been reported in humans, leptin receptor deficiency also presents with severe hyperphagia and weight gain. In addition, mild growth retardation and altered IGF-I secretion in these children suggest that the leptin receptor may interact with other hormonal systems.

Ghrelin, so named because of its action on the hypothalamus as a growth hormone–releasing peptide, is produced predominantly by parietal cells of the stomach, as well as in the intestines and pancreas in smaller amounts. Plasma ghrelin is increased by fasting and decreased by feeding, and levels are low in patients with obesity. Levels increase after caloric restriction, but not so much after gastric bypass surgery, suggesting that ghrelin may be in part responsible for the inability to decrease caloric restriction long term but may help to explain the reduced appetite seen in some patients after gastric bypass surgery. Ghrelin reaches the brain both by vagal innervations and through the blood–brain barrier. Ghrelin has the opposite effect of leptin in the CNS in that it stimulates food intake by activating neurons that produce NPY and AgRP and inhibits neurons that express POMC/CART.

Stimuli-Evoked Responses

The anticipatory responses to a meal are mediated by the CNS. Visual, olfactory, and auditory senses as well as the presence of food in the mouth can activate secretory responses from the salivary glands, stomach, and pancreas, and can initiate relaxation in the stomach, contraction of the gallbladder, and relaxation of the sphincter of Oddi. These actions prepare the GI tract to initiate digestion when the meal arrives. This preparation is important because digestive products of foodstuffs (e.g., amino acids, free fatty acids) are important stimuli in creating the maximum responses necessary to digest and absorb a meal. Thus, these nutrient products must be produced early in the meal. This cephalic phase of the meal is mediated through various brain centers, but the efferent signals all reach the gut through the vagus nerve. Once the meal enters the GI tract, the ENS becomes activated and works in concert with the CNS. For example, distention of the esophagus and/or stomach causes a contractile response mediated entirely by the ENS.

The most documented anticipatory CNS-mediated response is the cephalic phase of gastric secretion. Sensory input from the eye, nose, ear, and mouth send afferent signals to the dorsal vagal complex in the midbrain, where they are integrated and transmitted to GI organs by vagal efferent nerves. In the stomach, the response is to produce acid and pepsin. Acetylcholine release from the vagus stimulates pepsinogen release into the lumen of the stomach. In the distal stomach, the vagal efferent nerves activate the ENS to produce GRP and acetylcholine to release gastrin, stimulating acid and pepsinogen production. Thus, when food enters the stomach, some of the protein is rapidly converted to oligopeptides by the action of pepsin, produced from pepsinogen and activated in the presence of low pH. These oligopeptides stimulate the release of more gastrin to perpetuate the digestive process. In this process, as well as in other anticipatory responses, appetizing meals stimulate more response than bland or unappetizing meals. Thus, the higher centers of the CNS are important in regulating the initial response of the GI tract.

Although these anticipatory responses are clearly present at each meal, it is not certain to what degree they are essential for the assimilation of nutrients. For example, the stomach can be removed and digestion and absorption can proceed fairly completely. Anticipatory responses to a meal may be more important in determining the amount of food eaten at a meal than the absorption of nutrients. The loss of anticipatory relaxation of the proximal stomach allows only small volumes to be consumed at one time, and maintenance of sufficient food intake to maintain weight becomes difficult. Although this deficit can be overcome by cognitive training, the response to a meal is impaired. Impairment in the senses of sight, taste, and/or smell affects the cognitive drive that creates the desire to eat.

Mouth

Chewing and salivary secretion form the food into a round and smooth portion that can be swallowed. The mouth serves as the receptacle for these two functions: secretion and motility. Secretion into the oral cavity originates from the salivary glands and consists of fluid, electrolytes, and proteins. The structure and function of salivary glands, composed of acini that secrete their products through ducts, are analogous to the pancreas. Chloride (Cl) enters the lumen of the salivary gland through Cl channels, and Na enters paracellularly to maintain electroneutrality. In the ducts, the fluid is modified as Na and Cl leave the lumen; some Na is exchanged for K and some Cl is exchanged for HCO_3^-, thus producing a final salivary secretion rich in HCO_3^-. Stimulation of the parasympathetic nerves is the major factor in regulating salivary secretion by direct acinar and duct cell innervation and by altering the blood supply. However, vasoactive peptides are also released to regulate blood flow. Sympathetic nerve input also stimulates secretion, but to a much lesser extent.

Whole saliva is a complex solution of proteins, peptides, enzymes, hormones, sugars, lipids, and other compounds. It contains both salivary and nonsalivary components. The nonsalivary components include nasal and bronchial secretions, blood components, epithelial linings, food components, microorganisms, and gingival crevicular fluid. Salivary glands (parotid, submandibular glands, sublingual glands, and minor salivary glands) produce salivary secretions from acinar cells. Proteins present in salivary secretions are important during the initial stages of nutrient assimilation. The influence of salivary amylase on starch digestion in the mouth and esophagus is small because of the short residence time of food in the mouth. However, in the stomach, the attachment of amylase to its substrate protects the enzyme from inactivation at the slightly acid environment (pH of 5 to 6) of the stomach when it is buffered by food. Thus, the enzyme achieves a significant initial hydrolysis of dietary starch while still in the stomach. In addition, a non–bile salt-dependent triglyceride lipase is produced by Ebner glands at the base of the tongue. The amount of digestion of triglycerides by this lipase is

small, and the best dietary substrates for this enzyme are triglycerides that contain medium-chain fatty acids. The salivary glands also secrete haptocorrin (also known as R protein), a carrier protein that protects vitamin B_{12} from acid-peptic digestion in the stomach. Many other proteins are found in whole saliva, with some estimates of at least 2290 different proteins and significant overlap (27%) of proteins that are found in plasma. However, although the 22 most abundant proteins in plasma account for 99% of plasma's total protein content, only 40% of saliva's total protein content comes from the top 20 most abundant proteins in saliva (28). These proteins serve a variety of functions in addition to digestion, as outlined, including protecting against demineralization, aiding in remineralization, wound healing, immune defense, and protection from attack by oral microorganisms. The most abundant classes of salivary proteins include mucins, amylase, basic proline-rich proteins, acidic proline-rich proteins, glycosylated proline-rich proteins, "S" cystatin, histatin, IgA, IgG, and statherin (29). Saliva also may contain biomarkers of disease in the head and neck region, which may become useful in the future for early detection of disease.

The taste of food is an important regulator of food intake, and is governed both by input from smell (the olfactory bulb) and by taste receptors in the tongue. Seven transmembrane receptors (7TM) are now known to occur not only in the tongue but also in the GI tract, endocrine glands, and adipose tissue. These 7TMs are activated by amino acids, peptides, carbohydrates, or free fatty acids (30). Taste tissue in the tongue contains receptors responding to amino acids and peptides (T1R1/T1R3, GPRC6A, CaR), monosaccharides (T1R2/T1R3), and FFAs (GPR120, FFA1). The FFA transporter CD36 also functions as a taste receptor on the tongue (31).

The motility functions of the oral cavity are coordinated with the upper esophageal sphincter to propel the food bolus into the esophagus. This action requires the coordination of extrinsic muscles to modify the shape of the pharyngeal cavity and close the airways, and of intrinsic muscles to propel the bolus caudally. These two groups work in succession so that food does not reflux into the nose or larynx. These muscular units work in reverse order during the act of vomiting, again with the purpose of preventing the luminal contents from entering the airways.

Esophagus

The esophagus carries the food bolus from the mouth to the proximal stomach. Relaxation of the upper esophageal sphincter occurs immediately after swallowing, along with increased pharyngeal pressure. These pressure changes move the bolus into the esophagus. The esophagus is the first gut organ in which the phenomenon of peristalsis is encountered. Peristalsis along the length of the esophagus (primary peristalsis) is enhanced by distention in the esophagus produced by the food bolus (secondary peristalsis). The coordinated caudal movement of contraction and relaxation waves moves the food bolus along the length of the esophagus. The act of swallowing initiates both pharyngeal and esophageal peristalsis and relaxation of the lower esophageal sphincter, allowing the swallowed bolus to enter the proximal stomach. Immediately after a swallow, the lower esophageal sphincter pressure also decreases to that of the stomach, and remains low until the swallow is completed. At the end of the swallow, the lower esophageal sphincter contracts, stripping the end of the esophagus of any remaining food contents. The most important neurotransmitters for the motility pattern in the esophagus are acetylcholine (contraction) and VIP/NO (relaxation). Although the esophagus is often depicted as an open tube, the walls of the esophagus are actually approximated to each other during fasting conditions and in areas not distended by a food bolus during feeding. Thus, the bolus cannot travel down the esophagus in the absence of peristalsis. Surprisingly, gravity is not a significant factor in the function of the esophagus.

Stomach

The food bolus enters the stomach as large particles after chewing action in the mouth. In the stomach, the food is mixed and ground with secreted fluid and enzymes and converted to a suspension of particles small enough to pass the pylorus into the duodenum. In addition, fats are converted into an emulsion by mixing action, and small amounts of fatty acids and monoglycerides are formed. Protein and starch digestion also proceeds to create monomeric and oligomeric nutrients that can act further in the duodenum to potentiate the intestinal response to a meal. The two major components responsible for these overall actions of the stomach are motility and acid or peptic secretion.

The anticipatory cephalic phase and distention of the stomach by a meal both lead to receptive relaxation of the proximal stomach, thus accommodating the meal without increasing gastric pressure. Vagal afferent fibers in the gastric wall respond to changes in tension in the muscular coat of the stomach. These responses are processed in the dorsal vagal nucleus in the medulla and create vagal efferent responses that not only relax the proximal stomach but also increase gastrin, acid, and pepsinogen secretion; initiate antral and gallbladder contraction; relax the sphincter of Oddi; and stimulate pancreatic secretion. These vagovagal reflexes are important in the coordinated function of the organs of the upper GI tract (stomach, duodenum, gallbladder, and pancreas), and are part of the reason that these organs are considered as a cluster unit. The likely neural mediators of these reflexes are VIP and NO. Although the functions of the four upper GI organs are being considered separately, it is important to realize that these functions do not proceed in isolation but are part of a carefully programmed response involving the entire cluster unit.

Antral (distal stomach) contractions are initiated by distention of the stomach. The propulsion, grinding, and retropulsion action in the distal stomach serves to grind the meal into small pieces and mix it with gastric secretions rich in acid and pepsin. The food bolus is ground until the particle size becomes less than 2 mm so it can pass through the pylorus during the propulsive component. Peristalsis in the stomach is slow at a frequency of approximately three cycles per minute, mediated in large part by vagal and intrinsic gastric wall cholinergic neurons.

Gastric emptying is a closely regulated phenomenon and is modulated by factors other than particle size. The fastest rate of gastric emptying occurs with isotonic solutions. Most solid meals produce hypertonic solutions, and most liquids are either hypotonic or hypertonic. Thus, most meals will not be emptied at the fastest possible rate. The rate of gastric emptying after a meal is normally approximately 2 mL/minute. At this rate, the digestive and absorptive functions of the upper small intestine are not overwhelmed. Other inhibitory mechanisms affecting the rate of gastric emptying involve H^+ ion concentration and caloric load delivered to the duodenum.

Another major function of the stomach is to produce secretions rich in H^+ and pepsinogen. The parietal and chief cells are most responsible for the products entering the gastric lumen in response to a meal (Table 42.3) and occur in both the cephalic and gastric phases of gastric secretion as mentioned. Postprandially (gastric phase), the volume of gastric secretion increases and the ion concentration changes, almost entirely the result of parietal cell secretion. Nonparietal cell secretion from mucous and chief cells contributes HCO_3^--rich fluid in the fasting state. After a meal, H^+ is exchanged for Na^+, and Cl^- replaces HCO_3^- secretion. Most of these secretory changes occur during the gastric phase of acid secretion, which

TABLE 42.3	GASTRIC CELL SECRETORY PRODUCTS AND FUNCTION	
CELL TYPE	PRODUCT	FUNCTION
Surface cells	Mucus	Lubrication
Neck cells	Bicarbonate	Protection
	Trefoil peptides	
Parietal cells	Hydrogen ion	Protein digestion
	Intrinsic factor	Binding of cobalamin (vitamin B$_{12}$)
Chief cells	Pepsinogen	Protein digestion when activated
	Gastric lipase	Triglyceride digestion, not requiring bile salt, MCT > LCT
Endocrine cells	Gastrin	Release of histamine
	Histamine	Stimulation of acid secretion
	Somatostatin	Inhibition of acid secretion

LCT, long-chain triglyceride; MCT, medium-chain triglyceride.

occurs maximally about 60 to 90 minutes after ingestion of food. In healthy persons, the predominant proteins secreted into the stomach include pepsins A and C as well as gastric lipase and gastric intrinsic factor. However, in disease states such as gastric cancer or chronic gastritis, the range of secreted proteins become more complex and includes not only the pepsins and gastric lipase but also albumin, transthyretin, IgG, IgA, calgranulin A, and α_1-antitrypsin (32, 33).

The control of parietal cell secretion in the gastric phase involves multiple different cell types: parietal cells, enterochromaffinlike (ECL) cells, somatostatin (D) cells, ECs, and gastrin (G) cells. These cells are distributed in two different anatomic portions of the stomach; the parietal, ECL, and fundic D cells in the fundus, and the antral D cell and G cells in the antrum. Gastrin, acetylcholine, and histamine are the major stimulators of parietal cell acid secretion via receptors on the basolateral surface of the parietal cell. Although the histamine pathway is mediated by a different second messenger than the acetylcholine and gastrin pathway, they all result in stimulation of the proton pump on the apical membrane. In addition, histamine is the main determinant of gastric acid secretion, possibly through a potentiating effect on acetylcholine and gastrin. Gastrin also influences the production of histamine from ECL cells. Gastrin is released from the G cells in response to a meal by multiple mechanisms; acetylcholine and GRP acting through vagal and intrinsic nerves release gastrin during the cephalic and gastric phases of secretion, and luminal amino acids released by pepsin also stimulate gastrin release during the gastric phase. Gastrin acts in an endocrine fashion by binding to CCK-B receptors on the ECL cell causing histamine release by exocytosis. Somewhat later, synthesis of histidine decarboxylase is activated, causing additional histamine production. Finally, gastrin stimulates ECL cell growth. As a result of these three effects, ECL cell histamine production is increased and drives parietal cell activation and secretion. Gastrin accounts for approximately 70% of the stimulated histamine release, the remainder being driven by acetylcholine via muscarinic receptors, epinephrine via adrenergic receptors, and gastrin directly via CCK-B receptors. Acetylcholine stimulates acid secretion directly via M3 receptors on parietal cells and also indirectly by binding to M2 and M4 receptors on D cells, which inhibit somatostatin secretion. Ghrelin and coffee also stimulate acid secretion and glutamate indirectly (by inhibiting somatostatin secretion), but to a much smaller extent (4).

Gastric acid secretion is further regulated by feedback inhibition, mediated largely by somatostatin released from specialized endocrine (D) cells in the antrum and fundus (34). D cells typically act locally either through cytoplasmic processes or the local circulation; therefore, fundic D cells are more important than antral D cells in regulating histamine secretion from ECL cells and directly inhibiting acid secretion in the parietal cells, whereas antral D

cells exert their effects mainly on G cells and EC cells in the antrum. Different conditions may mediate the release of somatostatin from D cells in these two locations, and a host of factors are involved in the control of somatostatin secretion, including gastrin, GRP, VIP, pituitary adenylate–cyclase activation peptide (PACAP), $\beta2/\beta3$-adrenergic agonists, secretin, atrial natriuretic peptide (ANP), adrenomedullin, amylin, adenosine, and calcitonin gene–related peptide (CGRP), which stimulate secretion and acetylcholine, histamine, and interferon-γ inhibit somatostatin secretion. Gastric pH is also involved in the control of acid secretion. When the pH in the antral lumen falls to less than 3.0, somatostatin is released from antral D cells, thus inhibiting gastrin release from G cells by paracrine mechanisms. Moreover, luminal acid directly decreases gastrin release from G cells. This example of the regulation of gastric acid secretion after a meal is provided as one of the best-known examples of the intricate and complex coordination of GI function, using elements of the CNS, ENS, and GI hormones (34).

Gastric parietal cells also produce intrinsic factor, a carrier protein necessary for ileal absorption of vitamin B_{12}. Vitamin B_{12} fits into a hydrophobic pit of the intrinsic factor protein, forming the intrinsic factor–vitamin B_{12} complex that is the obligatory ligand for receptor-mediated absorption in the terminal ileum.

Duodenum

The duodenum is at the center of another elaborately coordinated regulatory process, integrating the functions of gastric emptying, bile formation, gallbladder and duodenal motility, and pancreatic and biliary secretion. For this reason, the concept of the duodenal cluster unit has been developed. This concept is also embryologically cogent. Each of the organs of the duodenal cluster unit (stomach, duodenum, liver, common bile duct, gallbladder, and pancreas) are derived from closely related structures at an early stage of fetal development. The liver, gallbladder, common bile duct, and ventral pancreas bud off together from the antimesenteric side of the duodenum, whereas the dorsal pancreatic bud develops from the mesenteric surface. The ventral pancreas then rotates to join the dorsal pancreas. It is not surprising, therefore, that sensors in the duodenum can regulate function in the other organs of the cluster unit.

The duodenum acts as both a simple mixing chamber and a regulatory center by containing cells and nerve endings that sense nutrient content, pH, osmolarity, and distention. The major hormones involved in regulating the duodenal cluster unit are CCK and secretin, although their effects are not exclusive. Moreover, the GI hormones that act in the duodenal cluster unit may act via an endocrine mechanism (through the bloodstream) or via paracrine mechanisms (locally within the intestinal mucosa). An acid pH leads to release of secretin and activation of extrinsic and intrinsic nerves to increase pancreatic and biliary secretion of water and HCO_3^- (35). The presence of digestive products of nutrients (amino acids, fatty acids, monosaccharides) leads to release of CCK and activation of extrinsic and intrinsic nerves, which inhibit gastric emptying and acid secretion, stimulate gallbladder contraction, stimulate pancreatic enzyme secretion, and initiate the small bowel motility pattern of the fed state. In addition, taste receptors have been found in the intestinal mucosa, where they act to trigger responses to nutrients (36, 37). G-protein–coupled receptors (GPCRs) for sweet, bitter, and umami (amino acid) taste have been found on enteroendocrine L cells and intestinal brush cells. The sweet sensors may stimulate secretion of GLP-1 and GIP. They may also enhance glucose absorption via up-regulation of mRNA encoding sodium-glucose cotransporter-1 (SGLT1) and T1R2/T1R3 sweet receptor-stimulated translocation of glucose transporter 2 (GLUT2) to the apical membrane of enterocytes, although further research in intact animals is needed to fully understand these interactions. Much less is known of the intestinal receptors involved in lipid sensing, although research suggests that T2R receptors on enteroendocrine cells may sense lipids either in addition to sensing bitter or by using bitter as a surrogate marker for lipids leading to release of CCK. Glutamate is involved in the sensing of amino acids, and one receptor for glutamate, mGluR1 has been found on the apical membranes of chief cells. In the duodenum, data suggest that glutamate stimulates the appearance of PepT1 (an oligopeptide transporter) with resultant rapid internalization of T1R1, T1R3 and α-gustducin; however, the significance of these findings is unclear (37).

Gastric acid secretion can be inhibited by the neural or hormonal systems originating in the duodenum (Table 42.4). This process is distinguished from inhibition by antral somatostatin in that the regulation of gastric acid secretion by duodenal acid, hyperosmolarity, and fatty acids also leads to inhibition of gastric emptying. In this

way the duodenal mucosa is doubly protected from an excessive influx of acid. GIP, formerly called gastric inhibitory polypeptide, released by the duodenum, inhibits gastric acid secretion and stimulates insulin release from pancreatic β cells.

The release of CCK from duodenal endocrine I cells after a meal is of crucial importance for meal digestion. CCK acts as a hormone to stimulate pancreatic secretion and increase antral, pyloric, and duodenal contractions. Moreover, CCK acting as a neurocrine peptide stimulates vagal afferent fibers that form part of the vagal efferent outflow after a meal, with subsequent effects on proximal gastric relaxation, increased acid output, gut motility, and pancreatic secretion. In fact, most of the effects of CCK after a meal may be mediated through its role as a neurocrine peptide. CCK is important in regulation of the biliary system and its components. The peptide stimulates gallbladder contraction and relaxes the sphincter of Oddi, allowing concentrated bile to enter the duodenum. This action is mediated by both the hormonal and the neurocrine functions of CCK. Stimulate the release of CCK, which in turn acts humorally on CCK-A receptors in the gallbladder. Moreover, in response to sensory afferent nerves activated by CCK, vagal efferent nerves mediated by acetylcholine contract the gallbladder, and vagal afferent nerves releasing VIP/NO relax the sphincter of Oddi.

A complex system regulates the release of CCK from endocrine I (CCK-secreting) cells in the duodenum. Luminal nutrients, especially protein, amino acids, and free fatty acids, initiate the signal. Protein in particular is involved in stimulating the release of three peptides that in turn release CCK-monitor peptide produced in pancreatic acinar cells, diazepam-binding inhibitor from porcine intestine, and CCK-releasing peptide produced in rat duodenal mucosal cells. Pancreatic phospholipase A_2 from pancreatic juice also may act as a secretin-releasing peptide (Table 42.5). Release of both peptides is mediated

TABLE 42.4	NEGATIVE REGULATION OF GASTRIC ACID SECRETION				
REGION	STIMULUS	MEDIATION	INHIBITS GASTRIN	DIRECTLY INHIBITS ACID
			Release	Secretion
Oxyntic gland area	Acid, CGRP, secretin, VIP	Somatostatin (endocrine)	Yes	Yes
Antrum	(pH <3.0)	Somatostatin (paracrine)	Yes	Yes
	Acid	Nervous reflex	No	Yes
		Decreases gastrin release from G cells	Yes	No
Duodenum	Hyperosmotic	Unidentified, might include CCK, peptide-YY, secretin, neurotensin, GLP-1 (peptides with enterogastrone activity)		
	Solutions, nutrients		No	Yes
Duodenum and jejunum	Fatty acids	GIP	Yes	Yes
		GLP-1, delayed gastric emptying		

CCK, cholecystokinin; CGRP, calcitonin gene–related peptide; GIP; glucose-dependent insulinotropic peptide; GLP, glucagon-like peptide; VIP, vasoactive intestinal polypeptide.

TABLE 42.5	PHASES OF PANCREATIC SECRETION AFTER A MEAL		
PHASES	PANCREATIC RESPONSE (%)	STIMULANTS	VAGAL-CHOLINERGIC PATHWAYS
Cephalic	25	Sight, smell, taste, eating	Cholecystokinin, secretin
Gastric	10	Distention	Enteropancreatic reflexes
Intestinal	50–75	Amino acids	Other hormones (?)
		Fatty acids	
		Calcium and hydrogen ions	Other hormones (?)

by parasympathetic (vagal) efferent nerves. Between meals these peptides are degraded by luminal trypsin that is highly concentrated. Thus, little CCK secretion occurs during fasting. However, as large quantities of protein enter the gut after a meal, the amount overwhelms luminal trypsin activity, and most of the putative regulatory peptides escape degradation. In this way the ingestion of protein regulates the release of CCK, which in turn stimulates the release of proteolytic enzymes from the pancreas, in conjunction with vagal efferent stimulation.

Another important role of the duodenal cluster unit is to neutralize the gastric acid delivered to the proximal duodenum and maintain a constant intraluminal pH. Multiple organs are involved in this regulation, including the duodenal mucosa, biliary system, and pancreas. The meal itself provides buffers, mostly in the form of peptides and fatty acids. Most of the neutralization comes from HCO_3^- secreted from the pancreas, biliary ducts, and duodenal mucosa. Secretin mediates the biliary and pancreatic response, whereas the ENS mediates the mucosal response. The major mucosal sensor is the endocrine secretin (S) cell, which is activated to release secretin when the luminal pH falls to less than 4.5. A low intraluminal pH stimulates duodenal HCO_3^- secretion via both central and enteric nerves, local prostaglandin production, and hormones. Mechanisms invoked can be cyclic adenosine monophosphate mediated (dopamine agonists, enteropeptide receptor agonists, VIP), cyclic guanosine monophosphate mediated (guanylin, uroguanylin), calcium mediated (muscarinic M_3 agonists, CCK_A agonists), or inhibition by neurotransmitters (α_2-adrenoceptor agonists, NPY receptor agonists, NO).

A final important role for the duodenum is to produce and maintain isotonicity of luminal contents thereby avoiding large shifts of fluid across the semipermeable membrane of the gut. This function is one performed by the duodenal mucosa alone, without other organs in the cluster unit. Most meals are either hypertonic or hypotonic. Thus, the duodenum must either add or absorb fluid and electrolytes. Remarkably, this adjustment is made within the duodenum. Under normal circumstances, however, the maximum rate of gastric emptying is about 2 mL/minute, so the proximal duodenum is not presented with larger volumes than it can accommodate for isotonic adjustment.

Enterocytes also produce brush-border membrane hydrolases (Table 42.6). These hydrolases are glycoproteins and are secreted from the cell and inserted into the brush-border membrane; the hydrophobic end attaches to the membrane, whereas the oligosaccharidase component projects into the lumen. Brush-border hydrolases are only expressed in villous enterocytes, predominantly in the duodenum and jejunum with decreased expression distally. Enzyme expression and activity are regulated by transcriptional, translational, and posttranslational processes, which are modified by dietary intake, pancreatic enzyme activity, trophic factors, and GI diseases.

Thus, passage through the duodenum changes the physical properties of the meal because of the contributions of the organs in the duodenal cluster unit. Large amounts of pancreatic hydrolases and bile salts are added, digesting nearly all ingested macromolecules (except dietary fiber) to oligomers or monomers solubilized in a form compatible with absorption. Intestinal fluid leaving the duodenum is more isosmotic, and the pH is made more neutral.

Liver and Biliary System

Bile is composed of both bile salts and excretory endogenous and exogenous compounds. Bile salts are crucial for solubilization and absorption of lipid soluble nutrients. Bile salts are synthesized and secreted by the liver, conjugated to either taurine or glycine to improve solubility, stored and concentrated in the gallbladder, and delivered to the duodenal lumen in response to a meal. Bile salts account for 61% of the total solute concentrations of bile. Other components include fatty acids, cholesterol, phospholipids, bilirubin, protein, and other compounds (e.g., drugs, environmental chemicals) (38). Bile salts are cofactors for pancreatic lipase and make lipids soluble by forming micelles. Between meals the gallbladder stores and concentrates the bile salts that are extracted by the

TABLE 42.6	INTESTINAL BRUSH-BORDER MEMBRANE HYDROLASE ACTIVITY IN NORMAL HUMAN BIOPSY SPECIMENS
HYDROLASE	APPROXIMATE ACTIVITY (UNITS/G PROTEIN)
Glucoamylase	250
Sucrase	100
α-Dextrinase	100
Lactase	45

liver from the blood. Two major factors regulate the supply of bile salts after a meal. First, CCK-stimulated contraction of the gallbladder and relaxation of the sphincter of Oddi release the gallbladder contents into the upper duodenum. This provides the first and immediate load of bile salts to enhance digestion by pancreatic lipase and fatty acid/monoglyceride and cholesterol solubilization. Second, bile salts subsequently move down the small intestine to the ileum, where they are absorbed by a receptor-mediated mechanism and returned to the liver via the bloodstream. The enterohepatic circulation (reabsorption in the ileum, uptake by the liver, and secretion back into the intestine) preserves bile salts and diminishes the need for new synthesis in the 1 to 2 hours after a meal. The entire body pool of bile salts (~3 to 4 g) is recirculated two to four times after each meal, providing 6 to 16 g of bile salts to the upper duodenum during the first hours after a meal. With a total luminal volume from diet and secretions of 2 to 3 L after each meal, this provides a large margin of safety for maintaining a luminal concentration above the critical micellar concentration of 2 to 4 mM needed for lipid solubilization and activation of pancreatic lipase.

Previously, very little was known about the proteins contained in bile because of difficulties in analysis because of the bile salt concentration and difficulties in obtaining samples from the biliary tree. Two hundred eighty-three proteins have been identified in bile, including potential biomarkers for biliary and pancreatic diseases (38).

Pancreas

Three phases of pancreatic secretion occur after a meal: cephalic, gastric, and intestinal (see Table 42.5). These phases have been described in an attempt to classify the multitude of events that occur postprandially. As seen in the other organs described earlier, pancreatic secretion is mediated by neural (vagal) efferent responses and by gut hormones (39). In humans, the cephalic phase of secretion is largely, if not exclusively, mediated by the vagus nerve. In this phase and in the gastric phase, the pancreas secretes mostly water and HCO_3^-. PP, located in specific PP cells in the pancreatic islets, acts as a negative feedback mechanism for the vagally stimulated portion of pancreatic secretion. PP is released in response to vagal efferent stimulation and inhibits the vagal effect on the pancreas.

In the intestinal phase, pancreatic enzymes are added to the large volume of fluid secreted. As noted, products of proteolysis and lipolysis stimulate the CCK (endocrine I) cells to release CCK, which likely acts neurally (through vagal stimulation of afferent pathways) and humorally on the pancreatic acinar cells to produce enzymes. Although the mechanism by which CCK senses these products remains unclear, it may involve a trypan sensitive CCK-releasing peptide, which leads to the release of 5-hydroxytryptamine from EC cell, which activates substance P neurons in the submucosa, turning the signal

into a cholinergic signal. This signal may then be transmitted to CCK-releasing peptide-producing cells, thus leading to the release of CCK. In fact, both CCK and 5-HT stimulate pancreatic secretion through vagal pathways and are the primary stimulators of postprandial pancreatic enzyme secretion (40). At the same time, H^+ ions stimulate the S cell to release secretin, which acts humorally on the pancreatic duct cells to secrete a HCO_3^--rich fluid necessary to neutralize gastric acid and allow pancreatic enzymes to be effective. Bile and fatty acids may also be able to stimulate secretin release, but these are likely much less important than acid in the physiologic stimulation of secretin release (40). In addition, enteropancreatic reflexes within the ENS, sensitive to distention, osmolarity, and various nutrients, stimulate pancreatic enzyme secretion mediated by gastrin, GRP, VIP, and NO (39, 40). Other neuropeptides that may increase pancreatic secretions include substance P, neurotensin, serotonin, and calcitonin gene–related peptide. In addition, insulin may modulate pancreatic secretion by potentiating the response of secretin and CCK.

Much less is known about the inhibition of pancreatic secretion compared with the stimulation of pancreatic secretion. It appears that both hyperglycemia and amino acid infusions can decrease pancreatic secretion, and it has been suggested that this effect is mediated by glucagon; however, this remains unclear. Somatostatin may also inhibit pancreatic secretions, possibly by blocking the effect of CCK at a central vagal site. CCK secretion and therefore pancreatic secretion can also be inhibited by nutrients in the colon. PYY (produced in the distal small bowel and colon) may also be involved in inhibiting pancreatic secretion via a cholinergic route (41) and hormonal route (42). GLP-1 also inhibits pancreatic secretion after ileal perfusion, which appears to be mediated through a central vagal mechanism (40). PP, localized to the islet of Langerhans, is also involved in inhibiting pancreatic secretions and likely modulates vagal efferent output to the pancreas via the CNS. Although the exact mechanism by which PP mediates that effect on the CNS is still unclear, it may be crossing the blood–brain barrier to interact with multiple sites in the brainstem (40). Ghrelin and leptin (a hormone produced by adipose tissue) also inhibit pancreatic secretion by a neurohormonal mechanism (42). It is also likely that a feedback mechanism exists with pancreatic enzymes and CCK secretion, possibly through a CCK-releasing factor protein, but this feedback mechanism is not completely understood in humans (40, 42). Bile and bile salts have also been postulated to be involved in a pancreatic secretion negative feedback loop; however, this remains controversial (42).

Approximately 0.7% to 10% of the pancreatic juice is protein. Most proteins secreted are enzymes and proenzymes, which are inactive precursor forms of enzymes that are cleaved to their active forms in the duodenal lumen. Most of the enzymes secreted by the pancreas are proteases and are secreted in an inactive precursor form to prevent

TABLE 42.7	PANCREATIC PROTEASES
PROTEASE	FUNCTION
Endopeptidases	
Trypsin	Cleaves internal bonds at lysine or arginine residues and cleaves other pancreatic proenzymes
Chymotrypsin	Cleaves bonds at aromatic or neutral amino acid residues
Elastase	Cleaves bonds at aliphatic amino acid residues
Exopeptidases	
Carboxypeptidase A	Cleaves aromatic amino acids from carboxy terminal end of protein and peptides
Carboxypeptidase B	Cleaves arginine or lysine from carboxy terminal end of proteins and peptides

digestion within the pancreas (Table 42.7). Trypsinogen accounts for 40% of the pancreatic protein secreted. In the intestinal lumen, trypsinogen is activated to trypsin by the enzyme enterokinase, produced by duodenal enterocytes. Trypsin, in turn, converts trypsinogen and all of the other proenzymes to their active form, and the intraluminal phase of intestinal digestion is initiated. Both CCK and insulin stimulate the production of pancreatic enzymes, which is thought to be mediated through an increase in translation because mRNA levels in the acinar cells do not increase after stimulation with CCK and insulin.

Pancreatic insulin secretion in response to a meal is enhanced by the release of GIP and GLP-1 from enteroendocrine cells in the duodenum (K and L cells, respectively). Although GIP was first recognized for its ability to inhibit gastric acid secretion, it was later found that the major function of this peptide is to mediate meal-stimulated insulin release from the pancreas. This observation led to changing the name of GIP from gastric inhibitory polypeptide to glucose insulinotropic polypeptide. Intraluminal glucose stimulates GIP and GLP-1 release, which acts humorally to augment the glucose-mediated release of insulin from β cells in pancreatic islets. This action of GIP helps to maintain blood glucose levels within a reasonable range after a meal and provides another example of the redundancy that is characteristic of the regulation of GI function after a meal. Evidence suggests that GLP-1 may also act on neurons in a similar manner as CCK. GLP-1 also has a second phase of secretion, when nutrients reach L cells in the distal small bowel, which is likely responsible for the other effects of GLP-1 including the ileal brake and appetite control (43).

NUTRIENT ABSORPTION

Fluid and Electrolytes

The GI tract absorbs large volumes of fluid each day. Approximately 9 L of water are delivered to the upper small intestine daily from dietary intake (2000 mL), saliva (1500 mL), gastric secretions (2500 mL), bile (500 mL), pancreatic secretions (1500 mL), and small intestinal secretions (1000 mL). Ninety-eight percent of the daily fluid load is absorbed, whereas only 100 to 200 mL/day is excreted in stool; approximately 85% (7.5 L) of water is absorbed in the jejunum and ileum and 13% (1.4 L) in the colon.

Water is absorbed passively throughout the intestine and is regulated primarily by active electrolyte absorption (44). Specific features of epithelial cells throughout the intestine are important in regulating fluid and electrolyte absorption. First, the apical (luminal) membrane contains specific electrolyte transporters and channels (45). Second, the basolateral (serosal) membrane contains an Na^+ pump that provides the drive for electrolyte absorption. Third, intestinal epithelial cells are linked to each other by tight junctions that are located close to the apical surface (46). The permeability of the intestinal epithelium depends on the number of tight junctions. The permeability of these intercellular junctions to solute, ion, and water movement decreases distally through the intestine. Therefore, the jejunum is more permeable or "leaky" than the ileum, which is more leaky than the cecum, which is more leaky than the rest of the colon.

Fluid and electrolytes are absorbed from the intestinal lumen directly through (transcellular pathway) or between (paracellular pathway) epithelial cells. Passive transport does not require energy and can occur transcellularly or paracellularly (47). The lipid content of the epithelial cell membrane prevents passive diffusion of charged electrolytes. Specialized proteins present in the apical membrane form channels or pores, which permit electrolyte transport. Passive transport through membrane channels is regulated by concentration and electrochemical gradients across the membrane. Ion channels are usually specific for certain ions and can be opened or closed by cellular messages. In the open state, more than 1 million ions can pass through per second, but no ions pass when the channel is closed. Passive transport can also occur via carriers, which are proteins located in the cell membrane. Carriers are specific for certain solutes or ions and facilitate their passive movement along a concentration or electrochemical gradient across the cell membrane. Carrier-mediated transport is much slower than movement through channels.

Active transport requires energy and permits the movement of a solute or ion against a concentration or electrochemical gradient. Active transport only occurs transcellularly and is mediated by a "pump" that moves ions in and out of the cell. The most important epithelial cell pump is the Na pump (also known as Na/K-ATPase) and moves three Na ions across the basolateral membrane in exchange for two K ions (Fig. 42.10). Therefore, the Na pump makes the intracellular Na concentration low and the intracellular potential difference negative compared with the extracellular environment.

research suggests that the microbiota diversity from the duodenum and jejunum vary from that found in the terminal ileum, with the most abundant genera coming from *Streptococcus*, *Veillonella*, and *Clostridium* in the proximal small bowel (79) and *Bacteroides*, *Firmicutes*, and *Proteobacteria* dominating the terminal ileum (85), as well as density of microbes increasing from proximal to distal small bowel (86). In the colon, the number of microorganisms increases 100,000-fold, consisting of nine different phyla, with *Firmicutes* and *Bacteroides* dominating (75). The ileocecal valve represents a physical barrier between the small and large intestine. Resection of the ileocecal valve permits translocation of bacteria flora from the colon to the remaining ileum, where the bacterial population becomes similar to that of the colon.

The interaction between enteric microflora and the host is complex. The presence of enteric organisms enhances the defense against pathogenic bacteria by stimulating antibody production, increasing cell-mediated immunity, and preventing the overgrowth of more pathogenic organisms. The mucosal barrier is a combined physicochemical complex function composed in part of mucus secretion, mucin glycoproteins, trefoil peptides, and surfactant phospholipids. It forms a separation of luminal contents from the mucosa and creates a framework for host–bacterial interactions. The innate immune system of the GI tract provides another set of defense mechanisms against pathogenic bacteria and parasites (see immune system section). Pattern recognition receptors (PPRs; also called Toll-like receptors) are present in some epithelial cells, and are more broadly expressed in macrophages and other immune cells. These receptors sense the presence of various bacterial macromolecules and initiate a nonspecific inflammatory response. Endogenous antimicrobial peptides, known as defensins, are produced by Paneth cells at the base of intestinal crypts and offer a broad spectrum of antimicrobial activity. Goblet cells also produce small cysteine-rich proteins, which have antihelminthic activity. Normal flora effectively competes for intraluminal fuels and adheres better to the intestinal wall, preventing pathogenic bacteria from establishing residence. The importance of this defense mechanism is illustrated by germ-free animals that cannot survive exposure to hostile microbes.

The gut microbiota also interacts with the host in nutrient metabolism. The gut microbiota is influenced by diet. Research suggests that carnivores, omnivores, and herbivores have different microbiota, and that the human microbiota resemble that of other omnivorous primates (87). Data from murine models demonstrate that a switch to a high-fat diet was associated with a change in the microbiota, with a decrease in *Bacteroides* and an increase in both *Firmicutes* and *Proteobacteria*. Intestinal bacteria also have important metabolic and nutritional functions, including hydrolysis of cholesterol esters, androgen, estrogen, and bile salts; use of carbohydrate, lipid, and protein; and consumption (vitamin B_{12} and folate) and production

TABLE 42.9	BIOCHEMICAL REACTIONS BY INTESTINAL BACTERIA
REACTION	REPRESENTATIVE SUBSTRATE
Hydrolysis	
Glucuronides	Estradiol-3-glucuronide
Glycosides	Cycasin
Sulfamates	Cyclamate, amygdalin
Amides	Methotrexate
Esters	Acetyldigoxin
Nitrates	Pentaerythritol trinitrate
Dehydroxylation	
C-Hydroxy groups	Bile acids
N-Hydroxyl groups	N-Hydroxyfluorenylacetamide
Decarboxylation	Amino acids
D-Demethylation	Biochanin A
Deamination	Amino acids
Dehydroxygenase	Cholesterol, bile acids
Dehalogenation	DDT
Reduction	
Nitro groups	*P*-Nitrobenzoid acid
Double bonds	Unsaturated fatty acids
Azo groups	Food dyes
Aldehydes	Benzaldehydes
Alcohols	Benzyl alcohols
N-Oxides	4-Nitroquinoline-1-oxide
Nitrosamine formation	Dimethylnitrosamine
Aromatization	Quinic acid
Acetylation	Histamine
Esterification	Galic aci

From Kim YS, Erickson RH. Role of peptidases of the human small intestine in protein digestion. Gastroenterology 1985;88:1071–3.

(biotin, folate, and vitamin K) of vitamins. All compounds that enter the alimentary tract by ingestion or intestinal secretion are potential substrates for bacterial metabolism (Table 42.9). Furthermore, the microbiota may influence and be influenced by obesity. Obese individuals have less diversity in their microbiota, a higher ratio of *Firmicutes* to *Bacteroides* (88), but also may have gut microbiota that are more efficient in nutrient harvest, degrading foodstuffs that would otherwise be indigestible to humans (80).

Given the multitude of interactions between the gut microbiota and the host, it is clear that the gut microbiome has implications on human health and that we can manipulate the microbiome to improve the health of the host. Several ways are currently used to influence the gut microbiota. Antibiotics have revolutionized our treatment of infectious disease, and have been used to treat pathogenic infections in the GI tract. They have also been used to treat small intestine bacterial overgrowth. Crohn's disease has also been treated with antibiotics (89, 90), and the success of antibiotics in Crohn disease may possibly be a result of increased *Escherichia coli* found in the intestines of patients with Crohn's disease (91). Antibiotics have also been used treat pouchitis in patients status post colon resection with ileal pouch-anal anastomosis (92). However, antibiotics can alter the gut microbiota in negative ways as well, sometimes leading to a state of dysbiosis (disruption of the gut microbiome) (93). The adult gut microbiota largely rebounds from the effects of antibiotics within 4 weeks, but antibiotic associated diarrhea can occur and the most common causative agent is *Clostridium difficile*. However, subtle changes in the gut microbiota may persist after antibiotic administration, the effects of which are unknown (93).

Other ways to influence the gut microbiota include probiotics and prebiotics (see the chapter on probiotics and prebiotics). Probiotics are live microorganisms that have beneficial effects on the GI tract, including down-regulating inflammatory cytokines, increasing IgA production, improving mucosal barrier function, and inhibiting pathogenic mucosal adherence (93). Probiotics have been successfully used to some extent in inflammatory bowel disease, irritable bowel syndrome, and antibiotic-associated diarrhea. Prebiotics are substances that are not digested by humans, but are fermented by gut microbiota and stimulate the growth or activity of the gut microbiota. Prebiotics are also resistant to gastric acid, hydrolysis by host enzymes, or absorption from the host GI tract. It is thought that prebiotics promote the growth of beneficial gut microbes, and they have been shown in mouse models to decrease proinflammatory cytokines (94).

Our knowledge of gut microbiota and host interactions as well as the effects on human health is still in its infancy. Further research into these interactions and the manipulation of the gut microbiome will further our ability to use the gut microbiome to improve human health.

IMMUNE SYSTEM

The alimentary tract houses a major portion of the body's immune system and is directed toward defending the host against bacterial, viral, parasitic, and food antigens that are constantly present in the intestinal lumen. The intestinal immune system consists of two arms, the innate and the adaptive immune system. These two systems share some components, and they work in concert together to protect the GI tract from pathogens. Components of the innate immune system include epithelial cells and specialized epithelial cells including Paneth cells, and goblet cells that secrete various defensive peptides, as well as antigen presenting cells. This arm of the immune system is more primitive and orchestrates a complex system of both defense and activation of the adaptive immune system as well as tolerance to protect but avoid unnecessary inflammation. This system also includes nonimmunologic components, including gastric acid, digestive enzymes, mucus, bile acids, and peristalsis; all of which make the GI tract less hospitable for many microbes. Moreover, mucosal cells are part of the innate system, including NK-T cells (shared with adaptive), phagocytes, mast cells, and myeloid cells. This system recognizes lipopolysaccharides, peptidoglycans, and lipoteichoic acids from pathogens. Receptors for the innate system are expressed

on monocytes, macrophages, dendritic cells, and B cells, as well as epithelial cells. These PPRs include TLRs and macrophage mannose receptors. The number of receptors are limited, as these recognize patterns, unlike adaptive immune cells that produce specific responses. The innate system responds rapidly within hours. The adaptive system takes days.

Paneth cells reside in the base of crypts near the multipotent stem cells. Paneth cells not only protect the crypt by producing both antimicrobial peptides and enzymes (α-defensins HD-5 and HD-6; group IIA phospholipase A_2, and lysozymes) but also produce inflammatory cytokines that attract antigen-presenting cells and lymphocytes, activating the adaptive immune response. Paneth cells are typically only found in the small intestine, but can be seen in the colon when it is inflamed (95).

Nonspecialized epithelial cells can also produce antimicrobial peptides and enzymes as well as inflammatory cytokines for activating the adaptive immune response; however, the types of peptides and enzymes are different (β-defensins, athelicidin, bactericidal/permeability-increasing protein). In addition, epithelial cells provide a barrier to pathogens and their toxins through intercellular junctions (tight junctions, adherens junctions, and desmosomes) (96).

Goblet cells secrete mucus, which is thought to provide a barrier at the mucosal surface of the intestine, and contains numerous antimicrobial compounds as well as compounds that may play a protective role in colitis, such as trefoil factor-3 (97).

Antigen-presenting cells are also an integral part of both the innate and adaptive immune response, essentially bridging the two components of the immune system. Multiple cell types can present antigens such as macrophages, B lymphocytes cells, basophils as well as epithelial cells. However, accumulated data have placed importance on a specialized macrophage called a dendritic cell, both with activation of an immune response as well as tolerance (98). It is unclear how these cells acquire antigen. Investigators have hypothesized that these cells may extend protrusions into the lumen to acquire antigen, recruit lymphocytes, induce Ig class switch, and stimulate Tregs (99), which play an important role in tolerance (98). However, this hypothesis may not be correct.

The adaptive immune system regulates antigen-specific immune responses and consists of the following components: (a) T lymphocytes, (b) B lymphocytes, (c) natural killer cells, (d) myelomonocytic cells (monocytes, neutrophils, eosinophils, and basophils), (e) cytokines, (f) antibodies (IgG, IgM and secretory IgA), and (g) gut-associated lymphoid tissue (GALT). Adaptive immunity also has two components, humoral and cellular. Antibodies from B lymphocytes defend against extracellular events. Cellular immunity from T cells protects against intracellular processes. Unlike innate, clonally distinct T cells maintain response to specific epitopes, determined by immunoglobulin receptors for B cells and T-cell receptors for T cells. Each cell can detect self from non-self. Adaptive immunity depends on tolerance, otherwise autoimmunity occurs. Autoimmunity in the intestine is not so common as for other organs, suggesting that the GALT can prevent activation of pathogenic clones. On repeated exposure the adaptive system responds more rapidly than on previous exposures. This system includes inductive sites where antigen is presented and effector sites in the mucosa where either stimulation or tolerance occurs depending on the antigens presented to the inductive site.

The secretion of the dimeric Ig, IgA, is an important GI tract protective mechanism. Secretory IgA, the predominant intestinal Ig, is produced by B lymphocytes in the lamina propria. Secretory IgA binds dietary antigens, thereby preventing their absorption, and can bind to pathogenic microorganisms, thereby preventing epithelial cell adherence and intestinal colonization.

GALT contains anatomically organized and nonorganized compartments within the submucosa, lamina propria, and epithelium to provide specialized host defense functions (Fig. 42.17). The nonorganized components include lymphocytes, plasma cells, macrophages in the lamina propria and epithelium, and mucosal and submucosal mast cells. The more organized structures include Peyer patches, isolated lymphoid follicles (ILFs), cryptopatches, and mesenteric lymph nodes.

Peyer patches are secondary lymphoid tissue in the GI tract. They develop during the prenatal period and are composed of three or more clusters of lymphoid aggregates that release lymphocytes after antigen processing (100, 101). Peyer patches do not contain afferent lymphatics; instead, they sample antigens with an overlying follicle-associated epithelium that contain M cells. M cells provide a selective site for sampling intraluminal antigens by permitting the transport of large molecules and microorganisms. These antigens come into contact with lymphocytes and macrophages located within an indented space below the M cell before entering Peyer patches. Activated lymphocytes from Peyer patches migrate to mesenteric lymph nodes, the systemic circulation, and back to specific mucosal sites, where they provide protective immunity from the offending antigen.

ILFs are non–Peyer patch B-lymphocyte containing aggregates, and in their mature form they look much like Peyer patches, except that they lack a discrete T-cell zone. This is thought to be because of how they form; ILFs are thought to be formed from cryptopatches (see the following) and therefore can develop or regress in response to changes in the intestinal flora (101).

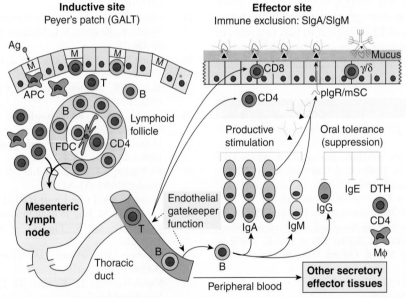

Fig. 42.17. Schematic depiction of the intestinal immune system. Inductive sites for mucosal T and B cells are constituted by gut-associated lymphoid tissue (GALT) such as Peyer patches with B-cell follicles and M cell (M)–containing follicle-associated epithelium through which exogenous antigens (Ag) are actively transported to reach professional antigen-presenting cells (APC), including dendritic cells, macrophages (MΦ), B cells, and follicular dendritic cells (FDCs). After being primed, naive T and B cells become memory/effector cells and migrate from GALT to mesenteric lymph nodes via efferent lymph and then via the thoracic duct to peripheral blood for subsequent extravasation at mucosal effector sites. This process is directed by the profile of adhesion molecules and chemokines expressed on the microvasculature—the endothelial cells thus exert a local "gatekeeper" function for mucosal immunity. The mucosal lamina propria (effector site) is illustrated with its various immune cells, including B cells (B), Ig-producing plasma cells, and CD4$^+$ T cells. The distribution of intraepithelial lymphocytes (mainly T-cell receptor α/β$^+$CD8$^+$ and some γ/δ$^+$ T cells) is also schematically depicted. Additional features are the generation of secretory IgA (SIgA) and secretory IgM (SIgM) via pIgR/membrane secretory component (mSC)–mediated epithelial export. The combined effect of oral tolerance mechanisms, mainly the action of regulatory T cells (not shown), provides a suppressive tone in the gut, normally keeping inflammation driven by IgG and IgE antibodies as well as cell-mediated (CD4$^+$ T cells and MΦ) delayed-type hypersensitivity (DTH) under control. (Reprinted with permission from Brandtzaeg P. Mucosal immunity: induction, dissemination, and effector functions. Scand J Immunol 2009;70:505–15.)

Cryptopatches are small clusters of cells that include dendritic cells, immature hematopoietic cells, very few T or B lymphocytes, and vascular cell adhesion molecule (VCAM) 1+ stromal cells. Some debate still occurs on the role of cryptopatches, but it is thought that cryptopatches are the precursor lymphoid aggregate that leads to the development of ILFs and may also generate lymphocytes (102). Furthermore, cryptopatches have yet to be found in humans; however, this may be because of the high prevalence of ILFs in the colon, where most of the biopsies studied from humans have been taken. Like Peyer patches, cryptopatches are thought to be formed early in life. Although the number of cryptopatches and ILFs may change throughout life, the sum of both cryptopatches and ILFs remains constant throughout life (101).

Mesenteric lymph nodes are found within the mesentery of the small bowel. They are activated within a few hours of oral antigen exposure. Although the mechanism by which they are activated is not completely understood, it likely involves multiple mechanisms, including activated T cells migrating to the mesenteric lymph node, dendritic cells migrating to the mesenteric lymph node–presenting antigen, and free antigen reaching the mesenteric lymph node (100). More recently, the roles, and regulation of Toll-like receptors and Nod-like receptors, collectively referred to as PRRs, which interact with microbial components (e.g., flagellin and lipopolysaccharide) and other ligands, have become increasingly understood in the intestine (103, 104). Intestinal PRRs appear to play key roles in host immunity, inflammatory responses, and also interact with the host microbiome to help maintain homeostasis between the intestine and its microbiota (104).

REFERENCES

1. Ham M, Kaunitz JD. Curr Opin Gastroenterol 2007;23: 607–16.
2. Del Valle JTA. Gastric secretion. In: Yamada T, Alpers DH, Kalloo AN et al, eds. Textbook of Gastroenterology. 5th ed. Oxford: Wiley-Blackwell, 2009:284–329.
3. Dimaline R, Varro A. Exp Physiol 2007;92:591–601.
4. Schubert ML. Curr Opin Gastroenterol 2010;26:598–603.
5. Rubin D. Small intestine: anatomy and structural anomalies. In: Yamada T, Alpers DH, Kalloo AN et al, eds. Textbook of Gastroenterology. 5th ed. Oxford: Wiley-Blackwell, 2009: 1085–107.
6. Kokrashvili Z, Rodriguez D, Yevshayeva V et al. Gastroenterology 2009;137:598–606.
7. Garrison AP, Helmrath MA, Dekaney CM. J Pediatr Gastroenterol Nutr 2009;49:2–7.
8. van der Flier LG, Clevers H. Annu Rev Physiol 2009;71: 241–60.
9. Cohn SM, Birnbaum EH, Friel CM. Colon: anatomy and structural anomalies. In: Yamada T, Alpers DH, Kalloo AN et al, eds. Textbook of Gastroenterology. 5th ed. Oxford: Wiley-Blackwell, 2009:1369–85.
10. Granger DN, Richardson PD, Kvietys PR et al. Gastroenterology 1980;78:837–63.
11. Geboes K, Geboes KP, Maleux G. Best Pract Res Clin Gastroenterol 2001;15:1–14.
12. Nowicki PT, Granger DN. Gastrointestinal blood flow. In: Yamada T, Alpers DH, Kalloo AN et al, eds. Textbook of Gastroenterology. 5th ed. Oxford: Wiley-Blackwell, 2009: 540–66.
13. Chou CC. Splanchnic and overall cardiovascular hemodynamics during eating and digestion. Fed Proc 1983;42:1658–61.
14. Dockray G. The brain-gut axis. In: Yamada T, Alpers DH, Kalloo AN et al, eds. Textbook of Gastroenterology. 5th ed. Oxford: Wiley-Blackwell, 2009;86–99.
15. Furness JB, Nguyen TV, Nurgali K et al. The enteric nervous system and its extrinsic connections. In: Yamada T, Alpers DH, Kalloo AN et al, eds. Textbook of Gastroenterology. 5th ed. Oxford: Wiley-Blackwell, 2009:15–39.
16. Hasler W. Motility of the small intestine and colon. In: Yamada T, Alpers DH, Kalloo AN et al, eds. Textbook of Gastroenterology. 5th ed. Oxford: Wiley-Blackwell, 2009:213–63.
17. Hasler W. The physiology of gastric motility and gastric emptying. In: Yamada T, Alpers DH, Kalloo AN et al, eds. Textbook of Gastroenterology. 5th ed. Oxford: Wiley-Blackwell, 2009:207–30.
18. Maljaars PWJ, Peters HPF, Mela DJ et al. Physiol Behav 2008;95:271–81.
19. Miller LJ. Gastrointestinal hormones and receptors. In: Yamada T, Alpers DH, Kalloo AN et al, eds. Textbook of Gastroenterology. 5th ed. Oxford: Wiley-Blackwell, 2009:57–89.
20. Field BCT, Chaudhri OB, Bloom SR. Nat Rev Endocrinol 2010;6:444–53.
21. Howarth GS. J Nutr 2003;133:2109–12.
22. Baggio LL, Drucker DJ. Gastroenterology 2007;132:2131–57.
23. Boguszewski CL, Paz-Filho G, Velloso LA. Endokrynol Pol 2010;61:194–206.
24. Fulton S. Front Neuroendocrinol 2010;31:85–103.
25. Suzuki K, Simpson KA, Minnion JS et al. Endocr J 2010; 57:359–72.
26. Zhang X, Shi T, Holmberg K et al. Proc Natl Acad Sci U S A 1997;94:729–34.
27. Abbott CR, Monteiro M, Small CJ et al. Brain Res 2005; 1044:127–31.
28. Loo JA, Yan W, Ramachandran P et al. J Dent Res 2010; 89:1016–23.
29. Messana I, Inzitari R, Fanali C et al. J Sep Sci 2008;31: 1948–63.
30. Wellendorph P, Johansen LD, Brauner-Osborne H. Vitam Horm 2010;84:151–84.
31. Abumrad NA. J Clin Invest 2005;115:2965–7.
32. Lee K, Kye M, Jang JS et al. Proteomics 2004;4:3343–52.
33. Liang CR, Tan S, Tan HT et al. Proteomics 2010;10: 3928–31.
34. Schubert ML, Peura DA. Gastroenterology 2008;134: 1842–60.
35. Nayeb-Hashemi H, Kaunitz JD. Curr Opin Gastroenterol Nov 2009;25:537–43.
36. Hyde R, Taylor PM, Hundal HS. Biochem J 2003;373:1–18.
37. Alpers DH. Curr Opin Gastroenterol 2010;26:134–9.
38. Farina A, Dumonceau JM, Lescuyer P. Exp Rev Proteom 2009;6:285–301.
39. Williams JA. Curr Opin Gastroenterol 2010;26:478–83.
40. Owyang CW, John A. Pancreatic secretion. In: Yamada T, Alpers DH, Kalloo AN et al, eds. Textbook of Gastroenterology. 5th ed. Oxford: Wiley-Blackwell, 2009:368–90.
41. Vona-Davis L, McFadden DW. Peptides 2007;28:334–8.
42. Morisset J. Pancreas 2008;37:1–12.
43. Parker HE, Reimann F, Gribble FM. Exp Rev Mol Med 2010;12:236–42.

information than thresholds about genotype-phenotype-diet-health connections (18). With good stimulus control, adding intensity to odor identification tasks tests for dysfunction and acuity. Intensity scales should be generalized to all sensations (not just chemosensations) or, for hedonic assessment, all pleasurable and unpleasurable activities. Participants should rate intensity of chemosensations relative to sensory modalities of comparison in a practice session to determine if they are able to correctly order the comparison series (e.g., weakest to brightest light). Experimenters can use the comparison intensity ratings to normalize the chemosensory ratings (19) or to covary in statistical analyses (20). The National Institutes of Health (NIH) Toolbox project has an odor identification task and taste intensity test to screen for smell and taste function.

TASTE

Any chemical that is soluble in the oral cavity watery medium (saliva, mucus) can stimulate taste—perceptual qualities of sweet, salty, sour, bitter, and umami (meaty/savory) via activating taste receptor cells. In general, sugars, alcohols, and some peptides are sweet; salts are salty; organic/inorganic acids are sour; many plant alkaloids, terpenoids, and flavonoids, and some salts and peptides are bitter; and certain amino acids are meaty/savory. Pleasure responses to sweetness and disliking for bitterness (and probably strong sour and umami) are present at birth (21) and not learned (22). Response to saltiness develops during the first year of life (23).

Within taste buds, taste receptor cells are discrete ovoid structures comprised of 50 to 150 cells arising from the epithelium, including basal cells (source of new taste cells) and elongated cells, with microvilli that extend through a pore into the oral cavity. Taste buds are found on the soft palate, pharynx, larynx, and epiglottis and within gustatory papillae on the tongue. After chemical activation and depolarization of receptor cells, afferent taste fibers within branches of three cranial nerves (CNs) transmit taste signals to the rostral nucleus of the solitary tract (gustatory NST), which also is involved in control of digestive, cardiovascular, and respiratory systems. The chorda tympani nerve (CTN), CN VII, innervates fungiform papillae on the tongue tip (Fig. 43.3). Foliate papillae on the posterior lateral tongue are innervated by the CTN (anterior papillae) and lingual nerve (CN IX, poster foliate papillae). The lingual nerve (CN IX) innervates circumvallate papillae (posterior tongue in a rearward facing V). The superficial petrosal nerve (CN VII) innervates soft palate taste buds, and the vagal nerve superior branch (CN X) innervates the epiglottis. All taste qualities are perceivable on all areas of CN innervation unless there is taste damage to a single CN (see later), making the "taste map"concept incorrect. Afferent taste fibers ending in the nucleus of the solitary tract synapse into second order neurons to the ventrobasal thalamus, then to the gustatory cortex, orbitofrontal cortex, amygdala, and lateral hypothalamus (24).

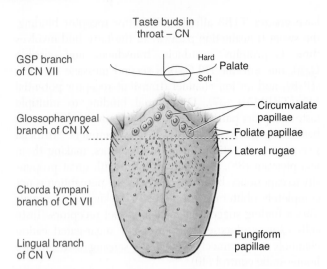

Fig. 43.3. Drawing showing cranial taste and trigeminal innervation of the tongue and throat as well as the taste papillae on the tongue. *CN*, cranial nerve.

Glutamate, an excitatory neurotransmitter, modulates information traveling from peripheral taste receptors to the brain; others likely regulate information carried from the brain to the peripheral taste system (25).

The density of fungiform papillae and their taste buds varies across individuals (26) and corresponds to taste intensity (18, 27–31). Conventional scaling (e.g., 9-point category scale) fails to show papillae density and taste intensity correlations (16), supporting that these scales do not capture differences in taste intensity (32). Five prototypical taste qualities are reviewed in the following subsections. Some evidence suggests metallic as a sixth taste. Humans can sense fatty acids in the oral cavity, but there is no unique taste percept to accompany fatty acid sensing.

Sweet

Various chemicals stimulate a singular perceptual experience that is qualitatively similar—low molecular weight, carbohydrate sweeteners, polyols, inorganic salts, and more than 25 different classes of synthetic noncaloric sweeteners (33). Multiple lines of psychophysical evidence exist for multiple sweet transduction mechanisms (34), including lack of cross-adaptation (sweeteners sharing similar binding would cross-adapt), inability to block sweetness of all sweeteners, and that sweetener combinations can produce greater than expected sweetness (i.e., synergy).

The primary sweet taste receptor, a heterodimer of two seven-transmembrane domain proteins, T1R2 and T1R3 (T1R2/T1R3) (35), has three or more sweet chemical binding sites. Humans carry three *TAS1R* taste receptor genes in a single cluster on chromosome 1. These proteins are part of class C GPCRs, which have large N-terminal Venus flytrap–like domains. Some sweeteners bind to the subunit T1R2 (e.g., aspartame, neotame), others to T1R3 (cyclamate). Sugars and sucralose bind to either but have greater T1R3 affinity (36). After receptor binding, the sweet transduction pathway in the taste bud involves three G proteins (gustducin, transducin, and possible $G_{i[2]}$), one enzyme ($PLC_{\beta 2}$), a second message receptor (IP_3R), and an ion channel (transient receptor potential M5 [TRPM5]) (37). Differential binding to multiple taste receptors partially explains flavor profile differences between sugar-based and artificial sweeteners. Artificial sweeteners also stimulate bitter receptors, making them less pleasant (38), especially to those with great propensity to experience bitterness. Sweet taste perception is not completely obliterated in T1R2/T1R3 knockout animals (39), a finding suggesting ancillary sweet receptors. Taste cells express glucose transporters or sugar-gated cation channels and connect sweet taste sensing with glucose homeostatic control (40).

Bitter

Multiple mechanisms and receptors respond to many chemicals with diverse structures that are bitter (33). The GPCRs for bitter taste are T2Rs (41, 42), with a family of approximately 25 membrane receptor genes (TAS2Rs) (43). Twenty-three are on 2 extended clusters on chromosomes 7q34–35 and 12p13.31–13.2, 1 is on chromosome 5p15.31, and another on 7q31.32. Bitter receptor genes are expressed in papillae in the oral cavity and extraorally in lung tissue, to respond to noxious compounds (44).

Most bitters likely stimulate multiple bitter receptors (i.e., broadly tuned). Although 70% of phenylthiocarbamide (PTC)/propylthiouracil (PROP) bitterness is mediated by TAS2R38 (18, 45), other receptors likely respond to these unique compounds. The bitter taste receptor structure is complex, with diverse binding sites. Bitter taste transduction involves a cascade of four intracellular signaling proteins, including the subunit α-gustducin, G-protein subunit G_{g13}, enzyme phospholipase $C_{\beta 2}$, IP_3 receptor type III, and TRPM5 ion channel (46, 47). Chemicals stimulate bitter taste via receptors or signaling proteins.

The bitter genes show high degrees of allelic variation. Evolutionary adaption to local plant environments may account for which alleles are favored (48). As natural toxins are often bitter, redundancy in bitter perception is evolutionarily advantageous. Feeney et al (49) reviewed the known *TAS2R2* single nucleotide polymorphisms (SNPs). Additionally, multiple SNPs for bitter receptors or salivary proline–rich proteins on chromosome 12 explained little variability in quinine bitterness (50); quinine is a promiscuous ligand, binding to at least nine different receptors, thus making it ideal for assessing taste function. Some coffee bitterness is explained by a haploblock across TAS2R3, TAS2R4, and TAS2R5; grapefruit juice bitterness and liking by TAS2R19 and possibly TAS2R60 (51). In vitro research suggests that hTAS2R39 responds to bitter tea catechins (52). Allelic variation in TAS2R31 and TAS2R44 explains differential response to saccharin and acesulfame-potassium (K).

Salty

Primarily added to foods as sodium chloride (NaCl), salt is important for saltiness, bitter blocking, flavor enhancement, and functional purposes (e.g., preservative). Sodium appetite homeostatically controls animals' sodium intake. In humans, early dietary experiences influence salt preference, including exposure to sodium-rich or sodium-depleted conditions during development (53). Children of mothers who experienced dehydration during pregnancy report greater salt preference during infancy (54) and adulthood (55). Females and males differ in affinity for salt (56), possibly because of sex hormones, as shown in pregnancy, when increasing salt preference is associated with the need to expand blood volume (57). Despite these examples, love of salt in humans is not really controlled by sodium appetite (55).

For human salt taste, some receptors are selective epithelial amiloride-sensitive sodium channels (ENaCs) (58). Sodium cations (Na^+) flux passively from the oral cavity to taste receptor cells through ENaCs. Na^+/K-adenosine triphosphatase (Na^+/K^+-ATPase) then pumps Na^+ back across the cell. The vanilloid receptor-1 (TRP cation channel, subfamily V, member 1 [TRPV1]) is a likely cation-nonspecific salt receptor (59). Salt evokes different qualities depending on concentration—weak concentrations taste sweet, higher concentrations are salty, and the highest are irritating (60).

Sour

Acids elicit sour taste by stimulating acid-seeking cells within taste buds and, if strong enough, elicit rejection. Specific receptors and transduction mechanisms for sour taste remain controversial, with several candidate receptors (61) or channels in which the hydrogen (H^+) from strong acids enter taste cells through ion channels (similar to NaCl), reducing intracellular pH. Weak acids pass through lipid soluble membranes. The pH reduction initiates a series of transduction and neural responses to sour stimuli (62).

Umami

Many classify umami, the savory flavor of monosodium glutamate (MSG), as the fifth basic taste. Free glutamates and Na^+ are found naturally in protein-rich foods and vegetables such as tomatoes. Initially, MSG was marketed as a flavor enhancer, adding mouth feel and flavor. Similar to sweet taste, there are multiple umami receptors (63)—a metabotropic glutamate receptor (taste-mGluR4) (64) and heterodimer of two seven-transmembrane domain proteins, T1R1 and T1R3 (35). The human umami receptor, a T1R1/T1R3 heterodimer, responds to glutamate, aspartate, and L-2-amino-4-phosphonobutyrate, with signal potentiation by purinic ribonucleotides inosine-5′-monophosphate and guanosine-5′-monophosphate (35). The mGluR4 may respond best to MSG threshold levels and T1R1/T1R3 best to concentrated MSG (65).

SNPs in TAS1R1 are associated with variation in umami sensitivity (49). There is in vitro functional variation in ability to bind MSG with amino acid substitutions in TAS1R1 and TAS1R3 receptor genes (66).

SMELL

Odors must be volatile, hydrophobic, single, or complex chemicals with relatively low molecular weight. The sense of smell, a dual sensory process, comprises transport of odors orthonasally via the nostrils and retronasally via the nasopharynx to olfactory receptors in the olfactory epithelium (Fig. 43.4). Brain activation differs with route of delivery (67). Hedonic responses to odors are not innate, but rather are learned through positive (e.g., pairing odors with energy, repetitive exposure) and negative (e.g., flavor aversions) conditioning.

The olfactory epithelium, the transduction site, sits behind the bridge of the nose, in the dorsal nasal cavity near the septum, and from superior to anterior middle turbinate. Orthonasal olfaction occurs passively with breathing—we may not think of eating until breathing in food smells. Sniffing increases the quantity and quality of odors reaching the olfactory receptors and stimulates neural activity throughout the olfactory system (68). Retronasal

olfaction is an active process in which the mouth, tongue, and swallowing movements work in synchrony to release and warm the volatiles and create a pressure differential that pumps them up through the oropharynx and nasopharynx to the olfactory epithelium (69). Food volatiles are integrated with taste and somatosensory sensations into a unitary percept in the orbitofrontal cortex (70) (see Fig. 43.4).

Olfactory receptor cells are bipolar neurons (giving rise to a dendrite on one side, an axon on the other) associated in the olfactory epithelium with supporting (mucus producing) and basal (for generating new neurons) cells. By diffusion and active transport via binding proteins, odors cross the mucus layer before binding with transmembrane GPCRs on long cilia of olfactory receptor neurons, dendritic side. Each olfactory receptor expresses 1 or 2 of the approximately 1000 different receptor types in most mammals (4). Humans, however, possess fewer than 400 functional olfactory receptor genes (71). The potential for coding odor quality is great, given the belief that each receptor binds several active chemical groups on different odor molecules (72). Diversity of receptor families implies diversity of responses to complex odors (73). The myth that humans distinguish 10,000 odors has no scientific basis (74). The active odor compounds in foods number

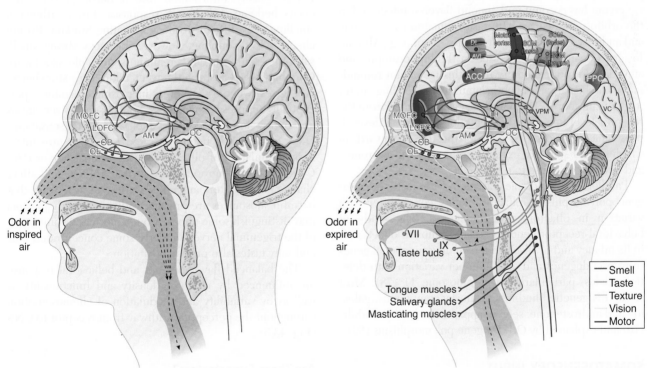

A   **B**

Fig. 43.4. A. Brain systems involved in smell perception during orthonasal olfaction (sniffing in). **B.** Brain systems involved in smell perception during retronasal olfaction (breathing out), with food in the oral cavity. Air flows indicated by *dashed and dotted lines; dotted lines* indicate air carrying odor molecules. *ACC,* accumbens; *AM,* amygdala; *AVI,* anterior ventral insular cortex; *DI,* dorsal insular cortex; *LH,* lateral hypothalamus; *LOFC,* lateral orbitofrontal cortex; *MOFC,* medial orbitofrontal cortex; *NST,* nucleus of the solitary tract; *OB,* olfactory bulb; *OC,* olfactory cortex; *OE,* olfactory epithelium; *PPC,* posterior parietal cortex; *SOM,* somatosensory cortex; *V, VII, IX, X,* cranial nerves; *VC,* primary visual cortex; *VPM,* ventral posteromedial thalamic nucleus. (Reprinted with permission from Shepherd G. Smell images and the flavour system in the human brain. Nature 2006;444:316–21.)

less than 1000 (http://www.flavornet.org), and individual ability to differentiate odors number in the hundreds (75).

Odor-receptor binding initiates the transduction cascade—activation of Gαolf, then adenylyl cyclase activation, and catalysis of cyclic adenosine 3′,5′-monophosphate (cAMP). A single CN (CN I) carries olfactory messages from the peripheral nervous system to the CNS. cAMP depolarizes the olfactory neuron; the action potential is carried by an unmyelinated axon through the cribriform plate of the ethmoid bone, where the axon synapses on second-order neurons located in olfactory bulb glomeruli (76). Differential activation of olfactory receptors produces spatially and temporally patterned activity across the glomeruli to form a unique percept, an odor image, similar to patterning in the visual system (77). Olfactory bulb microcircuits further enhance and sharpen odor images. Olfactory dysfunction occurs with loss of functional olfactory receptors, damage to olfactory neuron axons as they pass through the cribriform plate, and olfactory bulb reduction (68). Dysfunction is severe if the anatomic structures fail to regenerate. Odor quality is distorted if regeneration is incorrect.

The odor image is further modified with travel to the olfactory cortex, which refines, stores, and coordinates this image with complex behavioral responses. Through two more synapses, odor images are compared against templates of past experiences in the piriform cortex (e.g., this ice cream has coconut and almond flavors); integrated in the orbitofrontal cortex with taste, somatosensory, visual, and auditory sensations into a flavor percept (e.g., Almond Joy Ice Cream); and processed in the hippocampus and amygdala for odor memory (e.g., this ice cream reminds me of the beach) and hypothalamus as the feeding center (e.g., I want more). The odor image is modulated from the receptor level upward, in which odor adaptation desensitizes olfactory receptors, or from the top downward, in which hunger state, for example, influences the awareness and hedonic response to odors (77).

Parallel to phenotypic variation with taste receptor gene polymorphisms, olfactory acuity could differ with variation in olfactory receptor genes. The study of behavioral-receptor genotype relationships in olfaction is in its infancy and involves understanding functional genes from pseudogenes and copy-number variation with deletion alleles, particularly on chromosome 11 (78). Most studied is genetic blindness to musky compounds, galoxide and androstenone, seen in approximately 6% of adults (79) and explained by *OR7D4* gene polymorphisms (80).

SOMATOSENSORY INPUT

Touch, temperature, and chemesthesis are terms for somatosensation. Mechanoreceptors mediate touch and texture (e.g., particle size, mouthfeel, creaminess) by stimulating touch afferents in the trigeminal nerve, including those within fungiform papillae (81). On the posterior tongue, the glossopharyngeal nerve carries sensory fibers

for pain and temperature. Astringency is a dry, rough feeling caused when acids and polyphenols hinder salivary protein lubrication in the oral cavity. Thermoreceptors respond to food temperature. Noxious temperatures and irritants stimulate ion channels of the TRP family (82). Temperatures greater than 42°C, capsaicin (chili pepper), ethanol, and piperine (black pepper) stimulate TRPV1 (82). TRPM8 responds to cold (<25°C) and menthol or mint cooling. Because chemosensory irritation is polymodal and occurs via neurons that encode pain, heating or cooling, the term *chemesthesis* was created to describe chemical activation of somatosensation (83).

Individuals experience diminished touch sensations (numbness) and response to chemical irritants (desensitization). Chemical desensitization occurs through capsaicin application and removal (84), thus offering analgesia for peripheral oral pain (85). Individuals also perceive oral pain phantoms (e.g., burning mouth syndrome), described later.

INTEGRATION OF SMELL, TASTE, AND SOMATOSENSATION

In 1825, Brillat-Savarin wrote, "smell and taste are in fact but a single composite sense, whose laboratory is the mouth and its chimney the nose." The CNS integrates sensory information into a flavor percept that elicits hedonic and dietary responses. From orthonasal smelling, it is difficult to imagine eating Stinking Bishop cheese. Oral sampling, however, balances strong smell, salt-bitter-sour taste, and creaminess into a pleasant flavor. Coupling sweet taste with sweet odor (e.g., strawberry) synergizes sweetness, whereas increasing creaminess perceptually suppresses sweetness. Somatosensory sensations are tightly integrated with smell and taste sensations. Odor compounds, if concentrated enough, cause intranasal stimulation of olfactory and trigeminal nerves (86). Concentrated or noxious odors irritate the eye and affect change in respiratory and circulatory systems to warn that harmful substances are present. Individuals with anosmia may distinguish some odors through intranasal stimulation of the trigeminal nerve. Similarly, some concentrated sour and salty tastes also produce irritation.

The balanced flavor percept and behavioral response are influenced by receptor density and functionality as well as by variability and modulation of chemosensation throughout the perceptual pathway from receptor to CNS (Fig. 43.5).

Are There Supertasters?

Observations of individual variation in taste date to the nineteenth century (2). In the 1930s, Fox reported individual variation in ability to taste PTC bitterness (87), which was attributed to a genetic trait (88). (PROP is preferred as a safer and more pure stimulus.) Variation in PTC/PROP detection threshold has been studied

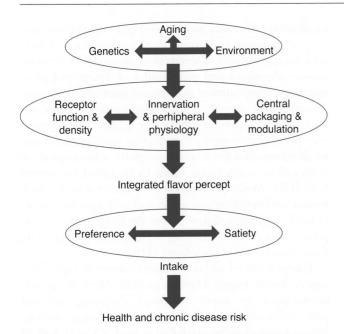

Fig. 43.5. Hypothesized pathway of associations among factors that influence variation in chemosensation to influence flavor perception, dietary behaviors, intake, and health outcomes.

hundreds of times with thousands of participants (89). In the 1960s, Fischer et al (3) connected quinine and PROP sensitivity to dietary preferences, smoking, and body weight, an observation suggesting that these bitter compounds captured broader differences in oral sensation.

Bartoshuk, who first used the supertaster label in print in 1991 (90), noticed that nontasters had a homogeneous response to PROP. Tasters were much more variable, including supertasters, who tasted PROP as intensely bitter. Suprathreshold identifies PROP supertasters (27), not threshold (91), originally by the ratio of perceived intensity of PROP to NaCl (27). Subsequent work indicated that supertasters tasted NaCl and PROP as more intense (56, 92). Thus, differential response to PROP bitterness reflected more than ability to sense the unique N-C=S moiety of PROP/PTC. Supertasters reported greater intensities from other basic tastes, retronasal odors, and somatosensory stimuli like irritation and texture (49, 81, 93, 94). Those who perceive more intense tastes and oral sensations, including PROP, have higher papillae density, unless damage to the taste system exists (16). Differential level of sensory input explains fundamental differences in cortical processing of taste (95). PROP tasting covaries with a gustin gene polymorphism (96). Nontasters have reduced salivary gustin levels. Future research will assess whether differences in salivary gustin levels explain orosensory differences between nontasters and supertasters based on taste bud density.

Supertasters are usually defined by PROP bitterness alone or PROP/NaCl ratio. (The ratio underestimates nontaster–supertaster differences; those who report both tastes as low or high are mathematically equated.) Because oral sensations are important to dietary behaviors and dietary

behaviors to health, could PROP bitterness or other chemosensations serve as biomarkers for diet-related chronic diseases (93)? PROP bitterness does not need to define supertasting (18, 97, 98). Other definitions have (96, 99, 100) and will be identified and tested for the ability to explain differences in dietary behaviors and health.

CHEMOSENSORY CHANGES WITH AGING AND ENVIRONMENTAL INSULTS

Genetic chemosensory predispositions are modified across life with maturation and exposure to pathogens and the environment. Females generally outperform males in taste and smell testing (101). Sex differences likely do not result from different allelic frequencies but from interactions among genotype, development, and the environment, as seen with *TAS2R38* (102). Relationships between sex hormones and chemosensory function are complex (81, 101). These senses may be heightened in women during childbearing age to ensure healthy pregnancies. Bitter perception rises across pregnancy to its first trimester peak and falls to its third trimester nadir (57). Aging is associated with chemosensory change with exposures to pathogens, chronic conditions, and environmental insults. Olfactory dysfunction, especially retronasal dysfunction, is more common than taste dysfunction.

Total taste loss (ageusia) is rare (103), and most "taste" disturbances are olfactory. Alteration from taste damage to a single CN is more common. Whole mouth tasting is preserved because of redundancy in the taste system. As discussed later, change in input from a single taste nerve may modify the integrated flavor percept associated with differences in food preference and dietary behaviors.

Most studied is taste alteration from the CTN, which changes the balance of taste, oral somatosensory, and retronasal olfactory input. One nineteenth-century example comes from Brillat-Savarin. As punishment, a prisoner had his anterior tongue cut off; after recovering, however, the prisoner did not complain of taste loss, but of intense, painful sensations from sour or bitter. The punishment eliminated CTN input (CN VII) to the CNS and released inhibition of inputs from other taste (CN IX and X) and trigeminal (CN V) nerves to maintain whole mouth taste and heighten pain from concentrated tastes (104).

Middle ear surgical procedures can change orosensation via CTN damage. In 1965, Bull (105) reported that after recovery from these operations, two of three patients complained of taste alterations, including inability to differentiate coffee from tea; foods such as bread were "doughy," and chocolate was "greasy." These complaints represent changes in the integrated flavor percept. CTN taste damage can occur with acoustic neuroma surgery (106), head trauma, upper respiratory tract infections, and middle ear infections. Experimental CTN anesthesia provides insight to clinical observations. Anesthesia abolishes anterior tongue taste while intensifying taste (especially bitterness) on the posterior tongue (107, 108), thus diminishing retronasal intensity and suggesting a mechanism for dysgeusia (107, 108) and oral pain phantoms. Burning mouth syndrome is associated with CTN taste damage, particularly in those with the most fungiform papillae (109). CTN depression of taste can heighten somatosensory sensations such as creaminess because papilla density and their trigeminal innervation are retained (13).

Olfactory functioning can be depressed (hyposmia) or absent (anosmia) for some (specific anosmia) or all odors (total anosmia) and altered in quality (parosmia). Age-related olfactory dysfunction is more common than whole mouth taste dysfunction, because olfactory information is carried by one CN versus three for taste. Individuals complain of taste loss. Oral sensory integration makes it difficult to distinguish taste from smell dysfunction. Careful questions and testing can characterize the type of chemosensory dysfunction (110).

Olfactory dysfunction results from alterations in peripheral and/or central processes (111). From more than 2400 residents (53 to 94 years old) of Beaver Dam, Wisconsin (112), olfactory dysfunction prevalence was 24.5%, which increased with age (62% greater than age 80), was greater in men and those reporting exposures to olfactory insults (see later). Asking individuals to self-report olfactory dysfunction underestimates the problem (113), especially among older adults (112). Olfactory and taste testing in future National Health and Nutrition Examination Surveys will provide nationally representative prevalence estimates of these disorders.

Upper respiratory tract infections, head trauma, inflammatory diseases (e.g., chronic nasal or sinus disease, allergic rhinitis) and neurodegenerative diseases (e.g., Alzheimer disease, Parkinson disease, Huntington disease, Down syndrome) (114) are the top causes of olfactory dysfunction in persons without major systemic diseases (115). These diseases diminish olfaction by (a) reducing odor transport to receptors, (b) damaging receptors that receive and transduce olfactory messages, and (c) damaging peripheral or central neurophysiologic systems. Direct exposure to toxins and infectious agents can damage olfactory receptor neurons. Head trauma can sever olfactory neurons passing through the ethmoid bone. Olfactory neurons can regenerate and produce replacement neurons, usually within 1 year after insult (116). Spontaneous improvement has been recorded in up to half of those seeking evaluation for olfactory dysfunction, greater recovery in those of younger age and less severe disturbance (117). Impaired oral health can decrease retronasal perception even if the olfactory system is intact (e.g., poorly fitting dentures, Sjögren syndrome).

Systemic diseases such as liver disease, kidney disease, diabetes mellitus, and diseases that influence mucus secretions (e.g., cystic fibrosis) can alter chemosensory function, with impairment related to the disease severity and complications, buildup of toxic metabolites (118), impaired nutritional status, and medication side effects (119). Some medication effects are pronounced and well documented (e.g., angiotensin-converting enzyme inhibitors); others are less clear because of inconsistent assessment of chemosensory alterations and complexities of dosing, polypharmacy, and drug–nutrient and disease interactions. Cancer therapies can directly impair chemosensory processes thus hindering stimulus transport (e.g., diminished mucus secretions) and changing transduction mechanisms. Some medications enter the mouth through the saliva to produce dysgeusia or reach blood levels to be tasted via venous taste (119). Medications can condition aversions in which nausea and vomiting are associated with specific flavors of food eaten immediately before the illness. Attention to patient reports and changing medications may alleviate these chemosensory complaints (119).

Except for head and neck cancer, cancer therapies (not cancer itself) impair chemosensation. Most frequently documented are mouth blindness, dysgeusia, and oral pain, presumably secondary to peripheral damage to taste nerves, intensifying orosensation in the CNS, as described earlier (120). Clinicians can improve dietary intake and quality of life by providing practical advice to patients with cancer who have chemosensory complaints (121).

Treatments for chemosensory disorders are sparse. Nasal or sinus disease is one of the few treatable causes of olfactory dysfunction. Treatment includes controlling the cause (e.g., allergens, nasal infections) and level of inflammation (e.g., systemic or topical corticosteroids) (122) (surgical interventions for severe sinusitis and nasal polyposis) (123). Experimental treatments targeting broad etiologic categories of chemosensory disorders may hold future promise (124).

Zinc requires special mention. Zinc supplementation fails to correct smell and taste dysfunction in normally nourished adults (125), and it is likely ineffective for older adults (126), unless they have zinc deficiency (127). Zinc supplementation may improve taste perception with zinc deficiency of chronic diseases (128, 129) and after radiation therapy for head and neck cancer (130). Zinc supplementation for olfactory functioning is questionable and potentially dangerous. Specifically, intranasal zinc gluconate, an over-the-counter alternative therapy for common cold prevention and treatment, causes hyposmia and anosmia, according to clinical, biologic, and experimental data (131).

CHEMOSENSORY VARIATION, NUTRITION, AND HEALTH

Figure 43.5 summarizes hypothesized associations among the integrated flavor percept, dietary intake, and health.

Food sensations stimulate physiologic responses before eating and through the mouth (cephalic phase responses), potentially to regulate food intake (132). For example, eating slowly decreases energy intake (133), possibly by promoting full flavor sensation, particularly retronasal olfaction, and satiating on the sensory signal to eat less.

Interactions between food sensations and intake are operationalized in the theory of sensory-specific satiety (SSS)—how liking of flavors of eaten food decreases relative to foods unconsumed (134). For example, there is desire to eat dessert even when full because of limited sweet satiation during the meal. Buffets promote overeating because of difficulty satiating on the diverse sensations, and monotonous diets limit flavor diversity to promote less intake (135). Chemosensory variation could influence SSS-intake relationships via differences in intensity, complexity, and preference for sensory signals (132, 136). SSS differences were not observed between anosmic and normosmic individuals (137), although smell was assessed orthonasally, a finding that may not reflect flavor messages relevant to eating (138). Taste receptors throughout the gastrointestinal tract are nutrient sensors to regulate release of gut neuropeptides that regulate hunger and satiety (139). Most research in this area involves animal models, but it certainly bears watching in the future (140).

The rest of this section reviews associations between orosensory variation and food preference, dietary behaviors, and chronic disease risk. The focus is adults—it is exceedingly difficult to scale chemosensation directly in children. Although early studies had inconsistent findings, evidence for these associations has grown through methodologic advances in characterizing chemosensory and hedonic experiences as well as orosensory phenotypes and genotypes. Implications of genetic variation in olfactory receptors on olfactory acuity, diet, and health are largely unknown. A family-based genome-wide analysis found some increased odds of early onset, extreme obesity in copy number variants on chromosome 11q11, a region of three olfactory receptor genes (OR4P4, OR4S2, and OR4C6), and many pseudogenes (141). Nutritional implications of age-related changes in olfaction and orosensation are reviewed elsewhere (110, 142).

Dietary Bitters

Many important phytonutrients are bitter, and ingestion decreases chronic disease risk (143). Most evidence associates PROP phenotype or genotype with vegetable consumption, initially focused on N-C=S vegetables, particularly Brassicaceae (94). PROP tasters by phenotype or genotype report these vegetables as more bitter (144) and consume them less frequently (145). Those who taste PROP as more bitter report sampled vegetables as more bitter, less sweet, and having a stronger retronasal flavor, which decreases preference for sampled vegetables and generalizes to less consumption of all vegetables (146). Individuals with a greater propensity to experience bitterness and limited prenatal and postnatal exposure to vegetable flavors (147) could experience the most negative vegetable sensations, which could generalize to overall vegetable disliking. Thus, taste genotype or phenotype could be a biomarker for habitual vegetable consumption

through vegetable preference and good candidates for Mendelian randomization studies of cancer and other health outcomes (145). Preliminary data support a link between PROP bitterness and colon cancer risk (148).

Chronic otitis media exposure in children (149) and CTN bitter taste impairment in adults (146) are associated with lower vegetable preference or intake. Attention to modifying vegetable tastes and balancing bitterness and sweetness could hold promise in conditioning preferences for sour- or bitter-tasting foods in children (150), especially supertaster children.

Explaining complex behavior with SNPs is problematic as a result of disconnects between phenotype and genotype (18, 151). Individuals vary in multiple genes or genetic–environmental influences that can mask single SNP, diet, and health associations. For example, two population-based studies did not find TAS2R38 and vegetable intake associations (152, 153). Another reported that fungiform papillae number exerts independent influences from TAS2R38 on vegetable intake (154). The genotype effect was attenuated in nontasters with fewer papillae compared with supertasters with more papillae (Fig. 43.6).

Taste genetics likely interact with environmental and metabolic factors to influence behaviors toward alcoholic beverages (155) and nicotine (156). Heightened bitter perception may confer protection against developing or maintaining high use. PROP supertasters taste alcoholic beverages as most bitter and least sweet, and they consume them least frequently (157). PROP/PTC nontasters are more likely to be chronic smokers (158, 159). TAS2R38 has been associated with alcohol intake or dependence (51, 160, 161) and nicotine dependence (162). TAS2R16 SNPs also have been associated with alcohol intake (51) and dependence (163).

Sweet Preference

Humans vary in perception of intensity of sweetness from sucrose (20), up to 33% attributable to heritability (164), as well as sweeteners such as aspartame (38). Variation in TAS1R2 has not been associated with differences in sweet sensitivity (165). Rare variants of SNPs in a noncoding region upstream from TAS1R3 explained variability in sucrose sensitivity, possibly influencing T1R3 transcription and functioning (165). PROP supertasters report greater sweetness from sucrose in water and milks that vary in fat (20).

The liking for sweet is innate and pronounced in childhood, possibly cueing an energy source to sustain growth. High sweetness exposure may elevate sweet preference later in life (22). What varies is preferred level of sweetness; 10% sucrose is optimal for some and 20% for others (166). Twin studies show a significant heritable component to sweet preference (164, 167). TAS1R2 has the highest genetic diversity, followed by TAS1R1 and TAS1R3 (168). Sweet liking, not sweetness, varies with TAS1R3

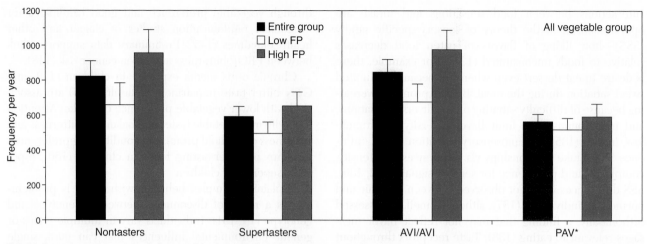

Fig. 43.6. Yearly consumption of all vegetables from the food frequency questionnaire (Mean ± SEM) among groups defined by phenotype (**left graph,** 3.2 mM propylthiouracil [PROP] bitterness) and genotype (**right graph,** *TAS2R38* receptor) for all subjects within that group *(black bar),* and for that group subdivided on the basis of fungiform papillae number median split, where *white bars* are below and *hatched bars* are above the median, respectively. Within nontasters (**left graph, left panel**) and AVI (alanine, valine, isoleucine) homozygotes (**right graph, left panel**), comparing intake across the low and high papillae groups revealed significant differences ($p < .05$); within the supertaster phenotype (**left graph, right panel**), the low/high papilla comparison was a trend ($p < .1$). For all subjects irrespective of papillae number *(black bars),* nontasters and AVI homozygotes ate vegetables more frequently ($p < .05$) than supertasters or PAV* (proline, alanine, valine), respectively. (Reprinted with permission from Duffy VB, Hayes JE, Davidson AC et al. Vegetable intake in college-aged adults is explained by oral sensory phenotypes and TAS2R38 genotype. Chemosens Percept 2010;3:137.)

polymorphisms (169). Variation in *TAS1R2* were associated with sugar consumption in two populations of overweight and obese individuals (170) and polymorphisms of three TAS2R9 SNPs, not TASR1 or TASR3, were associated with glucose homeostasis mechanisms (171).

Other taste genotypes and phenotypes likely interact with environmental influences to explain sweet preference. Bitterness of PROP or *TAS2R38* genotype is associated with sweet liking in children (94, 172). When controlling for weight and dietary restraint, PROP supertasters are more likely to be sweet dislikers (liking falls with growing sugar level) than likers (liking increases with growing sugar level) (31). The disliking is related to heightened sweetness related to higher fungiform papilla numbers (31, 169). Sweet or fat preference differs across individuals classified by fungiform papilla number and by PROP versus quinine bitterness (166). The impact of taste genetics on habitual sweet intake was suggested in a population-based study of children and adults, in which *TASR38* nontasters had a higher dental caries risk than did homozygous tasters (173). Future studies should carefully characterize taste phenotype or genotype and sweet preferences (13).

Salt and Sour Preference

Most sodium in the food supply is added during processing, and this may habituate us to higher levels. Some foods are consumed for saltiness (e.g., snacks). For others, salt is a flavor enhancer (e.g., cheese). Saltiness does not drive preference, except when it is missing, unpleasant sensations (e.g., bitterness) are heightened (174), especially

for supertasters (56). The level of added sodium varies greatly, more than twofold across regular-sodium soups. Perceived saltiness and liking for high-sodium foods vary across males and females and taste phenotype (56). NaCl levels can be reduced modestly in some foods (potato products, bread) without a negative impact on liking (9, 175), thus lowering sodium intakes and blood pressure. Savory seasonings improve palatability of low-sodium products. A total diet and behavioral approach aims to decrease blood pressure and cardiovascular risk (176). Public health experts suggest potassium chloride (KCl) as a salt substitute and to boost potassium intakes and benefit blood pressure control (176). Unfortunately, KCl is bitter, particularly to those with a propensity to taste bitterness.

Individuals vary in sour taste intensity and liking. From unpublished data in adults, 70% disliked 1-mM aqueous citric acid (ranged from weak to very strong disliking): the greater the intensity, the greater disliking. The intensity–hedonic relationship was weak among 30% who liked the solution (ranged from weak to strong liking). The citric acid solution was liked if it elicited a pure sour quality but disliked or rejected when it had bitter or irritation qualities. A twin study suggested that genetics may explain the 50% variation in citric acid intensity (177). Sour intensity and liking are associated with fruit consumption in infants (178) and children (179). Those liking intense sourness had the highest salivary flow rates to buffer the sourness (180).

Fat Preference

Texture is the primary oral sensory cue for fat, especially by fungiform papillae, which act as mechanical sensors as

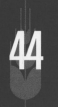

44 CONTROL OF FOOD INTAKE AND APPETITE[1]

SYED SUFYAN HUSSAIN, AKILA DE SILVA, AND STEPHEN ROBERT BLOOM

[1]**Abbreviations: 2-AG**, 2-arachidonoylglycerol; **α-MSH**, α-melanocyte-stimulating hormone; **AEA**, anandamide; **AgRP**, Agouti-related peptide; **AMP**, adenosine monophosphate; **AP**, area postrema; **ARC**, arcuate nucleus; **ATP**, adenosine triphosphate; **BDNF**, brain-derived neurotrophic factor; **CART**, cocaine- and amphetamine-regulated transcript; **CB1**, cannabinoid receptor type 1; **CCK**, cholecystokinin; **CNTF**, ciliary neurotrophic factor; **DMN**, dorsomedial nucleus; **DVC**, dorsal vagal complex; **DVN**, dorsal motor nucleus of the vagus; **GHS-R**, growth hormone secretagogue receptor; **GLP-1**, glucagon-like peptide-1; **LCFA**, long-chain fatty acids; **LepR**, leptin receptor; **LHA**, lateral hypothalamic area; **MC3R**, melanocortin receptor 3; **MC4R**, melanocortin receptor 4; **MCH**, melanin-concentrating hormone; **NPY**, neuropeptide Y; **NTS**, nucleus of the tractus solitarius; **OFC**, orbitofrontal cortex; **OXA**, orexin A; **OXB**, orexin B; **OXM**, oxyntomodulin; **PFA**, perifornical area; **POMC**, pro-piomelanocortin; **PP**, pancreatic polypeptide; **PYY**, peptide YY; **TRH**, thyrotropin-releasing hormone; **VMN**, ventromedial nucleus.

Traditionally, a distinction has been made between homeostatic and nonhomeostatic control of appetite and food intake. Homeostatic control refers to the alteration in consumption of food that follows sensing of energy balance. Following a meal, changes in circulating concentration of nutrients, in addition to activation of signaling pathways from the gut, lead to a reduction in subsequent feeding. Furthermore, adiposity signals that form long-term markers of energy balance also comprise important homeostatic controls of food intake. Appropriately matching food intake with metabolic need is achieved by the interaction of these inputs with key central neural appetite circuits.

Across species, food intake is also driven by factors other than basic physiologic or homeostatic need. Food appearance, flavor, timing and location of meals, and social, cultural, emotional, and economic influences affect food intake by nonhomeostatic mechanisms. Furthermore, nonhomeostatic control of food intake is modulated by hedonic mechanisms, reward pathways, and previous experience with food (mnemonic pathways).

Our understanding of the overall control of food intake and appetite has expanded, leading to the modern viewpoint that the distinction between homeostatic and nonhomeostatic pathways is, in fact, less rigid. Indeed, investigators recognize that nonhomeostatic pathways themselves modulate homeostatic pathways and lead to a network of hormonal and neural communication upstream of the overall outcome of feeding (Fig. 44.1).

CENTRAL CONTROLS OF FOOD INTAKE AND APPETITE

Coordination by the Hypothalamus

The hypothalamus is widely recognized as the "gate keeper" in the control of food intake and appetite. Peripheral signals of energy balance may act directly on the hypothalamus to control food intake, and this forms one important focus of current appetite research. Historically, the lateral hypothalamus was thought of as the "hunger center," and the medial hypothalamus was the "satiety center." This concept was based on lesioning experiments in animals; damage to the lateral hypothalamus produced anorexia, whereas damage to the medial hypothalamus led to hyperphagia (1). Although this view still largely holds true, it has been

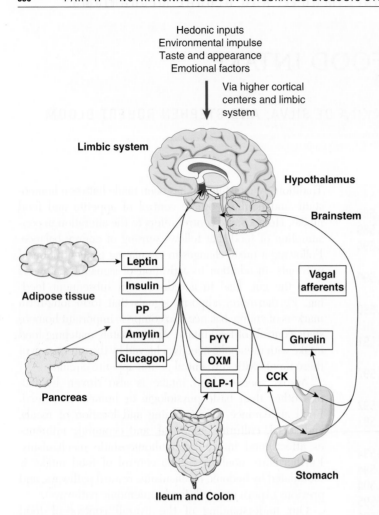

Fig. 44.1. An overview of the control of food intake and appetite. Peripheral signals are sensed and processed by the hypothalamus and brainstem. These signals are integrated with hedonic, mnemonic, emotional and environmental influences via higher cortical centers and the limbic system to generate feelings of satiety and hunger.

refined by our enhanced understanding of the role of individual nuclei within the hypothalamus and communication among them. The presence of a network of communication among the gut, pancreas, adipose tissue, brainstem, and hypothalamus to signal energy balance is also well established. Additionally, further communication exists between the hypothalamus and higher cortical centers pertaining to food memory and rewarding aspects of food, with resulting overall coordinated control of food intake.

Role of the Brainstem

The brainstem has a well-established role in the sensing of energy balance and modulation of food intake. Within the brainstem, the dorsal vagal complex (DVC) is the main organ responsible for facilitating the communication between peripheral signals of food intake and hypothalamic nuclei (2). The DVC consists of the nucleus of the tractus solitarius (NTS), the area postrema (AP), and the dorsal motor nucleus of the vagus (DVN). Vagal nerve afferents carry sensory information relaying hunger and satiety from the gut directly to the NTS. Transection of these gut sensory vagal nerve afferents results in increased meal size and duration (3). The absence of a complete blood–brain barrier in the AP also allows the brainstem to receive metabolic signals of energy balance (e.g., hormones and nutrients carried by the blood) directly.

The brainstem is then able to process these sensory inputs and relay them to the hypothalamus and higher cortical centers. In keeping with this, it is well established that neural projections are present from the brainstem to the hypothalamus (4). Efferent pathways also descend from the hypothalamus to the DVN (5). The DVN modulates efferent vagal nerve activity in the gastrointestinal tract and can alter gastric emptying, gastric motility, and pancreatic secretions. This function points to a role for the brainstem in modulating feeding-related activity as well as sensing energy balance.

Hypothalamic Nuclei Implicated in the Control of Food Intake

The arcuate nucleus (ARC) is thought to be the main hypothalamic area controlling food intake. It lies adjacent to the third ventricle and close to the median eminence, where an incomplete blood–brain barrier is thought to allow peripheral signals to gain access to the central nervous system. In mice, lesions of the ARC result in hyperphagia and obesity (6). Within the ARC, two groups of neurons are pivotal in regulating food intake. One group of neurons contains neuropeptide Y (NPY), and most of these also contain

Agouti-related peptide (AgRP). Activation of these neurons enhances food intake (i.e., these neurons are orexigenic). The second group is formed by neurons containing pro-opiomelanocortin (POMC) and cocaine- and amphetamine-regulated transcript (CART). Activation of these neurons reduces food intake (i.e., these neurons are anorexigenic).

Axons from NPY/AgRP and POMC/CART, neurons project from the ARC to other areas of the hypothalamus such as the paraventricular nucleus (PVN). Destruction of the PVN leads to hyperphagia and obesity in rats (7). In addition to the PVN, axons from the ARC also project to the ventromedial nucleus (VMN), dorsomedial nucleus (DMN), lateral hypothalamic area (LHA), and perifornical area (PFA) to modulate food intake.

Neuropeptides Implicated in the Control of Food Intake

Neuropeptide Y

NPY is the most powerful central stimulant of appetite, and most neurons expressing NPY are found within the ARC. Approximately 90% of NPY neurons coexpress AgRP. Central administration of NPY enhances food intake in rats (8). Furthermore, repeated daily injections of NPY into the hypothalamus result in chronic hyperphagia and weight gain in these animals (9). Conversely, ablation of NPY/AgRP neurons in mice leads to reduced body weight via reduced food intake (10). Of the six identified NPY receptors, the Y1 and Y5 receptors seem to mediate the orexigenic effect of NPY. Additionally, there appears to be local inhibition of anorexigenic POMC neurons in the ARC (11). NPY/AgRP neurons project within the hypothalamus from the ARC, to nuclei including the PVN, DMN, and LHA. In the PVN, direct stimulation of Y1 and Y5 receptors is thought to occur to increase food intake, in addition to inhibiting anorexigenic pathways by AgRP.

Agouti-Related Peptide

AgRP is a competitive antagonist of anorexigenic central melanocortin receptors (see later) in the PVN. Thus, AgRP increases food intake (12). A possible alternative mechanism of the orexigenic action of AgRP may involve action on orexin or opioid receptors (13).

Pro-opiomelanocortin and Melanocortins

POMC is the precursor of α-melanocyte-stimulating hormone (α-MSH). α-MSH is produced by cleavage of POMC and binds to the G-protein–coupled melanocortin receptor 4 (MC4R), which is highly represented in the hypothalamus, particularly in the PVN. α-MSH binding to the MC4R acts to reduce food intake (13). Consistent with this, mice lacking all POMC-derived peptides are hyperphagic and obese (14), as are MC4R knockout mice (15). In humans, nearly 100 different mutations of the *MC4R* gene are responsible for more than 5% of cases of morbid nonsyndromic obesity, and these individuals are hyperphagic (16). Furthermore, homozygous mutations in the *POMC* gene in humans result in early-onset obesity (17).

Diet-induced obesity in rats leads to up-regulation of POMC, followed by a reduction in food intake. This resultant anorexia is reversed by central administration of an MC4R antagonist (13). This finding highlights the role of POMC and melanocortins in responding to a state of positive energy balance by inducing anorexia. In contrast to the established role of MC4R, the role of melanocortin receptor 3 (MC3R) on food intake is less clear. Although MC3R-deficient mice show increased fat mass, administration of selective MC3R agonists appears not to alter food intake (18).

Cocaine- and Amphetamine-Regulated Transcript

CART is coexpressed by most POMC neurons in the ARC. Central intracerebroventricular administration of CART reduces food intake in rats whereas injection of CART antiserum does the opposite (19). In humans, a mutation of the *CART* gene that causes severe obesity has been described (20). The role of CART may vary in different brain regions, because CART injected directly into the ARC actually leads to an increase in food intake in fasted rats (21).

Hypothalamic Releasing Hormones

Corticotropin-releasing hormone and thyrotropin-releasing hormone (TRH) are expressed in PVN neurons. When these two hormones are administered centrally in rats, both inhibit food intake (22). TRH expression in the PVN is mediated by α-MSH and inhibited by NPY and AgRP (23), a finding consistent with the action of these peptides on food intake.

Orexins

Orexin A and B (OXA and OXB) activate G-protein–coupled receptors to increase food intake. OXA is more potent than OXB and is expressed in neurons of the DMN, PFA, and LHA, with additional projections to the NTS in the brainstem (24). In rats, central administration of an orexin antagonist inhibits feeding (25).

Melanin-Concentrating Hormone

Melanin-concentrating hormone (MCH) is an orexigenic signal expressed in neurons located in the LHA. Infusion of MCH in rats increases food intake and body weight (26). MCH knockout mice are resistant to diet-induced obesity (27). Two MCH receptors have been identified in humans whereas only one has been identified so far in rodents. MCH receptor knockout mice are resistant to diet-induced obesity (28).

Brain-Derived Neurotrophic Factor

Brain-derived neurotrophic factor (BDNF) is highly expressed in the VMN and acts via MC4R signaling to reduce food intake (29). Administration of BDNF into the lateral ventricles reduces food intake and body weight in rodents (30). Consistent with the foregoing, selective deletion of BDNF in the VMN and DMN of mice results in hyperphagia and obesity (31). ARC POMC neurons are thought to project to VMN BDNF neurons, thus activating them to lead to a reduction in food intake (29).

Ciliary Neurotrophic Factor

Ciliary neurotrophic factor (CNTF) is a cytokine expressed in several motor neuron populations. It induces an anorexigenic effect and weight loss, probably by inhibiting the expression and release of NPY in the hypothalamus (32). CNTF-mediated weight loss persists even after the cessation of treatment (33), a finding implying that it may alter the "set-point" of energy balance by inducing long-term changes in synaptic function.

The major hypothalamic nuclei and peptides implicated in the central control of food intake are shown in Figure 44.2.

Central Neurotransmitters Controlling Appetite and Food Intake

Neurotransmitters such as serotonin, norepinephrine, and dopamine act on central circuits to modulate appetite and food intake. Serotonin, produced in the dorsal raphe nucleus, reduces food intake and body weight (13). Norepinephrine, produced in the DVC and locus coeruleus, has differing effects on food intake depending on which of its receptors is stimulated; the action of norepinephrine on α_2 receptors stimulates food intake, whereas its action on α_1, β_2, and β_3 receptors reduces food intake (34).

In view of the foregoing findings, serotonin agonists (e.g., fenfluramine and dexfenfluramine) and serotonin and norepinephrine reuptake inhibitors (e.g., sibutramine) have been used as antiobesity agents. Although effective in reducing body weight, fenfluramine and dexfenfluramine have been withdrawn from the market because of serious cardiovascular side effects. Similarly, sibutramine, which was a treatment for obesity for several years, has been withdrawn because of serious cardiovascular side effects.

Dopamine appears to inhibit food intake in the ARC and LHA, whereas it has orexigenic action in the VMN (34). In addition to differing effects in different brain sites, dopamine exerts opposite effects on appetite, depending on which dopaminergic receptor subtype is stimulated. For example, the action of dopamine on D1 and D2 receptors reduces food intake, whereas stimulation of the D5 receptor is associated with reward pathways (35).

Hedonic Mechanisms and Corticolimbic Pathways Controlling Appetite and Food Intake

The word "hedonic" relates to pleasant (or unpleasant) sensations. It is apparent that visual, smell, and taste signals can override satiety signals to maintain food intake despite neutral or even positive energy balance. For example, the sweet taste of certain foods is associated with positive emotions that motivate animals to find food and continue consumption. These sensory signals are conveyed from visual, smell, and taste receptors to the NTS in the brainstem and are then relayed to corticolimbic reward centers implicated in appetite regulation. These sites include the hippocampus, amygdala, nucleus accumbens, ventral pallidum, ventral

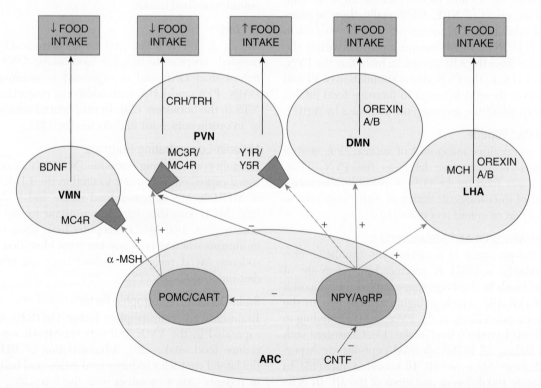

Fig. 44.2. The major hypothalamic nuclei and peptides implicated in the central control of food intake. *AgRP*, Agouti-related peptide; *α-MSH*, α-melanocyte-stimulating hormone; *ARC*, arcuate nucleus; *BDNF*, brain-derived neurotrophic factor; *CART*, cocaine- and amphetamine-regulated transcript; *CNTF*, ciliary neurotrophic factor; *CRH*, corticotropin-releasing hormone; *DMN*, dorsomedial nucleus; *LHA*, lateral hypothalamic area; *MC3R*, melanocortin receptor 3; *MC4R*, melanocortin receptor 4; *MCH*, melanin-concentrating hormone; *NPY*, neuropeptide Y; *POMC*, proopiomelanocortin; *PVN*, paraventricular nucleus; *TRH*, thyrotropin-releasing hormone; *VMN*, ventromedial nucleus.

tegmental area, and prefrontal cortex. Dopamine, serotonin, opioids, and norepinephrine have been implicated as important neurotransmitters involved in signaling within this network. The administration of an opioid μ-receptor agonist into the nucleus accumbens in fed rats elicits preferential intake of high-fat foods rather than carbohydrates (36).

Communication between reward centers and the hypothalamus (thought of as the main homeostatic controller of food intake, as discussed previously) culminates in overall coordination of food intake. Administration of an opioid μ-receptor agonist into the nucleus accumbens increases orexin neuron expression in the hypothalamus (37). Histochemical studies have also demonstrated connections between the cerebral cortex and MCH and orexin neurons in the LHA (38). Furthermore, in rats trained to associate the availability of food with the presentation of a food cup (resulting in conditioned food intake even when they are satiated), elimination of amygdala–hypothalamus connections completely abolishes this conditioned food intake (39). The preceding experiments highlight the importance of connections between homeostatic and nonhomeostatic centers controlling food intake.

Mnemonic Representations of Experience with Food

Past experience with specific foods forms an important contributor to continued consumption (if the previous experience was pleasant) or early cessation of intake (if the previous experience was unpleasant) regardless of satiety and energy balance. This phenomenon is referred to as conditioned preference or conditioned aversion, respectively. Evidence points to an important role for the orbitofrontal cortex (OFC), an area that receives converging sensory input in the nonhomeostatic control of food intake. The OFC is in contact with other cortical reward areas, such as the prefrontal, insular, perirhinal, entorhinal, and anterior cingulated cortices. Furthermore, the OFC communicates with the hippocampus and amygdala. Collectively, this group of brain

regions is thought to be important in the generation and maintenance of a working memory for food experiences (40).

Endocannabinoids

Endocannabinoids have been shown to produce a dose-dependent orexigenic effect (41). This effect is thought to occur via modulation of reward circuitry. The two main endocannabinoids in the brain are anandamide (AEA), derived from membranous phospholipids, and 2-arachidonoylglycerol (2-AG), derived from triglycerides. These substances are secreted by postsynaptic neurons and act in retrograde fashion, binding to cannabinoid receptor type 1 (CB1) receptors on presynaptic nerve terminals to inhibit the release of neurotransmitters.

CB1 receptors are colocalized with dopamine D1 and D2 receptors in the rat limbic forebrain; furthermore, dopamine receptor antagonists reduce the orexigenic effect of cannabinoid administration (42).

Endocannabinoids may also act directly on the hypothalamus to exert their orexigenic effect. In rodents, hypothalamic levels of 2-AG increase during fasting and then return to baseline after the animals are fed (43). Administration of AEA into the hypothalamic VMN results in hyperphagia that is reversible with administration of a CB1 receptor antagonist (44). Orexigenic neurons in the LHA express functional CB1 receptors (45), and stimulation of these receptors augments the OXA pathway (46) in addition to orexigenic MCH neurons (47) and NPY neurons (48).

Manipulation of the endocannabinoid system formed a therapeutic strategy in the treatment of obesity, namely, by using the CB1 receptor antagonist rimonabant. However, because of unacceptable and sometimes dangerous effects on mood, rimonabant was withdrawn from the market. The communications among peripheral inputs, the brainstem, hypothalamus, and higher brain centers in the control of appetite is shown in Figure 44.3.

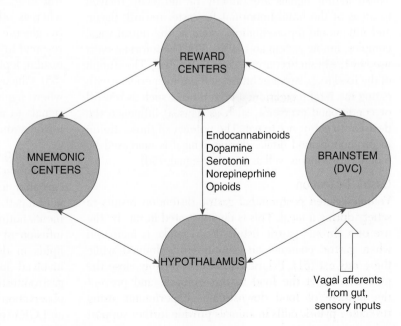

Fig. 44.3. Communication between the brainstem, hypothalamus, higher brain centers and peripheral neural inputs in the control of appetite.

PERIPHERAL CONTROLS OF FOOD INTAKE AND APPETITE

Neural, nutrient, and hormonal signals from the gastrointestinal system, endocrine organs, adipose tissue, and circulation all have essential roles in influencing food intake and appetite. These signals are triggered by mechanical and chemical effects of food on the digestive system and are also influenced by long-term energy stores, such as body fat. These peripheral signals specifically target areas of the hypothalamus and brainstem to regulate appetite by means of communicating information about the current state of energy balance. They include signals conveying a feeling of fullness (satiety signals), hunger (orexigenic signals), and pleasure or reward from the intake of food (hedonistic and positive-feedback signals). Appetite is the net result of the coordinated response to all these signals and achieves a balance between promoting efficient digestion and nutrient absorption in the gut and augmenting energy stores while food is available. These signals act in concert to control meal size and meal number, and they allow food intake, energy expenditure, and body adiposity to be homeostatically regulated (49).

Neural Signals

Orosensory and Optic Stimuli

Orosensory and optic stimuli provide the brain with sensory information regarding the nature of food. These stimuli include appearance, taste, smell, and textural stimuli. Visual information regarding the appearance of food is relayed via neural signals in the afferent optic fibers of cranial nerve I. Gustatory, olfactory, and orosensory information about food in contact with the tongue and palate is transduced into neural signals by the gustatory fibers of cranial nerves VII, IX, and X; olfactory fibers of cranial nerve I; and sensory fibers of cranial nerve V. These neural signals are directly or indirectly relayed to areas of the brain important for taste, reward, flavor, and mnemonic representations, such as the dorsal vagal complex, limbic system and OFC (50). The information is used by the brain to continue or to stop eating. The stimuli of the food (e.g., sweet or bitter) and prior experience with eating the food (conditioned preferences, such as reward or conditioned aversions, such as nausea) influence the decision to eat or not to eat. The potency of these stimuli in promoting food intake during a meal is increased by food deprivation as well as by other signals (50).

Gastric Distention

Volume-related postprandial gastric distention results in satiety during a meal. This is demonstrated in rats by the use of a chronic gastric fistula. Food intake is increased when gastric contents are continuously drained while these rats eat (51). Pyloric cuffs can reversibly close the pylorus, restrict the food to the stomach, and prevent the passage of food downstream. Experiments using reversible pyloric cuffs in animals provide further support

that gastric distention contributes to satiety during a meal (51, 52). These satiety signals arise from mechanical distention of the stomach rather than nutrient sensing (51). Mechanoreceptors in the stomach wall sense stretch, volume, and tension during a meal. This information is transmitted to the brain by afferent fibers of the vagal and spinal visceral nerves (53). Earlier gastric distention and satiety during a meal resulting from reduced stomach size forms the basis of restrictive bariatric surgical treatments (e.g., laparoscopic adjustable gastric banding) that are used in the management of severe obesity.

Nutrient Signals

Most nutrient signals exert their effects on the gastrointestinal system and induce the secretion of gastrointestinal hormones. However, changes in nutrients, such as blood glucose and lipids, are sensed by hypothalamic neurons in the brain involved in appetite regulation.

Glucose

The glucostatic theory of feeding was first proposed by Jean Mayer in 1952 (54). Although investigators have known for some time that peripheral and central glucoprivation (low glucose) can stimulate feeding (e.g., during hypoglycemia), the role of central glucosensing in affecting day-to-day food intake and the mechanisms involved in regulating this have been elucidated only more recently.

Glucose alters the firing rate of neurons in the ARC, LHA, and NTS (55). The cellular influx of glucose alters the ratio of adenosine monophosphate (AMP) to adenosine triphosphate (ATP) within the neuronal cell. This may affect ATP-dependent membrane channels that may influence neuronal depolarization, or it may alter the activity of important nutrient sensing enzymes (e.g., AMP-activated protein kinase), that have important roles in cellular processes relevant to energy homeostasis (56). Some neurons (e.g., ARC POMC neurons) are excited by glucose, whereas others (e.g., ARC NPY neurons) are inhibited by glucose (55). These glucose-sensitive neurons also respond to other hormonal and metabolic signals, such as insulin, leptin, lactate, ketone bodies, and free fatty acids (55). Glucose-sensitive neurons may represent focal points where signals converge to alter appetite and allow various signals to act in concert to influence the initiation and termination of meals.

Circulating Lipids

Circulating lipids such as long-chain fatty acids (LCFAs) can alter feeding behavior by directly activating central neural pathways (56). This was first highlighted by experiments noting a reduction in food intake after intravenous infusion of lipids (57). Further support for the role of lipids in directly activating central neuronal processes involved in appetite via mechanisms independent of gastrointestinal nutrient absorption was provided by the observation that intracerebroventricular administration of an LCFA (oleic acid) also decreased food intake (58).

The mechanisms by which neuronal cells sense alterations in circulating lipids are still under investigation. Investigators believe that key cellular processes relevant to energy homeostasis and influenced by other nutrients (e.g., glucose; see earlier) are also altered by the cellular influx of LCFAs (56). This concept may provide mechanisms for neuronal cells to integrate and respond to changes in circulating nutrients.

Gut Hormones

The gastrointestinal tract or gut is the largest endocrine organ in the body and secretes more than 30 different regulatory peptide hormones (59). These hormones influence certain important physiologic processes mainly related to digestion and absorption of nutrients, which are the primary roles of the gut. Some of these gut hormones are stimulated by gut nutrient content and interact with receptors at various points in the gut–brain axis (see Fig. 44.1) to affect short-term feelings of hunger and satiety (49). This process may indirectly control the delivery of nutrients to the gut to permit efficient digestion. These hormones are the subject of extensive research, given their potential as physiologic antiobesity therapies.

Cholecystokinin

Cholecystokinin (CCK) was the first gut hormone shown to influence food intake in animals and humans (60, 61). CCK is synthesized in the I cells of the small intestine. It is released postprandially in response to a meal to promote fat and protein digestion (62). It results in gallbladder contraction, relaxation of the sphincter of Oddi, somastostatin release, stimulation of pancreatic enzyme release, and slowed gastric emptying. Although delayed gastric emptying may augment gastric neural satiety signals via gastric mechanoreceptors, the mechanism by which CCK reduces food intake is thought to be primarily mediated via CCK1 receptors present on the afferent vagal nerve terminals (63). These afferent fibers transmit signals to the areas of the brain such as the NTS. The central melanocortin system has been implicated in mediating CCK's actions on reducing food intake (64).

Ghrelin

Ghrelin is the only known gut hormone that increases appetite. It is often referred to as the "hunger hormone." Ghrelin was first discovered as an endogenous ligand to the growth hormone secretagogue receptor (GHS-R) in the stomach. It is primarily produced by the A-cells of gastric fundus. Its other actions include increase in gastric motility and stimulation of growth hormone release. The metabolic effects of ghrelin include increased fat storage and decrease in fat use (65).

Plasma ghrelin levels rise before meals and decline after eating, thus implicating a role for ghrelin in controlling appetite. Peripheral and central administration of ghrelin potently increases food intake and body weight in rodents (62), a finding supporting its role as a hunger

hormone. These findings have been confirmed in several studies, and ghrelin is now considered as one of the most powerful physiologic orexigenic agents.

Ghrelin mediates its effects on food intake via the GHS-R. GHS-R–deficient mice are resistant to diet-induced obesity (66). The ARC NPY/AgRP neurons have been implicated in mediating ghrelin's central orexigenic effects. Ghrelin may reduce food intake by binding to the GHS-R on vagal afferent nerve terminals or in the neurons of the ARC and alter ARC NPY/AgRP neuronal activity (65).

Ghrelin levels are inversely correlated with body weight and may constitute a feedback mechanism to reduce appetite in obesity (62). Plasma ghrelin levels are also noted to increase on weight loss (62). This may be a factor resulting in poor adherence to diets and tendency to regain weight after initial weight loss.

Peptide YY

Peptide YY (PYY) is a member of PP fold family, which also includes NPY and pancreatic polypeptide. It is released by the L cells of the gastrointestinal tract and binds preferentially to the Y2 receptor (67).

PYY levels are low in the fasting state. PYY is released postprandially in proportion to the calories ingested and remains elevated for several hours (67). The release of PYY is augmented by dietary fat. PYY administration decreases food intake in rodents and humans (68, 69). PYY is one of the components of the ileal break effect, which inhibits food intake once nutrients are detected in the small intestine. PYY may reduce food intake by decreasing ARC NPY levels via the ARC Y2 receptor or via its effects on the vagus nerve (62), and it also delays gastric emptying.

Obese patients demonstrate a blunted postprandial rise in PYY that may contribute to reduced satiety and overeating (67). Gastric bypass surgery is one of the most effective treatments for obese patients. Sustained weight loss results from diminished appetite. Patients who have undergone gastric bypass demonstrate exaggerated postprandial PYY levels, and this may be an important factor in achieving prolonged weight loss (70). PYY-based antiobesity agents are currently under development.

Glucagon-like Peptide-1

Enteroendocrine L cells also synthesize preproglucagon that is processed into glucagon-like peptide-1 (GLP-1), glucagon-like peptide-2 (GLP-2), and oxyntomodulin. GLP-1 colocalizes with PYY and oxyntomodulin in the L cell. GLP-1 is released postprandially in proportion to calories ingested. It is an incretin, which results in increased glucose-dependent insulin release. It also reduces gastric emptying and gastric acid secretion and inhibits glucagon release. GLP-1 reduces food intake in animals and humans, as demonstrated by peripheral administration of GLP-1 in rodents and humans (71). Like PYY, GLP-1 is also one of the components of the ileal brake effect. Circulating GLP-1 exerts its effects on central feeding pathways via GLP-1 receptors in the hypothalamus (PVN), the brainstem, and the vagus nerve (62). Different long-acting analogs of GLP-1 are used in the treatment of type 2 diabetes and cause weight loss in this patient group. These analogs are currently undergoing clinical trials for the treatment of obesity.

Oxyntomodulin

Like GLP-1, oxyntomodulin is a product of preproglucagon and is secreted postprandially in proportion to caloric intake by the enteroendocrine L cell. It also binds to the GLP-1 receptor, although with reduced affinity (72). Not surprisingly, it has actions similar to those of GLP-1. It decreases gastric motility, has a weaker incretin effect, and reduces food intake with similar potency to GLP-1 when given peripherally to rodents and humans despite its lower receptor affinity (73, 74). Similar to PYY, oxyntomodulin levels rise after gastric bypass surgery and may be important in reducing appetite after this procedure (70).

Despite their similarities, GLP-1 and oxyntomodulin appear to have different roles in energy homeostasis. Oxyntomodulin also increases energy expenditure and may suppress ghrelin release (73, 74). Unlike GLP-1, it may act via the ARC (73). These differences may relate to different pharmacologic properties or different tissue specific actions. The therapeutic potential of oxyntomodulin in the treatment of obesity is currently under investigation.

Pancreatic Hormones

Hormones of the endocrine pancreas are secreted in response to gut nutrient content. The major function of the endocrine pancreas is to control glucose homeostasis in response to nutrient delivery, and insulin and glucagon is essential for this function. These hormones, as well as pancreatic polypeptide and amylin, also affect appetite through their direct and indirect effects on the brain.

Insulin

Insulin is released by the β cells of the pancreas in a glucose-sensitive manner and binds to the insulin receptor. The primary roles of insulin are to increase glucose uptake in peripheral tissues, decrease hepatic glucose production, and maintain glucose levels. Insulin release peaks postprandially in proportion to the glucose influx following a meal. Similar to leptin, insulin levels are also influenced by the amount of adipose tissue in the body, with higher levels in more obese individuals. Therefore, insulin is also considered an adiposity signal (75).

The most common effect on appetite mediated by insulin is seen in hypoglycemia after treatment with excess insulin in diabetes. In this situation, the increase in food intake is marked. This effect results from low blood glucose rather than from insulin directly (see the earlier discussion of glucostatic feeding). Insulin itself crosses the blood–brain barrier in a dose-dependent manner and

acts on ARC insulin receptors to decrease food intake (76). When insulin is centrally administered, a decrease in food intake and body weight is noted (77). The opposite is seen when insulin blocking antibodies are injected in the hypothalamus and when insulin receptor expression is selectively decreased in the ARC (78, 79). Insulin levels also augment the effect of other satiety signals, an effect also seen with leptin (75). Therefore, insulin provides signals to the brain that reflect circulating energy in the form of glucose and stored energy in the form of adipose tissue. These signals interact with other satiety signals to reduce food intake.

Glucagon

Glucagon is produced from preproglucagon cleavage in the α cells of the pancreas and binds to the glucagon receptor. It opposes insulin's actions on blood glucose and has an important role in maintaining blood glucose concentrations via increasing hepatic glycogenolysis, particularly as blood glucose levels fall. Glucagon levels increase postprandially, thus supporting a role in affecting food intake (75). Consistent with this, glucagon decreases meal size, and reduces overall food intake and body weight gain when administered to rodents (80). An increase in meal size is noted after intraperitoneal administration of a glucagon blocking antibody, a finding supporting a role for glucagon in satiation (81). Hepatic–portal infusions of glucagon affect food intake most potently, and this finding suggests that glucagon-induced satiation occurs via the liver. The afferent vagus nerve has been implicated in transducing glucagon's feeding-inhibitory effect from the liver to the NTS (75).

Co-agonists of glucagon and GLP-1 are currently being developed as potential antiobesity agents. Co-agonism with GLP-1 receptors reduces glucagon's detrimental effects on glucose homeostasis and may augment its anorexigenic effect. In rodents, initial studies have been promising (82).

Pancreatic Polypeptide

Along with NPY and PYY, pancreatic polypeptide (PP) belongs to the PP fold family. It is secreted by the PP cells in the periphery of the pancreatic islets. It binds preferentially to the Y4 and Y5 receptors (62). Like other satiety gut hormones, PP is secreted postprandially in proportion to calories ingested. It delays gastric emptying (83) and has also been shown to reduce appetite when given peripherally to mice and humans (84, 85). Investigators have postulated that PP exerts its effects via acting on the Y4 receptors in the ARC, in the AP, or via the vagus (62). The precise physiologic role of PP in appetite and the mechanism by which this occurs remains unclear.

Islet Amyloid Polypeptide

Islet amyloid polypeptide or amylin is cosecreted with insulin by the β cells of the pancreas in response to food intake. Amylin binds to AMY1, AMY2, and AMY3 receptors. Amylin is a satiety signal and reduces food intake. It also inhibits gastric secretion, delays gastric emptying, and improves glycemic control (86).

Peripheral administration of high-dose amylin reduces food intake and body weight (87) whereas antagonism of amylin has the opposite effect (75). This effect occurs via stimulation of neurons in the AP and NTS (75), with activation of the serotonin-histamine-dopaminergic system (88) and is independent of the vagus nerve (89). That amylin levels are proportional to body fat raises the possibility that, like leptin and insulin, amylin may also act as an adiposity signal (88).

A synthetic analog of amylin (Pramlintide, Amylin Pharmaceuticals, San Diego) is currently being used as adjunctive therapy in diabetes mellitus. Its use is associated with significant weight loss in patients with diabetes, and its utility as an antiobesity agent is under investigation (90).

GLP-2, glucose-dependent insulinotropic polypeptide, motilin, and somatostatin are other gastroenteropancreatic hormones with physiologic roles in the digestive system. At present, evidence is inconclusive to support a primary role for these hormones in regulating food intake.

Hormones from Adipose Tissue

The discovery of leptin in 1994 as a circulating protein produced by adipocytes (fat cells) regulating energy homeostasis represents a key milestone in understanding the complex systems that control appetite. Leptin provides a mechanism by which body fat can control food intake via a feedback system on the hypothalamus. This idea was initially proposed by Gordon Kennedy in 1953 as the "lipostatic theory" (91).

Leptin

Leptin is a hormone produced largely in the adipose tissue with levels proportional to fat stores and increased by overfeeding. Zhang et al demonstrated the absence of leptin in the inbred ob/ob strain of severely obese mice (92). Subsequently, human congenital leptin deficiency was identified in two severely obese cousins (93). The peripheral administration of leptin in both ob/ob mice and human congenital deficiency and central administration of leptin in ob/ob mice reversed the obese phenotype (94, 95). Therefore, leptin is a signal from the adipose tissue to the brain that reflects the state of energy stores and significantly influences appetite (96).

Leptin exerts its effects by acting on the leptin receptor (LepR). LepR mutations in mice (db/db strain mice) and humans are associated with severe obesity (96). Leptin acts on ARC LepR to stimulate POMC neurons and inhibit NPY/AgRP neurons to decrease food intake (96). Downstream signaling of leptin occurs via the MC4R (96). Leptin also acts on leptin receptors in other parts of the brain and has important effects on reward pathways, energy expenditure, pubertal development, fertility, and immune function (96).

Leptin levels are elevated in obese individuals, and administration of leptin in common obesity has a variable effect on food intake (96). This failure of leptin to diminish appetite in obesity is termed *leptin resistance* and is not completely understood.

Other Hormones

Thyroid hormones, gonadal steroids, and glucocorticoids regulate metabolic rate, reproductive state, and stress responses, respectively. These processes rely on adequate energy supplies. Therefore, it is not surprising that hormones regulating these processes are also involved in the endocrine regulation of appetite.

Thyroid Hormone

Thyroid hormone regulates basal metabolic state. Excess thyroid hormone in disease states such as hyperthyroidism is associated with increased food intake and decreased body weight from increased energy expenditure. Triiodothyronine is the active form of the thyroid hormone and is produced locally within tissues from the less active circulating thyroid hormone by the enzyme type 2 iodothyronine deiodinase. Triiodothyronine acts on the VMN and ARC to stimulate food intake and these effects are independent of energy expenditure (97, 98). It may mediate its affect by stimulating ARC NPY/AgRP neurons (99). The regulation of triiodothyronine levels locally within the hypothalamus may provide an additional control point for altering food intake (97).

Gonadal Steroids

Gonadal steroids influence appetite in a sex-specific manner. In rodents, orchiectomy (in males) decreases food intake, whereas ovariectomy (in females) increases food intake (100). Exogenous replacement of gonadal steroids reverses these changes (100). Hormone replacement therapy during menopause can reduce postmenopausal weight gain (101). Estrogen receptors have been identified in the ARC can influence POMC and NPY/AgRP neuronal signaling to alter appetite (102, 103). Estrogen also alters the satiating potency of other peripheral signals. In this regard, the effects on CCK have been best studied, and estrogen signaling in the NTS increases the sensitivity of CCK-induced satiation (100).

Glucocorticoids

Glucocorticoids are involved in the response to stress and mediate different tissue specific effects in various physiologic systems via glucocorticoid receptors that are widely expressed throughout the body, including the brain. Glucocorticoids generally stimulate food intake and weight gain. This is noted in diseases with glucocorticoid excess such as Cushing syndrome. Cortisol may influence the reward pathways promoting food intake and affect the ability of other signals, such as leptin, insulin, and NPY, to alter appetite (104).

Table 44.1 provides an overview of the major hormones, discussed in detail in this section, that influence appetite.

TABLE 44.1	SUMMARY OF MAIN HORMONES REGULATING FOOD INTAKE AND APPETITE				
	HORMONE	EFFECT ON FOOD INTAKE	MAIN SECRETION SITE	RECEPTOR	OTHER MAJOR ACTIONS
Satiety signals	Cholecystokinin	↓	I cells of small intestine	CCK 2 (CCK 1)	Contracts gallbladder, relaxes sphincter of Oddi, delays gastric emptying, releases pancreatic enzyme and somatostatin (Fat and protein digestion)
	Peptide YY	↓	L cells of GI tract	Y2	Delays gastric emptying
	GLP-1	↓	L cells of GI tract	GLP-1	Releases glucose-dependent insulin Decreases gastric motility
	Oxyntomodulin	↓	L cells of GI tract	GLP-1	Releases glucose-dependent insulin Decreases gastric motility
	Glucagon	↓	α cells of the pancreas	Glucagon	Increases blood glucose levels
	Pancreatic polypeptide	↓	PP cells of the pancreas	Y4 (Y5)	Delays gastric emptying
	Amylin	↓	β cells of the pancreas	AMY1–3	Inhibits gastric secretion Delays gastric emptying Decreases blood glucose levels
Orexigenic signals	Ghrelin	↑	A cells of gastric fundus	GHS-R	Increases gastric motility, growth hormone release
Adiposity signals	Leptin	↓	Adipocytes	Leptin	Regulates energy expenditure, reward, pubertal development, fertility, and immune function
	Insulin	↓	β cells of the pancreas	Insulin	Decreases blood glucose levels and increases glucose utilization
Other hormones	Thyroid	↑	Follicular cells of the thyroid gland	Thyroid	Increases basal metabolic rate
	Gonadal hormones	↑ (Men) ↓ (Women)	Testis Ovary	Androgen Estrogen	Regulates fertility
	Glucocorticoids	↑	Adrenal cortex	Glucocorticoid	Mediates responses to stress

CCK, cholecystokinin; GHS-R, growth hormone secretagogue receptor; GI, gastrointestinal; GLP-1, glucagon-like peptide-1.

Signals from the Immune System

Anorexia or decreased food intake during infectious, inflammatory, and neoplastic disease states is very evident. Anorexia appears to result from the action of cytokines in the brain.

Cytokines

Cytokines are small proteins secreted by cells of the immune system. Some cytokines potently inhibit food intake when given peripherally or centrally (105). Key cytokines implicated in illness-associated anorexia and weight loss are interleukin-1β, tumor necrosis factor-α, and interleukin-6. Cytokine-mediated suppression of food intake may occur by direct action of cytokines on the hypothalamus (e.g., ARC), via vagal afferents, or by induction of other hormones involved in appetite regulation (e.g., leptin) (105).

CONCLUSION

The regulation of food intake and appetite occurs through the integration of various central and peripheral signals of energy balance, as discussed in depth in this chapter. These signals interact at the level of the brainstem and hypothalamus to produce an overall response of hunger (and seeking of food) or fullness (and termination of the current meal) that alter food intake. Additionally, these neuronal networks are hugely modified by other influences such as sensory inputs, food memory, rewarding aspects of food, and numerous environmental and emotional factors. This modification is a particular feature of modern human eating behavior and may underpin the dysregulation of energy balance that is responsible for the current obesity epidemic. By means of ever-expanding current research fueled by the rise in obesity, it is hoped that our understanding of the complex and intricate signaling pathways governing appetite control will improve and pave the way for better antiobesity drug treatments.

ACKNOWLEDGMENTS AND DISCLOSURES

S.S.H. is funded by a Wellcome Trust Clinical Research Fellowship, and A.D.S. is funded by a Wellcome Trust/GlaxoSmithKline Translational Medicine Training Fellowship. The Department is funded by an Integrative Mammalian Biology (IMB) Capacity Building Award, an FP7-HEALTH-2009-241592 EurOCHIP grant, and funding from the National Institute for Health Research (NIHR) Biomedical Research Centre Funding Scheme.

S.R.B. declares an association with the following company: Pfizer Pharmaceuticals. S.R.B. is the inventor of patents describing the use of gut hormones and their analogs and derivatives in the treatment of obesity. A.D.S. and S.S.H. declare no competing interests.

REFERENCES

1. Mayer J, Thomas DW. Science 1967;156:328–37.
2. Bailey EF. Am J Physiol Regul Integr Comp Physiol 2008; 295:R1048–9.
3. Schwartz GJ. Nutrition 2000;16:866–73.
4. Ter Horst GJ, de Boer P, Luiten PG et al. Neuroscience 1989;31:785–97.
5. ter Horst GJ, Luiten PG, Kuipers F. J Auton Nerv Syst 1984; 11:59–75.
6. Olney JW. Science 1969;164:719–21.
7. Leibowitz SF, Hammer NJ, Chang K. Physiol Behav 1981; 27:1031–40.
8. Clark JT, Kalra PS, Crowley WR et al. Endocrinology 1984; 115:427–9.
9. Stanley BG, Kyrkouli SE, Lampert S et al. Peptides 1986; 7:1189–92.
10. Bewick GA, Gardiner JV, Dhillo WS et al. FASEB J 2005; 19:1680–2.
11. Roseberry AG, Liu H, Jackson AC et al. Neuron 2004;41: 711–22.
12. Rossi M, Kim MS, Morgan DG et al. Endocrinology 1998; 139:4428–31.
13. Schwartz MW, Woods SC, Porte D Jr et al. Nature 2000; 404:661–71.
14. Yaswen L, Diehl N, Brennan MB et al. Nat Med 1999;5: 1066–70.
15. Huszar D, Lynch CA, Fairchild-Huntress V et al. Cell 1997; 88:131–41.
16. Farooqi IS, Keogh JM, Yeo GS et al. N Engl J Med 2003; 348:1085–95.
17. Krude H, Biebermann H, Luck W et al. Nat Genet 1998; 19:155–7.
18. Abbott CR, Rossi M, Kim M et al. Brain Res 2000;869:203–10.
19. Kristensen P, Judge ME, Thim L et al. Nature 1998;393:72–6.
20. Yanik T, Dominguez G, Kuhar MJ et al. Endocrinology 2006;147:39–43.
21. Abbott CR, Rossi M, Wren AM et al. Endocrinology 2001; 142:3457–63.
22. Vettor R, Fabris R, Pagano C et al. J Endocrinol Invest 2002;25:836–54.
23. Fekete C, Marks DL, Sarkar S et al. Endocrinology 2004; 145:4816–21.
24. Rodgers RJ, Halford JC, Nunes de Souza RL et al. Regul Pept 2000;96:71–84.
25. Rodgers RJ, Halford JC, Nunes de Souza RL et al. Eur J Neurosci 2001;13:1444–52.
26. Qu D, Ludwig DS, Gammeltoft S et al. Nature 1996;380:243–7.
27. Kokkotou E, Jeon JY, Wang X et al. Am J Physiol Regul Integr Comp Physiol 2005;289:R117–24.
28. Chen Y, Hu C, Hsu CK et al. Endocrinology 2002;143:2469–77.
29. Xu B, Goulding EH, Zang K et al. Nat Neurosci 2003;6:736–42.
30. Pelleymounter MA, Cullen MJ, Wellman CL. Exp Neurol 1995;131:229–38.
31. Unger TJ, Calderon GA, Bradley LC et al. J Neurosci 2007; 27:14265–74.
32. Xu B, Dube MG, Kalra PS et al. Endocrinology 1998;139: 466–73.
33. Lambert PD, Anderson KD, Sleeman MW et al. Proc Natl Acad Sci U S A 2001;98:4652–7.
34. Ramos EJ, Meguid MM, Campos AC et al. Nutrition 2005; 21:269–79.
35. Pothos EN, Creese I, Hoebel BG. J Neurosci 1995;15:6640–50.
36. Zhang M, Gosnell BA, Kelley AE. J Pharmacol Exp Ther 1998;285:908–14.
37. Zheng H, Patterson LM, Berthoud HR. J Neurosci 2007; 27:11075–82.
38. Bittencourt JC, Presse F, Arias C et al. J Comp Neurol 1992;319:218–45.
39. Petrovich GD, Setlow B, Holland PC et al. J Neurosci 2002;22:8748–53.
40. Verhagen JV. Brain Res Rev 2007;53:271–86.
41. Williams CM, Kirkham TC. Physiol Behav 2002;76:241–50.
42. Verty AN, McGregor IS, Mallet PE. Brain Res 2004;1020: 188–95.
43. Hanus L, Avraham Y, Ben-Shushan D et al. Brain Res 2003; 983:144–51.
44. Jamshidi N, Taylor DA. Br J Pharmacol 2001;134:1151–4.
45. Cota D, Marsicano G, Tschop M et al. J Clin Invest 2003; 112:423–31.
46. Hilairet S, Bouaboula M, Carriere D et al. J Biol Chem 2003;278:23731–7.
47. Jo YH, Chen YJ, Chua SC Jr et al. Neuron 2005;48:1055–66.
48. Gamber KM, Macarthur H, Westfall TC. Neuropharmacology 2005;49:646–52.
49. Field BC, Chaudhri OB, Bloom SR. Nat Rev Endocrinol 2010;6:444–53.
50. Rolls ET. Philos Trans R Soc Lond B Biol Sci 2006;361:1123–36.
51. Smith GP. Pregastric and gastric satiety. In: Smith GP, ed. Satiation: From Gut to Brain. New York: Oxford University Press, 1998:10–39.
52. Ritter RC. Physiol Behav 2004;81:249–73.
53. Cummings DE, Overduin J. J Clin Invest 2007;117:13–23.
54. Mayer J. Bull N Engl Med Cent 1952;14:43–9.
55. Levin BE. Physiol Behav 2006;89:486–9.
56. Jordan SD, Könner AC, Bruning JC. Cell Mol Life Sci 2010; 67:3255–73.
57. Woods SC, Stein LJ, McKay LD et al. Am J Physiol 1984; 247:R393–401.
58. Obici S, Feng Z, Morgan K et al. Diabetes 2002;51:271–5.
59. Rehfeld JF. Physiol Rev 1998;78:1087–108.
60. Gibbs J, Young RC, Smith GP. J Comp Physiol Psychol 1973; 84:488–95.
61. Kissileff HR, Pi-Sunyer FX, Thornton J et al. Am J Clin Nutr 1981;34:154–60.
62. Chaudhri O, Small C, Bloom S. Philos Trans R Soc Lond B Biol Sci 2006;361:1187–209.
63. Bi S, Moran TH. Neuropeptides 2002;36:171–81.
64. Fan W, Ellacott KL, Halatchev IG et al. Nat Neurosci 2004; 7:335–6.
65. van der Lely AJ, Tschop M, Heiman ML et al. Endocr Rev 2004;25:426–57.
66. Zigman JM, Nakano Y, Coppari R et al. J Clin Invest 2005; 115:3564–72.
67. Renshaw D, Batterham RL. Curr Drug Targets 2005;6:171–9.
68. Batterham RL, Cowley MA, Small CJ et al. Nature 2002; 418:650–4.
69. Batterham RL, Cohen MA, Ellis SM et al. N Engl J Med 2003;349:941–8.
70. Vincent RP, le Roux CW. Clin Endocrinol (Oxf) 2008;69:173–9.
71. Drucker DJ. Cell Metab 2006;3:153–65.
72. Fehmann HC, Jiang J, Schweinfurth J et al. Peptides 1994; 15:453–6.
73. Dakin CL, Small CJ, Batterham RL et al. Endocrinology 2004;145:2687–95.
74. Cohen MA, Ellis SM, Le Roux CW et al. J Clin Endocrinol Metab 2003;88:4696–701.
75. Woods SC, Lutz TA, Geary N et al. Philos Trans R Soc Lond B Biol Sci 2006;361:1219–35.

76. Marks JL, Porte D Jr, Stahl WL et al. Endocrinology 1990;127:3234–6.
77. Woods SC, Seeley RJ. Int J Obes Relat Metab Disord 2001;25 Suppl 5:S35–8.
78. McGowan MK, Andrews KM, Grossman SP. Physiol Behav 1992;51:753–66.
79. Obici S, Feng Z, Karkanias G et al. Nat Neurosci 2002;5:566–72.
80. Geary N, Le Sauter J, Noh U. Am J Physiol 1993;264:R116–22.
81. Langhans W, Zeiger U, Scharrer E et al. Science 1982;218:894–6.
82. Day JW, Ottaway N, Patterson JT et al. Nat Chem Biol 2009;5:749–57.
83. Schmidt PT, Naslund E, Gryback P et al. J Clin Endocrinol Metab 2005;90:5241–6.
84. Asakawa A, Inui A, Yuzuriha H et al. Gastroenterology 2003;124:1325–36.
85. Batterham RL, Le Roux CW, Cohen MA et al. J Clin Endocrinol Metab 2003;88:3989–92.
86. Ludvik B, Kautzky-Willer A, Prager R et al. Diabet Med 1997;14 Suppl 2:S9–13.
87. Rushing PA, Hagan MM, Seeley RJ et al. Endocrinology 2000;141:850–3.
88. Reda TK, Geliebter A, Pi-Sunyer FX. Obes Res 2002;10:1087–91.
89. Lutz TA, Del Prete E, Scharrer E. Peptides 1995;16:457–62.
90. Hollander P, Maggs DG, Ruggles JA et al. Obes Res 2004;12:661–8.
91. Kennedy GC. Proc R Soc Lond B Biol Sci 1953;140:578–96.
92. Zhang Y, Proenca R, Maffei M et al. Nature 1994;372:425–32.
93. Montague CT, Farooqi IS, Whitehead JP et al. Nature 1997;387:903–8.
94. Friedman JM, Halaas JL. Nature 1998;395:763–70.
95. Farooqi IS, Jebb SA, Langmack G et al. N Engl J Med 1999;341:879–84.
96. Farooqi IS, O'Rahilly S. Am J Clin Nutr 2009;89:980S–4S.
97. Kong WM, Martin NM, Smith KL et al. Endocrinology 2004;145:5252–8.
98. Dhillo WS, Bewick GA, White NE et al. Diabetes Obes Metab 2009;11:251–60.
99. Coppola A, Liu ZW, Andrews ZB et al. Cell Metab 2007;5:21–33.
100. Asarian L, Geary N. Philos Trans R Soc Lond B Biol Sci 2006;361:1251–63.
101. Lopez M, Lelliott CJ, Tovar S et al. Diabetes 2006;55:1327–36.
102. Acosta-Martinez M, Horton T, Levine JE. Trends Endocrinol Metab 2007;18:48–50.
103. Gao Q, Mezei G, Nie Y et al. Nat Med 2007;13:89–94.
104. Adam TC, Epel ES. Physiol Behav 2007;91:449–58.
105. Buchanan JB, Johnson RW. Neuroendocrinology 2007;86:183–90.

SUGGESTED READINGS

Bellocchio L, Cervino C, Pasquali R et al. The endocannabinoid system and energy metabolism. J Neuroendocrinol 2008;20:850–7.

Chaudhri O, Small C, Bloom S. Gastrointestinal hormones regulating appetite. Philos Trans R Soc Lond B Biol Sci 2006;361:1187–209.

Obici S. Molecular targets for obesity therapy in the brain. Endocrinology 2009;150:2512–7.

Rolls ET. Brain mechanisms underlying flavour and appetite. Philos Trans R Soc Lond B Biol Sci 2006;361:1123–36.

Woods SC, D'Alessio DA. Central control of body weight and appetite. J Clin Endocrinol Metab 2008;93:S37–50.

45 NUTRITION AND THE IMMUNE SYSTEM[1]

CHARLES B. STEPHENSEN AND SUSAN J. ZUNINO

[1]**Abbreviations: AA**, arachidonic acid; **APC**, antigen-presenting cell; **BCR**, B-cell receptor; **CRP**, C-reactive protein; **CTL**, cytotoxic T lymphocyte; **DC**, dendritic cell; **DHA**, docosahexaenoic acid; **DTH**, delayed-type hypersensitivity; **EPA**, eicosapentaenoic acid; **HIV**, human immunodeficiency virus; **IFN**, interferon; **Ig**, immunoglobulin; **IL**, interleukin; **LPS**, lipopolysaccharide; **LTB**, leukotriene B; **MBL**, mannose-binding lectin; **NF-κB**, nuclear factor-κB; **NK**, natural killer; **PAMP**, pathogen-associated molecular pattern; **PGE$_2$**, prostaglandin E$_2$; **PUFA**, polyunsaturated fatty acid; **TCR**, T-cell receptor; **TGF**, transforming growth factor; **Th cell**, T-helper cell; **TLR**, Toll-like receptor, **Treg cell**, regulatory T cell; **VDR**, vitamin D receptor.

OVERVIEW OF THE IMMUNE SYSTEM

Functions

The principal function of the immune system is to protect the host from death and disability caused by infectious diseases (1). "Host," in this context, refers to a human or other animal infected by a potentially disease-causing (i.e., pathogenic) organism. Pathogens may be viruses, bacteria, fungi (or yeast), protozoa, or multicellular parasites including nematodes and flukes. Disease usually occurs when such organisms are specifically adapted to infect humans—the so-called professional pathogens. The names of many of these pathogens are well known: the measles virus, the cholera bacterium (*Vibrio cholerae*), the yeast *Candida albicans*, the malaria protozoa (*Plasmodium falciparum* and others of this genus), the hookworm nematodes (*Necator americanus* and *Ancylostoma duodenale*), and the liver fluke (*Schistosoma mansoni*). Most pathogens have evolved methods of evading the innate immune response and must be cleared by adaptive immunity. Some pathogens evade adaptive immunity as well (e.g., malaria protozoa or the human immunodeficiency virus [HIV]). The world is also full of opportunistic pathogens that may cause disease when the immune system is compromised by malnutrition, other infections (e.g., HIV), or advancing age. In addition, commensal organisms colonize the skin, intestine, and urogenital tracts and are benign or beneficial to the host. However, these organisms may also be harmful under certain circumstances and thus are also subject to control, but not elimination, by the immune system (2).

The immune system can also be activated by sterile injury that causes tissue damage but does not involve microorganisms (3). In this case, the innate immune system may be activated to stop bleeding and resolve tissue damage. Such sterile inflammation is an important factor in the development of many chronic inflammatory diseases (e.g., coronary artery disease) (4), discussed elsewhere in this book.

Innate and Adaptive Immunity

The immune system has two components: innate and adaptive (5), although the two work together as an integrated whole. The innate system is evolutionarily older, and it is fully functional at birth. Innate immune cells use a diverse group of receptors to recognize and respond to signature molecules from classes of microorganisms (e.g., flagella from some bacteria, cell wall carbohydrate from yeast, RNA from viral genomes). These responses are essentially the same for all individuals within a species. The adaptive system is different in that the host's response adapts to a specific pathogen (e.g., measles virus specifically and not RNA viruses in general) to develop immunologic memory that will respond more quickly and more efficiently the next time the same pathogen is encountered. Thus, individuals have different levels of adaptive immunity depending on their exposure history. The adaptive nature of this response explains why the first encounter with a childhood pathogen (e.g., measles) can make a child quite ill, but subsequent infections will likely go unnoticed.

Passive Protection of Infants

Infants have a full complement of innate immune cells at birth, although these cells respond less vigorously to microorganisms than do the same cell types from adults (6). In contrast, infants have not yet developed adaptive immunologic memory. However, infants transiently acquire some components of adaptive immunity from their mothers. For example, serum immunoglobulin G (IgG) antibody is transferred across the placenta to give infants protection against infections such as measles for up to 9 months (7). In addition, breast-fed infants receive secretory IgA antibody and many antimicrobial factors from colostrum and breast milk (8). This maternally derived protection for infants is important because the infant's adaptive immune system responds less robustly to pathogens than does the adult system (9, 10). This attenuated response may be beneficial because colonization of the gut and other epithelial surfaces with commensal microflora presents a major challenge to the developing immune system. Overresponding could be detrimental by causing tissue damage that could impede normal growth and development.

Organization of the Immune System

The immune system in humans and other mammals is made up of organs and tissues located strategically throughout the body to protect against invasion by microorganisms (1, 5). Primary organs, in which immune cells develop, include the bone marrow and thymus. All white blood cells (leukocytes) originate in the bone marrow (Table 45.1). One subset of lymphocytes, T lymphocytes, (also known as T cells) needs an additional maturation step in the thymus, however. In mammals, B lymphocytes (B cells) mature in the bone marrow, but in avian species, this step occurs in the bursa of Fabricius. The lymph nodes, spleen, and mucosa-associated lymphoid tissue (MALT) are secondary organs and tissues. These secondary sites are meeting places for immune cells that

are connected by the blood and lymphatic systems to allow transmission of information from the innate to the adaptive immune system.

The lymph nodes are located regionally (e.g., along lymphatic vessels draining specific regions of the body), and this information transfer occurs when an antigen-presenting cell (APC), after an encounter with invading microorganisms, travels through lymphatic vessels from peripheral tissues (e.g., skin, respiratory mucosa, gut) to enter the closest draining lymph node (1, 5). Because lymphatic vessels drain all tissues of the body, this APC-based surveillance system can deliver information from any site of infection to a regional lymph node. APC is a functional definition, and antigen presentation can be made by several cell types, including dendritic cells (DCs), macrophages, and B cells.

The spleen, like the lymph nodes, provides a site for APCs to transfer information to lymphocytes. The spleen also filters the blood. In the case of a breach of peripheral defenses, bloodborne microorganisms or infected erythrocytes (e.g., in the case of malaria) are removed from the blood by the spleen.

Intercellular Communication in the Immune System

Cells of the immune system aggregate in secondary lymphoid tissues and at sites of inflammation. These cells communicate with one another through cell-to-cell contact and soluble mediators to trigger changes in activity (e.g., chemotaxis) and gene expression. Cytokines, including interleukins, and chemokines are protein mediators produced by immune and other cells that trigger various responses in cells bearing the appropriate receptors. One large family of chemokines has a standard Cys-Cys or C-C motif, whereas a second family has a C-X-C motif. These chemokines are known as CC and CXC chemokines, respectively. The eicosanoid family of lipid-based mediators is synthesized primarily from arachidonic acid and also from eicosapentaenoic acid (EPA). The eicosanoids include leukotrienes produced from the 5-lipoxygenase enzymatic pathway as well as prostaglandins and thromboxanes from the cyclooxygenase pathway (5).

INNATE IMMUNITY

Epithelial Surfaces and Barrier Defenses

The innate immune system protects portal-of-entry sites used by pathogens to cause infections, including the skin, conjunctiva, respiratory tract, gut, and urogenital tract (1). Tissues at these portals are designed to protect against infection using various common mechanisms. These sites have a surface layer of epithelial cells interspersed with a few lymphoid or myeloid immune cells. The subepithelial tissue provides structure and contains blood vessels to provide entry into the epithelium for immune cells when needed, and lymphatic drainage to allow egress of APCs to the draining lymph node. Two interesting examples to consider are the skin and the intestine.

TABLE 45.1	CELLS OF THE IMMUNE SYSTEM

MYELOID CELLS

Common myeloid progenitor: Found in bone marrow; progenitor of all myeloid cells including monocyte lineage and granulocyte lineage cells

Monocyte lineage
Monocyte: Found in blood, differentiates to macrophage on entering tissues
Macrophage: Phagocytic cell found in tissues involved in defense against microorganisms and in "sterile" inflammation initiated by tissue damage (e.g., wound or plaque in coronary artery)
Immature dendritic cell: Found in blood, differentiates to dendritic cell in tissues
Dendritic cell: Functions as an antigen-presenting cell; delivers antigen from the periphery to lymphocytes in draining lymph nodes

Granulocyte lineage
Neutrophil: Principal phagocytic cell in blood; enters tissue in response to inflammation to kill invading bacteria by phagocytosis (ingestion), oxidative metabolism, and secretion of antibacterial peptides
Eosinophil: Found in blood; enters tissue to mediate inflammation in response to parasitic infections and allergies, including asthma
Basophil: Found in blood; enters tissue in response to parasitic infections
Mast cell: Found in tissues primarily at submucosal sites; responds to some antigens, including allergens, through immunoglobulin E molecules on mast cell surface; this activation causes a release of mediators that triggers local and systemic inflammation, including anaphylaxis

LYMPHOID CELLS

T cell: Normally found in blood and lymph nodes as well as in tissue at sites of inflammation; cell surface TCR recognizes peptide antigens; $CD8^+$ "killer" T cells recognize and kill virus-infected host cells; $CD4^+$ T-helper cells produce cytokines that stimulate development of $CD8^+$ T cells and B cells and stimulate protective responses of some myeloid cells, including macrophages
B cell: Normally found in blood and lymph nodes; cell surface BCR is a membrane-anchored immunoglobulin that recognizes foreign antigens: after antigenic stimulation, B cells develop into antibody-secreting plasma cells found in bone marrow and at submucosal surfaces
NK cell: Found in blood and tissues; does not have antigen-specific cell surface receptor; recognizes and kills virus-infected and other "stressed" or damaged cells through change in expression of cell surface receptors
NK T cell: Minor but diverse cell type that responds to nonpeptide "antigens" (typically lipid; presented by CD1 rather than MHC) through TCR of limited diversity; can be cytotoxic or regulatory

OTHER CELLS

Megakaryocyte: Found in bone marrow; precursor to small, nonnucleated platelets that are found in blood and mediate blood clotting
Erythroid progenitor cells: Found in bone marrow; progenitors for red blood cells

BCR, B-cell receptor; MHC, major histocompatibility complex; NK, natural killer; TCR, T-cell receptor.

The skin consists of two cellular layers, epidermis and dermis (11). The epidermis consists of four layers of keratinocytes interspersed with melanocytes and Langerhans cells, a professional APC and the principal immune cell of the uninfected epidermis. Some commensal microorganisms adhere to the epithelial surface and are adapted to persist in this niche (12). Pathogens, including strains of *Staphylococcus aureus*, may penetrate the skin by using special virulence factors (e.g., enzymes to break down extracellular matrix) to cause deeper infections that, if the local immune response is not sufficient, may become systemic (1, 13). The dermis contains blood capillaries and lymphatic drainage as well as various immune cells, the number and type varying depending on the immunologic challenge. Not all such challenges come from microorganisms. Inflammation in the skin may be triggered by irritants (e.g., chemicals, ultraviolet [UV] light), to which a person may become sensitized (e.g., poison ivy, which elicits an adaptive immune response).

The mucosal epithelium of the intestine consists of a single layer of absorptive epithelial cells interspersed with other cells, including (a) goblet cells that secrete a protective layer of mucus, (b) M cells that collect particulate antigen from the lumen for delivery to mucosa-associated APC in underlying lymphoid aggregates, (c) interdigitating DCs (a type of APC) that send cytoplasmic arms between epithelial cells to sample antigen from the gut lumen directly (2), and (d) Paneth cells in intestinal crypts that secrete antifungal α-defensins. The lamina propria underlying the gut epithelium contains abundant immune cells, particularly lymphocytes. Unlike in the dermis, many lymph nodes are present in the lamina propria (termed *Peyer patches*). These lymphocytes are localized to the lamina propria. Several factors including peristalsis, the mucus barrier, the relatively rapid turnover of epithelial cells, and secreted factors (e.g., IgA, antimicrobial peptides) help protect this epithelial barrier from microorganisms (14, 15). IgA and IgM are transported across intestinal epithelial cells and into the gut lumen by the polymeric Ig receptor (pIgR). The extensive network of APCs in the lamina propria, in concert with regulatory T (Treg) cells in the lamina propria, help the body differentiate commensal organisms from pathogens (16).

Other mucosal sites include the mouth, nasopharynx, trachea, esophagus, stomach, and urogenital tract. These sites have similar organizational features and functions (1). The lungs present a unique challenge in that alveoli are gas exchange surfaces and, because of the limits of gas diffusion, cannot be organized into multicellular layers. The final line of defense in the lungs is formed by the alveolar macrophages, which engulf and clear tiny particles and microorganisms (e.g., *Mycobacterium tuberculosis*).

Recognition of Pathogens by Innate Immune Cells

Epithelial cells are immune cells in that they can recognize and respond to pathogens (11) and thus are an integral part of the response to infection. Recognition of microorganisms occurs by pattern recognition receptors that recognize signature pathogen-associated molecular patterns (PAMPs) found in macromolecules common to groups of microorganisms but not typically found in mammals. The Toll-like receptors (TLRs) are the best studied and recognize PAMPs from different classes of bacteria, yeast, and viruses (17). For example, bacterial lipopolysaccharide (LPS) is recognized by TLR4, bacterial flagellin by TLR5, single-stranded RNA by TLR7, and repeated DNA sequences of the bases C and G (common in bacterial but not mammalian genomes) by TLR9. These same receptors are also used by APCs and macrophages.

Other receptors perform similar functions. For example, nucleotide-binding domain, leucine-rich repeat-containing (NLR) proteins also recognize PAMPs (18). These receptors are part of a multiprotein complex in the cytoplasm termed an *inflammasome* that results in cleavage of prointerleukin (pro-IL)-1β and pro-IL-18 to produce the active cytokines. This pathway can also be activated by nonmicrobial tissue irritants such as uric acid crystals, which accumulate in tissues of patients with gout, and the adjuvant alum, which is used in many human vaccines.

Local Inflammation

Binding of PAMPs to their cognate receptors activates cytoplasmic signal transduction pathways that initiate gene transcription in the nucleus. For example, the transcription of many proinflammatory cytokine and chemokines genes is regulated by the transcription factor nuclear factor-κB (NF-κB) (19). Genes induced by NF-κB include tumor necrosis factor (TNF)-α, IL-6, cyclooxygenase-2, and 5-lipoxygenase. Keratinocytes in the skin express TLRs that are activated during infections causing production of chemokines that attract T cells (e.g., CCL20 and CXCL9, 10 and 11) and neutrophils (CXCL1 and 8) (11) and cationic antimicrobial peptides (AMPs), such as cathelicidin and β-defensin (20), that mediate killing of invading bacteria and thus protect epithelial surfaces from infection.

The innate immune response can also protect against viral infections. Virus replication in most cells induces transcription of interferon-α, (IFN-α) and IFN-γ following recognition of double-stranded RNA by TLR3

or other sensors such as retinoic acid–inducible gene (RIG)-1 (21). These interferons bind to cell surface receptors on the same and adjacent cells and induce protective factors that degrade viral RNA or otherwise interfere with viral replication. IFN-α and IFN-γ also activate natural killer (NK) cells to kill target cells.

These initial responses to infection trigger a local inflammatory response involving cells already at the site and cells recruited to the site by soluble mediators (1, 5). Many tissues contain resident macrophages that also respond to infection by producing chemokines (CXCL8), cytokines (including IL-12, IL-1β, TNF-α, and IL-6), leukotrienes (including LTB$_4$ and LTE$_4$), prostaglandins (including prostaglandin E$_2$ [PGE$_2$]), and platelet-activating factor that mediate inflammation. The goal of this inflammation is to eliminate the pathogen or to minimize spread of the pathogen until adaptive immunity can produce a pathogen-specific response. The key events in inflammation include the following: (a) release of preformed mediators and rapid enzymatic production of mediators, followed by transcription and translation of chemokine and cytokine genes; (b) induction of cell adhesion molecules (e.g., intercellular adhesion molecule 1 [ICAM-1]) in the vascular endothelium in adjacent capillaries that slows the progress of leukocytes; (c) loosening of tight junctions between epithelial cells to allow egress of leukocytes along a chemokine gradient; (d) stimulation of blood clotting by activation of platelets to minimize "escape" of pathogens; (e) killing of microorganisms or infected cells by the leukocytes attracted to the site; and, (f) a recovery phase stimulates repair of damage caused by pathogens or the responding leukocytes.

Killing of bacteria by macrophages and neutrophils

Monocytes from the blood differentiate into macrophages following extravasation (22). Macrophages ingest invading microorganisms into phagocytic vesicles, the phagosome, by using several cell surface receptors. The phagosome fuses with lysosomes containing antibacterial peptides and enzymes (e.g., lysozyme). Following fusion, a respiratory burst involving nicotinamide adenine dinucleotide phosphate (NADPH) oxidase acidifies the phagolysosome and injects reactive oxygen species, which kill ingested microorganisms. Neutrophils are the most common white blood cell but are not found in healthy tissue. Their numbers at sites of inflammation increase rapidly during bacterial infections. Neutrophils kill engulfed bacteria in a manner similar to macrophages. The life span of the neutrophil is short, and these cells typically die after one round of phagocytosis and granule discharge. Macrophages live longer, have more cellular transcription machinery, and can regenerate phagosomes. Macrophages play a prominent role in responses to intracellular pathogens such as viruses and *M. tuberculosis*.

Opsonization and Complement-Mediated Killing

Some serum proteins (e.g., mannose-binding lectin [MBL]) and C-reactive protein (CRP), and secretory proteins such as surfactant proteins A and D produced in the lungs, bind to PAMPs on the surface of bacteria and enhance their uptake and killing by phagocytic cells (23). This activity is termed *opsonization*. The complement system of serum proteins opsonizes bacteria by binding to the bacterial surface directly or to MBL or antibody bound to the bacteria. Complement proteins undergo conformational change and enzymatic activation on binding, and a cascade of such events leads to formation of biologically active components such as C3a and C5a, which are chemoattractants for phagocytes, and C3b, which is an opsonin. In addition, accumulation of a several terminal complement components, known as a membrane attack complex, on the surface of a bacterial cell forms a pore that disrupts membrane integrity and kills the bacteria (5).

Systemic Inflammation and the Acute Phase Response

When production of TNF-α, IL-1β, and IL-6 at a site of inflammation is high, serum levels of these cytokines increase and systemic effects are triggered. These include fever, malaise, muscle aches, and decreased appetite. Fever is induced by PGE_2 acting on the hypothalamus. One early name for TNF-α was cachexin because it decreases appetite, an effect also mediated through the central nervous system. These cytokines also act on hepatocytes to increase synthesis of positive acute phase proteins, including ferritin, CRP, and MBL, and to decrease synthesis of negative acute phase proteins, including albumin and retinol-binding protein (RBP)—the serum transport protein for vitamin A. The positive acute phase proteins typically have a protective role in the innate immune response. They increase within a few hours and reach a peak at 10-fold to more than 100-fold their initial concentrations within a few days. CRP, for example, increases from approximately 1 mg/L to more than 100 mg/L during bacterial pneumonia and binds to cell wall polysaccharides, thus acting as an opsonin. The reason for decreased levels of negative acute phase proteins, which may drop by 25% to 50%, is not clear.

Serum iron, which is bound to the transport protein transferrin, also decreases during the acute phase response as a result of increased hepcidin synthesis (see also the chapter on iron). Hepcidin blocks normal recycling of transferrin-bound iron through macrophages and results in increased intracellular and decreased serum iron levels (24). Increased ferritin synthesis may facilitate intracellular iron storage. This sequestration of iron reduces its availability to opportunistic pathogens. Chronic inflammation may result in the anemia of chronic disease by decreasing the availability of iron for erythropoiesis. Serum zinc levels also decrease during the acute phase response to inhibit bacterial zinc acquisition.

Macronutrient metabolism is also altered during the acute phase response, with elevated levels of serum triglycerides, decreased β-oxidation of fatty acids, and increased gluconeogenesis. Neutrophils are also mobilized from bone marrow to increase availability at sites of inflammation, and TNF-α stimulates activation of APCs and their migration to lymph nodes.

Antigen-Presenting Cell Functions: Linking Innate to Adaptive Immunity

The mission of the APC is to stimulate an adaptive immune response by transferring information about a specific microorganism from the site of infection to the draining lymph node for presentation to T cells (5). At least three types of information are transferred. First, unique peptides from microbial proteins, or antigens, are displayed on the APC surface by major histocompatibility complex (MHC) molecules for presentation to naive T cells in the draining lymph node. This presentation leads to the formation of peptide-specific memory T cells that will respond to a specific pathogen, as discussed later. Some antigens stimulate development of memory B cells and an antibody response without T-cell help. Such T-cell–independent antigens may travel through the lymph in solution and bind to antigen-specific Ig molecules on the surface of naive B cells without APC help, thus stimulating the development of memory B cells and antibody-producing plasma cells. Memory B and T cells leave the lymph node through an efferent lymphatic vessel and eventually reach the bloodstream through the thoracic duct. From the bloodstream, these cells may recirculate to the initial site of infection, to specific tissues (e.g., mucosal sites or skin), or to lymph nodes.

The second type of information (or signal) transferred from APC to T cell is termed *costimulation* and involves activation of cell surface receptors on the T cell (e.g., cluster of differentiation 28 [(CD28]) by corresponding costimulatory molecules on the surface of the activated APC (e.g., B7 molecules, also known as CD80 and CD86). This costimulation enhances T-cell proliferation. The third type of information transmitted to the T cell by the APC is the differentiation signal, which consists principally of soluble mediators, typically cytokines, that help direct T-cell differentiation into a particular helper phenotype, as discussed later.

ADAPTIVE IMMUNITY

T cells and B cells are the principal cellular components of the adaptive immune system. The adaptive immune response develops more slowly after initial infection than does the innate response, but eventually it has a greater capacity to defend against the targeted pathogen. All mammals have similar adaptive immune systems, and laboratory mice are the favored model for research because of the availability of antibody reagents to characterize murine cells and molecules and because genetic manipulation of mice allows mechanistic studies in which specific genes can be targeted for decreased or enhanced expression.

T-Helper Lymphocytes

The T-lymphocyte pool (identified by expression of CD3 on the cell surface) consists of helper, cytotoxic, and regulatory cells (Fig. 45.1). The helper designation derives from the ability of these cells to help promote development of cytotoxic T-lymphocyte (CTL) and B-cell responses, but they also have effector functions in that they participate directly in the clearance of invading pathogens. Mature T-helper (Th) cells express CD4, whereas CTLs express CD8. Naive CD4$^+$ T cells differentiate into Th1, Th2, Th17, and Treg subtypes on activation, and each of these subtypes has different effector functions and mobilizes different cell types to remove invading pathogens (25–27) (see Fig. 45.1). These subtypes form persistent lineages represented in the memory response to different pathogens, although this commitment has some plasticity (28).

Th1 cells secrete cytokines that stimulate the activation of CTLs to enhance the clearance of intracellular pathogens. Th2 cells secrete cytokines that help activate B cells to synthesize Igs that, in turn, mediate protection and clearance of extracellular pathogens. Th2 cells also enhance responses against parasites that may include stimulating development of eosinophils, production of mucus, and peristalsis in the gut to clear pathogens. Th1 and Th2 lymphocytes develop in response to specific, differentiation-inducing cytokines (IL-12 and IL-18 for Th1 and IL-4 for Th2) produced by APCs or other cell types during initial exposure of a naive T cell to antigen. Mature Th1 and Th2 cells express signature transcription factors (T-box expressed in T cells [T-bet] for Th1 and GATA-binding factor 3 (GATA-3) for Th2), which help mediate and maintain their unique phenotypes, including distinct patterns of cytokine production. Th1 cells produce IL-2 (T-cell growth factor; naive T cells also produce IL-2), IFN-γ, and TNF-α. Th2 cells produce IL-4, IL-5, and IL-13 and may produce IL-6 and IL-10. IFN-γ produced by Th1 cells inhibits the generation of Th2 cells, whereas IL-4 produced by Th2 cells inhibits Th1 development. Th17 cells are a more recently discovered subset of CD4$^+$ T cells, and their development is stimulated by the cytokines IL-6 and transforming growth factor-β (TGF-β) (27), although in humans other cytokines may also play a role, including IFN-γ (29). Th17 cells are activated by a diverse number of extracellular bacterial and fungal pathogens not cleared well by a Th1 or Th2 response. Th1 and Th17 cells bridge the innate and adaptive immune responses by secreting IFN-γ and IL-17, respectively, which enhance innate effector mechanisms at sites of infection. IFN-γ activates macrophage-mediated killing of intracellular pathogens, whereas IL-17 induces neutrophil recruitment and the production of proinflammatory cytokines, chemokines, and metalloproteinases by epithelial cells to enhance resistance to extracellular bacteria.

Cytotoxic T Lymphocytes

CTLs are the principal type of adaptive immune cells that mediate the killing of cells infected with viruses (e.g., influenza, hepatitis B, and herpes simplex) and intracellular bacteria (e.g., *M. tuberculosis* and *Salmonella typhimurium*) (30) although evidence suggests a cytotoxic role for some CD4$^+$ T cells as well (31). CTLs also respond to intracellular parasitic infections caused by *Plasmodium* sp. (malaria), *Toxoplasma gondii* (toxoplasmosis), and *Trypanosoma cruzi* (Chagas disease). CTLs kill infected cells by the CD95 and perforin/granzyme-mediated lytic pathways (32, 33). NK cells of the innate immune system also kill cells by these mechanisms.

Regulatory T Lymphocytes

Treg cells play a critical role in the induction of self-tolerance and thereby significantly contribute to resistance to autoimmunity (34). They also play a role in immune

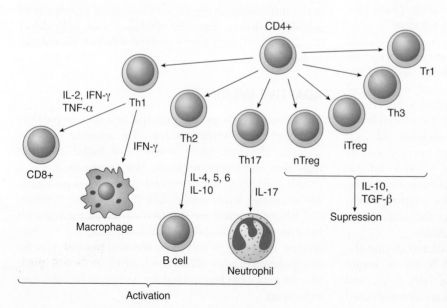

Fig. 45.1. CD4$^+$ T-helper and regulatory T cells. The figure shows the major subtypes described in the text, including major effector cytokines, cell types acted on by these cytokines, and the overall effect of the cell types, activation of pathogen clearance mechanisms, or suppression of cell-mediated responses. *IFN,* interferon; *IL,* interleukin; *TNF,* tumor necrosis factor; *TGF,* transforming growth factor; *Th,* T-helper cell.

homeostasis by suppressing excessive immune responses that may develop in response to infection and may be damaging to the host. Treg cells can be CD4$^+$ or CD8$^+$, although CD8$^+$ Treg cells have not been as extensively characterized (34, 35). The major class of CD4$^+$ Treg cells is characterized and identified by the expression of the signature transcription factor forkhead box P3 (FoxP3) and the surface marker CD25, which is the α chain of the IL-2 receptor.

B Lymphocytes

The primary role of B lymphocytes is to produce antibodies that are specific for a foreign antigen. Antibodies are Igs that have a basic unit, shaped like a Y, consisting of two identical heavy (H) and two identical light (L) polypeptide chains (Fig. 45.2). The C-terminus consists of the two heavy chains and denotes the constant (C) region. The two variable (V) regions formed at the N-terminal fork of the Y structure are composed of one heavy and one light chain each. The variable region is responsible for binding to foreign antigens. The five classes of Igs are IgM, IgD, IgG, IgA, and IgE. IgM exists as a pentamer of Ig units held together by a joining (J) chain peptide. IgA can form either a monomer or dimer joined by the J chain. Antibodies can bind directly to soluble, foreign antigen (e.g., to neutralize bacterial toxins) and to surfaces of microorganisms (as opsonins, to aggregate the microorganisms and to neutralize viruses) through the two antigen-binding sites on each molecule.

Diversity of T- and B-Lymphocyte Receptors

The specificity and diversity of both T-cell and B-cell responses are the result of somatic gene rearrangement and recombination events of Ig and receptor genes. The B-cell receptor (BCR) consists of an Ig unit, as described

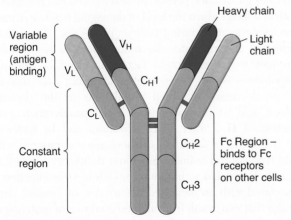

Fig. 45.2. Immunoglobulin structure: structure of the immunoglobulin (Ig) unit. The variable region (V) binds to antigen. The heavy chain (H) determines the class of Ig: IgM, IgD, IgG, IgA, or IgE. The Fc region can bind to Fc receptors and activate other immune cells to kill pathogens or induce internalization of the Ig–pathogen immune complex by phagocytosis. *C*, constant region; *L*, light chain.

earlier, associated with an α and β chain. The Ig genes are composed of V, D (diversity), J, and C gene segments. The light chain of the Ig is composed of recombined V, J, and C regions. The heavy chain recombines V, D, J, and C regions. The T-cell receptor (TCR) has an Ig-like structure, and the formation of the receptor is similar to that of Ig. Most T cells express TCRs composed of α and β chains. The α chain is composed of recombined V and J regions, and the β chain is composed of recombined V, D, and J regions. As with the BCR, the C region of both chains is spliced in during transcriptional processing. A few T cells have TCRs composed of γ and δ chains. These nonconventional T cells recognize nonpeptide antigens up-regulated by stressed cells and are important for clearance of extracellular and intracellular pathogens, tumor cells, and tissue healing (34).

IMPACT OF NUTRITION ON IMMUNITY

Vitamin A

Vitamin A deficiency causes squamous metaplasia at epithelial surfaces and thus can impair barrier defenses. Vitamin A deficiency also affects myelopoiesis and granulopoiesis in the bone marrow, thus impairing the activity of monocytes/macrophages and granulocytes (36) and the development and activity of NK cells (37). APC function is also altered by vitamin A deficiency and can impair antigen presentation (38), as well as enhance production of IL-12 (39), which may skew some adaptive responses away from the development of Th2 and toward that of Th1 cells. Antibody responses to T-cell–dependent antigens are impaired by vitamin A deficiency (40, 41); secretory IgA responses are particularly affected (36). Retinoic acid produced by some cells of the immune system, including APCs, appears to act in a paracrine manner to promote development of induced Treg (iTreg) cells in the intestine and may thus play a significant role in maintaining tolerant rather than inflammatory responses toward gut flora. Retinoic acid also enhances expression of α4β7 integrin and CCR9 on gut-derived lymphocytes (42). These molecules allow trafficking back to the gut for mature effector lymphocytes and IgA-producing plasma cells. Vascular endothelium in the gut expresses mucosal vascular addressin cell adhesion molecule 1 (MAdCAM-1), to which α4β7 binds, thus allowing extravasation. Epithelial and other cells in the gut express CCL25, which attracts CCR9-expressing cells.

Vitamin A deficiency increases the risk of death for infants and young children living in areas with a high burden of infectious diseases, and treatment of vitamin A deficiency with high-dose vitamin A capsules has been shown to reduce infant mortality when supplements are administered after 6 months of age (43). However, vitamin A supplementation can sometimes have adverse effects, such as increasing the severity of pneumonia (44) or increasing the risk of vertical transmission of HIV from mother to infant (45). These data suggest that vitamin A supplementation may have immune-modulating effects that are deleterious, depending on the type of response required for host protection. Thus, caution should be observed in providing such supplements during active infection.

Vitamin B6, Vitamin B12, and Folate

Vitamin B6, vitamin B12, and folate play critical roles in one-carbon metabolism and are essential for the synthesis of nucleic acids and proteins (46). Therefore, deficiency impairs both T-cell and B-cell function. Impairment of proliferative responses, decreased antibody synthesis, and reduced cytokine production have been observed in humans deficient for any of these nutrients.

Vitamin C

Human subjects fed a vitamin C–deficient diet had decreased delayed-type hypersensitivity (DTH) skin responses, which are mediated by the Th1 cytokine IFN-γ (47). Supplementation of these subjects with vitamin C normalized the DTH response, a finding indicating that vitamin C is involved in maintenance of Th1 function. In elderly subjects, vitamin C supplementation for 1 month increased the ex vivo proliferative responses of T cells to mitogen (48). Studies in a mouse model for asthma showed that high-dose supplementation with vitamin C increased the ratio of IFN-γ to IL-5 in bronchoalveolar fluid; again, this finding indicated that vitamin C promotes Th1 function (49). Neutrophils have high a cytoplasmic level of vitamin C and rapid regeneration of ascorbate (50), presumably to protect the host cell against the oxidative stress associated with bacterial killing.

Vitamin D

In the innate immune system, the active metabolite of vitamin D, calcitriol, can be produced by macrophages following TLR2-mediated expression of the 1-α-hydroxylase gene (51). Calcitriol can then act in an autocrine or paracrine fashion to increase expression of the antimicrobial peptides cathelicidin and β2-defensin, which mediate bacterial killing by macrophages. This activity may be a factor in host defense against tuberculosis (52) and suggests a mechanistic link between the observation of increased risk of vitamin D deficiency and certain vitamin D receptor (VDR) polymorphisms in patients with tuberculosis (53). These intriguing associations are a focus of current research efforts to determine whether vitamin D supplementation of humans can affect resistance to or recovery from infectious diseases (54). Vitamin D also affects development of other innate immune cells, including NK T cells (55).

Knockout of the VDR in mice enhances development of inflammatory bowel disease (56), which is mediated by an inflammatory T-cell response. Vitamin D3 treatment was also shown to inhibit the production of TNF-α and IFN-γ by Th1 cells and enhance expression of IL-4 by Th2 cells in a mouse model for experimental colitis (57). However, the enhancement of Th2 responses is controversial, because other investigators have shown that vitamin D3 inhibits IL-4 synthesis in mice and inhibits proliferation and synthesis of Igs, whereas it promotes apoptosis in human B cells (58). Vitamin D3 inhibits the generation of Th17 cells in vitro and impairs development of Th17 cells in vivo (59). Vitamin D3 increases the development of Treg cells and results in increased FoxP3 expression and IL-10 and TGF-β production (57). Vitamin D deficiency also increases the severity of experimental autoimmune encephalomyelitis (60), a mouse model of multiple sclerosis. The increase in Treg cell activity as well as number suggests that vitamin D3 may have an overall immunosuppressive activity toward the adaptive immune response, and a causal link has been postulated between vitamin D deficiency and the risk of autoimmune disease in humans, including multiple sclerosis (61).

Vitamin E

Vitamin E promotes Th1 responses in naive CD4+ T cells (62). Increases in DTH skin responses have been shown with vitamin E supplementation. In purified CD4+ T cells from young and old mice, vitamin E enhanced the formation of immune synapses between the TCRs and APCs (63). Many of the studies with vitamin E have been performed on elderly humans, and these data suggest that vitamin E supplementation may be important for improving the declining immune response in the aged and for decreasing the risk of some infections (64).

Selenium

Selenium is an essential component of the antioxidant enzymes glutathione peroxidase and thioredoxin reductase, both of which reduce the level of damaging reactive oxygen species generated during cellular processes. Thioredoxin reductase also regulates the redox potential key cellular enzymes and transcription factors involved in immune responsiveness (46). Selenoprotein knockout mice showed severe decreases of T-cell populations in the thymus, spleen, and lymph nodes (65). T-cell proliferation, production of IL-2 after TCR activation, and Ig synthesis by B cells were defective in these mice compared with wild-type control animals. Selenium deficiency (as well as vitamin E deficiency) in mouse models of virus infection is associated with an increased occurrence of virulent virus strains that may result from an increased rate of mutation of the viral genome or perhaps from increased virus replication and opportunity for mutation (66). Selenoproteins may play a prominent role in redox-mediated signaling from cell surface receptors (67), a mechanism that could be particularly important in activation of cells of the immune system.

Zinc

Studies in humans showed that deficiency of dietary zinc resulted in thymic atrophy, decreased numbers of peripheral T cells, and reduced IL-2 and IFN-γ production by T cells (68, 69). No effect on the Th2 cytokines IL-4 and IL-10 was reported. Zinc-deficient individuals have a decreased DTH response as a result of the reduction in IFN-γ production. Although Th2 cytokine expression does not appear to be affected by zinc deficiency, B cells have reduced antibody production, a finding indicating the importance of zinc in regulating both B-cell and T-cell activities. Frequent zinc supplementation of children at risk of zinc deficiency in developing countries has decreased not only the risk of infectious disease, particularly diarrhea, but also other infections (70).

Copper and Iron

Copper and iron are components of the antioxidant enzymes superoxide dismutase and catalase, respectively. These metals, along with selenium and zinc (also a component of superoxide dismutase), regulate the redox state and proliferative responses of T cells and B cells. T-cell proliferation is reduced in copper-deficient rats and humans (71). Iron is actively transported by the transferrin receptor that is up-regulated in activated T cells. Th1 cells are more sensitive to iron deficiency, which results in a reduction in IFN-γ production and decreased proliferation. Reduction of IFN-γ production leads to decreased CD8$^+$ CTL activation and DTH responsiveness.

Iron is required for the growth of microorganisms, and pathogens are specifically adapted to acquire iron in the relatively iron-poor environment of the human host (72). This need for iron by pathogens suggests that the decrease in serum iron seen during the acute phase is an attempt by the host to restrict iron availability to pathogens. This finding may explain the association of hemochromatosis (which results in increased tissue iron levels) with increased severity of invasive bacterial infections (73) and the increased risk of infectious diarrhea with use of iron supplements (74).

Omega-3 and Omega-6 Fatty Acids

Arachidonic acid (AA; C20:4, n-6) released by phospholipase A_2 activity from the membrane of monocytes, granulocytes, and, at times, lymphocytes is used as the precursor for synthesis of eicosanoid mediators of immune function including 2-series prostaglandins (e.g., PGE$_2$) (75) and 4-series leukotrienes (e.g., LTB$_4$) (76). Leukotrienes mediate inflammation by enhancing leukocyte chemotaxis, phagocytosis, and killing of bacteria by neutrophils and macrophages and by enhancing transcription of proinflammatory genes (77). PGE$_2$ has different effects, including enhancement of Th2 cytokines, promoting of IgG1 and IgE production, and diminishing of synthesis of proinflammatory cytokines (75). The marine fatty acid EPA (C20:5, n-3) is also a substrate for these enzymes, but the 3-series PG and 5-series LT products generally have different levels of activity. Diets in the United States are generally low in EPA. The use of supplements or consumption of EPA-rich marine foods increases the EPA/AA ratio in the membranes of monocytes and granulocytes, however, and results in relatively greater production of EPA-derived eicosanoids and changes in immune function (78). For example, increased EPA intake has anti-inflammatory effects in diseases such as rheumatoid arthritis (79), presumably because EPA-derived eicosanoids are less inflammatory than are AA-derived eicosanoids. For example, LTB$_5$ has lower activity than does LTB$_4$ to stimulate granulocyte chemotaxis (80), which could alleviate symptoms of arthritis. High levels of EPA intake may also have the unintended consequence of marginally decreasing bacterial killing by phagocytes (79). Intake of fish oil supplements is recommended to decrease the risk of cardiovascular disease, partly because of these anti-inflammatory effects that are thought to slow progression or stabilize arterial plaque (78).

In addition, another long-chain omega-3 fatty acid, docosahexaenoic acid (DHA; 22:5, n-3), has anti-inflammatory effects because it can be shortened to form EPA, whereas it also has independent effects related to production of novel anti-inflammatory immune mediators, resolvins and protectins (81). In addition, DHA can block TLR-mediated signaling initiated by LPS. Other polyunsaturated fatty acids (PUFAs) have similar but lesser effects (82). Saturated fatty acids can stimulate TLR-mediated signaling and can mimic, to a degree, the effect of TLR ligands such as LPS. The TLR-blocking effect of DHA and other PUFAs is independent of eicosanoid production and may be mediated by affecting lipid raft formation, which would influence TLR dimerization (in the case of TLR4) and could then induce signal transduction. A similar mechanism has been proposed for DHA-mediated decreases in TCR activation and T-cell proliferation (83).

REFERENCES

1. Mims CA, Nash A, Stephen J. Mims' Pathogenesis of Infectious Disease. 5th ed. San Diego: Academic Press, 2001.
2. Hill DA, Artis D. Annu Rev Immunol 2010;28:623–67.
3. Rock KL, Latz E, Ontiveros F et al. Annu Rev Immunol 2010;28:321–42.
4. Nahrendorf M, Pittet MJ, Swirski FK. Circulation 2010;121:2437–45.
5. Murphy KP, Travers P, Walport M et al. Janeway's Immunobiology. 7th ed. New York: Garland Science, 2008.
6. Marodi L. Clin Immunol 2006;118:137–44.
7. Hasselquist D, Nilsson JA. Philos Trans R Soc Lond B Biol Sci 2009;364:51–60.
8. Labbok MH, Clark D, Goldman AS. Nat Rev Immunol 2004;4:565–72.
9. Siegrist CA, Aspinall R. Nat Rev Immunol 2009;9:185–94.
10. Marchant A, Goldman M. Clin Exp Immunol 2005;141:10–8.
11. Nestle FO, Di Meglio P, Qin JZ et al. Nat Rev Immunol 2009;9:679–91.

12. Grice EA, Kong HH, Conlan S et al. Science 2009;324:1190–2.
13. Feng Y, Chen CJ, Su LH et al. FEMS Microbiol Rev 2008; 32:23–37.
14. Ogra PL. Mucosal Immunology. 2nd ed. San Diego: Academic Press, 1999.
15. Brandtzaeg P. Scand J Immunol 2009;70:505–15.
16. Izcue A, Coombes JL, Powrie F. Annu Rev Immunol 2009; 27:313–38.
17. Kawai T, Akira S. Curr Opin Immunol 2005;17:338–44.
18. Martinon F, Mayor A, Tschopp J. Annu Rev Immunol 2009; 27:229–65.
19. Kawai T, Akira S. Trends Mol Med 2007;13:460–9.
20. Yang D, Biragyn A, Hoover DM et al. Annu Rev Immunol 2004;22:181–215.
21. Diebold S. Immunol Lett 2009;128:17–20.
22. Serbina NV, Jia T, Hohl TM et al. Annu Rev Immunol 2008;26:421–52.
23. Bottazzi B, Doni A, Garlanda C et al. Annu Rev Immunol 2009;28:157–83.
24. Hugman A. Clin Lab Haematol 2006;28:75–83.
25. Mosmann TR, Cherwinski H, Bond MW et al. J Immunol 1986;136:2348–57.
26. Mosmann TR, Coffman RL. Annu Rev Immunol 1989;7:145–73.
27. Bettelli E, Korn T, Oukka M et al. Nature 2008;453: 1051–7.
28. Murphy KM, Stockinger B. Nat Immunol 2010;11:674–80.
29. Romagnani S, Maggi E, Liotta F et al. Mol Immunol 2009; 47:3–7.
30. Wong P, Pamer EG. Annu Rev Immunol 2003;21:29–70.
31. Brown DM. Cell Immunol 2010;262:89–95.
32. Russell JH, Ley TJ. Annu Rev Immunol 2002;20:323–70.
33. Chowdhury D, Lieberman J. Annu Rev Immunol 2008;26: 389–420.
34. Sakaguchi S, Yamaguchi T, Nomura T et al. Cell 2008;133: 775–87.
35. Lu L, Cantor H. Cell Mol Immunol 2008;5:401–6.
36. Stephensen CB. Annu Rev Nutr 2001;21:167–92.
37. Zhao Z, Murasko DM, Ross AC. Nat Immun 1994;13:29–41.
38. Duriancik DM, Lackey DE, Hoag KA. J Nutr 2010;140: 1395–9.
39. Cantorna MT, Nashold FE, Hayes CE. Eur J Immunol 1995;25:1673–9.
40. Pasatiempo AM, Kinoshita M, Taylor CE et al. FASEB J 1990;4:2518–27.
41. Ross AC. Vitam Horm 2007;75:197–222.
42. Iwata M, Hirakiyama A, Eshima Y et al. Immunity 2004;21: 527–38.
43. Black RE, Allen LH, Bhutta ZA et al. Lancet 2008;371: 243–60.
44. Stephensen CB, Franchi LM, Hernandez H et al. Pediatrics 1998;101:E3.
45. Fawzi WW, Msamanga GI, Hunter D et al. AIDS 2002;16: 1935–44.
46. Wintergerst ES, Maggini S, Hornig DH. Ann Nutr Metab 2007;51:301–23.
47. Jacob RA, Kelley DS, Pianalto FS et al. Am J Clin Nutr 1991; 54(Suppl):1302S–9S.
48. Kennes B, Dumont I, Brohee D et al. Gerontology 1983;29: 305–10.
49. Chang HH, Chen CS, Lin JY. J Agric Food Chem 2009;57: 10471–6.
50. Washko PW, Wang Y, Levine M. J Biol Chem 1993;268:15531–5.
51. Liu PT, Stenger S, Li H et al. Science 2006;311:1770–3.
52. Martineau AR, Wilkinson KA, Newton SM et al. J Immunol 2007;178:7190–8.
53. Wilkinson RJ, Llewelyn M, Toossi Z et al. Lancet 2000;355: 618–21.
54. Bruce D, Ooi JH, Yu S et al. Exp Biol Med (Maywood) 2010;235:921–7.
55. Yu S, Cantorna MT. Proc Natl Acad Sci U S A 2008;105: 5207–12.
56. Froicu M, Weaver V, Wynn TA et al. Mol Endocrinol 2003; 17:2386–92.
57. Daniel C, Sartory NA, Zahn N et al. J Pharmacol Exp Ther 2008;324:23–33.
58. Chen S, Sims GP, Chen XX et al. J Immunol 2007;179: 1634–47.
59. Tang J, Zhou R, Luger D et al. J Immunol 2009;182:4624–32.
60. Nashold FE, Spach KM, Spanier JA et al. J Immunol 2009;183:3672–81.
61. Cantorna MT. Nutr Rev 2008;66(Suppl):S135–8.
62. Meydani SN, Han SN, Wu D. Immunol Rev 2005;205:269–84.
63. Marko MG, Ahmed T, Bunnell SC et al. J Immunol 2007; 178:1443–9.
64. Meydani SN, Leka LS, Fine BC et al. JAMA 2004;292:828–36.
65. Shrimali RK, Irons RD, Carlson BA et al. J Biol Chem 2008; 283:20181–5.
66. Beck MA. J Nutr 2007;137:1338–40.
67. Hawkes WC, Alkan Z. Biol Trace Elem Res 2010;134:235–51.
68. Prasad AS. Curr Opin Clin Nutr Metab Care 2009;12:646–52.
69. Overbeck S, Rink L, Haase H. Arch Immunol Ther Exp (Warsz) 2008;56:15–30.
70. Fischer Walker C, Black RE. Annu Rev Nutr 2004;24:255–75.
71. Munoz C, Rios E, Olivos J et al. Br J Nutr 2007;98(Suppl 1): S24–8.
72. Bullen JJ, Rogers HJ, Spalding PB et al. J Med Microbiol 2006;55:251–8.
73. Khan FA, Fisher MA, Khakoo RA. Int J Infect Dis 2007; 11:482–7.
74. Gera T, Sachdev HP. BMJ 2002;325:1142.
75. Harris SG, Padilla J, Koumas L et al. Trends Immunol 2002; 23:144–50.
76. Radmark O, Werz O, Steinhilber D et al. Trends Biochem Sci 2007;32:332–41.
77. Peters-Golden M, Canetti C, Mancuso P et al. J Immunol 2005;174:589–94.
78. Adkins Y, Kelley DS. J Nutr Biochem 2010;21:781–92.
79. Fritsche K. Annu Rev Nutr 2006;26:45–73.
80. Moreno JJ. J Pharmacol Exp Ther 2009;331:1111–7.
81. Serhan CN, Chiang N, Van Dyke TE. Nat Rev Immunol 2008; 8:349–61.
82. Lee JY, Zhao L, Hwang DH. Nutr Rev 2010;68:38–61.
83. Kim W, Khan NA, McMurray DN et al. Prog Lipid Res 2010;49:250–61.

46 DEFENSES AGAINST OXIDATIVE STRESS[1]

DEAN P. JONES

---

[1]**Abbreviations: AMD**, age-related macular degeneration; **ATP**, adenosine triphosphate; **Cd**, cadmium; **CYP**, cytochrome P-450; **Cys**, cysteine; **CySSG**, cysteine-glutathione disulfide; **DRI**, dietary referintake; **ER**, endoplasmic reticulum; **Fe^{2+}**, ferrous iron; **Fe^{3+}**, feriron; **G6P**, glucose 6-phosphate; **GGT**, γ-glutamyltransferase; **GPX**, glutathione peroxidase; **GSH**, glutathione; **GSSG**, glutathione disulfide; **GST**, glutathione transfer; **H$_2$O$_2$**, hydrogen peroxide; **HNE**, 4-hydroxynonenal; **Met**, methio; **NAD$^+$**, oxidized nicotinamide adenine dinucleotide; **NADH**, reduced nicotinamide adenine dinucleotide; **NADP$^+$**, oxidized nicotinamide adenine dinucleotide phosphate; **NADPH**, nicotinamide adenine dinucleotide phosphate; **NO·**, nitric oxide; **NOS**, nitric oxide synthase; **Nox**, nitric oxide; **NOS**, nitric oxide synthase; **·OH**, hydroxyl radical; **PDI**, protein disulfide isomerase; **Prx**, peroxiredoxin; **PUFA**, polyunsaturated fatty acid; **RNS**, reactive nitrogen species; **ROS**, reactive oxygen species; **Sec**, selenocysteine; **SOD**, superoxide dismutase; **Trx**, thioredoxin; **UV**, ultraviolet.

OVERVIEW

Antioxidant defenses against oxidative stress have a rich history of scientific investigation, influenced by medicine, public health, commerce, and politics. Since 2000, considerable change in the scientific focus has occurred as results from large-scale, double-blind interventional trials with free radical scavenging antioxidants became available to show little to no benefit of these supplements to protect against human disease. The results of these antioxidant trials do not invalidate the substantial data associating oxidative stress with disease and antioxidants with protection against oxidative stress. Instead, the results indicate that oxidative stress is not adequately described as a simple imbalance between pro-oxidants and antioxidants.

This chapter surveys the sources and types of oxidative stress and the multiple systems that interact to maintain physiologic function and protect against disease. This is an active area of nutrition research, with important unknowns, uncertainty, and controversy. In addition to extensively studied mechanisms of oxidative damage to macromolecules, contemporary research emphasizes the importance of nutrition to support redox signaling. Redox signaling refers to pathways of cell and subcellular communication that involves oxidants; the associated signaling proteins are key sites of oxidative disruption in human diseases. Diet and nutrition are central to the function of these signaling systems, directly by maintaining the redox signaling components (e.g., enzymes, transporters, transcription factors) and indirectly by optimizing gene expression and epigenetic control of protective and repair systems.

Despite controversies and ongoing investigations, extensive research supports modern nutrition policies emphasizing adequacy of intake of the antioxidant vitamins C and E and the antioxidant mineral selenium as defined for their dietary reference intake (DRI) values. Zinc (Zn^{2+}), several vitamins (e.g., vitamin D and B vitamins), and some amino acids (methionine [Met], cysteine [Cys], glutamine) are important to maintain antioxidant functions dependent on glutathione (GSH). These indirect antioxidant functions can be important under some conditions and are addressed within DRIs, but they are not primary criteria for DRI values. At the same time, nutrition policies recognize a need to avoid excesses of some nutrients because of associated risks (e.g., vitamin E, selenium, iron in postmenopausal women and men, copper, and, in some cancer-prone populations, β-carotene). Ongoing research on nutrition and defenses against oxidative stress increasingly employs approaches that provide better spatial and temporal resolution of oxidative reactions within cells, focus on nonradical mechanisms, and integrate redox systems biology of the complete genome, epigenome, proteome, and metabolome.

DEFINITION OF OXIDATIVE STRESS

Oxidative stress is defined as an imbalance in pro-oxidant and antioxidant reactions that causes macromolecular damage or disrupts biologic redox signaling and control (1). This encompasses a broad spectrum of processes affecting the health of biologic systems, as depicted in Figure 46.1. All these processes involve electron transfer, or "redox," reactions, in which loss of one or more electrons (termed *oxidation*) occurs from a donor chemical, and gain of one or more electrons (termed *reduction*) occurs by an acceptor chemical. Conservation of matter requires that these processes be coupled (i.e., whenever something is oxidized, something else becomes reduced). The bias in use of oxidative stress, instead of reductive stress, is derived from life in an aerobic environment, where the carbon-, hydrogen-, nitrogen- and sulfur-containing chemicals are oxidized while O_2 serves as the electron acceptor, ultimately being reduced to water.

Pro-oxidants and Antioxidants

Pro-oxidants are agents that stimulate aberrant electron transfer in biologic systems and cause oxidative stress; these include both free radical oxidants and nonradical oxidant agents that initiate radical reactions, oxidize biologic components, or interfere with normal reductive and antioxidant functions. Free radicals (or more simply, radicals) are organic molecules or ions with an unpaired electron that are often reactive and function as pro-oxidants. Radicals support a unique chemistry in which chain reactions occur, such as those involved in polymerization of plastics. Nonradical oxidants are chemicals that participate in oxidation reactions not involving radical mechanisms. Antioxidants (Fig. 46.2) are agents that function at low concentrations to stop oxidative stress. These include radical-scavenging chemicals that accept or donate electrons to terminate radical chain reactions (see later) and chemicals and enzyme systems that eliminate or protect against oxidants, some of which are listed in Figure 46.3.

The term *antioxidant* is loosely defined and also includes agents that inactivate radical initiation and catalysis, such as metal ion chelators, agents that block radiation-induced

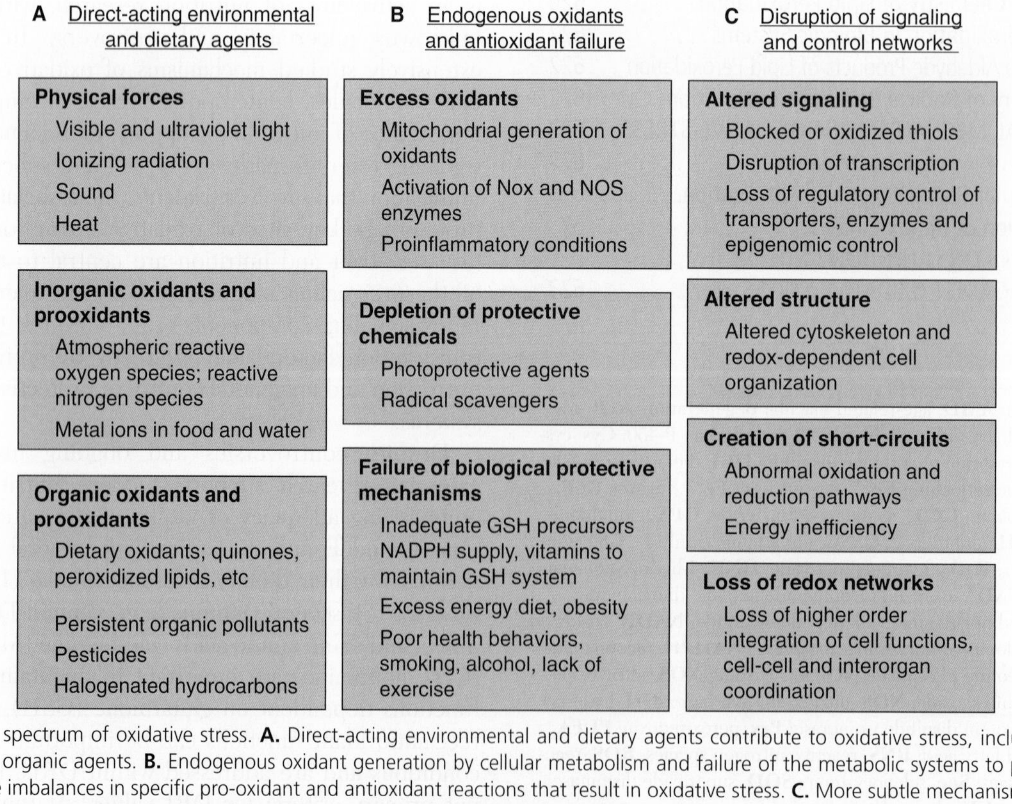

A Direct-acting environmental and dietary agents	B Endogenous oxidants and antioxidant failure	C Disruption of signaling and control networks
Physical forces Visible and ultraviolet light Ionizing radiation Sound Heat	**Excess oxidants** Mitochondrial generation of oxidants Activation of Nox and NOS enzymes Proinflammatory conditions	**Altered signaling** Blocked or oxidized thiols Disruption of transcription Loss of regulatory control of transporters, enzymes and epigenomic control
Inorganic oxidants and prooxidants Atmospheric reactive oxygen species; reactive nitrogen species Metal ions in food and water	**Depletion of protective chemicals** Photoprotective agents Radical scavengers	**Altered structure** Altered cytoskeleton and redox-dependent cell organization
Organic oxidants and prooxidants Dietary oxidants; quinones, peroxidized lipids, etc Persistent organic pollutants Pesticides Halogenated hydrocarbons	**Failure of biological protective mechanisms** Inadequate GSH precursors NADPH supply, vitamins to maintain GSH system Excess energy diet, obesity Poor health behaviors, smoking, alcohol, lack of exercise	**Creation of short-circuits** Abnormal oxidation and reduction pathways Energy inefficiency **Loss of redox networks** Loss of higher order integration of cell functions, cell-cell and interorgan coordination

Fig. 46.1. The spectrum of oxidative stress. **A.** Direct-acting environmental and dietary agents contribute to oxidative stress, including physical, inorganic, and organic agents. **B.** Endogenous oxidant generation by cellular metabolism and failure of the metabolic systems to protect against oxidants create imbalances in specific pro-oxidant and antioxidant reactions that result in oxidative stress. **C.** More subtle mechanisms of oxidative stress involve disruption of redox signaling and control mechanisms, such as occur by nonradical oxidants; these mechanisms may represent the most critical aspect of oxidative stress in chronic and age-related disease. *GSH*, glutathione; *NADPH*, nicotinamide adenine dinucleotide phosphate; *NOS*, nitric oxide synthase; *Nox*, nicotinamide adenine dinucleotide phosphate oxidase.

Antioxidants: agents that function at low concentrations to stop oxidative stress

1. Radical-scavenging chemicals that accept or donate electrons to terminate radical chain reactions (e.g., vitamin C)

2. Chemicals and enzyme systems that eliminate or protect against oxidants (e.g., GSH peroxidases)

3. Agents that prevent radical initiation (e.g., inhibitors of Cyp enzymes, radiation shields)

4. Agents that bind catalysts of oxidation (e.g., metal ion chelators)

5. Agents that counter oxidation of a substance with reduction (e.g., thiol antioxidants)

6. Agents that stabilize macromolecules against oxidation (e.g., Zn^{2+})

Fig. 46.2. Antioxidants refer to agents that act at low concentrations to stop oxidative stress. The term is loosely defined and can refer to radical scavengers as well as agents, such as zinc (Zn^{2+}), which interacts with thiols to decrease tendency toward oxidation. *Cyp*, cytochrome P-450; *GSH*, glutathione.

oxidation, and agents that counter oxidation of a substance with reduction. The term includes agents that protect against radical and nonradical oxidative mechanisms, and more specific terms such as "radical-scavenging antioxidant" or "thiol antioxidant" are used to discriminate these. The reactions of pro-oxidants and antioxidants have been extensively studied and provide a foundation to understand the biochemistry and biology of oxidative stress.

Challenges to Define Antioxidant Requirements

Knowledge about the chemistry of oxidative reactions is derived from studies with purified chemical systems. Extrapolation of this chemistry to biology and nutrition remains challenging because the simple models do not effectively describe complex systems. For most vitamins and minerals, support of specific proteins and biologic functions allows nutritional needs to be considered in

terms of the amounts needed for those respective functions. Because of the limited numbers of interaction sites on proteins, an amount of nutrient that is sufficient to saturate the sites or activities can be determined. However, such criteria do not exist for chemical reactions with high rate constants, such as those involved in free radical reactions associated with oxidative stress. For these reactions, one must extrapolate data from homogeneous chemical systems to nonhomogeneous biologic systems.

Within a compartment such as mitochondria or chromatin, the rate of reaction at a specific subcellular site is critical. Antioxidants that block radical reactions are consumed at such sites, with the result that the subcellular compartment becomes a "sink" for the antioxidant. Diffusion of an antioxidant to a sink varies as a function of the concentration difference (ΔC) between the source (e.g., blood) and the sink, according to the Fick equation (flux = diffusion coefficient $\times$ ΔC). In principle, there is no upper limit to the amount of antioxidant that could be beneficial. This is fundamentally different than for vitamins and minerals that saturate protein-dependent systems, and it represents an ongoing challenge to define antioxidant requirements. At the same time, recognition of this problem has led to an effort to develop more effective antioxidants by improving delivery to specific sites, such as design of specific mitochondrial antioxidants based on transport characteristics (2). Furthermore, beyond the problem of defining requirements for delivery to specific subcellular sites, defining antioxidant requirements is limited by overlapping and redundant activities. Multiple antioxidants block the same oxidative reactions. Thus, even though an overall antioxidant capacity may be needed, assignment of that requirement to an individual chemical is not possible.

Vitamin C and E Are the Only Antioxidants with Dietary Reference Intakes

Many naturally occurring antioxidant chemicals block free radical reactions, but only two, vitamins C (ascorbate) and E (α-tocopherol), have been found to have sufficient

Pro-oxidant Radicals		Nonradical oxidants	
Superoxide	$O_2^-\cdot$	Hydrogen peroxide	H_2O_2
Hydroxyl radical	$\cdot OH$	Hypochlorous acid	HOCl
Alkoxyl radicals	$RO\cdot$	Singlet oxygen	$^1O_2$
Peroxyl radical	$ROO\cdot$	Ozone	O_3
Nitric oxide	$NO\cdot$	Hydroperoxide	ROOH
Carbon-centered		Peroxynitrite	$ONOO^-$
radical	$\cdot CCl_3$	Alkylperoxynitrite	ROONO
		Nitrous acid	HNO_2
Stable radicals		Dinitrogen tetraoxide	N_2O_4
Ubisemiquinone		Disulfide	RSSR'
Semidehydroascorbate		Sulfenate	RSO^-
Vitamin E radical		Sulfinate	RSO_2^-

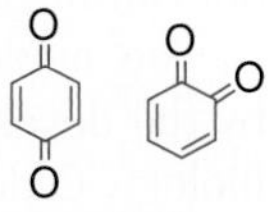

Quinones

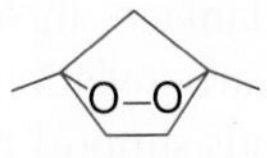

Endoperoxide

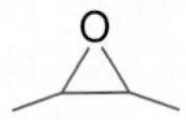

Epoxide

Fig. 46.3. Pro-oxidant radicals and nonradical oxidants in biologic systems. (See text for descriptions)

specificity for elimination of disease to warrant inclusion as vitamins (see the chapters on vitamin C and vitamin E). The DRI for ascorbate is based in part on the amount needed to support specific enzyme activities. Ascorbate does not show the characteristic of the hypothetic benefit of increased intake because it is water soluble, and its reabsorption by the kidneys is saturable. As a consequence, ascorbate ingested in excess of about 250 mg/day is directly lost in the urine. Establishment of DRI values for the fat-soluble α-tocopherol is less direct, but it similarly includes consideration of a specific α-tocopherol–binding protein in liver. Other antioxidants support the same types of radical-scavenging activities as vitamin C and E but do not have the same biochemical evidence to define a requirement. As indicated earlier, other chemicals have overlapping and redundant antioxidant activities so that requirements are difficult to establish and justify scientifically.

Contemporary Refinement in Definition

The contemporary definition of oxidative stress has been refined based on research findings since 2000 (1, 3–5). At this time, evidence became available to show that the principal thiol-disulfide systems controlling the oxidation-reduction states of proteins are not in a near-equilibrium state but rather are kinetically limited (6). Coupled with rapidly developing knowledge of redox-signaling nicotin-amide adenine dinucleotide phosphate (NADPH) oxi-dases, this discovery provided a framework to consider thiol redox circuits as a global system for regulation of cell and organ system function (7, 8). At the same time, results of large-scale, double-blind interventional studies with radical-scavenging antioxidants also began to appear in the literature (9–16). These studies showed that supplementa-tion with antioxidants (i.e., shifting the "balance" toward protection) had little or no health benefit in humans. Consequently, the original definition of oxidative stress has been qualified in the sense that an imbalance is now considered only in terms of specific reactions or pathways and not in terms of a "global" imbalance. In other words, in the current conceptualization, an imbalance in a spe-cific reaction or pathway can cause damage without an overall imbalance in the system, and a change in overall balance of pro-oxidants and antioxidants can occur with-out causing damage.

The modern view of oxidative stress is also affected by the development of "-omic" technologies and systems biology. Older criteria of oxidative stress were limited to gross measures, such as cell death (17) or macromolecular damage, including lipid peroxidation (18), global protein carbonylation (19), or DNA damage (20). Modern meth-ods support measures of expression of specific genes (21), modification of specific lipids (22), oxidation of specific proteins (23), and global effects on metabolic pathways (24, 25). These methods are enabling detailed understand-ing of the nutritional contributions to both radical and nonradical mechanisms of oxidative stress.

SPECTRUM OF OXIDATIVE STRESS

The spectrum of oxidative stress can be considered in terms of oxidants and pro-oxidants directly from the diet and environment (see Fig. 46.1A), oxidants generated endogenously with failure of endogenous protective sys-tems (see Fig. 46.1B), and more subtle disruption of redox signaling and control mechanisms (see Fig. 46.1C). For some of these, nutrition provides limited to no protection. For others, antioxidant defenses are clearly important and are affected by nutrition.

Environmental Causes of Oxidative Stress

Physical forces in the environment often represent an unavoidable source of oxidative stress. These forces are important in nutrition because they can affect the quality of food and nutritional supplements as well as have direct effects on human health. Oxidation during food storage and preparation adversely affects palatability and nutri-ent content. In general, this oxidation occurs by the same mechanisms described here, is managed within the food industries to maximize product shelf life, and is incorpo-rated in nutritional recommendations and food guides to account for such losses. Consequently, only the biologic effects of oxidative stress are addressed here.

Visible light can cause oxidative damage, but only the more intense blue light has been linked to disease. Blue light damages the retinal pigment epithelial cells in the sensory retina and contributes to age-related macular degeneration (AMD) (26). Ultraviolet (UV) light from the sun causes more extensive oxidative stress, such as oxidative damage to the skin, resulting in sunburn and skin cancers (27, 28). The evolution of humans as diurnal rather than nocturnal mammals, with relatively poor pro-tection by hair, has resulted in nutritional requirements that are distinct from requirements for other species. Ionizing radiation causes oxidative DNA damage and con-tributes to leukemias and other cancers (29, 30). Sound waves cause oxidative damage in lithotripsy of kidney stones and damage cochlear cells in hearing loss (31, 32). Heat increases oxidative reactions with resulting oxidative damage in thermal injury. Thus, exposures in the physical world include unavoidable causes of oxidative stress.

Few nutritional means are available to protect against these physical forces, but some exceptions exist. Some carotenoids accumulate in the retina and protect against light-induced damage. Lutein and zeaxanthin, in par-ticular, accumulate regionally in the macula and are currently being studied for protection against AMD at doses of 10 mg/day lutein and 2 mg/day zeaxanthin (26) in a double-blind randomized trial—the Age-Related Eye Disease Study-2 (AREDS2). Carotenoids function as intraocular filters to capture and dissipate light energy and scavenge singlet oxygen, a reactive form of molecular oxygen generated by photochemical activation (33). UV radiation is most effectively blocked by melanin, a natural polymer derived from tyrosine oxidation. Melanin production is deficient in albinism and is partially blocked by high phenylalanine in uncontrolled phenylketonuria. Pigmentation color is partially determined by Cys through a reaction that limits polymerization and results in reddish, rather than darker, pigments. For none of these reactions is nutrition very useful to enhance protection from UV radiation. Conversely, regular consumption of cocoa has been shown to protect against erythema from UV radiation, perhaps because of activation of endogenous antioxidant systems (34). Additionally, sulfur amino acids, lysine, zinc, vitamin C, and polyunsaturated fatty acids (PUFAs) used for inflammatory signaling may provide some benefit in the repair processes. Avoidance of sun exposure and use of commercial sunscreens are popular means to protect against UV light injury, but these limit natural synthesis of vitamin D in the skin.

Ionizing radiation from radioactive decay is similar to UV light in that nutrition is important in inflammatory signaling and repair but not by providing an ability to filter the radiation. For certain radiation exposures, however, supplemental iodine is thought to be beneficial by displacing and facilitating excretion of radioactive iodine. Precursors of GSH have been studied as means to protect

against side effects of radiation therapy in cancer; utility is limited because decreased tumoricidal activity accompanies protection of normal tissues. Consequently, common sense and avoidance are most important when confronting oxidative stress from physical exposures because of the limited benefits beyond sound nutritional strategies for health.

Direct-Acting Inorganic Chemicals and Xenobiotics

In addition to physical forces, direct-acting inorganic chemicals cause oxidative stress, especially affecting the respiratory and gastrointestinal systems. Atmospheric pollution contains certain reactive oxygen species (ROSs) and reactive nitrogen species (RNSs) that contribute to oxidative damage in the airways (35, 36). ROSs are oxygen-containing chemicals that are reactive with organic molecules and include superoxide anion radical, hydrogen peroxide (H_2O_2), lipid hydroperoxides, ozone, and related oxygen-centered radicals (Fig. 46.4). RNSs include nitric oxide (NO·), peroxynitrite, and other oxides of nitrogen. The terms *ROS* and *RNS* are commonly used because the chemistry is too complex and the analytic methods are insufficient to identify specific reactive species.

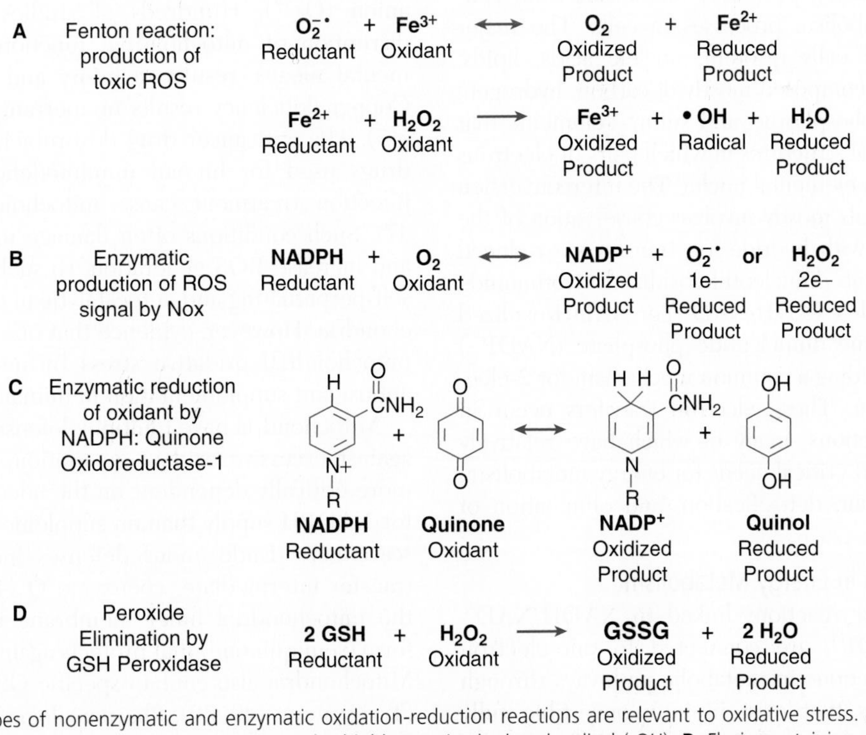

Fig. 46.4. Different types of nonenzymatic and enzymatic oxidation-reduction reactions are relevant to oxidative stress. **A.** The Fenton reaction is an iron-catalyzed Haber-Weiss reaction that generates the highly reactive hydroxyl radical (·OH). **B.** Flavin-containing enzymes, such as redox signaling proteins, nicotinamide adenine dinucleotide phosphate (NADPH) oxidase (Nox), catalyze both 1-electron and 2-electron transfers to O_2, thereby forming both $O_2^{-·}$ and hydrogen peroxide (H_2O_2). The most active NADPH oxidase, Nox-2, is present in phagocytic cells and activated to kill invading microorganisms. **C.** Two-electron transfer, shown for the detoxification enzyme NADPH:quinone reductase-1 (NQO1), is used to support chemical interconversions in intermediary metabolism. The niacinamide group shown for NADPH is identical to that in NADH and serves to transfer a pair of electrons as a hydride ion (H^-) without radical formation. **D.** Thiols are used as reductants to eliminate H_2O_2. In the reaction shown, glutathione (GSH) peroxidase catalyzes reduction of H_2O_2 to water without forming radicals as intermediates. The oxidized product formed from two GSH molecules is glutathione disulfide, GSSG. It is reduced back to GSH by an NADPH-dependent reductase (not shown), thus completing a detoxification cycle for peroxides. Fe^{2+}, ferrous iron; Fe^{3+}, ferric iron; *ROS*, reactive oxygen species.

Many transition metals catalyze electron transfer and also are important environmental sources of oxidative stress. Environmental dispersal of oxidative transition metals such as iron (37) and cadmium (Cd) (38–40) can cause acute toxicities. Cd is especially important as a contaminant in the diet because it is a common pollutant associated with industrialization and natural recycling of wastes as fertilizers. Cd was found to be increasing in some agricultural areas of southern Sweden at a rate of 1% per year. The biologic half-life of Cd in humans is about 20 years because of limited excretion. Pharmaceuticals (41), drugs of abuse, and chemicals from commercial products and industrial wastes (42, 43) also provide exogenous sources of oxidative stress. Ames (44) emphasized that natural toxicants in food pose a much greater risk than do manufactured sources. Although this may be generally true, the apparent increase in food borne toxicants, which cannot be compensated for by better nutrition, indicates an important need for nutrition and food scientists to limit sources of such contaminants.

Endogenous Superoxide and Peroxide Production

The most actively studied areas of nutrition and oxidative stress have involved endogenous oxidant generation and the failure of endogenous antioxidant defenses (see Fig. 46.1). This includes damaging processes that result from central oxidative metabolism processes in cells. The major macromolecules of cells (protein, nucleic acids, lipids, carbohydrates) are composed mostly of carbon, hydrogen, oxygen, nitrogen, phosphorus, and sulfur—elements that form stable chemical structures in which pairs of electrons are shared between elemental nuclei. The interconversion of these biochemicals mostly involves conservation of the pairs of electrons, with hydride ion transfer via reduced nicotinamide adenine dinucleotide/oxidized nicotinamide adenine dinucleotide ($NADH/NAD^+$) or NADH/oxidized nicotinamide adenine dinucleotide phosphate ($NADP^+$) (see Fig. 46.4) providing a common mechanism for 2-electron ($2\text{-}e^-$) transfer. These electron transfers occur in highly specific reactions, many of which have relatively high rates to support critical needs for energy metabolism, anabolism and repair, detoxification, and elimination of wastes.

Oxidant Production in Energy Metabolism

These $2\text{-}e^-$-transfer reactions linked to $NADH/NAD^+$ and $NADPH/NADP^+$ are connected to one-electron ($1\text{-}e^-$) transfer reactions in metabolic pathways through chemical structures that exist in interconvertible fully oxidized, $1\text{-}e^-$-reduced and $2\text{-}e^-$-reduced forms (see Fig. 46.4). These include hydroquinone/semiquinone/quinone and flavoprotein systems, with coenzyme Q providing an example of the former and the flavin mononucleotide (FMN) of mitochondrial NADH dehydrogenase providing an example of the latter. Living organisms use 1-electron chemistry in central energy capture and trans-fer reactions of photosynthesis and mitochondrial respiration. These $1\text{-}e^-$ transfers are physically contained within special membrane structures of chloroplasts and mitochondria. These features support the oxidation of macromolecular energy sources (fat, carbohydrate, and protein) through $2\text{-}e^-$ transfers with coupling to $1\text{-}e^-$ transfer pathways for production of adenosine triphosphate (ATP). The $1\text{-}e^-$ systems of mitochondria and chloroplasts are important in oxidative stress because these systems have very high electron transfer rates; are sensitive to visible and UV light, trace metals, oxidants, and reactive electrophiles; and cause extensive destruction to other biologic components.

Photosynthetic plants are rich sources of radical scavenging antioxidants, likely because of their need to control radical injury from sunlight while using the light-derived energy to drive photosynthesis and O_2 production. In contrast, mitochondria have high rates of electron transfer and require O_2 for ATP production. In both chloroplasts and mitochondria, damaged or malfunctioning electron transfer pathways represent a major source of endogenous oxidative stress.

Disruption of mitochondrial electron transfer has been extensively studied as a contributing mechanism in aging and disease. Damaged mitochondria have increased rates of $1\text{-}e^-$ transfer O_2 to produce the radical, superoxide anion ($O_2^{-\cdot}$). Hundreds of studies have shown that disruption of mitochondrial function, by many experimental means, results in injury and disease symptoms. Copper deficiency results in aberrant megamitochondria (45). The anticancer drug doxorubicin and antiretroviral drugs used for human immunodeficiency virus (HIV) infection treatment cause mitochondrial damage (46, 47). Such conditions often damage mitochondrial DNA, and increase ROS generation, so such conditions can be self-perpetuating and autocatalytic in destruction of mitochondria. However, evidence that one can protect against mitochondrial oxidative stress by nutritional or dietary antioxidant supplementation in humans is limited.

Mitochondria have multiple defense systems to protect against excessive oxidant generation, and these may be more critically dependent on the adequacy of precursors for NADPH supply than on supplementation with radical scavengers. Endogenous defenses include the electron transfer intermediate, coenzyme Q (48), which exists in the mitochondrial inner membrane in a stable, radical form (semiquinone) that protects against radical reactions. Mitochondria also contain specific GSH and thioredoxin (Trx) systems (49, 50). Pharmacologic forms of coenzyme Q show some promise of benefit in protecting mitochondria, but nutritional forms of coenzyme Q do not appear to be effectively delivered to mitochondrial inner membranes. Both GSH and Trx systems depend on adequate dietary selenium and riboflavin, although excesses of these are considered likely to be harmful, rather than to enhance activity further.

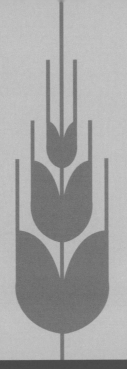

PART III

NUTRITIONAL NEEDS AND ASSESSMENT DURING THE LIFE CYCLE AND PHYSIOLOGIC CHANGES

48 BODY COMPOSITION[1]

SCOTT GOING, MELANIE HINGLE, AND JOSHUA FARR

A person's composition reflects his or her net lifetime accumulation of nutrients and other substrates acquired from the environment and retained in the body. These components, ranging from elements to tissues and organs, are the building blocks that give mass and shape and confer function to all living things. Body composition assessment methods allow scientists to describe how these components function and change with age, growth, and metabolic state. Clinicians rely on body composition measurements for diagnosis, judging disease risk, and determining efficacy of therapies to improve clinical outcomes. Serial body composition measurements are a reliable indicator of nutritional recovery from uncomplicated malnutrition or illness. Simple anthropometric measurements such as height (HT), weight (WT), and body mass index (BMI), as well as percent fat or lean mass, can be used to assess an individual's status against a standard, or relative to that person's "usual" over a specified period of time. These simple measures allow early detection of nutrient deficiencies or inadequate nutrient intake so that nutritional status can be improved through an individualized nutrition plan before disease occurs.

There is considerable interest in defining normal changes in human body composition during growth, maturation, and senescence. Defining normal is vital to understanding abnormal, which is associated with disease. This proposition is challenging, given the large variation that occurs within and among healthy individuals and the difficulty separating age-related from disease-related changes in older persons. Typically, descriptions of normal age trajectories have been based on a composite built on data from multiple studies that are usually cross-sectional, employ different methods, and are not population based (1). Few large-scale, population-based studies have been conducted to describe normal because of the cost and complexity of accurate body composition methods. Some reference data have been developed using anthropometry, dual-energy x-ray absorptiometry (DXA), and bioelectric impedance measurements obtained in the National Health and Nutrition Examination Survey (NHANES) (2). The anthropometric data have been used to describe age trajectories in the measured variables (e.g., HT, WT, and skinfolds) and estimates of composition. Chumlea et al (3) published reference data for body composition predicted using bioelectric impedance analysis (BIA) and Janssen et al (4) used BIA to develop reference data for predicted skeletal muscle (SM) mass. Laurson et al (5) developed percent body fat (PBF) growth curves for children and adolescents based on the NHANES III and IV surveys. These age trajectories should prove useful for defining typical changes in fatness in US boys and girls, although they are based on indirect, not direct, estimates of composition. Standards for adults are not well established.

---

[1]**Abbreviations: 3-MH**, 3-methylhistidine; **ADP**, air displacement plethysmography; **aLST**, appendicular lean soft tissue; **AT**, adipose tissue; **BCM**, body cell mass; **BD**, body density; **BIA**, bioelectric impedance analysis; **BM**, bone mineral; **BMI**, body mass index; **BV**, body volume; **CT**, computed tomography; **DXA**, dual-energy x-ray absorptiometry; **ECW**, extracellular water; **FFM**, fat-free mass; **FM**, fat mass; **HT**, height; **IBW**, ideal body weight; **ICW**, intracellular water; **LST**, lean soft tissue; **MRI**, magnetic resonance imaging; **NHANES**, National Health and Nutrition Examination Survey; **PBF**, percent body fat; **SAT**, subcutaneous adipose tissue; **SM**, skeletal muscle; **TBK**, total body potassium; **TBN**, total body nitrogen; **TBP**, total body protein; **TBW**, total body water; **UBW**, usual body weight; **VAT**, visceral adipose tissue; **WT**, weight.

BODY COMPOSITION

Five-Level Model

Approximately 50 elements in the body are organized into 100,000 chemical compounds, approximately 200 cell types, and 4 main tissues. The central model underlying body composition assessment is the five-level model (Table 48.1), in which body mass is considered as the sum of all components at atomic, molecular, cellular, tissue or organ, and whole body levels (6). Methods are available for measurement of components on each level, and the levels are interrelated so that components on one level can be used to estimate components on another level. Certain rules, reflecting these relationships, are inherent in the five-level model, and ultimately the accuracy of assessments depends on the validity of these rules.

Atomic Level

Body mass is composed of 11 major elements. Four of them—oxygen, carbon, hydrogen, and nitrogen—make up greater than 96% of body mass. The major elements are linked to higher level components. Other important elements are calcium, potassium, phosphorous, sulfur, sodium, chlorine, and magnesium. Most of these elements can be estimated in vivo by neutron activation analysis or whole body counting (7), research methods that are not widely used in clinical practice but are useful for establishing models underlying simpler methods. Total body carbon, total body nitrogen (TBN), and total body potassium (TBK) can be used with appropriate models to derive total

body fat (8), protein (8), and body cell mass (BCM) (9), although other approaches for estimating these components are more practical and widespread.

Molecular Level

The molecular level consists of six major components: water, lipid, protein, carbohydrates, bone minerals (BMs), and soft tissue minerals. Models having from two to six components can be created. The two-component, fat mass (FM) and fat-free mass (FFM) model, in which all nonlipid components are combined in FM, is most common. FFM is the actively metabolizing component and is often used as the reference for metabolic or functional indexes. Models with more than two compartments are called multicompartment models. These models divide the FFM into additional components that can be quantified in vivo. These models are used to minimize errors related to assumptions underlying the two-component model. In many situations, two-component models are not valid, such as in children, the elderly, and sick and infirm persons. Relying on fewer assumptions by measuring more components improves validity and accuracy, although they are more expensive, more burdensome, and the potential greater accuracy can be offset by greater measurement error if individual components are not measured accurately (10).

Cellular Level

Conceptually, the cellular level provides for multiple models based on different cell types. In practice, the most common model includes three components: extracellular

---

TABLE 48.1   MODELS AT DIFFERENT LEVELS OF BODY COMPOSITION AND RELATED EQUATIONS

LEVEL	MODEL	COMPONENTS (NO.)	EQUATION	REFERENCE (NO.)
Atomic	WT = 0 + C + H + N + Ca + P + K + S + Na + Cl + Mg	11		
Molecular	WT = F + W + P + M_s + M_o + G	6		
	WT = F + W + P + M	4	F = 2.747/BD − 0.714 (W) + 1.146 (M_o) − 2.0503	(117)
	WT = F + W + P + M	4	F = 2.75/BD − 0.714 (W) + 1.148 (M) − 2.05	(118)
	WT = F + W + solids	3	F = 2.118/BD − 0.78 (W) − 1.354	
	WT = F + M_o + residual	3	F = 6.386/BD + 3.961 (M) − 6.09	(40)
	WT = F + FFM	2	F = 4.95/BD − 4.50	(119)
		2	F = WT − TBK/2.66 (males); F = WT − TBK/2.51 (females)	
		2	F = WT − TBW/0.73	
Cellular	WT = CM + ECF + ECS	3		
	WT = FC + BCM + ECF + ECS	4	BCM = 0.00833 × TBK ECS = TBCa/0.177 ECF = (0.9 × TBC/plasma Cl)	
Tissue-system	WT = AT + SM + bone + blood + others			
Whole	WT = Head + neck + trunk + lower + extremities + upper extremities			

AT, adipose tissue; BCM, body cell mass; BD, body density; C, carbon; Ca, calcium; Cl, chloride; CM, cell mass; ECF, extracellular fluid; ECS, extracellular solids; F, fat; FC, fat cells; FFM, fat free mass; G, glycogen; H, hydrogen; K, potassium; M, mineral as a fraction of WT; Mg, magnesium; M_o, osseous mineral as a fraction of weight; M_s, cell mineral as a fraction of weight; N, nitrogen; Na, sodium; P, phosphorus; S, sulphur; SM, skeletal muscle; TBCa, total body calcium; TBK, total body potassium; TBW, total body water; W, water as a fraction of weight; WT, weight.

solids, extracellular fluid, and cells. The cellular mass can be divided further into two components, fat and BCM. BCM is the actively metabolizing component at the cellular level (11). The terms *fat* and *lipid* are often used interchangeably, although their meanings differ. In body composition assessment, lipid includes all of the biologic matter extracted with lipid solvents. These extracted lipids include triglycerides, phospholipids, and structural lipids that occur in small quantities in vivo (12). In contrast, fats refer to the specific family of lipids consisting of triglycerides (6). Based on reference man (13), approximately 90% of extractable lipids in healthy adults is triglyceride, although this proportion differs with dietary intake and illness (14). The remainder, approximately 10% of the total body lipid (nonfat lipid), are mainly composed of glycerophosphatides and sphingolipids.

Tissue–Organ Level

The major components on the tissue–organ level include adipose tissue (AT), SM, visceral organs, and bone. Some tissue–organ level components are single solid organs such as brain, heart, liver, and spleen. Others, such as SM and AT, are interspersed throughout the body. In common usage, fat and AT are often interchanged although they are distinct and on different levels, and the difference is important when measuring their mass and metabolic characteristics. Although fat is found primarily in AT, intracellular triglyceride pools are found in the liver, SM, and other organs, particularly in conditions such as hepatic steatosis and various forms of lipidosis. There are also small circulating extracellular pools of triglycerides, mainly as lipoproteins. AT consists of adipocytes, extracellular fluid, nerves, and blood vessels. AT compartments are distributed throughout the body, and their metabolic properties differ depending on location (15). AT compartments are closely linked with disease risk. Visceral AT (VAT) and its association with metabolic dysregulation and cardiovascular disease are perhaps the best studied, although ectopic fat in intramuscular and perivascular depots has also been linked to disease risk (15).

Whole Body Level

On the whole body level, composition is divided into regions such as appendages, trunk, and head. Rather than discrete components, trunk, and appendages are usually described by anthropometric measures such as circumferences, skeletal lengths, breadths, and skinfold thicknesses (16). Other whole body measures include body WT, volume, density, and electrical impedance. Anthropometric indexes have a long history of use as surrogates for body composition. Waist circumference, for example, has been used to predict obesity-related morbidity and mortality (17). Upper arm circumference, especially when corrected for subcutaneous AT, is a common index of nutritional status. Estimation of components on other levels (e.g., FM and FFM) is another common use of measures made on the whole body level.

The remainder of this chapter emphasizes description of the major components on the chemical, cellular, and tissue–organ levels, specifically body fat (or AT) and its anatomic distribution, and FFM, its main constituents, (BCM, water, SM, and bone), and the predominate methods used to measure them. These compartments have direct health and functional implications and some are used to index nutrient and energy needs. A comprehensive survey of other methods has been published in the literature (18). Anthropometric methods are discussed elsewhere in this volume.

Steady State

An important concept underlying body composition assessment is the notion that when body mass and energy stores are stable, the major components remain stable and thus maintain predictable interrelationships. Although components on the five levels are distinct, they are related and can be used to estimate components on the same and other levels. For example, assuming a constant ratio of total body protein (TBP) to TBN (TBP/TBN = 6.25), TBN (elemental level) can be used to estimate protein (chemical level). Similarly, BCM (cellular level) can be estimated from TBK (BCM = 0.00823 × TBK) and SM (tissue level) can be estimated from both TBK and TBN (SM = 0.0196 × TBK − 0.0261 × TBN). The premise of stable conversion factors used to estimate one component from another and the validity and accuracy of any method depends on the degree of departure from steady state.

HEIGHT AND BODY WEIGHT

Height

Skeletal size is a determinant of HT (19), which is correlated with FFM, the actively metabolizing cellular component and an important factor in estimating energy requirements. In adults, HT has been used to estimate ideal body WT (IBW) (20), which can be used to provide an estimate of daily nutrient needs to maintain a healthy WT for HT. Although body composition methods are needed to provide a precise estimate of metabolically active tissue, estimates such as these may be used to quickly calculate a reasonably accurate estimate of IBW in the field.

Body Weight

Body WT is used as an indirect measure of nutritional status because it is representative of body energy stores. Because of the tight regulation of carbohydrate and protein oxidation rates, any long-term changes in WT are assumed to reflect proportional changes in body fat stores. IBW is useful in establishing nutrient intake guidelines and setting parameters for a healthy WT range; however, an individual's usual body WT (UBW) (rather than IBW) may provide additional information useful for evaluating an individual's nutritional status. The difference between current and UBW or IBW may be compared against clinical parameters to determine risk of morbidity and mortality. Body WT typically varies less than ±0.1 kg/day in healthy adults. WT loss of more than 0.5 kg/day indicates negative energy or negative water balance or both. A clinically significant rate of WT loss is considered to be 1% to 2% over 1 week, 5% over 1 month, 7.5% over 3 months, or 10% or greater over 6 months (21). Severity of WT loss may also be evaluated by the absolute WT reduction, which also has prognostic value. An absolute WT of 85% to 95% of UBW (or 80% to 90% of IBW) indicates mild malnutrition, 75% to 84% of UBW (or 70% to 79% of IBW) indicates moderate malnutrition, and 75% or less of UBW (or ≤69% of IBW) indicates severe malnutrition (21). Absolute WT reduction to less than 55% to 60% of IBW places an individual at the limits of starvation (22). In infirm individuals, a WT loss between 10% and 20% of pre-illness WT over 6 months has been associated with functional abnormalities (23), whereas a loss of more than 20% of pre-illness WT suggests significant protein-energy malnutrition (23). The minimum survivable body WT in humans is between 48% and 55% of IBW or a BMI of approximately 13 kg/m^2.

Overconsumption of energy relative to requirements results in a positive energy balance which, if sustained, leads to WT gain and excess adiposity. Excess adiposity is associated with increased risk of morbidity and early mortality, because AT not only functions as a storage depot for excess energy, but also significantly influences endocrine function and metabolic and immune regulation. The maximum survivable body WT is approximately 500 kg (a BMI of ~150 kg/m^2) (24).

When using WT as an estimate of energy and protein needs, clinicians must consider factors that affect WT fluctuations or otherwise confound the assumption that WT is a surrogate of energy stores, such as rapid fluid shifts (intracellular to extracellular or intravascular to extravascular spaces) and accumulation of fluid secondary to inflammation. Edema and ascites and the medications used to treat them may cause fluid to shift to extracellular spaces, masking body composition changes and artificially increasing WT. Tumor growth or abnormal organ enlargement in disease states may cause an increase in WT and mask tissue loss (i.e., loss of fat or FFM). Morbidly obese individuals experiencing rapid, intentional WT loss may be at nutritional (and health) risk as WT (including lean mass and FM) decreases as a result of protein-calorie malnutrition and semistarvation. Finally, physical activity– or diet-induced changes in energy intake and expenditure affect glycogen mass (and its bound water) and body sodium, which is associated with fluid readjustment and WT fluctuations.

Body Mass Index

Ratios of WT to HT (WT/HT ratios) have a long history in studies of body habitus. BMI (WT, kg/HT, m^2) is the favored index because HT squared minimizes the relationship between HT and WT, at least in adults. Although not a direct measure of adiposity, BMI is a widely used surrogate for composition, based on the tenuous assumption that excess WT results from body fat. Although BMI and body fat are correlated, use of BMI as an "adiposity" index is confounded by differences in body proportions (e.g., trunk-to-leg length ratio), fat distribution, and composition relative to HT. Individuals with greater than average muscularity, for example, may be misclassified as overweight or obese, and elderly individuals may be considered normal WT obese (i.e., a normal WT despite muscle and bone loss because of added FM). In addition, composition and location of excess WT vary with gender, race, and age, information not captured by BMI (25). Despite these limitations, BMI predicts disease risk and standard definitions of overweight and obesity are in use (Table 48.2). Revised definitions have been proposed for Asians, who clearly have a different BMI–adiposity relationship (26).

TABLE 48.2	BODY MASS INDEX AND WAIST CIRCUMFERENCE CUTOFF POINTS AND RISK OF DISEASE		
BMI (kg/m^2)^a	OBESITY CLASS	MEN ≤102 cm (≤40 in) WOMEN ≤88 cm (≤35 in)	MEN >102 cm (>40 in) WOMEN >88 cm (>35 in)+
<16	Grade III protein-energy malnutrition	—	—
16.0–16.9	Grade II protein-energy malnutrition	—	—
17.0–18.5	Underweight (grade I protein-energy malnutrition)	—	—
18.5–24.9	Normal	—	—
25.0–29.9	Overweight	Increased	High
30.0–34.9	Class I obese	High	Very high
35.0–39.9	Class II obese	Very high	Very high
≥40	Class III severe obesity	Extremely high	Extremely high

BMI, body mass index.

^{a}BMI cutoff points represent World Health Organization standard for international classification, although cutoff points of 23, 27.5, 32.5, and 37.5 kg/m^2 have been suggested for Asian populations as points for public health action (26).

Adapted from the National Heart, Lung, and Blood Institute. Guidelines on Overweight and Obesity. Available at: http://www.nhlbi.nih.gov/guidelines/obesity/e_txtbk/txgd/4142.htm, with permission.

Differential changes in fat and FFM in boys and girls confound interpretation of BMI. Consequently, gender-specific, BMI-for-age percentiles are used in children and youth. Revised BMI growth charts for US youth were constructed with data from the NHANES surveys conducted before the rapid rise in pediatric obesity (27). The charts provide practical tools for clinicians to compare the growth of a child against the reference population and make inferences about nutritional status and risk with regard to overweight and obesity (28). In boys and girls less than 18 years old, underweight, overweight, and obesity are defined as age- and gender-specific BMI less than 5th, greater than 85th to less than 95th, and greater than or equal to 95th percentiles, respectively (29).

FAT FREE MASS

FFM is a heterogeneous compartment on the chemical level of analysis. Its primary constituents of intracellular and extracellular fluid, protein, and osseous and nonosseous minerals can be combined to form various models on which assessment methods are based (see Table 48.1). Historically, FFM has been estimated most commonly from body density (BD) estimated by underwater weighing (30), TBK estimated by whole body counting (7), and total body water (TBW) estimated by hydrometry (31). Each approach relies on a conversion factor based on an assumption of a constant relationship between the measured component and FFM. In healthy young adults, the assumption of chemical constancy introduces relatively little error. However, significant changes in FFM components with growth and maturation, aging, and illness are well described (1, 32–34) and introduce significant error unless appropriate adjustments are made. Gender and race or ethnicity differences are known (35) as well as effects of physical training (36). It is imperative that use of constants and equations be restricted to the groups for which they were developed unless their validity in another group has been shown. Alternatively, and especially when the condition of steady state is not met, application of multiple component models improves accuracy (37), although the requirement for more measures increases cost and patient burden and limits their use.

Densitometry

Historically, hydrodensitometry (underwater weighing) was used to estimate body volume (BV) and BD, which was converted to estimates of PBF and FFM (30). For young children, the elderly, and infirm, disabled, and other special populations, complete submersion in water is very difficult, if not impossible. An alternative approach, air displacement plethysmography (ADP), uses pressure–volume relationships to estimate BV and BD. The most recent form of ADP, the Bod Pod (COSMED USA, Inc. [formerly Life Measurements, Inc.], Concord, CA), provides a reliable means of determining BV (38, 39) and eliminates the need for submersion in water. The procedure can be performed by children and adults, although it does require a breathing maneuver to measure thoracic gas volume that may be difficult for young children and patients with pulmonary disease.

A major source of error in densitometry is the model used to convert BD to composition. In the classic two-component model, the densities of fat and FFM are assumed to be 0.9 and 1.1 g/mL, respectively. Using these densities, it is possible to derive an equation for estimating percent fat from BD (see Table 48.1). The density of FFM is derived from its primary constituents, water, protein, and mineral, as well as their respective fractions and densities (Table 48.3). The more closely the FFM components and their densities fit the individual being measured, the more accurate the result will be.

Many studies have demonstrated considerable variation in FFM composition and thus density attributed to growth and maturation (40), aging (41), and specialized

TABLE 48.3	FAT FREE BODY COMPOSITION AND DENSITY IN CHILDREN AND YOUTH					
	MALE			FEMALE		
AGE (y)	TBW/FFM (%)	M_O/FFM (%)	DFFM (g/cc)	TBW/FFM (%)	M_O/FFM (%)	DFFM (g/cc)
1	79.0	3.7	1.068	78.8	3.7	1.069
1–2	78.6	4.0	1.071	78.5	3.9	1.071
2–4	77.8	4.3	1.075	78.3	4.2	1.073
5–6	77.0	4.8	1.079	78.0	4.6	1.075
7–8	76.8	5.1	1.081	77.6	4.9	1.079
9–10	76.2	5.4	1.084	77.0	5.2	1.082
11–12	75.4	5.7	1.087	76.6	5.5	1.086
13–14	74.7	6.2	1.094	75.5	5.9	1.092
15–16	74.2	6.5	1.096	75.0	6.1	1.094
17–20	74.0	—	1.098	74.8	—	1.095
20–25	73.8	—	1.100	74.5	—	1.096

DFFM, density of fat free mass; FFM, fat free mass; M_o, osseous mineral as a fraction of weight; TBW, total body water.

Data from Boileau et al (120), Fomon et al (55), Haschke et al (121, 122), Lohman et al (123, 124), with permission, with some modifications of the estimates of Fomon et al (55) to provide for linear changes in body water and bone mineral with age.

training (42). Sex and racial differences also exist, and even within a population, considerable interindividual variation (37) invalidates the assumption of FFM chemical constancy. Consequently, multicomponent models (three-component and four-component models; see Table 48.1), which require fewer assumptions because more components are measured, are more accurate than the two-component model. In children and in patients with edema, combining a measure of TBW along with BD significantly improves estimation of FFM; similarly, in elderly patients and in patients with significant bone loss, combining a measure of body mineral with BD gives a more accurate estimate of FFM. When a multicomponent model is not feasible, accuracy can be improved by using a population-specific equation that has been adjusted for the anticipated changes that occur with growth, maturation, and aging (Table 48.4).

Whole Body Counting and Total Body Potassium

Potassium is mainly an intracellular ion that can be measured by whole body ^{40}K counting (7). Reproducibility of measurements is good, even in children weighing 20 to 25 kg (43). TBK is useful for estimating BCM, TBP (44–46), and SM mass (47, 48), although it is more commonly used to estimate FFM using a two-component model (25) in which TBK resides in FFM. This model assumes a stable TBK/FFM ratio; however, as the SM fraction of FFM increases during growth, the TBK/FFM ratio increases. These changes lead to complexities in developing appropriate model coefficients. In young healthy adults, the TBK/FFM ratios in men (2.66 g, K/kg FFM) and women (2.55 g, K/kg FFM) are well established and reasonably stable. In children, use of the adult TBK/FFM ratio underestimates FFM (49). In older adults, and the infirm with muscle loss (sarcopenia), a similar problem occurs.

Hydrometry and Total Body Water

On the molecular level, the water compartment consists of a singular molecular species, hydrogen oxide, which lends itself to the use of the isotope dilution principle for assessment of TBW. Although several tracers have been used, isotopes of water (radioactive tritium oxide, deuterium oxide, and oxygen-18 hydride) provide the most precise and accurate estimates of TBW (31). TBW is used in models to estimate body composition on the molecular, cellular, and tissue levels (see Table 48.1), although estimation of FFM based on the two-component model that restricts all water to FFM is the most common component estimated from TBW. Its calculation assumes constant hydration of FFM. This assumption is clearly incorrect in individuals who either are dehydrated or have abnormal water metabolism leading to edema. Among healthy adults, TBW is relatively constant and FFM is estimated assuming its water proportion is 73% (FFM = TBW/0.73). Infants and children have higher TBW/FFM ratios, and age-appropriate hydration constants must be used to estimate FFM (see Table 48.3). Malnourished patients with severe protein depletion may have hydration factors as high as 75% (50), and disease states that alter water metabolism producing edema also result in higher hydration constants (51). Some healthy groups also have higher TBW/FFM; for example, bodybuilders with expanded SM compartments have hydration constants elevated by 2% to 3% (52). This occurs not because of greater hydration in itself but because of a larger SM fraction of FFM. Pregnancy also results in an increase in hydration that depends on the trimester (53).

Dual-Energy X-Ray Absorptiometry

DXA is widely available and easily performed on most persons thus making it an attractive method for clinical studies. Because scan times are short and radiation exposure is low, this technique is acceptable for use in children, although very young children may need to be sedated. The main limitations are the WT limits of the scanners and errors related to larger patient size (54). Also, hardware and software differences exist across scanners, even from the same manufacturer, and longitudinal studies must be done using the same scanner and software (54).

The DXA method provides estimates of three main chemical level components: fat, lean soft tissue (LST), and BM. The LST includes two primary components at the cellular level, BCM and extracellular fluid. FFM is estimated as the sum of LST and BM. Both LST and BCM increase with age, although at different rates, such that the BCM component increases relative to LST with greater age during development (55, 56). Thus, LST is not metabolically homogeneous with respect to age in children, and results must be interpreted accordingly.

Like all indirect methods, DXA relies on assumptions of tissue constancy that may not always be accurate.

TABLE 48.4	EQUATIONS[a] FOR ESTIMATING PERCENTAGE OF FAT FROM BODY DENSITY IN CHILDREN AND YOUTH			
	MALES		FEMALES	
AGE (y)	C_1	C_2	C_1	C_2
1	5.72	5.36	5.69	5.33
1–2	5.64	5.26	5.65	5.26
3–4	5.53	5.14	5.58	5.20
5–6	5.43	5.03	5.53	5.14
7–8	5.38	4.97	5.43	5.03
9–10	5.30	4.89	5.35	4.95
11–12	5.23	4.81	5.25	4.84
13–14	5.07	4.64	5.12	4.69
15–16	5.03	4.59	5.07	4.64
18	4.95	4.50	5.05	4.62

[a]Adjusted for average changes in water, protein and mineral fractions of fat-free mass with growth and maturation (see Table 48.3). The C_1 and C_2 terms are derived from the general equation for estimating the percentage of fat from body density:

%Fat = $1/BD$ $[(d_1 d_2) / (d_1 - d_2)] - [d_2 / (d_1 - d_2)] \times 100$
where BD = body density, d_1 = density of fat-free mass, and d_2 = density of fat = 0.90 (g/cc) for all age groups, %Fat = $[C_1/BD - C_2] \times 100$

13. Snyder WS, Cook MJ, Nasset ES et al. Report of the Task Group on Reference Man. Oxford: Pergamon Press, 1984.

14. Comizio R, Pietrobelli A, Tan YX et al. Am J Physiol 1998;274:E860–6.

15. Going SB, Hingle M, De Meester F et al, eds. Physical activity in diet-induced disease causation and prevention in women and men. In: Modern Dietary Fat Intakes in Disease Promotion. Totowa, NJ: Humana Press, 2010:443–54.

16. Frisancho AR. Anthropometric Standards: An Interactive Nutritional Reference of Body Size and Body Composition for Children and Adults. Ann Arbor, MI: The University of Michigan Press, 2008.

17. Sardinha LB, Teixeira PJ. Measuring adiposity and fat distribution in relation to health. In: Heymsfield SB, Lohman TG, Wang ZM et al, eds. Human Body Composition. 2nd ed. Champaign, IL: Human Kinetics, 2005:177–201.

18. Heymsfield S, Lohman TG, Wang ZM et al, eds. Human Body Composition. 2nd ed. Champaign, IL: Human Kinetics, 2005:1–414.

19. Borisov BK, Marei AN. Health Phys 1974;27:224–9.

20. Hamwi G. Changing dietary concepts. In: Danowski TS, ed. Diabetes Mellitus: Diagnosis and Treatment, vol 1. New York: American Diabetes Association, 1964:73–8.

21. Blackburn GL, Bistrian BR, Maini BS et al. JPEN J Parenter Enteral Nutr 1977;1:11–22.

22. Heymsfield SB, Baumgartner RN, Pan SF. Nutritional assessment of malnutrition by anthropometric methods. In: Shils ME, Olson JA, Shike M. Modern Nutrition in Health and Disease. 9th ed. Baltimore: Lippincott Williams & Wilkins, 1999:903–21.

23. Pietrobelli A, Allison DB, Heshka S et al. Int J Obes Relat Metab Disord 2002;26:1339–48.

24. Heymsfield S, Baumgartner RN. Body composition and anthropometry. In: Shils ME, Shike M, Ross AC et al, eds. Modern Nutrition in Health and Disease. 10th ed. Baltimore: Lippincott Williams & Wilkins, 2005:751–70.

25. Forbes GB. Nutr Rev 1987;45:225–31.

26. World Health Organization. Lancet 2004;363:157.

27. National Center for Health Statistics (NCHS). CDC Growth Charts: United States. Available at: http://www.cdc.gov/growthcharts/background.htm. Accessed August 15, 2012.

28. Kuczmarski RJ, Ogden CL, Guo SS et al. Vital Health Stat 2002;11:1–190.

29. Barlow SE. Pediatrics 2007;120(Suppl 4):S164–92.

30. Going SB. Hydrodensitometry and air displacement plethysmography. In: Heymsfield SB, Lohman TG, Wang ZM et al, eds. Human Body Composition. 2nd ed. Champaign, IL: Human Kinetics, 2005:17–33.

31. Schoeller DA. Hydrometry. In: Heymsfield SB, Lohman TG, Wang ZM et al, eds. Human Body Composition. 2nd ed. Champaign, IL: Human Kinetics, 2005:35–49.

32. Sopher A, Shen W, Pietrobelli A. Pediatric body composition methods. In: Heymsfield SB, Lohman TG, Wang ZM et al, eds. Human Body Composition. 2nd ed. Champaign, IL: Human Kinetics, 2005:129–39.

33. Kotler DP, Engelson ES. Body composition studies in people with HIV. In: Heymsfield SB, Lohman TG, Wang ZM et al, eds. Human Body Composition. 2nd ed. Champaign, IL: Human Kinetics, 2005:377–87.

34. Janssen I, Roubenoff R. Inflammatory diseases and body composition. In: Heymsfield SB, Lohman TG, Wang ZM et al, eds. Human Body Composition. 2nd ed. Champaign, IL: Human Kinetics, 2005:389–400.

35. Malina RM. Variation in body composition associated with sex and ethnicity. In: Heymsfield SB, Lohman TG, Wang ZM et al, eds. Human Body Composition. 2nd ed. Champaign, IL: Human Kinetics, 2005:271–98.

36. Williams DP, Teixeira PJ, Going SB. Exercise. In: Heymsfield SB, Lohman TG, Wang ZM et al, eds. Human Body Composition. 2nd ed. Champaign, IL: Human Kinetics, 2005:313–30.

37. Wang Z, Shen W, Withers RT et al. Multicomponent molecular-levels models of body composition analysis. In: Heymsfield SB, Lohman TG, Wang ZM et al, eds. Human Body Composition. 2nd ed. Champaign, IL: Human Kinetics, 2005:163–75.

38. Dempster P, Aitkens S. Med Sci Sports Exerc 1995;27:1692–7.

39. Sly PD, Lanteri C, Bates JH. Pediatr Pulmonol 1990;8:203–8.

40. Lohman TG. Exerc Sport Sci Rev 1986;14:325–57.

41. Going S, Williams D, Lohman T. Exerc Sport Sci Rev 1995;23:411–58.

42. Modlesky CM, Cureton KJ, Lewis RD et al. J Appl Physiol 1996;80:2085–96.

43. Schneider S, Kolesnik JA, Wang J et al. Total body potassium (TBK) measurement: accuracy, efficiency, and reproducibility. Presented at the Experimental Biology meeting, San Francisco, April 1998.

44. Butte N, Heinz C, Hopkinson J et al. J Pediatr Gastroenterol Nutr 1999;29:184–9.

45. Butte NF, Hopkinson JM, Wong WW et al. Pediatr Res 2000;47:578–85.

46. Wang Z, Shen W, Kotler DP et al. Am J Clin Nutr 2003;78:979–84.

47. Wang ZM, Visser M, Ma R et al. J Appl Physiol 1996;80:824–31.

48. Wang Z, Zhu S, Wang J et al. Am J Clin Nutr 2003;77:76–82.

49. Lohman TG. Advances in Human Body Composition. Champaign, IL: Human Kinetics, 1992.

50. Beddoe AH, Streat SJ, Hill GL. Am J Physiol 1985;249:E227–33.

51. Keys A, Brozek J. Physiol Rev 1953;33:245–325.

52. Modlesky CM, Cureton KJ, Lewis RD et al. J Appl Physiol 1996;80:2085–96.

53. Sohlstrom A, Forsum E. Am J Clin Nutr 1997;66:1315–22.

54. Lohman TG, Chen Z. Dual-energy x-ray absorptiometry. In: Heymsfield SB, Lohman TG, Wang ZM et al, eds. Human Body Composition. 2nd ed. Champaign, IL: Human Kinetics, 2005:63–77.

55. Fomon SJ, Haschke F, Ziegler EE et al. Am J Clin Nutr 1982;35:1169–75.

56. Sopher A, Shen W, Pietrobelli A. Pediatric body composition methods. In: Heymsfield SB, Lohman TG, Wang ZM et al, eds. Human Body Composition. 2nd ed. Champaign, IL: Human Kinetics, 2005:129–39.

57. Pietrobelli A, Formica C, Wang Z et al. Am J Physiol 1996;271:E941–51.

58. Pietrobelli A, Faith MS, Allison DB et al. J Pediatr 1998;132:204–10.

59. Laskey MA, Flaxman ME, Barber RW et al. Br J Radiol 1991;64:1023–9.

60. Lohman TG, Harris M, Teixeira PJ et al. Ann N Y Acad Sci 2000;904:45–54.

61. Heyward VH, Stolarczyk LM. Applied Body Composition Assessment. 2nd ed. Champaign, IL: Human Kinetics, 2004.

62. Chumlea WC, Sun SS. Bioelectrical impedance analysis. In: Heymsfield SB, Lohman TG, Wang ZM et al, eds. Human Body Composition. 2nd ed. Champaign, IL: Human Kinetics, 2005:79–87.

63. Kushner RF, Roxe DM. Am J Kidney Dis 2002;39:154–8.

64. Sun SS, Chumlea WC, Heymsfield SB et al. Am J Clin Nutr 2003;77:331–40.

65. Lohman TG, Caballero B, Himes JH et al. Int J Obes Relat Metab Disord 2000;24:982–8.

66. O'Brien C, Young AJ, Sawka MN. Int J Sports Med 2002l;23:361–6.

67. Chen Z. Body composition and cancer. In: Heymsfield SB, Lohman TG, Wang ZM et al, eds. Human Body Composition. 2nd ed. Champaign, IL Human Kinetics, 2005:351–64.

68. Chertow GM, Lazarus JM, Lew NL et al. Kidney Int 1997;51: 1578–82.

69. Barak N, Wall-Alonso E, Cheng A et al. JPEN J Parenter Enteral Nutr 2003;27:43–6.

70. Bartok-Olson CJ, Schoeller DA, Sullivan JC et al. Ann N Y Acad Sci 2000;904:342–4.

71. Ellis KJ. Biol Trace Elem Res 1990;26–27:385–400.

72. International Commission on Radiological Protection. Report of the Task Group on Reference Man. ICRP report 23. New York: International Commission on Radiological Protection, 1984.

73. Burmeister W. Science 1965;148:1336–7.

74. Pierson RN Jr, Wang J. Mayo Clin Proc 1988;63:947–9.

75. Ellis KJ, Shukla KK, Cohn SH et al. J Lab Clin Med 1974;83:716–27.

76. Pierson RN Jr, Wang J, Heymsfield SB et al. Am J Physiol 1991;261:E103–.

77. Edelman IS, Leibman J. Am J Med 1959;27:256–77.

78. Schober O, Lehr L, Hundeshagen H. Eur J Nucl Med 1982;7:14–5.

79. Barac-Nieto M, Spurr GB, Lotero H et al. Am J Clin Nutr 1979;32:981–91.

80. Bulcke JA, Termote JL, Palmers Y et al. Neuroradiology 1979;17:127–36.

81. Mategrano VC, Petasnick J, Clark J et al. Radiology 1977;125:135–40.

82. Snyder WS, Cook MJ, Nasset ES et al. Report of the Task Group on Reference Man. Oxford: Pergamon Press, 1975.

83. Baumgartner RN, Koehler KM, Gallagher D et al. Am J Epidemiol 1998;147:755–63.

84. Talbot NB. Am. J. Dis. Child. 55:42.

85. Cheek DB. Human Growth: Body Composition, Cell Growth, Energy and Intelligence. Philadelphia: Lea & Febiger, 1968.

86. Elia M, Carter A, Smith R. Br J Nutr 1979;42:567–70.

87. Tomas FM, Ballard FJ, Pope LM. Clin Sci (Lond) 1979;56: 341–6.

88. Cohn SH, Vartsky D, Yasumura S et al. Am J Physiol 1980;239: E524–30.

89. Lukaski HC. Assessing muscle mass. In: Heymsfield SB, Lohman TG, Wang ZM, Going SB, eds. Human Body Composition. 2nd ed. Champaign, IL: Human Kinetics, 2005:203–18.

90. Rennie MJ, Millward DJ. Clin Sci (Lond) 1983;65:217–25.

91. Kvist H, Sjostrom L, Tylen U. Int J Obes 1986;10:53–67.

92. Sjostrom L. Int J Obes 1991;15(Suppl 2):19–30.

93. Tsubahara A, Chino N, Akaboshi K et al. Disabil Rehabil 1995;17:298–304.

94. Schick F, Machann J, Brechtel K et al. Magn Reson Med 2002;47:720–7.

95. Boesch C, Kreis R. Ann N Y Acad Sci 2000;904:25–31.

96. Boesch C, Slotboom J, Hoppeler H et al. Magn Reson Med 1997;37:484–93.

97. Goodpaster BH, Thaete FL, Simoneau JA et al. Diabetes 1997;46:1579–85.

98. Jacob S, Machann J, Rett K et al. Diabetes 1999;48:1113–9.

99. Perseghin G, Scifo P, De Cobelli F et al. Diabetes 1999; 48:1600–6.

100. Forbes GB. The companionship of lean and fat: some lessons from body composition studies. In: Whitehead RG, Prentice A, eds. New Techniques in Nutritional Research. New York: Academic Press, 1991.

101. Baumgartner RN. Ann N Y Acad Sci 2000;904:437–48.

102. Roubenoff R. Eur J Clin Nutr 2000;54(Suppl 3):S40–7.

103. Mott JW, Wang J, Thornton JC et al. Am J Clin Nutr 1999;69:1007–13.

104. Lohman TG. Advances in Body Composition Assessment. Current issues in exercise science series: monograph no. 3. Champaign, IL: Human Kinetics, 1992.

105. Laurson KR, Eisenmann JC, Welk GJ. Am J Prev Med 2011;41(4 Suppl 2):S87–92.

106. Jensen MD. Obesity (Silver Spring) 2006;14(Suppl 1):20S–24S.

107. Adams LA, Lymp JF, St Sauver J et al. Gastroenterology 2005;129:113–21.

108. Heaney RP, Abrams S, Dawson-Hughes B et al. Osteoporos Int 2000;11:985–1009.

109. Reid IR. Osteoporos Int 21008;9:595–606.

110. Gilsanz V, Chalfant J, Mo AO et al. J. Clin Endocrinol Metab 2009;94:3387–93.

111. Farr JN, Funk JL, Chen Z et al. J Bone Miner Res, 2011;26:2217–25.

112. Janghorbani M, Van Dam RM, Willett WC et al. Am J Epidemiol 2007;166:495–506.

113. Jensen LB, Quaade F, Sorensen OH. J Bone Miner Res 1994;9:459–63.

114. Wacker W, Barden HS. Pediatric Reference Data for male and female total body and spine BMD and BMC. Presented at ISCD Annual Meeting, Dallas, TX, March 2001.

115. Looker AC, Wahner HW, Dunn WL et al. Osteoporos Int 1998;8:468–89.

116. Assessment of fracture risk and its application to screening for postmenopausal osteoporosis. Report of a WHO Study Group. World Health Organ Tech Rep Ser 1994;843:1–129.

117. Selinger A. The body as a three component system. Doctoral dissertation. Urbana: The University of Illinois, 1977.

118. Siri WE. Body composition from fluid spaces and density: analysis of methods. In: Brozek J, Henschel A, eds. Techniques for Measuring Body Composition. Washington, DC: National Academy of Sciences, 1961:223–44.

119. Siri WE. The gross composition of the body. In: Tobias CA, Lawrence JH, eds. Advances in Biological and Medical Physics. New York: Academic Press, 1956:239–80.

120. Boileau RA, Lohman TG, Slaughter MH. Scand J Sports Sci 1987:17.

121. Haschke F, Fomon SJ, Ziegler EE. Pediatr Res 1981;15:847–9.

122. Haschke F. Acta Paediatr Scand 1983;307(Suppl):11.

123. Lohman TG, Boileau RA, Slaughter MH. Body composition in children and youth. In: Boileau RA, ed. Advances in Pediatric Sport Sciences. Champaign, IL: Human Kinetics, 1984:29–57.

124. Lohman TG, Slaughter MH, Boileau RA et al. Hum Biol 1984;56:667–79.

125. Janssen I, Heymsfield SB, Baumgartner RN et al. J Appl Physiol 2000;89:465–71.

SUGGESTED READINGS

Forbes GB. Human Body Composition. Growth, Aging, Nutrition, and Activity. New York: Springer, 1987.

Heymsfield SB, Lohman TG, Wang Z et al, eds. Human Body Composition. 2nd ed. Champaign, IL: Human Kinetics, 2005.

Heyward V, Wagner D. Applied Body Composition Assessment. 2nd ed. Champaign, IL: Human Kinetics, 2004.

49 USE AND INTERPRETATION OF ANTHROPOMETRY

YOUFA WANG, HYUNJUNG LIM, AND BENJAMIN CABALLERO

Anthropometry is defined as the measurement of humans for the purposes of understanding human physical variation. Anthropometric measures have been widely used for the assessment of nutritional and health conditions such as body composition (BC), malnutrition, and obesity. Changes in lifestyle, nutrition, and ethnic composition of populations lead to changes in body dimensions and BC. Anthropometric measures are more widely used in children than adults considering the routine needs of assessing growth (1, 2). The World Health Organization (WHO) has developed guidelines and growth references

to provide guidance on the use and interpretation of anthropometric measures (1, 2). At present, weight and height are the most widely used anthropometric measurements, and their derivative, the body mass index (BMI), is the most commonly used indirect indicator of obesity and body adiposity (3–5).

This chapter describes the most commonly used anthropometric measurements, the indices derived from them, and the use and interpretation of these. Advances in developing growth standards and reference charts are discussed. Another chapter provides a detailed description of BC techniques.

COMMONLY USED ANTHROPOMETRIC MEASURE INDICES

The commonly used anthropometric measures in adults and children include weight, height, waist circumferences (WC), skinfold thickness (measured on different body sites), and a set of weight-for-height indices such as BMI. Often such measures or a combination of them are used as indicators of BC, such as percentage of body fat (%BF). These measures and their strengths and limitations are summarized in Table 49.1. Note that underwater weighing and dual-energy x-ray absorptiometry (DXA) are considered the gold standards for BC assessment.

Several studies have assessed the validity of anthropometric measures such as BMI, WC, and skinfold thickness for estimating body fat using DXA as the reference method. Results indicate modest to excellent agreement, with correlations ranging from 0.37 to 0.99 in adults (6–8) and children (9). The agreement is stronger in healthy subjects ($R > .97$) (8). One study found that accuracy of most of the skinfold thickness equations for assessment of body fat at the individual level was poor in 13- to 17-year-old adolescents compared with DXA (10). Others found that skinfold thickness measures are better predictors of %BF than other simple anthropometric methods such as BMI (11). In Asian adolescents, clinical validity of weight- and height-based classification for obesity screening is poor when compared with that defined based on a %BF greater than or equal to the 95th percentile. According to Youden's index, a composite measure of accuracy indices indicating optimal sensitivity and

[1]**Abbreviations:** %BF, percentage of body fat; BC, body composition; BMI, body mass index; CDC, Centers for Disease Control and Prevention; CVD, cardiovascular disease; DXA, dual-energy x-ray absorptiometry; IDF, International Diabetes Federation; IOTF, International Obesity Task Force; LMS, least means squared; NCHS, National Center for Health Statistics; SD, standard deviation; WC, waist circumference; WHO, World Health Organization; WHtR, waist-to-height ratio.

TABLE 49.1	COMMONLY USED ANTHROPOMETRIC MEASURES AND THEIR MAIN STRENGTHS AND LIMITATIONS[a]		
	DEFINITION	STRENGTHS	LIMITATIONS
Weight	The sum of all body mass components	Predicting caloric expenditure and in indices of body composition Easy to use, inexpensive, safe	Not suitable for patients with some diseases such as kidney and heart diseases or liver cirrhosis with edema or ascites One needs to consider dehydration or amputation
Height	The distance from the heels to back of the head	Easy to measure Good indicator of child growth	Not suitable for young children <24 months old (should use length) or patients who cannot stand
Waist circumference	The distance around the smallest area below the rib cage and above the umbilicus using a nonstretched tape	Easy to measure Indicates abdominal fat contents Correlation with total fat mass and %BF Better predictor of many obesity-related diseases than BMI	Not useful for those <60 inches tall or with a BMI of ≥35 Different measurement protocols have been recommended, that is, how to position the tape
Skinfold thickness	The assessment of body fat amount (e.g., subcutaneous fat) at various body sites with caliper	The equipment is inexpensive and is portable Can indirectly estimate %BF or body composition using equations Correlate highly with hydrostatic weighing	Error of measurements depends on age, edema, muscle, several technical sources (e.g. examiner skill) Inaccurate if increasing obesity Not suitable for critical patients
BMI (kg/m^2)	A weight-for-height index, calculated as weight (kg)/height (m)^2	Cheap and easy to use High correlation with body fatness Good association with health outcomes Cut-points have been developed in adults and children	Cannot distinguish body fat mass and lean body mass May have different relationships with body fatness and health risk in different populations

[a]%BF, percentage of body fat; BMI, body mass index.

specificity rates, weight- and height-based classification only presented 48% in boys and 59% in girls (12).

A newer anthropometric index, the waist-to-height ratio (WHtR), has been proposed as a useful indicator of central obesity and for screening cardiovascular disease (CVD) risk (13, 14). The WHtR was strongly correlated with %BF and fat distribution, which are associated with increased CVD risks (15, 16). Some research has indicated that WHtR is independent of age and eliminates the need for percentiles for children (17, 18). A WHtR cut-point of 0.5 has been recommended to classify central obesity in adults and children and for different ethnic groups (14). For example, the optimal value for WHtR was 0.5 for Japanese adults and its sensitivities of various proposed obesity indices for identifying clustering of defined and other risk factors (13). Among children, the WHtR showed high sensitivity and specificity (>0.90) compared with WC in Chinese children (8 to 18 years old) (17). In a study of British children (5 to 16 years old), WHtR decreased with age (18); it also increased greatly during the past 10 to 20 years, and was found to be more closely related to morbidity than was BMI (18).

WC has been recommended by the WHO and the International Diabetes Federation (IDF) as a measure of central obesity, which is a key component for defining metabolic syndrome (19). Studies indicate that WC is a good predictor of the risks for a number chronic diseases, such as CVD and type 2 diabetes, and is often a better predictor than BMI (20). A set of sex- and ethnic-specific WC cut-points have been recommended for adults (19, 21–24); such as in men, 85 (Japan), 90 (by IDF for Asian and in countries such as China), 94 (Vietnam), 100 (France), and 102 (WHO international recommendation); and in women, 80 (by IDF), 85 (South Korea), 88 (WHO), and 90 (France and Japan). Previously, waist–hip ratio was used to measure central obesity, but later it was recommended that WC is adequate, whereas the ratio did not add much value.

DEVELOPMENT OF CUT-POINTS FOR ANTHROPOMETRIC MEASURES

One of the most common applications of anthropometric data is in the diagnosis or categorization of conditions such as underweight and overweight and the grading of their severity (3, 25–27). In addition, cutoff thresholds are used to elucidate variations in age, maturation, gender, ethnicity, and other "technical" factors that affect anthropometry "independently" or in conjunction with health or social causes or consequences as well as in applications such as policy formulation, social utility, and advocacy for particular problems and solutions (28). Different indicators and cut-points are needed for different application purposes. However, this notion may not be agreed by various user communities, because universal cut-points of simple

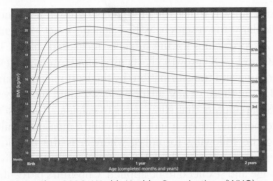

Fig. 49.1. The 2006 World Health Organization (WHO) growth standards: body mass index (BMI)-for-age percentiles for boys under 2 years old. (Reprinted with permission from http://www.who.int/childgrowth/standards/cht_bfa_boys_p_0_2.pdf.)

World Health Organization Growth References and Standards

Thus far, the WHO has published several versions of growth references recommended for international use to help assess children's growth and nutritional status (see Table 49.6). The three widely known versions are the 1978 WHO/NCHS Growth References (for children ≤10 years), the 1995 WHO Growth References (for children ≤19 years), and the 2006 WHO Growth Standards (for preschool children <6 years).

The 1978 World Health Organization/National Center for Health Statistics Growth References

In 1978, the WHO/NCHS produced a normalized version of the US growth curves, showing Z-scores. It has been widely used all over the world since then. However, it has a number of limitations (1). One main limitation is that the infant growth reference was developed based on data collected from the Fels Longitudinal Study, which followed mainly formula-fed infants in one area in the mid-west region of the United States. Moreover, these children were followed with large time intervals, which provided insufficient data to describe the rapid and changing rate of growth in early infancy (40). Additionally, the growth pattern of breast-fed infants differed from that of formula-fed infants (43). To overcome these limitations, new growth references and standards have been developed in the United States in 2000 and by the WHO in 2006, respectively (see the following).

The 1995 World Health Organization Growth References

In 1995, a WHO Expert Committee reviewed existing growth references and research findings and then re-endorsed the use of the 1978 WHO/NCHS Growth Charts. In addition, for adolescents, they recommended use of the sex- and age-specific BMI greater than or equal to the 85th percentile and both triceps and subscapular skinfold thickness greater than or equal to the 90th percentiles for classifying children as "at risk of overweight" and "overweight" (2). These percentiles were developed based on US data.

The committee acknowledged the weaknesses of these references, and recommended their use on a provisional basis until better references become available (2).

The 2006 World Health Organization Growth Standards for Preschool Children

In 2006, the WHO released new growth standards for children 0 to 5 years old. These growth charts were the first ever to be based on a prospective, detailed measurement of healthy children followed from birth—the Multicenter Growth Reference Study (41). The cohort included only affluent, exclusively breast-fed, and healthy infants and children whose mothers did not smoke during or after delivery, from six cities in Brazil, Ghana, India, Norway, Oman, and the United States. The data showed great similarities in growth across countries (44), and demonstrated that preschool children worldwide have the same growth potential if raised in an optimal environment. However, some countries, including the United States, still use their own growth references and standards.

The standards include a set of anthropometric indicators and sex-specific growth charts and tables of percentiles and Z-scores. In the Z-score growth charts, the curves for 0, ±2, and ±3 SD from the age-specific median of certain indicator are plotted. For percentile charts, five curves for the 3rd, 15th, 50th, 85th, and 97th percentiles are shown for each indicator. In the tables, the values of the indicator at 0, ±1, ±2, and ±3 SD, and for percentiles of 1st, 3rd, 5th, 15th, 25th, 50th, 75th, 85th, 97th, and 99th are provided for each age of month.

The 2007 World Health Organization Growth Reference for School-Age Children and Adolescents

In 2007 the WHO released a new growth reference for children 5 to 19 years old (45). The reference includes three indicators: BMI-for-age, weight-for-age, and height-for-age. For each indicator, charts and tables for percentiles and Z-scores were provided. The percentiled charts draw the 3rd, 15th, 50th, 85th, and 97th percentile curves, whereas the tables provide the values of anthropometric measures for more percentiles (e.g., 1st, 5th, 25th, 75th, 95th, and 99th). Regarding Z-scores of these three indicators, the curves for 0, ±1, ±2, and ±3 Z-scores from the median are shown on charts, and the values for these cut-points are provided in tables.

The WHO recommended the cut-points for overweight and obesity based on the BMI-for-age Z-scores. The analysis showed that the BMI-for-age Z-score equal to 1 at 19 years of age was 25.4 for boys and 25.0 for girls, which equals or is close to the WHO BMI cut-point of 25 used in adults. Thus, the reference curve of Z-score equal to 1 was recommended to classify overweight, whereas that of Z-score greater than 2 was recommended for classifying obesity based on the same idea. BMI-for-age Z-scores less than or equal to 2 and scores less than or equal to 3 were set as the cut-points for thinness and severe thinness, respectively. However, this reference is not widely used.

United States 2000 Centers for Disease Control and Prevention Growth Charts

These growth charts were developed based on different data sets and methods than for the one preceding it (40, 42). The 2000 Charts consist of a series of percentile curves of selected anthropometric measures, including weight-for-age, length-for-age, weight-for-length, and head circumference-for-age from birth to 36 months of age. The growth curves are laid out as two sets of charts—Individual Growth Charts and "Clinical Growth Charts. The growth charts and tables present the 3rd, 5th, 10th, 25th, 50th, 75th, 90th, 95th, and 97th percentile curves. The 85th percentile curve is in addition provided on the BMI-for-age and weight-for-stature growth charts for 2- to 20-year-old children and adults, recommended as cut-points for childhood overweight. Regarding the Z-score for the indicators, only tables provide the detailed corresponding values indicator-for-age at 0, ±0.5, ±1, ±1.5, and ±2.

Comparisons Using Different International and Local Growth References and Standards

Some studies attempted to test how comparable the results are if these growth references are applied on the same study population. Overall, they have shown that the estimated unhealthy growth status can vary when different growth references and standards are applied. For example, a study of US children 0 to 59 months old found disparity in the prevalence (percentage) of growth or nutritional status problems. Using the Centers for Disease Control and Prevention (CDC) 2000 reference, stunting prevalence was 3.7%; wasting was 5.0%; overweight was 9.2%; but according to the WHO Growth Standards, the figures were 7.0%, 2.8%, and 12.9%, respectively (46). One study found that according to the IOTF, US 2000 CDC, and Chinese BMI references, the obesity prevalence estimated for children 6 to 18 years old in Beijing varied between 5.8% and 9.8%, or 69% in relative terms (47). More research is needed to help understand and guide appropriate applications of such references in different populations.

How to Use Growth References and Standards in Practice

Growth references and standards are useful in clinical settings, population-based monitoring, and other research projects. To use a growth reference or standard to help assess individual or groups of children's growth and nutritional status, one must compare subjects' measures against the cut-points provided in the growth references or standards. For example, Figure 49.2 shows how to use the 2000 CDC Growth Charts to monitor a girl's growth in weight. This is a weight-for-age chart, and the girl's body weight measurements were plotted on the chart. These curves can be used to evaluate the position of a child's anthropometric measurement relative to the reference population.

Another way to use the more recent growth references, particularly for research, is to calculate exact percentile and Z-score values for the subjects' measured values. The WHO and CDC growth charts used similar techniques of smoothing and transformation (by the least means squared [LMS] method). They all provide sex- and age-specific LMS parameters that allow users to calculate the Z-score corresponding to each individual child's measured value, using the following formulas, where y is the individual observation, whereas the LMS parameters for the individual's age and sex need to be applied. Children's percentiles can be calculated after their Z-scores are obtained.

$$z = \frac{\left(y/M\right)^L - 1}{SL}$$

CONCLUSIONS

Anthropometry provides a group of useful, inexpensive, and noninvasive methods to assess the size, shape, and composition of the human body as well as health conditions such as malnutrition and obesity in adults and children. They are indirect measures of BC, whereas direct BC assessment methods such as DXA and air displacement plethysmography can provide accurate measures (e.g., total body fat, fat distribution). In general, the commonly used anthropometric measures such as BMI and WC have good validity in measuring body fat and predicting future health risks.

BC analysis, including anthropometry, has been used to study physiologic processes such as growth, development, and exercise physiology and is being applied increasingly to the study and clinical management of pathologic conditions. Whatever the reason for assessing BC, clinicians should have a general understanding of the most commonly used techniques for assessing BC as well as their main strengths and limitations.

At present, given its many strengths, BMI is the most widely used anthropometric measure in defining obesity and underweight; however, it has some limitations as an indirect measure. The cut-points of 25 and 30 are recommended by the WHO for classifying overweight and obesity, respectively, and these cut-points have been widely used since the late 1990s. However, there have been debates regarding whether population-specific BMI cut-points should be used. Different BMI cut-points have been developed and are used across countries. Lower BMI cut-points such as 23 and 25 were recommended for some Asian populations.

The use of BMI cut-points in children, which often are age- and sex-specific percentiles, is more complicated. Different percentiles that have been developed based on different data sets have been used across countries. At present, those in the 2006 WHO Growth Standards for preschool age children and those for children 2 to 18 years old in the IOTF BMI references are used worldwide. They can help facilitate international comparisons.

Case Study: Mary, Born Dec. 2, 1997

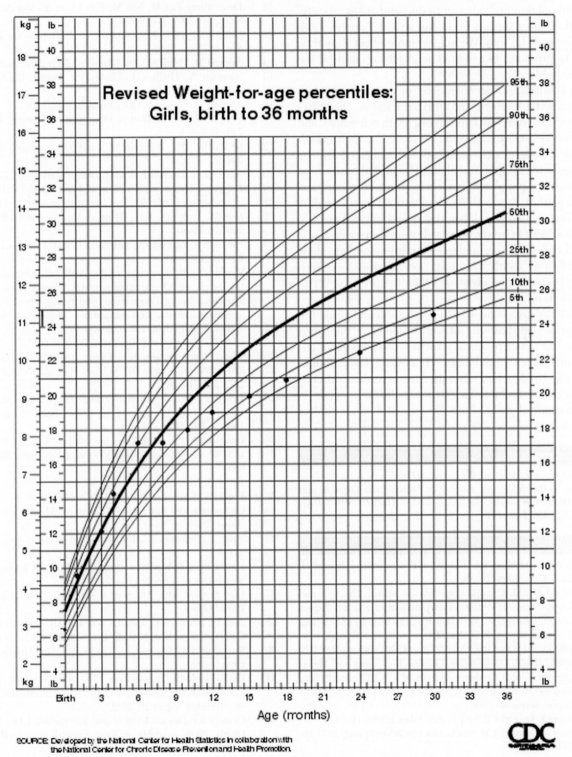

Revised Weight-for-age percentiles:
Girls, birth to 36 months

Age (months)

SOURCE: Developed by the National Center for Health Statistics in collaboration with
the National Center for Chronic Disease Prevention and Health Promotion.

CDC

Fig. 49.2. An example from the Centers for Disease Control and Prevention of how to use the growth chart to monitor an individual child's growth. This figure uses a case to show how to apply a growth chart to assess a child's growth trajectory and health status. It shows a girl who had experienced growth faltering after age of 6 months. More details are provided in the text. (Reprinted with permission from http://www.cdc.gov/nchs/images/nhanes/growthcharts/2000%20Chart.gif. Accessed August 10, 2012.)

Growing research suggests that WC is the best simple anthropometric predictor of body fat distribution (intraabdominal adipose tissue) and many obesity-related diseases such as CVD and type 2 diabetes, both in adults and children. We suggest more effort should be made to promote its use in clinical settings and by the general public.

For children, growth references (or standards) are useful to assess their growth and nutritional status. The WHO has developed different versions of growth references, and those before 2006 are based on US data. Usually a growth reference is developed based on data collected from a representative sample and shows the growth pattern of the reference population, which may not be an optimal growth pattern. A growth standard derived from a healthy and affluent child population can reflect optimal growth. The 2006 WHO Growth Standards were developed based on data collected from multiple countries, and help show how children should grow under optimal growth environment. It offers more advantages than the previous WHO growth references.

More research is needed to help assess and guide the appropriate applications of anthropometric measures and the use of international growth references and standards in different populations. Meanwhile, effort should be made to develop innovative new anthropometric measures and technologies to meet the new needs in the biomedical field, both for research and clinical purposes.

ACKNOWLEDGMENTS

This work was supported in part by research grants from the National Institutes of Health/National Institute of Diabetes and Digestive and Kidney Diseases (grant nos. R01DK81335-01A1, 1R03HD058077-01A1, and R03HD058077-01A1S1).

REFERENCES

1. Wang Y, Moreno LA, Caballero B et al. Food Nutr Bull 2006;27(Suppl):S175–88.
2. World Health Organization. Physical Status: The Use and Interpretation of Anthropometry. Report of a WHO Expert Committee. Geneva: World Health Organization, 1995:1–452. Technical Report Series No. 854.
3. Wang Y. Int J Obes Relat Metab Disord 2004;28(Suppl):S21–8.
4. World Health Organization. Obesity: Preventing and Managing the Global Epidemic. Report of a WHO consultation. Geneva: World Health Organization, 2000:1–253. Technical Report Series No. 894.
5. Wang Y, Lobstein T. Int J Pediatr Obes 2006;1:11–25.
6. Shea JL, Randell EW, Sun G. Obesity (Silver Spring) 2011;19:624–30.
7. Vasudev S, Mohan A, Mohan D et al. J Assoc Phys India 2004;52:877–81.
8. Wang ZM, Deurenberg P, Guo SS et al. Int J Obes Relat Metab Disord 1998;22:329–37.
9. El Taguri A, Dabbas-Tyan M, Goulet O et al. East Mediterr Health J 2009;15:563–73.
10. Rodriguez G, Moreno LA, Blay MG et al. Eur J Clin Nutr 2005;59:1158–66.
11. Sarria A, Garcia-Llop LA, Moreno LA et al. Eur J Clin Nutr 1998;52:573–6.
12. Deurenberg-Yap M, Niti M, Foo LL et al. Ann Acad Med Singapore 2009;38:3–6.
13. Hsieh SD, Ashwell M, Muto T et al. Metabolism 2010;59:834–40.
14. Ashwell M, Hsieh SD. Int J Food Sci Nutr 2005;56:303–7.
15. Nambiar S, Hughes I, Davies PS. Public Health Nutr 2010;13:1566–74.
16. Ashwell M, Gibson S. Obes Facts 2009;2:97–103.
17. Weili Y, He B, Yao H et al. Obesity (Silver Spring) 2007;15:748–52.
18. McCarthy HD, Ashwell M. Int J Obes (Lond) 2006;30:988–92.
19. Alberti KG, Zimmet P, Shaw J. Diabet Med 2006;23:469–80.
20. Lofgren I, Herron K, Zern T et al. J Nutr 2004;134:1071–6.
21. Japan Society for the Study of Obesity. Circ J 2002;66:987–92.
22. Lee SY, Park HS, Kim DJ et al. Diabetes Res Clin Pract 2007;75:72–80.
23. Hadaegh F, Zabetian A, Sarbakhsh P et al. Int J Obes (Lond) 2009;33:1437–45.
24. World Health Organization/International Association for the Study of Obesity/International Obesity Task Force. The Asia-Pacific Perspective: Redefining Obesity and Its Treatment. Health Communications. Melbourne, Australia: World Health Organization, 2000:1–56.
25. Chen X, Wang Y. Int J Epidemiol 2010;39:1045–7.
26. World Health Organization. Lancet 2004;363:157–63.
27. Zheng W, McLerran DF, Rolland B et al. N Engl J Med 2011;364:719–29.
28. Pelletier D. Food Nutr Bull 2006;27(Suppl):S224–36.
29. Power C, Lake JK, Cole TJ. Int J Obes Relat Metab Disord 1997;21:507–26.
30. Prentice AM, Jebb SA. Obes Rev 2001;2:141–7.
31. Ellis KJ, Abrams SA, Wong WW. Am J Epidemiol 1999;150:939–46.
32. Reilly JJ. Obes Res 2002;10:838–40.
33. Franklin M. Am J Clin Nutr 1999;70:157S–62S.
34. Okorodudu DO, Jumean MF, Montori VM et al. Int J Obes (Lond) 2010;34:791–9.
35. Wang J, Thornton JC, Burastero S et al. Obes Res 1996;4:377–84.
36. Deurenberg P, Yap M, van Staveren WA. Int J Obes Relat Metab Disord 1998;22:1164–71.
37. Low S, Chin MC, Ma S et al. Ann Acad Med Singapore 2009;38:66–9.
38. Cole TJ, Bellizzi MC, Flegal KM et al. BMJ 2000;320:1240–3.
39. Cole TJ, Flegal KM, Nicholls D et al. BMJ 2007;335:194.
40. Kuczmarski RJ, Ogden CL, Guo SS et al. Vital Health Stat 11 2002;1–190.
41. World Health Organization. The WHO Child Growth Standards. 2006. Available at: http://www.who.int/childgrowth/en/. Accessed August 10, 2012.
42. Centers for Disease Control and Prevention. CDC Growth Charts. 2000. Available at: http://www.cdc.gov/growthcharts/cdc_charts.htm. Accessed August 10, 2012.
43. de Onis M, Onyango AW. Acta Paediatr 2003;92:413–9.
44. World Health Organization. WHO Child Growth Standards: Length/Height-for-Age, Weight-for-Age, Weight-for-Length, Weight-for-Height and Body Mass Index-for-Age: Methods and Development. Geneva: World Health Organization, 2006:1–336.
45. de Onis M, Onyango AW, Borghi E et al. Bull World Health Org 2007;85:660–7.

46. Mei Z, Ogden CL, Flegal KM et al. J Pediatr 2008;153:622–8.

47. Shan XY, Xi B, Cheng H et al. Int J Pediatr Obes 2010; 5:383–9.

48. Poskitt EM. Acta Paediatr 1995;84:961–3.

49. Rolland-Cachera MF, Cole TJ, Sempe M et al. Eur J Clin Nutr 1991;45:13–21.

SUGGESTED READINGS

Wang Y. Epidemiology of childhood obesity—methodological aspects and guidelines: what is new? Int J Obes Relat Metab Disord 2004;28(Suppl):S21–8.

World Health Organization. Physical status: the use and interpretation of anthropometry. Report of a WHO expert committee. World Health Organ Tech Rep Ser 1995;854:1–452.

World Health Organization. Appropriate body-mass index for Asian populations and its implications for policy and intervention strategies. WHO expert consultation. Lancet 2004;363:157–63.

World Health Organization. The WHO Child Growth Standards. 2006. Available at: http://www.who.int/childgrowth/en/. Accessed August 10, 2012.

de Onis M, Garza C, Onyango AW et al. Comparison of the WHO child growth standards and the CDC 2000 growth charts. J Nutr 2007;137:144–8.

50 METABOLIC CONSEQUENCES OF STARVATION[1]

L. JOHN HOFFER

Starvation is the physical condition brought about by inadequate consumption, absorption, or retention of protein or dietary energy. The disease that eventually results from persistent starvation is *protein-energy malnutrition*. This chapter explains the physiology of starvation, which occurs both as a disease and in a nonpathologic form during therapeutic weight reduction. Pathologic starvation is usually caused by a general reduction of food intake; hence, it is commonly complicated by deficiencies of micronutrients as well as macronutrients (1, 2).

The physiology of starvation is central to human nutrition and many aspects of metabolism and medicine. Additional chapters in this edition deal with the clinical aspects of protein-energy malnutrition. This chapter explains the metabolic features of protein and energy insufficiency in humans, with the aim of establishing links between topics in physiology and clinical nutrition that are covered in other chapters in the text, including, among others, protein and energy metabolism, body composition, and nutritional assessment.

DEFINITIONS

Many terms have been used to describe starvation. In this chapter, starvation refers to states of negative protein or energy balance and their physiologic effects. A fast or total fast is a unique form of starvation in which all food energy is excluded. Terms such as *starvation, inanition, emaciation, wasting,* and *cachexia* have been used in the past interchangeably to describe the malnourished condition of famine victims, underfed prisoners, and people with chronic disease and important weight loss. In more recent years, cachexia has come to be used to refer specifically to the protein depletion induced by persistent, low-grade systemic inflammation or metabolic stress (3–6). Advancing old age is associated with loss of muscle mass and function, termed *sarcopenia* (4–6). Although potentially modifiable by diet and lifestyle, sarcopenia is not considered as a form of starvation in this chapter.

Starvation takes different forms. The cardinal feature of prolonged fasting is ketosis (7). Contrary to what has been claimed sometimes, ketosis is neither sensitive nor specific as an indicator of starvation. Moreover, mild ketonuria may be present in healthy lean young adults after the overnight fast and people subsisting on a fully adequate but carbohydrate-restricted diet. Ketosis is prevented or abolished by carbohydrate intakes as low as 100 g/day (8); hence, it is absent in most starving people.

PROLONGED FASTING

Carbohydrate Metabolism

A description of fasting metabolism best proceeds from the last meal before the fast begins. Characteristic of the

---

[1]**Abbreviations: ADP,** adenosine diphosphate; **BMI,** body mass index; **CED,** chronic energy deficiency; **FFM,** fat-free mass; **IGF,** insulinlike growth factor; **N,** nitrogen; **NPRQ,** nonprotein respiratory quotient; **REE,** resting energy expendi **SIRS,** systemic inflammatory response syndrome; **T₃,** triiodothy **T₄,** thyroxine.

fed state are increased blood concentrations of glucose, lipids, amino acids, and their metabolites. Carbohydrate and amino acid ingestion stimulates insulin secretion, which regulates their disposition within the tissues by stimulating glycogen, triglyceride, and protein synthesis while simultaneously inhibiting glycogenolysis, lipolysis, and proteolysis. Glucagon levels are unaltered or decreased after carbohydrate consumption, whereas protein consumption stimulates both glucagon and insulin secretion (7). Glucagon serves to stimulate liver glycogen breakdown and increase hepatic glucose output, thereby sustaining an adequate blood glucose concentration even as insulin stimulates glucose and amino acid uptake by peripheral tissues.

The fed state ends after the last nutrient has been absorbed and the transition to endogenous fuel consumption gets underway. The condition that exists after the overnight fast is convenient for study and is termed the *basal* or *postabsorptive* state. This state is characterized by the release, interorgan transfer, and oxidation of fatty acids and the net release of glucose from liver glycogen and amino acids from muscle; all these processes are activated by the relatively low circulating insulin concentration that prevails in this situation. The body's predominant postabsorptive fuel is fat. Thus, as indicated by the typical nonprotein respiratory quotient (NPRQ) of 0.8, fat oxidation typically accounts for two thirds of postabsorptive resting energy expenditure (REE) (9).

Under postabsorptive conditions, glucose enters the circulation and disappears into the tissues at a rate of 8 to 10 g/hour, replacing the body's extracellular free glucose pool of approximately 16 g every 2 hours (10). Glucose is normally the only fuel available to the brain. Any lowering of the blood (and cerebrospinal fluid) glucose concentration lower than a critical level promptly impairs consciousness, and if prolonged, can lead to neuron death. Given the brain's fixed and high metabolic requirement—approximately half the body's total glucose production rate—there is no room for error or delay in the delivery of glucose from the liver into the systemic circulation. The blood glucose concentration of healthy individuals is closely regulated by several physiologic control systems, chief of which are the insulin and glucagon systems.

In the period that follows metabolic disposition of a meal, continual extraction of circulating glucose by the tissues progressively lowers the blood glucose concentration. Insulin levels fall in concert, thereby automatically slowing the rate of glucose transport into muscle and fat cells, while stimulating hepatic glycogenolysis and inhibiting hepatic glycogen synthesis to assure the continued release of adequate amounts of glucose from the liver into the bloodstream.

Hepatic gluconeogenesis (the synthesis of glucose from lactate, amino acids, and glycerol) is a continuous process, even in the fed state (11). Early in the postabsorptive period, approximately half the glucose appearing in the circulation originates from gluconeogenesis and the other half from hepatic glycogenolysis (10, 12). The precise relative contributions of gluconeogenesis and glycogenolysis to the circulating glucose pool depend on the carbohydrate and protein content of the preceding diet, for these respectively determine the size of the liver's glycogen store and the rate at which glucogenic amino acids are reaching the liver to serve as a substrate for gluconeogenesis (13). As the fast is prolonged, glucose molecules derived from gluconeogenesis increasingly enter the circulation immediately rather than being sequestered in glycogen, and the liver gradually releases its entire glycogen store into the circulation. The kidneys are also gluconeogenic organs. Their fractional contribution to the circulating glucose pool increases as the liver's glycogen store is expended and total hepatic glucose output decreases (14).

A fast longer than 12 to 24 hours reduces insulin levels yet further, causing a substantial mobilization of free fatty acids and glycerol from adipose tissue and amino acids from muscle (15). Delivery of these molecules to the liver provides energy and the substrate for protein synthesis and gluconeogenesis. Plasma glucagon concentrations remain constant or increase, thus lowering the insulin–glucagon ratio to activate the liver to oxidize the increased amounts of fatty acids now being delivered to it. Once activated in this way, the liver's fatty acid oxidation rate is determined by the rate at which fatty acids are delivered to it (16). The rate of glucose conversion to coenzyme A, the entry substrate in the Krebs cycle, decreases importantly as the rate of fatty acid conversion to acetyl coenzyme A increases. Some of the acetyl coenzyme A produced from fatty acid oxidation is completely oxidized to carbon dioxide via the intrahepatic Krebs cycle, thereby serving as the liver's predominant energy source (17), but most of it is oxidized only as far as the four-carbon molecule, acetoacetic acid, which spontaneously interconverts with its oxidoreduction partner, β-hydroxybutyric acid, and, to a lesser extent, is irreversibly decarboxylated to acetone. These three molecules are collectively termed the *ketone bodies*. Under prolonged fasting conditions, the liver acts as a factory that absorbs fatty acids delivered to it from adipose tissue, converts their carbon into ketone bodies, and exports them into the general circulation.

A fast longer than 2 or 3 days completely exhausts the liver's approximately 80-g glycogen reserve (12, 18) and approximately half the glycogen in muscle (18, 19). The liver's gluconeogenic rate neither increases or decreases, and therefore accounts for an increasing fraction of its total glucose output rate (14), which decreases by 40% to 50% within the first few days of fasting (12, 20). Muscle cells do not export glucose, so their residual glycogen plays no role in steady-state whole body carbohydrate economy. Consequently, once the liver's glycogen store is completely exhausted, all the glucose that is oxidized in the body must be synthesized from three precursors: (1) the glucogenic amino acids; (2) glycerol released because of lipolysis;

and (3) lactate and pyruvate, molecules that, being the products of glycolysis, merely represent recycled glucose (21). The oxidation rate of preformed carbohydrate falls to zero, and as proof of this, the NPRQ falls to 0.7 (9).

Despite the marked reduction in hepatic glucose release, serum glucose concentrations decrease only moderately during fasting, because tissue glucose uptake and metabolism also decrease. Only part of this reduction in glucose metabolism is caused by reduced terminal glucose oxidation in muscle and adipose tissue, and none of it caused by a slower rate of lactate and pyruvate reconversion to glucose (the Cori cycle). An important reason for reduced tissue glucose use early in fasting, and the main reason for it in prolonged fasting, is a progressive switch by neural tissues to the use of ketone bodies as their energy supply (17, 22, 23). This phenomenon was elegantly demonstrated in a study of human subjects on a short-term fast in whom a combination of positron emission tomography and arterial–internal jugular vein sampling was used to measure glucose metabolism and β-hydroxybutyrate consumption. After 3.5 days of fasting, glucose consumption by the brain decreased by 25% and ketone body extraction increased correspondingly (24).

Ketosis

Ketosis (the presence of an abnormally high blood ketone body concentration) is the cardinal sign of prolonged fasting. Under nonfasting conditions acetoacetate oxidation furnishes only 2% to 3% of the body's total energy requirement (17), and blood ketone body concentrations are almost immeasurably low (25). Starvation ketosis is arbitrarily defined as being present when the blood acetoacetate concentration rises to 1.0 mmol/L and β-hydroxybutyrate to 2 to 3 mmol/L, as typically occurs by day 2 or 3 of fasting (17). Ketone bodies are usually absent from overnight fasting urine, but mild ketonuria is not abnormal in thin healthy persons and indicates a physiologically low basal insulin state (26, 27). After their release into the blood, acetoacetic acid and β-hydroxybutyric acid dissociate to form water-soluble anions. Some acetoacetic acid is decarboxylated to acetone, and by day 3 or 4 days of fasting, its characteristic sweet odor is detectable in the breath.

Two factors determine the liver's rate of ketone body synthesis. The first is the liver's maximum capacity for fatty acid β-oxidation when fully activated by a low-insulin state. This rate depends both on the mass of perfused metabolically active liver tissue and the rate at which adenosine diphosphate (ADP) becomes available from adenosine triphosphate (ATP) hydrolysis, which, in turn, depends on the liver's total energy expenditure rate (28). The second factor is the rate of adipose tissue triglyceride lipolysis, which determines the rate at which free fatty acids reach the liver.

The rate of ketogenesis is maximal as early as day 3 of fasting, but the blood ketone body concentration continues

to rise over the ensuing days and weeks. There are two explanations for this phenomenon. First, muscle decreases its rate of ketone body oxidation, shifting to fatty acids as its preferred fuel. Second, the renal tubules reabsorb ketone bodies with greater efficiency. After the first 4 to 7 days of a total fast, ketone body oxidation accounts for 30% to 40% of the body's total energy use. By week 3, a steady-state circulating ketone body concentration has been attained that is approximately twice the concentration that existed after the first 3 to 5 days. Because the brain uses ketone bodies in proportion to their delivery to it, brain ketone body oxidation steadily increases over this period as glucose oxidation decreases. After 3 to 5 weeks of fasting, brain glucose uptake is globally reduced by approximately 50% (17, 22). Moreover, by this time only 60% of the glucose taken up by the brain is fully oxidized to carbon dioxide and water, the rest being metabolized only as far as pyruvate and lactate, which return to the liver as gluconeogenic substrates (22). The combination of reduced terminal oxidation and increased local Cori cycling reduces the brain's rate of irreversible glucose oxidation by 75%, with an equivalent reduction in the body's requirement for gluconeogenesis from amino acids and glycerol.

Ketogenesis appears to be partly restrained by means of a negative feedback system which uses the circulating ketone body concentration as its sensor. Ketone bodies were long known to reduce lipolysis; but the mechanism for this effect was revealed more recently with the discovery of a G-protein–coupled receptor for niacin, a vitamin that, when administered in gram doses, potently inhibits lipolysis. The natural ligand for the niacin receptor has been identified as β-hydroxybutyrate (29). The physiologic mechanism that shifts muscle's fuel preference from ketone bodies to fatty acids, after approximately 2 weeks of fasting, remains unexplained (10). Perhaps there is a role for the niacin receptor in this process.

Biologic Significance of Ketosis

Mention of ketosis or ketoacidosis (ketosis severe enough to lower the serum bicarbonate concentration but still within its normal buffering capacity) brings diabetes mellitus to mind. In the most severe form of this disease, destruction of the pancreatic β cells results in nearly total insulin deficiency. The result is mobilization of fatty acids and a priming of the liver for ketone body production and gluconeogenesis, as occurs in simple fasting (16, 30). When carbohydrate is ingested without coordinated insulin secretion, little of the glucose appearing in the circulation is taken up by muscle and adipose tissue. The blood glucose concentration rises to high levels, greatly exceeding the renal threshold for glucose reabsorption. The result is glycosuria and an osmotic diuresis that depletes the body of water and extracellular fluid. In prolonged fasting by nondiabetic persons, ketone body levels seldom rise higher than 6 to 8 mmol/L, but they rise much higher in diabetic ketoacidosis, imposing an acid load too great for the body's buffering system to absorb and causing a dangerous fall in pH. This condition is known as ketoacidemia.

Why is the ketosis of simple fasting mild and clinically benign, whereas the ketoacidosis of diabetes commonly escalates into life-threatening ketoacidemia? Some understanding of the pathogenesis of severe ketoacidemia is provided by a consideration of the uncommon but well-documented syndrome called *nondiabetic ketoacidosis*. This life-threatening disease typically occurs when protracted vomiting and volume depletion follows an alcoholic drinking binge during which there has been no food consumption. The ketoacidemia that develops under these conditions may be as severe as diabetic ketoacidosis, even though the blood glucose concentration remains close to normal (31, 32). Nondiabetic ketoacidosis also occurs rarely in pregnancy. As with alcoholic nondiabetic ketoacidosis, gestational nondiabetic ketoacidosis occurs in a setting of fasting, physiologic severe hypoinsulinemia, and volume depletion or metabolic stress (33).

Two features distinguish severe ketoacidosis from the benign ketoacidosis of fasting: volume depletion and hypermetabolism. Volume depletion worsens existing ketoacidosis (and worsens hyperglycemia) in various ways: by reducing blood flow to the kidneys and brain, reducing brain and renal ketone body oxidation, and greatly reducing urinary ketone body excretion (32). Normal fasting is a hypometabolic phenomenon, whereas uncontrolled diabetes and hypermetabolic volume depletion are characterized by hyperglucagonemia and increased norepinephrine secretion. These hormones increase free fatty acid delivery to the liver (34, 35) and potentially increase its rate of energy consumption, thus making more ADP available and boosting its ketogenic capacity (28) under conditions in which volume depletion has reduced the glomerular filtration rate and hence reduced renal tubular sodium reabsorption and correspondingly reduced the kidneys' energy consumption and ketone body oxidation rate (32). The net effect is a large increase in circulating ketone bodies. During simple prolonged fasting, any stress-induced increase in the blood glucose concentration stimulates endogenous insulin release, which acts to reduce hepatic glucose release, restrain lipolysis, and inhibit ketogenesis (25). In severely volume-depleted states, this does not always happen, presumably because hyperadrenergic states inhibit insulin secretion (32). The notion that severe ketoacidosis arises in a setting of hypermetabolism was already appreciated in the preinsulin era. Before 1922, the only treatment that extended the life of insulin-dependent diabetic patients was a diet low in carbohydrate, which prevented hyperglycemia, glycosuria, and volume depletion, and a diet low in total energy, which reduced the patient's metabolic rate and hence the liver's ketogenic rate (36).

It is commonly repeated in the popular media that ketone bodies are toxic because the ketonuria associated with dietary carbohydrate restriction "damages the kidneys." This claim lacks a scientific basis. Perhaps the notion that ketone bodies are toxic arose because they partially inhibit the urinary excretion of urate (10), and this effect—especially in the setting of extracellular volume depletion, which increases renal tubular urate reabsorption (37, 38)—increases the serum uric acid concentration. Thus an attack of gout may occur in susceptible persons during total fasting or severe carbohydrate restriction. The possibility has been raised that hyperketonemia during pregnancy could adversely affect the fetal brain (27) or predispose to congenital malformations (39). It is certainly true that the rapid glucose use characteristic of late pregnancy predisposes to fasting hypoglycemia, hypoinsulinemia, mild ketosis, and ketonuria (40), and that ketone bodies are used as fuel by fetal tissues. However, no plausible mechanism has been advanced to explain why any of these effects would be harmful, and the clinical evidence linking ketonuria with adverse fetal outcomes is unconvincing (41). Nevertheless, it remains a common practice to counsel pregnant women to avoid periods of prolonged fasting (27).

In summary, prolonged fasting is characterized by a low blood glucose concentration, physiologic hypoinsulinemia, and moderate ketosis, whereas uncontrolled insulin-dependent diabetes is characterized by hyperglycemia, volume depletion, hypermetabolism, and severe ketosis, all of which are the direct or indirect result of severe insulin lack. Unlike diabetic ketoacidosis, fasting ketosis is physiologic and a manifestation of appropriate metabolic regulation. It does not evolve into a severe condition similar to diabetic ketoacidosis, except potentially in a setting of severe volume depletion and metabolic stress.

Protein and Energy Metabolism

Muscle proteolysis is normally held under restraint by circulating insulin. As insulin levels fall in the postabsorptive state, this restraint is partially relaxed, and muscle proteolysis increases and exceeds protein synthesis. The free amino acids liberated by this imbalance (many of them first partially degraded to nonessential amino acids) enter the bloodstream and travel to the splanchnic organs for use in gluconeogenesis and protein synthesis. As the fast is extended, insulin levels fall yet lower, further increasing net muscle proteolysis. The loss of skeletal muscle from the body is considerable. During the first 7 to 10 days of a total fast, whole body nitrogen (N) loss is in the range of 10 to 12 g/day, excreted chiefly as urinary urea (42, 43). Because proteins are 16% N by weight and the lean tissues are 75% to 80% water, the loss of 10 to 12 g/day N from the body is equivalent to the loss of 300 to 400 g/day of lean tissue (42, 44). If this rate of body N loss were to continue, the body's lean tissues would be lethally depleted within 3 weeks of continuous fasting. Instead, an adaptation takes effect after 7 to 10 days, which, by the end of 2 to 3 weeks, reduces the rate of N loss to less than one half of its initial rate. This incompletely understood adaptation is all the more remarkable when it is appreciated that approximately one half of urinary N by this time is in the form of ammonium that has been synthesized to buffer the protons generated by ketoacid production (7, 45). In experiments in which ammonium excretion was reduced to normal by providing an exogenous buffer, the rate of body N loss in prolonged "adapted" fasting was close to the "obligatory" rate of N loss considered to indicate the maximum efficiency of endogenous protein turnover (46–49).

Plasma branched-chain amino acid concentrations approximately double during the first 1 to 3 days of fasting, and their release from whole body proteins and subsequent oxidation increase by variable amounts (50–52). Urinary excretion of 3-methylhistidine, a marker of contractile protein breakdown, increases in the first few days of fasting (50, 53). However, by the 7- to 10-day mark, the initial increase in amino acid turnover is superseded, in some (50, 54) (although not all) studies (51), by a reduction in tracer-measured leucine or lysine (55) appearance into the circulation in a setting of continued significant urinary N excretion and whole body leucine oxidation. By the fourth week of fasting, urinary N excretion has greatly diminished, plasma leucine appearance further decreases (56, 57), and urinary 3-methylhistidine excretion is less than the prefasting rate (56).

The rapid rate of muscle protein loss in the first week of fasting is caused by a combination of reduced protein synthesis (owing to absent exogenous amino acids and the low-insulin state, because insulin normally stimulates protein synthesis) and the easing of insulin's normal restraint on muscle proteolysis (15, 58). What process reverses this catabolic process after approximately 2 weeks of fasting? Most authorities regard the shift in muscle fuel preference from ketone bodies to fatty acids (and the resulting sparing of ketone bodies for use by the brain) as crucial. As ketone bodies increasingly displace glucose as the brain's fuel, the body is not required to convert as much muscle protein into new glucose molecules, and the rate of net muscle proteolysis decreases.

But what is the specific metabolic signal that "tells" muscle cells to reduce their rate of net proteolysis at this point? Some studies suggest that hyperketonemia has a direct protein-sparing effect on skeletal muscle (59, 60), but an unequivocal demonstration of this effect is lacking (51). A role for free fatty acids in muscle protein sparing has been shown in short-term fasting humans (61). Perhaps increased fatty acid oxidation in muscle cells spares the branched-chain amino acids (which have structural similarity to fatty acids), and this sparing effect somehow mediates a reduction in net proteolysis (7, 62).

Weight Loss

During a prolonged total fast, both weight loss and N loss occur at a rate that is roughly proportional to the person's existing body weight and lean body mass (63, 64). Nonobese men with free access to water may lose 4 kg during the first 5 days of fasting and a further 3 kg over the next 5 days (42, 65) whereas very obese men lose roughly 50% more than this. In one extreme case, a patient with an initial body weight of 245 kg lost 32 kg after 30 days of fasting (63).

Water, not fat, accounts for most of the weight loss that occurs early in fasting (66). Approximately 65% of the total water lost from the body during the first 3 days is extracellular (65). This rapid mobilization of extracellular water and sodium is partly caused by a lack of dietary sodium and partly by a drop in circulating insulin concentration, which reduces insulin-mediated renal tubular sodium reabsorption (67). There is also a rapid loss of intracellular water caused by the dissolution of lean tissues (19 to 25 g water/g N), liver glycogen (2 to 3 g water/g glycogen) (68), and to a lesser extent, partial depletion of muscle glycogen (3 to 4 g water/g glycogen) (44, 69). However, after 3 days, liver glycogen is either gone or stabilized, and by 2 weeks extracellular fluid balance has been restored (63). Weight loss consequently slows greatly, for it is now solely due to lean tissue and adipose tissue loss, and their rates of loss are themselves slowed by adaptive protein sparing and reduced energy expenditure. Weight loss by a 3-week fasting, moderately obese person is typically approximately 350 g/day. This rate of weight loss is both clinically observed also predictable by means of simple calculation. Thus, a negative N balance of 4 g/day is equivalent to the loss of 125 g/day of hydrated lean tissue. Because adipose tissue is approximately 85% pure fat (70–72), a negative energy balance of approximately 1700 kcal/day is equivalent to the loss of approximately 200 g/day of adipose tissue. The calculated total weight loss is 325 g/day. The rate of weight loss continues to slow further as the body's lean tissue mass diminishes, in keeping with a first-order kinetic process.

Other Metabolic Effects

REE decreases within days of initiating a total fast; indeed, sleeping energy expenditure decreases within the first 48 hours (73). Some studies have reported a small *increase* in REE early in fasting (74, 75); this appears to result from catecholamine release that will occur if extracellular volume depletion is not prevented by generous sodium provision (76). After 2 weeks of fasting, REE has decreased by approximately 15% (77) and by 3 to 4 weeks by 25% to 35% lower than normal (65). The early reduction in REE is adaptive, being far too prompt to be accounted for by the loss of metabolically active tissues. Later reductions in REE are caused by the body's decreasing metabolic mass.

Serum albumin concentrations remain normal both in short-term and prolonged fasting, but concentrations of the rapidly turning over liver secretory proteins, transthyretin (thyroid-binding prealbumin) and retinol-binding protein promptly fall, as occurs even after simple

Protein Intake. N balance is improved by an increase in protein intake over a wide range of energy intakes from deficient to maintenance (120, 165), even in critical illness (166, 167). Adaptation to starvation increases the efficiency of retention of the protein in a given meal, so a meal high in protein will permit more absolute protein retention than one low in protein. Therefore, a high-protein starvation diet may be associated with protein equilibrium after only moderate lean tissue wasting, whereas a low-protein diet eventually may be compatible with the reestablishment of N equilibrium, but at a greater metabolic cost in terms of lean tissue wasting. Most, but not all (86), studies of therapeutic starvation suggest that a protein intake of 1.5 g protein/kg of normal body weight maintains N balance (85) or conserves FFM (168) better than lower intakes.

Stage of Starvation. As explained, prior protein depletion increases the efficiency of N retention at any protein and energy intake (56).

Exercise. Physical exercise maintains or mitigates loss of muscle mass during therapeutic weight reduction (136, 169).

Obesity. It has been claimed that obesity confers a protein-sparing effect during fasting and starvation (66, 170). Little good evidence supports this contention, given the confounding effects of differences in body stature, physical activity, and protein intake between therapeutically starving obese people and pathologically starving nonobese ones, the paucity of controlled studies, and the absence of a plausible biologic mechanism that would account for an obesity-specific protein-sparing phenomenon in starvation (171). Analysis of the composition of weight loss by weight-reducing obese patients fails to show slower loss of FFM in the more obese ones (172). Nor is such a finding unexpected. Some degree of lean tissue loss is inevitable during therapeutic weight reduction, for a lighter body needs less muscle to support and move it. Moreover, approximately 15% of the weight of adipose tissue consists of FFM that is obliged to be lost from the body when the adipose tissue mass decreases (70–72). Therefore, it is predictable that, to the extent that their lean tissue mass is greater than normal, the rate of N and FFM loss during starvation will be greater in more severely obese people (63, 173). Unlike in severe obesity, the lean tissue mass of moderately energy-restricted nonobese (or only mildly obese) people is, in fact, well maintained (174–176). This good preservation of the lean tissue mass of healthy, moderately energy-restricted people can be accounted for by their high level of physical activity (169), their usually generous protein intake, and their only modest adipose tissue unloading.

Other Factors. When weight loss persists despite conditions conducive to adaptation, attention should be directed to correctable factors such as dietary compliance, the level of protein intake, malabsorption, the adequacy of micronutrient provision (130, 177, 178), or an occult catabolic state. Even when all of such factors

are controlled or considered, the variation in individual responses to starvation is wide (179).

Characteristics of Successful Adaptation

Pathologic adaptation succeeds when metabolic adjustments and controlled lean tissue loss permit the body to reestablish energy and N equilibrium. The starving person survives, but at a metabolic and functional cost (115). The most apparent deficits are the loss of thermally insulating fat and muscle, with an associated loss of physical power. A hypometabolic state develops that is reminiscent of (but not identical to) hypothyroidism (180). Starving people tend to be hypothermic, and they fail to mount an appropriate thermic response to environmental cold (181). Their depleted muscle store diminishes their protein reserve; and this depletion, along with the slow rate of protein turnover in their remaining muscle (182), reduces options for protein remodeling in response to changing metabolic needs. Starving persons mount a blunted rise of protein turnover and a smaller catabolic response to metabolic stress (183).

Although muscle loss is the most obvious feature of starvation, deficits in central protein function may occur. The anatomic and functional consequences of severe clinical starvation are described in clinical (131, 184, 185) and medical reviews (2, 186–188). These deficits include anemia, altered heart muscle mass and function (189, 190), decreased respiratory muscle function and reduced ventilatory drive (191, 192), impaired healing of skin ulcers (193), altered gut anatomy and function (159, 194), altered drug metabolism (195), bone loss (196, 197), and immunodeficiency (198).

Weight-stable anorexia nervosa in an otherwise healthy person represents a rough conceptual paradigm of successful pathologic adaptation to starvation (199). More complex but similar examples can be observed daily in outpatient chronic disease clinics. The defining metabolic features of successful pathologic adaptation are less than critical total lean tissue depletion, weight stability, a normal plasma albumin level (in the absence of dehydration), a normal peripheral blood total lymphocyte count, and intact delayed cutaneous hypersensitivity (200).

Failed Adaptation

This should be suspected when a starving patient develops a catabolic state, as may be indicated by fever or a rapid heart rate. However, these responses to tissue injury or invasion may be blunted in starvation, and their absence does not rule out a catabolic stimulus nor does it exclude other factors that can reverse the adapted state. A more reliable sign of stress-induced protein wasting is an inappropriate rise in serum urea concentration and urinary urea excretion. The simplest indicator of the reversal of accommodation from any cause is the resumption of weight loss in a previously weight-stable, malnourished patient or failure to *gain* weight despite the development of edema. Either situation suggests that new lean tissue loss is occurring. The presence of factors that impair adaptation in an adapted-starving person should raise a red flag. These factors include further diminution of food intake, worsening of the primary disease (or the development of one of its complications), the onset of a new disease that imposes a metabolic stress, or the administration of a treatment (e.g., glucocorticoid therapy) that alters protein or energy metabolism (129).

Catabolic Stress.   The catabolic response to severe infection, trauma, or traumatic major surgery is the polar opposite of the adaptation to starvation, and reverses it (129), as does, to a lesser extent, the less intense inflammatory condition of cachexia, described later in this chapter.

Mineral Deficiency.   Mineral deficiencies, particularly those of potassium (177), phosphorus (177), zinc (130, 177, 178, 201, 202), and presumably magnesium, prevent maximal protein-sparing and may blunt or prevent an anabolic response to refeeding.

Metabolic Disease or the Administration of Hormones or Antimetabolites.   Hyperthyroidism, pheochromocytoma, glucagonoma, poorly controlled diabetes mellitus, and states of glucocorticoid excess (203) induce protein wasting. The presence of any of these diseases, or its new development, calls for attention to the starving patient's nutritional status, for in any of these situations a previously successful adaptation will be reversed and protein-energy malnutrition rapidly worsen. Evidence indicates that the efficiency of protein metabolism remains abnormal even during intense insulin treatment of insulin-dependent diabetes (204). Patients with insulin-dependent diabetes may be at especially increased risk of protein depletion during starvation.

Food Restriction too Severe.   The most common maladaptation to starvation is not really maladaptation, but simply the consequence of food deprivation that is so severe that adaptation to it is physiologically impossible. The result is continuous weight loss until death supervenes.

Clinical Significance of Serum Albumin

Hypoalbuminemia is an important predictor of an adverse clinical outcome, but contrary to common clinical assumption, it is neither sensitive nor specific as an indicator of protein deficiency or protein-energy malnutrition (5, 123, 124). Knowledge of a patient's serum albumin concentration is valuable in nutritional assessment for two reasons. First, a normal serum albumin concentration (in a volume-replete patient) strongly rules against the presence of an acute phase response and failed adaptation to starvation, and portends a favorable clinical outcome. Second, hypoalbuminemia, whatever its cause, almost always occurs in a clinical context of anorexia and inadequate food intake, and therefore alerts the clinician of the need for a comprehensive nutritional assessment and serious consideration of nutritional intervention.

Survival

The Minnesota experiment, among many others (205, 206), illustrated that body weight loss tracks lean tissue

loss in starving people whose starting body composition was normal. Approximately half of the total protein in the human body is extracellular and structural (mostly collagen). The other half is found within the lean tissues, which make up nearly half of total body weight in healthy people. Lean tissues are the site of N loss in starvation (207). It is commonly considered that 50% or greater depletion of the body's lean tissue mass is incompatible with survival (2, 89, 208). Body mass index (BMI, body weight in kilograms divided by the square of height in meters) is a better predictor of the certainty of death than body weight. Data analyzed by Henry (209) suggest that death is certain when the BMI falls to less than approximately 13 in men and 12 in women, although some subsequent experience indicates that a BMI of 10 is compatible with life in mature adults, and even lower BMIs have been tolerated by young adults (210). One fifth of starving adults more than 25 years old, and nearly one half of those less than 25 years old admitted to a medical unit in Somalia had a BMI less than 12. Survival with a BMI this low is rare in affluent countries, where advanced starvation typically occurs in elderly persons suffering from a primary medical or surgical condition. Such extraordinary tolerance to severe starvation by healthy young adults stands in marked contrast to conventional medical teaching, which dictates that any weight loss more than 10% lower than the patient's norm indicates potentially serious malnutrition (211). There is plainly an important interaction among malnutrition, age, and primary disease in starvation-related death.

In developed countries, where severe malnutrition is almost always attributable to a primary medical or surgical disease, the immediate causes of death are infectious pneumonia (related to decreased ventilatory mechanical function and drive, lung stasis, and ineffective cough), skin breakdown with local and systemic infection (related to inactivity, skin thinning, and edema), sepsis spreading from intravenous infusion catheters, diarrhea with dehydration, or synergistic worsening of the primary disease. Contributing to all these causes is starvation-induced immunodeficiency, itself the result of decreased intracellular protein stores, hypothermia, and micronutrient deficiencies (1, 2). In some patients, death is attributed to a cardiac arrhythmia (131, 212).

In summary, the nature and tempo of a patient's primary disease is a strong but not the only determinant of death in moderate, in-hospital starvation. As lean tissue depletion approaches and exceeds 40%, death directly owing to the complications of starvation becomes increasingly more certain, manifesting an immutable thermodynamic law that is unaffected by the number of diagnostic procedures, operative interventions, or antibiotic combinations administered to the patient, unless they are combined with an effective nutritional intervention (213).

Descriptions of needless death from starvation evoke feelings of dismay in most commentators. Particularly moving is Fliederbaum's description of the effects of severe starvation in the Warsaw ghetto (185):

> . . . Boys and girls from blooming like roses change into withered old people. One of the patients said, "Our strength is vanishing like melting wax candle." Active, busy, energetic people are changed into apathetic, sleepy beings, always in bed, hardly able to get up to eat or to go to the toilet. Passage from life to death is slow and gradual, like death from physiological old age. There is nothing violent, no dyspnea, no pain, no obvious changes in breathing or circulation. Vital functions subside simultaneously. Pulse rate and respiratory rate get slower and it becomes more and more difficult to reach the patient's awareness, until life is gone. People fall asleep in bed or on the street and are dead in the morning. They die during physical effort, such as searching for food, and sometimes even with a piece of bread in their hands.

HORMONAL MEDIATION OF THE ADAPTATION TO STARVATION

The foregoing discussion dealt with nutritional factors that affect the physiologic adaptation to starvation. This section briefly enumerates the biochemical mechanisms that mediate this adaptation.

Energy Metabolism

The adaptive reduction in REE in starvation is mediated by alterations in the peripheral metabolism of thyroxine (T_4), the hormone secreted by the thyroid gland, to its more active metabolite, triiodothyronine (T_3), and perhaps, to a lesser extent, by changes in sympathetic nervous system activity (85, 180, 214). Serum concentrations of thyrotropin, the pituitary hormone that regulates T_4 secretion, remain normal; but serum T_3 decreases within a few days (or even hours) after initiating a starvation diet. Serum levels of an inactive metabolite, reverse T_3, rise (215). Energy intake or, more specifically, the amount of carbohydrate consumed, directs this conversion process, apparently through its effect on insulin secretion (180, 216).

As long as volume depletion is prevented (76), catecholamine secretion and turnover decrease in uncomplicated starvation. The blood pressure, heart rate, and core temperature of starving people are reduced, as is their thermic response to cold or to a norepinephrine infusion. Pupil size, an indicator of basal sympathetic tone, is diminished (131, 137). As with T_4 to T_3 conversion, total energy and carbohydrate intake, at least in part because of their effect on insulin release, appear to be important regulators of these effects. The thyroid and catecholamine effects are interactive (217).

Plasma concentrations of leptin, a cytokine-like hormone released by adipocytes, decrease importantly both in short- and long-term energy restriction while also reflecting the magnitude of the body fat store in states of energy equilibrium (218, 219). Leptin interacts with insulin, which partly regulates its secretion (218).

Ghrelin is a peptide hormone secreted mainly by endocrine cells of the stomach. Circulating ghrelin concentrations increase before meals and are inhibited by food consumption, especially protein and carbohydrate. Ghrelin acts on the brain to modulate eating behavior and stimulate growth hormone secretion, coordinating the disposition of the ingested food. Plasma ghrelin concentrations increase in starvation (220–222).

Protein Metabolism

Insulin stimulates muscle and liver cells to increase protein synthesis and it inhibits protein breakdown in muscle and liver; insulin lack reduces protein synthesis in both tissues and markedly increases proteolysis in muscle (15, 223). In the splanchnic tissues, protein synthesis is increased by amino acid provision even in low insulin states, whereas muscle protein synthesis requires both insulin and an amino acid supply (224). Although not low enough to induce ketosis, insulin levels are reduced in starvation (175, 225). The combination of a low-insulin state and reduced dietary amino acid availability reduces muscle protein synthesis and, secondarily, proteolysis (105, 226). The combined effect of reduced insulin effect and diminished amino acid supply is expressed directly on the cells, but also may be expressed indirectly by diminishing the peripheral action of thyroid hormone (226).

Both protein or energy restriction and catabolic states lower circulating concentrations of the anabolic peptide hormone, insulinlike growth factor-I (IGF-I). IGF-I lowering occurs despite increased serum concentrations of growth hormone, which normally stimulates IGF-I release (216, 227). Structurally related to insulin, IGF-I stimulates net protein synthesis in a manner similar to insulin (15). Despite the complexity of IGF-I's autocrine and paracrine functions and its numerous plasma binding proteins (IGFBP), it is clear that IGF-I plays an important role in the adaptation of protein metabolism to altered nutritional states, acting in concert with insulin and thyroid hormone (228, 229). Both energy and protein intake affect plasma IGF-I concentrations and concentrations of its chief intravascular binding protein, IGFBP-3. When dietary energy is severely restricted, the amount of carbohydrate consumed is a major determinant of the circulating IGF-I response to growth hormone stimulation (227).

In summary, the level of protein intake appears to be the key external regulator of the adaptation of protein metabolism to starvation, because the ingested amino acids provide the main substrate for body protein synthesis. Both energy and protein restriction evoke an intricate, coordinated hormonal response, mediated by insulin, growth hormone, IGF-I, and thyroid hormone, which reorganizes amino acid traffic to bring about an orderly adaptation to the altered nutritional environment (230). Under favorable conditions this adaptation progressively reduces body protein loss until it matches the current level of protein intake, re-establishing zero body protein balance. The adaptation is partly automatic (because the lean tissue mass has decreased) and partly regulated, because a lower rate of protein synthesis and breakdown in the remaining lean tissues allows for more efficient processing of dietary protein and recycling of endogenous amino acids.

CHRONIC ENERGY DEFICIENCY

It is easy to recognize patients suffering from starvation in a clinic or hospital ward (129, 231), but far less obvious what the minimum acceptable food intake and corresponding nutritional state is in societies in which food is scarce and low body weight is common (208, 217, 232). To address this dilemma, a form of adapted protein-energy starvation called adult chronic energy deficiency (CED) has been defined (233, 234). This stable but undernourished condition is not necessarily pathologic, for it may be compatible with gainful employment, pregnancy, and other aspects of normal daily life. CED is defined as a subnormal BMI classified into three grades of severity: grade I, 17.0 to 18.4; grade II, 16.0 to 16.9; and grade III, less than 16 (233).

BMI reflects the body's fat store both in obesity and underweight. A BMI between 20 and 25 is generally regarded as normal (46). In the United States, Hungary, or Brazil, fewer than 5% of adults have a BMI less than 18.5, whereas 10% of Chinese, 20% of Congolese, 25% of Pakistani or Philippine adults, and nearly 50% of Indian adults have been reported in this category (233, 234). In otherwise healthy people, only grades II and III CED are associated with an increasing probability of days of illness, reduced physical work capacity, poorer reproductive function, and poorer lactation performance. Decreased voluntary physical activity has been shown only in grade III CED. Therefore, a BMI of 17.0 to 18.5 is compatible with normal function (235). Many normal persons—especially young adults—whose BMI is in this range could be incorrectly diagnosed as malnourished (233, 234).

In summary, it appears that young adults with no intercurrent disease can tolerate a BMI as low as 17 without physiologic dysfunction, even though they lack nutritional reserves. Even BMIs less than 17, although associated with disability, may be tolerable in well-adapted CED. At the other extreme, BMIs greater than 18.5 do not rule out severe protein-energy malnutrition, because an increased adipose or extracellular fluid mass may conceal serious lean tissue depletion. Better criteria than body weight or BMI alone are plainly required to identify dangerous protein or protein-energy starvation. The best clinical criteria currently available are ones that point to failed adaptation to starvation, namely, continuing weight loss, functional disability, and hypoalbuminemia, the latter indicating the presence of a catabolic state that will predictably impair adaptation (3, 236). It is usually possible to distinguish between normalcy and CED in someone with a low but stable body weight. The normal person will report normal appetite and food intake, a normal level of physical function, and adequate muscle mass on physical examination.

CACHEXIA

Patients with severe tissue injury develop a hypermetabolic response termed the *systemic inflammatory response syndrome* (SIRS), which has been defined as the presence of two or more of the following: fever (or profound hypothermia), tachycardia, tachypnea, and leukocytosis (or increased numbers of band forms) (237). Other defining features of the SIRS are changes in acute phase serum protein concentrations (238), anorexia, increased energy expenditure, increased whole body protein turnover, and protein wasting (237). Protein wasting may be regarded as the metabolic cost of rapidly mobilizing amino acids for wound healing and the synthesis of immune cells and proteins (239).

A milder inflammatory condition is highly prevalent on the general medical and surgical wards of hospitals. This syndrome, termed *cachexia* (3–6), develops in the presence of chronic infection, inflammatory disease, neoplastic disease (when associated with continuous involuntary weight loss), and in many forms of end-organ disease including chronic renal failure and end-stage heart disease (240–243). Cachexia is characterized by anorexia, the anemia of chronic disease, and abnormal concentrations of the acute phase serum proteins (238) (some of which, such as C-reactive protein, fibrinogen, ferritin and haptoglobin, are increased, whereas others, such as transferrin, transthyretin and albumin, are decreased).

It has been proposed that cachexia not be considered as a form of malnutrition, on the grounds that it is neither caused by inadequate nutritional intake nor cured by supplemental nutrition (3, 244). However, unlike SIRS, in which protein catabolism predominates, the major contributor to body weight and lean tissue loss in most cachectic syndromes is cytokine-induced anorexia and reduced food consumption combined with impaired adaptation. Anorexia and the inhibition of anabolic signals caused by cytokines hinder nutritional rehabilitation, and the constitutional symptom of fatigue limits mobility and the muscular exercise people need to maintain or rebuild their lean tissues (245). Nevertheless, protein and energy balance can be maintained and improved in many cases if an appropriate nutritional and exercise strategy can be implemented (241, 246–248).

REFEEDING

The refeeding syndrome develops in severely wasted patients during the first week of nutritional repletion (96, 249). Expansion of the extracellular fluid volume is rapid and considerable, and not infrequently leads to dependent edema. Refeeding edema results from the combined effects of increased sodium intake (in a sodium-depleted person) and the antinatriuretic effect of insulin, levels of which increase in response to increased carbohydrate consumption. Refeeding edema can be minimized by limiting sodium and carbohydrate intake during refeeding (96, 128, 249). Carbohydrate refeeding may stimulate enough glucose-6-phospate and glycogen synthesis to seriously lower serum phosphate concentrations. Refeeding also increases REE, and, when protein is included, stimulates N retention, new cell synthesis, and cellular rehydration (128, 250). Depletion of phosphate, potassium, magnesium, zinc, and vitamins used in metabolic pathways is common (130, 177, 178, 201, 202, 249, 251). Unless mineral status is judiciously monitored during refeeding, acute deficiencies will develop, especially of phosphorus and potassium. Mild deficiencies may merely prevent an anabolic response to refeeding (177, 178, 201). Left heart failure may occur in predisposed patients (252). The ingredients for heart failure are an abrupt increase of intravascular volume, increased REE (which increases demands for cardiac output), an atrophic left ventricle with a poor stroke volume (131, 253), and myocardial deficiencies of potassium, phosphorus, or magnesium. Cardiac arrhythmias may occur (254). Acute thiamine deficiency is a potential hazard (249).

REE returns toward normal as the result of two processes. First, the hypometabolic state of adapted starvation is reversed, and REE increases substantially during the first week of refeeding (250, 255). REE then increases more gradually as the lean tissue mass rebuilds. Circulating IGF-I, which is reduced in all forms of starvation, increases rapidly within days to a week of refeeding and is associated with improving N balance (227, 256, 257). The specific changes in body composition that occur during refeeding depend on the existing metabolic state and body composition, and importantly, on the composition of the refeeding diet. A diet high in sodium and carbohydrate predisposes to large increases in extracellular volume and refeeding edema. A high-energy, low-protein diet produces fat gain but does not increase the lean tissue mass (128). A high-protein diet (e.g., 2 g/kg body weight/day) can arrest ongoing N losses even when energy balance is negative (157). A high-energy, high-protein diet repletes both fat and lean tissue stores at a rate that can be predicted reasonably accurately from the resulting energy and N balances, both of which can be measured or estimated. Physical activity stimulates muscle accretion. Malnourished patients who remain immobile increase their central protein stores upon refeeding—an important benefit—but do not regain much muscle mass. Ongoing inflammation can reduce or prevent lean tissue regain even when the energy balance is positive, and hence merely induce fat accumulation.

Many features of the refeeding process are illustrated by a clinical trial in which two protein levels were sequentially provided to severely starved men (128). When the diet was generous in energy (2250 kcal/day) but low in protein (27 g/day), the patients' weight, body fat, and serum cholesterol increased, but N balance remained nearly zero; their serum albumin, blood hematocrit, and urinary creatinine excretion (a measure of the body's muscle mass)

failed to increase even after 45 days of refeeding. When the protein content of the diet was increased to 100 g/day, daily N balance became strongly positive. After 45 days of consuming this diet, BMI had increased to normal, serum albumin was nearly normal, and creatinine excretion had increased by 40%. Ninety days of the 100-g protein diet were required before serum albumin, BMI, and blood hemoglobin were fully normalized.

The following steps are recommended when refeeding severely malnourished patients. Once fluid volume and electrolyte disorders have been corrected (and kept normal, if necessary, by continuing supplementation), a mixed diet is provided at the estimated maintenance energy level to establish tolerance and avoid the refeeding syndrome. Close clinical monitoring and judicious administration of carbohydrate continue until blood electrolyte concentrations and the patient's clinical status have stabilized (251). Even at a maintenance level of energy provision, N balance becomes positive in nonstressed patients (165). Energy intake is then increased to promote adipose tissue restoration and accelerate protein accretion. A generous protein intake (1.5 to 2.0 g/kg of dry body weight) promotes the most rapid repletion of body protein at any energy level (165). Greater protein intakes than this confer no additional advantage to the nonstressed adult (210).

REFERENCES

1. Golden MHN, Jackson AA. Chronic severe undernutrition. 5th ed. In: Olson RE, Brosquist HP, Chichester CO et al, eds. Present Knowledge in Nutrition. Washington, DC: Nutrition Foundation, 1984:57–67.
2. Rivers JPW. The nutritional biology of famine. In: Harrison GA, ed. Famine. Oxford: Oxford University Press, 1988: 57–106.
3. Evans WJ, Morley JE, Argilés J et al. Clin Nutr 2008;27:793–9.
4. Thomas DR. Clin Nutr 2007;26:389–99.
5. Jensen GL, Bistrian B, Roubenoff R et al. JPEN J Parenter Enteral Nutr 2009;33:710–6.
6. Muscaritoli M, Anker SD, Argiles J et al. Clin Nutr 2010;29: 154–9.
7. Cahill GF Jr. Clin Endocrinol Metab 1976;5:397–415.
8. Aoki TT, Muller WA, Brennan MF et al. Am J Clin Nutr 1975;28:507–11.
9. Lusk G. The Science of Nutrition. Philadelphia: Saunders, 1928.
10. Felig P. Starvation. In: DeGroot LJ, Cahill GF Jr, Odell WD et al, eds. Endocrinology. New York: Grune & Stratton, 1979:1927–40.
11. Radziuk J, Pye S. Diabetes Metab Res Rev 2001;17:250–72.
12. Rothman DL, Magnusson I, Katz LD et al. Science 1991;254:573–6.
13. Jungas RL, Halperin ML, Brosnan JT. Physiol Rev 1992;72:419–48.
14. Nuttall FQ, Ngo A, Gannon MC. Diabetes Metab Res Rev 2008;24:438–58.
15. Kettelhut IC, Wing SS, Goldberg AL. Diabetes Metab Rev 1988;4:751–72.
16. Foster DW, McGarry JD. N Engl J Med 1983;309:159–69.
17. Owen OE, Caprio S, Reichard GA Jr et al. Clin Endocrinol Metab 1983;12:359–79.

18. Hultman E, Nilsson LH. Nutr Metab 1975;18(Suppl):45–64.

19. Sugden MC, Sharples SC, Randle PJ. Biochem J 1976;160: 817–9.

20. Nair KS, Woolf PD, Welle SL et al. Am J Clin Nutr 1987; 46:557–62.

21. Katz J, Tayek JA. Am J Physiol 1998;275:E537–42.

22. Owen OE, Morgan AP, Kemp HG et al. J Clin Invest 1967; 46:1589–95.

23. Redies C, Hoffer LJ, Beil C et al. Am J Physiol 1989;256: E805–10.

24. Hasselbalch SG, Knudsen GM, Jakobsen J et al. J Cereb Blood Flow Metab 1994;14:125–31.

25. Balasse EO, Fery F. Diabetes Metab Rev 1989;5:247–70.

26. Haymond MW, Karl IE, Clarke WL et al. Metabolism 1982;31:33–42.

27. Rudolf MC, Sherwin RS. Clin Endocrinol Metab 1983;12: 413–28.

28. Halperin ML, Cheema-Dhadli S. Diabetes Metab Rev 1989; 321–36.

29. Guyton JR. Curr Opin Lipidol 2007;18:415–20.

30. McGarry JD, Woeltje KF, Kuwajmi M et al. Diabetes Metab Rev 1989;5:271–84.

31. Fulop M. Diabetes Metab Rev 1989;5:365–78.

32. Halperin ML, Cherney DZI, Kamel KS. Ketoacidosis. In: DuBose TD Jr, Hamm LL, eds. Acid–Base Disorders: A Companion to Brenner and Rector's The Kidney. Philadelphia: Saunders, 2002:67–82.

33. Mahoney CA. Am J Kidney Dis 1992;20:276–80.

34. Schade DS, Eaton RP. Diabetes 1979;28:5–10.

35. Miles JM, Haymond MW, Nissen SL et al. J Clin Invest 1983;71:1554–61.

36. Bliss M. The Discovery of Insulin. Toronto: McLelland & Stewart, 1982.

37. Weinman EJ, Eknoyan G, Suki WN. J Clin Invest 1975;55: 283–91.

38. Feinstein EI, Quion-Verde H, Kaptein EM et al. Am J Nephrol 1984;4:77–80.

39. Eriksson UJ. Diabetes Metab Rev 1995;11:63–82.

40. Laffel L. Diab/Metab Res Rev 1999;15:412–26.

41. Toohill J, Soong B, Flenady V. Cochrane Database Syst Rev 2008;(3):CD004230.

42. Krzywicki HJ, Consolazio CF, Matoush LO et al. Am J Clin Nutr 1968;21:87–97.

43. Hammarqvist F, Andersson K, Luo JL et al. Clin Nutr 2005;24:236–43.

44. Reifenstein EC Jr, Albright F, Wells SL. J Clin Endocrinol 1947;5:367–95.

45. Sapir DG, Chambers NE, Ryan JW. Metabolism 1976;25: 211–20.

46. Food and Agriculture Organization/World Health Organization/ United Nations University. Energy and Protein Requirements: FAO/WHO/UNU Expert Consultation. Geneva: World Health Organization, 1985. Technical Report Series 724.

47. Crim MC, Munro HN. Proteins and amino acids. In: Shils ME, Olson JA, Shike M, eds. Modern Nutrition in Health and Disease. 8th ed. Philadelphia: Lea & Febiger, 1994:3–35.

48. Lariviere F, Kupranycz D, Chiasson JL et al. Am J Physiol 1992;263:E173–9.

49. Raguso CA, Pereira P, Young VR. Am J Clin Nutr 1999;70: 474–83.

50. Lariviere F, Wagner DA, Kupranycz D et al. Metabolism 1990;39:1270–7.

51. Umpleby AM, Scobie IN, Boroujerdi MA et al. Eur J Clin Invest 1995;25:619–26.

52. Afolabi PR, Jahoor F, Jackson AA et al. Am J Physiol 2007; 293:E1580–9.

53. Giesecke K, Magnusson I, Ahlberg M et al. Metabolism 1989; 38:1196–200.

54. Vazquez JA, Morse EL, Adibi SA. J Clin Invest 1985;76: 737–43.

55. Henson LC, Heber D. J Clin Endocrinol Metab 1983;57:316–9.

56. Hoffer LJ, Forse RA. Am J Physiol 1990;258:E832–40.

57. Winterer J, Bistrian BR, Bilmazes C et al. Metabolism 1980;29:575–81.

58. Jefferson LS. Diabetes 1980;29:487–96.

59. Palaiologos G, Felig P. Biochem J 1976;154:709–16.

60. Nair KS, Welle SL, Halliday D et al. J Clin Invest 1988;82: 198–205.

61. Norrelund H, Nair KS, Nielsen S et al. J Clin Endocrinol Metab 2003;88:4371–8.

62. May ME, Buse MG. Diabetes Metab Rev 1989;5:227–45.

63. Drenick EJ. Weight reduction by prolonged fasting. In: Bray GA, ed. Obesity in Perspective: John E. Fogarty International Center for Advanced Study in the Health Sciences. DHEW publication no. NIH 75–708. Bethesda, MD: National Institutes of Health, 1973:341–60.

64. Contaldo F, Presto E, Di Biase G et al. Int J Obes 1982;6: 97–100.

65. Drenick EJ. The effects of acute and prolonged fasting and refeeding on water, electrolyte, and acid-base metabolism. In: Maxwell MH, Kleeman CR, eds. Clinical Disorders of Fluid and Electrolyte Metabolism. New York: McGraw-Hill, 1980:1481–501.

66. Van Itallie TB, Yang MU. N Engl J Med 1977;297:1158–61.

67. Hood VL. Fluid and electrolyte disturbances during starvation. In: Kokko JP, Tannen RL, eds. Fluids and Electrolytes. Philadelphia: Saunders, 1986:712–41.

68. Nilsson LH. Scand J Clin Lab Invest 1973;32:317–23.

69. Olsson KE, Saltin B. Acta Physiol Scand 1970;80:11–8.

70. Grande F, Keys A. Body weight, body composition and calorie status. In: Goodhart RS, Shils ME, eds. Modern Nutrition in Health and Disease. 6th ed. Philadelphia: Lea & Febiger, 1980:3–34.

71. Garrow JS. Am J Clin Nutr 1982;35:1152–8.

72. Waki M, Kral JG, Mazariegos M et al. Am J Physiol 1991;261:E199–203.

73. Weyer C, Vozarova B, Ravussin E et al. Int J Obes 2001;25: 593–600.

74. Elia M. Effect of starvation and very low calorie diets on protein-energy interrelationships in lean and obese subjects. In: Scrimshaw N, Schurch B, eds. Protein-Energy Interactions. Lausanne: Nestlé Foundation, 1992:249–84.

75. Zauner C, Schneeweiss B, Kranz A et al. Am J Clin Nutr 2000;71:1511–5.

76. Welle S. Am J Clin Nutr 1995;62:1118S–22S.

77. Tracey KJ, Legaspi A, Albert JD et al. Clin Sci 1988;74:123–32.

78. Shetty PS, Watrasiewicz KE, Jung RT et al. Lancet 1979;2:230–2.

79. Hoffer LJ, Bistrian BR, Young VR et al. Metabolism 1984;33:820–5.

80. Barrett PVD. JAMA 1971;217:1349–53.

81. Corvilain B, Abramowicz M, Fery F et al. Am J Physiol 1995;269:G512–7.

82. Peters A, Rohloff D, Kohlmann T et al. Blood 1998;91:691–4.

83. Gamble JL. Harvey Lectures 1947;43:247–73.

84. O'Connell RC, Morgan AP, Aoki TT et al. J Clin Endocrinol Metab 1974;39:555–63.

85. Gelfand RA, Hendler R. Diabetes Metab Rev 1989;5:17–30.

86. Vazquez JA, Kazi U, Madani N. Am J Clin Nutr 1995;62: 93–103.

87. Bolinger RE, Luker BP, Brown RW et al. Arch Intern Med 1966;118:3–8.

88. Leiter LA, Marliss EB. JAMA 1982;248:2306–7.

89. Elia M. Clin Nutr 2000;19:379–86.

90. Korbonits M, Blaine D, Elia M et al. Eur J Endocrinol 2007;157:157–66.

91. Friedl KE, Moore RJ, Martinez-Lopez LE et al. J Appl Physiol 1994;77:933–40.

92. Thomson TJ, Runcie J, Miller V. Lancet 1966;2:992–6.

93. Barnard DL, Ford J, Garnett ES et al. Metabolism 1969;18:564–9.

94. Stewart WK, Fleming LW. Postgrad Med J 1973;49:203–9.

95. Devathasan G, Koh C. Lancet 1982;Nov.13:1108–9.

96. Crook MA, Hally V, Panteli JV. Nutrition 2001;17:632–7.

97. Waterlow JC. What do we mean by adaptation? In: Blaxter K, Waterlow JC, eds. Nutritional Adaptation in Man. London: John Libbey, 1985:1–11.

98. Hoffer LJ. Evaluation of the adaptation to protein restriction in humans. In: El-Khoury AE, ed. Methods for the Investigation of Amino Acid and Protein Metabolism. Boca Raton, FL: CRC Press, 1999:83–102.

99. Food and Agriculture Organization/World Health Organization/United Nations University. Protein and Amino Acid Requirements in Human Nutrition: Report of a Joint WHO/FAO/UNU Expert Consultation. World Health Organization, 2007. WHO Technical Report Series 935.

100. Carpenter KJ. Protein and Energy: A Study of Changing Ideas in Nutrition. New York: Cambridge University Press, 1994.

101. Young VR, Marchini JS. Am J Clin Nutr 1990;51:270–89.

102. Durnin JV, Garlick P, Jackson AA et al. Eur J Clin Nutr 1999; 53(Suppl):S174–S176.

103. Krebs HA. Adv Enzyme Regul 1972;10:397–420.

104. Young VR, Moldawer LL, Hoerr R et al. Mechanisms of adaptation to protein malnutrition. In: Blaxter K, Waterlow JC, eds. Nutritional Adaptation in Man. London: John Libbey, 1985:189–217.

105. Eisenstein RS, Harper AE. J Nutr 1991;121:1581–90.

106. Young VR, Meredith C, Hoerr R et al. Amino acid kinetics in relation to protein and amino acid requirements: the primary importance of amino acid oxidation. In: Garrow JS, Halliday D, eds. Substrate and Energy Metabolism in Man. London: John Libbey, 1985:119–34.

107. Klasing KC. J Nutr 2009;139:11–2.

108. Millward DJ, Rivers JPW. Eur J Clin Nutr 1988;42:367–93.

109. Hamadeh MJ, Hoffer LJ. Am J Physiol 2001;280:E857–E866.

110. Hoffer LJ, Bistrian BR, Young VR et al. J Clin Invest 1984; 73:750–8.

111. Quevedo MR, Price GM, Halliday D et al. Clin Sci 1994;86:185–93.

112. Forslund AH, Hambraeus L, Olsson RM et al. Am J Physiol 1998;275:E310–E320.

113. Arnal MA, Mosoni L, Boirie Y et al. Am J Physiol 2000;278:E902–E909.

114. Hoerr RA, Matthews DE, Bier DM et al. Am J Physiol 1993;264:E567–E575.

115. Waterlow JC. Annu Rev Nutr 1986;6:495–526.

116. Panel on Macronutrients, Subcommittees on Upper Reference Levels of Nutrients and Interpretation and Uses of Dietary Reference Intakes, Standing Committee on the Scientific Evaluation of Dietary Reference Intakes. Dietary Reference Intakes for Energy, Carbohydrate, Fiber, Fat, Fatty Acids, Cholesterol, Protein, and Amino Acids (Macronutrients). Washington, DC: Food and Nutrition Board, Institute of Medicine, National Academy Press, 2005.

117. Ihle BU, Becker G, Whitworth JA et al. N Engl J Med 1989;321:1773–7.

118. Castaneda C, Charnley JM, Evans WJ et al. Am J Clin Nutr 1995;62:30–9.

119. Castaneda C, Dolnikowski GG, Dallal GE et al. Am J Clin Nutr 1995;62:40–8.

120. Munro HN. General aspects of the regulation of protein metabolism by diet and hormones. In: Munro HN, Allison JB, eds. Mammalian Protein Metabolism, vol 1. New York: Academic Press, 1964:381–481.

121. Latham MC. Protein-energy malnutrition. In: Brown ML, ed. Present Knowledge in Nutrition. Washington, DC: International Life Sciences Institute-Nutrition Foundation, 1990:39–46.

122. Ahmed T, Rahman S, Cravioto A. Indian J Med Res 2009;130:651–4.

123. Franch-Arcas G. Clin Nutr 2001;20:265–9.

124. Ballmer PE. Clin Nutr 2001;20:271–3.

125. Barac-Nieto M, Spurr GB, Lotero H et al. Am J Clin Nutr 1978;31:23–40.

126. Lunn PG, Morley CJ, Neale G. Clin Nutr 1998;17:131–3.

127. Jackson AA, Phillips G, McClelland I et al. Am J Physiol 2001;281:G1179–87.

128. Barac-Nieto M, Spurr GB, Lotero H et al. Am J Clin Nutr 1979;32:981–91.

129. Hoffer LJ. CMAJ 2001;165:1345–9.

130. Golden BE, Golden MH. Eur J Clin Nutr 1992;46:697–706.

131. Keys A, Brozek J, Henschel A et al. The Biology of Human Starvation. Minneapolis: The University of Minnesota Press, 1950.

132. Kalm LM, Semba RD. J Nutr 2005;135:1347–52.

133. Ravussin E, Lillioja S, Anderson TE et al. J Clin Invest 1986;78:1568–78.

134. Foster GD, Wadden TA, Kendrick ZV et al. Med Sci Sports Exerc 1995;27:888–94.

135. Rosenbaum M, Vandenborne K, Goldsmith R et al. Am J Physiol 2003;285:R183–92.

136. Prentice AM, Goldberg GR, Jebb SA et al. Proc Nutr Soc 1991;50:441–58.

137. Shetty PS, Kurpad AV. Eur J Clin Nutr 1990;44(Suppl):47–53.

138. Toth MJ. Curr Opin Clin Nutr Metab Care 1999;2:445–51.

139. Leibel RL, Rosenbaum M, Hirsch J. N Engl J Med 1995;332:621–8.

140. Rosenbaum M, Hirsch J, Murphy E et al. Am J Clin Nutr 2000;71:1421–32.

141. Heyman MB, Young VR, Fuss P et al. Am J Physiol 1992;263:R250–7.

142. Weinsier RL, Schutz Y, Bracco D. Am J Clin Nutr 1992;55:790–4.

143. McClave SA, Snider HL. Curr Opin Clin Nutr Metab Care 2001;4:143–7.

144. Soares MJ, Piers LS, Shetty PS et al. Clin Sci 1994;86:441–6.

145. Ravussin E, Bogardus C. Am J Clin Nutr 1989;49:968–75.

146. Luke A, Schoeller DA. Metabolism 1992;41:450–6.

147. Scalfi L, Di Biase G, Coltorti A et al. Eur J Clin Nutr 1993;47:61–7.

148. Grande F. Man under caloric deficiency. In: Dill DB, ed. Handbook of Physiology, Section 4: Adaptation to the Environment. Washington, DC: American Physiological Society 1964:911–37.

149. Lusk G. Physiol Rev 1921;1:523–52.

150. Smith SR, Pozefsky T, Chhetri MK. Metabolism 1974;23:603–18.

151. Hamadeh MJ, Schiffrin A, Hoffer LJ. Am J Physiol 2001;281:E341–8.

152. Waterlow JC. Annu Rev Nutr 1995;15:57–92.

153. Rennie MJ, Harrison R. Lancet 1984;1:323–5.

154. Wykes LJ, Fiorotto M, Burrin DG et al. J Nutr 1996;126:1481–8.

155. Garlick PJ, Clugston GA, Waterlow JC. Am J Physiol 1980;238:E235–44.

156. Tessari P, Garibotto G, Inchiostro S et al. J Clin Invest 1996;98:1481–92.

157. Hoffer LJ. Am J Clin Nutr 2003;78:906–11.

158. Kurpad AV, Regan MM, Raj T et al. Am J Clin Nutr 2003;77:101–8.

159. Winter TA. Curr Opin Clin Nutr Metab Care 2006;9:596–602.

160. Elwyn DH, Gump FE, Munro HN et al. Am J Clin Nutr 1979;32:1597–611.

161. Pellett PL, Young VR. The effects of different levels of energy intake on protein metabolism and of different levels of protein intake on energy metabolism: a statistical evaluation from the published literature. In: Scrimshaw N, Schurch B, eds. Protein-Energy Interactions. Lausanne: Nestlé Foundation, 1992:81–121.

162. Munro HN. Physiol Rev 1951;31:449–88.

163. Kinney JM, Elwyn DH. Annu Rev Nutr 1983;3:433–66.

164. Goranzon H, Forsum E. Am J Clin Nutr 1985;41:919–28.

165. Shaw SN, Elwyn DH, Askanazi J et al. Am J Clin Nutr 1983;37:930–40.

166. Dickerson RN. Curr Opin Clin Nutr Metab Care 2005;8:189–96.

167. Singer P. Wien Klin Wochenschr 2007;119:218–22.

168. Piatti PM, Monti F, Fermo I et al. Metabolism 1994;43:1481–7.

169. Ballor DL, Poehlman ET. Int J Obes 1994;18:35–40.

170. Elia M, Stubbs RJ, Henry CJ. Obes Res 1999;7:597–604.

171. Hoffer LJ, Bistrian BR. J Obes Weight Reduction 1984;3:35–47.

172. Donnelly JE, Jacobsen DJ, Whatley JE. Am J Clin Nutr 1994;60:874–8.

173. Henry RR, Wiest-Kent TA, Scheaffer L et al. Diabetes 1986;35:155–64.

174. Velthuis-te Wierik EJM, Westerterp KR, van den Berg H. Int J Obes 1995;19:318–24.

175. Friedl KE, Moore RJ, Hoyt RW et al. J Appl Physiol 2000;88:1820–30.

176. Weyer C, Walford RL, Harper IT et al. Am J Clin Nutr 2000;72:946–53.

177. Rudman D, Millikan WJ, Richardson TJ et al. J Clin Invest 1975;55:94–104.

178. Knochel JP. Adv Int Med 1984;30:317–35.

179. Passmore R, Strong JA, Ritchie FJ. Br J Nutr 1958;12:113–22.

180. Danforth E Jr, Burger AG. Annu Rev Nutr 1989;9:201–27.

181. Golden MHN. Marasmus and kwashiorkor. In: Dickerson JWT, Lee MA, eds. Nutrition and the Clinical Management of Disease. 2nd ed. London: Edward Arnold, 1988:88–109.

182. Millward DJ. Proc Nutr Soc 1979;38:77–88.

183. Tomkins AM, Garlick PJ, Schofield WN et al. Clin Sci 1983;65:313–24.

184. Helweg-Larsen P, Hoffmeyer H, Kieler J et al. Acta Med Scand 1952;144(Suppl):1–460.

185. Fliederbaum J. Clinical aspects of hunger disease in adults. In: Winick M, ed. Hunger Disease: Studies by the Jewish Physicians in the Warsaw Ghetto. New York: John Wiley & Sons, 1979:11–44.

186. Owen OE. Starvation. In: DeGroot LJ, Besser GM, Cahill GF Jr et al, eds. Endocrinology. 2nd ed. Philadelphia: Saunders, 1989:2282–93.

187. Grant JP. Clinical impact of protein malnutrition on organ mass and function. In: Blackburn GL, Grant JP, Young VR, eds. Amino Acids: Metabolism and Medical Applications. Boston: John Wright, 1983:347–58.

188. Mora RJF. World J Surg 1999;23:530–5.

189. de Simone G, Scalfi L, Galderisi M et al. Br Heart J 1994;71:287–92.

190. Cooke RA, Chambers JB. Br J Hosp Med 1995;54:313–7.

191. Baier H, Somani P. Chest 1984;85:222–5.

192. Pingleton SK. Clin Chest Med 2001;22:149–63.

193. Thomas DR. Nutrition 2001;17:121–5.

194. Stacher G. Scand J Gastroenterol 2003;38:573–87.

195. Speerhas R. Cleve Clin J Med 1995;62:73–5.

196. Schurch MA, Rizzoli R, Slosman D et al. Ann Intern Med 1998;128:801–9.

197. Spence LA, Weaver CM. Am J Clin Nutr 2003;133:850S–1S.

198. Woodward B. Nutr Rev 1998;56:S84–S92.

199. Polito A, Cuzzolaro M, Raguzzini A et al. Eur J Clin Nutr 1998;52:655–62.

200. Bistrian BR. Nutritional assessment of the hospitalized patient: a practical approach. In: Wright RA, Heymsfield S, eds. Nutritional Assessment. Boston: Blackwell, 1984:183–205.

201. Wolman SL, Anderson GH, Marliss EB et al. Gastroenterol 1979;76:458–67.

202. Khanum S, Alam AN, Anwar I et al. Eur J Clin Nutr 1988;42:709–14.

203. Garrel DR, Delmas PD, Welsh C et al. Metabolism 1988;37:257–62.

204. Hoffer LJ. J Nutr 1998;128:333S–6S.

205. McWhirter JP, Pennington CR. Br Med J 1994;308:945–8.

206. Martin AC, Pascoe EM, Forbes DA. J Paediatr Child Health 2009;45:53–7.

207. James HM, Dabek JT, Chettle DR et al. Clin Sci 1984;67:73–82.

208. James WPT, Ferro-Luzzi A, Waterlow JC. Eur J Clin Nutr 1988;42:969–81.

209. Henry CJK. Eur J Clin Nutr 1990;44:329–35.

210. Collins S. Nature Med 1995;1:810–4.

211. ASPEN Board of Directors and the Clinical Guidelines Task Force. JPEN J Parenter Enteral Nutr 2002;26:1SA–138SA.

212. Isner JM, Roberts WC, Heymsfield SB et al. Ann Intern Med 1985;102:49–52.

213. Kotler DP, Tierney AR, Wang J et al. Am J Clin Nutr 1989;50:444–7.

214. Palmblad J, Levi L, Burger A et al. Acta Med Scand 1977;201:15–22.

215. Bianco AC, Salvatore D, Gereben B et al. Endocr Rev 2002;23:38–89.

216. Becker DJ. Annu Rev Nutr 1983;3:187–212.

217. Shetty PS. Nutr Res Rev 1990;3:49–74.

218. Coleman RA, Herrmann TS. Diabetologia 1999;42:639–46.

219. Prentice AM, Moore SE, Collinson AC et al. Nutr Rev 2002;60:S56–S67.

220. Foster-Schubert KE, Overduin J, Prudom CE et al. J Clin Endocrinol Metab 2008;93:1971–9.

221. Ashitani J, Matsumoto N, Nakazato M. Peptides 2009;30:1951–6.

222. Karczewska-Kupczewska M, Straczkowski M, Adamska A et al. Eur J Endocrinol 2010;162:235–9.

223. Abumrad NN, Williams P, Frexes-Steed M et al. Diabetes Metab Rev 1989;5:213–26.

IL-6 concentrations (65), and this attenuation coincides with preservation of central nervous system structure and motor function to resemble a more youthful phenotype (66, 67). In a long-term study in lean humans, CR resulted in 81% lower C-reactive protein levels, 47% lower TNF-α levels, and 17% lower concentrations of transforming growth factor-β_1 (TGF-β_1; stimulates tissue fibrosis), as compared with control subjects. These cytokine levels coincided with a significantly lower atherosclerosis risk profile and with improved diastolic cardiac function (14, 17). Collectively, both animal and human studies suggest that CR reduces systemic inflammation, at least when energy intake is sufficiently restricted. In light of the role of inflammation in the pathogenesis of numerous diseases and aging, these changes could be responsible for some of the life span–prolonging effects of CR.

Hormesis

Hormesis is a biologic phenomenon by which a low-intensity stressor increases resistance to another, more intense stressor. The hormetic response seems to be an evolutionarily acquired survival mechanism that allows an organism to adapt to modestly adverse external conditions so that it can better survive during more severe adverse conditions. Examples of hormetic responses are vaccination, in which administration of killed or inactivated pathogens stimulates immune defense activity against disease, and radiation hormesis, in which exposure of mice to low-levels of ionizing radiation protects against cancer when the mice are exposed to higher levels of radiation (68). Hormesis has also been proposed to play a role in aging and in mediating some of the antiaging effects of chronic CR (69). The hypothesis is that CR is a low-grade stressor that causes a survival response in the organism by activating antiaging pathways (69). In support of this notion, CR has been shown to increase serum levels of corticosterone and to enhance the expression of heat shock proteins, both of which may help the organism deal with a large array of acute stressors and toxic agents (70–72). Furthermore, calorie-restricted animals are more resistant to a wide range of external stresses (e.g., radiation, surgery, exposure to heat) (69–73). Finally, CR has been shown to enhance DNA repair systems and to up-regulate endogenous enzymatic and nonenzymatic antioxidative defense mechanisms (74, 75). These findings provide evidence that hormetic adaptations to CR prepare the organism to better handle stresses that cause oxidative damage.

Oxidative Stress

Macronutrients are metabolized to yield energy for the synthesis of ATP, which is the immediate energy source used in most energy-requiring processes in animals and humans. During macronutrient metabolism, activity of the electron transport chain generates free radical molecules, primarily superoxide anion, hydrogen peroxide, and nitric oxide, which are often called reactive oxygen species. Free radicals are highly reactive molecules that readily participate in oxidation reactions with molecules, such as protein, lipid, and DNA, and thereby cause oxidative damage to these molecules and the structures in which they are located.

One theory on the causes of aging suggests that the age-associated increase in the accumulation of oxidative damage to nuclear and mitochondrial DNA is largely responsible for the deterioration in tissue structure and function that occurs during aging and ultimately causes functional deterioration and death of the organism (76). CR has been shown to reduce oxidative stress and the age-associated accumulation of oxidative damage (77). Mitochondrial free radical production, which normally increases with age, is attenuated in mice undergoing CR (78).

Antioxidant enzyme levels are elevated in calorie-restricted rats, and this increase coincides with lower levels of oxidative damage markers (79, 80). Studies have also demonstrated that mitochondrial uncoupling protein (UCP) levels increase with CR (81, 82). Although UCPs (at least UCP3) appear to contribute to lower levels of oxidative stress (82), the mechanism for this effect, and for the longevity-enhancing effects of UCPs, is not clear (83). Most of the data in support of the oxidative damage hypothesis of aging are correlative, however, and data from several studies do not support the theory that oxidative stress under normal conditions plays a key role in modulating aging and life span in mammals.

Supplementation with antioxidants does not increase life span in mice (84, 85), and prospective trials in humans suggest that antioxidant supplementation does not protect against age-related disease (86–88) and may even increase disease risk (89, 90). Moreover, whereas only one rodent study demonstrated life span–prolonging effects of over-expressing human catalase localized to mitochondria (91), most mice overexpressing antioxidant enzymes (e.g., various combinations of copper zinc superoxide dismutase, catalase, and manganese superoxide dismutase) showed no effect on life span (92). Finally, mice with genetic deletion of several antioxidant enzymes (e.g., $Sod2^{+/-}$, $Prxd1^{+/-}$, and $Sod1^{+/-}$ mice) do not have a shorter life span, despite having elevated oxidative stress and increased cancer incidence (93).

SUMMARY AND CONCLUSIONS

Both CR and decreases in the activity of nutrient-sensing pathways slow aging and increase maximal life span in a wide range of model organisms (e.g., yeast, worms, flies, rodents). Studies of rodents have shown that CR without malnutrition has powerful, cancer-protective effects (up to 62% reduction in cancer incidence), and it increases maximal life span by as much as 60%. Animal studies also show that it is possible to slow aging and protect against cancer by partially inhibiting activity in molecular pathways that are down-regulated by CR. Prevention or delays in incidence and progression of other disease such as cardiovascular disease, kidney disease, and neurodegenerative disease are also common findings in calorie-restricted animals. Moreover, data from postmortem pathologic studies demonstrated that 30% to 50% of calorie-restricted rodents, and also long-lived mutant mice (e.g., dwarf and GH receptor mice), died when they are very old, without any evidence of lethal disease at death; this finding suggests that in mammals, aging and the development of chronic diseases are not inexorably linked (9, 29, 94).

Data are accumulating on the long-term effects of CR without malnutrition in nonhuman and human primates. In both, CR with adequate nutrition protects against obesity, type 2 diabetes, hypertension, and cardiovascular diseases, which are by far the primary causes of death in developed countries. The risk of developing and dying of cancer is also reduced in calorie-restricted monkeys. CR in humans reduces metabolic and hormonal factors that are associated with increased cancer risk (95).

Although the precise mechanisms for these beneficial effects of CR are not clear, substantial insights regarding mechanisms and metabolic adaptations have been gained. Mechanisms likely to be involved in these adaptations include neuroendocrine alterations, reductions in anabolic signaling through the insulin/IGF-I/TOR pathways, reductions in inflammation and oxidative stress, hormesis, and up-regulation of autophagy. These insights into the adaptive responses to CR provide important information about the way in which CR may help prevent age-related disease and maintain a more youthful health state into old age. Equally important, however, is that this information helps in understanding the basic biologic processes of aging and what governs them.

ACKNOWLEDGMENTS

Drs. Weiss and Fontana are recipients of research support from the National Institutes of Health and the Longer Life Foundation and have no disclosures to report.

REFERENCES

1. Pugh TD, Klopp RG, Weindruch R. Neurobiol Aging 1999;20:157–65.
2. McCay CM, Crowell MF, Maynard LA. J Nutr 1935;10:63–79.
3. Fontana L, Partridge L, Longo VD. Science 2010;328:321–6.
4. Lawler DF, Larson BT, Ballam JM et al. Br J Nutr 2008;99:793–805.
5. Weindruch R, Walford RL. Science 1982;215:1415–8.
6. Weindruch R, Walford RW. The Retardation of Aging and Disease by Dietary Restriction. Springfield, IL: Charles C Thomas, 1988.
7. Masoro EJ. Mech Ageing Dev 2005;126:913–22.
8. Fontana L, Klein S. JAMA 2007;297:986–94.
9. Shimokawa I, Higami Y, Hubbard GB et al. J Gerontol B Psychol Sci Soc Sci 1993;48:B27–B32.
10. Anderson RM, Shanmuganayagam D, Weindruch R. Toxicol Pathol 2009;37:47–51.
11. Colman RJ, Anderson RM, Johnson SC et al. Science 2009;325:201–4.
12. Colman RJ, Beasley TM, Allison DB et al. J Gerontol A Biol Sci Med Sci 2008;63:556–9.
13. Messaoudi I, Warner J, Fischer M et al. Proc Natl Acad Sci U S A 2006;103:19448–53.
14. Fontana L, Meyer TE, Klein S et al. Proc Natl Acad Sci U S A 2004;101:6659–63.
15. Fontana L, Klein S, Holloszy JO. Age (Dordr) 2010;32:97–108.
16. Hofer T, Fontana L, Anton SD et al. Rejuvenation Res 2008;11:793–9.
17. Meyer TE, Kovacs SJ, Ehsani AA et al. J Am Coll Cardiol 2006;47:398–402.
18. Heilbronn LK, de Jonge L, Frisard MI et al. JAMA 2006;295:1539–48.
19. Fontana L, Klein S, Holloszy JO et al. J Clin Endocrinol Metab 2006;91:3232–5.
20. Cangemi R, Friedmann AJ, Holloszy JO et al. Aging Cell 2010;9:236–42.
21. Sonntag WE, Lynch CD, Cefalu WT et al. J Gerontol A Biol Sci Med Sci 1999;54:B521–B538.
22. Fontana L, Weiss EP, Villareal DT et al. Aging Cell 2008;7:681–7.
23. Dunn SE, Kari FW, French J et al. Cancer Res 1997;57:4667–72.
24. Stewart CE, Rotwein P. Physiol Rev 1996;76:1005–26.
25. Butt AJ, Firth SM, Baxter RC. Immunol Cell Biol 1999;77:256–62.
26. Flurkey K, Papaconstantinou J, Miller RA et al. Proc Natl Acad Sci U S A 2001;98:6736–41.
27. Holzenberger M, Dupont J, Ducos B et al. Nature 2003;421:182–7.
28. Kurosu H, Yamamoto M, Clark JD et al. Science 2005;309:1829–33.
29. Ikeno Y, Bronson RT, Hubbard GB et al. J Gerontol A Biol Sci Med Sci 2003;58:291–6.
30. Bartke A, Chandrashekar V, Bailey B et al. Neuropeptides 2002;36:201–8.
31. Bluher M, Kahn BB, Kahn CR. Science 2003;299:572–4.
32. Selman C, Lingard S, Choudhury AI et al. FASEB J 2008;22:807–18.
33. Taguchi A, Wartschow LM, White MF. Science 2007;317:369–72.
34. Braverman LE, Utiger RD, eds. Werner and Ingbar's The Thyroid: A Fundamental and Clinical Text. 9th ed. New York: Lippincott Williams & Wilkins, 2004.
35. Weiss EP, Villareal DT, Racette SB et al. Rejuvenation Res 2008;11:605–9.
36. Stager JM. J Appl Physiol 1983;54:1115–9.
37. Ortega E, Pannacciulli N, Bogardus C et al. Am J Clin Nutr 2007;85:440–5.
38. Terman A, Kurz T, Navratil M et al. Antioxid Redox Signal 2010;12:503–35.
39. Stadtman ER. Ann N Y Acad Sci 2001;928:22–38.
40. Levine B, Kroemer G. Cell 2008;132:27–42.
41. Mizushima N, Levine B, Cuervo AM et al. Nature 2008;451:1069–75.
42. Cuervo AM, Bergamini E, Brunk UT et al. Autophagy 2005;1:131–40.
43. Vellai T, Takacs-Vellai K, Sass M et al. Trends Cell Biol 2009;19:487–94.
44. Eisenberg T, Knauer H, Schauer A et al. Nat Cell Biol 2009;11:1305–14.

45. Simonsen A, Cumming RC, Brech A et al. Autophagy 2008; 4:176–84.

46. Donati A, Recchia G, Cavallini G et al. J Gerontol A Biol Sci Med Sci 2008;63:550–5.

47. Cavallini G, Donati A, Gori Z et al. Exp Gerontol 2001;36: 497–506.

48. Melendez A, Talloczy Z, Seaman M et al. Science 2003;301: 1387–91.

49. Weiss EP, Racette SB, Villareal DT et al. Am J Clin Nutr 2006;84:1033–42.

50. Parr T. Gerontology 1997;43:182–200.

51. Liu HY, Han J, Cao SY et al. J Biol Chem 2009;284:31484–92.

52. Bergamini E, Del Roso A, Fierabracci V et al. Exp Mol Pathol 1993;59:13–26.

53. Bergamini E, Cavallini G, Donati A et al. Biomed Pharmacother 2003;57:203–8.

54. Feghali CA, Wright TM. Front Biosci 1997;2:d12–d26.

55. Hansson GK. N Engl J Med 2005;352:1685–95.

56. Coussens LM, Werb Z. Nature 2002;420:860–7.

57. Eikelenboom P, Veerhuis R. Exp Gerontol 1999;34:453–61.

58. Pickup JC. Diabetes Care 2004;27:813–23.

59. Araya J, Nishimura SL. Annu Rev Pathol 2010;5:77–98.

60. Eddy AA. Pediatr Nephrol 2000;15:290–301.

61. Marra F, Aleffi S, Galastri S et al. Semin Immunopathol 2009;31:345–58.

62. Serrano AL, Munoz-Canoves P. Exp Cell Res 2010.

63. Matsuzaki J, Kuwamura M, Yamaji R et al. J Nutr 2001;131: 2139–44.

64. Ershler WB, Sun WH, Binkley N et al. Lymphokine Cytokine Res 1993;12:225–30.

65. Willette AA, Bendlin BB, McLaren DG et al. Neuroimage 2010;51:987–94.

66. Bendlin BB, Canu E, Willette A et al. Neurobiol Aging 2010.

67. Kastman EK, Willette AA, Coe CL et al. J Neurosci 2010; 30:7940–7.

68. Mitchel RE. Dose Response 2007;5:284–91.

69. Masoro EJ. Interdiscip Top Gerontol 2007;35:1–17.

70. Sabatino F, Masoro EJ, McMahan CA et al. J Gerontol 1991;46:B171–B179.

71. Klebanov S, Diais S, Stavinoha WB et al. J Gerontol A Biol Sci Med Sci 1995;50:B78–B82.

72. Heydari AR, Wu B, Takahashi R et al. Mol Cell Biol 1993;13:2909–18.

73. Berg TF, Breen PJ, Feuers RJ et al. Food Chem Toxicol 1994;32:45–50.

74. Weraarchakul N, Strong R, Wood WG et al. Exp Cell Res 1989;181:197–204.

75. Cho CG, Kim HJ, Chung SW et al. Exp Gerontol 2003;38: 539–48.

76. Harman D. J Gerontol 1956;11:298–300.

77. Sohal RS, Weindruch R. Science 1996;273:59–63.

78. Sohal RS, Ku HH, Agarwal S et al. Mech Ageing Dev 1994; 74:121–33.

79. Rao G, Xia E, Nadakavukaren MJ et al. J Nutr 1990;120: 602–9.

80. Hyun DH, Emerson SS, Jo DG et al. Proc Natl Acad Sci U S A 2006;103:19908–12.

81. Liu D, Chan SL, Souza-Pinto NC et al. Neuromolecular Med 2006;8:389–414.

82. Bevilacqua L, Ramsey JJ, Hagopian K et al. Am J Physiol 2005;289:E429–E438.

83. Dietrich MO, Horvath TL. Pflugers Arch 2010;459:269–75.

84. Holloszy JO. Mech Ageing Dev 1998;100:211–9.

85. Lee CK, Pugh TD, Klopp RG et al. Free Radic Biol Med 2004;36:1043–57.

86. Rautalahti MT, Virtamo JR, Taylor PR et al. Cancer 1999;86:37–42.

87. Liu S, Ajani U, Chae C et al. JAMA 1999;282:1073–5.

88. Heart Protection Study Collaborative Group. Lancet 2002; 360:23–33.

89. Bjelakovic G, Nikolova D, Simonetti RG et al. Lancet 2004;364: 1219–28.

90. Bairati I, Meyer F, Gelinas M et al. J Natl Cancer Inst 2005;97: 481–8.

91. Schriner SE, Linford NJ, Martin GM et al. Science 2005;308: 1909–11.

92. Perez VI, Van Remmen H, Bokov A et al. Aging Cell 2009;8: 73–5.

93. Muller FL, Lustgarten MS, Jang Y et al. Free Radic Biol Med 2007;43:477–503.

94. Vergara M, Smith-Wheelock M, Harper JM et al. J Gerontol A Biol Sci Med Sci 2004;59:1244–50.

95. Longo VD, Fontana L. Trends Pharmacol Sci 2010;31:89–98.

SUGGESTED READINGS

Fontana L, Klein S. Aging, adiposity, and calorie restriction. JAMA 2007;297:986–94.

Fontana L, Partridge L, Longo VD. Extending healthy lifespan: from yeast to humans. Science 2010;328:321–6.

Masoro EJ. Overview of caloric restriction and ageing. Mech Ageing Dev 2005;126:913–22.

Anderson RM, Weindruch R. Metabolic reprogramming, caloric restriction and aging. Trends Endocrinol Metab 2010;21:134–41.

52 NUTRITION IN PREGNANCY[1]

R. ELAINE TURNER

Optimal nutrition is integral to a healthy pregnancy, which can be described as "without physical or psychological pathology in mother or fetus, results in delivery of a healthy baby" (1). Although the influence of poor nutritional status on adverse pregnancy outcome was documented early in the twentieth century, retrospective studies considering the effects of food shortages in the Netherlands during World War II clearly identified the influence of diet on pregnancy outcome (2–4). Nutrition can affect the mother's health and risk of pregnancy complications; it also affects the growth and development of the fetus, risk of birth defects, and health of the infant at delivery. Further studies have linked both undernutrition and overnutrition during pregnancy to increased risks of obesity, coronary heart disease, hypertension, diabetes, metabolic syndrome, and psychiatric disorders in the children; these findings suggest a persistent change in gene expression in response to the intrauterine environment (5–8).

CURRENT PUBLIC HEALTH OBJECTIVES RELATED TO PREGNANCY AND NEONATAL HEALTH

Maternal and infant health are important predictors of the future health of the nation's citizens. As identified in *Healthy People 2020*, a major public health goal is to "improve the health and well-being of women, infants, children, and families" (9). Public health issues related to maternal and child health include morbidity and mortality of pregnant and postpartum women; fetal, perinatal, and infant mortality; birth outcomes; prevention of birth defects; and access to preventive care. Progress has been made toward objectives related to fetal, infant, and maternal deaths; prenatal care; and prevention of neural tube defects (NTDs); however, the percentages of low birth weight (LBW) and preterm delivery have increased (10). Healthy People 2020 objectives continue to emphasize the importance of nutrition, prenatal care, and preconception health in improving the health of mothers and infants (8).

---

[1]**Abbreviations: AI**, adequate intake; **BEE**, basal energy expenditure; **BMI**, body mass index; **DHA**, docosahexaenoic acid; **DRI**, dietary reference intake; **EAR**, estimated average requirement; **FAS**, fetal alcohol syndrome; **GDM**, gestational diabetes mellitus; **GWG**, gestational weight gain; **IOM**, Institute of Medicine; **IUGR**, intrauterine growth restriction; **LBW**, low birth weight; **LGA**, large for gestational age; **NTD**, neural tube defect; **PKU**, phenylketonuria; **RDA**, recommended dietary allowance; **TEE**, total energy expenditure; **UL**, tolerable upper intake level.

PRECONCEPTION HEALTH

Nutritional status before pregnancy is a key factor in overall maternal health and in the risk of birth defects. Women who are contemplating pregnancy can make dietary and lifestyle changes that will reduce the risk of poor pregnancy outcome. The Centers for Disease Control and Prevention identified preconception risk factors for poor pregnancy outcomes (Table 52.1) and developed 10 recommendations to improve preconception health (11). Folic acid supplements before and during the early stages of pregnancy reduce the risk of NTDs and other birth defects. Ideally, all women of childbearing age should be consuming 400 µg/day of folic acid in addition to folate provide through foods (12) because nearly one half of all pregnancies in the United States are unplanned (13). Women following vegan or other strict vegetarian diets should also take supplemental vitamin B_{12} because the status of this vitamin is another risk factor for NTDs (12).

Preconception iron status is important to reducing the risk during pregnancy of iron deficiency and anemia, which, in turn, can lead to intrauterine growth restriction (IUGR) and preterm birth (14). Preconception care should include screening for iron deficiency anemia. Multivitamin and mineral supplementation may help to improve nutritional status in women who are following inappropriate diets, are avoiding numerous foods or groups of foods, are underweight, are trying to lose weight, or are abusing alcohol.

Achieving a healthy weight before pregnancy can improve chances of conception and pregnancy outcome and may improve lactation (13, 15). Women who are obese at the start of pregnancy are at greater risk of gestational diabetes mellitus (GDM) and preeclampsia and of experiencing induced labor and cesarean section. Obese women may also have more difficulty initiating

breast-feeding (15–17). Infants born to women who were obese before pregnancy are at increased risk of congenital abnormalities, NTDs, stillbirth, macrosomia, and obesity later in life (15). Physical activity can help to improve weight and nutritional status; however, the amount of physical activity needed daily for weight management, chronic disease risk reduction, and enhanced physical fitness varies (18–20).

Management of preexisting chronic disease is another important element of preconception planning. Women with hypertension are at risk of maternal, fetal, and neonatal morbidity and mortality. The severity of hypertension and the presence of preeclampsia affect pregnancy outcomes (21).

Diabetes increases the risk of birth defects, especially defects of the heart and central nervous system, and it also increases the risk of spontaneous abortion (21). Attaining good blood glucose control before conception and during organogenesis can substantially reduce risks.

Approximately 3000 to 4000 women of childbearing age in the United States have phenylketonuria (PKU) without severe mental retardation (22). To prevent mental retardation, microcephaly, and congenital heart disease in the infant, pregnant women with PKU must resume a low-protein, amino acid–modified diet during pregnancy (22). Ideally, women with PKU should resume the diet before conception to regain control of blood phenylalanine and then maintain continued tight control throughout pregnancy.

MATERNAL PHYSIOLOGIC CHANGES DURING PREGNANCY

Numerous anatomic, biochemical, and physiologic changes occur during pregnancy to maintain a healthy environment for the growing fetus without compromising the mother's health. Many of these changes begin in the early weeks of pregnancy, and together they regulate maternal metabolism, promote fetal growth, and prepare the mother for labor, birth, and lactation. A review of the physiologic changes during pregnancy sets the stage for understanding the changes in nutrient requirements that accompany pregnancy.

Maternal plasma volume begins to expand near the end of the first trimester, with a total increase in volume of 50% by 30 to 34 weeks of gestation. Red blood cell production is stimulated with a total increase in red blood cell mass of approximately 33%. Hematocrit levels decline until the end of the second trimester, by which time red blood cell synthesis is synchronized with plasma volume increase. Declining concentrations of plasma proteins and other nutrients are expected because of the expansion of blood volume. Poor plasma volume expansion predicts a poorly growing fetus and poor pregnancy outcome (23).

Cardiac output increases approximately 30% to 50% during pregnancy. Elevated cardiac output occurs in response to increased tissue demands for oxygen and

TABLE 52.1	PRECONCEPTION RISK FACTORS FOR POOR PREGNANCY OUTCOME

Alcohol misuse
Antiepileptic drug use
Diabetes (preconception)
Folic acid deficiency
Hepatitis B infection
Human immunodeficiency infection/acquired immunodeficiency syndrome
Hypothyroidism
Isotretinoin use
Maternal phenylketonuria
Rubella seronegativity
Obesity
Oral anticoagulant use
Sexually transmitted diseases
Smoking

From Johnson K, Posner SF, Biermann J et al. Recommendations to improve preconception health and health care: United States: a report of the CDC/ATSDR Preconception Care work group and the Select Panel on Preconception Care. MMWR Morb Mortal Wkly Rep 2006;55:1–23, with permission.

is accompanied by an increase in stroke volume. The size of the heart increases by approximately 12%, probably because of the increased blood volume and cardiac output. Systemic blood pressure declines slightly during pregnancy, with the majority of the change occurring in diastolic pressure (5 to 10 mm Hg). Diastolic pressure returns to prepregnancy levels near term.

Respiratory changes support increased maternal and fetal requirements for oxygen. As the uterus enlarges, the diaphragm is elevated, which reduces lung capacity by about 5%, and residual volume is reduced by approximately 20%. Tidal volume increases as pregnancy progresses, resulting in increased alveolar ventilation and more efficient gas exchange, given that oxygen consumption increases only 15% to 20%. Respiration rate increases only slightly.

The kidneys increase slightly in both length and weight during pregnancy; and the ureters elongate, widen, and become more curved. Glomerular filtration rate increases by approximately 50%, and renal plasma flow rate increases by 25% to 50%. Renin levels increase early in the first trimester and continue to rise until term. Most pregnant women are resistant to the pressor effects of the resulting elevation of angiotensin II levels, but enhanced renin secretion may help to explain preeclampsia. A marked increase in excretion of glucose, amino acids, and water-soluble vitamins occurs, probably because the higher glomerular filtration rate presents higher levels of nutrients than the tubules can reabsorb.

Changes along the gastrointestinal tract support the increased demand for nutrients during pregnancy. Appetite increases, although initially this may be offset by nausea and vomiting. Motility of the gastrointestinal tract is reduced by increased levels of progesterone that, in turn, decrease the production of motilin, a hormone that stimulates smooth muscle in the gastrointestinal tract. Elongation in gastrointestinal transit time occurs largely in the third trimester of pregnancy and is not accompanied by a change in gastric emptying time (24). Gallbladder emptying time is reduced and often incomplete.

The basal metabolic rate rises by the fourth month of gestation and is usually increased by 15% to 20% by term. An elevated basal metabolic rate reflects the increased demand for and consumption of oxygen. Most (50% to 70%) of the energy needs of the fetus are provided by glucose, with approximately 20% coming from amino acids and the remainder derived from fat. Use of fatty acids for fuel is enhanced in the mother to conserve glucose for use by the fetus.

WEIGHT GAIN

Optimal birth weight is influenced by maternal weight gain. In 2009, the Institute of Medicine (IOM) released updated recommendations for gestational weight gain (GWG) (23). These recommendations, based on prepregnancy body mass index (BMI), reflect the GWG and rate of weight gain associated with best pregnancy outcome (Table 52.2).

Determinants of Gestational Weight Gain

Numerous factors potentially influence the amount of weight gained during pregnancy, including environmental factors, maternal genetics and body size, medical and psychologic conditions, and behavioral factors. Limited evidence is available to ascertain the strength of most of these relationships (23). Prepregnancy BMI is likely the best independent predictor of GWG (23). A review of several studies showed that mean weight gain by underweight (BMI <18.5 kg/m^2) and normal weight (BMI 18.5 to 24.9 kg/m^2) women was within the new IOM recommendations, whereas mean GWG of overweight (25.0 to 29.9 kg/m^2) and obese (≥30 kg/m^2) women was higher than the new recommendations (23).

Effect on Fetal and Maternal Outcomes

Studies show a linear relationship between GWG and birth weight for gestational age. Poor weight gain is associated with poor fetal growth, LBW, small for gestational age birth weight, and risk of preterm delivery (23, 25). Carmichael and Abrams (25) found that a marked acceleration or deceleration of gain toward the end of pregnancy was associated with lower gestational age and risk of spontaneous preterm delivery. Low GWG is also associated with failure to initiate breast-feeding (23).

TABLE 52.2	GESTATIONAL WEIGHT GAIN RECOMMENDATIONS		
WEIGHT CATEGORY	PREPREGNANCY BODY MASS INDEX (kg/m^2)	TOTAL WEIGHT GAIN (kg)	RATE OF WEIGHT GAIN[a] (MEAN; kg/wk)
Underweight	<18.5	12.5–18.0	0.51
Normal weight	18.5–24.9	11.5–16.0	0.42
Overweight	25.0–29.9	7–11.5	0.28
Obese	≥30.0	5–9	0.22

[a]Second and third trimesters

Adapted with permission from Institute of Medicine, National Research Council. Weight Gain During Pregnancy: Reexamining the Guidelines. Washington, DC: National Academies Press, 2009.

Excessive weight gain affects infant growth, increases the chance of large for gestational age (LGA) birth weight and cesarean delivery, and is associated with higher body fatness in childhood. Women who are overweight or obese are more likely than women of normal weight to gain more weight than is recommended (26), and exceeding recommendations was found to be more likely in low-income women (27). Excessive GWG is further associated with postpartum weight retention and future overweight or obesity (23).

Ideally, weight gain recommendations should be individualized to promote best outcomes while reducing risk for excessive postpartum weight retention and reducing the risk of later chronic disease in the child. The most effective approach for reducing negative outcomes associated with GWG is for women to be within the normal range for BMI at the time of conception (23). Even small weight gains between pregnancies increase the risk of maternal complications and stillbirth (28). Further, advice about appropriate GWG should be given during prenatal care, with tracking of actual weight gain and referral to services for counseling on diet and physical activity as needed (23).

ENERGY AND NUTRIENT NEEDS

To support the growth of the fetus and the health of the mother, requirements for energy and for most vitamins and minerals are higher during pregnancy.

Energy

Energy is needed to support basal energy expenditure (BEE), physical activity, the thermic effect of food, and, in pregnant women, growth of the fetus and deposition of maternal tissues. BEE increases because of the enhanced metabolism of the uterus and fetus and the increased work of the heart and lungs. Increased BEE represents the major component of increased energy requirements. Studies estimate the cumulative increase in BEE at 106 to 180 kcal/day, although variation among subjects is substantial (26). Late in pregnancy, the fetus uses approximately 56 kcal/kg/day, which represents about one half of the increment of BEE.

The theoretic energy cost of energy deposition can be estimated from the amount of protein and fat deposited (19). Mean total energy deposition is 39,862 kcal (180 kcal/day). Analysis of studies employing the doubly labeled water method shows a median change in total energy expenditure (TEE) of 8 kcal/gestational week. The estimated energy requirement for pregnancy is thus derived from the sum of TEE for a nonpregnant woman plus 8 kcal/gestational week plus 180 kcal/day for energy deposition. This increase in recommended energy intake is suggested only for the second and third trimesters because TEE changes little in the first trimester, and weight gain is minimal. Therefore, during the second trimester, an additional 340 kcal/day greater than nonpregnant energy requirements is recommended. This increase climbs to 452 kcal/day extra in the third trimester.

Ultimately, the best method for assessing the adequacy of energy intake is to monitor GWG. The recommended balance of energy sources during pregnancy is the same as for nonpregnant women: 10% to 35% as protein, 45% to 65% as carbohydrate, and 20% to 35% of kcal as fat (19). IOM recommendations for nutrient intake during pregnancy are summarized in Table 52.3.

Protein

During pregnancy, whole body protein turnover increases, and substantial amounts of protein are accumulated by the growth of the fetus, uterus, blood volume, placenta, amniotic fluid, and maternal skeletal muscle (19). Considering protein deposition over the last two trimesters, the recommended dietary allowance (RDA) increases by 25 g/day. For a reference woman weighing 57 kg, this is an additional 0.27 g/kg/day for a total of 1.1 g/kg/day during pregnancy.

Carbohydrate

The fetus uses glucose as its major energy source. The transfer of glucose from mother to fetus is estimated at 17 to 26 g/day. By the end of pregnancy, all this glucose is thought to be used by the fetal brain (19). The estimated average requirement (EAR) for carbohydrate increases from 100 g/day to 135 g/day, which translates to an RDA for carbohydrate for pregnant women of 175 g/day.

Fat

Fat is a major source of energy for the body and aids in the absorption of fat-soluble vitamins and carotenoids. Some studies have shown lower maternal concentrations of arachidonic acid in plasma and red blood cell phospholipids (19). However, no evidence indicates that supplementation with n-6 fatty acids has any beneficial effect on fetal growth and development. The developing brain accumulates large amounts of docosahexaenoic acid (DHA) during prenatal and postnatal development, continuing through the first 2 years of life. Fetal tissue has active desaturases to allow DHA formation from α-linolenic acid. No evidence has been found of physiologic benefit to the infant of increasing DHA intake during pregnancy if the diet meets n-3 and n-6 requirements. Therefore, adequate intake (AI) values for essential fatty acids during pregnancy are based on median intakes among pregnant women in the United States: 13 g/day for linoleic acid and 1.4 g/day for α-linolenic acid.

Fat-Soluble Vitamins

Vitamin A is important for regulation of gene expression and for cell differentiation and proliferation, particularly for the development of the vertebrae and spinal cord, the

TABLE 52.3	RECOMMENDED DIETARY ALLOWANCE, ADEQUATE INTAKE, OR ACCEPTABLE MICRONUTRIENT DISTRIBUTION RANGE AND TOLERABLE UPPER INTAKE LEVEL FOR NUTRIENTS DURING PREGNANCY

VITAMINS	RECOMMENDED DIETARY ALLOWANCE, ADEQUATE INTAKE, OR ACCEPTABLE MICRONUTRIENT DISTRIBUTION RANGE	TOLERABLE UPPER INTAKE LEVEL
Vitamin A (μg/d)	770	3,000
Vitamin C (mg/d)	85	2,000
Vitamin D (μg/d)	15	100
Vitamin E (μg/d)	15	1,000
Vitamin K (μg/d)	90[a]	
Thiamin (mg/d)	1.4	
Riboflavin (mg/d)	1.4	
Niacin (mg/d)	18	35
Vitamin B6 (mg/d)	1.9	100
Folate (μg/d)	600	1,000[c]
Vitamin B12 (μg/d)	2.6	
Pantothenic Acid (mg/d)	6[a]	
Biotin (μg/d)	30[a]	
Choline (mg/d)	450[a]	3,500
MINERALS		
Calcium (mg/d)	1,000	2,500
Chromium (μg/d)	30[a]	
Copper (μg/d)	1,000	10,000
Fluoride (mg/d)	3[a]	10
Iodine (μg/d)	220	1100
Iron (mg/d)	27	45
Magnesium (mg/d)	350	350[d]
Manganese (mg/d)	2.0[a]	11
Molybdenum (μg/d)	50	2000
Phosphorus (mg/d)	700	3500
Selenium (μg/d)	60	400
Zinc (mg/d)	11	40
Potassium (g/d)	4.7[a]	
Sodium (g/d)	1.5[a]	2.3
Chloride (g/d)	2.3[a]	3.6
MACRONUTRIENTS		
Carbohydrate (g/d)	175	
Total fiber (g/d)	28[a]	
Total fat (g/d)	20–35[b]	
n-6 Polyunsaturated fatty acids (g/d)	13[a]	
n-3 polyunsaturated fatty acids (g/d)	1.4[a]	
Protein (g/d)	71	

[a]Adequate intake
[b]Acceptable micronutrient distribution range
[c]In the form of folic acid
[d]As pharmacological agents only

From Food and Nutrition Board, Institute of Medicine. Dietary Reference Intake Reports. Available at: http://www.nap.edu. Accessed July 22, 2012, with permission.

limbs, heart, eyes, and ears. Direct studies of vitamin A status are lacking, but the increase in maternal requirement of 70 μg/day as retinol activity equivalents is estimated based on the amount of vitamin A assumed to be accumulated by the fetal liver (29).

Excess retinol intake is a known human teratogen. The most critical period for damage appears to be in the

first trimester, resulting in spontaneous abortions and birth defects affecting the cardiovascular system, central nervous system, craniofacial area, and thymus (30). The threshold for risk remains controversial (30–33); however, teratogenicity was used as the critical adverse effect for women of childbearing age in determining the tolerable upper intake level (UL) of 3000 μg/day of

contaminants including mercury, because methylmercury crosses the placenta and can cause significant neurodevelopmental abnormalities (61). Specifically, pregnant women should avoid large predatory fish such as shark, swordfish, tilefish, king mackerel; they should eat up to 12 oz/week of a variety of other seafood and limit albacore tuna consumption to no more than 6 oz; and they should check local advisories regarding locally caught seafood (57, 62). A study of seafood consumption during pregnancy and neurodevelopmental outcomes in children suggests that restriction of fish consumption may increase the risk of suboptimal development (63).

Vegetarian Diets

During pregnancy, nutrient needs for vegetarians are the same as for nonvegetarians except for a higher recommendation for iron intake (29). Analysis of available studies suggests that pregnant vegetarians consume lower levels of protein, vitamin B$_{12}$, calcium, and zinc, but no evidence indicates detrimental outcomes for mother or fetus (64). Vegetarian diets can be planned that meet the needs for all nutrients, with special attention to vitamin B$_{12}$, vitamin D, calcium, iron, and zinc (64).

Caffeine

The need to restrict or eliminate caffeine intake during pregnancy remains controversial. Caffeine is metabolized more slowly in pregnant women and passes readily through the placenta to the fetus. Epidemiologic studies investigating a link between caffeine intake and risk of spontaneous abortion or LBW have been inconclusive and results are likely affected by confounders such as smoking and alcohol use. In a prospective study, caffeine intake of >100 mg/day throughout pregnancy was associated with risk of fetal growth restriction, with smokers at higher risk than non-smokers (65). An intervention study to reduce caffeine intake beginning in the second trimester reduced LBW risk in women who smoked (66). It is prudent for pregnant women to limit their caffeine consumption, especially since most caffeine-containing foods are low in nutritional value.

Alcohol

In the United States, approximately 12% of pregnant women report alcohol use, and nearly 3% are binge drinkers (1). Alcohol use can cause numerous adverse effects on the fetus, the most severe outcomes being mortality and fetal alcohol syndrome (FAS) (67). However, the specific amount of alcohol exposure required to cause FAS has not been determined. Dose, timing, duration of exposure, genetic factors, and protective factors are all contributors (67). Studies suggest that approximately 9 to 10 of every 1000 live births are negatively affected by alcohol consumption during pregnancy.

According the IOM, the diagnosis of FAS requires (a) confirmed maternal exposure, (b) the presence of a characteristic pattern of facial anomalies, (c) growth retardation, and (d) central nervous system neurodevelopmental abnormalities (68). The characteristic facial features include short palpebral fissures, epicanthal folds, midface hypoplasia, a depressed wide nasal bridge, anteverted nares, a long hypoplastic philtrum, and a thin upper vermilion border (69). Central nervous system abnormalities can include decreased head size, brain structure abnormalities, impaired fine motor skills, hearing loss, poor tandem gait, and poor hand–eye coordination. Growth retardation typically continues after delivery and often persists into adolescence (70).

The only preventive measure for FAS and milder versions of the disorder known as partial FAS is the complete abstinence from alcohol during pregnancy. Longitudinal data suggest that deficits in height, weight, head circumference, palpebral fissures, and skinfold thickness are apparent even among light drinkers consuming up to 1.5 drinks/week (71).

Herbal and Other Dietary Supplements

Although many pregnant women benefit from supplementation with vitamins and minerals to achieve the recommended nutrient intakes in pregnancy, less is known about the benefits or risks of herbal and other dietary supplements. Very few studies have examined the efficacy and safety of alternative therapies during pregnancy (1), and so it is most prudent to consider these remedies as suspect until proven safe. Remedies promoted to pregnant women are often for easing gastrointestinal distress (72). Although ginger has been shown to be effective in reducing pregnancy-induced nausea (73), other botanical therapies such as red raspberry, peppermint, and wild yam have not been formally studied.

Many herbal products have been identified as potentially unsafe for use during pregnancy (1). Safety issues range from potential embryotoxicity to the more likely hormonal effects and drug interactions (74). Given the lack of premarket requirements for proof of safety and efficacy for dietary supplements, pregnant women should discuss such supplements with their health care providers before they continue to use them. Unfortunately, sometimes advice of the health care provider carries its own risks. Finkel and Zarlengo (75) reported a case of a woman advised by her obstetrician to drink a tea made from blue cohosh, an herb used in Native American medicine to induce labor. Two days after delivery, the infant suffered a stroke, and the cocaine metabolite benzoylecgonine was detected in the infant's urine and in the mother's bottle of blue cohosh. It was not known whether benzoylecgonine is also a metabolite of blue cohosh, whether the supplement was contaminated with cocaine, or whether toxicologic testing could have identified a cross-reacting substance.

Smoking

Cigarette smoking during pregnancy is linked to preterm delivery, spontaneous abortion, and LBW. Carbon monoxide and nicotine from cigarettes increase fetal carboxyhemoglobin and reduced placental blood flow, thus limiting oxygen delivery to the fetus (1). In a 2007 survey, nearly 27% of women reported smoking before pregnancy, whereas less than 16% smoked during the last 3 months of pregnancy (76). Smoking rates are higher in older teens and women in their early 20s, and in white, non-Hispanic women with less than a high school education (77).

Illicit Drugs

In addition to alcohol and tobacco, illicit drugs such as marijuana, cocaine, and heroin can have devastating effects on a developing fetus. Approximately 5% of pregnant women use illicit drugs (78); rates of drug use are lower in nonpregnant women with the exception of 15 to 17 year olds. Marijuana accounted for 75% of the illicit drug use, but many pregnant women also used cigarettes and alcohol. Although it is often difficult to isolate the effects of an illicit drug from concurrent use of alcohol or tobacco, marijuana and cocaine have been linked to reduced fetal growth (1). Cocaine use has also been associated with premature labor and spontaneous abortion. Exposure to heroin and other opiates leads to a withdrawal syndrome that affects the central nervous, autonomic nervous, and gastrointestinal systems (79). Although most outcomes of prenatal illicit drug use are limited to the early postnatal period, results are emerging from longitudinal studies that suggest longer term effects on language function and academic achievement (80, 81).

NUTRITION-RELATED COMPLICATIONS AND PROBLEMS

Gastrointestinal Problems

Among the most common problems during early pregnancy are nausea and vomiting. So-called morning sickness affects 70% to 85% of pregnant women. Early nausea is associated with gastric dysrhythmias and hormonal changes that slow gastrointestinal motility (82). Studies in humans and animals associated reduced energy intakes in early pregnancy with higher placental weight, thus leading to the hypothesis that secretion of human chorionic gonadotropin and thyroxine results in morning sickness and decreased energy intake which, in turn, lowers maternal secretion of anabolic hormones (83). Suppressing maternal tissue synthesis may favor nutrient partitioning to the developing placenta. Management of nausea and vomiting depends on the severity of symptoms; most women with mild episodes are helped by eating smaller, more frequent meals, avoiding offending odors, and drinking adequate fluids.

Heartburn is another common gastrointestinal complaint experienced by approximately two thirds of pregnant women. The main factor in heartburn is lowered pressure across the lower esophageal sphincter caused by increased progesterone secretion. Serious reflux complications are rare during pregnancy (84). Heartburn is generally relieved by eating smaller, more frequent meals, avoiding lying down after eating, elevating the head while sleeping, and avoiding known irritants (1).

Constipation resulting from slowed gastrointestinal motility can be aggravated by high-dose iron supplements. Including generous amounts of fiber, adequate fluids, and regular exercise can help to relieve constipation (1).

Low Birth Weight

Infants who are born with LBW (<2500 g) can be divided into two categories: those born too early and those with IUGR. In developed countries, approximately 50% of all LBW infants are preterm, whereas in developing countries, most LBW infants are affected by IUGR. Approximately 7% of live births in the United States are LBW, with 3.6% of LBW infants born full term (85). LBW is the risk factor most closely associated with neonatal death; therefore, improving birth weight has a significant effect on infant mortality.

Poor nutrition is a known cause of LBW, especially in developed countries. Other contributing factors include smoking, infections, hypertension, and environmental factors. In the United States, an estimated 20% to 30% of LBW is attributable to smoking and its impact on IUGR. Low weight gain in either the second or third trimester increases the risk of IUGR, as does low prepregnancy BMI and young age (1). Longitudinal studies are beginning to shed light on the influence of birth weight on cognitive function and the future risk of chronic disease. Consistent, early prenatal care can help improve nutrition and identify patterns of weight gain that pose a risk of LBW.

Gestational Diabetes Mellitus

GDM affects approximately 4% of all pregnant women (85). Numerous risk factors are associated with increased incidence of GDM, the strongest of which are age, prepregnancy weight, family history of diabetes mellitus, and ethnicity. Maternal complications associated with GDM include higher rates of hypertensive disorders, cesarean delivery, recurrent GDM, and future development of type 2 diabetes mellitus. For the fetus, GDM increases the risk of macrosomia, hyperbilirubinemia, hypoglycemia, and erythremia. Macrosomia (usually defined as a birth weight >4000 g) is the most common fetal complication and is associated with high prepregnancy BMI and previous GDM (86). Diabetes and nutrition counseling, along with intensive self-monitoring of blood glucose and insulin therapy, is effective in reducing the negative outcomes associated with GDM.

Hypertensive Disorders

Gestational hypertension is defined as hypertension (blood pressure ≥140 mm Hg systolic or 90 mm Hg diastolic) without proteinuria occurring after 20 weeks' gestation (1). Approximately 25% of women with gestational hypertension will develop *preeclampsia,* which is defined as hypertension with proteinuria (>300 mg/24 hours) after 20 weeks' gestation. Preeclampsia may progress to *eclampsia,* a condition marked by seizures that is life threatening to both mother and infant. Preeclampsia affects 3% to 5% of pregnancies in the United States and is associated with substantial risks including IUGR, death, preterm delivery, and maternal renal failure, seizures, pulmonary edema, stroke, and death (87). Currently, the cause of preeclampsia is unknown, and accurate screening tests are not available. Risk factors include primiparity, obesity, obesity with GDM, history of preeclampsia, chronic hypertension, older age, and African-American race (1, 15).

Preeclampsia is thought to be a two-stage disease: reduced placental perfusion is followed by hypertension and proteinuria. In addition to these maternal features, reduced perfusion extends to virtually all organs and is caused by vasoconstriction, microthrombi formation, and reduced circulating plasma volume. Endothelial dysfunction is also present and appears to predate clinical symptoms.

Because of an increased incidence of preeclampsia noted in women of low socioeconomic status, nutritional factors have long been suggested as contributing to the disorder. Energy intake, macronutrient balance, n-3 fatty acids, calcium, sodium, zinc, iron, magnesium, and folate have all been studied for causal or preventive roles; however, conclusive links between nutrient intake and preeclampsia have not been found. Future directions for research include the role of nutrients in the inflammatory response, in insulin resistance, and in oxidative stress, all thought to be contributing factors to the development of preeclampsia (1).

Neural Tube Defects

NTDs are the most common major congenital malformations of the central nervous system and represent varying degrees of disturbance of the embryonic process of neurulation. NTDs include anencephaly, meningomyelocele, meningocele, and craniorachischisis. Neurulation is the first organogenetic process to be initiated and completed (12). The process begins approximately 21 days after conception and is completed by day 28.

The etiology of NTDs includes heredity, probably related to multiple genes influenced by environmental factors. The relationship between folate and NTDs was first suggested by Hibbard in 1964 (12). Observational studies show reduced risk of NTDs with increased dietary folate intake (88, 89). Studies of folic acid supplements generally support a 70% to 80% risk reduction with 400 μg/day of folic acid (12, 39). The mechanism by which folate could reduce NTDs is still unknown; improved folate status may possibly overcome deficiency in production of proteins or DNA at the time of neural tube closure.

As a result of the accumulated evidence, the US Public Health Service recommended in 1992 that all women capable of becoming pregnant consume 400 μg/day of folic acid, a recommendation echoed in the 1998 DRI report on water-soluble vitamins (12). In an effort to improve folic acid intake, mandatory fortification of enriched cereal grains began in 1998. The required level of fortification (1.4 mg folic acid/kg grain) was estimated to increase folic acid intake by 100 μg/day. Data from population-based surveillance systems show a 30% reduction in the prevalence of NTDs from 1995 to 2005 (90).

SUMMARY

Healthy outcomes for both mother and baby can result from preconception assessment, good nutrition, healthy lifestyle choices, adequate weight gain, and early prenatal care. Prenatal care is important for nutrition assessment, evaluation of risk factors, and follow-up to ensure optimal outcomes. Early screening can identify physiologic or psychologic problems and initiate appropriate therapy. As the United States strives toward new objectives in Healthy People 2020, researchers must continue to identify nutritional intervention strategies that are effective at improving pregnancy outcomes.

REFERENCES

1. Kaiser L, Allen LH, American Dietetic Association. J Am Diet Assoc 2008;108:553–61.
2. Stein Z, Susser M. Pediatr Res 1975;9:70–6.
3. Stein Z, Susser M. Pediatr Res 1975;9:76–83.
4. Rosebook TJ, Painter RC, van Abeelen AF, et al. Maturitas 2011;70:141–5.
5. Kyle UG, Pichard C, Curr Opin Clin Nutr Metab Care 2006;9:388–94.
6. Wadhwa PD, Buss C, Entringer S et al. Semin Reprod Med 2009;27:358–68.
7. Barker DJ, Osmond C, Kajantie E et al. Ann Hum Biol 2009;36:445–58.
8. Tamashiro KL, Moran TH. Physiol Behav 2010;100:560–6.
9. US Department of Health and Human Services. HealthyPeople.gov. Available at: http://healthypeople.gov/2020. Accessed July 22, 2012.
10. US Department of Health and Human Services. Health People 2010 Final Review. Available at: http://www.cdc.gov/nchs/healthy_people/hp2010/hp2010_final_review.htm. Accessed July 22, 2012.
11. Johnson K, Posner SF, Biermann J et al. MMWR Morb Mortal Wkly Rep 2006;55:1–23.
12. Food and Nutrition Board, Institute of Medicine. Dietary Reference Intakes for Thiamin, Riboflavin, Niacin, Vitamin B_6, Folate, Vitamin B_{12}, Pantothenic Acid, Biotin, and Choline. Washington, DC: National Academy Press, 1998.

13. Moos MK, Dunlop AL, Jack BW et al. Am J Obstet Gynecol 2008;199(Suppl 2):S280–9.

14. Gardiner PM, Nelson L, Shellhaas CS et al. Am J Obstet Gynecol 2008;199(Suppl 2):S345–56.

15. Siega-Riz AM, King JC, American Dietetic Association. J Am Diet Assoc 2009;109:918–27.

16. Jevitt C, Hernandez I, Groer M. J Midwifery Womens Health 2007;52:606–13.

17. Nommsen-Rivers LA, Chantry CJ, Peerson JM et al. Am J Clin Nutr 2010;92:574–84.

18. US Department of Health and Human Services, US Department of Agriculture. Nutrition and Your Health: Dietary Guidelines for Americans. 6th ed. Washington, DC: US Government Printing Office, 2005.

19. Food and Nutrition Board, Institute of Medicine. Dietary Reference Intakes for Energy, Carbohydrate, Fiber, Fat, Fatty Acids, Cholesterol, Protein, and Amino Acids. Washington, DC: National Academy Press, 2002.

20. US Department of Health and Human Services. 2008 Physical Activity Guidelines for Americans. Washington, DC: US Government Printing Office, 2008. ODPHP Publication No. U0036.

21. Dunlop AL, Jack BW, Bottalico JN et al. Am J Obstet Gynecol 2008;199(Suppl 2):S310–27.

22. Brown AS, Fernhoff PM, Waisbren SE et al. Genet Med 2002;4:84–9.

23. Institute of Medicine, National Research Council. Weight Gain During Pregnancy: Reexamining the Guidelines. Washington, DC: National Academies Press, 2009.

24. Chiloiro M, Darconza G, Piccioli E et al. J Gastroenterol 2001;36:538–43.

25. Carmichael SL, Abrams B. Obstet Gynecol 1997;89:865–73.

26. Strychar IM, Chabot C, Champagne F et al. J Am Diet Assoc 2000;100:353–6.

27. Schieve LA, Cogswell ME, Scanlon KS. Matern Child Health J 1998;2:111–6.

28. Villamor E, Cnattingius S. Lancet 2006;368:1164–70.

29. Food and Nutrition Board, Institute of Medicine. Dietary Reference Intakes for Vitamin A, Vitamin K, Arsenic, Boron, Chromium, Copper, Iron, Manganese, Molybdenum, Nickel, Silicon, Vanadium, and Zinc. Washington, DC: National Academy Press, 2001.

30. Simpson JL, Bailey LB, Pietrzik K et al. J Matern Fetal Neonatal Med 2011;24:1–24.

31. Voyles LM, Turner RE, Lukowski MJ et al. J Am Diet Assoc 2000;100:1068–70.

32. Rothman KJ, Moore LL, Singer MR et al. N Engl J Med 1995;333:1369–73.

33. Miller RK, Hendricks AG, Mills JL et al. Reprod Toxicol 1998;12:75–88.

34. Hollis BW, Wagner CL. CMAJ 2006;174:1287–90.

35. Food and Nutrition Board, Institute of Medicine. Dietary Reference Intakes for Calcium, Phosphorus, Magnesium, Vitamin D, and Fluoride. Washington, DC: National Academy Press, 1997.

36. Nesby-O'Dell S, Scanlon K, Cogswell M et al. Am J Clin Nutr 2002;76:187–92.

37. Hollis BW, Wagner CL. Am J Clin Nutr 2004;79:717–26.

38. Food and Nutrition Board, Institute of Medicine. Dietary Reference Intakes for Vitamin C, Vitamin E, Selenium, and Carotenoids. Washington, DC: National Academy Press, 2000.

39. Simpson JL, Bailey LB, Pietrzik K et al. J Matern Fetal Neonatal Med 2010;23:1323–43.

40. Caudill MA, Cruz AC, Gregory JF et al. J Nutr 1997;127:2363–70.

41. Zempleni J, Mock DM. Proc Soc Exp Biol Med 2000;223:14–21.

42. Takechi R, Taniguchi A, Ebara S et al. J Nutr 2008;138:680–4.

43. Food and Nutrition Board, Institute of Medicine. Dietary Reference Intakes for Water, Potassium, Sodium, Chloride, and Sulfate. Washington, DC: National Academy Press, 2004.

44. Prentice A. J Nutr 2003;133(Suppl):1693S–9S.

45. Leverett DH, Adair SM, Vaughan BW et al. Caries Res 1997;31:174–9.

46. Allen LH. Am J Clin Nutr 2000;71(suppl):1280S–4S.

47. Turner RE, Langkamp-Henken B, Littell RC et al. J Am Diet Assoc 2003;103:461–6.

48. King JC. Am J Clin Nutr 2000;71(suppl):1334S–43S.

49. Scholl TO, Hediger ML, Schall JI et al. Am J Epidemiol 1993;137:1115–24.

50. Goldenberg RL, Tamura T, Neggers Y et al. JAMA 1995;274:463–8.

51. Caulfield LE, Zavaleta N, Figueroa A et al. J Nutr 1999;129:1563–8.

52. Merialdi M, Caulfield LE, Zavaleta N et al. Obstet Gynecol Surv 2005;60:13–5.

53. Merialdi M, Caulfield LE, Zavaleta N et al. Am J Obstet Gynecol 2004;190:1106–12.

54. Barr SI, Murphy SP, Poos MI. J Am Diet Assoc 2002;102:780–8.

55. Turner RE, Langkamp-Henken R, Littell R. J Am Diet Assoc 2003;103:563.

56. Institute of Medicine. Nutrition During Pregnancy: Part II. Nutrient Supplements. Washington, DC: National Academy Press, 1990.

57. US Department of Agriculture. Health & Nutrition Information for Pregnant & Breastfeeding Women. Available at http://www.choosemyplate.gov/pregnancy-breastfeeding.html. Accessed July 22, 2012.

58. James DC, Lessen R. J Am Diet Assoc 2009;109:1926–42.

59. American College of Gynecologists and Obstetricians. Obstet Gynecol 2002;99:171–3.

60. Dye TD, Knox KL, Artal R. Am J Epidemiol 1997;146:961–5.

61. Mozaffarian D, Rimm EB. JAMA 2006;296:1885–99.

62. Nesheim MC, Yaktine AL, eds. Seafood Choices: Balancing Benefits and Risks. Washington, DC: National Academies Press, 2007.

63. Hibbeln JR, Davis HM, Steer C et al. Lancet 2007;369:578–85.

64. Craig WJ, Mangels AR, American Dietetic Association. J Am Diet Assoc 2009;109:1266–82.

65. CARE Study Group. BMJ 2008;337:a2332.

66. Bech BH, Obel C, Henriksen TB et al. BMJ 2007;384:409.

67. Lupton C, Burd L, Harwood R. Am J Med Genet 2004;127C:42–50.

68. Stratton K, Howe C, Battaglia F. Fetal Alcohol Syndrome: Diagnosis, Epidemiology, Prevention and Treatment. Washington, DC: National Academy Press, 1996:17–20.

69. Stoler JM, Holmes LB. Am J Med Genet C Semin Med Genet 2004;127C:21–7.

70. Day NL, Leech SL, Richardson GA et al. Alcohol Clin Exp Res 2002;26:1584–91.

71. Day NL, Richardson GA. Am J Med Genet C Semin Med Genet 2004;127C:28–34.

72. Westfall RE. Complement Ther Nurs Midwifery 2004;10:30–6.

73. White B. Am Fam Physician 2007;75:1689–91.

74. Rousseaux CG, Schachter H. Birth Defects Res B Dev Reprod Toxicol 2003;68:505–10.

75. Finkel RS, Zarlengo KM. N Engl J Med 2004;351:302–3.

76. Reinold C, Dalenius K, Smith B et al. Pregnancy Nutrition Surveillance 2007 Report. Atlanta: Centers for Disease Control and Prevention, 2009.

77. Ventura SJ, Hamilton BE, Mathews TJ et al. Pediatrics 2003;111:1176–80.

78. Substance Abuse and Mental Health Services Administration. Results from the 2008 National Survey on Drug Use and Health: National Findings. Office of Applied Studies, NSDUH series H-36, DHHS publication no. SMA 09-4434. Rockville, MD, 2009. Available at: http://www.oas.samhsa.gov/NSDUH/2k8NSDUH/2k8results.cfm#Ch2. Accessed August, 15, 2010.

79. Chiriboga CA. Neurologist 2003;9:267–79.

80. Minnes S, Singer LT, Kirchner HL. Neurotoxicol Teratol 2010;32:443–51.

81. Linares TJ, Singer LT, Kirchner HL. J Pediatr Psychol 2006;31:85–97.

82. Jednak MA, Shadigian EM, Kim MS et al. Am J Physiol 1999;277:G855–61.

83. Huxley RR. Obstet Gynecol 2000;95:779–82.

84. Richter JE. Gastroenterol Clin North Am 2003;32:235–61.

85. Reinold C, Dalenius K, Brindley P et al. Pregnancy Nutrition Surveillance 2008 Report. Atlanta: Centers for Disease Control and Prevention, 2010.

86. Van Wootten W, Turner RE. Am J Diet Assoc 2002;102:241–3.

87. Solomon CG, Seely EW. N Engl J Med 2004;350:641–2.

88. Shaw GM, Schaffer D, Verlie EM et al. Epidemiology 1995;6:219–26.

89. Werler MM, Shapiro S, Mitchell AA. JAMA 1993;269:1257–61.

90. National Birth Defects Prevention Network. Available at: http://www.nbdpn.org. Accessed August 15, 2010.

SUGGESTED READINGS

Kaiser L, Allen LH, American Dietetic Association. Position of the American Dietetic Association: nutrition and lifestyle for a healthy pregnancy outcome. J Am Diet Assoc 2008;108:553–61.

Poston L, Harthoorn LF, Van Der Beek EM. Obesity in pregnancy: implications for the mother and lifelong health of the child. A consensus statement. Pediatr Res 2011;69:175–80.

Reinold C, Dalenius K, Brindley P et al. Pregnancy Nutrition Surveillance 2009 Report. Atlanta: Centers for Disease Control and Prevention, 2011.

53

NUTRITION IN LACTATION[1]

DEBORAH L. O'CONNOR AND MARY FRANCES PICCIANO[†]

Human milk, a complex food, provides both nutrition and bioactive components that confer benefits for the growth, development, and health of infants. In recognition of this, the World Health Organization (WHO), the American Academy of Pediatrics (AAP), and Health Canada all recommend exclusive breast-feeding for the first 6 months of life. At 6 months, it is advised that infants be introduced to nutrient-rich, solid foods and breast-feeding be continued for the first 12 to 24 months of life and beyond (1–3). Exclusive breast-feeding is

defined as not receiving any solids or liquids other than breast milk (4). Despite these recommendations, only 33% and 13% of infants in the United States are exclusively breast-fed through 3 or 6 months, respectively (5). In fact, only 43% of infants are fed any human milk at all at 6 months. Initiation rates are somewhat more encouraging, with 75% of US women initiating breast-feeding. The US Healthy People 2020 objectives are to increase the proportion of US mothers who breast-feed (any breast-feeding) their babies to 82% in the early postpartum period and to 61% at 6 months, as well as to increase exclusivity of breast-feeding at 3 and 6 months to 46% and 26%, respectively (6). Few contraindications to breast-feeding exist. Generally, women who test positive for human immunodeficiency virus (HIV), have active and untreated tuberculosis, have human T-cell lymphotropic virus type 1 or type 2, or use either illegal drugs or certain prescribed drugs, such as chemotherapeutic drugs for cancer treatment, should not breast-feed (4). Infants with galactosemia should not be breast-fed. In developing countries, however, a safe alternative to breast-feeding may not be available, and evaluation of the relative risks of infant feeding choices may be necessary.

Human milk is a unique food that provides much more than nutrition for the infant. In addition to macronutrients and micronutrients, an impressive body of evidence indicates that human milk contains a host of other components—including anti-inflammatory agents, immunoglobulins, antimicrobials, antioxidants, oligosaccharides, cytokines, hormones, and growth factors—that have biologic activities related to development, metabolic regulation, inflammation, and pathogenesis (7). The combined effects of these bioactive components may result in the observed protection that human milk provides breast-feeding infants against infectious diseases, allergic disorders, and chronic diseases with an immunologic basis (8).

This chapter summarizes information on the prevalence of lactation, its physiologic aspects, and the composition of human milk. In addition, it highlights the possible beneficial impact of lactation on both the breast-fed, full-term infant and the breast-feeding mother and suggests directions for future lactation research.

---

[1]**Abbreviations: AAP**, American Academy of Pediatrics; **AHRQ**, Agency for Healthcare Research and Quality; **ALA**, α-linolenic acid; **ARA**, arachidonic acid; **BMD**, bone mineral density; **DHA**, docosahexaenoic acid; **HIV**, human immunodeficiency virus; **LA**, linoleic acid; **LC-PUFA**, long-chain polyunsaturated fatty acid; **NHANES**, National Health and Nutrition Examination Survey; **OR**, odds ratio; **PROBIT**, Promotion of Breastfeeding Intervention Trial; **RR**, relative risk; **UNICEF**, United Nations Children's Fund; **WHO**, World Health Organization; **WIC**, Special Supplemental Nutrition Program for Women, Infants, and Children.

[†]Deceased. With the passing of Dr. Picciano, she unfortunately was unable to review the revision of this chapter.

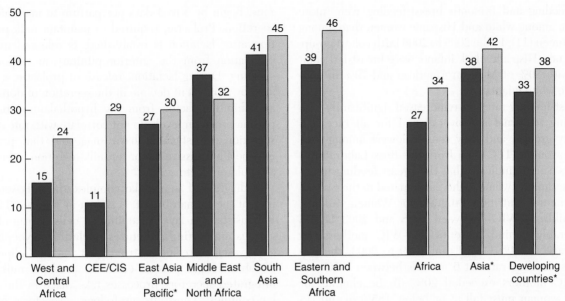

Fig. 53.1. Trends globally, from 1995 to 2008, in the percentage of infants less than 6 months who were exclusively breast-fed. *Asterisks,* excluding China; CEE/CIS, Central and Eastern Europe/Commonwealth of Independent States region. (Data from UNICEF. UNICEF Global Databases 2010, from Multiple Indicator Cluster Surveys, Demographic Health Surveys, and Other National Surveys. Available at: http://www.childinfo.org/breastfeeding_progress.html. Accessed June 28, 2011, with permission.)

PREVALENCE OF BREAST-FEEDING

Throughout the World

The WHO Global Data Bank on Breastfeeding provides surveillance data, primary from national and regional surveys, from 94 countries or 65% of the world's infant population (<12 months) (9). These data suggest that initiation rates for breast-feeding in the United States are similar to those of the United Kingdom (76%) and Germany (77%) but lower than those of Canada (93%) and Austria (93%). The percentage of mothers who exclusively breast-feed to 4 months in the United States (33%) is lower than in Canada (51%), but the exclusivity to 6 months is low in the United States (14%), Canada (14%), Germany (22%), and Austria (22.4%). The United Nations Children's Fund (UNICEF) provides exclusivity of breast-feeding data globally by geographic region (10). Rates for exclusive breast-feeding of infants from 0 to 5 months of life have been estimated to be highest in East Asia and the Pacific region (43%) and in Eastern and Southern Africa (41%), and lowest in West and Central Africa (20%) and in Central and Eastern Europe and the Commonwealth of Independent States (22%) (Fig. 53.1). The global average of exclusive breast-feeding from 0 to 5 months reported by UNICEF was 37%.

In the United States

The prevalence of breast-feeding in the United States has been estimated by several large national surveys, including the Ross Laboratories Mothers Survey, the National Health and Nutrition Examination Survey (NHANES, 1996 to 2006), and the Centers for Disease Control and Prevention National Immunization Survey (5, 11, 12). The Ross Laboratories Mothers Survey was initiated in 1954 and has expanded considerably since then. It was designed to determine patterns of milk feeding during infancy. The reported percentage of mothers who ever breast-fed increased from low levels in the 1950s and 1960s to a high point in 1982, declined throughout the 1980s, but then increased through the 1990s (Table 53.1) (12, 13).

According to NHANES, the percentage of infants who were ever breast-fed increased from 60% among infants born in 1993 to 1994 to 77% among infants born in 2005 to 2006 (11). In contrast, no significant change in the rate of breast-feeding at 6 months of age occurred for infants born between 1993 and 2004. Both in-hospital

TABLE 53.1	IN-HOSPITAL AND 6-MONTH BREAST-FEEDING RATES ACCORDING TO PARTICIPATION IN THE SPECIAL SUPPLEMENTAL NUTRITION PROGRAM FOR WOMEN, INFANTS, AND CHILDREN			
	IN-HOSPITAL BREAST-FEEDING (%)		BREAST-FEEDING AT 6 MO (%)	
YEAR	WIC	NON-WIC	WIC	NON-WIC
1978	34.4	48.1	10.0	20.0
1982	45.3	65.0	16.1	29.4
1984	39.9	67.6	12.0	28.5
1990	33.7	62.9	8.2	23.6
2002	58.8	79.2	22.1	42.7
2003	54.3	76.1	21.0	42.7

WIC, Special Supplemental Nutrition Program for Women, Infants, and Children.

Data from Ryan AS, Zhou W. Lower breastfeeding rates persist among the Special Supplemental Nutrition Program for Women, Infants, and Children participants, 1978–2003. Pediatrics 2006;117:1136–46, with permission. Some data extrapolated from figures.

breast-feeding and 6-month breast-feeding were more common among white and Hispanic women than among black women (11). In the 2005 to 2006 birth cohort group, 65% of non-Hispanic black infants were breast-fed compared with 80% of Mexican-American and 79% of non-Hispanic white infants.

Breast-feeding rates have increased significantly with increasing maternal age overall and for all race and ethnicity groups, and they remain lowest among low-income women (11). Data from the Ross Laboratories Mothers Survey indicate that the breast-feeding initiation rates among women who participated in the Special Supplemental Nutrition Program for Women, Infants, and Children (WIC) between 1978 and 2003 lagged considerably behind those of non-WIC mothers, by an average of 24% (13). From 1999 to 2003, the gap in breast-feeding rates at 6 months between WIC and non-WIC mothers exceeded 20%. To be eligible for WIC, a woman must fall at or below 185% of the US poverty income guidelines, or she or a family member must receive some form of financial assistance from the government. WIC revised their food packages to enhance the monetary value of the breast-feeding packages, which were thought to be a disincentive to breast-feeding. Before these changes, the market value of the food package for an exclusive formula-feeding mother and infant was approximately $1380 compared with $670 for a mother who decided to breast-feed exclusively for the first year.

MAMMARY GLAND AND REGULATION OF MILK SECRETION

The mature breast of nonpregnant, nonlactating women has a treelike pattern of branching ducts that extends from the nipple to the edges of the fat pad. Alveolar clusters exist in a dynamic state, with growth and complexity increasing and decreasing in response to the hormonal changes of the menstrual cycle. During pregnancy, lobular alveolar complexes expand dramatically in response to progesterone, prolactin, and placental lactogen. Secretory differentiation occurs around midpregnancy (stage 1 lactogenesis), but milk secretion is inhibited by high progesterone levels (14, 15).

Lactogenesis and lactation are regulated through complex endocrine system control mechanisms that coordinate the actions of various hormones, including the reproductive hormones prolactin, progesterone, placental lactogen, oxytocin, and estrogen (15, 16). Although it is known that progesterone suppresses active milk secretion during lactogenesis 1, hormonal regulation during this stage is not well understood (16). After parturition, lactogenesis 2, also called secretory activation, is initiated through progesterone withdrawal, combined with high levels of prolactin; this process results in secretion of colostrum ("early milk") and then milk. Initiation of lactogenesis 2 does not require infant suckling, but suckling

must begin by 3 to 4 days postpartum to maintain milk secretion. Prolactin, required to maintain milk production after lactation is established, is released into the circulation from the anterior pituitary in response to suckling. During lactation, release of prolactin is mediated by a transient decline in the secretion of dopamine, an inhibiting factor, from the hypothalamus. Because plasma prolactin levels do not correlate with rate of milk secretion, investigators have suggested that prolactin may be a permissive factor for milk secretion rather than a regulatory factor (16).

A diagram of an alveolar complex, the milk-secreting unit of the human breast, is shown in Figure 53.2 (17). It consists of a layer of epithelial cells surrounded by various supporting structures, including myoepithelial cells, vasculature, and a stroma that contains adipocytes, fibroblasts, and plasma cells. To produce milk, four integrated secretory processes take place in the alveolar complex. These are as follows: exocytosis of milk protein, lactose, and other components of the aqueous phase via Golgi-derived secretory vesicles; fat synthesis and secretion through milk fat globules; secretion of ions, water, and glucose; and transcytosis of immunoglobulins and other substances from the interstitial spaces. Milk is secreted into the alveolar lumina and stored there until ejection by contraction of the myoepithelial cells (14). Although milk secretion is a continuous process, the amount produced is regulated primarily by infant demand.

Suckling causes neural impulses to be sent to the hypothalamus; this triggers oxytocin release from the posterior pituitary. Oxytocin brings about contraction of the myoepithelial cells and thus forces milk into the ducts of the nipple so it is available for the infant. This response (let-down) also can be triggered simply by seeing the infant or hearing the infant cry. When milk is removed from the breast after parturition, milk volume increases significantly within several days postpartum. During lactation, the typical daily volume of milk transferred to the infant increases from 0.50 mL on day 1, to 500 mL by day 5, to 650 mL by 1 month, and to 750 mL by 3 months. Most women are capable of secreting considerably more milk than needed by a single infant. When milk is not removed, either by infant suckling or other means, involution of the mammary epithelium occurs, and milk secretion stops within 1 to 2 days.

COMPOSITION OF HUMAN MILK

Human milk is a remarkably complex biologic fluid. It is composed of thousands of constituents that are dispersed throughout various phases, including an aqueous phase with true solutions (87%), colloidal dispersions of casein molecules (0.3%), emulsions of fat globules (4%), fat globule membranes, and live cells. Milk composition changes substantially as early milk develops the characteristics of mature milk that are evident by day 10 of lactation.

WHO Collaborative Study Team demonstrated that infants in less developed countries who are not breast-fed have a sixfold greater risk of dying of infectious diseases in the first 2 months of life than do infants who are breast-fed (59). A growing body of evidence also suggests that breast-feeding, mediated by several of the bioactive components of human milk, can reduce morbidity in developed countries (4).

The Agency for Healthcare Research and Quality (AHRQ) published a report in 2007 that summarized the evidence from systematic reviews and meta analyses on breast-feeding and maternal and infant health outcomes in developed countries (60). The AHRQ concluded that breast-feeding was associated with reduction in risk of acute otitis media, nonspecific gastroenteritis, severe lower respiratory tract infections, atopic dermatitis, asthma (young children), obesity, type 1 and 2 diabetes, childhood leukemia, sudden infant death syndrome, and necrotizing enterocolitis. The excess risk of each of these health outcomes as a result of not breast-feeding is summarized in Table 53.4. Although these findings are suggestive, the authors of this report cautioned that almost all the data in their review were gathered from observational studies. Therefore, one should not infer causality based on these findings. Another limitation of this evidence-based review was the wide variation in quality of the body of evidence across health outcomes.

IMPACT OF LACTATION ON THE MOTHER

Just as for the infant, evidence indicates that breast-feeding has several direct health benefits for the mother. Exclusive breast-feeding to 6 months, for example, has

been shown to be associated with a delay in postpartum resumption of menses and hence improved birth spacing (61). The AHRQ evidence report on breast-feeding and maternal and infant health outcomes in developed countries found that breast-feeding was associated with reduced risk of maternal type 2 diabetes and of breast and ovarian cancer (60). No relationship was found between a history of lactation and the risk of osteoporosis. The effect of breast-feeding on postpartum weight loss was unclear. Early cessation of breast-feeding or not breast-feeding was associated with an increased risk of maternal postpartum depression, but whether breast-feeding alters the risk of depression or whether postpartum depression leads to early cessation of breast-feeding is unclear.

Fertility

Breast-feeding is accompanied by a period of amenorrhea and infertility that results from suckling-induced suppression of ovarian activity. Suckling interferes with the normal pulsatile secretion pattern of hypothalamic gonadotrophin-releasing hormone and, consequently, with the secretion of luteinizing hormone and follicle-stimulating hormone (gonadotropins) stimulated by gonadotropin-releasing hormone. Normal secretion of follicle-stimulating hormone returns early in lactation, and ovarian follicles may develop; luteinizing hormone secretion, however, remains suppressed by suckling. Because ovarian follicles do not produce normal levels of estradiol while luteinizing hormone remains suppressed, ovulation also is suppressed by suckling and lactational amenorrhea is the result (62). In fact, the Bellagio consensus of 1988 postulated that full or nearly full breast-feeding during lactational amenorrhea provides approximately 98% protection from pregnancy in the first 6 months after childbirth (63).

This estimate of contraceptive efficacy was confirmed by prospective studies of lactating women in both developing and developed countries (64, 65). A study of more than 4000 mother–infant pairs reported that, for full breast-feeding, cumulative pregnancy rates during lactational amenorrhea ranged from 0.9% to 1.2% in the first 6 months postpartum, but they increased to 6.6% to 7.4% at 12 months postpartum (64). A decline in sucking stimulus appears to be the critical factor that determines when postpartum ovulation will resume (62). Thus, supplementation with formula or solid foods during breast-feeding likely will hasten the return of fertility. Kramer and Kakuma, in their Cochrane systematic review, reported that women who exclusively breast-fed for 6 months or longer had more prolonged amenorrhea, compared with those who began mixed breast-feeding 3 to 4 months postpartum (61). Mixed breast-feeding was defined as the introduction of complementary liquid or solid foods at 3 to 4 months, with continued breast-feeding thereafter through 6 months.

TABLE 53.4	EXCESS HEALTH RISKS ASSOCIATED WITH NOT BREAST-FEEDING
OUTCOME	**EXCESS RISK[a] (%)**
Acute ear infection (otitis media)	100
Eczema (atopic dermatitis)	47
Diarrhea and vomiting (gastrointestinal infection)	178
Hospitalization for lower respiratory tract disease in the first year	257
Asthma, with family history	67
Asthma, no family history	35
Childhood obesity	32
Type 2 diabetes mellitus	64
Acute lymphocytic leukemia	23
Acute myelogenous leukemia	18
Sudden infant death syndrome	56
Among preterm infants	
Necrotizing enterocolitides	138
Among mothers	
Breast cancer	4
Ovarian cancer	27

[a]The excess risk is approximated by using the odds ratios reported in the referenced studies.

From US Department of Health and Human Services. The Surgeon General's Call to Action to Support Breastfeeding. Washington, DC: US Department of Health and Human Services, 2011. #Available at: http://www.surgeongeneral.gov. Accessed June 22, 2011, with permission.

Weight Retention and Type 2 Diabetes

In North America, most women enter pregnancy either overweight or obese, and at least half will gain more weight during pregnancy than recommended (66). Although many women express a desire to lose weight after childbirth and return to their prepregnancy weight, postpartum weight loss is highly variable. Weight gained during pregnancy and not lost postpartum no doubt contributes to overweight and obesity in women of childbearing age. A woman who is lactating has the same requirement for regulating body weight as one who is not lactating, except that she is producing a continuous supply of milk and thus creating much higher energy output. The total energy cost to a woman who is exclusively breast-feeding an infant to 6 months postpartum is estimated to be 500 kcal/day. If energy intake and physical activity remain unchanged, theoretically you could expect a 0.5 kg/week weight loss. The AHRQ review concluded, however, that the overall effect of breast-feeding on return to prepregnancy weight was negligible (<1 kg) (60). The review concluded that other factors likely have a greater effect on postpartum weight retention including income, prepregnancy body mass index, ethnicity, gestational weight gain, and energy intake. In general, women included in the studies reviewed did not adhere to recommendations to breast-feed exclusively for 6 months, and it has been argued that breast-feeding of sufficient intensity and duration is necessary to promote accelerated postpartum weight loss.

One of the risk factors for unsuccessful initiation of breast-feeding is obesity, which complicates assessment of the possible impact of breast-feeding on postpartum weight retention (66). Baker et al (67) showed that breast-feeding had a significant independent contribution to postpartum weight loss among women from the Danish National Birth cohort ($n = 36,030$) who had reasonable pregnancy weight gains (~12 kg) and who breast-fed as recommended (exclusive breast-feeding to 6 months and to any extent to 12 months). In fact, by 6 months, postpartum weight retention was eliminated.

Evidence indicates that breast-feeding has a beneficial effect on maternal glucose and lipid metabolism (60). In women with gestational diabetes, lactation has been associated with improved pancreatic β-cell function. The AHRQ review concluded that, among women without a history of gestational diabetes, longer duration of lifetime breast-feeding is associated with a reduced risk of developing type 2 diabetes.

Breast and Ovarian Cancers

Several reviews focused on the numerous epidemiologic studies that investigated a possible link between breast-feeding and breast cancer risk (68–70). The findings, from both a qualitative literature review (70) and a metaanalysis of appropriate published studies (69), suggested that breast-feeding reduces risk, especially among premenopausal women, and that risk reduction is directly related to lifetime duration of breast-feeding. For ever breast-feeding versus never breast-feeding, the metaanalysis (random effects model) reported adjusted ORs of 0.84, 0.76, and 0.83 for all women, non menopausal women, and menopausal women, respectively, and noted that various studies adjusted for different covariates (69). For all women, breast-feeding for longer than 12 months reduced breast cancer risk by 28% (not adjusted for covariates) compared with breast-feeding for 0 to 6 months. A more recent reanalysis of data from 47 epidemiologic studies in 30 countries reported a relative risk (RR) of 0.96 for ever breast-feeding versus never breast-feeding, and breast cancer risk decreased by 4.3% for every 12 months of breast-feeding. Risk reduction did not differ significantly by menopausal status, age, parity, ethnicity, or various other personal characteristics (68). Several biologic mechanisms for a protective effect of breast-feeding on breast cancer have been proposed, including the following: delay in reestablishing ovulation, which reduces exposure to reproductive hormones; removal of estrogens through breast fluid; physical changes in the mammary epithelial cells that accompany milk production (maximum differentiation); and production of growth factors during lactation such as transforming growth factor-β1, shown to be a negative growth factor in human breast cancer cells (69–71).

Epithelial ovarian cancers, which account for approximately 90% of all ovarian cancers, have significant histologic differences, findings suggesting that these cancers may have heterogeneous causes. Some evidence indicates that reproduction-related risk factors are inversely related to risk for nonmucinous tumors (e.g., serous, endometrioid, clear cell) but not for mucinous tumors (72–74). One multiethnic, case-control study reported that, compared with never breast-feeding, ever breast-feeding lowered the risk of all types of epithelial ovarian cancer, except for invasive mucinous tumors. In addition, duration of breast-feeding was significantly associated with decreased risk of nonmucinous tumors (RR = 0.4 for >16 months), but not mucinous tumors (RR = 0.9 for >16 months) (74). In another study, ever breast-feeding was associated with significant decreased risk only for endometrioid/clear cell tumors (RR = 0.4), and the risk decreased with breast-feeding duration (73). Some other investigations, however, did not find significant differences in risk among histologic types of epithelial ovarian cancer in relation to breast-feeding practices (72, 75). Suppression of ovulation, which results in less chronic trauma to the ovarian epithelium, has been proposed as one potential mechanism through which breast-feeding may reduce ovarian cancer risk (73).

Osteoporosis

Calcium resorbed from the bones of the lactating woman is the primary source of calcium in human milk (76, 77), and evidence indicates that increasing calcium intake through either diet or supplementation does not prevent resorption (31, 78, 79). However, studies consistently show that the skeletal calcium lost during lactation is rapidly regained after weaning (76, 77). The recovery of bone mineral density (BMD) after weaning appears to be influenced by the duration of lactation and postpartum amenorrhea, and recovery varies among skeletal sites (76). For example, greater BMD increases have been found in the lumbar spine than in the femoral neck during the first 6 months after weaning (76, 80). Bone recovery is complete for most women and occurs even with multiple and closely spaced pregnancies and periods of lactation (80, 81). A study that measured BMDs for 30 grand multiparous Finnish-American women who had borne at least 6 children and who breast-fed each child for at least 6 months found that repeated pregnancies and lactation, without a recovery interval, were not associated with either lowered BMD or osteoporosis or osteopenia in these women. Moreover, women with 10 or more children did not have lower BMD than did women who had 6 to 9 children (81). In general, duration of lactation does not appear to be associated with increased fracture risk or with osteoporosis later in life (76).

FUTURE RESEARCH DIRECTIONS

Breast-feeding clearly provides optimal nutrition and other health benefits for the newborn as well as health benefits for the lactating mother. Not yet clear are the extent of these benefits and the mechanisms responsible. Very little is known about either the synthesis or regulation of already identified bioactive components in milk or their relation to maternal diet. In fact, many more bioactive components will probably be identified in human milk, and extensive research will be essential to investigate not only their origins but also their specific roles in contributing to potential health benefits for the infant.

Comprehensive, carefully designed prospective studies that rigorously adjust for confounding variables must be carried out to define possible existing relationships between breast-feeding, especially duration of breast-feeding, and specific outcomes for infants—including cognitive development and risk of acute disease in infancy, as well as chronic disease in childhood and beyond. Similarly, research must focus on clarifying associations between breast-feeding and consequences for maternal health. For example, can breast-feeding influence genetic susceptibility with regard to a woman's risk of hormone-related cancers? Considerable work needs to be done to understand the factors related to the lower incidence and duration of breast-feeding among obese women to develop, implement, and evaluate strategies to overcome this issue. In all studies, identifying the biologic mechanisms underlying these relationships is paramount.

Controlled clinical trials that randomize individual mother–infant pairs to either breast-feeding or no breast-feeding are not possible because of ethical considerations, and alternative trial designs must be considered. One such example of an alternative trial design would be the randomization approach adopted by the PROBIT trial in Belarus (82). Investigators used a cluster randomization approach to assign one set of maternity hospitals and their associated clinics in the country to a breast-feeding promotion program (intervention group) and a second set to receive the usual practices and policies with regard to breast-feeding (control). The intervention resulted in an increase in both the incidence and duration of breast-feeding. The investigators went on successfully to assess the degree of breast-feeding and the occurrence of various infant health outcomes including gastrointestinal tract infection, respiratory tract infection, atopic eczema, neuro development, and obesity.

It is reasonable to expect that breast-feeding recommendations may differ depending on whether an infant is ill or is at increased risk of disease because of environmental factors, genetic susceptibility, or maternal factors (e.g., viral infection); and on whether the mother is at increased risk of acute disease, as are malnourished or HIV-infected mothers, or for chronic diseases, such as hormone-related cancers. Finding answers to the many questions regarding the potential short-term and long-term health benefits of breast-feeding, for both mother and infant, will help to determine how best to optimize these benefits for mother–child pairs in various circumstances, whether in developing or developed countries.

REFERENCES

1. Health Canada. Exclusive Breastfeeding Duration: 2004 Health Canada Recommendation. Available at: http://www.hc-sc.gc.ca/fn-an/nutrition/infant-nourisson/excl_bf_dur-dur_am_excl-eng.php. Accessed June 22, 2011.
2. World Health Organization. The Optimal Duration of Breastfeeding: Results of a WHO Systematic Survey. Geneva: World Health Organization, 2001. Available at: http://www.who.int/inf-pr-2001/en/note2001-07.html. Accessed June 22, 2011.
3. Kleinman RE, ed. Pediatric Nutrition Handbook. 6th ed. Elk Grove Village, IL: American Academy of Pediatrics, 2004.
4. US Department of Health and Human Services. The Surgeon General's Call to Action to Support Breastfeeding. Washington, DC: US Department of Health and Human Services, Office of the Surgeon General, 2011. Available at: http://www.surgeongeneral.gov. Accessed June 22, 2011.
5. Centers for Disease Control and Prevention. Breastfeeding Among U.S. Children Born 1999–2007. CDC National Immunization Survey. Available at: http://www.cdc.gov/breastfeeding/data/NIS_data/index.htm. Accessed June 22, 2011.
6. US Department of Health and Human Services. Health People.gov. Available at: http://www.healthypeople.gov/2020. Accessed May 10, 2012.
7. Chirico G, Marzollo R, Cortinovis S et al. J Nutr 2008;138:1801S–6S.

8. Newburg DS, ed. Bioactive Components of Human Milk. New York: Kluwer Academic/Plenum Publishers, 2001.

9. World Health Organization. Global Data Bank on Breastfeeding. Geneva: World Health Organization. Available at: http://www.who.int/nutrition/databases/infantfeeding/en/. Accessed June 23, 2011.

10. United Nations Children's Fund. Breastfeeding and Complementary Feeding. Geneva: World Health Organization, 2001. Available at: http://www.childinfo.org/breastfeeding_iycf.php. Accessed June 22, 2011.

11. McDowell MA, Wang CY, Kennedy-Stephenson J. Breastfeeding in the United States: Findings from the National Health and Nutrition Examination Surveys 1999–2006. NCHS data briefs no. 5. Hyattsville, MD: National Center for Health Statistics, 2008.

12. Ryan AS, Wenjun Z, Acosta A. Pediatrics 2002;110:1103–9.

13. Ryan AS, Zhou W. Pediatrics 2006;117:1136–46.

14. Neville MC. Pediatr Clin North Am 2001;48:13–34.

15. Neville MC, Morton J. J Nutr 2001;131:3005S–8S.

16. Neville MC, McFadden TB, Forsyth I. J Mammary Gland Biol Neoplasia 2002;7:49–66.

17. McManaman JL, Neville MC. Adv Drug Deliv Rev 2003; 55:629–41.

18. Picciano MF. Pediatr Clin North Am 2001;48:263–4.

19. Food and Nutrition Board, Institute of Medicine. Dietary Reference Intakes for Thiamin, Riboflavin, Niacin, Vitamin B_6, Folate, Vitamin B_{12}, Pantothenic Acid, Biotin, and Choline. Washington, DC: National Academy Press, 1998.

20. Food and Nutrition Board, Institute of Medicine. Dietary Reference Intakes for Vitamic C, Vitamin E, Selenium, and Carotenoids. Washington, DC: National Academy Press, 2000.

21. Food and Nutrition Board, Institute of Medicine. Dietary Reference Intakes for Vitamin A, Vitamin K, Arsenic, Boron, Chromium, Copper, Iodine, Iron, Manganese, Molybdenum, Nickel, Silicon, Vanadium, and Zinc. Washington, DC: National Academy Press, 2001.

22. Food and Nutrition Board, Institute of Medicine. Dietary Reference Intakes for Energy, Carbohydrate, Fiber, Fat, Fatty Acids, Cholesterol, Protein, and Amino Acids. Washington, DC: National Academy Press, 2005.

23. Kodentsova VM, Vrzhesinskaya OA. Bull Exp Biol Med 2006;141:323–7.

24. Motil KJ, Sheng HP, Montandon CM et al. J Pediatr Gastroenterol Nutr 1997;24:10–7.

25. Jensen RG. Lipids 1999;34:1243–71.

26. Jensen RG. Handbook of Milk Composition. San Diego: Academic Press, 1995.

27. Hamosh M. Pediatr Clin North Am 2001;48:69–86.

28. Haskell MJ, Brown KH. J Mammary Gland Biol Neoplasia 1999;4:243–57.

29. Paediatr Child Health 2007;12:583–98.

30. Wagner CL, Greer FR. Pediatrics 2008;122:1142–52.

31. Food and Nutrition Board, Institute of Medicine. Dietary Reference Intakes: Calcium and Vitamin D. Washington, DC: National Academy Press, 2011.

32. Picciano MF. Pediatr Clin North Am 2001;48:53–67.

33. Institute of Medicine. Nutrition During Pregnancy. Washington, DC: National Academy Press, 1990.

34. von Schenck U, Bender-Gotze C, Koletzko B. Arch Dis Child 1997;77:137–9.

35. Delange F. Proc Nutr Soc 2000;59:75–9.

36. Grosvenor CE, Picciano MF, Baumrucker CR. Endocr Rev 1993;14:710–28.

37. Hosea Blewett HJ, Cicalo MC, Holland CD et al. Adv Food Nutr Res 2008;54:45–80.

38. World Health Organization, Department of Nutrition for Health and Development. WHO Child Growth Standards: Length/Height-for-Age, Weight-for-Age, Weight-for-Length, Weight-for-Height and Body Mass Index-for-Age Methods and Development. Geneva: World Health Organization, 2006.

39. Baker RD, Greer FR. Pediatrics 2010;126:1040–50.

40. Dewey KG. Pediatr Clin North Am 2001;48:87–104.

41. Anderson JW, Johnstone BM, Remley DT. Am J Clin Nutr 1999;70:525–35.

42. Kramer MS, Aboud F, Mironova E et al. Arch Gen Psychiatry 2008;65:578–84.

43. O'Connor DL, Jacobs J, Hall R et al. J Pediatr Gastroenterol Nutr 2003;37:437–46.

44. Vohr BR, Poindexter BB, Dusick AM et al. Pediatrics 2007;120:e953–9.

45. Jain A, Concato J, Leventhal JM. Pediatrics 2002;109: 1044–53.

46. Kris-Etherton PM, Innis S, American Dietetic Association et al. J Am Diet Assoc 2007;107:1599–611.

47. Delgado-Noguera MF, Calvache JA, Bonfill Cosp X. Cochrane Database Syst Rev 2010;(12):CD007901.

48. Bergmann KE, Bergmann RL, Von Kries R et al. Int J Obes Relat Metab Disord 2003;27:162–72.

49. Dewey KG. J Hum Lact 2003;19:9–18.

50. Monasta L, Batty GD, Cattaneo A et al. Obes Rev 2010; 11:695–708.

51. Kramer MS, Matush L, Vanilovich I et al. J Nutr 2009;139: 417S–21S.

52. Read JS. Pediatrics 2003;112:1196–205.

53. Georgeson JC, Filteau SM. AIDS Patient Care STDS 2000;14:533–9.

54. Willumsen JF, Newell ML, Filteau SM et al. AIDS 2001; 15:1896–8.

55. American Academy of Pediatrics Committee on Pediatric AIDS. Pediatrics 2008;122:1127–34.

56. Canadian Paediatric Society. Can J Infect Dis Med Microbiol 2006;17:270–2.

57. Phadke MA, Gadgil B, Bharucha KE et al. J Nutr 2003;133: 3153–7.

58. World Health Organization. Guidlines on HIV and Infant Feeding. Geneva: World Health Organization, 2010.

59. WHO Collaborative Study Team on the Role of Breastfeeding on the Prevention of Infant Mortality. Lancet 2000;355: 451–5.

60. Ip S, Chung M, Raman G et al. Evid Rep Technol Assess (Full Rep) 2007;(153):1–186.

61. Kramer MS, Kakuma R. Cochrane Database Syst Rev 2002;(1):CD003517.

62. McNeilly AS. J Mammary Gland Biol Neoplasia 1997;2: 291–8.

63. Kennedy KI, Rivera R, McNeilly AS. Contraception 1989; 39:477–96.

64. Fertil Steril 1999;72:431–40.

65. Kennedy KI, Visness CM. Lancet 1992;339:227–30.

66. Institute of Medicine, National Research Council. Weight Gain During Pregnancy: Reexamining the Guidelines. Washington, DC: National Academies Press, 2009.

67. Baker JL, Gamborg M, Heitmann BL et al. Am J Clin Nutr 2008;88:1543–51.

68. Collaborative Group on Hormonal Factors in Breast Cancer. Lancet 2002;360:187–95.

69. Bernier MO, Plu-Bureau G, Bossard N et al. Hum Reprod Update 2000;6:374–86.

70. Lipworth L, Bailey LR, Trichopoulos D. J Natl Cancer Inst 2000;92:302–12.

71. Newcomb PA, Egan KM, Titus-Ernstoff L et al. Am J Epidemiol 1999;150:174–82.

72. Purdie DM, Siskind V, Bain CJ et al. Am J Epidemiol 2001;153:860–4.

73. Titus-Ernstoff L, Perez K, Cramer DW et al. Br J Cancer 2001;84:714–21.

74. Tung KH, Goodman MT, Wu AH et al. Am J Epidemiol 2003;158:629–38.

75. Modugno F, Ness RB, Wheeler JE. Ann Epidemiol 2001; 11:568–74.

76. Kalkwarf HJ, Specker BL. Endocrine 2002;17:49–53.

77. Kovacs CS. J Clin Endocrinol Metab 2001;86:2344–8.

78. Kalkwarf HJ, Specker BL, Ho M. J Clin Endocrinol Metab 1999;84:464–70.

79. Prentice A, Jarjou LM, Stirling DM et al. J Clin Endocrinol Metab 1998;83:1059–66.

80. Karlsson C, Obrant KJ, Karlsson M. Osteoporos Int 2001;12:828–34.

81. Henderson PH 3rd, Sowers M, Kutzko KE et al. Am J Obstet Gynecol 2000;182:1371–7.

82. Kramer MS, Chalmers B, Hodnett ED et al. JAMA 2001;285:413–20.

SUGGESTED READINGS

Hosea Blewett HJ, Cicalo MC, Holland CD et al. The immunological components of human milk. Adv Food Nutr Res 2008;54:45–80.

Jensen RG. Handbook of Milk Composition. San Diego: Academic Press, 1995.

WHO Collaborative Study Team on the Role of Breastfeeding on the Prevention of Infant Mortality. Effect of breastfeeding on infant and child mortality due to infectious diseases in less developed countries: a pooled analysis. Lancet 2000;355:451–5.

Ip S, Chung M, Raman G et al. A summary of the Agency for Healthcare Research and Quality's evidence report on breastfeeding in developed countries. Breastfeed Med 2009;4(Suppl 1): S17–30.

US Department of Health and Human Services. The Surgeon General's Call to Action to Support Breastfeeding. Washington, DC: US Department of Health and Human Services, 2011.

54 NUTRITIONAL REQUIREMENTS OF INFANTS AND CHILDREN[1]

WILLIAM C. HEIRD

The nutritional requirements of infants and children reflect this population's unique maintenance needs as well as the needs for growth and developmental changes in organ function and body composition. Moreover, because the metabolic rate of infants and children is greater and the turnover of nutrients more rapid than those of the adult, the unique nutrient needs for growth and development are superimposed on higher maintenance requirements than those of the adult. In addition, the potential impact of intake during early life on later development and health must be considered. Finally, provision of these greater needs, particularly to the smaller members of this population, is hindered by their lack of teeth as well as their limited digestive and metabolic processes.

In this chapter, the nutrient needs of normal infants and children, as well as factors of importance in meeting these needs, are discussed, as are the nutritional needs of low birth weight (LBW) infants and ways of providing these needs. The nutrient needs of infants and children with acute or chronic diseases affecting nutrient needs or management are discussed in another chapter, which also includes a general discussion of approaches to providing the nutritional needs of compromised infants and children and a detailed discussion of parenteral nutrition in infants and children.

NUTRIENT NEEDS OF THE NORMAL INFANT AND CHILD

The estimated average requirement (EAR) of a specific nutrient is the amount of that nutrient that results in some predetermined physiologic end point. In infants, the major end point is maintenance of satisfactory rates of growth and development and prevention of specific nutrient deficiencies. The EAR is usually defined experimentally, often over a relatively short period and in a relatively small study population. By definition, the EAR meets the needs of roughly half of the population in which it was established, but not necessarily the needs of the other half. For some, it may be excessive, whereas for others it may be inadequate.

The recommended intake or recommended dietary allowance (RDA) of a nutrient, conversely, is the intake deemed by a scientifically knowledgeable group to meet the "requirement" of most healthy members of a population.

---

[1]**Abbreviations: AI**, adequate intake; **DRI**, dietary reference intake; **EAR**, estimated average requirement; **EER**, estimated energy requirement; **FDA**, Food and Drug Administration; **LBW**, low birth weight; **LC-PUFA**, long-chain polyunsaturated fatty acid; **PUFA**, polyunsaturated fatty acid; **RDA**, recommended dietary allowance; **UL**, tolerable upper intake level.

In general, if the EAR of a specific population is known and is normally distributed, the RDA is set at the EAR plus two standard deviations. RDAs are useful for assessing the nutrient intakes of individuals; that is, the usual intake of a nutrient at or higher than its RDA has a low probability of being inadequate. RDAs are less useful for assessing the adequacy of the nutrient intake of a group.

In recognition of the lack of a valid EAR for many nutrients and the uncertainty of an RDA based on limited information, the latest recommendations of the Food and Nutrition Board of the Institute of Medicine (1–6), are designated dietary reference intakes (DRIs). These include RDAs for those nutrients for which an EAR has been established; therefore, an RDA can be established reliably, as well as other "reference intakes," including adequate intake (AI) and tolerable upper intake level (UL).

The AI of a specific nutrient is the daily intake of that nutrient by a group of healthy individuals. It is based on the group's observed or approximated intake of that nutrient. Thus, a mean intake of a nutrient at or high than the AI has a low probability of being inadequate. The content of specific nutrients in the average volume of milk consumed by healthy, normally growing, breast-fed infants is considered an AI of most nutrients for infants less than 6 months of age. This definition is consistent with national and international recommendations for exclusive breast-feeding for the first 6 months of life (7, 8). For the 7- to 12-month-old infant, the AI of many nutrients is set at the amount of the nutrient in the average volume of human milk plus the average amount of complementary foods consumed by healthy, normally growing 7- to 12-month-old infants. The AIs of other nutrients for the 7- to 12-month-old infant are extrapolated from that of the 0- to 6-month-old infant or that of the older child or adult. An EAR for a few nutrients has been established for the 7- to 12-month old child as well as older infants and children, either directly or by extrapolation from EARs of adults or older children. For these, an RDA can be (and has been) established.

The UL is the highest daily intake of a specific nutrient that is likely to pose no risk. It is not a recommended level of intake but rather an aid for avoiding excessive intakes and adverse effects secondary to such intakes.

The most recent reference intakes of various nutrients proposed by the Food and Nutrition Board of the Institute of Medicine for infants and children less than 8 years of age are summarized in Table 54.1. ULs of those nutrients for which one has been established are summarized in Table 54.2. The DRIs of some nutrients for the 0- to 6-month old infant, the 7- to 12-month-old infant, the 1- to 3-year-old child, and the 4- to 8-year-old child are discussed briefly in the sections that follow.

Energy

Per unit of body weight, the normal infant and young child require at least twice as much energy as the adult (i.e., 80 to 100 kcal/kg/day versus 30 to 40 kcal/kg/day).

This greater need reflects primarily the infant's higher resting metabolic rate and special needs for growth and development.

The estimated energy requirement (EER) of the infant and young child proposed by the Food and Nutrition Board of the Institute of Medicine (5), that is, the energy intake predicted to maintain energy balance (which is not the same as EAR), is based on analysis of total energy expenditure data obtained by the doubly labeled water method (TEE = 88.6 × weight − 99.4) plus an allowance for energy deposition incident to growth as determined from measurements of weight gain and body composition of normally growing infants and young children (9).

Equations for predicting the EER (kcal/day) of infants and children less than 3 years of age are as follows:

- 0 to 3 months (88.6 × weight of infant − 99.4) + 175
- 4 to 6 months (88.6 × weight of infant − 99.4) + 56
- 7 to 12 months (88.6 × weight of infant − 99.4) + 22
- 1 to 3 years (88.6 × weight of child − 99.4) + 22

The EER of the infant younger than 6 months of age determined in this way is very close to the mean energy intake of exclusively breast-fed infants.

The EER of the 3- to 8-year-old child also is based on total expenditure measured by the doubly labeled water method plus an allowance for growth (20 kcal/day) and an adjustment for physical activity level. For this age group, the equation predicting TEE differed between boys and girls and included age, height, and weight. This was adjusted for physical activity level (PC, 1.0 for sedentary to 1.42 [boys] or 1.56 [girls] if very active). For 3- to 8-year-old boys, the equation for EER (kcal/day) is as follows:

$$\text{EER} = 88.5 - 61.9 \times \text{age [years]} + \text{PC} \times (26.7 \times \text{weight [kg]} + 903 \times \text{height [m]}) + 20$$

For girls it is the following:

$$\text{EER} = 135.3 - 30.8 \times \text{age [years]} + \text{PC} \times (10 \times \text{weight [kg]} + 934 \times \text{height [m]}) + 20$$

With respect to the source of energy, no evidence exists that either carbohydrate or fat is superior, provided total energy intake is adequate. Sufficient carbohydrate to avoid ketosis or hypoglycemia is required (~5.0 g/kg/day), as is enough fat to avoid essential fatty acid deficiency (0.5 to 1.0 g/kg/day of linoleic acid plus a smaller amount of α-linolenic acid).

The AIs of carbohydrate and fat proposed by the Food and Nutrition Board of the Institute of Medicine (5) for the 0- to 6-month-old (i.e., 60 g/day [~10 g/kg/day] and 31 g/day [~5 g/kg/day], respectively) are based on the carbohydrate and fat contents of an average intake of human milk. The AIs for the 7- to 12-month-old infant (i.e., 95 g/day [~10.5 g/kg/day] and 30 g/day [~3.3 g/kg/day], respectively) are based on the average consumption of carbohydrate and fat from human milk plus complementary foods. An EAR for carbohydrate for the older child was

TABLE 54.1	DIETARY REFERENCE INTAKES OF NUTRIENTS FOR NORMAL INFANTS[a]

	REFERENCE INTAKE PER DAY			
NUTRIENT	0–6 mo (6 kg)	7–12 mo (9 kg)	1–3 y (13 kg)	4–8 y (22 kg)
Energy (kcal [kJ]/24 h)	550 (2,310)	750 (3,013)	1,074 (4,494)	See text
Fat (g/24 h)	31	30	—	—
Linoleic acid (g/24 h)	4.4	4.6	7	10
α-Linolenic acid (g/24 h)	0.5	0.5	0.7	0.9
Carbohydrate (g/24 h)	60	95	130	130
Protein (g/24 h)	9.3	11[a]	13.7[a]	21[a]
Electrolytes and minerals				
Calcium (mg/24 h)	210	270	500	800
Phosphorus (mg/24 h)	100	275	460[a]	500[a]
Magnesium (mg/24 h)	30	75	80[a]	130[a]
Sodium (mmol/24 h)	5	6	42	53
Chloride (mmol/24 h)	5	16	42	53
Potassium (mmol/24 h)	10	18	77	97
Iron (mg/24 h)	0.27	11[a]	7[a]	10[a]
Zinc (mg/24 h)	2	3[a]	3[a]	5[a]
Copper (μg/24 h)	200	220	340[a]	440[a]
Iodine (μg/24 h)	110	130	90[a]	90[a]
Selenium (μg/24 h)	15	20	20[a]	30[a]
Manganese (mg/24 h)	0.003	0.6	1.2	1.5
Fluoride (mg/24 h)	0.01	0.5	0.7	1.0
Chromium (μg/24 h)	0.2	5.5	11	15
Molybdenum (μg/24 h)	2	3	17[a]	22[a]
Vitamins				
Vitamin A (μg/24 h)	400	500	300[a]	400[a]
Vitamin D (μg/24 h)	5	5	5	5
Vitamin E (mg α-TE/24 h)	4	6	6[a]	7[a]
Vitamin K (μg/24 h)	2.0	2.5	30	55
Vitamin C (mg/24 h)	40	50	15[a]	25[a]
Thiamin (mg/24 h)	0.2	0.3	0.5[a]	0.6[a]
Riboflavin (mg/24 h)	0.3	0.4	0.5[a]	0.6[a]
Niacin (mg NE/24 h)	2	4	6[a]	8[a]
Vitamin B₆ (μg/24 h)	0.1	0.3	0.5[a]	0.6[a]
Folate (μg)	65	80	150[a]	200[a]
Vitamin B₁₂ (μg/24 h)	0.4	0.5	0.9[a]	1.2[a]
Biotin (μg/24 h)	5	6	8	12
Pantothenic acid (mg/24 h)	1.7	1.8	2	3
Choline (mg/24 h)	125	150	200	250
Water (L/24 h)	0.7	0.8	1.3	1.7

α-TE, α-tocopherol equivalent; NE, niacin equivalent.

[a]Recommended dietary allowance; other intakes are adequate intake.

Data from references 1 to 6, with permission.

established by extrapolation from adult requirements. It is 100 g/day for both the 1- to 3-year-old (8.3 g/kg/day) and the 4- to 8-year-old (5 g/kg/day) child. The RDA is 130 g/day (10.8 and 6.5 g/kg/day, respectively, for the younger and older child). AIs for fat beyond 1 year of age have not been determined.

The AIs of n-6 polyunsaturated fatty acids (PUFAs; primarily linoleic acid) and n-3 PUFAs (primarily α-linolenic acid) proposed for the 0- to 6-month-old, based on the average consumption of these fatty acids by exclusively breast-fed infants, are 4.4 g/day (~0.73 g/kg/day) and 0.5 g/day (~83 mg/kg/day), respectively (5). Those for the 7- to 12-month-old child, based on the average consumption of these fatty acids from human milk plus complementary foods, are 4.6 g/day (~0.5 g/kg/day) and 0.5 g/day (~56 mg/kg/day), respectively (5). AIs of these

fatty acids for the 1- to 3-year-old and the 4- to 8-year-old child are based on the median intakes of these fatty acids by children of these age groups reported by the Continuing Survey of Food Intake by Individuals. They are 7 and 10 g/day (0.58 and 0.5 g/kg/day), respectively, for n-6 PUFAs and 0.7 and 0.9 g/day (58 mg/kg/day and 45 mg/kg/day), respectively, for n-3 PUFAs. On average, AIs of these two fatty acid groups account for 5% to 7% and 0.5% to 1.0% of the EER, respectively.

Concern exists that infants may also require a preformed intake of at least some of the longer-chain, more unsaturated derivatives of linoleic and α-linolenic acids (e.g., arachidonic and docosahexaenoic acids). These fatty acids are present in human milk but, until recently, were not present in formulas. Further, the contents of these fatty acids in plasma and erythrocyte lipids are lower in infants fed unsupplemented

| TABLE 54.2 | TOLERABLE UPPER INTAKE LEVELS OF NUTRIENTS FOR INFANTS AND YOUNG CHILDREN |

	INTAKE PER DAY			
NUTRIENT	0–6 mo (6 kg)	7–12 mo (9 kg)	1–3 y (13 kg)	4–8 y (22 kg)
Energy (kcal [kJ]/24 h)	ND	ND	ND	ND
Fat (g)	ND	ND	ND	ND
Carbohydrate	ND	ND	ND	ND
Protein (g/24 h)	ND	ND	ND	ND
Electrolytes and minerals				
Calcium (mg/24 h)	ND	ND	2,500	2,500
Phosphorus (g/24 h)	ND	ND	3	3
Magnesium (mg/24 h)	ND	ND	65	110
Sodium (mg/24 h)	ND	NA	65	83
Chloride (mg/24 h)	ND	ND		
Potassium (mg/24 h)	ND	ND	ND	ND
Iron (mg/24 h)	40	40	40	40
Zinc (mg/24 h)	4	5	7	12
Copper (μg/24 h)	ND	ND	1,000	3,000
Iodine (μg/24 h)	ND	ND	200	300
Selenium (μg/24 h)	45	60	90	150
Manganese (mg/24 h)	ND	ND	2	3
Fluoride (mg/24 h)	0.7	0.9	1.3	2.2
Chromium (μg/24 h)	ND	ND	ND	ND
Molybdenum (μg/24 h)	ND	ND	300	600
Vitamins				
Vitamin A (μg/24 h)	600	600	600	900
Vitamin D (μg/24 h)	25 (1,000 IU)	50 (2,000 IU)	50 (2,000 IU)	
Vitamin E (mg α-TE/24 h)	ND	ND	200	300
Vitamin K (μg/24 h)	ND	ND	ND	ND
Vitamin C (mg/24 h)	ND	ND	400	650
Thiamin (mg/24 h)	ND	ND	ND	ND
Riboflavin (mg/24 h)	ND	ND	ND	ND
Niacin (mg/24 h)	ND	ND	10	15
Vitamin B$_6$ (μg/24 h)	ND	ND	30	40
Folate (μg)	ND	ND	300	400
Vitamin B$_{12}$ (μg/24 h)	ND	ND	ND	ND
Biotin (μg/24 h)	ND	ND	ND	ND
Pantothenic acid (mg/24 h)	ND	ND	ND	ND
Choline (mg/24 h)	ND	ND	1	1
Water (L/24 h)	ND	ND	ND	ND

α-TE, α-tocopherol equivalent; IU, international units; ND, data are insufficient to establish a tolerable upper intake level for normal individuals.

Data from references 1 to 6, with permission.

formulas versus breast-fed infants (10, 11) or those fed formulas supplemented with these fatty acids. The brain content of docosahexaenoic but not arachidonic acid also is lower in infants fed unsupplemented formula than in breast-fed infants (12, 13). However, the results of functional outcome studies of breast-fed versus formula-fed infants and infants fed formulas with and without arachidonic and docosahexaenoic acid are inconclusive (14–16). Overall, these studies provide little evidence that the absence of these fatty acids in term infant formulas is problematic provided intakes of both linoleic and α-linolenic acid are adequate (17). There also is no convincing evidence that the amounts of long-chain PUFAs (LC-PUFAs) in available supplemented formulas pose safety concerns, and a convincing argument can be made for the likelihood that some infants may benefit from the supplemented fatty acids.

In toto, the specific needs for carbohydrate and fat, including LC-PUFA, amount to no more than 30 kcal (125.5 kJ)/kg/day, or only approximately one third of infant and young child's EER. Whether the remainder should consist predominantly of carbohydrate, predominantly of fat, or equicaloric amounts of each is not known. Human milk and most currently available formulas contain roughly equicaloric amounts of each. Because a higher percentage of energy as carbohydrate increases osmolality and a higher percentage as fat may exceed the infant's ability to digest and absorb fat, roughly equicaloric amounts of each seems reasonable.

In concert with the recommendation that the dietary fat intake of the general population be reduced to improve cardiovascular health, it has been suggested that this guideline be applied to infants and young children. However, because fat is a major source of energy as well as the only source of essential fatty acids, concern exists that such diets may limit growth. Thus, groups responsible for making recommendations for infants and young children have not endorsed this recommendation for those less than 2 years of age (18). However, little reason exists not to reduce intake of cholesterol and saturated fat. The Acceptable Macronutrient Distribution Range of fat suggested for the 1- to 3-year-old child by the Panel on Macronutrients of the Food and Nutrition Board of the Institute of Medicine (5) is 30% to 40% of energy. The range suggested for the 4- to 8-year-old child is 25% to 35% of energy (5% to 10% of n-6 and 0.6% to 1.2% as n-3 fatty acids).

Until recently, few actual data concerning growth of infants and young children receiving "low-fat" diets were available, but a study in Finland suggests that the fear of growth failure with such diets may be overrated (19). In this study of more than 1000 infants, half of whom received dietary counseling to limit saturated fat and cholesterol intakes and half of whom did not, growth of the 2 groups did not differ. Although energy and fat intake of the intervention group was somewhat lower than that of the control group, the mean fat intake of both groups was close to 30% of total energy. The intervention group also had lower serum cholesterol concentrations at 3 years of age or on termination of the study.

Protein

The protein needs of the infant and young child, per unit of body weight, also are greater than those of the adult, reflecting primarily the infant's and young child's additional needs for growth. The AI of protein established by the Food and Nutrition Board of the Institute of Medicine (5) for the 0- to 6-month-old infant, 9.3 g/day or approximately 1.5 g/kg/day (assuming a mean weight of 6 kg), is based on the observed mean protein intake of infants fed principally with human milk.

EARs for protein intake were established for the 7- to 12-month old infant as well as the 1- to 3-year-old and 4- to 8-year-old child (5). These values are based on maintenance protein needs plus the additional need for protein deposition as determined by measurements of body composition of normally growing infants and children, assuming an efficiency of deposition of dietary protein intake of 56%. The EAR for the 7- to 12-month-old infant is 0.98 g/kg/day. That for the 1- to 3-year-old child is 0.86 g/kg/day and for the 4- to 8-year-old child is 0.76 g/kg/day. Because the calculated coefficient of variation is approximately 12%, RDAs are 1.24 × EAR: 1.2 g/kg/day for the 7- to 12-month-old infant, 1.05 g/kg/day for the 1- to 3-year-old child, and 0.95 g/kg/day for the 4- to 8-year-old child.

The required intake of protein is a function of its quality, which usually is defined as how closely its indispensable amino acid pattern resembles that of human milk protein. It also follows that the overall quality of a specific protein can be improved by supplementing it with the lacking (or limiting) indispensable amino acid(s). An example is soy protein, which, in its native state, has insufficient methionine, but when fortified with methionine approaches or equals the overall quality of human milk protein (20).

TABLE 54.3	DIETARY REFERENCE INTAKES (mg/kg/d) OF ESSENTIAL AMINO ACIDS FOR INFANTS AND CHILDREN			
AMINO ACID	0–6 mo[a]	7–12 mo[b]	1–3 y[b]	4–8 y[b]
Aromatic amino acids	120	61	46	38
Isoleucine	78	36	28	25
Leucine	139	71	56	47
Lysine	95	66	51	43
Sulfur amino acids	52	32	25	21
Threonine	65	36	27	22
Tryptophan	25	10	7	6
Valine	77	42	32	27

[a]Adequate intake.
[b]Recommended dietary allowance.

AIs of the essential amino acids for the 0- to 6-month-old infant are set at the amounts of each in the amount of human milk protein equal to the AI of protein. For the 7- to 12-month-old, 1- to 3-year-old, and 4- to 8-year-old child, EARs of the essential amino acids are based on the pattern of these amino acids in body protein and the EAR of protein. The AIs of the essential amino acids for the 0- to 6-month-old infant and the EARs of the older infant and young child are shown in Table 54.3.

Minerals

Calcium accounts for 1% to 2% of the weight of the adult, and approximately 99% of this is in teeth and bones. Accretion of calcium during infancy and early childhood ranges from 60 to 100 mg/day in children 2 to 5 years of age to 100 to 160 mg/day for those 6 to 8 years of age. Because percent absorption is quite variable, an AI obviously is important. The AIs of calcium set by the Food and Nutrition Board of the Institute of Medicine for the 0- to 6-month-old and 7- to 12-month-old infant are based, respectively, on the amount of calcium in the average intake of principally breast-fed infants and the average intakes of calcium from human milk plus complementary foods (3) (i.e., 210 and 270 mg/day, respectively). Calcium absorption of formula-fed infants is less than that of breast-fed infants, but the calcium content of formulas is higher; thus, calcium retention of breast-fed and formula-fed infants differs minimally if at all. The AI of calcium for the 4- to 8-year-old child, 800 mg/day, is based on balance studies showing that an intake of 800 to 900 mg/day results in a mean calcium accretion of 174 mg/day. There being no similar balance data for the 1- to 3-year-old, the AI of this age group, 500 mg/day, is based on extrapolation from the AI of the 4- to 8-year-old child. Assuming 20% retention, this intake should result in accretion of approximately 100 mg/day.

The AI of phosphorus is 100 mg/day for the 0- to 6-month-old infant and 275 mg/day for the 7- to 12-month-old infant (3). These values are based on the average intake of the 0- to 6-month-old breast-fed infant and the combined intake of breast milk and complementary foods of the 7- to 12-month-old infant. EARs of phosphorus were established for the 1- to 3-year-old and 4- to 8-year-old child, based on factorial estimates; these are 380 and 405 mg/day, respectively. RDAs (EAR × 1.20) are 460 and 500 mg/day, respectively.

Trace Minerals and Vitamins

DRIs have been established for all trace minerals except arsenic, boron, nickel, silicon, and vanadium, as well as for all vitamins (2, 4). These recommendations are summarized in Table 54.1. DRIs of major importance are iron, zinc, and vitamin D.

Although in theory the normal infant has sufficient stores of iron at birth to meet requirements for 4 to 6 months, iron deficiency during infancy is quite common. This probably reflects the marked variability in both iron stores and iron absorption among infants. Despite the low iron content of human milk, the Food and Nutrition Board of the Institute of Medicine set the AI of iron for the 0- to 6-month-old infant at the intake of iron by the principally breast-fed infant (4) at 0.27 mg/day. Moreover, the iron content of human milk is much more bioavailable than that of formulas. For this reason, only iron-fortified formulas are recommended. The EARs of iron for the 7- to 12-month-old infant, the 1- to 3-year-old child, and the 4- to 8-year-old child are based on a factorial approach accounting for obligatory losses as well as increases in hemoglobin mass, tissue iron, and storage iron. Assuming 10% bioavailability for the 7- to 12-month-old infant and 18% for the 1- to 8-year old child, EARs were set at 6.9, 3.0, and 4.1 mg/day, respectively, for the 7- to 12-month-old infant, the 1- to 3-year-old child, and the 4- to 8-year-old child. RDAs are 11, 7, and 10 mg/day, respectively.

Zinc is a component of as many as 100 enzymes with quite diverse functions (e.g., RNA polymerases, alcohol dehydrogenase, carbonic anhydrase, alkaline phosphatases). It also is important for the structural integrity of proteins and in regulation of gene transcription. Because of the participation of zinc in such a wide range of vital metabolic processes, symptoms of deficiency, even mild deficiency, are quite diverse. A primary feature of zinc deficiency is impaired growth velocity, which can occur with only modest degrees of restriction and circulating zinc concentrations that are indistinguishable from normal. Other features of zinc deficiency include alopecia, diarrhea, delayed sexual maturation, eye and skin lesions, and impaired appetite. Because of these diverse features of deficiency and the lack of reliable clinical or functional indicators of zinc status, adequate zinc intake is of primary importance.

As for other nutrients, the AI of zinc for the 0- to 6-month-old infants is based on the mean zinc intake of exclusively breast-fed infants (4). Because the zinc concentration of human milk falls from approximately 4.0 mg/L at 2 weeks postpartum to approximately 1.0 mg/L at 6 months postpartum, the AI, 2 mg/day, reflects an average intake of human milk of 0.78 L and a zinc concentration of 2.5 mg/L. EARs of zinc for the 7- to 12-month-old infant, the 1- to 3-year-old child, and the 4- to 8-year-old child are based on factorial analysis or extrapolation from the adult EAR, both of which are similar (2.5 mg/day for the 7- to 12-month-old infant and the 1- to 3-year-old child; 4 mg/day for the 4- to 8-year-old child). RDAs reflect a coefficient of variation or 10% (i.e., 1.2 × EAR).

The major function of vitamin D is to maintain serum calcium and phosphorus concentrations within the normal range by enhancing their absorption from the small intestine. Vitamin D is present in very few foods naturally; rather, it is synthesized from sterols in skin by the action of sunlight. Provided sunlight exposure is adequate, neither the breast-fed nor the formula-fed infant requires vitamin D. Some infants and children who live in northern latitudes or whose exposure to sunlight is otherwise limited (e.g., use of sun blocks or avoiding sunlight to prevent cancer; extensive clothing for religious or modesty reasons) may require supplemental vitamin D. The AIs established by the Food and Nutrition Board of the Institute of Medicine, 200 IU/day for the 0- to 6-month-old and 7- to 12-month-old infant as well as the 1- to 3-year-old and 4- to 8-year-old child, are based on the assumption that no vitamin D is obtained by exposure to sunlight (3). These intakes maintain normal serum 25-hydroxy-vitamin D values and are not associated with evidence of vitamin D deficiency. Although available infant formulas provide as much as 400 IU/day, this amount is not thought to be excessive.

Water and Electrolytes

The AI of water for the normal infant is based on the average fluid intake of the predominantly breast-fed 0- to 6-month-old child (~700 mL/day) and the average intake of human milk and complementary foods (including juices and other fluids) by the 7- to-12-month-old child (~800 mL/day). However, because of higher obligate renal, pulmonary, and dermal water losses as well as a higher overall metabolic rate, the infant is more susceptible to development of dehydration, particularly with vomiting or diarrhea. Thus, provision of 150 mL/kg/day is often recommended.

Intakes of electrolytes by the breast-fed and formula-fed infant as well as children between 1 and 8 years of age fed conventional foods, appear to approximate the DRIs of each (see Table 54.1).

FEEDING THE INFANT

The DRIs are for individual nutrients. However, these nutrients are not provided individually but rather as components of the diet. For the infant, who experiences considerable growth as well as developmental advances, providing the foods necessary to meet specific needs for all nutrients sometimes can be challenging. Some of the most important issues in meeting this challenge are discussed in the sections that follow.

Breast-Feeding

One of the first decisions that must be made is whether the infant will be breast-fed or formula fed. In this regard, human milk is uniquely adapted to the human infant's needs and hence is the most appropriate milk. In addition, it contains bacterial and viral antibodies that are thought to provide local gastrointestinal immunity against organisms entering the body by this route. These antibodies probably account, at least partially, for the lower prevalence of diarrhea as well as otitis media, pneumonia, bacteremia, and meningitis during the first year of life in infants who are exclusively breast-fed versus formula fed for the first 4 to 6 months of life (7, 8). Some evidence also indicates that breast-fed infants may have a lower frequency of food allergies and a lower incidence of chronic diseases in later life.

The psychologic advantages of breast-feeding for both mother and infant are well recognized. The mother is personally involved in the nurturing of her baby, thus resulting both in a feeling of being essential and a sense of accomplishment while the infant is provided with a close and comfortable physical relationship with the mother.

The first 2 weeks after birth are crucial for establishing successful breast-feeding. Daily weight gains of the infant, although important for ascertaining the volume of milk produced, should not be overly emphasized during this time. Further, supplemental bottle feedings to achieve weight gain may compromise attempts at breast-feeding and therefore should be limited.

Provided the mother's milk supply is ample, her diet is adequate, and she is not infected with human immunodeficiency virus, no disadvantages of breast-feeding exist for the healthy term infant. Allergens to which the infant is sensitized can be conveyed in the milk, but the presence of such allergens is rarely a valid reason to stop breast-feeding. Rather, an attempt should be made to identify the offending allergen and remove it from the mother's diet.

Maternal contraindications to breast-feeding also are few. Markedly inverted nipples may be troublesome, as may fissuring or cracking of the nipples, but the latter usually can be avoided by preventing engorgement. Mastitis also may be alleviated by continued and frequent nursing on the affected breast to keep it from becoming engorged, but local heat applications and antibiotics may be necessary occasionally. Acute maternal infection may contraindicate breast-feeding if the infant does not have the same infection; otherwise, no need exists to stop nursing unless the condition of either the mother or the infant necessitates it. If the mother's condition does not permit breast-feeding, the breast may be emptied and the milk given to the infant by bottle or cup. Mothers with septicemia, active infections, or breast cancer should not breast-feed. Substance abuse and severe neuroses or psychoses may also be contraindications to breast-feeding.

Formula Feeding

Objective studies of growing infants less than 4 to 6 months of age show minimal, if any, differences in rate of growth, blood constituents, metabolic performance or body composition between breast-fed infants and infants fed modern iron-supplemented formulas. Thereafter, growth of the formula-fed infant usually is somewhat more rapid than that of the breast-fed infant. Such investigations attest to the ability of both breast milk and modern infant formulas to support normal growth and development of the infant. Thus, the mother who is unable or does not wish to nurse her infant need not have a lesser sense of accomplishment or affection for her baby than the nursing mother. Moreover, the quality of attachment and mothering as well as the degree of security and affection provided the infant need not be different with formula feeding versus breast-feeding. Further, the clear economic advantages and microbiologic safety of breast-feeding are of lesser importance for affluent developed societies with ready access to a clean water supply and refrigeration than for less developed and less affluent societies. Thus, a reasonable and conservative approach is to allow the mother to make an informed choice about how she wishes to feed her infant and support her in that decision. As stated by Fomon (21), "In industrialized countries, any woman with the least inclination toward breast-feeding should be encouraged to do so, and all assistance possible should be provided. At the same time, there is little justification for attempts to coerce women to breast-feed. No woman in an industrialized country should be made to feel guilty because she elects not to breast-feed her infant."

The nutrient content of infant formulas marketed in the United States is regulated by the Infant Formula Act and enforced by the Food and Drug Administration (FDA). Most industrialized and many developing countries have similar regulations. All formulas must contain minimum amounts of all nutrients known or thought to be required by infants, and increasing emphasis is placed on avoiding specified maximum amounts of each. The most recent recommendations for the minimum and maximum nutrient contents of term infant formulas marketed in the United States are shown in Table 54.4 (22). The minimum recommended amount of each nutrient is greater than the amount of that nutrient in human milk and hence greater than the DRI of that nutrient for infants less than 1 year old (see Table 54.1).

In addition to assuring the FDA that each marketed formula contains the minimum recommended amount and no more than the maximum amount of each nutrient for the intended shelf-life of the formula, manufacturers

TABLE 54.4	LIFE SCIENCES RESEARCH ORGANIZATION RECOMMENDATIONS FOR TERM INFANT FORMULAS[a]	
	MINIMUM	**MAXIMUM**
Energy (kcal/day):	63	71
Fat (g)	4.4	6.4
Linoleic acid (%)	8	35
α-Linolenic acid (%)	1.75	4
LA/ALA ratio	16:1	6:1
Carbohydrate (g)	9	13
Protein (g)	1.7	3.4
Electrolytes and minerals		
Calcium (mg)	50	140
Phosphorus (mg)	20	70
Magnesium (mg)	4	17
Sodium (mg)	25	50
Chloride (mg)	50	160
Potassium (mg)	60	160
Iron (mg)	0.2	1.65
Zinc (mg)	0.4	1.0
Copper (μg)	60	160
Iodine (μg)	8	35
Selenium (μg)	1.5	5
Manganese (μg)	1.0	100
Fluoride (μg)	0	60
Chromium	0	0
Molybdenum	0	0
Vitamins		
Vitamin A (IU)	200	500
Vitamin D (IU)	40	100
Vitamin E (mg α-TE)	0.5	5.0
Vitamin K (μg)	1	25
Vitamin C (mg)	6	15
Thiamin (μg)	30	200
Riboflavin (μg)	80	300
Niacin (μg)	550	2,000
Vitamin B_6 (μg)	30	130
Folate (μg)	11	40
Vitamin B_{12} (μg)	0.08	0.7
Biotin (μg)	1	15
Pantothenic acid (μg)	300	1,200
Other ingredients		
Carnitine (mg)	1.2	2.0
Taurine (mg)	0	12
Inositol (mg)	4	40
Choline (mg)	7	30
Nucleotides (mg)	0	16

ALA, α-linolenic acid; α-TE, α-tocopherol equivalent; LA, linoleic acid.

[a]Amounts = 100 kcal unless indicated otherwise.

Adapted with permission from Raiten DJ, Talbot JM, Waters JH. Assessment of nutrient requirements for infant formulas. J Nutr 1998:128:2059S–293S.

of infant formulas also must assure that the formula was manufactured safely and hygienically. Thus, each batch of manufactured formula is assayed continually throughout its shelf-life. Manufacturers also are responsible for assuring the FDA that each marketed formula, as the sole source of nutrition, supports normal growth and development of infants for at least the first 4 months of life. This is usually done by conducting growth studies of a new formula during the first 4 months of life in a sufficient number of infants to detect a 3 g/day difference in rate of weight gain. The efficacy and safety of substituting

alternative sources of various nutrients also must be demonstrated by appropriate studies.

Numerous formulas are available for feeding the normal infant. The composition of the most commonly used formulas is shown in Table 54.5. Most are available in ready-to-use, concentrated liquid, and powdered forms. Powdered formulas are somewhat lower in cost and are used with increasing frequency.

The most commonly used formulas contain various mixtures of bovine milk proteins. The protein concentration of all is approximately 1.5 g/dL. Thus, the infant who receives a sufficient volume to provide the EER, approximately 90 kcal/kg/day or approximately 135 mL/kg/day, receives a protein intake of approximately 2.0 g/kg/day. This is approximately 50% more than the intake of the breast-fed infant and hence the AI of protein for the 0- to-6-month-old child; it is approximately 70% more than the RDA of protein for the 7- to-12-month-old child.

Unmodified bovine milk protein has a whey-to-casein ratio of 18:82, whereas modified bovine milk protein can have various ratios; historically, the most common has been 60:40. Both modified and unmodified bovine milk proteins appear to be equally efficacious for the normal term infant, but the lower curd tension of the whey-predominant proteins is thought to be preferable. Formulas containing soy protein, as well as formulas containing partially hydrolyzed bovine milk proteins, are available for feeding infants who are intolerant of bovine milk or soy protein (Table 54.6).

Although lactose-free bovine milk formulas are available, the major carbohydrate of the most commonly used formulas is lactose. The most commonly used soy protein formulas contain either sucrose or a glucose polymer. Thus, these formulas or lactose-free bovine milk protein formulas are useful for the infant with either transient or congenital lactase deficiency.

The fat content of both bovine milk and soy protein formula usually comprises approximately 50% of the nonprotein energy. In general, intestinal absorption of the blend of vegetable oils present in current formulas is at least 90%. Formulas supplemented with the LC-PUFAs, docosahexaenoic acid and arachidonic acid, have become available.

The electrolyte, mineral, and vitamin contents of most formulas are similar and, when formulas are fed in adequate amounts, provide the DRIs for minerals and vitamins. Both iron-supplemented (~12 mg/L) and non-supplemented (~1 mg/L) formulas are available, but iron-supplemented formulas are recommended.

FEEDING THE OLDER INFANT

The goal of both breast-feeding and formula feeding is to deliver enough nutrients to support adequate growth. Exclusive breast-feeding is thought to do so for the first 6 months, and certainly the first 4 months of life, whereas exclusive formula feeding can do so for at least the first

TABLE 54.5	NUTRIENT CONTENT OF SOME COMMON TERM INFANT FORMULAS[a]		
COMPONENT	SIMILAC[b]	ENFAMIL[c]	GOOD START[d]
Energy (kcal/L)	676	680	676
Protein (g)	2.07 (52% casein, 48% whey)	2.1 (40% casein; 60% whey)	2.4 (100% whey)
Fat (g)	5.4 (high-oleic safflower, coconut, and soy oils)	5.3 (palm olein, soy, coconut, and high-oleic sunflower oils)	5.1 (palm olein, soy, coconut, and high-oleic safflower oils)
Carbohydrate (g)	10.8 (lactose)	10.7 (lactose)	11.0 (lactose, corn maltodextrin)
Electrolytes and minerals			
Calcium (mg)	78	78	64
Phosphorus (mg)	42	53	36
Magnesium (mg)	6.1	8	7.1
Iron (mg)	1.8	1.8	1.5
Zinc (mg)	0.75	1	0.8
Manganese (μg)	5	15	7.1
Copper (μg)	90	75	80.5
Iodine (μg)	6.1	10	12
Selenium (μg)	—	—	—
Sodium (mg)	24	27	24
Potassium (mg)	105	107	101
Chloride (mg)	65	63	65.5
Vitamins			
Vitamin A (IU)	300	2,094	302
Vitamin D (IU)	60	60	60
Vitamin E (IU)	1.5	2	2
Vitamin K (μg)	8	8	8.0
Thiamin (μg)	100	80	60
Riboflavin (μg)	150	140	141
Vitamin B$_6$ (μg)	60	60	75
Vitamin B$_{12}$ (μg)	0.25	0.3	0.25
Niacin (μg)	1,050	1,000	750
Folic acid (μg)	15	16	15
Pantothenic acid (μg)	450	500	453
Biotin (μg)	4.4	3	2.2
Vitamin C (mg)	9	12	9
Choline (mg)	16	12	12
Inositol (mg)	4.7	6	18

[a]Amount/100 kcal unless noted otherwise.
[b]Ross Laboratories, Columbus, OH.
[c]Mead-Johnson Nutritionals, Evansville, IN.
[d]Carnation Nutritional Products, Glendale, CA.

year of life. As a rule of thumb, the normal term infant's weight should double by 4 to 5 months of age and triple by 12 months of age.

By 6 months of age, the infant's previously compromised capacity to digest and absorb a variety of dietary components as well as to metabolize, use, and excrete the absorbed products of digestion is near the capacity of the adult (23). Moreover, the infant is more active, has good head control, is beginning to sit alone, and is beginning to explore his or her surroundings. Hence, during this interval, diet plays numerous roles other than delivery of required nutrients. Various concerns also emerge during this period. With the eruption of teeth, the role of diet in development of dental caries must be considered (24). The long-term effects of inadequate or excessive intakes during infancy also must be considered, as does the psychosocial role of foods during development and the impact of feeding practices during this period on subsequent feeding behavior.

These considerations are the basis for most of the recommendations for feeding during the second 6 months of life (Tables 54.7 and 54.8), particularly for the formula-fed infant whose nutrient needs during this period can be met with reasonable amounts of currently available infant formulas. The exclusively breast-fed infant, however, requires additional nutrients (e.g., iron) after 4 to 6 months of age.

Infant Formula versus Bovine Milk

Current recommendations are to avoid intake of bovine milk, particularly low-fat or skimmed milk, before at least 1 year of age. However, surveys have shown that many infants older than 6 months of age, albeit fewer than before 2000, and even some younger infants are fed homogenized bovine milk, rather than infant formula, and many of these infants are fed low-fat or skimmed milk (25).

TABLE 54.6   NUTRIENT CONTENT (AMOUNT/100 kcal) OF SOY FORMULAS AND HYDROLYZED FORMULAS

COMPONENT	ISOMIL[a,b]	PROSOBEE[c]	ALIMENTUM[a]
Energy (kcal/L)	676	680	676
Protein (g)	2.45 (soy protein isolate; L-methionine)	2.5 (soy protein isolate; L-methionine)	2.75 (casein hydrolysate)
Fat (g)	5.3 (soy high-oleic safflower; coconut oils)	5.3 (palm olein; soy; coconut and high-oleic sunflower oils)	5.5 (67% LCT; 33% MCT)
Carbohydrate (g)	10.3 (corn syrup; sucrose)	10.6 (corn syrup solids)	10.2
Electrolytes and minerals			
Calcium (mg)	105	104	105
Phosphorus (mg)	75	82	75
Magnesium (mg)	7.5	11	7.5
Iron (mg)	1.8	1.8	1.8
Zinc (mg)	0.75	1.2	0.75
Manganese (μg)	25	25	8
Copper (μg)	75	75	75
Iodine (μg)	15	15	15
Selenium (μg)	—	—	—
Sodium (mg)	44	35	44
Potassium (mg)	108	120	120
Chloride	62	80	80
Vitamins			
Vitamin A (IU)	300	294	300
Vitamin D (IU)	60	60	45
Vitamin E (IU)	1.5	2	3
Vitamin K (μg)	11	8	15
Thiamin (μg)	60	80	60
Riboflavin (μg)	90	90	90
Vitamin B$_6$ (μg)	60	60	60
Vitamin B$_{12}$ (μg)	0.45	0.3	0.45
Niacin (μg)	1,350	1,000	1,350
Folic acid (μg)	15	16	15
Pantothenic acid (μg)	754	500	754
Biotin (μg)	4.5	3	4.5
Vitamin C (mg)	9	12	9
Choline (mg)	8	8	8
Inositol (mg)	5	6	5

LCT, long-chain triglyceride; MCT, medium-chain triglyceride.

[a]Ross Laboratories, Columbus, OH.
[b]Isomil-SF (sucrose free) has similar composition with exception that glucose polymers are substituted for corn syrup and sucrose.
[c]Mead Johnson Nutritionals, Evansville, IN.

TABLE 54.7   FOOD GUIDELINES

FOOD GROUP	SERVINGS/DAY	SERVING SIZE
Grain	6–11	1 slice bread ½ cup rice (cooked) ½ cup pasta
Fruit	2–4	¼ medium melon 1 whole fruit ¾ cup juice ½ cup canned fruit ½ cup berries, grapes
Vegetables	3–5	½ cup raw or cooked
Milk	2–3	1 cup milk, yogurt 2 oz cheese
Meat	2–3	2–3 oz lean, cooked ½ cup dried beans[a] 1 egg[a]
Fats/sweets	Limit	

[a]These amounts are equal to 1 oz lean meat. Two servings are equal to one meat serving.

TABLE 54.8   SERVINGS OF VARIOUS FOOD GROUPS NEEDED TO PROVIDE DIFFERENT DAILY ENERGY INTAKES

	SERVINGS NEEDED FOR DAILY ENERGY INTAKES		
FOOD GROUP	1,600 kcal	2,200 kcal	2,800 kcal
Bread	6	9	11
Fruits	2	3	4
Vegetables	3	4	5
Meat	5 oz	6 oz	7 oz
Milk	2–3	2–3	2–3
Total fat (g)	53	73	83
Added sugar (tsp)	6	12	18

The consequences of these practices are not known with certainty. However, bovine milk contains roughly three times as much protein and about twice as much sodium as the most commonly used infant formulas but less than half as much linoleic acid. Ingestion of bovine milk also increases intestinal blood loss and hence contributes to development of iron deficiency anemia (26). The protein and sodium intakes of infants fed skimmed rather than whole bovine milk are even higher, the iron intake is equally low, and the intake of linoleic acid is very low.

Whether the high protein and sodium intakes of infants fed either whole or skimmed milk are problematic is not known with certainty. Clearly, the low iron intake is undesirable, but medicinal iron supplementation should prevent development of deficiency. The low intake of linoleic acid may be more problematic. Although signs and symptoms of essential fatty acid deficiency appear to be uncommon in infants fed either whole or skimmed milk, an exhaustive search for such symptoms has not been made. Moreover, biochemical evidence of essential fatty acid deficiency without overt signs and symptoms has been reported in both younger and older infants fed formulas with a low content of linoleic acid (27). In contrast, infants who were breast-fed or fed formulas with high linoleic acid content earlier in life may have sufficient body stores to limit the consequences of a low intake later.

Resolving the issues concerning the use of bovine milk in feeding the infant is important for economic as well as health reasons. Because the cost of bovine milk is considerably less than that of infant formula, replacing formula with homogenized bovine milk before 1 year of age obviously has important economic advantages for most families. In addition, if the various food assistance programs could provide homogenized bovine milk rather than formula to infants, even infants older than 6 months of age, the programs' current funds would permit expansion of benefits to many more needy infants. Clearly, this cannot be recommended without further data concerning the consequences of feeding bovine milk versus formula.

Complementary Feeding

Some investigators distinguish between complementary foods (i.e., foods that do not displace breast milk intake) and replacement foods (i.e., foods that displace breast milk intake). However, any energy-containing food will displace breast milk. Thus, all foods are referred to as complementary foods. These foods should be introduced in a stepwise fashion to both breast-fed and formula-fed infants, beginning about the time the infant is able to sit unassisted, which is usually between 4 and 6 months of age (28). Iron-supplemented cereals are usually the first such foods given. Vegetables and fruits are usually introduced next, followed shortly by meats and, finally, by eggs. Historically, the order in which foods are introduced has received considerable attention. However, this is no longer considered crucial, and many experts now recommend introducing meats, a good source of iron and zinc, as one of the first complementary foods. Only one new food should be introduced at a time, and additional new foods should be spaced by at least 3 days, both to allow detection of any adverse reactions to newly introduced food and to permit the infant to become familiar with the taste and texture of the new food. New foods may be introduced even more slowly if a family history of food or other allergies exists.

Either home-prepared or manufactured complementary foods are acceptable. The latter are convenient. Further, many such products have supplemental nutrients (e.g., iron, zinc, some vitamins). These foods also are available in different consistencies to match the infant's ability to tolerate larger size particles as he or she matures.

Prepared dinners and soups containing meat and one or more vegetables are quite popular. However, the protein content of these products is not as high as that of strained meat. Puddings and desserts also are popular items, but aside from their milk and egg contents, they are poor sources of nutrients other than energy; thus, intakes of these should be limited. Moreover, intake of egg-containing products generally should be delayed, especially if a family history of food or other allergies exists, until after the infant has demonstrated tolerance of eggs (either a mashed hard-boiled egg yolk or a commercial egg yolk preparation).

Historically, juices have been considered a necessary item in the infant's diet. However, aside from their vitamin content, they provide minimal nutrients other than energy, which may interfere with AIs of other nutrients. Considering this, current recommendations are to limit juice intake to 4 oz (120 mL)/day. Sweetened flavored drinks, of course, should be avoided (29).

Although feeding practices vary widely during the second half of the first year of life, most surveys indicate that infants fed according to current practices receive AIs of most nutrients (30).

FEEDING THE TODDLER

By the end of the first year of life, most infants have adapted to a schedule of three meals a day plus about two snacks. Although considerable latitude in the diet of each infant should be permitted, to allow for personal idiosyncrasies and family habits, parents should be given an outline of the basic daily dietary needs. Equally important, parents should be aware of what to expect in terms of eating behavior as the child matures.

Reduced Food Intake

Toward the end of the first year of life, the rate of growth decreases, and the child's intake decreases or fails to increase as rapidly as during the first year of life. Further, it is not unusual for the child to have temporary periods of not being interested in certain foods or, indeed, in any

permitting the roughly 10% to 15% of body weight usually lost over the first several days of life to be recouped more rapidly and also possibly reducing the duration and hence the cost of hospitalization. Proponents of the former view advocate feeding human milk because of its demonstrated and theoretic nonnutritional benefits, such as enhanced maternal–infant bonding, protection against infection and necrotizing enterocolitis, and better neurodevelopmental outcome. These proponents also point out that the lower protein content of human milk is less likely to overwhelm the LBW infant's limited capacity to catabolize excess protein. Proponents of the latter view stress the potential advantages of catch-up growth and point out that protein intakes well in excess of those from human milk do not appear to tax the LBW infant's ability to catabolize protein.

Ongoing findings of a multicenter study that began in the early 1980s in England (47) provide some insight into this long-standing controversy. In this study, infants whose mothers elected to provide milk for feeding their infants were assigned randomly to receive supplements of either banked human milk or formula; and infants whose mothers elected not to provide milk were assigned randomly, at some centers, to receive either a preterm formula or banked human milk and, at others, to receive a preterm or term formula. Infants fed human milk, either as the sole diet or with formula, had a lower incidence of both necrotizing enterocolitis and infections during the neonatal period (48). In addition, although developmental indices at 18 months and later (49, 50) were higher in infants assigned to the preterm versus the term formula (i.e., higher versus lower intakes of protein and other nutrients) during the immediate neonatal period, those infants assigned to banked human milk versus preterm formula did not differ, and those assigned to banked human milk, which provided less protein than term formula, were less adversely affected than those who received term formula (51). Moreover, neurodevelopmental indices of infants fed their own mother's milk during hospitalization showed a neurodevelopmental advantage at 7 to 8 years of age (52) as well as later.

Energy Requirements

The usual assumption is that LBW infants require approximately 120 kcal/kg/day—75 kcal/kg/day for resting expenditure and the remainder for specific dynamic action (10 kcal/kg/day), replacement of inevitable stool losses (10 kcal/kg/day), and growth (25 kcal/kg/day). The usual allotment for resting needs (75 kcal/kg/day) includes the resting energy requirement (50 to 60 kcal/kg/day) and additional allotments for activity and response to cold stress. However, LBW infants are relatively inactive, and, with careful control of environmental temperature, energy expenditure in response to cold stress is minimal. Most studies in relatively inactive infants maintained in a strictly thermoneutral environment suggest that the resting energy requirement (i.e., the basal requirement plus requirements for activity and response to cold stress) is little more than 60 kcal/kg/day

(53–56). Fecal losses of nutrients, especially fat, are inevitable in the fed LBW infant. The extent of these losses is a function of the infant's stage of development and the nature of the fat intake (see the later section on fat requirements), but infants fed either human milk or modern formulas rarely experience stool fat losses exceeding 10% of the fat intake, or 5% of the nonprotein energy intake.

The energy requirement for growth includes two components: the energy cost of synthesizing new tissue, which is included in the measurement of resting expenditure; and the energy value of stored nutrients. Values of 3 to 6 kcal/g weight gain have been quoted for the latter component. Because deposition of calorically dense fat tissue requires more calories than deposition of lean body mass, such a range is not surprising. The calculated energy value of tissue deposited by the normally growing fetus between 30 and 38 weeks of gestation is 2.0 to 2.5 kcal/g (see Table 54.9), whereas the calculated energy value of tissue deposited by the normally growing term infant between birth and 4 months of age is approximately 4.5 kcal/g (57).

Clearly, the energy requirement of LBW infants varies considerably. Aside from growth, the factors of greatest quantitative importance are the activity state and the environmental conditions under which the infant is nursed. Although an energy intake as high as 165 kcal/kg/day has been recommended (see Table 54.10) an energy intake of 120 kcal/kg/day is adequate for most LBW infants.

Protein Requirements

Until approximately 1940, most LBW infants were fed human milk, but this practice was largely abandoned following demonstration that a higher protein intake than provided by human milk resulted in a greater rate of weight gain (58). However, the high-protein formula used in this study also contained more electrolytes and minerals than human milk, and many investigators argued that the greater rate of weight gain was simply the result of water retention secondary to the greater electrolyte or mineral intake rather than to deposition of lean mass secondary to the greater protein intake. This debate was eventually resolved by studies showing a direct relationship between protein intake and deposition of lean body mass, as well as between solute intake and deposition of extracellular fluid (59, 60).

In general, a protein intake of approximately 3 g/kg/day appears to support intrauterine rates of weight gain and nitrogen retention (61, 62). Conversely, higher intakes are well tolerated metabolically and support greater rates of weight gain and nitrogen retention (63, 64). The protein, of course, must provide sufficient amounts of all essential amino acids (65). The minimum and maximum contents of each recommended by the Life Sciences Research Organization (LSRO) Expert Panel on Nutrient Contents of Preterm Infant Formulas (45) are shown in Table 54.12. These are based on the amounts of essential amino acids in human milk protein if fed at the minimum and maximum amounts recommended (see Table 54.11).

TABLE 54.12	MINIMUM AND MAXIMUM CONTENTS OF ESSENTIAL AMINO ACIDS (mg/100 kcal) RECOMMENDED FOR PRETERM INFANT FORMULAS BY LIFE SCIENCES RESEARCH ORGANIZATION PANEL ON NUTRIENT CONTENTS OF PRETERM INFANT FORMULAS

AMINO ACID	MINIMUM	MAXIMUM
Histidine	53	76
Isoleucine	129	186
Leucine	252	362
Lysine	182	263
Sulfur amino acids	85	123
Aromatic amino acids	196	282
Threonine	113	163
Tryptophan	38	55
Valine	132	191
Arginine	72	104

Adapted with permission from Klein CJ. Nutrient requirements for preterm infant formulas. J Nutr 2002;132:1395S–577S.

Current LBW infant formulas contain modified bovine milk protein (60% whey proteins and 40% caseins); however, little evidence indicates that this protein is more efficacious than unmodified bovine milk protein (18% whey proteins and 82% caseins), particularly with respect to growth (66). Of theoretic interest is that plasma threonine concentrations of infants fed modified bovine milk formulas are approximately double those observed in infants fed unmodified bovine milk protein formulas, whereas plasma tyrosine concentrations are higher in infants fed unmodified bovine milk formulas.

Most LBW infants currently are fed either "fortified" human milk or an LBW infant formula, both providing protein intakes of 3.2 to 3.6 g/kg/day. Despite these protein intakes, which support intrauterine rates of protein accretion and growth, 90% of infants who weigh less than 1250 g at birth weigh less than the 10th percentile of intrauterine growth standards at discharge (34, 67), a finding illustrating the inadequacy of these intakes to support sufficient catch-up growth. For this reason, more recent recommendations for protein intake of LBW infants approach 4.5 g/kg/day (46). Unfortunately, formulas and human milk fortifiers providing these higher recommended intakes are not available and have not been thoroughly studied (Table 54.13).

Because most LBW infants remain growth retarded at discharge, "postdischarge" formulas have been introduced. These formulas provide more protein and somewhat more energy than standard term infant formulas,

TABLE 54.13	COMPOSITION (AMOUNT/100 kcal) OF STANDARD FORMULAS FOR LOW BIRTH WEIGHT INFANTS

COMPONENT	SIMILAC SPECIAL CARE[a]	ENFAMIL PREMATURE[b]
Energy (kcal/L)	806	810
Protein (g)	2.73 (bovine milk; whey)	3 (bovine milk; whey)
Fat (g)	5.43 (50% medium-chain triglycerides; 20% soy oil; 20% coconut oil)	5.1 (40% medium-chain triglycerides; 40% soy oil; 20% coconut oil)
Carbohydrate (g)	10.7 (40% lactose; 60% glucose polymers)	11.1 (50% lactose; 50% glucose polymers)
Electrolytes and minerals		
Calcium (mg)	181	165
Phosphorus (mg)	91	83
Magnesium (mg)	12.4	6.8
Iron (mg)	0.4[c]	0.25
Zinc (mg)	1.5	1.5
Manganese (mg)	12.4	6.3
Copper (μg)	252	125
Iodine (μg)	6.2	25
Selenium (μg)	—	—
Sodium (mg)	43	40
Potassium (mg)	131	101
Chloride (mg)	84	85
Vitamins		
Vitamin A (IU)	1,250	1,250
Vitamin D (IU)	150	272
Vitamin E (IU)	4	6.3
Vitamin K (μg)	12	8
Thiamin (μg)	250	200
Riboflavin (μg)	620	300
Vitamin B6 (μg)	250	150
Vitamin B12 (μg)	0.55	0.25
Niacin (μg)	5,000	4,000
Folic acid (μg)	37	35
Pantothenic acid (μg)	1,900	1,200
Vitamin C (mg)	37	20
Biotin (μg)	37	4
Choline (mg)	10	12
Inositol (mg)	6	17

[a]Ross Laboratories, Columbus, OH.
[b]Mead Johnson Nutritionals, Evansville, IN.
[c]Iron content of low-iron formula.

with the intent of supporting continued catch-up growth after discharge. Based on the limited data available, these formulas support some catch-up growth, but this appears to be true for only a short period after discharge (68–71). However, the growth advantage achieved during this period persists through 18 months of age.

Fat Requirements

Fat accounts for approximately half of the nonprotein energy content of human milk and most infant formulas, including those designed for LBW infants. Nonetheless, the only known requirement for fat in human nutrition other than a source of energy is to provide essential fatty acids. Formerly, investigators thought that this requirement could be met by provision of 2% to 4% of the total energy intake as linoleic acid, but it is now clear that some α-linolenic acid also is required. Evidence also indicates that LBW infants may benefit from supplementation with the longer-chain, more unsaturated n-6 and n-3 fatty acids, for example, arachidonic acid and docosahexaenoic acid. These fatty acids rather than their precursors, linoleic and α-linolenic acids, accumulate in the retina and brain during development. However, plasma and erythrocyte lipid levels of these fatty acids are lower in infants who do not receive an exogenous source of these fatty acids, and most available studies suggest that supplementation of LBW infant formula with these fatty acids may have at least transient beneficial effects on visual function or neurodevelopmental indices (72–74). Both fatty acids are present in human milk but in varying amounts. Most modern LBW infant formulas also contain these fatty acids in amounts approximating their average content in human milk.

Carbohydrate Requirements

The central nervous system and the hematopoietic tissue depend primarily on glucose as a metabolic fuel, which, in the term infant and adult, can be produced from either exogenously administered protein or endogenous protein stores (i.e., gluconeogenesis). Thus, in contrast to requirements for specific amino acids and fatty acids, no absolute requirement for carbohydrate appears to exist. However, exogenous glucose is necessary to prevent hypoglycemia, particularly in preterm infants.

Carbohydrates, like fat, comprise approximately half of the nonprotein energy content of both human milk and LBW infant formulas. Although the predominant carbohydrate of human milk is lactose, LBW infant formulas usually contain a mixture of lactose and glucose polymers (see Table 54.13). Even though development of intestinal lactase activity lags behind development of other disaccharidases, most viable infants tolerate lactose quite well.

Fluid and Electrolyte Requirements

Recommended water intakes of LBW infants range from 138 to 200 mL/kg/day (see Table 54.10). These include allotments for insensible water loss, obligatory renal losses, other losses and growth, all of which are quite variable and affected by numerous physiologic factors (e.g., body temperature, ambient temperature, ambient humidity, activity, and respiratory rate).

Insensible water loss varies considerably among LBW infants. Moreover, both pulmonary and cutaneous components of insensible water loss are related inversely to ambient humidity. Under usual nursery conditions, the insensible water loss of term infants is approximately 30 mL/kg/day, but the very small infant's altered skin permeability to water may result in much greater cutaneous losses. Phototherapy also increases insensible water losses (75). Nursing the infant in relatively high humidity, conversely, tends to decrease cutaneous losses as well as pulmonary losses. In general, the insensible water losses of LBW infants usually are at least twofold greater than those of the term infant, and those of the most immature LBW infants may be severalfold greater.

Obligatory renal water losses of LBW infants also are quite variable. Although even very immature infants can regulate the volume of urine excreted according to the solute load and the available water, both renal concentrating and diluting mechanisms are somewhat limited (76). In general, allowance for a urinary volume of 50 to 60 mL/kg permits excretion of the usual range of solute loads at urine concentrations of 150 to 450 mOsm/L, which are easily achieved, even by a very immature kidney.

In unfed infants, fluid losses through the gastrointestinal tract are minimal, but in fed infants, approximately 10% of the fluid intake is lost in stool. Infants receiving phototherapy experience even greater stool losses of water (75).

The fluid requirement for growth is a function of both the rate of growth and the water content of the newly synthesized tissue. The water content of tissue deposited during the last trimester of gestation is approximately 70% (see Table 54.9), whereas the water content of the tissue deposited by the term infant between birth and 4 months of age is only 40% to 45% (57). An estimate of 50% to 60% for the growing LBW infant seems reasonable.

The water requirements for insensible (30 to 60 mL/kg/day) and obligatory losses (50 to 60 mL/kg/day) as well as for growth (10 to 20 mL/kg/day) are reduced by the endogenously produced water of oxidation (i.e., approximately 12 mL/kg/day). Thus, the LBW infant, like the term infant, seems to have a minimum water requirement of approximately 100 mL/kg/day; however, the very immature infant and the infant undergoing phototherapy may require much more. In general, a fluid intake of 140 mL/kg/day is well tolerated by most infants after the first few days of life. Intakes higher than this amount are thought to increase the likelihood of developing patent ductus arteriosus (77).

Recommendations for sodium, chloride, and potassium intakes of LBW infants are 2.0 to 3.0/mEq/kg/day of each. These intakes should replace obligatory losses and support reasonable rates of growth. The quantities of potassium and chloride present in the volumes of both human milk and commonly used formulas usually ingested are sufficient to provide the recommended amounts. However, the sodium content of human milk (~1.2 mEq/100 kcal), even if completely absorbed, may be low.

Mineral Requirements

Early studies of calcium and phosphorus needs of infants, including LBW infants, were directed toward defining the intakes necessary to prevent hypocalcemia. Because this condition develops more commonly in infants fed formulas with a high content of phosphorus relative to calcium (i.e., a low calcium-to-phosphorus ratio), the ratio of calcium to phosphorus intake, rather than the absolute intakes of either, was emphasized. Experience has shown that a ratio of roughly 1.5 to 2.0 is satisfactory.

The amount of calcium retained during the latter part of normal intrauterine growth is approximately 5 mmol (200 mg)/kg/day (see Table 54.9). The calcium content of human milk is sufficient to provide only about 10% of this amount. Thus, if the LBW infant's requirement for calcium is assumed to be the amount necessary to support continuation of the intrauterine rate of accumulation, human milk obviously contains inadequate calcium. The phosphorus content of human milk also is somewhat low. Moreover, LBW infants fed unsupplemented human milk have less dense skeletons radiographically than those fed formulas containing large amounts of calcium and many develop rickets and/or fractures (78, 79). Thus, LBW infants fed human milk, including those fed their own mother's milk, require supplemental calcium and phosphorus for optimal skeletal mineralization. The calcium content of modern preterm infant formulas appear to be adequate.

Iron requirements depend on the existing body stores and the rate of growth. The LBW infant obviously has more limited stores of iron than the term infant, and therefore is more susceptible to the development of iron deficiency, especially during periods of rapid growth. Investigators have estimated that the "average" LBW infant's endogenous stores of iron will be depleted sometime during the second or third month of life rather than during the fourth or fifth month of life, as occurs in the term infant. However, most LBW infants experience further depletion of iron stores secondary to blood loss from biochemical monitoring. Thus, the LBW infant should receive iron supplements or iron-fortified formulas as early as possible. Such supplements, however, may increase the infant's need for vitamin E, especially when formulas high in PUFAs are fed (see later). In addition, the bactericidal properties of the iron-binding proteins of human milk (i.e., lactoferrin and lactoglobulin) are neutralized if saturated with iron (80). Current LBW infant formulas appear to contain adequate amounts of PUFAs, vitamin E, and iron.

Little information is available concerning the LBW infant's requirements for other trace minerals. In general, the recommended intakes of these minerals are based either on the amounts provided by human milk or the amounts that accumulate in utero during the last trimester of pregnancy. The amounts listed in Table 54.10 appear to be adequate.

A zinc intake of 500 μg/100 kcal, assuming 50% absorption from the gastrointestinal tract, should allow accumulation of zinc at the intrauterine rate. The concentration of zinc in human milk is approximately 3 to 5 mg/L; thus, it provides minimally adequate zinc to allow accumulation at the intrauterine rate. Conversely, the zinc content of human milk is absorbed more efficiently than that of bovine milk (81).

The recommended copper intake (see Table 54.10) is approximately the amount present in human milk and may not allow accumulation of copper at the intrauterine rate. Thus, some investigators recommend a higher copper intake. Because hepatic stores of copper are quite large at birth, this probably is not necessary.

Vitamin Requirements

Recommendations concerning either requirements or advisable allowances of vitamins for LBW infants are based largely on recommendations for term infants, and these appear to be reasonable. Infants fed sufficient amounts of either human milk or currently available formulas to produce adequate growth receive sufficient amounts of all vitamins, although human milk may be deficient in vitamin D. Nonetheless, because the consumption of sufficient volumes of formula to satisfy vitamin requirements may not be attained for several weeks, a supplement containing vitamins A, C, and D is often recommended. In addition, the LBW infant may have special needs for vitamin E.

Vitamin E functions as an antioxidant to prevent peroxidation of PUFAs in various cell membranes. Thus, inadequate vitamin E intake results in erythrocyte hemolysis (82). Because the PUFA content of all membranes is related to intake of these fatty acids, infant formulas containing vegetable oils with a high PUFA content impose a greater vitamin E requirement. Such formulas therefore should have a higher vitamin E content. In general, the aim should be to provide at least 1 IU of vitamin E per gram of PUFAs; that is, an E/PUFA ratio of 1. This may need to be reevaluated now that formulas supplemented with LC-PUFAs are available; however, these fatty acids comprise no more than 1% of the total fat content.

LBW infants fed formulas containing PUFAs and given therapeutic doses of iron also have a greater incidence of erythrocyte hemolysis and lower serum vitamin E levels than do infants fed formulas containing less iron and PUFAs (83). Thus, the relationship between the vitamin E and iron contents of the formula and the relationship

stimulate maturation of the gonads and production of the sex steroid hormones, testosterone, responsible for the development of secondary sex characteristics that occur in boys; and estrogen, responsible for the development of secondary sex characteristics in girls. Estrogen and progesterone (synthesized in the corpus luteum and released in response to LH) control the menstrual cycle and development of secondary sex characteristics in girls.

Undernutrition has long been recognized as a key regulator of sexual maturation in both males and females (5). The discovery of leptin, a peptide hormone secreted from adipocytes, has shed light on this relationship (6). Animals and humans with a defect in the gene that secretes leptin are both extremely obese and infertile. This is in part because leptin is necessary for function of the gonadotropin-releasing hormone pulse generator that is responsible for pulsatile secretion of sex hormones (7). Undernourished boys and girls experience delays in sexual maturation that can in part be explained by reductions in leptin as a response to low body fat. In contrast, the relationship between overnutrition (e.g., in obesity) and sexual maturation is less clear. Although several studies suggested that obesity is associated with early sexual maturation in girls (2), this relationship has proved more complicated in boys. Some studies identified that higher levels of body fat are associated with later puberty in boys (8, 9), whereas others showed that the age of pubertal onset had declined by 3 months since the 1990s (10). Because the prevalence of obesity has increased in children over this period, investigators have hypothesized that increasing adiposity may positively influence the onset of puberty in boys by stimulating the hypothalamic-pituitary axis, similar to what has been proposed in girls. The extent to which puberty onset is the result of obesity itself or to the effects of hormones released from adipocytes is unclear.

Sexual Maturity Ratings: Tanner Stages

Although the timing of major pubertal milestones in girls and boys varies substantially, the sequence of events that occur during puberty are consistently observed. To illustrate the importance of this variation for determining nutrient needs, one can compare two girls, both 12 years of age, but girl A has completed her growth spurt whereas girl B is still in the prepubertal stage. Girl A would likely require less energy for growth, but she may require additional micronutrients, such as iron, to account for blood losses during menstruation, compared with girl B. As one quickly realizes, chronologic age is irrelevant because of the substantial variation in onset and timing of pubertal events. During puberty, sexual maturation is more important in assessing nutrient needs, growth, and development than chronologic age.

One of the most common methods by which health professionals and researchers assess development is by evaluating Tanner stages, named for James Tanner, the pediatrician who first described these stages (11). These scales rate pubertal development based on secondary sex characteristics: testicular and penile development and appearance of pubic hair in boys and breast development and appearance of pubic hair in girls. Tanner stage 1 signifies the prepubertal stage, Tanner stages 2 to 5 depict various stages of puberty, and Tanner stage 5 indicates the completion of puberty (Table 55.1).

TABLE 55.1	TANNER STAGING IN ADOLESCENT GIRLS AND BOYS

GIRLS		
STAGE	BREAST DEVELOPMENT	PUBIC HAIR GROWTH
1	Prepubertal; nipple elevation only	Prepubertal; no pubic hair
2	Small, raised breast bud	Sparse growth of hair along labia
3	General enlargement of/raising of breast and areola	Pigmentation, coarsening and curling, with an increase in amount
4	Further enlargement with projection of areola and nipple as secondary mound	Hair resembles adult type, but not spread to medial thighs
5	Mature, adult contour, with areola in same contour as breast and only nipple projecting	Adult type and quantity, spread to medial thighs

BOYS		
STAGE	GENITAL DEVELOPMENT	PUBIC HAIR GROWTH
1	Prepubertal; no change in size or proportion of testes, scrotum, and penis from early childhood	Prepubertal; no pubic hair
2	Enlargement of scrotum and testes; reddening and change in texture in skin of scrotum; little or no penis enlargement	Sparse growth of hair at base of penis
3	Increase first in length, then width of penis; growth of testes and scrotum	Darkening, coarsening and curling, increase in amount
4	Enlargement of penis with growth in breadth and development of glands; further growth of testes and scrotum, darkening of scrotal skin	Hair resembles adult type, but not spread to medial thighs
5	Adult size and shape genitalia	Adult type and quantity, spread to medial thighs

Reprinted with permission from Tanner JM. Growth at Adolescence. 2nd ed. Oxford: Blackwell Scientific, 1962.

The onset and length of the Tanner stages have ethnic variations, particularly in girls. Non-Hispanic black girls enter puberty at an earlier age than non-Hispanic white girls (12). Nearly 50% of non-Hispanic black girls are reported to be in Tanner stage 2 by 8 years of age. However, by menarche, the age of the first menstrual period, the differences between non-Hispanic black and non-Hispanic white girls are less pronounced (12). Early puberty is a risk factor for future development of insulin resistance (IR), cardiovascular disease (CVD), and other chronic diseases (13); determining the reasons for early puberty therefore has clinical relevance. Another consideration in accurate determination of Tanner stage is the increasing prevalence of obesity. When obesity coincides with accumulation of fat in the breasts, self-assessment of Tanner stage can be compromised (14).

Body Composition Changes

Marked changes occur in both height and body composition during adolescence, both of which have major implications for determining energy and nutrient requirements and may subsequently affect body image and food choices. During this time, boys' muscle mass increases and shoulders broaden, whereas girls increase body fat and develop rounder hips and smaller waists. The pattern and rate of development in body composition differ in boys and girls. Girls attain peak height growth velocity at a younger age than boys, at 11.5 years of age versus 13.5 years of age (3), but boys attain a higher maximal height growth velocity and increased height for a longer period of time.

Girls gain fat mass (FM) steadily through age 16. Boys have an initial increase in FM between age 8 and 14 years, then a decline between ages 14 and 16 years, followed by a plateau (15). The distribution of FM also changes: in boys, increased deposition of subcutaneous adipose tissue (SAT) occurs in the trunk area, whereas in girls, SAT is deposited in the gluteal–femoral region. This results in the characteristic body composition patterns of adult men and women in which men have more upper body fat and women have wider hips and more lower body fat. Patterns of change in fat-free mass (FFM) also differ: girls increase in FFM until age 15 years, and boys increase in FFM through age 18 years, with the most rapid increase occurring between 12 and 15 years (15). The composition of FFM also changes during this time, from 80% water in young childhood to approximately 73% water by ages 10 to 15 years (16). The rise in density of FFM is caused by accretion of protein and minerals in the FFM compartment during growth.

For girls, a negative relationship has been observed among age at menarche, body mass index (BMI), and body fatness (15). Girls who are more pubertally advanced tend to be taller and have more FM, bone mineral content, and FFM compared with same-age girls at a lower stage of pubertal development (15). Girls with early growth spurts reach Tanner stage 2 and menarche earlier than girls with average and late growth spurts (17). Further, girls with early menarche are fatter at the end of puberty than girls with late menarche. This is of concern because tracking of FM into adulthood is strong: girls in the highest FM category have a 55% chance of staying within that category 10 years later, whereas girls in the lowest FM category in adolescence have a 77% change of staying within their category (18).

Bone's response to forces and its capacity for growth are greatest during adolescence. Endogenous estrogens and androgens independently exert effects on bone acquisition and upkeep. Estrogen lowers the bone remodeling threshold, and girls experience greater gains in bone mass during puberty than boys (19). Bone acquisition and metabolism are influenced by hormonal, dietary, and lifestyle factors. In addition to the sex hormones, growth hormone, IGF-I, cortisol, thyroid hormones, parathyroid hormone, vitamin D, and leptin may influence bone metabolism during puberty (20). Physical activity during puberty has positive effects on bone accrual and turnover. Increased lean mass improves bone mass strength, and bone metabolism is influenced by dietary intakes of high-quality protein, calcium, magnesium, phosphorus, and vitamins D, K, and C (20).

Changes in body composition that occur during adolescence guide nutrient recommendations: growth increases energy demands and protein requirement, and bone accrual requires protein, minerals, and vitamins. The adolescent period and the changes in body composition that occur can pose emotional and psychologic distress, which can lead to unhealthy eating patterns, affect subsequent health in adulthood, and set the stage for increased metabolic risk.

DAILY RECOMMENDED INTAKES FOR ADOLESCENTS

Dietary Guidelines for Americans

The Dietary Guidelines for Americans (DGA) were updated in 2010 (21). The main concept included in those guidelines was that Americans of all ages should balance calories to maintain and sustain a healthy body weight. For children and adolescents, this is defined as sex-specific BMI for age between the 5th and 85th percentile. For those who are overweight and obese, BMI for age between the 85th and 95th percentile and 95th percentile or greater, respectively, recommendations are to reduce calorie intakes from foods and beverages, increase physical activity, and reduce sedentary behavior. Other specific recommendations include limiting sodium intakes to less than 2300 mg/day or less than 1500 mg/day for non-Hispanic blacks and adolescents with hypertension, T2D, or chronic kidney disease; and limiting intakes of solid and *trans*-fats, added sugars, and foods with refined grains, particularly those that also contain solid fats, added sugars, and sodium.

Dietary Reference Intakes for Adolescents

The DRIs are established and published by the US Department of Agriculture. Committees consisting of US and Canadian experts on specific nutrients review the scientific literature, consider the roles of nutrients in reducing disease risk, evaluate indicators of adequacy, and estimate average requirements for each nutrient. This information is interpreted in light of current intakes by various North American population groups.

The DRIs consist of four types of reference values. The estimated average requirement (EAR) is the amount of a nutrient that would meet the requirements of 50% of healthy individuals of different sex and age groups. This value is used for calorie and macronutrient recommendations. The recommended dietary allowance (RDA) is calculated from the EAR to meet the needs of 97% to 98% of healthy individuals. The adequate intake (AI) is established when an EAR cannot be determined from available data. It is based on experimental data or determined from

estimated intakes of a group of healthy individuals. The underlying assumption is that the amount of the nutrient consumed by these people is adequate to sustain health. The tolerable upper intake level is the highest amount of a nutrient that can be consumed without posing a risk of adverse side effects for almost all individuals.

For setting nutrient intake guidelines, the Institute of Medicine defines adolescence as ages 9 to 18 years. DRIs for adolescents account for variability in requirements related to growth rates. Table 55.2 shows the nutritional goals set forth by the DGA based on DRI and dietary guidelines recommendations.

DIETARY BEHAVIORS OF ADOLESCENTS

Skipping Meals

The transition from childhood to adolescence is a time when eating habits are changing, and the patterns developed during adolescence tend to continue into adulthood (22).

TABLE 55.2 NUTRITIONAL GOALS FOR AGE–GENDER GROUPS BASED ON DIETARY REFERENCE INTAKES AND DIETARY GUIDELINES RECOMMENDATIONS

NUTRIENT (UNITS)	SOURCE OF GOAL	FEMALE 9–13 y	MALE 9–13 y	FEMALE 14–18 y	MALE 14–18 y
Protein (g)	RDA	34	34	46	52
% of calories	AMDR	10–30	10–30	10–30	10–30
Carbohydrates (g)	RDA	130	130	130	130
% of calories	AMDR	45–65	45–65	45–65	45–65
Total fiber (g)	IOM	22	25	25	31
Total fat (% of calories)	AMDR	25–35	25–35	25–35	25–35
Saturated fat (% of calories)	DG	<10	<10	<10	<10
Linoleic acid (g)	AI	10	12	11	16
% of calories	AMDR	5–10	5–10	5–10	5–10
α-Linolenic acid (g)	AI	1.0	1.2	1.1	1.6
% of calories	AMDR	0.6–1.2	0.6–1.2	0.6–1.2	0.6–1.2
Cholesterol (mg)	DG	<300	<300	<300	<300
Calcium (mg)	RDA	1,300	1,300	1,300	1,300
Iron (mg)	RDA	8	8	15	11
Magnesium (mg)	RDA	240	240	360	410
Phosphorus (mg)	RDA	1,250	1,250	1,250	1,250
Potassium (mg)	AI	4,500	4,500	4,700	4,700
Sodium (mg)	UL	<2,200	<2,200	<2,300	<2,300
Zinc (mg)	RDA	8	8	9	11
Copper (μg)	RDA	700	700	890	890
Selenium (μg)	RDA	40	40	55	55
Vitamin A (μg RAE)	RDA	600	600	700	900
Vitamin D (μg)	RDA	15	15	15	15
Vitamin E (mg AT)	RDA	11	11	15	15
Vitamin C (mg)	RDA	45	45	65	75
Thiamin (mg)	RDA	0.9	0.9	1.0	1.2
Riboflavin (mg)	RDA	0.9	0.9	1.0	1.3
Niacin (mg)	RDA	12	12	14	16
Folate (μg)	RDA	300	300	400	400
Vitamin B_6 (mg)	RDA	1.0	1.0	1.2	1.3
Vitamin B_12 (μg)	RDA	1.8	1.8	2.4	2.4
Choline (mg)	AI	375	375	400	550
Vitamin K (μg)	AI	60	60	75	75

AI, adequate intake; AMDR, acceptable macronutrient distribution range; AT, α-tocopherol; DG, dietary guidelines; IOM, Institute of Medicine; RAE, retinoic acid equivalents; RDA, recommended dietary allowance; UL, upper limit.

Adapted with permission from US Departments of Agriculture and of Health and Human Services. Report of the Dietary Guidelines Advisory Committee on the Dietary Guidelines for Americans, 2010. Washington, DC: US Government Printing Office, 2010.

Data from the National Longitudinal Study of Adolescent Health (23) showed that regular breakfast consumption in adolescence significantly predicted young adulthood breakfast patterns. Breakfast is a common meal skipped by many adolescents, and its consumption tends to decrease with age during adolescence (24). In the National Health and Nutrition Examination Survey (NHANES) from 1999 to 2006, 20% of children 9 to 13 years old skipped breakfast compared with 32% of 14 to 18 year olds (25). This finding has implications for the health of adolescents because low meal frequency, breakfast skipping, and high consumption of sugar-sweetened beverages (SSBs) have been identified as factors associated with obesity (26).

Several studies have reported that breakfast consumption is associated with lower BMI or protection against obesity (23–25). In the School Nutrition Dietary Assessment Study, BMI decreased by 0.15 points for every additional breakfast meal consumed per week (27). This effect was strongest among non-Hispanic whites and was not observed among Hispanics. Daily breakfast consumers also gain less weight over time than adolescents who do not eat breakfast regularly (28). In addition, breakfast consumption has an important impact on nutrient intakes, particularly fiber and calcium (24); and adolescents who skip breakfast have lower intakes of most vitamins and minerals, including B vitamins, folate, calcium, phosphorus, magnesium, iron, and zinc than those who eat ready-to-eat cereal for breakfast (25).

Familial factors play a role in establishing healthful dietary patterns in adolescence. Adolescent breakfast consumption is associated with having at least one parent at home in the morning (23), and breakfast skipping is more prevalent in single-parent or low-income families (25).

Beverage Consumption

Another dietary behavior that has important nutritional implications for adolescents is beverage consumption (29). Overall, in the United States, children and adolescents drink more SSBs and less milk than they did in 1977 (30, 31). In 2005 to 2006, adolescents were drinking approximately 175 mL of milk daily compared with 606 mL of SSBs (31). Patterns of beverage intakes also change dramatically between childhood and adolescence. Intakes of both milk and fruit juice decline by approximately 30% over the 10-year period spanning childhood to middle adolescence (32). Furthermore, the proportion of children consuming soda remains stable, but the amount of soda consumed increases (32), whereas daily milk consumption continues to decline by approximately 0.5 servings in adolescents from ages 15 to 20 years (33).

Trends in beverage consumption affect the nutritional adequacy of adolescent diets. Soda consumers at age 5 or 7 years have been shown to have lower percentage of total dietary energy intakes from protein and lower fiber, calcium, magnesium, phosphorus, vitamin K, and vitamin D and higher intakes of added sugars than do nonsoda consumers through midadolescence (32). In Project EAT (Eating Among Teens), more than 72% of 15-year-old girls and 55% of boys had calcium intakes lower than the AI for their age (33). Over the 5-year follow-up, intakes decreased such that 68% of women and 53% of men consumed less than the AI, even though the AI is 300 mg lower for calcium at age 20 years compared with age 15 years. Low intake of dietary calcium can result from low milk consumption, and this may increase risk for both low mineral content and density (34). Further, greater intakes of SSBs are also associated with higher body fat, waist circumference, and weight status among girls throughout the 5- to 15-year age period (35).

As with breakfast consumption, family environment is also related to beverage consumption patterns. In non-Hispanic white girls, high SSB intake was related to lower parental income and education level and higher parental BMI (35). Availability of milk at meals is positively associated with daily calcium intakes (33).

Diet Nutrient Density

Our current food environment has been described as "obesogenic" because of the ready availability of large portions; the high quantity and variety of energy-dense snacks, sweets, and fast foods; and the low accessibility of whole grains and fresh fruits and vegetables. Adolescent dietary patterns are affected by this food environment. Adolescents are eating excess amounts of energy-dense, nutrient-deplete foods, and their diets are lacking in whole grains, fruits, and vegetables. Data from NHANES revealed that the top sources of energy were grain desserts, pizza, and soda in 2 to 18 year-olds (36). Consumption of "empty calories," or energy sources that provide no major vitamins or minerals, was far in excess of the recommended allowances. Intervening during this time is important because the dietary patterns of adolescence often track into adulthood (37).

The National Heart, Lung, and Blood Institute Growth and Health Study followed a cohort of 2371 non-Hispanic black and white 9- to 10-year-old girls for 10 years. Dietary patterns that were most common during this time showed high intakes of processed grains, lunch meats, pizza, fried potatoes, sweet breads, and fruit and a low intake of vegetables. Only 12% of girls met the requirements of a "healthy" diet: rich in fruits, green salads and other vegetables, unprocessed whole grains, baked or steamed meat and poultry, and low-fat, unflavored dairy (38). High intake of fast food is a common dietary pattern, particularly problematic in late adolescence, because this is when individuals have more autonomy and money to purchase food (39). These dietary patterns are of concern from a nutritional perspective because they contain excess fat, sodium, and added sugars and lack dietary fiber, folic acid, calcium, and potassium.

Snacking has increased in adolescents since the 1970s. In 1977 to 1978, 61% of adolescents reported snacking on any given day, whereas in 2005 to 2006, 83% did. In addition, snacking frequency has also increased; the percentage of adolescents who report consuming three or more snacks daily has more than doubled. Snack foods provide 23% of total daily calorie requirements, approximately 526 kcal, for adolescents. In general, snack foods for this age group are high in sugars, solid fats, or both, and contain fewer vitamins and minerals than foods consumed at meal times. Although snacking has been associated with increased total energy intake, the relationship with BMI has been inconsistent. On a positive note, because fruits such as apples, oranges, bananas, and orange juice are common snacks, snacking fulfills more than 25% of vitamin E and C requirements and 23% of magnesium requirements. In addition, 20% of daily calcium requirements are reportedly achieved through snacking. Clearly, cutting out snacks entirely is not advisable, but improving the quality of these snacks by reducing "empty calorie" sources and increasing dairy, high-quality protein, fiber and whole grains, and nutrient-rich fruits and vegetables is warranted (http://www.ars.usda.gov/ba/bhnrc/fsrg).

Adolescents who tend to follow healthier eating patterns share certain characteristics. First, eating dinners together as a family may protect against the development of obesity (40), and it has been associated with increased consumption of fruits and vegetables and reduced intakes of SSBs and fried foods (41). Having healthy foods available in the home and modeling healthy eating behaviors have been associated with improvements in adolescent eating behavior (42). Reducing the amount of unhealthy foods that are available and easily accessible at home can also improve adolescents' diets (43). Even though adolescents may strive for independence at this time, they still need continued parental involvement and support to assist with the development of healthful, lifelong eating behaviors.

When adolescents fill up on energy-dense foods that lack nutrients, the possibility that their diets will lack the vitamins and minerals needed for growth is high. Diets of adolescent girls are often lacking in folate, vitamin A, vitamin E, vitamin B_6, calcium, iron, zinc, magnesium, and fiber. Adolescent boys generally achieve higher nutrient adequacy, but folate, vitamin E, calcium, magnesium, and fiber intakes are low (44). Iron is a mineral of concern for adolescent girls. Although the rapid growth and increased blood volume that occur during this time increase the body's demands for iron, girls are particularly susceptible to iron deficiency anemia because of blood losses that occur during menstruation. Girls also tend to consume fewer red meats than do boys, and meats contain the most bioavailable source, heme iron, as opposed to nonheme iron found in green leafy vegetables. Reduced meat consumption can also limit dietary sources of zinc, a mineral that is critical for growth and sexual development. Finally, reduced folate intake can be a special concern for adolescent girls who are pregnant because this vitamin is essential for proper fetal development and closure of the neural tube (44).

SPECIAL CONSIDERATIONS

Eating Disorders

Eating disorders are the third most common chronic disease in adolescence, with only obesity and asthma occurring at higher rates (45). Eating disorders share two common features: disturbed eating (e.g., undereating, overeating, eating the wrong things) and distorted body image (e.g., feeling fat, extreme fear of weight gain). The best-known eating disorders are anorexia nervosa and bulimia nervosa. According to the *Diagnostic and Statistical Manual of Mental Disorders,* fourth edition, *anorexia nervosa* is defined as a refusal to maintain a healthy BMI (BMI ≥ 18.5), an intense fear of gaining weight, a disturbance in one's body image, and a failure to menstruate for three or more cycles (46). In *bulimia nervosa,* eating patterns are disrupted such that individuals show repeated patterns of bingeing, followed by compensatory behaviors to avoid weight gain, such as excessive exercise or purging. The prevalence of these disorders is 0.5% and 1.5% for anorexia and bulimia, respectively. However, up to 14% of adolescents have disordered eating patterns without meeting all the diagnostic criteria, and some individuals present with symptoms of both anorexia and bulimia (47). Eating disorders were once thought to affect primarily only non-Hispanic white girls of higher socioeconomic status, but more recent evidence suggests that the prevalence is increasing among boys (48) and minority populations (49).

Adolescents are vulnerable to developing eating disorders for several reasons. First, the physical changes that occur during puberty may often be accompanied by feelings of dissatisfaction with one's body, and, as a result, adolescents may attempt to diet. Dieting is an independent risk factor for developing eating disorders, and consequently, childhood overweight is a risk factor for developing eating disorders later in life (50). Media use in adolescents is another factor that may predispose adolescents to eating disorders. Adolescents spend more than 7 hours/day watching television, reading magazines, and searching the Internet (51), and girls who read fashion magazines are more likely to develop distorted images about their own bodies (52). Proanorexia and probulimia websites on the Internet that contain strategies for hiding eating disorders from parents, pictures of famous celebrities with exceedingly thin figures, and unhealthy tips for teenagers to manage body weight have increased (53). Exposure to these websites has been associated with low self-esteem, poor body image, and increased concern about body weight compared with individuals who viewed control websites (54). A third reason why eating disorders often appear during adolescence has been attributed to an epigenetic effect, or an interaction between genes and the environment that influences the onset of disordered eating traits. Twin studies have demonstrated moderate levels of heritability of eating disorders (55). However, genetic effects on the development of eating disorders vary by age: eating disorders that develop before adolescence have low heritability, whereas those that develop in early adolescence through adulthood are more likely to be heritable (56). These findings are intriguing, but the exact mechanisms by which the events of puberty trigger the onset of eating disorders have not been determined.

Although eating disorders are primarily considered psychologic disorders, nutrition plays an integral role in determining their medical complications and treatment outcomes. The medical complications of eating disorders can be widespread and affect all body systems (57), but most symptoms resolve after medically supervised refeeding (58). However, depending on the severity and timing of the energy restriction, adolescents suffer from some complications that are thought to be irreversible, such as a loss of bone mineral density (BMD) and growth retardation (59). In addition, puberty can often be delayed in individuals with eating disorders, particularly in those who lose significant amounts of body fat (60).

Teenage Athletes

Adolescent participation in organized sports in the United States has increased (61). Young athletes have added nutritional requirements based on the increased energy expenditure incurred in sports participation. In general, fluid intake should be 0.5 to 1 L/day greater than baseline requirements to compensate for added fluid lost in sweat (62), and energy intakes should be increased above and beyond the needs for normal growth and basal metabolic requirements (61). If energy intakes are adequate to support growth and development while compensating

for the added expenditure from sports participation, then adolescents should meet all their nutrient needs. In other words, although absolute protein and carbohydrate needs are higher in teenage athletes than in their nonathletic counterparts, the recommendations are the same in terms of percentage of energy intake: 12% to 15% of energy for protein and at least 50% for carbohydrates (61). Athletes do not need additional vitamins and minerals and, because of their greater food intake, generally achieve or approach daily recommended intakes for vitamins and minerals more readily than do nonathletic teenagers (61).

Nutritional issues can arise if the teenage athlete adopts a vegetarian diet or does not consume adequate calories or hydration. Voluntary dehydration is used in some sports to meet a weight category requirement and can cause an athlete to enter a competition in a dehydrated state. This situation can lead to hyponatremia and impaired performance. Chronic inadequate calorie intake has implications for amenorrhea, low BMD, and impaired growth and performance. This is part of a phenomenon known as the *female athlete triad*. Vegetarian diets can also pose nutritional issues if they are not well planned or are overly restrictive (63). Iron absorption from plant foods is lower than that from animal foods and can lead to low iron status. Vitamin B_{12} is found only in animal products, and deficiency of this nutrient can cause macrocytic anemia. Finally, because of the high bulk, or low energy density, of vegetarian diets, it may be difficult for teenage athletes to meet their energy requirements (63).

In 2007, the American College of Sports Medicine published a position paper that defined the female athlete triad as an interrelationship of low energy availability, amenorrhea, and osteoporosis (Fig. 55.1) that may occur in the absence of disordered eating and that allows inadequate

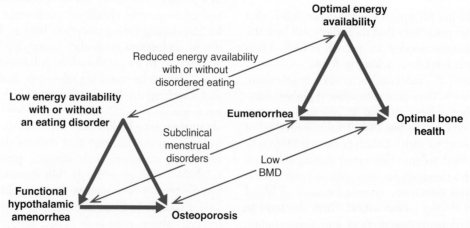

Fig. 55.1. Female athlete triad. The spectrums of energy availability, menstrual function, and bone mineral density (BMD) along which female athletes are distributed *(narrow arrows)*. An athlete's condition moves along each spectrum at a different rate, in one direction or the other, according to her diet and exercise habits. Energy availability, defined as dietary energy intake minus exercise energy expenditure, affects BMD both directly by metabolic hormones and indirectly by effects on menstrual function and thereby estrogen *(thick arrows)*. (Reprinted with permission from Nattiv A, Loucks AB, Manore MM et al. American College of Sports Medicine position stand: the female athlete triad. Med Sci Sports Exerc 2007;39:1867–82.)

available energy for use in cellular maintenance, thermo-regulation, growth, and reproduction (64). *Amenorrhea* is the absence of menstrual cycles for more than 3 months, and osteoporosis is reflected by a BMD Z-score lower than −1. In female athletes, chronic low energy intakes result in low FM, which leads to low circulating leptin levels. Low leptin is proposed to reduce LH pulse frequency and increase its pulse amplitude, thus resulting in disturbance or loss of menstruation (65). Low energy intakes can also reduce bone formation (65). Athletes at greatest risk are those who restrict their intake, exercise for long periods, or adopt restrictive vegetarian diets (64). Dieting, psychologic predisposition, low self-esteem, family dysfunction, abuse, and biologic and genetic factors have been identified as contributors to the female athlete triad (64).

Although exercise in adolescence is healthy and can lead to the establishment of lifelong physical activity habits, some associated behaviors and dietary habits must be monitored. Adequate energy intakes for growth and the added demands of exercise are essential to the athlete for both optimal performance and growth and maturation.

Pregnancy

Pregnancy during adolescence continues to be a major public health challenge in the United States. In 2008, 41.5 of 1000 total live births were attributed to girls between the ages of 15 and 19 years (http://www.cdc.gov). Pregnancy places additional nutritional demands on adolescents, who already have increased energy requirements to meet the demands of their own rapid growth. An additional complication is the lack of cognitive maturity to appreciate the sacrifices involved with caring for a growing fetus and, subsequently, infant. Teen pregnancy is more common in minority populations who have lower socio-economic means, and as a result, the social and medical support for a pregnant teen may be limited. It is therefore not surprising that infants born to adolescent mothers younger than 15 years are twice as likely to be low birth weight and are three times as likely to suffer infant mortality compared with infants born to adult mothers. Younger mothers are also at higher risk of pregnancy complications, such as pregnancy-induced hypertension, abnormally high weight gains, anemia, and renal disease (66).

Reviews of dietary surveys suggest that pregnant adolescents consume inadequate amounts of a variety of nutrients, including total energy, iron, folate, calcium, vitamin E, and magnesium (67). These nutrients all play critical roles in fetal growth. Pregnant non-Hispanic black girls from lower socioeconomic status households are at even greater risk than other ethnic groups of consuming poor quality diets (68), incurring excessive weight gain (69), and neglecting intake of prenatal vitamins (70). In addition, the dietary patterns that are common in adolescence, such as skipping meals and high SSB intake, are particularly detrimental during pregnancy. Support for pregnant adolescents must be multidisciplinary to address the social, behavioral, medical, and nutritional issues faced during this time. In addition, nutrition education to help adolescents achieve appropriate weight gain for their BMI is crucial for ensuring the healthy birth weight of the infant, as well as the optimal growth and development of the adolescent mother (71). Low-income mothers can gain nutritional support and receive supplemental sources of protein, vitamins, and minerals by joining the Special Supplemental Nutrition Program for Women, Infants, and Children.

Obesity and Metabolic Disorders

The prevalence of obesity has been on the rise in the United States and worldwide over the past several decades in both children and adults. Data from the 1999 to 2004 NHANES survey show that approximately one third of 8 to 19 year olds are overweight, and approximately 17% are obese (72). Of concern is the sharp rise in the prevalence of severe obesity, BMI 99th percentile or greater for sex and age, among children and adolescents. A 300% increase in the prevalence of severe obesity occurred in 2 to 19 year olds between NHANES 1976 to 1980 and 1999 to 2004 (73). This increase was mostly seen in non-Hispanic blacks and Mexican Americans and was related to poverty.

The high rates of overweight and obesity among adolescents are of concern for several reasons. First, body composition in adolescence tracks into adulthood, thereby increasing the odds of remaining overweight or obese as adults. Second, adult obesity is associated with a range of metabolic disorders including T2D, CVD, hypertension, cancers, sleep disorders, osteoarthritis, and breathing problems. Third, obesity in adolescence also increases the risk of developing metabolic syndrome and T2D in adolescence. *Metabolic syndrome* is a constellation of risk factors for CVD and T2D that include large waist circumference or obesity, dyslipidemia (low high-density lipoprotein cholesterol [HDL-C] and/or high triglycerides), elevated fasting glucose levels or IR, elevated blood pressure, and, in some cases, inflammation, microalbuminemia, and thrombosis (74).

High body fatness in adolescence is a clear risk factor for T2D and CVD. In adolescents, progression of IR to T2D actually occurs more quickly than in adults, for whom the period of IR can persist for decades before T2D develops (75). In addition, adverse CVD risk profiles are observed in adolescents. Data from the Bogalusa Heart Study showed that, among 5 to 17 year olds, the prevalence of having two metabolic syndrome risk factors, whether high sum of skinfolds (adiposity), triglycerides, low-density lipoprotein cholesterol, fasting insulin, and blood pressure or low HDL-C, was 59% in those with severe obesity, whereas it was 5% in those with a BMI lower than the 25th percentile (76). The prevalence of having three or more metabolic risk factors was present in 7% of obese and 33% of severely obese adolescents (73).

Puberty itself has been shown to lead to a state of IR. Insulin-stimulated glucose uptake is reported to be approximately 30% lower in adolescents in Tanner stages 2 to 4 compared with those in Tanner stage 1, and insulin sensitivity is reduced by 25% to 30% (75). The timing of lowest insulin sensitivity seems to be in Tanner stage 3, and insulin sensitivity recovers in Tanner stage 5. Moreover, the rise in fasting plasma glucose, fasting plasma insulin, and the acute insulin response to glucose during this period is similar across sex and ethnic groups, and the relative changes are equivalent between lean and obese adolescents (75). However, controversy exists concerning the role of change in body fat on the transient IR observed during puberty. Some investigators reported that it was not associated with changes in body fat, visceral fat, sex steroid hormones, or IGF-I (75), whereas others suggested that it likely is caused by changes in total and distribution of body fat and hormone release (77). Nonetheless, it is agreed that transient IR, during puberty, is a natural occurrence (75) that may possibly help promote growth (77).

Sleep is another factor that may affect obesity and metabolic disorders during adolescence. A wide array of literature shows an inverse association between sleep duration and prevalence of obesity in both children and adults (78, 79). Sleep needs vary with age, and, during adolescence, recommended sleep duration ranges between 8.5 and 9.25 hours/night. The Sleep in America Poll 2010 revealed that adolescents aged 13 to 18 years sleep, on average, 7 hours 26 minutes on weekdays, and 61% get inadequate sleep on weekdays. These statistics cause concern because a study of 16- to 19-year-olds reported that short sleep, less than 8 hours/night, was associated with high caloric intakes from snacks (80).

SUMMARY

Adolescence is a critical period of development because of the rapid changes in physical, cognitive, and psychologic growth that occur. During this time, eating behaviors change as children grow and begin taking more autonomy over their feeding. Offering adolescents appropriate levels of support can improve their chances of maintaining healthful dietary behaviors into adulthood. This is particularly critical for adolescents who have additional needs, including athletes, pregnant teens, and those who have disordered eating behaviors. Finally, the prevalence of obesity and metabolic diseases has been increasing throughout the population, including adolescents. Comprehensive nutrition support for this age group needs to include a strong focus on weight gain prevention.

ACKNOWLEDGMENTS

We are recipients of research support from the National Institutes of Health and the Obesity Society.

REFERENCES

1. Yamaki K, Rimmer JH, Lowry BD et al. Res Dev Disabil 2011; 32:280–8.
2. Rosenfield RL, Lipton RB, Drum ML. Pediatrics 2009; 123:84–8.
3. Veldhuis JD, Roemmick JN, Richmond EJ et al. Endocr Rev 2005;26:114–46.
4. Giustina A, Veldhuis D. Endocr Rev 1998;19:717–97.
5. Vermeulen A. Environ Health Perspect 1993;101:91–100.
6. Rosebaum M, Leibel RL. N Engl J Med 1999;341:913–5.
7. Apter D, Butzow TL, Laughlin GA et al. J Clin Endocrinol Metab 1994;79:119–25.
8. Wang Y. Pediatrics 2002;110:903–10.
9. Lee JM, Kaciroti N, Appugliese D et al. Arch Pediatr Adolesc Med 2010;164:139–44.
10. Sorenson K, Aksglaede L, Petersen JH et al. J Clin Endocrinol Metab 2010;95:263–70.
11. Tanner JM. Growth at Adolescence. 2nd ed. Oxford: Blackwell Scientific, 1962.
12. Hermann-Giddens ME, Slora EJ et al. Pediatrics 1997;99: 505–11.
13. Solorzano CMB, McCartney CR. Reproduction 2010;140: 399–410.
14. Bonat S, Pathomvanich A, Keil MF et al. Pediatrics 2002; 110:743–7.
15. Siervogel RM, Demerath EW, Schubert C et al. Horm Res 2003;60:36–45.
16. Wang Z, Deurenberg P, Wang W et al. Am J Physiol 1999;276: E995–E1003.
17. Buyken A, Bolzenius K, Karaolis-Danckert N et al. Am J Hum Biol 2011;23:216–24.
18. Vink EE, van Coeverden SCCM, van Mil EG et al. Obesity 2010;18:1247–51.
19. Schiessl H, Frost HM, Jee WS. Bone 1998;22:1–6.
20. Perez-Lopez FR, Chedraui P, Cuadros-Lopez JL. Curr Med Chem 2010;17:453–66.
21. US Departments of Agriculture and of Health and Human Services. Report of the Dietary Guidelines Advisory Committee on the Dietary Guidelines for Americans, 2010. Washington, DC: US Government Printing Office, 2010.
22. Story M, Neumark-Sztainer D, French S. J Am Diet Assoc 2002;102:S40–51.
23. Merten MJ, Williams AL, Shriver LH. J Am Diet Assoc 2009;109:1384–91.
24. Affenito SG, Thompson DR, Barton BA et al. J Am Diet Assoc 2005;105:938–45.
25. Deshmukh-Taskar PR, Nicklas TA, O'Neil CE et al. J Am Diet Assoc 2010;110:869–78.
26. Moreno LA, Rodriguez G, Fleta J et al. Crit Rev Food Sci Nutr 2010;50:106–12.
27. Gleason PM, Dodd AH. J Am Diet Assoc 2009;109:S118–28.
28. Timlin MT, Pereira MA, Story M et al. Pediatrics 2008;121: e638–45.
29. St-Onge MP, Keller KL, Heymsfield SB. Am J Clin Nutr 2003; 78:1068–73.
30. Nielsen SJ, Popkin BM. Am J Prev Med 2004;27:205–10.
31. Popkin BM. Physiol Behav 2010;100:4–9.
32. Fiorito LM, Marini M, Mitchell MC et al. J Am Diet Assoc 2010;110:543–50.
33. Larson NI, Neumark-Sztainer D, Harnack L et al. J Nutr Educ Behav 2009;41:254–60.
34. Black RE, Williams SM, Jones IE et al. Am J Clin Nutr 2002; 76:675–80.

35. Fiorito LM, Marini M, Francis LA et al. Am J Clin 2009; 90:935–42.
36. Reedy J, Krebs-Smith SM. J Am Diet Assoc 2010;110:1477–84.
37. Mikkila V, Rasanen L, Raitakari OT et al. Br J Nutr 2005; 93:923–31.
38. Ritchie LD, Spector P, Stevens MJ et al. J Nutr 2007;137: 399–406.
39. Cutler GJ, Flood A, Hannan P et al. J Nutr 2009;139:323–8.
40. Taveras EM, Rifas-Shiman SI, Berkey CS et al. Obes Res 2005;13:900–6.
41. Gillman MW, Rifas-Shiman SI, Frazier AL et al. Arch Fam Med 2000;9:235–40.
42. Cutler GJ, Flood A, Hannan P et al. J Am Diet Assoc 2011; 111:230–40.
43. Vereecken C, Haerens L, De Bourdeaudhuij I et al. Public Health Nutr 2010;13:1729–35.
44. Story M, Stang J, eds. Guidelines for Adolescent Nutrition Services. Minneapolis: University of Minnesota, 2005. Available at: http://www.epi.umn.edu/let/pubs/adol_book.shtm. Accessed June 2, 2011.
45. Reijonen JH, Prat HD, Patel DR et al. J Adolesc Res 2003; 8:209–22.
46. American Psychiatric Association. Diagnostic and Statistical Manual of Mental Disorders. 4th ed. Washington, DC: American Psychiatric Association, 1994.
47. Kohn MR, Golden N. Pediatr Drugs 2001;3:91–99.
48. Dominé F, Berchtold A, Akré C et al. J Adolesc Health 2009;44:111–7.
49. Bryn Austin S, Spadano-Gasbarro J, Greaney ML et al. J Adolesc Health 2011;48:109–12.
50. Kotler LA, Cohen P, Davies M et al. J Am Acad Child Adolesc Psychiatry 2001;40:1434–40.
51. Strasburger VC, Jordan AB, Donnerstein E. Pediatrics 2010;125:756–67.
52. Hogan MJ, Strasburger VC. Adolesc Med State Art Rev 2008;19:421–546.
53. Borzekowski DLG, Schenk S, Wilson J et al. Am J Public Health 2010;100:1526–34.
54. Bardone-Cone AM, Cass KM. Int J Eat Disord 2007;40: 537–48.
55. Bulik CM, Sullivan PF, Wade TD et al. Int J Eat Disord 2000;27:1–20.
56. Klump KL, Burt SA, Spanos A et al. Int J Eat Disord 2010: 43:679–88.
57. Rosen DS. Pediatrics 2010;126:1240–53.
58. Brambilla F, Monteleone P. In: Maj M, Halmi K, Lopez-Ibor JJ et al, eds. Eating Disorders. Chichester, UK: Wiley, 2003:139–92.
59. Katzman DK. Int J Eat Disord 2005;37:S52–9.
60. Misra M, Aggarwal A, Miller KK et al. Pediatrics 2004:114: 1574–83.
61. Petrie H, Stover EA, Horswill CA. Nutrition 2004;20: 620–31.
62. Bonci L. Pediatr Ann 2010;39:300–6.
63. Barr SI, Rideout CA. Nutrition 2004;20:696–703.
64. Nattiv A, Loucks AB, Manore MM et al. Med Sci Sports Exerc 2007;39:1867–82.
65. Warren MP, Chua AT. Ann N Y Acad Sci 2008;1135: 244–52.
66. Lenders CM, McElrath TF, Scholl TO. Curr Opin Pediatr 2000;12:291–6.
67. Moran VH. Br J Nutr 2007;97:411–25.
68. Grunbaum J, Kann L, Kinchen SA et al. MMWR Morb Mortal Wkly Rep 2002;51:1–58.
69. Chang SC, O'Brien KO, Nathanson MS et al. J Pediatr 2003; 103:1653–7.
70. Stang J, Story MT, Harnack L et al. J Am Diet Assoc 2000; 100:905–10.
71. Nielsen JN, Gittelsohn J, Anliker J et al. J Am Diet Assoc 2006;106:1825–40.
72. Flegal KM, Ogden CL, Yanovski JA et al. Am J Clin Nutr 2010;91:1020–6.
73. Skelton JA, Cook SR, Auinger P et al. Acad Pediatr 2009;9:322–9.
74. Lévesque J, Lamarche B. J Nutrigenet Nutrigenomics 2008;1:100–8.
75. Goran MI, Ball GDC, Cruz ML. J Clin Endocrinol Metab 2003;88:1417–27.
76. Freedman DS, Zuguo M, Srinivasan SE et al. J Pediatr 2007;150:12–7.
77. Roemmich JN, Clark PA, Lusk M et al. Int J Obes 2002; 26:701–9.
78. Patel SR, Hu FB. Obesity 2008;16:643–53.
79. Chen X, Beydoun MA, Wang Y. Obesity 2008;16:265–74.
80. Weiss A, Xu F, Storfer-Isser A et al. Sleep 2010;33:1201–9.

SUGGESTED READINGS

Cutler GJ, Flood A, Hannan P et al. Multiple sociodemographic and socioenvironmental characteristics are correlated with major patterns of dietary intake in adolescents. J Am Diet Assoc 2011;111:230–40.

Larson NI, Neumark-Sztainer D, Story M. Weight control behaviors and dietary intake among adolescents and young adults: longitudinal findings from Project EAT. J Am Diet Assoc 2009;109:1869–77.

Nattiv A, Loucks AB, Manore MM et al. The female athlete triad. Med Sci Sports Exerc 2007;39:1867–82.

Ritchie LD, Spector P, Stevens MJ et al. Dietary patterns in adolescence are related to adiposity in young adulthood in black and white females. J Nutr 2007;137:399–406.

Rosenfield RL, Bordini B. Evidence that obesity and androgens have independent and opposing effects on gonadotropin production from puberty to maturity. Brain Res 2010;1364:186–97.

56 NUTRITION IN OLDER ADULTS[1]

CONNIE WATKINS BALES AND MARY ANN JOHNSON

---

[1]**Abbreviations: AD**, Alzheimer disease; **AI**, adequate intake; **CHD**, coronary heart disease; **CKD**, chronic kidney disease; **CVD**, cardiovascular disease; **DRI**, dietary reference intake; **EAR**, estimated average requirement; **H2RA**, histamine H_2 receptor antagonist; **IDA**, iron deficiency anemia; **NHANES**, National Health and Nutrition Examination Survey; **OAA**, Older Americans Act; **PPI**, proton pump inhibitor; **RDA**, recommended dietary allowance; **USDA**, United States Department of Agriculture; **VMS**, vitamin and/or mineral supplement.

OVERVIEW

Between the years 2000 and 2050, the number of adults aged 60 years and older will double in the United States and more than triple worldwide (1, 2). The "graying" of the world's population brings a considerable burden of chronic diseases, and many, if not most, of these diseases have a strong nutritional component. Thus, this chapter reviews the impact of diet on chronic health conditions and selected nutrients of concern as well as the infrastructure in the United States for meeting the food and nutrient needs of older adults in the continuum of care in community and long-term care settings. Although knowledge of how nutrition supports health throughout life is growing, much remains to be learned and applied in numerous areas, including the following: (a) the behavioral sciences, concerning ways to improve eating habits and thus lessen the burden of chronic disease; (b) the policy arena, to ensure that all older people have access to safe and nutritious foods at all times; and (c) the basic and clinical sciences, to delineate the role of specific foods and nutrients further in maximizing health and minimizing the adverse consequences of sarcopenia, weight loss, nutritional frailty, and other age- and nutrition-related concerns.

Current and Future Demographics of Aging

In 2009, 12.9% of the US population was at least 65 years of age; in several states, the proportion exceeded 15% (Florida, Maine, Pennsylvania, and West Virginia). On average, approximately 4.1% of older adults lived in institutional settings, but this number increased with age from 0.9% for those 65 to 74 years old, to 3.5% for those 75 to 84 years old, and to 14.3% for those 85 years old or older. An additional 2.4% lived in senior housing with at least one supportive service. Eleven states had more than 50% of the nation's older adults, each with more than 1 million older people: California, Florida, Georgia, Illinois, Michigan, New Jersey, New York, North Carolina, Ohio, Pennsylvania, and Texas. Approximately 38.8% of older women and 18.7% of older men lived alone, and the proportion of persons living alone increased with advanced age. The median income of older adults was $25,877 for men and $15,282 for women in 2009, and approximately 8.9% were below the poverty level (10.7% of women and 6.6% of men) (3).

The number of individuals in the United States who are 65 years old and older will more than double from 40 million in 2010 to 88 million in 2050, whereas those aged 85 years old and older will increase by more than three-fold to 19 million (3). Ethnic and racial diversity is also increasing. Between 2010 and 2050, the number of older Hispanics will increase from 2.8 million to 17.5 million, whereas the number of older blacks will increase from 3.3 million to 9.9 million (3). In 2007, life expectancy in the United States at birth was 77.9 years; it was 30.9, 18.6, and 6.5 years at ages 50, 65, and 85, respectively (4). This population shift is a global phenomenon; in fact, the United States ranks only forty-ninth in life expectancy worldwide (5).

In summary, major demographic shifts will be associated with particularly large increases in the oldest old (>85 years of age) and of racial and ethnic minorities. These trends bring new challenges in health care, especially for preventive and therapeutic nutritional care for older adults.

Physiologic and Other Changes Affecting Nutritional Risk

Certain physiologic and metabolic changes inherent in the aging process have the potential to increase nutritional risk. The requirements for some, but not all, nutrients can be altered by these changes. Some of these factors and their potential influences on nutrient needs and intakes are shown in Table 56.1. Additionally, medical comorbidities and a host of other factors, including economic, geographic, and psychosocial concerns, can also affect diet behaviors and thus nutritional status.

Assessment of Nutritional Status

Nutritional screening and assessment should be part of the standard of care for all older adults (6). The goal of nutritional screening is to identify individuals who are at increased risk of being undernourished or malnourished. For those found to be at nutritional risk, a full assessment is warranted. Although biochemical indicators can signal a nutritional problem at the subclinical level, blood markers of nutritional status are far from specific. Serum albumin, the most commonly measured parameter, declines slightly with age (0.8 g/L/decade after age 60 years) and is influenced by a host of pathologic changes that are frequent in older adults, including chronic inflammation, advanced liver disease, heart failure, and nephrotic syndrome. Additionally, albumin is unlikely to be responsive to protein repletion in a timely manner (7).

Assessment of status for micronutrients is not routinely conducted unless a specific deficiency is suspected. Micronutrients most likely to be assessed in older persons include vitamins B_{12} (cobalamin concentration should be >350 pg/mL) and D 25[OH]D_3; concentration should be >50 nmol/L or 20 ng/L) and markers of iron status (ferritin should be 12 to 300 ng/mL in men and 12 to 150 ng/mL in women; hemoglobin should be 14.0 to 17.5 g/dL in men and 12.3 to 15.3 g/dL in women.)

Proposed guidelines entitled "Adult Starvation and Disease-Related Malnutrition" from an international consensus guideline committee may also be applicable to older adults in the medical setting (8). The biochemical and body composition cut points are in development, but the guidelines propose that malnutrition can occur under different situations, requiring differing interventions: (a) pure chronic starvation without inflammation, (b) chronic disease or conditions that impose sustained inflammation to a mild to moderate degree, and (c) acute disease or injury states with a marked inflammatory response.

In the community setting and in long-term care, the challenge is to achieve early identification of risk factors and signs of impending problems relating to food intake so that appropriate interventions can be optimally effective.

TABLE 56.1	POTENTIAL PHYSIOLOGIC AND METABOLIC DETERMINANTS OF NUTRIENT NEEDS AND INTAKES IN OLDER ADULTS	
	FACTOR OR CONDITION	**EFFECT ON DIETARY REQUIREMENTS**
Physiologic changes	Decreased total energy expenditure and reduced physical activity	Decreased energy requirement; increased importance of nutrient dense diet
	Decreased muscle mass and strength	Possible increased protein requirement; functional impairments could limit food access.
	Decreased immune competence	Possible increased requirement for iron, zinc, other nutrients
	Detrimental oral changes	Decreased amount and/or quality of nutrient intake
	Gastrointestinal: atrophic gastritis	Increased requirements for folate, calcium, vitamin K, vitamin B_{12}, and iron
	Menopause	Decreased requirement for iron
Metabolic changes	Reduced skin synthesis of previtamin D_3; impaired renal activation of and reduced gut response to 1,25(OH)$_2$D	Increased requirements for vitamin D and calcium
	Increased retention of vitamin A; altered hepatic metabolism	Decreased requirement for vitamin A
	Decreased ability to regulate fluid balance	Fluid needs possibly increased or decreased; fluid monitoring required

A physical examination can reveal signs of clinical nutritional deficiencies, including skin changes, fatigue, weakness, changes in ability to taste or smell, and gastrointestinal complaints (poor appetite, oral problems, nausea, vomiting, diarrhea, constipation). Changes in mental or emotional status may also be associated with an inadequate nutritional state (9). However, the single most important clinical measure of undernutrition in older adults is that of current body weight and any recent changes. The Long-Term Care Minimum Data Set considers a weight loss of 5% of usual body weight in 30 days or 10% in 180 days as a trigger for activating clinical assessment protocols (10). Unintentional recent weight loss is associated with increased mortality (11). Even with a stable body weight, older adults may have a marked reduction in fat-free mass or increases in fat mass (12).

Dietary assessments can be problematic in some older adults (13) because underreporting and memory problems may diminish accuracy. However, important questions about the number of meals eaten or skipped, the types and amounts of foods and nutritional supplements ingested, and potential barriers to consuming a nutritionally adequate diet can be very helpful in guiding subsequent interventions. Given the lack of any one gold standard measure of nutritional status, the use of indices that combine several variables is common. The best known of these indices intended for use in older adults is the Mini Nutritional Assessment (14). This validated tool has been widely used and shown to be predictive of adverse clinical events and mortality (15); a short version has also been validated (14).

Dietary Reference Intakes for Older Adults

Dietary recommendations for intakes of essential nutrients by age and gender are set by the Food and Nutrition Board of the Institute of Medicine. These recommendations, along with typical intakes of older adults, are shown in Table 56.2. Some dietary reference intake (DRI) recommendations are

TABLE 56.2	RECOMMENDATIONS AND INTAKES OF SELECTED NUTRIENTS FOR OLDER ADULTS (NHANES)[a]							
	RDA (EAR) OR AI[a]				INTAKES FROM FOOD[b] (UNLESS OTHERWISE INDICATED)			
	MEN 50–70 y	MEN >70 y	WOMEN 50–70 y	WOMEN >70 y	MEN 60–69 y[b] or 51–70 y[c,d]	MEN ≥70 y[b] or ≥71 y[c,d]	WOMEN 60–69 y[b] or 51–70 y[c,d]	WOMEN ≥70 y[b] or ≥71 y[c,d]
Energy (kcal)[b]					2,140	1,837	1,597	1,491
Protein (g)[b]	56 (46)	56 (46)	46 (38)	46 (38)	84.5	72.7	61.4	56.9
Dietary fiber (g)[b]	30	30	21	21	17.4	17.0	14.9	14.1
Sodium (mg)[b]	1,300	1,200	1,300	1,200	3,517	3,012	2,674	2,364
Potassium (mg)[b]	4,700	4,700	4,700	4,700	2,891	2,728	2,378	2,189
Calcium (mg)[c]	1,000 (800)	1,200 (1,000)	1,200 (1,000)	1,200 (1,000)	951	871	788	748
Diet + supplements (mg)[c,e]					1,092	1,087	1,186	1,139
Vitamin D (μg)[c,e]	15 (10)	20 (10)	15 (10)	20 (10)	5.1	5.6	3.9	4.5
Diet + supplements (μg)[c,e]					8.8	10.7	10.1	10.0
Magnesium (mg)[b]	420 (350)	420 (350)	320 (265)	320 (265)	310	280	253	233
Iron (mg)[b]	8 (6)	8 (6)	8 (5)	8 (5)	16.8	15.6	12.9	12.6
Zinc (mg)[b]	11 (9.4)	11 (9.4)	8 (6.8)	8 (6.8)	13.0	11.5	9.6	9.0
Folate (μg DFE)[e]	400 (320)	400 (320)	400 (320)	400 (320)	583	558	460	454
Diet + supplements (μg DFE)[d]					938	935	900	797
Vitamin B12 (μg)[b]	2.4 (2.0)	2.4 (2.0)	2.4 (2.0)	2.4 (2.0)	6.01	5.40	4.31	4.37
"Added" vitamin B12 (μg)[b]					0.94	1.14	0.87	0.94
Vitamin B6 (mg)[b]	1.7 (1.4)	1.7 (1.4)	1.5 (1.3)	1.5 (1.3)	2.06	1.97	1.60	1.54
Vitamin A (μg RAE)[b]	900 (625)	900 (625)	700 (500)	700 (500)	650	706	651	616
Vitamin E (mg)[b]	15 (12)	15 (12)	15 (12)	15 (12)	7.6	7.1	6.5	6.2
Vitamin K (μg)[b]	120	120	90	90	97.7	96.6	104.5	95.0

AI, adequate intake; DFE, dietary folate equivalent; EAR, estimated average requirement; NHANES, National Health and Nutrition Examination Survey; RAE, retinol activity equivalents; RDA, recommended dietary allowance.

[a]Recommendations for intake are from the Dietary Reference Intakes (22, 33, 43, 155–157).
[b]Data from Agricultural Research Service, US Department of Agriculture, National Health and Nutrition Examination Survey, 2007 to 2008. What we Eat in America. Nutrient Intakes from Food: Mean Amounts Consumed per Individuals, One Day, 2007–2008. Available at: http://www.ars.usda.gov/Services/docs.htm?docid=18349. Accessed April 16, 2011.
[c]Data from Bailey RL, Dodd KW, Goldman JA et al. Estimation of total usual calcium and vitamin D intakes in the United States. J Nutr 2010;140:817–22.
[d]Data from Bailey RL, Dodd KW, Gahche JJ et al. Total folate and folic acid intake from foods and dietary supplements in the United States: 2003–2006. Am J Clin Nutr 2010;91:231–7.
[e]Multiply micrograms of vitamin D by 40 to obtain international units.

higher for men compared with women, such as DRIs for protein, fiber, magnesium, zinc, vitamin B_6, vitamin A, and vitamin K. DRI recommendations increase with age for vitamin D and decrease with age for sodium (16, 17).

As already indicated, a host of physiologic and psychosocial factors can influence food intake and determine whether diets consumed by older adults actually meet nutritional needs. As illustrated in Table 56.2, results of National Health and Nutrition Examination Survey (NHANES) surveys show that average intakes from diet alone exceeded recommendations for protein, fiber, sodium, iron, zinc, folate, vitamin B_{12}, vitamin B_6, and vitamin A. Nutrients for which dietary intakes were generally lower than recommendations included potassium, magnesium, calcium, and vitamins D and E. The intakes of most nutrients were consistently higher in persons 60 to 69 years old compared with those 70 years old or older, except for intakes of vitamin D, vitamin A, vitamin K, and "added" vitamin B_{12}; however, vitamin D intakes remained much lower than recommendations for all age groups.

Dietary Guidelines for Older Americans

Along with the DRIs, the Dietary Guidelines for Americans are used to assist with meal planning for congregate and home-delivered meals and in institutional settings, as well as for general dietary guidance (18). Food-based recommendations at various energy intakes facilitate meal planning (e.g., the recommended servings of fruit, vegetables, whole grains, meat equivalents, and milk products). Specific recommendations relevant to older adults emphasize consuming "added" vitamin B_{12} from fortified foods or supplements and the health benefits of limiting sodium intake (to <1500 mg/day). Across the life span, the nutrients of concern were identified as vitamin D, calcium, potassium, and dietary fiber.

NUTRIENT-SPECIFIC CONCERNS IN OLDER ADULTS

Energy, Protein, Fiber, and Fluid

Energy requirements as well as intakes decrease with advancing age. A gradual reduction of approximately 7 and 10 kcal/year for women and men, respectively, occurs (19). Similarly, protein intakes decrease with age. However, the current recommended dietary allowance (RDA) for protein is not changed with age; it is 0.80 g/kg/day of high-quality protein (20). Most community-dwelling individuals are not at high risk for protein or protein-calorie malnutrition, but home-bound (21) and hospitalized older adults (see subsequent section) as well as nursing home residents are all at risk of protein insufficiency. Reduced food intake resulting from the anorexia of aging may also jeopardize the adequacy of protein and other essential nutrients. Frailty secondary to poor nutritional intake is addressed in a subsequent section.

Fiber intake is inversely associated with the risk of several age-related diseases; the adequate intake (AI) for fiber is based on prospective studies of fiber and coronary heart disease (CHD) (22). Although no tolerable upper intake limit (UL) for dietary fiber has been established, the functional fibers added to some foods, beverages, and supplements may increase the risk of adverse effects (22). The AI for total fiber is based on energy intake and not on age itself (22). Fiber intake is much lower than the AI, and fiber is considered a nutrient of concern (18). Fiber is only one of numerous factors related to constipation (23). Aging is associated with a shift toward less healthful intestinal microflora, so there is interest in how fiber, other dietary components, and probiotics influence intestinal health.

Appropriate hydration can be a challenge for older adults, with the most common concerns focused on risks for dehydration (24). More recently, however, the potential negative effects of excessive water consumption have also been noted, including dilutional hyponatremia (water intoxication) and increased nocturia (25). Consumption of six to eight glasses of fluid a day is likely adequate for healthy elderly people except during stressful situations that are likely to increase fluid loss (e.g., severely hot weather, heavy exertion) (26).

Alcohol

Although light to moderate alcohol intake has been linked with several health benefits in midlife, in later life the risks of alcohol may outweigh the health-promoting effects (27). Health risks associated with alcohol use in older adults include increased risk of falling, adverse cognitive effects, drug–alcohol interactions, and nutrient displacement in the diet (28). Ethanol tolerance is often lower in older adults because of physiologic changes, central nervous system alterations, and pharmaceutical use. Thus, fewer drinks than expected may lead to intoxication, adverse events, accidents, and fatalities. This is also true for alcohol toxicity (to brain and liver) as a result of changes in ethanol metabolism, distribution, and elimination; these findings emphasize the importance of moderation with regard to alcohol use in this age group (29).

Current estimated rates of moderate and heavy alcohol use among older adults in the United States are 56% and 9% for men and 40% and 2% for women, respectively (27, 30). Individuals in the Baby Boom generation report higher alcohol use than in earlier cohorts; if they continue their level of use at older ages, rates of moderate and heavy drinking in the older population will be even higher in future years. Problems with heavy alcohol use and abuse in older populations may be precipitated by psychosocial challenges in late life, including depression, social isolation, and bereavement. Moreover, it may be difficult to assess the level of alcohol use because of different perceptions about what constitutes "a drink," as well as poor memory and underreporting (31). Specific nutritional concerns in heavy drinkers include the potential for B-vitamin deficiencies, especially of folate and vitamin B_{12}, and increased antioxidant nutrient requirements (from increased oxidative stress with heavier alcohol consumption) (27).

Vitamin D and Calcium

Calcium and vitamin D are involved in numerous biologic functions, the best known of which is skeletal health (32, 33). In NHANES 2001 to 2006, the prevalence of serum 25-hydroxyvitamin D (25[OH]D) concentrations lower than 30 nmol/L (risk of deficiency) was 6%, 7%, 11%, and 11% in men 51 to 70 years old, men more than 70 years old, women 51 to 70 years old, and women more than 70 years old, respectively, whereas the prevalence of serum 25(OH)D concentrations of 30 to 49 nmol/L (risk of inadequacy) was 25%, 24%, 28%, and 27% in men 51 to 70 years old, men more than 70 years old, women 51 to 70 years old, and women more than 70 years old, respectively (34). Even after 80 years of age, risk factors such as advanced age, race (black versus white), season, and nonuse of dietary supplements were associated with poor vitamin D status (35).

In NHANES 2003 to 2006, mean intake of calcium from the diet exceeded the estimated average requirement (EAR) only for men 60 to 69 years old, but the intake of calcium from supplements increased intakes to higher than the EAR for all age groups (see Table 56.2.) (16). Among supplement users who were men 51 to 70 years old, men 71 years old or older, women 51 to 70 years old, and women 71 years old or older, the intake of supplemental calcium was 268, 372, 578, and 608 mg/day, respectively, and of supplemental vitamin D was 9.4, 10.9, 11.2, and 10.7 µg/day, respectively (16). Supplements of oral vitamin D_3 or D_2 with or without calcium were associated with reduction in fracture risk in institutionalized individuals, but the benefits were inconsistent in community-dwelling individuals (33). Very high single annual doses of vitamin D (12,500 µg or 500,000 IU) may decrease fall and fracture risk (36, 37).

Vitamin B_{12}, Folate, and Vitamin B_6

The increased prevalence of vitamin B_{12} deficiency with aging is attributed mainly to atrophic gastritis, which occurs in approximately 10% to 30% of older adults and impairs digestion of protein-bound vitamin B_{12} from animal foods (38, 39). Other potential causes of protein-bound vitamin B_{12} malabsorption include gastric resection and gastric infection with *Helicobacter pylori* (40), as well as the long-term use of drugs that block gastric acid secretion (histamine H_2 receptor antagonists [H2RAs] and proton pump inhibitors [PPIs]). These pharmacologic agents are commonly used for the treatment of gastroesophageal reflux and peptic ulcer disease (7, 8). Most, although not all, of the available evidence to date supports

an association between the long-term use of H2RAs and PPIs and vitamin B_{12} deficiency in older adults (9).

Even after the age of 80 years, risk factors such as advanced age, atrophic gastritis, nonuse of dietary supplements, and race (white race) were associated with poor vitamin B_{12} status (41). Approximately 1% to 2% of older adults have pernicious anemia, which results from a loss of the intrinsic factor needed for intestinal absorption of vitamin B_{12}; vitamin B_{12} status in these individuals is maintained by monthly injections or daily oral doses (1000 to 2000 µg daily, (42). People 51 years old and older should meet the recommendation from "added" vitamin B_{12} in fortified foods or dietary supplements (43). In NHANES 2007 to 2008, total dietary intakes of vitamin B_{12} were more than double the RDA, but the intake of added vitamin B_{12} from dietary sources was only approximately 1 µg/day (see Table 56.2.).

The EAR and RDA for vitamin B_6 are higher in older compared with younger people, based on assessment of biochemical markers of vitamin B_6 status during depletion and repletion studies (43). In NHANES 2007 to 2008, average dietary intakes of vitamin B_6 were much higher than the EAR and RDA (Table 56.2.); however, low intakes and poor status are common in studies of older adults in the United States and elsewhere (44). In NHANES 2003 to 2006, among persons 65 years old and older, the prevalence of low plasma pyridoxal 5'-phosphate was 24% in those who did not use supplements and 6% in supplement users (<20 nmol/L, index of adequacy) (45).

The EAR and RDA for folate are similar for older and younger adults, except no specific recommendation exists for older adults to consume folic acid (43). Dietary intake alone is much higher than the EAR and RDA (see Table 56.2). In NHANES 2005 to 2006, red blood cell folate concentrations were higher in older (≥60 years) compared with younger adults, and the overall prevalence of low folate status was very low across the population (46). Following folic acid fortification of the food supply in the United States in 1998, benefits to older adults may include decreased risk of stroke (47, 48), but concerns exist about increased risks of certain health problems such as impaired cognition (49).

Serum homocysteine concentrations are positively associated with several health conditions and are inversely associated with folate, vitamin B_{12}, and vitamin B_6 status. However, additional prospective studies and randomized controlled trials are needed to elucidate the role of homocysteine and these B vitamins in age-associated health conditions such as cardiovascular disease (CVD) (50), neurologic and psychiatric diseases (51), Alzheimer disease (AD) (52), and osteoporosis (53).

Iron

Aging decreases iron requirements for older women (cessation of menstruation) such that iron recommendations are the same for older men and women; iron intakes generally exceed the EAR and RDA (see Table 56.2.) (54).

In NHANES 1999 to 2000, among those 70 years old and older, the prevalence of iron deficiency was 3% in men and 6% in women, and the prevalence of iron deficiency anemia (IDA) was 1% (55). Although iron stores (e.g., ferritin) increase with age, evidence is inconclusive for a causal role of high iron status or high iron stores with CVD or cancer, except that liver iron accumulation is a risk factor for hepatocellular carcinoma in hemochromatosis (56). At least 20% of anemia in older adults is attributed to iron deficiency; the most common cause of IDA is blood loss related to a gastrointestinal disorder, and distinguishing IDA from other anemias is necessary (57).

Vitamins A, E, and K

Vitamin A intakes from food are generally higher than the EAR but lower than the RDA in older adults (see Table 56.2.) (56). Although vitamin A intake recommendations do not change with age (56), advanced age may predispose to vitamin A intoxication (58). High vitamin A status as a risk factor for poor bone health remains uncertain (56). Studies showed that vitamin A status and fractures were associated positively only in persons with lower vitamin D intake (59), were not associated (60), or had a U-shaped relationship such that both high and low vitamin A status increased the risk of fractures (61).

Although no evidence indicates that either absorption or use changes with age, reported intakes of vitamin E are often less than the EAR (see Table 56.2.), possibly because of efforts to cut intakes of high-fat foods or underreporting of these foods. Marginal vitamin E status could compromise the ability of older adults to defend against oxidative damage. However, increasing the intakes of vitamin E (to ≥400 IU) using supplements is not likely to be beneficial (62) and has been linked to an increase in the risk of hemorrhagic stroke (63).

The requirement for vitamin K does increase with aging, and intakes of this vitamin are generally adequate in older adults (see Table 56.2.), perhaps because of generous intakes of vegetable sources (64). Vitamin K status could be important for bone health in older adults, through its role in posttranslational modification of osteocalcin. However, studies to date are not in agreement about a bone benefit in older adults (65). Additionally, the vitamin has the potential to interact with anticoagulant medications that are commonly used by older adults (66).

Magnesium

Magnesium recommendations remain the same for all adults after the age of 30 years, and men have higher requirements than women (32). Magnesium intakes were lower than the EAR in older adults (see Table 56.2.). With advancing age, there may be decreased magnesium absorption, increased urinary excretion, and concern about high intakes in patients with renal failure (32). Magnesium has been associated with numerous age-related conditions (32, 67), including poor functional status in older adults (68).

Zinc

The interaction of aging with zinc requirements is poorly understood; moreover, dependable markers of true zinc status are lacking. Average zinc intakes are higher than the RDA in community-dwelling older adults (see Table 56.2.), but evidence indicates that zinc insufficiency could be common in nursing home residents (69). The immunoregulatory role of zinc is particularly important in older adults because immune function declines with age; thus, mild-to-moderate zinc deficiency could impair resistance to infection and response to immunizations and contribute to increasing susceptibility to illness. For example, Prasad et al (70) demonstrated a reduction in the number of infections experienced by healthy elderly subjects receiving zinc supplementation. Thus, further studies are needed to explore whether correction of zinc deficiency could reduce infection rates and all-cause mortality in older adults (71).

Micronutrient Supplements

Supplements of micronutrients (vitamins and/or minerals; VMS) have two important and distinct potential applications for older adults. The first is the repletion of a confirmed clinical or subclinical deficiency, an important and well-accepted therapeutic application. The second is the reason that most older VMS users choose to take them, and that is for the preservation of health or prevention of disease. Most surveys indicate a higher use of VMS among older adults compared with the general population. VMS use is more likely in women than men and is typically linked to strong health-seeking behaviors (72, 73). Although the most commonly used type of VMS is a multivitamin-mineral preparation, in fact, limited scientific support exists for either the health-related efficacy or adverse effects of long-term use of this type of supplement. Controlled trials are needed to define the potential benefits and risks of VMSs more clearly (72).

Nutrients with antioxidant activity are commonly supplemented and have been extensively studied because of epidemiologic findings linking dietary consumption of these nutrients with health benefits. However, the results for vitamins A, C, E, and β-carotene for the prevention of CVD (74) or cancer have been largely disappointing and do not support the use of supplements of these nutrients. Some evidence indicates benefits of antioxidant supplements for delaying progression of age-related macular degeneration (75) and of selenium for cancer prevention (76, 77), although further research is needed before recommendations can be made. The experience with supplements of B vitamins is parallel to that with antioxidants.

Despite compelling epidemiologic evidence linking the amino acid homocysteine with negative health outcomes and the demonstrated ability of the B vitamins folate, vitamin B_{12}, and vitamin B_6 to lower homocysteine concentrations, evidence from large randomized controlled trials has shown little benefit of these vitamins for delaying CVD (78) or age-related cognitive changes (51). Moreover, in studies of folic acid supplements, the evidence of benefit in cancer prevention is coupled with concerns about enhancing the growth of existing undiagnosed cancers (79, 80) and with promotion of CVD (81). In contrast, as already discussed, strong evidence supports the benefits of supplements of calcium and vitamin D for reducing the risk of fractures (both nutrients together) and falls (vitamin D). However, dietary sources of calcium need to be emphasized to minimize the number of pills taken per day, thus enhancing compliance and reducing the likelihood of side effects, such as constipation and arterial calcification (82). Clear cardiovascular health benefits have been shown with modest increases in consumption of fatty fish or fish oil supplements, including lowering of serum triglyceride concentrations (83) and reduction in the risk of death and sudden cardiac death (84).

NUTRITION-RELATED HEALTH CONCERNS AND COMMUNITY-BASED SERVICES

Physical Activity and Obesity

Participation in regular physical activity declines with age; and this change, along with age-associated decreases in energy requirements, contributes to a gradual accumulation of body fat mass. Inactivity is associated with elevated risk for chronic diseases (e.g., CVD, hypertension, certain cancers, and type 2 diabetes), metabolic syndrome, and premature mortality and is one of the strongest predictors for physical disability in older adults (85). Not unexpectedly, obesity, defined as a body mass index of 30 kg/m^2 or greater, is becoming increasingly prevalent (86) and is associated with increased risks of CVD, diabetes, cancer, cognitive decline, and mortality in older adults (87). However, the advisability of weight loss interventions in this population has been questioned out of concerns about potential losses of lean muscle or bone mass, the "reverse benefit" of obesity in the event of acute inflammatory disease (88) or other serious illness (89), and evidence linking lower body mass index to higher overall mortality.

Nonetheless, intervention trials showed clinically significant benefits of weight reduction with regard to osteoarthritis, physical function, diabetes, and CHD (90). When exercise is combined with weight loss, it may promote conservation of lean body mass (91) as well as improved cardiorespiratory function and balance. Further study is needed to identify the safest and most effective intervention strategies for obese older adults who are experiencing functional or metabolic complications as a result of excessive adiposity (92).

Osteoporosis

Osteoporosis is diagnosed based on low bone mineral density or the presence of fragility fractures, such as vertebral or hip fractures. In 2005, the estimated number of fractures in adults 50 years old or older was more than 2 million, including hip fractures in 222,753 older women and in 73,857 older men (93). Although many dietary factors influence bone health throughout life (94), the primary diet-related recommendations for the general population are AI of calcium (1200 mg/day) and vitamin D (20 to 25 μg/day) as well as avoidance of excess alcohol for fall prevention (95). Vitamin D with calcium reduces hip fractures in older adults (96). Fall prevention becomes increasing important for prevention of hip fractures in older adults (95), and vitamin D supplements reduce the rate of falls in nursing home residents (97).

Diabetes

Among adults 60 years old or older in the United States in 2007, 23.1% had diabetes, and this age group had 51.6% of all diabetes cases (98). Adiposity and weight gain in midlife contribute to the development of diabetes in later life (99), and lifestyle improvements in persons at high risk for diabetes reduced the risk of a diabetes diagnosis more in older compared with younger people (100). Diabetes contributes to the disablement process, so consideration of self-management abilities and frailty is important in diabetes care in older people (101). Diabetes was among the stronger health-related predictors of nursing home admission (also high blood pressure, cancer, and stroke) (102). In NHANES 1999 to 2004, only approximately half of older adults with diabetes attained treatment goals, and rates of meeting these goals decreased with increasing age (103).

Cardiovascular Disease and Chronic Heart Failure

About 40.4 million of the estimated 82.6 million US residents with one or more types of CVD are 65 or more years of age (104). According to NHANES 1999 to 2004, older adults are undertreated for hypertension, dyslipidemia, and diabetes, which are among the major risk factors for CVD (103). Investigators have speculated that some of the "treatment gap" may be related to a more conservative approach to CVD prevention and management, because of practitioner concerns about adverse drug reactions, comorbidities, impaired cognition, vision, or hearing, and socioeconomic status (105). However, secondary prevention interventions to control risk factors in older people with CHD appear to be as effective as in younger people (106).

Chronic hypertension and CHD account for more than 70% of heart failure cases (107). A complex array of neurohormonal, immunologic, and metabolic derangements contribute to the progression of CHF, including increased basal metabolic rate, changes in protein and

84. Mozaffarian D, Rimm EB. JAMA 2006;296:1885–99.

85. Stuck A, Walthert J, Nikolaus T et al. Soc Sci Med 1999;48: 445–69.

86. Federal Interagency Forum on Aging-Related Statistics. Older Americans 2008: Key Indicators of Well-Being. Available at: http://www.agingstats.gov/Main_Site/Data/2008_Documents/OA_2008.pdf. Accessed May 11, 2012.

87. Houston DK, Nicklas BJ, Zizza CA. J Am Diet Assoc 2009;109:1886–95.

88. Kalantar-Zadeh K, Abbott KC, Salahudeen AK et al. Am J Clin Nutr 2005;81:543–54.

89. Bouillanne O, Dupont-Belmont C, Hay P et al. Am J Clin Nutr 2009;90:505–10.

90. Bales C, Buhr G. J Am Med Dir Assoc 2008;9:302–12.

91. Avila JJ, Gutierres JA, Sheehy ME et al. Eur J Appl Physiol 2010;109:517–25.

92. Jensen GL, Hsiao PY. Evid Based Med 2010;15:41–2.

93. Burge R, Dawson-Hughes B, Solomon DH et al. J Bone Miner Res 2007;22:465–75.

94. Ontjes DA, Anderson JJ. Nutritional and pharmacological aspects of osteoporosis. In: Bales CW, Ritchie CS, eds. Handbook of Clinical Nutrition and Aging. 2nd ed. New York: Humana, 2009:417–38.

95. National Osteoporosis Foundation. Clinician's Guide to Prevention and Treatment of Osteoporosis. Available at: http://www.nof.org/sites/default/files/pdfs/NOF_ClinicianGuide2009_v7.pdf . Accessed May 11. 2012.

96. Avenell A, Gillespie WJ, Gillespie LD et al. Cochrane Database Syst Rev 2009;(2):CD000227.

97. Cameron ID, Murray GR, Gillespie LD et al. Cochrane Database Syst Rev 2010;(1):CD005465.

98. Centers for Disease Control and Prevention. Diabetes Public Health Resource. Available at: http://www.cdc.gov/diabetes/pubs/pdf/ndfs_2011.pdf. Accessed May 11, 2012.

99. Biggs ML, Mukamal KJ, Luchsinger JA al. JAMA 2010; 303:2504–12.

100. Knowler WC, Barrett-Connor E, Fowler SE et al. N Engl J Med 2002;346:393–403.

101. Bourdel Marchasson I, Doucet J, Bauduceau B et al. J Nutr Health Aging 2009;13:685–91.

102. Gaugler JE, Duval S, Anderson KA et al. BMC Geriatr 2007;7:13.

103. McDonald M, Hertz RP, Unger AN et al. J Gerontol A Biol Sci Med Sci 2009;64:256–63.

104. American Heart Association 2012 Statistical Fact Sheet: Older Americans and Cardiovascular Diseases. Dallas: American Heart Association, 2012. Available at: http://www.heart.org/idc/groups/heart-public/@wcm/@sop/@smd/documents/downloadable/ucm_319574.pdf. Accessed May 31, 2012.

105. Kriekard P, Gharacholou SM, Peterson ED. Clin Geriatr Med 2009;25:745–55, x.

106. Williams MA, Fleg JL, Ades PA et al. Circulation 2002;105: 1735–43.

107. Holley C, Rich MW. Chronic heart failure. In: Bales CW, Ritchie CS, eds. Handbook of Clinical Nutrition and Aging. 2nd ed. New York: Humana, 2009:333–54.

108. Scharver CH, Hammond CS, Goldstein LB. Post-stroke malnutrition and dysphagia. In: Bales CW, Ritchie CS, eds. Handbook of Clinical Nutrition and Aging. 2nd ed. New York: Humana, 2009:479–98.

109. Dennis MS, Lewis SC, Warlow C. Lancet 2005;365:764–72.

110. Abbott KC, Glanton CW, Trespalacios FC et al. Kidney Int 2004;65:597–605.

111. Beddhu S. Nutrition and chronic kidney disease. In: Bales CW, Ritchie CS, eds. Handbook of Clinical Nutrition and Aging. 2nd ed. New York: Humana, 2009:403–16.

112. Pilotto A, Sancarlo D, Franceschi M et al. Am J Nephrol 2010;23(Suppl 15):S5–10.

113. de Pablo P, McAlindon TE. Osteoarthritis. In: Bales CW, Ritchie CS, eds. Handbook of Clinical Nutrition and Aging. 2nd ed. New York: Humana, 2009:439–78.

114. DeFrances CJ, Lucas CA, Buie VC et al. Natl Health Stat Report 2008;5:1–20.

115. Murphy L, Schwartz TA, Helmick CG et al. Arthritis Rheum 2008;59:1207–13.

116. Blagojevic M, Jinks C, Jeffery A et al. Osteoarthritis Cartilage 2010;18:24–33.

117. Plassman BL, Langa KM, Fisher GG et al. Neuroepidemiology 2007;29:125–32.

118. Alzheimer's Association. Alzheimers Dement 2009;5:234–70.

119. Grodstein F. Alzheimers Dement 2007;3(Suppl):S16–22.

120. Middleton LE, Yaffe K. Arch Neurol 2009;66:1210–5.

121. Middleton LE, Yaffe K. J Alzheimers Dis 2010;20:915–24.

122. Li L, Lewis TL. Alzheimer's disease and other neurodegenerative disorders. In: Bales CW, Ritchie CS, eds. Handbook of Clinical Nutrition and Aging. 2nd ed. New York: Humana, 2009:499–522.

123. Nord MA, Coleman-Jensen A, Andres M, Carson S. Household Food Security in the United States, 2009. Available at: http://www.ers.usda.gov/Publications/ERR108/ERR108.pdf. Accessed May 11, 2012.

124. Lee JS, Fischer JG, Johnson MA. J Nutr Elder 2010;29: 116–49.

125. Ziliak J, Gundersen C. Senior Hunger in The United States: Differences across States and Rural and Urban Areas. 2009. Available at: http://www.mowaa.org/document.doc?id=193. Accessed May 31, 2012.

126. Ziliak J, Gundersen C, Haist M. The Causes, Consequences, and Future of Senior Hunger in America. 2008. Available at: http://www.mowaa.org/document.doc?id=13. Accessed May 31, 2012.

127. Bengle R, Sinnett S, Johnson T et al. J Nutr Elder 2010;29: 170–91.

128. Brewer DP, Catlett CS, Porter KN et al. J Nutr Elder 2010;29: 150–69.

129. Kamp BJ, Wellman NS, Russell C. J Am Diet Assoc 2010;110: 463–72.

130. US Department of Agriculture. Nutrition Assistance Programs. Available at: http://www.fns.usda.gov/fns/. Accessed May 11, 2012.

131. Administration on Aging. Home and Community Based Long-Term Care. Available at: http://www.aoa.gov/AoARoot/AoA_Programs/HCLTC/Nutrition_Services/index.aspx. Accessed May 31, 2012.

132. O'Shaughnessy CV. The Aging Services Network: Accomplishments and Challenges in Serving a Growing Elderly Population. National Health Policy Forum, 2008. Available at: http://www.nhpf.org/library/details.cfm/2625. Accessed May 11, 2012.

133. Johnson MA, Fischer JG, Park S. J Nutr Elder 2008;27:29–46.

134. Lee JS, Sinnett S, Bengle R et al. J Appl Gerontol 2010;30: 587–606.

135. Heersink JT, Brown CJ, Dimaria-Ghalili RA et al. J Nutr Elder 2010;29:4–41.

136. Gariballa S, Forster S. Clin Nutr 2007;26:466–73.

137. Edington J, Boorman J, Durrant ER et al. Clin Nutr 2000;19:191–5.

138. Singh H, Watt K, Veitch R et al. Nutrition 2006;22:350–4.

139. Arvanitakis M, Coppens P, Doughan L et al. Clin Nutr 2009;28:492–6.

140. Locher JL, Wellman NS. J Nutr Gerontol Geriatr 2011; 30:24–8.

141. Sloane PD, Ivey J, Helton M et al. J Am Med Dir Assoc 2008;9:476–85.

142. Bales CW, Ritchie CS. Redefining nutritional frailty: interventions for weight loss due to undernutrition. In: Bales CW, Ritchie CS, eds. Handbook of Clinical Nutrition and Aging. 2nd ed. New York: Humana, 2009:157–82.

143. Evans WJ, Morley JE, Argiles J et al. Clin Nutr 2008; 27:793–9.

144. Janssen I. Sarcopenia. In: Bales CW, Ritchie CS, eds. Handbook of Clinical Nutrition and Aging. 2nd ed. New York: Humana, 2009:183–206.

145. Engel JH, Siewerdt F, Jackson R et al. J Am Geriatr Soc 2011;59:482–7.

146. Locher JL, Robinson CO, Roth DL et al. J Gerontol A Biol Sci Med Sci 2005;60:1475–8.

147. Reuben DB, Hirsch SH, Zhou K et al. Am Geriatr Soc 2005;53:970–5.

148. Niedert KC. J Am Diet Assoc 2005;105:1955–65.

149. Milne AC, Potter J, Avenell A. Cochrane Database Syst Rev 2002;(3):CD003288.

150. Candy B, Sampson EL, Jones L. Int J Palliat Nurs 2009; 15:396–404.

151. Evans BD. J Hosp Palliat Nurs 2002;4:91–9.

152. Heuberger RA. J Nutr Elder 2010;29:347–85.

153. Ritchie CS, Kvale E. Nutrition at the end of life: ethical issues. In: Bales CW, Ritchie CS, eds. Handbook of Clinical Nutrition and Aging. 2nd ed. New York: Humana, 2009:235–44.

154. Eggenberger SK, Nelms TP. J Clin Nurs 2004;13:661–7.

155. Food and Nutrition Board, Institute of Medicine. Dietary Reference Intakes for Vitamin C, Vitamin E, Selenium, and Carotenoids. Washington, DC: National Academy Press, 2000.

156. Food and Nutrition Board, Institute of Medicine. Dietary Reference Intakes for Vitamin A, Vitamin K, Arsenic, Boron, Chromium, Copper, Iodine, Iron, Manganese, Molybdenum, Nickel, Silicon, Vanadium, and Zinc. Washington, DC: National Academy Press, 2001:115, 182, 340–4.

157. Food and Nutrition Board, Institute of Medicine. Dietary Reference Intakes for Water, Potassium, Sodium, Chloride, and Sulfate. Washington, DC: National Academy Press, 2004.

SUGGESTED READINGS

Bales CW, Ritchie CS, ed. Handbook of Clinical Nutrition and Aging. 2nd ed. New York: Humana, 2009.

Buhr G, Bales CW. Nutritional supplements for older adults: review and recommendations. Part I. J Nutr Elder 2009;28:5–29.

Buhr G, Bales CW. Nutritional supplements for older adults: review and recommendations. Part II. J Nutr Elder 2010;29:42–71.

Hausman DB, Fischer JG, Johnson MA. Nutrition in centenarians. Maturitas 2011;68:203–9.

Heuberger R. Artificial nutrition and hydration at the end of life: a review. J Nutr Elder 2010;29:347–85.

Johnson MA, Dwyer JT, Jensen GL et al. Challenges and new opportunities for clinical nutrition interventions in the aged. J Nutr 2011;141:535–41.

Lee JS, Fischer JG, Johnson MA. Food insecurity, food and nutrition programs, and aging: experiences from Georgia. J Nutr Elder 2010;29:116–49.

CLINICAL MANIFESTATIONS OF NUTRIENT DEFICIENCIES AND TOXICITIES[1]

DOUGLAS C. HEIMBURGER

Nutritional disorders result from imbalances between the body's requirements for nutrients and energy sources and the supplies of these substrates of metabolism. These imbalances may take the form of either deficiency or excess and may be attributable to inappropriate intake or to defective utilization or, frequently, a combination of both.

---

[1]**Abbreviations: ATP**, adenosine triphosphate; **DRI**, dietary reference intake; **HDN**, hemolytic disease of the newborn; **TPN**, total parenteral nutrition.

Despite our extensive understanding of human nutritional requirements for maintenance of health, malnutrition continues to be one of the main causes of morbidity and mortality in low- and middle-income countries, especially in young children (1). In technologically advanced societies, undernutrition resulting from dietary restriction no longer constitutes a major hazard to health, but it continues to occur in hospitalized patients and in other especially vulnerable groups. However, deficiency states continue to arise in patients with certain cultural or religious precepts, long-term alcohol or drug abuse, debilitating disease, or food faddism. Vigilance is needed to detect secondary undernutrition resulting from malabsorption; failure in transport, storage, or cellular utilization; excessive losses; or inactivation by genetic mutations of essential metabolic pathways that increase needs. The improper use of nutrient supplements, often because of ignorance about proper dosage or by failure of excretion through renal failure with continued nutrient intake, has been a major cause of toxicity (2).

This chapter addresses clinical manifestations of nutritional disorders related to vitamins, minerals, and essential fatty acids. It has been included because the chapters concerned with the individual nutrients do not uniformly discuss clinical aspects of deficiencies and excesses. Descriptions of clinical symptoms of deficiency of each nutrient are followed by brief consideration of who is likely to be at risk of deficiency and, if relevant, who is likely to be at risk of toxic levels.

VITAMINS

Vitamin A (Retinol)

Deficiency

The symptoms and signs of vitamin A deficiency have been studied in greater detail than those of any other nutritional deficiency disorder (3, 4). The eye is primarily involved, and the condition, given the general name of xerophthalmia, predominantly affects young children. Impaired dark adaptation or night blindness (i.e., decreased vision in dim light) is an early symptom and can be elicited by a careful history and some simple tests in a poorly illuminated room (5). Photopic and color vision, mediated by the retinal cones, is usually unaffected.

Dryness (xerosis) and unwettability of the bulbar conjunctiva follow. Conjunctival impression cytology is abnormal at this stage. Bitot spot, an accumulation of desquamated cells most commonly seen in the interpalpebral fissure on the temporal aspect of the conjunctiva, is another sign (Fig. 57.1A). In older children and adults, Bitot spots may be stigmata of past deficiency, or they may be entirely unrelated to vitamin A deficiency when local trauma is responsible. Corneal involvement, starting as a superficial punctate keratopathy (6) and proceeding to xerosis (see Fig. 57.1B) and varying degrees of "ulceration" and liquefaction (keratomalacia) (see Fig. 57.1C), frequently results in blindness. Punctate degenerative changes in the retina (xerophthalmic fundus) are rare signs of chronic deficiency usually seen in older children (7). Corneal scars may have many causes, but those that are bilateral in the lower and outer part of the cornea of a person with a history of past malnutrition or measles, or both, often signal earlier vitamin A deficiency.

Extraocular manifestations include perifollicular hyperkeratosis, an accumulation of hyperkeratinized skin epithelium around hair follicles most commonly seen on the lateral aspects of the upper arms and the thighs. This finding is also seen in starvation and has been attributed to a deficiency of B-complex vitamins or essential fatty acids. Other changes may occur, including impaired taste, anorexia, vestibular disturbance, bone changes with pressure on cranial nerves, increased intracranial pressure, infertility, and congenital malformations (8).

Toxicity (Hypervitaminosis A)

Most of the features relate to a rise in intracranial pressure: nausea, vomiting, headache, vertigo, irritability, stupor, fontanel bulging (in infants), papilledema, and pseudotumor cerebri (mimicking brain tumor) (9). Pyrexia and peeling of the skin also occur.

Chronic poisoning produces a bizarre clinical picture that is often misdiagnosed because of failure to consider excessive vitamin A intake (9). It is characterized by anorexia, weight loss, headache, blurred vision, diplopia, dry and scaling pruritic skin, alopecia, coarsening of the hair, hepatomegaly, splenomegaly, anemia, subperiosteal new bone growth, cortical thickening (especially bones of hands and feet and long bones of the legs), and gingival discoloration. The x-ray appearance may assist in making a correct diagnosis. Cranial sutures are widened in the young child.

Vitamin A and other retinoids are powerful teratogens in both pregnant experimental animals and women (9). Birth defects have been reported in the children of women receiving 13-*cis*-retinoic acid (isotretinoin) during pregnancy (10). An increased risk of birth defects is present in infants of women taking more than 10,000 IU/day of supplementary preformed vitamin A before the seventh week of gestation (11). Significant evidence indicates that long-term intake of larger-dose supplements of retinol is associated with increased risk of bone fractures in older

Swedish men (12) and women (13) as well as in women in the United States (14).

Hypercarotenosis

Excessive intake of carotenoids can cause hypercarotenosis. Yellow or orange discoloration of the skin (xanthosis cutis, carotenoderma) affects areas where sebum secretion is greatest——nasolabial folds, forehead, axillae, and groin——and keratinized surfaces such as the palms and soles (see Fig. 57.1F). The sclerae and buccal membranes are not affected——a feature that distinguishes this condition from jaundice, in which these tissues are yellowed. No toxicity is apparent, and the discoloration gradually disappears with reduction of intake.

Vitamin D (Calciferol)

Deficiency

Vitamin D deficiency is manifested as rickets in children and osteomalacia in adults. Persons with those forms not resulting from primary vitamin D or calcium deficiency—previously termed *metabolic rickets*—also exhibit signs and symptoms of the underlying disease and hypocalcemia.

Rickets. The rachitic infant is restless and sleeps poorly. Craniotabes, softening of the bones of the skull and their ready depression on palpation, is often the earliest sign; but it must be present away from the suture lines to be diagnostic of rickets. Frontal bossing occurs, and the fontanels close late. Sitting, crawling, and walking are all delayed. If the disease is active when these activities occur, weight bearing results in bowing of the arms, knock-knees (genu valgum), or outward bowing (genu varum) (Fig. 57.2A and B). The characteristic x-ray appearance usually precedes clinical signs. Bone morphology is discussed elsewhere in this text.

Occasionally, stridor and intermittent sudden airway obstruction resulting from laryngospasm may manifest in infancy as a result of hypocalcemia accompanying biochemical and x-ray evidence of rickets but without the classic bony physical signs (15). A few instances of congenital cataract appeared to be caused by vitamin D deficiency in the mother (16).

Osteomalacia. The main features of osteomalacia are bone pain and tenderness, skeletal deformity, and weakness of the proximal muscles. Muscle weakness is a subtle indicator of vitamin deficiency (17). In severe cases, all the bones are painful and tender, often enough to disturb sleep. Tenderness may be particularly marked over Looser zones (Milkman lines), usually occurring in the long bones, pelvis, ribs, and around the scapulae in a bilaterally symmetric pattern. These radiotranslucent zones are sometimes termed *pseudofractures*. True fractures of the softened bones are common. The proximal muscle weakness, the cause of which is uncertain, is more marked in some forms of osteomalacia than in others. Osteomalacia usually results in a waddling gait and in difficulty going up and down the stairs. In elderly persons, it may simulate paraplegia; in younger persons, it may simulate muscular dystrophy.

headache (38). Liver dysfunction manifesting as elevated serum liver enzymes is reasonably common, and liver failure can occur. Diabetic patients also require special monitoring of glucose because niacin may worsen insulin resistance. Sustained-release forms of niacin are used to minimize these effects.

Pyridoxine (Vitamin B₆)

Deficiency

Pyridoxine deficiency induced by poor intake in adults is rarely severe enough to produce signs or symptoms. Volunteers receiving a deficient diet and a pyridoxine antagonist became irritable and depressed. Seborrheic dermatitis affected the nasolabial folds, cheeks, neck, and perineum. Several subjects also developed glossitis, angular stomatitis, blepharitis, and peripheral neuropathy.

Pyridoxine deficiency can also manifest as microcytic anemia, particularly in infants (39–41). An uncommon form of sideroblastic anemia, often severe, has been reported to respond in some instances to pyridoxine, but most cases appear to result from dependency rather than deficiency (42). An inherited error in the vitamin B₆–dependent enzyme cystathionine β-synthase leads to severe abnormalities at an early age.

Toxicity

Megadoses of pyridoxine (>200 mg/day) can cause sensory neuropathy, including progressive sensory ataxia and profound lower limb impairment of position and vibration sense (43). Touch, temperature, and pain perception are less affected. The tolerable upper limit for adults is 100 mg/day.

Biotin

Deficiency

Biotin deficiency has occasionally been induced in patients who consumed large amounts of raw egg white over a prolonged period. Egg white contains avidin, which antagonizes the action of biotin. The skin of the face and hands becomes dry, shiny, and scaly. The oral mucosa and tongue are swollen, magenta, and painful.

The most clear-cut cases of biotin deficiency occurred in children and adults maintained on long-term TPN before biotin was included in commercial vitamin formulations. An infant with short gut syndrome received TPN from 5 months of age. Five months later, the infant lost all body hair and developed a waxy pallor, irritability, lethargy, mild hypotonia, and an erythematous rash. Biotin deficiency was confirmed biochemically, and all signs were reversed by supplementation (44). Two adult patients receiving home parenteral nutrition after extensive gut resection developed hair loss that was reversed by 200 μg biotin given intravenously daily (45). Another adult with alopecia, rash, and metabolic acidosis responded to 60 μg of biotin added to parenteral fluids (see Fig. 57.2D).

Toxicity

No reports of adverse effects of biotin intake up to 200 mg orally or 20 mg intravenously have been published.

Vitamin B₁₂ (Cobalamin)

Deficiency

Deficiency may be primary or secondary, as in pernicious anemia.

Pernicious Anemia. Pernicious anemia, an autoimmune disorder resulting in a deficiency of intrinsic factor, usually manifests after middle age, especially in persons with prematurely gray hair and blue eyes. A slight female preponderance exists. The most common complaints—those associated with anemia—ordinarily do not arise until the anemia is well advanced. Neurologic changes may long precede the hematologic changes. The tongue may be red, smooth, shiny, and painful. Anorexia, weight loss, indigestion, and episodic diarrhea are all usually present. In advanced cases, patients usually have pyrexia, enlargement of the liver and spleen, and occasionally bruising resulting from thrombocytopenia. Older patients may present with congestive cardiac failure.

Distal sensory neuropathy with stocking-glove sensory loss, paresthesias, and areflexia may occur in isolation or more commonly together with a form of myelopathy known as subacute combined degeneration of the spinal cord. In this condition, the initial symptom is symmetric paresthesias of the feet or, occasionally, of the hands. A combination of weakness and loss of postural sense makes walking increasingly difficult. Psychiatric disturbances, especially mild dementia, may be the presenting or only feature. Visual loss from optic atrophy is common. Congenital lack of intrinsic factor manifests before the age of 2 years with irritability, vomiting, diarrhea, weight loss, and megaloblastic anemia.

Primary Dietary Deficiency. When dietary lack or malabsorption is the cause of deficiency, megaloblastic anemia is usually the most prominent feature, but glossitis, optic atrophy, and subacute combined degeneration of the spinal cord have also been described. Hyperpigmentation of the skin of the forearms has been reported. Megaloblastic anemia developed in an infant who was exclusively breast-fed by a vegan mother (46).

Folic Acid

Deficiency

The anemia of folic acid deficiency has morphologic features indistinguishable from those of vitamin B₁₂ deficiency, but it develops much more rapidly. Subacute combined degeneration of the spinal cord does not occur, but approximately 20% of patients may have peripheral neuropathy. The tongue may be red and painful in the acute stage. In chronic deficiency, the tongue papillae atrophy, leaving a shiny, smooth surface. Hyperpigmentation of the skin similar to that occasionally seen in vitamin B₁₂ deficiency has been noted.

Folic acid therapy before conception is now accepted as protective against neural tube defects in infants of families in which these abnormalities have previously arisen (47). Low plasma folate levels were associated with an increased risk of early spontaneous abortion (48).

Toxicity

The required addition of 400 μg per serving of ready-to-eat cereals has raised the question of excess. Using data from the Food and Drug Administration, the Food and Nutrition Board of the Institute of Medicine stated, "It is unlikely that intake of folate added to foods or as supplements would regularly exceed 1000 μg for any of the life stage or gender groups" (49).

Administration of folate for megaloblastic anemia should be given only after ruling out cobalamin deficiency as the primary cause, because folate administration may improve the hematologic manifestations of vitamin B_{12} deficiency without arresting its neurologic effects.

Caution should be exercised in the use of nitrous oxide anesthesia because of the possibility of the presence of a rare and severe methylene tetrahydrofolate reductase deficiency that may lead, as it did in the case of a child, to death associated with high homocysteine and low methionine blood levels (50, 51).

Vitamin C (Ascorbic Acid)

Deficiency

Scurvy tends to affect either the very young or the elderly. The clinical picture differs in these two groups.

Infantile Scurvy (Barlow Disease). The onset of infantile scurvy, usually in the second half of the first year of life, is preceded by a period of fretfulness, pallor, and loss of appetite. Localizing signs are tenderness and swelling, most marked at the knees or ankles. These signs result from characteristic bone changes demonstrable by radiograph.

The infant often adopts the "pithed frog" position of maximum comfort, with the legs flexed at the knees and the hips partially flexed and externally rotated. The arms are less commonly involved. Hemorrhage and spongy changes in the gums are confined to the sites of teeth that have recently erupted or are about to do so. Bleeding may occur anywhere in the skin (the orbit is a frequent site) or from mucous membranes, including the renal tract. In infancy, intracranial hemorrhages are rapidly progressive if treatment is delayed, and death may occur. Petechiae and ecchymoses, usually found in the region of the bone lesions, are less common than in the adult. Microcytic hypochromic anemia is common, whereas a normochromic normocytic picture is less so. Older children may develop the perifollicular hemorrhages and hair changes seen in the adult.

Adult Scurvy. Early symptoms of adult scurvy are weakness, easy fatigue, and listlessness, followed by shortness of breath and aching bones, joints, and muscles,

especially at night. These symptoms are followed by characteristic changes in the skin (52). Acne, indistinguishable from that of adolescence, precedes defects in the hairs of the body. These defects consist of broken and coiled ("corkscrew") hairs and a "swan-neck" deformity. Perifollicular hemorrhages and perifollicular hyperkeratosis are common, especially on the thorax, forearms, thighs, legs, and anterior abdominal wall (see Fig. 57.2E and F).

Frank bleeding is a late feature of scurvy. The classic gum changes are associated only with natural teeth or buried roots and are enhanced by poor dental hygiene and advanced caries. The interdental papillae become swollen and purple and bleed with trauma. In advanced scurvy, the gums are spongy and friable, bleeding freely. Secondary infection leads to loosening of the teeth and to gangrene. Patients who are edentulous or whose teeth are in good repair have little or no evidence of scorbutic gingivitis. Hemorrhage commonly occurs deep in muscles and into joints, as well as over large areas of the skin in the form of ecchymoses. Multiple splinter hemorrhages may form a crescent near the distal ends of the nails. Old scars break down, and new wounds fail to heal. Bleeding into viscera or the brain leads to convulsions and shock; death may occur abruptly.

Toxicity

Long-term supplementation of vitamin C in excess of the tolerable upper limit can cause diarrhea, kidney stones, and excess iron absorption.

Choline

The feeding of a choline-deficient diet restricted in methionine resulted in decreased choline stores in a large number of species ranging from rodents to baboons and caused liver dysfunction in most. Many also had growth retardation, renal dysfunction, hemorrhage, or bone abnormalities (53).

A low-choline diet ingested for 3 weeks by healthy men resulted in decreased plasma choline levels and some abnormal liver functions as indicated by a liver function test (54). In a placebo-controlled study of patients receiving parenteral feeding that compared a choline- and lipid-free formula plus placebo with a similar formula with choline, results of liver chemistry studies became elevated, with evidence of liver steatosis. No changes in total bilirubin, hemoglobin, hematocrit, white blood cells, platelets, or other blood chemistry studies were noted (55). In a pilot study of patients receiving TPN, evidence indicated that a low-choline formula caused verbal and visual impairment (56).

However, evidence of a choline requirement in experimental laboratory animals occurred only in those with reduced dietary methionine. This finding is relevant because of the close relationships of choline, methionine, folate, and vitamin B_{12}. The human studies did not examine the role of added methionine or cysteine or of the

Molybdenum

Deficiency

An autosomal recessive molybdenum cofactor deficiency resulting in deficiencies of xanthine oxidase and sulfite oxidase was reported in more than 20 patients (86). Patients had severe brain damage and frequent convulsions, and about half failed to survive beyond early infancy.

Only one clear-cut case related to prolonged TPN has been reported, involving tachycardia, tachypnea, headache, night blindness, central scotomas, nausea, vomiting, lethargy, disorientation, and coma (87). These manifestations were reversed by 300 μg/day of molybdenum, and the urinary excretion of abnormal amounts of methionine was dramatically decreased.

Toxicity

Elevated blood levels of molybdenum secondary to intakes of 10 to 15 mg/day were associated with hyperuricemia and a goutlike syndrome in Armenia in 1961 (88). However, other investigators were unable to confirm this effect of molybdenum (26).

Manganese

Deficiency

One unsubstantiated case of human manganese deficiency was reported to have occurred when manganese was inadvertently omitted from an experimental diet fed to a volunteer. Clinical signs included weight loss, transient dermatitis, nausea and vomiting, changes in hair color, and slow growth of hair (89).

Toxicity

Manganese toxicity is usually reported in persons who mine or refine ore. Initial signs include insomnia, depression, and delusions, followed by anorexia, arthralgias, and weakness. Eventually changes occur resembling parkinsonism or Wilson disease. Well water with high manganese content may be responsible for occurrence of a parkinsonian syndrome (90). Manganese accumulates in the basal ganglia of patients with biliary obstruction and cirrhosis of the liver, and investigators have suggested that this may be associated with the occurrence of encephalopathy in these patients (91). The excess manganese is associated with high signal intensity in the basal ganglion on a magnetic resonance imaging scan.

REFERENCES

1. Black RD, Allen LH, Bhutta ZA et al. Lancet 2008;371:243–60.
2. Hathcock JN. Am J Clin Nutr 1997;66:427–37.
3. McLaren DS. Nutritional Ophthalmology. New York: Academic Press, 1980.
4. Sommer A, West KP Jr. Vitamin A Deficiency, Health, Survival and Vision. New York: Oxford University Press, 1996.
5. Sommer A, Hussaini G, Muhilal et al. Am J Clin Nutr 1980;33: 887–91.
6. Sommer A, Emran N, Tamba T. Am J Ophthalmol 1979; 87:330–3.
7. Teng KH. Ophthalmologica 1959;137:81–5.
8. International Vitamin A Consultative Group. The Symptoms and Signs of Vitamin A Deficiency and Their Relationship to Applied Nutrition. Washington, DC: International Vitamin A Consultative Group, 1981.
9. Hathcock JN, Hattan DG, Jenkins MY et al. Am J Clin Nutr 1990;52:183–202.
10. Lammer EJ, Chen DT, Hoar RM et al. N Engl J Med 1985; 313:837–41.
11. Rothman KJ, Moore LL, Singer MR et al. N Engl J Med 1995; 333:1369–73.
12. Michaelsson K, Lithel H, Vessly B et al. N Engl J Med 2003; 384:287–94.
13. Melhus H, Michaelsson K, Kindmark A et al. Ann Intern Med 1998;129:770–8.
14. Feskanich D, Singh V, Willett C et al. JAMA 2002;287:47–54.
15. Train JJA, Yates RW, Sury MRJ. BMJ 1995;310:48–9.
16. Blau EB. Lancet 1996;347:626.
17. Glenrup H, Mikkelsen K, Poulsen L et al. Calcif Tissue Int 2000;66:419–24.
18. Black JA, Bonham Carter JE. Lancet 1963;2:745–9.
19. Rosenberg RN. N Engl J Med 1995;333:1351–2.
20. Johnson L, Bowen FW Jr, Abbasi S et al. Pediatrics 1985;75: 619–38.
21. Miller ER 3rd, Pastor-Barriuso R, Dalal D et al. Ann Intern Med 2005;142:37-46.
22. Shearer MJ. Lancet 1995;345:229–34.
23. American Academy of Pediatrics Committee on Fetus and Newborn. Pediatrics 2003;112:191–2.
24. Pettifor JM, Benson R. J Pediatr 1975;86:459–62.
25. Feskanich D, Weber P, Willett WC et al. Am J Clin Nutr 1999; 69:74–9.
26. Food and Nutrition Board, Institute of Medicine. Dietary Reference Intakes for Vitamin A, Vitamin K, Arsenic, Boron, Chromium, Copper, Iodine, Iron, Manganese, Molybdenum, Nickel, Silicon, Vanadium, and Zinc. Washington, DC: National Academy Press, 2001:187.
27. Campbell CH. Lancet 1984;2:446–9.
28. Jeffrey FE, Abelmann WH. Am J Med 1971;50:123–8.
29. Haas RH. Annu Rev Nutr 1988;8:483–515.
30. Editorial. Lancet 1990;2:912–3.
31. Victor M, Adams RD, Collins GH. The Wernicke-Korsakoff Syndrome. Oxford: Blackwell, 1971.
32. Seehra H, MacDermott N, Lascelles RG et al. BMJ 1996; 312:434.
33. Jelliffe DB. Infant Nutrition in the Tropics and Subtropics. 2nd ed. Geneva: World Health Organization, 1968.
34. Food and Nutrition Board, Institute of Medicine. Dietary Reference Intakes for Thiamin, Riboflavin, Niacin, Vitamin B6, Folate, Vitamin B12, Pantothenic Acid, Biotin, and Choline. Washington, DC: National Academy Press, 2000:81.
35. Stephens JM, Grant R, Yeh CS. Am J Emerg Med 1992;10:61–3.
36. Lopez R, Cole HS, Montoya MF et al. J Pediatr 1975;87:420–2.
37. Food and Nutrition Board, Institute of Medicine. Dietary Reference Intakes for Thiamin, Riboflavin, Niacin, Vitamin B6, Folate, Vitamin B12, Pantothenic Acid, Biotin, and Choline. Washington, DC: National Academy Press, 2000:115.
38. Hankes LV, Nicotinic acid and nicotinamide. In: Machlin LJ, ed. Handbook of Vitamins. New York: Marcel Dekker, 1984: 329–77.
39. Mueller JE, Vilter RW. J Clin Invest 1950;29:193–201.
40. Snyderman SE, Holt LE, Carretero R et al. Am J Clin Nutr 1953;1:200.
41. Bessey OA, Adam DJ, Hansen AE. Pediatrics 1957;20:33–44.

42. Weintraub LR, Conrad ME, Crosby WH. N Engl J Med 1966; 275:169–76.

43. Schaumberg H, Kaplan J, Windebank A et al. N Engl J Med 1983;309:445–8.

44. Mock DM, DeLorimer AA, Leberman WM et al. N Engl J Med 1981;304:820–3.

45. Innis SM, Allardyce DB. Am J Clin Nutr 1983;37:185–7.

46. Higginbottom MC, Sweetman K, Nyhan WL. N Engl J Med 1978;299:317–20.

47. MRC Vitamin Study Research Group. Lancet 1991;338:131–7.

48. George L, Mills JL, Johansson ALV et al. JAMA 2002;288:1867–73.

49. Food and Nutrition Board, Institute of Medicine. Dietary Reference Intakes for Thiamin, Riboflavin, Niacin, Vitamin B$_6$, Folate, Vitamin B$_{12}$, Pantothenic Acid, Biotin, and Choline. Washington, DC: National Academy Press, 2000:283.

50. Rothenberg SP, daCosta MP, Sequeira J et al. N Engl J Med 2004;350:134–42.

51. Erbe RW, Salis RJ. N Engl J Med 2003;349:5–6.

52. Hodges RF, Hood J, Canham JE et al. Am J Clin Nutr 1971; 24:432–43.

53. Food and Nutrition Board, Institute of Medicine. Dietary Reference Intakes for Thiamin, Riboflavin, Niacin, Vitamin B$_6$, Folate, Vitamin B$_{12}$, Pantothenic Acid, Biotin, and Choline. Washington, DC: National Academy Press, 2000:396.

54. Zeisel SH, da Costa KA, Franklin PD et al. FASEB J 1991; 5:2093–98.

55. Buchman AC, Ament ME, Sobel M et al. JPEN J Parenter Enteral Nutr 2001;25:260–68.

56. Buchman AL, Sobel M, Brown M et al. JPEN J Parenter Enteral Nutr 2001;25:30–35.

57. Fleming CR, Smith LM, Hodges RE. Am J Clin Nutr 1976; 29:976–83.

58. Holman RT, Johnson SB, Hatch TF. Am J Clin Nutr 1982; 35:617–23.

59. Anderson GJ, Connor WE. Am J Clin Nutr 1989;49:585–7.

60. Bentur L, Alon U, Berant M. Pediatr Rev Commun 1987;1: 291–310.

61. Bishop N. N Engl J Med 1999;341:602–4.

62. Thacher TD, Fischer PR, Pettifor JM et al. N Engl J Med 1999;341:563–8.

63. Weinsier RL, Krumdieck CL. Am J Clin Nutr 1981;34:393–9.

64. Knochel JP. N Engl J Med 1985;313:447–9.

65. Berner YM, Shike M. Annu Rev Nutr 1988;8:121–48.

66. Britton J, Pavord I, Richards K et al. Lancet 1994;344:357–62.

67. Hetzel BS, Hay ID. Clin Endocrinol 1979;11:445–60.

68. Hetzel BS, Dunn JT. Annu Rev Nutr 1989;9:21–38.

69. Andersen HT, Barkve H. Scand J Clin Lab Invest Suppl 1970; 25:1–62.

70. Slotzfus RJ, Kvalsvig JD, Chwaya HN et al. BMJ 2001;323: 1389–96.

71. Danks DM. Annu Rev Nutr 1988;8:235–57.

72. Prasad AS. BMJ 2003;326:409–10.

73. Hambidge KM, Krebs NF, Walravens PA. Nutr Res 1985;1: 306–16.

74. Goldenberg RL, Tamura T, Neggers Y. JAMA 1995;274:463–8.

75. Younaszai HD. JPEN J Parenter Enteral Nutr 1983;7:72–4.

76. Golden MHN, Golden BE. Am J Clin Nutr 1981;34:900–8.

77. National Research Council. Health Effects of Ingested Fluoride. Washington, DC: National Academy Press, 1993.

78. Chen X, Yang G, Chen J et al. Biol Trace Elem Res 1980;2: 91–107.

79. Mo D. Pathology and selenium deficiency in Kashin-Beck disease. In: Combs GF Jr, Levander OA, Oldfield JE, eds. Selenium in Biology and Medicine. New York: Van Nostrand Reinhold, 1987:924–33.

80. Moreno-Reyes R, Mathieu F, Boelaert M et al. Am J Clin Nutr 2003;78:137–44.

81. Vinton NE, Dahlstrom KA, Strobel CT et al. J Pediatr 1987; 111:711–7.

82. Yang G, Wang S, Zhou R et al. Am J Clin Nutr 1983;37: 872–81.

83. Centers for Disease Control. MMWR Morb Mortal Wkly Rep 1984;33:157–8.

84. Jeejeebhoy KN, Chu RC, Marliss EB et al. Am J Clin Nutr 1977;30:531–8.

85. Verhage AH, Cheong WK, Jeejeebhoy KN. JPEN J Parenter Enteral Nutr 1996;20:123–7.

86. Rajagopalan KV. Annu Rev Nutr 1988;8:401–27.

87. Abumrad NN, Schneider AJ, Steele D et al. Am J Clin Nutr 1981;34:2551–9

88. Kovalski VV, Yatovaya GA, Shmavonyau DM. Zh Obshch Biol 1961;22:179.

89. Doisy EA Jr. Effects of deficiency in manganese upon plasma and cholesterol in man. In: Hoekstra WG, Suttie JW, Ganther HE et al, eds. Trace Element Metabolism in Animals, vol 2. Baltimore: University Park Press, 1974:668–70.

90. Kondakis XG, Makris N, Leotsinidis M et al. Arch Environ Health 1989;44:175–8.

91. Krieger D, Krieger S, Jansen O et al. Lancet 1995;346:270–4.

SUGGESTED READINGS

Black RD, Allen LH, Bhutta ZA et al. Maternal and child undernutrition: global and regional exposures and health consequences. Lancet 2008;371:243–60.

McLaren DS. A Colour Atlas and Text of Diet-Related Diseases. 2nd ed. London: Wolfe, 1992.

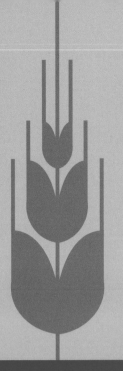

PREVENTION AND MANAGEMENT OF DISEASE

PART IV

PREVENTION AND MANAGEMENT OF DISEASE

Genetic Heritability of Body Weight

In family studies, BMI is correlated between first-degree family members (38), and having an overweight parent increases the risk that the children will become overweight (39, 40). In adoption studies, genetic factors account for 20% to 60% of the variation in BMI (41). The BMIs of the biologic, not adoptive, parents is more strongly correlated with the adult weight of the adoptive child (42). In data from numerous twin studies (>25,000 pairs), genetic factors explain 50% to 90% of the variance in BMI, especially in identical twins (41), regardless of whether twins were raised separately or apart (43).

Genetic Disorders Causing Obesity

Susceptibility to obesity appears to be a polygenic trait (related to more than one gene) in most people (44, 45); however, several rare monogenic (single gene) disorders have been identified where severe, early-onset obesity is often the predominant feature. Mutations or deficiency in genes that regulate body fat, body weight, or satiety have been associated with severe, early-onset obesity and include leptin (46), the leptin receptor (47), the melanocortin-4 receptor (MCR4) (48), proopiomelanocortin (POMC) (48, 49), and prohormone convertase 1 (PC1) (50). MCR4 mutations are the most common, accounting for up to 6% of cases (51).

Pleiotropic syndromes have multiple, widespread effects resulting from a single gene defect. The most common pleiotropic obesity syndrome is Prader-Willi syndrome (PWS), occurring in 1 in 25,000 births (52). PWS results from an abnormality on chromosome 15q11.2 and produces infantile myotonia, mental retardation, hypogonadism, overeating, and early-onset obesity (53). Other obesity syndromes include Bardet-Biedl syndrome, Albright hereditary osteodystrophy, fragile X syndrome, Börjeson-Forssman-Lehmann syndrome, Cohen syndrome, and Alström syndrome (53).

Genetic Influences on Common Susceptibility to Obesity

Susceptibility to obesity in most of the population is likely caused by input of multiple genes that influence food intake and energy expenditure, with additional interactions between genes and environment. Numerous genes have been identified that appear to be associated, either directly or indirectly, with the regulation of body weight (54). These susceptibility genes likely code for metabolic and hormonal factors that regulate aspects of energy intake, energy use, and energy expenditure. Common variants (or polymorphisms) of these genes could affect individual susceptibility to obesity. Through natural selection, these genes may have become more common because of the evolutionary advantage that they offer by promoting energy storage to survive periods of food deprivation. Within our current environment, these genes are now associated with an increased risk of obesity and associated metabolic diseases, such as type 2 diabetes (55). Identification of new genes, their role in weight gain, and their interactions with the environment is a rapidly progressing area of research. Polymorphisms

within the fat mass and obesity-associated gene (*FTO*) on chromosome 16 became the first to be associated reproducibly with the risk of being overweight or obese in multiple populations (56). Studies have yet to identify the exact mechanism of action, but they suggest that the FTO gene product may be involved in controlling food intake.

An emerging field called epigenetics also explains some of the impact of genes on the development of obesity. Epigenetics is the study of gene function alterations, induced without DNA sequence modifications, that are heritable (57). Epigenetic marks can affect different biologic processes such as imprinting. Imprinted disorders such as PWS, discussed in the previous section, often include obesity among their clinical characteristics (57).

Medical Conditions That Can Contribute to Development of Obesity

Numerous medical conditions are associated with obesity. Endocrine disorders associated with weight gain include Cushing's syndrome, hypothyroidism, adult growth hormone deficiency, and polycystic ovarian syndrome (58). Psychiatric conditions include binge eating disorder (59), night eating syndrome, and depression (60). Injury to the ventromedial or paraventricular regions of the hypothalamus or the amygdala leads to hyperphagia and obesity. Iatrogenic weight gain is often caused by medication use with certain drug classes, such as steroid hormones, antidepressants, and antidiabetic agents. Weight gain with these drugs is generally modest, except with high-dose corticosteroids, which can produce true obesity (58). Drugs that may promote weight gain and their therapeutic alternatives are shown in Table 58.2.

Environmental Influences on Obesity

Kelly Brownell was one of the first people to postulate that certain environmental factors can promote obesity. The food environment in developed countries facilitates increased food intake because of the overabundance of inexpensive, calorie-dense foods (61). In addition, the physical activity environment discourages physical activity because it is no longer commonly required for transportation or for securing food and shelter (61). The end result is an environment that serves to increase energy intake and reduce energy expenditure. A summary of environmental factors providing a constant pressure toward positive energy balance and an increase in body fat mass is shown in Figure 58.4. More recently, additional environmental factors such as prenatal and early postnatal influences, environmental toxins, viruses, smoking cessation, and sleep deprivation have also been hypothesized to be involved in promoting the development of obesity.

Environmental Influences on Energy Intake

The environment can influence behaviors surrounding the amount and composition of the food we eat. Factors related to diet composition, portion size, dietary variety, and cost

TABLE 58.2	DRUGS THAT MAY PROMOTE WEIGHT GAIN AND THERAPEUTIC ALTERNATIVES

DRUGS THAT MAY PROMOTE WEIGHT GAIN	DRUGS THAT ARE WEIGHT NEUTRAL OR PROMOTE WEIGHT LOSS
Psychiatric/neurologic medications	Alternative psychiatric/neurologic medications
Antipsychotic drugs	Antipsychotic drugs
Olanzapine, clozapine	Ziprasidone, risperidone, quetiapine
Antidepressants	Antidepressants
SSRIs, TCAs, MAOIs	Bupropion, nefazodone
Antiepileptic drugs	Antiepileptic drugs
Gabapentin, valproate, carbamazepine	Topiramate, lamotrigine
Lithium	Alternatives to steroid hormones
Steroid hormones	Barrier contraceptive methods
Hormonal contraceptives	NSAIDs
Corticosteroids	Weight loss
Progestational steroids	Alternative antidiabetic agents
Antidiabetic agents	Metformin
Insulin	Acarbose, miglitol
Sulfonylureas	Orlistat, sibutramine
Thiazolidinediones	Decongestants, inhalers
Antihistamines	Alternative antihypertensive agents
Antihypertensive agents	ACE inhibitors, calcium channel blockers
α- and β-Adrenergic blockers	
Protease inhibitors[a]	

ACE, angiotensin-converting enzyme; MAOI, monoamine oxidase inhibitor; NSAID, nonsteroidal anti-inflammatory drug; SSRI, selective serotonin reuptake inhibitor; TCA, tricyclic antidepressant.

[a]May cause weight gain, but less than the drugs they replace.

Reprinted with permission from Aronne LJ, Segal KR. Weight gain in the treatment of mood disorders. J Clin Psychiatry 2003;64(Suppl):22–9.

and convenience of food may all affect energy intake and thus the propensity to positive energy balance and obesity.

Dietary Fat
Diets high in fat have been suggested to increase the risk of obesity. Sedentary animals given unrestricted access to high-fat diets gain weight and become obese as compared with those given unrestricted access to a low-fat diet (62). Because human subjects also tend to eat a constant weight of food on both high- and low-fat diets, high-fat diets seem to increase the risk for overeating and excessive caloric intake (62). A comprehensive review of the epidemiologic literature on the relationship between dietary fat intake and body weight (63) concluded that although the data are not entirely consistent, it appears that that the more dietary fat humans consume, the greater their body weight.

Energy Density
Energy density is the "amount of energy [calories or joules] in a given weight [grams] of food (kcal/g or kJ/g)" (64).

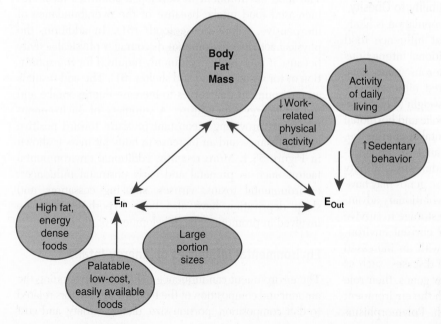

Fig. 58.4. Environmental factors providing a constant pressure toward positive energy (*E*) balance and an increase in body fat mass. (Reprinted with permission from Hill JO, Wyatt HR, Melanson EL. Genetic and environmental contributions to obesity. Med Clin North Am 2000;84:333–46.)

discrimination contribute to low self-esteem and depression among obese people who seek treatment. Notable also are the greater social stigma borne by obese women compared with obese men in the United States and the higher prevalence of obesity among those of low socioeconomic status, African-Americans, Latinos, and Native Americans. For example, approximately 80% of middle-aged African-American women in the United States are overweight or obese. Compelling evidence shows health benefits associated with even modest weight loss, a finding suggesting that people who are obese should be encouraged to lose weight (15–18).

This chapter aims to provide an overview of the assessment and treatment of obesity, with the primary focus on dietary and exercise interventions. Pharmacologic and surgical therapies are a second-line option in the treatment of obesity and are reviewed in less depth.

EVALUATING OBESITY

Physical Assessment

Classification of obesity was proposed by an expert panel convened by the National Institute of Health, National Heart, Lung, and Blood Institute (NHLBI) in 1998 after extensive review of health complications associated with this condition (19). The panel classified obesity and overweight status based on BMI and waist circumference. Associated disease risk is shown in Table 59.1 (20). Obesity is technically defined as an excess of body fat (>25% of body weight for men and >30% for women), rather than an excess of body weight in itself (19). However, the measurement of percentage of body fat is more difficult to obtain and is not as intuitive as body weight. Thus, relative weight is a reasonable surrogate measure for adiposity. Measuring weight adjusted for height, or BMI, defined as weight in kilograms divided by the square of the height in meters, is usually the first step in assessing obesity and is very useful for diagnosing and grading the severity of the condition and its attendant risks (see Table 59.1). Although BMI is the standard measure of relative weight, it may

overstate the actual degree of adiposity in very muscular people (e.g., certain types of athletes and laborers), and it may understate adiposity in very sedentary individuals with little muscle mass. The latter is called *sarcopenic obesity*, characterized by a normal or low BMI with increased percentage of body fat and reduced lean body mass. A BMI of 25 to 30 kg/m^2 is defined as overweight, 30 to 40 kg/m^2 as obese, and 40 kg/m^2 or higher as severely or morbidly/grade III obese (20).

Waist circumference is the second step in the assessment of obesity. A waist circumference larger than 88 cm (35 in) in women and larger than 102 cm (40 in) in men constitutes abdominal or visceral obesity and is associated with an increased risk of health complications (20). Waist circumference can be easily measured with a tape rule around the widest point above the hips. In the case of abdominal fat deposition, even mild excess adiposity may pose medical complications, such as increased risk of hypertension, dyslipidemias, and type 2 diabetes (10, 20–22). Visceral obesity can exist even in the absence of overall obesity (i.e., at BMIs below the cutoff points for obesity or overweight) (10, 20–22). With visceral obesity, even with a normal BMI, it is probably best to encourage weight loss for medical reasons, especially if the patient already suffers from complicating medical conditions or has a strong family history of diabetes, cardiovascular, or cerebrovascular disease. For patients with cosmetic or trivial obesity, the benefits (and motivators) for successful weight loss are more psychosocial than medical. These patients should be encouraged to focus on a healthier diet (with low refined carbohydrate, low saturated fat, and high fiber) and increased physical fitness rather than just the number on the scale.

Psychosocial and Behavioral Assessment

A psychosocial and behavioral assessment should be performed because it can provide considerable information about the patient's readiness to lose weight as well as identify disordered eating behaviors. Obese individuals commonly exhibit depression, with the degree of severity often greater with severe obesity (23–25). A behavioral

TABLE 59.1	CLASSIFICATION OF OVERWEIGHT AND OBESITY BY BODY MASS INDEX, WAIST CIRCUMFERENCE, AND ASSOCIATED DISEASE RISK				
			DISEASE RISK RELATIVE TO NORMAL WEIGHT AND WAIST CIRCUMFERENCE		
WEIGHT CATEGORY	BMI	OBESITY CLASS	MEN <102 cm (<40 in) WOMEN <88 cm (<35 in)	MEN >102 cm (>40 in) WOMEN >88 cm (>35 in)	
Underweight	<18				
Normal	18.5–24.9				
Overweight	25.0–29.9		Increased	High	
Obesity	30.0–34.9	I	High	Very high	
	35.0–39.9	II	Very high	Very high	
Extreme obesity	>40.0	III	Extremely high	Extremely high	

BMI, body mass index.

Adapted with permission from National Institutes of Health, National Heart, Lung, and Blood Institute. Clinical Guidelines on the Identification, Evaluation, and Treatment of Overweight and Obesity in Adults—The Evidence Report. National Institutes of Health.

psychologist or other skilled professional can inquire into depressive symptoms by asking about the patient's mood and related symptoms and signs or assessing depression with formal tests (26). Obese persons with significant depression should be provided appropriate treatment (cognitive behavior therapy or pharmacotherapy) before or during weight reduction efforts.

Approximately 30% of obese individuals who seek weight reduction suffer from *binge eating disorder* (27). Binge eating is characterized by consumption of large amounts of food until one is uncomfortably full and eating alone when not hungry. In addition, patients have a loss of control over eating behavior and a negative emotional state after the binge (27). Other clues to the presence of an eating disorder or binge eating disorder include altered body image (believing one is obese when one is not) and obsession with one's body weight (recurring thoughts or weighing oneself multiple times daily). When purging (vomiting or using laxatives or diuretics) or compulsive exercise is used following binging to control weight, *bulimia nervosa,* rather than binge eating disorder, is the likely diagnosis. Although anorexia nervosa and bulimia nervosa are commonly recognized as serious eating disorders (28), binge eating disorder is more common and often occurs in those who are overweight or obese rather than underweight. Merely prescribing a diet is usually not helpful and may even be counterproductive in an obese patient suffering from this disorder. Referral to a specialized treatment program may be helpful. Specific cognitive behavioral therapies have been developed for the treatment of binge eating disorder (29); however, the condition often responds favorably to a structured, individualized weight loss program along with behavioral therapy. Behavioral evaluation also may identify situations, feelings, or other issues that lead to inappropriate eating (i.e., eating that is not triggered by hunger).

Evaluating Dietary and Activity Habits

A complete dietary and physical assessment is helpful in evaluating the contribution of these factors to weight gain in an obese individual (30). This assessment can identify problem areas related to diet and exercise that may need modification to lose weight. Formal methods of assessing diet intake including 24-hour recall, 7-day food records, food frequency questionnaires (FFQs), and structured interviews (31–33) can help to determine the obese person's current food choices and eating habits. Moreover, general discussions such as talking about past dieting experiences (if applicable) and asking the reason the patient thinks that he or she was not successful in the past can help in learning more about the patient's motivations, needs, and barriers to change.

It is important also to ask about current medications, including over-the-counter or prescription drugs, herbs, and vitamin or mineral supplements if any. This information can help assess for potential food–drug interactions,

assess daily intake in relation to nutrient requirements, and assist in the evaluation of methods used to address weight and nutritional issues by the patient. Often, an obese person reveals more information to a dietitian when specifically probed to answer these questions than when meeting with a primary health care provider. Any food allergies or intolerances (e.g., gluten, lactose) also should be covered.

Different dietary assessment methods have their strengths and limitations. For example, a 24-hour diet recall is helpful in assessing food and beverage intake, including the type and amount of food, brand names of foods, cooking methods, time of day, and location of eating (31–33). Multiple-day food records or food diaries assess food and beverage consumption over a period of typically 3 to 7 days, and intake is recorded either before or after eating. It is helpful for both the patient and the clinician to discuss how to measure or estimate food portions appropriately to create accurate accounts of food consumed and to document as many aspects of the food as possible (e.g., method of food preparation, type and amount of condiments used, name brands, restaurant names). Behaviorally relevant information also can be recorded in multiple-day food diaries, including an assessment of hunger levels before and after eating, in addition to feelings, thoughts, and situations surrounding the eating event. Nutritional information and calculations can be included, such as calories, fat grams, carbohydrate servings, sodium, and others. Accuracy depends on the person's memory, completeness of reporting, and the interviewing and communication skills of both the patient and the evaluator.

The data gleaned from any dietary assessments should be interpreted with caution, however, because retrospective and even prospective underreporting and overreporting are common. FFQs are self-administered tests with multiple questions about frequency of consumption and portion size of many different foods over the prior 1 month or 3 months. Questions in FFQs also may include information on food purchasing and preparation methods. FFQs can help identify inadequacy or overconsumption of specific food groups, or patterns of specific foods or preparation methods. Like the food diary, the FFQ can offer a more real-life assessment of the patient's typical food choices because it can be completed outside of the provider's office.

Reduced levels of physical activity can be a major factor in the etiology of obesity and may be a direct result of acute or chronic illness, job change or retirement, or just sedentary lifestyles in general, such as more television viewing or screen time (34–37). An inventory of the person's usual physical activity and preferred forms of exercise can identify opportunities for increasing the level of energy expended through physical activity. Food record forms can include a place for physical activity, which can be helpful in discussing exercise habits and goals. However, the provider must recognize and communicate that exercise alone is, unfortunately, not an effective method for losing weight. It is difficult for the untrained person to do enough of it, and most, if not all, of the expended energy may be compensated by increased caloric intake. Exercise is a very good way to maintain a lower weight after weight loss, thus enabling a person to eat somewhat more than a nonexerciser and maintain weight. Regular aerobic exercise and strength training also will improve cardiovascular fitness, trim inches, and promote growth of metabolically more active muscle tissue.

The exercise assessment should include a record of the usual degree of physical activity, any limiting factors such as joint disease or previous injuries, types of activity the patient finds enjoyable, and a measurement, preferably by an exercise physiologist or certified trainer of the current fitness level. Physical activity level can be assessed broadly by inquiring about the amount of walking done in a day, flights of stairs climbed, and hours of television watched (38). More formal assessment can be conducted using a pedometer to determine the number of steps walked daily, or an accelerometer, which also can assess the intensity of activity.

A rule of thumb in prescribing an exercise regimen is to use a phased-in approach. Most obese patients start out with a limited capacity to exercise. Rather than suggesting a type or level of activity that is unlikely to maximize adherence, make sure that the plan fits the patient's current abilities, schedule, and lifestyle. The first phase often consists of increasing the amount of everyday physical activity, so-called lifestyle activity, without introducing a formal exercise regimen. Lifestyle activities include taking the stairs in gradually increasing fashion, parking the car farther away from the destination, walking to the mailbox, and the like. This phase alone may double the level of physical activity in a very sedentary person.

The next phase is a walking plan. People are most likely to comply with such a plan if the walk is scheduled during typically available times, such as a break or lunchtime during work hours. Scheduling exercise when the individual's daily energy level is the highest (e.g., early morning for many people) is often more effective than at the end of a long day. Having a companion to walk with and a place to walk indoors also are helpful in increasing adherence.

One half hour is a good minimum time to recommend that a patient should make available for each session of exercise. An hour or longer is best for weight control. The intensity of the exercise is not critical to the burning of calories: walking at a leisurely pace for 1 hour is roughly equal to walking briskly for half an hour. Allow the patient to set the pace. Initially, it may be quite slow, but in the absence of severe pulmonary, cardiovascular, or joint disease, most patients soon find the going easier and faster. Goal setting can strengthen this reinforcement. Having the patient keep a log of the time spent walking and the distance covered after each session is useful. The patient can then see the progress being made and can set the goal a bit higher as warranted.

In the next phase of a progressive exercise plan, the types of activities performed should be broadened.

Walking or jogging can and should remain a feature at this stage, but with the addition of other forms of aerobic exercise. Perhaps recommend aerobics classes, stationary or outdoor bicycling, swimming, a cross-country skiing machine, or just about anything else that will burn calories and be enjoyable to the patient. Team or racquet sports and golf can be suggested to provide social interaction, as well as to increase energy expenditure. Again, the most important criterion for a good exercise plan is one that the patient is likely to follow and be comfortable with as a lifelong habit.

Weight Loss Readiness

Successful weight loss can be achieved and maintained when the obese individual is determined and motivated. For this, the provider must assess and evaluate the readiness state of the individual. It is essential for the obese individual to be motivated to make lasting lifestyle changes; however, internal self-motivation is more sustainable than external motivators such as a spouse's demands or the anticipation of a special event. The stages of change model for behavior change intervention may be useful in assessing where an individual is with regard to making behavior changes and in helping the individual move along the continuum from precontemplation to action stages (39). Although internal motivation is the key to successful weight loss and maintenance, external stimuli, such as support from friends and family, and environmental factors, such as easy access to healthful foods and safe places to walk and run, also play important roles. Garnering these support systems can assist the individual to be mentally ready to move along the path of the action stage of weight loss and then weight maintenance efforts.

The provider should assist the obese individual to set goals that are "smart goals" (i.e., ones that are specific, measurable, achievable, realistic, and timely) because such goals are more likely to be achieved. Social support from family and friends also can improve the likelihood of success in making behavior changes. Enlisting help from others (e.g., in keeping trigger foods outside the house and in trying healthier foods) has been shown to improve the chances of success (40). In addition to support from family and friends, online or local weight loss support groups provide opportunities for discussing challenges and giving or receiving support. These can improve a patient's outcome both during and after initial treatment.

SELECTING THE RIGHT TREATMENT

Initial weight loss should be achieved with a comprehensive program that includes dietary changes, increased physical activity, and behavior modification. The recommended rate of weight loss depends on the degree of obesity, the presence or absence of comorbid conditions, the results of behavioral assessment, and patient preference. According to NHLBI guidelines (20), overweight individuals (BMI = 25 to 29.9 kg/m^2) without any associated risk factors should be encouraged to prevent further weight gain or lose weight with simple dietary modifications. However, if this condition is accompanied by one or more cardiovascular risk factors, lifestyle modification is recommended in which diet, exercise, and behavior therapy may be helpful. Similarly, for individuals with moderate obesity (BMI >30 kg/m^2) and no additional risk factors, lifestyle modifications are beneficial, aiming for a rate of weight loss of 1 to 1.5 lb/week (a calorie deficit of 500 to 750 kcal/day), a rate that is generally safe and rapid enough to sustain motivation. However, for individuals with BMI greater than 30 kg/m^2, or greater than 27 with medically important comorbid conditions, if lifestyle modifications alone are not successful, pharmacologic interventions may be an option. For individuals with severe obesity (BMI >35 kg/m^2 with comorbidities, or >40 kg/m^2 without), more aggressive energy restriction under medical supervision may be preferable. In the presence of significant comorbid conditions for individuals with severe obesity, bariatric surgery is an option to be considered as well.

DIETARY INTERVENTION

Weight gain is always a result of excess energy intake compared with energy expenditure. This creates a state of positive energy balance, eventually resulting in obesity or in greater obesity for those already obese (41). Although certain circumstances can increase energy intake and decrease energy expenditure, in the United States typically, volitional or semivolitional increases in food intake along with sedentary lifestyle are what throw off the balance between energy input and energy output.

Although diet therapy remains the cornerstone of weight loss (42), adherence to diet is often difficult for those trying to lose weight, with failure to follow the recommended diet consistently. Although the diet often recommended contains 50% to 55% of calories from carbohydrates, less than 30% from fat, and 15% from protein (42), low satiety, palatability issues, and lack of variety are often experienced, resulting in low adherence to standard, heart-healthy diets (42). A low-fat, low-refined carbohydrate diet allows for less restriction in the volume of food consumed because fatty and processed foods are more energy dense.

To lose weight at 1 to 2 lb/week, a healthy rate of weight loss as recommended by NHLBI guidelines (20), a calorie deficit of 500 to 1000 calories/day is required. Both dietary intake restriction and increased exercise can contribute to the energy deficit required (3500 calories = 1 lb of fat). Low-calorie diets (LCDs) contain 800 to 1500 kcal/day; on occasion, very-low-calorie diets (VLCDs), which contain fewer than 800 kcal/day, may be necessary to lose weight adequately among individuals with severe obesity, especially when they have serious comorbid conditions. VLCDs should be used under medical supervision (20).

Moderate Energy-Deficit Diets

Moderate energy-deficit diets (1500 to 1800 kcal/day) follow the guidelines laid out by the US Department of Agriculture *Dietary Guidelines for Americans* (43). A caloric deficit of 500 calories/day can be created to achieve approximately 1 lb of weight loss/week. The provider can design a low-calorie, food-based diet that has either a balanced deficit (reducing total number of calories while keeping proportions from carbohydrate, fat, and protein roughly the same as before) or a fat deficit (with most of the caloric reduction resulting from restriction of fat intake). The fat-deficit approach may be preferable for individuals consuming too much fat, especially saturated fat. In addition, a greater volume of food can be eaten on a diet that emphasizes complex and vegetable-source carbohydrates and reduces fat to less than 30% of calories consumed.

Restricting dietary fat is an approach that can serve to minimize hunger while maximizing satiety by replacing dietary fat with complex carbohydrates such as fruits, vegetables, and whole grains, which are less energy-dense (lower calorie), higher in fiber and water content, and more filling than foods with higher energy density, which tend to be higher in fat and sugar content. Moreover, research shows that the US population consumes diets that are high in fat and sugar and low in fiber (44–46), which are associated with high energy density and subsequent weight gain (47–50). This dietary approach to reduce weight often works, at least short term; because gram for gram, fat has more than double the calories of carbohydrates or proteins (9 versus 4 calories/g). For this reason, teaching individuals how to eat a larger volume of food for any given number of calories by focusing on a combination of complex carbohydrates and lean proteins is invaluable. In addition, lowering fat intake can help boost metabolism because fewer calories are used to convert dietary fat into body fat compared with carbohydrates and proteins. A relatively low-fat diet can improve cholesterol and reduce risk for chronic disease as well. Finally, these diets may be easier to adhere to because small changes are required in eating habits (e.g., cutting out hidden fats and simple sugars).

Low-Calorie Diets

For patients with BMIs between 25 and 34.9, especially those with comorbidities such as type 2 diabetes or high blood pressure, an LCD (800 to 1500 kcal/day) is appropriate as a first-line approach. This diet provides 800 to 1500 kcal/day. Research shows that for those with a starting BMI greater than 30, these diets are helpful in producing a typical loss of more than 8% of initial body weight over 3 to 6 months of treatment, with substantial health benefits (51–53). However, diet therapy combined with intense behavioral therapy and support is essential to losing and maintaining the weight loss. These diets can vary in protein, carbohydrate, and fat content (53).

Very-Low-Calorie Diets

Individuals with severe or morbid obesity (BMI ≥40) can benefit from a moderately restricted diet; however, it typically will take at least 1 year of steady dieting to lose 50 lb with this modest level of energy restriction. Few individuals can sustain even a moderately restrictive diet for this long. Thus, it may be reasonable for such patients to begin with a period of more severe energy restriction under medical monitoring. VLCDs, defined as containing fewer than 800 kcal/day, may be food based or may use meal replacements, often in the form of soy, egg, or milk-based high protein, low-carbohydrate, low-fat shakes or bars, containing vitamins and minerals to prevent nutrition deficiencies.

This approach can be quite useful if it is monitored and accompanied by a comprehensive program of behavior modification and physical activity. Initial, but usually temporary, side effects may include hunger, fatigue, and lightheadedness; later on, constipation and intolerance to cold may occur. The increased risk of developing gallstones (54) may be transient. Studies show that weight loss of 10% to 20% can be achieved initially with VLCDs (55–60); however, adherence for more than several months may not be sustainable. A high protein content consumed during a VLCD may minimize muscle wasting as the rapid weight loss occurs (61). The main drawback of VLCDs is frequently rapid weight regain after the weight loss phase (62). Thus, use of VLCDs is most effective in the context of a well-rounded, multidisciplinary approach to weight loss and long-term weight control. Careful attention to a weight maintenance program is essential following a VLCD. VLCD programs should encourage exercise and provide ongoing support, perhaps with groups, classes, or individual sessions.

Low-Carbohydrate, High-Protein Diets

Low-carbohydrate diets typically recommend up to 20 g of carbohydrate at the onset of the diet (e.g., the Atkins diet), with a high intake of protein and fat (63). This diet typically involves three phases. The first phase is called the induction phase, which is the weight loss initiation phase and includes no more than 5% of energy from carbohydrate, 35% from protein, and 60% from fat (63). The second phase, called the ongoing phase, is a continuation of weight loss, with the proportions of carbohydrate (9%), protein (33%), and fat (58%) slightly liberalized. The third phase is the maintenance phase, in which carbohydrate intake increases to no more than 20% of total energy with 25% to 27% protein and approximately 52% fat.

Any restrictive diet can cause diuresis in the initial 1 to 2 weeks, resulting in 2% to 4% weight loss largely because of water loss (64). Evidence from several studies indicates that low-carbohydrate diets are initially more effective compared with diets low in fat and calories for weight loss and improving cardiovascular risk factors associated with

obesity (65–69). However, no significant differences are present between diets after 1 year (65–69). Lower attrition rates also are observed with the low-carbohydrate diets, perhaps because of higher satiety associated with high intakes of protein (70).

Diuresis may possibly result in the more rapid weight loss seen with low-carbohydrate diets in the early phase. No truly long-term studies have been conducted to date. Although benefits of low-carbohydrate diets have been reported on markers of cardiovascular risk factors, concerns exist regarding high intake of fat in the diet. High fat intake, particularly saturated fat in the diet, is associated with health problems such as certain types of cancers and cardiovascular disease (71, 72). Other health concerns, including cognitive impairment, constipation, diarrhea, dizziness, halitosis, headaches, insomnia, kidney stones, and nausea, have been reported in individuals with low-carbohydrate intakes (73–76).

Low-Fat, Low-Energy-Density Diets

A typical US diet is moderately high fat and energy dense. Several studies show that energy-dense food intake is associated with higher BMI and body weight (77–82). Weight gain from high intake of energy-dense foods such as fats has been attributed to passive overconsumption, likely because of the relatively low satiety value and high palatability of such foods (83). Reducing the energy density of the diet by replacing fat with more fruits and vegetables and grains can be an effective strategy to lose weight because fat, at 9 kcal/g, provides more than double the calories provided by carbohydrates (4 kcal/g) and proteins (4 kcal/g). Moreover, several studies have shown that lower energy-density foods such as fruits, vegetables, and whole grains lower energy intake because of increased satiety of the diet (84–86) that translates into lower BMI (77–82). Typically, low-fat, low-energy diets concentrate on reducing overall calories in the diets. Studies using this approach have reported significant weight loss in obese individuals compared with low-fat high-carbohydrate diets, which are not calorically controlled (87, 88). However, more long-term studies are needed to see whether those who lose weight on these diets compensate for lower calories or maintain the weight lost.

Low-Glycemic-Index Diets

The *glycemic index of foods* refers to the metabolic effects produced by carbohydrate-rich foods on blood glucose and insulin levels (89). Ingestion of high-glycemic-index foods such as potatoes and white bread produce rapid increases in blood glucose and insulin levels (89). These changes in blood glucose and insulin levels result in short sustenance of satiety, low levels of fat oxidation, and subsequent weight gain secondary to poor appetite regulation caused by the rapid rise and fall in blood glucose and insulin (89). Diets that are low glycemic index contain more fruits and vegetables, which are high in fiber and are lower in foods high in simple carbohydrates such as sugar, refined foods, and starchy vegetables (89).

Several studies examined the effects of low-glycemic-index foods on weight loss (90–93) and showed promise in the use to these diets for the treatment of obesity. One study showed that lowering the glycemic load of an energy-restricted diet significantly reduced body weight, increased fat oxidation, and decreased fat regain after weight loss (90). A low-glycemic-index, energy-restricted diet may yield greater benefits than a reduced-fat energy-restricted diet (91, 92). Low-glycemic-index diets may attenuate reductions in resting energy expenditure (91), commonly seen in obese individuals following energy-restricted diets. Moreover, low-glycemic-index diets have been shown to improve satiety and improve cardiovascular disease risk factors (91, 92). The Zone diet and Weight Watchers diet are based primarily on low-glycemic-index foods, as are the later phases of the South Beach diet.

Balanced Deficit/Portion-Controlled Diets

A balanced-deficit diet involves balanced restrictions in the major food groups from the food guide pyramid. It may emphasize a limitation of fat to 20% to 25% of total calories consumed. This approach generally allows less restriction in the volume of food consumed because fatty foods are more compact and energy dense. For example, a small piece of cheese may contain 250 calories, whereas a large tomato and a head of lettuce total only 125 calories. In addition, reducing serving sizes from each food group can allow for a calorie restriction of 300 to 500 kcal/day, resulting in weight loss of up to 1 lb/week. However, this weight loss may not be consistent and may frustrate in individuals trying to lose weight quickly. In balanced-deficit diets, the goal is to achieve caloric deficit working in the context of unchanged initial dietary choices. Therefore, adherence to this diet may be better because the diet involves only portion changes, rather than avoidance of specific foods that may be favorites. Foods rich in fats and sugar need not be replaced in a balanced-deficit diet. A related approach to a balanced-deficit diet is a portion-controlled diet.

US diets today are not only high in saturated fats and sugars, but also often contain huge portion sizes, which result in increased energy intake (94). Several studies showed that portion-controlled diets lead to mean weight loss of up to 10% of initial body weight (95–99). One study reported that portion-controlled diets were beneficial in achieving weight loss among diabetic obese individuals as compared with American Diabetes Association standard dietary recommendations (96). Those who controlled portion sizes in the study lost 2.59 kg as compared with those in the control group, who gained 2.15 kg (96). Pedersen et al (97) reported that obese diabetic patients following a portion-controlled diet were able to reduce medications for diabetes and lost 1.8% of body weight, compared with

1% in the control group. Similarly, one study reported 6.5% of initial body weight loss and 3.6 kg of fat mass loss in overweight or obese women with portion-controlled entrees, as compared with controls (99).

It may be possible for individuals to adhere better to portion-controlled diets. However, nutrition education needs to be provided to understand portion sizes. Individuals should be encouraged to use measuring cups and spoons, food scales, and or familiar objects (e.g., a deck of cards or the palm of the hand), both to estimate their dietary intake and to serve themselves. Three ounces provide a serving of protein (meat, chicken, or fish), one half cup counts as one serving of cooked starch (rice, pasta, or potatoes), and one teaspoon (or thumb tip) is a serving of fat (oil). Checking labels for serving size and number of servings per package is imperative to understanding exactly how much of a food is being consumed. One package does not necessarily equal one serving.

Meal Replacement Diets

Meal replacement diets may be a good choice when conventional LCDs have not worked or for those seeking rapid initial weight loss. This approach can enhance motivation to continue losing weight. Typically, meal replacement diets include one or more meals replaced by commercial dietary formulations, which are nutritionally balanced and macronutrient and calorie controlled (800 to 1600 cal/day) (100). One metaanalysis of six randomized controlled trials reported that meal replacements for weight loss induced significantly greater weight loss (~6 lb) compared with conventional LCDs at 3 months and 1 year (101). Similarly, Ashley et al (102) reported that dieters using meal replacements lost weight and met essential nutrient intakes adequately compared with those who lost weight by a standard LCD.

Another study found that a diet containing meal replacements (five meals daily totaling 1000 kcal/day) helped obese individuals lose more than 10% of initial body weight in 16 weeks versus a loss of 6.9% on a whole food-based diet (103). However, those on the meal replacement diet regained more during the maintenance phase (24 weeks) compared with those on a food-based diet (103). Thus, several studies conducted to test the efficacy of meal replacements as compared with standard LCDs have reported greater benefits for initial weight loss (101–104).

Although meal replacement diets are a good approach for initial, rapid weight loss, have good nutritional quality, and may even avoid nutritional inadequacies that can arise from conventional LCDs, weight maintenance on a long-term basis, as with most all dietary approaches to weight loss, has not been well studied or demonstrated.

In summary, no one dietary approach appears to be substantially better or worse than the others. Although several diets have been reported superior for achieving weight loss, the choice of a specific dietary approach needs to be based on an individual's goals, medical needs, and preferences. Many people are motivated to lose weight faster during the initial phases of weight control, and this can help guide the choice of dietary approach toward a more aggressive level of energy restriction, if medically appropriate. In contrast, for some clients, long-term weight control is the more motivating factor, and then standard dietary approaches at a more modest level of energy restriction may be preferable. The general health of the obese individual, including the presence or absence of specific comorbid conditions, also plays an important role in selecting a dietary approach. The provider and the client therefore must have an ongoing, long-term relationship in which a long-term, multidisciplinary approach can be used. Interventions that include increased levels of social support and self-regulatory methods such as goal setting and self-monitoring, along with increased contact with providers, have been shown to be more effective, irrespective of the mode of intervention (105).

PHYSICAL ACTIVITY FOR WEIGHT LOSS

As discussed, to lose 1 lb of fat/week, a 500-calorie deficit/ day must be sustained. Creating and adhering to a level of deficit by diet alone can be challenging in our obesogenic environment. Combining physical activity with an LCD can ease achieving this level of energy deficit and also can be sustained more readily in the long term. According to a joint panel of experts from the American College of Sports Medicine (ACSM) and the Centers for Disease Control and Prevention (106), healthy adults should engage in at least 30 minutes of moderate-intensity (defined as 3 to 6 metabolic equivalents [METs]) physical activity, preferably every day. These recommendations were further updated by a joint panel of experts from the ACSM and American Heart Association by detailing the types of activity and amounts needed to maintain health and prevent weight gain (107).

These specifications are for a minimum of 30 minutes of moderate-intensity physical activity (e.g., brisk walking) for 5 days/week or vigorous-intensity (>6 METs; e.g., jogging) exercise for 3 days/week. However, for obese individuals, a review of evidence from research studies by the ACSM indicates that more than 60 minutes of moderate-intensity physical activity for at least 4 days/ week can help in achieving clinically significant weight loss without dietary caloric restriction (108). However, when moderate-intensity physical activity (between 30 and 60 minutes/day for 5 days/week) is coupled with energy restriction from the diet, weight loss is easier to achieve (108). For weight maintenance or prevention of weight regain, moderate-intensity physical activity of more than 60 minutes/day for at least 5 days is needed (108).

Effect of Exercise on Weight Loss

The level of physical activity recommended by the ACSM to lose weight may seem like a daunting task for many overweight and obese individuals. However, when just starting an exercise program, it is worthwhile to start with small goals and increase the level and intensity of exercise gradually to reach ACSM recommendations. One study reported that, at the end of 1 year, caloric restriction plus more than 200 minutes of physical activity/week resulted in significantly greater weight loss among sedentary obese participants, along with improved cardiovascular fitness, compared with those who were physically active for less than 150 minutes/week. This study reported no significant effect of the exercise intensity level on change in body weight (109).

Although adding physical activity to a weight loss regimen can help in achieving a desired level of caloric restriction more easily, another study reported no added effect of physical activity plus calorie restriction on body weight loss, fat loss, and visceral fat loss after 6 months of intervention (110). In this study, the control group (on a dietary energy restriction of 25%) had lost more than 18 lb, approximately 6 kg of fat mass, and approximately 1 kg of visceral fat, whereas the intervention group (12.5% reduced energy intake and 12.5% increased energy expenditure through exercise) loss was approximately 18 lb, approximately 6.5 kg, and approximately 1 kg, respectively (110). However, those who exercised along with dietary calorie restriction showed improved cardiovascular fitness (110). Similar to these results, Nicklas et al (111), reported no significant differences in body weight and visceral fat loss among those who used a weight loss regimen that included calorie restriction with or without moderate- and vigorous-intensity exercise. However, those who lost weight and visceral fat on the calorie restriction along with vigorous activity preserved lean body mass better (111).

Thus, several studies showed beneficial effects of energy restriction plus exercise on body composition changes, but without added weight loss benefits through including exercise (109–112). However, exercise along with calorie restriction appears to enhance cardiovascular health benefits and preserve lean body mass (108–112), and this approach is therefore advisable to include in a weight loss regimen unless physical conditions contraindicate exercise.

Exercise and Weight Maintenance

Weight regain is very common and often rapid once a strict weight loss regimen is ended. This regain can be attributed to low adherence to maintenance levels of exercise and dietary compliance (113). Many factors contribute to this relapse, including low motivation and diminished or terminated support from the provider. One study showed that after the initial weight loss phase (2 months; mean weight loss achieved ~14 kg), subjects regained on average more than 60% of the weight lost by the end of an 8- to 31-month unsupervised weight maintenance phase. This weight regain was accompanied by significant gains in fat mass and waist circumference, along with decreased levels of physical activity (113).

Although weight regain is very difficult to prevent entirely, continuation of some form of exercise may slow and diminish its degree (113, 114). One study showed that after a 12-week weight loss regimen, those who continued walking at moderate intensity regained weight and fat at a slower pace than those who were sedentary during the 40-week maintenance phase (114). Those who exercised regained approximately 7 lb less in body weight and had a 3.8-cm smaller waist circumference compared with those who did not exercise (114). A supervised weight maintenance regimen can help in slowing weight and fat mass regain significantly (113). Borg et al (113) reported the benefits of supervised walking or resistance training for 6 months after weight loss. Subjects incorporating walking or resistance training regained less (~4 lb) or no weight and maintained fat mass (113). Other studies showed that physical activity alone may not help in maintaining weight loss, though (115, 116). Dietary restraint along with physical activity may prove to be more successful in maintaining weight loss and slowing or preventing weight regain than physical activity alone (115). Restricting calories from fat along with high physical activity may prove to be the most effective strategy to maintain weight loss on a long-term basis (116).

Resistance Training for Weight Loss and Maintenance

Resistance (strength) training can be added to an aerobic exercise regimen and has been shown to help preserve muscle mass (106, 107, 113). Studies have shown that resistance training along with aerobic exercise, in addition to calorie-restricted diet, results in weight loss along with muscle strength preservation and improvements in physical functioning (117). One study reported that those who incorporated resistance training during the weight maintenance phase were likely to regain fat mass at a slower pace or were less likely to regain fat mass compared with those who did not, in spite of overall body weight regain (113). Resistance training may not correlate with body weight changes during the weight loss phase or may result in weight gain because muscle mass (which is denser than fat) increases with resistance training (107, 118). Resistance training is associated with lower levels of visceral fat, which, in turn, is associated with a higher risk of cardiovascular disease (118).

Although emphasis has been placed on aerobic training to lose body weight and fat, combining resistance training with calorie-restricted regimen for weight loss can indirectly aid in weight loss by improving muscle mass, strength, and endurance (118, 119). Moreover, these changes are associated with health benefits, such as increased insulin sensitivity in type 2 diabetes (118, 120). One study reported that resistance training improved insulin sensitivity and weight loss more than aerobic training in an African-American population (120). In addition, resistance training appears to decrease bone loss, which

can be seen in those who lose weight by caloric restriction alone (121), and improves basal metabolic rate (BMR) (122) which is associated with more fat-free mass in obese individuals (123).

Summary

Physical activity along with caloric restriction appears to be a better approach to losing weight and maintaining the weight loss. Calorie restriction alone for weight loss may lower BMR and fat-free mass and adversely affect bone parameters. Adding endurance and resistance training to calorie restriction may mitigate these weight loss–associated issues. Exercise, when used along with calorie restriction, should be performed at least five times a week for more than 240 minutes to lose weight and thereafter at least five times a week for 150 to 240 minutes to help maintain the weight loss. Although cutting back on calories and simultaneously increasing energy expenditure may seem like an intimidating task, planning an exercise schedule that is based on enjoyable activities may help ease this set of behavior changes. Encouraging individuals to add more movement into their daily lives (e.g., taking the stairs rather than the elevator), brainstorming how they can exercise with family and friends, and helping them add variety to their routines to avoid boredom are all useful tools. Exercise should start slowly and be increased progressively based on individuals' tolerance level to enhance adherence.

BEHAVIOR THERAPY

Behavior therapy to treat obesity aims to identify events and stimuli that trigger inappropriate behaviors associated with excess caloric intake and to develop approaches to control these behaviors. Behavioral interventions focus on modifying cognitive, emotional, and social events that influence the individual's choices that result in weight gain. Studies show that behavior therapy as an adjunct to exercise and diet therapy to lose weight produces significantly better results than exercise and diet alone (124, 125).

Several components of behavior therapy can help the individual develop skills to achieve weight loss and successfully maintain it. These include setting goals, identifying the process to achieve these goals based on individual needs, monitoring the progress, removing barriers, building support from friends and family, and controlling stimuli to inappropriate behaviors (126). Weight loss and maintenance for obese individuals requires long-term lifestyle changes; thus, behavior modifications should aim at setting realistic and measurable goals. Interventions that include group sessions rather than individualized sessions can be more effective treatment modalities for obesity (127–129). Studies show that group treatment can produce significantly greater weight loss (~13%) than individual sessions (>11%) (128) and is more likely to help maintain weight loss (129). The known benefits of social support may explain the superiority of group sessions over individual sessions.

Weight regain is another issue that behavior modification can help address, especially by focusing on reinforcements that can help to maintain higher adherence to changes in lifestyle. One study showed that teaching individuals to take responsibility for weight maintenance by developing problem-solving skills to overcome setbacks improves weight loss maintenance (130). These techniques and skills include providing incentives for motivation, learning how to preplan weekly low-calorie meals and control portions, providing additional support from peers, increasing provider and patient contact, encouraging self-monitoring, and others. Social support, along with these techniques, improves weight maintenance after initial weight loss (130). Thus, several studies suggested that behavior therapy beyond the initial weight loss phase is important in maintaining the weight loss (129–132).

In summary, because the long-term results of attempts at weight loss are often poor, it is important to expose the individual, at the beginning of treatment, to the attitudes and behaviors that are likely to foster long-term maintenance of weight loss. Some key components of a successful behavior modification approach for weight control include the following:

1. Readiness: The timing for change is vital. If the individual is not yet convinced of the need to modify weight, or is in the midst of a stressful life event such as divorce, the chances of success are poor.
2. Setting reasonable goals: Aiming for an attainable rather than an "ideal" body weight is advisable. A reasonable long-term goal may be the lowest weight the patient has successfully maintained for 1 year or more during the previous 10 years.
3. Reliable support systems: Obtaining help from others enhances both weight loss and maintenance. This usually involves seeking out a friend or relative who knows how to listen and not just give advice.
4. Building in maintenance: Planning and executing behavioral changes from day 1 are essential. Helping patients become invested in their goals by teaching them how to talk to themselves in a positive way to enhance commitment to self-set objectives is a useful technique.
5. Making gradual changes: Modifying food choices and level of physical activity reduces the sense of deprivation and may make the process of change easier (and the changes themselves more likely to be sustained).
6. Keeping records: Recording weight, foods eaten, exercise, and precipitants of inappropriate eating is an excellent way to identify problem areas and to spot a relapse before it gets out of hand.
7. Making it enjoyable: It is much easier to comply with the new behaviors if they can be enjoyed. If the individual cannot stand to exercise, do not tell him or her to do it anyway. Instead, suggest walking around the mall to people-watch. The achievement of a positive change in lifestyle is, by itself, very reinforcing and should not be discounted as a source of satisfaction and enjoyment.
8. Being flexible: This applies to both the care provider and the patient. If an approach that has been given a fair trial is not working, or if the patient's circumstances change, the weight loss plan may need to change, too. Helping individuals lose weight and keep it off requires a comprehensive and sustained effort. Although it is true that only the individual can do it, this is one area in which the diligent and caring provider can make a real difference.

PHARMACOLOGIC TREATMENT FOR WEIGHT LOSS

Lifestyle modifications discussed earlier form the cornerstone and first stage of any weight loss plan. Adjunctive anorectic medications may be useful, if this approach (lifestyle modification including diet, exercise, and behavior therapy) alone does not result in weight loss. Pharmacotherapy may be helpful when compliance to lifestyle modification begins to waver or physical hunger becomes an issue during dieting. There is little doubt that such medications significantly increase weight loss during the period in which they are used, and they may help with maintaining weight loss (although weight tends to be regained even with continued drug use) (133). However, pharmacologic treatments are best suited for those who are severely obese (BMI >40 kg/m^2) or who have two or more significant medical comorbidities (20).

The most commonly used weight loss drugs that have been approved by the FDA are orlistat and phentermine (133). Sibutramine (Meridia) was withdrawn from the market in 2010. In addition to these medications, several combination pharmacologic treatments are being developed to target the neuronal pathways associated with energy homeostasis in the hypothalamus and involve hormones such as leptin, ghrelin, and insulin (133, 134). The discovery of leptin unveiled several neurohormonal targets for pharmacologic treatments that include inhibition of neuropeptide Y, which stimulates food intake, and stimulation of the melanocortin-4 receptor, which inhibits food intake (133). Although several therapies are now focusing on developing pharmacologic treatments that can decrease food intake and/or increase energy expenditure, this discussion covers the most commonly prescribed, FDA-approved weight loss medications: orlistat and phentermine.

Orlistat

Orlistat (Xenical) is an inhibitor of gastrointestinal lipases that prevents the intestinal hydrolysis of triglycerides into the absorbable free fatty acids and monoacylglycerols. It induces weight loss by reducing nutrient absorption, specifically dietary fat, by up to 30% (133), and several studies of 1 to 2 years' duration established its efficacy in inducing moderate weight loss compared with placebo (4.7% to 10% versus 3.0% to 6.1%). In general, 120 mg of orlistat three times a day before meals, along with a calorie-restricted diet is associated with approximately 5% to 10% initial weight loss and improved weight mainte- nance (135–140). Finer et al (136) reported a mean 8.5% initial weight loss in obese individuals taking orlistat com- pared with 5.4% in the placebo group at the conclusion of a 12-month intervention period (136). The orlistat group also experienced more improvement in metabolic mark- ers, including total cholesterol, low-density lipoprotein cholesterol, and the ratio of low-density lipoprotein to high-density lipoprotein, but they reported a 26% higher frequency of transient gastrointestinal events (136).

One study by Sjöström et al (137) suggested that orli- stat may help to maintain weight loss. This study enrolled 743 patients into a 4-week, hypocaloric diet (caloric deficit ~600 kcal/day) and then randomized them to orlistat (120 mg three times daily) or placebo for 1 year. The orlistat group lost 10.2 % body weight compared with 6.1% in the placebo group. After the first year, patients were rerandom- ized to orlistat or placebo but on a eucaloric (weight mainte- nance) diet. Those continuing on orlistat regained on average half as much weight as those who were switched to placebo. Those switched from placebo to orlistat lost an additional 0.9 kg compared with a mean regain of 2.5 kg in patients con- tinuing on placebo (137). Several studies have shown similar effects of orlistat on weight loss in interventions of 6 months (139, 140), 1 year (136, 140), and 2 years (137).

In addition to weight loss, orlistat has been shown to improve cardiovascular risk factors, blood pressure, and insulin sensitivity in type 2 diabetes (137–140). For indi- viduals taking orlistat, which blocks absorption of fats of all kinds, a daily fat-soluble vitamin supplement (and not at the same time as taking orlistat) is needed to prevent deficiency of vitamins A, D, E and K (136). Although gastrointestinal side effects such as diarrhea, bloating, flatulence, fecal urgency and incontinence, and steatorrhea are common with orlistat, these effects are generally mild to moderate and decrease with duration of treatment (135–141).

Because of reports of adverse effects of orlistat on the liver, the FDA issued updated safety concerns in September 2009, although the drug is now also available over the counter in a lower strength dose of 60 mg (133). A few short-term studies (16 to 24 weeks) reported ben- eficial effects of even low doses of orlistat (60 mg once or three times a day) on weight loss (~5% reduction) and improvements in metabolic risk factors (142, 143). One study reported significant benefits of low-dose orlistat on weight loss and metabolic markers even in overweight but not obese (BMI 25 to 28 kg/m^2) adults when accompanied by lifestyle modification (143).

Phentermine

Phentermine is a noradrenergic compound approved by the FDA in 1959 for "short-term" use, generally defined as a period of less than 12 weeks (133). One long-term study examined data from 300 patients treated with phen- termine, 15 to 75 mg/day, and found significant weight loss and maintenance of more than 10% of initial weight loss for up to 8 years (144). In general, participants did not report feeling hungry and reported better control over food intake and cravings; this control tended to dimin- ish over time but could often be regained if doses were increased progressively. Common adverse effects reported included dry mouth and insomnia (144).

One randomized controlled trial of 24-week intervention with a combination of pramlintide and phentermine (37.5 mg) reported a weight loss of 11.3 % (145). Increases in heart rates (4.5 beats/minute) and diastolic blood pressure (3.5 mm Hg) also were observed (145). In combination with fenfluramine (removed from the market in 1997), phenter- mine use was shown to cause valvular heart disease (146). However, phentermine alone has not been implicated. Phentermine use is common in the United States because of its generic availability at low cost. However, administra- tion of phentermine for more than 12 weeks is still consid- ered "off-label" use in the United States; in Europe, the drug is not licensed for use at all (133).

In summary, pharmacologic therapy for the treatment of obesity holds promise and can be a useful adjunct to diet and lifestyle change. Moreover, when lifestyle modification has been ineffective or stalls, pharmacologic treatment as an adjunct therapy may be helpful. However, given that various side effects are associated with pharma- cologic therapies, these drugs should be prescribed and monitored regularly by medical practitioners. There also is a slight chance of abuse with the use of these medications. Although combinations of medications will undoubtedly be more effective than individual agents (145), these com- binations do have the potential to cause more side effects (146). In addition, pharmacologic interventions alter eat- ing behaviors; this situation is far more complicated and variable than alteration of physiologic parameters (e.g., blood pressure), thus making development of pharmaco- logic treatments to assist weight loss challenging.

SURGICAL TREATMENT

Although lifestyle modifications that include combinations of diet, exercise, behavior therapy, and pharmacologic agents for severely obese people can produce changes in body weight, these changes may prove to be insig- nificant and have insufficient health benefits. In these patients, weight-loss surgery is a second-stage approach. The National Institutes of Health consensus conference on gastrointestinal surgery for severe obesity concluded that weight-loss surgery may be an appropriate option for those who are severely obese (BMI >40 kg/m^2) or those who have a BMI greater than 35 kg/m^2 with two or more obesity related comorbidities (20, 147). Moreover, weight- loss surgery in such individuals has the potential to resolve associated medical comorbidities completely (147).

The first surgical approach to obesity was jejuno-ileal bypass, first performed in the early 1950s (148). Two other procedures were introduced in the late 1960s by Dr. Mason: the Roux-en-Y gastric bypass and vertical gastric banding (148). Dr. Scopinaro introduced another option, biliopancreatic diversion, in the late 1970s. In the 1990s, a procedure was introduced, first in Europe, in which the size of the stomach was reduced by adjustable gastric banding, followed by laparoscopic sleeve gastrectomy, introduced in 2002 by Dr. Gagner (148).

Before an obese individual decides on surgery to lose weight, or before the physician decides to recommend surgery as an option, the patient must be assessed using a multidisciplinary approach. This ideally should involve not only the surgeon and referring physician but also dietitians, psychologists, nurses, and an anesthesiologist. The patient's medical and nutritional history must be evaluated as well as a psychologic assessment to understand any underlying issues more clearly before a decision is reached regarding suitability for surgery (148). Contraindications include issues that can hinder adherence to the recommended postoperative care needed to achieve expected outcomes. These issues include psychologic disturbances, medical problems that may worsen or contraindicate major surgery, and a nonsupportive environment (148).

Surgical treatments are the most efficacious option for individuals who have morbid obesity, and these treatments produce weight loss that is superior to other approaches. However, the rate of success following bariatric surgery is highly variable, and risks of postoperative complications are present. Therefore, a multidisciplinary approach needs to be adopted so that proper evaluation and selection of the patients occurs preoperatively and long-term postoperative care and monitoring are ensured. For a detailed discussion of bariatric surgery procedures, see the chapter on bariatric surgery.

CONCLUSIONS

Obesity management is perhaps the greatest challenge faced by health care professionals today. With the rise in obesity rates comes a plethora of medical complications. Although increasing research in obesity has provided some clarity on the causes of the obesity epidemic and has helped to develop effective treatment modalities, further research is needed to understand the basis of certain behaviors adopted by obese individuals and ways to modify these behaviors effectively to achieve long-term weight management. Almost all adults who become obese do so not because of a specific medical or metabolic condition but because of lifestyle behaviors leading to increased food consumption or decreased energy expenditure.

Therefore, to prevent obesity or slow its progression, efforts should be devoted to improving environmental factors and personal behavior. Examples include improving school meals and snacks, educating individuals on the importance of healthy foods, providing resources to improve physical activity, and educating parents on ways to enhance healthy eating and physical activity behaviors in their children.

Although the obesity treatment modalities discussed in this chapter can be successfully applied to obese individuals, changing or improving our environment is the key to preventing and reversing this public health epidemic.

REFERENCES:

1. Wang Y, Beydoun MA, Liang L et al. Obesity 2008;16:2323–30.
2. Ogden CL, Carroll MD, Curtin LR et al. JAMA 2010;303:242–9.
3. Hill JO. Endocr Rev 2006;27:750–61.
4. Kelly T, Yang W, Chen CS et al. Int J Obes 2008;32:1431–7.
5. Popkin BM. Nutr Rev 2004;62:S140–3.
6. Du H, Feskens E. Acta Cardiol 2010;65:377–86.
7. Giskes K, van Lenthe F, Avendano-Pabon M et al. Obes Rev 2011;12:e95–e106.
8. Feng J, Glass TA, Curriero FC et al. Health Place 2010;16:175–90.
9. Field AE, Coakley EH, Must A et al. Arch Intern Med 2001;161:1581–6.
10. Janssen I, Katzmarzyk PT, Ross R. Arch Intern Med 2002;162:2074–9.
11. Finkelstein EA, Brown DS, Wrage LA et al. Obesity (Silver Spring) 2010;18:333–9.
12. Puhl RM, Andreyeva T, Brownell KD. Int J Obes 2008;32:992–1000.
13. Carr D, Jaffe KJ, Friedman MA. Obesity (Silver Spring) 2008;16:S60–8.
14. Latner JD, Stunkard AJ, Wilson GT. Obes Res 2005;13:1226–31.
15. Look AHEAD Research Group, Wing RR. Arch Intern Med 2010;170:1566–75.
16. Williamson DF, Thompson TJ, Thun M et al. Diabetes Care 2000;23:1499–504.
17. Gregg EW, Williamson DF. The relationship of intentional weight loss to disease incidence and mortality. In: Wadden TA, Stunkard AJ, eds. Handbook of Obesity Treatment. New York: Guilford Press, 2002:125–43.
18. Knowler WC, Barrett-Connor E, Fowler SE et al. N Engl J Med 2002 ;346:393–403.
19. Rush EC, Goedecke JH, Jennings C et al. Int J Obes (Lond) 2007;31:1232–9.
20. National Institutes of Health, National Heart, Lung, and Blood Institute. Obes Res 1998;6:51S–209S.
21. Janssen I, Katzmarzyk PT, Ross R. Arch Intern Med 2002;162:2074–9.
22. Janssen I, Katzmarzyk PT, Ross R. Am J Clin Nutr 2004;79:379–84.
23. Ma J, Xiao L. Obesity (Silver Spring) 2010;18:347–53.
24. Onyike CU, Crum RM, Lee HB et al. Am J Epidemiol 2003;158:1139–47.
25. Zhao G, Ford ES, Dhingra S et al. Int J Obes (Lond) 2009;33:257–66.
26. Steer RA, Brown GK, Beck AT et al. Psychol Rep 2001;88:1075–6.
27. de Zwaan M. Int J Obes Relat Metab Disord 2001;25:S51–5.
28. Sim LA, McAlpine DE, Grothe KB et al. Mayo Clin Proc 2010;85:746–51.
29. Hay PP, Bacaltchuk J, Stefano S et al. Cochrane Database Syst Rev 2009;(4):CD000562.
30. Wadden TA, Phelan S. Behavioral assessment of the obese patient. In: Wadden TA, Stunkard AJ, eds. Handbook of Obesity Treatment. New York: Guilford Press, 2002:186–226.

31. Øverby NC, Serra-Majem L, Andersen LF. Br J Nutr 2009;102:S56–63.

32. Cade J, Thompson R, Burley V et al. Public Health Nutr 2002; 5:567–87.

33. Poslusna K, Ruprich J, de Vries JH et al. Br J Nutr 2009; 101(Suppl 2):S73–85.

34. Abbott RA, Davies PS. Eur J Clin Nutr 2004;58:285–91.

35. Jackson DM, Djafarian K, Stewart J et al. Am J Clin Nutr 2009; 89:1031–6.

36. Centers for Disease Control and Prevention. MMWR Morb Mortal Wkly Rep 2011;60:614–8.

37. Slingerland AS, van Lenthe FJ, Jukema JW et al. Am J Epidemiol 2007;165:1356–63.

38. Andersen RE, Wadden TA, Bartlett SJ et al. JAMA 1999;281:335–40.

39. Di Noia J, Prochaska JO. Am J Health Behav 2010;34:618–32.

40. Anderson ES, Winett RA, Wojcik JR et al. J Health Psychol 2010;15:21–32.

41. Zheng H, Lenard NR, Shin AC et al. Int J Obes (Lond) 2009;33:S8–13.

42. Abete I, Astrup A, Martínez JA et al. Nutr Rev 2010;68:214–31.

43. US Department of Agriculture, US Department of Health and Human Services. Dietary Guidelines for Americans, 2010. 7th ed. Washington, DC: US Government Printing Office, 2010.

44. Bleich SN, Wang YC, Wang Y et al. Am J Clin Nutr 2009; 89:372–81.

45. Bachman JL, Reedy J, Subar AF et al. J Am Diet Assoc 2008; 108:804–14.

46. Drewnowski A. Am J Prev Med 2004;27:154–62.

47. Savage JS, Marini M, Birch LL. Am J Clin Nutr 2008;88:677–84.

48. Bes-Rastrollo M, van Dam RM, Martinez-Gonzalez MA et al. Am J Clin Nutr 2008;88:769–77.

49. Howarth NC, Murphy SP, Wilkens LR et al. J Nutr 2006; 136:2243–8.

50. Kant AK, Graubard BI. Int J Obes (Lond) 2005;29:950–6.

51. Bischoff SC, Damms-Machado A, Betz C et al. Int J Obes 2012;36:614–24.

52. Riecke BF, Christensen R, Christensen P et al. Osteoarthritis Cartilage 2010;18:746–54.

53. Noakes M, Keogh JB, Foster PR et al. Am J Clin Nutr 2005; 81:1298–306.

54. Broomfield PH, Chopra R, Sheinbaum RC et al. N Engl J Med 1988;319:1567–72.

55. Arai K, Miura J, Ohno M et al. Am J Clin Nutr 1992;56:275S–6S.

56. Ryttig KR, Flaten H, Rössner S. Int J Obes Relat Metab Disord 1997;21:574–9.

57. Ryttig KR, Rössner S. J Intern Med 1995;238:299–306.

58. Lantz H, Peltonen M, Agren L et al. J Intern Med 2003; 254:272–9.

59. Miura J, Arai K, Tsukahara S et al. Int J Obes 1989;13:73–7.

60. Rössner S, Flaten H. Int J Obes Relat Metab Disord 1997; 21:22–6.

61. Wadden TA, Berkowitz RI. Very-low-calorie diets. In: Fairburn CG, Brownell KD, eds. Eating Disorders and Obesity. New York: Guilford Press, 2001:529–33.

62. Saris WH. Obes Res 2001;9:295S–301S.

63. Last AR, Wilson SA. Am Fam Physician 2006;73:1942–8.

64. Shils M, Olson J, Shike M et al, eds. Modern Nutrition in Health and Disease. 9th ed. Baltimore: Lippincott Williams & Wilkins, 1999.

65. Hession M, Rolland C, Kulkarni U et al. Obes Rev 2009;10: 36–50.

66. Nordmann AJ, Nordmann A, Briel M et al. Arch Intern Med 2006;166:285–93.

67. Brehm BJ, Seeley RJ, Daniels SR et al. J Clin Endocrinol Metab 2003;88:1617–23.

68. Foster GD, Wyatt HR, Hill JO et al. N Engl J Med 2003; 348:2082–90.

69. Yancy WS Jr, Olsen MK, Guyton JR et al. Ann Intern Med 2004;140:769–77.

70. Soenen S, Westerterp-Plantenga MS. Curr Opin Clin Nutr Metab Care 2008;11:747–51.

71. Lichtenstein AH, Kennedy E, Barrier P et al. Nutr Rev 1998; 56:S3–19.

72. Weisburger JH. J Am Diet Assoc 1997;97:S16–23.

73. Reddy ST, Wang CY, Sakhaee K et al. Am J Kidney Dis 2002; 40:265–74.

74. Breslau NA, Brinkley L, Hill KD et al. J Clin Endocrinol Metab 1988;66:140–6.

75. Wing RR, Vazquez JA, Ryan CM. Int J Obes Relat Metab Disord 1995;19:811–6.

76. Johnston CS, Tjonn SL, Swan PD et al. Am J Clin Nut 2006; 83:1055–61.

77. Vergnaud AC, Estaquio C, Czernichow S et al. Br J Nutr 2009; 102:302–9.

78. Savage JS, Marini M, Birch LL. Am J Clin Nutr 2008;88:677–84.

79. Bes-Rastrollo M, van Dam RM, Martinez-Gonzalez MA et al. Am J Clin Nutr 2008;88:769–77.

80. Howarth NC, Murphy SP, Wilkens LR et al. J Nutr 2006; 136:2243–8.

81. Ello-Martin JA, Roe LS, Ledikwe JH et al. Am J Clin Nutr 2007;85:1465–77.

82. Ledikwe JH, Blanck HM, Kettel Khan L et al. Am J Clin Nutr 2006;83:1362–8.

83. Westerterp KR. Physiol Behav 2006;89:62–5.

84. Ledikwe JH, Blanck HM, Khan LK et al. J Am Diet Assoc 2006;106:1172–80.

85. Rolls BJ, Roe LS, Meengs JS. Am J Clin Nutr 2010;91:913–22.

86. Rolls BJ, Roe LS, Meengs JS. J Am Diet Assoc 2004;104: 1570–6.

87. Schlundt DG, Hill JO, Pope-Cordle J et al. Int J Obes Relat Metab Disord 1993;17:623–9.

88. Jeffery RW, Hellerstedt WL, French SA et al. Int J Obes Relat Metab Disord 1995;19:132–7.

89. Brand-Miller JC, Holt SH, Pawlak DB et al. Am J Clin Nutr 2002;76:281S–5S.

90. Abete I, Parra D, Martinez JA. Clin Nutr 2008;27:545–51.

91. Pereira MA, Swain J, Goldfine AB et al. JAMA 2004;292: 2482–90.

92. Ebbeling CB, Leidig MM, Feldman HA et al. JAMA 2007;297:2092–102.

93. Ebbeling CB, Leidig MM, Sinclair KB et al. Arch Pediatr Adolesc Med 2003;157:773–9.

94. Ello-Martin JA, Ledikwe JH, Rolls BJ. Am J Clin Nutr 2005;82:236S–241S.

95. Faucher MA, Mobley J. J Midwifery Womens Health 2010; 55:60–4.

96. Gupta AK, Smith SR, Greenway FL et al. Diabetes Obes Metab 2009;11:330–7.

97. Pedersen SD, Kang J, Kline GA. Arch Intern Med 2007; 167:1277–83.

98. Wadden TA, Butryn ML, Wilson C. Gastroenterology 2007; 132:2226–38.

99. Hannum SM, Carson L, Evans EM et al. Obes Res 2004; 12:538–46.

100. Ditschuneit HH. Nestle Nutr Workshop Ser Clin Perform Programme 2006;11:171–9.

101. Ashley JM, Herzog H, Clodfelter S et al. Nutr J 2007;6:12.

102. Ashley JM, Herzog H, Clodfelter S et al. Nutr J 2007;6:12.
103. Davis LM, Coleman C, Kiel J et al. Nutr J 2010;9:11.
104. Allison DB, Gadbury G, Schwartz LG et al. Eur J Clin Nutr 2003;57:514–22.
105. Greaves CJ, Sheppard KE, Abraham C et al. BMC Public Health 2011;11:119.
106. Pate RR, Pratt M, Blair SN et al. JAMA 1995;273:402–7.
107. Haskell WL, Lee IM, Pate RR et al. Med Sci Sports Exerc 2007;39:1423–34.
108. Donnelly JE, Blair SN, Jakicic JM et al. Med Sci Sports Exerc 2009;41:459–71.
109. Chambliss HO. Clin J Sport Med 2005;15:113–5.
110. Redman LM, Heilbronn LK, Martin CK et al. J Clin Endocrinol Metab 2007;92:865–72.
111. Nicklas BJ, Wang X, You T et al. Am J Clin Nutr 2009;89:1043–52.
112. Cox KL, Burke V, Morton AR et al. Metabolism 2003;52:107–15.
113. Borg P, Kukkonen-Harjula K, Fogelholm M et al. Int J Obes Relat Metab Disord 2002;26:676–83.
114. Fogelholm M, Kukkonen-Harjula K, Nenonen A et al. Arch Intern Med 2000;160:2177–84.
115. Vogels N, Westerterp-Plantenga MS. Int J Obes 2005;29:849–57.
116. Leser MS, Yanovski SZ, Yanovski JA. J Am Diet Assoc 2002;102:1252–6.
117. Anton SD, Manini TM, Milsom VA et al. Clin Interv Aging 2011;6:141–9.
118. Hills AP, Shultz SP, Soares MJ et al. Obes Rev 2010;11:740–9.
119. Walberg JL. Sports Med 1989;7:343–56.
120. Winnick JJ, Gaillard T, Schuster DP. Ethn Dis 2008;18:152–6.
121. Daly RM, Dunstan DW, Owen N et al. Osteoporos Int 2005;16:1703–12.
122. Dolezal BA, Potteiger JA. J Appl Physiol 1998;85:695–700.
123. Lazzer S, Bedogni G, Lafortuna CL et al. Obesity 2010;18:71–8.
124. Shaw K, O'Rourke P, Del Mar C et al. Cochrane Database Syst Rev 2005;(2):CD003818.
125. Avenell A, Broom J, Brown TJ et al. Health Technol Assess 2004;8:iii-iv, 1–182.
126. Lang A, Froelicher ES. Eur J Cardiovasc Nurs 2006;5:102–14.
127. Renjilian DA, Perri MG, Nezu AM et al. J Consult Clin Psychol 2001;69:717–21.
128. Miller WM, Franklin BA, Nori Janosz KE et al. Metab Syndr Relat Disord 2009;7:441–6.
129. Cresci B, Tesi F, La Ferlita T et al. Eat Weight Disord 2007;12:147–53.
130. Perri M, Corsica J. Improving the maintenance of weight lost in behavioral treatment of obesity. In: Wadden TA, Stunkard A, eds. Handbook of Obesity. New York: Guilford Press, 2002:357–94.
131. Leermakers E, Perri M, Shigaki C et al. Addict Behav 1999;24:219–7.
132. Wadden TA, Vogt RA, Foster GD, et al. J Consult Clin Psychol 1998;66:429–33.
133. Vetter ML, Faulconbridge LF, Webb VL et al. Nat Rev Endocrinol 2010;6:578–88.
134. Jéquier E. Ann N Y Acad Sci 2002;967:379–88.
135. Hauptman J. Endocrine 2000;13:201–6.
136. Finer N, James WP, Kopelman PG et al. Int J Obes Relat Metab Disord 2000;24:306–13.
137. Sjöström L, Rissanen A, Andersen T et al. Lancet 1998;352:167–72.
138. Halpern A, Mancini MC, Suplicy H et al. Diabetes Obes Metab 2003;5:180–8.
139. Muls E, Kolanowski J, Scheen A et al. Int J Obes Relat Metab Disord 2001;25:1713–21.
140. Derosa G, Mugellini A, Ciccarelli L et al. Clin Ther 2003;25:1107–22.
141. Acharya NV, Wilton LV, Shakir SA. Int J Obes (Lond) 2006;30:1645–52.
142. Smith SR, Stenlof KS, Greenway FL et al. Obesity (Silver Spring) 2011;19:1796–803.
143. Anderson JW, Schwartz SM, Hauptman J et al. Ann Pharmacother 2006;40(10):1717–23.
144. Hendricks EJ, Greenway FL, Westman EC et al. Obesity (Silver Spring) 2011;19:2351–60.
145. Aronne LJ, Halseth AE, Burns CM et al. 2010;18:1739–46.
146. Connolly HM, Crary JL, McGoon MD et al. N Engl J Med 1997;337:581–8.
147. Brolin RE. Nutrition 1996;12:403–4.
148. Kissane NA, Pratt JS. Best Pract Res Clin Anaesthesiol 2011;25:11–25.

60 BARIATRIC SURGERY[1]

KEVIN TYMITZ, THOMAS MAGNUSON, AND MICHAEL SCHWEITZER

Obesity is a significant health concern in this country. It is a disease that is created by a multitude of genetic and environmental factors. The consequences of obesity are as equally complex as its etiology, affecting every organ system in the human body as well as imposing serious psychological stress often associated with social isolation, depression, and numerous other psychologic comorbidities. Medical management, unfortunately, usually fails to achieve sustained weight loss; and currently, bariatric surgical procedures are the most effective means to achieve sustained weight loss and also provide durable treatment of obesity-associated morbidities.

Weight-loss surgery is not a simple "cure" for this very complex and debilitating disease. It does, however, provide a powerful tool for patients to achieve success. A successful long-term outcome depends on the patient's commitment to a lifetime of dietary and lifestyle changes. For this reason, there must be a multidisciplinary approach that

includes surgeons, primary care physicians, psychologists, nurses, and dietitians to provide critical instructions to help patients adhere to the dietary and lifestyle changes consistent with the surgery.

The several types of bariatric surgery differ in expected outcomes in terms of weight loss and the likelihood of predisposing patients to nutritional deficiencies postoperatively. To understand these deficiencies and their appropriate management fully, it is imperative to understand the origin of the deficit. The purpose of this chapter is to review the various surgical procedures currently offered and the potential nutritional deficiencies that may ensue. Health care professionals must be aware of these deficiencies and the practice guidelines that must be followed to prevent these deficiencies because some of them may have serious consequences.

OVERVIEW

The prevalence of obesity continues to increase at an alarming rate throughout industrialized nations. Obesity is a disease that affects 34% of adults 20 years old and older in the United States, and this amounts to more than 72 million people. Approximately 33.3% of US men and about 35.3% of US women are obese. Nearly 6% of adults are classified as morbidly obese, with a body mass index (BMI) greater than 40 (1).

Obesity is a leading preventable cause of death worldwide, with increasing prevalence in adults and children. It is viewed as one of the most serious public health problems of the twenty-first century. Obesity is stigmatized in much of the modern world (particularly in the Western world), although it was widely perceived as a symbol of wealth and fertility at other times in history and still is in some parts of the world.

Health care professionals need to be concerned about the prevalence of obesity because of the well-established relationships between excess body weight and serious medical conditions such as type 2 diabetes, hypertension, and heart disease, just to name a few. These relationships have long been established in the adult obese population and more recently also have been observed at an increasing rate in the adolescent population.

Unfortunately, no single solution to prevent or treat obesity is beneficial for everyone. Treatment of obesity

---

[1]**Abbreviations: BMI,** body mass index; **D-RYGB,** distal Roux-en-Y gastric bypass; **DS-BPD,** duodenal switch with biliopancreatic diversion; **IF,** intrinsic factor; **JIB,** jejunoileal bypass; **LAGB,** laparoscopic adjustable gastric band; **LVSG,** laparoscopic vertical sleeve gastrectomy; **RYGB,** Roux-en-Y gastric bypass; **TPN,** total parenteral nutrition.

may include a combination of diet, exercise, behavior modification, and medications. For most patients, although these methods may provide a moderate amount of weight loss, the benefits are usually short lived. Hence, bariatric surgery has evolved over the past couple of decades and has been shown to be effective in reducing obesity-related comorbidities, improving the quality of life, and decreasing the number of sick days, monthly medication costs, and overall mortality. With the increasing rates of weight loss procedures, the quality, efficacy, and surgical outcomes have improved with the creation of Bariatric Centers of Excellence designated by the American Society of Metabolic and Bariatric Surgery and the American College of Surgeons. The benefits of bariatric procedures in morbidly obese patients outweigh the risks. With the advent of minimally invasive surgical procedures, bariatric surgery is a reasonable treatment option in those who strongly desire substantial weight loss and have life-threatening comorbid conditions.

Definition of Morbid Obesity

The definition and classification of obesity are based on calculation of the BMI—calculated as weight in kilograms divided by height in meters squared. For the majority of the population (except athletes), BMI provides a reliable indicator of the body fat composition. It is used to stratify patients into categories that may lead to health problems. Patients with a BMI of 30 to 35 kg/m^2 are considered to have class I obesity, a BMI of 35 to 40 kg/m^2 is class II, and a BMI higher than 40 kg/m^2 is class III. Morbid obesity is defined as a BMI of 40 kg/m^2 or higher or a BMI of 35 kg/m^2 or higher in patients with comorbidities. Patients are defined as suffering from superobesity or megaobesity if their BMI is higher than 50 or 70 kg/m^2, respectively.

Indications

The National Institutes of Health issued a consensus statement in 1991 (2) regarding the effectiveness of bariatric surgery. The statement outlined patient selection criteria that are still in place today (Table 60.1). Patients are considered candidates for bariatric surgery if they have a BMI of 40 kg/m^2 or greater or a BMI between 35 and 40 kg/m^2 if an obesity-related comorbid

---

TABLE 60.1	INDICATIONS FOR BARIATRIC SURGERY FOR MORBID OBESITY

1. BMI ≥40 kg/m^2
2. BMI 35–40 kg/m^2 with significant obesity-related comorbidities (hypertension, diabetes)
3. Unsuccessful attempt at weight loss by nonoperative means
4. Clearance by dietitian and mental health professional
5. No medical contraindications to surgery

BMI, body mass index.

---

condition exists, such as diabetes or hypertension. In general, appropriate candidates for surgery should demonstrate prior unsuccessful attempts at medically supervised weight reduction programs and should have realistic expectations regarding the long-term outcomes achieved with the surgery. Relative contraindications include an inability to comply with postoperative requirements and follow-up, active alcohol or substance abuse, and uncontrolled psychiatric disease.

Preoperative Assessment of the Obese Patient

The evaluation of potential patients for bariatric surgery should involve a multidisciplinary team approach. This team should include a dietitian and a mental health professional familiar with bariatric surgery. Their purposes are to obtain a complete past dietary and behavioral eating history, educate the patient on postoperative dietary expectations, examine the social support structure, and ensure that any psychiatric or behavioral disorders are optimally controlled. At the Johns Hopkins Center for Bariatric Surgery in Baltimore, all patients are required to attend a multidisciplinary preoperative education seminar. Postoperative participation in support groups is also encouraged.

Nutritional Deficits in the Obese Patient

Nutritional assessment must be an essential part of the preoperative evaluation of the obese patient. Despite the increased caloric intake of the obese population, many suffer from various nutritional deficiencies, particularly the morbid obese with a BMI higher than 40. Consumption of excess calories does not usually correlate with overconsumption of fresh fruits and vegetables or high-quality, nutrient-dense foods. Instead, this more likely correlates with the consumption of higher calorie processed foods that are of low nutritional quality that is very common in developed countries such as the United States. In fact, it is estimated that 27% to 30% of the daily caloric intake of the average US adult or child consists of these low-nutrient-dense food sources, with sweeteners and desserts contributing an estimated 18% to 24% of the total (3, 4).

As the obesity epidemic continues to flourish, obesity should be recognized as a risk factor for many nutrient deficiencies. For example, obese individuals tend to have lower mean levels of vitamin D and calcium compared with lean subjects (5). There are many theories behind this observation including decreased consumption of vitamin D–fortified milk, sedentary lifestyle, reduced exposure to sunlight, and sequestration of the lipid-soluble vitamin in the excess adipose tissue, which can be verified by studies that show serum 25-hydroxyvitamin D (25[OH]D) levels to be inversely proportional to increasing fat mass (6, 7). Decreased vitamin D levels can have deleterious effects on the immune system and may play a role in increasing the risk of cancers, diabetes mellitus, autoimmune diseases, and cardiovascular disease (8). It is estimated that 25% to 80% of adult patients before bariatric surgery may have baseline vitamin D deficiency (9, 10). Other studies looking at baseline nutritional deficits of adults presenting for bariatric surgery also showed decreased levels of the other fat-soluble vitamins A, K, and E (11, 12).

Low vitamin B_{12} levels have been reported in up to 18% of severely obese adults (13), and vitamin B_1 (thiamin) deficiency has been noted in up to 29% of patients undergoing bariatric surgery (9). Deficiencies of other B vitamins are not currently known because they are not frequently included in screening. Unfortunately, depending on the type of surgical procedure and compliance with postoperative supplementation, these deficiencies can become highly exacerbated.

TYPES OF PROCEDURES

The dramatic growth in bariatric surgical procedures performed over the past couple of decades can be attributed to many factors. Increased patient acceptance is one major factor, and it can be attributed in large part to the introduction of laparoscopic and minimally invasive surgical techniques. Significant advantages are offered with laparoscopic and minimally invasive surgery such as less pain, fewer wound complications, and early recovery with relatively low complication rates. Advances in anesthesia, critical care, and parenteral nutrition are other milestones in the success of bariatric procedures.

The bariatric surgical options can be classified into the following three categories: restrictive procedures, malabsorptive procedures, and combined restrictive and malabsorptive procedures. Purely restrictive procedures depend on restriction of the amount of food that enters the foregut. In contrast, malabsorptive procedures depend on the malabsorption of nutrients by bypassing various segments of the small intestine. Combined restrictive and malabsorptive procedures are a combination of the two.

Purely Restrictive Procedures

The laparoscopic adjustable gastric band (LAGB) received Food and Drug Administration approval in 2001 and has been in clinical use in the United States since that time. The LAGB is the only device that is adjustable after surgery, thus allowing for tightening or loosening of the band through a subcutaneous port placed for fluid injection. Other advantages of the band include relative ease of placement, lack of operative staple lines or need for bowel transection, and reversibility. The band does require, however, an average of five to six adjustments in the first year after surgery; and its success depends in part on patient compliance and close follow-up.

Dissection for the LAGB (Fig. 60.1) is first performed bluntly at the angle of His, thus freeing up attachments for

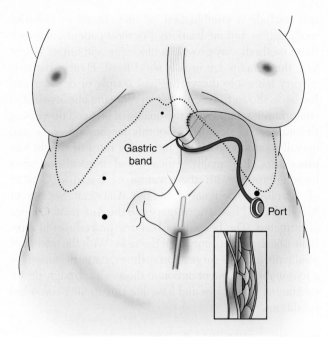

Fig. 60.1. Laparoscopic adjustable gastric band. (Courtesy Johns Hopkins University.)

later insertion of the band. The gastrohepatic ligament is then opened, and the plane posterior to the gastroesophageal junction is bluntly dissected. The adjustable band is placed in the abdomen through a trocar in the left upper quadrant and is secured around the gastroesophageal junction, with a slightly diagonal orientation up toward the angle of His. One to four sutures are then placed from the fundus to the proximal stomach around the band, to secure the band in place and minimize the possibility of band migration or herniation. The band tubing is brought out through the left upper quadrant trocar site, where it is secured to the subcutaneous injection port. Fascia is cleared in this area, and the port is secured to the fascia with care taken not to entrap or kink the band tubing. The band is left empty until 6 weeks postoperatively, when patients receive their first fill. Frequent office visits are usually necessary, especially over the first year, for fluid fills or removal to obtain an appropriate restriction with food ingestion to sustain an appropriate weight loss.

Of the commonly performed bariatric procedures, the laparoscopic vertical sleeve gastrectomy (LVSG) is the most recently introduced, and only limited outcomes data (5 years) are available. Unlike the band, the LVSG does not involve an implanted foreign body that can potentially erode or migrate, and it does not require frequent adjustments. The sleeve resection may also achieve weight loss by affecting satiety. Serum levels of ghrelin, a proappetite hormone produced in the fundus, are reduced after the LVSG because that area of the stomach has been resected. In addition, the sleeve procedure is not reversible because a partial gastrectomy is performed, but it can be converted to a gastric bypass or duodenal switch later if greater weight loss is desired.

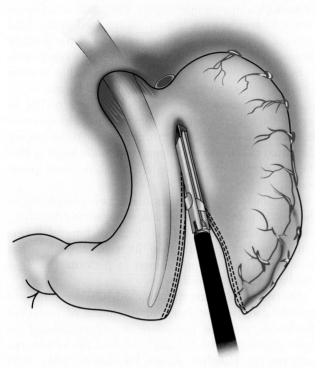

Fig. 60.2. Laparoscopic vertical sleeve gastrectomy. (Courtesy Johns Hopkins University.)

The LVSG (Fig. 60.2) is performed by first dividing the short gastric vessels along the greater curve of the stomach beginning near the antrum and extending to the angle of His. A 40F bougie is placed in the stomach and is directed along the lesser curve. The stomach is then divided with the laparoscopic stapler by using the bougie as a guide, beginning 6 cm from the pylorus on the greater curve side and continuing up to the angle of His. The lateral stomach specimen is then removed from one of the trocar sites.

Malabsorptive Procedures

Jejunoileal bypass (JIB) is a purely restrictive procedure that was very common in the 1960s and 1970s despite lack of scientific study of its mechanism of action. This particular procedure bypasses approximately 90% of the small intestine. The proposed mechanism of action was induced weight loss by a surgically induced short gut syndrome. This procedure is based on canine studies performed in the mid-1950s that showed that 50% of the small intestine in dogs can be removed without apparent effects, with profound interference with fat absorption associated with weight loss (14). Many complications were associated with bypassing a large portion of the small intestine, however. Patients suffered frequent flatulence and diarrhea secondary to bypassing the site of bile acid reabsorption. Electrolyte deficiencies were common secondary to loss of potassium, calcium, and magnesium. Various vitamin deficiencies frequently led to neuropathies, bone demineralization, and protein malnutrition. Exposure of colonic mucosa to excessive bile salts created

calcium oxalate renal stones. In addition, bacterial overgrowth in the bypassed small intestine led to hepatic decomposition and arthritis. It was later determined that the actual mechanism of action of weight loss from this procedure was learned behavior. The rectal complications and intense anal irritation from the diarrhea led to patients' changes in eating habits (15). Patients learned very quickly that, to function in society, they had to consume only minimal fat and nutrients before venturing away from their homes. For these reasons, the JIB procedure has long been abandoned, but it did pave the way for the more recent techniques of bariatric surgery.

The laparoscopic duodenal switch with biliopancreatic diversion (DS-BPD) is predominantly a malabsorptive operation that involves preservation of the gastric pylorus and creation of a short, 100-cm ileal "common channel," where food and biliopancreatic enzymes are allowed to mix. Because of the potential for malabsorption-related nutritional deficiencies and the complexity of the operation, DS-BPD is the least common bariatric operation performed (5% to 10% overall).

The first step in the DS-BPD (Fig. 60.3) involves dividing the small bowel 250 cm from the ileocecal valve. The proximal end of the bowel is then anastomosed to the distal ileum

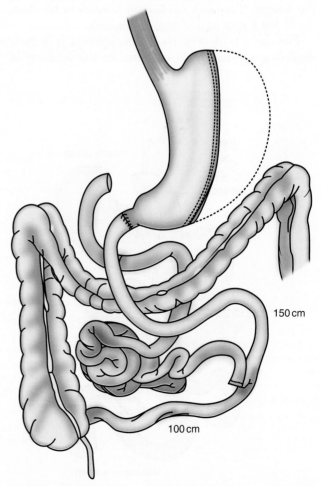

150 cm

100 cm

Fig. 60.3. Duodenal switch with biliopancreatic diversion. (Courtesy Johns Hopkins University.)

100 cm from its juncture with the cecum. A vertical sleeve gastrectomy is then performed over a 48F bougie to reduce the size of the stomach, thus providing some restriction as well. The duodenum is divided approximately 3 to 4 cm distal to the pylorus with a laparoscopic stapler. The Roux limb is then brought antecolic up to the end of the proximal duodenum, and a side-to-side anastomosis is performed.

Combined Restrictive and Malabsorptive Procedures

Roux-en-Y gastric bypass (RYGB) is the most common bariatric procedure performed in the United States (60% to 70% overall). It has been demonstrated in numerous reports to achieve durable long-term weight loss and remission of metabolic disease with a reasonably low complication rate. The procedure-related rate of remission of type 2 diabetes is among the highest of the bariatric procedures: 84% to 98%, depending on the preoperative severity and duration of the diabetes (16, 17). Normoglycemia often occurs within days after the operation well before significant weight loss has occurred (18). This finding suggests that the resolution of type 2 diabetes is related not only to restriction of caloric intake but also to changes in gut peptide secretion secondary to bypassing a portion of the foregut. The exact mechanism remains to be elucidated, but it is an area of ongoing research.

For the RYGB (Fig. 60.4), the jejunum is initially divided approximately 60 cm distal to the ligament of

Treitz with a laparoscopic stapler. The proximal biliopancreatic limb of jejunum is then anastomosed to the distal segment of jejunum 75 to 100 cm distal to the point of division. This anastomosis is performed in a side-to-side fashion. The mesenteric defect is closed with a running suture to help minimize the risk of internal hernia.

Next, dissection is performed at the angle of His, to expose the left crus, and at the gastrohepatic ligament, to gain access to the lesser sac. Multiple staple cartridges are then used to transect the stomach up to the angle of His, thus creating a vertically oriented, 20-mL proximal gastric pouch.

The Roux limb of jejunum is routinely brought up to the gastric pouch in an antecolic-antegastric orientation. This seems to reduce the incidence of internal hernia and is simpler to perform than the retrocolic-retrogastric approach. The gastrojejunostomy is performed using a standard side-to-side technique.

Outcomes following the standard RYGB continue to provide good weight loss and resolution of comorbid conditions, and the procedure is still considered by most surgeons to be the gold standard for weight-loss surgery (19). However, weight loss failure (BMI >35) can and still does occur, reportedly in 15% to 35% of cases (20–22). This outcome is more commonly seen in superobese patients. It is common for these patients to seek additional surgery to attain their goals. One way to do this is to convert to a distal Roux-en-Y gastric bypass (D-RYGB). With this procedure, conversion is made to a 100- to 150-cm common limb, therefore promoting further malabsorption.

POTENTIAL NUTRIENT DEFICITS AFTER BARIATRIC SURGERY

As previously mentioned, early attempts at bariatric surgery, such as the JIB, shed light on the potential nutritional consequences of bypassing a significant portion of the small intestine. Even as the surgical techniques have evolved and improvements made, very specific guidelines still must be followed to prevent serious complications.

As the number of people who undergo bariatric surgery increases, more patients are being followed up by general practitioners who need to be aware of these preventable complications. The type and the frequency of the nutritional deficiency are related to the type of operation performed. Purely restrictive procedures, such as the LAGB and LVSG, have the least impact on vitamin and mineral absorption because none of the small intestine is bypassed. DS-BPD is the procedure performed today with the greatest impact on nutrients because a large portion of the small bowel is bypassed with only a short common channel for absorption. Regardless of the procedure, patients must constantly be monitored for the development of nutritional deficiencies and receive the appropriate supplementation.

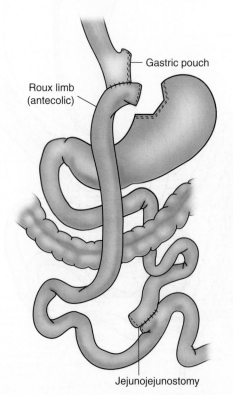

Fig. 60.4. Roux-en-Y gastric bypass. (Courtesy Johns Hopkins University.)

Gastric pouch

Roux limb (antecolic)

Jejunojejunostomy

Pathophysiology of Diabetes

In the fed state, insulin is secreted from the pancreatic β cells in response to the increased circulating glucose concentrations, thus promoting glycogen synthesis in liver and muscle, lipid formation in adipocytes, and amino acid uptake and protein synthesis in most cells. In the postabsorptive state, during starvation, and in response to stress, decreased insulin levels and increased glucagon contribute to glycogen breakdown, lipolysis, hepatic ketogenesis, and decreased synthesis and increased degradation of protein. This decline in insulin levels also results in an increased hepatic release of glucose into the systemic circulation to maintain glucose levels (66, 67).

In DM, decreased insulin action poses a range of metabolic abnormalities that span from the effects of mild insulin deficiency, as seen in hyperglycemia, to the effects of insulinopenia, as seen in diabetic ketoacidosis (DKA) associated with fluid and electrolyte depletion (68). In postabsorptive or fasted states, hyperglycemia does not resolve and often worsens. Low insulin activity results in exaggerated counterregulatory responses that normally serve to protect against the development of hypoglycemia (69). The result of decreased insulin action and elevated counterregulatory hormones (glucagon, catecholamines and to a lesser extent, growth hormone and cortisol) includes, initially, the conversion of stored glycogen to glucose. Glucagon is a potent activator of glycogenolysis and gluconeogenesis (in the liver) and is able to increase endogenous glucose production.

In DM, relative or absolute insulin deficiency leads to a marked decrease in activity of the glucose transporter-4 (GLUT4) largely as a consequence of decreased insulin-stimulated GLUT4 localization to the surface membranes of skeletal muscle. The results are a decrease in the normal postmeal flux of glucose into skeletal muscle and increased circulating plasma glucose (65).

DM is also associated with increased activity of enzymes involved in gluconeogenesis and decreased activity of glycolytic and oxidative enzymes. In addition, DM is often associated with relative or absolute hyperglucagonemia, resulting from loss of the suppressive effect of insulin on glucagon secretion by the pancreatic α cell.

COMPLICATIONS

DM is a chronic disease that can cause complications leading to significant morbidity and premature death, particularly if it is not well treated.

Acute Complications

Symptoms of hyperglycemia include increased polyuria (frequent urination), polydipsia (excessive thirst), fatigue, irritability, blurred vision, and weight loss. Blurry vision results from osmolar shifts from hyperglycemia within the lens (67). Polyuria and polydipsia occur when blood glucose increases above the urinary filtering threshold of 180 mg/dL. In normal glucose states, all glucose filtered at the glomerulus is reabsorbed by the tubules. However, the elevated plasma glucose in DM may lead to an increase in the filtered load of glucose that exceeds the maximum tubular reabsorptive capacity, and large amounts of glucose may be excreted (71). For the same reason, large amounts of ketones may also appear in the urine. These urinary losses further deplete the body of nutrients and lead to weight loss. Far worse, however, is the effect of these solutes on sodium and water excretion.

DKA and the hyperglycemic hyperosmolar state (HHS) are acute complications of DM. DKA was formerly considered a hallmark of type 1 DM, but it may also rarely occur in type 2 DM (72). HHS is primarily seen in individuals with type 2 DM. Both disorders are associated with absolute or relative insulin deficiency, volume depletion, and acid–base abnormalities. In DKA, the osmotic force exerted by unreabsorbed glucose and ketones leads to retention of water in the tubule, thereby preventing its reabsorption and leading to fluid depletion. Sodium reabsorption is also retarded, and the net result is marked excretion of sodium and water, which can lead in worst cases to hypotension, brain damage, and death if left untreated (73).

The most frequent complication in diabetic persons who are treated with insulin is hypoglycemia. However, hypoglycemia can also occur in patients who are not taking insulin but are using hypoglycemic agents such as insulin secretagogues.

Chronic Complications

Chronic complications occur over years or decades of hyperglycemia and are often difficult or impossible to reverse. Examples include microvascular complications (i.e., small vessel disease) such as retinopathy, neuropathy, and nephropathy or macrovascular complications (i.e., large vessel disease) such as coronary heart disease, peripheral vascular disease, or stroke. The pathophysiologic features of both microvascular and macrovascular complications are similar; both types of complications are secondary to oxidative damage from long-term, uncontrolled hyperglycemia, resulting in plaque formation and narrowing of small and large blood vessels and ischemic damage to end organ tissues. The risk of CVD is increased two to four times in patients with DM, and CVD can be fatal.

Chronic microvascular complications of DM can be delayed or prevented by optimal glycemic control (i.e., hemoglobin A1c <7%), as demonstrated in several key studies including the DCCT in type 1 DM and the UK Prospective Diabetes Study (UKPDS) in type 2 DM. These landmark trials concluded that achieving and maintaining serum glucose levels in this range slowed the onset and progression of eye, kidney, and nerve diseases caused by DM. Macrovascular complications of DM such as heart disease can be reduced both with optimal glycemic control, as demonstrated in the long-term follow-up of studies such as the DCCT and UKPDS, and with cardiovascular

TABLE 61.3	CHRONIC COMPLICATIONS OF DIABETES MELLITUS

I. Microvascular
  A. Retinopathy (nonproliferative or proliferative)
    a. Macular edema
  B. Neuropathy
    a. Peripheral
    b. Autonomic
  C. Nephropathy
II. Macrovascular
  A. Cardiovascular disease
  B. Peripheral vascular disease
  C. Cerebrovascular disease
III. Other less common complications
  A. Gastrointestinal diseases (e.g., gastroparesis, diarrhea)
  B. Genitourinary diseases (e.g., uropathy, sexual dysfunction)
  C. Dermatologic or musculoskeletal diseases (e.g., shin spots, osteoporosis)
  D. Infectious diseases (e.g., osteomyelitis, zygomycoses)
  E. Hematologic or malignant diseases (e.g., anemia, pancreatic cancer)
  F. Neurologic or psychiatric diseases (e.g., dementia, depression)

risk factor modification of comorbidities such as hypertension and dyslipidemia.

Other common complications include poor wound healing, increased susceptibility to infections, erectile dysfunction, and gastroparesis. In addition, many comorbidities associated with DM may influence DM management, including human immunodeficiency virus infection, cystic fibrosis, polycystic ovarian syndrome, postpancreatectomy DM, and Cushing syndrome. Sleep apnea and depression are also common (Table 61.3). This list is by no means inclusive.

DM is manageable. Its complications are not inevitable with optimal glycemic control and cardiovascular risk factor management, and they can be treated if they occur.

GOALS FOR MEDICAL NUTRITION THERAPY

MNT is a vital component in the prevention and management of DM. MNT varies with the type of DM and the age of the individual. In general, MNT promotes healthy eating habits, helps control blood glucose and lipid levels, and helps with weight management by making lifestyle modifications. MNT has been seen to be effective with reported decreases in hemoglobin A1c of 1% to 2%, depending on the type and duration of DM (74, 75). MNT has the greatest impact at the initial diagnosis of DM and continues to be an effective intervention at any time throughout the disease process (76–78).

Once the diagnosis of DM is established, treatment includes a medical nutrition plan, pharmacologic therapy (oral agents, noninsulin injectables, insulin, or a combination of these), regular monitoring by health care professional

team, and, most important, self-monitoring and continuing education of the patient or caregiver about managing DM. MNT should be offered in several phases, based on the individual's comprehension and readiness to learn. Just as the disease process has different stages, the individual's ability to understand also has different levels. During the initial treatment, basic principles, such as identifying sources of carbohydrates and prevention and treatment of hypoglycemia, may be introduced. During later sessions, in-depth self-management guidance, such as carbohydrate counting and adjusting insulin-to-carbohydrate ratios, is provided. Throughout the treatment process, individualization is the key. Table 61.4 depicts the ADA goals for MNT for various circumstances in which treatment should be tailored to achieve these goals (79).

Nutritional Plan

To achieve these goals, formal process steps include a nutrition assessment, nutrition diagnosis, and intervention, followed by monitoring and evaluation. Nutrition management includes monitoring of blood glucose, medications, physical activity, education, behavior modification, and evaluation of cardiovascular and renal status, to

TABLE 61.4	AMERICAN DIABETES ASSOCIATION GOALS FOR MEDICAL NUTRITION THERAPY

For those at risk for diabetes or prediabetes:
• To decrease the risk of diabetes and cardiovascular disease by promoting healthy food choices and physical activity and thus facilitating loss of excess body weight
For those individuals with diabetes:
• Achieve and maintain
  • Blood glucose levels in the normal range or as close to normal as safely possible
  • A lipid and lipoprotein profile that reduces the risk for vascular disease
  • Blood pressure levels in the normal range or as close to normal as safely possible
• To prevent, or at least slow, the rate of development of the chronic complications of diabetes by modifying nutrient intake and lifestyle
• To address individual nutrition needs, by taking into account personal and cultural preferences and willingness to change
• To maintain the pleasure of eating by limiting food choices only when indicated by scientific evidence
For those with specific situations:
• For youth with type 1 diabetes, youth with type 2 diabetes, pregnant and lactating women, and older adults with diabetes, to meet the nutritional needs of these unique times in the life cycle
• For individuals treated with insulin or insulin secretagogues, to provide self-management training for safe conduct of exercise, including the prevention and treatment of hypoglycemia, and diabetes treatment during acute illness

Adapted with permission from the American Diabetes Association. Nutrition recommendations and interventions for diabetes: a position statement of the American Diabetes Association. Diabetes Care 2008;31:S61–78.

rogate carbohydrate sources rather than as an addition. However, it is difficult for persons to do this without adding additional calories and carbohydrates.

Nonnutritive sweeteners can be beneficial to persons with DM because these substances add flavor without adding calories or eliciting a glycemic response. The nonnutritive sweeteners are derived from substances of several different chemical classes that interact with taste receptors, and they typically exceed the sweetness of sucrose by a factor of 30 to 13,000 times (117). Currently, six nonnutritive sweeteners are approved by the US Food and Drug Administration (FDA) regulated as food additives for use in DM that report no effect on changes in glycemic response. In addition, some are heat resistant and can be used for cooking and baking. See Table 61.6 for a comparative summary on individual nonnutritive sweeteners.

Results from some studies suggest that users of nonnutritive sweeteners may tend to consume more calories and even gain weight because of specific effects of the sweetener on appetite. However, the data on this issue are controversial (118–120), and a definitive conclusion awaits further research.

Food Exchanges

Patients and most health professionals have shifted away from the use of traditional exchange lists for meal planning. These traditional exchange lists estimated not only carbohydrates but also proportions of fats and proteins in similar foods. Food exchanges are still helpful in identifying carbohydrate amounts for common foods, such as ½ cup of vegetables, which quantifies carbohydrate servings into 15-g exchanges. The trend therefore is to emphasize the total carbohydrate in gram amounts or by carbohydrate "choices" in which one choice is equal to 15 g of carbohydrate. Examples of a 15-g carbohydrate choice include one slice of bread, ⅓ cup of pasta or rice, or one small apple. Fat intake should also be addressed, with more emphasis on the types of fats, saturated versus monounsaturated and polyunsaturated. This shift in teaching allows for more emphasis on specific carbohydrate and fat awareness, rather than lumping mixed foods together in exchanges.

Carbohydrate Counting

Carbohydrate counting and carbohydrate awareness are essential because carbohydrate intake is the primary nutrient affecting postprandial blood glucose levels (121). Carbohydrate counting also allows flexibility in food choices and helps promote glycemic control (122). Other methods for estimating carbohydrate intake are the exchange system and experience-based estimations (123). Carbohydrate awareness is helpful for all persons with DM, but it is essential in treating type 1 DM, so the patient knows the effect of the meal on blood glucose and can better match food intake to insulin doses.

The model of carbohydrate counting is a nutrition strategy that requires the patient to have knowledge of carbohydrate amounts in food and is highly dependent on the patient's ability to monitor blood glucose levels and perform mathematical conversions to determine the amount of carbohydrate in meals. The three levels of carbohydrate counting (basic, intermediate, and advanced) can be evolved through by a motivated individual with DM once carbohydrate amounts and equivalents in foods are maintained at consistent blood glucose levels (Table 61.7).

Carbohydrate counting uses a grouping method to place foods in categories of similar carbohydrate equivalency. Carbohydrate counting estimates intake either by total grams of carbohydrate or by one serving, which is considered 15 g (Table 61.8). For example, one carbohydrate serving is equal to a 15-g carbohydrate serving of starch, grain, fruit, or milk. A patient's ability to follow this method will allow for a greater variety in food choices (124).

Micronutrients

Continual interest exists in supplementation with various vitamins, minerals, and trace elements. Investigators are interested in trace elements and minerals such as chromium, potassium, magnesium, vanadium, and zinc and their effects on blood glucose control in DM. The evidence, however, is slim and unconvincing that supplementation of any of these trace elements has a beneficial effect, except perhaps in true deficiency.

TABLE 61.7	LEVELS OF CARBOHYDRATE COUNTING	
LEVEL	DIABETES TYPE	DESCRIPTION
Level I: Basic	Type 1, type 2, or gestational	Key concept of carbohydrate counting: awareness of which foods contain carbohydrates, portion sizes, avoidance of sweets and sweetened beverages, and carbohydrate consistency
Level II: Intermediate	Type 1, type 2, or gestational	Understanding of how blood glucose levels are affected and managed by food, medications, and physical activity; focused on pattern management and reducing weight gain if necessary
Level III: Advanced	Type 1	Teaching how to calculate carbohydrate-to-insulin ratios when using multiple daily injections or insulin infusion pumps to match short-acting insulin to carbohydrate
Portion control emphasized in all three levels		

Adapted with permission from Gillespie SJ, Kulkarni KD, Daly AE. Using carbohydrate counting in diabetes clinical practice. J Am Diet Assoc 1998;98:897–905.

TABLE 61.8	EXAMPLES OF 15-GRAM CARBOHYDRATE SERVINGS IN FOOD GROUPS CONTAINING CARBOHYDRATES			
STARCH OR GRAIN	FRUIT	MILK	SWEETS	COMBINATION FOODS
¼ large bagel	1 small fresh fruit	1 cup white milk	2-in square piece	½ cup casserole
1 slice bread	½ banana	½ cup chocolate milk	of cake or brownie	½ sandwich
1 6-in tortilla	½ canned fruit in light	1 cup soy milk	without icing	1 cup meat stew with
½ cup cooked cereal	syrup	1 cup plain yogurt	2 small cookies	vegetables
⅓ cup pasta	2 tbsp dried fruit		5 vanilla wafers	1 small taco
⅓ cup rice	17 small grapes		½ cup sugar-free	
1 cup coup	1 cup melon		pudding	
½ cup corn	¾–1 cup berries		1 tbsp sugar or honey	
½ cup mashed			½ cup plain ice cream	
potatoes			¼ cup sherbet or sorbet	
5 crackers				
3 cups popcorn				
¾ oz potato or				
tortilla chips				
½ cup cooked beans				
or lentils				

When an individual is in poor glucose control or taking diuretic medications, serum magnesium levels may be low. Serum magnesium blood testing is recommended to determine whether a deficiency exists.

Routine supplementation of vitamins E and C and carotene is not advised because of lack of evidence of efficacy and concern related to long-term safety. Vitamin E supplementations were found to have no beneficial effects on cardiovascular outcomes, microvascular complications, or on glycemic control in persons with DM and CVD (125). Vitamins B_1, B_6, and B_{12} are sometimes used to treat diabetic peripheral neuropathy, but without much strong supporting evidence of benefit.

Chromium may have positive effects on glucose metabolism; however, studies have yielded conflicting results, and routine supplementation is not currently recommended. Supplements are indicated for vitamins, minerals, and trace elements when a deficiency is suspected or likely. High-risk populations include elderly persons, pregnant or lactating women, strict vegetarians, or persons on a calorie-restricted diet, with poor glycemic control, or taking medications that alter micronutrient metabolism. Folate supplementation is well documented to improve the outcome of pregnancy, with or without DM.

In addition, deficiencies in vitamin D in many populations have been reported as a result of decreased sun exposure, aging, and/or lactose intolerance (decrease in milk fortified with vitamin D consumption). The literature suggests an association between vitamin D insufficiency and glycemic control (126), although further studies are needed. Calcium supplementation is indicated, particularly in elderly persons, if daily intake is less than 1.0 to 1.5 g.

In summary, evidence is weak that vitamin, mineral, or trace element supplementation benefits patients with DM without a true deficiency, and none of these supplements have clear benefits on glucose control. It would obviously be attractive if simple oral supplements could facilitate normoglycemia. If the diet is adequate, supplementation has little or no role in the control of DM, and general nutritional guidelines for vitamins and trace elements should be followed.

PHYSICAL ACTIVITY

The American College of Sports Medicine (ACSM) defines physical activity as "bodily movement that is produced by the contraction of skeletal muscle and that substantially increases energy expenditure." Regular physical activity is strongly encouraged in all persons with DM and should be incorporated into the daily lifestyle. The ADA and ACSM currently recommend 150 minutes/week of moderate to vigorous aerobic activity over at least 3 days a week, and 2 to 3 days/week of moderate to vigorous resistance exercises (127). Exercise has beneficial effects on glycemic control, body composition, hypertension, hyperlipidemia, and obesity, as well as psychologic effects (128–130). Snowling and Hopkins (129) reported an average hemoglobin A1c reduction of −0.8% after 130 to 270 minutes/week of exercise for 6 months, within the range to promote significant reductions in microvascular, macrovascular, and nonvascular complications in persons with DM. Physical activity also increases insulin sensitivity, so adjustments to prevent low blood glucose, such as exercise after meals, additional carbohydrate intake, or less insulin than usual (≤50%) are recommended depending on the intensity and duration of exercise.

Special precautions must be considered in prescribing an exercise plan. Because patients with DM are also known to be at a higher risk of developing CVD, neuropathy, nephropathy, and retinopathy, further evaluation may be warranted to determine whether these complications exist and/or the degree of progression to ascertain an appropriate physical activity program. For example,

CVD is the major cause of mortality for people with DM; therefore, a careful cardiac assessment should be performed before any fitness program is initiated in high-risk individuals. This assessment may include a graded exercise stress test. It is routinely advised for any individual to consult a physician before initiating an exercise program.

ADDITIONAL CONSIDERATIONS

Children

Primary goals of nutrition therapy for children with DM are to promote normal growth and development, achieve good glycemic control, prevent hypoglycemia, and decrease the risk of complications. The nutritional management of type 1 and type 2 DM in children varies because most children with type 1 DM are thin at diagnosis, whereas most children with type 2 DM are overweight.

Type 1 Diabetes

Providing enough calories for growth has always been a concern when developing the nutrition plan for children with DM. Parents and children with type 1 DM need to be guided in adjusting the insulin dose to the child's increasing energy needs and be warned against withholding food or substituting noncaloric foods in an effort to keep blood glucose levels under control. Adequate growth should be monitored several times a year to ensure appropriate growth for the child's age and gender, especially in the first few years after the diagnosis. As with adults, the nutrition plan should be customized to the child's needs and preferences and carefully evaluated and readjusted as the child grows. The ADA recommends progressively stricter hemoglobin A1c goals for type 1 DM with age: 0 to 6 years, 7.5% to 8.5%; 6 to 12 years, less than 8%; 13 to 19 years, less than 7.5%,; older than 19 years, less than 7% (29). Care and education should be provided by a DM team with a pediatric endocrinologist, a nurse, a dietitian, and a mental health counselor who are familiar with the normal stages of childhood and adolescent development and how they affect DM management (131).

Type 2 Diabetes

The increasing prevalence of type 2 DM in youth is related to the increasing obesity epidemic in children. Obesity, which causes insulin resistance, is the strongest modifiable risk factor for type 2 DM in children 10 to 19 years old. The increased incidence of type 2 DM, especially in minority ethnic groups (e.g., African-Americans), is related to the increased prevalence of obesity in children. Treatment involves medications to normalize glycemia, lifestyle modifications in food intake and physical activity to promote weight loss, and control of comorbidities (132). Currently, only insulin and metformin are approved for use in children by the FDA.

Elderly Patients

Type 2 DM in persons more than 65 years old is a major public health problem. Normal aging is associated with impaired insulin sensitivity (133–135), possibly because of lower density of the glucose carrier GLUT4 in the muscle that could contribute to insulin resistance (136). Biologic changes associated with aging may also contribute to impaired insulin sensitivity, including increased abdominal fat mass, decreased physical activity, mitochondrial dysfunction, hormonal changes, increased oxidative stress, and inflammation (137). The presence of comorbidities, cognitive dysfunction, and functional disabilities affects the management of DM, especially in elderly persons. Depression and dementia are more common in older adults with DM and are associated with difficulties in self-management that lead to poor glycemic control. Older adults with DM are two to three times more likely to have functional disabilities, including difficulties walking a quarter mile, lifting heavy objects, doing housework, or participating in leisure activities, compared with their nondiabetic counterparts (138).

Lifestyle interventions are recommended for clinical treatment. Weight loss recommendations for older adults who are overweight and obese are appropriate. In contrast, debilitated nursing home residents may not be good candidates for weight loss (139). The hemoglobin A1c goal of less than 7% for otherwise healthy older adults with type 2 DM and a life expectancy of more than 5 years is recommended by the ADA (29). However, elderly persons with multiple comorbidities, functional disabilities, and/or limited expected life expectancy may benefit from less stringent hemoglobin A1c goals (i.e., <8%) although more studies are needed (140) One serious complication of DM treatment in elderly patients is hypoglycemia. Factors associated with hypoglycemia include renal impairment, coadministration of insulin sensitizers or insulin, exercise, skipped meals, calorie restriction, recent hospitalization polypharmacy, and therapy with salicylates, sulfonamides, fibric acid derivatives, and warfarin (141).

PHARMACOLOGY

Diet and exercise may be enough to control blood glucose levels for persons with type 2 DM. However, for those who are not able to meet hemoglobin A1c goals, modern pharmacologic regimens for DM lend themselves to a variety of combinations tailored to an individual's needs. Currently, seven classes of oral medications are available for DM: metformins, sulfonylureas, meglitinides, D-phenylalanine derivatives, thiazolidinediones, α-glucosidase inhibitors, and dipeptidyl peptidase-4 (DPP-4) inhibitors (Table 61.9), as well as combination products. Insulin carries the greatest risk for hypoglycemia. In contrast, the risk of experiencing the symptoms of hypoglycemia for a person not taking any DM medications

| TABLE 61.9 | ORAL AND INJECTABLE BLOOD GLUCOSE–LOWERING MEDICATIONS | | | |

CLASSIFICATION MEDICATION	ROUTE	MECHANISM OF ACTION	TIME AND DOSE	COMPLICATIONS OR COMMENTS
Sulfonylureas • Glimepiride (Amaryl) • Glipizide (Glucotrol) • Glipizide ER (Glucotrol XL) • Glyburide (DiaBeta, Micronase)	Oral	Stimulate first-phase insulin secretion by binding to and causing closure of potassium-ATP channels on pancreatic β-cell membranes, with consequent membrane depolarization, calcium influx, and insulin exocytosis	One or two times a day	Contraindicated in diabetic ketoacidosis; not to be used for therapy in type 1 diabetes mellitus; patients should avoid excessive alcohol use (increased risk for hypoglycemia); may cause weight gain, nausea, diarrhea, or heartburn; check liver function tests
Biguanides • Glucophage (Metformin) • Glucophage XR (Metformin XL)	Oral	Decreases hepatic glucose production, and decreases intestinal absorption of glucose	Two to three times a day; XR once a day	Well tolerated if taken with or after meals (reduces GI upset); not be used in patients with mild renal insufficiency (creatinine >1.4–1.5 mg/dL); excessive alcohol use (increases risk of lactic acidosis) should be avoided; may cause nausea, vomiting, diarrhea, flatulence, abdominal pain, cobalamin (vitamin B_{12}) deficiency, or asthenia (physical weakness or loss of strength)
α-Glucosidase inhibitors • Miglitol (Glyset) • Acarbose (Precose)	Oral	Competitively and reversibly inhibit enzymes (α-glucoside hydrolases) that break down complex sugars in the small intestinal brush border; cause delayed absorption of simple sugars from the gut, thus reducing postprandial hyperglycemia	Take before each meal; swallow with first bite of food	Contraindicated in GI conditions such as inflammatory bowel disease, intestinal obstruction or ileus, conditions potentially exacerbated by increased intestinal gas, conditions associated with digestion or absorption, or colonic ulcerations; GI disturbances (flatulence, diarrhea, bloating, abdominal pain) can occur (in ≤74%).
Thiazolidinediones • Rosiglitazone (Avandia) • Pioglitazone (Actos)	Oral	Increase insulin-dependent glucose disposal primarily by decreasing insulin resistance in the periphery; also affect fatty acid metabolism	Once or twice daily with or without food	Liver damage possible; enzymes to be monitored carefully; can lead to weight gain or heart failure; not to be used in persons with congestive heart failure (NYHA class III or IV heart failure); rosiglitazone black box warning for cardiovascular mortality, and access severely restricted by FDA in 2010
Meglitinides • Repaglinide (Prandin) • Senaglinide (nateglinide; Starlix)	Oral	Increases insulin secretion by pancreatic β cells; short-acting	5–30 min before meals	Better control of postprandial hyperglycemia and associated with a lower risk of delayed hypoglycemic episodes; hypoglycemia, headache, nausea, vomiting, diarrhea, upset stomach, joint pain possible
DPP-IV inhibitors • Sitagliptin (Januvia) • Saxagliptin (Onglyza) • Linagliptin (Tradjenta)	Oral	Inhibit the degradation of incretins such as GLP-1 by inhibiting the enzyme IV (DPP-IV); prolonged incretin effect enhancing glycemic control through various mechanisms	Usually once a day	Possible nasopharyngitis or upper respiratory tract infections, headache, nausea, diarrhea, abdominal pain, urinary tract infections, peripheral edema; weight neutral
Incretin mimetics • Exenatide (Byetta) • Liraglutide (Victoza) • Exenatide ER (Bydureon)	Injectable	Stimulate glucose-dependent insulin secretion, slow gastric emptying; inhibit glucagon secretion; suppress appetite	Once or twice a day; inject within an hour of meals	Nausea, usually improving over time; hypoglycemia, especially with sulfonylureas; may be associated with weight loss
Antihyperglycemic agent • Pramlintide (Symlin)	Injectable	Slows gastric emptying; suppresses an exaggerated rise in postprandial glucagon; induces satiety	Inject before major meals	Reduced insulin dosage needed with drug initiation to avoid severe hypoglycemia

ATP, adenosine triphosphate; DPP-IV, dipeptidyl peptidase IV; FDA, Food and Drug Administration; GI, gastrointestinal; GLP-1, glucagon-like peptide-1; NYHA, New York Heart Association.

is rare. Patients and health professionals must understand the effects of meals and medications on hypoglycemia and glycemic control.

Insulin Therapy

Insulin therapy is indicated for everyone with diagnosed type 1 DM. Even in people whose glucose levels are nearly normal ("honeymoon" period or latent autoimmune diabetes of adulthood), if type 1 DM is diagnosed, the current evidence recommends starting insulin immediately, both in anticipation of diminished β-cell function and to preserve some islet function. Given the liability of type 1 DM, generally both long-acting and short- or fast-acting insulin should be started. Frequent self-monitoring of blood glucose by the patient guides therapy (142). Patients may be recommended to test before meals (goal blood glucose, 70 to 130 mg/dL), occasionally also 2 hours after meals (goal blood glucose, 140 to 180 mg/dL), at bedtime (goal blood glucose, 100 to 140 mg/dL), with symptoms of hyperglycemia or hypoglycemia, and occasionally overnight. Most insulin dose adjustments should be in 10% to 20% increments, depending on the degree of glucose abnormality. Table 61.10 contains a summary of currently available insulins.

Herbal Supplements or Complementary and Alternative Medicine

Herbal supplements, or complementary and alternative medicine therapy, are commonly used in many cultures for the treatment of DM. Herbal supplements should not be used in place of conventional medical therapy for DM. Although the benefits of some of these compounds have been observed, current data are insufficient to recommend any herbal remedies in the treatment of DM, and in some cases, these remedies can have adverse effects. In addition, although generally well tolerated at the doses reported, some compounds have significant herb–drug interactions that may interfere with the efficacy of the drug (143). For example, one of the most popular medicinal herbs, especially in Asia, is ginseng (*Panax ginseng*). The active compounds are thought to be ginsenosides, which, in some preclinical studies, suggested improvements in insulin resistance. Human models, however, failed to prove that oral ginseng products or ginsenoside RE improved glucose homeostasis, treated type 2 DM, or improved β-cell function or insulin sensitivity (144). The more alarming issue is the herb and drug interaction. Concomitant administration of ginsenosides with

TABLE 61.10	TYPES OF INSULIN				
TYPE	GENERIC NAME (BRAND NAME)	ONSET	PEAK	DURATION	COMMENTS
Rapid-acting insulin	Insulin aspart (NovoLog) Insulin glulisine (Apidra) Insulin lispro (Humalog)	10–20 min	2 h	4 h	Fastest-acting insulins on the market; can be taken right before or during a meal
Short-acting insulin	Regular insulin (Humulin R, Novolin R)	30–60 min	2–4 h	6–8 h	Injected 30 min before meals to cover the sugars absorbed from food
Intermediate-acting insulin	NPH insulin (Humulin N, Novolin N)	1–3 h	4–10 h	10–16 h	Often used in combination with rapid- or short-acting insulin; can also be given in combination with oral agents in type 2 diabetes; usually given twice a day
Long-acting insulin	Insulin glargine (Lantus) Insulin detemir (Levemir)	1–3 h	Theoretically peakless (glargine); 6–8 h (detemir)	20–24 h (glargine); 6–24 h (detemir)	Often used with a rapid- or short-acting insulin to cover the sugars absorbed from food at mealtimes; can also be given in combination with oral agents in type 2 diabetes; given once or twice a day (detemir)
Mixtures	Novolin 70/30, Humulin 70/30, NovoLog mix 70/30, Humalog mix 75/25, Humalog mix 50/50	Varies according to type	Varies according to type	Varies according to type	Convenient for people who use a mixture of short- or rapid-acting insulin and long-acting insulin by providing both in one syringe; helpful for those with poor dexterity or eyesight or for anyone who has problems drawing up insulin from two different bottles or reading the instructions and dosages on bottle labels

NPH, neutral protamine Hagedorn.

warfarin appears to reduce warfarin's therapeutic effect (145). The ADA discourages the use of concurrent use of herbal supplements with prescription medications without the physician's knowledge.

Several other herbal supplements may have some benefits, although not enough evidence is available to warrant recommendations. Cinnamon (*Cinnamon cassia*) has mixed results on the ability to enhance insulin signaling and increase glycogen synthase activity. Human trials investigated the use of 1 to 6 g /day. Modest effect on reducing fasting blood glucose (5% to 24%) with short-term administration was reported; however, the results were mixed (146). A few other herbal therapies used in Ayurvedic medicine have also been observed to have some glycemic benefits. Bitter melon (*Momordica charantia*) may improve insulin resistance through activation of adenosine monophosphate kinase; however, in the studies reviewed, no sufficient evidence was found, and gastrointestinal distress was reported (147, 148). Fenugreek (*Trigonella foenum-graecum*) contains 4-hydroxyisoleucine, which may enhance insulin secretion (149). However, Basch et al (150) reported mixed results, as well as adverse effects of transient diarrhea, flatulence, and dizziness. Gymnema (*Gymnema sylvestre*) leaves are used to treat DM, cholesterol issues, and obesity in Ayurvedic medicine and had some benefit noted in small trials of limited quality (decrease of ~0.6% hemoglobin A1c) in doses of 200 to 400 mg twice daily of the leaf extract.

Although benefits of some of these compounds have been described, current data are insufficient to recommend any herbal remedies in the treatment of DM. In addition, the purity and advertised amounts of the active ingredients of many dietary supplements have been questioned. Further research is needed to establish the role of herbal medicines adequately in management of DM.

CONCLUSION

DM is a chronic disease with a global prevalence that continues to grow and is associated with both a significant individual and public health burden. Lifestyle modifications including medical nutritional therapy remain the cornerstones of successful management of DM, in conjunction with glucose-lowering medications when indicated. In addition, education on the principles of physical activity, on the need for self-monitoring of blood glucose, and on adjustment of appropriate medications during times of illness, for example, is also vital to the person with DM. The multidisciplinary health care team should work together with the patient with DM to achieve good glycemic control, attain optimal serum lipid levels and blood pressure, and maintain a desirable body weight, as well as other risk factor modifications to prevent the development of long-term complications of DM and reduce the morbidity and mortality associated with this chronic disease.

ACKNOWLEDGMENTS

The assistance of Emily Borsch, BS, and the constructive feedback of Emily Loghmani, MS, RD, CDE, are greatly appreciated.

REFERENCES

1. Cowie, CC, Rust KF, Ford ES et al. Diabetes Care 2009; 32:287–94.
2. Cowie, CC, Rust KF, Byrd-Holt DD et al. Diabetes Care 2010;33:562–8.
3. Centers for Disease Control and Prevention. National Diabetes Fact Sheet, 2011. Available at: http://www.cdc.gov/diabetes/pubs/pdf/ndfs_2011.pdf. Accessed June 10, 2012.
4. World Health Organization. Diabetes. Fact sheet no. 312. 2011. Available at: http://www.who.int/mediacentre/factsheets/fs312/en. Accessed June 10, 2012.
5. Xu JQ, Kochanek KD, Murphy SL et al. Natl Vital Stat Rep 2010;827.
6. Zhang X, Saaddine JB, Chou CF et al. JAMA 2010;304: 649–56.
7. Li Y, Burrows N, Gregg L. Declining trends in hospitalizations for non-traumatic lower extremity amputation in the diabetic population: United States, 1988–2006. Abstract presented at: 70th Scientific Sessions of the American Diabetes Association; Orlando, Florida, June 2010.
8. United States Renal Data System. Renal Data Extraction and Referencing System. 2010 Annual Data Report Dataset. Available at: http://www.usrds.org/2010/view/default.asp
9. Gregg EW, Sorlie P, Paulose-Ram R et al. Diabetes Care 2004;27:1501–97.
10. Eastman RC. Neuropathy in diabetes. In: National Diabetes Data Group, eds. Diabetes in America. 2nd ed. Washington, DC: US Department of Health and Human Services, National Institutes of Health, National Institute of Diabetes and Digestive and Kidney Diseases, 1995:339–48. NIH publication 95–1468.
11. Gorina Y, Lentzer H. Multiple Causes of Death in Old Age. Aging Trends no. 9. Hyattsville, MD: National Center for Health Statistics, 2008.
12. Geiss LS, Herman WH, Smith PJ. Mortality in non–insulin-dependent diabetes. In: National Diabetes Data Group, eds. Diabetes in America. 2nd ed. Washington, DC: US Department of Health and Human Services, National Institutes of Health, National Institute of Diabetes and Digestive and Kidney Diseases, 1995:233–57. NIH publication 95–1468.
13. Kuller LH. Stroke and diabetes. In: National Diabetes Data Group, eds. Diabetes in America. 2nd ed. Washington, DC: US Department of Health and Human Services, National Institutes of Health, National Institute of Diabetes and Digestive and Kidney Diseases, 1995:449–56. NIH publication 95–1468.
14. Knowler WC, Barrett-Connor E, Fowler SE et al. N Engl J Med 2002;346:393.
15. Franz MJ, Monk A, Barry B et al. J Am Diet Assoc 1995;95: 1009–17.
16. Diabetes Control and Complications Trial Research Group. N Engl J Med 1993;329:977–86.
17. Zajac J, Shrestha A, Patel P et al. The main events in the history of diabetes mellitus. In: Poretsky L, ed. Principles of Diabetes Mellitus. 2nd ed. New York: Springer, 2010: 3–16.
18. Ahmed A. Saudi Med J 2002;23:373–8.

19. Chalmers K. Medical nutrition therapy. In: Kahn R, King G, Moses, A et al. Joslin's Diabetes Mellitus. 14th ed. Baltimore: Lippincott Williams & Wilkins, 2005:611–632.

20. American Diabetes Association. Diabetes Care 1994;17: 490–518.

21. Expert Committee on the Diagnosis and Classification of Diabetes Mellitus. Diabetes Care 2003;26:S5–20.

22. National Diabetes Data Group. Diabetes 1979;28:1039–57.

23. World Health Organization. Diabetes Mellitus: Report of a WHO Study Group. Geneva: World Health Organization, 1985. Technical Report Series No. 727.

24. American Diabetes Association. Diabetes Care 2011;34: S62–9.

25. World Health Organization. Report of a WHO/IDF Consultation: Definition and Diagnosis of Diabetes Mellitus and Intermediate Hyperglycemia. Geneva: World Health Organization Document Production Services, 2006:1–46.

26. Huang ES, Basu A, O'Grady M et al. Diabetes Care 2009; 32:2225–9.

27. Shaw JE, Sicree RA, Zimmet PZ. Diabetes Res Clin Pract 2010;87:4–14.

28. Dall TM, Zhang Y, Chen Y et al. Health Aff 2010;29:297–303.

29. American Diabetes Association. Diabetes Care 2011;34: S11–61.

30. Roglic G, Unwin N. Diabetes Res Clin Pract 2010;87:15.

31. Zhang P, Zhang X, Brown J et al. Diabetes Res Clin Pract 2010;87:293–301.

32. DIAMOND Project Group. Diabet Med 2006;23:857–66.

33. Borchers AT, Uibo R, Gershwin ME. Autoimmun Rev 2010; 9:A355–65.

34. Soltesz G, Patterson C, Dahlguist G et al. Pediatr Diabetes 2007;8:6–14.

35. Dahlguist G, Ivarsson SA, Lindstrom B et al. Diabetes 1995;44:408–13.

36. Hyoty H, Hiltunen M, Knip M et al. Diabetes 1995;44:652–7.

37. Dahlquist GG, Boman JE, Juto P. Diabetes Care 1999;22: 364–5.

38. Hiltunen M, Hyoty H, Knip M et al. J Infect Dis 1997;175: 54–60.

39. Viskari HR, Koskela P, Lonnrot M et al. Diabetes Care 2000;23: 414–6.

40. Wagener DK, Laporte RE, Orchard TJ et al. Diabetologia 1983;225:82–5.

41. Patterson CC, Carson DJ, Hadden DR et al. Diabetes Care 1994;17:376–81.

42. McKinney PA, Parslow R, Gurney K et al. Diabetologia 1997;40:933–9.

43. Dahlquist G. Nutritional factors. In: Leslie RDG, ed. Causes of Diabetes: Genetic and Environmental Factors. Chichester, UK: Wiley, 1993:125–132.

44. Vaarala O, Knip M, Paronen J et al. Diabetes 1999;48: 1389–94.

45. Akerblom HK, Virtanen SM, Ilonen J et al. Diabetologia 2005;48:829–37.

46. EURODIAB Substudy 2 Study Group. Diabetologia 1999; 42:51–4.

47. Patterson CC, Dahlquist G, Gyurus E et al. Lancet 2009;373: 2027–33.

48. Chan JM, Rimm E, Colditz G et al. Diabetes Care 1994; 17:961–9.

49. Nicholson W, Asao K, Brancati F et al. Diabetes Care 2006; 29:2349–54.

50. Koppes L, Dekker J, Hendrick H et al. Diabetes Care 2005; 28:719–25.

51. Willi C, Bodenman P, Ghali W et al. JAMA 2007;298:2654–64.

52. Yeh H, Duncan B, Schmidt M et al. Ann Intern Med 2010; 152:10–7.

53. Golden S. Curr Diabetes Rev 2007;3:252–9.

54. Avila-Curiel A, Shamah-Levy T, Galindo-Gomez C et al. Rev Invest Clin 2007;59:246–55.

55. Schootman M, Andresen E, Wolinsky F et al. Am J Epidemiol 2007;166:379–87.

56. Shai I, Jiang R, Manson J et al. Diabetes Care 2006;29: 1585–90.

57. Larsson S, Wolk A. J Intern Med 2007;262:208–14.

58. Nettleton J, Lutsey P, Wang Y et al. Diabetes Care 2009;32:688–94.

59. Zimmet P, Alberti KG, Shaw J. Nature 2001;414:782.

60. Ramachandran A, Snehalatha C, Latha E et al. Diabetologia 1997;40:232–37.

61. National Center for Health Statistics, Centers for Disease Control and Prevention. 2005–2008 National Health and Nutrition Examination Survey (NHANES). Available at: http://www.cdc.gov/nchs/nhanes.htm. Accessed June 10, 2012.

62. Jovanovic L, Pettitt DJ. JAMA 2001;286:2516–18.

63. Bellamy L, Casas J, Hingorani A et al. Lancet 2009;373: 1773–79.

64. Kim C, Berger DK, Chamany S. Diabetes Care 2007;30: 1314–9.

65. McCowen KC, Deaconess BI, Smith RJ. Classification and chemical pathology: diabetes mellitus. In: Caballero B, ed. Encyclopedia of Human Nutrition. 2nd ed. London: Elsevier, 2005:543–51.

66. Shrayyef MZ, Gerich JE. Normal Glucose Homeostasis. In: Poretsky L, ed. Principles of Diabetes Mellitus. 2nd ed. New York: Springer, 2010:19–35.

67. Vander A, Sherman J, Luciano D. Regulation of organic metabolism, growth, and energy balance. In: Nunes I, Schauck D, Bradley J. Human Physiology. 5th ed. New York: McGraw-Hill, 1990:555–600.

68. Woerle HJ, Meyer C, Dostou JM et al. Am J Physiol Endocr Metab 2003;284:E716–25.

69. Gosmanov NR, Szoke E, Israelian Z et al. Diabetes Care 2005;28:1124–31.

70. Ruder NB, Myers MG Jr, Chipkin SR, Tornhein K. Hormone-fuel interrelationships: fed state, starvation, and diabetes mellitus. In: Kahn C, King G, Moses A et al, eds. Joslin's Diabetes Mellitus. 14th ed. Philadelphia: Lippincott Williams & Wilkins, 2005:127–44.

71. Fonseca V, Pendergrass M, McDuffie R. Complications of diabetes. In: Fonseca V, Pendergrass M, McDuffie R. Diabetes in Clinical Practice. London: Springer, 2010: 41–57.

72. Umpierrez G, Casals M, Gebhart S et al. Diabetes 1995;44: 790–5.

73. Feng Y, Fleckman A. Acute hyperglycemia syndromes: diabetic ketoacidosis and the hyperosmolar state. In: Poretsky L, ed. Principles of Diabetes Mellitus. 2nd ed. New York: Springer, 2010:281–95.

74. Pastors J, Franz M, Warshaw H et al. J Am Diet Assoc 2003; 103:827–31.

75. Pastors J, Warshaw H, Daly A et al. Diabetes Care 2002;25: 608–13.

76. Monk A, Barry B, McClain K et al. J Am Diet Assoc 1995;95: 999–1006.

77. Delahanty L. J Am Diet Assoc 1998;98:28–30.

78. Franz M, Boucher J, Green-Pastors J et al. J Am Diet Assoc 2008;108:S52–8.

79. American Diabetes Association, Bantle J, Wylie-Rosett J et al. Diabetes Care 2008;31:S61–78.

80. Franz MJ, Powers MA, Leontos C et al. J Am Diet Assoc 2010;110:1852–89.

81. Connor H, Annan F, Bunn E et al. Diabet Med 2003;20:786–807.

82. Kulkarni K, Castle G, Gregory R et al. Diabetes Spectrum 1997;10:248–56.

83. Sacks F, Bray G, Carey V et al. N Engl J Med 2009;360:859–73.

84. Garg A, Bantle J, Henry R et al. JAMA 1994;271:1421–8.

85. Gerhard G, Ahmann A, Meeuws K et al. Am J Clin Nutr 2004;80:668–73.

86. Delahanty L, Nathan D, Lachin J et al. Am J Clin Nutr 2009;89:518–24.

87. Food and Nutrition Board, Institute of Medicine. Dietary Reference Intakes for Energy, Carbohydrate, Fiber, Fat, Fatty Acids, Cholesterol, Protein, and Amino Acids (Macronutrients). Washington, DC: National Academy Press, 2005.

88. Loghmani E, Rickard K, Wahsburne L et al. J Pediatr 1991;119:53.

89. Wolever TMS, Hamad S, Chiasson JL et al. J Am Coll Nutr 1999;18:242–7.

90. Boden G, Sargrad K, Homko C et al. Ann Intern Med 2005;142:403–11.

91. Nielsen JV, Jonsson E, Ivarsson A. Ups J Med Sci 2005;110:267–73.

92. Hession M, Rolland C, Kulkarni U et al. Obes Rev 2009;10:36–50.

93. Brand-Miller JC, Stockmann K, Atkinson F et al. Am J Clin Nutr 2009;87:97–105.

94. Foster-Powell K, Holt S, Brand-Miller J. Am J Clin Nutr 2002;76:5–56.

95. Jenkins D, Kendal C, Augustin LS et al. Am J Med 2002;113:30S–7S.

96. Hansen H, Christensen P, Tauer-Lassen E et al. Kidney Int 1999;55:621–8.

97. Raal FJ, Kalk WJ, Lawson M et al. Am J Clin Nutr 1994;60:579–85.

98. Meloni C, Morosetti M, Suraci C et al. J Renal Nutr 2002;12:96–101.

99. Meloni C, Tatangelo P, Cipriani S. J Renal Nutr 2004;14:208–13.

100. Azadbakht L, Shakerhosseini R, Atabak S. Eur J Clin Nutr 2003;57:1292–4.

101. Martinez-Gonzalez M, de la Fuente-Arrillaga C, Nunez-Cordoba J et al. BMJ 2008;336:1348–51.

102. Wang C, Harris WS, Chung M et al. Am J Clin Nutr 2006;84:5–7.

103. Marlett JA. Dietary fiber and cardiovascular disease. In: Cho SS, Dreher ML, eds. Handbook of Dietary Fiber. New York: Marcel Dekker, 2001:17–30.

104. Jensen MK, Koh-Banerjee P, Ju FB et al. Am J Clin Nutr 2004;80:1492–9.

105. Brown L, Rosner B, Willett W et al. Am J Clin Nutr 1999;69:30–42.

106. Van Horn L, McCoin M, Kris-Etherton P et al. J Am Diet Assoc 2008;108:287–331.

107. Chandalia M, Garg A, Lutjohann D et al. N Engl J Med 2000;342:1392–8.

108. Hagander B, Asp NG, Efendic S et al. Am J Clin Nutr 1988;47:852–8.

109. Giacco R, Parillo M, Rivellese A. Diabetes Care 2000;23:1461–6.

110. Slavin JL. J Am Diet Assoc 2008;109:1716–31.

111. Bolin TD, Stanton RA. Eur J Surg 1998;582:115–8.

112. Tomlin J, Lowis C, Read NW. Gut 1991;32:665–9.

113. American Dietetic Association. J Am Diet Assoc 2004;104:255–75.

114. Bloomgarden ZT. Diabetes Care 2011;34:e46–51.

115. Coulston A, Hollenbeck C, Donner C et al. Metabolism 1985;34:962–6.

116. Chong MFF, Fielding BA, Frayn KN. Am J Clin Nutr 2007;85:1511–20.

117. Whitehouse C, Boullata J, McCauley, L. AAOHN J 2008;56:251–9.

118. Ludwig DS. JAMA 2009;302:2477–8.

119. Mattes, R, Popkin B. Am J Clin Nutr 2009;89:1–14.

120. Pepino M, Bourne C. Curr Opin Clin Nutr Metab Care 2011;14:391–5.

121. Sheard N, Clark N, Brand-Miller J et al. Diabetes Care 2004;27:2266–71.

122. Chiesa G, Piscopo M, Rigamonti A et al. Acta Biomed 2005;76:44–8.

123. Wheeler ML, Pi-Sunyer FX. J Am Diet Assoc 2008;108:S34–9.

124. Gillespie SJ, Kulkarni KD, Daly AE. J Am Diet Assoc 1998;98:897–905.

125. Lonn E, Dagenais G, Yusuf S et al. Diabetes Care 2002;25:1919–27.

126. Pittas A, Lau N, Hu F et al. J Clin Endocrinol Metab 2007;92:2017–29.

127. Colberg S, Sigal R, Fernhall B et al. Diabetes Care 2010;33:e147–67.

128. Marwick T, Hordern M, Miller T et al. Circulation 2009;119:3244–62.

129. Snowling NJ, Hopkins WG. Diabetes Care 2006;29:2518–62.

130. Williamson D, Rejeski J, Lang W et al. Arch Intern Med 2009;169:163–71.

131. Silverstein J, Klingensmith G, Copeland K et al. Diabetes Care 2005;28:186–212.

132. Rosenbloom A, Silverstein J, Amemiya S et al. Pediatr Diabetes 2009;10:17–32.

133. Røder M, Schwartz R, Prigeon R et al. J Clin Endocrinol Metab 2000;85:2275–80.

134. DeFronzo RA. Diabetes Care 1981;4:493–501.

135. Elahi D, Muller D, Egan J et al. Novartis Found Symp 2002;242:222–42.

136. Houmard J, Weidner M, Dolan P et al. Diabetes 1995;44:555–60.

137. Goulet E, Hassaine A, Dionne I et al. Exp Gerontol 2009;44:740–4.

138. Kalyani R, Saudek C, Brancati F et al. Diabetes Care 2010;33:1055–60.

139. Wedick N, Barrett-Connor E, Knoke J et al. J Am Geriatr Soc 2002;50:1810–5.

140. Brown A, Mangione C, Saliba D et al. J Am Geriatr Soc 2003;51:S265–80.

141. Neumiller J, Setter S. Am J Geriatr Pharmacother 2009;7:324–42.

142. Hirsh I, Bode B, Childs B et al. Diabetes Technol Ther 2008;10:419–39.

143. Yeh G, Eisenberg D, Kaptchuk T et al. Diabetes Care 2003;26:1277–94.

144. Reeds D, Patterson B, Okunade A et al. Diabetes Care 2011;34:1071–6.

145. Yuan C, Wei G, Dey L et al. Ann Intern Med 2004;141: 23–7.
146. Kirkham S, Akilen R, Sharma S et al. Diabetes Obes Metab 2009;11:1100–3.
147. Cheng H, Huang H, Chang C et al. J Agric Food Chem 2008;56:6835–43.
148. Miura T, Itoh C, Iwamoto N et al. J Nutr Sci Vitaminol (Tokyo) 2001;47:340–4.
149. Sauvaire Y, Petit P, Broca C et al. Diabetes 1998;47: 206–10.
150. Basch E, Ulbricht C, Kuo G et al. Altern Med Rev 2003; 8:20–7.

SUGGESTED READINGS

American Diabetes Association. Standards of medical care in diabetes: 2011. Diabetes Care 2011;34:S11–61.

American Diabetes Association, Bantle J, Wylie-Rosett J et al. Nutrition recommendations and interventions for diabetes: a position statement of the American Diabetes Association. Diabetes Care 2008;31:S61–78.

National Guideline Clearinghouse. Guideline synthesis: nutritional management of diabetes mellitus. In: National Guideline Clearinghouse. Rockville (MD): Agency for Healthcare Research and Quality (AHRQ); 2009 Mar (revised 2012 April) Available at: http://www.guideline.gov/synthesis/index.aspx. Accessed May 12, 2011.

62 METABOLIC SYNDROME: DEFINITION, RELATIONSHIP WITH INSULIN RESISTANCE, AND CLINICAL UTILITY[1]

DOMINIC N. REEDS

The term *metabolic syndrome* (MS) is used to describe a cluster of metabolic disorders: insulin resistance (IR) or hyperglycemia, abdominal obesity, dyslipidemia (high very-low-density lipoprotein-triglyceride [VLDL-TG] concentration and low plasma high-density lipoprotein cholesterol [HDL-C]), and essential hypertension (HTN). These factors are important because each component increases the risk of development of type 2 diabetes mellitus (DM) and cardiovascular disease (CVD). Recognition of the association between the components of MS with both DM and CVD has been known since the 1930s. Progress in understanding the pathogenesis of the syndrome has been hindered by the challenge of understanding the complex relationships among features of MS, IR or insulin sensitivity, pancreatic β-cell function, and host factors.

HISTORICAL CONTEXT

Until the 1960s, the prevailing belief was that an absolute insulin deficiency was the primary metabolic defect in type 2 DM. This belief persisted despite studies performed

---

[1]**Abbreviations: BMI**, body mass index; **CHD**, coronary heart disease; **CVD**, cardiovascular disease; **DM**, diabetes mellitus; **FA**, fatty acid; **FFA**, free fatty acid; **HDL-C**, high-density lipoprotein cholesterol; **HIV**, human immunodeficiency virus; **HR**, hazard ratio; **HTN**, hypertension; **IFG**, impaired fasting glucose; **IGT**, impaired glucose tolerance; **IHTG**, intrahepatic triglyceride; **IR**, insulin resistance; **LDL-C**, low-density lipoprotein cholesterol; **MS**, metabolic syndrome; **TG**, triglyceride; **VAT**, visceral adipose tissue; **VLDL-TG**, very-low-density lipoprotein-triglyceride; **WC**, waist circumference; **WHO**, World Health Organization.

as early as the 1930s that indicated that resistance to insulin-mediated stimulation of glucose clearance was present in subjects with type 2 DM (1–5). The availability of the insulin immunoassay, developed by Yalow and Berson in 1960, established that most patients with DM had higher plasma insulin levels than healthy subjects (6). This new ability to measure both plasma glucose and insulin concentration allowed the development of oral glucose tolerance testing (7) and the glucose clamp techniques (8). Various glucose clamp techniques exist; however, the most commonly performed is probably the euglycemic hyperinsulinemic clamp. In this protocol, a constant infusion of insulin is administered to the subject to cause hyperinsulinemia, and the rate of glucose infusion (glucose disposal) necessary to maintain euglycemia is determined. Concomitant infusion of stable isotope–labeled tracers of amino acids, glucose, and fatty acids (FAs) during clamps may be performed to allow for calculation of glucose production, amino acid deposition, VLDL-TG synthesis, and lipolysis, among other metabolic measures (9–13). These methods have proved critical in dissecting the complex relationships between organ-specific IR and insulin secretion.

Subsequent studies showed that most subjects with type 2 DM had resistance to insulin action in adipose tissue (inhibition of lipolysis), liver (inhibition of glucose production), and skeletal muscle (stimulation of glucose disposal) (14–16). Curiously, insulin-mediated stimulation of amino acid deposition may be normal in subjects with DM, but it is impaired in subjects with other forms of IR, such as that of the human immunodeficiency virus (HIV)–associated MS (17). It is widely believed in the United States that IR almost always precedes the development of DM. This paradigm is supported by studies that have shown that IR is seen at an early age in first-degree relatives of people with type 2 DM (18), and IR indicates an increased risk of development of DM (19–23).

The relationship between IR and insulin secretion is complex. In general, IR causes increased insulin secretion and reduced hepatic insulin clearance, resulting in systemic hyperinsulinemia. Although a focus is often placed on insulin as a regulator of blood glucose, insulin plays a key role in the regulation of lipid and protein metabolism, in addition to cellular growth and development. Seminal studies by Hollenbeck and Reaven and Yeni-Komshian et al (24, 25) systematically examined IR in nondiabetic individuals. Insulin-mediated glucose uptake was found to vary by up to eightfold in healthy subjects.

These and subsequent studies showed that more insulin-resistant subjects had greater plasma insulin concentration, VLDL-TG, and plasma glucose during the oral glucose tolerance test than did insulin-sensitive subjects, findings supporting the relationship between IR and MS (26). During his Banting lecture, Reaven proposed that DM was not the only adverse outcome associated with hyperinsulinemia, but that elevated insulin concentrations could activate metabolic pathways and result in dyslipidemia and HTN (27). He termed this collection of metabolic disturbances syndrome X. Subsequently, several articles described the associations among IR, dyslipidemia, HTN, elevated waist circumference (WC), and the risk of CVD and DM (28–32).

The first formal definition of MS was by the World Health Organization (WHO) in 1998 (Table 62.1) (33). This initial definition focused on IR as the main contributor to the syndrome and *required* the presence of IR in addition to two of the following: obesity, HTN, high TG, low HDL-C, or microalbuminuria. In 2001, the report of the Adult Treatment Panel III (ATP III) of the National Cholesterol Education Program also noted the relationship between IR and known CVD risk factors (Table 62.2) (34). The committee suggested that these lipid and nonlipid abnormalities were all metabolically related and used the term *metabolic syndrome*. In contrast to the WHO, this definition did not require the presence of IR, but rather a focus was placed on abdominal obesity, thus suggesting an additional risk posed by abdominal fat.

Since these initial definitions, MS has entered the clinical vernacular and is used to define a clinical state associated with an increased risk for the development of CVD and

DM. Reaven himself *did not* propose syndrome X for use as a diagnostic entity but rather to provide a framework for understanding the complex relationships among abdominal obesity, IR, and the adverse consequences of hyperinsulinemia. The rest of this chapter describes the components of MS, a critical appraisal of the role of IR as the pathogenic factor for MS, and the utility of MS in clinical practice.

Waist Circumference

Obesity (body mass index [BMI] ≥ 30 kg/m^2) is associated with an increased risk of CVD and DM (35, 36) (Table 62.3). Upper body obesity, in particular visceral obesity, may confer a greater cardiometabolic risk than obesity alone. Because precise measurement of abdominal fat requires expensive imaging techniques, WC is often used as a marker of both obesity and increased

TABLE 62.2	NATIONAL HEART, LUNG, AND BLOOD INSTITUTE AND AMERICAN HEART ASSOCIATION DEFINITION OF METABOLIC SYNDROME

	ATP III
HDL-C (mg/dL)	<40 (men), <50 (women)
TG (mg/dL)	>150
Waist circumference (in)	>40 (men), >35 (women)
BP (mm Hg)	Systolic ≥130 and/or diastolic ≥85
FBG (mg/dL)	≥110

ATP III, Adult Treatment Panel III; BP, blood pressure; FBG, fasting blood glucose; HDL-C, high-density lipoprotein cholesterol; TG, triglyceride concentration.

From Grundy SM. Definition of metabolic syndrome: report of the National Heart, Lung, and Blood Institute/American Heart Association conference on scientific issues related to definition. Circulation 2004;109:433–8, with permission.

TABLE 62.1	WORLD HEALTH ORGANIZATION METABOLIC SYNDROME CRITERIA

Insulin resistance identified by one of the following:
  Type 2 diabetes
  FBG >110 mg/dL
  IGT >140 mg/dL
  FBG <110 mg/dL but in lowest quartile of glucose disposal during hyperinsulinemic, euglycemic conditions
And any two of the following:
  TG ≥150 mg/dL
  HDL-C <35 mg/dL (men), <39 mg/dL (women)
  BMI >30 kg/m^2 and/or waist-to-hip ratio >0.9 (men), >0.85 (women)
  Urinary albumin excretion rate ≥20 μg/min or albumin-to-creatinine ratio ≥30 mg/g

BMI, body mass index; FBG, fasting blood glucose; HDL-C, high-density lipoprotein cholesterol; IGT, impaired glucose tolerance; TG, triglycerides.

From Grundy SM. Definition of metabolic syndrome: report of the National Heart, Lung, and Blood Institute/American Heart Association conference on scientific issues related to definition. Circulation 2004;109:433–8, with permission.

TABLE 63.3	HARMONIZED METABOLIC SYNDROME CRITERIA

MEASURE	CATEGORY CUTOFF POINTS
Elevated waist circumference	Population and country specific definitions
Plasma TG or drug treatment	≥150 mg/dL
Plasma HDL-C or drug treatment	<40 (men) mg/dL, <50 (women) mg/dL
BP (mm Hg) or drug treatment	Systolic ≥130 and/or diastolic ≥85
FBG or drug treatment	≥100 mg/dL

BP, blood pressure; FBG, fasting blood glucose; HDL-C, high-density lipoprotein cholesterol; TG, triglyceride.

Adapted from Grundy SM. Harmonizing the metabolic syndrome: a joint interim statement of the International Diabetes Federation Task Force on Epidemiology and Prevention; National Heart, Lung, and Blood Institute; American Heart Association; World Heart Federation; International Atherosclerosis Society; and International Association for the Study of Obesity. Circulation 2009;120:1640–5.

abdominal fat (37–39). Currently, no uniform approach for measurement of WC exists; however, the reproducibility of WC measurement is high when performed by trained technicians (40). The most commonly used sites for measurement of WC are the midpoint between the lowest rib and the iliac crest, the umbilicus, and the site of the narrowest measured WC. WC correlated well with abdominal fat in large studies (41). The cutoff values for WC were obtained following regression analysis of the relationship between BMI and WC in a large Scottish study. A WC value of 40 in. in men and 35 in. in women was chosen because these values corresponded to a BMI of 30 kg/m².

The reasons for the close relationships among WC, visceral adiposity, and cardiometabolic risk are unknown; however, several mechanisms have been proposed. IR has been closely linked to adipose tissue macrophage content in both human and animal studies. Immune cells, in particular macrophages, may be trafficked into fat tissue by increases in interstitial and/or plasma FA concentration (42, 43). These cells may release various factors such as tumor necrosis factor-α and interleukin-6 that act directly on surrounding adipocytes, thus impairing insulin action and promoting release of FAs. Curiously, animal studies suggest that inhibition of this inflammatory response protects against obesity-associated IR (44).

Another hypothesis centers on the belief that visceral adipose tissue (VAT) has a direct effect on insulin sensitivity, lipid metabolism, and blood pressure. The venous drainage of abdominal visceral fat leads directly to the hepatic portal vein, so that FA released by the visceral fat depot would dramatically increase hepatic FA delivery (see Fig. 62.3). FA delivered to the liver can be exported as VLDL-TG, oxidized, or stored. Failure to export or oxidize these FA would therefore promote hepatic steatosis and, as a result, hepatic IR. This process would be exacerbated by mild hyperglycemia because elevated blood glucose concentration reduces hepatic FA oxidation. Elegantly performed studies showed that a greater proportion of FA delivery to the liver originates from VAT and that hepatic free FA (FFA) delivery increases with increasing VAT mass (45).

Because intrahepatic triglyceride (IHTG) and VAT are strongly correlated with one another, it is not clear whether increased WC (and by imputation, increased VAT) or increased IHTG are independent risk factors for dyslipidemia and IR. Fabbrini et al (46) measured insulin sensitivity using euglycemic hyperinsulinemic clamps (Fig. 62.1) and VLDL-TG production (Fig. 62.2) in a cohort of obese subjects. Subjects were then separated into groups by matching on visceral fat mass and in a second analysis on IHTG content. VLDL-TG production rates were increased, and insulin sensitivity in liver, muscle, and adipose tissue was impaired in subjects with high IHTG. In contrast, VLDL-TG production and insulin sensitivity were not impaired when subjects were matched for IHTG and then divided into high and low VAT. This finding suggests that differences in hepatic

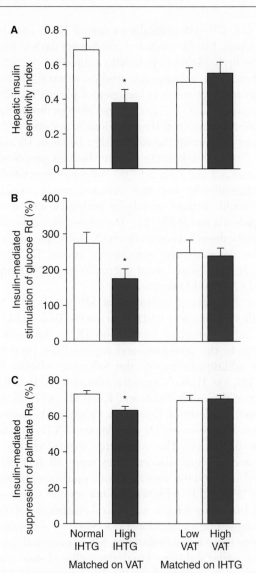

Fig. 62.1. Hepatic **(A)**, skeletal muscle **(B)**, and adipose tissue **(C)** insulin sensitivity in subjects matched on visceral adipose tissue (VAT) volume with either normal or high intrahepatic triglyceride (IHTG) content and subjects matched on IHTG content who had either low or high VAT volume. AU, arbitrary units. Values are means ± SEM. *, value is significantly different from the corresponding value in the normal IHTG group, $p < .05$. Hepatic insulin sensitivity was determined by calculating the reciprocal of the product of basal endogenous glucose production rate, in micromoles per kilogram of fat free mass (FFM) per minute, and fasting plasma insulin concentration in milliunits per liter). *Ra,* rate of appearance; *Rd,* rate of disappearance. (Reprinted with permission from Fabbrini E, Magkos F, Mohammed BS et al. Intrahepatic fat, not visceral fat, is linked with metabolic complications of obesity. Proc Natl Acad Sci U S A 2009;106:15430–5.)

FA handling (i.e., FFA oxidation versus storage) and resultant hepatic steatosis play major roles in determining whether abdominal obesity causes metabolic abnormalities.

In light of these data, investigators have proposed that differences in the capacity of adipocytes to expand in size, number, and function in response to excess caloric intake determine whether excess caloric delivery and abdominal obesity cause IR and hyperlipidemia. Failure to be able

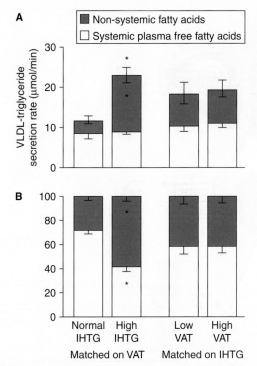

Fig. 62.2. Very low-density lipoprotein-triglyceride (VLDL-TG) secretion rate **(A)** and the relative contribution of systemic (generated primarily by lipolysis of subcutaneous adipose tissue triglycerides) and nonsystemic fatty acids (generated primarily by lipolysis of intrahepatic triglycerides) to VLDL-TG production **(B)** in subjects matched on visceral adipose tissue (VAT) volume with either normal or high intrahepatic triglyceride (IHTG) content and subjects matched on IHTG content who had either low or high VAT volume. Values are means ± SEM. *, value is significantly different from corresponding value in the normal IHTG group, *p* < 0.001. (Reprinted with permission from Fabbrini E, Magkos F, Mohammed BS et al. Intrahepatic fat, not visceral fat, is linked with metabolic complications of obesity. Proc Natl Acad Sci U S A 2009;106:15430–5.)

to expand adipose tissue depots and adequately sequester fat in adipocytes may cause increased plasma FFA concentration and deposition in ectopic sites such as liver and skeletal muscle (lipotoxicity). FAs are taken up generally in relation to their plasma concentration, so that increases in FFA supply will inhibit glucose uptake and oxidation and cause glucose intolerance (47–49). This process may be further exacerbated by increased expression of CD36, an FA transporter, on target organ membranes (46). Increased plasma FFA concentration and accumulation of FAs in liver and muscle are strongly associated with impaired insulin sensitivity in these organs (46).

Whether WC is a better predictor of IR and cardiometabolic risk than that predicted by BMI alone is debated. Several studies indicated that WC is a more reliable indicator of CVD risk than BMI. In a study involving 27,000 subjects, WC predicted MI in both genders and across a wide variety of ethnic groups, whereas BMI as a predictor was weaker and far less consistent overall (50). Furthermore, when controlled for other factors, WC but not BMI was predictive of MI risk. Similarly, WC but not

BMI was predictive of risk for transient ischemic attack and stroke (51). Conversely, the International Day for the Evaluation of Abdominal Obesity Study conducted in 168,000 patients found that the association between CVD and either obesity or WC was comparable, with odds ratios in men of 1.6 for WC and 1.32 for BMI (36).

The predictive power of WC for risk of DM and dyslipidemia is less clear. A sample of approximately 2000 subjects from the Dallas Heart Study found that in men, but not women, WC was a better predictor of DM risk and dyslipidemia (52). A consensus statement (and excellent review of the clinical data for WC) issued in 2007 by the Obesity Society, the American Society for Nutrition, and the American Diabetes Association stated that WC provides "incremental value in predicting diabetes mellitus, coronary heart disease, and mortality rate above and beyond that provided by BMI" (41).

In conclusion, WC can be reliably measured in a clinical setting with a high degree of reproducibility. Although increased WC identifies people with greater amounts of abdominal fat, it is not clear that VAT itself is responsible for development of MS, but rather hepatic FA handling is critical. WC identifies people at higher risk of development of DM, dyslipidemia, and CVD than BMI alone; however, the magnitude of this difference is variable. Furthermore, WC may be most helpful in studies conducted in differing racial and ethnic groups because of differences in normal BMI values and distributions among populations.

Dyslipidemia

Dyslipidemia is common in patients with other features of MS and indicates IR in liver, adipose tissue, and skeletal muscle in many disease entities, including HIV infection (53). A schema for the relationships among visceral fat, skeletal muscle, and the liver with respect to lipid metabolism is shown in Figure 62.3. In insulin-resistant subjects, low plasma HDL-C and hypertriglyceridemia are more common than elevations in low-density lipoprotein cholesterol (LDL-C). However, treatment of elevated LDL-C is of paramount importance. When dyslipidemia occurs in the setting of IR, it is associated with elevated levels of small dense LDL-C, which may be especially atherogenic (54). Somewhat surprisingly, serum lipids may directly affect insulin secretion. HDL-C may actually stimulate insulin secretion and inhibit apoptosis of pancreatic β cells, thus underlining the intimate relationship between dyslipidemia and IR (55, 56). Abundant data link low HDL-C and, to a lesser degree, hypertriglyceridemia, with subsequent development of CVD. Although reducing LDL-C is of clear benefit in patients with cardiac risk factors, fewer data support interventions to increase HDL-C and lower triglycerides.

Hypertriglyceridemia

High plasma VLDL-TG concentrations result from increased production, reduced clearance, or a combination

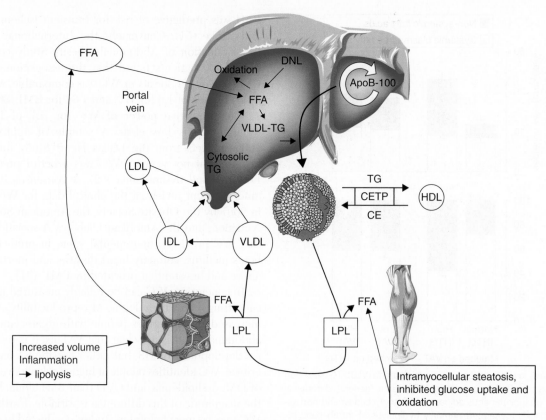

Fig. 62.3. Schema for very-low-density lipoprotein (VLDL)-triglyceride (TG) and free fatty acid (FFA) metabolism. Increased FFA release from visceral fat depots as a result of many causes, increases hepatic FFA availability, increased VLDL-TG synthesis, and as a result, increases high-density lipoprotein (HDL) clearance. Increased peripheral FFA supply from the action of lipoprotein lipase (LPL) on VLDL-TG antagonized glucose uptake and oxidation by peripheral tissues and promotes ectopic deposition of FFA. Hyperglycemia inhibits FFA oxidation. Apo B-100, apolipoprotein B-100; *CE*, cholesterol ester; *CETP*, cholesterol ester transfer protein; *DNL*, de novo lipogenesis; *IDL*, intermediate-density lipoprotein; *LDL*, low-density lipoprotein. (Courtesy of Bettina Mittendorf.)

of both factors. Increased production of VLDL-TG, rather than reduced clearance, is the most common defect in clinical practice because inborn errors of metabolism resulting in a primary defect in VLDL-TG clearance are uncommon. VLDL-TGs are synthesized from FFAs obtained either from hepatic de novo lipogenesis or circulating FFA released from subcutaneous fat (systemic FFA), VAT, or intrahepatic lipid stores (nonsystemic FFA).

Rates of FFA release are often elevated in insulin-resistant states, in particular during nocturnal hours, despite prevailing hyperinsulinemia (57). In response to increased FFA availability and chronically elevated plasma insulin concentration, hepatic production of the VLDL-TG associated protein apolipoprotein-B-100 may be increased. An increase in the VLDL-TG pool, under the influence of cholesterol ester transfer protein, will promote transport of triglyceride bound in VLDL-TG particles to HDL-C, increasing HDL-C clearance (58). As a result, typically, an inverse relationship exists between plasma VLDL-TG and HDL-C concentrations.

Weight loss typically reduces VLDL-TG levels, mainly because of a reduction in the contribution of "nonsystemic" FFA to VLDL-TG synthesis (59). This finding implies

that VLDL-TG levels decline owing to a combination of reduced IHTG stores, de novo synthesis of FFA, and release of FFA from VAT. Pharmacologic interventions that reduce lipolysis, such as acipimox, reduce VLDL-TG levels and raise HDL, but they also appear to improve insulin sensitivity in insulin-resistant subjects, thus emphasizing the close relationship between plasma FFA concentration and glucose and lipid metabolism (60, 61). Data regarding the clinical utility of reducing TG to reduce CVD risk are not robust (see later), although when plasma VLDL-TG concentrations are greater than 500 mg/dL despite adequate glycemic control, pharmacologic therapy for TG control may be necessary to reduce the risk of pancreatitis.

High-Density Lipoprotein

Lifestyle interventions, including weight loss, in particular loss of abdominal fat, and resistance or aerobic exercise, are modestly effective at increasing HDL-C concentrations and improve insulin sensitivity. The cardiometabolic benefits of drug interventions to increase HDL-C are unclear, particularly in the setting of IR. The Helsinki Heart Study and the Veterans Affairs HDL Intervention Trial (VA-HIT) showed an approximate 34% reduction in CVD risk in patients treated with gemfibrozil; however, these benefits were most pronounced in those with low HDL-C rather than hypertriglyceridemia (62, 63). Curiously, those with the highest plasma insulin concentration at study entry had the greatest benefit. In stark contrast, the Fenofibrate Intervention and Event Lowering in Diabetes (FIELD) and the Action to Control Cardiovascular Risk in Diabetes (ACCORD) lipid study failed to show a CVD risk reduction with the use of fenofibrate in patients with DM (64, 65). Although the implications of these studies remain debated, it seems reasonable to assume that pharmacotherapy to increase HDL-C should not be the initial therapy in high-risk patients; rather, interventions to reduce LDL-C should be the primary goal of initial care. Furthermore, it is likely that all HDL-C is not created equal and that the physiologic function of circulating HDL-C is critical to its role in reducing CVD risk (66).

Glucose

Impaired fasting glucose (IFG) is common in patients with HTN, dyslipidemia, and abdominal obesity; and it increases the risk of developing DM and CVD. Approximately 5% of patients with IFG per year progress to DM, although the risk increases exponentially as FBG approaches 125 mg/dL. The cutoff of 100 mg/dL is relatively arbitrary, and the relationship of DM risk and FBG should be viewed as a continuum. Lifestyle intervention, metformin, and pioglitazone have all been shown to reduce the rate of progression to DM in people with impaired glucose tolerance (IGT) and IFG (67, 68).

IGT and DM are far more common in patients with IR. However, the threshold at which IR is sufficient to cause DM is highly variable. As many as 25% of healthy, nondiabetic subjects have IR comparable to that seen in DM (69). This finding reflects the wide variation in insulin-stimulated glucose disposal among individuals and variations in the capacity of β cells and end organs to adapt to worsening IR (24). Although specific, fasting blood glucose is relatively insensitive for identification of patients at risk for MS and DM. Indeed, a study found that IFG was only 28% sensitive in women and 48% sensitive in men for identifying subjects with IR (70). Therefore, a normal FBG value should not be viewed as reassuring in patients with risk factors for DM and CVD, and a high index of suspicion for the presence of underlying DM should remain. Oral glucose tolerance testing is more sensitive for detection of patients at increased risk of DM, although it is rarely performed clinically because of cost and time considerations. As such, many patients with prediabetes are missed because of reliance on FBG levels.

Use of plasma insulin concentration to identify subjects at risk for DM is also problematic. The capacity and durability of the β-cell response are critical in determining the threshold at which IR overwhelms the adaptive β-cell response. Indeed, many subjects with profound hyperinsulinemia do not have DM. For example, insulin sensitivity was examined in a cohort of extremely obese women (BMI = 49 kg/m^2) with evidence of IR (acanthosis nigricans) (71). Despite normal fasting plasma glucose concentration (87 ± 5 mg/dL) and normal oral glucose tolerance, plasma insulin concentrations were sixfold higher than in lean control subjects, and rates of glucose disposal during euglycemic hyperinsulinemic clamps were 50% lower. These data clearly illustrate the capacity of the pancreatic β cell to adapt to IR and extreme obesity and the critical role of this adaptation in the prevention of DM. Furthermore, despite being almost universally hyperinsulinemic, most obese patients never develop DM.

Blood Pressure

Essential HTN is extremely common in patients with other features of MS. Several lines of evidence suggest that IR may directly contribute to development of HTN. Both patients with HTN and their first-degree relatives are more likely to be insulin resistant than are normotensive patients without a family history of HTN (72, 73). IR appears to be a major risk factor for subsequent development of HTN. Modan et al (74) systematically examined the relationship between HTN and oral glucose tolerance (using a 100 g glucose load) in a cohort of 2475 subjects of Israeli origin. Glucose tolerance and HTN were strongly associated ($p < .001$), even at the mildest levels of both conditions. This association was independent of age, obesity, and antihypertensive medication use. Several factors in this study strongly support the role of IR in HTN: (a) 83% of hypertensive subjects were insulin resistant or obese; (b) HTN was strongly associated with both fasting and postglucose hyperinsulinemia; and (c) the effects of HTN, glucose tolerance, and obesity were linearly additive to the total serum insulin concentration.

The effects of insulin itself on blood pressure are complicated and cannot be fully addressed in this chapter. Insulin increases renal sodium retention, thus promoting fluid retention. Indeed, initiation of insulin therapy frequently causes mild edema in patients with previously poorly controlled DM. Insulin infusion increases heart rate and sympathetic nervous system activity, which, in turn, increases myocardial contractility and vascular tone and promotes salt retention via secretion of renin. Conversely, intravenous insulin may also dilate peripheral blood vessels, although this effect is blunted in DM (75).

Obesity may contribute to HTN through release of adipocyte-related factors. Adipocytes contain angiotensinogen, which may not only induce IR and HTN but may also stimulate aldosterone secretion (76, 77). Components or metabolites of FAs may also contribute, such as an epoxy-keto derivative of linoleic acid, which is capable of stimulating aldosterone secretion (78).

If IR and hyperinsulinemia directly contribute to HTN, then interventions that improve insulin sensitivity would be expected to improve blood pressure. Lifestyle interventions, specifically weight loss and aerobic exercise, reduce IR and improve blood pressure and all other features of MS. Conversely, drugs that improve insulin action, such as thiazolidinediones or metformin, do not appear to improve blood pressure. Because of the other metabolic actions of these agents, it is difficult to determine whether potential blood pressure benefits from either agent are obscured by their side effects.

Essential HTN is clearly relevant to the development of CVD. Pharmacologic interventions to treat HTN clearly reduce morbidity and mortality, although the specific blood pressure targets remain debated. HTN is probably most clinically relevant when it occurs in the setting of dyslipidemia. The Copenhagen Male Study divided 3000 male participants into tertiles based on HDL-C and TG concentration (79). Surprisingly, CVD risk was not increased in participants with essential HTN and normal HDL-C and VLDL-TG concentration, but CVD risk was greatly increased in those with the lowest HDL-C and highest VLDL-TG concentrations.

Is Metabolic Syndrome Caused by Insulin Resistance?

MS was initially developed as a diagnostic tool to amalgamate a cluster of closely related metabolic disorders that were postulated to occur as a result of IR. Although MS is strongly associated with IR because of the inclusion of elevated fasting blood glucose, it is unlikely that IR is the sole cause of MS and increased CVD risk. Many (80–85) but by no means have all studies (86–88) found that IR increased CVD risk, however. Indeed, the assessment of what actually constitutes IR is difficult to determine. As discussed, insulin-stimulated glucose disposal rates vary so widely that it is impossible to classify subjects as insulin resistant based only on glucose disposal alone (24, 25). Similarly, absolute insulin concentrations are also widely variable (27, 89), in part because of the differences in the methods used to measure insulin concentration. Variations in the affinity of anti-insulin antibodies used in radioimmunoassay or enzyme-linked immunosorbent assays for cross-reactive peptides such as proinsulin may also contribute to these interlaboratory differences.

Matters become more complex when measures of IR and hyperinsulinemia are applied to large patient populations. Although most obese subjects are hyperinsulinemic and insulin resistant, one fourth may have IR without hyperinsulinemia, and another one fourth may have hyperinsulinemia but lack IR (89). These data suggest that hyperinsulinemia and IR each probably captures slightly different populations at risk of MS (90, 91). Although most people with MS are insulin resistant, this is because of inclusion of elevated fasting glucose. Abundant data indicate that most adults and children with evidence of IR do not meet criteria for MS (91–93). Indeed, it can be argued that IR is not the sole or perhaps even the primary defect in patients with DM or MS.

Although the classic studies by Reaven showed, in nondiabetic subjects, that IR was strongly associated with features of MS (24), many individuals in the least insulin-sensitive quartile had IR that was at least as severe as that of subjects with IGT or type 2 DM (69). These data strongly imply that β-cell function or host adaptation to underlying IR is a critical determinant of whether IR results in metabolic abnormalities or causes hyperinsulinemia alone (i.e., without concomitant development of features of MS). This idea is supported by abundant experimental evidence. β-cell dysfunction is identifiable in patients at high risk for development of type 2 DM, such as those with a family history of DM (94, 95), prior gestational diabetes (96), or polycystic ovarian syndrome (94), even when they still have normal glucose tolerance. A study by Villareal et al (97) suggested that genetic defects in insulin secretion may be associated with host adaptations that increase peripheral insulin sensitivity. This finding suggests that host differences in the capacity to respond to insulin secretory defects may also play a role in determination of when IR or pancreatic failure causes development of DM or MS.

In summary, it is challenging to determine which subjects fulfill criteria for IR. Indeed, studies that relate IR to CVD risk are all associative. Insulin affects innumerable metabolic pathways; therefore, IR or hyperinsulinemia probably would be statistically associated with the features of MS. Failure of other metabolic pathways to adapt to IR clearly plays a critical role in developing MS. For hyperglycemia to result, many other regulatory mechanisms that influence glucose homeostasis must fail. Similarly, it is likely that multiple other steps within the metabolic pathways involved in MS must dysfunction before IR is able to cause metabolic disturbances. Therefore, MS represents a collection of statistically associated factors that individually and collectively confer an increased CVD risk; and whether they all share a similar pathogenic factor is unclear.

CLINICAL UTILITY OF METABOLIC SYNDROME

That patients with MS are at increased risk for development of DM and CVD is generally accepted. This is logical, given that the components of MS each individually increase the risk of CVD. The main clinical question that arises when considering MS is whether MS itself confers a greater risk for CVD than would be expected for any combination of its components (i.e., is the whole greater than the sum of its parts?)

In examining the contribution of MS to coronary heart disease (CHD) risk, it is clear that people with DM should be excluded from analysis. DM so dramatically increases CVD risk that it overwhelms the value of any other indices for risk assessment. For example, Malik et al (98), using the Second National Health and Nutrition Examination Survey (NHANES II) data set, found that DM conferred a fivefold hazard ratio for CHD compared with a hazard ratio of 3.5 of MS. In patients with known CVD, the addition of DM increased CHD risk 11-fold (98).

the inflammatory process by acting, for example, as chemoattractants. Some of the inflammatory mediators may escape the inflammatory site into the circulation and from there exert systemic effects. For example, the cytokine interleukin-6 (IL-6) induces hepatic synthesis of the acute phase protein C-reactive protein (CRP), whereas the cytokine tumor necrosis factor-α (TNF-α) elicits metabolic effects within skeletal muscle, adipose tissue, and bone.

Characteristics of Inflammatory Conditions

Inflammation is a recognized contributor to the pathology of many conditions. In some cases, such as rheumatoid arthritis (RA), inflammatory bowel diseases (IBD), asthma, and psoriasis, the central role of inflammation to the pathologic features is well recognized. Persons with these conditions have heavy infiltration of inflammatory cells at the site of disease activity (e.g., joints, intestinal mucosa, lungs, skin), and they have elevated concentrations of inflammatory mediators at those sites and in the systemic circulation. These conditions are treated with varying levels of success by anti-inflammatory drugs. In other cases, such as atherosclerosis and obesity, the role of inflammation has emerged more recently, and its contribution to the pathologic features alongside the many other relevant factors is less clear. Persons with these conditions show infiltration of inflammatory cells at the site of disease activity (e.g., blood vessel wall, adipose tissue) and have moderately elevated levels of inflammatory mediators in the systemic circulation.

Chronic Inflammation of the Joints: Rheumatoid Arthritis

RA is a common autoimmune disease characterized by chronic inflammation of the synovium of the joints (2). It can lead to long-term joint damage, resulting in chronic pain, loss of function, and disability. The main risk factors for the disease include genetic susceptibility, sex (it is two to three times more common in women than in men), age, smoking, and certain infectious agents. The main predisposing genetic factor is human leukocyte antigen (HLA)-DR4, although other genetic factors have been discovered, such as genetic polymorphisms in the lymphoid protein tyrosine phosphatase (3), which result in altered T-lymphocyte reactivity. In RA, the synovium (or synovial membrane) becomes hypertrophic and edematous. Angioneogenesis, recruitment of inflammatory cells resulting from production of chemokines, local retention, and cell proliferation contribute to the accumulation of cells in the inflamed synovium. Locally expressed degradative enzymes (matrix metalloproteases) digest extracellular matrix and destroy articular structures.

The synovial membrane that extends to the cartilage and bone is known as pannus. It actively invades and destroys the periarticular bone and cartilage at the margin between synovium and bone. T cells are actively involved in the pathogenesis of RA. Activated T cells, which are abundantly present in the inflamed joints of patients with RA, can stimulate other cells (e.g., B cells, macrophages, and fibroblastlike synoviocytes) (4). These T cells are found to participate in the complex network of cell- and mediator-driven events that lead to inflammation and joint destruction. B cells are the source of autoantibodies produced in RA and contribute to immune complex formation and complement activation in the joints (5).

The major effector cells in the pathogenesis of arthritis are synovial macrophages and fibroblasts. Activated macrophages are critical in RA, not only because of macrophage-derived cytokines (in particular, TNF-α and IL-1) in the synovial compartments but also because of their localization at strategic sites within the destructive pannus tissue. Evidence indicates proliferation and expression of inflammatory cytokines and chemokines by fibroblast-like synovial cells in inflamed synovia.

Chronic Inflammation of the Gastrointestinal Mucosa: Inflammatory Bowel Diseases

Ulcerative colitis (UC) and Crohn disease (CD) are the two main forms of IBD. CD can affect any part of the gastrointestinal tract, whereas UC primarily affects the colon (6, 7). IBDs are multifactorial conditions with both genetic and environmental components; the final outcome is driven by an aberrant immune response to normal commensal microbiota in individuals who have a weakened gut epithelial barrier (8).

Although a genetic component is known to be involved in IBD, stronger evidence indicates a genetic link in CD: a mutation in the *NOD2/CARD-15* (called IBD-1) gene has been found in 30% of patients with CD (9). NOD2 is a cytoplasmic receptor for certain peptides found in bacterial cell walls that may reduce the ability of patients with CD who have this mutation to clear invasive bacteria. Indeed, evidence indicates microbial involvement in both forms of IBD, with disturbed interaction between the mucosal immune system and the commensal gut microbiota. In both forms of IBD, large infiltrates of neutrophils are present in the inflamed tissue. The T-cell response profiles associated with UC and CD are different in that a helper T-cell (Th1) pattern of cytokine formation develops in CD with increased production of TNF-α, interferon (IFN)-γ, IL-12, IL-6, and IL-1β, whereas UC more resembles a modified Th2 profile in which cytokines including IL-5 and IL-10 are up-regulated, although IL-4 is not. In addition to this change in cytokine profile, intestinal B lymphocytes produce large amounts of immunoglobulin G (IgG). TNF-α is expressed in the intestinal mucosa of patients with IBD and triggers inflammation through a nuclear factor κB (NF-κB)–dependent signaling cascade.

Many of the cytokines involved act on the signal transducers and activators of transcription (STAT) family. STAT-3 signaling has been found in UC and CD, in which it has been shown to be confined to areas of active inflammation, infiltrating macrophages, and T cells. STAT-3 induces transcription of the proinflammatory cytokine IL-6, which can increase resistance of T cells to apoptosis and lengthen the chronicity of CD as a result of the accumulation of reactive T cells. Other factors implicated in CD include generation of matrix metalloproteinases, which can degrade extracellular matrices and cause ulceration and tissue destruction.

Chronic Inflammation of the Airways: Asthma

Asthma, a chronic inflammatory disease of the lungs, is traditionally classified as allergic or nonallergic. Allergic asthma is the most common form in children, whereas in adults, asthma without known allergen triggers is more common. However, the distinction depends on the demonstration of triggering allergens and is somewhat unclear. Various "nonspecific" irritants may aggravate asthma and trigger an asthmatic attack.

Asthma has chest tightness, wheeze, cough, and dyspnea as prominent symptoms; and it is functionally characterized as reversible bronchial obstruction, caused by contraction of the smooth muscle layer in the mucosa of the bronchi, by mucus production, mucosal edema, and mucosal inflammation. Airway hyperresponsiveness (oversensitivity and overreactivity to stimuli) is typically present in asthma.

A prominent cell in the asthmatic inflammation is the eosinophil, together with lymphocytes. Granulocytes other than eosinophils may be present to varying degrees. The inflammation may lead to destruction and shedding of the epithelial cell layer. Over time, structural changes take place in asthma—so-called remodeling. Inflammation becomes permanent and more severe, and reversibility of the airway obstruction is less complete.

Several genes have been implicated in asthma (e.g., *ADAM33*) (10). Investigators have estimated that more than a dozen polymorphic genes regulate features of asthma such as the inflammatory response, IgE synthesis, cytokine and chemokine production, airway remodeling, and airway function (11). At the heart of the allergic reaction is the interaction between IgE molecules bound to specific receptors on the membrane of mast cells and their corresponding allergens. When the IgE molecules are cross-linked by allergen, the mast cell is triggered to release the potent inflammatory mediators contained in its cytoplasmic granules, and the allergic inflammatory response develops. This response has two phases: an early virtually immediate reaction and a late response developing after several hours. Mast cells are the key cells in the early response, whereas eosinophils are the predominant cell in the late response. Increased levels of the Th2 cytokines IL-4, IL-5, IL-9, and IL-13 have been demonstrated in the asthmatic airway (12). This Th2-driven inflammation has two arms: one through B cells activated by IL-4 to produce IgE, which triggers the mast cell–mediated allergic inflammation; and the other through IL-4, but mainly by IL-13–mediated direct effects on epithelium and bronchial smooth muscle (13). TNF-α has also been reported to play an important role in severe asthma (14).

Chronic Inflammation of the Skin: Psoriasis

Psoriasis is a common inflammatory disease of the skin, although joint symptoms can also be a feature. A genetic susceptibility and associations with other inflammatory conditions are known. Streptococcal infections and physical trauma to the skin may also be involved. The pathophysiology involves an interaction between the immune system and the skin. Psoriasis is characterized by an infiltrate of T lymphocytes into the dermis, formation of clusters of neutrophils in the epidermis, involvement of two or three layers of the epidermis in proliferation, and greatly accelerated but incomplete differentiation. Activation of the innate immune system by streptococcal products and, most likely, as yet unidentified factors induces release of cytokines including IFN-α and IFN-γ. The cellular source of these cytokines is unclear, but it may be dendritic cells. These cytokines activate keratinocytes to proliferate and to produce angiogenic factors that induce proliferation of dermal microvessels.

Chronic Inflammation of the Vascular Wall: Atherosclerosis

Atherosclerosis or "hardening of the arteries" is the major cause of cardiovascular disease. Endothelial dysfunction is the key underlying event, and this is characterized by altered endothelial function, enhanced adhesion molecule expression, and impaired endothelium-dependent vasodilator responses. Leukocytes become attached to the dysfunctional endothelium and subsequently accumulate within the subendothelial space. Monocyte-derived macrophages are converted to lipid-laden foam cells within the artery wall, thus giving rise to a lesion termed the *fatty-streak*. The conversion of the fatty streak into a fibrous atherosclerotic plaque necessitates the recruitment and proliferation of vascular smooth muscle cells (15).

Atherosclerosis is now considered to be a chronic inflammatory disease, and at every stage of its evolution it is characterized by monocyte-macrophage and T-lymphocyte infiltration (16). The possible stimuli to this inflammatory process include oxidized low-density lipoproteins, homocysteine, free radicals generated from cigarette smoking, and infectious microorganisms. The T-cell infiltrates are predominantly T-helper (i.e., CD4$^+$) cells, and cells derived from human lesions react to antigens derived from oxidized low-density lipoproteins, heat shock proteins, and microorganisms (16). The cytokine milieu within atherosclerotic lesions is thought to promote a Th1-dominated response associated with macrophage activation and the production of IFN-γ and IL-1β. The ongoing inflammation involves various growth factors and cytokines, which lead to intimal thickening by stimulating smooth muscle cell migration, proliferation, and extracellular matrix generation.

Chronic Inflammation of Adipose Tissue: Obesity

Obesity is characterized by an expansion of the mass of adipose tissue and dramatic changes in its distribution in the body. A mechanistic link between obesity and low-grade inflammation was first proposed by Hotamisligil et al (17), who showed that white adipose tissue synthesizes and releases TNF-α. The range of inflammatory proteins produced by adipose tissue is now known to be extremely wide and includes leptin, adiponectin, some acute phase proteins, cytokines (including IL-1, IL-6, and TNF-α), chemokines (including IL-8, monocyte chemoattractant protein-1 [MCP-1], RANTES [now known as chemokine (C-C motif) ligand CCL5], and macrophage inflammatory protein-1α and -1β [now known as CCL3 and CCL4, respectively]), and complement factors (including C3) (18). Obesity is associated with chronic elevation of the circulating concentrations of inflammatory proteins including several acute phase inflammatory proteins such as CRP, proinflammatory and anti-inflammatory cytokines, and soluble adhesion molecules (18).

Adipose tissue is a heterogeneous tissue composed of several cell types: mature adipocytes, preadipocytes, fibroblasts, endothelial cells, mast cells, granulocytes, lymphocytes, and macrophages. Because of the heterogeneity of cells in the adipose tissue, the cellular source of the inflammatory factors secreted by the tissue into the circulation remains unknown. However, both adipocytes and classic inflammatory cells, especially macrophages, seem likely to be involved. T lymphocytes appear to play a key early role in adipose tissue inflammation (19). Many mediators synthesized by the adipose tissue are candidates to attract inflammatory cells. Leptin induces adhesion proteins, thus facilitating the migration of monocytes. Conversely, adiponectin may inhibit this process. MCP-1 is a strong chemoattractant and is thought to be a major player in macrophage accumulation within the adipose tissue. Local hypoxia could also play an important role in the attraction and retention of macrophages within the adipose tissue.

Common Features of Chronic Inflammatory Processes

Although inflammation-induced tissue damage occurs in an organ-specific manner (joints, gut, lungs, skin, blood vessel wall, adipose tissue) in different diseases or conditions, some commonality exists among the responses seen in the different organs (summarized in Table 63.2). In general, the inflammatory response observed is normal, but it occurs in the wrong context; this relates to inappropriate barrier function (epithelial or endothelial), inappropriate triggering (i.e., a response to a normally benign stimulus equivalent to a loss of tolerance), lack of down-regulation to control the response, and tissue destruction with a loss of function. In some cases, the inflammation is the result of exogenous triggers such as allergens or microbes. In other

TABLE 63.2	SUMMARY OF THE CHARACTERISTICS OF INFLAMMATORY DISEASE STATES						
	RHEUMATOID ARTHRITIS	CROHN DISEASE	ULCERATIVE COLITIS	ASTHMA	PSORIASIS	ATHEROSCLEROSIS	OBESITY
Organ affected	Joints	Entire gastrointestinal tract	Colon and rectum	Lungs	Skin	Vascular wall	Adipose tissue
Predisposing genetic factors	HLA-DR4 subtypes	*NOD2;* IBD locus	IBD locus; *MUC3;* HLA-DR subtypes?	*ADAM33;* Th2 gene cluster	*PSORS1*	Several, including apolipoprotein E4	Several suggested
Triggering factor(s)	Not known	Commensal gut microbes	Commensal gut microbes	Allergens; irritants	Skin streptococci	Endothelial injury; oxidized low-density lipoprotein	Energy intake in excess of expenditure
Clinical features	Joint swelling, pain, and erosion	Gut ulceration; diarrhea; abdominal pain; weight loss; malaise	Gut ulceration; bloody diarrhea; abdominal pain; urgency to defecate	Wheeze; mucus; breathlessness; impaired lung function	Dry skin	Plaque formation; ultimately myocardial infarction, stroke, and so forth from plaque rupture	Weight gain; insulin resistance
Cells involved	Th1 cells; fibroblasts; B cells; macrophages; synoviocytes	Th1 cells	Th1 and Th2 cells (Th2 dominant); granulocytes	Th2 cells; mast cells; eosinophils	Th1 cells; NK cells; granulocytes; keratinocytes	Macrophages; T cells; platelets; endothelial cells	Adipocytes; macrophages
Mediators involved	TNF-α, IL-1, IL-6, IL-17, PGs, LTB$_4$, MMPs	TNF-α, IL-6, IL-12, PGs, MMPs	TNF-α, IL-5, IL-13, PGs	TNF-α, IL-5, IL-13, cysLTs	Th1 type cytokines, LTB$_4$, angiogenic factors	MCP-1 in plaque formation; MMPs in plaque rupture	MCP-1

cysLT, cysteinyl leukotriene; HLA, human leukocyte antigen; IBD, inflammatory bowel disease; IL, interleukin; LT, leukotriene; MCP, monocyte chemoattractant protein; MMP, matrix metalloproteinase; NK, natural killer; PG, prostaglandin; Th, helper T cell; TNF, tumor necrosis factor.

Modified with permission from Calder PC, Albers R, Antoine JM et al. Inflammatory disease processes and interactions with nutrition. Br J Nutr 2009;101:S1–45.

cases, it is secondary to tissue damage caused by endogenous molecules such as oxidized low-density lipoprotein.

The involvement of different triggers is also reflected in the distinct associations with polymorphisms in receptors involved in pattern recognition such as NOD2 in CD or with other molecules involved in specific adaptive immune responses such as HLA-DR subtypes in UC and RA (see Table 63.2). However, although trigger, localization, and resulting clinical symptoms are different, many of the processes, cells, and molecules involved in the actual inflammatory response are remarkably similar (see Table 63.2).

Most, if not all, of the chronic inflammatory diseases considered here are characterized by overproduction of cytokines (TNF-α, IL-1β, IL-6, IFN-γ), chemokines (IL-8, MCP-1), eicosanoids (prostaglandin E$_2$, 4-series leukotrienes), and matrix metalloproteinases. Elevated levels of these mediators act to amplify the inflammatory process (e.g., by attracting further inflammatory cells to the site) and contribute to tissue destruction (see Fig. 63.1) and to the clinical symptoms observed. Many of these mediators are positively regulated through NF-κB, and some are negatively regulated through peroxisome proliferator-activated receptors (PPARs) and liver X receptors. Entry of inflammatory cells to sites of inflammatory activity is facilitated by up-regulation of adhesion molecules on the endothelium, a process that is promoted by inflammatory cytokines and by a range of inflammatory triggers, frequently acting through NF-κB. The continuous process of tissue injury, healing, and repair, in response to the release of cytokines, chemokines, and growth factors by infiltrating inflammatory cells, as well as resident tissue cells, results in tissue remodeling.

Why resolution of inflammation is absent or abnormal in so many pathophysiologic processes remains largely unknown, although several mechanisms may be considered. First, persistent insult (i.e., chronic infection, continued exposure to triggering stimuli) may provide a continued proinflammatory stimulus. Second, the inflammatory response results in tissue damage, and loss of barrier function may lead to exposure of antigens and loss of tolerance to autoantigens or components of the microbiota, which then provide a trigger to drive prolonged inflammation. Third, local overproduction of survival factors such as IL-5, granulocyte-macrophage colony-stimulating factor, and IL-1β may result in prolonged survival and activity of granulocytes. Finally, negative feedback (control) mechanisms that lead to loss of inflammatory control may be deficient. Although the relative importance may differ, these mechanisms seem to contribute to most of the conditions described here.

FOOD, NUTRITION, AND INFLAMMATORY PROCESSES: SOME GENERAL CONSIDERATIONS

It is clear that "classic" inflammatory diseases (e.g., RA, IBD, asthma, psoriasis) occur as a result of an interaction between a genetic predisposition, which may not be fully understood, and environmental factors. Diet is likely to feature as an environmental factor to differing extents in different inflammatory conditions. The emerging "metabolic" inflammatory diseases (e.g., atherosclerosis, obesity) clearly have a strong dietary component, but inflammation is a less obvious, and only relatively recently recognized, feature of these conditions. Thus, the impact of diet on the inflammatory component of these diseases is difficult to separate from the impact of diet on the other components.

Irrespective of the nature of the inflammation, it is important to distinguish between dietary factors as direct causal factors (i.e., triggers or stimulators) of the inflammatory response and dietary factors as modifiers or regulators of the inflammatory response to another trigger or stimulant. Examples in which diet is a direct causal factor include asthma triggered by exposure to a food allergen (e.g., cows' milk protein, peanut protein) and celiac disease, an inappropriate adverse immunologic response to gluten and gluten-like proteins of some grains (wheat, rye, barley) that results in chronic inflammation of the small intestinal mucosa (20). In these conditions, avoidance of foods that contain the trigger of the inflammation is the obvious key to treatment.

Other examples of dietary components that act as direct triggers of inflammation are emerging. In vitro experiments showed that saturated fatty acids can activate inflammatory cells through Toll-like receptor 4 and the NF-κB pathway in the same way as bacterial lipopolysaccharide (21, 22). This finding raises the possibility that exposure of inflammatory cells to certain nonesterified saturated fatty acids could be an important factor in driving inflammation; this could be very important in metabolic inflammation as seen in obesity, type 2 diabetes, nonalcoholic fatty liver disease, and atherosclerosis. Advanced glycated end products (AGEs) are formed by chemical reactions between glucose and amino acid residues during food processing and in cooking; they are also formed in vivo. Inflammatory cells express receptors for AGEs (RAGE), and RAGE induces inflammatory signaling. Thus, AGEs from foods or formed endogenously may possibly trigger inflammation (23).

Breakdown of barrier function is a key factor in some inflammatory diseases such as IBD. An inadequate or inappropriate diet may possibly contribute to a breakdown in the gastrointestinal barrier, which, in genetically predisposed individuals and perhaps in the presence of other factors, influences the initiation, progression, and severity of the disease. Furthermore, one key "environmental" factor contributing to IBD is now recognized to be the composition of the gut microbiota; diet clearly can influence the gut microbiota and therefore may have an indirect influence on IBD in this way. Thus, diet can be seen to be one step removed from direct causal factors (gut barrier breakdown; microbiota composition) of the initiation, progression, and severity of IBD.

A strong interaction occurs between oxidative stress and inflammation. The generation of oxidants (e.g., superoxide radicals, hydrogen peroxide) is part of the host inflammatory response. Oxidants can damage components of host cells. In turn, oxidants and oxidized cell components, acting through transcription factors such as NF-κB, induce production of inflammatory eicosanoids and cytokines, among other mediators (Fig. 63.2). Thus, dietary components that contribute to oxidative stress (e.g., oxidized lipids that result from heating cooking oils to high temperature) could promote inflammatory responses, whereas dietary components that inhibit or quench oxidative stress (various antioxidants) could decrease the strength of inflammatory responses.

The nature of the diet can affect the concentrations of hormones (e.g., insulin, leptin, cortisol) that, in turn, affect inflammatory processes. Some dietary components act as substrates for biosynthesis of inflammatory mediators (e.g., arginine is the precursor of nitric oxide and the n-6 fatty acid arachidonic acid is the precursor of inflammatory prostaglandins). Thus, diet could play a key role in maintaining availability of such substrates to fuel the inflammatory response. Finally, some dietary components act as regulators of various aspects of inflammatory cell responses. For example, marine n-3 fatty acids influence signaling pathways in inflammatory cells through actions at the membrane, the cytosol, and the nucleus (24–26), and therefore they act to modify the responses initiated by various inflammatory triggers.

DIETARY APPROACHES TO PREVENTING OR AMELIORATING INFLAMMATION

Caloric Restriction and Weight Loss

Weight loss is accompanied by decreased concentrations of circulating markers of inflammation (27), but whether this effect is secondary to the weight loss itself or to the nature of the diet used to induce weight loss is difficult to determine. However, it seems likely that reduced secretion of proinflammatory mediators from adipocytes or activated macrophages of adipose tissue contributes to the effect of weight loss. Conversely, calorie restriction itself may play an anti-inflammatory role (28). Key mediators of the effect are proteins of the sirtuin and FoxO families, which are induced or activated during states of limited energy supply. The sirtuins are oxidized nicotinamide adenine dinucleotide (NAD^+)–dependent deacetylases of substrates ranging from histones to transcriptional regulators. As a consequence, metabolic efficiency is improved, cell defenses against stress are strengthened, and inflammatory activities are dampened, notably by decreasing the activation of

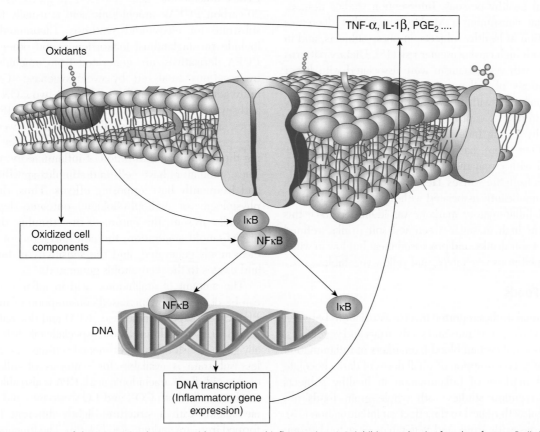

Fig. 63.2. Representation of the interaction between oxidant stress and inflammation. *IκB*, inhibitory subunit of nuclear factor κB; *IL*, interleukin; *NFκB*, nuclear factor κB; *PG*, prostaglandin; *TNF*, tumor necrosis factor. (Reproduced with permission from Calder PC, Albers R, Antoine JM et al. Inflammatory disease processes and interactions with nutrition. Br J Nutr 2009;101:S1–45.)

NF-κB (29, 30). FoxO proteins are transcription factors that regulate the expression of genes involved in energy homeostasis, cell survival, and inflammatory responses including NF-κB (31, 32). Reducing energy intake appears to be more important than the nature of low-calorie food; decreased concentrations of inflammatory markers are observed with a low-calorie, fat-rich diet as well as with a low-calorie, carbohydrate-rich diet (33). However, it is conceivable that some dietary components are better regulators of sirtuin or FoxO activity than others.

Dietary Patterns

Epidemiologic studies examined the associations between particular dietary patterns or intake of specific types of foods and measures of inflammation. These studies usually focused on blood markers of inflammation (e.g., plasma concentrations of CRP or cytokines) and were conducted largely in the context of the low-grade chronic inflammation associated with cardiovascular disease, insulin resistance, and overweight and obesity. Epidemiologic associations must be confirmed through intervention studies.

Greater adherence to the traditional Mediterranean diet (rich in fruits, vegetables, whole grains, legumes, nuts, fish, and low-fat dairy products, with moderate consumption of wine, and with olive oil as the principal source of fat) is associated with lower blood concentrations of inflammatory markers in healthy persons. Intervention studies demonstrated that consuming a Mediterranean diet decreases inflammation in healthy subjects, in obese subjects, and in subjects with high cardiovascular risk (18). Dietary patterns consistent with vegetarianism were associated with lower concentrations of inflammatory markers in the bloodstream compared with nonvegetarian diets (18). Healthy eating patterns, as captured by scoring systems such as the Healthy Eating Index, the Diet Quality Index, or the Prudent Diet Score, have all been shown to be inversely associated with circulating markers of inflammation (18). Using data from the Nurses' Health Study, a dietary pattern that was significantly associated with higher concentrations of several inflammatory markers was identified (34); this pattern was high in sugar-sweetened soft drinks, refined grains, diet soft drinks, and processed meat but low in wine, coffee, cruciferous vegetables, and yellow vegetables.

Specific Foods

Observational studies reported inverse associations between intake of whole grains, nuts and seeds, fruits and vegetables, fish, and tea and certain blood biomarkers of inflammation (18). Regular consumption of small doses of dark chocolate decreased markers of inflammation in healthy subjects (35). Intervention studies with whole grain foods are inconsistent with regard to the effect on inflammation (18). Interventions with fruits and vegetables as a food group have been successful at reducing the blood concentrations of inflammatory proteins (18). However, studies focusing on a single variety of vegetable or fruit have been inconsistent (18). Soy protein appears not to affect circulating markers of inflammation, but one study with soy nuts reported reduced plasma CRP, TNF-α, IL-18, and E-selectin concentrations (18). Intervention trials of drinking black tea, green tea, or coffee have not yielded a clear picture regarding a possible anti-inflammatory effect (18).

SELECTED NUTRIENTS THAT MAY PREVENT OR AMELIORATE INFLAMMATION

Observations that healthy diets and their components (whole grains, nuts and seeds, fruits and vegetables, and fish) are associated with reduced inflammation have focused attention on the nutrients provided by those diets and foods as having anti-inflammatory properties. Key among these nutrients are antioxidant vitamins (C, E, and carotenoids), flavonoids, and marine n-3 fatty acids.

Marine n-3 Polyunsaturated Fatty Acids

Mechanism of Action

The key link between fatty acids and inflammation is that eicosanoids, which act as mediators and regulators of inflammation, are generated from 20-carbon polyunsaturated fatty acids (PUFAs). Because inflammatory cells typically contain a high proportion of the n-6 PUFA arachidonic acid and low proportions of other 20-carbon PUFAs, arachidonic acid is usually the major substrate for eicosanoid synthesis. Eicosanoids, which include prostaglandins, leukotrienes, and other oxidized PUFA derivatives, are generated from arachidonic acid by reactions catalyzed by cyclooxygenase (COX) and lipoxygenase (LOX) enzymes. At least two COX enzymes and several LOX enzymes are expressed in different cell types, according to different conditions; between them, they produce a range of mediators involved in modulating the intensity and duration of inflammatory responses. These mediators have cell- and stimulus-specific sources and frequently have opposing effects. Thus, the overall physiologic (or pathophysiologic) outcome depends on the cells present, the nature of the stimulus, the timing of eicosanoid generation, the concentrations of different eicosanoids generated, and the sensitivity of target cells and tissues to the eicosanoids generated.

The amount of arachidonic acid in inflammatory cells can be decreased by increased consumption of marine n-3 PUFAs (eicosapentaenoic acid [EPA] and docosahexaenoic acid [DHA]) found in seafood, especially oily fish, and usually given as fish oil in experimental settings (24–26). Thus, less substrate is available for synthesis of inflammatory eicosanoids from arachidonic acid. EPA is also able to act as a substrate for both COX and LOX enzymes and produces eicosanoids with a structure slightly different from that formed from arachidonic acid (24–26). The functional significance of this finding is that the mediators formed from EPA are typically less potent than those formed from arachidonic acid. A novel family of mediators, termed E- and D-series resolvins, formed from EPA and DHA, respectively, by the sequential actions of COX-2 and LOX enzymes has been identified. These resolvins have been shown to exert potent anti-inflammatory and inflammation-resolving actions (36). Thus, one anti-inflammatory mechanism of action of marine n-3 PUFAs is antagonism of production of inflammatory eicosanoids from arachidonic acid coupled with the generation of less potent EPA-derived eicosanoids and anti-inflammatory resolvins from EPA and DHA. Altered eicosanoid and resolvin profiles may have downstream effects because these lipid mediators regulate production of inflammatory cytokines. However, eicosanoid-independent effects of marine n-3 PUFAs also seem likely. These PUFAs have been shown to decrease activation of the proinflammatory transcription factor NF-κB to activate the anti-inflammatory transcription factor PPAR-γ, and to alter key structural and functional aspects of the plasma membrane (24–26).

As a result of these actions, marine n-3 PUFAs have been shown to alter leukocyte chemotaxis, adhesion molecule expression, and production of inflammatory cytokines (24, 25). Observational studies demonstrated an inverse association between intake or status of marine n-3 PUFAs and circulating inflammatory marker concentrations (18). Intervention studies with marine n-3 PUFAs showed reduced production of inflammatory eicosanoids and cytokines by isolated inflammatory cells (24–26). Anti-inflammatory actions of plant n-3 PUFA α-linolenic acid appear to require its conversion to the more biologically active EPA (18).

Effects on Clinical Outcomes in Inflammatory Conditions

Rheumatoid Arthritis. Dietary fish oil showed improvements in animal models of RA (37). Several studies reported anti-inflammatory effects of fish oil in patients with RA, such as decreased leukotriene B_4 production by neutrophils and monocytes, decreased IL-1 production by monocytes, decreased plasma IL-1β concentrations, decreased serum CRP concentrations, and normalization of the neutrophil chemotactic response (37). Several randomized, placebo-controlled, double-blind studies of fish oil in RA have been reported (37–40). The dose of marine n-3 PUFAs used in these trials was between 1.6 and 7.1 g/day and averaged approximately 3.5 g/day. Almost all these trials showed some benefit of fish oil, including reduced duration of morning stiffness, reduced number of tender or swollen joints, reduced joint pain, reduced time to fatigue, increased grip strength, and decreased use of nonsteroidal anti-inflammatory drugs. One study reported greater efficacy of fish oil against a background diet designed to be low in arachidonic acid. Metaanalyses of the trials of marine n-3 PUFAs in RA concluded that clinical benefit does exist (38, 39), including reduced requirements for corticosteroids (40).

Inflammatory Bowel Diseases. Dietary fish oil showed improvements in animal models of IBD (41). Indications exist that a diet high in n-6 and low in n-3 PUFAs is associated with increased incidence of IBD (41).

Marine n-3 PUFAs are incorporated into gut mucosal tissue of patients with IBD who supplement their diet with fish oil, and this results in anti-inflammatory effects, such as decreased eicosanoid production by colonic mucosa and by isolated leukocytes (41). Several randomized, placebo-controlled, double-blind studies of fish oil in IBD have been reported (40, 41). The dose of marine n-3 PUFAs used in these trials was between 2.7 and 5.6 g/day and averaged approximately 4.5 g/day. Some of these trials indicated benefits of fish oil that included improved clinical score, improved gut mucosal histology, improved sigmoidoscopic score, lower rate of relapse, and decreased use of corticosteroids, although findings were not consistent across studies (40, 41). A metaanalysis concluded that the requirement for corticosteroids may be reduced (40).

Asthma. Several studies reported anti-inflammatory effects of fish oil in patients with asthma, such as decreased 4-series leukotriene production and leukocyte chemotaxis (25). Some randomized, placebo-controlled, double-blind studies of fish oil in asthma have been reported (25). A systematic review concluded that no consistent effect was noted on lung function, asthma symptoms, asthma medication use, or bronchial hyperreactivity (42), whereas a more recent report covering 26 studies (both randomized, placebo-controlled and others) concluded that no definitive conclusion could be drawn regarding the efficacy of marine n-3 fatty acid supplements as a treatment for asthma in children and adults (43). However, one study in children showed improved lung function and reduced asthma medication use with fish oil (44).

Psoriasis. Dietary supplementation studies with fish oil did not present a clear picture although some of these studies reported clinical benefit (45).

Cardiovascular Disease. Substantial evidence from ecologic, epidemiologic, and case-control studies indicates that consumption of fish, fatty fish, and marine n-3 PUFAs reduces the risk of cardiovascular mortality (46–49). Secondary prevention studies using marine n-3 PUFAs in myocardial infarction survivors showed a reduction in total mortality and cardiovascular mortality, with an especially potent effect on sudden death (50). Marine n-3 PUFAs were shown to influence several cardiovascular risk factors (46, 47), but the extent to which a reduction in inflammation protects against growth of the atherosclerotic plaque and decreases the risk and severity of cardiovascular events was not clear. However, more recent studies suggested that marine n-3 PUFAs may act to stabilize advanced atherosclerotic plaques, perhaps through their anti-inflammatory effects (51, 52).

Antioxidant Vitamins

Mechanisms of Action

Strong interaction occurs between oxidative stresss and inflammation. The generation of oxidants is part of the the host inflammatory response. Oxidants can damage components of host cells. In turn, oxidants and oxidized cell components, acting through transcription factors such as NF-κB, induce production of inflammatory eicosanoids and cytokines (see Fig. 63.2). Thus, one mechanism to diminish inflammatory mediator production may be to prevent oxidative stress. This is accomplished through enhancing antioxidant defense mechanisms, including increasing the concentrations of antioxidant vitamins such as vitamin C (ascorbate), vitamin E (tocopherols and tocotrienols), and carotenoids (β-carotene, lycopene, lutein, astaxanthin).

Antioxidant vitamins act to reduce exposure to oxidants and thereby decrease activation of NF-κB and subsequent production of inflammatory cytokines, eicosanoids, and so on (1). Inflammatory cells maintain high intracellular concentrations of vitamin C, although these concentrations become depleted during acute activation. At the site of inflammation, the ratio of oxidized to reduced ascorbate is increased (1). Observational studies reported inverse relationships between intake or status of antioxidant vitamins (vitamin C, lutein, lycopene) and various circulating markers of inflammation (18). Intervention with a diet of carotenoid-rich fruits and vegetables reduced CRP concentration (53), whereas a tomato-based drink (providing lycopene, β-carotene, phytoene, phytofluene, and α-tocopherol) decreased blood TNF-α concentrations (54).

Effects in Inflammatory Conditions

Rheumatoid Arthritis. Evidence of ascorbate oxidation has been seen in RA, and low antioxidant status was a risk factor for RA over 20 years of follow-up of a case-control study (1). Low intake of some carotenoids has been linked with increased risk of RA (1). Vitamin E in the form of α-tocopherol decreased inflammation and improved pathologic features and disease severity in animal models of RA (1). Vitamins C and E (α-tocopherol) have been shown to decrease RA severity in patients (1).

Inflammatory Bowel Diseases. Serum and leukocyte ascorbate and serum carotenoid concentrations are low in patients with CD (1). Inflamed colonic tissue from patients with CD or UC has a lower ascorbate content than uninflamed tissue (1), a finding consistent with the use of ascorbate as the result of inflammatory reactions. In a rat model of colitis, lycopene decreased the inflammatory response and mucosal damage (1).

Asthma. Asthmatic patients have lower vitamin C concentrations in plasma, leukocytes, and lung fluid than controls (1). In addition, oxidized glutathione is increased in lung fluid, a finding suggestive of oxidative stress in the airways (1). Cross-sectional studies showed an inverse relation between plasma vitamin C and lung inflammation and suggested that high vitamin C intakes or plasma concentrations promoted better lung function (1). Clinical trials showed that vitamin C supplements (typically 2 g/day) exert protective effects on airway responsiveness and allergens (1).

Flavonoids

Polyphenols are secondary metabolites of plants. They include flavanones, flavones, flavanols, and flavonols. In vitro studies suggested that flavonoids have anti-inflammatory activity through several mechanisms, including the following: decreased eicosanoid production through inhibition of phospholipase A2, COX, and LOX; inhibition of inducible nitric oxide synthase; and inhibition of inflammatory cytokine production (1). These effects all seem to involve inhibition of activation of key proinflammatory transcription factors such as NF-κB and activator protein-1 (1). Although some flavonoids were shown to have effects in animal models of inflammatory processes (1), human studies investigating the effect of flavonoids on markers of inflammation are scarce, and most of them focus on the use of flavonoid-rich foods and not on pure molecules. For example, the effects of red wine (55) and chocolate (35) on inflammatory markers are believed to result from their constituent flavonoids. Bioavailability of polyphenols is poor, and circulating concentrations are low and are often much lower than those used in the in vitro experiments that demonstrated strong anti-inflammatory effects. Very little information on flavonoids exists in relation to inflammatory disorders.

GUT MICROBIOTA AND INFLAMMATION

Gut Microbiota

Up to 10^{14} microorganisms are contained in the adult human body (10 times more microbial cells than human cells), and most of these microorganisms are located in the gastrointestinal tract (56). More than 1 kg of bacteria is present in the gut, and feces typically comprise 50% bacteria. This means that humans excrete 50 to 100 g of bacteria each day. Microorganisms are at their lowest numbers ($<10^3$ colony-forming units [CFU]/g) in the stomach because of its low pH and fast transit time, but they reach levels as high as 10^{12} CFU/g in the colon, a reflection of the colon's much slower transit time, less acidic pH, and low oxygen levels. At least 500 different bacterial species have been cultured from feces (including lactobacilli and bifidobacteria), yet just 40 species account for 99% of those that have been identified. The microbial inhabitants of the intestinal microbiota are still not fully identified because of the limitations of identification techniques and individual variations. Newer molecular typing methods are now enabling identification of further gut-associated species.

The major function of the colonic microbiota is the fermentation of dietary substances that have passed undigested through the small intestine and of mucus produced within the gut. Saccharolytic fermentation produces short-chain fatty acids such as acetate, propionate, and butyrate, which are essential nutrients for the colonocytes. Interactions also occur between gut microbiota and inflammatory cells present within and beyond the gut epithelium (57); these interactions can be chemical or may involve direct cell-to-cell contact. Investigators believe that such interactions play an important role in defining the inflammatory response in the gut wall.

Prebiotics and Probiotics

Prebiotics are "nondigestible food ingredients that beneficially affect the host by selectively stimulating the growth, and/or activity, of one or a limited number of beneficial bacteria in the colon and thus improve host health" (58). Prebiotics are typically carbohydrates that escape digestion by mammalian enzymes in the small intestine but are hydrolyzed by microbial enzymes in the colon (58). Prebiotics include fructooligosaccharides and galactooligosaccharides. These typically promote growth of lactobacilli and bifidobacteria. Probiotics are "live microorganisms which when administered in sufficient amounts confer a health benefit to the host" (59).

Lactic acid–producing bacteria, including lactobacilli and bifidobacteria of human intestinal origin, are the most commonly used probiotics. Probiotic bacteria modulate the gastrointestinal microenvironment and release antimicrobial factors such as defensins (60). Several probiotics successfully preserve epithelial barrier function by induction of mucin secretion, maintenance of cytoskeletal integrity, tight junction protein phosphorylation, or induction of heat shock proteins. Potential anti-inflammatory effects of probiotic bacteria, including lactobacilli and bifidobacteria, seem to be based on their direct interaction with intestinal epithelial cells, which have a key role in sensing danger signals within the luminal microenvironment. Some probiotic bacteria antagonize NF-κB activation and thereby decrease production of proinflammatory cytokines (1). Some probiotic strains (or their components) interact with gut-residing dendritic cells to induce their maturation and secretion of IL-10, which is thought to favor the induction of regulatory T cells (1).

Effects in Inflammatory Bowel Diseases

Prebiotics and probiotics, alone or in combination, have been shown to induce anti-inflammatory effects and histologic improvements in animal models of IBD (1). In addition, prebiotics and probiotics improve inflammatory markers, gut histology, and disease severity in patients with IBD, although not all studies of probiotics demonstrated these findings (1, 61, 62), most likely because specific organisms or combinations of organisms are required to be effective. Furrie et al (63) showed that a combination of fructooligosaccharides and the probiotic *Bifidobacterium longum* up-regulated mucosal β-defensins, decreased mucosal inflammatory cytokines, and improved gut histology in patients with UC. Taken together, the human study results demonstrate that therapeutic intervention with prebiotics or probiotics in IBD is encouraging but not as straightforward as expected from the findings of the experimental animal models of colitis. A combination of different lactobacilli and bifidobacteria or a combination of probiotics and prebiotics appears to be required for effective treatment of IBD.

SUMMARY AND CONCLUSIONS

Inflammation is a stereotypical physiologic response to infections and tissue injury. It initiates pathogen killing as well as tissue repair processes and helps to restore homeostasis at infected or damaged sites. Acute inflammatory reactions are usually self-limiting and resolve rapidly. This process involves the activation of negative feedback mechanisms such as the secretion of immunoregulatory cytokines (e.g., IL-10 and transforming growth factor-β), inhibition of proinflammatory signaling cascades, receptor shedding, and activation of regulatory cells. Inflammatory responses that fail to regulate themselves can become chronic and contribute to the perpetuation and progression of disease. Characteristics typical of chronic inflammatory responses underlying the pathophysiology of several disorders include loss of barrier function, responsiveness to a normally benign stimulus, infiltration of inflammatory cells into compartments where they are not normally found in such high numbers, and overproduction of oxidants, cytokines, chemokines, eicosanoids, and matrix metalloproteinases. The levels of these mediators amplify the inflammatory response, are destructive, and contribute to the clinical symptoms.

A healthy eating pattern characterized by consumption of whole grains, nuts and seeds, fruits and vegetables, and fish is associated with reduced inflammation, a finding suggesting candidate anti-inflammatory dietary components. However, the number of studies assessing therapeutic benefits of dietary interventions in established inflammatory disorders is still fairly limited. Nevertheless, good evidence indicates efficacy of marine n-3 PUFAs in RA; the evidence in CD and psoriasis is less strong, and it is rather weak in UC and asthma. These fatty acids are also beneficial in established cardiovascular disease, but the extent to which this benefit is attributable to their anti-inflammatory effects is not clear. Dietary antioxidants represent a crucial line of defense against oxidative and inflammatory insult common to the development of many pathologic disorders, and a potentially protective role of dietary antioxidants in disease prevention is supported by extensive basic scientific evidence. The common mechanism of oxidative stress development in most of the disorders considered here makes the role of dietary antioxidants crucial for optimal preventive and therapeutic actions.

Despite these considerations, trials in patients suggest limited clinical benefit from antioxidant vitamins in the disorders considered here, although some evidence indicates benefit from vitamins C and E in RA and vitamin C in asthma. The intestinal flora is in intimate contact with the most highly developed immunologic organ of the human body embedded in the intestinal tract. Continuous interaction occurs between the intestinal bacterial ecosystem and the host. The composition of this microbiota can be modified by intake of prebiotics or of probiotics. Evidence indicates that prebiotics and probiotics lead to clinical improvement in IBD, but the effects of probiotics are strain and species dependent. Studies with different dietary components in various models and clinical settings have demonstrated that dietary constituents modulate pathways involved in controlling inflammation, including intracellular signaling pathways, transcription factor activity, and generation of inflammatory mediators.

REFERENCES

1. Calder PC, Albers R, Antoine JM et al. Br J Nutr 2009;101: S1–45.
2. Lee DM, Weinblatt ME. Lancet 2001;358:903–11.
3. Firestein GS. Nature 2003;423:356–61.
4. Panayi GS, Lanchbury JS, Kingsley GH. Arthritis Rheum 1992;35:729–35.
5. Weyand CM, Seyler TM, Goronzy JJ. Arthritis Res Ther 2005;7(Suppl 3):S9–12.
6. Farrell RJ, Peppercorn MA. Lancet 2002;359:331–40.
7. Shanahan F. Lancet 2002;359:62–9.
8. Duchmann R, Kaiser I, Hermann E et al. Clin Exp Immunol 1995;102:448–55.
9. Ogura Y, Bonen DK, Inohara N et al. Nature 2001;411:603–6.
10. Van Eerdewegh P, Little RD, Dupuis J et al. Nature 2002;418:426–30.
11. Fahy JV, Corry DB, Boushey HA. Curr Opin Pulm Med 2000;6:15–20.
12. Ray A, Cohn L. J Clin Invest 1999;104:985–93.
13. Barrios RJ, Kheradmand F, Batts L et al. Arch Pathol Lab Med 2006;130:447–51.
14. van Oosterhout AJ, Bloksma N. Eur Respir J 2005;26:918–32.
15. Ross R. Nature 1993;362:801–9.
16. Hansson GK. N Engl J Med 2005;352:1685–95.
17. Hotamisligil GS, Shargill NS, Spiegelman BM. Science 1993;259:87–91.
18. Calder PC, Ahluwalia N, Brouns F et al. Br J Nutr 2011;106(Suppl 3):S5–78.
19. Kintscher U, Hartge M, Hess K et al. Arterioscler Thromb Vasc Biol 2008;28:1304–10.
20. Kagnoff MF. Gastroenterology 2005;128(Suppl):S10–8.
21. Lee JY, Sohn KH, Rhee SH et al. J Biol Chem 2001;276: 16683–9.
22. Weatherill AR, Lee JY, Zhao L et al. J Immunol 2005;174: 5390–7.
23. Lin L, Park S, Lakatta EG. Front Biosci 2009;14:1403–13.
24. Calder PC. Lipids 2003;38:342–52.
25. Calder PC. Am J Clin Nutr 2006;83:1505S–19S.
26. Calder PC. Eur J Pharmacol 2011;668(Suppl 1):S50–8.
27. Esposito K, Pontillo A, Di Palo C et al. JAMA 2003;289: 1799–804.
28. Holloszy JO, Fontana L. Exp Gerontol 2007;42:709–12.
29. Guarente L, Picard F. Cell 2005;120:473–82.
30. Dali-Youcef N, Lagouge M, Froelich S et al. Ann Med 2007;39:335–45.
31. Salminen A, Ojala J, Huuskonen J et al. Cell Mol Life Sci 2008;65:1049–58.
32. Kim DH, Kim JY, Yu BP et al. Biogerontology 2008;9:33–47.
33. Sharman MJ, Volek JS. Clin Sci 2004;107:365–9.
34. Schulze MB, Hoffmann K, Manson JE et al. Am J Clin Nutr 2005;82:675–84.
35. di Giuseppe R, Di Castelnuovo A, Centritto F et al. J Nutr 2008;138:1939–45.
36. Serhan CN, Chiang N, van Dyke TE. Nature Rev Immunol 2008;8:349–61.
37. Calder PC. Proc Nutr Soc 2008;67:409–18.
38. Fortin PR, Lew RA, Liang MH et al. J Clin Epidemiol 1995;48:1379–90.
39. Goldberg RJ, Katz J. Pain 2007;129:210–33.
40. MacLean CH, Mojica WA, Morton SC et al. Effects of Omega-3 Fatty Acids on Inflammatory Bowel Disease, Rheumatoid Arthritis, Renal Disease, Systemic Lupus Erythematosus, and Osteoporosis. Rockville, MD: Agency for Healthcare Research and Quality, 2004.
41. Calder PC. Mol Nutr Food Res 2008;52:885–97.
42. Woods RK, Thien FC, Abramson MJ. Cochrane Database Syst Rev 2002;(3):CD001283.
43. Schachter H, Reisman J, Tran K et al. Health Effects of Omega-3 Fatty Acids on Asthma. Rockville, MD: Agency for Healthcare Research and Quality, 2004.
44. Nagakura T, Matsuda S, Shichijyo K et al. Eur Respir J 2000;16:861–5.
45. Ziboh V. The role of n-3 fatty acids in psoriasis. In: Kremer J, ed. Medicinal Fatty Acids in Inflammation. Basel: Birkhauser, 1998:45–53.
46. Bucher HC, Hengstler P, Schindler C et al. Am J Med 2002;112:298–304.
47. Studer M, Briel M, Leimenstoll B et al. Arch Intern Med 2005;165:725–30.
48. Calder PC. Clin Sci 2004;107:1–11.
49. Calder PC, Yaqoob P. Cell Mol Biol 2010;56:28–37.
50. Anonymous. Lancet 1999;354:447–55.
51. Thies F, Garry JM, Yaqoob P et al. Lancet 2003;361:477–85.
52. Cawood AL, Ding R, Napper FL et al. Atherosclerosis 2010;212:252–9.
53. Watzl B, Kulling SE, Möseneder J et al. Am J Clin Nutr 2005;82:1052–8.
54. Riso P, Visioli F, Grande S et al. J Agric Food Chem 2006;54:2563–6.
55. Zern TL, Wood RJ, Greene C et al. J Nutr 2005;135:1911–7.
56. Holzapfel WH, Haberer P, Snel J et al. Int J Food Microbiol 1998;41:85–101.
57. Preidis GA, Versalovic J. Gastroenterology 2009;136:2015–31.
58. Gibson GR, Roberfroid MB. J Nutr 1995;125:1401–12.
59. Food and Agriculture Organization, World Health Organization. Health and nutritional properties of probiotics in food including powder milk with live lactic acid bacteria, a joint FAO/WHO expert consultation. Cordoba, Argentina, 1–4 October 2001:1–34. Available at: http://www.who.int/foodsafety/publications/fs_management/probiotics/en/index.html. Accessed May 25, 2012.
60. Penner R, Fedorak RN, Madsen KL. Curr Opin Pharmacol 2005;5:596–603.
61. Lomax AR, Calder PC. Br J Nutr 2009;101:633–58.
62. Lomax AR, Calder PC. Curr Pharm Des 2009;15:1428–518.
63. Furrie E, Macfarlane S, Kennedy A et al. Gut 2005;54: 242–9.

SUGGESTED READINGS

Calder PC, Ahluwalia N, Brouns F et al. Dietary factors and low-grade inflammation in relation to overweight and obesity. Br J Nutr 2011; 106(Suppl 3):S5–78.

Calder PC, Albers R, Antoine JM et al. Inflammatory disease processes and interactions with nutrition. Br J Nutr 2009;101:S1–45.

Gibson GR, Roberfroid MB. Dietary modulation of the human colonic microbiota: introducing the concept of prebiotics. J Nutr 1995;125:1401–12.

Tilg H, Moschen AR. Adipocytokines: mediators linking adipose tissue, inflammation and immunity. Nat Rev Immunol 2006;6:772–783.

64

NUTRIENT AND GENETIC REGULATION OF LIPOPROTEIN METABOLISM[1]

EDWARD A. FISHER, RAANAN SHAMIR, AND ROBERT A. HEGELE

The relationships among different dietary components and lipoprotein metabolism have been long recognized on both an experimental and an observational basis. For example, the INTERHEART study showed, among many other findings, that across many ethnic groups and areas of the world, cardiovascular disease (CVD) risk was inversely related to the consumption of "heart-healthy" foods: indeed, approximately 30% of the population-attributable risk of CVD was accounted for by an unhealthy dietary intake (1). In classic studies (2–4), the relationships between dietary cholesterol and specific characteristics of fats (particularly the degree of fatty acid saturation) and plasma levels of low-density lipoprotein (LDL) cholesterol (LDL-C) and high-density lipoprotein (HDL) cholesterol (HDL-C) were established by careful clinical experimentation. Over the subsequent years, additional studies were conducted in animals and humans to show that the other macronutrients, protein and carbohydrate, as well as other dietary components, also had effects on plasma lipid and lipoprotein levels (5).

As cell and molecular biologic techniques advanced in the last quarter of the twentieth century, a battery of studies was conducted to elucidate the mechanistic underpinnings of the clinical observations and intervention results. These studies were greatly expanded in scope by the revolution in molecular genetic manipulation of the mouse genome, which allowed the development of models in which candidate genes implicated in the response to nutritional factors could be inserted by transgenesis or inactivated by homologous recombination in the context of normal and abnormal backgrounds and conditions (e.g., atherosclerosis). The sequencing of the human genome, coupled with high-throughput technologies, led to

---

[1]**Abbreviations: ABCA1,** adenosine triphosphate–binding cassette protein A1; **ABL,** abetalipoproteinemia; **ADH,** autosomal dominant hypercholesterolemia; **ANGPTL,** angiopoietin-like protein; **Apo,** apolipoprotein; **ARH,** autosomal recessive hypercholesterolemia; **CAD,** coronary artery disease; **CE,** cholesteryl ester; **CETP,** cholesterol ester transfer protein; **CVD,** cardiovascular disease; **FCH,** familial combined hyperlipidemia; **FDB,** familial defective apolipoprotein-B; **FH,** familial hypercholesterolemia; **FHBL,** familial hypobetalipoproteinemia; **GLGC,** Global Lipids Genetics Consortium; **GWAS,** genome-wide association study; **HDL,** high-density lipoprotein; **HDL-C,** high-density lipoprotein cholesterol; **HL,** hepatic lipase; **HMG-CoA,** hydroxymethyl-glutaryl-coenzyme A; **IDL,** intermediate-density lipoprotein; **LCAT,** lecithin:cholesterol acyltransferase; **LDL,** low-density lipoprotein; **LDL-C,** low-density lipoprotein cholesterol; **LDLR,** low-density lipoprotein receptor gene; **LDLRAP1,** low-density lipoprotein receptor adapter protein 1; **LIPC,** hepatic lipase gene; **LPL,** lipoprotein lipase; **miRs,** micro-RNAs; **MTP,** microsomal triglyceride transfer protein; **PCSK9,** proprotein convertase subtilin/kexin type 9; **RCT,** reverse cholesterol transport; **TG,** triglyceride; **VLDL,** very-low-density lipoprotein.

the next phase of discovery in many areas of physiology and pathophysiology. For lipoprotein metabolism, by 2010 (6), genome-wide association studies (GWASs) had established 95 genetic loci associated with the plasma concentrations of total lipids (cholesterol, triglycerides [TGs]) and the individual lipoprotein fractions. Some of these loci were known from previous evidence to be functional players in lipid and lipoprotein metabolism, and the regulation of many of these was known to be subject to a component of the diet. Other loci found by GWASs were completely novel discoveries, with their roles and regulation still to be established. This chapter summarizes the major genetic factors that are known to determine or have strong influence on human lipoprotein metabolism. For a detailed summary of the impact of specific nutrients on human lipoprotein plasma levels, the reader is referred to the chapter on nutrition in the prevention of coronary heart disease and in the management of lipoprotein disorders.

HIGH PLASMA LEVELS OF TOTAL AND LOW-DENSITY LIPOPROTEIN CHOLESTEROL

High blood cholesterol, especially LDL-C, is associated with increased risk of premature CVD. Measurement of serum total cholesterol is a reflection of the amount of cholesterol contained within circulating very-low-density lipoproteins (VLDLs), LDLs, HDLs, and chylomicrons (although chylomicron levels are essentially nil when cholesterol is measured in the fasting state). Thus, a fasting lipoprotein profile is needed when hypercholesterolemia is identified or suspected. Hypercholesterolemia with either a monogenic or multifactorial basis affects approximately 5% of the population, but increased risk of premature atherosclerosis has been mainly established for the monogenic disorders that result in elevated LDL (7).

LDL is rich in cholesteryl esters (CEs), and each particle contains a single molecule of apolipoprotein-B-100 (Apo-B-100). LDL is derived from VLDL, and it serves as a carrier of cholesterol made in the liver to peripheral tissues. Cellular uptake of LDL-C depends on binding of LDL, through Apo-B, to the LDL receptor. Currently, three monogenic disorders causing autosomal dominant hypercholesterolemia (ADH) have been identified, as well as one autosomal recessive form (Table 64.1). Mutations in the LDL receptor gene (*LDLR*) are the most common among these, whereas mutations in other genes (e.g., in *APOB*, resulting in defective Apo-B and in propro-tein convertase subtilisin/kexin type 9 [*PCSK9*] encoding PCSK9 enzyme account for a minor fraction of patients presenting with ADH.

TABLE 64.1	MONOGENIC DISORDERS CAUSING ELEVATED LOW-DENSITY LIPOPROTEIN CHOLESTEROL LEVELS				
DISORDER	ESTIMATED INCIDENCE	LDL SERUM LEVELS	CLINICAL FINDINGS	GENE DEFECT	TREATMENT
Heterozygous familial hyper-cholesterolemia (HeFH)	1:500[a]	Usually >200 mg/dL; can be lower in children	Tendon xanthomata (hallmark), xanthelasma, corneal arcus	Autosomal dominant (ADH) mutations in LDL receptor gene	Dietary treatment[b]; drug treatment[c]
Homozygous familial hyper-cholesterolemia (HoFH)	1 per million	LDL >400 mg/dL (average >600 mg/dL)	Planar, tendon, and tuberous xanthomata by age 6 y; death from coronary disease as early as 10 y age; irreversible aortic valve involvement by age 10 y if untreated	Mutations in LDL receptor gene in both alleles	Dietary treatment; drug treatment when some LDL receptor activity present; LDL apheresis; liver transplantation
PCSK9 mutations	≤3% of cases with ADH[d]	Similar to HeFH	Similar to HeFH	ADH; gain of func-tion mutations	Similar to HeFH
Familial defec-tive Apo-B	≤7% of cases with ADH[d]	Similar to HeFH	Similar to HeFH	ADH; Apo-B gene mutations in LDL receptor binding domain	Similar to HeFH
Autosomal recessive hyper-cholesterolemia (ARH)	Few cases	Similar to HoFH; on average, ~100–150 mg/dL lower than HoFH	Similar to HoFH, with less aortic valve involvement and slower progression	Mutations in adaptor protein that is essen-tial, in the liver, for clathrin-mediated endocytosis of LDL	Dietary treatment; response to statin therapy

ADH, autosomal dominant hypercholesterolemia; Apo-B, apolipoprotein B; LDL, low-density lipoprotein.

[a]Can be more frequent than 1:100 in various populations because of a founder effect.

[b]Restriction of dietary saturated fat and dietary cholesterol can reduce LDL serum levels but are insufficient to achieve normal values. They have an added effect with drug therapy.

[c]Statins are the main treatment. Combination of statins with ezetimibe further lowers LDL blood levels. Combination of statins with bile acid resins also has a synergistic effect.

[d]As reported in Rahalkar AR, Hegele RA. Monogenic pediatric dyslipidemias: classification, genetics and clinical spectrum. Mol Genet Metab 2008;93:282–94.

although symptoms such as pancreatitis usually occur when TG levels are higher than 2500 mg/dL (>30 mmol/L) (40). LDL-C and HDL-C levels are often lower than normal (41). Plasma appears milky and turbid, or lipemic, because of its high TG content (39).

Genetic causes of fasting chylomicronemia include homozygous defects in one of several proteins that are involved in vascular hydrolysis of TG-containing lipoproteins. These defects in one way or another undermine the normal activity of LPL, which is the key enzyme in vascular endothelium that hydrolyzes TG-rich lipoproteins. Familial chylomicronemia is rare (1 in 10^6 people) and is most often caused by defective activity of LPL resulting from homozygous loss of function mutations in the *LPL* gene (41). Even less common causes are homozygous mutations in *APOC2* encoding Apo-C-II, which is a cofactor for the activation of LPL (41); *APOA5* encoding Apo-A-V (42), which is thought to stabilize LPL-mediated hydrolysis; *GPIHBP1* encoding glycosylphosphatidylinositol-anchored HDL-binding protein, which mediates transcytosis of LPL to the capillary surface (43); and *LMF1* encoding lipase maturation factor 1, which is

important for the proper folding and assembly of LPL (44). In the past, the diagnosis of LPL deficiency was guided by biochemical demonstration of a compromise in the lipolytic activity of postheparin plasma, but genomic DNA sequence analysis has become the current standard method for diagnosis.

Genetic Causes of Hypertriglyceridemia without Fasting Chylomicronemia

Several genetic causes of this condition are listed in Table 64.5.

Familial Combined Hyperlipidemia

The defining lipoprotein abnormalities in familial combined hyperlipidemia (FCH) are increased VLDL and LDL with depressed HDL, associated with an abnormal lipoprotein profile in at least one first-degree relative (37). This relatively common phenotype affects approximately 1 in 40 people. Patients may sometimes have xanthomata, as seen in FH (discussed earlier), and also increased CVD risk. Investigators suggested that FCH in some families is monogenic, with the causative gene purported to be

TABLE 64.5	GENETIC CAUSES OF HIGH TRIGLYCERIDES WITHOUT FASTING CHYLOMICRONEMIA				
DISORDER	ESTIMATED INCIDENCE	LIPID LEVELS	ASSOCIATED FINDINGS	GENE DEFECT	DIETARY AND OTHER THERAPY
Familial combined hyperlipidemia (hyperlipoproteinemia type 2B)	1 in 40	Total cholesterol ≤400 mg/dL; LDL cholesterol ≤320 mg/dL; TG levels ≤800 mg/dL; HDL cholesterol 30–45 mg/dL	Tendon xanthomata, xanthelasmas; early cardiovascular disease a common feature	Complex trait, cumulative susceptibility of small-effect common alleles and rare mutations of multiple genes; some monogenic forms, including *USF1* gene	Restrictions in dietary fat, reduction of high glycemic index food, cessation of alcohol; higher doses or combinations of drug treatment required to lower both LDL cholesterol and TG
Dysbetalipoproteinemia (hyperlipoproteinemia type 3)	1 in 10,000	Total cholesterol average 450 mg/dL with TG 700 mg/dL; direct measurements of LDL disproportionately low (e.g., 120 mg/dL); this LDL includes IDL particles; most TG-rich lipoproteins are β-VLDL	Palmar xanthomata, tuberous and tuberoeruptive xanthomata; premature atherosclerosis	Cumulative susceptibility of small-effect common alleles of multiple genes as above concurrent with homozygosity for *APOE* E2/E2 isoform; several mutations in the *APOE* gene can produce a dominantly inherited phenotype	Weight loss can cause remission of the overt lipoprotein disorder; high-fat meals worsen dyslipidemia; reduced-fat diet reduces chylomicron production, improving fasting lipids; control of diabetes or hypothyroidism improves the dyslipidemia
Familial hypertriglyceridemia (hyperlipoproteinemia type 4)	1 in 20	TG levels ≤800 mg/dL and HDL cholesterol levels 30–45 mg/dL; some have near normal levels	None	Complex trait, cumulative susceptibility of small-effect common alleles and rare mutations of multiple genes, including *LPL* and *APOA5*, occurring together in the same patient	Not formally studied; restrictions in dietary fat, reduction of high glycemic index food, cessation of alcohol, and avoidance of high-fat splurges expected to reduce TG levels

APO, apolipoprotein; HDL, high-density lipoprotein; IDL, intermediate-density lipoprotein; LDL, low-density lipoprotein; TG, triglyceride; VLDL, very-low-density lipoprotein.

USF1, which encodes an upstream stimulatory factor (45). However, more recent findings suggested that FCH represents a spectrum of disorders for which a range of common and rare genetic variants contributes to susceptibility (46).

Familial Dysbetalipoproteinemia (Hyperlipoproteinemia Type 3)

Dysbetalipoproteinemia has a population prevalence of approximately 1 in 10,000 (37). The main lipoprotein abnormality is an increase in TG-rich lipoprotein remnants, also known as IDLs or β-VLDLs. Affected people often have tuberous or tuberoeruptive xanthomata on the extensor surfaces of their extremities (elbows and knees), planar or palmar crease xanthomata, and increased CVD risk. People with this disorder typically are homozygous for the LDL receptor binding-defective *APOE* E2 isoform. In addition, a range of common and rare genetic variants contributes to susceptibility to this disorder (46). Disease expression often requires accompanying factors such as obesity, type 2 diabetes, or hypothyroidism. The rare disorder, HL deficiency resulting from homozygous mutations in the *LIPC* gene encoding HL, shares some clinical and biochemical features in common with familial dysbetalipoproteinemia (47).

Familial Hypertriglyceridemia

The less severe familial hypertriglyceridemia is relatively common, 1 in 20 adults, based on the definition of fasting plasma TG exceeding the 95th percentile of the population distribution (37). In contrast to the rare monogenic defects that underlie chylomicronemia syndromes, less severe hypertriglyceridemia represents a molecularly heterogeneous group of disorders. Careful study of the genomic DNA of hypertriglyceridemic patients showed a significant excess both of alleles of certain common single nucleotide polymorphisms (SNPs) and of more severe rare heterozygous mutations (46). This complex genetic architecture suggests that an individual who carries an excess of specific common and rare susceptibility variants is more likely, in the context of adverse secondary factors (e.g., obesity, poor diet, high alcohol intake, poorly controlled diabetes, and hypothyroidism), to develop common hypertriglyceridemia. Treatment includes management of secondary factors contributing to the trait together with improved diet.

LOW PLASMA LEVELS OF CHOLESTEROL OR TRIGLYCERIDES

Genetic conditions associated with low plasma TG are listed in Table 64.6.

Abetalipoproteinemia

This rare disorder is an autosomal recessive disease that results from mutations in the microsomal TG transfer protein (*MTP*) gene encoding the VLDL assembly factor, MTP. In the homozygous state, very little Apo-B in either the liver or intestine can be lipidated in the endoplasmic reticulum. The poorly folded Apo-B protein is directed to the proteasome pathway for degradation (48). Thus, few Apo-B–containing lipoproteins can be assembled and secreted, resulting in low plasma levels of chylomicrons, VLDLs, and LDLs. The patients also have failure to thrive because of fat malabsorption, which results from the failure to form chylomicrons and from deficient absorption and transport of vitamin E. The deficiency of vitamin E results in a neurologic disorder characterized by sensory loss and ataxia. Deficiency of vitamin A underlies atypical retinitis pigmentosa, whereas deficiency of vitamin D can lead to osteomalacia, rickets, and/or osteoporosis. Vitamin K deficiency underlies easy bruising and bleeding. In addition, the red blood cells in abetalipoproteinemia (ABL) have a characteristic deformity referred to as acanthocytosis, which, together with low LDL-C, is pathognomonic.

Once the diagnosis of ABL is made, these multiplex clinical problems can be arrested and ameliorated by administration of water-soluble forms of vitamin E, together with high oral doses of other fat-soluble vitamins, which are absorbed through the medium-chain TG pathway into the portal circulation. In the heterozygous state, such as obligate heterozygote parents, plasma levels of Apo-B–containing lipoproteins are essentially normal, and the spectrum of clinical features seen in homozygotes is completely absent (49).

Familial Hypobetalipoproteinemia

Familial hypobetalipoproteinemia (FHBL) most often results from mutations in the *APOB* gene encoding Apo-B. Heterozygotes have low plasma levels (lower than the 5th percentile) of either LDL-C or Apo-B. Homozygotes can have virtually absent LDL-C and Apo-B–containing lipoproteins and can manifest the same eye, bone, blood, and neurologic manifestations as patients with ABL. The main differentiating feature is that obligate heterozygote parents of a homozygous child with FHBL have half-normal LDL-C and Apo-B levels.

The most common cause of FHBL is the inheritance of a mutated *APOB* gene containing a nonsense mutation resulting in a premature stop codon, although numerous missense mutations have been reported more recently. In contrast to the *APOB* mutations in the receptor-binding domain that cause FDB, the FHBL mutations in *APOB* result in the production of carboxy-truncated forms of Apo-B that can vary in length from 2% to 89% of normal of the full length hepatically produced Apo-B-100. The intestine normally produces a shorter Apo-B isoform that arises from editing of the *APOB* mRNA, called Apo-B48, that is 48% of the hepatic protein. Depending on the position of the truncation mutation, patients have reduced production of Apo-B as well as increased clearance from the plasma of lipoproteins containing the truncated

TABLE 64.6	**LOW PLASMA LEVELS OF CHOLESTEROL OR TRIGLYCERIDES**				
DISORDER	**ESTIMATED INCIDENCE**	**LIPID LEVELS**	**ASSOCIATED FINDINGS**	**GENE DEFECT**	**DIETARY AND OTHER THERAPY**
Abetalipoproteinemia (ABL)	<120 cases described	Total cholesterol and TG <50 mg/dL	Fat malabsorption, including vitamin E, deficiency of which leads to ataxia, sensory loss, and retinitis pigmentosa; obligate heterozygotes have no biochemical or clinical phenotype	Autosomal recessive with loss of function mutations in the *MTP* gene, whose product is required for Apo-B lipoprotein assembly in intestine and liver	Fat-reduced diet or substitute medium-chain TG; vitamin E supplementation
Familial hypobetalipo-proteinemia (FHBL)	For the forms related to the *APOB* gene: homozygous form very rare; heterozygous 1:3,000; also rare are 3 other forms not linked to the *APOB* gene	Patients homozygous for truncating mutations of Apo-B have lipid levels similar to ABL; for heterozygotes and those with the non–Apo-B forms, milder (~50%–70%) reductions in plasma Apo-B or LDL-C noted	For homozygotes with Apo-B truncations, same as in ABL; some compound heterozygotes may also have less severe fat malabsorption. Hepatic steatosis may also be present in both homozygotes and heterozygotes; Obligate heterozygotes have reduced plasma LDL and Apo-B; Most heterozygotes are generally asymptomatic	For the *APOB* gene–associated forms, truncating protein mutations. For the other forms, there is 1) linkage to chromosome locus 3p21; 2) loss of function mutation of *PCSK9*; or, 3) a familial form that remains unassociated with a gene or chromosomal locus	For the homozygotes with Apo-B truncations, same as for ABL; some heterozygotes also need vitamin E supplementation and dietary fat restriction; no therapies currently recommended for the other forms
Familial combined hypolipidemia[a]	Rare (a few families for each variant)	Heterozygotes: TG <65 mg/dL, LDL-C <75 mg/dL, HDL-C normal; compound heterozygotes: TG <25 mg/dL, LDL-C <35, HDL-C <20 (based on data for patients with *ANGPTL3* mutations)	None	Nonsense mutation in *ANGPTL3*	None described

APOB, apolipoprotein-B; HDL-C, high-density lipoprotein cholesterol; LDL-C, low-density lipoprotein cholesterol; TG, triglyceride.

[a]Data from Romeo S, Yin W, Kozlitina J et al. Rare loss-of-function mutations in ANGPTL family members contribute to plasma triglyceride levels in humans. J Clin Invest 2009;119:70–9; and Musunuru K, Pirruccello JP, Do R et al. Exome sequencing, ANGPTL3 mutations, and familial combined hypolipidemia. N Engl J Med 2010;363:2220–7.

Other data from Denke MA. Nutrient and genetic regulation of lipoprotein metabolism. In: Shils ME, Shike M, Ross AC et al, eds. Modern Nutrition in Health and Disease. 10th ed. Baltimore: Lippincott Williams & Wilkins, 2006; and Schonfeld G, Lin X, Yue P. Familial hypobetalipoproteinemia: genetics and metabolism. Cell Mol Life Sci 2005;62:1372–8.

species. The defective allele exerts a negative effect on the production of Apo-B encoded by the normal allele, thus giving rise to the dominant nature of the defect.

The heterozygous state is found in 1 in 3000 individuals, and the homozygous state is exceedingly rare, probably as rare as ABL. Simple heterozygotes have low plasma total cholesterol and LDL-C as well as reduced TG levels and are usually asymptomatic, although they can have fatty liver. In contrast, compound heterozygotes or homozygotes may suffer from fat malabsorption and other

features of ABL, although even patients with the most severe forms of FHBL are usually less clinically affected than are patients with ABL (50). At least three additional non-*APOB* gene–related forms of FHBL are also recognized (see Table 64.6).

PCSK9 Deficiency

In contrast to the very high levels of LDL-C that are seen with gain of function mutations in *PCSK9*, heterozygous loss of function mutations in *PCSK9* result in increased levels of the LDL receptor and enhanced clearance of LDL particles. Heterozygotes for loss of function mutations in *PCSK9* have markedly depressed levels of LDL-C and of Apo-B, and they also have a markedly reduced lifetime risk of CAD. Only a handful of homozygotes for loss of function mutations in *PCSK9* mutations have been reported, and the main feature of these mutations is biochemical, with very low plasma but not absent LDL-C and Apo-B, without any of the multisystem manifestations of ABL or homozygous FHBL.

Familial Combined Hypolipidemia

Previous studies had linked rare loss of function mutations in angiopoietin-like proteins (ANGPTLs; particularly 3 and 4) to low plasma TG levels (51). In an exome-sequencing approach in which members of one family with inherited hypobetalipoproteinemia—but no mutations in *MTP*, *APOB*, or *PCSK9*—were analyzed, investigators found that nonsense mutations in *ANGPTL3* were associated with low plasma levels of LDL-C and TGs in simple heterozygotes and extremely low plasma levels of LDL-C, HDL-C, and TGs in compound heterozygotes (52). These patients had no other clinical features. From preclinical studies, a potential mechanism contributing to these changes was proposed to be the loss of function of ANGPTL3, an inhibitor of lipoprotein and endothelial lipases, resulting in greater remodeling of Apo-B–containing lipoproteins and HDL.

FUTURE DIRECTIONS

Most areas of human biology and medicine have been affected by the progress resulting from the human genome project and related initiatives. Lipoprotein metabolism is no exception. The field has already benefited and will continue to benefit from progress in the genomic and postgenomic research era.

Genome-Wide Association Studies

The GWASs research strategy is based on the idea that common genetic variants in the population exert subtle effects on a quantitative trait and cumulatively produce a penetrant phenotype, such as dyslipidemia. Thus, GWASs employ genome-wide SNP microarrays (or gene chips) to evaluate the association between common genetic variants from across the genome and plasma lipids or lipoproteins (37). The definitive GWAS from the Global Lipids Genetics Consortium (GLGC) reported a metaanalysis of genetic determinants of plasma lipids in more than 100,000 subjects from multiple ethnic groups and with a range of lipid and cardiovascular phenotypes (6). The GLGC analysis identified 95 loci that contribute to variation in plasma lipid and lipoprotein concentrations. About half of these loci had no prior connection

to lipid and lipoprotein metabolism. It is very likely that some of the new proteins and pathways that were identified by the GWAS approach will be new targets for therapy.

Genetic Risk Prediction of Dyslipidemia and Atherosclerosis

Early identification of subjects at risk for developing dyslipidemia could provide an opportunity for early lifestyle modification or evidence-based pharmacologic interventions capable of decreasing the prolonged burden of exposure to a suboptimal lipid profile and other risk factors. It is now becoming feasible to integrate all relevant genetic risk variants to determine a patient's overall "genetic risk score" for specific dyslipidemias and atherosclerosis (6). Genetic variables may improve risk determinations derived from existing risk prediction algorithms such as the Framingham risk score.

Next-Generation DNA Sequencing

Next-generation sequencing of whole exomes (i.e., all coding regions) or whole genomes will generate extensive new information about interindividual DNA differences. Accounting for both common and rare deleterious or protective alleles could help to assign risk for development of dyslipidemia or atherosclerosis more accurately and may help with identification of subgroups of patients who are more likely to respond to particular drug interventions. This active area of study is called pharmacogenomics. Genetic information is also included as a covariate in studies of lipoprotein responsiveness to dietary interventions in the evolving area of nutrigenomics. Tailored dietary advice, in addition to other lifestyle interventions, may one day be offered to dyslipidemic patients based on their particular genetic profile.

Challenges and Opportunities Arising from Emerging Genomic Technologies

The need for a mechanistic understanding of how the new genes found in GWASs cause deviations in plasma lipoproteins will challenge our experimental capacity, but it is essential to develop new approaches to understand gene function (functional genomics) rapidly. In addition, the potential exists for unforeseen ethical, legal, and social issues that may arise when complete human genomic information becomes part of a patient's medical record. Taking full advantage of the opportunities that have arisen through the discoveries from genetic studies will require analogous technologic advances allowing high-throughput, reliable, and robust functional validation at all stages: in vitro, in vivo in nonhuman species and humans, and, ultimately, clinical trials of diet and other therapies.

REFERENCES

1. Iqbal R, Anand S, Ounpuu S et al. Circulation 2008;118:1929–37.
2. Ahrens EH Jr, Insull W Jr, Blomstrand R et al. Lancet 1957; 272:943–53.
3. Hegsted DM, McGandy RB, Myers ML et al. Am J Clin Nutr 1965;17:281–95.
4. Anderson JT, Grande F, Keys A. Am J Clin Nutr 1976;29:1184–9.
5. Hegsted DM, Kritchevsky D. Am J Clin Nutr 1997;65:1893–6.
6. Teslovich TM, Musunuru K, Smith AV et al. Nature 2010; 466:707–13.
7. Varret M, Abifadel M, Rabes JP et al. Clin Genet 2008; 73:1–13.
8. Cohen H, Shamir R. Lipid disorders in children and adolescents. In: Lifshitz F, ed. Pediatric Endocrinology. London: Informa Healthcare, 2006:279–90.
9. Durrington P. Lancet 2003;362:717–31.
10. Rahalkar AR, Hegele RA. Mol Genet Metab 2008;93:282–94.
11. Daniels SR, Greer FR. Pediatrics 2008;122:198–208.
12. Lambert G. Curr Opin Lipidol 2007;18:304–9.
13. Cohen JC, Boerwinkle E, Mosley TH Jr et al. N Engl J Med 2006;354:1264–72.
14. Innerarity TL, Weisgraber KH, Arnold KS et al. Proc Natl Acad Sci U S A 1987;84:6919–23.
15. Defesche JC, Pricker KL, Hayden MR et al. Arch Intern Med 1993;153:2349–56.
16. Garcia CK, Wilund K, Arca M et al. Science 2001;292:1394–8.
17. Soutar AK. IUBMB Life 2010;62:125–31.
18. Weissglas-Volkov D, Pajukanta P. J Lipid Res 2010;51:2032–57.
19. Lewis GF, Rader DJ. Circ Res 2005;96:1221–32.
20. Kastelein JJ, van Leuven SI, Burgess L et al. N Engl J Med 2007; 356:1620–30.
21. Matsuura F, Wang N, Chen W et al. H J Clin Invest 2006;116: 1435–42.
22. Rayner KJ, Suarez Y, Davalos A et al. Science 2010;328:1570–3.
23. Franceschini G, Werba JP, D'Acquarica AL et al. Clin Pharmacol Ther 1995;57:434–40.
24. McPherson R, Frohlich J, Fodor G et al. Can J Cardiol 2006; 22:913–27.
25. Assmann G, von Eckardstein A, Brewer HB. Familial analphalipoproteinemia: Tangier disease. In: Scriver CR, Beaudet AL, Sly Ws et al, eds. The Metabolic and Molecular Bases of Inherited Disease. 8th ed. New York: McGraw-Hill, 2001:2937–60.
26. Bodzioch M, Orso E, Klucken J et al. Nat Genet 1999;22:347–51.
27. Brooks-Wilson A, Marcil M, Clee SM et al. Nat Genet 1999;22:336–45.
28. Rust S, Rosier M, Funke H et al. Nat Genet 1999;22:352–5.
29. Vedhachalam C, Duong PT, Nickel M et al. J Biol Chem 2007; 282:25123–30.
30. Nofer JR, Remaley AT. Cell Mol Life Sci 2005;62:2150–60.
31. Fredrickson DS. J Clin Invest 1964;43:228–36.
32. Serfaty-Lacrosniere C, Civeira F, Lanzberg A et al. Atherosclerosis 1994;107:85–98.
33. Soumian S, Albrecht C, Davies AH et al. Vasc Med 2005; 10:109–19.
34. Kuivenhoven JA, Pritchard H, Hill J et al. J Lipid Res 1997; 38:191–205.
35. Gigante M, Ranieri E, Cerullo G et al. J Nephrol 2006;19: 375–81.
36. von Eckardstein A. Atherosclerosis 2006;186:231–9.
37. Hegele RA. Nat Rev Genet 2009;10:109–21.
38. Stroes ES, Nierman MC, Meulenberg JJ et al. Arterioscler Thromb Vasc Biol 2008;28:2303–4.
39. Yuan G, Al-Shali KZ, Hegele RA. CMAJ 2007;176:1113–20.
40. Brunzell JD, Bierman EL. Med Clin North Am 1982;66: 455–68.
41. Fojo SS, Brewer HB. J Intern Med 1992;231:669–77.
42. Talmud PJ. Atherosclerosis 2007;194:287–92.
43. Beigneux AP, Franssen R, Bensadoun A et al. Arterioscler Thromb Vasc Biol 2009;29:956–62.
44. Peterfy M, Ben-Zeev O, Mao HZ et al. Nat Genet 2007;39: 1483–7.
45. Lee JC, Lusis AJ, Pajukanta P. Curr Opin Nat Genet 2010; 42:684–7.
47. Connelly PW, Hegele RA. Crit Rev Clin Lab Sci 1998;35:547–72.
48. Fisher EA, Ginsberg HN. J Biol Chem 2002;277:17377–80.
49. Kane JP, Havel RJ. Disorders of the biogenesis and secretion of lipoproteins containing the B apolipoproteins. In: Scriver CR, Beaudet AL, Sly WE, Valle DS, eds. The Metabolic and Molecular Basis of Inherited Disease, 8th ed. New York: McGraw-Hill, 1995:1860–66.
50. Schonfeld G, Lin X, Yue P. Cell Mol Life Sci 2005;62:1372–8.
51. Romeo S, Yin W, Kozlitina J et al. J Clin Invest 2009;119:70–9.
52. Musunuru K, Pirruccello JP, Do R et al. N Engl J Med 2010;363:2220–7.

SUGGESTED READINGS

Hegele R. Plasma lipoproteins: genetic influences and clinical implications. Nat Rev Genet 2009;10:109–21.

Johansen CT, Wang J, Lanktree MB et al. Excess of rare variants in genes identified by genome-wide association study of hypertriglyceridemia. Nat Genet 2010;42:684–7.

Rahalkar AR, Hegele RA. Monogenic pediatric dyslipidemias: classification, genetics and clinical spectrum. Mol Genet Metab 2008;93: 282–94.

Schonfeld G, Lin X, Yue P. Familial hypobetalipoproteinemia: genetics and metabolism. Cell Mol Life Sci 2005;62:1372–8.

Teslovich TM, Musunuru K, Smith AV et al. Biological, clinical and population relevance of 95 loci for blood lipids. Nature 2010;466: 707–13.

NUTRITION IN THE PREVENTION OF CORONARY HEART DISEASE AND THE MANAGEMENT OF LIPOPROTEIN DISORDERS[1]

ERNST J. SCHAEFER

Coronary heart disease (CHD) is a leading cause of death and disability in Western societies. Both increased plasma low-density lipoprotein (LDL) cholesterol (LDL-C; >160 mg/dL or 4.2 mmol/L) and decreased high-density lipoprotein (HDL) cholesterol (HDL-C; <40 mg/dL or 1.0 mmol/L), along with aging, elevated systolic blood pressure (>140 mm Hg), cigarette smoking, and diabetes (fasting glucose >125 mg/dL), have all been defined as independent risk factors for CHD. CHD is caused by atherosclerosis, a process in which the coronary arteries as well as other arteries become occluded.

The characteristics of this process in the artery wall are the presence of cholesterol-laden macrophages or foam cells, proliferation of smooth muscle cells with excess connective tissue, calcification, and sometimes thrombosis as the terminal event occluding the artery. A heart attack or myocardial infarction (MI) occurs when one or more of the three major coronary arteries becomes blocked (1). A stroke occurs when one or more of the arteries supplying the brain becomes occluded. CHD and stroke together are known as cardiovascular disease (CVD), which accounts for about half of all mortality in developed societies including the United States.

Aging, high blood pressure, diabetes, and smoking can all damage the lining of the artery wall. Moreover, LDLs can be deposited in the artery wall, especially at sites of damage. Therefore high levels of LDL-C (>160 mg/dL or 4.2 mmol/L) associated with high total cholesterol values (>240 mg/dL or 6.2 mmol/L) are a significant risk factor for CHD. In addition, HDLs serve to remove cholesterol from the artery wall. Low levels of HDL-C (<40 mg/dL or 1.0 mmol/L) are a significant CHD risk factor (2). Diets high in animal fat, dairy products, eggs, sugar, and salt have been associated with excess obesity, elevated blood cholesterol, and high age-adjusted CHD mortality rates (1). Family history of premature CHD and age are also significant risk factors for CHD (2, 3).

NATIONAL GUIDELINES

United States Dietary Guidelines

Every 5 years, the federal government updates dietary guidelines for the United States. In the 2010 version (4), the following four initial recommendations were made with the goal of preventing chronic disease and promoting health:

1. Prevent or reduce overweight or obesity through improved eating and physical activity behaviors.
2. Control total calorie intake to manage body weight. For people who are overweight or obese, this will mean fewer calories from foods and beverages.
3. Increase physical activity and reduce time spent in sedentary behaviors.
4. Maintain appropriate calorie balance during each stage of life: childhood, adolescence, adulthood, pregnancy and breast-feeding, and older age.

---

[1]**Abbreviations: Apo,** apolipoprotein; **ATP,** Adult Treatment Panel; **CETP,** cholesterol ester transfer protein; **CHD,** coronary heart disease; **CRP,** C-reactive protein; **CVD,** cardiovascular disease; **DHA,** docosahexaenoic acid; **EPA,** eicosapentaenoic acid; **HDL,** high-density lipoprotein; **HDL-C,** high-density lipoprotein cholesterol; **IVUS,** intravascular ultrasound; **JELIS,** Japan Eicosapentaenoic Acid Lipid Intervention Study; **LCAT,** lecithin:cholesterol acyltransferase; **LDL,** low-density lipoprotein; **LDL-C,** low-density lipoprotein cholesterol; **Lp(a),** lipoprotein(a); **LPL,** lipoprotein lipase; **MI,** myocardial infarction; **MTP,** microsomal transfer protein; **NCEP,** National Cholesterol Education Program; **NHLBI,** National Heart, Lung, and Blood Institute; **TLC,** therapeutic lifestyle change; **VLDL,** very-low-density lipoprotein.

Dietary guidelines for the general population focus on building long-term eating patterns that promote health maintenance. The guidelines include specific recommendations, which include the following: balancing caloric intake and physical activity to reduce overweight and obesity; restricting sodium to less than 2300 mg/day; reducing saturated fat to less than 10% of calories, with replacement by monounsaturated and polyunsaturated fats, and limiting cholesterol to less than 300 mg/day; restricting intakes of *trans*-fats, solid fats, sugars, refined grains, and sugars; and limiting consumption of alcohol (no more than one drink per day in women and no more than two drinks per day in men). In those with LDL-C levels higher than 160 mg/dL after ruling out secondary causes, further restriction of saturated fat to less than 7% of calories and cholesterol to less than 200 mg/day is recommended. Additionally, specific foods or food groups to increase or decrease are also recommended for the general population (Table 65.1). Additional guidelines for special groups including pregnant and lactating women and persons more than 50 years old have also been established.

Guidelines of the National Cholesterol Education Program

The National Heart, Lung, and Blood Institute (NHLBI) launched the National Cholesterol Education Program (NCEP) in 1985, with the goal of reducing CHD deaths in the United States by reducing the percentage of US residents with high blood cholesterol levels. The NCEP released three sets of guidelines for treatment of adults, referred to as Adult Treatment Panel (ATP) guidelines, in 1988 (ATP I), 1994 (ATP II), and 2001 (ATP III), with an optional update in 2004 (2, 3). Newer guidelines are expected in 2012. The NCEP recommends that lipids be measured on several occasions after an overnight fast to assess total cholesterol, triglycerides, HDL-C, and calculated LDL-C. Calculated LDL-C is equivalent to total cholesterol minus HDL-C minus triglycerides divided by 5, provided the subject is fasting and triglyceride values are less than 400 mg/dL) (5).

The following values have been classified as optimal with regard to CHD risk:

1. Total cholesterol lower than 200 mg/dL
2. Triglycerides lower than 150 mg/dL

TABLE 65.1	SUMMARY OF UNITED STATES DIETARY GUIDELINES, 2010, RELEVANT TO ATHEROSCLEROSIS PREVENTION IN THE GENERAL POPULATION

I. Recommendations to prevent chronic disease and promote health
1. Prevent or reduce overweight or obesity through improved eating and physical activity behaviors.
2. Control total calorie intake to manage body weight. For people who are overweight or obese, this will mean fewer calories from foods and beverages.
3. Increase physical activity and reduce time spent in sedentary behaviors.
4. Maintain appropriate calorie balance during each stage of life: childhood, adolescence, adulthood, pregnancy and breast-feeding, and older age.

II. Foods to decrease
1. Reduce daily sodium intake to less than 2,300 mg, and further reduce intake to 1,500 mg in those who are 51 years old and older and those of any age who are African-American or have hypertension, diabetes, or chronic kidney disease. The 1,500-mg recommendation applies to about half of the US population, including children, and the majority of adults.
2. Consume less than 10% of calories from saturated fat by replacing them with monounsaturated and polyunsaturated fatty acids.
3. Consume less than 300 mg/day of dietary cholesterol.
4. Keep *trans*-fatty acid consumption as low as possible by limiting foods that contain synthetic sources of *trans*-fats, such as partially hydrogenated oils, and by further limiting solid fats.
5. Reduce the intake of calories from solid fats and sugars.
6. Limit the consumption of foods that contain refined grains, especially grain foods that contain solid fats, added sugars, and sodium.
7. If alcohol is consumed, it should be consumed in moderation—up to one drink per day in women and two drinks per day in men—and only by adults of legal drinking age.

III. Foods to increase
1. Increase vegetable and fruit intake.
2. Eat a variety of vegetables, especially dark green and red and orange vegetables, and beans and peas.
3. Increase intake of fat-free or low-fat milk and milk products, such as milk, yogurt, cheese, or fortified soy beverages.
4. Choose a variety of protein foods, which include seafood, lean meat, and poultry, eggs, beans and peas, soy products, and unsalted nuts and seeds.
5. Increase the amount and variety of seafood consumed by choosing seafood in place of some meat and poultry.
6. Replace protein foods that are higher in solid fats with choices that are lower in solid fats and calories and/or are sources of oils.
7. Use oils to replace solid fats where possible.
8. Choose foods that provide more potassium, fiber, calcium, and vitamin D, which are nutrients of concern in US diets. These foods include vegetables, fruits, whole grains, and milk and milk products.

Data from US Department of Agriculture. Dietary Guidelines for Americans 2010. Available at: www.dietaryguidelines.gov. Accessed June 15, 2012, with permission.

3. Non–HDL-C lower than 130 mg/dL
4. LDL-C lower than 100 mg/dL
5. HDL-C higher than 50 mg/dL

The following values have been classified as abnormal and are associated with increased CHD risk:

1. Total cholesterol higher than 240 mg/dL
2. Triglycerides higher than 150 mg/dL
3. Non–HDL-C (total cholesterol − HDL-C) higher than 190 mg/dL
4. LDL-C higher than 160 mg/dL
5. HDL-C lower than 40 mg/dL in men and lower than 50 mg/dL in women

Before therapy is initiated, secondary causes of lipid abnormalities should be excluded. These causes include the following: diabetes mellitus, hypothyroidism, liver disease, and renal failure; and the use of drugs that increase LDL-C or decrease HDL-C (progestins, anabolic steroids, and corticosteroids). In addition, in patients without CHD or diabetes, the 10-year risk of developing CHD should be calculated using the point system shown in Tables 65.2 and 65.3 or by accessing the NHLBI website (6). Using the website is more accurate because it treats variables continuously rather than with intervals. The point system separates subjects by gender, and then the 10-year risk of developing CHD is estimated from age, total cholesterol, smoking status, HDL-C, and systolic blood pressure.

The ATP III established the following categories of risk and LDL-C goals of therapy in 2001, and these recommendations were modified in 2004 (2, 3), as follows:

High risk: High risk has been defined as having CHD, including a history of MI, unstable or stable angina, coronary artery angioplasty or bypass surgery, or evidence of myocardial ischemia, or having a CHD risk equivalent based on evidence of peripheral vascular disease, abdominal aortic aneurysm, carotid artery disease, stroke, transient ischemic attacks, diabetes, or two or more CHD risk factors and a 10-year risk of hard CHD end points of more than 20% based on the Framingham risk assessment (see Tables 65.2 and 65.3). CHD risk factors have been defined by ATP III as cigarette smoking, hypertension (blood pressure >140/90 mm Hg or the use of antihypertensive medication), low HDL-C (<40 mg/dL), family history of premature heart disease (CHD in a male first-degree relative <55 years old, CHD in a female first-degree relative <65 years old), and age (men >45 years old, women >55 years old). In high-risk patients as defined earlier, the current NCEP ATP III LDL-C goal is less than 100 mg/dL, with an optional goal of less than 70 mg/dL, using both dietary therapy and medications as treatments (2, 3).
Moderately high risk: In subjects with two or more CHD risk factors as listed earlier and a 10-year risk

of hard CHD end points of 10% to 20% based on the Framingham risk score (see Tables 65.2 and 65.3), the current NCEP ATP III LDL-C goal is less than 130 mg/dL using both dietary and drug therapy (2, 3).
Moderate risk: In subjects with two or more CHD risk factors as listed earlier and a 10-year risk of hard CHD end points of less than 10% based on the Framingham risk score (see Tables 65.2 and 65.3), the current NCEP ATP III LDL-C goal is less than 130 mg/dL using both dietary and drug therapy (2, 3).
Low risk: In subjects with one or no CHD risk factors as listed earlier and a 10-year risk of hard CHD end points of less than 10% based on the Framingham risk score (see Tables 65.2 and 65.3), the current NCEP ATP III LDL-C goal is less than 160 mg/dL using both dietary and drug therapy (2, 3).

Risk Assessment Methods

As previously mentioned, the Framingham risk assessment score is recommended by NCEP ATP III. Risk can be calculated electronically by accessing the NHLBI website (6) or by using the point system provided in the guidelines and found in Tables 65.2 and 65.3 (2). An alternative is the Reynolds Risk Score, which incorporates the same risk factors as the Framingham score and also includes family history of CHD before age 60 years and levels of C-reactive protein (CRP). This score can be accessed at the Reynolds Risk Score website (7), and it is based on two large population studies (8, 9). Another option used by some physicians is to assess the cardiac calcium score, a 30-second test performed using computed tomography (10). This test provides clear information about the presence of calcified plaque in the coronary arteries; the cardiac calcium score is the most powerful available CHD risk factor (10). Most physicians do not actually calculate risk assessment by these methods, but they often use their own clinical judgment about whether any form of therapy (lifestyle and medication) is indicated. This approach often causes physicians to overtreat low-risk patients and undertreat high-risk patients.

Therapeutic Lifestyle Changes Diet

The cornerstone of therapy to help patients achieve their LDL-C goal remains lifestyle modification. For the general population, the NCEP recommended a diet containing less than 10% of calories as saturated fat and less than 300 mg/day of dietary cholesterol (2). For those with elevated total cholesterol levels (especially >240 mg/dL with an LDL-C value >160 mg/dL), greater change is needed, and the recommended therapeutic lifestyle changes (TLC) of the NCEP ATP III are more stringent, as listed in Table 65.4. If after 6 weeks of dietary modification the LDL-C goal has not been achieved, ATP III recommended the addition of stanol or sterol margarine (two servings per day) and/or viscous fiber.

between 1959 and 1965, whereas between 1965 and 1971, the hospitals were crossed over, with hospital N subjects receiving the usual Finnish diet and hospital K receiving the experimental diet. The goal was to replace the dairy and butter fat in the usual Finnish diet with skimmed milk "filled" with soybean oil instead of full-fat milk and replacing butter with margarine high in soybean oil in the experimental diet (38–40). Both diets contained about 2800 calories, with approximately 110 g of fat (35% of calories). However, the usual Finnish diet contained about 19% of calories as saturated fat and about 4.5% as polyunsaturated fat, with 480 mg of cholesterol per day. For the experimental diet, these parameters were about 9% saturated fat and 14% polyunsaturated fat, with 280 mg of cholesterol per day, respectively. In subsets of individuals, the fatty acid content of adipose tissue for linoleic acid and myristic acid was measured and determined to be about 10% and 4.3% of total fatty acids on the usual diet and about 30% and 1.5% of total fatty acids on the experimental diet, respectively.

Mean CHD mortality rates were significantly ($p = .002$) lower by 53% on the experimental diet than on the usual diet. For hospital K, these rates were 50.6% lower on the experimental diet versus the usual Finnish diet, whereas for hospital K, these rates were 56.1% lower. Blood cholesterol levels were also significantly lower by 12% for hospital K (236 versus 268 mg/dL) and by 19% for hospital N (216 versus 267 mg/dL) on the experimental diet than on the usual diet (38–40). Similar effects were observed in women, with a 34% mean reduction in CHD mortality rates in favor of the experimental diet group, but these differences did not reach statistical significance, in part because of substantially lower event rates in women overall as compared with men of similar ages (40).

Minnesota Mental Hospital Study. In this open-label randomized study, 9057 men and women of all ages at six mental hospitals and one nursing home in Minnesota were placed on diets containing about 40% fat, but differing in polyunsaturated fat content (5% versus 15%), saturated fat (18% versus 9%), and dietary cholesterol (466 versus 166 mg/day) (41). The treatment group had 14% lower serum cholesterol levels, but no significant difference was noted in CHD morbidity or mortality among the groups (41). This negative result may have resulted from the relatively normal mean serum cholesterol of the study population (207 mg/dL at baseline), the relatively young age of the study population in which the largest single age group was less than 30 years, or the relatively short duration of the test diets (mean, 384 days) (41). The shorter duration of the study resulted from discharges from the mental hospital in part because of the introduction of the medication chlorpromazine (Thorazine).

Lyon Diet Heart Trial. This trial was a secondary prevention study in 605 men and women who had a prior MI. Study subjects were randomized to a usual French diet or a more "Mediterranean diet" in which all subjects also received 2 servings per day of a specially prepared margarine high in α-linolenic acid (42). After a 44-month average follow-up, the diet group had a 76% decrease in cardiac deaths (with 6 deaths in the treatment group versus 19 deaths in the control group; $p < .01$) (42). The benefit in this trial was related to increases in levels of plasma α-linolenic acid (42).

Women's Health Initiative. The largest dietary intervention trial to have ever been conducted using dietary modification instead of supplements was the Women's Health Initiative trial. In this trial, 48,835 postmenopausal women aged 50 to 79 years were randomly allocated to a diet low in fat (40% of total or 19,541) versus their usual diet (60% of total or 29,294). All subjects in the control group received a copy of *Dietary Guidelines for Americans*. The dietary intervention was implemented by holding group classes and individual interview sessions that included dietary assessments using food frequency questionnaires (43). The goals of the intervention were to decrease total fat intake to 20% of calories and to increase the intake of vegetables and fruits to 5 servings per day and grains to 6 servings per day (43).

The investigators reported that the subjects in the active dietary arm of the study, at 6 years of follow-up, had a total fat intake of 28.8% of calories (versus 37.0% in the control group), saturated fat intake of 9.5% (versus 12.4% in the control group), monounsaturated fat intake of 10.8% (versus 14.2% in the control group), and polyunsaturated fat intake of 6.1% (versus 7.5% in the control group) (44). They had increased their vegetable and fruit intake by 1.1 servings per day and their grain intake by 0.5 servings per day (44). One of the confounding features of the study was that of those participating in the active dietary arm, 8052 women also participated in the hormone replacement arm of the Women's Health Initiative, and 5017 participated in the calcium and vitamin D arm of this study (44).

The primary aim of the study was to ascertain whether a low-fat diet would reduce the risk of breast cancer. Over 8.1 years of follow-up, 0.42% women per year developed breast cancer in the diet group versus 0.45% per year in the control group (45). Therefore, subjects in the active diet group lowered their risk of developing invasive breast cancer by 9% (hazards ratio, 0.91; confidence interval, 0.83 to 1.01; $p = .07$) (45). The investigators also assessed the impact of the dietary intervention on CVD (44).

After 8.1 years of follow-up, the risk of CHD was reduced 3% (hazards ratio, 0.97; confidence interval, 0.90 to 1.06), and the risk of stroke was increased by 2% (hazards ratio, 1.02; confidence interval, 0.90 to 1.15) (44). The dietary intervention also had no significant impact on risk of colorectal cancer or the development of diabetes (46, 47). The diet group did significantly ($p < .05$) reduce LDL-C by 3.55 mg/dL, lower systolic blood pressure by 0.31 mm Hg, and reduce factor VIIC by 4.29%, as compared with the control group (44). However, in a subgroup analysis of those women who achieved less than 6.1% of calories as saturated fat, the risk of CHD was reduced

19% (hazards ratio, 0.81; confidence interval, 0.69 to 0.95; $p < .01$) (44). Such differences were also observed in those subjects in the diet group who had the lowest *trans*-fatty acid intake (hazards ratio, 0.81; confidence interval, 0.69 to 0.95) (44).

Dietary Intervention Studies Using Omega-3 Fatty Acid Supplements

Diet Atherosclerosis and Reinfarction Trials. The Diet Atherosclerosis and Reinfarction Trials (DART) in the United Kingdom in more than 2000 patients with established CHD documented beneficial effects of fish consumption or the use of 2 fish oil capsules per day in reducing CHD death by 29% (48). However, this finding was not confirmed in a follow-up study, possibly because of much greater aspirin use in the second study (49).

Gruppo Italiano per lo Studio della Sopravvivenza nell'Infarto miocardico-Prevenzione. In Gruppo Italiano per lo Studio della Sopravvivenza nell'Infarto miocardico-Prevenzione (GISSI-Prevenzione), a large Italian study of 11,323 patients who had a history of MI, the use of 1 g/day of concentrated fish oil (containing 465 mg of eicosapentaenoic acid [EPA] and 375 mg of docasahexaenoic acid [DHA]) was associated with a reduction in overall recurrence of CHD as well as a very striking 53% reduction in sudden death in the first 4 months after MI in those persons receiving the active supplement versus the control group (50, 51). This product is now marketed in the United States as a triglyceride-lowering agent known as Lovaza, given at 4 g/day, and it often lowers triglycerides significantly ($\leq$50% or more) in combination with statin therapy in patients with triglyceride levels higher than 500 mg/dL (52).

Japan Eicosapentaenoic Acid Lipid Intervention Study. The Japan Eicosapentaenoic Acid Lipid Intervention Study (JELIS) was a study in which 15,000 male and female subjects without CHD and 3645 subjects with CHD between 40 and 75 years of age, with total cholesterol levels greater than 250 mg/dL, were all placed on statin and then randomized to receive EPA 1800 mg/day group or no additional treatment. The primary end point was a major cardiovascular event (sudden death, fatal or nonfatal MI, unstable angina, angioplasty, or coronary artery bypass surgery). After 4.6 years of follow-up, the rate of events was 19% lower in the EPA group ($p = .011$) (53). No differences were noted in sudden death rates between the groups. In patients with earlier CHD, events were also reduced 19% by EPA versus no treatment ($p = .048$), whereas in patients with a history of earlier MI, the event risk was reduced with EPA by 27% ($p = .033$) (54). No effect on stroke risk was noted, except in subjects with an earlier stroke, in whom the use of EPA resulted in a 20% relative risk reduction in recurrent stroke ($p < .05$) (55).

In the overall JELIS study, the most striking benefit was noted in those subjects with triglyceride levels higher than 150 mg/dL and HDL-C levels lower than 40 mg/dL, in whom the use of EPA reduced CHD events by 53% ($p = .043$) (56). The use of EPA also reduced CHD risk by 22% ($p < .05$) in subjects with impaired glucose tolerance (fasting glucose >110 mg/dL) (57). EPA use was not associated with any significant effects on lipid levels; however, its use was associated with marked increases in plasma EPA, and study subjects with levels greater than 150 µg/mL had the lowest risk in the trial (58).

Alpha Omega Trial. A more recent study of 4837 patients after MI who were randomized to placebo margarine, margarine containing 2 g of α-linolenic acid, margarine containing a total of 400 mg of combined EPA and DHA, or margarine containing the combination of these fatty acids was carried out over 40 months (59). No significant effects were noted on CVD end points. However, this study may have been underpowered, and the dose of omega-3 fatty acids given may have been too low.

Conclusions from Dietary Interventions Trials

The overall data from the dietary intervention studies support the concept of decreasing saturated fat to less than 7% of calories and dietary cholesterol to less than 200 mg/day and increasing polyunsaturated fatty acids to more than 10% of calories (ideally ~12%), as well as increasing the intake of fish, fish oil, or the omega-3 fatty acids, especially EPA. In the Women's Health Initiative, the women in the control group were consuming 14% of calories as monounsaturated fat, 12.5% as saturated fat, and 7.5% of calories as polyunsaturated fat. Benefit was noted when saturated fat intake was reduced to less than 6.1% of calories (44). However, in the most successful dietary intervention studies such as the Finnish Mental Hospital Study, saturated fat was replaced by polyunsaturated fat and not by carbohydrate (38–40). Therefore, if the women in the Women's Health Initiative had been instructed to increase their intake of polyunsaturated fatty acids from vegetable oil such as soybean oil or canola oil significantly, it is possible they would have had a much greater benefit in terms of CHD risk reduction (44).

The ideal diet for CHD risk reduction may well be one containing less than 7% of calories as saturated fat and less than 200 mg of cholesterol per day, with about 10% to 15% of calories from monounsaturated fat and about 10% to 15% of calories as polyunsaturated fat from vegetable oils such as soybean or canola oil, along with three or more servings of oily fish per week or two fish oil capsules per day. Under controlled conditions such diets will lower LDL-C by 15% or more, associated with enhanced LDL-Apo-B fractional catabolism. With the addition of almost daily servings of fish, triglyceride levels are also lowered, associated with decreased very-low-density lipoprotein (VLDL) Apo-B production (1). Large, randomized, placebo-controlled trials have not shown any significant benefit in terms of CHD risk reduction associated with the use of vitamin E, vitamin C, a mixture of antioxidant vitamins, the potent antioxidant probucol or analogs, or the combination of folate and vitamins B_6 and B_{12} (60–64).

5. Friedewald WT, Levy RI, Fredrickson DS. Clin Chem 1972; 18:499–502.

6. National Heart, Lung, and Blood Institute. Third Report of the Expert Panel on Detection, Evaluation, and Treatment of High Blood Cholesterol in Adults (Adult Treatment Panel III). Available at: http://www.nhlbi.nih.gov/guidelines/cholesterol. Accessed June 15, 2012.

7. Reynolds Risk Score. Available at: http://www.reynoldsriskscore.org. Accessed June 15, 2012.

8. Ridker PM, Buring JE, Rifai N et al. JAMA 2007;297:611–19.

9. Ridker PM, Paynter NP, Rifai N et al. Circulation;2008:2243–51.

10. Budoff MJ Shaw LJ, Lou ST et al. J Am Coll Cardiol 2007; 49:1860–70.

11. Schaefer EJ, Lichtenstein AH, Lamon-Fava S et al. Arterioscler Thromb Vasc Biol 1995;15:1079–85.

12. Schaefer EJ, Lichtenstein AH, Lamon-Fava S et al. Am J Clin Nutr 1996;63:234–41.

13. Lichtenstein AH, Ausman LM, Jalbert SM et al. J Lipid Res 2002;43:264–73.

14. Lichtenstein AH, Ausman LM, Carrasco W et al. Atheroscler Thromb 1994;14:168–75.

15. Lichtenstein AH, Ausman LM, Jalbert SM et al. N Engl J Med 1999;340:1933–40.

16. Hegsted DM, Ausman LM, Johnson JA et al. Am J Clin Nutr 1993;57:875–83.

17. Mensink RP, Katan MB. Arterioscler Thromb 1992;12:911–19.

18. Yu S, Derr J, Etherton TD et al. Am J Clin Nutr 1995;61: 1129–39.

19. Schaefer EJ, Lamon-Fava S, Ausman LM et al. Am J Clin Nutr 1997;65:823–30.

20. Li Z, Otvos JD, Lamon-Fava S et al. J Nutr 2003;133:3428–33.

21. Lopez-Miranda J, Ordovas JM, Mata P et al. J Lipid Res 1994;35:1965–75.

22. Talati R, Sobieraj DM, Makanji SS et al. J Am Diet Assoc 2010;110:719–26.

23. Olson BH, Anderson SM, Becker MP et al. J Nutr 1997; 127:1973–80.

24. Stanhope Kl, Schwartz JM, Keim NL et al. J Clin Invest 2009;119:1322–34.

25. Keys A. Circulation 1970;41:1162–75.

26. Kato H, Tillotson J, Nichaman JZ et al. Am J Epidemiol 1973;97:372–83.

27. Stamler J. Population studies. In: Levy RI, Dennis BR, Ernst N eds. Nutrition, Lipids, and Coronary Heart Disease. New York: Raven Press, 1979:25–88.

28. Schaefer EJ, Augustin JL, Schaefer MM et al. Am J Clin Nutr 2000;71:746–51.

29. Yusuf S, Hawken S, Ounpuu S et al. Lancet 2004;364:937–52.

30. Leren P. Acta Med Scand 1966;466:1–92.

31. Leren P. Circulation 1970;42:935–42.

32. Hjermann I, Velve Byre K et al. Lancet 1981;2:1303–10.

33. Hjermann I, Holme I, Leren P. Am J Med 1986;80:7–11.

34. Dayton S, Pearce ML, Goldman H et al. Lancet 1968;2:1060–2.

35. Dayton S, Pearce ML, Hashimoto S. Circulation 1969; 34(Suppl II):1–63.

36. Pearce ML, Dayton S. Lancet 1971;1:464–7.

37. Sturdevant RA, Pearce ML, Dayton S. N Engl J Med 1973; 288:24–7.

38. Turpeinen O. Circulation 1979;59:1–7.

39. Turpeinen O, Karvonen MJ, Pekkarinen M et al. Int J Epidemiol 1979;8:99–118.

40. Miettinen M, Turpeinen O, Karvonen MJ et al. Int J Epidemiol 1983;12:7–25.

41. Frantz ID Jr, Dawson EA, Ashman PL et al. Arteriosclerosis 1989;9:129–35.

42. de Lorgeril M, Salen P, Martin JL et al. Circulation 1999; 99:779–85.

43. Patterson RE, Kristal AR, Tinker LF et al. Ann Epidemiol 1999;9:178–87.

44. Howard BV, Van Horn L, Hsia J et al. JAMA 2006;295:655–66.

45. Prentice RL, Chlebowski RT, Patterson R et al. JAMA 2006; 295:629–42.

46. Beresford SM, Johnson KC, Ritterberg C et al. JAMA 2006; 295:643–54.

47. Tinker LF, Bonds DE, Margolis KL et al. Arch Intern Med 2008;168:1500–11.

48. Burr ML, Gilbert JF, Holliday RM et al. Lancet 1989;2:757–61.

49. Burr ML. Proc Nutr Soc 2007;66:9–15.

50. GISSI Prevenzione Investigators. Lancet 1999;354:447–55.

51. Marchioli R, Barzi F, Bomba E et al. Circulation 2002; 105:1897–903.

52. Davidson MH, Stein EA, Bays HE et al. Clin Ther 2007; 29:1354–67.

53. Yokoyama M, Origasa H, Matzuzaki M et al. Lancet 2007; 370:1090–8.

54. Matsuzaki M, Yokoyama M, Saito Y et al. Circ J 2009; 73:1283–90.

55. Tanaka K, Ishikawa Y, Yokoyama M et al. Stroke 2008; 39:2052–58.

56. Saito Y, Yokoyama M, Origasa H et al. Atherosclerosis 2008; 200:135–40.

57. Oikawa S, Yokoyama M, Origasa H et al. Atherosclerosis 2009;206:535–9.

58. Itakura H, Yokoyama M, Matsuzaki M et al. J Atheroscler Thromb 2011;18:99–107.

59. Kromhout D, Giltay EJ, Geleijnse JM. N Engl J Med 2010;363:2015–26.

60. Bleys J, Miller ER 3rd, Pastor-Barriuso R et al. Am J Clin Nutr 2006;84:880–7.

61. Mead A, Atkinson G, Albin D et al. J Hum Nutr Diet 2006; 19:401–19.

62. Tardif JC, McMurray JJ, Klug E et al. Lancet 2008;371:1761–8.

63. Study of the Effectiveness of Additional Reductions in Cholesterol and Homocysteine (SEARCH) Collaborative Group, Armitage JM, Bowman L et al. JAMA 2010;303: 2486–94.

64. Clarke R, Halsey J, Lewington S et al. Arch Intern Med 2010;170:1622–31.

65. Cholesterol Treatment Trialists (CTT) Collaborators, Baigent C, Blackwell L et al Lancet 2005;366:1267–78.

66. Cholesterol Treatment Trialists' (CTT) Collaborators, Baigent C, Blackwell L et al. Lancet 2010;376:1670–81.

67. Ridker PM, Danielson E, Fonseca FA et al. N Engl J Med 2008;359:2195–207.

68. Ridker PM, Danielson E, Fonseca FA et al. Lancet 2009; 373:1175–82.

69. Nicholls SJ, Tuzcu EM, Sipahi I et al. JAMA 2007;297:499–508.

70. Nicholls SJ, Ballantyne CM, Barter P et al. N Engl J Med 2011;365:2078–87.

71. Niemi M, Pasanen MK, Neuvonen PJ. Pharmacol Rev 2011; 63:157–81.

72. Akao H, Polisecki E, Kajinami K et al. Atherosclerosis 2012; 220:413–7.

73. SEARCH Collaborative Group. N Engl J Med 2008;359: 789–99.

74. Voora D, Shah SH, Spasojevic I et al. J Am Coll Cardiol 2009;54:1609–16.

75. Sattar NJ, Davis BR, Pressel SL, at al. Lancet 2010;375:735–42.

76. Culver AL, Ockene JS, Balasubramanian R et al. Arch Intern Med 2012;172:144–52.

77. Thongtang N, Ai M, Otokozawa S et al. Am J Cardiol 2011; 107:387–92.

78. Cholesterol Treatment Trialists' (CTT) Collaborators, Kearney PM, Blackwell L et al. Lancet 2008;371:117–25.

79. Lamon-Fava S, Diffenderfer MR, Barrett PH et al. J Lipid Res 2007;48:1746–53.

80. Asztalos BF, LeMaulf F, Dallal GE et al. Am J Cardiol 2007;99:681–85.

81. Asztalos BF, Cupples LA, Demissie S et al. Arterioscler Thromb Vasc Biol 2004;24:2181.

82. Staels B, Dallongeville J, Auwerx J et al. Circulation 1998; 98:2088–93.

83. Schaefer EJ, Lamon-Fava S, Cole T et al. Atherosclerosis 1996;127:113–22.

84. Asztalos BF, Collins D, Horvath KV et al. Metabolism 2008; 57:77–83.

85. Saku K, Gartside PS, Hynd BA et al. J Clin Invest 1985; 75:1702–12.

86. Watts GF, Barrett PH, Ji J et al. Diabetes 2003;52:803–11.

87. Millar JS, Dufy D, Gadi R et al. Arterioscler Thromb Vasc Biol 2009;29:140–46.

88. Manninen V, Elo O, Frick HH et al. JAMA 1988;260:641–51.

89. Robins SJ, Collins D, Wittes JT et al. JAMA 2001;285: 1585–91.

90. Rubins HB, Robins SJ, Collins D et al. Arch Intern Med 2002;162:2597–604.

91. DAIS Investigators. Lancet 2001;357:1890–95.

92. Keech AC, Simes RJ, Barter P et al. Lancet 2005;366: 1849–61.

93. Keech AC, Mitchell P, Summanen PA et al. Lancet 2007; 370:1687–97.

94. Rajamani K, Colman PG, Li LP et al. Lancet 2009;373: 1780–88.

95. ACCORD Study Group, Ginsberg HN, Elam MB et al. N Engl J Med 2010;362:1563–74.

96. Tonkin AM, Chen L. Circulation 2010;122:850–52.

97. Lamon-Fava S, Diffenderfer MR, Barrett PHR et al. Arterioscler Thromb Vasc Biol 2008;28:1672–8.

98. Canner PL, Berge KG, Wenger NK et al. J Am Coll Cardiol 1986;8:1245–55.

99. Berge KG, Canner PL. Eur J Clin Pharm 1991;40(Suppl 1): S49–51.

100. Canner PL, Furberg CD, Terrin ML et al. Am J Cardiol 2005;95:254–7.

101. Canner PL, Furberg CD, McGovern ME. Am J Cardiol 2006; 97:477–9.

102. Brown GB, Zhao XQ, Chait A et al. N Engl J Med 2001; 345:1583–92.

103. Asztalos BF, Batista M, Horvath KV et al. Arterioscler Thromb Vasc Biol 2003;23:847–52.

104. AIM-HIGH Investigators, Boden WE, Probstfield JL et al. N Engl J Med 2011;365:2255–67.

105. Treatment of HDL to Reduce the Incidence of Vascular Events (HPS2-THRIVE). Available at: http://www.clinicaltrials.gov. Accessed June 15, 2012.

106. Altmann SW, Davis HR Jr, Zhu LJ et al. Science 2004; 303:1201–4.

107. Davis HR Jr, Basso F, Hoos LM et al. Atheroscler Suppl 2008; 9:77–81.

108. Sudhop T, Lutjohann D, Kodal A et al. Circulation 2002; 106:1943–8.

109. Pearson TA, Ballantyne CM, Veltri E et al. Am J Cardiol 2009; 103:369–74.

110. Lipid Clinics Coronary Primary Prevention Trial results. JAMA 1984;251:365–74.

111. Fonseca VA, Rosenstock J, Wang K et al. Diabetes Care 2008; 31:1479–84.

112. Genest JJ, Martin-Munley S, McNamara JR et al. Circulation 1992;85:2025–33.

113. van Himbergen T, Otokozawa S, Matthan NR et al. Arterioscler Thromb Vasc Biol 2010;30:1113–20.

114. Lamon-Fava S, Marcovina SM, Albers JJ et al. J Lipid Res 2011;52:1181–7.

115. Schaefer EJ, Santos RD, Asztalos BF. Curr Opin Lipidol 2010;21:289–97.

116. Spady DK, Kearney DM, Hobbs HH. J Lipid Res 1999; 40:1384–94.

SUGGESTED READINGS

Davidson MH, Stein EA, Bays HE et al. Combination prescription omega 3 fatty acids with simvastatin (COMBOS). Clin Ther 2007;29:1354–67.

Expert Panel. Executive summary of the third report of the National Cholesterol Education Program (NCEP) Expert Panel on Detection, Evaluation, and Treatment of High Blood Cholesterol in Adults (Adult Treatment Panel III). JAMA 2001;285:2486–97.

Howard BV, Van Horn L, Hsia J et al. Low-fat dietary pattern and risk of cardiovascular disease. JAMA 2006;295:655–66.

Marchioli R, Barzi F, Bomba E et al. Early protection against sudden death by n-3 polyunsaturated fatty acids after myocardial infarction: time course analysis of the results of the Gruppo Italiano per lo Studio della Sopravvienza nell' infarto Miocardico (GISSI)–Prevenzione. Circulation 2002;105:1897–903.

Mead A, Atkinson G, Albin D et al. Dietetic guidelines on food and nutrition in the secondary prevention of cardiovascular disease: evidence from systematic reviews of randomized controlled trials (second update, January 2006). J Hum Nutr Diet 2006;19:401–19.

Schaefer EJ. Lipoproteins, nutrition, and heart disease. Am J Clin Nutr 2002;75:191–212.

the setting of either the DASH diet (32) or a high dietary potassium intake.

Observational studies have examined the relationship of sodium intake with CV outcomes. Substantial methodologic issues, often related to accuracy of sodium measurement, have made it methodologically challenging to find direct evidence of a relationship between sodium intake and CV disease (40). Despite these challenges, a metaanalysis of prospective observational studies found an association between higher sodium intake and increased risk of stroke and CV disease (41). Still, other studies (42, 43) have documented paradoxic findings, likely related to methodologic issues, especially given consistent findings of benefit in the few available trials with clinical outcomes (36, 44, 45).

To date, three moderate-sized trials have examined the effects of a reduced sodium intake on clinical CV events (36, 44, 45). Two of these trials tested reduced-sodium lifestyle interventions, and one trial looked at the effects of a reduced-sodium/high-potassium salt substitute. Each trial found a 21% to 41% reduction (significant in two studies [44, 45]) in clinical CV disease events among the persons who received the intervention. Consequently, direct evidence from trials, although limited, corroborates the benefits of sodium reduction on BP.

A reduced sodium intake could have other health benefits. Potential benefits include a reduced risk of subclinical CV disease (i.e., left ventricular [LV] hypertrophy, ventricular fibrosis, and diastolic dysfunction), kidney damage, gastric cancer, and disordered mineral metabolism (i.e., increased urinary calcium excretion, potentially leading to osteoporosis) (46). In particular, LV mass is directly associated with sodium intake in cross-sectional studies, and one small trial in the early 1990s documented that sodium reduction can reduce LV mass (47). A reduced sodium intake has been associated with reduced risk of heart failure (48). However, in patients with advanced heart failure, abrupt sodium reduction, especially in the setting of high-dose diuretic therapy, may be harmful (49).

In addition to the many benefits of a reduced sodium intake, there is no convincing or consistent evidence of harm. Although some sodium intake is necessary, there is no evidence that insufficient sodium intake is a public health concern. Extreme sodium reduction (<20 mmol/day) could potentially cause adverse effects on blood lipids and insulin resistance; however, moderate sodium reduction has no such effects (30, 50). A reduced sodium intake may increase plasma renin activity (PRA), as does the DASH diet (51). However, the clinical relevance of a modest increase in PRA remains unclear. In fact, thiazide diuretics, a class of antihypertensive drug therapies that raises PRA, reduce CV disease risk (52).

The 2005 and 2010 Dietary Guidelines for Americans, as well as numerous other organizations, recommend a population-wide reduction in sodium intake. Current dietary guidelines recommend no more than 2300 mg/day of sodium for the general population and no more than 1500 mg/day for blacks, middle-aged and older persons, and individuals with hypertension, diabetes, or chronic kidney disease (CKD); combined, these groups represent nearly half of all US adults. Because such a large portion of the population falls under the latter recommendation level, the American Heart Association set 1500 mg (65 mmol) of sodium as the recommended upper limit of daily intake for all the US population (53). Survey data indicate that most children and adults vastly exceed this recommended amount.

In summary, existing data strongly support the current, population-wide recommendations to decrease sodium intake, both by choosing foods with low sodium levels and by limiting the amount of sodium added to food. However, because more than 75% of sodium consumption comes from processed foods (54), any meaningful approach to reducing sodium intake must involve food manufacturers and restaurants. Professional organizations have recommended that the food industry should progressively cut the amount of sodium added to foods in half over the next 10 years (55). Because these voluntary recommendations have failed to yield meaningful reductions in sodium intake, an Institute of Medicine report has recommended a national approach, implemented through the Food and Drug Administration, to achieve population-wide reductions in sodium intake (56).

Increased Potassium Intake

Another dietary factor that lowers BP is high potassium intake. Evidence of this relationship has been documented in animal studies, observational studies, clinical trials, and meta-analyses of these trials. Although data from individual trials have had inconsistent findings, three meta-analyses each found a significant inverse relationship between potassium intake and BP in hypertensive patients and equivocal effects in nonhypertensive individuals (57). A 1997 meta-analysis found that a net increase in urinary potassium excretion of 2 g/day (50 mmol/day) was associated with average SBP/DBP reductions of 4.4/2.5 mm Hg in hypertensive individuals and 1.8/1.0 mm Hg in nonhypertensive individuals (58). Increased potassium intake has beneficial effects on BP regardless of absolute potassium intake level, with benefits noted in both a low-potassium intake setting (e.g., 1.3 to 1.4 g/day, or 35 to 40 mmol/day) and a much higher intake setting (e.g., 3.3 g/day, or 84 mmol/day) (59). Increased potassium intake lowers BP to a greater extent in blacks compared with whites and therefore should be a valuable tool to reduce health disparities related to elevated BP and its complications.

The best way to increase potassium intake is to consume foods that are rich in potassium, such as fruits and vegetables. In the DASH trial, the two groups that increased fruit and vegetable consumption, and thereby increased potassium intake, both lowered BP (32, 60). The DASH diet provides roughly 4.7 g/day (120 mmol/day) of potassium. Another trial documented that increased fruit and vegetable intake lowers BP, but it did not specify the amount of potassium that was consumed (61).

Potassium and sodium interact such that the effects of potassium on BP depend on the concurrent intake of sodium and vice versa. Specifically, a reduced sodium intake has greater BP-lowering effects when potassium intake is low and has lesser BP-reducing effects when potassium intake is high. In addition, increased potassium intake has greater BP-lowering effects when sodium intake is high and has lesser BP-reducing effects when sodium intake is low. For example, in one trial, a high potassium intake (120 mmol/day) diminished the pressor response to increased sodium consumption in nonhypertensive black men and, to a lesser extent, in nonblacks (Fig. 66.5) (62).

The lack of dose-response studies precludes a firm recommendation for a specific potassium intake level to reduce BP, although an Institute of Medicine committee set a recommended intake of 4.7 g/day (120 mmol/day) (63). This level is similar to the average total potassium intake in clinical trials, the highest dose in the one available dose-response trial, and the potassium content of the DASH diet (60).

Among healthy individuals with normal kidney function, a potassium intake from foods that is greater than 4.7 g/day (120 mmol/day) does not pose a risk because excess potassium is readily excreted. However, in individuals whose urinary potassium excretion is impaired, such as by drugs or medical conditions, an intake less than 4.7 g/day (120 mmol/day) is advised because of the risk of adverse cardiac effects (dysrhythmias) from hyperkalemia.

Angiotensin-converting enzyme inhibitors, angiotensin receptor blockers, nonsteroidal anti-inflammatory drugs, and potassium-sparing diuretics are drugs that may impair potassium excretion. Impaired renal excretion of potassium is associated with certain medical conditions, such as diabetes, CKD, end stage renal disease, severe heart failure, and adrenal insufficiency. In addition, elderly individuals are at increased risk of hyperkalemia. Although CKD may impair renal excretion of potassium, available evidence is insufficient to identify the level of kidney function below which hyperkalemia will result from a high dietary intake of potassium. Because of this uncertainty, an expert panel set a wide range of recommended potassium intake (2000 to 4000 mg/day) in patients with advanced (stage 3 or 4) CKD (64).

Moderation of Alcohol Consumption

A direct, dose-response relationship between alcohol consumption and BP has been documented through observational and experimental studies, especially in the setting of more than two alcoholic drinks per day (65). This relationship is independent of potential confounders such as age, obesity, and sodium intake (66). Although some studies have shown that the alcohol–BP relationship also extends into the "light drinking" range of two or fewer drinks per day, this is the range in which alcohol may reduce the risk of CHD.

A meta-analysis of 15 randomized trials reported that reduced alcohol consumption (median self-reported alcohol intake reduction of 76%; range, 16% to 100%) lowered BP by 3.3/2.0 mm Hg (65). BP reductions appeared to be dose dependent, and the magnitude of the reductions was similar in nonhypertensive and hypertensive individuals.

Overall, available evidence supports moderation of alcohol intake (among those who drink) as an effective approach to lower BP. The general consensus is that alcohol consumption should be limited to no more than two alcoholic drinks per day in men and to no more than one alcoholic drink per day in women and lighter-weight persons. One drink is defined as 12 oz of regular beer, 5 oz of wine (12% alcohol), or 1.5 oz of 80 proof distilled spirits.

Dietary Patterns

Vegetarian Diets

Certain dietary patterns, particularly vegetarian diets, have been associated with low BP. Vegetarians have strikingly lower BP than nonvegetarians in industrialized countries, where elevated BP is widespread. Strict vegetarians residing in Massachusetts have some of the lowest BP levels observed in the industrialized world. Individuals who consume a vegetarian diet may also experience a slower, age-related rise in BP.

Several aspects of a vegetarian lifestyle could potentially affect BP, including nondietary factors (e.g., physical activity), established dietary risk factors (e.g., sodium,

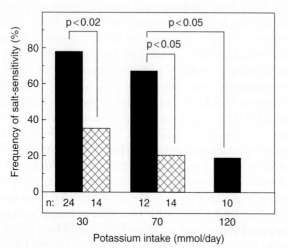

Fig. 66.5. Prevalence of sodium sensitivity in normotensive individuals (blacks, *solid bars;* whites, *cross-hatched bars*) at three levels of potassium intake. Sodium sensitivity is defined by a sodium-induced increase in mean arterial pressure of at least 3 mm Hg. (Reprinted with permission from Morris RC Jr, Sebastian A, Forman A et al. Normotensive salt sensitivity: effects of race and dietary potassium. Hypertension 1999;33:18–23.)

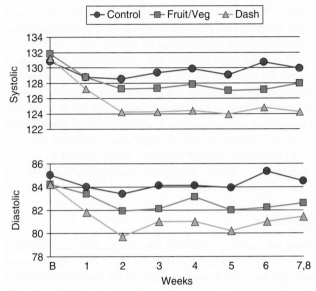

Fig. 66.6. Blood pressure by week during the Dietary Approaches to Stop Hypertension (DASH) feeding study in three diets (control diet, fruits and vegetables diet, and the DASH diet.) (Adapted with permission from Appel LJ, Moore TJ, Obarzanek E et al. A clinical trial of the effects of dietary patterns on blood pressure: DASH Collaborative Research Group. N Engl J Med 1997;336:1117.)

potassium, weight, alcohol), and other aspects of a vegetarian diet (e.g., high fiber, no meat). To a limited extent, observational studies have controlled for the well-established dietary determinants of BP. In two clinical trials, one in nonhypertensive persons (67) and another in hypertensive individuals (68), lacto-ovovegetarian diets reduced SBP by about 5 mm Hg but had equivocal effects on DBP.

Dietary Approaches to Stop Hypertension Diet

In the DASH trial, participants were randomized to one of three diets, and the effects of each diet on BP were studied (60). The most effective diet, now termed the *DASH diet*, emphasized fruits, vegetables, and low-fat dairy products; it included whole grains, poultry, fish and nuts; and it was reduced in fats, red meat, sweets, and sugar-containing beverages. It was rich in potassium, magnesium, calcium, and fiber, and it was low in total fat, saturated fat, and cholesterol; it was also slightly increased in protein. Participants following the DASH diet significantly reduced their BP by a mean of 5.5/3.0 mm Hg compared with the control group. The reductions in BP resulting from the diets occurred rapidly, taking 2 weeks or less to manifest (Fig. 66.6).

In subgroup analyses (60), the DASH diet significantly lowered BP in all major subgroups (men, women, African-Americans, non–African-Americans, hypertensive persons, and nonhypertensive individuals). However, the effects of the DASH diet in the African-American participants were most striking, with average BP reductions of 6.9/3.7 mm Hg. These observed reductions were significantly larger than the corresponding reductions in white

participants (3.3/2.4 mm Hg). The beneficial effects of the DASH diet in hypertensive individuals (BP reductions of 11.6/5.3 mm Hg) have obvious clinical significance, and the corresponding effects in nonhypertensive individuals (3.5/2.2 mm Hg) have major public health implications (see Fig. 66.1). The DASH-Sodium trial (described earlier) (32) documented that the DASH diet significantly lowered BP at each of three sodium levels (see Fig. 66.4), with the combination of the DASH diet and the lowest sodium intake yielding the greatest reductions in BP.

A third trial, OmniHeart, examined whether altering macronutrient intake could also improve the DASH diet and its BP-lowering effects (12). This feeding study tested three variants of the DASH diets: a first diet rich in carbohydrate (58% of total calories), a second diet rich in protein (about half from plant sources), and a third diet rich in unsaturated fat (predominantly monounsaturated fat). Each diet was similar to the original DASH diet in that each was reduced in saturated fat, cholesterol, and sodium and rich in fruit, vegetables, fiber, and potassium at recommended levels. Although all three OmniHeart diets lowered SBP (Fig. 66.7), substituting some of the carbohydrate (~10% of total kcal) with either protein or unsaturated fat further lowered BP.

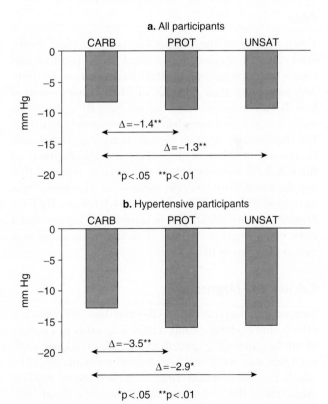

Fig. 66.7. Effects of three healthy dietary patterns tested in the OmniHeart feeding study on systolic blood pressure (CARB, similar to the DASH diet; PROT, rich in protein, about half from plant sources; and UNSAT, rich in monounsaturated fat) in all participants **(A)** and in hypertensive participants **(B)**. (Reprinted with permission from Appel LJ, Brands MW, Daniels SR et al. Dietary approaches to prevent and treat hypertension: a scientific statement from the American Heart Association. Hypertension 2006;47:296–308.)

There has been a great deal of conjecture about those components of DASH-style diets that may be responsible for the BP-lowering effects. The diet high in fruits and vegetables resulted in BP reductions that were nearly half of the total effect of the DASH diet (see Fig. 66.6). Fruits and vegetables are rich in many nutrients, including potassium, magnesium, and fiber. Of these nutrients, evidence on the BP-lowering effects of potassium is most persuasive, particularly in hypertensive individuals and African-Americans. Because the fruits and vegetables diet accounted for approximately half of the BP-lowering effects of the DASH diet, some other component of the DASH diet must be responsible for further reducing BP. Compared with the fruits and vegetables diet, the DASH diet provided more vegetables, low-fat dairy products, and fish while containing less red meat, sugar, and refined carbohydrates.

The DASH diet is considered safe and appropriate for the general population. However, it is not recommended for persons with advanced CKD because of its relatively high potassium, phosphorus, and protein content (64).

DIETARY FACTORS WITH LIMITED OR UNCERTAIN EFFECTS

Fiber

Fiber consists of the indigestible parts of plant foods. Observational studies and several trials provide evidence that increased fiber intake may decrease BP (69). Although more than 40 trials of fiber supplementation have been conducted, most did not have BP as their primary outcome, and many had a multicomponent intervention. Additionally, findings from these trials are obfuscated by the use of different definitions and classifications of fiber. A 2005 meta-analysis of the 24 trials reported that supplemental fiber (average increase of 11.5 g/day) was associated with a net BP reduction of 1.1/1.3 mm Hg (70). Overall, data are insufficient to recommend supplemental fiber or an increased intake of dietary fiber alone as a means of lowering BP.

Calcium and Magnesium

Increased dietary calcium intake may have BP-reducing effects, and evidence of this relationship exists in a variety of studies, including animal studies, observational studies, trials, and meta-analyses. A 1995 meta-analysis (71), which examined results from 23 observational studies, documented this inverse association between dietary calcium intake and BP. However, the effect size was relatively small, and there was evidence of publication bias and heterogeneity across studies. Meta-analyses of randomized trials of calcium supplementation (400 to 2000 mg/day) noted modest reductions in SBP of 0.9 to 1.9 mm Hg and DBP of 0.2 to 1.0 mm Hg (72–75). There is speculation that the level of dietary calcium intake may affect the presser response to sodium, as evidenced by a few small trials showing that calcium supplementation mitigated the effects of high sodium intake on BP.

The evidence implicating magnesium intake as a major determinant of BP is inconclusive. Many observational studies, often cross-sectional, have found an inverse association between dietary magnesium intake and BP. However, a meta-analysis of 20 randomized trials found no clear effect of increased magnesium intake on BP (76).

In summary, current evidence is insufficient to recommend either calcium or magnesium supplementation as a means to reduce BP.

Fat Intake

Total fat includes saturated fat, omega-3 polyunsaturated fat, omega-6 polyunsaturated fat, and monounsaturated fat. Although early studies focused on the effects of total fat intake on BP, there is a plausible biologic basis to hypothesize that certain types of fat (e.g., omega-3 polyunsaturated fat) may lower BP, whereas other types of fat (e.g., saturated fat) may raise it.

Omega-3 Polyunsaturated Fat

Several small trials and metaanalyses of these trials (77) have found evidence that high-dose, omega-3 polyunsaturated fatty acid (commonly termed *fish oil*) supplements can lower BP in hypertensive individuals. In nonhypertensive individuals, BP reductions resulting from fish oil supplements tend to be small or nonsignificant. The effect appears to be dose dependent, with BP reductions occurring at relatively high doses of fish oil, namely, 3 g/day or more. In hypertensive individuals, average SBP/DBP reductions were 4.0/2.5 mm Hg (78). Because of side effects, such as a fishy taste and belching, and the high dose required to lower BP, fish oil supplements cannot be routinely recommended as a means to lower BP.

Saturated Fat

The effect of saturated fat on BP in adults has been examined in several observational studies and a few clinical trials (79). In most of these trials and the two prospective observational studies, the Nurses' Health Study and the Health Professionals Follow-up Study, saturated fat intake was not associated with onset of hypertension (80, 81). In the few available trials, diet interventions that focused on lowering saturated fat intake did not affect BP (79). Because most trials tested diets that concurrently reduced saturated fat and increased polyunsaturated fat, the lack of a BP effect also suggests no benefit from polyunsaturated fat. In a large randomized controlled trial, healthy infants who received a reduced saturated fat dietary intervention had significantly reduced SBP and DBP, each by 1 mm Hg lower than control, over 7 months to 15 years of age (82). These findings of an early effect of reduced saturated fat intake on BP suggest that dietary saturated fat intake may be useful in preventing hypertension.

Omega-6 Polyunsaturated Fat

Dietary intake of omega-6 polyunsaturated fat (mostly linoleic acid in Western diets) has been shown to have little or no effect on BP (79). An overview of cross-sectional studies that correlated BP with tissue or blood levels of omega-6 polyunsaturated fat found no apparent relationship. Prospective observational studies and clinical trials have been equally unsupportive.

Monounsaturated Fat

Although early trials did not support an association between monounsaturated fat intake and BP, subsequent trials found that diets rich in monounsaturated fats modestly lower BP (83). However, an increase in monounsaturated fat is often linked to a reduction in carbohydrate consumption, potentially with a change in the type of carbohydrate as well (84). Therefore, it remains unclear whether the effects of increased monounsaturated fat intake reflect an increase in this nutrient and/or a decrease in carbohydrate intake or change in the type of carbohydrate.

Carbohydrate

Both the amount and type of carbohydrate consumed may affect BP, but the existing evidence is inconclusive. Globally, many populations that consume carbohydrate-rich, low-fat diets have lower BP levels than do Western countries (85). Still, the findings of observational studies have been inconsistent (86). Increasing carbohydrate intake by decreasing total fat typically did not reduce BP in small early trials. In contrast, the OmniHeart feeding trial documented that partial exchange of carbohydrate with monounsaturated fat or protein (roughly half from plant sources) lowers BP (12). (Figure 66.7)

Although uncertain, more recent evidence shows promise of a link between increased intake of added sugars and elevated BP. Studies include animal studies in which rats were fed high doses of fructose, acute ingestion studies in which humans were fed high doses of different sugars, and more recently, epidemiologic studies. In cross-sectional studies, drinking more sugar-sweetened beverages was associated with elevated BP in adolescents (87). In prospective observational studies, consumption of more than one soft drink per day significantly increased the odds of developing high BP (88). In another cohort study, intake of sugar-sweetened beverages and artificially sweetened beverages was directly associated with risk of hypertension; the effects appeared unrelated to fructose intake (89). In post hoc analyses of a completed trial, there was a direct relationship between reductions in sugar-sweetened beverage intake and reductions in BP (90). Nonetheless, randomized trials in humans have found inconsistent results (91). In a meta-analysis of trials that isocalorically substituted fructose for other sugars, a 1.5 mm Hg net reduction in DBP and no effect on SBP were reported (92). Overall, further research is necessary before recommendations

can be made about modifying the amount and type of carbohydrate intake as a means to lower BP.

Cholesterol

To date, few studies have examined the effects of dietary cholesterol on BP. In observational analyses of the Multiple Risk Factor Intervention Trial, there were significant, positive associations between cholesterol intake and both SBP and DBP. In longitudinal analyses from the Chicago Western Electric Study, there were significant direct relationships of change in SBP over 8 years with dietary cholesterol, as well as the Keys score (86). Despite these findings, the dearth of evidence precludes any firm recommendations regarding dietary cholesterol as a way to reduce BP.

Protein

Evidence from numerous observational studies has consistently documented an inverse association between protein intake (93), especially protein from plants, and BP. Two major observational studies, the International Study on Macronutrients and Blood Pressure (INTERMAP) and the Chicago Western Electric Study, noted significant inverse relationships between protein intake and BP (86, 93). In both these studies, diets higher in protein from plant sources were associated with lower BP, whereas diets higher in protein from animal sources had no significant effect on BP.

In contrast to the vast evidence from observational studies, few trials have tested the effects of increased protein intake on BP. Two trials found that increased protein intake from soy supplements can reduce BP. In one trial of individuals taking antihypertensive agents (94), supplemental soy protein (total of 25% kcal protein, half from soy) reduced average 24-hour BP by 5.9/2.6 mm Hg. In a large trial conducted in the People's Republic of China (95), supplemental soy protein, which increased total protein intake from 12% to 16% kcal, lowered average BP by 4.3/2.7 mm Hg, net of a supplemental carbohydrate control group. Overall, clinical trials and observational studies support the hypothesis that an increased intake of protein from plant sources can lower BP, although further evidence is needed before recommendations can be made.

Vitamin C

Laboratory, observational, and depletion-repletion studies suggest that increased vitamin C intake and higher vitamin C levels are associated with lower BP. A 1997 systematic review noted that that most cross-sectional studies reported an inverse association between plasma vitamin C levels and BP (96). A large number of randomized trials, often with small samples or methodologic limitations, tested whether vitamin C supplements lower

BP. In a meta-analysis of 29 controlled trials, vitamin C supplementation lowered SBP/DBP by 3.8/1.5 mm Hg (97). Still, because of poor quality of many trials, it remains unclear whether an increased intake or supplementation of diet with vitamin C lowers BP.

GENE–DIET INTERACTIONS

An emerging body of evidence indicates that genetic factors affect BP levels and the BP response to dietary modifications. Most of the existing research has focused on genetic factors that influence the BP response to dietary sodium intake. Several genotypes that affect BP have been identified, most of which influence the renin-angiotensin-aldosterone axis or renal sodium handling. A line of research focusing on Mendelian diseases related to either high or low BP has identified six genes associated with higher BP and eight genes associated with lower BP (98). Of considerable importance is the fact that each of these genes regulates renal sodium handling, and mutations in these genes increase or decrease net sodium chloride reabsorption, resulting in raised or reduced BP, respectively.

A few trials have examined the interactive effects of dietary modifications for individuals with specific genotypes on changes in BP. In trials, genetic variation of the angiotensinogen gene modified the BP response to weight change (99), to changes in sodium intake in whites (33, 99), and to the DASH diet (100). Polymorphism of the α-adducin gene also appears to affect the BP response to sodium chloride (101). Finally, the angiotensin-converting enzyme insertion/deletion (ACE I/D) polymorphism may also affect the BP response to weight change (102).

EFFECTS OF MULTIPLE DIETARY CHANGES

Despite the potential for large BP reductions from implementing several concurrent dietary modifications, few trials have examined the total BP effects of multicomponent interventions. In general, multicomponent intervention trials have shown subadditivity, meaning the BP reductions of interventions with two or more dietary changes are less than the sum of BP reductions from separate interventions implementing each component alone. Despite subadditivity, the BP-lowering effects of multicomponent interventions are often sizeable and clinically relevant. One small but well-controlled trial tested the effects of a comprehensive program of supervised exercise with provision of prepared DASH-style meals to accomplish weight loss and sodium reduction among medication-treated hypertensive adults (103). The diet and exercise program greatly reduced daytime ambulatory BP by 12.1/6.6 mm Hg, net of control. Subsequently, a behavioral intervention trial, PREMIER, also tested the effects of these recommended lifestyle modifications (weight loss, sodium reduction, increased physical activity, and the DASH diet) (104).

In nonhypertensive individuals, mean BP reductions were 9.2/5.8 mm Hg (3.1/2.0 mm Hg, net of control). In hypertensive individuals, none of whom were taking medication, corresponding BP reductions were 14.2/7.4 mm Hg (6.3/3.6 mm Hg, net of control).

SPECIAL POPULATIONS

Children

The problem of elevated BP manifests early in life, perhaps in utero, and many observational studies have noted that childhood BP levels are associated with BP levels in adulthood (105). Therefore, strategies to reduce BP in children and lessen the age-related rise in BP seem prudent, even though there is limited evidence from clinical trials. The evidence that BP levels and the prevalence of obesity in children and adolescents have increased between National Health and Nutrition Examination Surveys (NHANES) conducted in 1988 to 1994 and 1999 to 2000 further emphasizes the importance of efforts to lower BP in children (21). A meta-analysis of trials in children, in which reduced dietary sodium interventions lowered BP, highlights the value of sodium intake reduction in children (106). In addition, observational studies have found that children in the United States have BP levels that exceed BP levels of middle-aged adults in populations exposed to a low-sodium diet (14).

Aside from these few studies, research on the effects of dietary elements on BP in children is sparse and has methodologic limitations, including small sample size, suboptimal BP measurements, and minimal dietary contrast (107). Consequently, the effects of diet on BP in children and adolescents are extrapolated from studies conducted in adults. Such extrapolations are reasonable because of the chronic nature of elevated BP that results from the insidious rise in BP throughout childhood and adulthood.

Older Persons

Dietary modifications to lower BP should be particularly beneficial as adults age. The age-related rise in BP is especially noticeable in middle-aged and older persons, and the incidence of BP-related CV disease is markedly high in older persons. Although most diet trials examined the effects on BP in middle-aged persons, several were conducted in older individuals (25, 108) whereas others presented results stratified by age. Several important findings have emerged. First, the evidence that older persons can implement and maintain dietary changes, specifically dietary sodium reduction and weight loss, is extraordinarily consistent. Second, the BP reduction from dietary changes is greater in older persons than in middle-aged individuals (34, 35). Third, because of high attributable risk related to elevated BP in elderly persons, the benefits of dietary modifications on BP should reduce CV disease risk considerably.

African-Americans

African-Americans, on average, have higher BP and are at greater risk of BP-related complications, especially stroke and kidney disease, than are whites. As reported previously, in rigorously controlled efficacy trials, African-Americans achieve greater BP reductions than whites from several nonpharmacologic therapies, particularly decreased sodium intake, increased potassium intake, and the DASH diet (see earlier). The potential benefits of interventions targeting these dietary changes are augmented because survey data indicate that, on average, African-Americans consume higher levels of sodium and lower levels of potassium than do whites (63). Given these dietary trends, healthy dietary modifications could lead to substantial benefits that may provide a means to reduce racial disparities in BP and its CV and renal complications (109).

CONCLUSION

A compelling body of evidence supports the concept that several dietary factors affect BP. Dietary changes known to lower BP effectively are weight loss, reduced sodium intake, increased potassium intake, moderation of alcohol intake (among those who drink), and DASH-style dietary patterns. Although other dietary elements may also affect BP, existing evidence is inconclusive, and/or their effects are small.

Given the direct, progressive relationship of BP with clinical outcomes, strategies to lower BP in both nonhypertensive and hypertensive individuals are warranted. Such efforts will require individuals to make behavioral modifications and society to make substantial environmental changes that facilitate rather than impede desirable behavioral modification by individuals.

REFERENCES

1. Kearney PM, Whelton M, Reynolds K et al. Lancet 2005;365:217–23.
2. Lawes CM, Vander Hoorn S, Rodgers A et al. Lancet 2008; 371:1513–8.
3. World Health Organization. Global Health Risks: Mortality and Burden of Disease Attributable to Selected Major Risks. Geneva: World Health Organization Press, 2009.
4. Centers for Disease Control and Prevention. MMWR Morb Mortal Wkly Rep 2011;60:103–8.
5. Egan BM, Zhao Y, Axon RN. JAMA 2010;303:2043–50.
6. Intersalt Cooperative Research Group. BMJ 1988;297:319–28.
7. Vasan RS, Beiser A, Seshadri S et al. JAMA 2002;287:1003–10.
8. Chobanian AV, Bakris GL, Black HR et al. Hypertension 2003;42:1206–52.
9. Lewington S, Clarke R, Qizilbash N et al. Lancet 2002;360: 1903–13.
10. Stamler J, Stamler R, Neaton JD. Arch Intern Med 1993;153: 598–615.
11. Vasan RS, Larson MG, Leip EP et al. N Engl J Med 2001;345:1291–7.
12. Appel LJ, Sacks FM, Carey VJ et al. JAMA 2005;294:2455–64.
13. Stamler J. Hypertension 1991;17:I16–20.
14. Appel LJ. J Clin Hypertens (Greenwich) 2008;10:7–11.
15. Appel LJ. Hypertension: A Companion to Braunwald's Heart Disease 1st ed. Philadelphia: Saunders, 2007:202–12.
16. Sacks FM, Campos H. N Engl J Med 2010;362:2102–12.
17. Appel LJ, Brands MW, Daniels SR et al. Hypertension 2006;47:296–308.
18. Appel LJ, Giles TD, Black HR et al. J Am Soc Hypertens 2010;4:79–89.
19. Flegal KM, Carroll MD, Kit BK et al. JAMA 2012;307:491–7.
20. Ogden CL, Carroll MD, Kit BK et al. JAMA 2012;307: 483–90.
21. Muntner P, He J, Cutler JA et al. JAMA 2004;291:2107–13.
22. Neter JE, Stam BE, Kok FJ et al. Hypertension 2003;42: 878–84.
23. Stevens VJ, Obarzanek E, Cook NR et al. Ann Intern Med 2001;134:1–11.
24. Trials of Hypertension Prevention Collaborative Research Group. Arch Intern Med 1997;157:657–67.
25. Whelton PK, Appel LJ, Espeland MA et al. JAMA 1998; 279:839–46.
26. Knowler WC, Barrett-Connor E, Fowler SE et al. N Engl J Med 2002;346:393–403.
27. Svetkey LP, Stevens VJ, Brantley PJ et al. JAMA 2008; 299:1139–48.
28. Look AHEAD Research Group, Wing RR. Arch Intern Med 2010;170:1566–75.
29. Sjostrom CD, Peltonen M, Wedel H et al. Hypertension 2000;36:20–5.
30. He FJ, MacGregor GA. J Hum Hypertens 2002;16:761–70.
31. Pimenta E, Gaddam KK, Oparil S et al. Hypertension 2009;54:475–81.
32. Sacks FM, Svetkey LP, Vollmer WM et al. N Engl J Med 2001;344:3–10.
33. Johnson AG, Nguyen TV, Davis D. J Hypertens 2001;19:1053–60.
34. Vollmer WM, Sacks FM, Ard J et al. Ann Intern Med 2001;135:1019–28.
35. Bray GA, Vollmer WM, Sacks FM et al. Am J Cardiol 2004;94:222–7.
36. Appel LJ, Espeland MA, Easter L et al. Arch Intern Med 2001;161:685–93.
37. Obarzanek E, Proschan MA, Vollmer WM et al. Hypertension 2003;42:459–67.
38. He FJ, Markandu ND, MacGregor GA. Hypertension 2001;38:321–5.
39. Johnson RJ, Herrera-Acosta J, Schreiner GF et al. N Engl J Med 2002;346:913–23.
40. Appel LJ. BMJ 2009;339:b4980.
41. Strazzullo P, D'Elia L, Kandala NB et al. BMJ 2009;339: b4567.
42. Stolarz-Skrzypek K, Kuznetsova T, Thijs L et al. JAMA 2011;305:1777–85.
43. O'Donnell MJ, Yusuf S, Mente A et al. JAMA 2011;306: 2229–38.
44. Chang HY, Hu YW, Yue CS et al. Am J Clin Nutr 2006;83: 1289–96.
45. Cook NR, Cutler JA, Obarzanek E et al. BMJ 2007;334:885.
46. Frohlich ED. Hypertension 2007;50:161–6.
47. Jula AM, Karanko HM. Circulation 1994;89:1023–31.
48. He J, Ogden LG, Bazzano LA et al. Arch Intern Med 2002;162:1619–24.
49. Paterna S, Gaspare P, Fasullo S et al. Clin Sci (Lond) 2008;114:221–30.
50. Harsha DW, Sacks FM, Obarzanek E et al. Hypertension 2004;43:393–8.

51. Chen Q, Turban S, Miller ER et al. J Hum Hypertens 2011 Nov 3 [Epub ahead of print].

52. Psaty BM, Lumley T, Furberg CD et al. JAMA 2003;289: 2534–44.

53. Lloyd-Jones D, Hong Y, Labarthe D et al. Circulation 2010;121:586–613.

54. Mattes RD, Donnelly D. J Am Coll Nutr 1991;10:383–93.

55. Dickinson BD, Havas S, Council on Science and Public Health, American Medical Association. Arch Intern Med 2007;167:1460–8.

56. Institute of Medicine. Strategies to Reduce Sodium Intake in the United States. Washington, DC: National Academy Press, 2010.

57. Geleijnse JM, Kok FJ, Grobbee DE. J Hum Hypertens 2003;17:471–80.

58. Whelton PK, He J, Cutler JA et al. JAMA 1997;277:1624–32.

59. Naismith DJ, Braschi A. Br J Nutr 2003;90:53–60.

60. Appel LJ, Moore TJ, Obarzanek E et al. N Engl J Med 1997;336:1117–24.

61. John JH, Ziebland S, Yudkin P et al. Lancet 2002;359: 1969–74.

62. Morris RC Jr, Sebastian A, Forman A et al. Hypertension 1999;33:18–23.

63. Food and Nutrition Board, Institute of Medicine. Dietary Reference Intakes: Water, Potassium, Sodium Chloride, and Sulfate. Washington, DC: National Academy Press, 2004.

64. National Kidney Foundation. Am J Kidney Dis 2004(Suppl 1); 43:S1–29.

65. Xin X, He J, Frontini MG et al. Hypertension 2001;38:1112–7.

66. Okubo Y, Miyamoto T, Suwazono Y et al. Alcohol 2001;23: 149–56.

67. Rouse IL, Beilin LJ, Armstrong BK et al. Lancet 1983;1:5–10.

68. Margetts BM, Beilin LJ, Vandongen R et al. Br Med J (Clin Res Ed) 1986;293:1468–71.

69. Whelton SP, Hyre AD, Pedersen B et al. J Hypertens 2005;23:475–81.

70. Streppel MT, Arends LR, van 't Veer P et al. Arch Intern Med 2005;165:150–6.

71. Cappuccio FP, Elliott P, Allender PS et al. Am J Epidemiol 1995;142:935–45.

72. Allender PS, Cutler JA, Follmann D et al. Ann Intern Med 1996;124:825–31.

73. Bucher HC, Cook RJ, Guyatt GH et al. JAMA 1996;275: 1016–22.

74. Griffith LE, Guyatt GH, Cook RJ et al. Am J Hypertens 1999;12:84–92.

75. van Mierlo LA, Arends LR, Streppel MT et al. J Hum Hypertens 2006;20:571–80.

76. Jee SH, Miller ER 3rd, Guallar E et al. Am J Hypertens 2002;15:691–6.

77. Geleijnse JM, Giltay EJ, Grobbee DE et al. J Hypertens 2002;20:1493–9.

78. Appel LJ, Miller ER 3rd, Seidler AJ et al. Arch Intern Med 1993;153:1429–38.

79. Morris MC. J Cardiovasc Risk 1994;1:21–30.

80. Ascherio A, Rimm EB, Giovannucci EL et al. Circulation 1992;86:1475–84.

81. Ascherio A, Hennekens C, Willett WC et al. Hypertension 1996;27:1065–72.

82. Niinikoski H, Jula A, Viikari J et al. Hypertension 2009;53: 918–24.

83. Ferrara LA, Raimondi AS, d'Episcopo L et al. Arch Intern Med 2000;160:837–42.

84. Shah M, Adams-Huet B, Garg A. Am J Clin Nutr 2007;85:1251–6.

85. Sacks FM, Rosner B, Kass EH. Am J Epidemiol 1974;100: 390–8.

86. Stamler J, Liu K, Ruth KJ et al. Hypertension 2002;39: 1000–6.

87. Bremer AA, Auinger P, Byrd RS. J Nutr Metab 2010;2010: 196476 [Epub 2009 Sep 6].

88. Dhingra R, Sullivan L, Jacques PF et al. Circulation 2007;116:480–8.

89. Cohen L, Curhan G, Forman J. J Gen Intern Med 2012 Apr 27 [Epub ahead of print].

90. Chen L, Caballero B, Mitchell DC et al. Circulation 2010;121:2398–406.

91. Visvanathan R, Chen R, Horowitz M et al. Br J Nutr 2004;92:335–40.

92. Ha V, Sievenpiper JL, de Souza RJ et al. Hypertension 2012;59:787–95.

93. Elliott P, Stamler J, Dyer AR et al. Arch Intern Med 2006;166:79–87.

94. Burke V, Hodgson JM, Beilin LJ et al. Hypertension 2001;38:821–6.

95. He J, Gu D, Wu X et al. Ann Intern Med 2005;143:1–9.

96. Ness AR, Chee D, Elliott P. J Hum Hypertens 1997;11: 343–350.

97. Juraschek SP, Guallar E, Appel LJ et al. Am J Clin Nutr 2012;95:1079–88.

98. Lifton RP, Wilson FH, Choate KA et al. Cold Spring Harb Symp Quant Biol 2002;67:445–50.

99. Hunt SC, Cook NR, Oberman A et al. Hypertension 1998;32:393–401.

100. Svetkey LP, Moore TJ, Simons-Morton DG et al. J Hypertens 2001;19:1949–56.

101. Grant FD, Romero JR, Jeunemaitre X et al. Hypertension 2002;39:191–6.

102. Kostis JB, Wilson AC, Hooper WC et al. Am Heart J 2002;144:625–9.

103. Miller ER 3rd, Erlinger TP, Young DR et al. Hypertension 2002;40:612–8.

104. Appel LJ, Champagne CM, Harsha DW et al. JAMA 2003; 289:2083–93.

105. Dekkers JC, Snieder H, Van Den Oord EJ et al. J Pediatr 2002;141:770–9.

106. He FJ, MacGregor GA. Hypertension 2006;48:861–9.

107. Simons-Morton DG, Obarzanek E. Pediatr Nephrol 1997;11:244–9.

108. Applegate WB, Miller ST, Elam JT et al. Arch Intern Med 1992;152:1162–6.

109. Erlinger TP, Vollmer WM, Svetkey LP et al. Prev Med 2003;37:327–33.

C. PEDIATRIC AND ADOLESCENT DISORDERS

67 PEDIATRIC FEEDING PROBLEMS[1]
RICHARD M. KATZ, JAMES K. HYCHE, AND ELLEN K. WINGERT

Undernutrition is a major problem in the world and certainly a major contributor to disease and poor growth in vulnerable populations. Prolonged undernutrition affects the physical health as well as the mental and social development of children. In addition, it exacts a heavy cost to their families and society at large. Primary causes of undernutrition are availability of food and the ability or willingness to consume available nutrition. This chapter focuses on feeding disorders as an increasingly common source of undernutrition in young children.

Feeding disorders is a term used to describe children experiencing difficulty in consuming adequate nutrition by mouth (impaired feeding), those who eat too much (hyperphagia), and those who eat inappropriate items (pica). The term is often mistaken for eating disorders such as anorexia and bulimia, but it is unrelated to the risk factors in adolescent bulimia and anorexia nervosa.

Most normally developing children learn to accept and consume a well-balanced, healthful diet to sustain growth and health (1). They develop the capacity for self-regulation and adapt to various parent and environmental changes. Satter (2) has expanded this concept and outlined the role of the child and the parent during feeding. However, biologic, personal, and social factors can interfere with the principle of self-regulation.

Nearly 25% of infants and children are affected by feeding disorders at some point in their development. The rate is much higher, nearly 80%, among children with

developmental disabilities. Further breakdown of the prevalence indicates 52% of toddlers are not consistently hungry at mealtimes, 42% end meals after a brief session, 35% are picky eaters, and 33% show food selectivity (3). However, severe feeding problems are noted in children (3% to 10%), (4) with greater prevalence in children with physical disabilities (26% to 90%) and among those with medical illness and prematurity (10% to 49%) (5–7).

The consequences of undernutrition on growth and development are well documented (8–10) and cause substantial morbidity and mortality. Feeding disorders affect the whole family resulting in significant stress and strain in the caregiver–child relationship (11). Two thirds of a caregiver's waking time may be spent in attending to a child with disordered feeding (12), and this intense involvement of a primary caregiver takes time away from other family and household duties.

Feeding disorders have multiple etiologies, including medical, nutritional, behavioral, psychologic, and environmental factors (8, 9). Table 67.1 presents examples of common childhood feeding problems. Children with developmental disabilities, medical conditions, and severe behavior problems are unlikely to outgrow their feeding problems without intervention. Therefore, it is important that caregivers and care providers recognize a child's feeding problem early and have an evaluation to offer early intervention to arrest the downward spiral of the child's feeding problem.

Children with feeding disorders are a heterogeneous group. They range from those without medical problems to those who have gastrointestinal (GI) tract disorders, systemic illness, developmental delay, and physical disabilities. Forty-five percent of children with normal development have mealtime problems (13). Most of these children's feeding concerns were reported as one of poor appetite, and in 23% of cases the children were of normal weight and height.

A child's feeding progresses from a strictly biologic need to a process combining maturation and learning in a nurturing social environment. Thus, feeding disorders should be conceptualized as biopsychosocial problems. Interactions among the three mechanisms pose a challenge to the differential diagnosis and evaluation and treatment. Many, but not all, persistent feeding difficulties in children

---

[1]**Abbreviation: GI**, gastrointestinal.

TABLE 67.1	COMMON FEEDING PROBLEMS

Total food refusal
Food refusal by volume
Food refusal by texture
Food refusal by type
Bottle dependency
Lengthy meals
Maladaptive behaviors
Adipsia

TABLE 67.2	OPTIMIZING THE FEEDING ENVIRONMENT

Quiet room with limited distractions
Developmentally appropriate positioning
Stable and supportive chair
Developmentally appropriate utensils
Child demonstration of readiness cues for feeding
Stable routine and schedules
Caregiver positioned at eye level

may have an associated underlying structural, neurologic, or physiologic disorder. Yet, in most children with significant feeding disorders, no clear etiology becomes apparent with even the most thorough evaluation.

Feeding is a complex task requiring a sequential progression of a repertoire of skills to be successful. Guidance to families based on developmental progressions observed in normal children are inappropriate for children with cerebral palsy, failure to thrive, syndromic disorders, and muscular and neuromuscular problems. Poor coordination of oral structures may interfere with the ability to move food in the mouth, chew, or swallow in a safe and effective manner. Delayed motor skills may interfere with self-feeding.

Successful feeding often is perceived by parents as a measure of parenting competence. Effective feeding is contingent on the ability of both the adult and child to give, read, and interpret the others' cues. Neurologic impairment may interfere with the ability to give clear hunger or satiety cues.

Children usually refuse food after negative experiences. These negative or aversive experiences may include pain in the act of eating or being fed, painful experiences around the facial–oral area, or adverse oral–sensory reactions. Subsequently, when food is presented, anticipatory anxiety arises and the child may refuse to eat at all, refuse to eat an adequate amount, or refuse to eat certain foods. Parents need to know that this is a learned response. Caregivers should be helped to understand that food refusal behaviors are an expression of anxiety or fear, rather than indicative that the child is "bad" or "difficult," or that their fear "is all in their head." Often, problems are worsened unintentionally by caregiver mismanagement. It is important to educate parents and caregivers regarding how the child's feeding problem developed and what they can learn to do to change their child's feeding behavior (14). In many instances, caregivers experience guilt about their contribution, real or imagined, to the child's feeding problems. They need assurance that a few behavioral changes (e.g., making mealtime pleasant) may improve their child's eating behavior (Table 67.2).

Feeding disorders include various feeding behaviors and characteristics. These behaviors can be categorized into ability (unable to perform) and motivational deficits (unwilling) (15). A child with low energy or fine motor deficits may not self-feed. A child reported as having poor appetite and reduced consumption may have swallow dys-

function, taste aversion, texture sensitivity, dental problems, recurring ear infections, or many other disorders. A child with severe gastroesophageal reflux may actively gag or vomit to relieve the discomfort. Total food refusal is uncommon in normal healthy children, except during illness or transiently when they are emotionally upset. However, a comprehensive assessment is still necessary to rule out physical causes of food refusal.

As proposed by the American Psychiatric Association Task Force for Revision of the *Diagnostic and Statistical Manual for Mental Disorders*, Fifth edition (*DSM*), children with feeding disorders can be broadly divided into three categories: children who do not eat enough or show little interest in eating; children who exhibit severe food selectivity and accept only a limited diet in relation to sensory features; and children whose food refusal is related to aversive experiences. In addition, children with feeding disorders include those who are healthy, have digestive disorders, and have special needs. Feeding difficulties in healthy children often are transitional and resolve spontaneously. However, in some children the problem persists and may require professional care. Suboptimal calorie intake, food selectivity by type, disruptive mealtime behaviors, and excessive meal duration are commonly seen feeding problems in healthy children. Table 67.3 presents ideas on how to improve mealtime behaviors in a child who is a picky eater.

Diagnosing medical disorders in children with feeding difficulties is a challenge, especially in infants and toddlers who are unable to report on their condition. Table 67.4 lists examples of medical conditions commonly seen in children with complex feeding difficulties.

TABLE 67.3	STRATEGIES TO IMPROVE MEALTIME BEHAVIORS OF "PICKY EATERS"

Cut down grazing.
Keep junk foods out of view.
Caregivers should model eating novel foods.
Offer small amounts at each serving.
Present the same novel food for 10 to 20 meals.
Make the foods attractive.
Food consistency should suit the child.
Add condiments and sauces that the child likes.
Add other foods to boost calories, such as grated cheese, cream, gravy, and butter.
Aim for high-density, low-volume foods.
Reinforce appropriate feeding behaviors.

TABLE 67.4	MEDICAL CONDITIONS SEEN IN FEEDING PROBLEMS

Anatomic abnormalities
  Cleft lip or palate
Pierre Robin sequence
CHARGE association
Cardiopulmonary effects
Complex congenital heart disease
Chronic lung disease
Aspiration pneumonia
Neuromuscular disorders
  Cerebral palsy
  Cranial nerve anomalies
  Pseudobulbar palsy
  Intracranial mass lesion
Disorders of esophageal phase of swallowing
  Cricopharyngeal achalasia
  Tracheoesophageal fistula/esophageal atresia repair
  Esophageal mass, stricture, web
  Vascular rings
  Foreign bodies
Motility disorders
Lumen disorders
  Gastroesophageal reflux disease
  Peptic esophagitis/gastritis
  Inflammatory bowel disease
Genetic disorders
  Prader-Willi syndrome
  Trisomy 21
  Velocardiofacial syndrome (22q11.2 deletion syndrome)
Metabolic disorders
Miscellaneous
  Constipation
  Food allergies

CHARGE, coloboma, heart disease, atresia choanae, retarded growth and retarded development and/or CNS anomalies, genital hypoplasia, and ear anomalies and/or deafness.

In most cases, a team of experienced professionals from several disciplines including gastroenterology, nutrition, occupational therapy or speech therapy, and psychology are necessary to establish a differential diagnosis of the presenting symptoms to specify the cause or function. In an interdisciplinary team, the physician treats underlying medical causes; the dietician determines calories needed, appropriate foods and required nutrients; the occupational or speech therapist evaluates oral motor and pharyngeal skills, positioning for feeding, the need for adaptive equipment, and self-feeding skills; and the psychologist works to develop strategies in the treatment plan to decrease the child's mealtime anxiety and related food refusal behaviors, increase the motivation to eat and drink, and eliminate disruptive feeding behaviors. Ultimately, for treatment to be effective over the long term, parents and other caregivers must be trained to implement all feeding recommendations in the home, daycare, and school environments. All referral concerns, no matter how simple or unimpressive, should be addressed, which allays caregiver concerns and averts more serious problems. Prognosis with early intervention is very favorable for most cases. Early intervention increases the effectiveness of therapy.

ASSESSMENT

The process of understanding the origin of feeding disorders involves identifying symptoms and behaviors as well as determining the predisposing, precipitating, and perpetuating factors. Child characteristics such as temperament, recurrent illness, low resilience, and parent characteristics of depression or poor coping ability can act as predisposing factors. Precipitating factors include acute or chronic illness, injury, pain, and child maltreatment. Perpetuating factors include continued pain and discomfort as well as reinforcement derived from well-meaning but faulty behavior management. Identification of these factors has strong treatment implications.

Five major areas should be evaluated when assessing children with feeding disorders: history, physical examination (including oral and pharyngeal assessment), nutritional assessment, anthropometric assessment, and behavioral observation.

History

A detailed history helps to formulate the nature of the problem, especially for the conditions that affect nutritional status and feeding care. Focus also should be on the child's developmental level and the caregiver's understanding and knowledge of appropriate feeding regimens, textures, volumes, and methods. Possible medication effects on a child's feeding include depressed appetite, nausea, GI irritation, and constipation. Some of the medications and their effects on the GI system and potential for feeding difficulties are presented in Table 67.5. In young children, the prenatal risk factors and neonatal history should be obtained, especially in premature infants or those with a complicated neonatal course. Surgical history is vital, particularly GI surgery, but any surgery in childhood could result in disordered eating. Finally, a family history could elicit other evidence of feeding and eating disorders.

A profile of the child's feeding history should include the onset, course, frequency, intensity, duration, and variability of feeding behaviors across time, settings, and personnel. A profile of the caregiver's temperament, knowledge of child development and feeding practices, their own feeding history, attitude toward the child, coping skills, and resources also should be gathered. The

TABLE 67.5	MEDICATIONS CAUSING INTERFERING SIDE EFFECTS

MEDICATION	POSSIBLE GASTROINTESTINAL EFFECTS
Iron	Nausea, vomiting
Amoxicillin	Nausea, vomiting, pain
Nonsteroidal anti-inflammatory drugs	Mucosal injury
Psychotropics	Lethargy, dysphagia

role of the family, particularly the primary caregiver (whether the mother, father, grandparent, or babysitter), and the daycare worker is paramount in the management of feeding difficulties. In a typical feeding situation, the parent decides what to serve the child and the child eats to satisfaction. Caregiver temperament, knowledge, resources, motivation, mental, and physical health status can affect feeding interactions and outcomes during meals profoundly. A determination as to whether the child's feeding pattern is normal for age and developmental levels should be made. Often, children's behaviors of concern to parents could be developmental variations, such as poor self-feeding or messy eating at 1 year of age. Caregivers who fail to understand developmental variations become anxious and devise novel feeding techniques, often creating a conflict between parent compulsion and child capacity. Variability in eating between meals is common in children between the ages of 2 to 5 years. These children are active, easily distracted, and resist being confined in the high chair for very long. They demand independence and control and insist on certain utensils and foods. In fact, weight gain slows down and children of this age do not require the same calories as they did as infants. The slope in the National Center for Health Statistics growth chart reflects this decrease in growth velocity.

Anthropometry

Measurements of height, weight, and weight-to-height ratio are indispensable in determining nutrition and growth status. Much can be learned about the child's growth and development by plotting serial points of these values. A thorough analysis of the serial points can help establish the onset and course as well as the precipitating and perpetuating factors of the feeding problem. Children below the 5th percentile should not be assumed to have a problem. Weight gain should be a concern only if the child's growth velocity falters and falls off the growth curve. However, even well-nourished children often need assistance because they may exhibit feeding behaviors that interfere with routines and are a source of stress and concern for caregivers.

Physical Examination

A thorough physical examination should be conducted to rule out organic causes. Any organ or system of the body, especially the GI system, can act as a precipitating factor for feeding problems. Patient observation should focus on child temperament, tactile responses, motor control, oral integrity, coordination, suck/swallow competency, positioning, and signs of pain and discomfort. A physician may observe parts of the feeding anatomy and function that are accessible to clear the patient for safe oral feeding. Speech and occupational therapists may conduct feeding trials to explore oral motor functioning, positioning, sensation, swallow efficiency, muscle strength,

suck-swallow-breathing coordination, and self-feeding skills. Instrumental evaluations can be used along with the clinical assessment. The modified barium swallow study is the most common assessment for evaluating the dynamic phases of swallowing function. This evaluation provides information regarding structural and functioning findings, the risk of aspiration, and the effectiveness of treatment techniques. Fiberoptic endoscopic evaluation of swallowing uses a flexible endoscope passed transnasally to allow visualization of the nasal, pharyngeal, and laryngeal structures (16). Ultrasound as an imaging tool visualizes the relationships between movement patterns of the oral and pharyngeal structures (16).

Nutritional assessment of the child's dietary intake is critical. Dietary information can be used to determine calories consumed and nutritional components of the diet. Diet history should include both current and past practices and feeding patterns. Dietary information may be obtained through caregiver recall; however, this may be inaccurate. Children's feeding varies among meals and days. Assessing a single meal or a day's calorie count does not reveal the child's true nutritional status. Therefore, analysis of a 3-day food diary provides the most valid estimate of the child's true intake variations in food types eaten and amounts consumed. Nutritional strategies given to families should consider family preferences, resources, culture, ethnicity, and education. Parents should be reassured if their children are receiving adequate nutrition and are following their growth curve, no matter how small or thin the child may appear.

Feeding disorders in children with medical problems are complex because they interact with behavioral and social factors, making differential diagnoses more challenging. The most common clinical symptoms suggestive of medical conditions are dysphagia, gastroesophageal reflux, diarrhea, and constipation. GI disorders interfere with the process of consumption, retention, digestion, absorption, and elimination (Table 67.6), frequently resulting in weight loss, lethargy, illness, and feeding disorders.

In some cases, seemingly functional disorders may later reveal underlying organic causes of the feeding disorder. For example, delayed gastric emptying without evidence of systemic disease may develop in healthy children (17). Similar findings of latent physical problems without clinical evidence were identified by Staiano et al (18) in their study of upper GI motility in children with progressive

---

TABLE 67.6 | **GASTROINTESTINAL DISORDERS AFFECTING THE PROCESS OF NUTRITION ASSIMILATION**

Consumption: appetite, dysphagia, aspiration, craniofacial abnormalities
Retention: emesis, diarrhea
Digestion: food allergy, lactose intolerance
Absorption: celiac disease, dumping syndrome
Elimination: constipation, Hirschsprung disease

TABLE 67.7	SYMPTOMS OF GASTROESOPHAGEAL REFLUX

Vomiting	Coughing
Frequent swallowing	Regurgitation
Dental erosion	Food refusal
Stricture	Barrett esophagus
Anemia	Bleeding
Stridor	Hoarseness
Arching	Posturing

TABLE 67.9	PARENT–CHILD INTERACTION

PARENT: POSITIVE BEHAVIORS AND SKILLS	PARENT: NEGATIVE BEHAVIORS
Affectionate	Distant
Enthusiastic	Passive
Supportive	Overcontrolling
Engaging	Harsh, irritable
Rewarding	Punitive
Calm	Anxious
Interprets the child's cues correctly	Preoccupied
Copes with stress and frustration	Overwhelmed
Sets limits	Undercontrolling

muscular dystrophy. It is common for symptoms of a motility disorder, food allergy, and lactose intolerance to emerge once children are taught to eat larger volumes and an increased variety of foods. Presumably, the child was self-regulating and avoided the "toxic" substance through food refusal. Most often a diagnostic evaluation is needed to confirm presumed clinical diagnoses. Food allergies are an increasingly common problem in infants and children. Most food allergies do not manifest with classic immunoglobulin E–mediated symptoms such as urticaria or pruritus, but they often manifest with mild-to-moderate GI distress that can lead to food refusal behaviors (19, 20). Therefore, most children with food refusal should have allergy evaluations. GI tract disorders beyond gastroesophageal reflux disease can play a role in maladaptive feeding behaviors. Anomalies such as malrotation, esophageal stenosis, vascular anomalies, and motility disorders of the esophagus, stomach, and duodenum all have been associated with food refusal (21, 22).

Emesis is a common presenting symptom in children with GI tract disorders, food allergies, conditioned aversion, rumination, or other underlying disorder. Most common, however, is gastroesophageal reflux. Symptoms of reflux are presented in Table 67.7. Children with such symptoms should be referred to a gastroenterologist for diagnosis and therapy.

Dysphagia can occur in one or more phases of swallowing, including the oral phase, initiation of the swallow, pharyngeal phase, and esophageal phase (16). Causes of dysphagia may include neurologic disorders, anatomic abnormalities, pulmonary disease, and genetic syndromes (23). Clinical manifestations of dysphagia include oral motor delays, poor suck-swallow-breathe coordination, respiratory distress, food refusals, and food selectivity (23). Table 67.8 presents common symptoms of dysphagia in children.

Behavioral Observation

Observation of feeding is of critical value and provides direct evidence and insight into the feeding problem. Parent and child behavior during feeding is reciprocal. The child's feeding behaviors affects the caregiver's attitude and feeding methods toward the child; just as the parent's temperament and feeding techniques affect the child's response to the feeding situation. Observation of the parent–child dyad in the clinic may not represent their natural behaviors. Videotaping of home meal sessions, when possible, offer a more realistic performance. The important elements of parent–child behaviors to be observed during meal trials are presented in Tables 67.9 and 67.10.

Feeding disorders manifested by children with normal growth parameters may manifest as restricted food variety, inappropriate food consistency, and disruptive mealtime behaviors. Children, who missed the opportunity to experience foods and textures at certain developmental stages, the "critical" or "sensitive" periods, are more resistant to new foods and higher textures. Texture difficulty, in the absence of oral–motor dysfunction can result from dental problems, developmentally inappropriate food textures, or avoidance because of an aversive experience of gagging and choking. Children diagnosed with autism spectrum disorder tend to demonstrate difficulty with food textures without presenting with delayed oral motor skills or pharyngeal difficulties (23).

Environment

Environmental factors often are given little importance in the assessment of feeding disorders. Yet overwhelming

TABLE 67.8	SYMPTOMS OF DYSPHAGIA

Drooling
Chewing difficulty
Food pocketing
Gagging with textures
Coughing during and after swallowing
Wet voice quality after swallowing

TABLE 67.10	PARENT–CHILD INTERACTION

CHILD: POSITIVE BEHAVIORS	CHILD: NEGATIVE BEHAVIORS
Attentive	Distracted
Pleasant	Irritable
Cooperative	Resistant
Accepts limits	Throws tantrums
Responsive	Defiant

evidence indicates their significance in the development, maintenance, and/or exacerbation of feeding problems (13, 24). Thus, a planned assessment and observation of the feeding environment during the assessment phase is important. The child's natural feeding environment can provide critical information in understanding the parents' priorities, available resources, and settings that affect the child's feeding behaviors. Children do not feed for nutritional values. Rather, they are motivated by taste, smell, color, and social reinforcement. Functional analysis to determine their likes and dislikes will reveal why children accept some foods, eat well at certain meals, or feed with one caregiver and not another.

TREATMENT

Medical

Treatment is rarely straightforward, even in situations in which the etiology and functional causes of the feeding disorder have been identified. Gastroenterologists have developed many noninvasive techniques for the evaluation of GI functions (25). Medical treatment is extensive for organically based feeding difficulties. Occasionally, hospitalization may be needed for objective clinical observation when initial assessment does not provide the answer to the problem or when caregiver report and child status are incongruent. In many cases, management using alternative routes of delivering nutrition may be needed. Enteral feedings should be considered in children who cannot consume sufficient calories by mouth, those who tire easily from the effort to chew and swallow, require undue amount of caregiver time, become ill frequently, are medically unsafe, or cannot safely drink liquids. Children with severe malnutrition and failure to thrive and those with severe food allergies also may benefit from enteral feeding. Even when a child is on enteral feedings, nonnutritive and nutritive stimulation should be initiated at the earliest possible opportunity.

Behavioral

Applied behavior analysis has been successfully applied in treating feeding problems including disruptive mealtime behaviors (25), food refusal (26, 27), and food preference (28). Feeding disorders in children resulting from behavioral and caregiver mismanagement can be treated effectively using applied behavioral techniques. Children diagnosed with severe food selectivity require focused intervention using behavioral and/or cognitive behavioral strategies to (1) decrease anxiety, (2) break the task of eating novel foods into small manageable steps that are taught sequentially, or (3) decrease or eliminate disruptive meal escape/avoidance behaviors. Initial treatment always should be aimed at making changes to the feeding routine, schedules, feeding environment, and caregiver feeding skills. What occurs outside of feeding sessions—including sleep deprivation, poor bowel habits, lethargy,

and irritability—can affect children's feeding behaviors significantly. Intervention should be focused on teaching the parent to understand the child's temperament, set limits, and facilitate the child's internal regulation of feeding (29). This includes dieticians' instructions about foods with good nutritional values, food preparation and storage techniques, as well as tube feeding management, which always should be attempted before more intrusive treatment procedures.

Oral–Motor

The goal of oral–motor intervention is to improve the quality of feeding skills within the child's functional ability. As part of the therapeutic process, the occupational/speech therapist develops oral motor exercises to strengthen muscles, reduce postural effort with proper positioning, and provide adaptive equipment to improve self-feeding skills. In addition, textures may be modified to improve bolus control and swallowing abilities or control the size or flow rate of bolus delivery. Treatment techniques always should include caregiver training to ensure consistent carryover at meals. In most cases, there exist effective therapeutic techniques to treat pediatric feeding problems. Treatment techniques are individualized to the child's feeding difficulties and adapted to the caregiver's ability to follow through with the recommendations.

SUMMARY

Feeding disorders are surprisingly common. The incidence of feeding disorders will continue to rise as sick children survive because of advances in medical technology. Feeding disorders occur as a result of medical, sensory, physical, personal, social, and environmental dynamics. These factors rarely operate independently. Prolonged feeding problems have grave consequences for the child's physical, cognitive, and social health, and lead to caregiver stress and family dysfunction. The multifactorial etiology of feeding disorders demands a multidisciplinary feeding team to treat the whole child as well as their caregivers effectively.

Caregiver education and training are indispensable to maintenance and generalization and to avoid regression and the revolving door phenomenon. Most children with feeding disorders can be treated effectively, in the absence of an active medical problem, by an experienced feeding team.

REFERENCES

1. Davis, CM Can J Med Assoc 1939;41:257–61.
2. Satter E. J Pediatr 1990;117:181–9.
3. Reau NR, Senturia YD, Lebailly SA et al. J Dev Behav Pediatr 1966;17:149–53.
4. Lindberg L, Bohlin G, Hagekull B. Int J Eat Disord 1991; 10:395–405.
5. Reilley S, Skuse D, Problete X. J Pediatr 1996;129:877–82.
6. Douglas JE, Bryon M. Arch Dis Child 1985;75:304–8.
7. Thommessen M, Heidberg A, Kasse BF et al. Acta Paediatr 1991;80:527–33.

8. Riordan MM, Iwata BA, Wohl KM et al. Appl Res Ment Retard 1980;1:95–112.

9. Babbitt RL, Hoch TA, Coe DA et al. J Dev Behav Pediatr 1994; 15:278–91.

10. Barett DE, Radke-Yarrow M, Klein RE. Dev Psychol 1984; 18:541–56.

11. Greer AJ, Gulotta CS, Laud RBJ. Pediatr Psychol 2008; 33:612–20.

12. Chase HP, Martin H. N Engl J Med 1970; 933–9.

13. Linscheid TR. Disturbances of eating and feeding. In: Magrab PR, ed. Psychological Problems in Early Life, Early Life Conditions and Chronic Diseases Chronic Diseases. Baltimore: University Park Press, 1978:191–218.

14. Fischer E, Silverman A. Semin Speech Lang 2007;28:223–31.

15. Manikam R, Perman J. J Clin Gastroenterol 2000;11:34–46.

16. Arvedson JC. Dev Disabil Res Rev 2008;14:118–27.

17. Marchi M, Cohen P. J Am Acad Child Adolesc Psychiatry 1990; 29:112–7.

18. Staiano A, Giudice E, Romano A et al. J Pediatr 1992; 121:720–4.

19. Haas AM. Curr Allerg Asthma Rep 2010;10:258–64.

20. Garcia-Careaga M Jr, Kerner JA Jr. Nutr Clinc Pract 2005; 5:526–35.

21. Zangen T, Cairla C, Zangen S et al. J Pediatr Gastroenterol Nutr 2003;37:225–7.

22. Cucchiara S. Int Semin Paediatr Gastroenterol Nutr 1998;7:2.

23. Lefton-Greif MA. Phys Med Rehabil Clin North Am 2008; 19:837–51.

24. Palmer S, Horn S. Feeding problems in children. In: Palmer S, Ekvall S, eds. Pediatric Nutrition in Developmental Disorders. 6th ed. Springfield, IL: Charles C Thomas, 1978:107–29.

25. O'Brian F, Azrin NH. J Appl Behav Anal 1972;5:389–99.

26. Ahearn WH, Kerwin ME, Eicher PS et al. J Appl Behav Anal 1996;29:321–32.

27. Thompson RJ, Palmer S. J Nutr Educ 1974;6:63–6.

28. Chatoor I, Hirsch R, Persinger M. Infant Young Child 1997; 9:12–22.

29. Martin AW. Dysphagia 1991;16:129–34.

68 PROTEIN-ENERGY MALNUTRITION[1]

MANUEL RAMIREZ-ZEA AND BENJAMIN CABALLERO

The term *malnutrition* technically includes both undernutrition and overnutrition (obesity), but it continues to be used by most organizations to define nutrient deficiencies or inadequate body weight for age or relative to height. This chapter uses the term *protein-energy malnutrition* (PEM) to describe the condition in which the most salient elements are a depletion of body energy stores and of tissue proteins, observed over a range of combinations and severity, and usually accompanied by micronutrient deficiencies. PEM can be the direct result of inadequate food intake (primary PEM), or caused by recurrent illnesses associated with gastrointestinal malabsorption, reduced appetite, and/or increased nutrient needs (secondary PEM). This chapter discusses primary PEM.

HISTORICAL BACKGROUND

Although undernutrition has existed since ancient times, the condition was not clinically described until the seventeenth century, when Soranio coined the term *marasmus* to describe emaciated children (1). In 1865, Hinojosa in Mexico described a syndrome associated with edema, skin and mucosal lesions, hair discoloration, and apathy (2). The syndrome was attributed to multiple vitamin deficiencies (3) until 1932, when Cicely Williams, working in West Africa, correctly linked it with deficient protein intake and named it *kwashiorkor*, or disease of the weaned child (4). Numerous studies described the same syndrome under a variety of names: Seller (1906) in Germany as "Mehinahrschaden," Patron-Correa (1908) in Mexico as "culebrilla," Marfan (1910) in France as "dystrophoie desfarineux," Frontali (1927) in Italy as "distrofia de farine," Lieurade (1932) in Cameroon as "les enfants rouges," Williams (1932) in England as kwashiorkor, Oropeza y Castillo (1937) in Venezuela as "síndrome de carencia: avitaminosis," Trowell (1937) in Uganda as "infantile pellagra," and Scroggie (1941) in Chile as "síndrome pluricarencial de la infancia"; it has rightly been called the disease of the 100 names (5, 6).

Between 1949 and 1953, the Food and Agriculture Organization and the World Health Organization (WHO) commissioned several teams to study the disease in Africa (John Brock and Marcel Autret), Central America and Mexico (Moises Behar and Marcel Autret), and Brazil (John Waterlow and Arturo Vergara). This initiative was the beginning of intense research activity during the following 20 years that resulted in consistent definition of the syndrome and of treatment approaches (6). Key discoveries included the association of kwashiorkor with low concentration of serum proteins, with low protein quality, and with extensive and cyclic interactions between undernutrition and infection (7, 8).

In the last third of the twentieth century to the present time, severe cases of undernutrition were seen mostly in refugee and emergency camps. World attention switched to moderate forms of undernutrition (moderate acute

---

[1]**Abbreviations: ART**, antiretroviral therapy; **DALYs**, disability-adjusted life years; **HA**, height for age; **HIV**, human immunodeficiency virus; **IUGR**, intrauterine growth restriction; **MUAC**, midupper arm circumference; **NG**, nasogastric; **ORS**, oral rehydration solution; **OTP**, outpatient therapeutic program; **PEM**, protein-energy malnutrition; **PUFA**, polyunsaturated fatty acid; **ReSoMal**, rehydration solution for malnutrition; **RUSF**, ready-to-use supplementary food; **RUTF**, ready-to-use therapeutic food; **SC**, stabilization center; **SFP**, supplementary feeding program; **SPEM**, severe protein-energy malnutrition; **UNICEF**, United Nations Children's Fund; **WA**, weight for age; **WH**, weight for height; **WHO**, World Health Organization.

undernutrition, moderate or severe stunting) as well as to their long-term consequences (e.g., Barker hypothesis).

EPIDEMIOLOGY

The most vulnerable period during the life course for stunting and acute undernutrition is early childhood, as a result of the high nutritional requirements relative to body size. Frequent acute infections aggravate the problem by further increasing nutrient demands or gastrointestinal losses. The prevalence of severe wasting is usually highest in the first 2 years of life, and it declines thereafter. The prevalence of stunting has been shown to increase progressively until reaching a plateau around 24 months (Fig. 68.1) (9).

In 2005, about 36 million (6.5%) children less than 5 years old who were living in developing countries had moderate wasting, and another 19 million (3.5%) had severe wasting or severe protein-energy malnutrition (SPEM). Approximately 69% of severely wasted children lived in Asia, 29% in Africa, and 2% in Latin America. This is part of the reason that 99% of deaths in children younger than 5 years old occur in those continents (10). This prevalence varies substantially within countries and is highest for the poorest segments of the population.

In 2010, there were 171 million (26.7%) stunted children worldwide, of whom 97.5% lived in developing countries (11). Although this represented a relative decrease of 33% since 1990, when the percentage was 39.7%, stunting remains a public health problem in many developing countries. Approximately 90% of stunted children live in just 36 countries (21 in Africa, 13 in Asia, and 2 in Latin America)

(10). Of all stunted children, 58% live in Asia (half in India), 35% in Africa, and 7% in Latin America. The relative decrease between 1990 and 2010 has been remarkable in Asia (43%, from 48.6% to 27.6%) and Latin America (43%, from 23.7% to 13.5%), but in Africa the decrease was only 5% (from 40.3% to 38.2%). If these trends continue as anticipated, there will be the same number of stunted children in Asia and Africa by 2020 (11).

Undernutrition often starts during pregnancy as a result of dietary deficiencies and concurrent increases in nutrition requirements of the pregnant woman. Low birth weight infants secondary to intrauterine growth restriction (IUGR; at term babies who weighed <2500 g) represent around 11% of all live births each year in developing countries—12.8 million in 2004 (10). The prevalence of acute undernutrition in older children (>5 years of age) is lower than in younger children, and the condition tends to be less severe. Stunting can be highly prevalent in children over 5 years of age, but because it is usually an irreversible condition related to undernutrition in the first two years of life.

Acute primary PEM in adolescents and adults is rare and is usually associated with a primary illness that compromises food intake or increases intestinal losses. Acute PEM may result from chronic deprivation caused by medical conditions or by protracted food scarcity.

In developed countries, primary undernutrition is an uncommon condition, seen mainly among young children of the lowest socioeconomic groups, elderly persons who live alone, and adults addicted to alcohol and drugs. Some cases are also associated with food faddism or extreme nutritional practices (12).

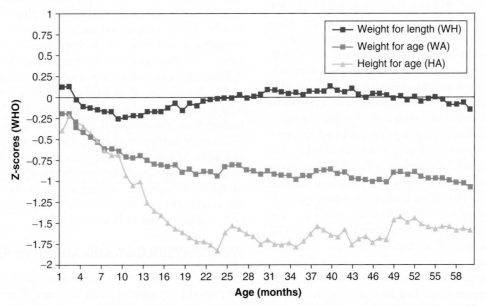

Fig. 68.1. Time course of changes in anthropometric indicators from birth to 60 months, relative to the World Health Organization (WHO) standards, in children from developing countries. Data represents the average from national anthropometric surveys from 54 countries. HA begins below the standard, falls considerably until 24 months of age, and increases slightly after 24 months. WA declines moderately until 24 months and remains fairly stable after that. WH drops slightly until 9 months, raises up to reach the standard mean around 24 months and remains reasonably stable after that. (From Victora CG, de Onis M, Hallal PC, Blossner M, Shrimpton R. Worldwide timing of growth faltering: revisiting implications for interventions. Pediatrics 2010;125:e473-80.)

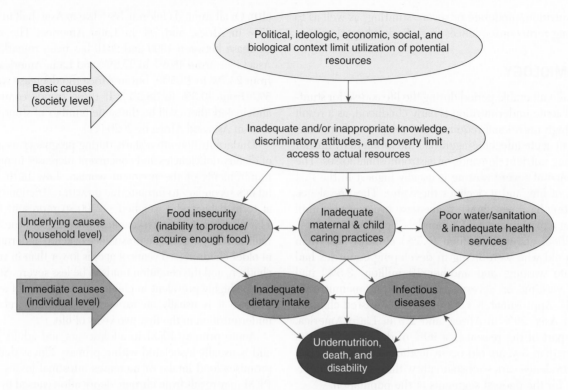

Fig. 68.2. Conceptual framework of undernutrition. Causes are categorized in three: basic (society level), underlying (household level), and immediate (individual level). Undernutrition has also a potentiating effect on infections, leading to a vicious cycle. (Adapted with permission from United Nations Children's Fund [UNICEF]. Strategy for Improved Nutrition of Children and Women in Developing Countries. New York: UNICEF, 1990.)

ETIOLOGY

The conceptual framework of malnutrition developed by the United Nations Children's Fund (UNICEF) in 1990 is still valid (Fig. 68.2) (13). Inadequate dietary intake and repeated infectious diseases are *immediate causes* of undernutrition. Infections are a major factor in the etiology of undernutrition as a result of increased nutrient demands, greater nutrient losses, and disruption of metabolic equilibrium. Conversely, the potentiating effects of undernutrition on infections, particularly diarrhea and acute lower respiratory infections, explain most deaths of children between 6 to 59 months of age in developing countries (14–16). For example, each episode of diarrhea in the first 24 months has been shown to increase the adjusted odds of stunting by a factor of 1.05 (10). This leads to a vicious cycle, in which undernutrition is a health outcome as well as a risk factor for disease and exacerbation of undernutrition (17).

Immediate causes of undernutrition are associated with environmental, economic, and sociopolitical factors, considered underlying and basic causes (see Fig. 68.2). *Underlying causes* are those that take place at the household level and can be categorized into three main factors: food insecurity; defective maternal and child caring practices; and unsafe water, poor sanitation, and inadequate health services. The first factor leads to inadequate dietary intake, the last cluster to disease, whereas the intermediate factor may contribute to both immediate causes.

Underlying causes are directly influenced by *basic causes* such as limited education, poverty, and marginalization. The status of women in particular (education, income) tends to influence infant and child feeding. Food security is related to a complex interaction of factors that include agricultural and food production policies, regulation of food marketing and advertisement, and food subsidies. Additionally, sociocultural elements such as religious beliefs and traditions can affect food preferences and net energy intake. A key biologic factor for childhood PEM is maternal malnutrition, resulting in IUGR and low birth weight (18).

In each particular context, the dynamic interrelation among basic and underlying causes can vary. For example, in an environment where enough energy is supplied and sanitation is improved, wasting may be reduced, but stunting could still be constrained by other limiting factors (e.g., micronutrient deficiencies) (19).

PATHOPHYSIOLOGY AND ADAPTIVE RESPONSES

Stunting and acute undernutrition develop gradually over weeks or months, with a series of metabolic and behavioral adjustments that result in decreased nutrient demands and a nutritional equilibrium compatible with a lower level of cellular nutrient availability. If the supply of nutrients is persistently low, the individual can no longer adapt and may die. When undernutrition develops slowly, as is usually the case in stunting, moderate wasting, and marasmus, individuals are better adapted to their current nutritional status and have a less fragile metabolic equilibrium than do those with more acute undernutrition, as in kwashiorkor of rapid onset.

Observational and experimental evidence increasingly supports an association between undernutrition during fetal and early postnatal life and increased susceptibility to chronic diseases later in life. The mechanisms underlying this relationship are related to epigenetics, which refers to the ways in which the developmental environment can influence the mature phenotype (20). Epigenetic processes, such as DNA methylation and histone modification, are induced by cues from the developmental environment, thus modulating gene expression (developmental plasticity). Maternal and early postnatal undernutrition can induce a series of thrifty phenotypes as a defensive response of the developing fetus or infant against an immediate challenge. For example, maternal undernutrition reduces the number of nephrons in the child, and this may be related to low mRNA expression resulting from a mutation of the paired box gene 2 (*PAX2*) during kidney development (21). Fewer nephrons have been related to hypertension later in life (22). Protein-restricted diets have been associated with reduced promoter methylation and increased expression in the liver of the transcription factor peroxisome proliferator-activated receptor-α (PPAR-α), which causes an increase in circulating concentrations of the ketone β-hydroxybutyrate and glucose (23, 24). Even mild undernutrition can cause phenotypic modifications that affect physiology to aspects of the predicted adult environment (e.g., sparse environment) more precisely (25). If the adaptive change is not appropriate for the subsequent environment (e.g., energy-rich environment), the risk of disease increases.

Mild and Moderate Protein-Energy Malnutrition

In the first stages of PEM, a decrease in energy intake is followed by an adaptive reduction in energy expenditure. This includes a decrease in playtime and physical activity in children, which may subsequently develop into overt apathy and unresponsiveness (26–29). In adults, the need for longer periods of rest is increased, and the capacity for prolonged physical work is reduced (30, 31). When the decrease in energy expenditure cannot compensate for the insufficient intake, energy is mobilized from fat depots, thus leading to weight loss (31). Mobilization of energy from lean body mass also occurs as skeletal muscle protein catabolism contributes energy via conversion of glucogenic amino acids, such as alanine. In children, an additional critical adaptive response is reduction in or cessation of longitudinal growth, which results in chronic undernutrition (stunting). These changes are usually associated with multiple micronutrient deficiencies of variable severity.

As protein and energy deficits progress, the initial adaptation evolves into *accommodation*, a term coined by Waterlow to describe a response in which normal functions are present but operating at a reduced level (adaptation); survival is achieved at the cost of suppressing or severely reducing certain key physiologic functions (accommodation). For example, protein catabolism is an adaptive mechanism to provide glucose during periods of fasting, such as nighttime sleep. Similarly, prolongation of the half-life of plasma albumin is an adaptive mechanism to reduce protein synthesis. However, if protein synthesis is further curtailed, plasma albumin concentration will fall to abnormal concentrations, thus resulting in clinical edema (32, 33). Similar transitions from adaptation to accommodation can be described for blood pressure, skin characteristics, glomerular filtration rate, and others.

Severe Protein-Energy Malnutrition

Immunity defense responses are diminished in children with SPEM because many immune proteins (e.g., immunoglobulins, complement components, acute phase proteins) are reduced or depleted. Similarly, lymph nodes, adenoids, and the thymus may be reduced in size (34, 35). Phagocytosis, chemotaxis, and intracellular functions are also impaired. As a consequence, the usual clinical signs of infection (inflammation, fever) may not be present in the child with SPEM suffering an acute infectious episode. Instead, signs of the failure of homeostasis, such as hypoglycemia or hypothermia, may appear.

Reduction in hemoglobin concentration and red cell mass almost always accompanies PEM, as a result of bone marrow suppression and reduced oxygen needs, the latter related to depleted skeletal muscle mass (36). These adaptive responses are reversed when and if nutritional rehabilitation is successful. Administration of hematinics to a SPEM patient will not induce a hematopoietic response until dietary treatment produces an increase in lean body mass. Giving iron early in treatment can increase free iron, with promotion of free radicals and their damaging effects, and can also make some infections worse.

Total body potassium decreases in SPEM because of the reduction in muscle proteins and increased urinary and fecal losses. At least one third of the cell's energy expenditure results from the sodium/potassium-adenosine triphosphatase (Na^+/K^+-ATPase) pump. In patients with SPEM, this pump slows down because of the diminished energy substrates (ATP). This leads to potassium loss and increased intracellular sodium (37). Water accompanies the sodium influx, and intracellular overhydration may occur. These alterations in cell electrolytes and energy sources may explain, at least in part, the increased fatigability and reduced strength of skeletal muscle, which can even affect respiratory muscles.

Cardiac output, heart rate, and blood pressure decrease; and central circulation takes precedence over peripheral circulation (38, 39). Cardiovascular reflexes are altered, leading to postural hypotension and diminished venous return. These circulatory changes also impair heat generation and loss. Peripheral circulatory failure com-

TABLE 68.1 CLASSIFICATION OF SEVERITY OF CURRENT (WASTING) AND PAST OR CHRONIC (STUNTING) PROTEIN-ENERGY MALNUTRITION

	WASTING			STUNTING
	0–5 y	5–18 y	ADULTS	0–18 y
	WH[a]	BMI FOR AGE[b]	BMI[c]	HA[d]
Mild	−1.1−−2.0 Z	−1.1−−2.0 Z	17.0–18.4	−1.1−−2.0 Z
Moderate	−2.1−−3.0 Z	−2.1−−3.0 Z	16.0–16.9	−2.1−−3.0 Z
Severe	<−3.0 Z	<−3.0 Z	<16.0	<−3.0 Z

BMI, body mass index; HA, height for age; WH, weight for height.

[a]Based on the 2006 World Health Organization (WHO) child growth standards for 0 to 5 years (47).
[b]Based on the 2007 WHO growth reference data for 5 to 19 years (48).
[c]Based on the classification proposed by James et al (88).
[d]Based on the 2006 WHO child growth standards for 0 to 5 years and the 2007 WHO growth reference data for 5 to 19 years (47, 48).

parable to hypovolemic shock may occur. The reduced kidney filtration capacity may result in volume overload and heart failure under relatively moderate water loads.

Impaired intestinal absorption of lipids and carbohydrates and decreased glucose absorption are relatively frequent (40, 41), but they can be partially compensated for by higher intake, to permit nutritional recovery (42). However, reduced intestinal motility and intestinal bacterial overgrowth may predispose patients to diarrhea.

The adaptive response of energy homeostasis involves several endocrine changes (43). Insulin secretion is reduced and glucagon and epinephrine release are increased in response to reduced plasma glucose and free amino acid concentrations. These changes lead to decreases in muscle protein synthesis, lipogenesis, and growth and increases in lipolysis and glycogenolysis. Insulin resistance at the periphery increases, probably from the increase in plasma free fatty acids. Secretion of human growth hormone is stimulated, and insulinlike growth factor activity is reduced, as a response to low plasma concentration of amino acids. These changes also decrease muscle protein synthesis and glucose uptake by tissues and growth as well as increase lipolysis and visceral protein synthesis. The stress induced by persistent starvation, further amplified by infections, stimulates epinephrine and cortisol secretion. These changes also increase lipolysis, glycogenolysis, muscle protein catabolism, and visceral protein turnover. SPEM early in life may result in impaired brain growth, nerve myelination, neurotransmitter production, and nerve conduction velocity.

The metabolic factors leading to edematous SPEM (kwashiorkor) are not yet fully understood, but severe protein deficiency is an important causal factor. Lack of vitamins and minerals present in protein foods of animal origin is also important. Other factors that may contribute to kwashiorkor, with its characteristic edema, hypoalbuminemia, and enlarged fatty liver, are as follows: overloading of a severely malnourished person with carbohydrates; metabolic stress induced by infections; lower adrenocortical response that reduces the efficiency to preserve visceral proteins; and effects of free radicals, which are increased by infections, toxins, sunlight, trauma, and catalysts such as iron (44–46).

DIAGNOSIS

The diagnostic criteria of PEM are based on its severity (mild, moderate, severe) and time course (acute, chronic) and are determined primarily by anthropometry. Other clinical and biochemical findings become evident later in the progression of the disease. The WHO developed child growth reference standards that can be used across different countries to estimate growth adequacy or to diagnose underweight (47, 48).

In children less than 5 years of age, weight for height (WH) is an index of current nutritional status, and lower values indicate recent depletion of body mass (wasting). In older children and adolescents, the body mass index (BMI)-for-age is used instead of WH. Height for age (HA) indicates long-term growth retardation (stunting), but often with adequate weight relative to height (49). Weight for age (WA) indicates growth delay, but it cannot discriminate recent body mass depletion from low stature resulting from chronic undernutrition. For a detailed discussion on the use of anthropometric measurements, see the chapter on anthropometry. The cutoff points to assess severity and duration of PEM are shown in Table 68.1. The unit measure used in children is the Z-score, which defines standard deviations from the reference median value.

The diagnostic criteria for SPEM in children aged 6 to 60 months may include two additional indicators: midupper arm circumference (MUAC) and bilateral edema (Table 68.2). MUAC is included because weight and height measures may not be feasible in large-scale

TABLE 68.2 DIAGNOSTIC CRITERIA FOR SEVERE PROTEIN-ENERGY MALNUTRITION IN CHILDREN 6 TO 60 MONTHS OLD

INDICATOR	MEASURE	CUTOFF
Severe wasting	Weight for height	<−3.0 Z
Severe wasting	Midupper arm circumference	<115 mm
Bilateral pitting edema	Clinical sign	

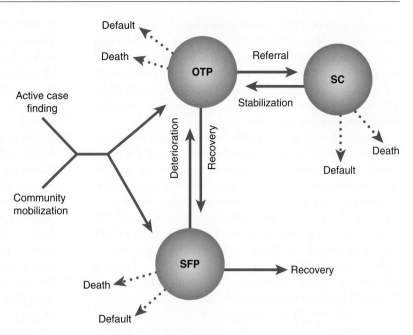

Fig. 68.3. Components of a community-based management of undernutrition program. OTP, outpatient therapeutic program; SFP, supplementary feeding program; SC, stabilization center. Children with PEM are identified through community mobilization and active case-finding. Those with moderate PEM are admitted into the SFP and receive regular dry rations for consumption at home until fully recovered. Those with SPEM with no medical complications are admitted into the OTP and receive weekly RUTF and medicines to treat simple medical conditions for consumption at home. Those with SPEM and medical complications are referred to the SC for inpatient treatment until well enough to return to outpatient care in the OTP and when the condition has improved, discharged into the SFP for supplementary feeding until fully recovered. (From Valid International. Community Based Therapeutic Care: A Field Manual. Oxford: Valid International, 2006.)

community-based programs. Both WFH and MUAC cutoffs have a specificity of more than 99%. However, only 40% of cases selected by one criterion are also selected by the other (50). This difference is partly explained because children with low MUAC tend to be younger than those with WFH lower than −3.0 Z. This phenomenon deserves further research.

Edematous malnutrition (kwashiorkor) is characterized by soft, pitting, painless edema, usually in the feet and legs, but sometimes extending to the perineum, upper extremities, and face. Most patients have skin lesions, often confused with pellagra, in the areas of edema. The epidermis peels off in large scales, exposing underlying tissues that are easily infected. Weight deficit, after accounting for the weight of edema, is usually not as severe as in marasmus. Differential diagnosis on nonnutritional causes of edema must be made through the clinical history, physical examination, and urinalysis.

TREATMENT

Management and treatment of PEM must adapt to the local situation and resources. In countries where acute undernutrition prevails, the ideal model is a community-based approach (Fig. 68.3). This model aims to achieve the greatest possible coverage and allows accessibility to appropriate care for the highest possible proportion of the population. This strategy can reduce to 10% to 15% the number of patients who need inpatient care. Individuals with moderate acute PEM and no medical complications may be admitted to a supplementary feeding program (SFP) that provides dry take-home rations. Those with SPEM and no medical complications may be referred to an outpatient therapeutic program (OTP). Cases with serious medical complications are treated in an inpatient

stabilization center (SC) until they are well enough to be discharged into the OTP and eventually to the SFP (51).

Impact analysis of 21 programs implemented in Malawi, Ethiopia, and Sudan showed that more than three fourths of severely undernourished patients were treated as outpatients, with coverage rates of 73%, recovery rates of 79% and mortality rates of 4.1% (52). The mean length of stay at an OTP was between 40 and 50 days, and the rates of weight gain were between 4 and 5 g/kg/day. This rapid weight gain is possible by providing high energy (>150 kcal/kg/day) and protein (4 to 6 g/kg/day) intakes and micronutrients. Options used for community-based therapy include short-stay day-care or residential nutrition centers (<4 weeks), treatment at home (no food provided) with home or clinic visits, and treatment at home with ready-to-use therapeutic food (RUTF) with home or clinic visits (53). RUTF can reduce the burden of caregivers and health staff, but its cost and logistics for procurement and distribution may not be sustainable. Advantages of community-based management are lower exposure to hospital-acquired infections and reduced time caregivers spend away from home.

Mild and Moderate Protein-Energy Malnutrition

Mild and moderate PEM is usually treated in ambulatory settings (e.g., SFPs). Admission criteria can also be based on MUAC in emergency or relief situations (<125 mm in children and <210 mm in pregnant and lactating women with a baby <6 months of age) (51). Accelerated linear growth is a better indicator of nutritional adequacy and recovery for a child with mild or moderate undernutrition than is weight gain. The younger the age at which stunting is identified, the easier is its reversal (54). Children can gain height at a rate at least three times the normal rate of height gain (55, 56). Investigators have estimated that a severely stunted (<-3 Z HFA) 6-month old child can gain 2 Z-score units in 28 days, and a 24-month old child can take 72 days (57). Some experts have proposed a critical window of opportunity to effect recovery growth while minimizing its potential adverse consequences, probably within the first 2 years of life.

A general rule is to provide a total intake, including the home diet, of at least twice the protein and 1.5 times energy requirements. Nutrient requirements for moderately undernourished children have been estimated to be between the recommended nutrient intakes for normal Western children and the nutrient density in the F-100 formula used for rehabilitation of children with SPEM (57). For growth nutrients (protein, sulfur, potassium, sodium, magnesium, phosphorus, and zinc), a factorial method was used to determine the increment that should be added to allow rates of weight gain of at least 5 g/kg/day, enough energy to synthesize mixed tissue (fat and lean, 5 kcal/g) and to regain the weight deficit in 30 days or less. For protective nutrients (calcium, iron, copper, selenium, iodine, thiamin, riboflavin, niacin, pyridoxine, cobalamin, folic acid, ascorbic acid, vitamin E, retinol, vitamin D, vitamin K, biotin, pantothenic acid, essential fatty acids), increments were based on the additional needs to counteract oxidative and other stresses associated with unhygienic, polluted conditions.

Foods with energy densities between 1 and 1.5 kcal/g are recommended for children with stunting and between 1.5 and 2 kcal/g for moderate undernutrition (58). Energy density can be increased by adding oil to the food. The fat energy percentage of diets for moderately undernourished children should be kept between 35% and 45%, with at least 4.5% n-6 polyunsaturated fatty acid (PUFA) and 0.5% n-3 PUFA. About one third of the protein intake should come from high-quality, high–amino acid score proteins, typically from animal sources. Fiber, particularly insoluble fiber, phytate, and polyphenol intakes should be kept as low as possible since interfere in nutrient and energy digestibility. To cover the high mineral and vitamin requirements, fortification or supplementation may be necessary. Sugar should not exceed 10% of energy, although up to 20% for a few weeks may be acceptable. There is no demonstrable need to add salt to recovery diets.

Dietary management in food-secure populations can be achieved by nutritional counseling about improving the existing diets and better use of food resources. In cases of food insecurity, food supplements should be considered and instructions for their use provided, if these supplements represent a less expensive option for providing all nutrients needed that cannot be easily supplied by local foods (59). Three alternatives have been used so far:

1. Fortified blended foods (e.g., corn-soy blend or wheat-soy blend with a micronutrient premix) have been distributed particularly by the World Food Program, UNICEF, and the US Agency for International Development. However, this may not be the best option for refeeding because these foods do not contain all nutrients required, contain relatively high quantities of antinutrients and fiber, are low in essential fatty acids, do not contain milk, and do not provide enough energy.

2. Ready-to-use supplementary foods (RUSFs) have been formulated for moderately undernourished children. These are basically modifications of RUTFs, such as Supplementary Plumpy (replaced dried milk by whey and soy protein isolates to reduce costs), Project Peanut Butter (peanut-soybean paste), Indian ready-to-use food for children, and baked biscuits. These products may be better than fortified blended foods, although their impact needs to be assessed.

3. Complementary food supplements are food-based complements added to foods just before consumption to improve nutritional value. Several provide essential micronutrients, amino acids, fatty acids, and/or enzymes (micronutrient powders; powdered supplements of protein, amino acids, and micronutrients), but they contain little additional energy. Others provide a substantial amount of energy (industrially produced complementary foods, 45-g [250-kcal] and 90-g [500-kcal] lipid-based nutrient supplements typically contain milk powder, oil, peanut paste, sugar, and micronutrients). Few data exist on their impact (60, 61), and cost-effectiveness is a challenge.

Severe Protein-Energy Malnutrition

If both options are available, management of children with SPEM can be based on ambulatory or inpatient programs, depending on status on admission (Table 68.3) (62). The presence of poor appetite or medical complications usually requires inpatient management. When inpatient programs are the only option, the goal is to achieve -1 Z WFH before discharge, which usually requires 2 to 6 weeks in a successful treatment regimen.

Patients in the OTP receive 200 kcal/kg/day of RUTF to eat at home in small frequent feedings (up to eight times a day) before eating other foods, except for breast milk if the mother is still breast-feeding. Children less than 6 months of age should not receive RUTF but breast-feeding and milk-based diets. All patients should also receive a course of oral broad-spectrum antibiotics, anthelmintic treatment, folic acid, and, if appropriate, vitamin A, measles vaccination, and antimalarial drugs. Patients should attend the OTP every week or two for medical evaluation, additional medical treatment if needed, and to receive enough RUTF to last until the next appointment (52). Health education given to caregivers is essential to ensure the child's recovery. When criteria for discharge have been met (see Table 68.3), OTP discharges should be sent to the SFP, where patients should stay for a minimum of 2 months.

TABLE 69.1	CORE AND SECONDARY TARGETS OF INBORN ERRORS OF METABOLISM WITH ONLINE MENDELIAN INHERITANCE IN MAN NUMBER RECOMMENDED FOR NEWBORN SCREENING, MARKER ANALYTES USED WITH TANDEM MASS SPECTROMETRY SCREENING, AND NUTRITION SUPPORT DURING DIAGNOSIS AND ACUTE THERAPY

INBORN ERROR (OMIM NO.)	MARKER ANALYTE	NUTRITION SUPPORT DURING DIAGNOSIS AND ACUTE ILLNESS
Core targets		
Amino acid disorder		
Argininosuccinic acidemia (No. 207900)	CIT	Rapid intervention is required Blood NH_3 >200 μmol/L Delete protein 1–2 d only; increase L-ARG and/or L-CIT if not arginase deficient If necessary, IV glucose and electrolytes at 150 mL/kg/24h to supply 10 mg/kg/min Give Pedialyte and sugar-sweetened, caffeine-free soft drinks with added Polycose or Moducal to maintain energy intake at 125%–150% of RDA Initiate oral medical food and complete diet as rapidly as tolerated Sodium benzoate, phenylbutyric acid, or phenylacetic acid is used to help decrease blood NH_3
Citrullinemia (No. 215700)	CIT	Rapid intervention is required Blood NH_3 >200 μmol/L Delete protein 1–2 d only; increase L-ARG if not arginase deficient If necessary, give IV glucose and electrolytes at 150 mL/kg/24h to supply 10 mg/kg/min Give Pedialyte and sugar-sweetened, caffeine-free soft drinks with added Polycose or Moducal to maintain energy intake at 125%–150% of RDA Initiate oral medical food and complete diet as rapidly as tolerated Sodium benzoate, phenylbutyric acid, or phenylacetic acid is used to help decrease blood NH_3
Homocystinuria (No. 236200)	MET	Maintain adequate hydration Administer 25–100 mg/kg pyridoxine in addition to usual infant formula for 1 mo to determine if patient is vitamin B_6 responsive If patient is not vitamin B_6 responsive, restrict MET (20 mg/kg) with medical food, folate, betaine, and complete diet at end of 1 mo
Maple syrup urine disease (MSUD) (Nos. 248600, 248611, 248610, 238339)	LEU ± VAL	Rapid intervention is required Delete BCAAs 1–2 d Correct metabolic acidosis and electrolyte abnormalities Provide adequate energy to suppress endogenous protein catabolism (125%–150% of RDA for age) Monitor hydration status, electrolyte status, and clinical symptoms carefully to prevent neurologic crisis. Add L-ILE to therapy within 1–2 d when plasma ILE concentration reaches ≈105 μmol/L Plasma LEU concentration remains elevated for prolonged period if either ILE or VAL is deficient Suspect concurrent sepsis Initiate oral medical food and complete diet as soon as tolerated
Phenylketonuria (PKU) (No. 261600)	PHE, PHE/TYR	Delete dietary PHE 1–2 d *only* For infant, offer Pedialyte with added Polycose to maintain electrolyte balance if needed If necessary, give IV glucose, electrolytes at 150 mL/kg/24h to supply a glucose infusion rate of 10 mg/kg/min, and amino acids free of PHE to maintain anabolism Give sugar-sweetened, caffeine-free soft drinks with added Polycose or Moducal to maintain energy intake at 100% of RDA Initiate oral medical food and complete diet as rapidly as tolerated
Tyrosinemia type I (TyrI) (No. 276700)	TYR	Rapid intervention is required Delete dietary PHE, TYR, 1–2 d *only* For infant, offer Pedialyte with added Polycose to maintain electrolyte balance if needed

(Continued)

TABLE 69.1	CORE AND SECONDARY TARGETS OF INBORN ERRORS OF METABOLISM WITH ONLINE MENDELIAN INHERITANCE IN MAN NUMBER RECOMMENDED FOR NEWBORN SCREENING, MARKER ANALYTES USED WITH TANDEM MASS SPECTROMETRY SCREENING, AND NUTRITION SUPPORT DURING DIAGNOSIS AND ACUTE THERAPY *(Continued)*

INBORN ERROR (OMIM NO.)	MARKER ANALYTE	NUTRITION SUPPORT DURING DIAGNOSIS AND ACUTE ILLNESS
		If necessary, give IV glucose and electrolytes at 150 mL/kg/24h to supply a glucose infusion rate of 10 mg/kg/min, and amino acids free of PHE and TYR to maintain anabolism Give sugar-sweetened, caffeine-free soft drinks with added Polycose or Moducal to maintain energy intake at 120%–130% of RDA Initiate oral medical food and complete diet as rapidly as tolerated
Fatty acid oxidation disorders		
Carnitine uptake deficiency (CUD) (No. 212140)	CO	Give uncooked cornstarch as needed to help prevent hypoglycemia if ≥6 mo of age Avoid fasting If necessary, give IV glucose at 150 mL/kg to supply a glucose infusion rate of 10 mg/kg/min At home, give frequent feedings of fluids containing 2.5 g carbohydrate per fluid ounce Initiate oral diet as rapidly as possible
Long-chain-hydroxy-acyl-CoA dehydrogenase deficiency (LCHAD) (No. 609016)	C16-OH; C18:1-OH,	Give uncooked cornstarch as needed to help prevent hypoglycemia if ≥6 mo of age Avoid fasting If necessary, give IV glucose at 150 mL/kg to supply a glucose infusion rate of 10 mg/kg/min At home, give frequent feedings of fluids containing 2.5 g carbohydrate per fluid ounce Initiate oral diet as rapidly as possible
Medium-chain acyl-CoA dehydrogenase deficiency (MCAD) (No. 201450)	C8/C10 ± C6, C10:1, C8	Give uncooked cornstarch as needed to help prevent hypoglycemia if ≥6 mo of age Avoid fasting If necessary, give IV glucose at 150 mL/kg to supply a glucose infusion rate of 10 mg/kg/min At home, give frequent feedings of fluids containing 2.5 g carbohydrate per fluid ounce Initiate oral diet as rapidly as possible Avoid medium-chain triglycerides
Trifunctional protein (TFP) deficiency (No. 609015)	C16-OH, C18:1-OH	Give uncooked cornstarch as needed to help prevent hypoglycemia if ≥6 mo of age Avoid fasting If necessary, give IV glucose at 150 mL/kg to supply a glucose infusion rate of 10 mg/kg/min At home, give frequent feedings of fluids containing 2.5 g carbohydrate per fluid ounce Initiate oral diet as rapidly as possible
Very-long-chain acyl-CoA dehydrogenase deficiency (VLCAD) (No. 201475)	C14:1, C14:1/C12:1 ± C14, C16, C18:1	Give uncooked cornstarch as needed to help prevent hypoglycemia if ≥6 mo of age Avoid fasting If necessary, give IV glucose at 150 mL/kg to supply a glucose infusion rate of 10 mg/kg/min At home, give frequent feedings of fluids containing 2.5 g carbohydrate per fluid ounce Initiate oral diet as rapidly as possible
Organic acid disorders		
β-Ketothiolase (BKT) deficiency[a] (No. 248600)	C5:1, ± C5OH	Delete dietary ILE 1–2 d only Administer L-carnitine Offer Pedialyte with Polycose to maintain electrolyte balance if needed Give IV glucose and electrolytes at 150 mL/kg/24h to supply a glucose infusion of 10 mg/kg/min, if required Give sugar-sweetened, caffeine-free soft drinks with added Polycose or Moducal to maintain energy intake at 100%–125% of RDA Initiate oral medical food and complete diet as rapidly as possible

TABLE 69.1	CORE AND SECONDARY TARGETS OF INBORN ERRORS OF METABOLISM WITH ONLINE MENDELIAN INHERITANCE IN MAN NUMBER RECOMMENDED FOR NEWBORN SCREENING, MARKER ANALYTES USED WITH TANDEM MASS SPECTROMETRY SCREENING, AND NUTRITION SUPPORT DURING DIAGNOSIS AND ACUTE THERAPY *(Continued)*

INBORN ERROR (OMIM NO.)	MARKER ANALYTE	NUTRITION SUPPORT DURING DIAGNOSIS AND ACUTE ILLNESS
β-Methylcrotonyl-CoA carboxylase (3MCC) deficiency[a] (No. 210200)	C5-OH, ± C5:1	Delete dietary LEU 1–2 d only Administer IV L-carnitine Provide vigorous fluid replacement Correct metabolic acidosis and electrolyte abnormalities Provide adequate energy to suppress catabolism (125%–150% of RDA for age) If necessary, give IV glucose, lipid, and L-amino acids free of LEU Initiate oral medical food and complete diet as rapidly as tolerated
Cobalamin A and B (Cbl A, B) defects[a] (Nos. 251100, 251110)	C3, C3/C2	Delete ILE, MET, THR, VAL 1–2 d *only* Initiate oral diet as rapidly as possible and administer pharmacologic doses of folate and IM hydroxycobalamin
Glutaric acidemia type I[a] (GA-I) (No. 231670)	C5-DC	Delete LYS and TRP 1–2 d *only* For infant, offer Pedialyte with added Polycose to maintain electrolyte balance if needed If necessary, give IV glucose and electrolytes at 150 mL/kg/24h to supply a glucose infusion of 10 mg/kg/min, and amino acids free of LYS and TRP Give sugar-sweetened, caffeine-free soft drinks with added Polycose or Moducal to maintain energy intake at 100% Initiate oral medical food and complete diet as rapidly as tolerated
HMG-CoA lyase deficiency[a] (No. 246450)	C5-OH, ± C6-DC	Rapid intervention is required Delete LEU 1–2 d only Limit fat intake Administer L-carnitine Vigorous replacement of fluids Correct severe metabolic acidosis and electrolyte abnormalities Provide adequate energy to suppress endogenous protein catabolism (125%–150% of RDA for age) Suspect concurrent sepsis: have a low threshold to treat after obtaining appropriate cultures Initiate oral medical food and complete diet as rapidly as tolerated
Isovaleric acidemia[a] (IVA) (No. 243500)	C5	Delete dietary LEU 1–2 d *only* Administer GLY and L-carnitine For infant, offer Pedialyte with Polycose to maintain electrolyte balance if needed Give sugar-sweetened, caffeine-free soft drinks with added Polycose or Moducal to maintain energy intake at 100%–125% of RDA If necessary, give IV glucose and electrolytes at 150 mL/kg/24h to supply a glucose infusion rate of 10 mg/kg/min, and amino acids free of LEU. Initiate oral medical food and complete diet as rapidly as tolerated
Methylmalonic acidemia[a] (MUT) (No. 251000)	C3, C3/C2	Rapid intervention is required Delete ILE, MET, THR, VAL 1–2 d *only* Administer L-carnitine Provide vigorous replacement of fluids Correct severe metabolic acidosis and electrolyte abnormalities; provide adequate energy to suppress endogenous protein catabolism (125%–150% of RDA for age) Suspect concurrent sepsis: have a low threshold to treat after obtaining appropriate cultures
Multiple carboxylase deficiency[a] (MCD) (No. 253260)	C5-OH, ± C3	Biotin, 10–20 mg/d For infant, offer Pedialyte with added Polycose to maintain electrolyte balance if needed If necessary, give IV glucose and electrolytes at 150 mL/kg/24h to supply a glucose infusion rate of 10 mg/kg/min Give sugar-sweetened, caffeine-free soft drinks with added Polycose or Moducal to maintain energy at 100%–125% of RDA Initiate complete diet as rapidly as tolerated

(Continued)

TABLE 69.1	CORE AND SECONDARY TARGETS OF INBORN ERRORS OF METABOLISM WITH ONLINE MENDELIAN INHERITANCE IN MAN NUMBER RECOMMENDED FOR NEWBORN SCREENING, MARKER ANALYTES USED WITH TANDEM MASS SPECTROMETRY SCREENING, AND NUTRITION SUPPORT DURING DIAGNOSIS AND ACUTE THERAPY *(Continued)*

INBORN ERROR (OMIM NO.)	MARKER ANALYTE	NUTRITION SUPPORT DURING DIAGNOSIS AND ACUTE ILLNESS
Propionic acidemia[a] (PPA) (No. 606054)	C3, C3/C2	Rapid intervention is required Delete ILE, MET, THR, VAL 1–2 d Administer L-carnitine Provide vigorous replacement of fluids Correct severe metabolic acidosis and electrolyte abnormalities Provide adequate energy to suppress endogenous protein catabolism (125%–150% of RDA for age) Suspect concurrent sepsis: have a low threshold to treat after obtaining appropriate cultures Initiate complete diet as rapidly as tolerated
Other disorders		
Biotinidase (BIOT deficiency (No. 253260)	±C5-OH, C5:1	Biotin, 10–20 mg/d For infant, offer Pedialyte with added Polycose to maintain electrolyte balance if needed Give sugar-sweetened, caffeine-free soft drinks with added Polycose or Modual to maintain energy at 100%–125% of RDA If necessary, give IV electrolytes and glucose at 150 mL/kg/24h to supply a glucose infusion rate of 10 mg/kg/min Initiate infant formula as rapidly as tolerated
Cystic fibrosis (CF) (No. 219700)		Refer to pediatric gastroenterologist
Galactose-1-phosphate uridyltransferase (GALT) deficiency[b] (No. 606999)		Avoid lactose- and galactose-containing infant formulas. Avoid drugs containing galactose or lactose
Secondary targets		
Amino acid disorders		
Argininemia (No. 107830)	ARG	Rapid intervention is required Blood NH$_3$ >200 μmol/L Delete protein 1–2 d *only* Give Pedialyte and sugar-sweetened, caffeine-free soft drinks with added Polycose or Modual to maintain energy intake at 125%–150% of RDA If necessary, give IV glucose and electrolytes at 150 mL/kg/24h to supply glucose at 10 mg/kg/min Initiate oral medical food and complete diet as rapidly as tolerated Sodium benzoate, phenylbutyric acid, or phenylacetic acid is used to help decrease blood NH$_3$
Biopterin regeneration (BIOPT REG) deficiency (No. 261630)	PHE, PHE/TYR	
Biopterin synthesis (BS) defect (No. 261630)	PHE, PHE/TYR	
Citrin deficiency (No. 603471)	CIT	High-protein, low-carbohydrate diet
Hypermethioninemia (No. 250850)	MET	Delete MET 1–2 d *only* Initiate oral medical food and complete diet as rapidly as tolerated
Hyperphenylalaninemia (No. 261630)	PHE	Delete dietary PHE 1–2 d *only* For infant, offer Pedialyte with added Polycose to maintain electrolyte balance if needed If necessary, give IV glucose, electrolytes at 150 mL/kg/24h to supply a glucose infusion rate of 10 mg/kg/min, and amino acids free of PHE to maintain anabolism Give sugar-sweetened, caffeine-free soft drinks with added Polycose or Modual to maintain energy intake at 100% of RDA Initiate oral medical food and complete diet as rapidly as tolerated

TABLE 69.1	CORE AND SECONDARY TARGETS OF INBORN ERRORS OF METABOLISM WITH ONLINE MENDELIAN INHERITANCE IN MAN NUMBER RECOMMENDED FOR NEWBORN SCREENING, MARKER ANALYTES USED WITH TANDEM MASS SPECTROMETRY SCREENING, AND NUTRITION SUPPORT DURING DIAGNOSIS AND ACUTE THERAPY *(Continued)*

INBORN ERROR (OMIM NO.)	MARKER ANALYTE	NUTRITION SUPPORT DURING DIAGNOSIS AND ACUTE ILLNESS
Tyrosinemia type II (TyrII) (No. 276600)	TYR	Delete dietary PHE, TYR, 1–2 d *only* For infant, offer Pedialyte with added Polycose to maintain electrolyte balance if needed; give sugar-sweetened, caffeine-free soft drinks with added Polycose or Moducal to maintain energy intake at 120%–130% of RDA If necessary, give IV glucose and electrolytes at 150 mL/kg/24h to supply a glucose infusion rate of 10 mg/kg/min, and amino acids free of PHE and TYR to maintain anabolism Initiate oral medical food and complete diet as rapidly as tolerated
Tyrosinemia type III (TyrIII) (No. 276710)	TYR	Delete dietary PHE, TYR, 1–2 d *only* For infant, offer Pedialyte with added Polycose to maintain electrolyte balance if needed If necessary, give IV glucose and electrolytes at 150 mL/kg/24h to supply a glucose infusion rate of 10 mg/kg/min, and amino acids free of PHE and TYR to maintain anabolism Give sugar-sweetened, caffeine-free soft drinks with added Polycose or Moducal to maintain energy intake at 120%–130% of RDA Initiate oral medical food and complete diet as rapidly as tolerated
Fatty acid oxidation disorders		
Carnitine acylcarnitine transporter (CACT) defect (No. 212138)	C16:1; C18:1	Rapid intervention is required Avoid fasting If necessary, give IV electrolyte and glucose at 150 mL/kg to supply a glucose infusion rate of 10 mg/kg/min. Give uncooked cornstarch as needed to help prevent hypoglycemia if ≥6 mo of age At home, give frequent feedings of fluids containing 2.5 g carbohydrate per fluid ounce Initiate oral diet as rapidly as possible
Carnitine palmitoyl-transferase I (CPT IA) defect (No. 600528)	Carnitine	Give uncooked cornstarch as needed to help prevent hypoglycemia if ≥6 mo of age Avoid fasting If necessary, give IV glucose at 150 mL/kg to supply a glucose infusion rate of 10 mg/kg/min At home, give frequent feedings of fluids containing 2.5 g carbohydrate per fluid ounce Initiate oral diet as rapidly as possible
Carnitine palmitoyl-transferase II (CPT II) defect (No. 255110)	C16:1, C18:1	Give uncooked cornstarch as needed to help prevent hypoglycemia if ≥6 mo of age Avoid fasting If necessary, give IV glucose at 150 mL/kg to supply a glucose infusion rate of 10 mg/kg/min At home, frequent feedings of fluids containing 2.5 g carbohydrate per fluid ounce Initiate oral diet as rapidly as possible
Dienoyl-CoA reductase deficiency (DE RED) (No. 222745)		Give uncooked cornstarch as needed to help prevent hypoglycemia if ≥6 mo of age Avoid fasting If necessary, give IV glucose at 150 mL/kg to supply a glucose infusion rate of 10 mg/kg/min At home, frequent feedings of fluids containing 2.5 g carbohydrate per fluid ounce Initiate oral diet as rapidly as possible
Glutaric acidemia type II[a] (GA-II) (Multiple acyl-CoA dehydrogenase deficiency) (No. 231680)	C4, C5, C5-DC, C6, 8, 12, 14, 16	Delete LYS and TRP 1–2 d *only* Restrict fat Administer L-carnitine and GLY Administer riboflavin Maintain anabolism, electrolyte balance and hydration Initiate oral medical food and complete diet as rapidly as tolerated

(Continued)

TABLE 69.1 CORE AND SECONDARY TARGETS OF INBORN ERRORS OF METABOLISM WITH ONLINE MENDELIAN INHERITANCE IN MAN NUMBER RECOMMENDED FOR NEWBORN SCREENING, MARKER ANALYTES USED WITH TANDEM MASS SPECTROMETRY SCREENING, AND NUTRITION SUPPORT DURING DIAGNOSIS AND ACUTE THERAPY *(Continued)*

INBORN ERROR (OMIM NO.)	MARKER ANALYTE	NUTRITION SUPPORT DURING DIAGNOSIS AND ACUTE ILLNESS
Medium-chain ketoacyl-CoA thiolase deficiency (MCKAT) (No. 602199)	C8, C8/C10, ±C6, C6, C10:1	Give uncooked cornstarch as needed to help prevent hypoglycemia if ≥6 mo of age Avoid fasting If necessary, give IV glucose at 150 mL/kg to supply a glucose infusion rate of 10 mg/kg/min At home, give frequent feedings of fluids containing 2.5 g carbohydrate per fluid ounce Initiate oral diet as rapidly as possible
Medium-/short-chain hydroxyacyl-CoA dehydrogenase deficiency (M/SCHAD) (No. 300256)	C4-OH	Give uncooked cornstarch as needed to help prevent hypoglycemia if ≥6 mo of age Avoid fasting If necessary, give IV glucose at 150 mL/kg to supply a glucose infusion rate of 10 mg/kg/min At home, give frequent feedings of fluids containing 2.5 g carbohydrate per fluid ounce Initiate oral diet as rapidly as possible
Short-chain acyl-CoA dehydrogenase deficiency (SCAD) (No. 201470)	C4	Give uncooked cornstarch as needed to help prevent hypoglycemia if ≥6 mo of age Avoid fasting If necessary, give IV glucose at 150 mL/kg to supply a glucose infusion rate of 10 mg/kg/min At home, give frequent feedings of fluids containing 2.5 g carbohydrate per fluid ounce Initiate oral diet as rapidly as possible
Organic acid disorders		
2-Methyl-3-hydroxybutyric acidemia (2M3HBA)	C5, C5:1, C5-OH	Delete dietary ILE 1–2 d *only* Administer L-carnitine Offer Pedialyte with Polycose to maintain electrolyte balance if needed Give IV glucose and electrolytes at 150 mL/kg/24h to supply a glucose infusion rate of 10 mg/kg/min, if required Give sugar-sweetened, caffeine-free soft drinks with added Polycose or Modual to maintain energy intake at 100%–125% of RDA Initiate oral medical food and complete diet as rapidly as tolerated
2-Methylbutyryl-CoA dehydrogenase deficiency (2MBG) (No. 600006)	C5	? LEU restriction
3-Methylglutaconyl hydratase deficiency[a] (3MGA) (No. 250950)	C5-OH	Delete dietary LEU 1–2 d *only* Administer IV L-carnitine Provide vigorous fluid replacement Correct metabolic acidosis and electrolyte abnormalities Provide adequate energy to suppress catabolism (125%–150% of RDA for age) If necessary, give IV glucose, lipid, and L-amino acids free of LEU Return to oral medical food and complete diet as rapidly as tolerated
Cobalamin C and D (Cbl C, D) defects[a] (Nos. 277410, 277400)	C3/C2	Delete ILE, MET, THR, VAL 1–2 d *only* Initiate oral diet as rapidly as possible and administer pharmacologic doses of folate and IM hydroxycobalamin
Isobutyryl-CoA dehydrogenase deficiency (IBG) (No. 611283)	C4	Delete dietary LEU 1–2 d *only* Increase GLY, VAL and L-carnitine For infant, offer Pedialyte with Polycose to maintain electrolyte balance if needed If necessary, give IV glucose and electrolytes at 150 mL/kg/24h to supply a glucose infusion rate of 10 mg/kg/min, and amino acids free of LEU Give sugar-sweetened, caffeine-free soft drinks with added Polycose or Modual to maintain energy intake at 100%–125% of RDA Initiate oral medical food and complete diet as rapidly as tolerated

TABLE 69.1	CORE AND SECONDARY TARGETS OF INBORN ERRORS OF METABOLISM WITH ONLINE MENDELIAN INHERITANCE IN MAN NUMBER RECOMMENDED FOR NEWBORN SCREENING, MARKER ANALYTES USED WITH TANDEM MASS SPECTROMETRY SCREENING, AND NUTRITION SUPPORT DURING DIAGNOSIS AND ACUTE THERAPY *(Continued)*	
INBORN ERROR (OMIM NO.)	**MARKER ANALYTE**	**NUTRITION SUPPORT DURING DIAGNOSIS AND ACUTE ILLNESS**
Malonic (MAL) acidemia (No. 248360)	C3	Restrict fat Administer L-carnitine and medium-chain triglycerides Avoid fasting Give uncooked cornstarch as needed to help prevent hypoglycemia if ≥6 mo of age If necessary, give IV glucose at 150 mL/kg to supply a glucose infusion rate of 10 mg/kg/min At home, give frequent feedings of fluids containing 2.5 g carbohydrate per fluid ounce Initiate oral diet as rapidly as possible
Other disorders		
Galactokinase (GALK) deficiency[b] (No. 230200)		Same as for normal infant Avoid formula, food, and drugs containing galactose or lactose Initiate oral diet as rapidly as tolerated
Galactose epimerase (GALE) deficiency[b] (No. 230350)		Same as for normal infant Avoid formula, food, and drugs containing galactose or lactose Initiate oral feedings as soon as tolerated

Colon (:) followed by number, double bonds; ARG, arginine; BCAA, branched-chain amino acid; C, acyl group or carbon chain; CIT, citrulline; CoA, coenzyme A; DC, dicarboxyl; GLY, glycine; HMG-CoA, 3-hydroxy-3-methylglutaryl-coenzyme A; ILE, isoleucine; IM, intramuscular; IV, intravenous; LEU, leucine; LYS, lysine; MET, methionine; NH3, ammonia; O, oxygen; OH, hydroxy; OMIM, Online Mendelian Inheritance in Man; PHE, phenylalanine; RDA, recommended dietary allowance; THR, theronine; TRP, tryptophan; TYR, tyrosine; VAL, valine.

[a]One or more amino acids involved in disorder.
[b]Screened for by measuring blood galactose.

Data from references 2 and 12 to 20, with permission.

produced by mutant proteins. This therapeutic mechanism is exemplified in PKU, homocystinuria, and MSUD. Tetrahydrobiopterin (BH$_4$ [Kuvan]) is available as a drug for therapy of patients with non-PKU hyperphenylalaninemia to enhance PAH activity (37). Pharmacologic intake of vitamin B$_6$ in homocystinuria or vitamin B$_1$ in MSUD increases intracellular pyridoxal phosphate or thiamin pyrophosphate (TPP) and increases the specific activity of CβS or BCKAD complex, respectively (38–41). Another approach is to provide chemical chaperones to stabilize mutant proteins. For example, excess intravenous infusion of D-galactose has increased defective α-galactosidase in the cardiac variant of Fabry disease (42).

8. Replacing deficient coenzymes. Various vitamin-dependent disorders are caused by blocks in coenzyme production and are "cured" by lifetime pharmacologic intake of a specific vitamin precursor. This mechanism presumably involves overcoming a partially impaired enzyme reaction by mass action. If reactions that are required to produce methylcobalamin (CH$_3$-B$_{12}$) or adenosylcobalamin are impaired, homocystinuria or methylmalonic aciduria (or both) will result. Daily intake of milligram quantities of vitamin B$_{12}$ may cure both disorders (43). In biotinidase deficiency, the coenzyme biotin is not released from its covalently bound state. Reviews of "vitamin-dependency syndromes" have been published (39–41).

9. Artificially inducing enzyme production. If the structural gene or enzyme is intact, but suppressor, enhancer, or promoter elements are not functional, abnormal amounts of enzyme may be produced. It should be possible to "turn on" or "turn off" the structural gene and enable normal enzymatic production to occur. PAH activity has been induced in patients diagnosed with PKU when they received PHE loading for 3 days with intact protein (44, 45). Polyethylene glycol–coated phenylalanine ammonia lyase is undergoing clinical studies in patients with PKU to determine efficacy and allergenicity (46). In the acute porphyria of type I tyrosinemia, excessive δ-aminolevulinic acid (δ-ALA) production may be reduced by suppressing transcription of the δ-ALA synthase gene with excess glucose (GLU) and hematin (Figs. 69.1 and 69.2). In type I tyrosinemia, the overproduction of succinylacetone may be "turned off" by blocking an earlier enzyme *p*-OH-phenylpyruvate oxidase with the drug NBTC.

10. Replacing enzymes. Many attempts to replace deficient enzymes by plasma infusion and microencapsulation have been tried, with limited success. The use of polyethylene glycol coating of adenosine deaminase significantly prolonged the biologic half-life of this enzyme in treating severe combined immunodeficiency (47). The engineering of β-glucosidase with a high mannan receptor site enables intravenous use of

TABLE 69.2 CHROMOSOMAL LOCATION, GENE SIZE, NUMBER OF MUTATIONS, TISSUE DISTRIBUTION OF GENES, AND GENOTYPE/PHENOTYPE CORRELATIONS

ENZYME	CHROMOSOMAL LOCATION	GENE SIZE (kb)	NUMBER OF MUTATIONS	TISSUE DISTRIBUTION	GENOTYPE/ PHENOTYPE CORRELATION
Enzymes of amino acid metabolism					
Phenylalanine hydroxylase	12q22-q24.1	>90	>500	Liver, kidney	Genotype broadly predicts metabolic and clinical phenotype
Dihydropteridine reductase	4p15.1-p16.1		21	Liver, fibroblasts, erythrocytes, leukocytes, platelets	?
Guanosine triphosphate cyclohydrolase	14q22.1-q22.2	30	42	Liver	None
6-Pyruvoyltetrahydropterin synthase	11q22.3-q23.3	?	>28	Liver, erythrocytes	Genotype associated with phenotype
Pterin-4 α-carbinolamine dehydratase	10q22		7	Lymphocytes, scalp hair root cells	Mild phenotypes
Fumarylacetoacetate hydrolyase	15q23-q25		34	Liver, renal tubules, lymphocytes, erythrocytes	Genotype not clearly associated with phenotype
Maleylacetoacetate isomerase	14q24.3	?	3	Liver, fibroblasts, kidney	?
Tyrosine aminotransferase	16q22.1	10.9	15	Liver, kidney	None
4-Hydroxyphenylpyruvate dioxygenase	12q24-qter	21	?	Liver	?
Cystathionine β-synthase	21q22.3	30	30	Liver, fibroblasts, brain, phytohemagglutinin-stimulated lymphocytes, amniotic fluid cells, chorionic villus cells	Genotype associated with phenotype I278T: vitamin B_6 responsive T353M: African, not vitamin B_6 responsive G307S: Celtic, not-vitamin B_6 responsive
Methionine-S-adenosyltransferase	10q22	20	17	Liver (22, 28)	Genotype not clearly associated with phenotype
Enzymes of organic acid metabolism					
Branched-Chain α-Ketoacid Dehydrogenase Complex					
E1α (decarboxylase)	19q13.3	55	12	Liver, fibroblasts, leukocytes, muscle	Y393W (Mennonite) (classic phenotype)
E1β (stabilizes E1α)	6q1.4	100	4	Liver, fibroblasts, leukocytes, muscle	11bp del → stop
E2 (transacylase)	1p31	68	6	Liver, fibroblasts, leukocytes, muscle	E163X R183P, common in Ashkenazi?
E3 (lipoamide dehydrogenase)	7p22	20	10	Liver, fibroblasts, leukocytes, muscle	Affects pyruvate and α-ketoglutarate dehydrogenases as well
E1α kinase (inactivating)	16p13.12	40	2	Liver, fibroblasts, leukocytes, muscle	Inhibited by tumor necrosis factor α and produces cancer cachexia
E1α phosphatase (activating)	?	?	?	Liver, fibroblasts, leukocytes, muscle	Actives branched-chain-α-ketoacid dehydrogenase complex
Isovaleryl-CoA dehydrogenase	15q14-q15	2.1–4.6	20	Liver, fibroblasts	Genotype not associated with phenotype
3-Methylcrotonyl-CoA carboxylase	?	?	?	Fibroblasts, lymphocytes	Genotype associated with phenotype
3-Methylglutaconyl-CoA-hydratase (type 1)	?	?	?	Fibroblasts, lymphocytes	?
3-Hydroxy-3-methylglutaryl-CoA lyase (HMG-CoA lyase)	1p35.1.36.1	?	?	Liver	Genotype associated with phenotype

ENZYME	CHROMOSOMAL LOCATION	GENE SIZE (kb)	NUMBER OF MUTATIONS	TISSUE DISTRIBUTION	GENOTYPE/ PHENOTYPE CORRELATION
2-Methylbutyryl-CoA dehydrogenase (Acyl-CoA dehydrogenase-SBCAD)	10q26.13	20	>12	Fibroblasts (15, 21)	None reported
Multiple carboxylase (Holocarboxylase synthetase)	?	?	>30	Liver, fibroblasts, leukocytes (32)	Genotype associated with phenotype
Glutaryl-CoA dehydrogenase	19p13.2	7	>90	Liver, kidney, fibroblasts, leukocytes, amniotic fluid cells, chorionic villus cells.	None between genotype and clinical severity Specific mutations correlate with severity of organic aciduria
Propionyl-CoA carboxylase				Heart, kidney, liver cells	None
α-Subunit	13q32	100	?		
β-Subunit	3q13.3q22	?	?		
Methylmalonyl-CoA mutase	6p12-p21.2	?	22	Kidney, liver, placenta cells	Genotype associated with phenotype
Biotinidase	3p25	?	>100	Serum leukocytes, fibroblasts (25)	None reported
β-Ketothiolase (mitochondrial acetoacetyl-CoA thiolase)	11q22.3-q23.1	1.5	>40	Liver (26)	None reported
2-Methyl-3-hydroxybutyryl-CoA dehydrogenase	XP11.2 H517B10 gene (35)	1.3	?	All human tissue Highest in liver and kidney	?
Isobutyrl-CoA dehydrogenase	ACAD8gene			Fibroblasts	
Malonyl-CoA decarboxylase	MLYCD gene (30)		22	Fibroblasts (29)	None reported
Cobalamin A	4q31.21	?	?	Liver, skeletal muscle (24)	?
Cobalamin B	12q24 (24)	1.1	?	Liver, skeletal muscle, fibroblasts (36)	?
Cobalamin C	1P34.1 MMACHC protein (34)	?	>42	Fibroblasts	None reported
Cobalamin D	2q23.2 MMADHC protein (23)			Fibroblasts (27)	None reported
Enzymes of nitrogen metabolism					
Mitochondrial					
Carbamylphosphate synthetase 1	2q35	122	>32	Liver, intestine, kidney (trace)	Genotype associated with phenotype
N-acetylglutamate synthetase	17q21.31	?	?	Liver, intestine, kidney (trace), spleen	Genotype associated with phenotype
Ornithine transcarbamylase	Xp21.1	73	>230	Liver, intestine, kidney (trace)	Genotype associated with phenotype
Citrin	7q21.3	?	30	Liver, kidney, heart, small intestine (31, 33)	?
Cytosol					
Argininosuccinate synthetase	9q34.1 (many pseudogenes) 7cen-q11.2	53	14	Liver, kidney, fibroblasts, brain (trace)	Genotype associated with phenotype
Argininosuccinate lyase	?	?	12	Liver, kidney, brain, fibroblasts	Genotype associated with phenotype
Arginase	6q23	13	2	Liver, erythrocytes, lens, brain (trace)	Genotype associated with phenotype
Enzymes of galactose metabolism					
Galactose-4-epimerase	1p36-35	4	9	Erythrocytes, fibroblasts, liver	Unclear
Galactokinase	17p24	7.3	13	Liver	Cataracts only
Galactose-1-phosphate uridyltransferase	9p13	4.3	>150	Erythrocytes, leukocytes, fibroblasts, intestinal mucosa, liver	Genotype associated with phenotype Q188R (white) S135L (black), Δ5 kb (Ashkenazi)

CoA, coenzyme A.

TABLE 69.3	APPROXIMATE DAILY REQUIREMENTS FOR SELECTED NUTRIENTS[a] BY INFANTS AND CHILDREN WITH SELECTED INHERITED DISORDERS OF AMINO ACID AND ORGANIC ACID METABOLISM

		AGE						
NUTRIENT	UNIT	0 < 6 mo	6 < 12 mo	1 < 4 y	4 < 7 y	7 < 11 y	11 < 15 y	15 < 19 y
Energy	kcal/kg	145–95	135–80	—	—	—	—	—
	kcal/d	—	—	1,300	1,700	2,400	2,200–2,700	2,100–1,800
	(range)			900–1,800	1,300–2,300	1,650–3,300	1,500–3,700	1,200–3,900
Fluid	mL/kg[b]	160–135	145–120	95	90	75	50–55	50–65
Protein[c]	g/kg	3.5–3.0	3.0–2.5	—	—	—	—	—
	g/d	—	—	30–55	35–65	40–75	50–90	50–95
Fat	g/d	31	30	—	—	—	—	—
Linoleic acid	g/d	4.4	4.6	7.0	10	10–12	16	16
α-Linolenic acid	g/d	0.5	0.5	0.7	0.9	1.0–1.2	1.0–1.2	1.1–1.6
Isoleucine[d]								
MSUD[d]	mg/kg	90–30	90–30	85–20	80–20	30–20	30–20	30–10
PPA/MMA[d]	mg/kg	100–70	90–60	80–50	70–40	60–30	50–25	40–20
Leucine[d]								
MSUD[d]	mg/kg	100–60	75–40	70–40	65–35	60–30	50–30	41–15
Isovaleric acidemia[d]	mg/kg	150–70	130–70	100–60	90–50	80–40	70–30	60–25
Lysine[d]								
GA-I[d]	mg/kg	100–70	90–40	80–30	75–25	65–25	60–20	55–15
Methionine[d]								
HCU[d]	mg/kg	35–20	35–15	30–10	20–10	20–10	20–10	10–5
PPA/MMA[d]	mg/kg	50–30	45–25	40–20	35–15	30–10	25–10	20–10
Phenylalanine[d],								
PKU[d]	mg/kg	70–20	50–15	40–15	35–15	30–15	30–15	30–10
Tyrosinemias[d]	mg/kg	95–45	90–35	85–30	80–25	70–20	70–20	65–15
Threonine[d]								
PPA/MMA[d]	mg/kg	80–50	70–40	60–30	55–25	50–25	45–25	40–25
Tyrosine[d]								
PKU[d]	mg/kg	350–300	300–250	230	175	140	110–120	110–120
Tyrosinemias	mg/kg	95–45	75–30	60–30	50–25	40–20	30–15	30–10
Tryptophan[d]								
GA-I	mg/kg	40–10	30–10	20–10	15–8	10–6	8–5	8–4
Valine[d]								
MSUD	mg/kg	95–40	60–30	85–30	50–30	30–25	30–20	30–15
PPA/MMA	mg/kg	85–50	80–45	75–45	70–40	60–30	60–30	50–30

GA-I, glutaric acidemia type I; HCU, homocystinuria; MMA, methylmalonic acidemia; MSUD, maple syrup urine disease; PKU, phenylketonuria; PPA, propionic acidemia.

[a]All known essential amino acids, essential fatty acids, minerals, and vitamins must be provided in adequate amounts.

[b]At least 1.5 mL of fluid should be offered for each kilocalorie of energy ingested by the infant and 1 mL/kcal by children and adults.

[c]Mean daily protein intake by physiologically normal children by age is as follows: 2 < 4 years, 54.9 g; 4 < 9 years, 66.1 g; 9 < 4 years, 80.9 g; 14 < 19 ayears, 96.5 g.

[d]After 1 to 2 days of deleting appropriate amino acids, introduce those amino acids at the maximum noted for age. Monitor plasma concentrations frequently, and modify the amino acid prescription appropriately.

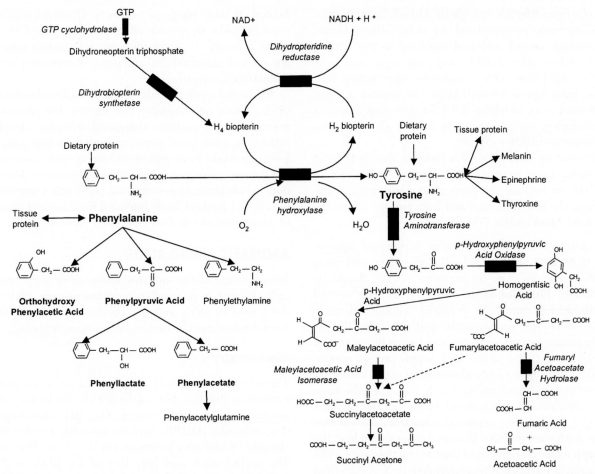

Fig. 69.1. Metabolism of aromatic amino acids. The metabolic flow and nutrient interaction in disorders of phenylalanine and tyrosine are diagrammed. The *black bars* represent impaired enzymes in biopterin biosynthesis, phenylketonuria, and tyrosinemia. *GTP,* guanosine triphosphate; *NAD,* nicotinamide adenine dinucleotide (NADH is the reduced form).

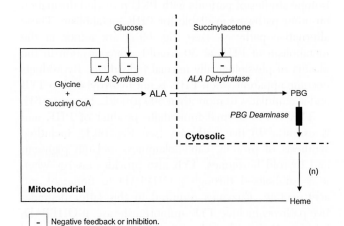

☐ – Negative feedback or inhibition.

Fig. 69.2. Inhibition site in heme biosynthesis of relevance to diagnosis and treatment of tyrosinemia type I. The *black bar* represents the partial block in acute intermittent porphyria with resultant overproduction of δ-aminolevulinic acid (δ-ALA) and porphobilinogen (PBG) with decreased heme biosynthesis. In type I tyrosinemia, succinylacetone is produced and inhibits δ-ALA dehydratase with accumulation of δ-ALA alone, which is neurotoxic. δ-ALA accumulation can be reduced by addition of excess dietary glucose (GLU) and by hematin infusions that negatively control δ-ALA synthase at levels of both enzyme and gene expression. *CoA,* coenzyme A.

alglucerase (Ceredase) to treat type I Gaucher disease. Human α-galactosidase A replacement therapy in Fabry disease reverses substrate storage in the lysosome (42). Recombinant human α-glucosidase can prevent progression and improve cardiac and muscle function in Pompe disease (48). Polyethylene glycol–coated phenylalanine ammonia lyase is undergoing clinical studies in patients with PKU to determine efficacy and allergenicity (46).

11. Transplanting organs. Liver transplantation in a host of inherited metabolic disorders benefits systemic metabolism; the return of organ function replaces deficient enzyme activity (49, 50). Bone marrow and kidney transplantations are also of benefit.

12. Correcting the underlying defect in DNA so the body can manufacture its own functionally normal enzymes. The DNA for many proteins that are functionally deficient such as adenosine deaminase, hypoxanthine-guanine phosphoribosyl transferase, and ornithine transcarbamylase (OTC) and the low-density lipoprotein cholesterol receptor have been cloned, and retroviral constructs containing their cDNA have been transfected into dividing somatic

cells from affected individuals. Human gene therapy is currently contemplated for these inborn errors, although several technical problems in the toxicity of vectors, gene stability, and gene expression must be solved first. Other molecular approaches such as homologous recombination to correct mutant sequences or to inhibit RNA for dominant disorders producing antagonism to the normal allele are also future possibilities (51, 52).

13. Preventing absorption of a nutrient that is toxic in excess. Large neutral amino acids (LNAAs) free of PHE are available for preventing absorption of PHE from the intestinal tract and from passage across the blood–brain barrier (53).

Nutrition management remains a principal component in treating all these inherited disorders, and some practical considerations for nutrition support should be considered. Foremost is the need to maintain normal growth, which cannot be achieved without adequate intake of energy, amino acids, and nitrogen. Energy requirements are greater than normal when intact protein is restricted and free amino acids supply protein equivalent (54). Free amino acids administered in one daily dose are oxidized to a much greater extent than when the same dose is divided and administered throughout the day (55). Nitrogen balance was improved considerably when free amino acids were ingested in several doses throughout the day with intact protein rather than in one dose (56). With total protein intakes (protein equivalent [g N × 6.25 from free amino acids = g protein equivalent] plus intact protein) 25% or more greater than RDA for intact protein for age (1) and closer to actual intakes by physiologically normal children in the United States (57), patients with PKU in the United States have grown normally in height (58). If adequate energy and amino acids cannot be ingested to support normal growth through oral feedings, then nasogastric, gastrostomy, or parenteral feedings should be used. Failure to adapt nutrient intake to the individual needs of each patient can result in mental retardation, metabolic crises, neurologic crises, growth failure, and, with some inherited metabolic diseases, death. When specific amino acids or nitrogen require restriction, total deletion of the toxic nutrient for 1 to 3 days in the presence of excess energy intake is the best approach to initiating therapy. Longer deletion or overrestriction may precipitate deficiency of the amino acids or nitrogen. Because the most limiting nutrient in the diet determines growth rate, overrestriction of an amino acid, nitrogen, or energy will result in further intolerance of the toxic nutrients.

Diet restrictions to correct imbalances in metabolic relationships require the use of elemental medical foods. These medical foods must be accompanied by small amounts of intact protein that supply the restricted amino acids. Intact proteins seldom supply more than 50%, and often supply much less, of the protein requirements of patients. Nitrogen-free foods that provide energy are limited in their range of nutrients. Consequently, care must be taken to provide all nutrients required in adequate amounts (1), particularly because certain minerals are not well absorbed (59) and some vitamins may not be metabolized normally.

Elemental medical foods consist of small molecules that often provide an osmolality that exceeds the physiologic tolerance of the patient. Abdominal cramping, diarrhea, distention, nausea, and vomiting result from hyperosmolar feedings. Aside from gastrointestinal distress, more serious consequences can occur, such as hypertonic dehydration, hypovolemia, hypernatremia, and death. Osmolalities of selected medical foods intended for inherited diseases of amino acid metabolism have been published (60).

AROMATIC AMINO ACIDS

Inborn errors of the aromatic amino acids were historically the first to respond to nutrition support. PKU was discovered in 1933, and the prevention of its resultant mental retardation by dietary intervention is classic.

Biochemistry

The essential amino acid PHE is used for tissue protein synthesis and hydroxylation to form TYR. The hydroxylation reaction requires PAH, oxygen (O_2), BH_4, dihydropteridine reductase (DHPR), and nicotinamide adenine dinucleotide (NAD) plus hydrogen ion (H+) (see Fig. 69.1). The normal adult uses only 10% of the RDA for PHE for new protein synthesis, and approximately 90% is hydroxylated to form TYR. The growing child uses 60% of the required PHE for new protein synthesis, and 40% is hydroxylated to form TYR. Mass spectrometry and stable isotope studies of patients with PKU provide information on other pathways available for PHE metabolism. These alternative pathways (see Fig. 69.1) are minor in the metabolism of PHE at 50 μmol/L concentration in the plasma of physiologically normal individuals. Byproducts become apparent when PHE is not hydroxylated to TYR and accumulates to more than 500 μmol/L, however (61).

TYR is the normal immediate product of PHE and is essential to five pathways (see Fig. 69.1), including synthesis of protein, catecholamines, melanin pigment, and thyroid hormones. TYR also provides energy when it is catabolized through p-OHPPAD to fumarate and acetoacetate. Enzymes required in this latter degradative pathway include TYR aminotransferase, p-OHPPAD, homogentisic acid oxidase, and fumarylacetoacetic acid hydrolase (FAH) (see Fig. 69.1).

Phenylketonuria

PKU is a group of inherited disorders of PHE metabolism caused by impaired PAH activity. The disease is expressed at 3 to 6 months of age and is characterized by developmental delay, microcephaly, abnormal electroencephalogram (EEG), eczema, musty odor, and

differentiating between ingestion of inadequate calories and excess PHE intake, respectively.

PHE deficiency associated with inadequate PHE intake has three specific stages of development (96, 97). The first stage is characterized biochemically by decreased blood and urine PHE. Clinically, the child may appear normal, lethargic, or anorectic and may fail to gain length or weight. In the older child, increases in blood alanine and β-hydroxybutyric and acetoacetic acidemia result from muscle alanine production and β-lipolysis. In the second stage, blood PHE concentrations increase as a result of muscle protein degradation, although blood TYR concentrations may be low. BCAA concentrations may increase with decreases in other plasma amino acids. Aminoaciduria appears because of renal tubular malabsorption. In this stage, body protein stores are catabolized, energy sources are depleted, and active membrane transport functions are impaired. Eczema is common. In the third stage of PHE deficiency, blood PHE concentration is lower than normal, as are concentrations of other amino acids. Accompanying clinical manifestations include failure to grow, osteopenia, anemia, sparse hair, and, finally, death if the deficiency is not corrected by supplemental dietary PHE and TYR.

Insufficient protein intake results in an inadequate supply of essential amino acids or nitrogen for growth. When protein synthesis is decreased, PHE is no longer used for growth and accumulates in the blood. When catabolism occurs because of a prolonged lack of nitrogen or amino acid intake, the blood PHE concentration increases because tissue protein contains some 5.5% PHE. In instances of protein insufficiency, medical food intake should be increased to supply the required nitrogen or essential amino acids.

Energy, the first requirement of the body, is necessary for growth. When energy is provided as carbohydrate and fat, and if adequate nitrogen is available, nonessential amino acids may be synthesized from their ketoacid precursors. Further, carbohydrate ingestion leads to insulin secretion; and insulin promotes amino acid transport into the cell and consequent protein synthesis (97). When energy intake is inadequate, tissue catabolism occurs to meet energy needs. Such catabolism releases PHE, thus leading to an elevated blood PHE concentration. Sufficient energy must be provided through generous but not excess use of nonprotein and low-protein foods to ensure a normal growth rate.

A low blood PHE concentration (<25 μmol/L) may lead to depressed appetite (98), decreased growth (99), and if prolonged, mental retardation (84). Low blood PHE concentrations are often caused by inadequate prescription of PHE. In such cases, the prescription for PHE can be increased by the addition of measured amounts of intact protein.

Assessment of Nutrition Support.   Along with biweekly assessment of growth through measurement

of length, weight, and head circumference (HC) and evaluation of development, the adequacy of PHE and TYR intake is determined by twice-weekly quantitation of plasma PHE and TYR concentrations during the first 6 months and weekly thereafter until the child is 1 year of age. The first year is the period of most rapid growth and of greatest vulnerability to nutrition insult. After 1 year of age, weekly blood tests suffice for monitoring the diet. If plasma PHE concentrations exceed 300 μmol/L (5 mg/dL), the prescription for PHE is decreased, and frequent blood tests are done until plasma PHE concentrations are between 60 and 300 μmol/L.

For blood tests to be of use in adjusting the prescription, laboratory analyses must be both accurate and prompt. Fluorometric, ion-exchange, high-performance liquid chromatography, and MS/MS methods are quantitative and are preferred to monitor plasma PHE and TYR concentrations. If properly instructed, parents may be given responsibility for obtaining the specimens on filter paper or in microcapillary tubes and mailing them to a central laboratory.

A record of food ingested before blood sampling for PHE and TYR measurement is essential and should be kept by the child's caregiver. The correlation among (a) the child's intake of PHE, TYR, protein, and energy; (b) the child's clinical status; and (c) the plasma PHE and TYR concentrations is considered when the diet is altered.

Results of Therapy.   Early diagnosis and treatment (before 2 weeks of age) of infants with PKU with a nutritionally adequate, PHE-restricted, TYR-supplemented diet promotes normal growth and prevents mental retardation. A national study showed that mean height, weight, HC, IQ scores of children who were treated early were the same as those of physiologically normal children at 4 years of age (100, 101). Trefz et al (81) reported that when blood PHE concentration was maintained at less than 360 μmol/L, no difference was observed in mean IQ by genotype of 9-year-old children.

The semisynthetic nature of the PHE-restricted diet has led to questions concerning its adequacy. Mean serum carnitine (total and free) of treated patients was in the reference range when patients were fed medical foods containing carnitine (102, 103). Medical foods containing increased amounts of L-TYR have alleviated the problem of low plasma TYR concentrations (104, 105). After an overnight fast, the concentrations of plasma GLY were elevated in patients, one group of whom received a GLY-free medical food (Periflex; Nutricia North America, Gaithersburg, MD) (106). Treated patients with PKU often have lower-than-normal concentrations of transthyretin when they are fed the RDA for protein (107). Arnold et al (108) and Acosta et al (95) reported a positive correlation between height and plasma transthyretin with concentrations less than 200 mg/L associated with poor linear growth.

Depressed plasma concentrations of total cholesterol have been reported in treated children and untreated adults with PKU (109–111). Pregnant women with PKU whose serum cholesterol concentrations failed to increase during early gestation often had a spontaneous abortion (112), possibly because of an inadequate hormonal response to pregnancy. Castillo et al (113) reported inhibition of brain and liver 3-hydroxy-3-methylglutaryl-CoA (HMG-CoA) reductase and mevalonate-5-pyrophosphate decarboxylase in experimental hyperphenylalaninemia. According to Artuch et al (114), elevated plasma PHE concentrations resulted in decreased serum ubiquinone 10 concentrations. Hargreaves et al (115), however, found no difference in mononuclear cell coenzyme Q_{10} concentrations among control, treated, and untreated patients with PKU. Lower-than-normal plasma and erythrocyte docosahexaenoic acid concentrations and higher-than-normal n-6 series fatty acid concentrations have been found in patients undergoing therapy for PKU (116, 117). The significance of these differences is unclear, but they appear to be the result of the low fat content of the medical food (118, 119).

Iron deficiency has been reported in children undergoing therapy for PKU despite intakes greater than the RDA (120, 121). A poor selenium status has been found in children with PKU who were receiving medical foods without added selenium (122). Patients with PKU and low selenium concentrations had elevated concentrations of thyroxine and reverse triiodothyronine, which decreased significantly with selenium supplementation (123). Plasma retinol concentrations of children with PKU are often lower than concentrations in normal children (107), but they are within reference ranges with adequate medical food intake (91).

Bone changes were reported as early as 1956 in treated children with PKU. Preschool children with plasma PHE concentrations within treatment range had normal bone mineralization (124–127). Greeves et al (128) reported that 25% of patients with PKU, most of whom were more than 8 years of age, had a history of fractures compared with 18% of physiologically normal siblings. Untreated PKU mice (PAH^{enu-2}) had reduced mean femur weight compared with treated and control mice and shorter mean femur length than control mice. Femur strength was greater in treated mice compared with control mice (129). Elevated serum prolactin concentrations in patients with poorly controlled PKU resulted in a high prevalence of menstrual irregularities in the girls (130). As blood PHE concentration increased in older patients under poor dietary control, values for bone mineral content and bone density were always lower than control values. Amino acid imbalances, inadequate protein intake, the need for phosphorus to buffer organic acids made from excess dietary PHE, and inadequate estrogen because of excess prolactin secretion could have contributed to bone abnormalities (131). Mussa et al (132) reported that as plasma PHE concentrations increased, osteoclastogenesis increased, leading to bone damage.

Mean plasma concentrations of immunoglobulin A and immunoglobulin M were significantly lower in patients with PKU undergoing therapy (133) than in physiologically normal children.

Diet Discontinuation.   In the past, certain clinicians suggested that the diet could be discontinued at 4, 6, or 12 years of age with no adverse effects (134–137). Investigators questioned this possibility because studies showed significant differences in performance and intelligence in children (101, 138) and in neurologic function in adults who discontinued the diet and in those who remained on the diet. Severe agoraphobia (139), reversible by a return to the PHE-restricted diet, was also reported in adults. Vitamin B_{12} deficiency resulting in hematologic changes and neurologic disease occurs in off-diet patients who refuse foods of animal origin but who fail to ingest PHE-free medical foods (140, 141). Vegan-type methylmalonic aciduria from vitamin B_{12} deficiency is the most likely pathophysiologic mechanism.

In studies using the patient as his or her own control, elevated plasma PHE concentrations prolonged the performance time on neuropsychologic tests of higher integrative function, reduced the mean power frequency of the EEG, and decreased urinary dopamine excretion and plasma L-DOPA in older treated patients with PKU (142, 143). A correlation was found among high plasma PHE concentrations, prolonged performance time on neuropsychologic tests, and decreased urinary dopamine in 10 patients. In a study of eight additional patients, statistically significant decreases were found in the mean power frequency of the EEG and in plasma L-DOPA when plasma PHE concentration increased (143). EEG slowing occurred in PKU heterozygotes at concentration changes of blood PHE induced by aspartame ingestion (150 μmol/L) (75). These effects were reversible and correlated in the reverse direction when the plasma PHE concentration was reduced. Severe neurologic deterioration occurred in several off-diet patients with PKU (74, 144). Reversal of most of the symptoms occurred in a patient who returned to a PHE-restricted diet that contained medical food (74).

Maternal Phenylketonuria

Pregnant women with PKU who are untreated at conception and during gestation have children with intrauterine growth retardation, microcephaly, and congenital anomalies, often severe and incompatible with life. Mental retardation is common in children of mothers whose plasma PHE concentration is higher than the normal range (145). The pathogenesis of the fetal damage is uncertain but is believed to be related to elevated maternal blood PHE concentration (146) because PHE is actively transported across the placenta to the fetus (147). Fetal plasma PHE concentrations are one and one half to two times those of maternal blood (148). Such elevated fetal plasma PHE concentrations are again concentrated twofold to fourfold by the fetal blood–brain barrier (149). Intraneuronal PHE concentrations of 600 μmol interfere with brain development by one or more of the several previously described mechanisms, including abnormal oligodendroglial migration and myelin and other protein synthesis (150). Thus, it is extremely important to maintain normal plasma PHE concentrations in the reproductive-age woman with PKU before conception and throughout gestation. Surviving children of untreated women fail to grow and develop normally (151). In fact, Kirkman (152) predicted that if the fertility of these women is normal and they are not treated with dietary control of PHE intake, the incidence of PKU-related mental retardation could return to the prescreening level after only one generation.

In 1984, the Maternal Phenylketonuria Collaborative Study (MPKUCS) was initiated to answer questions related to diet and reproductive outcome in women with PKU (153). Results of the MPKUCS supported the premise that a PHE-restricted diet, plasma PHE concentrations lower than 360 μmol/L, and the gestational age at which the diet is initiated affect reproductive outcome (154).

Nutrition Support of Maternal Phenylketonuria. The PHE-restricted diet should be initiated at least 3 months before a planned pregnancy by women who have PKU, if they have previously discontinued the diet. The objectives of therapy for pregnant women with PKU are a healthy mother and a normal, healthy newborn. To obtain adequate protein and fat storage in early pregnancy to support third-trimester fetal growth, careful attention

must be paid to diet and nutrition status. Although the plasma PHE concentration most likely to yield the best reproductive outcome is unknown, one group of investigators suggested that these objectives may be achieved by a PHE-restricted diet that maintains plasma PHE concentration between 60 and 180 μmol/L (155). Plasma PHE concentrations lower than 60 μmol/L may lead to maternal muscle wasting and poor fetal growth. The recommended PHE intake to prescribe for initiating therapy is given in Table 69.7 (1, 112, 116). Other indices of nutrition status should be in the normal range for pregnant women. After initiation of diet with the minimum recommended PHE prescription (see Table 69.7), the plasma PHE concentration should be monitored twice weekly to maintain the targeted plasma PHE concentration.

Even after the plasma PHE concentration is stabilized in the treatment range, frequent changes in the individualized diet prescription are required as pregnancy progresses, based on concentrations of plasma PHE, TYR, and other amino acids and on weight gain. PHE and TYR requirements of each pregnant woman depend on genotype, age, state of health, protein intake, and trimester of pregnancy (112). At approximately midpregnancy, PHE tolerance increases considerably.

As noted for the child with PKU, the amount of protein prescribed (see Table 69.7) exceeds the RDA because of the use of free amino acids as the primary source of protein equivalent. A PHE-free medical food (see Table 69.5) is used to provide most of the protein

TABLE 69.7	**RECOMMENDED PHENYLALANINE, TYROSINE, PROTEIN, FAT, ESSENTIAL FATTY ACID, AND ENERGY INTAKES FOR PREGNANT WOMEN WITH PHENYLKETONURIA**							
	NUTRIENTS							
TRIMESTER AND AGE (y)	PHENYLALANINE[a,b] (mg/d)	TYROSINE[b] (mg/d)	PROTEIN (g/d)	FAT[c] (g/d)	LINOLEIC ACID (g/d)	α-LINOLENIC ACID (g/d)	ENERGY[c] (kcal/d)	
							MEAN	RANGE
Trimester 1 (0 < 14 wk gestation)								
15 < 19	200 < 820	≥7,600	≥76	36–132	13	1.4	2,500	1,600–3,400
19 < 24	180 < 800	≥7,400	≥74	47–124	13	1.4	2,500	2,100–3,200
≥ 24	180 < 800	≥7,400	≥74	47–132	13	1.4	2,500	2,100–3,400
Trimester 2 (14 < 27 wk gestation)								
15 < 19	200 < 1000	≥7,600	≥76	36–132	13	1.4	2,500	1,600–3,400
19 < 24	180 < 1000	≥7,400	≥74	47–124	13	1.4	2,500	2,100–3,200
≥ 24	180 < 1000	≥7,400	≥74	47–132	13	1.4	2,500	2,100–3,400
Trimester 3 (27 < 41 wk gestation)								
15 < 19	330 < 1200	≥7,600	≥76	36–132	13	1.4	2,500	1,600–3,400
19 < 24	310 < 1200	≥7,400	≥74	47–124	13	1.4	2,500	2,100–3,200
≥ 24	310 < 1200	≥7,400	≥74	47–132	13	1.4	2,500	2,100–3,400

[a]Recommended range of phenylalanine (PHE) intake covered approximately 80% of women studied in the Maternal Phenylketonuria Collaborative Study (MPKUCS). Initiate the diet with the lowest amount recommended for the trimester and age. Frequent monitoring of plasma PHE is essential to prevent deficiency or excess. Modify the prescription based on the following: frequent plasma PHE and tyrosine (TYR) concentrations; intakes of PHE, TYR, protein, and energy; and maternal weight gain. Recommended iron intake is from MPKUCS data in Acosta PB, Michals-Matalon K, Austin V et al. Nutrition findings and requirements in pregnant women with phenylketonuria. In: Platt LD, Koch R, de la Cruz F, eds. Genetic Disorders and Pregnancy Outcome. New York: Parthenon, 1997:21–32.
[b]L-TYR is very insoluble in water. Consequently, any supplemental L-TYR should be mixed with fruit purees, mashed potatoes, or soup for ingestion. Recommended intake is from MPKUCS data in Acosta PB, Michals-Matalon K, Austin V et al. Nutrition findings and requirements in pregnant women with phenylketonuria. In: Platt LD, Koch R, de la Cruz F, eds. Genetic Disorders and Pregnancy Outcome. New York: Parthenon, 1997:21–32.
[c]Modified from Otten JJ, Hellwig JP, Meyers LD. Dietary Reference Intakes: The Essential Guide to Nutrient Requirements. Washington, DC: National Academies Press, 2006. For some women, energy requirements may be greater than the upper limit of the range given to obtain appropriate weight gain.

prescribed; and nitrogen-free foods, such as pure sugars and fats, are used to supply the remaining energy needs.

Birth measurements of neonates of women with PKU are negatively correlated with maternal plasma PHE concentrations and are positively correlated with maternal energy and protein intakes and weight gain during pregnancy. The 5-year mean HC Z-scores of children of women who attained plasma PHE concentrations lower than 360 μmol/L by 10 weeks' gestation and throughout pregnancy were 0.50 ± 1.53 versus 0.30 ± 0.88 at birth, whereas the mean HC Z-scores of children of women with a plasma PHE concentration by 10 weeks' gestation and throughout the remainder of gestation of 360 to 600 μmol/L declined from -0.65 ± 0.87 to -0.87 ± 1.97. The 5-year HC of children of women with plasma PHE concentrations greater than 600 μmol/L throughout pregnancy decreased from -1.46 ± 1.08 at birth to -2.09 ± 1.57. Over the 5 years, catch-up growth did not occur in height of children of women with plasma PHE concentrations greater than 360 μmol/L (156). The plasma PHE concentration of the pregnant woman with PKU is negatively correlated with total protein intake (157), a finding suggesting that total protein intake should minimally be at the amount recommended in Table 69.7 for better control of plasma PHE.

Appropriate maternal weight gain is related to height and prepregnancy weight and is greater for underweight women than for women of normal weight. Data in Table 69.8 (158) describe recommended pregnancy weight gain for underweight, normal-weight, and overweight women.

Two families of fatty acids, linoleic (C18:2, n-6) and α-linolenic (C18:3, n-3), are essential for humans (1). Adequate intakes of linoleic and α-linolenic acids are suggested to be 13 and 1.4 g/day, respectively, during pregnancy (1). Women in the MPKUCS who had a good reproductive outcome had a greater fat intake throughout pregnancy than did women with a poor outcome (112). Whether the poor outcome was caused by inadequate essential fatty acids is not clear. Because some of the medical foods are devoid of or contain very little fat and essential fatty acids, the fat used to supply 30% to 40% of

energy in the diet should be obtained from cooking and salad oils, margarines, salad dressing, and shortenings with either unhydrogenated canola oil or soybean oil as the first ingredient (94).

PHE-free medical foods that provide the prescribed protein equivalent (nitrogen × 6.25) for the pregnant woman with PKU also provide the required amounts of minerals and vitamins. Therefore, a prenatal vitamin capsule containing vitamins A and D should not be prescribed for women ingesting adequate amounts of PHE-free medical food. In fact, supplementation may provide vitamin A at levels approaching those that are teratogenic (159). Those women who do not ingest adequate medical food before and during gestation should be given supplements of folic acid and vitamin B_{12} to help decrease the incidence of congenital heart defects in children, however (160).

Monitoring Nutrition Support. Ongoing monitoring of women with PKU involves measuring plasma concentrations of PHE and TYR, maternal weight gain, and concentrations of other plasma amino acids, transthyretin, ferritin, and zinc. Because pregnant women with PKU are at risk for premature delivery, they should be treated as high-risk patients, even if their plasma PHE concentrations are in the targeted treatment range. Multiple ultrasound studies, beginning at 16 to 20 weeks' gestation, may be requested to monitor fetal head size and intrauterine growth patterns. A level II ultrasound to scan for heart defects and other malformations may also be ordered.

Tyrosinemias

Several known disorders of TYR metabolism (Table 69.9) may be amenable to nutrition support (see Fig. 69.1). Precise biochemical diagnosis is important because disorders such as liver disease, scurvy, and prematurity may produce increases in blood TYR concentrations that are not caused by permanent specific enzyme defects in TYR metabolism.

Seven clinical forms of hereditary tyrosinemia have been reported (see Table 69.9). Type Ia is caused by a primary defect of hepatic FAH with the production of an abnormal metabolite, succinylacetone (161). The gene for FAH has been localized to chromosome 15q23-25 (see Table 69.2) (161). Succinylacetone is formed from the accumulated substrate fumarylacetoacetate (FAA) (see Fig. 69.1). FAA, at subapoptotic doses, has been reported to induce spindle disturbances and segregational defects in both rodent and human cells, a finding leading to the speculation that FAA functions as a thiol-reacting agent that disturbs the organelle/mitotic spindle (162). If maleylacetoacetic acid isomerase is functional, succinylacetone is also formed from maleylacetoacetate. Succinylacetone is extremely toxic and is associated with impaired active transport function and disordered hepatic enzymes, including p-OHPPAD and δ-ALA dehydratase (161). Decreased activity of both hepatic and erythrocyte δ-ALA dehydratase has been reported in these patients

TABLE 69.8	RECOMMENDED WEIGHT GAIN DURING PREGNANCY FOR WOMEN WITH PHENYLKETONURIA	
WEIGHT STATUS AT CONCEPTION	RECOMMENDED WEIGHT GAIN	
	First Trimester (kg)	Total (kg)
Normal weight	1.6	11.4–15.9
Underweight	2.3	12.7–18.2
Overweight	0.9	6.8–11.4
Obese		5.0– 9.1

From Rasmussen KM, Catalano PM, Yaktine AL. New guidelines for weight gain during pregnancy: what obstetrician/gynecologists should know. Curr Opin Obstet Gynecol 2009;21:521–6.

TABLE 69.9	INHERITED DISORDERS PRODUCING INCREASED PLASMA TYROSINE	
DESIGNATION	ENZYME DEFECT	CLINICAL FEATURES
Hepatorenal tyrosinemia (type Ia)	Fumarylacetoacetate hydrolyase	Cirrhosis Renal Fanconi syndrome Acute porphyria (succinylacetone) Hepatocellular carcinoma
Hepatorenal tyrosinemia (type Ib)	Maleylacetoacetate isomerase	Liver failure Fanconi syndrome Psychomotor retardation (no succinylacetone)
Oculocutaneous tyrosinemia (type II)	Hepatic cytosol tyrosine aminotransferase	Eye and skin disorders with variable mental retardation Hydroxyphenylpyruvic acidemia
Primary p-OHPPAD deficiency (type IIIa)	p-OHPPAD	Neurologic abnormalities Mental retardation
Hawkinsinuria (type IIIb)	p-OHPPAD	Metabolic acidosis Microcephaly
Transient neonatal (type IIIc)	p-OHPPAD	Prematurity, possibly benign
Tyrosinosis (Medes)	Possibly type Ia	Myasthenia (possibly acute porphyric attack)

p-OHPPAD, 4-hydroxyphenylpyruvic acid dioxygenase.

and is postulated to be the mechanism for development of acute porphyric-like episodes (see Fig. 69.2) (161). Using the drug NTBC to inhibit p-OHPPAD activity has prevented acute porphyric episodes and decreased rates of progression of cirrhosis and Fanconi syndrome (163).

Tyrosinemia type Ia is characterized by a generalized renal tubular impairment with hypophosphatemic rickets, progressive liver failure producing cirrhosis and hepatic cancer, hypertension, episodic behavioral and peripheral nerve deficiencies, and elevated concentrations of blood PHE and TYR with succinylacetone and δ-ALA excretion in urine (161). The most common mutant allele is a splice donor site gain in intron 12 (IVS12G A + 5). Many other missense and nonsense mutations are known (see Table 69.2). Reversion of the IVS12 mutation to normal in noncancerous hepatic nodules is described. FAH is expressed in amniotic and chorionic villus cells, and prenatal diagnosis is available by biochemical or molecular techniques (161).

Tyrosinemia type Ib, believed to be caused by a deficiency of maleylacetoacetate isomerase, has been reported in one infant (161). Liver failure, renal tubular disease, and progressive psychomotor retardation occurred before the child's death at 1 year of age. Succinylacetone did not accumulate. If this finding is confirmed, the pathophysiology of tyrosinemia type I will require reevaluation.

Tyrosinemia type II is characterized by greatly elevated concentrations of blood and urine TYR and increases in urinary phenolic acids, N-acetyltyrosine, and tyramine. A deficiency of hepatic cytosolic TYR aminotransferase has been demonstrated (161). Characteristic physical findings include stellate corneal erosions and plaques and bullous lesions of the soles and palms. Persistent keratitis and hyperkeratosis occur on the fingers and palms of the hands and on the soles of the feet (164). These skin abnormalities respond to restriction of dietary PHE and TYR. Intracellular crystallization of TYR is thought to cause these inflammatory responses. Mental retardation may occur. The TYR aminotransferase gene is located on human chromosome 16q22.1 (see Table 69.2). Missense, deletions, nonsense, and splice site mutations are known.

Three clinical subsets of type III tyrosinemia result from dysfunctions of p-OHPPAD (see Fig. 69.1 and Table 69.9). The most severe is type IIIa with no hepatic p-OHPPAD. Neurologic abnormalities including seizures, ataxia, and mental retardation have been reported in untreated patients with type IIIa (165). Hawkinsinuria (type IIIb) is named for the 2-L-cysteinyl 5-1,4-dihydroxycyclohexenyl-acetic acid that presumably is formed from an intermediate of impaired p-OHPPAD reaction. Metabolic acidosis, failure to thrive, and an odor resembling a swimming pool odor are described. PHE and TYR restriction improves the critical condition.

Type IIIc is neonatal tyrosinemia, associated with increased plasma and urinary concentrations of TYR and its metabolites. It occurs in 0.2% to 10% of neonates (161). Short-term protein restriction to 1.5 to 2.0 g/kg body weight/day has lowered plasma TYR concentrations in most patients within 4 weeks of life. Whether added ascorbate will stabilize and increase the activity of p-OHPPAD in this disorder is not clear. Persistence of hypertyrosinemia in this disorder may lead to impaired mental function (166), and short-term diet and ascorbate therapy are recommended.

Diagnosis

Differential diagnosis, imperative for institution of appropriate therapy, requires quantitation of plasma amino acids by ion-exchange chromatography and of urinary organic acids by GC/MS. The more severe tyrosinemia type I may not be detected by newborn screening using the bacterial inhibition assay because newborn blood TYR concentrations may not be higher than 8 mg/dL (440 µmol/L). If blood TYR exceeds 8 mg/dL (440 µmol/L) at 14 days of age, renal tubular and hepatic function are evaluated, as well as urine, by organic acid analysis for the presence of *p*-hydroxyphenyl acids and succinylacetone. Prenatal diagnosis of hereditary tyrosinemia type I has been made by measurement of succinylacetone in amniotic fluid (167), by measurement of FAH activity in cultured amniotic fluid cells, and by molecular analyses. Tyrosinemia type II results in a marked increase in urinary *p*-OH-phenylacids and blood TYR (161). It increases with increasing age of the infant, whereas type IIIc decreases. Hawkinsinuria is measured by its ninhydrin reaction using ion-exchange chromatography.

Treatment

Therapy of the hereditary tyrosinemias requires a firm diagnosis because the approaches to treatment among the various types are different. The objective of nutrition support for the hereditary tyrosinemias is to provide a biochemical environment that allows normal growth and development of intellectual potential. Nutrition management alone prevents pathophysiologic changes only in types II and III, for which the prognosis is excellent. Plasma PHE concentration should be maintained between 40 and 80 µmol/L, and plasma TYR concentration should be between 50 and 150 µmol/L. 2-(2-Nitro-4-trifluoromethylbensylate)-1,3-cyclohexanedione therapy in tyrosinemia type Ia, with concomitant nutrition management to maintain plasma TYR concentration at less than 500 µmol/L (168), has prevented acute porphyria episodes, decreased rates of progression of cirrhosis and Fanconi syndrome, greatly improved the survival of patients, and reduced the need for liver transplantation during early childhood. The homeostatic effects of NTBC on succinylacetone production also decrease but do not eliminate the risk for hepatocarcinoma.

Renal impairment, if present, must also be treated in tyrosinemia type Ia. Generalized renal tubular failure may result in metabolic acidosis, hypophosphatemia, rickets, and hypokalemia unless replacement of bicarbonate, phosphate, 1,25-dihydroxycholecalciferol, and potassium is instituted. Rapid treatment of infections is required to prevent a catastrophic catabolic state with overproduction of succinylacetone.

Many of the porphyric symptoms are caused by overproduction of δ-ALA secondary to the inhibitory effect of succinylacetone on δ-ALA dehydratase or decreased heme biosynthesis (see Fig. 69.2). Parenteral nutrition with 20% to 25% dextrose solution may control these acute porphyric attacks (169). Continued or progressive loss of energy-requiring functions that involve loosely bound heme to heme-protein (plasma membrane transporters, cytochrome P-450) may be caused by rapid turnover and insufficient heme biosynthesis (see Fig. 69.2). Infusions of hematin have produced transient decreases in δ-ALA and have improved acute attacks of intermittent porphyria, but this invasive therapy is not recommended unless NTBC is unavailable (7, 170). Hepatocellular carcinoma, however, is not prevented and requires liver transplantation to prevent metastases (161). The drug NTBC, which inhibits the activity of *p*-OHPPAD in the treatment of tyrosinemia type I, reduces the need for liver transplantation, and diet therapy is an indicated adjunct to drug therapy (168). An excellent mouse model exists (171). Whether newborn or infant treatment of tyrosinemia type I with diet and NTBC will prevent hepatocarcinoma is not clear. Follow-up of liver α-fetoprotein and enzymes, as well as hepatic sonography, are indicated. Hepatic transplantation may be required.

Nutrient Requirements. A prescription that recommends daily amounts of PHE, TYR, protein, energy, and fluid should be written. The prescription for PHE and TYR is based on blood analyses correlated with intake that indicate the child's requirement or tolerance for each amino acid (see Table 69.3).

Because a large portion of PHE is normally hydroxylated to form TYR, PHE must also be restricted in the diet of patients with tyrosinemia. PHE requirements appear to be greater for children with tyrosinemia than for children with PKU. In general, the more distal is the block in the catabolic pathway, the more normal is the amino acid requirement. The TYR needs of children with tyrosinemia have been inadequately described and vary with the metabolic state of the child and the accumulation of succinylacetone. When plasma TYR is inadequately controlled in NTBC-treated patients, symptoms of tyrosinemia type II occur (168).

Because the primary protein source used for infants is a free amino acid mix, the recommended intake is greater than for physiologically normal infants (see Table 69.3). For tyrosinemia type Ia, when NTBC is administered, energy needs are similar to those of physiologically normal infants (1).

Fat, essential fatty acids, mineral and vitamin recommendations are the same as in the patient with PKU (see Table 69.3).

Medical Foods Free of Phenylalanine and Tyrosine. Adequate protein cannot be obtained from intact protein without ingesting excess PHE and TYR (proteins contain, by mass, 1.4% to 5.8% TYR) (94). Thus, special medical foods are used that contain no PHE or TYR. Several medical foods free of PHE and TYR and containing minerals and vitamins are available to provide protein. Sources of medical foods are given in Table 69.5.

Other Foods. Composition of foods as supplied by USDA is available in reference 94.

Initiation of Nutrition Support. The most rapid decline of blood TYR concentration at the time of diagnosis may be obtained by feeding a 20 kcal/oz (67 kcal/dL) PHE- and TYR-free formula with no added sources of PHE and TYR. Total energy intake greater than 120 kcal/kg/day is required to prevent a catabolic phase. Laboratory results of blood PHE and TYR concentrations should be rapidly available or deficiency of PHE and TYR (172) could be precipitated. Catabolism, caused by inadequate intake of protein, energy, PHE, or TYR, is particularly undesirable in treating tyrosinemia type I because a catabolic phase with overproduction of succinylacetone will worsen the clinical state. Intact protein sources containing 20 to 70 mg PHE and 60 to 80 mg TYR/kg body weight/day are usually required after 1 to 2 days of total restriction in the newborn period in the patient with tyrosinemia type II or III. Patients with tyrosinemia type Ia may tolerate more dietary PHE and TYR if they are managed with NTBC.

Assessment of Nutrition Support. Frequency of assessment is dictated by the type of tyrosinemia and the clinical course of the patient. In tyrosinemia type I, vital signs, height, weight, HC, neurologic examination, and development are documented weekly for the first 3 months; biweekly for the second 3 months; and monthly between 6 months and 1 year of life. Plasma amino acids are quantitated by ion-exchange chromatography or MS/MS, and succinylacetone and p-hydroxyphenyl organic acids are quantitated by GC/MS. Additional laboratory studies include urinary δ-ALA, blood and urine assessment of renal losses (bicarbonate [HCO_3^-], potassium [K^+], and sodium [Na^+]), and liver status (α-fetoprotein and liver function tests). Clinical status, dietary intake, and laboratory data should be monitored and correlated in managing tyrosinemia type Ia at intervals indicated previously. Application for eventual liver transplantation should be initiated within the first year of life for patients with type Ia tyrosinemia.

Outcomes of Nutrition Support. Outcomes to date have been variable with tyrosinemia type Ia (161). Some of this variation is caused by the lack of clear diagnostic criteria in the past to delineate the various types of tyrosinemia. Early detection and diagnosis using GC/MS, PHE and TYR restriction, hematin infusions, and early replacement of renal tubular losses bring success at early ages in patients with treated tyrosinemia type Ia. Although NTBC may be the ultimate treatment for tyrosinemia type Ia, institution of the treatment immediately after birth may be necessary to prevent hepatocellular carcinomas, and hepatic transplantation will be required if liver nodules progress on hepatic sonography or if the liver α-fetoprotein concentration rises suddenly (163). The PHE- and TYR-restricted diet has been successful in several patients with tyrosinemia types II and III, with rapid resolution of clinical signs and symptoms (161). Neonatal tyrosinemia requires early but transient protein restriction. The efficacy of oral ascorbate at 50 mg/day is unclear. Controlled outcome data are not yet available.

SULFUR-CONTAINING AMINO ACIDS

The biochemistry and nutrition requirements for sulfur-containing amino acids have been largely elucidated in humans by studies of inherited blocks in their metabolic pathways.

Biochemistry

Intact protein contains approximately 0.3% to 5.0% MET (94). Some dietary MET is used by the body for tissue protein synthesis, but most is used through the transsulfuration pathway to form adenosylmethionine, adenosylhomocysteine, homocysteine, cystathionine, α-ketobutyrate, cysteine, and their derivatives (Fig. 69.3). The first step in the transsulfuration pathway is the synthesis of S-adenosylmethionine (SAM), a reaction catalyzed by MET-S-adenosyltransferase (MAT). Impaired MAT results in hypermethioninemia and variable clinical expression from sulfurous breath odor to mental retardation. The hepatic isoform of MAT only is deficient (28). In this reaction, the adenosyl portion of adenosine triphosphate (ATP) is transferred to MET. Biologically important compounds that obtain their methyl group from SAM include creatine, choline, phosphatidylcholine, methylated DNA and RNA, and epinephrine. Decarboxylated SAM is the source of the three carbon moieties of spermidine and spermine. S-adenosylhomocysteine is formed as an intermediary product in this pathway and is hydrolyzed to homocysteine.

Homocysteine has four possible pathways open to it. Homocysteine reacts with serine in the presence of CβS, found in liver and brain, to form cystathionine (see Fig. 69.3). CβS requires pyridoxal phosphate as a coenzyme. Homocysteine can also be remethylated to form MET through two different enzymatic reactions. In one reaction, the methyl group is derived from betaine and is catalyzed by betaine-homocysteine methyltransferase. The second reaction requires N^5-methyltetrahydrofolate as a methyl donor to CH_3-B_{12} (see Fig. 69.3) and is catalyzed by 5-methyltetrahydrofolate-homocysteine methyltransferase. Finkelstein (173) used an in vitro system that approximated in vivo conditions in rat liver to measure the simultaneous product formation by the three enzymes that use homocysteine. In this control system, 5-methyltetrahydrofolate-homocysteine methyltransferase, betaine homocysteine methyltransferase, and CβS accounted for 27%, 27%, and 46% of the homocysteine consumed, respectively. The fourth pathway open to homocysteine is spontaneous oxidation to homocystine (see Fig. 69.3). This reaction occurs inside cells only when homocysteine is present in abnormal amounts. It is essentially irreversible because the disulfide bond of homocystine is covalent. Homocystine is not further metabolized. CβS metabolizes most homocysteine with high affinity to cystathionine, by using serine as a cosubstrate and pyridoxal phosphate as a stabilizing active coenzyme. Cystathionine is then hydrolyzed to cysteine and α-ketobutyrate. The enzyme cystathioninase, which also uses pyridoxal phosphate as a coenzyme, is required for this reaction (see Fig. 69.3). A deficiency of cystathioninase results in cystathioninuria,

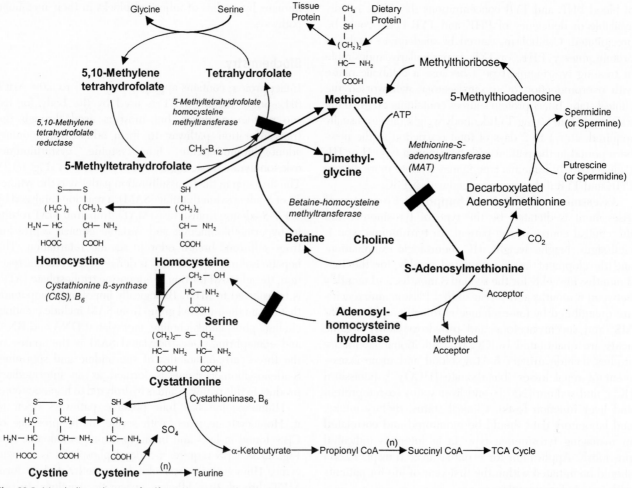

Fig. 69.3. Metabolic pathways of sulfur amino acids. The *black bars* represent impaired reactions in three inherited metabolic disorders resulting in hyperhomocyst(e)inemia. *CoA*, coenzyme A; *TCA*, tricarboxylic acid.

which has no pathologic consequence. α-Ketobutyrate is converted to propionyl-CoA, which is carboxylated to methylmalonyl-CoA and isomerized to succinyl-CoA, a Krebs cycle intermediate. L-Cysteine is catabolized to pyruvate, ammonia (NH_3), and hydrogen sulfide (H_2S).

Three analytes suggesting inherited disorders of MET metabolism are currently part of newborn screening: MET for homocystinuria and hypermethioninemia and C3 with C3/C2 for cobalamin defects.

Homocystinuria

Defects in the function of CβS or 5-methyltetrahydrofolate-homocysteine methyltransferase result in classic homocystinuria. Impaired activity of the latter enzyme may be caused by failure to synthesize CH_3-B_{12} from vitamin B_{12} or by a deficiency in 5,10-methylenetetrahydrofolate reductase, as well as by mutations in the apoenzyme CβS. Several different defects impair the uptake, transfer, and conversion of dietary vitamin B_{12} to CH_3-B_{12} (39, 174). Both hydroxycobalamin and folate are required to treat these disorders.

The most common form of homocystinuria is caused by a deficiency of CβS. The human CβS locus has been

mapped to chromosome 21q-22.3 (175). The gene has been cloned, and more than 90 mutations are characterized in expression systems. Although phenotypes vary for the same genotype, some mutations respond to vitamin B_6 (I278T, P145L, A114V), and others do not (G307S) (176). Severely impaired enzyme function produces accumulation of plasma homocyst(e)ine and MET and decreased cyst(e)ine in cells and physiologic fluids. If this biochemical circumstance is not treated early in life, skeletal changes, dislocated lenses, intravascular thromboses, osteoporosis, malar flushing, and, in some patients, mental retardation will occur.

The skeletal changes and dislocated lenses are presumably caused by a structural defect in collagen formation produced by α-homocystine interaction with aldose groups on collagen (28) or by irreversible inhibition of lysyl oxidase by homocysteine thiolactone (177). Intravascular thromboses may occur at any age and have been found in coronary, renal, carotid, and intracranial arteries. The natural history of homocystinuria caused by CβS deficiency was clarified in a large series of patients (178). Investigators suggested, however, that in Denmark, most homozygotes for mutation C.833T > C(p.12787) are unaffected or are diagnosed following thromboembolic events occurring in the third decade of life (179). Heterozygosity for some mutations in CβS (or in tetrahydrofolate reductase) may predispose patients to the development of premature occlusive arterial disease (180).

It is not known to what degree the mental retardation seen in homocystinuria is attributable to a metabolic sequela, such as a deficiency of cystathionine in myelin formation, or results from multiple small cerebrovascular thromboses. Mental deficiency may occur in patients with severely impaired CβS as a consequence of multiple cerebral arteriolar obstructions if homocystinemia is not controlled by diet.

Screening

CβS deficiency is inherited as an autosomal recessive disease. Accurate estimates of the incidence for homocystinuria are not available, but newborn screening in 13 countries found 1 case in 344,000 infants screened (28). Homocystinuria occurs in many ethnic groups, but it has a higher frequency in persons of Irish descent (1 in 58,000) than in other ethnic groups (28). This finding may be a bias of ascertainment because of the original description of and continued screening for this disorder in the Irish population. Vitamin B_6–responsive mutations in CβS are probably not ascertained by neonatal screening for elevated blood MET concentrations.

Selective screening uses the inexpensive urinary nitroprusside reaction. In this reaction, excessive amounts of reduced homocysteine and cysteine form a stable red color with nitroprusside. This selective screening test for sulfur amino acids should be included in the evaluation of any patient with an unknown cause of arterial thrombosis, dislocated lens, marfanoid habitus, or mental retardation. This test result is also positive in cystinuria, and this test should be included as a screen for patients with nephrolithiasis.

In a large survey of patients with homocystinuria caused by CβS deficiency, only 13% had a response to vitamin B_6 (28). Most of these patients had "leaky mutations" with residual CβS activity and disease that was expressed in adolescence or young adulthood rather than in early childhood. Response to vitamin B_6 occurs in several mutations, with some residual enzyme activity. The mechanism involves stabilizing CβS to biologic degradation (28). The more residual enzyme activity is present, the more dramatic is the response to vitamin B_6. Hypermethioninemia may not be present in the newborn if CβS activity exceeds 15% of normal. Some patients with CβS deficiency have no activity in the fibroblasts, yet they appear to have a vitamin B_6 response (176).

Diagnosis

Positive results in a newborn screen by bacterial inhibition assay for MET must be followed by an assay of plasma amino acids using ion-exchange chromatography or MS/MS because many environmental and genetic variations cause neonatal hypermethioninemia. In patients with a CβS defect, homocystine, cysteine-homocysteine, and MET concentrations are all elevated in plasma and increase with increased protein intake (see Fig. 69.3). Demonstration of significantly decreased CβS, folate, CH_3-B_{12}, or homocysteine methyltransferases is necessary to confirm the diagnosis and to implement appropriate therapy. MET may be elevated in the absence of homocystinemia in liver disease and in specific impairment of SAM. By contrast, in defects of homocysteine remethylation to MET, MET is low or normal, whereas homocysteine concentrations are elevated. Hyperhomocysteinemia caused by disorders of cobalamin methylation to CH_3-B_{12} or the two homocysteine methyltransferases are not detected by nonselective newborn screening for elevated blood MET but by elevated C3 and the ratio of C3 to C2. Similarly, vitamin B_6–responsive mild CβS deficiency is missed by newborn screening. Thus, selective screening using urinary nitroprusside reaction or plasma amino acid analysis is indicated for all children or adults with ectopic lens, unexplained vascular occlusions, marfanoid habitus, and mental delay.

Management of CH_3-B_{12} deficiency or impaired methyl transfer with homocystinuria does not include MET-restricted diets. Rather, pharmacologic amounts of vitamin B_{12}, folate, choline, or betaine are added depending on the primary defect. Liver biopsy specimens, transformed lymphoblasts, or cultured skin fibroblasts express CβS and are used to confirm the most common cause of homocystinuria; and molecular screening and sequencing of the CβS gene are useful in predicting management. Prenatal diagnosis can be provided by direct enzyme assay of amniotic fluid cells or by DNA analysis if the mutations are known (28, 176).

Treatment

If homocystinuria is caused by CβS deficiency expressed in the newborn, the clinical objectives are (a) to prevent the development of skeletal and ocular abnormalities, (b) to prevent intravascular thromboses, and (c) to ensure normal intellectual development.

Pharmacologic doses of pyridoxine should be tried in all patients with hypermethioninemia and homocystinemia (28, 176). Some mutations are known to be responsive (see Table 69.3). In newborns and early childhood, 25 to 100 mg/day should be tried for 4 weeks before MET restriction. Older children and adults should be given oral pyridoxine (1 g/day). The effect of pyridoxine on plasma MET and homocystine concentrations is monitored weekly on a constant protein intake. Because enzyme stabilization is the most common mechanism of vitamin responsivity, weeks may be required for a biochemical response to occur. If the plasma MET and homocysteine concentrations are reduced, the amount of pyridoxine should be gradually lowered until the minimum dose required to maintain biochemical normality is reached. Doses of 25 to 750 mg/day have been required for some patients. Excess vitamin B_6 for prolonged periods may cause peripheral neuropathy (181) and liver injury (182); consequently, if vitamin B_6 is not helpful, it should be discontinued. Betaine supplements (6 g/day) help to maintain postprandial plasma homocysteine concentrations in the nearly normal range in vitamin B_6–responsive individuals (183).

Patients whose condition does not respond completely to pyridoxine require a MET-restricted diet supplemented with L-cysteine. Cysteine becomes an essential amino acid in homocystinuria (see Fig. 69.3). If plasma folate concentrations are lower than normal owing to excess use in remethylating homocysteine to MET, folate should be added as a supplement.

Betaine is used as adjunctive therapy in patients who are not responsive to vitamin B_6. Doses required range from 120 to 150 mg/kg/day and are divided into three doses per day. Total plasma homocyst(e)ine should be followed as the parameter of effective therapy because both free MET and free homocysteine in plasma may decrease to normal, whereas total plasma homocyst(e)ine remains elevated and in concentrations that increase risks of vascular occlusion (184). Adverse events from betaine treatment are rare but have been reported. According to one group of investigators (185), one child who was noncompliant with diet restriction and who had a plasma MET concentration of 3000 μmol/L developed cerebral edema that resolved when betaine was discontinued. Van Calcar (186) described inherited disorders of sulfur amino acid metabolism as well as their nutrition management.

Nutrient Requirements. In prescribing and implementing nutrition care plans for infants and children with homocystinuria caused by CβS deficiency, one must consider energy, protein, MET, cysteine, folate, vitamins B_6 and B_{12}, betaine, and fluid needs. Younger infants have a greater MET requirement per kilogram of body weight than do older infants. Suggested daily MET intakes range from 35 mg/kg in the young infant to 5 mg/kg in the 15- to 19-year-old patient. Suggested beginning energy, protein, MET, and fluid intakes for infants and children of different ages are given in Table 69.3. If the medical food mixture provides more than 24 kcal/oz, extra fluid should be offered between feedings to prevent dehydration.

Calcium cystinate, a soluble form of L-cystine, should supplement the MET-restricted diet at all ages. The young infant should be offered 300 mg/kg body weight. This amount may be decreased to 200 mg/kg at 6 months of age and 100 mg/kg at 3 years of age and thereafter. The calcium cystinate should be mixed with the MET-free medical food to provide even distribution throughout the day. Older children can sprinkle it in applesauce or other low-protein solids.

Methionine-Free Medical Foods. Several medical foods have been developed as protein sources for patients with homocystinuria. Sources of these products are given in Table 69.5.

Other Foods. MET may be provided for the young infant by addition of specified amounts of proprietary infant formula to the MET-free medical foods. As growth and development proceed, intact protein-containing foods should be added at the usual ages to supply essential MET. The MET requirement is small, and most foods contain moderate amounts in relation to the requirement (94). The amount of intact protein that can be ingested therefore is small. See reference 66 for nutrient composition of foods that may be used to help supply MET and other nutrients. A sample diet for a neonate is given in Table 69.10.

Assessment of Nutrition Support. After the introduction of the diet and stabilization, plasma MET and cystine concentrations should be monitored twice weekly until 3 months of age. Weekly monitoring is suggested until 6 months of age and twice monthly thereafter if blood MET concentrations are stable. Because free MET and homocystine in plasma may revert to normal, whereas total plasma homocyst(e)ine remains elevated, measurement of plasma cystine is recommended when the free MET is normal or the free homocystine is not measurable. After a diet change, plasma MET and cysteine should be measured after 3 days have elapsed. A 3-day diet diary before each blood sample is necessary to evaluate plasma MET and cysteine. Plasma MET should be maintained between

TABLE 69.10	SAMPLE DIET: HOMOCYSTINURIA (2 WEEKS OF AGE), WEIGHT 3.25 KG				
PRESCRIPTION	TOTAL	PER kg			
Methionine (mg)	98	30			
Cystine (mg)	975	300			
Protein (g)	11.4	3.5			
Energy (kcal)	390	120			
Water to make (mL)	600				
MEDICAL FOOD	AMOUNT	METHIONINE (mg)	CYSTINE (mg)	PROTEIN (g)	ENERGY (kcal)
XMET Analog[a,b]	52 g	0	183	6.8	247
Enfamil Lipil Powder	47 g	99	61	4.6	221
L-Cystine, 10 mg/mL	73 mL	0	730	0	0
Water to make	600 mL				
Total		99	974	11.4	468

[a]Nutricia North America.
[b]Other medical foods that may be used for infants are Hominex-1 (Abbott Nutrition) and HCY-1 (Mead Johnson Nutritionals).

15 and 45 μmol in 2- to 4-hour postfeeding plasma. Little or no homocystine should be present in blood and urine. Total plasma homocyst(e)ine should approach 10 μM/L. Growth and development as well as clinical evaluation of the pulses, skeletal growth, and ocular lenses, are routinely assessed.

Results of Nutrition Support. In a retrospective study of 629 patients with CβS deficiency, MET restriction initiated neonatally prevented mental retardation, decreased the frequency of lens dislocation, and reduced the incidence of seizures. Pyridoxine treatment of late-detected vitamin B_6–responsive patients decreased the rate of thromboembolic events (178). Hispanic male twins born at 38 weeks' gestation with homocystinuria grew well during the entire first year of life while on nutrition support. The protein intake of these two patients averaged 3.7 g/kg/day during the first 6 months of life and 2.6 g/kg/day during the second 6 months. Energy intake averaged 131 kcal/kg during the first 6 months and 100 kcal/kg during the second 6 months. Patients with poorly controlled plasma homocysteine concentrations may have excessive growth in height. Optimal metabolic control may prevent overgrowth (187).

Cysteine deficiency manifested as abnormally low plasma cystine concentrations, elevated plasma MET, and weight loss in a 3-year-old boy with homocystinuria who received 32 mg/kg/day of L-cysteine was reported (188). The Hispanic twins referred to earlier received 58 to 118 mg cystine/kg/day, which resulted in plasma cystine concentrations of 19 to 30 μmol/L. Up to 150 mg L-cystine/kg/day may be required to maintain normal plasma cystine concentrations.

Elevated plasma copper and ceruloplasmin concentrations were found in 15 patients with homocystinuria, compared with concentrations found in age- and gender-matched physiologically normal controls. No relationship with plasma homocysteine could be found (189). The twins mentioned earlier had elevated serum copper concentrations of 151 and 144 μg/dL at approximately 13 months of age. Low plasma selenium concentration (approximately 15 μmol/L) and erythrocyte glutathione peroxidase activity (approximately 3 U/g hemoglobin) were found in a child with homocystinuria who was treated with a medical food free of selenium (190). Administration of 50 μg selenium (in selenium-enriched yeast) every other day was required to maintain normal indices of selenium status. The twins mentioned earlier ingested, on average, 26 μg selenium (as sodium selenite) daily throughout the first year of life. Serum selenium concentrations ranged between 60 and 72 μg/L, very similar to values reported for physiologically normal babies fed human milk (191).

Vitamin A absorption tests were carried out in eight untreated patients with homocystinuria by measuring the elevation in serum after administration of vitamin A alcohol (retinol). The explanation proposed for the resulting subnormal serum vitamin A elevation was that retinol was oxidized by −SH groups excreted into the gut (192).

Of the eight plasma retinol values obtained on the twins studied, one was less than 20 μg/dL and five were between 20 and 30 μg/dL. According to parental report, vitamin A intake was always more than adequate (1.20 to 5.58 times the RDA for age). Serum transthyretin concentrations were all less than 20 mg/dL (marginal), and two of the four values obtained were less than 15 mg/dL (deficient).

Fasting serum folate concentrations in eight untreated patients with homocystinuria were found to be abnormally low (4 ng/mL compared with 8 ng/mL in control subjects). Two of these subjects were treated with 20 mg/day folate, which led to a decrease in urinary homocystine excretion (193). Severe folate deficiency was found in an untreated infant with homocystinuria who was receiving diluted boiled cow's milk for an episode of gastroenteritis. Excessive use of 5-methyltetrahydrofolate in the remethylation of homocysteine to form MET is proposed as a reason for folate deficiency in untreated patients (194). The twins in our study had adequate hemoglobin concentrations after 4 months of age, and mean corpuscular volume was normal.

Termination of Nutrition Support. Most clinicians who treat individuals with homocystinuria believe that patients should be kept on the diet indefinitely. Termination of the diet after growth is achieved may lead to thromboembolisms and ciliary muscle laxity with lens dislocation. Yap et al (195) reported that appropriate homocysteine-lowering therapy significantly reduced the vascular risk in patients with homocystinuria. When initiation or maintenance of nutrition support is not possible, acetylsalicylic acid (1 g/day) and dipyridamole (100 mg/day) increase platelet survival time and decrease thrombotic events (196). Pharmacologic doses of vitamin E may reduce oxidative stress and platelet activation in patients with homocystinuria (197). Vitamin B_6 in pharmacologic doses should be continued in vitamin B_6–responsive patients.

Reproductive Performance

Fewer conceptions are reported for both men and women whose condition does not respond to vitamin B_6 than for those whose condition does. Children of male patients do not suffer excess losses and are generally reported to be physiologically normal. A study showed that higher rates of fetal loss occurred in presumptive heterozygous fetuses carried by CβS-deficient mothers than occurred in physiologically normal women (178). Good reproductive outcome was reported in children of a woman who had tight metabolic control during pregnancy (198). Whether hypermethioninemia, homocysteinemia, or other metabolic variations in MET metabolism are teratogenic is unclear, but a teratogenic mechanism as defined for maternal PKU is possible. In addition, folate-responsive neural tube defects may involve hyperhomocyst(e)inemia as a pathophysiologic mechanism.

Carrier State

Heterozygotes for CβS deficiency may be at risk for premature vascular occlusion. The physician's duty to diagnose, inform, and treat extended family members of probands with CβS deficiency awaits further definition of this risk and outcomes of intervention (199).

ORGANIC ACIDS

Several essential amino acids contribute to the synthesis of the acyl groups of organic acids. Among these are the following: the BCAAs, ILE, LEU, and VAL; the sulfur amino acid MET; the hydroxy amino acid threonine (THR); and the dibasic amino acids lysine (LYS) and TRP (see Figs. 69.3 and 69.4).

Biochemistry

The BCAAs, ILE, LEU, and VAL are essential nutrients. In the newborn, 75% of the amounts ingested is used for protein synthesis. That present in excess of need for synthetic purposes is degraded through many steps to provide energy (see Fig. 69.4). When acetyl-CoA and succinyl-CoA are not formed from the appropriate BCAA, they are not available

to enter the tricarboxylic acid cycle to yield energy because the organic acids are excreted in the urine. The initial step in catabolism is reversible transamination, requiring a specific transaminase and the coenzyme pyridoxal phosphate. The second step is irreversible oxidative decarboxylation, which uses the BCKAD complex. This complex is located in the inner mitochondrial membrane and requires the coenzymes TPP, lipoic acid, CoA, and NAD^+ (200–204). Figure 69.4 diagrams this overall reaction. At least six proteins are involved: E1α, E1β, E2, E3, a kinase, and phosphatase.

Isovaleryl-CoA, synthesized from α-ketoisocaproic acid by BCKAD, is catalyzed to 3-methylcrotonyl-CoA by isovaleryl-CoA dehydrogenase (IVD), a mitochondrial enzyme that requires flavoprotein and uses electron transfer factor (ETF) (see Fig. 69.4). Mutations in the gene for IVD result in isovaleric acidemia (see Table 69.2) (205). According to Xu et al (206), approximately 14% of α-ketoisocaproate is catabolized to hydroxymethylbutyrate in homogenized rat and human liver by cytosolic α-ketoisocaproate dehydrogenase. No in vivo data to support this pathway have been published, however.

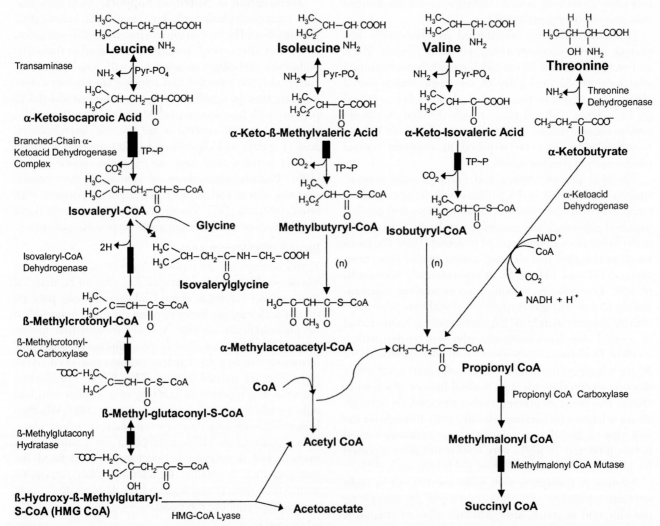

Fig. 69.4. Metabolism of branched-chain amino acids and threonine. The *black bars* indicate sites of enzyme defects. *CoA,* coenzyme A; *(n),* several steps; *NAD,* nicotinamide adenine dinucleotide (NADH is the reduced form).

3-Methylcrotonyl-CoA is carboxylated at the 4-carbon by 3-methylcrotonyl-CoA carboxylase to form 3-methylglutaconyl-CoA (see Fig. 69.4). This enzyme, associated with the inner mitochondrial membrane, contains covalently bound biotin. Mutations in the gene for 3-methylcrotonyl-CoA carboxylase result in 3-methylcrotonylglycinuria (see Table 69.2).

3-Methylglutaconyl-CoA hydratase, presumably located in the mitochondria, hydrates 3-methylglutaconyl-CoA to HMG-CoA. HMG-CoA is cleaved by HMG-CoA lyase to acetoacetic acid and acetyl-CoA (see Fig. 69.4). Mutations in the gene for 3-methylglutaconyl-CoA hydratase result in 3-methylglutaconic aciduria, whereas mutations in the gene for HMG-CoA lyase result in hydroxymethylglutaric aciduria (see Table 69.2).

Complete catabolism of ILE through its major degradative pathway results in the synthesis of acetyl-CoA and succinyl-CoA (see Fig. 69.4). After synthesis of 2-methylbutyryl-CoA by BCKAD, this organic acid is catalyzed by a dehydrogenase to tiglyl-CoA, which is acted on by a hydratase to form 2-methyl-3-hydroxybutyryl-CoA. This compound is used by a dehydrogenase to form 2-methylacetoacetyl-CoA. Mitochondrial acetoacetyl-CoA thiolase (β-ketothiolase) interconverts 2-methylacetoacetyl-CoA to acetyl-CoA plus propionyl-CoA. Propionyl-CoA plus HCO_3^-, in the presence of ATP, biotin, and magnesium (Mg^+), is acted on by propionyl-CoA carboxylase to form D-methylmalonyl-CoA. The biotin molecule is responsible for the transfer of the carboxyl group. Isolated deficiency of the propionyl-CoA carboxylase, caused by mutations in the genes encoding its nonidentical α- and β-subunits (see Table 69.2), results in propionic acidemia (PPA) (207).

Methylmalonyl-CoA racemase converts D-methylmalonyl-CoA to L-methylmalonyl-CoA, which is isomerized to succinyl-CoA by methylmalonyl-CoA mutase. This dimer contains 1 mol of tightly bound adenosylcobalamin per mole of subunit. Mutations in the gene encoding for methylmalonyl-CoA mutase, as well as those encoding for mitochondrial glutathionylcobalamin reductase and adenosylreductase, result in methylmalonic acidemia (MMA) (see Table 69.3 and Fig. 69.4). Cytosolic cobalamin reductase/β-ligand transferase deficiency results in homocystinuria and MMA (207).

After synthesis of isobutyryl-CoA from 2-ketoisovaleric acid by BCKAD (see Fig. 69.4), it is acted on by isobutyryl-CoA dehydrogenase (208), followed by a hydratase, a deacylase, and two further dehydrogenases to form propionyl-CoA (207). A deficiency of isobutyryl-CoA dehydrogenase results in difficulty metabolizing essential VAL.

Two other amino acids, MET and THR, as well as odd-chain fatty acids, thymine, uracil, and the side chain of cholesterol, are catabolized to propionyl-CoA (see Figs. 69.3 and 69.4). The transamination of MET becomes most prominent when plasma MET concentrations exceed 350 μmol/L and seems to function as a spillover pathway that accounts for only a minor portion of total MET catabolism (209). Even in the fasting state with plasma MET concentrations in the normal range, however, some MET is transaminated and decarboxylated to form 3-methylthiopropionate (210, 211), and the α-ketobutyrate formed by the transsulfuration pathway is also used to synthesize propionyl-CoA (see Fig. 69.3).

The major pathway of THR catabolism is through oxidation of the hydroxyl group by a specific dehydrogenase to form α-amino-β-ketobutyrate, which subsequently forms acetyl-CoA plus GLY. Another lesser used pathway of catabolism is through serine (THR) dehydrogenase and deamination to form α-ketobutyrate (212), which is acted on by α-ketoacid dehydrogenase to form propionyl-CoA (213) (see Fig. 69.4). Energy, normally obtained from the oxidation of succinyl-CoA in the tricarboxylic acid cycle, is lost in the urine as propionic acid and methylmalonic acid in PPA and MMA, respectively.

Two essential amino acids contained in food and body protein, LYS and TRP, are precursors of glutaric acid (Fig. 69.5). The metabolism of TRP does not resemble that of any other metabolite (212). Its principal degradative pathway occurs in the liver and leads to the formation of nicotinic acid, usually classified as a vitamin, and many byproducts that accumulate under normal circumstances. TRP metabolism also leads to serotonin. The initial reaction in the main pathway is oxygenation to form formylkynurenine. The enzyme, TRP oxygenase, contains an iron porphyrin. The formate of N-formylkynurenine is handled as a C_1 fragment by the H_4 folate system. Kynurenine is a branch point; the main pathway continues with a mixed-function oxygenase that includes flavin adenine dinucleotide and uses NAD or NAD phosphate (NADP) as the cosubstrate in the synthesis of 3-hydroxykynurenine. One side branch splits off the bulk of the side chain as alanine through the action of the pyridoxal phosphate enzyme kynureninase, and another side branch removes the α-amino group by transamination (also using pyridoxal phosphate), but the keto group forms a Schiff base with the aromatic amine to form the stable aromatic compound kynurenate. Kynurenate has been found in the brain, where it antagonizes the effects of excitatory amino acids.

3-Hydroxykynurenine is also a branch point. The main pathway now uses the kynureninase that caused a branch earlier to remove alanine but to produce 3-hydroxyanthranilate. The branch is again caused by transamination, which also results in a quinoline ring to form xanthurenic acid. A third oxygenase cleaves 3-hydroxyanthranilate to an unstable intermediate, 2-amino-3-carboxymuconic 6-semialdehyde. This unstable intermediate cyclizes to a Schiff base to form quinolinate. An enzyme, picolinic carboxylase, competes with the formation of quinolinate and decarboxylates the intermediate to one that forms picolinate. Most of the decarboxylated material is caught by a dehydrogenase, however, that converts the aldehyde to an acid

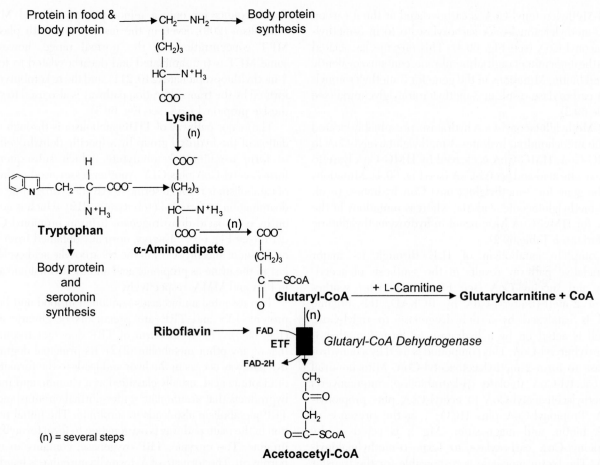

Fig. 69.5. Metabolism of lysine and tryptophan. The *black bar* indicates the site of the enzyme defect in glutaric acidemia type I. *L-Carnitine* enhances urinary excretion of glutaric acid. *ETF* is the electron transfer factor that, when impaired, may cause glutaric aciduria and the accumulation of other substrates using ETF. *CoA,* coenzyme A; *FAD,* flavin adenine dinucleotide.

and leads through α-ketoadipate and glutaryl-CoA to acetoacetyl-CoA (see Fig. 69.5).

LYS is one of two essential amino acids that have an α-amino group that does not equilibrate with the body pool of amino groups; the other is THR. The amino group of LYS is transferred to other amino acids, but the reverse does not occur. Most degradation of LYS occurs by a unique pathway in which a secondary amine is formed between the ε-amino group and the carbonyl group of α-ketoglutarate. The product, saccharopine, is formed by an enzyme that reduces the hypothetical Schiff base with NADP. Normally, saccharopine does not accumulate but is oxidized by another dehydrogenase that splits the linkage on the other side of the bridge nitrogen. The sum of the reduction-oxidation reactions is effectively a transamination yielding glutamate and α-aminoadipic semialdehyde. The latter can form a Schiff base, but with the double bond on the side of the nitrogen atom away from the carboxylate. This compound can be oxidized by another dehydrogenase to become α-aminoadipate. A transamination converts this homolog of glutamate to the corresponding α-ketoadipate. In a reaction analogous to the oxidation of α-ketoglutarate to succinyl-CoA,

glutaryl-CoA is formed (see Fig. 69.5). Another oxidation introduces a double bond, forming glutaconyl-CoA, which is decarboxylated to crotonyl-CoA. This unsaturated fatty acyl-CoA is an intermediate in the normal oxidation of fatty acids, and subsequent reactions of the material derived from LYS are those of fatty acid oxidation leading to acetoacetyl-CoA (212).

Branched-Chain α-Ketoaciduria (Maple Syrup Urine Disease)

MSUD is a group of inherited disorders of ILE, LEU, and VAL metabolism. These disorders result from several different gene mutations that impair various components of the multienzyme BCKAD (see Fig. 69.6 and Table 69.2). These genes are *E1α, E1β, E2,* and *E3* (200). *E1α* is inactivated by a kinase and activated by its phosphatase (see Table 69.2). The BCKAD-specific kinase and phosphate have not been cloned nor do they have chaperonin proteins involved in their mitochondrial assembly process. Almost all mutations in these proteins that produce MSUD are private. The only one common among Mennonites is the one in the E1α protein, and it is a substitution of asparagine for

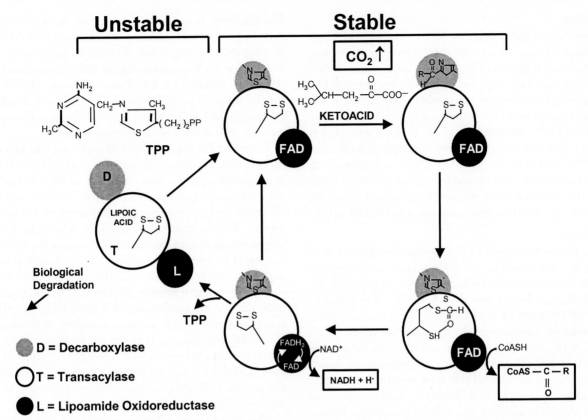

Fig. 69.6. Model for stabilization of branched-chain α-ketoacid dehydrogenase by thiamin pyrophosphate (TPP). The multienzyme complex branched-chain α-ketoacid dehydrogenase has a configuration that is more stable to degradation when TPP binding sites on its decarboxylase moiety are occupied. *CoASH,* coenzyme A; *FAD,* flavin adenine dinucleotide (FADH is the reduced form); *NAD,* nicotinamide adenine dinucleotide (NADH is the reduced form).

TYR at amino acid 393 (Y393N) (see Table 69.2). Although most mutant enzymes are immunologically present, one reported patient had absent branched-chain acyltransferase (E2) as a cause of thiamin-resistant MSUD (202, 214, 215). An autosomal recessive mode of inheritance was found in all reported cases, a finding supporting a nuclear rather than a mitochondrial origin of these proteins. The cellular mechanisms involved in assembling the products of these nuclear genes into a multienzyme complex in mitochondria are of considerable clinical and fundamental importance and remain unresolved.

Infants with MSUD appear normal at birth and are clinically well until after they eat a protein-containing feeding. The most severely impaired enzymes may produce seizures, apnea, and death within 10 days of birth. The disorder is characterized by elevated blood, urine, and cerebrospinal fluid concentrations of the BCKAs, their amino acid precursors, and the pathognomonic alloisoleucine. Progressive neurologic dysfunction and production of fragrant urine with the odor of burnt sugar (caramel) or maple syrup follow. The sweet smell may be evident only in earwax and is easily sensed after otoscopic examination. Neurologic impairment in the newborn is manifested by poor sucking, irregular respiration, rigidity alternating with periods of flaccidity, opisthotonos, progressive loss of the Moro reflex, and seizures.

Several variants covering a spectrum of impaired mitochondrial BCKAD complexes have been reported. Clinical manifestations are expressed intermittently on protein loading or with febrile illness in patients with partial enzyme activity between 5% and 20% of normal. Patients with 3% to 30% BCKAD complex activity express an intermediate form of the disease. A thiamin-responsive form with expression similar to the intermediate form has been described (200). Whole body LEU-1-^{13}C oxidation to $^{13}CO_2$ may be the best method of ascertaining total body needs because peripheral cells may not reflect liver and renal BCKAD function (202, 203).

Untreated patients with classic MSUD (<2% BCKAD complex activity) who survive beyond early infancy have retarded physical and mental development (214, 215). Early diagnosis and therapy lead to normal growth and development (8). If death occurs in the first few days of life, few unique abnormalities are seen in the brain. With prolonged survival, deficient myelination is thought to be caused by enzymes involved in myelin formation, inhibition of amino acid transport, and inhibition by BCKAs of oxidative phosphorylation (214, 215). Jouvet et al (216) reported that increased concentrations of BCKAs, in particular of α-ketoisocaproic acid, induced apoptosis in glial and neuronal cells in culture and in vivo after intracerebral injection into the developing rat brain.

Screening

Because apnea and death may be the first clinical manifestations of the classic disorder, newborn screening, retrieval, and initiation of therapy are urgent; and all four processes must be completed within the first week of life. Nonselected screening of the newborn population is currently in progress (in some states) using an MS/MS assay for blood LEU concentrations (217). Bedside screening in selected children uses the urinary dinitrophenylhydrazine (DNPH) reaction for branched-chain α-ketoaciduria. This reaction can also be used to monitor dietary progress. International newborn screening indicates that the incidence of MSUD is approximately 1 in 185,000 (217).

Diagnosis

Any infant with a blood LEU concentration greater than 4 mg/dL (305 μmol/L) on the newborn screening test should be immediately evaluated. Most infants with the classic disease have more than 8 mg/dL (610 μmol/L) LEU at 72 hours of age. Diagnosis is confirmed using ion-exchange chromatography to quantitate plasma ILE, LEU, VAL, and alloisoleucine and GC/MS to identify urinary BCKAs. The extent of enzyme impairment should be determined on cultured cells such as dermal fibroblasts to enable future prenatal diagnosis, because prenatal monitoring is available if the cellular phenotype is confirmed in fibroblasts cultured from the patient's skin (218). Total body LEU oxidation using stable isotopes and the $^{13}CO_2$ breath test is the most reliable diagnostic tool for establishing dietary needs, including thiamin responsivity, however (203). Except in Mennonites, molecular analysis is useful only for research purposes.

Treatment

Relatively little help in managing MSUD has resulted from advances in mutation analysis, except for the role of pharmacologic coenzymes. When TPP saturates its site on E1α, the biologic turnover of BCKAD is decreased (see Fig. 69.6). Increasing thiamin ingestion increases intracellular TPP, and the TPP binding sites on the decarboxylase (E1) moiety of the BCKAD complex become saturated. When these TPP binding sites are occupied, the multienzyme complex undergoes a conformational change that makes it more resistant to chymotrypsin and heat degradation. The biologic half-life of the enzyme and overall activity are increased when a new equilibrium of enzyme synthesis and degradation is reached. This model has been tested and is supported by clinical, functional, and structural studies (202, 204, 218, 219) (see Fig. 69.6).

Although hemodialysis with nitrogen-free dialysate or exchange transfusion may be required when diagnosis is delayed, if screening, retrieval, and diagnosis are completed within 8 to 10 days of life, these actions are seldom necessary. Because hemodialysis superimposes iatrogenic risk and prolongs a catabolic phase, it is not recommended. BCAA-free orogastric feeding of protein and energy should begin as soon as the diagnosis is made.

The objective is to produce anabolism in the infant and thereby prevent accumulation of neurotoxic BCKAs (220). If orogastric feeding is not acceptable, gastrostomy or a central line for hyperalimentation with dextrose and lipid should be initiated for initial care of classic MSUD during the neonatal period. Except during illness, restricting protein intake to 1.5 g/kg/day may be adequate therapy for patients with 20% or more of enzyme activity.

Long-term therapy for MSUD is dietary. The objective of long-term nutrition support in the child with MSUD is to maintain plasma concentrations of BCAAs that will allow maximal development of intellect while supplying adequate energy, protein, and other nutrients for optimal growth. Plasma concentrations of BCAAs (3 to 4 hours after a meal) should be maintained within the following ranges: ILE, 40 to 90 μmol/L; LEU, 80 to 200 μmol/L; and VAL, 200 to 425 μmol/L. ILE deficiency results in skin lesions that resemble acrodermatitis enteropathica (221, 222). With a deficiency of ILE or VAL, the plasma concentration of LEU remains elevated. With deletion of the BCAAs, plasma ILE returns to normal first, followed by VAL. When adequate dietary ILE and VAL are then added to maintain normal plasma concentrations, the plasma LEU concentration returns to normal in 5 to 10 days (223).

The objectives of nutrition support are met by using a combination of medical foods (see Table 69.5 for sources of medical foods and reference 94 for nutrient composition of other foods) and intact protein. Most patients with MSUD who have detectable BCKAD multienzyme complex by immunoassay respond to oral thiamin administration of 100 to 1000 mg daily (202, 203, 219). Supraphysiologic amounts of oral thiamin should be added for at least a 3-month trial period because they stabilize the enzyme complex (see Fig. 69.6). Increased residual specific activity of mitochondrial membrane-bound enzymes may require this prolonged period because of the biologic half-life of this subcellular organelle. During this period, decreased sensitivity to dietary BCAAs is usually observed, and more can be added to the diet. Evaluation of total body LEU oxidation before and during thiamin administration gives direct evidence of responsivity (203). In classic MSUD, thiamin is only an adjunct therapy, and dietary restriction of ILE, LEU, and VAL is needed.

In one report, orthoptic liver transplantation resulted in a clear increase in whole body BCKA oxidation to at least the level of MSUD variants. These patients no longer required BCAA restriction, and the risk of metabolic decompensation during catabolism was abolished (224).

Nutrient Requirements. Data in Table 69.4 outline the suggested amounts of BCAAs, protein, energy, and fluid to offer the infant or child with MSUD. Because the BCAAs are essential, they cannot be deleted from the diet without producing growth failure and death. In planning nutrition support of the infant or child with MSUD, a prescription should be written that includes recommended

Biochemistry

Central dogma holds that ammonia is converted to urea in the liver through the Krebs-Henseleit cycle (Fig. 69.7) and is excreted in the urine. The first three enzymes of the cycle and N-acetylglutamate synthetase are mitochondrial. N-acetylglutamate synthetase catalyzes the conversion of acetyl-CoA plus glutamate to N-acetylglutamate, an essential cofactor for carbamylphosphate synthesis. Carbamylphosphate synthetase I catalyzes the conversion of ammonia, ATP, and bicarbonate to carbamylphosphate. OTC uses carbamylphosphate and ornithine (ORN) as cosubstrates to form citrulline (CIT), which is exported from mitochondria to the cytoplasm, where cytosolic reactions are linked to those three mitochondrial functions. CIT and aspartate form argininosuccinic acid, a reaction catalyzed by argininosuccinic acid synthetase. Fumarate is cleaved from argininosuccinic acid by argininosuccinic acid lyase, yielding arginine (ARG). Urea is then formed by the action of arginase, regenerating cytosolic ORN, which is transported back into the mitochondria to react with OTC.

Citrin is an isoform of the mitochondrial aspartate-glutamate carrier in the inner mitochondrial membrane and is responsible for the exchange of aspartate for cytosolic glutamate and H^+ ion. Patients with a deficiency of citrin (CTNL2) have mutations on chromosome 7q21.3 (33) and elevated plasma CIT concentrations; and in neonates, intrahepatic cholestasis and secondary argininosuccinic acid synthetase deficiency are observed. Coma and death may result from brain edema (31).

Urea Cycle Enzyme Deficiencies

Disorders of the urea cycle comprise a group of inherited defects in the six enzymes that produce urea (see Fig. 69.7) (308). With the exception of OTC deficiency, all these disorders have an autosomal recessive mode of inheritance. OTC deficiency is inherited as an X-linked dominant trait that is usually lethal in male patients. Many of the genes for these enzymes have been localized to the human genome, have been cloned, and have had mutations defined. *OTC*, a 73-kb gene containing 10 exons, is located on Xp21.1. More than 230 mutations have been defined with some genotype–phenotype relationships (309). For example, the generation of stop codons from R109X and R109Q results in no residual liver enzyme and a severe neonatal presentation. By contrast, the R129-to-histidine mutation, also present in the *spf-ash* mouse model of OTC deficiency, has a milder phenotype and residual liver enzyme activity (310). Carbamylphosphate synthetase is located on 2q35, argininosuccinic acid synthetase is located on 9q34, argininosuccinic acid lyase is located on 7q11, and arginase is present on 6q23. All are primarily expressed in liver, and all these genes have defined mutations in their respective disorders (see Table 69.2) (308, 309, 311, 312). Argininosuccinic acid synthetase has several pseudogenes that confound DNA analysis (308). In OTC deficiency, defects in the protein include disordered mitochondrial uptake and immunologically absent protein in this organelle (310). Arginase has two genes with differential expression in liver and erythrocytes. In addition to these defects in ureagenesis, a seventh cause of hyperammonemia is the

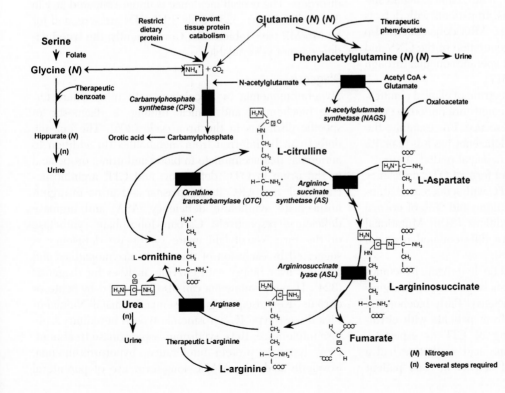

Fig. 69.7. Inborn errors in the urea cycle and nutrition approaches to their management. Ammonia fixation and urea production are metabolically cycled, with inherited blocks producing hyperammonemia indicated by *black bars*. Important nitrogen molecules and the biochemical origins are outlined in *boxes*. Mitochondrial enzymes in urea synthesis are carbamylphosphate synthetase, N-acetylglutamate synthetase, and ornithine transcarbamylase. Use of benzoate, phenylacetate, and phenylbutyrate is indicated to provide alternate pathways for nitrogen excretion. Dietary arginine is added to provide urea cycle substrate distal to genetically impaired reactions. Restriction of dietary protein and addition of dietary energy to prevent protein catabolism are also indicated. CoA, coenzyme A.

hyperammonemia, homocitrullinemia, hyperornithinemia syndrome, which is caused by defective mitochondrial uptake of ORN (313).

Hyperammonemia is a biochemical manifestation of all disorders of the urea cycle. Other biochemical characteristics of each defect follow: carbamylphosphate synthetase I defect causes decreased plasma CIT; OTC deficiency results in orotic aciduria and X-linked patterns of transmission; argininosuccinate synthetase deficiency is associated with increased plasma CIT accompanied by orotic aciduria; argininosuccinate lyase deficiency (ASA) causes increased argininosuccinate in plasma and urine; and arginase deficiency is characterized by increased ARG in plasma and urine. Clinical features in the newborn suggesting urea cycle enzyme deficiency (UCED) occur with protein ingestion. In increasing order of severity, these defects include poor feeding, vomiting, lethargy, hypotonia, stupor, bleeding diatheses, convulsions, coma, shock, and death (308, 314). Mental retardation occurs in survivors of these disastrous newborn episodes, but successful control of hyperammonemia in the newborn may prevent this sequela.

Clinical Phenotypes

Hyperammonemia and its clinical sequelae of vomiting, lethargy, and coma relate to excessive protein intake, catabolism, or valproate therapy (315) and are observed in all the UCEDs. Biochemical and phenotypic manifestations differ in the individual enzyme deficiencies, however. In ASA, a specific hair abnormality, trichorrhexis nodosa, is evident. This condition is related to ARG deficiency and the relatively high ARG content of normal hair protein. Hair reverts to normal with ARG supplementation. Adult siblings with ASA may have few, if any, clinical manifestations despite identical mutations. In patients with defects in one of the first four enzymes, ARG deficiency is also associated with progressive degeneration of the CNS and a peculiar rash with control of hyperammonemia through protein restriction alone (316, 317).

Each enzyme defect has a spectrum of clinical manifestations ranging from death in the newborn period to cyclic vomiting and migraine in adolescence. For example, the typical male patient with OTC deficiency has less than 5% normal activity and dies in the neonatal period. A surviving male child with the late-onset form of OTC deficiency has immunologically present OTC with a decreased affinity for ORN, a shift of pH optimum, and 25% of normal activity under physiologic conditions (318). Mutational analyses of the *OTC* gene have differentiated neonatal from late-onset phenotypes (308).

Enzymatic evidence of genetic heterogeneity comes from kinetic studies in fibroblasts of patients with argininosuccinic acid synthetase deficiency. Early biochemical studies showed that enzymes from patients with citrullinemia had decreased binding of CIT or aspartate, but the residual argininosuccinic acid synthetase had a distinct and different curve of activity in each patient

(319). Analyses of RNA in citrullinemic patients showed heterogeneity, and more than 20 different mutations are now defined (308).

Expression of the Heterozygous State for Ornithine Transcarbamylase Deficiency. The female heterozygote of OTC deficiency may have mild protein intolerance manifested clinically by migraine in adults and by cyclic vomiting with intermittent hyperammonemia in children. When protein or ammonium chloride loads were administered to 15 children with migraine and cyclic vomiting, 9 had abnormally high baseline plasma ammonium levels; the tests produced marked hyperammonemia in 8 children, and 6 developed migraine symptoms. Enzyme assay in 7 girls with cyclic vomiting showed 3 with deficient OTC activity. Heterozygous female patients with OTC deficiency may be asymptomatic or as severely affected as hemizygous male patients (320).

Screening

Nonselected screening of all newborns for UCEDs was routinely conducted in Massachusetts using a bacterial auxotroph that required ARG. Among the children tested, 9 of 700,000 newborns were found to be homozygous affected or heterozygous for ASA (321). Problems associated with analysis of ammonia in blood were described by Barsotti (322). This method can be readily adopted in offices and hospitals for selective screening. Its lack of use in the United States is related to cost and demand. Several states now screen for citrullinemia and argininosuccinic aciduria using MS/MS.

The true incidence of UCEDs is not known because population-based screening has not been conducted, and many undiagnosed deaths may be caused by these disorders. The overall incidence is underestimated at 1 in 30,000 live births (323). Only 3 UCEDs are screened for by MS/MS (see Table 69.1). Consequently, the true incidence is not yet available.

Diagnosis

Hyperammonemia in association with other characteristic biochemical and clinical findings is diagnostic of specific disorders in the urea cycle (308). The enzyme defect can be inferred from metabolites (in addition to ammonia) that accumulate in blood and urine: orotic acid in the urine in OTC deficiency; and CIT, argininosuccinic acid, and ARG in the plasma and urine in argininosuccinate synthetase deficiency, ASA, and arginase deficiency, respectively. Carbamylphosphate synthetase or the rare N-acetylglutamate synthetase deficiency is suggested by exclusion of these four enzymopathies and requires liver biopsy with enzyme analyses for diagnosis (324). Hyperammonemia can also be caused by acute or chronic liver diseases, galactosemia, neonatal Niemann-Pick disease type IC, tyrosinemia type I, hereditary fructose intolerance, Reye syndrome, asparaginase treatment, PPA, lysinuric protein intolerance, hyperornithinemia, isovaleric acidemia, MMA, long-term use of parenteral

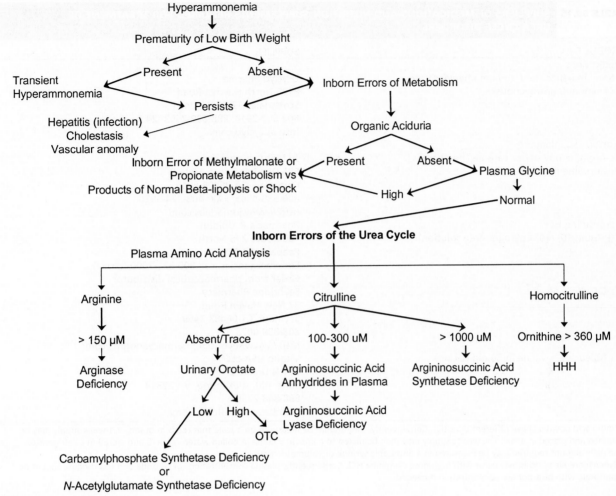

Fig. 69.8. Algorithm for differential diagnosis of urea cycle disorders. *HHH,* hyperornithinemia, homocitrullinemia, and hyperammonemia; *OTC,* ornithine transcarbamylase.

amino acids, and many different infectious agents in infancy. Definitive diagnosis depends on clinical acumen followed by appropriate laboratory studies (314). A suggested algorithm for differential diagnosis of UCEDs is given in Figure 69.8. A suspected UCED is a medical emergency and requires immediate intervention.

Treatment

The treatment of inherited urea cycle enzymopathies can be divided into short-term and long-term therapy and depends on the specific diagnosis (325). Valproate therapy should be avoided in patients with UCEDs because the use of this agent may enhance hyperammonemia (264, 315).

Short-Term Therapy.   The preferred approach is to begin orogastric perfusion with high energy intake (150 kcal/kg/day) but no protein. Pro-Phree (Abbott Nutrition) or PFD1 (Mead Johnson Nutritionals) is useful for this approach (see Table 69.5). L-ARG (350 to 500 mg/kg/day) should be added to this formulation. Sodium benzoate (300 mg/kg/day) can successfully reduce acute hyperammonemia in the neonatal period by conjugation of benzoic acid with GLY to form hippurate. Phenylbutyric acid or

phenylacetic acid (500 mg/kg/day) is also given to form phenylacetylglutamine, which is excreted in the urine, thus eliminating from the body two nitrogen atoms per molecule (see Fig. 69.7 and Table 69.15). Urinary potassium loss is enhanced by the excretion of hippurate and phenylacetylglutamine. Consequently, plasma potassium concentrations should be monitored, and supplements should be given if needed (325).

Hemodialysis may be useful in the presence of coma in reducing plasma ammonium concentrations. Peritoneal dialysis for 7 days in a male neonate with OTC deficiency removed 50 times more ammonia than did a single exchange transfusion. Peritoneal dialysis includes risks such as *Candida* peritonitis and continued catabolism, however. If dialysis is used, parenteral L-ARG HCl and sodium phenylbutyrate should be given as well. Continued intravenous protein-free energy is also recommended.

A priority of newborn therapy is to force the neonate into an anabolic phase with high-energy feedings (Table 69.16). Peripheral venous hyperalimentation with 10% to 20% GLU and lipid (2 to 4 g/kg) may be necessary if gavage is not tolerated. As gavage feedings are

TABLE 69.15	SUPPLIERS OF MEDICATIONS AND NUTRITION SUPPLEMENTS REQUIRED FOR TREATMENT OF UREA CYCLE DISORDERS

PRODUCT	SUPPLIER
Medications	
Sodium benzoate + sodium phenylacetate (Ammonul) (intravenous)	Ucyclyd Pharma 8125 North Hayden Road Scottsdale, AZ 85258-2463 602-667-3914, 888-829-2593 (24 h) http://ucyclyd.com/
Nutrition supplements	
L-Arginine powder or capsule (free base) L-Citrulline powder[a]	Jo Mar Laboratories 583 Division Street, Suite B Campbell, CA 95008-6915 800-538-4545; FAX: 408-374-5920 http://www.jomarlabs.com/
L-Arginine HCl[b] (R-Gene-10) (10% pyrogen-free solution)	Pharmacia & Upjohn 100 Route 206 North Peapack, NJ 07977 For emergencies, call 800-821-7000 (direct) Order from pharmaceutical distributor
L-Citrulline powder[a]	Seybridge Pharmacy 37 New Haven Road Seymour, CT 06483-3469 203-888-0073 http://www.seybridgepharmacyandgifts.com/
L-Isoleucine, L-valine in 50-mg packets	Vitaflo USA LLC 211 N Union St Suite 100, Alexandria, VA 22314 888-848-2356 http://www.vitaflousa.com/

[a]Amino acid powders have different densities. Consequently, they should be measured on a scale that reads in grams. A 1-week supply may be weighed and placed in a vial. The week's supply may then be mixed to a known volume in boiled water, capped, and stored in a refrigerator. The daily amount required may be measured in a disposable syringe or volumetric flask.

[b]Hyperchloremic acidosis may occur with high-dose L-arginine HCl. Consequently, plasma concentrations of chloride and bicarbonate should be monitored, with bicarbonate administration if needed.

increased, peripheral alimentation should be decreased. After 1 to 2 days of no-protein, high-energy, L-ARG HCl–supplemented and benzoate-supplemented feedings, blood ammonia concentrations should revert to nearly normal. Cautious addition of 1.0 to 1.5 g/kg/day of protein is then necessary.

Long-Term Therapy. The objectives of therapy in a child with a UCED are to maintain plasma concentrations of ammonia as close to normal as possible and to supply protein and other essential amino acids and nutrients that will allow maximal intellectual development and optimal growth. Four major approaches are used in treating individuals with UCEDs (see Fig. 69.7): (a) reducing precursors of ammonia (protein intake), (b) correcting ARG deficiency, (c) enhancing alternate mechanisms of waste nitrogen loss, and (d) accelerating renal excretion of accumulated intermediates (325).

Methods used to reduce ammonia precursors include protein restriction, prevention of body protein catabolism, and use of essential and semiessential amino acids. Any time that intake of protein or essential amino acids is severely restricted, precursors for synthesis of carnitine (LYS, MET), glutathione (cysteine, glutamate), and taurine (cysteine) may be limiting. Restricted MET intake

may result in a decrease in the available pool of labile methyl groups required for synthesis of important metabolic compounds.

L-ARG base supplementation is required in all the UCEDs except arginase deficiency. To maintain normal or slightly elevated plasma ARG concentrations, 100 to 500 mg/kg of body weight daily are used (326). L-ARG can then produce ORN for ammonia fixation and drive the cycle to CIT and argininosuccinate (see Fig. 69.7). These two amino acids are poorly absorbed by the kidney and allow nitrogen loss. Acceleration of renal excretion of accumulated intermediates in the impaired cycle is sought. ARG supplementation increases CIT and argininosuccinic acid excretion in argininosuccinic acid synthetase and ASA, deficiencies respectively.

Waste nitrogen urinary loss can be enhanced by the use of sodium benzoate, phenylacetate, or phenylbutyrate (326) (see Fig. 69.7). GLY conjugates with benzoate through GLY-N-acylase, which leads to excretion of a nearly stoichiometric quantity of nitrogen as hippurate (see Fig. 69.7). Toxicity is low on 200 to 500 mg/kg/day. Folate must be administered to provide a source of one-carbon fragments for synthesis of GLY from serine to prevent GLY depletion. Pyridoxine is necessary for transamination.

TABLE 69.16	RECOMMENDED DAILY NUTRIENT INTAKES (RANGES) FOR INFANTS AND CHILDREN WITH UREA CYCLE DISORDERS

AGE	NUTRIENT		
	L-ARGININE[a] (g/kg)	PROTEIN[b] (g/kg)	ENERGY[b,c] (kcal/kg)
Months			
0 < 1	500–100	2.2–1.5	155–120
1 < 2	500–100	2.0–1.5	150–115
2 < 3	500–100	1.9–1.3	145–110
3 < 4	400–100	1.5–1.2	140–105
4 < 5	400–100	1.4–1.0	135–100
5 < 6	400–100	1.3–1.0	130–95
6 < 7	400–100	1.2–0.89	125–90
7 < 8	300–100	1.1–0.8	120–85
8 < 9	300–100	1.1–0.8	115–80
9 < 10	300–100	1.0–0.8	110–80
10 < 11	300–100	1.0–0.8	105–80
11 < 12	300–100	1.0–0.8	105–80
Years			
1 < 2	300–100	1.3–0.8	110–105
2 < 3	300–100	1.2–0.8	105–100
3 < 4	300–100	1.1–0.8	100–95
4 < 7	300–100	1.0–0.7	95–85
7 < 11	300–100	1.0–0.7	85–65
11 < 19	300–100	1.0–0.6	60–40

[a]Not used with arginase deficiency.
[b]Based on the 50th percentile weight for age. Modify as needed to maintain normal linear growth and plasma ammonia concentrations <10 μmol/L.
[c]Supply at least 1.5 mL fluid/kcal to infants and 1.0 mL/kcal to children.

Pantothenic acid (4 mg/L) in tissue culture media enhanced CoA and hippurate concentrations to a greater extent than did smaller or greater amounts (327). Phenylbutyrate and phenylacetate increase urinary nitrogen excretion as phenylacetylglutamine. The suggested dose is 500 mg/kg of body weight. This efficient alternative pathway removes two molecules of nitrogen per molecule of phenylacetylglutamine and requires monitoring of protein intake to prevent deficiency. Excess use of these nitrogen-binding drugs can lead to nitrogen deficiency and poor growth.

Further, the use of phenylbutyrate leads to excretion of glutamine as phenylacetylglutamine and increased LEU oxidation in normal adults (328). Plasma BCAA concentrations and protein synthesis are also decreased with the administration of phenylbutyrate at 10 g/day with a protein intake of 0.4 g/kg body weight/day (329).

Patients with CIT II deficiency require a diet very different from that fed in other UCEDs. This diet for CIT II must be high protein (17% to 21% of energy), high fat (40% to 47% of energy) and low carbohydrate (33% to 40% of energy), with L-ARG supplements (see Table 69.3) (31, 325).

Catabolism during a febrile illness or because of poor appetite may lead to life-threatening elevations in blood ammonia. In addition to prompt diagnosis and treatment of the infection, decreased protein intake (0 g for

1 to 2 days), increased energy intake, and peritoneal dialysis may all be required. Gastrostomy feedings may be required to ensure adequate intake and to prevent inadequate growth or catabolism.

In planning nutrition support of the infant or child with a UCED, a formal prescription should be written that includes recommended amounts of protein, energy, fluid, and L-ARG, and drugs that enhance nitrogen loss. The prescription for protein should be based on the specific diagnosis, degree of impaired urea cycle, and blood ammonia concentrations and correlated with various parameters of growth, including rates of height and weight increase and hair, nails, teeth, and skin changes.

Protein intake suggested in Table 69.16 are based on amount required to cover obligatory nitrogen losses and growth needs (330) and are modified based on unpublished data from 10 infants with 1 of 4 different enzyme defects diagnosed within the first 10 days of life. Intake may need to be increased if the child does not grow adequately on the recommended intake or if sodium benzoate, phenylacetate, or phenylbutyrate is administered. Overrestriction of protein may lead to catabolism and impaired renal activity to excrete ammonium (NH_4^+). TRP intake should be at the minimal requirement for growth to prevent excess serotonin synthesis that suppresses appetite (331).

Energy intakes recommended in Table 69.16 are somewhat higher than those for physiologically normal infants and children, to provide ketoacid precursors from carbohydrate for synthesis of nonessential amino acids and to prevent protein degradation. Carbohydrate should not provide more than 50% of the energy because of frequently elevated plasma triacylglycerol concentrations.

In any situation in which protein-restricted diets are fed, L-carnitine supplements may be necessary. Recommended amounts of supplemental L-carnitine are 50 to 100 mg/kg/day. L-Carnitine supplements are reported to lower blood ammonium concentrations (332, 333). Citrate deficiency was reported in patients with ASA, and supplementation was recommended (334, 335).

Medical Foods for Urea Cycle Disorders. Nutrition support of UCEDs requires restricting nitrogen intake, which is best accomplished by providing approximately two thirds the prescribed protein in the form of essential amino acids only (medical foods). Sources of medical foods for UCEDs are given in Table 69.5. Cyclinex-1 and Cyclinex-2 (Abbott Nutrition) contain 25 mg of L-carnitine per gram of protein, as well as ample BCAAs.

Other Foods. The nutrient content of foods containing intact protein are available from USDA (94). Table 69.17 provides a sample diet for an infant with a UCED.

Assessment of Nutrition Support. Frequency of assessment is in part dictated by the clinical course of the patient. Blood ammonia concentrations should be monitored routinely and maintained at less than 50 μM. Plasma concentrations of amino acids should be monitored

TABLE 69.17	SAMPLE DIET: UREA CYCLE ENZYME DEFECT (2 WEEKS OF AGE), WEIGHT 3.25 kg			
PRESCRIPTION	TOTAL	PER kg		
L-Arginine (mg)	975	300		
Protein (g)	7.2	2.2		
Energy (kcal)	470	145		
Water to make (mL)	600			
MEDICAL FOOD	AMOUNT	L-ARGININE (mg)	PROTEIN (g)	ENERGY (kcal)
Cyclinex-1 Powder[a,b]	69 g	0	5.2	352
Similac Advance Infant with Iron Powder[a]	20 g	65	2.2	104
Polycose liquid[a]	7 mL	0	0.0	14
L-Arginine[c], 10 mg/mL	92 mL	920	0.0	0
Water to make	600 mL			
Total		985	7.2	470

[a]Abbott Nutrition.
[b]Another medical food that may be used for infants is WND (Mead Johnson Nutritionals).
[c]DO NOT use with arginase deficiency.

and maintained in the normal range. Plasma albumin and globulin concentrations are indices of protein status and should be evaluated frequently. Plasma transthyretin and retinol-binding protein have shorter half-lives than albumin and can provide information on protein status at an earlier stage in deficiency than can albumin. Caretakers should provide diet diaries and records of health status in tandem with blood tests for ammonia and plasma amino acid determinations. Growth and development should be routinely assessed. If evidence of protein deficiency occurs or if growth is not maintained, increased protein intake will be necessary.

Results of Nutrition Support. Results of therapy in infants with complete or nearly complete enzyme deficiencies have been less than optimal, with delayed death and subnormal development. If serious brain swelling and coma are prevented in the neonatal period or if the onset of disease expression is delayed, physical growth and mental development will be more nearly normal with nutrition and pharmacologic support (308, 336–338). In one report, better protein intake improved both growth and protein status without a concomitant increase in plasma ammonia concentrations (339). If the diagnosis is anticipated and treatment is begun during the neonatal period in children with affected siblings with citrullinemia or argininosuccinic acidemia, a relatively normal outcome is observed even in patients with severe enzyme defects (340). Coma may occur postpartum in the woman with OTC deficiency unless a protein-restricted diet and phenylbutyrate are administered (341). Female patients with symptomatic OTC deficiency have fewer hyperammonemic episodes and a reduced risk of further cognitive decline if they are treated with a protein-restricted diet and drugs that enhance waste nitrogen excretion (336, 342, 343). A successful pregnancy outcome was reported in a woman with ASA (344). Phenylbutyrate and a protein-restricted diet in a female patient with OTC deficiency resulted in a normal infant (345).

GALACTOSE

Biochemistry

Because lactose from milk is the principal carbohydrate and energy source for infants and young children, galactose (GAL) maintains a central metabolic role in human nutrition. Lactose is hydrolyzed in the intestine by lactase to GLU and GAL, and 0.5 to 1.0 mg GAL/kg per minute is produced endogenously (346). GAL is converted to uridine diphosphate (UDP) GAL and GLU-1-phosphate (GLU-1-P). UDP-GAL and UDP-GLU are essential building blocks for the posttranslational trafficking and function of membrane bound and secreted proteins. GLU-1-P is converted to energy. This evolutionarily conserved pathway occurs primarily in the liver (Fig. 69.9). First, GAL enters cells by a permease. Then GAL is phosphorylated to GAL-1-phosphate (GAL-1-P) by galactokinase (GALK). Classic galactosemia is caused by impaired GAL-1-P uridyl transferase (GALT). GALT is highly conserved from *Escherichia coli* to humans in its catalytic structure and function. UDP-GLU binds and releases GAL-1-P by dissociation reactions. Then the UMP-GALT complex binds GAL-1-P, releases UDP-GAL, and frees GALT for a subsequent set of bimolecular reactions. UDP-GAL and UDP-GLU are important precursors for glycoproteins and glycolipids; UDP-GAL and UDP-GLU are interconverted by epimerase (see Fig. 69.9).

Galactosemia

Elevated blood GAL levels may occur because of deficient functioning of GALK, GALT, or UDP-GAL-4-epimerase (347) (see Fig. 69.9). Patients with GALK deficiency produce excess galactitol and galactonic acid through alternate pathways and have only cataracts without hepatocellular dysfunction. GALK deficiency does not produce the acute hepatotoxic manifestations or

372. Elsas LJ, Dembure PP, Langley S et al. Am J Hum Genet 1994;54:1030–6.
373. Fridovich-Keil JL, Langley SD, Mazur LA et al. Am J Hum Genet 1995;56:640–6.
374. Beutler E, Baluda MC. J Lab Clin Med 1966;68:137–41.
375. Elsas LJ. Prenat Diagn 2001;21:302–3.
376. Jakobs C, Kleijer WJ, Allen J et al. Eur J Pediatr 1995; 154(Suppl):S33–6.
377. Acosta PB. Nutrition management of patients with inherited metabolic disorders of galactose metabolism. In: Acosta PB, ed. Nutrition Management of Patients with Inherited Metabolic Disorders. Sudbury, MA: Jones and Bartlett, 2010:343–67.
378. Singh RH, Kennedy MJ, Jonas CR et al. J Inherit Metab Dis 2003;26:123A.
379. Panis B, Gerver WJ, Rubio-Gozalbo ME. Eur J Pediatr 2007;166:443–6.
380. Kaufman FR, Loro ML, Azen C et al. J Pediatr 1993;123: 365–70.
381. Rubio-Gozalbo ME, Hamming S, van Kroonenburgh MJ et al. Arch Dis Child 2002;87:57–60.
382. Berry GT, Nissim I, Gibson JB et al. Eur J Pediatr 1997;156 (Suppl 1):S43–9.
383. Berry GT, Singh RH, Mazur AT et al. Pediatr Res 2000;48: 323–8.
384. Zlatunich CO, Packman S. J Inherit Metab Dis 2005;28: 163–8.
385. Portnoi PA, MacDonald A. J Hum Nutr Diet 2009;22:400–8.
386. Gross KC, Acosta PB. J Inherit Metab Dis 1991;14:253–8.
387. Gropper SS, Gross KC, Olds SJ. J Am Diet Assoc 1993;93: 328–30.
388. Cerbulis J. Arch Biochem Biophys 1954;49:442–50.
389. Gitzelmann R, Auricchio S. Pediatrics 1965;36:231–5.
390. Koch R, Acosta P, Ragsdale N et al. J Am Diet Assoc 1963; 43:212–5.
391. Ning C, Reynolds R, Chen J et al. Pediatr Res 2000;48:211–7.
392. Holton JB. Galactosemia. In: Schaub J, van Hoof F, Vis HL, eds. Inborn Errors of Metabolism. New York: Raven Press, 1991:169–80.
393. Lineback DR, Ke CH. Cereal Chem 1975;52:334–7.
394. Acosta PB, Gross KC. Eur J Pediatr 1995;154(Suppl):S87–92.
395. Kumar A, Weatherly MR, Beaman DC. Pediatrics 1991; 87:352–60.
396. Harju M. Milchwissenschaft 1990;45:411–5.
397. Segal S. Int Pediatr 1992;7:75–82.
398. Wiesmann UN, Rose-Beutler B, Schluchter R. Eur J Pediatr 1995;154(Suppl):S93–6.
399. Weese SJ, Gosnell K, West P et al. J Am Diet Assoc 2003; 103:373–5.
400. Rubio-Gozalbo ME, Panis B, Zimmermann LJ et al. Mol Genet Metab 2006;89:316–22.
401. Asp NG. Biochem J 1971;121:299–308.
402. Andersson L, Bratt C, Arnoldsson KC et al. J Lipid Res 1995;36:1392–400.
403. Donnell GN, Bergren WR, Perry G et al. Pediatrics 1963;31:802–10.
404. Kaufman FR, Xu YK, Ng WG et al. J Pediatr 1988;112: 754–6.
405. Shield JP, Wadsworth EJ, MacDonald A et al. Arch Dis Child 2000;83:248–50.
406. Webb AL, Singh RH, Kennedy MJ et al. Pediatr Res 2003;53:396–402.
407. Ng WG, Xu YK, Kaufman FR et al. J Inherit Metab Dis 1989;12:257–66.
408. Gibson JB, Reynolds RA, Palmieri MJ et al. Metabolism 1995;44:597–604.
409. Manis FR, Cohn LB, McBride-Chang C et al. J Inherit Metab Dis 1997;20:549–55.
410. Rubio-Gozalbo ME, Gubbels CS, Bakker JA et al. Hum Reprod Update 2010;16:177–88.
411. Rutherford PJ, Davidson DC, Matthai SM. J Hum Nutr Diet 2002;15:39–42.
412. Berry GT. Eur J Pediatr 1995;154(Suppl):S53–64.
413. Lai K, Tang M, Yin X et al. Biosci Hypotheses 2008;1:263–71.
414. Wehrli SL, Berry GT, Palmieri M et al. Pediatr Res 1997; 42:855–61.
415. Komrower GA. J Inherit Metab Dis 1982;5(Suppl 2):96–104.

70 INHERITED LIPID DISORDERS OF β-OXIDATION[1]

JERRY VOCKLEY, LYNNE A. WOLFE, AND DEBORAH L. RENAUD

---

[1]**Abbreviations: ABC**, adenosine triphosphate–binding cassette; **ACAD**, acyl-CoA dehydrogenase; **ACD**, acyl-coenzyme A dehydrogenase; **AFLP**, acute fatty liver of pregnancy; **ATP**, adenosine triphosphate; **CACT**, carnitine-acylcarnitine translocase; **CoA**, coenzyme A; **CPT**, carnitine palmitoyltransferase; **DHA**, docosahexaenoic acid; **EFA**, essential fatty acid; **ETF**, electron transfer flavoprotein; **FAD**, flavin adenine dinucleotide; **GA**, glutaric aciduria; **HELLP**, hemolysis, elevated liver enzymes, low platelet; **HMG**, hydroxymethylglutaryl; **LCAD**, long-chain acyl-coenzyme A dehydrogenase; **LCHAD**, long-chain 3-hydroxyacyl-coenzyme A dehydrogenase; **MADD**, multiple acyl-coenzyme A dehydrogenation disorder; **MCAD**, medium-chain acyl-coenzyme A dehydrogenase; **MCT**, medium-chain triglyceride; **MRI**, magnetic resonance imaging; **PKU**, phenylketonuria; **PTS**, peroxisomal targeting signal; **RCDP**, rhizomelic chondrodysplasia punctata; **SCAD**, short-chain acyl-coenzyme A dehydrogenase; **SCOT**, succinyl-coenzyme A:3-ketoacid coenzyme A transferase; **SIDS**, sudden infant death syndrome; **TFP**, trifunctional protein; **VLCAD**, very-long-chain acyl-coenzyme A dehydrogenase; **VLCFA**, very-long-chain fatty acid; **X-ALD**, X-linked adrenoleukodystrophy.

β-Oxidation, which results in sequential cleavage of two carbon units from fatty acids, represents an important source of energy for the body during times of fasting and metabolic stress. Free fatty acids released into the blood by catabolism of fat stores or from dietary sources are metabolized in the mitochondria. β-Oxidation also functions as a degradative route for complex lipids in a different subcellular compartment, the peroxisomes (sometimes referred to as microbodies). Peroxisomes are subcellular organelles bounded by a single lipid bilayer membrane (1). They are ubiquitously distributed in tissues but are particularly abundant in liver and kidney (2).

All peroxisomal proteins are encoded in the nuclear genome, synthesized on free cytoplasmic polyribosomes, and transported to the organelle posttranslationally. This process is mediated by specific targeting sequences on proteins and a variety of specific receptor proteins on the peroxisomes (3–6). The most common is the presence of a serine-lysine-leucine amino acid motif at the carboxy terminus of the protein. This peroxisomal targeting signal (PTS1), present in more than 95% of proteins destined for the peroxisomal matrix, binds to the cytosolic receptor protein Pex5p. A second mechanism uses an amino terminus targeting signal (PTS2) that binds to the receptor protein Pex7p. The PTS-receptor complexes are stabilized and transported to the peroxisomal membrane, where they interact with the docking machinery and are then translocated into the peroxisomal matrix. To date, 32 proteins involved in these processes, encoded by *PEX* genes and known as peroxins, have been identified and characterized.

Mitochondria are bounded by two lipid bilayer membranes (the inner and outer mitochondrial membranes) (7). The intermembrane space constitutes a distinct compartment within the mitochondria, whereas the space bounded by the inner mitochondrial membrane is known as the matrix. Mitochondria are unique organelles in animals in that they contain their own genetic information and are solely maternally inherited (8). Most proteins found in the mitochondria, however, are nuclear encoded and thus are inherited in a standard Mendelian fashion. In general, they are synthesized in a larger precursor form containing information in an amino terminal signal peptide necessary for targeting the proteins to the mitochondria (9, 10). These signal sequences are usually removed after import

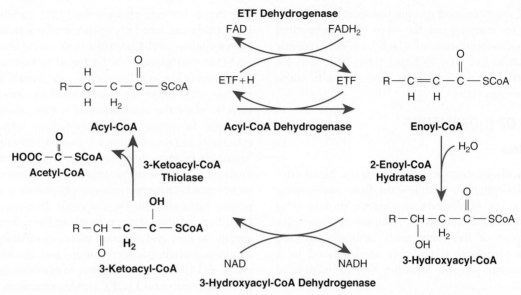

Fig. 70.1. Pathway of enzyme and transporter proteins involved in mitochondrial β-oxidation. *CoA,* coenzyme A; *ETF,* electron transfer flavoprotein; *FAD,* flavin adenine dinucleotide; *NAD,* nicotinamide adenine dinucleotide. (Modified and reprinted with permission of the Mayo Clinic and Foundation from Vockley J. The changing face of disorders of fatty acid oxidation. Mayo Clin Proc 1994;69:249–57.)

of the protein into the mitochondrion (11). More than one targeting signal may be necessary to direct the imported protein to the correct mitochondrial space or membrane.

Peroxisomes and mitochondria arise by division of previously existing organelles and are randomly distributed to daughter cells on cellular division (12, 13). Peroxisomes interact with mitochondria at multiple levels. They share common fission factors, which are involved in the division of both peroxisomes and mitochondria. Peroxisomes are metabolically linked to mitochondria through the β-oxidation of fatty acids and the metabolism of reactive oxygen species. Secondary mitochondrial changes occur in some peroxisomal biogenesis defects (14, 15).

Mitochondrial β-oxidation is predominantly responsible for the oxidation of fatty acids of carbon length 20 or less (16, 17). β-Oxidation is a complex process involving transport of activated acyl-coenzyme A (CoA) moieties into the mitochondria and sequential removal of 2 carbon acetyl-CoA units (Fig. 70.1) (18). The pathway of mitochondrial fatty acid oxidation is initiated by activation of fatty acids to acyl-CoA esters in the cytosol. The fatty acids are then transferred across the mitochondrial membrane bound to carnitine. Within the mitochondrial matrix, the acylcarnitines are converted back to acyl-CoAs. The 4 steps of the β-oxidation cycle then sequentially remove 2 carbons until the acyl-CoA (n carbons) is fully converted to n/2 acetyl-CoA molecules. In peripheral tissues, the acetyl-CoA is terminally oxidized in the Krebs cycle for adenosine triphosphate (ATP) production. In the liver, the acetyl-CoA from fatty acid oxidation can instead be used for the synthesis of ketones, 3-hydroxybutyrate, and acetoacetate, which are then exported for final oxidation by brain and other tissues (Fig. 70.2) (19).

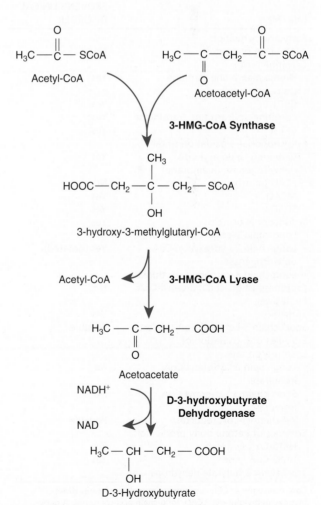

Fig. 70.2. Generation of ketone bodies from the products of β-oxidation. *CoA,* coenzyme A; *HMG,* hydroxymethylglutaryl; *NAD,* nicotinamide adenine dinucleotide.

At least 25 enzymes and specific transport proteins are responsible for carrying out the steps of mitochondrial fatty acid metabolism, some of which have only recently been recognized (see Fig. 70.1 and Table 70.1) (10). Of these, defects in at least 22 have been shown to cause disease in humans (10).

ENZYMES OF β-OXIDATION

Mitochondria

Free fatty acids are transported through the blood after intestinal absorption or mobilization from endogenous stores by the use of albumin as a carrier protein or in the form of triacylglycerols in lipoprotein complexes (20). Transport of free fatty acids intracellularly and through the cytoplasm is probably accomplished by a specific transport process; however, the mechanism of

TABLE 70.1	ENZYMES INVOLVED IN MITOCHONDRIAL FATTY ACID OXIDATION

ENZYME	PROVEN CLINICAL DISORDER
Fatty acid activation	
Acyl-CoA synthetase	No
Carnitine cycle	
Plasma membrane carnitine transporter	Yes
CPT I	Yes
Carnitine-acylcarnitine translocase	Yes
CPT II	Yes
Mitochondrial β-oxidation spiral	
Very long-chain acyl-CoA dehydrogenase (membrane)	Yes
LCAD (matrix)	No
MCAD	Yes
SCAD	Yes
Trifunctional protein	Yes
Long-chain 2-enoyl CoA hydratase	
Long-chain 3-hydroxyacyl-CoA dehydrogenase	Yes (isolated)
Long-chain 3-ketoacyl-CoA thiolase	
Crotonase (short-chain 2-enoyl-CoA hydratase)	No
SCHAD	Yes
Short-chain 3-ketoacyl-CoA thiolase	Possible
Enzymes of β-oxidation of unsaturated fats	
Long-chain Δ^3,Δ^2-enoyl-CoA isomerase	No
Short-chain Δ^3,Δ^2-enoyl-CoA isomerase	No
2,4-Dienoyl-CoA reductase	Possible
Enzymes of ketone body production	
HMG-CoA synthase	Yes
HMG-CoA lyase	Yes
D-3-Hydroxybutyrate dehydrogenase	

CoA, coenzyme A; CPT, carnitine palmitoyltransferase; HMG, hydroxymethylglutaryl; LCAD, long-chain acyl-coenzyme A dehydrogenase; MCAD, medium-chain acyl-coenzyme A dehydrogenase; SCHAD, short-chain 3-hydroxyacyl-coenzyme A dehydrogenase; SCAD, short-chain acyl-coenzyme A dehydrogenase;.

this step is not well characterized (21). Before undergoing β-oxidation, free fatty acids must be activated to their corresponding acyl-CoA thioesters. Long-chain specific acyl-CoA synthetases can be found in various subcellular locations but are thought to arise from a single gene product (22). Short- and medium-chain carboxylic acids directly enter the mitochondrial matrix, where they are activated. In contrast, long-chain fats are activated in the cytoplasm and require active transport into mitochondria. Transport of long-chain acyl-CoAs requires at least two enzymes, a transporter protein and the use of carnitine as an intermediate carrier molecule. Carnitine is itself transported intracellularly by a specific transporter protein (23). Two carnitine transporters have been described, one specific to liver and a second with a more ubiquitous distribution, including kidney, muscle, and fibroblasts. Long-chain acyl-CoAs are conjugated to carnitine by carnitine palmitoyltransferase I (CPT I). This enzyme is located on the inner aspect of the outer mitochondrial membrane. Tissue-specific isoforms of this enzyme exist for muscle, liver, and brain (23). Long-chain acylcarnitines are then passed to carnitine palmitoyltransferase II (CPT II) in the inner mitochondrial membrane by a translocase.

Once present in the mitochondrial matrix, acyl-CoAs of all chain lengths undergo a series of enzymatic reactions that results in the release of the two carbon unit acetyl-CoAs and a new acyl-CoA molecule that is two carbons shorter. The first step in this cycle is the dehydrogenation of the acyl-CoA to 2-enoyl-CoA. This reaction is catalyzed by a family of related enzymes, the acyl-CoA dehydrogenases (ACAD) (24). Four different members of this family are active in β-oxidation: very-long-, long-, medium-, and short-chain acyl-CoA dehydrogenases (very-long-chain acyl-CoA dehydrogenase [VLCAD], long-chain acyl-CoA dehydrogenase [LCAD], medium-chain acyl-CoA dehydrogenase [MCAD], and short-chain acyl-CoA dehydrogenase [SCAD], respectively), which differ in their chain length specificity. The role of LCAD in fatty acid β-oxidation is unclear. LCAD is present in much lower concentrations than VLCAD in tissues where the two have been separated and thus would appear to play a minor role in the flux of fatty acids through β-oxidation. However, LCAD has significant activity toward long, branched-chain substrates, unlike VLCAD, and thus may be more important in their metabolism (25, 26). A final long-chain ACAD, designated ACAD9, is more active toward unsaturated substrates than saturated ones, but its full role in cellular metabolism is not yet clear (27).

The acyl-coenzyme A dehydrogenases (ACDs) differ from most other dehydrogenases because they use electron transfer flavoprotein (ETF) as a final electron acceptor and thus can channel electrons directly into the ubiquinone pool of the electron transport machinery by way of ETF:ubiquinone oxidoreductase (ETF dehydrogenase) (28). The ACDs are homotetramers (except VLCAD and ACAD9, which are homodimers) whose monomers are synthesized in a larger precursor form in the cytoplasm from nuclear encoded transcripts and are then transported into mitochondria (24, 29). Once inside the mitochondrial matrix, the leader peptide is removed by a specific protease; and the mature subunits assemble into the active multimer. One molecule of flavin adenine dinucleotide (FAD) is noncovalently attached to each ACD subunit. cDNAs for each of these proteins have been cloned, and sequence analysis shows that they are approximately 30% to 35% conserved, a finding suggesting evolution from a common primordial gene (29). Four other members of this gene family are involved in the metabolism of branched-chain amino acids, lysine, and tryptophan rather than in β-oxidation (30).

The 2-enoyl-CoA moieties produced by the ACDs are hydrated to 3-hydroxyacyl-CoAs. These, in turn, undergo 2,3-dehydrogenation to 2-ketoacyl-CoAs, followed by cleavage of the thioester bond (31). This releases acetyl-CoA and completes one turn of the recursive β-oxidation cycle. The exact mechanism of these steps varies for substrates of differing chain length. The mitochondrial trifunctional protein (TFP) contains 2-enoyl-CoA hydratase, 3-hydroxyacyl-CoA dehydrogenase, and 3-ketoacyl-CoA thiolase activities for longer chain acyl-CoA substrates (32). This complex is an octamer consisting of 4α and 4β subunits. Long-chain 3-hydroxyacyl-coenzyme A dehydrogenase deficiency (LCHAD) and 3-enoyl-CoA hydratase activities reside on the α subunit, whereas 3-ketoacyl-CoA thiolase activity resides on the β subunit.

In contrast, individual proteins that catalyze these reactions for shorter chain substrates have single activities. These proteins include a short- to medium-chain 3-hydroxyacyl-CoA dehydrogenase (S/MCHAD), a short-chain enoyl-CoA hydratase (also called crotonase), and distinct medium- and short-chain 3-ketoacyl-CoA thiolases (31, 33). The substrate specificities of many of these enzymes overlap, and additional enzymes with yet different substrate optima likely exist for some steps of β-oxidation. Enzymes catalyzing several additional sets of reactions are necessary for the complete oxidation of unsaturated fatty acyl-CoA molecules including a 2,4-dienoyl-CoA reductase (34) and a Δ^3-, Δ^2-enoyl-CoA isomerase (26). In odd-chain (carbon number) fatty acid oxidation, the final three carbon intermediate propionyl-CoA is metabolized by propionyl-CoA carboxylase. Evidence suggests that VLCAD, ACAD9, and TFP associate with the inner mitochondrial membrane and may interact with the acyl-carnitine transport and respiratory chain complexes to allow channeling of substrate directly from one enzyme to the next. Ketone bodies are produced exclusively in the liver from acetyl-CoA generated by β-oxidation (see Fig. 70.2). Hydroxymethylglutaryl (HMG)-CoA synthase forms 3-hydroxy-3-methylglutaryl-CoA (HMG-CoA) from acetoacetyl-CoA and acetyl-CoA. Acetyl-CoA and acetoacetate are then produced by cleavage of HMG-CoA by HMG-CoA lyase (19, 35). Finally, acetoacetate is reduced

to D-3-hydroxybutyrate by D-3-hydroxybutyrate dehydrogenase within mitochondria (36).

Several alternative metabolic pathways become important when mitochondrial β-oxidation is impaired. Peroxisomal β-oxidation allows continued metabolism of longer-chain fats, whereas ω-oxidation in the cytosol (which proceeds from the opposite end of the fatty acid) results in the production of the characteristic dicarboxylic acids often present in these disorders. In addition, deacylation of acyl-CoA by cytosolic thioesters and conjugation of acyl-CoAs to glycine and carnitine become important mechanisms of CoA scavenging and detoxification, respectively.

PEROXISOMES

β-Oxidation in peroxisomes and mitochondria similarly involves four steps: dehydrogenation, hydration of the double bond, a second dehydrogenation, and then thiolytic cleavage. However, the β-oxidation cycle in peroxisomes differs from mitochondria in several important ways (37–39). The peroxisomal cycle results only in partial-chain shortening rather than complete oxidation of fatty acids. As a result, ATP production from peroxisomal substrates is less efficient because electrons produced by peroxisomal oxidases are donated directly to molecular oxygen for hydrogen peroxide production rather than to the respiratory chain. Carnitine plays a role in the export of chain-shortened fatty acids from the peroxisome but is not involved in fatty acid uptake.

Four peroxisomal half ATP-binding cassette (ABC) transporters have been described, including ALDP, ALDRP, PMP70, and PMP69 (40). The best characterized of these half transporters is ALDP, which is involved in the transport of acyl-CoA esters across the peroxisomal membrane. X-linked adrenoleukodystrophy (X-ALD) is caused by mutations in the *ABCD1* gene coding for ALDP (40). The activation of fatty acids to fatty acyl-CoAs is accomplished by acyl-CoA synthetases in the peroxisomal membrane (41). The first step of the β-oxidation cycle in the peroxisomal matrix is oxidation by straight-chain acyl-CoA oxidase (also called palmitoyl-CoA oxidase), leading to production of an enoyl-CoA (6, 39) (Fig. 70.3). Additional oxidases can perform similar reactions using 2-methyl branched-chain acyl-CoAs and CoA intermediates of bile acids as substrates (branched-chain acyl-CoA oxidases). Because the branched-chain acyl-CoA oxidases are stereospecific, 2-methyl-CoA racemase converts (2R)-methyl fatty acids to their (2S) diastereomers for oxidation. The second and third steps of the β-oxidation cycle are carried out by a bifunctional protein complex containing enoyl-CoA hydratase and 3-hydroxyacyl-CoA dehydrogenase activities associated with the inner aspect of the peroxisomal membrane (42, 43). Peroxisomal specific 3-ketoacyl-CoA thiolases catalyze the final step of the cycle, to produce acetyl-CoA and regenerate an acyl-CoA (38, 39).

Multiple carnitine acyltransferases with different chain-length specificities catalyze the conversion of acetyl-CoA and acyl-CoAs to acetylcarnitine and acylcarnitines, thus

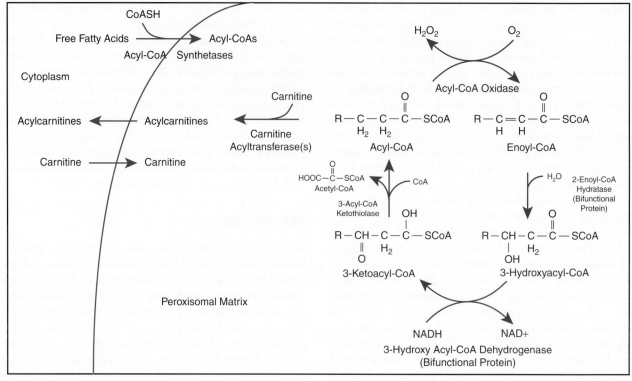

Fig. 70.3. β-Oxidation of fatty acids in the peroxisome. *CoA*, coenzyme A; *NAD*, nicotinamide adenine dinucleotide.

facilitating their export from the peroxisome (41). The chain-shortening step of the synthesis of docosahexaenoic acid (DHA) (C22:6) is achieved by a single cycle of peroxisomal β-oxidation (41). Additional enzymes involved in the metabolism of unsaturated long-chain fats in peroxisomes include organelle-specific 2,4-dienoyl-CoA reductase, 3/2 enoyl-CoA isomerase, 2-enoyl-CoA hydratase, 2,5 enoyl-CoA reductase, and 3, 5/2, 4-dienoyl-CoA isomerase.

In addition to β-oxidation, peroxisomes are involved in several important metabolic pathways, including α-oxidation of phytanic acid and other fatty acids, ether-phospholipid biosynthesis (including plasmalogens), detoxification of glyoxylate, pipecolic acid oxidation, biosynthesis of cholesterol, and other isoprenoids and the metabolism of reactive species (6, 38).

DEFECTS OF MITOCHONDRIAL FATTY ACID METABOLISM

Defects of the Carnitine Cycle

Defects identified in this pathway include that of a specific plasma membrane carnitine transporter protein, CPT I, and CPT II, as well as the carnitine-acylcarnitine translocase (CACT). A single report of two patients with an undefined defect in fatty acid oxidation and free fatty uptake in fibroblasts has been published (44).

Deficiency of the plasma membrane carnitine transporter represents primary carnitine deficiency (23). Carnitine is freely filtered by the kidney and must be reabsorbed from the proximal tubules to preserve plasma levels. Because the transporter for carnitine is deficient in kidney as well as in muscle and liver, tissues whose carnitine content is highest, this defect results in defective renal reabsorption and reduced tissue storage of carnitine (23). This leads to a deficiency of carnitine in end organs and an impairment of long-chain fatty acid metabolism. Patients with carnitine transporter deficiency can present with severe hypoglycemia and dilated cardiomyopathy in infancy or childhood. Alternatively, they may show onset of hypertrophic cardiomyopathy, progressive muscle weakness, and muscle lipid storage with mild elevations of creatine kinase. Hypertrophic cardiomyopathy has been reported in middle-aged carriers of *OCTN2* mutations. Fetal hydrops secondary to this disorder has been reported.

Multiple reports of asymptomatic, affected mothers have been identified when newborn screening of their affected or carrier children have tested positive for severely low free carnitine levels. Plasma carnitine levels are extremely low or undetectable in these children, but they rise dramatically with supplementation with pharmacologic doses of carnitine (100 to 400 mg/kg/day). Patients' symptoms also show dramatic resolution with therapy. Outcome is likely to be good if diagnosis is promptly made and therapy is instituted. Carnitine transporter deficiency can be diagnosed by uptake studies using cultured fibroblast or direct molecular analysis of the *OCTN2* gene.

Deficiency of liver CPT I has been reported. Severe disease is usual, but milder variants have been identified in geographically restricted populations. Diagnosis is based on enzymatic and mutation analysis. Severe symptoms include episodic hypoketotic hypoglycemia beginning in infancy and multiorgan system failure (45–47). Muscle and cardiac symptoms are not present. In one case, an apparently healthy girl aged 2 years and 9 months developed hepatomegaly and coma following a viral illness and died (48). Organic aciduria is not prominent in this disorder, but hyperammonemia may be present. Plasma carnitine is normal or elevated with a high free fraction. Elevated levels of creatine kinase were seen in siblings from one family. Analysis of samples from patients with CPT I deficiency has revealed normal CPT I levels in muscle but low activity in other tissues, including liver (47). Patients thus far have not responded well to therapy with carnitine, but presymptomatic treatment in subsequent affected siblings and infants identified through expanded newborn screening programs may change this observation.

Molecular analysis of patients with CPT I deficiency has identified common mutations in the *CPT1A* gene in the Hutterite and Canadian First Nation and Inuit populations (49, 50). Identified through newborn screening programs, affected individuals have, for the most part, been well. Patients with isolated muscle CPT I deficiency have not been reported.

Deficiency of the CACT was initially reported in newborns who had a nearly uniform poor outcome, presenting with severe hypoketotic hypoglycemia and cardiac arrhythmias or hypertrophy (51). All these infants had a grossly elevated acylcarnitine-to-free carnitine ratio, whereas dicarboxylic aciduria was reported in one. Carnitine supplementation did not appear to improve clinical symptoms. More recently, patients with a milder clinical course have been identified who responded well to modest carnitine supplementation and dietary therapy (23). Two affected siblings have been reported in which the younger sibling was prospectively treated and had not developed any sequelae 2 years later (52). These patients appear to have a higher level of residual enzyme activity than the more severely affected patients. Specific diagnosis of this disorder can be made by direct enzyme or molecular analysis.

CPT II deficiency is the most common of this group of disorders. It classically manifests in late childhood or early adulthood as episodes of recurrent exercise- or stress-induced myoglobinuria (23, 53). Episodes can be severe enough to lead to acute renal failure. Patients are typically well between episodes. They have no tendency to develop hypoglycemia. Weakness and muscle pain are reported. The characteristic diagnostic finding in these patients is a low total plasma carnitine level with increased acylcarnitine fraction and no dicarboxylic aciduria. Long-chain acylcarnitines may be elevated (23).

A more severe variant of CPT II deficiency manifesting with symptoms similar to those of CPT I deficiency has been appreciated. In these patients, the presenting symptoms were neonatal hypoglycemia, hepatomegaly,

and cardiomyopathy. A severe reduction of CPT II activity was found in all tissues tested, including liver, heart, muscle, and fibroblasts, although CPT I activity was normal. Plasma carnitine levels were not increased.

Mutations in the cDNA for CPT II have been described, and expression studies of mutant CPT II alleles suggest that the level of residual function of the mutant enzyme may be responsible for determining the clinical phenotype (54). Carnitine supplementation does not benefit the severe form of CPT II deficiency (23). Familial phenotypic variation has been reported (55). A common mutation has been reported to account for half of mutant alleles in the late onset form of the disease (56). A common coding polymorphism has also been reported in the CPT II coding region that may predispose to clinical symptoms under some (unknown) circumstances. Occasional families with apparent autosomal dominant transmission of partial CPT II deficiency have been described, and at least one case appears to be related to a mutation on one CPT II allele (55–57). Why these patients exhibit symptoms is unknown, although a dominant negative effect on tetramer assembly and modifying gene effects have been postulated (58, 59).

Defects of Acyl-Coenzyme A Dehydrogenases

The first patient with VLCAD deficiency presented with ventricular fibrillation and respiratory arrest at 2 days of age and exhibited massive dicarboxylic aciduria (60). It is now clear that VLCAD deficiency can manifest with a spectrum of symptoms, including early-onset cardiac and skeletal myopathy, hypoketotic hypoglycemia, hyperammonemia, and hepatocellular failure (61). Recurrent rhabdomyolysis and myopathy beginning in adolescence have also been described (62). 3-Hydroxy-dicarboxylic acids or saturated dicarboxylic acids may be present in the urine (60, 63). Cloning of the gene for VLCAD has allowed identification of various genetic defects, but no common mutations have emerged (64). Some correlation of specific genotypes with phenotype exists, although it is imperfect. Fibroblast studies suggest that VLCAD enzyme targets different fatty acid chain lengths with different phenotypes, but this finding has not been supported in vivo (17).

One report of three cases of ACAD9 deficiency has been published (65). The first patient was a 14-year-old, previously healthy boy who died of a Reye-like episode and cerebellar stroke triggered by a mild viral illness and ingestion of aspirin. The second patient was a 10-year-old girl who first presented at age 4 months with recurrent episodes of acute liver dysfunction and hypoglycemia, with otherwise minor illnesses. The third patient was a 4.5-year-old girl who died of cardiomyopathy and whose sibling also died of cardiomyopathy at age 21 months. Mild chronic neurologic dysfunction was reported in all three patients. Defects in *ACAD9* mRNA were identified in the first two patients, and all patients manifested marked defects in ACAD9 protein. Despite a significant overlap of substrate specificity, it appears that ACAD9 and VLCAD are unable to compensate for each other in patients with either deficiency.

Putative LCAD deficiency has been reported, but all the patients originally categorized as LCAD deficient subsequently were proved to have a deficiency of VLCAD instead (66). Thus, there are no known patients with bona fide LCAD deficiency.

Numerous patients with SCAD deficiency have been reported (67, 68). Clinical findings have included episodes of intermittent metabolic acidosis, neonatal hyperammonemic coma, neonatal acidosis with hyperreflexia, multicore myopathy, infantile-onset lipid storage myopathy with failure to thrive, and hypotonia. Hypoglycemia has been a rare finding in this disorder. The characteristic metabolites of ethylmalonic and methylsuccinic acids of SCAD deficiency were also detected in individuals with normal SCAD activity in fibroblasts (67). The presence of one of two relatively common variants of SCAD (625 G>A and 511 C>T) predisposes to excessive ethylmalonic acid production but it probably is not clinically important. These polymorphisms subtly affect the function of the purified proteins encoded by these variants, although both are still active (69). Few patients identified on the basis of elevated ethylmalonic acid excretion, neuromuscular symptoms, and deficient SCAD activity in fibroblasts carried two pathogenic mutations (70). The remaining patients were double heterozygous for a pathogenic mutation and the previously identified 625 G>A variation, homozygous for one of the variations, 625 G>A or 511 C>T, or double heterozygous for both.

In general, it is clear that most patients with complete SCAD deficiency identified through newborn screening have been well, whereas numerous symptoms continue to be ascribed to the deficiency in patients identified through clinical testing later in life (68, 71). The full clinical spectrum of this deficiency and the clinical relevance of common polymorphisms remain to be defined (67).

MCAD deficiency has emerged as one of the most common inborn errors of metabolism in the United States and Western Europe, and it has been extensively reviewed (17, 72, 73). The most frequent clinical presentation is one of intermittent hypoketotic hypoglycemia with onset in the second year of life (74). Mild hyperammonemia and coma may or may not be present. These findings often lead to the nonspecific diagnosis of Reye syndrome. The patient is usually well between attacks. Dicarboxylic aciduria is extensive during the attacks, but it can be undetectable by routine means when the patient is well. Similarly, microvesicular and macrovesicular hepatic steatosis, muscle weakness, and lipid excess in muscle present during the acute illness may resolve between acute episodes. Most patients who die of MCAD deficiency do so after having survived an initial episode. Thus, recurrent Reye syndrome–like episodes especially should trigger suspicion of this disorder.

Sudden death in a previously healthy child has been described in numerous cases of MCAD deficiency. This can occur as early as the first day of life, and it has been seen in a previously healthy adult who was being calorie restricted after abdominal surgery. In the appropriate age range, such deaths are often misattributed to sudden infant death syndrome (SIDS). Autopsy usually demonstrates the characteristic microvesicular and macrovesicular steatosis and should suggest the diagnosis. Analysis of the acylcarnitine and acylglycine profile from a bile specimen, as well as enzyme assay in cultured fibroblast (which may be recovered from deep tissues such as the fascia lata of the thigh up to 48 hours postmortem), may be helpful in proving it. Finally, completely asymptomatic individuals have been identified in the course of family studies of patients. The diagnosis of MCAD deficiency in asymptomatic individuals is possible by metabolite analysis of various bodily fluids (75).

Remarkable progress has been made in our understanding of the molecular mechanisms responsible for MCAD deficiency. Following cloning of the cDNA for MCAD, several groups simultaneously reported that a single common mutant allele was responsible for up to 90% of mutant alleles in patients with this disorder (76, 77). The substitution of a G for an A residue at position 985 (985 A>G) results in the replacement of a lysine by a glutamic acid residue and production of an unstable protein (78). Furthermore, screening of newborn blood samples has revealed a high carrier frequency for this disorder in some populations. Allele frequencies for the 985 A>G mutation range from 1 in 20 in northern European populations to less than 1 in 100 in Asian and some southern European populations. In the United States, the estimated carrier frequency for all mutations in whites is 1 in 60 (76). This translates into a predicted disease frequency of 1 in 15,000. MCAD deficiency is much less frequent in the African and Asian populations. The predicted incidence for MCAD based on these studies is similar to or greater than that for phenylketonuria (PKU).

Deficiency of Other β-Oxidation Enzymes

Long-Chain 3-Hydroxyacyl-Coenzyme A Dehydrogenase Deficiency

Patients with a deficiency of this enzyme tend to fall into two clinical subclasses (79–81). One group presents primarily with symptoms of cardiomyopathy, myopathy, and hypoglycemia. Peripheral neuropathy and recurrent myoglobinuria may be present. These patients are deficient in all three enzymatic activities of the TFP. The other group, deficient only in LCHAD activity, has hepatocellular disease with hypoglycemia with or without pigmentary retinopathy. Cholestasis and fibrosis may also be present (82). Considerable overlap in these groups has been described, however, and LCHAD deficiency has also been reported in patients with recurrent Reye syndrome–like symptoms and in sudden infant death (83). Milder cases with adolescent onset of recurrent rhabdomyolysis have been reported (84).

In a large series of patients with isolated LCHAD deficiency, the mean age of clinical presentation was 5.8 months, and seven patients presented in the neonatal period (80). Thirty-nine patients presented with hypoketotic hypoglycemia, whereas 11 presented with chronic problems, consisting of failure to thrive, feeding difficulties, cholestatic liver disease, or hypotonia. Mortality in this series was high; 38% died within 3 months of diagnosis. Morbidity in the surviving patients was also high, with recurrent metabolic crises and muscle problems despite therapy.

In a series of 21 patients with TFP deficiency, 9 presented with rapidly progressive clinical deterioration. Six of these patients had hypoketotic hypoglycemia (81). The remaining 12 patients presented with nonspecific chronic symptoms, including hypotonia (100%), cardiomyopathy (73%), failure to thrive, or peripheral neuropathy. Ten patients presented in the neonatal period. Mortality was high (76%) and was mostly attributable to cardiac disease. Two patients who were diagnosed prenatally died despite treatment.

Defects in the α-subunit destabilize the TFP and result in the multiple enzymatic deficiencies seen in some patients (81, 85–87). A common G to C mutation at nucleotide position 1528 (1528 G>C) accounts for approximately 60% of mutant alleles identified thus far. Heterozygosity for TFP α-subunit deficiency has been implicated in the development of acute fatty liver of pregnancy (AFLP) or hemolysis, elevated liver enzymes, low platelet (HELLP) syndrome (see later). Mutations in the β-subunit of TFP have been less well characterized, but they can also lead to destabilization of TFP (88). Patients with primary defects in respiratory chain function can have a secondary decrease of LCHAD activity or a less specific decrease in fibroblast oxidation of radiolabeled palmitate (89). Thus, care must be taken to differentiate these patients appropriately from those with primary LCHAD deficiency.

One patient was reported to have a potential defect in the enzyme 2,4-dienoyl-CoA reductase (90). This patient presented in the newborn period with persistent hypotonia. She was found to have elevated lysine and decreased carnitine in plasma. 2-trans,4-cis-Decadienenoylcarnitine was identified in plasma and urine, and reduced activity of 2,4-dienoyl-CoA reductase was found in liver and muscle. The patient died at 4 months of age of respiratory acidosis. A mouse model of this deficiency leads to severe hypoglycemia (91). Confirmation of the clinical significance of this defect awaits the identification of additional patients.

Multiple Acyl-Coenzyme A Dehydrogenation Disorder

Abnormalities of ETF or ETF:ubiquinone oxidoreductase (ETF dehydrogenase) deficiency lead to an in vivo deficiency of all the dehydrogenases that use ETF as an electron acceptor (28). These include the ACDs discussed earlier, as well as isovaleryl-CoA dehydrogenase, 2-methylbutyryl-CoA dehydrogenase, isobutyryl-CoA dehydrogenase, glutaryl-CoA

dehydrogenase, dimethylglycine dehydrogenase, and sarcosine dehydrogenase—enzymes involved in the intermediate metabolism of branched-chain amino acids, tryptophan, lysine, and choline. Accumulation of intermediate compounds related to blockages in all these pathways is seen. Because of the presence of glutaric acid in the urine of some patients, this disorder is frequently referred to as glutaric aciduria type II (GA II), to distinguish it from a primary deficiency of glutaryl-CoA dehydrogenase (GA I).

Clinical manifestations of multiple acyl-CoA dehydrogenation disorder (MADD) are extremely heterogeneous (92, 93). A neonatal form can be seen with severe hypotonia, dysmorphic features, and cystic kidneys. These infants also exhibit metabolic acidosis and hypoglycemia. Milder variants are common, manifesting with nonspecific neurologic signs, lipid storage myopathy, fasting hypoketotic hypoglycemia, or intermittent acidosis. In some patients, only fasting hypoketotic hypoglycemia or intermittent acidosis is seen and can be of late onset (92, 94). In these cases, the organic acid profile in times of illness is usually dominated by ethylmalonic and adipic acids, thus leading to the alternate name of ethylmalonic-adipic aciduria for this disorder. Structural brain abnormalities are common, including agenesis of the cerebellar vermis, hypoplastic temporal lobes, and focal dysplasia of cerebral cortex (95). Neuronal migration abnormalities may be present. Neonatal fatal cardiomyopathy has been reported (96). Some patients with MADD respond dramatically to riboflavin with normalization of clinical symptoms and biochemical markers (92, 97, 98).

Analysis of fibroblasts from patients with MADD has revealed defects in both protein subunits of ETF and in ETF dehydrogenase (99). Cell lines with and without immunologically cross-reactive material have been described. cDNAs for both subunits of ETF and ETF dehydrogenase have been cloned, and direct mutational analysis has revealed various defects in patients (92). For the most part, riboflavin-responsive patients have been found to have mutations in the *ETFDH* gene that presumably affect either protein folding or FAD binding. Otherwise, correlation of the mutation identified with severity of clinical symptoms has not been possible.

Disorders of Ketone Bodies

The patients with 3-ketoacyl-CoA thiolase deficiency were originally described with developmental delay and muscle weakness; one of them died of a Reye-like illness with urine metabolite findings suggestive of a defect in mitochondrial 3-ketoacyl-CoA thiolase (100). Definitive enzyme testing was not performed. Since then, more than 30 patients have been identified with mutations in this gene, also known as short-chain 3-ketoacyl-CoA thiolase. Most patients have had a presentation of recurrent episodes of acidosis exacerbated by intercurrent illness, but with a characteristic persistence of the presence of ketone bodies in blood and urine when they are well (72). Hypoglycemia has not been common. A single patient with medium-chain 3-ketoacyl-CoA thiolase deficiency had metabolic acidosis, liver dysfunction, and rhabdomyolysis that was associated with vomiting and dehydration.

Deficiency of HMG-CoA lyase, which is also active in the metabolism of leucine and ketone synthesis, has been reported in almost 100 patients (101). It manifests with hypoketotic hypoglycemia with hyperammonemia and acidosis in the first year of life. Seizures and white matter abnormalities were described in one child and one adult subsequently diagnosed with HMG-CoA lyase deficiency (102, 103). Identification of hydroxymethyl glutaric acid in the urine is diagnostic. Common mutations exist in Saudi Arabia as well as in Spain and Portugal (101). Multiple variants have been found in apparently asymptomatic adults.

Succinyl-CoA:3-ketoacid CoA transferase (SCOT) functions in conjunction with mitochondrial acetoacetyl-CoA thiolase to generate ketones in extrahepatic tissues. SCOT deficiency manifests as persistent ketonuria in the first 1 to 2 years of life, whereas acetoacetyl-CoA thiolase deficiency manifests with variable clinical symptoms and exaggerated ketoacidosis in response to minor physiologic stress (36, 104). HMG-CoA synthase deficiency has been reported in six patients who presented with coma, hypoglycemia, and dicarboxylic aciduria with very low ketones (105). Their acylcarnitine profiles were reported as normal.

Multiple Defects in Energy Metabolism

Inborn errors of fatty acid metabolism show considerable variation in the severity of symptoms. This variation is often ascribed to the differential effects of specific mutations on gene and enzyme function, but such genotype and phenotype correlations are usually imprecise. In addition, in some patients with clinical and biochemical findings consistent with a defect in energy metabolism (especially recurrent hypoglycemia or rhabdomyolysis), it is ultimately impossible to arrive at a precise molecular or enzymatic diagnosis. Investigators have estimated that 2% to 3% of the US population is heterozygous for various β-oxidation disorders (87). The identification of concurrent partial defects in β-oxidation with or without partial deficiencies in other energy metabolism pathways has been reported (58, 59, 106). The development of symptoms consistent with reductions in energy metabolism related to the compound effects of these partial defects has been termed *synergistic heterozygosity* (59). Based on the relatively high frequencies of known disorders of energy metabolism, this may represent a previously unrecognized, relatively common mechanism of disease of potentially great clinical relevance.

Pregnancy-Induced Symptoms in β-Oxidation Defects

Numerous reports have described LCHAD-deficient patients born following pregnancies with various complications (107). Twenty-one pregnancies complicated

by AFLP or HELLP syndrome have been reported. The 1528 G>C mutation was present on at least one allele of the TFP α-subunit gene in all 12 affected infants in whom molecular genetic studies were done. Three patients with CPT I deficiency, 1 patient with CACT deficiency, 1 patient each with MCAD and SCAD deficiency, and more than 1 patient with complete TFP deficiency were born to mothers who developed liver disease during their pregnancies (108–110).

β-Oxidation is now recognized as critical to the normal development and function of the placental–fetal unit (111). During the last trimester of pregnancy, there is an increase in long-chain fatty acids considered critical to generating ketones to meet increasing fetal energy demands. A relative deficiency of maternal plasma carnitine also occurs. This may contribute to the development of liver-related complications of pregnancy in carriers of β-oxidation disorders. In a retrospective case-control study, a greater than 18% increase in pregnancy-related liver disease across the entire β-oxidation spectrum was found (112). Low birth weight and premature delivery are also reported in carriers of β-oxidation disorders (111, 112). Thus, pregnancies complicated by AFLP or HELLP should trigger an evaluation for a β-oxidation defect in the baby following delivery. It may also be reasonable to provide known carriers of β-oxidation disorders carnitine supplementation, especially during the last trimester of pregnancy. No clinical studies have identified whether prenatal carnitine supplementation has any impact on preventing liver-related complications or the outcome of the fetus.

PEROXISOMAL DEFECTS

Defects of Peroxisomal Biogenesis

Defects of peroxisomal biogenesis with a resulting failure to import all or a subset of matrix enzymes are more common than single enzyme deficiencies (Table 70.2). Apparent absence or significant reduction in the number

TABLE 70.2	**ENZYMES OF PEROXISOMAL β-OXIDATION**

Acyl-CoA synthetases
Acyl-CoA oxidases (straight chain and branched chain)
Acyl-CoA thioesterases
Bifunctional protein
  2-Enoyl-CoA hydratase
  3-Hydroxyacyl-CoA dehydrogenase
  3-Ketoacyl-CoA thiolases
Carnitine acyltransferases
  2-Methyl-CoA racemase
Enzymes of β-oxidation of unsaturated fats
  2,4-Dienoyl-CoA reductase
  3,2-*Trans*-enoyl-CoA isomerase
  2-Enoyl-CoA hydratase
  2,5-Enoyl-CoA reductase
  Delta-3,5-delta2,4-Dienoyl-CoA isomerase

CoA, coenzyme A.

propionyl-CoA in the final cycle of β-oxidation. The anaplerotic effect of the propionyl-CoA may ameliorate the secondary tricarboxylic acid cycle deficiency that can occur in patients with long-chain β-oxidation defects. Uncontrolled studies have reported promise in this regard, but definitive studies have yet to be performed (150–152).

DHA deficiency may develop in patients with LCHAD deficiency, and it has been hypothesized as a cause for retinal degeneration in these patients (153). One study demonstrated improved vision outcomes in LCHAD patients with higher DHA levels and lower 3-hydroxya-cylcarnitines (142).

Commercially available medical foods provide formulations composed of modified fats, concentrated proteins, and multivitamins. Formulas that contain a high percentage of calories from MCT oil have been suggested for use to manage patients with long-chain fatty acid oxidation disorders. When prescribed in conjunction with sufficient EFA supply, this approach can meet the essential nutrient needs of patients. Other strategies include a combination of available formulas to produce a diet high in complex carbohydrates, low in fat, and adequate in vitamin and mineral content (147). No clinical studies have been performed to assess the long-term efficacy of these formulas for the unique requirements of patients with β-oxidation disorders.

Increased caloric intake from carbohydrates may be necessary during intercurrent illness because of increased metabolic demands on the body. This need can be met by oral intake or nasogastric tube administration of an appropriate formula intravenous fluid if oral intake is inadequate. Intravenous infusion of glucose (8 to 10 mg/kg/minute) can be used when oral intake is interrupted or during acute episodes associated with infection (146, 147).

Carnitine supplementation has long been used in the treatment of disorders of β-oxidation, based on the rationale that it allows repletion of the intramitochondrial carnitine pool and accelerates the removal of toxic fatty acid intermediates (148). Carnitine use, however, remains controversial and of unproven value except in carnitine transporter deficiency (146, 154). Carnitine supplementation has been reported to normalize plasma carnitine levels and increase urinary excretion of acylcarnitine esters; however, it does not always prevent the accumulation of toxic medium-chain free fatty acids in plasma, prevent spontaneous episodes of hypoglycemia, or reduce symptoms of lethargy, hypoglycemia, and vomiting (155). Conversely, short periods of carnitine supplementation have been suggested to increase ketogenesis and reduce symptoms during periods of fasting hypoglycemia (156). Concern over the arrhythmogenic potential of long-chain acylcarnitine intermediates remains (157). Recommended doses range from 50 mg/kg/day in children to 150 mg/kg/day in adults (147).

Riboflavin is the precursor to FAD, an essential cofactor for the ACDs, ETF, and ETF dehydrogenase. Several patients with biochemical abnormalities suggestive of

β-oxidation defects have been described who responded with clinical improvement to pharmacologic doses of riboflavin (100 to 200 mg/day). One of these groups had a variant of ETF dehydrogenase with an as yet undefined defect in interaction with FAD (92). Increasing intramitochondrial concentrations of FAD by administration of riboflavin apparently allows enough cofactor binding to restore activity. A second set of patients with a picture of late-onset lipid storage myopathy and muscle weakness showing some level of hepatic dysfunction has been described (158). Again, these patients appeared to respond to therapy with riboflavin, but their defect remains undefined. Marked clinical heterogeneity within each group has been documented.

Bezafibrate has been shown to up-regulate oxidation rates of long-chain fats with decreased muscle pain and increased physical activity in some patients with long-chain β-oxidation disorders, even those with severe VLCAD missense mutations (159–162).

Peroxisomes

Treatment of patients with defects in peroxisomal β-oxidation has been difficult. Therapy for X-ALD has received the most attention (163). Adrenal hormone replacement for adrenal insufficiency is required in the majority of male patients with X-ALD and in 1% to 2% of female carriers. Several inhibitors of VLCFA synthesis have been used in an attempt to control excess accumulation of VLCFAs in patients. These include oleic acid, glycerol trioleate, and glycerol trierucate, popularly known as "Lorenzo's oil." The first extensive therapeutic trial to address the efficacy of Lorenzo's oil employed a diet that provided 10% of calories as fat, with less than 10 to 15 mg of C26:0 fatty acid per day (164). In addition, 1.7 g/kg body weight/day of glycerol trioleate oil and 0.3 g/kg body weight/day of glycerol trierucate were also given, along with 10 to 15 mL of safflower oil and 2 g fish oil (to avoid a deficiency of EFAs). Using this regimen, VLCFA levels were normalized in patients with either adrenoleukodystrophy or adrenomyeloneuropathy, but little or no clinical improvement could be documented (164).

A more recent study showed similar results (165). This study, however, raised significant safety concerns about Lorenzo's oil, thus prompting a recommendation not to prescribe Lorenzo's oil routinely to patients with X-ALD who already have neurologic deficits. Prospective evaluation of asymptomatic boys with biochemically proved X-ALD and with a normal neurologic examination and MRI scans at enrollment was performed. Lorenzo's oil delayed the onset of neurologic and MRI abnormalities in the group of patients whose plasma C26:0 concentrations normalized on treatment compared with historical controls (125). The protective effect was partial; 24% of patients in this group developed MRI abnormalities, and 11% developed both neurologic and MRI abnormalities.

Twelve patients with X-ALD treated with lovastatin for 3 to 12 months had an initial decline in VLCFAs, which was variably sustained. No conclusion about clinical efficacy was possible from this small study (166). Studies to determine whether lovastatin may be protective in asymptomatic boys are ongoing.

Hematopoietic stem transplantation has shown the most promise for boys with the childhood cerebral form of X-ALD (167–172). Short-term stabilization of clinical findings and MRI abnormalities have been demonstrated in patients when hematopoietic stem transplantation or cord blood transplantation was performed early in the course. Transplantation of autologous hematopoietic stem cells genetically altered to express ALDP may be an option for boys who do not have a human leukocyte antigen (HLA)–matched donor or adults with cerebral disease who are at significant risk of mortality with conventional allogeneic hematopoietic stem cell transplantation (173). There continues to be no effective treatment for boys with advanced disease. N-Acetyl-L-cysteine in conjunction with stem cell transplantation may improve outcome in boys with advanced cerebral disease (174). Specific therapy for the other single enzyme defects of peroxisomal β-oxidation has not been reported.

Treatment of the disorders of peroxisomal biogenesis has been problematic because of the multisystemic involvement and the numerous metabolic pathways affected in these individuals. In addition to reduction of VLCFA intake, patients may benefit from a reduction of phytanic acid intake (<10 mg/day) as in adult Refsum disease (132). Dairy products, ruminant fats, and ruminant meats are the prime dietary sources of phytanic acid. Green vegetables, originally excluded from the diet, are no longer believed to contribute significantly to the physiologic phytanic acid load. Unfortunately, limited information is available on many food items. It is difficult to reduce dietary intake of phytanic acid less than 10 to 20 mg/day.

Benefits in uncontrolled studies have been reported for supplementation of patients with oral formulations of ether lipids, cholic (100 mg/day) and deoxycholic acids (100 mg/day), and DHA (250 mg/day) (175–177). Five patients with peroxisomal biogenesis disorders whose DHA levels were normalized with supplementation (200 to 600 mg/day) were found to have some clinical improvement in vision and muscle tone (178). Progression in myelination on MRI scans was noted during DHA supplementation. The largest reported series to date describes 20 patients treated with DHA ethyl ester (100 to 500 mg/day) for 6 weeks to 9 years (179). All patients received an age-appropriate diet, limiting green leaves and white fat in meat, and supplemented with vitamins A, D, E, and K. Liver function studies improved in all patients, and VLCFA levels decreased in 18 of 20 patients. An improvement in vision was observed in 12 of 20 children. Muscle tone was believed to be improved in 13 of 20. Progression in myelination on MRI scans was observed in 9 of the 12 patients for whom data were available.

One study examined the effect of DHA supplementation on ophthalmology parameters in 23 patients: 2 with classical Zellweger syndrome, 19 with milder Zellweger syndrome spectrum phenotypes, and 2 with bifunctional protein deficiency (180). Nystagmus improved in all patients. Stabilization or improvement in vision and retinal function was seen in the majority of patients with the milder phenotypes. The improvement in vision noted with normalization of blood DHA levels may be related to the role of DHA in the visual pathway. DHA-containing phospholipids bilayers within the retina optimize the kinetics of the metarhodopsin II–G-protein–coupled signaling pathway (181). Correction of DHA deficiency in patients with peroxisomal biogenesis defects should be initiated as early as possible. Supplementation of vitamins A, D, E, and K, as well as carnitine, may be indicated. Bile acid supplementation may be beneficial in patients with liver dysfunction. Patients should be monitored for adrenal insufficiency and treated accordingly. Patients with seizures, when present, should be treated with anticonvulsant medications. Patients with milder phenotypes may benefit from hearing aids, glasses, and developmental services. Detailed prospective studies to evaluate the effectiveness of treatment in these patients are needed.

REFERENCES

1. Lazarow PB, Moser HW. Disorders of peroxisome biogenesis. In: Scriver C, Beaudet AL, Sly W et al, eds. The Metabolic and Molecular Basis of Inherited Disease. New York: McGraw-Hill, 1995:2287–324.
2. Molzer B, Bernheimer H, Budka H et al. J Neurol Sci 1981;51:301–10.
3. Brosius U, Gartner J. Cell Mol Life Sci 2002;59:1058–69.
4. Girzalsky W, Saffian D, Erdmann R. Biochim Biophys Acta 2010;1803:724–31.
5. Purdue PE, Lazarow PB. Annu Rev Cell Dev Biol 2001;17:701–52.
6. Wanders RJA. Lipobiology 2004;33:295–317.
7. Schatz G. FEBS Letts 1979;103:203–11.
8. Wallace DC, Lott MT, Shoffner JM et al. J Inherit Metab Dis 1992;15:472–9.
9. Volchenboum SL, Vockley J. J Biol Chem 2000;275:7958–63.
10. Vockley J, Whiteman DA. Neuromuscul Disord 2002;12:235–46.
11. Isaya G, Sakati WR, Rollins RA et al. Genomics 1995;28:450–61.
12. Benard G, Bellance N, James D et al. J Cell Sci 2007;120:838–48.
13. Diaz F, Moraes CT. Cell Calcium 2008;44:24–35.
14. Delille HK, Alves R, Schrader M. Histochem Cell Biol 2009;131:441–6.
15. Thoms S, Gronborg S, Gartner J. Trends Mol Med 2009;15:293–302.
16. Chegary M, Brinke HT, Ruiter JP et al. Biochim Biophys Acta 2009;1791:806–15.
17. Vockley J, Singh RH, Whiteman DA. Curr Opin Clin Nutr Metab Care 2002;5:601–9.

18. Vockley J. Mayo Clin Proc 1994;69:249–57.

19. Fukao T, Song XQ, Mitchell GA et al. Pediatr Res 1997; 42:498–502.

20. McGarry JD, Foster DW. Annu Rev Biochem 1980;49:395–420.

21. Stremmel W, Strohmeyer G, Berk PD. Proc Natl Acad Sci U S A 1986;83:3584–8.

22. Abe T, Fujino T, Fukuyama R et al. J Biochem 1992;111:123–8.

23. Longo N, Amat di San Filippo C, Pasquali M. Semin Med Genet 2006;142:77–85.

24. Gregersen N, Andresen BS, Pedersen CB et al. J Inherit Metab Dis 2008;31:643–57.

25. Battaile KP, McBurney M, Van Veldhoven PP et al. Biochim Biophys Acta 1998;1390:333–8.

26. Lea WP, Abbas AS, Sprecher H et al. Biochim Biophys 2000;31:2–3.

27. Ensenauer R, He M, Willard JM et al. J Biol Chem 2005; 280:32309–16.

28. Frerman FE, Goodman SI. PNAS 1985;82:4517–20.

29. Tanaka K, Matsubara Y, Indo Y et al. The acyl-CoA dehydrogenase family: homology and divergence of primary sequence of four acyl-CoA dehydrogenases and consideration of their functional significance. In: Tanaka K, Coates PM, eds. Fatty Acid Oxidation: Clinical, Biochemical and Molecular Aspects. New York: Alan R. Liss, 1990:577–98.

30. Vockley J, Ensenauer R. Semin Med Genet 142:95–103.

31. Houten SM, Wanders RJ. J Inherit Metab Dis 2010;33:469–77.

32. Orii KE, Orii KO, Souri M et al. J Biol Chem 1999;274:8077–84.

33. Filling C, Keller B, Hirschberg D et al. Biochem Biophys Res Commun 2008;368:6–11.

34. Helander HM, Koivuranta KT, Horellikuitunen N et al. Genomics 1997;46:112–9.

35. Mitchell GA, Fukao T. Inborn errors of ketone body metabolism. In: Scriver C, Beaudet AL, Sly W et al, eds. The Metabolic and Molecular Basis of Inherited Disease. New York: McGraw-Hill, 2001:327–56.

36. Kassovskabratinova S, Fukao T, Song XQ et al. Am J Hum Genet 1996;59:519–28.

37. Wanders RJ. Mol Genet Metab 2004;83:16–27.

38. Wanders RJ, Waterham HR. Biochim Biophys Acta 2006;1763:1707–20.

39. Poirier Y, Antonenkov VD, Glumoff T et al. Biochim Biophys Acta 2006;1763:1413–26.

40. Wanders RJ, Visser WF, van Roermund CW et al. Pflugers Arch 2007;453:719–34.

41. Ramsay RR. Am J Med Sci 1999;318:28–35.

42. Palosaari PM, Vihinen M, Mantsala PI et al. J Biol Chem 1991;266:10750–3.

43. Palosaari PM, Hiltunen JK. J Biol Chem 1990;265:2446–9.

44. Odaib AA, Shneider BL, Bennett MJ et al. N Engl J Med 1998;339:1752–7.

45. Ijlst L, Mandel H, Oostheim W et al. J Clin Invest 1998;102:527–31.

46. Bennett MJ, Boriack RL, Narayan S et al. Mol Genet Metab 2004;82:59–63.

47. Wieser T, Deschauer M, Olek K et al. Neurology 2003;60:1351–3.

48. Vianey-Saban C, Mousson B, Bertrand C et al. Eur J Pediatr 1993;152:334–8.

49. Prasad C, Johnson JP, Bonnefont JP et al. Mol Genet Metab 2001;73:55–63.

50. Park JY, Narayan SB, Bennett MJ. Clin Chem Lab Med 2006;44:1090–1.

51. Stanley CA, Hale DE, Berry GT et al. N Engl J Med 1992;327:19–23.

52. Pierre G, Macdonald A, Gray G et al. J Inherit Metab Dis 2007;30:815.

53. Engel AG, Angelini C. Science 1973;173:899–902.

54. Bonnefont JP, Taroni F, Cavadini P et al. Am J Hum Genet 1996;58:971–8.

55. Vladutiu GD, Bennett MJ, Fisher NM et al. Muscle Nerve 2002;26:492–8.

56. Taggart RT, Smail D, Apolito C et al. Hum Mutat 1999;13:210–20.

57. Vladutiu GD, Bennett MJ, Smail D et al. Mol Genet Metab 2000;70:134–41.

58. Vladutiu GD. Mol Genet Metab 2001;74:51–63.

59. Vockley J, Rinaldo P, Bennett MJ et al. Mol Genet Metab 2000;71:10–8.

60. Bertrand C, Largilliere C, Zabot MT et al. Biochim Biophys Acta 1993;1180:327–9.

61. Aoyama T, Souri M, Ueno I et al. Am J Hum Genet 1995;57:273–83.

62. Ogilvie I, Pourfarzam M, Jackson S et al. Neurology 1994; 44:467–73.

63. Aoyama T, Uchida Y, Kelley RI et al. Biochem Biophys Res Commun 1993;191:1369–72.

64. Andresen BS, Olpin S, Poorthuis B et al. Am J Hum Genet 1999;64:479–94.

65. He M, Rutledge S, Kelly D et al. Am J Hum Genet 2007; 81:87–103.

66. Yamaguchi S, Indo Y, Coates PM et al. Pediatr Res 1993;34:111–3.

67. Jethva R, Bennett MJ, Vockley J. Mol Genet Metab 2008;95:195–200.

68. van Maldegem BT, Wanders RJ, Wijburg FA. J Inherit Metab Dis 2010;12:923–30.

69. Nguyen T, Riggs C, Babovic-Vuksanovic D et al. Biochemistry 2002;41:11126–33.

70. Pedersen CB, Kolvraa S, Kolvraa A et al. Hum Genet 2008;124:43–56.

71. van Maldegem BT, Duran M, Wanders RJ et al. JAMA 2006; 296:943–52.

72. Bennett MJ, Rinaldo P, Strauss AW. Crit Rev Lab Sci 2000; 37:1–44.

73. Rinaldo P, Matern D, Bennett MJ. Annu Rev Physiol 2002;64:477–502.

74. Iafolla AK, Thompson RJ, Roe CR. J Pediatr 1994;124:409–15.

75. Rinaldo P, Cowan TM, Matern D. Genet Med 2008;10:151–6.

76. Tanaka K, Yokota I, Coates PM et al. Hum Mutat 1992;1:271–9.

77. Andresen BS, Bross P, Udvari S et al. Hum Mol Genet 1997;6:695–707.

78. Yokota I, Saijo T, Vockley J et al. J Biol Chem 1992; 267:26004–10.

79. Strauss AW, Bennett MJ, Rinaldo P et al. Semin Perinatol 1999;23:100–12.

80. den Boer ME, Wanders RJ, Morris AA et al. Pediatrics 2002;109:99–104.

81. den Boer MEJ, Dionisi-Vici C, Chakrapani A et al. J Pediatr 2003;142:684–9.

82. Odievre MH, Sevin C, Laurent J et al. Acta Pediatr 2002; 91:719–22.

83. Pons R, Roig M, Riudor E et al. Pediatr Neurol 1996;14:236–43.

84. Miyajima H, Orii KE, Shindo Y et al. Neurology 1997;49:833–7.

85. Spiekerkoetter U, Khuchua Z, Yue Z et al. Pediatr Res 2004;55:190–6.

86. Angdisen J, Moore VD, Cline JM et al. Curr Drug Targets Immune Endocr Metabol Disord 2005;5:27–40.

87. Rector RS, Payne RM, Ibdah JA. Adv Drug Del Rev 2008; 60:1488–96.

88. Ushikubo S, Aoyama T, Kamijo T et al. Am J Hum Genet 1996;58:979–88.

89. Enns GM, Bennett MJ, Hoppel CL et al. J Pediatr 2000; 136:251–4.

90. Roe CR, Millington DS, Kodo NN et al. J Clin Invest 1990; 85:1703–7.

91. Miinalainen IJ, Schmitz W, Huotari A et al. PLoS Genet 2009;5:e1000543.

92. Olsen RKJ, Andresen BS, Christensen E et al. Hum Mutat 2003;22:12–23.

93. Frerman FE. Biochem Soc Trans 1988;16:416–8.

94. Gregersen N, Bross P, Andresen BS. Eur J Biochem 2004; 271:470–82.

95. Takanashi J, Fujii K, Sugita K et al. Pediatr Neurol 1999; 20:142–5.

96. Singla M, Guzman G, Griffin AJ et al. Pediatr Cardiol 2008; 29:446–51.

97. Gregersen M, Rhead W, Christensen E. Riboflavin responsive glutaric aciduria type II. In: Tanaka K, Coates PM, eds. Fatty Acid Oxidation: Clinical, Biochemical, and Molecular Aspects. New York: Alan R. Liss, 1990:477–94.

98. Wen B, Dai T, Li W et al. J Neurol Neurosurg Psychiatry 2010; 81:231–6.

99. Loehr JP, Goodman SI, Frurman FE. Pediatr Res 1990; 27:311–5.

100. Bennett MJ, Sherwood WG. Clin Chem 1993;39:897–901.

101. Pie J, Lopez-Vinas E, Puisac B et al. Mol Genet Metab 2007; 92:198–209.

102. Yylmaz Y, Ozdemir N, Ekinci G et al. Pediatr Neurol 2006; 35:139–41.

103. Bischof F, Nägele T, Wanders RJA et al. Ann Neurol 2004; 56:727–30.

104. Song XQ, Fukao T, Mitchell GA et al. Biochim Biophys Acta Mol Basis Dis 1997;1360:151–6.

105. Kayser R, Heyde CE. Orthopade 2006;35:306–18.

106. Vladutiu G. Muscle Nerve 2000;23:1157–9.

107. Ibdah JA, Dasouki MJ, Strauss AW. J Inherit Metab Dis 1999; 22:811–4.

108. Walter JH. J Inherit Metab Dis 2000;23:229–36.

109. Matern D, Hart P, Murtha AP et al. J Pediatr 2001;138: 585–8.

110. Matern D, Schehata BM, Shekhawa P et al. Mol Genet Metab 2001;72:265–8.

111. Shekhawat PS, Matern D, Strauss AW. Pediatr Res 2005; 57:78R–86R.

112. Browning MF, Levy HL, Wilkins-Haug LE et al. Obstet Gynecol 2006;107:115–20.

113. Tager JM, Van der Beek WA, Wanders RJ et al. Biochem Biophys Res Commun 1985;126:1269–75.

114. Lazarow PB. J Neuropathol Exp Neurol 1995;54:720–5.

115. Zellweger H. Dev Med Child Neurol 1987;29:821–9.

116. Thomas GH, Haslam RH, Batshaw ML et al. Clin Genet 1975;8:376–82.

117. Gatfield PD, Taller E, Hinton GG et al. Can Med Assoc J 1968;99:1215–33.

118. Steinberg SJ, Dodt G, Raymond GV et al. Biochim Biophys Acta 2006;1763:1733–48.

119. Moser AB, Rasmussen M, Naidu S et al. J Pediatr 1995;127: 13–22.

120. Moser HW. Mol Genet Metab 1999;68:316–27.

121. Suzuki Y, Shimozawa N, Imamura A et al. J Inherit Metab Dis 2001;24:151–65.

122. Steinberg S, Chen L, Wei L et al. Mol Genet Metab 2004; 83:252–63.

123. Wanders RJA. Single peroxisomal enzyme deficiencies. In: Scriver C, Beaudet AL, Sly W et al, eds. The Metabolic and Molecular Basis of Inherited Disease. New York: McGraw-Hill, 2001:3219–56.

124. Mosser J, Lutz Y, Stoeckel ME et al. Hum Mol Genet 1994; 3:265–71.

125. Moser HW, Raymond GV, Lu SE et al. Arch Neurol 2005; 62:1073–80.

126. Moser HW, Mahmood A, Raymond GV. Nat Clin Pract Neurol 2007;3:140–51.

127. Clayton PT. Biochem Soc Trans 2001;29:298–305.

128. Ferdinandusse S, Denis S, Hogenhout EM et al. Hum Mutat 2007;28:904–12.

129. Ferdinandusse S, Barker S, Lachlan K et al. J Neurol Neurosurg Psychiatry 2010;81:310–2.

130. Buoni S, Zannolli R, Waterham H et al. Brain Dev 2007;29:51–4.

131. Thompson SA, Calvin J, Hogg S et al. J Neurol Neurosurg Psychiatry 2008;79:448–50.

132. Steinberg D. Refsum disease. In: Scriver C, Beaudet AL, Sly W et al eds. The Metabolic and Molecular Basis of Inherited Disease. New York: McGraw-Hill, 1995:2351–69.

133. Wanders RJ, Komen JC. Biochem Soc Trans 2007;35:865–9.

134. Saudubray JM, Martin D, de Lonlay P et al. J Inherit Metab Dis 1999;22:488–502.

135. Smith EH, Matern D. Curr Prot Hum Genet 2010;17:1–20.

136. Chace D, Barr J, Duncan M et al. Clin Lab Stand Inst Doc 2007;27:1–79.

137. Wilcken B. J Inherit Metab Dis 2010;75:1079–83.

138. Moser AB, Kreiter N, Bezman L et al. Ann Neurol 1999; 45:100–10.

139. Bennett MJ, Rinaldo P. Clin Chem 2001;47:1145–6.

140. Gillingham M, Van Calcar S, Ney D et al. J Inherit Metab Dis 1999;22:123–31.

141. Gillingham MB, Connor WE, Matern D et al. Mol Genet Metab 2003;79:114–23.

142. Gillingham MB, Weleber RG, Neuringer M et al. Mol Genet Metab 2005;86:124–33.

143. Gillingham MB, Scott B, Elliott D et al. Mol Genet Metab 2006;89:58–63.

144. Gillingham MB, Purnell JQ, Jordan J et al. Mol Genet Metab 2007;90:64–9.

145. Gillingham MB, Matern D, Harding CO. Top Clin Nutr 2009;24:359–65.

146. Catzeflis C, Bachmann C, Hale DE et al. Eur J Pediatr 1990;149:577–81.

147. Solis JO, Singh RH. J Am Diet Assoc 2002;102:1800–3.

148. Kerner J, Hoppel C. Ann Rev Nutr 1998;18:179–206.

149. Uauy R, Treen M, Hoffman DR. Semin Perinatol 1989;13: 118–30.

150. Roe CR, Roe DS, Wallace M et al. Mol Genet Metab 2007;92:346–50.

151. Roe CR, Mochel F. J Inherit Metab Dis 2006;29:332–40.

152. Roe CR, Sweetman L, Roe DS et al. J Clin Invest 2002; 110:259–69.

153. Harding CO, Gillingham MB, van Calcar SC et al. J Inherit Metab Dis 1999;22:276–80.

154. Howat AJ, Bennett MJ, Uren S et al. Br Med J 1985;290:1771–3.

155. Rinaldo P, Schmidtsommerfeld E, Posca AP et al. J Pediatr 1993;122:580–4.

156. Nyhan W, Ozand P. Disorders of fatty acid oxidation. In: Shils ME, ed. Atlas of Metabolic Diseases. London: Chapman and Hall, 1998:223–30.

Vitamin B5 (Pantothenic acid) (µg)	1,230 (750)	500	500	1,040	750	1,043	800	500	421	620
Vitamin B6 (Pyridoxal PO4) (µg)	98 (60)	60	60	208	60	250	100	60	84.2	123.5
Vitamin B7 (Biotin) (µg)	7.50 (4.5)	3	3	7.8	4.5	18.8	9	3	4.2	3.1
Vitamin B9 (Folic acid) (µg)	24.6 (15)	16	16	15.6	15	25	25	16	29.5	10.2
Vitamin B12 (Cobalamin) (µg)	0.74 (0.4)	0.3	0.3	0.62	0.45	0.6	0.4	0.3	0.4	0.26
Vitamin C (Ascorbic acid) (mg)	14.8 (9)	12	12	8.1	9.0	10	15	12	9	9.26
Choline (mg)	19.3 (12)	24	24	13	12	35	16	24	15	13.1
Inositol (mg)	8.0 (5)	17	17	4.7	5	8.3	35	17	5.1	23.3

MCT, medium chain triglyceride; RCF, Ross Carbohydrate Free.

[a]Abbott Nutrition, Columbus, OH.

[b]Note that this formula contains no carbohydrate, which accounts for its markedly different nutrient content vs. the other formulas shown. However, if 13 fl oz (390 ml) RCF is reconstituted with 54 g carbohydrate, e.g., glucose, and 12 fl oz (360 ml) water as the manufacturer recommends, the alternate values listed in (parentheses) will result, which approximates the carbohydrate content of most other formulas shown (i.e., approximately 2 g carbohydrate/fl oz of formula). As noted (see text), if other formulas are poorly tolerated (i.e., result in the resumption of diarrhea), the authors recommend initially reconstituting RCF with 12 g carbohydrate, e.g., glucose, and 12 fl oz (360 ml) water (i.e., approximately 0.5 g carbohydrate/fl oz of formula), before gradually increasing carbohydrate content, progressively reconstituting RCF with additional increments of 12 g carbohydrate, e.g., glucose, per 12 fl oz (360 ml) water, daily or every other day as tolerance for carbohydrate increases. Once full carbohydrate content (i.e., approximately 2 g carbohydrate/fl oz of formula) is tolerated, the patient usually can be switched to a carbohydrate-containing formula.

[c]Mead Johnson Nutrition, Evansville, IN.

[d]Note that this formula is designed for preterm infants.

[e]Nutricia North America, Gaithersburg, MD.

[f]Note that these formulas are hypoallergenic.

liquid milk–based diet, and/or a dry, solid, ready to use therapeutic food that can be eaten without adding water (e.g., Plumpy'nut; Nutriset, Malaunay, France), to minimize the risk of bacterial contamination (36). A Working Group Report from the First World Congress of Pediatric Gastroenterology, Hepatology, and Nutrition summarizes the latest advances in this field (37).

In general, the most common cause of acute diarrhea in developed countries is viral infection, chiefly resulting from contact with infected individuals; less common is bacterial infection, related either to socioeconomic dislocation or foreign travel (38, 39). Therefore, a stool culture to detect a specific pathogen usually is not helpful. The pathophysiology of most toxicogenic (i.e., enteropathogenic) bacterial diarrheas (e.g., *Salmonella, Shigella,* and *Campylobacter* spp., enteropathogenic *Escherichia coli* serotype O157:H7) is secretory diarrhea resulting from stimulation of the adenylate cyclase system, as occurs in cholera) (40); by contrast, the pathophysiology of most viral diarrheas (e.g., rotavirus) is both osmotic (inhibition of glucose transport as described for rotavirus) (41) and secretory. As such, testing the stool for pH and the presence of reducing substances may be very helpful, because a low pH (<6.0) and the presence of reducing substances suggest carbohydrate intolerance, hence a viral origin. The stool is best tested after a period of adequate intake of a reducing sugar (e.g., a 5% glucose solution or ORS); in addition, the water content of the stool, rather than any solid matter, should be tested.

Carbohydrate malabsorption in acute diarrhea is common but fortunately transient in most cases. Malabsorption of all carbohydrates, including glucose, may occur. However, this should not preclude administration of ORS in acute diarrhea. Occasionally, the carbohydrate malabsorption persists, and the patient develops postinfectious gastroenteritis. Young infants in lower growth percentiles who present with metabolic acidosis are particularly vulnerable to postinfectious gastroenteritis. Before the inception of total parenteral nutrition (TPN), this entity carried a high case fatality rate. However, this condition can now be managed successfully in most cases with nutritional support through the parenteral route with careful introduction of elemental or semielemental formulas.

If the origin of the diarrhea seems to be osmotic, and reintroduction of a carbohydrate-containing formula results in resumption of the diarrhea, a carbohydrate-free formula (see Table 71.1) usually is well tolerated. However, such formulas can result in ketosis and occasionally hypoglycemia; thus, some carbohydrate intake is necessary. In the hospitalized child, this can be provided intravenously. Most children who do not require hospitalization usually tolerate at least some sugar intake by the enteral route. In general, 0.5 g of glucose or sucrose per ounce of formula, provided intake is adequate but not excessive, is well tolerated and prevents ketosis and hypoglycemia. If this preparation is tolerated, the amount of carbohydrate can be increased daily or every other day as tolerance for carbohydrate increases. Once full carbohydrate content (i.e., approximately 2 g/oz) is tolerated, the patient usually can be switched to a carbohydrate-containing formula.

If the origin of the diarrhea is secretory, feeding usually does not affect the volume of stool output. In many cases, in fact, a glucose-electrolyte solution (e.g., ORS) seems to decrease the volume of stool output. In any event, fluid and electrolyte replacement must keep pace with intestinal losses until the diarrhea abates. Therefore, decisions concerning feeding must be based on clinical experience in such patients.

Regardless of the cause of the diarrhea, the tendency to avoid feedings containing lactose, especially breast milk, in most infants with diarrhea is unnecessary. In fact, continued breast-feeding should be encouraged. If stool pH is normal when the child is first seen and reducing substances are not present, lactase deficiency is an unlikely contributor to the diarrhea.

In a few patients, the acute episode of diarrhea does not resolve in the usual 4 to 5 days. In these patients, nutritional management becomes a much more important consideration. Although most infants can tolerate a 4- to 5-day period with little or no nutritional intake, few can tolerate a period of more than 2 weeks without becoming malnourished and developing secondary intestinal changes caused by both persistent diarrhea and malnutrition. Such infants are much more likely to develop secondary deficiencies of mucosal disaccharidases (e.g., lactase deficiency, and less commonly, sucrase deficiency). Monosaccharide intolerance may also develop. In these infants, management without hospitalization is difficult. Choice of formula again must be made on the basis of the suspected or culture-proven cause of the diarrhea; in addition, the much greater likelihood of secondary mucosal hydrolase deficiencies must be taken into account. If small volumes of a particular formula are reasonably well tolerated, it frequently is possible to deliver sufficient amounts to meet nutritional needs by use of a continuous infusion technique (41). Again, in small infants, this usually requires hospitalization.

Chronic Diarrhea

Noninfectious causes of chronic diarrhea result from a spectrum of congenital or acquired abnormalities that include changes in villous structure (e.g., celiac disease), ultrastructural abnormalities (e.g., microvillous inclusion disease), and abnormalities at the molecular level (e.g., congenital chloride diarrhea). If not managed appropriately, these disorders frequently result in the same secondary changes in mucosal function observed in acute diarrheas. The nutritional management of the two most common illnesses associated with chronic diarrhea, celiac disease and inflammatory bowel disease, are described here. Nutritional management of other chronic diarrheas, in general, is similar to that described earlier and must be

relatively low dose of 0.5 g/kg/day and increased gradually to a maximum dose of 3 g/kg/day. In all patients, the emulsion should be infused continuously throughout the day.

The 20% soybean oil emulsion seems to be cleared more rapidly than the 10% emulsion and therefore is less likely to cause hypertriglyceridemia (159). Hyperphospholipidemia and hypercholesterolemia, both of which occur routinely in patients receiving the 10% soybean emulsion, do not occur with use of the 20% emulsion (159). The explanation presumably is the lower phospholipid-triglyceride ratio of the 20% versus the 10% emulsion.

Because the size of the lipid particles of the emulsions (0.4 to 0.5 μm) exceeds the pore size of an effective filter (0.22 μm), filters should not be used for the infusion of fat emulsions, nor should the emulsions be mixed directly with other components of the infusate. This practice, which seems to be relatively common, may not destroy the emulsion, but it certainly inhibits detection of chemical incompatibilities within the complicated infusate (e.g., precipitation of calcium phosphate). The potential hazards of the latter possibility are compounded by the fact that filters cannot be used.

Complications of Total Parenteral Nutrition

TPN is associated with numerous complications, both catheter or infusion related and metabolic.

Catheter-related complications include arterial catheter insertion, pneumothorax, hemothorax, injury to an artery, and hematoma at the time of catheter insertion. Thrombosis, dislodgment, perforation, infusion leaks (pericardial, pleural, mediastinal), and infections also may occur reported during use of central vein catheters. The most common infusion-related problem of central vein TPN is infection. The most frequent complications of peripheral vein TPN are phlebitis and soft tissue sloughs. All these complications can be controlled, but it is difficult to prevent them entirely. Although the catheter- and infusion-related complications of central TPN are potentially more serious, the actual per diem complication rates of central and peripheral TPN are equivalent. Careful attention to care of the central catheter, including frequent dressing changes, is particularly important for controlling infection. Careful and frequent observation of the infusion site is necessary to prevent infiltration of infusates delivered by peripheral vein, as well as to ensure proper long-term function of central vein catheters.

Metabolic complications result either from the limited metabolic capacity of the patient for the various components of the nutrient infusate or from the infusate itself. The metabolic complications most commonly observed and their probable causes are listed in Table 71.6. One of the more troublesome of these is the occurrence of abnormal plasma amino acid patterns with use of many of the currently available amino acid mixtures (160). Cyst(e)ine and tyrosine, both of which are thought to be essential amino acids for the newborn, and perhaps for all patients receiving parenteral nutrients, are unstable or only sparingly soluble; hence, none of the currently marketed mixtures contains

TABLE 71.6	METABOLIC COMPLICATIONS OF TOTAL PARENTERAL NUTRITION AND THEIR PROBABLE CAUSES
COMPLICATION	**PROBABLE CAUSE**
Disorders related to metabolic capacity of patient	
Hyperglycemia	Excessive intake (either excessive concentration or infusion rate), change in metabolic state (e.g., infection, surgical stress)
Hypoglycemia	Sudden cessation of infusion
Azotemia	Excessive nitrogen intake
Electrolyte disorders	Excessive or inadequate intake
Mineral disorders	Excessive or inadequate intake
Vitamin disorders	Excessive or inadequate intake
Essential fatty acid deficiency	Failure to provide essential fatty acids
Hyperlipidemia	Excessive intake, change in metabolic state (e.g., stress, sepsis)
Disorders related to infusate components	
Metabolic acidosis	Use of hydrochloride salts of amino acids (e.g., cysteine)
Hyperammonemia	Inadequate arginine intake
Abnormal plasma aminograms	Amino acid pattern of nitrogen source
Hepatic disorders	Unknown; suggested etiologies include prematurity, malnutrition, sepsis, inadequate stimulation of bile flow, toxic effects of amino acids, specific amino acid deficiency, excessive amino acid and/or carbohydrate intake, and nonspecific response to lack of feeding

appreciable amounts of these amino acids (see Table 71.3). Further, all result in very low plasma cyst(e)ine and tyrosine concentrations (158). Many available mixtures also have large amounts of only a few nonessential amino acids (e.g., glycine) rather than a mixture of all nonessential amino acids (see Table 71.3); as a result, extremely high plasma concentrations of the amino acids present in excess are commonly seen.

Whether these abnormal plasma amino acid patterns are hazardous, or even undesirable, is not known. However, considering the well-known relationship between abnormally high plasma amino acid concentrations and mental retardation in infants with inborn errors of metabolism (e.g., phenylketonuria), as well as the relationship between inadequate intake of a specific amino acid and a low plasma concentration of that amino acid, normalization of plasma amino acid patterns seems warranted. Some of the newer amino acid mixtures (e.g., TrophAmine; B. Braun, Irvine, CA) accomplish this to a large extent (161).

Although some of the metabolic complications are unavoidable, many can be controlled by careful monitoring and appropriate adjustment of the infusate. A suggested monitoring schedule is given in Table 71.7. The monitoring required to ensure safe and efficacious use of lipid emulsions is the most problematic. The most common practice (i.e., inspection of the plasma for turbidity) may not reliably detect elevated plasma triglyceride and free fatty acid concentrations (162). For this purpose, actual chemical determinations are

TABLE 71.7	SUGGESTED MONITORING SCHEDULE DURING TOTAL PARENTERAL NUTRITION	
VARIABLES TO BE MONITORED	SUGGESTED FREQUENCY (per wk)[a]	
	INITIAL PERIOD[a]	LATER PERIOD[a]
Growth variables		
Weight	7	7
Length	1	1
Head circumference	1	1
Metabolic variables		
Plasma electrolytes	3–4	2
Plasma calcium, magnesium, phosphorus	2	1
Blood acid–base status	3–4	1
Blood urea nitrogen	2	1
Plasma albumin	1	1
Liver function studies	1	1
Serum lipids[b]		
Hemoglobin	2	2
Urinary glucose	2–6/d	2/d
Variables for detection of infection		
Clinical observations (activity, temperature, etc.)	Daily	Daily
White blood cell count	As indicated	As indicated
Cultures	As indicated	As indicated

[a]Initial period is the time during which the desired energy intake is being achieved or the time(s) of metabolic instability.
[b]See text.

required. Because this usually is not practical, a reasonable compromise is to observe the plasma frequently (at least three times per day initially) for evidence of lipid accumulation (primarily triglyceride) and to measure triglyceride and free fatty acids less frequently. Careful monitoring is particularly important while the lipid dose is being increased, while the infant is unstable, and when a change in the infant's condition occurs. If turbidity of the plasma is observed, the rate of infusion should be decreased or the infusion stopped completely until the turbidity clears. Usually, the infusion can then be resumed at a lower rate. Once the desired dose of intravenous fat is achieved, serum turbidity should be checked once per day (unless the patient becomes unstable), and actual determinations of serum triglyceride and free fatty acid concentrations should be made weekly.

Liver disease remains the most frequent complication of long-term parenteral nutrition. As stated, secondary biliary cirrhosis, hepatic failure, end stage liver disease, and death may result. The origin remains uncertain but is likely to be multifactorial. Treatment modalities are empiric and include employing a choleretic agent (i.e., ursodeoxycholic acid), cycling the infusate, treating intestinal bacterial overgrowth, ensuring vigilant catheter care, minimizing the amount of lipid infused, and, in refractory cases, performing biliary irrigation (see earlier).

Weaning Infants from Total Parenteral Nutrition

In most infants, administration of parenteral nutrients need not interfere with introducing enteral feedings as soon as

they are likely to be tolerated. Once started, the volume of enteral feedings can be advanced as tolerated by the infant and the volume of the parenteral nutrition infusate can be decreased. During the period of combined enteral and parenteral nutrition, care should be taken to ensure both that nutrient requirements are met as nearly as possible and that tolerance for both fluids and nutrients is not exceeded. This requires careful attention to the total (parenteral plus enteral) intake and frequent adjustment downward of the parenteral intake as enteral intake increases.

Home Parenteral Nutrition

Today, most patients who require parenteral nutrients for a long period leave the hospital and receive this therapy at home. Considering the many difficulties of in-hospital parenteral nutrition (see earlier), the potential problems of TPN at home seem formidable. Nonetheless, both patients who can tolerate some enteral intake and patients who can tolerate only parenteral nutrients have been treated successfully at home for several months to years. In many cases, sufficient nutrients can be administered during only a portion of the day, thus allowing the older patient to pursue reasonably normal daytime activities and the younger patient (as well as his or her parents) to sleep with little danger of accidental disconnection of the infusion system. Small portable infusion pumps are available such that the necessary apparatus can be enclosed in vests, backpacks, and so on, to allow even the patient who requires constant infusion of parenteral nutrients to lead a reasonably normal life. Obviously, home parenteral nutrition is more likely to be successful for the older child, adolescent, or adult. However, with careful patient (and parent) selection, young infants also can be managed quite successfully at home.

In general, the catheter used for home TPN is the Broviac catheter, which can be used for several months, and frequently for years. Standard nutrient infusates are obtained from the hospital pharmacy or from commercial concerns and are stored in a small home refrigerator. Catheter care is managed by the patient or a family member after careful training before patient discharge.

All the usual metabolic and catheter-related complications of parenteral nutrition can occur at home as well as in the hospital. However, patients who can be managed successfully with home parenteral nutrition usually have reached the point at which requirements are reasonably stable. Thus, less frequent monitoring is sufficient. Nonetheless, successful home parenteral nutrition, particularly for the young pediatric patient, requires frequent outpatient visits and frequent telephone contact. Some commercial home parenteral nutrition services include frequent home visits by a nurse.

Overall, administration of parenteral nutrients at home has been much more successful than initially envisioned. Certainly, the practice improves the quality of life for patients who require long-term parenteral nutrition. However, the purpose of parenteral nutrition is to provide the necessary nutrients transiently while the compromised gastrointestinal function necessitating use of parenteral nutrition recovers. Some patients may never be able to survive without parenteral nutrition, but attempts to increase enteral intake must continue. Unfortunately, this is not always the case; rather, discharge from the hospital often is viewed as the goal of therapy, and once it is achieved, attempts to increase the tolerance of enteral intake slows or stops. It is important that this attitude not become more common.

SUMMARY

The nutritional management of infants and children with specific diseases and other conditions must take into account both the increased nutrient requirements occasioned by the presence of these disorders and the decreased nutrient intake that so often accompanies them. The method of delivery of these increased nutrients may vary, but conventional feeding is preferred to enteral feeding, which, in turn, is preferred to parenteral feeding, although appropriate supplementation may be required if the chosen method is insufficient to meet the dietary needs of the patient.

REFERENCES

1. Menon G, Poskitt EME. Arch Dis Child 1985;60:1134–9.
2. Thommessen M, Heiberg A, Kase BF. Eur J Clin Nutr 1992;46:457–64.
3. Romholt Hansen S, Dorup I. Acta Paediatr 1993;82:166–72.
4. Mitchell IM, Logan RW, Pollock JCS et al. Br Heart J 1995;73:277–83.
5. Cameron JW, Rosenthal A, Olson AD. Arch Pediatr Adolesc Med 1995;149:1098–102.
6. Varan B, Tokel K, Yilmaz G. Arch Dis Child 1999;81:49–52.
7. Barton JS, Hindmarsh PC, Scrimgeour CM et al. Arch Dis Child 1994;70:5–9.
8. Salzer HR, Haschke F, Wimmer M et al. Pediatr Cardiol 1989;10:17–23.
9. Bougle D, Iselin M, Kahyat A et al. Arch Dis Child 1986;61:799–801.
10. Schwarz SM, Gewitz MH, See CC et al. Pediatrics 1990;86:368–73.
11. Jackson M, Poskitt EME. Br J Nutr 1991;65:131–43.
12. Unger R, DeKleermaeker M, Gidding SS et al. Arch Pediatr Adolesc Med 1992;146:1078–84.
13. Hofner G, Behrens R, Koch A et al. Pediatr Cardiol 2000;21:341–6.
14. Schuumans FM, Pulles-Heintzberger CFM, Gerver WJM et al. Acta Paediatr 1998;87:1250–5.
15. Bines JE, Truby HD, Armstrong DS et al. J Pediatr 2002;140:527–33.
16. Erskine JM, Lingard CD, Sontag MD et al. J Pediatr 1998;132:265–9.
17. Lai H-C, Kosorok MR, Laxova A et al. Pediatrics 2000;105:53–61.
18. Zemel BS, Jawad AF, FitzSimmons S et al. J Pediatr 2000;137:374–80.
19. Peterson ML, Jacobs DR, Milla CE. Pediatrics 2003;112:588–92.
20. Konstan MW, Butler SM, Wohl MEB et al. J Pediatr 2003;142:624–30.
21. Mansell AL, Andersen JC, Muttart CR et al. J Pediatr 1984;109:700–5.
22. McPhail GL, Acton JD, Fenchel MC et al. J Pediatr 2008;153:752–7.
23. Farrell PM, Kosorok MR, Rock MJ et al. Pediatrics 2001;107:1–13.
24. Stark LJ, Mulvihill MM, Jelalian E et al. Pediatrics 1997;99:665–71.
25. Powers SW, Patton SR, Byars KC et al. Pediatrics 2002;109:e75.
26. Nasr SZ, Durry D. Pediatr Pulmonol 2008;43:209–19.
27. Hardin DS, Rice J, Ahn C et al. J Pediatr 2005;146: 324–8.
28. Schnabel D, Grasemann C, Staab D et al. Pediatrics 2007;119:e1230–8.
29. Hardin DS, Ellis KJ, Dyson M et al. J Pediatr 2001;139:636–42.
30. Eubanks V, Koppersmith N, Wooldridge N et al. J Pediatr 2002;140:439–44.
31. McNaughton SA, Shepard RW, Greer RG et al. J Pediatr 2000;136:188–94.
32. Wilson DC, Rashid M, Durie PR et al. J Pediatr 2001;138:851–5.
33. Couper R, Belli D, Durie P et al. J Pediatr Gastroenterol Nutr 2002;35:S213–33.
34. Borowitz D, Baker RD, Stallings V. J Pediatr Gastroenterol Nutr 2002;35:246–59.
35. Alam NH, Hamadani JD, Dewan N et al. J Pediatr 2003;143:614–9.
36. Diop EHI, Dossou NI, Ndour MM et al. Am J Clin Nutr 2003;78:302–7.
37. Udall JN, Bhutta ZA, Firmansyah A et al. J Pediatr Gastroenterol Nutr 2002;35:S173–9.
38. Cohen MB. J Pediatr 1991;118:S34–9.
39. Ethelberg S, Olesen B, Neimann J et al. Epidemiol 2006;17:24–30.
40. Sack RB. Bacterial and parasitic agents of acute diarrhea. In: Bellanti JA, ed. Acute Diarrhea: Its Nutritional Consequences in Infancy. New York: Raven Press, 1983:53–65.
41. Hamilton JR. Viral enteritis: a cause of disordered small intestinal epithelial renewal. In: Lebenthal E, ed. Chronic Diarrhea in Children. New York: Raven Press, 1984:269–76.
42. Hill I, Fasano A, Schwartz R et al. J Pediatr 2000;136:86–90.
43. Hoffenberg EJ, MacKenzie T, Barriga KJ et al. J Pediatr 2003;143:308–14.
44. Catassi C, Fabiani E, Iacono G et al. Am J Clin Nutr 2007;85:160–6.
45. Fabiani E, Taccari LM, Ratsch IM et al. J Pediatr 2000;136:841–3.
46. Hoffenberg EJ, Haas J, Drescher A et al. J Pediatr 2000;137:361–6.
47. Kalayci AG, Kansu A, Girgin N et al. Pediatrics 2001;108:E89.
48. Mora S, Borera G, Beccio S et al. J Pediatr 2001;139:516–21.
49. Kavak US, Yuce A, Kocak N et al. J Pediatr Gastroenterol Nutr 2003;37:434–6.
50. Hill ID, Bhatnagar S, Cameron DJS et al. J Pediatr Gastroenterol Nutr 2002;35:S78–88.
51. Castile RG, Telander RL, Cooney DR et al. J Pediatr Surg 1980;15:462–9.
52. Markowitz J, Grancher K, Rosa J et al. J Pediatr Gastroenterol Nutr 1993;16:373–80.
53. Sentongo TA, Semeao EJ, Piccoli DA et al. J Pediatr Gastroenterol Nutr 2000;31:33–40.

54. Rosenthal SR, Snyder JD, Hendricks KM et al. Pediatrics 1983;72:481–90.

55. Motil KJ, Grand RJ, Davis-Kraft L et al. Gastroenterology 1993;105:681–91.

56. Kanof ME, Lake AM, Bayless TM. Gastroenterology 1988;95:1523–7.

57. Belli DC, Seidman E, Bouthillier L et al. Gastroenterology 1988;94:603–10.

58. Polk DB, Hattner JA, Kerner JA. JPEN J Parenter Enteral Nutr 1992;16:499–504.

59. Hueschkel RB, Menache CC, Megerian JT et al. J Pediatr Gastroenterol Nutr 2000;31:8–15.

60. Johnson T, Macdonald S, Hill SM et al. Gut 2006;55:356–61.

61. Day AS, Whitten KE, Lemberg DA et al. J Gastroenterol Hepatol 2006;21:1609–14.

62. Dziechciarz P, Horvath A, Shamir R et al. Aliment Pharmacol Ther 2007;26:795–806.

63. Hartman C, Berkowitz D, Weiss B et al. Isr Med Assoc J 2008;10:503–7.

64. Ruemmele FM, Roy CC, Levy E et al. J Pediatr 2000;136:285–91.

65. Buller H, Chin S, Kirschne B et al. J Pediatr Gastroenterol Nutr 2002;35:S151–8.

66. Rudolph CD, Mazur LJ, Liptak GS et al. J Pediatr Gastroenterol Nutr 2001;32(Suppl):S1–31.

67. Pareek N, Fleisher DR, Abell T. Am J Gastroenterol 2007;102:2832–40.

68. Pfau BT, Li BUK, Murray RD et al. Pediatrics 1996;97:364–8.

69. Wilmore DW. J Pediatr 1972;80:88–95.

70. Cooper A, Floyd TF, Ross AJ et al. J Pediatr Surg 1984;19: 711–8.

71. Parker P, Stroop BS, Greene H. J Pediatr 1981;99:360–4.

72. Kurkchubasche AG, Rowe MI, Smith SD. J Pediatr Surg 1993;28:1069–71.

73. Sondheimer JM, Cadnapaphornchai M, Sontag M et al. J Pediatr 1998;132:80–4.

74. Bines J, Francis D, Hill D. J Pediatr Gastroenterol Nutr 1998;26:123–8.

75. Andorsky DJ, Lund DP, Lillehei CW et al. J Pediatr 2001;139:27–33.

76. Kollman KA, Lien EL, Vanderhoof JA. J Pediatr Gastro-enterol Nutr 1999;28:41–5.

77. Weiming Z, Ning L, Jieshou L. JPEN J Parenter Enteral Nutr 2004;28:377–81.

78. Byrne TA, Wilmore DW, Iyer K et al. Ann Surg 2005;242: 655–61.

79. Kaufman SS, Loseke CA, Lupo JV et al. J Pediatr 1997;131:356–61.

80. Farrell MK, Balistreri WF. Clin Perinatol 1986;13:197–212.

81. Cooper A, Betts JM, Pereira GR et al. J Pediatr Surg 1984;19:462–6.

82. Meehan JJ, Georgeson KE. J Pediatr Surg 1997;32:473–5.

83. Sondheimer JM, Asturias E, Cadnapaphornchai M. J Pediatr Gastroenterol Nutr 1998;27:131–7.

84. Cooper A, Ross AJ, O'Neill JA et al. J Pediatr Surg 1985;20:772–4.

85. Teitelbaum DH, Tracy TF, Aouthmany MM et al. Pediatrics 2005;115:1332–40.

86. Gura KM, Duggan CP, Collier SB et al. Pediatrics 2006;118:e197–201.

87. Le HD, deMeijer VE, Robinson EM et al. Am J Clin Nutr 2011;94:749–758.

88. Kohl M, Wedel T, Entenmann A et al. J Pediatr Gastroenterol Nutr 2007;44:237–44.

89. Shin JI, Namgung RM Park MS et al. Eur J Pediatr 2008;167:197–202.

90. Diamond IR, deSilva NT, Tomlinson GA et al. J Parental Enteral Nutr 2011;35:596–602.

91. Walker-Smith J, Barnard J, Bhutta Z et al. J Pediatr Gastroenterol Nutr 2002;35:S98–105.

92. Williams DM, Sreedhar SS, Mickell JJ et al. Arch Pediatr Adolesc Med 2002;156:893–900.

93. Fiaccadori E, Maggiore U, Giacosa R et al. Kidney Int 2004; 65:999–1008.

94. Maxvold NJ, Smoyer WJ, Custer JR et al. Crit Care Med 2000; 28:1161–5.

95. Rees L, Shaw V. Pediatr Nephrol 2007;22:1689–702.

96. Wingen AM, Mehls O. Pediatr Nephrol 2002;17:111–20.

97. Furth SL, Hwang W, Yan C et al. Pediatr Nephrol 2002; 17:450–5.

98. Tom A, McCauley L, Bell L et al. J Pediatr 1999;134:464–71.

99. Kari J, Gonzalez C, Ledermann et al. Kidney Int 2000;57: 1681–7.

100. Ledermann SE, Shaw V, Trompeter RS. Pediatr Nephrol 1999;13:870–5.

101. National Kidney Foundation Kidney Disease Outcomes and Quality Initiative (K/DOQI). Am J Kidney Dis 2000; 35(Suppl):S1–40.

102. Salusky I, Fine RN, Nelson P et al. Am J Clin Nutr 1983;38: 599–611.

103. Edefonti A, Picca M, Damiani B et al. Pediatr Nephrol 1999; 13:253–8.

104. McKinney RE, Robertson WR, Duke Pediatric AIDS Clinical Trials Unit. J Pediatr 1993;123:579–82.

105. Miller TL, Evans S, Orav EJ et al. Am J Clin Nutr 1993;57: 588–92.

106. Falloon F, Eddy J, Pizzo PA. J Pediatr 1989;144:1–30.

107. Miller TL, Evans SE, Vasquez I et al. Pediatr Res 1997;41:85A.

108. Miller TL, Orav EJ, Colan S et al. Am J Clin Nutr 1997;66: 660–4.

109. Kabue MM, Kekitiinwa A, Maganda A et al. AIDS Patient Care STDs 2008;22:245–51.

110. Henderson RA, Saavedra JM, Perman JA et al. J Pediatr Gastroenterol Nutr 1994;18:429–34.

111. Miller TL, Awnetwant EL, Evans S et al. Pediatrics 1995;96: 696–702.

112. Clarick RH, Hanekom WA, Yogev R et al. Pediatrics 1997; 99:354–7.

113. Guarino A, Spagnuolo MI, Giocomet V et al. J Pediatr Gastroenterol Nutr 2002;34:366–71.

114. Miller TL, Easley KA, Zhang W et al. Pediatrics 2001;108: 1287–96.

115. Trois L, Cardoso EM, Miura E. J Trop Pediatr 2008;54: 19–24.

116. Jirapinyo P, Brewster D, Succi RC et al. J Pediatr Gastroenterol Nutr 2002;35:S134–42.

117. Mehta NM, Compher C, ASPEN Board of Directors. JPEN J Parenter Enteral Nutr 2009;33:260–76.

118. Duffy B, Pencharz P. Pediatr Res 1986;20:32–5.

119. Keshen TH, Miller RG, Jahoor F et al. J Pediatr Surg 1997;32:958–62.

120. Hunter DC, Jaksic T, Lewis D et al. Br J Surg 1988;75:875–8.

121. Coss-Bu JA, Jefferson LS, Walding D et al. Am J Clin Nutr 1998;67:74–80.

122. Joosten KF, Verhoeven JJ, Hazelet JA. Nutrition 1999;15:444–8.

123. Coss-Bu JA, Klish WJ, Walding D et al. Am J Clin Nutr 2001;74:664–9.

124. Hardy CM, Dwyer J, Snelling LK et al. Nutr Clin Pract 2002;17:182–9.

125. Mehta NM, Bechard LJ, Leavitt K et al. JPEN J Parenter Enteral Nutr 2009;33:336–44.

126. Chwals WJ, Bistrian BR. Crit Care Med 2000;28:2655–6.

127. Jaksic T, Shew SB, Keshen TH et al. J Pediatr Surg 2001; 36:63–7.
128. Mehta NM, Bechard LJ, Dolan M et al. Pediatr Crit Care Med 2011;12:398–405.
129. Friedman Z, Danon A, Stahlman MT et al. Pediatrics 1976;58:640–9.
130. van Aerde JE, Sauer PJ, Pencharz PB et al. Am J Clin Nutr 1994;59:659–62.
131. Patterson BW, Nguyen T, Pierre E et al. Metabolism 1997;46: 573–8.
132. Hart DW, Wolf SE, Herndon DN et al. Ann Surg 2002;235: 152–61.
133. Schwarz SM, Corredor J, Fisher-Medina J et al. Pediatrics 2001;108:671–6.
134. Rommel N, DeMeyer AM, Feenstra L et al. J Pediatr Gastroenterol Nutr 2003;37:75–84.
135. Cooper A, Heird WC. Am J Clin Nutr 1982;35:1132–41.
136. Baker JP, Detsky AS, Wesson DE et al. N Engl J Med 1982;306:969–72.
137. Flegal KM, Wei R, Ogden C. Am J Clin Nutr 2002;75: 761–6.
138. Waterlow JC. Br Med J 1972;3:566–9.
139. Chellis MJ, Sanders SV, Webster H et al. JPEN J Parenter Enteral Nutr 1996;20:71–3.
140. Briassoulis GC, Zavras NJ, Hatzis MT. Pediatr Crit Care Med 2001;2:113–21.
141. Briassoulis G, Zavras N, Hatzis T. Nutrition 2001;17:548–57.
142. deLucas C, Moreno M, Lopez-Herce J et al. J Pediatr Gastroenterol Nutr 2000;130:175–80.
143. Kawagoe JY, Segre CA, Pereira CR et al. Am J Infect Control 2001;29:109–14.
144. Meert KL, Daphtary KM, Metheny NA. Chest 2004;126: 872–8.
145. Sanchez C, Lopez-Herce J, Carrillo A et al. Nutrition 2007; 23:16–22.
146. Horn D, Chaboyer W. Am J Crit Care 2003;12:461–8.
147. Horn D, Chaboyer W, Schluter PJ. Aust Crit Care 2004;17: 98–103.
148. Heird WC. Justification of total parenteral nutrition. In: Yu VYH, MacMahon RA, eds. Intravenous Feeding of the Neonate. London: Edward Arnold, 1992:166–75.
149. Kashyap S, Heird WC. Protein requirements of low birth-weight, very low birthweight, and small for gestational age infants. In: Räihä NCR, ed. Protein Metabolism During Infancy. Nestlé Nutrition Workshop Series, vol 33. New York: Raven Press, 1995:133–51.
150. Collins JN, Hoope M, Brown K et al. J Pediatr 1991;118:921–7.
151. Greene HL, Hambidge KM, Schanler R et al. Am J Clin Nutr 1988;48:1324–42.
152. Paulsrud JR, Pensler L, Whitten CF et al. Am J Clin Nutr 1972;25:897–904.
153. Shennan AT, Bryan MD, Angel A. J Pediatr 1977;91:134–7.
154. Park W, Paust H, Brösicke H et al. JPEN J Parenter Enteral Nutr 1986;10:627–30.
155. Greene HL, Hazlett D, Demree R. Am J Clin Nutr 1976; 29:127–5.
156. Friedman Z, Marks MH, Maisels J et al. Pediatrics 1978;61: 694–8.
157. Loo LS, Tang JP, Kohl S. J Infect Dis 1982;146:64–70.
158. Odell GTB, Cukier JO, Ostrea EM Jr et al. J Lab Clin Med 1977;89:29–307.
159. Haumont D, Deckelbaum RJ, Richelle M et al. J Pediatr 1989;115:787–93.
160. Winters RW, Heird WC, Dell RB et al. Plasma amino acids in infants receiving parenteral nutrition. In: Green HL, Holliday MA, Munro HN, eds. Clinical Nutrition Update: Amino Acids. Chicago: American Medical Association, 1977: 147–54.
161. Heird WC, Dell RB, Helms RA et al. Pediatrics 1987;80: 401–8.
162. Schreiner RL, Glick MR, Nordschow CW et al. J Pediatr 1979;94:197–200.

FOOD INSECURITY IN CHILDREN: IMPACT ON PHYSICAL, PSYCHOEMOTIONAL, AND SOCIAL DEVELOPMENT[1]

72

RAFAEL PÉREZ-ESCAMILLA

Decades of research have conclusively shown that child malnutrition has a negative impact on the physical and intellectual development of children (1, 2). The consequences of household food insecurity (FI) on child development have just begun to be understood, however. This discrepancy is explained in part by the fact that global consensus on the definition of household FI was reached only at the end of the twentieth century. This chapter examines the influence of household FI on the development, health, and well-being of children and youth and discusses potential mediators, specifically maternal depression.

FOOD INSECURITY DEFINITION

Household food security has been defined as "access by all people at all times to enough food for an active, healthy life and includes, at a minimum, (a) the ready availability of nutritionally adequate and safe foods and (b) an assured availability to acquire acceptable foods in socially acceptable ways (e.g., without resorting to emergency food

supplies, scavenging, stealing, or other coping strategies)." Thus, FI exists in situations with "limited or uncertain availability of nutritionally adequate and safe foods or limited or uncertain ability to acquire acceptable foods in socially acceptable ways" (3).

FOOD INSECURITY MEASUREMENT

The five commonly used methods for assessing FI directly or indirectly are as follows: (a) the Food and Agricultural Organization (FAO) method for estimating average calories available per capita, (b) household income and expenditure surveys, (c) dietary intake surveys, (d) maternal-child anthropometry, and (e) experience-based FI scales (4). Experience-based scales were originally developed in the United States, and their use has spread globally (4, 5). These scales are strongly grounded on qualitative research conceptualizing FI as a "managed" household process that moves through a series of stages. This process starts with a state of worry or anxiety related to the uncertainty about future access to food and is followed by sacrificing dietary quality and eventually reducing the amount of food consumed, first among adults and then among children (4).

FI scales include questions that examine each stage or one specific stage of FI. Questions are usually answered by an adult who knows about the food situation in the household, and for each household a total summative score is estimated based on the number of affirmative responses. These scores can then be converted into FI categories (i.e., food security, mild FI, moderate FI, severe FI) based on cutoff points that discriminate among the different stages of FI experienced by households. The US Household Food Security Survey Module (HFSSM) was found to have adequate psychometric behavior and validity for use in both large-scale surveys and smaller studies in the United States, and this tool has been adapted and validated in other developed and several developing countries (5–7).

Experience-based FI scales directly measure the phenomenon of interest, are easy to apply, and have been well accepted by both target communities and policy makers (4, 6). These scales do not capture all the dimensions of the FI construct, however. For example, they do not assess the safety of the food supply accessed by the household or measure issues related to water security.

---

[1]**Abbreviations: BMI**, body mass index; **C-SNAP**, Children's Sentinel Nutrition Assessment Project; **ECLS**, Early Childhood Longitudinal Study; **ECLS-B**, Early Childhood Longitudinal Study-Birth Cohort; **FAO**, Food and Agricultural Organization; **FI**, food insecurity; **HFSSM**, Household Food Security Survey Module; **IDA**, iron-deficiency anemia; **NHANES**, National Health and Nutrition Examination Survey; **SEM**, structural equation model; **USDA**, US Department of Agriculture.

In addition, the measure captures FI at the household level but cannot identify individuals within the same household experiencing different degrees of FI (6).

This chapter reviews evidence focused on experience-based FI scales because of the following: (a) these FI scales are constructed around the consensus definition of household food security adopted by the international community; (b) they represent a direct measurement of the phenomena of interest; and (c) a substantial body of evidence evaluating the impact of FI on child nutrition and health outcomes, based on these scales, is available.

GLOBAL FOOD INSECURITY TRENDS

The US Census Bureau reports annual household FI rates since 1995 estimated from the 18-item HFSSM applied through the December Current Population Survey Food Security Supplement. The reference time period of the HFSSM is the 12 months preceding the survey, and households are classified as having food security, low food security, or very low food security, based on the number of affirmative answers to the HFSSM items (6). In 2008, 14.6% of US households were food insecure (i.e., with either low or very low food security). This rate, which translates into 17.1 million households, is the highest ever recorded since 1995. US households are more likely to be food insecure if they are poor, are headed by a single woman, have a head of household who reports being Hispanic or African-American, and they have children. Indeed, according to the US Department of Agriculture (USDA) (8), households with children had almost twice the rate of FI as those without children (21% versus 11.3%, respectively). Thus, normal development of a substantial number of low-income children in the United States may be at risk, to the extent that development is influenced by FI.

Household FI estimates based on experience-based scales are difficult to compare across countries because different scales, time frames, and classification algorithms have been used. One exception is the work by Nord and Hopwood (9), who demonstrated that national adult

TABLE 72.1	PERCENTAGE OF INDIVIDUALS IN CANADA AND THE UNITED STATES WHO LIVE IN FOOD-INSECURE HOUSEHOLDS[a-c]	
	CANADA	UNITED STATES
	PERCENTAGE OF INDIVIDUALS (%)	
All Individuals	7.0	12.6
Adults	6.6	10.8
Children	8.3	17.9

[a]Estimates derived from US household food security classification methodology using the past 12 months as a reference period. Based on data from 2004 Canadian Community Health Survey, cycle 2.2; and 2003–2005 US Current Population Survey Food Security Supplements.
[b]*Food insecure* refers to households with "low" and "very low" food security.
[c]All differences between Canada and the United States are statistically significant (*p* < .05).

Adapted with permission from Nord M, Hopwood HA. A Comparison of Household Food Security in Canada and the United States. Report ERR-67. Washington, DC: Economic Research Service, US Department of Agriculture, 2008.

and child FI rates, estimated with the HFSSM, are significantly lower in Canada than in the United States even after investigators controlled for key socioeconomic and demographic confounders (Table 72.1). Differences in social policies in both countries may partly explain these findings.

Perez-Escamilla et al (10) documented that household FI was substantially worse in Mexico than in Uruguay when these investigators applied the Latin American and Caribbean Household Food Security Scale (ELCSA) (7) and used similar tool application and nationally representative sampling procedures (Fig. 72.1).

Regional and global estimates derived from a standardized FI experience-based scale are still not available. Therefore, one must rely on other FI indicators to estimate the magnitude of the problem. The FAO estimates that approximately 1 billion individuals worldwide experience caloric undernutrition (11). The problem is more severe in sub-Saharan Africa and in South and Southeast Asia (Table 72.2). This figure largely underestimates the magnitude of the FI problem because hundreds of

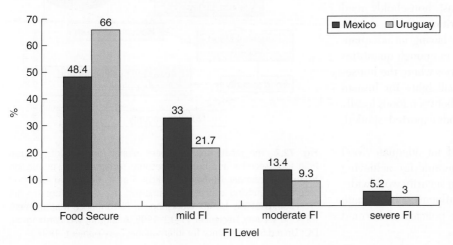

Fig. 72.1. Household food insecurity (FI) levels in Mexico and Uruguay assessed with the 16-item Latin American and Caribbean Household Food Security Scale (ELCSA) (7) through nationally representative public opinion polls in 2007 (Mexico) and 2009 (Uruguay). (Adapted with permission from Pérez-Escamilla R, Parás P, Acosta MJ et al. FASEB J 2011;25:226–8).

TABLE 72.2	**PREVALENCE OF CALORIC UNDERNOURISHMENT[a] IN TOTAL POPULATIONS ACROSS TIME**			
COUNTRY GROUPS/WORLD REGIONS	1990–1992 (%)	1995–1997 (%)	2000–2002 (%)	2005–2007 (%)
World	16	14	14	13
Developed countries	—	—	—	—
Developing world	20	17	17	16
Asia and the Pacific[b]	20	16	16	16
East Asia	18	12	10	10
Southeast Asia	24	18	17	14
South Asia	22	20	21	22
Central Asia	8	9	18	10
Western Asia	41	27	15	7
Latin America and the Caribbean	12	11	10	8
North and Central America	8	8	7	7
Caribbean	26	28	22	24
South America	12	10	10	8
Near East and North Africa	6	8	8	7
Near East	7	11	10	9
North Africa	—	—	—	—
Sub-Saharan Africa	34	33	31	28
Central Africa	32	49	55	53
East Africa	45	44	39	34
Southern Africa	43	41	38	33
West Africa	20	15	14	10

[a]*Undernourishment* refers to the condition of people whose dietary energy consumption is continuously below a minimum dietary energy requirement for maintaining a healthy life and carrying out a light physical activity with an acceptable minimum body weight for attained height.
[b]Includes Oceania.

From Food and Agricultural Organization. Food Security Statistics. Available at: http://www.fao.org/economic/ess/ess-fs/en. Accessed November 23, 2011, with permission.

millions of individuals who may have access to sufficient or even excessive amounts of calories may not have access to diets of adequate nutritional quality (4).

CONCEPTUAL FRAMEWORK

Nutrition security, a condition that occurs when the body tissues are exposed to optimal amounts of nutrients and other essential substances, is the result of household food security, health care access security, and access to other basic human needs, including adequate sanitation. Food security and the other determinants of nutrition security interact with each other (12). For example, a household with limited resources for purchasing food may decide to not bring a child to the doctor and not to purchase needed medications. For food security to exist, households need to have access to healthy and nutritious foods. Access to these foods, in turn, depends on having an adequate income and for foods to be available in enough quantities in the country, region, and communities where the households are located. National food availability for human consumption represents the balance between foods locally grown and foods imported, minus foods exported, spoiled, or fed to animals (Fig. 72.2).

Thus, ultimately, maintenance of an adequate food supply at the global level is paramount for achieving household food security and nutrition security worldwide. Global food supplies are strongly influenced by climate change, agricultural commodity price policies, and armed conflicts (13).

Household FI can affect a child's physical, mental, social, and psychoemotional development through different pathways (Fig. 72.3). One biologic pathway involves the direct link among FI, poorer dietary intakes, nutritional status, and overall well-being. A second psychoemotional pathway involves the worry or anxiety, feeling of

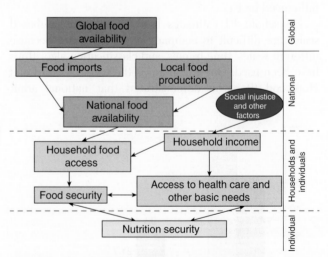

Fig. 72.2. The relationships between global food security, household food security, and nutrition security. (Adapted with permission from Frankenberger TR, Frankel L, Ross S et al. Household livelihood security: a unifying conceptual framework for CARE programs. In: Proceedings of the USAID Workshop on Performance Measurement for Food Security, December 11–12, 1995, Arlington, VA. Washington, DC: United States Agency for International Development, 1997.)

health problems of 23% versus 31% versus 37%, respectively ($p < .05$). In this study, behavioral or mental health problems were defined as aggressiveness, anxiety, depression, lack of concentration, or hyperactivity.

NHANES III results showed that 6- to 11-year-old children from food insufficient (as opposed to food sufficient) households had lower arithmetic scores and were more likely to have repeated a grade, to have seen a psychologist, and to have more difficulty getting along with their peers. In addition to the last two outcomes, food insufficient adolescents were also more likely to be have been suspended from school (67). NHANES III analyses also revealed that 15- to 16-year-old adolescents from food insufficient households were more likely to have experienced dysthymia, thoughts of death, and a desire to die and also to have attempted suicide (62).

Longitudinal SEMs applied to the ECLS-Birth Cohort (ECLS-B) data showed that FI at 9 months of age predicted lower maternal attachment and lower mental development at 2 years of age. For both outcomes, this association was mediated by maternal depression and poorer parenting practices at 9 months (61). Another longitudinal analysis of the ECLS-B data documented that FI is likely to impair child academic and social development, although several effects may be gender specific (29). FI in kindergarten predicted lower mathematics scores and social skills in third grade among girls, but not boys. Similarly, girls (but not boys) from persistently food-insecure households (i.e., those households that were food insecure both in kindergarten and in third grade) had lower increases in reading scores compared with their persistently food-secure counterparts. Children (both boys and girls) living in households that were food secure in kindergarten and then became food insecure by third grade had lower increases in reading scores compared with those children whose households were persistently food secure. Transitioning from FI to food security during the same period of time was associated with improved social skills among girls only (29).

In summary, the studies reviewed in this section strongly suggest that FI in children represents not only a biologic but also a psychoemotional and developmental challenge. This challenge, in turn, is likely to translate into poor academic performance and intellectual achievement later in life. All these studies were conducted in the United States, and most included Hispanic children. Thus, improving food security in Hispanic households is likely to improve the overall well-being of the children belonging to the fastest growing population group in the country. These conclusions need to be confirmed through additional longitudinal studies because most evidence to date is cross-sectional.

Maternal Depression

Studies have consistently found an independent association between FI and maternal depression (68, 69). Pregnant women from North Carolina who were food insecure (as opposed to food secure) were more likely to have higher levels of perceived stress, trait anxiety, and depressive symptoms (68). These dose-response relationships were a function of FI severity. Pregnant Latinas living in Connecticut were also more likely to have elevated levels of depression symptoms if they lived in food-insecure (as opposed to food secure) households (69). As previously indicated, findings from the ECLS data showed that FI at 9 months of age was associated with maternal depression, which, in turn, mediated the association between FI and poorer health and mental development, as well as obesity, outcomes at 2 years of age (33, 61). The C-SNAP study found that maternal depressive symptoms were associated not only with FI but also with worse child health indicators and less likelihood to remain enrolled in a food assistance program (70). The study conducted by Whitaker et al (66) also found that FI was independently and positively associated, in a dose-response fashion, with maternal clinical depression and anxiety symptoms. As previously reported, this study showed a dose-response relationship between FI severity and child behavioral or mental health problems (i.e., aggressiveness, anxiety, depression, lack of concentration, or hyperactivity) among children who were an average of 3 years old.

From the child development perspective, these findings are of concern because maternal depression has been associated with lower quality care and maternal-child interactions, less attachment to the child, and even child neglect and abuse (44). Thus, maternal depression may be one of the factors mediating the relationship of FI with worse child psychosocial development.

CONCLUSIONS

The preponderance of the evidence suggests that household FI has a strong influence on children's dietary quality, psychobehavioral and intellectual development, and health status. The plausibility of the developmental findings is high because FI has been shown not only to influence nutritional status but also to represent a major psychoemotional stressor to both children and their caretakers. The impact of FI on child underweight and overweight is mixed and appears to be context specific.

Several limitations of the currently available evidence are important to recognize. First, most study designs have been cross-sectional. Second, different scales, cutoff points, and reference time periods have been used to classify households into different food (in)security categories. For example, although some studies have examined different levels of FI severity, others have classified households only as food secure or food insecure (i.e., dichotomous). Similarly, the use of different scales is a cause for concern because findings may be influenced by the choice of scale (71). Third, most studies have used multivariate main effects models without taking into account that several of the key "confounders" included are likely to be mediators or effect modifiers of the relationship between FI and child development or health outcomes. More theory-based hypothesis testing statistical models such as SEMs are needed for a better understanding of the pathways by which FI adversely affects child well-being. This knowledge is needed to inform policy and to develop evidence-based, effective interventions.

POLICY IMPLICATIONS

Policies that are effective at reducing poverty and FI are likely to translate into improved human development. Because human development is the foundation for social capital, which, in turn, is the engine that drives national development, investing in these programs should be a top priority for governments worldwide. Funding is needed to conduct the research needed to understand more precisely the pathways by which FI affects human development. The generation of this knowledge is essential for the identification of intervention points to buffer children from the negative consequences of FI. Given the demonstration of the internal validity of experience-based scales in diverse settings, it is important to support efforts that seek to harmonize household FI scales for application at the regional (7) or even the global (72) level.

ACKNOWLEDGMENTS

I am grateful to Drs. Amber Hromi-Fiedler and Donna J. Chapman for their editorial review and substantive feedback on this chapter. I was partially supported through the Connecticut National Institutes of Health (NIH) Project EXPORT Center for Eliminating Health Disparities among Latinos (NIH-NCHMD P20MD001765). The views expressed in this chapter are mine and do not necessarily represent those of the NIH or its National Center on Minority Health and Health Disparities. This chapter is dedicated to Ernesto Pollitt, my mentor, colleague, and friend.

REFERENCES

1. Pollitt E. J Nutr 2000;130(Suppl):350S–3S.
2. Victora CG, Adair L, Fall C et al. Lancet 2008;371:340–57.
3. Anderson SA. J Nutr 1990;120:1557–1600.
4. Perez-Escamilla R, Segall-Corrêa AM. Rev Nutr (Brazil) 2008;21(Suppl):15–26.
5. Coates J, Frongillo EA, Rogers BL et al. J Nutr 2006;136(Suppl):1438S–48S.
6. National Research Council. Food Insecurity and Hunger in the United States: An Assessment of the Measure. Washington, DC: National Academies Press, 2006:1–114.
7. Pérez-Escamilla R, Melgar-Quiñonez H, Nord M et al. Perspect Nutr Hum (Colombia) 2007(Suppl):117–34.
8. US Department of Agriculture Food Security Data. Available at : http://www.ers.usda.gov/Briefing/FoodSecurity. Accessed November 23, 2011
9. Nord M, Hopwood HA. A Comparison of Household Food Security in Canada and the United States. Report ERR-67. Washington, DC: Economic Research Service, US Department of Agriculture, 2008.
10. Pérez-Escamilla R, Parás P, Acosta MJ et al. FASEB J 2011; 25:226–8.
11. Food and Agricultural Organization. Food Security Statistics. Available at: http://www.fao.org/economic/ess/ess-fs/en. Accessed November 23, 2011.
12. Frankenberger TR, Frankel L, Ross S et al. Household livelihood security: a unifying conceptual framework for CARE programs. In: Proceedings of the USAID Workshop on Performance Measurement for Food Security, December 11–12, 1995, Arlington, VA. Washington, DC: United States Agency for International Development, 1997.
13. Brown L. Sci Am 2009;300:50–7.
14. Dave JM, Evans AE, Saunders RP et al. J Am Diet Assoc 2009;109:697–701.
15. Rosas LG, Harley K, Fernald LC et al. J Am Diet Assoc 2009;109:2001–9.
16. Oh SY, Hong MJ. Eur J Clin Nutr 2003;57:1598–604.
17. Knueppel D, Demment M, Kaiser L. Public Health Nutr 2010;13:360–7.
18. Pérez-Escamilla R, Segall-Corrêa AM, Kurdian Maranha L et al. J Nutr 2004;134:1923–8.
19. Melgar-Quiñonez HR, Zubieta AC, MkNelly B et al. J Nutr 2006;136(Suppl):1431S–7S.
20. Rafiei M, Nord M, Sadeghizadeh A et al. Nutr J 2009;8:28.
21. Hackett M, Melgar-Quiñonez H, Alvarez MC. Rev Panam Salud Publica 2009;25:506–10.
22. Isanaka S, Mora-Plazas M, Lopez-Arana S et al. J Nutr 2007;137:2747–55.
23. Alvarado BE, Zunzunegui MV, Delisle H. Cad Saude Publica 2005;21:724–36.
24. Gomes Pimentel P, Sichieri R, Salles-Costa R. R Bras Estud Popul 2009;26:283–94.
25. Oliveira JS, Cabral de Lira PI, Maia SR et al. Rev Bras Saude Mater Infant 2010;10:237–45.
26. Frongillo EA, Nanama S. J Nutr 2006;136(Suppl):1409S–19S.
27. Baig-Ansari N, Rahbar MH, Bhutta ZA et al. Food Nutr Bull 2006;27:114–27.
28. Rose D, Bodor JN. Pediatrics 2006;117:464–73.
29. Jyoti DF, Frongillo EA, Jones SJ. J Nutr 2005;135:2831–9.
30. Alaimo K, Olson CM, Frongillo EA Jr. Arch Pediatr Adolesc Med. 2001;155:1161–7.
31. Casey PH, Simpson PM, Gossett JM et al. Pediatrics 2006;118:e1406–13.
32. Gundersen C, Garasky S, Lohman BJ. J Nutr 2009;139: 1173–8.
33. Bronte-Tinkew J, Zaslow M, Capps R et al. J Nutr 2007;137: 2160–5.
34. Dubois L, Farmer A, Girard M et al. Soc Sci Med 2006;63: 1503–16.
35. Matheson DM, Varady J, Varady A et al. Am J Clin Nutr 2002;76:210–7.
36. Kaiser LL, Melgar-Quiñonez HR, Lamp CL et al. J Am Diet Assoc 2002;102:924–9.
37. Buscemi J, Beech BM, Relyea G. J Immigr Minor Health 2009 May 29 [Epub ahead of print].
38. Martin KS, Ferris AM. J Nutr Educ Behav 2007;39:31–6.
39. Ortiz-Hernández L, Acosta-Gutiérrez MN, Núñez-Pérez AE et al. Rev Invest Clin 2007;59:32–41.
40. Shrewsbury V, Wardle J. Obesity 2008;16:275–84.
41. Burns C, Jones SJ, Frongillo EA. Poverty, household food insecurity and obesity in children. In: Waters E, Swinburn B, Seidell J et al. eds. Preventing Childhood Obesity. Oxford: Wiley Blackwell, 2010:129–37.
42. Dinour LM, Bergen D, Yeh MC. J Am Diet Assoc 2007;107: 1952–61.
43. Mirza M, Fitzpatrick-Lewis D, Thomas H. Is There a Relationship between Food Insecurity and Overweight/Obesity? Hamilton, Ontario, Canada: Effective Public Health Practice Project, 2007.
44. Cook JT, Frank DA. Ann N Y Acad Sci 2008;1136:193–209.

45. Peterman JN, Wilde PE, Liang S et al. Am J Public Health 2010;100:1930–7.

46. Olson CM, Bove CF, Miller EO. Appetite 2007;49:198–207.

47. Park K, Kersey M, Geppert J et al. Public Health Nutr 2009;12:2120–8.

48. Skalicky A, Meyers AF, Adams WG et al. Matern Child Health J 2006;10:177–85.

49. Eicher-Miller HA, Mason AC, Weaver CM et al. Am J Clin Nutr 2009;90:1358–71.

50. Pasricha SR, Black J, Muthayya S et al. Pediatrics 2010;126:e140–9.

51. Pérez-Escamilla R, Dessalines M, Finnigan M et al. J Nutr 2009;139:2132–8.

52. Cook JT, Frank DA, Berkowitz C et al. J Nutr 2004;134:1432–8.

53. Chilton M, Black MM, Berkowitz C et al. Am J Public Health 2009;99:556–62.

54. Alaimo K, Olson CM, Frongillo EA Jr, Briefel RR. Am J Public Health. 2001;91:781–6.

55. Radimer K. Public Health Nutr 2002;5:859–64.

56. Perez-Escamilla R. La inseguridad alimentaria: marco conceptual e implicaciones para la niñez [Food insecurity: conceptual framework and implications for the child]. In: Vasquez-Garibay E, Romero-Velarde E, eds. La Nutrición Pediátrica en América Latina. Nestlé Nutrition Institute Workshop LATAM, vol 1. Mexico City: Nestec (Vevey, Switzerland) and Intersistemas (Mexico City), 2008:25–48.

57. Sampaio MFA, Kepple AW, Segall-Corrêa AM et al. Segur Aliment Nutr (Campinas, Brazil) 2006;13:64–77.

58. Wehler CA, Scott RI, Anderson JJ. J Nutr Educ 1992;24(Suppl):29S–35S.

59. Casey PH, Szeto KL, Robbins JM et al. Arch Pediatr Adolesc Med 2005;159:51–6.

60. Rose-Jacobs R, Black MM, Casey PH et al. Pediatrics 2008;121:65–72.

61. Zaslow M, Bronte-Tinkew J, Capps R et al. Matern Child Health J 2009;13:66–80.

62. Alaimo K, Olson CM, Frongillo EA. J Nutr 2002;132:719–25.

63. Kleinman RE, Murphy JM, Little M et al. Pediatrics 1998;101:e3.

64. Weinreb L, Wehler C, Perloff J et al. Pediatrics 2002;110:e41.

65. Murphy JM, Wehler CA, Pagano ME et al. J Am Child Adolesc Psychiatry 1998;37:163–71.

66. Whitaker RC, Phillips SM, Orzol SM. Pediatrics 2006;118:e859–68.

67. Alaimo K, Olson CM, Frongillo EA Jr. Pediatrics. 2001;108:44–53.

68. Laraia BA, Siega-Riz AM, Gundersen C et al. J Nutr 2006;136:177–82.

69. Hromi-Fiedler A, Bermúdez-Millán A, Segura-Pérez S et al. Matern Child Nutr 2010 Aug 23 [Epub ahead of print].

70. Casey P, Goolsby S, Berkowitz C et al. Pediatrics 2004;113:298–304.

71. Kaiser LL, Townsend MS, Melgar-Quiñonez HR et al. Am J Clin Nutr 2004;80:1372–8.

72. Hadley C, Maes K. Lancet 2009;374:1223–4.

73 NUTRITION AND DENTAL MEDICINE[1]

RIVA TOUGER-DECKER, DIANE RIGASSIO RADLER, AND DOMINICK P. DEPAOLA

CELLULAR AND STRUCTURAL CHARACTERISTICS OF THE ORAL TISSUES

Distinctive characteristics of oral tissues, such as the inability of enamel to remodel and the high cellular turnover rate of oral mucosa, the rates of alveolar bone growth, and the production of saliva, make oral tissues a unique indicator of physiologic perturbations. The oral cavity is a site of symptoms of many chronic diseases including dental caries, periodontal disease, acquired immunodeficiency syndrome (AIDS), nutritional anemias, herpes, salivary gland disorders, osteoporosis, diabetes, and cancer. Congenital anomalies such as cleft lip and palate are birth defects that have a complex genetic and environmental etiology linked to maternal nutrient status, folate in particular.

The linkages between oral disease and systemic health are expanding in depth and breadth with some profound observations. Within the past two decades, clear linkages have been established between periodontal disease and cardiovascular disease, diabetes, stroke, and adverse pregnancy outcomes. For example, periodontal disease is associated with increased risk of cardiovascular disease (1) and preterm delivery (2, 3). The inherent nature of oral infectious diseases requires an adequately functioning immune and cellular repair system, and unequivocal data link nutrient intake and these host defense mechanisms. The relationships among oral health, systemic health, and nutrition require the careful attention of all health professionals including physicians, dentists, registered dietitians, and nurses (3).

To fully appreciate these complex relationships, it is vital to understand the structure and function of the craniofacial-oral-dental complex. Teeth are specialized structures necessary for the initial processing of food and are composed of three mineralized tissues: enamel, dentin, and cementum, which encase the highly vascular dental pulp or "nerve." These relationships can be seen in the schematic cross section of a tooth in Figure 73.1. The teeth are retained in their bony sockets by means of a fibrous structure termed the *periodontal membrane* or *ligament*. Factors such as bacteria and the inflammatory immune response can affect the integrity of this structure and bone surrounding the socket, resulting in periodontal disease that may progress sufficiently to cause loosening and loss of the teeth (4).

---

[1]**Abbreviations: ADA**, American Dental Association; **AIDS**, acquired immunodeficiency syndrome; **CRA**, caries risk assessment; **DMFS**, decayed-missing-filled surfaces; **ECC**, early childhood caries; **GI**, gastrointestinal; **HIV**, human immunodeficiency virus; **NHANES**, National Health and Nutrition Examination Survey; **NIDR**, National Institute of Dental Research.

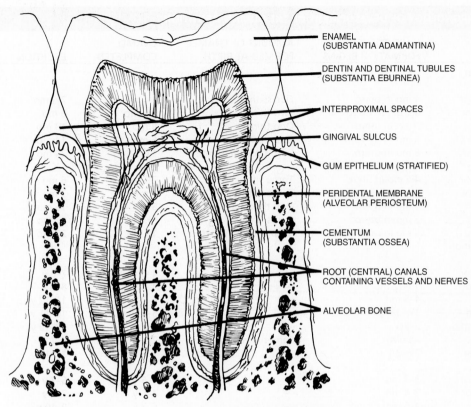

ENAMEL
(SUBSTANTIA ADAMANTINA)

DENTIN AND DENTINAL TUBULES
(SUBSTANTIA EBURNEA)

INTERPROXIMAL SPACES

GINGIVAL SULCUS

GUM EPITHELIUM (STRATIFIED)

PERIDENTAL MEMBRANE
(ALVEOLAR PERIOSTEUM)

CEMENTUM
(SUBSTANTIA OSSEA)

ROOT (CENTRAL) CANALS
CONTAINING VESSELS AND NERVES

ALVEOLAR BONE

Fig. 73.1. Schematic illustration of teeth in contact with the alveolar bone.

Each tooth develops from a tooth bud or germ located in the jaws. The bud consists of an epithelial component that arises as an invagination from the surface and produces enamel. The mesenchymal component consists of the dental papilla, which produces the tooth pulp and dentin, and the dental follicle, which produces the cementum and periodontal ligament once the tooth has formed. Table 73.1 details the chronology of the formation of the human dentition. The primary teeth begin forming at approximately 6 weeks in utero when cells in the primitive oral cavity differentiate to form the dental lamina, which is the site of tooth bud development. The formation of the crown of the tooth begins with the secretion of a dentin matrix containing collagen fibrils. Mineral ions then enter the matrix to form small crystals on or between the collagen fibrils. Enamel formation begins as soon as the first dentin layer has been laid down. This mineralization process constitutes the maturation of enamel and continues after the matrix is fully formed. As can be seen in Table 73.1, the mineralization process begins as early as 4 months in utero and continues into late adolescence. After the tooth erupts into the oral cavity, it continues to incorporate minerals (including fluoride) into its structure from saliva, food, and drinking fluids (5).

The life history of a tooth may be divided into three main eras: (a) the period during which its crown is forming and mineralizing in the jaw, (b) the period of maturation when the tooth is erupting into the oral cavity and its root or roots are forming, and (c) the maintenance period while it is functioning in the oral cavity (5). During the preeruptive period, the developing enamel and dentin are subject to nutritional deficiencies or imbalances in the same manner as any other developing tissues. Nutrient deficiencies can affect the secretory and the maturation stages of enamel formation. Following eruption into the oral cavity, the enamel is bathed in saliva and is exposed to oral microorganisms and their byproducts as well as food, so nutritional deficiencies or excesses and dietary habits may affect teeth in a local manner (5).

At least three striking differences exist between the mineralized tissues of teeth and other tissues of the body. First, enamel contains no capillary or lymphatic vessels to act as transport systems; however, the intimate relationships between the organic and the inorganic components of enamel suggest that pathways in the enamel exist for diffusion of ions and small molecules from saliva, and possibly from blood. Although the dentin likewise contains no vascular elements, it is more readily permeable to the passage of extracellular fluids from the blood, by way of the dentinal tubules that traverse the dentin. The interchange among elements in the enamel takes place through the bathing of its external surface with saliva. In contrast, the interchange in the dentin occurs by the movement of ions present in the blood supply to the pulp or periodontal membrane (4). Second, because of the

TABLE 73.1	CHRONOLOGY OF DEVELOPMENT OF THE HUMAN DENTITION				
TOOTH	HARD TISSUE FORMATION BEGINS	AMOUNT OF ENAMEL FORMED AT BIRTH	ENAMEL COMPLETED	ERUPTION	ROOT COMPLETED
Primary dentition					
Maxillary					
Central incisor	4 mo in utero	Five sixths	1½ mo	7½ mo	1½ y
Lateral incisor	4½ mo in utero	Two thirds	2½ mo	9 mo	2 y
Cuspid	5 mo in utero	One third	9 mo	18 mo	3¼ y
First molar	5 mo in utero	Cusps united	6 mo	14 mo	2½ y
Second molar	6 mo in utero	Cusp tips still isolated	11 mo	24 mo	3 y
Mandibular					
Central incisor	4½ mo in utero	Three fifths	2½ mo	6 mo	1½ y
Lateral incisor	4½ mo in utero	Three fifths	3 mo	7 mo	1½ y
Cuspid	5 mo in utero	One third	9 mo	16 mo	3¼ y
First molar	5 mo in utero	Cusps united	5½ mo	12 mo	2¼ y
Second molar	6 mo in utero	Cusp tips still isolated	10 mo	20 mo	3 y
Permanent dentition					
Maxillary					
Central incisor	3–4 mo	—	4–5 y	7–8 y	10 y
Lateral incisor	10–12 mo	—	4–5 y	8–9 y	11 y
Cuspid	4–5 mo	—	6–7 y	11–12 y	13–15 y
First bicuspid	1½–1¾ y	—	5–6 y	10–11 y	12–13 y
Second bicuspid	2–2¼ y	—	6–7 y	10–12 y	12–14 y
First molar	At birth	Sometimes a trace	2½–3 y	6–7 y	9–10 y
Second molar	2½–3 y	—	7–8 y	12–13 y	14–16 y
Mandibular					
Central incisor	3–4 mo	—	4–5 y	6–7 y	9 y
Lateral incisor	3–4 mo	—	4–5 y	7–8 y	10 y
Cuspid	4–5 mo	—	6–7 y	9–10 y	12–14 y
First bicuspid	1¾–2 y	—	5–6 y	10–12 y	12–13 y
Second bicuspid	2¼–2½ y	—	6–7 y	11–12 y	13–14 y
First molar	At birth	Sometimes a trace	2½–3 y	6–7 y	9–10 y
Second molar	2½–3 y	—	7–8 y	11–13 y	14–5 y

absence of cells, mineralized dental tissues do not have a microscopically or chemically detectable ability to repair improperly formed or mineralized areas, and the tooth does not have the ability to repair itself after a portion has been destroyed by tooth decay or mechanical injury. An exception is the remineralization of slightly demineralized, superficial areas of the enamel where the organic matrix and surface integrity are still intact, commonly referred to as "white spots." In addition, secondary dentin is formed by the odontoblasts, which persist throughout life on the pulpal surface of the dentin, in response to chemical stimuli from an advancing carious lesion in an effort to mitigate the noxious influence. Lack of ability to repair dental tissues is in direct contrast to bone, with its continual turnover and ability to remodel (4). Third, unlike other tissues, the mineralized tissues of teeth undergo a partial change of environment. When the tooth begins to emerge into the oral cavity, the vascular supply to the enamel organ is severed, and the enamel surface comes in contact with a complex mixture of saliva, microorganisms, food debris, and epithelial remnants. Thus, instead of a pure systemic environment, the erupted tooth has, in addition, an oral or external environment. As a consequence, the enamel and cementum surfaces on which

carious lesions are initiated by microbial action are largely outside the influences of humoral immune systems, so immune relationships with the caries process are primarily limited to those in saliva (4).

The development and maintenance of the soft tissues and bone that support the teeth are also subject to nutrient defects. The periodontium, as seen in Figure 73.1, comprises the gingiva; the periodontal ligament (peridental membrane), which joins the root cementum to the alveolar bone; the root cementum, which is a specialized, mineralized tissue similar to bone that covers the root of the tooth; and the alveolar bone, which forms and supports the sockets of the teeth. The alveolar bone grows in response to dental eruption, is modified by dental changes, and resorbs when teeth are lost. The finite space between the tooth and the gingiva, known as the gingival sulcus, is lined by a nonkeratinized epithelium. In addition, dental plaque, one of the primary agents responsible for the initiation of both dental caries and gingivitis, contains a high concentration of bacteria, which, in the gingival sulcus, are juxtaposed with a "naked" epithelium. Thus, bacteria and their byproducts or antigens can permeate the gingival epithelium and precipitate a classic inflammatory response that denotes periodontal disease. In fact, an intact immune system, which is highly dependent on nutrient status, is vital to maintain periodontal health. The diversity of hard and soft tissues that comprise the oral structures and the distinctive nutritional needs of each contribute to the uniqueness of the mouth as an external reflection of past and present nutritional problems (3, 6).

ROLE OF NUTRITION IN CRANIOFACIAL AND ORAL TISSUE DEVELOPMENT

Nutrient deficits can result in defects in tooth and salivary gland development. The most commonly studied conditions and nutrients that have affected tooth integrity, enamel solubility, and salivary flow and composition in animal models include protein-calorie malnutrition, ascorbic acid, vitamin A, vitamin D, calcium and phosphorus, iron, zinc, and fluoride. Malnutrition—deficiencies of vitamin A, ascorbic acid, vitamin D, and iodine—and fluoride excess have been demonstrated to affect human dentition (Table 73.2). The reader is also encouraged to review relevant sections of chapters in this text on each specific nutrient mentioned.

Enamel hypoplastic defects and hypomineralization have been the hallmarks of undernutrition and overnutrition during tooth development (7, 8). Vitamin A deficiency has been implicated as a critical factor in tooth health because it frequently accompanies protein-calorie malnutrition and is known to affect epithelial tissue

development, tooth morphogenesis, and odontoblast differentiation (9). The interference with calcification is manifested clinically by enamel hypoplasia (10). Additionally, vitamin A excess, when present during the first trimester of pregnancy, can result in severe craniofacial and oral clefts and limb defects (11).

Vitamin D, calcium, and phosphorus deficiencies all result in significant effects on tooth development and decreased resistance to dental caries. If a vitamin D deficiency occurs in utero or young infants, there may be delays in tooth eruption and quality of enamel is delayed, thereby increasing caries risk (12). Leaver demonstrated that extreme calcium and phosphorus deficiencies may result in hypomineralization of developing teeth (13). The deficit, however, must be severe enough to reduce plasma levels of calcium and phosphorus. The highly effective homeostatic mechanisms in humans that mobilize calcium from the skeleton to maintain normal plasma calcium levels make the chances of this occurring rare. Bawden postulated that vitamin D hypovitaminosis may be more important in considering hypomineralization resulting from inadequate calcium transport into developing dental tissues (14). Vitamin D deficiency has also been shown to affect tooth structure and to delay eruption patterns of teeth (15).

In childhood vitamin D deficiency, teeth are characterized microscopically by a widened layer of predentin, by the presence of interglobular dentin, and by interference

TABLE 73.2	EFFECTS OF NUTRIENT DEFICIENCIES ON TOOTH DEVELOPMENT		
NUTRIENT	EFFECT ON TISSUE	EFFECT ON CARIES	HUMAN DATA
Protein-calorie malnutrition	Tooth eruption delayed Tooth size Enamel solubility decreased Salivary gland dysfunction	Yes	Yes
Vitamin A	Decreased epithelial tissue development Tooth morphogenesis dysfunction Decreased odontoblast differentiation Increased enamel hypoplasia	Yes	Yes
Vitamin D/calcium/ phosphorus	Lowered plasma calcium Hypomineralization (hypoplastic defects) Tooth integrity compromised Delayed eruption patterns	Yes	Yes
Ascorbic acid	Dental pulpal alterations Odontoblastic degeneration Aberrant dentin	No	No
Fluoride	Stability of enamel crystal (enamel formation) Inhibition of demineralization Stimulation of remineralization Mottled enamel (excess) Inhibition of bacterial growth	Yes	Yes
Iodine	Delayed tooth eruption Altered growth patterns Malocclusion	No	Yes
Iron	Slow growth Tooth integrity Salivary gland dysfunction	Yes	No

with enamel formation (hypoplastic defects) (16). Young children with rickets have delayed eruption of the deciduous teeth, and the sequence of eruption is altered. The permanent incisors, cuspids, and first molars are usually affected because their development coincides with the age at which rickets is most common. Vitamin D–resistant rickets results in more frequent and severe tooth defects relative to primary rickets, including large pulps with developmental "exposures" of the pulp.

Vitamin C deficiency has also been demonstrated to affect tooth development and eruption. Deciduous and permanent teeth of scorbutic infants contain minute pulpal hemorrhages attributable to vitamin C deficiency. In older vitamin C–deficient children, the dental pulp undergoes hyperemia, edema, necrosis, and aberrant calcification, whereas the dentin shows odontoblastic degeneration and irregular formation (17). The relationship between vitamin C deficiency and dental caries is poorly defined, however. Although it is likely that the primary mechanism of vitamin C deficiency–induced tooth, gingival, and bone disease is mediated through the disruption of collagen biosyntheses, no study has clearly demonstrated the relationship between scurvy and dental caries (18). In areas where goiter is endemic, children born to mothers with severe iodine deficiency are characterized by marked mental and physical growth retardation. Eruption of the primary and secondary teeth is often greatly delayed and precluded. Malocclusion may occur because of the altered patterns of craniofacial growth and development.

Nutritional status during development can have profound effects on oral disease when malnutrition is present. Several studies have demonstrated that tooth eruption is delayed, tooth integrity is compromised (especially enamel surface solubility), and the incidence of dental caries is increased in chronically malnourished animals and children (19, 20). In Lima, Peru, Alvarez et al demonstrated significant delays in tooth eruption and exfoliation in three groups of malnourished children; such delays were associated with and appeared to be the direct cause of a significant temporal delay in caries development in the primary teeth (21). These data support previous studies on malnourished children in India and Guatemala (22, 23).

The development of teeth and salivary glands is intimately associated with the nutrient supply. Teeth subjected to nutritional insult during critical stages of development show a diminished ability to withstand caries and thus are at a higher risk for decay. Menaker and Navia found that impaired salivary function has accompanied the morphologic changes in teeth, which may be a primary factor in the subsequent increase in caries susceptibility (24). These data also explain in part the positive association between socioeconomic status and the prevalence of dental caries in deciduous but not permanent teeth (20). Nutritional injuries early in life may affect tooth formation and may result in increased caries susceptibility, and, depending on when malnutrition occurs in childhood, will impact caries risk.

Malnutrition early in life delays tooth development; hence, teeth erupt later and caries will occur in the older child (20). As is discussed in the section under dental caries, the incidence of caries is more prevalent among economically deprived population groups, which also have a high risk of poor diets. As such, one may see concurrent increases in caries and malnutrition risk; in cases such as this, it may be difficult to determine which came first, the caries or the malnutrition, but both warrant immediate intervention using a team-based approach (5). Thus, in understanding any cross-sectional survey on caries prevalence, the nutritional and diet history must be taken into account.

On a broader scale, 3% of babies born in the United States each year have some birth defect evident at birth or later (25, 26). Prominent among these defects are structural, functional, or biochemical abnormalities involving the craniofacial complex. The most common of these malformations are cleft lip and cleft palate, affecting, 1 in 600 white infants, with the incidence higher among Asians, Native Americans, and Inuit and lower among blacks (25, 27). In addition, select other craniofacial oral-dental disorders such as craniosynostosis, hemifacial microsomia, anodontia, amelogenesis imperfecta, dentinogenesis imperfecta, osteogenesis imperfecta, chondrodystrophies, and juvenile periodontitis represent major challenges to human oral health (28). Neural tube defects are among the most common birth defects despite the decline in incidence with folate fortification of grain products (29); they range in severity and can result in incomplete formation of cranial bones. Many of these malformations and disorders have a genetic basis or an environmental cause. Certain nutrients given in excess, especially early in pregnancy (e.g., retinoic acid, and other lipophilic molecules such as vitamins K and E) are known to induce craniofacial oral-dental malformations.

The regulatory genes and gene products functioning as transcriptional factors for the bronchial arches that give rise to the midface and lower face are being discovered, and their interaction with nutrients (e.g., retinoic acid via its specific receptors) has been found to be critical to craniofacial oral-dental morphogenesis (30). Excess exogenous retinoic acid produces significant craniofacial malformations associated with clefting, dental development, hemifacial microsomia, spina bifida, eye defects, and limb morphogenesis (31). A striking illustration of the need to understand the effects of nutrition on birth defects are the data that demonstrated that folate supplements provided around the time of conception significantly reduced the recurrence of neural tube defects among high-risk persons in the United Kingdom and elsewhere (29, 32, 33). Similar data are being established relating folic acid or multivitamins in congenital craniofacial malformations such as cleft lip and/or cleft palate (29, 33). Taparia et al advocated for the role of adequate folate for its protection against neurotubular and craniofacial defects and hypothesize roles for folate receptors in these disorders (33).

often high levels of fluoride. To reduce the risk of infants receiving too much fluoride, beginning in 1979, infant formula manufacturers voluntarily reduced the amount of fluoride in formulas. Soy-based formulas appear to have higher fluoride levels than milk-based formulas because the soy products contain components that bind fluoride. The Iowa Fluoride Study, which is the longest longitudinal study of fluoride exposure (diet or nondiet), fluorosis and caries conducted in the US to date, recruited new mothers between 1992 and 1995 and followed them and their infants through age 9 months, periodically assessing dental status and conducting food frequency questionnaires to assess fluoride consumption (96). Supplemental use of fluoride along with amounts of fluoride in toothpaste were also recorded. In infants aged 3 to 9 months, the majority of fluoride came from reconstituted infant formulas and other beverages with added water that was fluoridated. In toddlers (aged 16–36 months), dentifrices contributed a substantial amount of fluoride. Fluoride intake of those with mild fluorosis was higher than those without fluorosis. Almost all of the identified cases of fluorosis in this longitudinal study of 600 children with data through age 9 months were mild. The authors found no evidence to recommend avoidance of fluoridated water for reconstituting infant formulas. They suggested that individuals concerned about risk of mild fluorosis who use powdered infant formulas normally reconstituted with fluoridated water should consult their dentists or physician for recommendations regarding use of water with lower fluoride levels and that parents should supervise use of fluoridated toothpastes to ensure that no more than a "pea-sized" amount is used and it is expectorated rather than swallowed (96).

Given continued concerns about dental fluorosis and use of infant formulas, additional research was conducted by the ADA Foundation Research Institute (95), and evidence-based clinical recommendations regarding fluoride intake and infant formula (97) were developed by the ADA Council on Scientific Affairs. Siew et al analyzed fluoride concentrations of milk and soy-based formulas, testing both powdered and liquid forms (95). The formulas themselves had low concentrations of fluoride, with soy-based having slightly higher amounts than milk-based formulas for all types. The amounts of fluoride in the formulas were compared with the adequate intake and tolerable upper levels for fluoride recommended by the Institute of Medicine (100). Fluoride concentrations of reconstituted formulas varied with the level of fluoride in the water used for reconstitution. The authors found that if infants were given only powdered or concentrate formulas reconstituted with fluoridated water that contains 0.7 to 1.2 ppm, they would likely exceed the tolerable upper level for fluoride and thus increase risk of fluorosis (95). Risk of exceeding the tolerable upper limit would be minimal if the fluoride concentration of water used to reconstitute formulas was less than 0.5 ppm. Ready-to-feed formulas do not require water dilution and did not

contain high levels of fluoride (95). It is important to note if an infant was fed only formula reconstituted with water containing no fluoride, the fluoride intake would likely be suboptimal.

In early 2011, the ADA Council on Scientific Affairs released evidence-based clinical recommendations regarding fluoride intake and infant formula (97). For infants fed exclusively powdered or liquid concentrate formulas that require water dilution for use, the clinical recommendations are consistent with the findings of Levy et al (96) and the ADA Research Foundation study (95). The recommendations supported "the continued use of powdered or liquid concentrate infant formulas reconstituted with optimally fluoridated drinking water" provided individuals are aware of the risk of dental fluorosis (p84, ref 97), emphasized the importance of consulting with dentists and physicians about use of fluoridated water and infant formulas, and advised use of fluoride-free water (or water with low fluoride concentrations) for reconstituting formulas when there was concern about the risk of fluorosis, provided one consults with a physician or dentist (97). These recommendations had evidence grades of "D" and "C" respectively (97). In general, the current studies reviewed regarding risk of fluorosis and use of infant formulas consistently indicate that parents should consult their dentist and physician when using formulas requiring reconstitution with fluoridated water about the risk of fluorosis for their infants. It is also prudent to consider other sources of fluoride consumed by toddlers and children such as reconstituted foods and fluids made with fluoridated water and use of fluoridated dentifrices, and consult with dentists and physicians about individual concerns regarding fluorosis.

EFFECT OF NUTRITION ON ORAL SOFT TISSUES

The integrity of the teeth, oral mucosa, and tongue may be compromised by nutrient deficiencies and excesses, local oral diseases, and oral manifestations of systemic diseases, as discussed in other sections of this chapter. Clinicians must be adept at combining physical examination findings with a comprehensive diet and nutrition history as well as medical and medication history, to determine possible causes of oral lesions and other alterations in the integrity of the oral mucosa or tongue. Although it is not the role of nondentist practitioners to diagnose oral diseases, it is incumbent on these professionals to screen for and detect conditions that are not normal and to refer patients appropriately to dentists for comprehensive care (49, 101). Clinical signs of deficiencies of B-vitamins and iron in particular may manifest in the oral cavity (see specific chapters on individual nutrients elsewhere in text).

Oral screening for nutritional deficits and excesses can be easily done by dietetic, medical, nursing, and other health professionals (49, 101–103). An intraoral and extraoral screen as part of a dietetic professional's usual patient assessment should identify existing or potential problems with one or more of the following:

1. Oral manifestations of a nutritional disorder
2. Oral manifestations of a systemic disease that affects diet and nutritional status such as diabetes
3. Local oral conditions interfering with ingestion, mastication, swallowing ability, taste, and saliva
4. Dietary influences on the oral cavity and their contributions to oral diseases (49, 104)

Once any or all of these finding are determined, the professional should consult with and refer patients to general dentists or appropriate dental specialists for diagnosis and care as well as provide appropriate diet intervention and nutritional care.

NUTRIENT DEFICIENCIES

The oral mucosa is particularly susceptible to physiologic or anatomic changes resulting from nutritional deficit or toxicity. Because the turnover rate of oral mucosal cells is relatively rapid (gingival sulcular epithelial cells have a turnover rate of 3 to 7 days), sufficient nutrients must be available at the appropriate times and in the correct concentration for DNA replication, protein synthesis, and cell and tissue maturation to occur. The oral epithelium acts as an effective barrier against the invasion of toxic substances, particularly antigens derived from oral microbes, into the underlying collagenous connective tissue. Inadequate nutrition can compromise the integrity of the oral epithelia, thus increasing the tissue's susceptibility to infectious disease.

For these reasons, the oral cavity is one of the first regions of the body to exhibit clinical signs of nutrient deficits and malnutrition. Virtually every classic nutrient deficiency or toxicity, including scurvy, beriberi, and pellagra, has signs and symptoms in the oral cavity and surrounding structures. The lips, tongue, oral mucosa, and gingiva may all reflect nutritional aberrations long before signs are apparent elsewhere in the body (Table 73.4).

The dorsum of the tongue may undergo changes in size or color, and taste changes may result from atrophy or hypertrophy of tongue papillae. Long-standing nutrient deficiencies may lead to atrophy of the papillae and denudation of the dorsum. A bright red, painful tongue and swelling of the oral mucosa may be early symptoms of pernicious anemia resulting from a lack of vitamin B_{12}. Inflammation, a burning sensation, and tenderness of the tongue or palate may be caused by a deficiency of B vitamins, protein, or iron (105). The mucosa may become pale in iron-, folic acid–, or vitamin B_{12}–induced anemias. Atrophy of the filiform papillae of the tongue (glossitis) is a sign of malnutrition usually resulting from multiple nutritional deficiencies.

In ascorbic acid deficiency, the classic oral signs of scurvy are first seen in the oral cavity and include red swollen interdental papillae that bleed readily and inflamed and swollen marginal and attached gingiva. Although no longer a public health problem, ascorbic acid deficiency may occur most likely secondary to increased losses combined with dietary deficiency. No scientifically sound evidence supports a direct relationship between periodontal disease and ascorbic acid status in any population other than smokers, and even there the evidence is weak. No evidence has been found that consumption of ascorbic acid in excess of the dietary reference intakes is associated with increased oral health (106).

TABLE 73.4	NUTRITION RISK FACTORS TO CONSIDER IN PHYSICAL EXAMINATION	
BODY AREA	**NUTRITION RISK SYMPTOMS**	**NUTRITION IMPLICATIONS**
Hair	Dull, shedding, easily pluckable	Generalized protein calorie malnutrition
Face	a. Malar pigmentation (dark skin over cheeks and under eyes) Bitemporal wasting	Niacin, B vitamins, malnutrition
	b. Nasolabial seborrhea	Niacin, riboflavin, vitamin B_6
	c. Edematous	Protein deficiency
	d. Moon face	Corticosteroid impact
	e. Lack of color	Inadequate iron, undernutrition
Eyes	Pale eye membranes	Inadequate iron
	Bitot spots, conjunctival xerosis, keratomalacia, corneal xerosis	Inadequate vitamin A
Lips	Cheilosis (red/swelling)	Inadequate niacin, riboflavin
	Angular fissures	Inadequate niacin, vitamin B_6, riboflavin, iron
Gingiva	Spongy, bleeding, abnormal redness	Inadequate vitamin C
Tongue	a. Glossitis (red, raw, fissured)	Inadequate folate, niacin, riboflavin, iron, vitamins B_6, and B_{12}
	b. Pale, atrophic, smooth/slick (filiform papillary atrophy)	Inadequate iron, vitamin B_{12}, niacin, folate
	c. Magenta color	Inadequate riboflavin
Nails	Spoon shaped, brittle, ridged	Inadequate iron
Back muscles	Bony prominences along shoulder girdle Tendons prominent to palpation	Malnutrition

Reprinted with permission from Touger-Decker R. Clinical and laboratory assessment of nutrition status. Dent Clin North Am 2003:47:259–78.

TABLE 73.5	FUNCTIONAL ORAL NUTRITION RISK EVALUATION[a]	
STRUCTURE	**PATIENT-FOCUSED EXAMINATION**	**MANAGEMENT**
Lips	Dryness; sensation; cracking or fissuring, swelling; history of blisters or ulcers	Alter diet texture and consistency
Gingiva and oral mucosa	Soreness/pain; bleeding spontaneously, change in appearance; swelling, growths, discharge; bad taste; halitosis	Alter diet texture, temperature, and consistency
	Red or white patches/lesions	Screen for oral cancer, nutrient deficiencies
	Erosion/ulceration; focal pigmentation; erythema	
Teeth	Toothache/pain; looseness and mobility; dental prosthesis (removable or fixed); edentulism	Adjust diet, consistency; evaluate caries risk; consider altered taste/smell
Tongue	Soreness/pain; burning; rough patches; dryness; cracking or fissuring; growths; changes in taste; ulcers	Screen for systematic disease, nutrient deficiencies; alter diet texture
Temporomandibular joint	Difficulty or painful opening; grinding sounds on joint opening/chewing with limited range or pain; weakness of chewing muscles	Change diet consistency, food "hardness"; limit "chewy" foods
Salivary glands	Mucosal dryness; too little or too much saliva; drooling; change in color, consistency,; difficulty swallowing dry food; altered taste; dry eyes; gland pain or swelling	Increase fluids; evaluate for dysgeusia, dysphagia; limit spices, "hard" foods; review changes in prescriptions; evaluate zinc status
Neck	Tender/swollen lymph nodes, other swellings	Medical consultation
Skin	Change in appearances; rashes, sores, lumps, itching	Medical consultation

[a]For each section, ask about patient complaints, duration of symptoms, and any changes in appearance, size, acuity, frequency, and pain.

Reprinted with permission from Touger-Decker R, Sirois D. Approaches to oral nutrition health risk assessment. In: Touger-Decker R, Sirois DA, Mobley CC, eds. Nutrition and Oral Medicine. Totowa, NJ: Humana Press, 2005.

No clinical sign is of significance by itself, however, because several etiologic factors usually contribute to a differential diagnosis. For example, inflammation or cracking of the lips may be caused by allergies, licking of the lips, or drooling, as well as by nutritional aberrations. Angular cheilosis can result not only from vitamin deficiencies but also when overclosure of the jaw in denture wearers allows the skin folds at the corners of the mouth to provide a moist area for bacterial or fungal infections to develop. Table 73.5 provides a functional oral assessment tool that can be used as a broad clinical examination guide for nondentist health providers.

NUTRIENT EXCESSES

Nutrient excesses can also affect the oral cavity. Vitamin A toxicity can impair the proper development of the oral mucosal epithelium and can result in a variety of oral changes including delayed wound healing (107, 108). Rebound scurvy is a condition in which scurvy develops as an adaptation result of fast withdrawal after chronic high intake levels of vitamin C in animals (109). Its existence in human populations has not been determined; but, historically, some supportive evidence exists (110), which has been reported clinically in patients who abruptly terminated a habit of megadosing on vitamin C.

PERIODONTAL DISEASE

Periodontal disease is a general term describing bacterial infection of either the gingiva (that part of the oral mucosa that covers the root and the apical portion of the crown) or both the gingiva and the attachment apparatus

(ligamentous attachment of the tooth to the surrounding alveolar bone). If the infection is confined to the gingival unit, the resulting disease is called gingivitis. If the infection involves the destruction of the tissue attaching tooth to bone, the disease is termed *periodontitis* or *periodontal disease*. The two diseases are not a continuum of the same process but are in fact two separate diseases, each associated with different plaque flora. The cause of gingivitis is relatively simple, whereas the etiology of periodontitis is extremely complex. Although bacterial plaque is the major etiologic agent in both conditions, other local and systemic factors—many still emerging in the scientific understanding of the disease—play a large role as well. Most forms of periodontitis result in a slow loss of attachment of the tooth from the surrounding alveolar bone, resulting in loosening of the teeth and eventually edentulism.

The reaction of the periodontal tissues to microbial antigens and byproducts is a classic chronic inflammatory-immune response like that observed in infectious diseases in general. Optimal functioning of the host's cellular and humoral immune system and phagocytic system and the integrity of the oral mucosa (particularly the gingival sulcular epithelium) are important to the maintenance of periodontal health and the prevention of periodontal disease.

The associations among dietary intake, nutrition status, and periodontal disease have been fraught with limited scientific evidence and many claims for curative roles of nutrients. Clearly, relationships exist between periodontal disease and wound healing, nutrition status, and immune response; and relationships also exist between periodontal disease and individual nutrients (food and supplement forms) and select host defense and health variables. Deficiencies of select nutrients may compromise the systemic response to inflammation and infection and may further exacerbate nutrient needs (111, 112). Although limited research has demonstrated that persons who smoke and consume a diet low in vitamin C had significantly higher levels of periodontal disease, no recommendations have been made for smokers to take supplemental doses of vitamin C for prevention or treatment of periodontal disease (111). Nutrient deficiencies can compromise the associated inflammatory response and wound healing, given the direct influence of nutritional well-being on the synthesis and release of cytokines and their action (112). Malnutrition can cause adverse alterations in the volume and antibacterial and physiochemical properties of saliva. Supplemental intake of any nutrients beyond the dietary reference intakes is not recommended for the prevention or treatment of periodontal disease (106). Boyd and Madden have summarized the nutrient effects on the periodontium in Table 73.6 (113).

Diabetes mellitus (types 1 and 2) and osteoporosis (discussed in detail in the next section) are associated with increased risk of periodontal disease. Likewise, so are menopause and pregnancy, for which the relationship is most likely hormonal in nature. However, here too the inflammatory process is likely involved. Strong evidence exists of associations between periodontal disease and systemic health such as metabolic syndrome, cardiovascular disease, other chronic disease states, and genetic predisposition (1, 114–116). The relationship between periodontal disease and chronic systemic disease has not been fully elucidated; however, suggested mechanisms include the role of bacteria (*Porphyromonas gingivalis*) or the systemic effect of chronic infection and inflammation. As the nature of the association and causal links continue to be explored, it is important for all health professionals to encourage positive oral and systemic health behaviors aimed at reducing risk of periodontal and cardiovascular diseases, respectively. Links between chronic obstructive pulmonary disease and periodontal disease are being explored, with the origin being bacterial in nature. Elevated systemic inflammatory markers such as C-reactive protein (CRP), which is also a notable marker for cardiovascular disease, have been correlated with periodontal disease (117).

Choi et al explored the relationships among impaired fasting glucose, diabetes, and chronic periodontitis using NHANES III data (115). Using pocket depths as a measure of periodontal disease, this group found that the "highest quintile of pocket depths were positively associated with impaired fasting glucose . . . and diabetes . . . compared with the lowest quintile" (115). Although longitudinal data are lacking on improved outcomes following periodontal disease treatment, health care providers can be advocates in educating patients about the oral and systemic health connection (118).

DIABETES AND ORAL HEALTH

It is important to recognize the relationship between diabetes mellitus and oral health as management of blood glucose control impacts the health of the oral cavity, and disease, of the oral cavity may make glucose control more challenging. Oral implications of poorly controlled diabetes mellitus may include, but are not limited to, increased risk and incidence of soft tissue infection, poor wound healing, increased incidence and severity of caries, candidiasis, periodontal disease, xerostomia, alterations in taste, and burning mouth or tongue (117, 119). The oral manifestations in such patients are most likely related to the results of polyuria, altered response to infection, microvascular changes, and, possibly, salivary hyperglycemia (increased glucose in saliva). Caries risk may be related to the inherent increased risk of infection, salivary hyperglycemia, and xerostomia. Candidiasis, often presenting on the tongue, is a fungal infection often associated with hyperglycemia, impaired immune response, and diminished salivary flow (117). Periodontal disease has been referred to as the "sixth complication of diabetes mellitus" (120) because persons with diabetes are at greater risk of developing periodontal disease, and the severity of the disease is relative to the glucose control and duration of the disease. Dysgeusia may result from altered salivary chemistry (from poorly controlled diabetes), xerostomia, burning mouth or tongue, and/or candidiasis. All potential causes should be explored to determine whether the patient has any other underlying disorder.

Careful evaluation and monitoring of glycemic control is critical in determining the risk assessment for progression to the oral complications of diabetes. Persons with type 1 or type 2 diabetes who complain of dry mouth, burning tongue, or altered taste, as well as those presenting with candidiasis, should be evaluated for their glycemic control. Appropriate intervention includes management of diabetes and of oral health in such patients. With proper management techniques, both oral health and diabetes can be managed with lifestyle modifications, treatment, and routine maintenance. A regimen of controlled diet, conscientious and effective oral hygiene, and topical fluoride and smoking cessation, when indicated, can maintain oral health integrity throughout life (119, 121).

ALVEOLAR BONE HEALTH, OSTEOPOROSIS, AND DENTATE STATUS

One of the more dramatic clinical signs of severe periodontal disease is resorption of alveolar bone, which ultimately results in tooth loss. The literature has long speculated that calcium deficiency and osteoporosis are etiologic factors in periodontitis, and that periodontal disease may be a harbinger of systemic metabolic bone disorders (122, 123), which would then lead to tooth loss.

TABLE 73.6	NUTRIENT EFFECTS ON THE PERIODONTIUM		
NUTRIENT	FUNCTIONAL CHANGES RESULTING FROM INADEQUATE INTAKE	GROUPS AT RISK OF INADEQUATE INTAKE	FOOD SOURCES OF NUTRIENT
Protein	Compromised antibacterial properties of saliva Impaired acute-phase response to infection ↓Neutrophil function Lag period in the initiation of wound healing ↓Collagen synthesis	Persons with poorly controlled diabetes Patients with advanced cancer Patients with advanced AIDS Patients fasting ≥4 d or those with chronic poor nutrient intakes	Meat Dairy Legumes
Vitamin A	↓Production of γ-interferon ↓Collagen synthesis ↓Epithelialization Incidence of infection	Patients with cystic fibrosis Patients with advanced AIDS Persons with GI conditions with malabsorption Persons taking weight-loss medication: orlistat	Fortified dairy foods Dark green leafy vegetables Meat and dairy
B-complex vitamins	Inability to produce adequate energy ↓Protein synthesis, including DNA and RNA Breakdown of the mucosal barrier to pathogens	Persons with HIV infection Elderly vegans (vitamin B_{12}) Postgastrectomy patients Patients taking medications: H_2 blockers, phenytoin, methotrexate	Enriched breads and cereals Green leafy vegetables Meat and dairy
Vitamin C	↓Neutrophil function Breakdown of the mucosal barrier to pathogens ↓Collagen synthesis	Smokers Substance abusers Elderly persons Persons with chronic disease People who avoid fruits and vegetables	Citrus fruits Dark green leafy vegetables Potatoes Cantaloupe
Vitamin D	Impaired absorption of calcium	Elderly women in northern latitudes; those with little sun exposure	Fortified milk Eggs Liver
Vitamin E	↓Overall immune response ↓Antibody production	Persons with GI conditions with malabsorption Patients with advanced AIDS	Nuts and seeds Polyunsaturated oils Whole grains
Vitamin K	↓Bone density and possibly bone strength	Persons receiving anticoagulant therapy	Green leafy vegetables Liver
Boron	Impaired wound healing Possible association with bone calcification		Legumes Fruits, especially dried Vegetables
Calcium	Inadequate formation of peak bone mass Accelerated bone loss postmenopausally Osteoporosis Possible association with tooth loss	Young women Postmenopausal women	Milk and milk products Tofu processed with calcium Legumes Dried fruit
Copper	↓Tensile strength of collagen ↑Bone fragility ↓Proliferation neutrophils	Persons with an increased intake of antacids Persons taking megadoses of iron/zinc Alcohol abusers Patients with cystic fibrosis Patients with short bowel syndrome Postgastric bypass patients Persons taking medications: dexamethasone, penicillamine	Green leafy vegetables Whole grains Nuts Meats Whole grains Shellfish Chocolate Organ meats
Iron	↓Neutrophil phagocytic activity ↓Proliferation lymphocytes	Young children Women of childbearing age	Meat Eggs Legumes Dried fruit
Magnesium	More rapid development of osteopenia	Persons with chronic alcoholism Medications: diuretics Elderly persons Postmenopausal women Persons with diabetes	Green leafy vegetables Whole grains Nuts
Zinc	↑Susceptibility to infection ↓Protein synthesis, including DNA and RNA	Elderly persons? Persons with alcoholism	Meats Whole grains

AIDS, acquired immunodeficiency syndrome; GI, gastrointestinal; HIV human immunodeficiency virus.

Adapted with permission from Boyd LD, Madden TE. Nutrition and the periodontium. In: Palmer CA, ed. Diet and Nutrition in Oral Health. Englewood Cliffs, NJ: Prentice-Hall 2003:202–12.

Given that currently one in two women and one in eight men older than 65 years have osteoporosis and the predictions of the 2004 Surgeon General's report on bone health and osteoporosis, which states that by the year 2020 one in two US adults older than 50 years will have or be at high risk of developing osteoporosis, the relationship between this disease and periodontal disease deserves attention (124).

The alveolar process (crest of the maxilla and mandible) is composed primarily of trabecular bone. Histologically, it is the same type of bone found in the distal radius, neck of the femur, and vertebrae. When negative calcium balance occurs in the body, calcium is more easily mobilized from skeletal sites consisting of trabecular rather than cortical bone. Thus, the alveolar bone provides a potential labile source of calcium available to meet other tissue needs. Because the alveolar process is thought to undergo resorption before other bones, change detected in the alveolar process may be used for early diagnosis of osteoporosis. In women, a high correlation has been shown between dental bone mass and total bone mass; women with low bone density have fewer teeth. Women with severe residual ridge resorption have osteopenia on the iliac crest, and those with severe postmenopausal osteoporosis are three times more likely to be edentulous than physiologically normal control subjects (125).

Longitudinal, cross-sectional, and epidemiologic studies (126–130) have demonstrated significant relationships among tooth loss, periodontal disease, low calcium intake, and osteoporosis in older men and women who are at increased risk of both osteoporosis and periodontal disease. Dietrich found that higher serum $25(OH)D_3$ levels were associated with decreased loss of tooth attachment in adults more than 50 years old (129). Payne et al examined changes in alveolar bone height in postmenopausal women with and without osteoporosis over 24 months (130). The relationship between alveolar bone loss and bone mineral density was significant. Women with osteoporosis lost significantly more alveolar bone than those without the condition. Jabbar et al (131), in a cohort of postmenopausal women, found that periodontal disease was more frequent in women with osteoporosis than in a matched cohort without osteoporosis. A common denominator for both diseases is bone loss, which is more often seen in women in the peri- and postmenopausal years. According to Krall, "the available evidence supports the hypothesis that poor systemic bone status contributes to tooth loss and periodontal disease but is not conclusive" (132). Prospective clinical trials are needed, using men and women at varying stages of adulthood to determine whether a causal relationship exists, and, if so, whether treatment of the underlying causative condition affects the other. For example, if osteoporosis is found to cause periodontal disease, then, what is the impact of that on the periodontal disease?

Resorption of the alveolar process is a widespread problem among patients with dentures. Remodeling of the alveolar bone occurs in response to occlusal forces associated with chewing. With the loss of teeth, the alveolar bone is no longer required for tooth support; as a consequence, bone resorption is accelerated, and bone height is diminished. Bone loss is greatest during the first 6 months following tooth extractions. The reduction in residual ridge height is more pronounced in women than in men, and resorption is greater in the mandible than in the maxilla. Severe mandibular resorption makes it difficult to construct a mandibular denture with good stability and retention. Bone resorption and loss are common denominators of both periodontal disease and osteoporosis, and a low calcium intake may compound bone loss in denture wearers (133). In a study of postmenopausal women, researchers described an association between calcium and vitamin D supplementation and reduced risk of tooth loss; those who experienced tooth loss were significantly more likely to experience systemic bone loss (134). Problems associated with small sample sizes, varying definitions of periodontal disease and osteoporosis, and the lack of prospective data have been cited as reasons for inconclusive results; longitudinal studies are advocated (133, 134). Positive calcium balance may be especially important along with adequate nutrition status to help preserve the integrity of the residual ridges of edentulous postmenopausal women.

Although an intact dentition is not absolutely essential to maintain nutritional health, loss of teeth or the supporting periodontium can affect food selection and subsequent nutritional status. Periodontal disease, with its associated tissue soreness, pain, tooth sensitivity, bone resorption, and tooth mobility, can lead to a preference for foods of low nutritional value and the avoidance of foods requiring chewing. The same may be true of persons with severe dental caries and those with dentures.

Missing teeth, the absence of natural posterior occluding tooth surfaces, or ill-fitting dentures may impair biting and chewing and resultant dietary intake and nutritional status, often manifesting in a diet with less fruit, vegetable, and fiber intake and altered macronutrient consumption than in people with more teeth (135–140). Oral pain and discomfort also may influence daily activities, which, in turn, may affect dietary intake and quality of life (136, 141).

Dentures can also affect taste and swallowing ability, especially if they are maxillary (upper) dentures. A maxillary denture can also impede swallowing. When the hard palate is covered, it is difficult for the tongue to determine the location of food in the mouth, form a bolus, and swallow, which may contribute to dysphagia.

The dentally impaired can maintain good dietary intake and adequate nutrition status by making appropriate food selections and adapting gradually to new dentures. Persons receiving new dentures should be counseled on

47. Milgrom P, Zero DT, Tanzer JM. Academic Pediatrics 2009; 9:404–9.

48. Moynihan P. Bulletin of the World Health Organization. 2005; 83:694–9.

49. Touger-Decker R, Mobley C. J Am Diet Assoc 2007;107: 1418–28.

50. Johnson RK, Frary C. J Nutr 2001;131:2766S–71S.

51. Touger-Decker R, van Loveren C. Am J Clin Nutr 2003; 78(Suppl):881S–92S.

52. Van Horn L, Johnson RK, Flickinger BD et al. Circulation 2010;122:2470–90.

53. Lingstrom P, van Houte J, Kashket S. Crit Rev Oral Biol Med 2000;11:366–80.

54. Cleaton-Jones P, Richardson BD, Sinwel R et al. Caries Res 1984;18:472–7.

55. Persson LA, Stecksen-Blicks C, Holm AK. Commun Dent Oral Epidemiol 1984;12:390–7.

56. Burt BA, Pai S. J Dent Educ 2001;65:1017–24.

57. Anderson CA, Curzon ME, Van Loveren C et al. Obesity Reviews 2009;10(Suppl 1):41–54.

58. Konig KG, Navia JM. Am J Clin Nutr 1995;62:275S–83S.

59. Kantor KS. A Dietary Assessment of the US Food Supply: Comparing per Capita Food Consumption with Food Guide Pyramid Serving Recommendations. Food and Rural Economics Division, Economics Research Service. US Department of Agriculture, Agricultural Economic Report no. 772. Washington, DC: US Government Printing Office, 1998.

60. Krebs-Smith SM. J Nutr 2001;131:527S–35S.

61. Harris R. J Dent Res 1963;42:1387–99.

62. Rugg-Gunn AJ, Hackett AF, Appleton DR. Caries Res 1987;21:464–78.

63. Stephan RJ. J Am Dent Res 1940;27:718–23.

64. Birkhed D. Caries Res 1984;18:120–7.

65. Lussi A, Jaeggi T. Clin Oral Invest 2008;12(Suppl 1):S5–S13.

66. Ehlen LA, Marshall TA, Qian F et al. Nutr Res 2008;28:299–303.

67. Hildebrandt GH, Sparks BS. J Am Diet Assoc 2000;131:909–16.

68. Ly KA, Milgrom P, Rothen M. J Am Dent Assoc 2008;139: 553–63.

69. Milgrom P, Ly KA, Rothen M. Adv Dent Res 2009;21:44–7.

70. Soderling E, Hirvonen A, Karjalainen S et al. Eur J Dent 2011;5:24–31.

71. Tanzer JM, Slee AM. J Am Dent Assoc 1983;106:331–3.

72. Lout RK, Messer LB, Soberay A et al. Caries Res 1988;22: 237–41.

73. Mundorff SA, Featherstone JDB, Bibby BC et al. Caries Res 1990;24:344–55.

74. Pollard MA, Imfeld T, Higham SM et al. Caries Res 1996; 30:132–7.

75. Lussi A, Jaeggi T, Zero D. Caries Res 2004 38(Suppl 1):34–44.

76. Kashket S, van Houte J, Lopez LR et al. J Dent Res 1991; 70:1314–9.

77. Kashket S, Zhang J, van Houte J. J Dent Res 1996;75:1885–91.

78. Silva MF, Jenkins GN, Burgess RC et al. Caries Res 1986; 20:263–9.

79. DePaola DP, Kashket S. Nutr Rev 2002;60:97–103.

80. DePaola DP. J Dent Res 1986;65:1540–3.

81. Schachtele CF, Harlander SK. J Can Dent Assoc 1984;50:213–9.

82. Ritter AV, Shugars DA, Bader JD. Community Dent Oral Epidemiol 2010;38:383–97.

83. van Houte J, Jordan R, Laraway R et al. J Dent Res 1990; 69:1463–8.

84. Papas AS, Palmer CA, Rounds MC et al. Ann N Y Acad Sci 1989;561:124–42.

85. Billings RJ. J Public Health Dent 1996;56:37.

86. O'Sullivan DV, Tinanoff N. J Dent Res 1993;72:1577–8.

87. Ripa LW. Pediatr Dent 1988;10:268–82.

88. Palmer CA, Kent R, Loo CY et al. J Dent Res 2010;89:1224–9.

89. Ismail AI, Hasson H. J Am Dent Assoc 2008;139:1457–68.

90. Rozier RG, Adair S, Graham F et al. J Am Dent Assoc 2010;141:1480–89.

91. US Department of Health and Human Services, Proposed HHS Recommendations for Fluoride Concentration in Drinking Water for Prevention of Dental Caries. January 2011. Available at: http://www.hhs.gov/news/press/2011pres/01/pre_pub_frn_fluoride.html. Accessed June 3, 2011.

92. Dean HT. Epidemiological studies in the United States. In: Moulton FR, ed. Dental Caries and Fluoride. Washington, DC: American Association for Advancement of Science, 1946.

93. Murray JJ, Rugg-Gunn AJ. Fluorides and Dental Caries. 2nd ed. Bristol, UK: John Wright & Sons, 1982.

94. Brunelle JA. Carlos JP. J Dent Res 1990;69:723–7.

95. Siew C, Strock S, Ristic H et al. J Am Dent Assoc 2009; 140:1228–36.

96. Levy S, Broffit B, Marshall TA et al. J Am Dent Assoc 2010;141:1190–1201.

97. Berg J, Gerweck C, Hujoel PP et al. J Am Dent Assoc 2011;142:79–87.

98. Beltran-Aguilar ED, Barker L, Dye BA. Prevalence and Severity of Enamel Fluorosis in the United States, 1986–2004. NCHS data brief no 53. Hyattsville, MD: National Center for Health Statistics. 2010a. Available at: http://www.cdc.gov/nchs/data/databriefs/db53.htm. Accessed March 5, 2012.

99. Ismail Al, Messer JG. J Public Health Dent 1996;56:22–7.

100. Food and Nutrition Board, Institute of Medicine. Dietary Reference Intakes for Calcium, phosphorus, magnesium, vitamin D and Fluoride, Washington, DC: National Academies Press, 1997:218–313.

101. Radler DR, Touger-Decker R. Top Clin Nutr 2005;20:181–8.

102. American Dietetic Association. International Dietetics and Nutrition Terminology (IDNT) Manual, 3rd ed. Chicago: American Dietetic Association, 2011.

103. Mackle T, Touger-Decker R, O'Sullivan Maillet J et al. J Am Diet Assoc 2004;103;1632–8.

104. Touger-Decker R. Dent Clin North Am 2003 47:259–78.

105. Moynihan PJ, Lingstrom P. Oral consequences of nutritional well-being. In: Touger-Decker R, Sirois DA, Mobley CC, eds. Nutrition and Oral Medicine. Totowa, NJ: Humana Press, 2005:107–125.

106. Food and Nutrition Board, Institute of Medicine. Dietary Reference Intakes for Vitamin C, Vitamin E, Selenium and Carotenoids. Washington, DC: National Academies Press, 2000.

107. Hathcock J, Hattan DC, Jenkins M et al. Am J Clin Nutr 1990;52:183–202.

108. Food and Nutrition Board, Institute of Medicine. Dietary Reference Intakes for Vitamin A, Vitamin K, Arsenic, Boron, Chromium, Copper, Iodine, Iron, Manganese, Molybdenum, Nickel, Silicon, Vanadium and Zinc. Washington, DC: National Academies Press, 2001.

109. Tsao CS, Leung PY. J Nutr 1988;118:895–900.

110. Omaye ST, Skala JH, Jacob RA. Am J Clin Nutr 1988;48:379–81.

111. Nishida M, Grossi SG, Dunford RG et al. J Periodontol 2000;71:1215–23.

112. Enwonwu CO. Am J Clin Nutr 1995;61(Suppl):430S–6S.

113. Boyd LD, Madden TE. Nutrition and the periodontium. In: Palmer CA, ed. Diet and Nutrition in Oral Health. Englewood Cliffs, NJ: Prentice-Hall, 2003:202–12.

114. D'Aiuto F, Sabbah G, Donos N et al. J Clin Endocrinol Metab 2008;3989–94, 2008.

115. Choi YH, McKeown RE, Mayer-David EJ et al. Diabetes Care 2011;34:381–6.

116. Shaefer AS, Richter GM, Nothnagel M et al. J Dent Res 2010;89:384–8.

117. Lamster IB, Lalla E, Borgnakke WS et al. J Am Dent Assoc 2008;139:19S–24S.

118. Hein C. The role of the professional in educating the public about the importance of oral health. In: Genco RJ, Williams RC, eds. Periodontal Disease and Overall Health: A Clinician's Guide. Yardley, PA: Professional Audience Communications, 2010:288–304.

119. Lalla E, Hsu WC, Lamster IB. Dental and medical comanagement of patients with diabetes. In: Genco RJ, Williams RC, eds. Periodontal Disease and Overall Health: A Clinician's Guide. Yardley, PA: Professional Audience Communications, 2010:216–34.

120. Loe H. Diabetes Care 1993;16:329–34.

121. Li S, Williams PL, Douglas CV. J Am Dent Assoc 2011;142: 28–37.

122. Whalen J, Krook L. Nutrition 1996;12:53–4.

123. Kribbs PJ. J Prosthet Dent 1990;63:86–9.

124. US Department of Health and Human Services. Bone Health and Osteoporosis: A Report of the Surgeon General. Rockville, MD: Office of the Surgeon General. Available at: http://www.surgeongeneral.gov/library/bonehealth/content.html. Accessed June 2, 2011.

125. Jeffcoat MK, Chesnut C. J Am Dent Assoc 1993;124:49–56.

126. Krall E, Wehler C, Garcia RI et al. Am J Med 2001;111:452–6.

127. Nishida M, Grossi SG, Dunford RG et al. J Periodontol 2000;71:1057–66.

128. Yoshihara A, Seida Y, Hanada N et al. J Clin Periodontol 2004;21:680–4.

129. Dietrich T. Am J Clin Nutr 2004;80:108–13.

130. Payne JB, Reinhardt RA, Nummikoski PV et al. Osteoporosis Int 1999;10:34–40.

131. Jabbar S, Drury J, Fordham J et al. J Periodont Res 2011;46:97–104.

132. Krall E. Osteoporosis. In: Touger-Decker R, Sirois DA, Mobley CC, eds. Nutrition and Oral Medicine. Totowa, NJ: Humana Press, 2005:261–70.

133. Wactawski-Wende J. Ann Periodontol 2001;6:197–208.

134. Krall EA, Wehler C, Garcia RI et al. Am J Med 2001:111:452–6.

135. Marshall TA, Warren, JJ, Hand, JS et al. J Am Dent Assoc 2002;133:1369–79.

136. Polzar I, Schlimmel M, Muller F et al. Int Dent J 2010;60: 143–55.

137. Savoca MR, Arcury TA, Leng Z et al. J Am Geriatr Soc 2010; 58:1225–32.

138. Nowjack-Raymer RE, Sheiham A. J Dent Res 2003;82:123–6.

139. Tsakos G, Herrick K, Sheiham A et al. J Dent Res 2010;89: 462–7.

140. Sahyoun NR, Lin CL, Krall E. J Am Diet Assoc 2003;103:61–6.

141. Allen F. Health Qual Life Outcomes 2003;1:40.

142. Kademani, D, Glick M. Quintessence Int 1998;29:523–34.

143. Narani N, Epstein JB. J Clin Periodontol 2001;28:137–45.

144. Patel A, Glick M. Human immunodeficiency virus. In: Touger-Decker R, Sirois D, Mobley C, eds. Nutrition and Oral Medicine. Totowa, NJ: Humana Press, 2005: 241–60.

145. Sirois DA. Mt Sinai J Med 1998;65:322–32.

146. Das KM. Dig Dis Sci 1999;44:1–13.

147. Siegel MA, Jacobsen JJ, Braun RJ. Diseases of the gastrointestinal tract. In: Greenberg MS, Glick M, eds. Burket's Oral Medicine Diagnosis and Treatment. 10th ed. Hamilton, Ontario, Canada: BC Decker, 2003:389–406.

148. Chainani-Wu N. Nutr Cancer 2002;44:104–26.

149. World Cancer Research Fund/American Institute for Cancer Research. Food, Nutrition, Physical Activity, and the Prevention of Cancer: A Global Perspective. Washington, DC: American Institute for Cancer Research, 2007. Available at: http://www.dietandcancerreport.org/. Accessed August 18, 2012.

150. Davidson P, Touger-Decker R. Nut Clin Pract 2009;24:250–60.

151. Morse DE. Oral and pharyngeal cancer. In: Touger-Decker R, Sirois DA, Mobley CC, eds. Nutrition and Oral Medicine. Totowa, NJ: Humana Press, 2005:205–22.

152. Franceschi S, Favero A, Conti E et al. Br J Cancer 1999; 80:614–20.

153. Tavani A, Gallus S, La Vecchia C et al. Eur J Cancer Prev 2001;10:191–5.

154. Negri E, Franceschi S, Bosetti C et al. Int J Cancer 2000; 86:122–7.

155. Petridou E, Zavras A, Lefatzis D et al. Cancer 2002;94:2981–8.

156. National Cancer Institute. Oral Complications of Chemotherapy and Head/Neck Radiation Available at: http://www.cancer.gov/cancertopics/pdq/supportivecare/oralcomplications/HealthProfessional/Page5#Section_337. Accessed May 15, 2011.

157. Elliott L, Molseed L, Davis-McCallum P et al. The Clinical Guide to Oncology Nutrition. 2nd ed. Chicago, American Dietetic Association: 2006.

158. Brown C, Wingard J. Semin Oncol Nurs 2004;20:16–21.

159. Ghezzi EM, Ship JA. J Dent Res 2003;82:844–8.

160. Grisius MM, Fox PC. Salivary gland diseases. In Greenberg MS, Glick M, eds. Burket's Oral Medicine Diagnosis and Treatment. 10th ed. Hamilton, Ontario, Canada: BC Decker, 2003:235–70.

161. Turner MD, Ship JA. J Am Dent Assoc 2007;138(Suppl):15S–20S.

162. Turner M, Jahangiri L, Ship J. J Am Dent Assoc 2007;139: 146–50.

163. Heft MW, Baum BJ. J Dent Res 1984;63:1182–5.

164. Faine MP. Dent Clin N Am 2003;47:395–410.

165. Aranha ACC, Eduardo CP, Cordas TA. J Contemp Dent Pract 2008;9:73–81.

166. Russo LL, Campisi G, Fede OD et al. Oral Diseases 2008; 14:479–84.

167. Frydrych AM, Davies GM, McDermott BM. Aust Dent J 2005;50:6–15.

168. Gross KBW, Brough KM, Randolph PM. J Dent Child 1986;53:378–81.

169. Federal Agency Forum on Aging-Related Statistics. AgingStats.gov. Available at: http://www.aoa.gov/agingstatsdotnet/Main_Site/Data/2010_Documents/Population.aspx. Accessed May 15, 2011.

170. Moynihan P, Bradbury J. Nutrition 2001;17:177–8.

171. Moynihan P. J Am Dent Assoc. 2007;138:493–7.

172. Savocca MR, Arcucry TA, Leng X et al. Public Health Nutr 2009;13:486–74.

173. Brodeur JM, Laurin D, Vallee R et al. J Prosthet Dent 1993;70:468–73.

SUGGESTED READINGS

Anderson CA, Curzon ME, Van Loveren C et al. Sucrose and dental caries: a review of the evidence. Obes Rev 2009;10(Suppl 1):41–54.

Institute of Medicine of the National Academies. Advancing Oral Health in America. Washington, DC: National Academies Press, 2011.

Savoca MR, Arcury TA, Leng X et al. Association between dietary quality of rural older adults and self-reported food avoidance and food modification due to oral health problems. J Am Geriatr Soc 2010;58:1225–1232.

Touger-Decker R. Clinical and laboratory assessment of nutrition status in dental practice. Dent Clin North Am 2003;47:259–278.

Touger-Decker R, Mobley CC, American Dietetic Association. Position of the American Dietetic Association: oral health and nutrition. J Am Diet Assoc 2007;107:1418–1428.

74 ESOPHAGUS AND STOMACH[1]

MARK H. DELEGGE

The esophagus and stomach are critical structures involved in the process of oral intake and digestion. Absorption of nutrients in these organs is minimal. Without a properly functioning esophagus and stomach, the ability to eat and initially digest can be significantly impaired. Additionally, partial or total surgical resection of the esophagus or stomach, for symptomatic disease states, also can markedly affect a person's ability to eat or drink. Physiologic and anatomic aspects of the esophagus and stomach are covered in detail in the chapter on the nutritional physiology of the alimentary tract.

ESOPHAGUS

Anatomy

The esophagus is a tubular structure that is approximately 30 cm in length (1) (Fig. 74.1). The organ is artificially divided into the proximal, mid, and distal esophagus. This structure is extremely muscular, which correlates to its major function, propulsion. The funnel-shaped pharynx joins the mouth to the esophagus. Where the pharynx connects to the esophagus is a ring of tissue known as the upper esophageal sphincter (UES). The sphincter opens to allow food or fluids to pass with a swallowing effort. The upper esophagus consists of striated muscle. There is an inner circular layer and an outer longitudinal layer of muscle. At the level of the aortic arch, the esophageal striated muscle transforms into smooth muscle. A

[1]**Abbreviations: DS**, dumping syndrome; **ENS**, enteric nervous system; **GERD**, gastroesophageal reflux disease; **LES**, lower esophageal sphincter; **UES**, upper esophageal sphincter.

ring of thick smooth muscle called the lower esophageal sphincter (LES) sits at the bottom of the esophagus and is approximately 40 cm from the incisors (teeth). The LES serves to allow food and fluids to flow from the esophagus when it is in a relaxed state and to prevent regurgitation of gastric materials back into the esophagus when it is in a contracted state. The muscle of the esophagus receives its innervation from cranial nerve X (2). This nerve originates in the dorsal motor nucleus of the vagus nerve and synapses on the myenteric plexus (esophageal nerve system).

Disease

When disease of the esophagus exists, it generally involves a process that affects the esophageal lining (mucosa) or the muscular component of the esophagus.

Muscular (Motor)

The classic muscle disorder of the esophagus is known as achalasia (3). The primary features are lack of esophageal muscle contractions (peristalsis) in combination with failure to relax the LES. This leads to the inability of materials to flow from the mouth through the esophagus and into the stomach. If a diagnostic radiogram is obtained, it will show a dilated esophagus and a tight LES resulting in what radiologist's term a classic "bird's beak" sign. Interestingly, these patients have a 2% to 7% risk of squamous cell cancer of the esophagus. Treatment consists of medications (very poor results) or the use of a large balloon or surgery to tear the LES. This treatment attempts to eliminate the LES barrier to food and fluid movement through the esophagus to the stomach. Because of their poor esophageal propulsion, these patients are very dependent on gravity and must remain upright after eating to allow materials to pass from the mouth to the stomach. These patients can regurgitate food back into their mouth with the risk for aspiration, especially at night when they are lying down. In some cases, patients are unable to consume enough calories and protein by mouth and require a gastrostomy tube for enteral nutrition, assuming their stomach functions appropriately.

Hypomotility (decreased muscle contractions) of the esophagus can occur with systemic disease in which the muscle and/or nerves of the esophagus are affected, resulting in reduced or absent peristalsis (4). This occurs

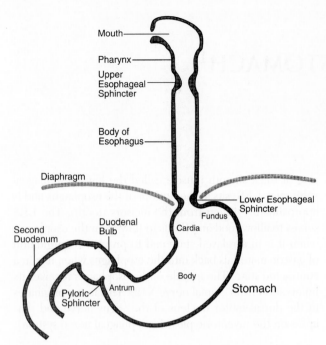

Fig. 74.1. Anatomy of the human upper gastrointestinal tract.

commonly in scleroderma and other connective tissue diseases. Other diseases that can lead to hypomotility disorders of the esophagus include diabetes mellitus, amyloidosis, or hypothyroidism. There are no known effective treatments for hypomotility disorder effects on the esophagus. Patients will attempt to modify their diet (more liquids in their diet). Failure to be able to consume enough nutrition orally should result in the placement of a gastrostomy tube for enteral nutrition support. (Please see the chapter on enteral feeding for tube feeding strategies.)

Inflammation and Cancer

Mucosal-based disease also can affect a person's ability to eat. The best example of this is cancer of the esophagus. Adenocarcinoma is now the most common cause of esophageal cancer in the United States. Deficiency or low intake of specific nutrients (vitamins A, B₆, C, E, and folate) has been epidemiologically associated with esophageal cancer (5). Dietary fiber has been suggested to be protective against the development of adenocarcinoma in such studies. Adenocarcinoma of the esophagus is believed to be secondary to chronic gastroesophageal reflux disease (GERD). This leads to the development of a histologic precursor of adenocarcinoma of the esophagus, known as Barrett esophagus (6).

Worldwide, squamous cell cancer of the esophagus is the most common esophageal cancer. It is caused by tobacco and alcohol use most frequently. Other less common associations include achalasia, lack of trace metals (especially selenium), lye ingestion, ionizing radiation, and human papillomavirus. Deficiency of vitamins A and C also is associated with the development of squamous cell

cancer of the esophagus. Overall, cancer of the esophagus is more common in men by a 3:1 ratio (7).

In patients with esophageal cancer, oral intake can be compromised because of esophageal obstruction. The tumor itself can be shrunk temporarily with the use of endoscopic therapies, including tumor tissue ablation. The placement of an esophageal stent across the tumor also can temporarily open the esophagus (8). Frequently, the patient cannot eat or drink enough to maintain his or her nutritional status and requires a gastrostomy feeding tube. Some surgeons prefer a jejunostomy feeding tube over a gastrostomy feeding tube for patients who will receive surgery because they do not want a hole in the stomach to repair before pulling it up into the thoracic cavity after esophagectomy (9).

Treatment of esophageal cancer is poor if surgery is not an option for cure. Radiation is rarely used as monotherapy for esophageal cancer. Chemotherapy can be used as monotherapy but is more commonly used as systemic therapy for patients with metastatic disease. Combined radiotherapy and chemotherapy are used for patients with regional metastasis. Esophagectomy is the primary treatment for esophageal cancer and generally is reserved for patients who have an optimal chance of being completely cured (10). Ivor-Lewis esophagectomy entails removal of most of the esophagus and a pull-up of the stomach into the thoracic cavity and the attachment of the esophagus to the very upper portion of the esophagus just below the UES. This surgery carries a 5% to 10% mortality rate. Morbidity from this surgery can include anastomotic leakage, pulmonary problems, and coronary events. Patients can develop anastomotic strictures, gastroparesis, and regurgitation after surgery. This problem can become significant enough to require a feeding tube. In these situations, a jejunal feeding tube is required.

Inflammation and ulceration of the esophagus also can impair oral intake. Generally, this is secondary to the pain of inflammation, but it also can be secondary to the chronic problems seen with esophageal mucosal inflammation, such as esophageal strictures, leading to partial or complete esophageal obstruction.

The definition of GERD is damage to the esophageal mucosa from the regurgitation of gastric contents. Approximately 18% of the US population reports GERD symptoms weekly (11). Increasing age increases the frequency of GERD. Patients with GERD may have impaired quality of life because of intermittent pain and nausea. Although very effective medical treatment strategies for GERD exist, approximately 5% to 10% of patients are recalcitrant to the medications. Corrective surgical therapy may be required for these patients. The most common surgery is a Nissen fundoplication (12).

Anorexia may develop with GERD because chronic discomfort and nausea resulting from reflux can affect appetite. In addition, if the GERD symptoms are worse with eating, this will also result in a reduced oral intake.

It has been shown that GERD can be a cause of anorexia in elderly persons. More severe manifestations of GERD are esophageal ulceration and stricture formation (13). GERD-based strictures are more commonly seen in the distal esophagus. These strictures may require balloon dilation with the use of an endoscope. The "obstruction" caused by these strictures can lead to a change in diet or a markedly reduced oral intake resulting in malnutrition and weight loss.

STOMACH

Anatomy

The stomach is a large tubular structure that has the ability to expand significantly to accept both fluids and food (see Fig. 74.1). It is divided into four separate components; the cardia, the fundus, the body, and the antrum (proximal to distal stomach, respectively). Histologically, the muscle cells in the antrum are the densest. At the top of the stomach is the LES described previously. At the bottom of the stomach is another valve, the pylorus, which regulates movement of material from the stomach into the small intestine. The stomach itself, in addition to expanding to accommodate ingested materials, grinds food into smaller particles by the "crushing" action of the antrum.

The stomach wall consists of four layers: the mucosa, submucosa, muscularis, and serosa (14). The submucosal layer consists of connective tissue interlaced with the enteric nervous plexus (the nerve system of the stomach). It is known that the origin of electrical activity in the stomach (pacemaker) exists in the body of the stomach at the greater curvature. Digestive events in the stomach are linked to the functional capacity of different cell populations of the gastric epithelial lining. The gastric lining consists of thick folds, each of which contains microscopic gastric pits (14). The mucosa of the body and fundus of the stomach contains oxyntic glands (Fig. 74.2). Oxyntic glands are lined by parietal cells that secrete gastric acid and intrinsic factor and by chief cells that secrete pepsinogen and gastric lipase (14). In contrast, the pyloric glands that form the antral mucosa contain few parietal cells or chief cells, but rather contain mucus-secreting cells and G cells, which produce the hormone gastrin (see Fig. 74.2).

Motor Function (Contraction)

Motor function of the gastrointestinal tract depends on the contraction of smooth muscle cells and integration and modulation by enteric and extrinsic nerves. Derangements of the mechanisms that regulate gastrointestinal motor function may lead to altered gut motility. The nervous system controlling gastric motility includes both the central nervous system and the enteric nervous system (ENS) (15). The ENS is the gut's intrinsic neural system. It consists of approximately 100 million neurons organized into ganglionic plexuses.

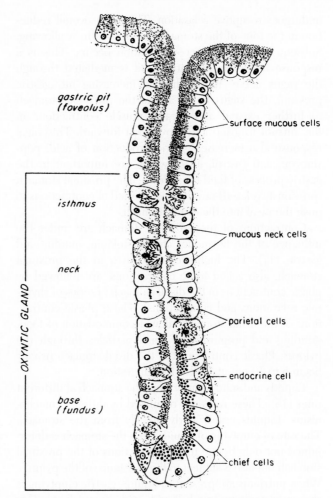

Fig. 74.2. Gastric gland from the body of a mammalian stomach. (Reprinted with permission from Ito S, Winchester RJ. The fine structure of the gastric mucosa in the bat. J Cell Biol 1963;16:541–77.)

The motor (propulsive) function of the stomach is characterized by distinct neuromuscular function in the fasting and fed state. The fasting (or interdigestive) period is characterized by distinct motor waves. In a 60- to 90-minute period in the interdigestive phase, three distinct motor (muscle contraction) wave patterns exist (16): phase 1 (quiescent), phase 2 (intermittent pressure waves), and phase 3 (high-pressure waves). Phase 3 contractions drive food particles effectively from the stomach down through the small intestine. Sometimes they are called "housekeeper waves."

In the postprandial period, the interdigestive waves are replaced by a very irregular series of pressure waves. The duration of this postprandial period is approximately 1 hour for every 200 kcal of nutrients that are consumed. This is then followed by the previously mentioned interdigestive wave patterns. After food ingestion, the stomach undergoes several relaxations and contractions to accommodate ingested food and move it forward into the small intestine. The proximal stomach, in response to a meal, undergoes receptive relaxation. This is an overall reduction in the tone of the stomach in response to swallowing. Subsequently, gastric accommodation occurs. This is a response to gastric distention and is mediated through the vagus nerve. Responding to increasing intragastric pressure, the vagus nerve allows the proximal stomach to further expand and creates muscle contractions in the antrum to grind and move food forward. This vagal response also increases gastric production of acid, pepsinogen, and gastrin, all of which are important in the gastric process of food breakdown. The proximal stomach (previously relaxed) now begins a period of contractions to push the meal into the distal stomach.

Contractions of the proximal stomach are under the influence of the hormones cholecystokinin, motilin, and gastrin (17). The high-pressure waves in the proximal stomach, also called tonic contractions, are followed by phasic contractions in the distal stomach (a series of rhythmic relaxations and contractions). These phasic contractions of the distal stomach allow accommodation of food, grinding and propulsion of small particles through the pylorus. Phasic contractions of the distal stomach usually begin 5 to 10 minutes after food ingestion.

Liquids and solids empty from the stomach at different rates (18). These rates are regulated by different mechanisms. Liquids empty fairly quickly from the stomach. The rate of emptying of liquids from the stomach is determined not only by the tonic contractions of the proximal stomach but also is subject to the resistance of the pylorus. When nutrients are present in liquids, gastric emptying is slower as compared with liquids without nutrients. This is as a result of a hormonal feedback response from the small intestine. The higher the concentration of nutrients in a liquid, the slower is the gastric emptying (19). In addition, the lower the pH of a solution, the slower is the gastric emptying. Solids empty at a slower rate from the stomach than do liquids. Ingested food substances must be reduced to a 1- to 2-mm particle size to pass through the pylorus into the small intestine. There is a lag phase between when food is ingested and when it is reduced to a small enough particle size to pass through the pylorus into the small intestine. The smaller the food particle size originally ingested, the shorter is this lag phase.

Disease

When disease of the stomach exists, generally it involves a process that affects the gastric lining (mucosa; inflammatory diseases) or the neuromuscular component of the stomach. Diseases of the gastric lining include peptic ulcer disease, gastritis, and cancer. Diseases of the neuromuscular component include gastroparesis and postsurgical gastric emptying abnormalities.

Inflammatory Diseases

Gastritis and Ulceration. This is an inflammatory reaction in the gastric mucosa that has a variety of clinical features, etiologies, and histology (20). Acute gastritis is generally erosive or neutrophilic. Acute erosive gastritis is usually secondary to a chemical injury of the gastritis lining from substances such as alcohol, aspirin, bile reflux, acid, or severe trauma and sepsis. In trauma and sepsis, gastritis is a result of underperfusion of the gastric mucosa. Acute neutrophilic gastritis is from infectious infestation of the gastric mucosa, usually from *Helicobacter pylori* infection (21). In general, a patient's appetite and caloric intake may be affected by these diseases because of pain and nausea. No specific dietary causes or diet-based treatments have been rigorously studied in gastritis or gastric ulceration, and patients are simply advised to avoid foods and dietary patterns that cause symptoms.

Chronic gastritis conditions also exist and are also known as atrophic gastritis. The chronicity of the inflammation can lead to atrophy of mucosal-based cells. Atrophic gastritis can be of an "autoimmune type" that is associated with severe atrophy of the stomach acid–producing cells (22). This can be seen in old age and with systemic autoimmune disorders such as pernicious anemia, Hashimoto thyroiditis, Addison disease, diabetes mellitus, or Sjögren syndrome. In general, these patients do not make stomach acid and therefore are at risk for vitamin B_{12} deficiency resulting from the resultant atrophy of the gastric parietal cells, which make the intrinsic factor essential for vitamin B_{12} absorption. There is also an increased risk of gastric cancer in these conditions. A second common form of chronic gastritis is a result of *H. pylori* infection known as multifocal atrophic gastritis (23). The existence of chronic gastritis can result in symptoms of pain and nausea that intensifies with eating, resulting in a reduced calorie intake. Less common forms of gastritis include infectious gastritis (bacterial, fungal, or viral) or eosinophilic from extensive eosinophil infiltration into all layers of the stomach (24).

More severe forms of gastric mucosal inflammation lead to actual ulcer formation. This is usually owing to acid injury after breakdown of the gastric mucosal protective layer from nonsteroidal anti-inflammatory medications, alcohol, acid, bile, pepsin, and *H. pylori* infection. Patients may develop abdominal pain, early satiety, and nausea, resulting in a reduced appetite and oral intake. There is a form of extreme acid overproduction in the stomach from elevated levels of serum gastrin or histamine resulting in "super high" gastric acid concentrations. This can result in extreme gastric or duodenal ulcer formation known as Zollinger-Ellison syndrome (25). The extreme acid production not only leads to peptic ulceration but also to malabsorption of nutrients as a result of degradation of pancreatic enzymes by acid (26). Again, no specific dietary treatments have been shown to improve gastric ulceration; thus, patients are advised to avoid food items that cause symptoms.

Cancer. Gastric cancer is the second most common cancer worldwide and the second most common cause of cancer-related deaths (27). Approximately 20,000 cases of gastric cancer are discovered in the United States

of a registered dietician to determine details of habitual nutrient intake and to work with the physician and patient on appropriate food and nutrient intake strategies. This may require specific oral nutrient supplements to correct or prevent macronutrient or micronutrient depletion (e.g., complete liquid or solid nutritional supplements, specific calorie or protein supplements, specific or complete vitamin, mineral, and trace element supplements). In severe cases, a specialized nutrition support service may be needed to help initiate and manage use of complete parenteral nutrition formulations and/or intravenous hydration and micronutrient/electrolyte administration (see later chapters in the section on the alimentary tract). In all cases, serial evaluation of body weight and physical examination changes indicative of nutrient depletion/repletion, serial laboratory tests of specific micronutrient concentrations in blood, and stool analysis as outlined in the preceding is important to monitor the efficacy of therapy in patient management.

REFERENCES

1. Naveh Y, Ken-Dror A, Zinder O et al. J Pediatr Gastroenterol Nutr 1986;5:210–13.
2. Simko V. Am J Gastroenterol 1981;75:204–8.
3. Amann ST, Josephson SA, Toskes PP. Am J Gastroenterol 1997;92:2280–4.
4. Stein J, Purschian B, Bieniek U et al. Eur J Gastroenterol Hepatol 1994;6:889–94.
5. Mylvaganam K, Hudson PR, Ross A et al. Gut 1986;27:1347–52.
6. Stein J, Purschian B, Zeuzem S et al. Clin Chem 1996;42:309–12.
7. Larvela IE. Ann Med 2005;37:179–85.
8. Corazza GR, Benati G, Strocchi A et al. J Lab Clin Med 1994;124:695–700.
9. Romagnuolo J, Schiller D, Bailey RH. Am J Gastroenterol 2002;97:1113–26.
10. Craig RM, Ehrenpreis ED. J Clin Gastroenterol 1999;29:143–50.
11. Ehrenpreis ED, Salvino M, Craig RM. J Clin Gastroenterol 2001;33:36–40.
12. Schmidt PN, Blirup-Jensen S, Svendsen PJ et al. Scand J Clin Lab Invest 1995;55:35–45.
13. Umar SB, DiBaise JK. Am J Gastroenterol 2010;105:43–9.
14. Strygler B, Nicor MJ, Santangelo WC et al. Gastroenterology 1990;99:1380–7.
15. Takeda H, Nishise S, Furukawa M et al. Dig Dis Sci 1999;44:2313–8.
16. Seok JW, Kim S, Lee SH et al. Clin Nucl Med 2002;27:431–3.
17. Fernandez-Banares F, Esteve M, Salas A et al. Am J Gastroenterol 2007;102:2520–8.
18. Nyhlin H, Merrick MV, Eastwood MA et al. Gastroenterology 1983;84:63–8.
19. Brydon WG, Nyhlin H, Eastwood MA et al. Eur J Gastroenterol Hepatol 1996;8:117–23.
20. Maiden L, Elliott T, McLaughlin SD et al. Dig Dis Sci 2009;54:1280–3.
21. May A, Färber M, Aschmoneit I et al. Am J Gastroenterol 2010;105:575–81.
22. Maurino E, Capizzano H, Niveloni S et al. Dig Dis Sci 1993;38:2028–33.
23. Siegel LM, Stevens PD, Lightdale CJ et al. Gastrointest Endosc 1997;46:226–30.
24. Cammarota G, Cesaro P, Cazzato A et al. J Clin Gastroenterol 2009;43:244–8.
25. Rubio-Tapia A, Murray JA. Gastrointest Endosc 2007;66:382–6.
26. McHugh JB, Appelman HD, McKenna BJ. Am J Gastroenterol 2007;102:1084–9.
27. Choueiri NE, Balci NC, Alkaade S et al. Curr Gastroenterol Rep 2010;12:114–20.
28. Owens SR, Greenson JK. Histopathology 2007;50:64–82.
29. Hopper AD, Cross SS, Sanders DS. Endoscopy 2008;40:219–24.
30. DiBaise JK. Pract Gastroenterol 2008;32:15–28.
31. Khoshini R, Dai SC, Lezcano S et al. Dig Dis Sci 2008;53:1443–54.
32. Riordan SM, McIver CJ, Walker BM et al. Am J Gastroenterol 1996;91:1795–803.
33. Dave-Verma H, Moore S, Singh A et al. Curr Probl Diagn Radiol 2008;37:279–87.
34. Zuccaro P, Stevens T, Repas K et al. Pancreatology 2009;9:764–9.
35. Liu NF, Lu Q, Wang CG et al. Lymphology 2008;41:111–5.
36. Braden B. Best Pract Res Clin Gastroenterol 2009;23:337–52.
37. Corazza GR, Menozzi MG, Strocchi A et al. Gastroenterology 1990;98:302–9.
38. King CE, Toskes PP, King CE et al. Gastroenterology 1986;91:1447–51.
39. Riordan SM, McIver CJ, Duncombe VM et al. Am J Gastroenterol 1995;90:1455–60.
40. Domínguez Muñoz JE. Best Pract Res Clin Gastroenterol 2010;24:233–41.
41. Stevens T, Conwell DL, Zuccaro Jr G et al. Am J Gastroenterol 2006;101:351–5.
42. Stevens T, Conwell DL, Zuccaro Jr G et al. Gastrointest Endosc 2008;67:458–66.
43. Stevens T, Conwell DL, Zuccaro Jr G et al. Am J Gastroenterol 2007;102:297–301.
44. Luth S, Teyssen S, Forssmann K et al. Scand J Gastroenterol 2001;36:1092–9.
45. Chen WL, Morishita R, Eguchi T et al. Gastroenterology 1989;96:1337–45.

SUGGESTED READINGS

DiBaise JK. Nutritional consequences of small intestinal bacterial overgrowth. Pract Gastroenterol 2008;32:15–28.

Fernandez-Banares F, Esteve M, Salas A et al. Systematic evaluation of the causes of watery diarrhea with functional characteristics. Am J Gastroenterol 2007;102:2520–8.

Owens SR, Greenson JK. The pathology of malabsorption: current concepts. Histopathology 2007;50:64–82.

Romagnuolo J, Schiller D, Bailey RH. Using breath tests wisely in gastroenterology practice: an evidence-based review of indications and pitfalls in interpretation. Am J Gastroenterol 2002;97:1113–26.

Umar SB, DiBaise JK. Protein-losing enteropathy: case illustrations and clinical review. Am J Gastroenterol 2010;105:43–9.

76 DIET AND INTESTINAL DISACCHARIDASES[1]

STEVE HERTZLER, YEONSOO KIM, RUBINA KHAN, MICHELLE ASP, AND DENNIS SAVAIANO

Disaccharides are a significant source of carbohydrates in the diet. The major disaccharides include sucrose (O-α-D-glucopyranosyl-[1→2]-β-fructofuranoside), lactose (O-β-D-galactopyranosyl-[1→4]-β-glucopyranose), maltose (O-α-D-glucopyranosyl-[1→4]-α-glucopyranose), and trehalose (O-α-D-glucopyranosyl-[1→1]-α-glucopyranose). Lactose is the primary carbohydrate in human milk, which contains approximately 7% lactose by weight, among the highest of all mammalian milks (Table 76.1). Sucrose, lactose, and maltose comprise approximately 30%, 6%, and 1% to 2%, respectively, of the total carbohydrate in the diet (1). The majority of the maltose present in the intestine is derived from starch digestion, with only small amounts being contributed from grains and fermented beverages. The only significant dietary sources of trehalose are mushrooms and other fungi.

Because the small intestine is normally impermeable to disaccharides, intestinal disaccharidase activity is required for absorption of their component monosaccharides (2). In humans and other mammals, four known enzymes or enzyme complexes exist for disaccharide digestion: sucrase-isomaltase (SI), lactase-phlorizin hydrolase (LPH; lactase), maltase-glucoamylase, and trehalase (3). In contrast to the other enzymes that hydrolyze alpha-glucosidic bonds, lactase hydrolyzes beta-glucosidic bonds. Low levels of any of these enzymes in the intestinal mucosa results in carbohydrate malabsorption that also may be associated with clinical symptoms such as diarrhea, abdominal pain, and flatulence.

DEVELOPMENT OF BRUSH-BORDER DIGESTIVE ENZYMES

The carbohydrate-digesting enzymes of the small intestine are anchored in the brush border. The disaccharidases present include sucrase, lactase, glucoamylase, isomaltase, and trehalase. The substrates and products of each disaccharidase are shown in Table 76.2 (4). SI activity at 34 weeks of gestation reaches 70% of the adult level, rising to the adult level at birth (5). Glucoamylase and trehalase activities are detected at 13 weeks of gestation (6). Lactase activity develops later in gestation. The lactase activity is only 30% that of a full-term infant at 34 weeks of gestation and is still just 70% of the full-term level by 35 to 38 weeks (5).

The activity of disaccharidases in the brush border is recognized as the rate-limiting step in disaccharide digestion (7). Thus, congenital or acquired enzyme deficiencies cause poor absorption of disaccharides. In addition, loss of disaccharidase activity can occur secondary to damage to the intestinal mucosa because of certain diseases (e.g., alcoholism, celiac disease), infections, medications, surgery, or radiation exposure (8).

LACTASE-PHLORIZIN HYDROLASE

Location and Functions

The highest activity of LPH in humans is found in the jejunum, approximately 50 to 200 cm distal to the ligament of Treitz. Its activity is 25% lower at Treitz's ligament and is minimal in the ileum (9). The gene for LPH is located on chromosome 2 and it directs the synthesis of a pre-pro form of LPH in the enterocytes. The pre-pro LPH is processed intracellularly (and possibly by pancreatic proteases) into the mature form that is anchored in the cell membrane at the brush border.

---

[1]**Abbreviations: LNP**, lactase nonpersistence; **LPH**, lactase-phlorizin hydrolase; **PBS**, phosphate-buffered saline; **PNG**, pyridoxine-5′-β-D-glucoside; **RER**, rough endoplasmic reticulum; **SI**, sucrase-isomaltase; **SNP**, single nucleotide polymorphism.

TABLE 76.1	**LACTOSE CONTENT OF SELECTED DAIRY FOODS**	
FOOD	TYPICAL SERVING SIZE	LACTOSE CONTENT PER SERVING (g)
Whole milk	245 g (1 cup)	11
2% reduced-fat milk	245 g (1 cup)	9–13
Nonfat milk	245 g (1 cup)	12–14
Lactose-reduced milk		
70% lactose reduced	245 g (1 cup)	3–4
100% lactose reduced	245 g (1 cup)	0–1
Low-fat yogurt	245 g (1 cup)	11–15
Cheese		
Blue, parmesan	56.7 g (2 oz)	1–2
Camembert	56.7 g (2 oz)	0–1
Cheddar, gouda	56.7 g (2 oz)	1–2
Cottage cheese	210 g (1 cup)	7–8
Ice cream—10% fat	133 g (1 cup)	9–10
Ice cream—16% fat	148 g (1 cup)	9–10
Ice milk	132 g (1 cup)	9–10

Adapted with permission from Moore BJ. Dairy foods: are they politically correct? Nutr Today 2003;38:82–90.

The human enzyme has two catalytic sites, both on the luminal side of the enterocyte cell membrane. These active sites, β-galactosidase (EC 3.2.1.23) and phlorizin hydrolase (EC 3.2.1.62), comprise Glu1749 in domain IV and Glu1273 in domain III, respectively (10). The β-galactosidase portion is able to hydrolyze lactose, cellobiose, o-nitro-phenyl-β-glucopyranoside, and o-nitro-phenyl-β-galactopyranoside (10). Phlorizin hydrolase is able to hydrolyze phlorizin, β-glycopyranosyl-ceramides, and m-nitro-phenyl-β-glucopyranoside (10).

Beyond its well-recognized role in lactose digestion, evidence indicates that LPH could be involved in the hydrolysis of other nutritionally important β-glucosides. For example, although the glycosylated forms of isoflavones and flavonoids occur in nature, only the aglycone forms can be absorbed from the intestine. It was previously assumed that the colonic microflora was mainly responsible for this deconjugation. However, two studies

(11, 12) demonstrated that the lactase catalytic site of LPH is able to hydrolyze glycosylated isoflavones and flavonoids, making them available for absorption in the small intestine. Similarly, the hydrolysis of a β-glucosidic linkage is necessary to release pyridoxine from pyridoxine-5'-β-D-glucoside (PNG), an important step in increasing the bioavailability of this form of vitamin B_6 that provides roughly 15% of the total vitamin B_6 in a mixed diet (13). Mackey et al (13) reported that LPH purified from rat small intestinal mucosa possesses the capability to hydrolyze PNG in vitro.

Types of Hypolactasia and Lactase Nonpersistence

Full-term infants, regardless of racial or ethnic background, generally possess high levels of lactase activity. Congenital lactase activity is the rare condition in which lactase is absent at birth. Even in Finland, where the condition is most common, only 42 cases were reported from 1966 to 1998 (14). In these infants, lactase activity in jejunal biopsy specimens is reduced to 0 to 10 IU/g protein, and severe diarrhea results from unabsorbed lactose (14). Treatment with a lactose-free formula eliminates the diarrhea and promotes normal growth and development. Congenital lactase deficiency is a separate clinical entity from congenital lactose intolerance. Congenital lactose intolerance is a rare and serious disease with vomiting, failure to thrive, dehydration, disacchariduria including lactosuria, renal tubular acidosis, aminoaciduria, liver damage, and cataracts as possible clinical sequelae (15–18). The cause of this disorder is not lactase deficiency but rather the gastric absorption of intact lactose (16). Although this condition can be fatal in early infancy if not recognized, a milk-free diet leads to rapid recovery; and often, patients may be able to tolerate a normal diet (with milk) after 6 months of age (15).

The loss of intestinal lactase activity (hypolactasia) is either congenital or acquired, and lactase is the only digestive enzyme for which greatly reduced activity in adulthood is common. Acquired hypolactasia is subdefined as primary or secondary. Primary hypolactasia (also referred

TABLE 76.2	**ROLE OF BRUSH-BORDER ENZYMES IN DIGESTION OF DISACCHARIDES AND STARCH**		
ENZYME	ENZYMATIC ACTIVITY	SUBSTRATE	PRODUCTS
Lactase	β-(1-4) Galactosidase	Lactose	Glucose, galactose
Sucrase	α-(1-4) Glucosidase Hydrolysis of the α-1, β-2 glucose-fructose bond in sucrose	Sucrose, maltose, maltotriose, α-limit dextrins with terminal α 1-4 links	Glucose, fructose, maltooligosaccharides with terminal α 1-6 linkages
Glucoamylase	α-(1-4) Glucosidase	Maltose, maltotriose, Maltooligosaccharide	Glucose, maltooligosaccharide with terminal α 1-6 linkage
Isomaltase	α-(1-6) Glucosidase	Maltose, isomaltose, α-limit dextrins (maltooligosaccharide with terminal α 1-6 links)	Glucose, maltooligosaccharides
Trehalase	α- and β-Glucosidase (tested on renal trehalase)	Trehalose	Glucose

Adapted with permission from Treem WR. Congenital sucrase-isomaltase deficiency. J Pediatr Gastroenterol Nutr 1995;21:1–14.

to as lactase nonpersistence [LNP]) is a genetically programmed, irreversible loss of the majority (90% to 95%) of intestinal lactase activity that occurs sometime after weaning, probably between 3 and 5 years of age (19, 20). LNP affects approximately 75% of the world's population (Table 76.3). Interestingly, most Northern Europeans and a few pastoral tribes in African and the Middle East maintain high lactase levels throughout life (21). Because the loss of lactase is the normal pattern in mammalian physiology (humans are the only known mammalian species to have a subpopulation that retains lactase activity) and is not pathogenic, the use of the term "lactase deficiency" to describe the primary loss of lactase is incorrect. Last, the terms lactase nonpersistence and lactose intolerance should not be used interchangeably. The former term simply describes the loss of lactase activity, whereas the latter pertains to the development of clinical symptoms resulting from lactose maldigestion. Two major hypotheses exist to explain the pattern of LNP distribution in the world population. The first—the geographic hypothesis—was proposed by Simoons in 1978 (22). According to this hypothesis, mutations for lactose persistence occurred several thousand years ago, during the origin of dairying. In those geographic regions where dairy farming was practiced, individuals with the mutation coding for lactose digestion had improved tolerance to milk and gained a selective advantage over their counterparts, especially when living under marginal nutritional conditions.

More recently, the malaria hypothesis has been proposed by Anderson and Vullo (23). The authors suggest that malaria selected for LNP. Noting that LNP is common in geographic areas of world that are endemic for malaria, the authors posit that the genetic tendency for LNP would cause lactose maldigestion and intolerance symptoms leading to a corresponding decline in milk intake in affected individuals. Because milk products are excellent sources of riboflavin, it is further proposed that

many of these individuals may have had marginal riboflavin deficiency. A state of marginal riboflavin deficiency that could be tolerated by the person and yet still lead to localized flavin deficiency in the erythrocytes, is theorized to inhibit the multiplication of malaria parasites and, thus, reduce mortality from malaria. Although this hypothesis is interesting, a study conducted in Northern Sardinia showed no differences in the prevalence of LNP in villages with a past history of low, intermediate, or high malaria morbidity and mortality (24). A further commentary on this study (25) points out that, in contrast to the data on LNP, the frequencies of glucose-6-phosphate dehydrogenase deficiency and β-thalassemia trait (two disorders that are known to be selected for by malaria) were strikingly higher in the areas with a high past malarial endemicity versus the area with low malarial endemicity. Thus, the limited evidence presented so far does not support the malaria hypothesis.

In LNP individuals, lactase activity in the jejunal enterocytes is found in a mosaic-type pattern, meaning that some jejunal enterocytes produce high levels of lactase, whereas others, even those sharing the same villus, do not produce lactase (26, 27). Thus, rather than a uniform reduction in lactase production among all enterocytes, LNP individuals may have a patchy distribution of lactase-producing enterocytes that are low in number relative to the non–lactase-producing enterocytes. However, in lactase-persistent individuals, all enterocytes may produce lactase.

The molecular basis for LNP has received much attention. LNP is an autosomal recessive trait and the gene for human LPH is located on chromosome 2q21 (28). Initial studies suggested that alterations in the posttranslational modifications of LPH were responsible for the low lactase activity in hypolactasia (29, 30). Rossi et al (26) found that intestinal biopsies of hypolactasic individuals in Southern Italy had substantial levels of lactose mRNA. Thus, it was thought that hypolactasic persons do synthesize the lactase protein, but that posttranslational modifications cause it to be either malfolded and enzymatically inactive or result in its intracellular degradation (31). Sebastio et al (32) studied individuals with the hypolactasic phenotype and the lactase-persistent phenotype. There was no clear difference in the lactase mRNA levels in the intestinal biopsies of individuals with either phenotype. The authors concluded that expression of lactase is controlled at the posttranscriptional level.

Despite this evidence, the current opinion is that lactase regulation is primarily at the level of transcription. Numerous studies (33–35) have demonstrated the importance of the presence of an adequate lactase mRNA level to have expression of LPH activity. Krasinski et al (36) found that LPH mRNA levels in rats were abundant before weaning but declined twofold to fourfold during weaning. The LPH activity observed in the rats corresponded with the protein and mRNA levels at the different life stages. Thus, transcriptional mechanisms

TABLE 76.3	PREVALANCE OF LACTASE NONPERSISTENCE IN VARIOUS ETHNIC GROUPS	
GROUP	**PREVALENCE (%)**
Northern European	2–7
White (United States)	6–22
Central European	9–23
Indian (Indian subcontinent)	
Northern	20–30
Southern	60–70
Hispanics	50–80
Ashkenazi Jews	60–80
African-American	60–80
Black African	70–95
Native American	80–100
Asian	85–100

Adapted with permssion from Srinivasan R, Minocha A. When to suspect lactose intolerance: symptomatic, ethnic, and laboratory clues. Postgrad Med 1998;104:109–23. Also contains information from Sahi T. Genetics and epidemiology of adult-type hypolactasia. Scand J Gastroenterol 1994;29(Suppl 202):7–20.

were thought to be responsible for regulation of lactase biosynthesis. Escher et al (37) studied lactase specific activity and lactase mRNA levels in Asian, black, and white patients. They observed that lactase activity always corresponded with the lactase mRNA levels, thereby suggesting that transcriptional regulation is responsible for variable lactase activity. Further, studies of the porcine LPH gene have identified a sequence CE-LPH1 in the promoter region, which binds a *trans*-acting nuclear factor NF-LPH1. High levels of NF-LPH1 were found in enterocytes of newborn pigs that had high lactase activity, whereas the levels were lower in adult pigs that had low lactase activity. It was suggested that the nuclear factor NF-LPH1 could be implicated in the lowering of lactase activity at weaning and could provide an explanation for the molecular regulation of hypolactasia (38). Subsequent studies have shown that other nuclear factors also may interact with the CE-LPH1 promoter region (39).

The newer finding in the area of the genetics of lactose intolerance is the discovery of single nucleotide polymorphisms (SNP) that appear to define individuals who will maintain or lose lactase activity after weaning. The first of these to be discovered is C/T-13910, in European populations (40). A one base-pair polymorphism 13.9 kb upstream from the lactase gene on chromosome 2 appears to be responsible for determining lactose digestion status in many European populations. The location of the SNP appears to be the binding site for the transcription factor Oct-1. The expression of the lactase gene is severalfold higher for the T-13910 allele. Both T/T-13910 and C/T-13910 allow enough transcription binding that nonpersistence is seen only with the homozygous C/C-13910 allele. This is a plausible molecular explanation for the dominance of tolerance long observed in lactose genetics. A second essential finding is that SNPs vary by racial group around the world. Initial thought was that maybe three different SNPs existed for Europeans, Middle Eastern populations, and Africans. However, to date, at least eight unique SNPs have been identified (41). It is possible that much of the variation around age at onset and degree of intolerance could be related to the specific SNPs.

Secondary acquired hypolactasia occurs because of enterocyte damage resulting from disease, medication, surgery, or radiation (42). Table 76.4 lists some of the causes of secondary hypolactasia. In one study of malnourished patients, lactase was reduced to a greater degree than other disaccharidases and was the last of the disaccharidases to recover (43). A possible explanation is that the activity of lactase is only about 50% as high as the other disaccharidases, even in lactase persistent individuals (44). A key issue in the management of secondary hypolactasia is lactose restriction in the diet. Although removing lactose-containing dairy foods may improve clinical tolerance, it also may deprive a malnourished patient of the nutritional value of these foods. Secondary hypolactasia can be reversed once the underlying problem has been resolved, but the process is slow and can take 6 months or longer (42).

Clinical Assessment of Lactase Activity

Lactase activity is assessed by either direct or indirect methods. The direct measurement of the lactase activity obtained by a small intestinal mucosal biopsy or intestinal perfusion is the most accurate, but these methods are invasive and carry risk for complications, such as intestinal bleeding (45). Thus, direct methods are rarely performed clinically.

Indirect methods for assessing the digestion of a dose of lactose include breath tests (hydrogen, $^{13}CO_2$, $^{14}CO_2$), blood tests (glucose and galactose), urine tests (galactose, lactose/lactulose ratio), fecal tests (pH, reducing substances) and intolerance symptoms. Of these methods, the breath hydrogen test is currently the most widely used. The test is based on the principle that lactose, which escapes digestion in the small intestine, is fermented by the colonic bacteria, resulting in the generation of hydrogen gas (the only known source of molecular hydrogen in the body). A portion of this hydrogen gas diffuses into the blood and is excreted via the lungs. The method has excellent sensitivity and specificity, but careful attention to the test protocol is required (44).

TABLE 76.4	**POTENTIAL CAUSES OF SECONDARY HYPOLACTASIA**	
DISEASES		
SMALL BOWEL	**MULTISYSTEM**	**IATROGENIC**
HIV enteropathy	Carcinoid syndrome	Chemotherapy
Regional enteritis (e.g., Crohn disease)	Cystic fibrosis	Radiation enteritis
Sprue (celiac and tropical)	Diabetic gastropathy	Surgical resection of intestine
Whipple diseases (intestinal lipodystrophy)	Protein energy malnutrition	Medications
Ascaris lumbricoides infection	Zollinger-Ellison syndrome	Colchicine (antigout)
Blind loop syndrome	Alcoholism	Neomycin (antibiotic)
Giardiasis	Iron deficiency	Kanamycin (antibiotic)
Infectious diarrhea		Aminosalicylic acid (antibiotic)
Short gut		

Reprinted with permission from Savaiano D, Hertzler S, Jackson KA et al. Nutrient considerations in lactose intolerance. In: Coulston AM, Rock CL, Monsen ER, eds. Nutrition in the Prevention and Treatment of Disease. San Diego: Academic Press, 2001:563–75.

Lactose Maldigestion and Symptoms of Lactose Intolerance

The well-documented high prevalence of LNP in much of the world's population has unfortunately misled many to believe that lactose intolerance is equally common. However, a large body of evidence now exists demonstrating that symptoms of lactose intolerance in response to physiological amounts of lactose (8 to 16 fl oz of milk) affect only a small fraction of lactose maldigesters (46). An example is a study by Carroccio et al (47). In this study, 323 Sicilian adults (72 children aged 5 to 16 years, 141 adults aged 17 to 64 years, and 110 elderly adults aged 65 to 85 years) underwent breath hydrogen testing with a 25-g lactose dose (1 g/kg for children) to determine lactose digestion status and were queried for the presence of lactose intolerance in the ensuing 24-hour period. Of the 323 individuals, 117 (36%) were classified as lactose maldigesters. Just 13 of the lactose maldigesters experienced symptoms of lactose intolerance, which was 4% of the total study group and 11% of the lactose maldigesters.

Another concern is that many individuals may self-diagnose lactose intolerance when they may not be lactose maldigesters. Two studies by Suarez et al and another by Johnson et al (48–50) demonstrated that 30% to 33% of subjects who claim to have lactose intolerance are, in fact, lactose digesters. Of the 49 subjects in the Carroccio et al study (47) who had self-reported milk intolerance at entry into the study, just five were both lactose maldigesters and lactose intolerant. It is likely that some individuals who self-diagnose with lactose intolerance may have an underlying bowel. The findings indicate that diagnosing lactose intolerance solely on the basis of reported symptoms after milk ingestion is unreliable. Objective tests of lactose maldigestion, or the evaluation of symptoms in a double-masked, placebo-controlled study are necessary (51).

Symptoms of lactose intolerance include flatulence, cramping, abdominal pain, nausea, distention, bloating, and diarrhea (52), and appear to be related to the ability of the colonic microflora to process undigested lactose (53). Differences in the types of bacteria and/or their metabolic activities affect how lactose is fermented. It has been proposed that a dominance of lactic acid bacteria in the colon would improve the fermentation of lactose into short-chain fatty acids and other products that are absorbed easily from the colon (54). Thus, the potential for osmotic diarrhea caused by unfermented lactose would diminish. Further, lactic acid bacteria also may reduce intestinal gas production either directly or indirectly. Lactic acid bacteria are able to ferment lactose without producing hydrogen (55) and the pH-lowering effect of lactic acid may inhibit bacteria that are major hydrogen producers (e.g., clostridia, *Escherichia coli*) (56, 57). Given that hydrogen gas can account for 50% or more of total colonic gas during active fermentation (58), reducing hydrogen production should appreciably lower the volume of gas

produced and, therefore, reduce flatulence. However, some studies suggest that subjective symptoms may result from an individual's increased sensitivity to gas, not an increase in the absolute volume of gas (59, 60).

It is common for many lactose-maldigesting individuals to believe that any amount of lactose will cause intolerance symptoms. However, the relationship between lactose maldigestion and the development of lactose intolerance is complex. The symptom response is influenced by several physiologic and psychosocial factors including dose, transit, residual lactase, and colonic capacity.

Dietary Approaches for Overcoming Lactose Intolerance

Dose of Lactose

Historically, a 50-g lactose challenge (equivalent to 1 L of milk) has been used in lactose tolerance testing. Between 80% and 100% of lactose maldigesters experience intolerance symptoms when such an unphysiologic amount of lactose is fed on an empty stomach (19). However, the symptom responses to a typical serving of milk (e.g., 8 fl oz of milk [240 mL] containing 12 g lactose) are typically much lower and are often absent in lactose maldigesters. Residual lactase activity may help to explain tolerance to smaller lactose loads. Bond and Levitt (61), using an intestinal intubation technique, demonstrated that lactose maldigesters may absorb anywhere from 42% to 75% of a 12.5-g lactose dose. The combination of the relatively small amount of lactose, coupled with residual lactase activity, usually results in negligible symptom responses at lactose doses of 12 g or less. Some studies (62–64) have identified a small number of individuals who may be sensitive to as little as 3 to 5 g lactose. However, one study (62) did not have appropriate masking of treatment identities, whereas another double-blind study (63), found that only 3/59 lactose maldigesters had a positive symptom response to 3 g lactose, a number that was not different from the 0-g lactose placebo. Further, a double-blind study by Suarez et al (48) found that even subjects who claimed to be severely lactose intolerant did not report more symptoms when 8 fl oz per day of regular versus 100% lactose-hydrolyzed milk was fed for 7 days. Hertzler et al (65), using breath hydrogen analysis, determined that a 2-g lactose dose was completely absorbed, whereas there was some evidence of lactose maldigestion (without symptoms) at a 6-g dose. Good tolerance to doses of lactose up to 7 g has been confirmed (66).

Larger but still physiologic loads of lactose (e.g., 15 to 25 g) cause symptoms in approximately 50% of lactose maldigesters (67). In general, 12 g or greater of lactose can cause abdominal pain in some lactose maldigesters, whereas significant increases in flatulence symptoms may not be present until the lactose dose reaches 20 g (65, 68). However, if a total of approximately 25 g lactose is consumed as two separate doses of 12 g each at breakfast and dinner, symptoms are minimal (49). Lactose maldigesters

28. Grand RJ, Montgomery RK, Chitkara DK et al. Gut 2003; 52:617–19.
29. Witte J, Lloyd M, Lorenzsonn V et al. J Clin Invest 1990; 86:1338–42.
30. Lorenzsonn V, Lloyd M, Olen WA. Gastroenterology 1993; 105:51–9.
31. Naim HY. Histol Histopathol 2001;16:553–61.
32. Sebastio G, Villa M, Sartorio R et al. Am J Hum Genet 1989;45:489–97.
33. Montgomery RK, Büller HA, Rings EH et al. FASEB J 1991;5:2824–32.
34. Lloyd M, Mevissen G, Fischer M et al. J Clin Invest 1992; 89:524–9.
35. Fajardo O, Naim HY, Lacey SW. Gastroenterology 1994; 106:1233–41.
36. Krasinski SD, Estrada G, Yeh KY et al. Am J Physiol 1994;267:G584–G94.
37. Escher JC, de Koning ND, van Engen CG et al. J Clin Invest 1992;89:480–3.
38. Troelsen JT, Olsen J, Norén O et al. J Biol Chem 1992; 267:20407–11.
39. Troelsen JT, Mitchelmore C, Spodsberg N et al. Biochem J 1997;322:833–8.
40. Enattah NS, Sahi T, Savilahti et al. Nat Genet 2002;30:233–7.
41. Tishkoff SA, Reed FA, Ranciaro A et al. Nat Genet 2007; 39:31–40.
42. Scrimshaw NS, Murray EB. Am J Clin Nutr 1988;48:1083–159.
43. Khambadkone MR, Jain MK, Ganapathy S. Ind Pediatr 1994; 31:1351–5.
44. Gray G. Gastroenterology 1993;105:931.
45. Arola H. Scand J Gastroenterol 1994;29(Suppl):26–35.
46. McBean LD, Miller GD. J Am Diet Assoc 1998;98:671–6.
47. Carroccio A, Montalto G, Cavera G et al. J Am Coll Nutr 1998; 17:631–6.
48. Suarez FL, Savaiano DA, Levitt MD. N Engl J Med 1995; 333:1–4.
49. Suarez FL, Savaiano DA, Arbisi P et al. Am J Clin Nutr 1997; 65:1502–6.
50. Johnson AO, Semenya JG, Buchowski MS et al. Am J Clin Nutr 1993;57:399–401.
51. Suarez F, Levitt M. Gut 1997;41:715–6.
52. Srinivasan R, Minocha A. Postgrad Med 1998;104:109–23.
53. Vonk RJ, Priebe MG, Koetse HA et al. Eur J Clin Invest 2003;33:70–5.
54. Hill MJ. Bacterial adaptation to lactase deficiency. In: Delmont J, ed. Milk Intolerances and Rejection. New York: Karger 1983:22–6.
55. Ballongue J. Bifidobacteria and probiotic action. In: Selminen S, von Wright A, eds. New York: Marcel Dekker, 1993:369–71.
56. Perman J, Modler S, Olson AC. J Clin Invest 1981;67:643–50.
57. Vogelsang H, Ferenci P, Frotz S et al. Gut 1988;29:21–6.
58. Tomlin J, Lowis C, Read NW. Gut 1991;32:665–9.
59. Hammer HF, Petritsch W, Pristautz H et al. Wien Klin Wochenschr 1996;108:175–9.
60. Levitt MD, Furne J, Olsson S. Ann Intern Med 1996;124: 422–4.
61. Bond JH, Levitt MD. Gastroenterology 1976;70:1058–62.
62. Bedine MS, Bayless TM. Gastroenterology 1973;65:735–43.
63. Newcomer AD, McGill DB, Thomas PJ et al. Gastroenterology 1978;74:44–6.
64. Gudmand–Høyer E, Simony K. Dig Dis 1977;22:177–81.
65. Hertzler SR, Huynh B-C, Savaiano DA. J Am Diet Assoc 1996;96:243–6.
66. Vesa TH, Korpela RA, Sahi T. Am J Clin Nutr 1996;64:197–201.

67. Savaiano DA, Levitt MD. J Dairy Sci 1987;70:397–406.
68. Gremse DA, Greer AS, Vacik J et al. Clin Pediatr 2003;42:341–5.
69. Suarez FL, Adshead J, Furne JK et al. Am J Clin Nutr 1998;68:1118–22.
70. Hertzler SR, Savaiano DA. Am J Clin Nutr 1996;64:232–6.
71. Ladas S, Papanikos J, Arapakis G. Gut 1982;23:968–73.
72. Labayen I, Forga L, Gonzalez A et al. Aliment Pharmacol Ther 2001;15:543–9.
73. Solomons NW, Guerrero AM, Torun B. Am J Clin Nutr 1985;41:199–208.
74. Martini MC, Savaiano DA. Am J Clin Nutr 1988;47:57–60.
75. Dehkordi N, Rao DR, Warren AP et al. J Am Diet Assoc 1995;95:484–6.
76. Vesa TH, Marteau PR, Briet FB et al. J Nutr 1997;127:2316–20.
77. Vesa TH, Marteau PR, Briet FB et al. Am J Clin Nutr 1997;66:123–6.
78. Peuhkuri K, Vapaatalo H, Nevala R et al. Scand J Clin Invest 2000;60:75–80.
79. Leichter JL. Am J Clin Nutr 1973;26:393–6.
80. Cavalli-Sforza LT, Strata A. Hum Nutr Clin Nutr 1986;40C: 19–30.
81. Vesa TH, Lember M, Korpela R. Eur J Clin Nutr 1997;51: 633–6.
82. Lee CM, Hardy CM. Am J Clin Nutr 1989;49:840–4.
83. Jarvinen RMK, Loukaskorpi M, Uusitupa MIJ. Eur J Clin Nutr 2003;57:701–5.
84. Gallagher CR, Molleson AL, Caldwell JH. J Am Diet Assoc 1974;65:418–9.
85. Kolars JC, Levitt MD, Aouji M et al. N Engl J Med 1984; 310:1–3.
86. Savaiano DA, Abou El Anouar A, Smith DE et al. Am J Clin Nutr 1984;40:1219–23.
87. Lerebours E, Ndam CND, Lavoine A et al. Am J Clin Nutr 1989;49:823–7.
88. Martini MC, Lerebours EC, Lin WJ et al. Am J Clin Nutr 1991;54:1041–6.
89. Gilliland SE, Kim HS. J Dairy Sci 1984;67:1–6.
90. Răsic J, Kurmans JA. The nutritional-physiological value of yoghurt. In: Yogurt: Scientific Grounds, Technology, Manufacture, and Preparations. Copenhagen: Technical Dairy Publishing, 1978:99–137.
91. Martini MC, Bollweg GL, Levitt MD et al. Am J Clin Nutr 1987;45:432–6.
92. Martini MC, Kukielka D, Savaiano DA. Am J Clin Nutr 1991;53:1253–8.
93. Shermak MA, Saavedra JM, Jackson TL et al. Am J Clin Nutr 1995;62:1003–6.
94. Martini MC, Smith DE, Savaiano DA. Am J Clin Nutr 1987;46:36–40.
95. Hertzler SR, Clancy SM. J Am Diet Assoc 2003;103:582–7.
96. Newcomer AD, Park HS, O'Brien PC. Am J Clin Nutr 1983;38:257–63.
97. Mc Donough FE, Hitchins AD, Wong NP. Am J Clin Nutr 1987;45:570–4.
98. Lin MY, Savaiano DA, Harlander S. J Dairy Sci 1991;74:87–95.
99. Onwulata CI, Rao DR, Vankineni P. Am J Clin Nutr 1989; 49:1233–7.
100. Saltzman JR, Russell RM, Golner B et al. Am J Clin Nutr 1999;69:140–6.
101. Montes RG, Bayless TM, Saavedra JM et al. J Dairy Sci 1995;78:1657–64.
102. Kim HS, Gilliland SE. J Dairy Sci 1983;66:959–66.
103. Jiang T, Mustapha A, Savaiano DA. J Dairy Sci 1996;79:750–7.
104. Mustapha A, Jiang T, Savaiano DA. J Dairy Sci 1997;80:1537–45.

105. Geel TM, McLaughlin PM, de Leij LF et al. Mol Genet Metab 2007;92:299–307.

106. Land O Lakes. Dairy Ease Nutritional Information. Available at: http://www.dairyease.com/benefits/nutritional_whole.html. Accessed on July 12, 2012.

107. Lactaid. Lactaid products. Available at: http://www.lactaid.com. Accessed on July 12, 2012.

108. Rosado JL, Morales M, Pasquetti A et al. La Rev Invest Clin 1988;40:141–7.

109. Biller JA, King S, Rosenthal A et al. J Pediatr 1987;111:91–4.

110. Payne-Bose D, Welsh JD, Gearhart HL et al. Am J Clin Nutr 1977;30:695–7.

111. Payne DL, Welsh JD, Manion CV. Am J Clin Nutr 1981; 34:2711–5.

112. Pedersen ER, Jensen BH, Jensen HJ. Scand J Gastroenterol 1982;17:861–4.

113. Brand JC, Holt S. Am J Clin Nutr 1991;54:148–51.

114. Turner SJ, Daly T, Hourigan JA et al. Am J Clin Nutr 1976; 29:739–44.

115. Paige DM, Bayless TM, Mellits ED et al. J Agric Food Chem 1979;27:677–80.

116. Cheng AHR, Brunser O, Espinoza J et al. Am J Clin Nutr 1979;32:1989–93.

117. Rosado JL, Morales M, Pasquetti A. JPEN J Parenter Enteral Nutr 1989;13:157–61.

118. Nagy L, Mozsik G, Garamszegi M et al. Acta Med Hung 1983;40:239–45.

119. Reasoner J, Maculan TP, Rand AG et al. Am J Clin Nutr 1981;34:54–60.

120. Ramirez FC, Lee K, Graham DY. Am J Gastroenterol 1994; 89:566–70.

121. Gao KP, Mitsui T, Fujiki K et al. Nagoya J Med Sci 2002; 65:21–8.

122. Lin MY, DiPalma JA, Martini MC et al. Dig Dis Sci 1993; 38:2022–7.

123. Sanders SW, Tolman KG, Reitburg DP. Clin Pharmacol 1992;11:533–8.

124. DiPalma JA, Collins MS. J Clin Gastroenterol 1989;11:290–3.

125. Moskovitz M, Curtis C, Gavaler J. Am J Gastroenterol 1987; 82:632–5.

126. Suarez FL, Zumarraga LM, Furne JK et al. J Am Diet Assoc 2001;101:1447–52.

127. Nielsen OH, Schiotz PO, Rasmussen SN et al. J Pediatr Gastroenterol Nutr 1984;3:219–23.

128. Gilat F, Russo S, Gelman-Malachi E, Aldor TA. Gastro-enterology 1972;62:1125–7.

129. Keusch GT, Troncale FJ, Thavaramara B et al. Am J Clin Nutr 1969;22:638–41.

130. Reddy V, Pershad J. Am J Clin Nutr 1972;25:114–9.

131. Habte D, Sterky G, Hjalmarsson B. Acta Paediatr Scand 1973;62:649–54.

132. Greenfield H. Nutr Today 2003;38:77–81.

133. Johnson AO, Semenya JG, Buchowski MS et al. Am J Clin Nutr 1993;58:879–81.

134. Pribila BA, Hertzler SR, Martin BR et al. J Am Diet Assoc 2000;100:524–28.

135. Briet F, Pochart P, Marteau P et al. Gut 1997;41:632–5.

136. During MJ, Xu R, Young D et al. Nat Med 1998;4:1131–5.

137. West LF, Davis MB, Green FR et al. Ann Hum Genet 1988;52:57–61.

138. Green F, Edwards Y, Hauri HP et al. Gene 1987;57:101–10.

139. Lloyd ML, Olsen WA. N Engl J Med 1987;316:438–42.

140. Jacob R, Zimmer KP, Schmitz J et al. J Clin Invest 2000; 106:281–7.

141. Ouwendijk J, Moolenaar CEC, Peters WJ et al. J Clin Invest 1996;97:633–41.

142. Moolenaar CEC, Ouwendijk J, Wittpoth M et al. J Cell Sci 1997;110:557–67.

143. Rosensweig NS, Herman RH. J Clin Invest 1968;47: 2253–62.

144. Schmitz J, Odievre M, Rey J. Gastroenterology 1972;62: 389–92.

145. Muldoon C, Maguire P, Gleeson F. Am J Gastroenterol 1999;94:2298–9.

146. Ringrose RE, Preiser H, Welsh JD. Dig Dis Sci 1980;25:384–7.

147. Cooper BT, Scott J, Hopkins J et al. Dig Dis Sci 1983;28:473–7.

148. Gudmand-Høyer E, Fenger HJ, Kern-Hansen P et al. Scand J Gastroenterol 1987;22:24–8.

149. Lebenthal E, Khin-Maung U, Zheng BY et al. J Pediatr 1994;124:541–6.

150. Nichols BL, Avery SE, Karnsakul W et al. J Pediatr Gastroenterol Nutr 2002;35:573–9.

151. Karsakul W, Luginbuehl U, Hahn D et al. J Pediatr Gastroenterol Nutr 2002;35:551–6.

152. Treem WR, McAdams L, Stanford L et al. J Pediatric Gastroenterol Nutr 1999;28:137–42.

153. Treem WR, Ahsan N, Sullivan B et al. Gastroenterology 1993;105:1061–8.

154. Gudmand-Høyer E, Fenger HJ, Skovbjerg H et al. Scand J Gastroenterol 1988;23:775–8.

155. Eze LC. Biochem Genet 1989;27:487–95.

156. Arola H, Koivula T, Karvonen AL et al. Scand J Gastroenterol 1999;898–903.

157. Oku T, Nakamura S. Eur J Clin Nutr 2000;54:783–8.

158. Yoshida K, Mizukawa H, Haruki E. Clin Chim Acta 1993; 215:123–4.

SUGGESTED READINGS

Arola H. Diagnosis of hypolactasia and lactose malabsorption. Scand J Gastroenterol Suppl 1994;202:26–35.

Carroccio A, Montalto G, Cavera G et al. Lactose intolerance and self-reported milk intolerance: relationship with lactose maldigestion and nutrient intake. Lactase Deficiency Study Group. J Am Coll Nutr 1998;17:631–6.

Gudmand-Høyer E, Skovbjerg H. Disaccharide digestion and maldigestion. Scand J Gastroenterol Suppl 1996;216:111–21.

Martini MC, Lerebours EC, Lin WJ et al. Strains and species of lactic acid bacteria in fermented milks (yogurts): effect on in vivo lactose digestion. Am J Clin Nutr 1991;54:1041–6.

Southgate DA. Digestion and metabolism of sugars. Am J Clin Nutr 1995;62(Suppl):203S–10S.

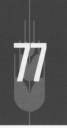

77 SHORT BOWEL SYNDROME[1]

KHURSHEED N. JEEJEEBHOY

DEFINITION

A consensus paper (1) provided the following definitions: Short-bowel syndrome results from surgical resection, congenital defect, or disease-associated loss of absorption and is characterized by the inability to maintain protein-energy, fluid, electrolyte, or micronutrient balances when on a conventionally accepted, normal diet. Intestinal failure results from obstruction, dysmotility, surgical resection, congenital defect, or disease-associated loss of absorption and is characterized by the inability to maintain protein-energy, fluid, electrolyte, or micronutrient balance. The major difference between intestinal failure and short bowel is that intestinal failure is the result of a variety of conditions such as chronic intestinal obstruction, whereas short bowel implies a reduction of functional intestinal surface area for absorption.

ETIOLOGY

The principal causes of short bowel syndrome are outlined in Table 77.1. The two major causes of surgical short bowel are inflammatory bowel disease and vascular disease. The risk factors for vascular disease leading to resection of the intestine are the same as those for other vascular diseases: increasing age, smoking, cardiac disease leading to low output or predisposing to embolization, hypercoagulable states, diabetes, and vasculitis.

---

[1]**Abbreviations: CI**, confidence interval; **DFD**, defined formula diet; **EGF**, epidermal growth factor; **GH**, growth hormone; **GLP**, glucagon-like peptide; **HEN**, home enteral nutrition; **HGH**, human growth hormone; **HPN**, home parenteral nutrition; **IGF-I**, insulinlike growth factor-I; **IT**, intestinal transplantation; **ORS**, oral rehydration solution; **PN**, parenteral nutrition; **SCFA**, short-chain fatty acid; **TGF-α**, transforming growth factor-α.

TABLE 77.1	CAUSES OF SHORT BOWEL SYNDROME

Intestinal resection
  Ileal resection
  Ileocolic resection
  End jejunostomy
Mucosal disease
  Celiac disease
  Whipple disease
  Lymphoma
  Ulcerative jejunoileitis
  Abetalipoproteinemia
Small bowel disease
  Radiation injury and chemotherapy
  Inflammatory bowel disease
  Neoplasms
  Autoimmune disease
  Infection (e.g., human immunodeficiency virus)
Gut bypass
  Intestinal fistulas
  Surgical bypass

PATHOPHYSIOLOGIC CONSIDERATIONS

To understand and treat this condition, it is necessary to understand normal function and how it is altered by the short bowel syndrome.

Gastric Emptying

The rate at which a meal enters the intestine is regulated by the rate of gastric emptying. Gastric emptying of liquids depends on their osmolarity. For digestible solids, the emptying is regulated by the particle size. However, intestinal contents entering the distal intestine inhibit gastric emptying (2). Gastric hypersecretion occurs after significant small bowel resection and reduces nutrient absorption by inactivating pancreatic enzymes.

Small Bowel

Small bowel motility is three times slower in the ileum than in the jejunum (3). In addition, the ileocecal valve may slow transit, especially when the ileum has been resected (4).

The adult small bowel receives about 5 to 6 L of endogenous secretions and 2 to 3 L of exogenous fluids per day. It reabsorbs most of this volume in the small bowel. The amount reabsorbed in the small intestine depends on the nature of the meal (5). With a meat- and salad–based meal, most of the fluid is absorbed in the jejunum, whereas with a milk and doughnut meal, less is absorbed proximally and more distally. In addition, the absorptive processes are different in the jejunum as compared with the ileum. These differences depend partly on the nature of the electrolyte transport processes and partly on the permeability of the intercellular junctions. In general, water absorption is a passive process resulting from the active transport of nutrients and electrolytes. The transport of sodium creates an electrochemical gradient and also drives the uptake of carbohydrates and amino acids across the intestinal mucosa. In addition, the ileum has neutral sodium chloride absorption. However, the net absorption depends not only on these processes but also on the extent of back diffusion of the transported material into the intestinal lumen through leaky intercellular junctions. In the jejunum, these junctions are very leaky, and thus jejunal contents are always isotonic.

Fluid absorption in this region of the bowel is very inefficient when compared with the ileum. It has been estimated that the efficiency of water absorption is 44% and 70% of the ingested load in the jejunum and ileum, respectively. For sodium, the corresponding estimates are 13% and 72% (5). Hence, the ileum is important in the conservation of fluid and electrolytes.

Unique Functions of the Ileum

The terminal ileum uniquely absorbs vitamin B_{12} and bile salts. Bile salts are essential for the efficient absorption of fats and fat-soluble vitamins. Normally, the demand for bile salts imposed by fat absorption cannot be met by synthesis alone. This full need is met only by ileal resorption of bile salts, which are then recycled into the intestine. With ileal resection, the loss of bile salts increases and is not met by an increase in synthesis. The bile salt pool is depleted, and fat absorption is reduced. In addition, loss of bile salts into the colon affects the colonocytes and reduces the ability of the colon to reabsorb salt and water. The result is increased diarrhea. In the colon, bile salts are also dehydroxylated to deoxy bile salts that induce colonic water secretion.

Colon

The colon has the slowest transit, varying between 24 and 150 hours. The intercellular junctions are the tightest in this part of the bowel, and the efficiency of water and salt absorption in the colon exceeds 90% (6). In addition, carbohydrate is fermented in the colon to short-chain fatty acids (SCFAs) having two important actions. First SCFAs enhance salt and water absorption (7). Second, the energy content of malabsorbed carbohydrates is salvaged by being absorbed as SCFAs. Data suggest that in patients with short bowel syndrome, this salvage may be greater than in physiologically normal persons (8). Thus, the colon becomes an important organ for fluid and electrolyte conservation and for the salvage of malabsorbed energy substrates in patients with a short bowel.

EFFECTS OF INTESTINAL RESECTION

Motility

Gastric motility is enhanced following small bowel resection (9). Whereas proximal resection does not increase the rate of intestinal transit, ileal resection significantly accelerates intestinal transit (9, 10). In this situation, the colon aids in slowing intestinal transit so that in patients with a short bowel without a colon, a marker fed by mouth was completely excreted in a few hours (11).

Absorption of Fluid and Electrolytes

The effect of intestinal resection depends on the extent and site of resection. Proximal resection results in no bowel disturbance because the ileum and colon absorb the increased fluid and electrolyte load efficiently. The remaining ileum continues to absorb bile salts, and thus there is little reaching the colon to impede salt and water resorption. In contrast, when the ileum is resected, the colon receives a much larger load of fluid and electrolytes and also receives bile salts that reduce its ability to absorb salt and water, with resulting diarrhea. In addition, if the colon is resected, the ability to maintain fluid and electrolyte homeostasis is severely impaired (12).

Absorption of Nutrients

Absorption of nutrients occurs throughout the small bowel, and the removal of the jejunum alone causes the ileum to take over most of the lost function. In this situation, no significant malabsorption occurs (13). In contrast, even a loss of a 100 cm of ileum causes steatorrhea (14). The degree of malabsorption increases with the length of small bowel resection, and the variety of nutrients malabsorbed increases (15, 16). Balance studies of energy absorption showed that the absorption of fat and carbohydrate was equally reduced to between 50% and 75% of intake (17). However, nitrogen absorption was reduced to a lesser extent, namely, to 81% of intake (17). In the study of Ladefoged et al (16), the degrees of calcium, magnesium, zinc, and phosphorus absorption were reduced but did not correlate with the remaining length of bowel; and it was recommended that parenteral nutrition (PN) be mandatory in these patients. Other studies showed similar reduction in absorption, but only half the patients required parenteral replacement.

Data recalculated from Nightingale et al (18) in patients with a jejunostomy indicate that fluid balance can be maintained by the oral route if the remaining small bowel exceeds 110 cm (Fig. 77.1), but nutrient balance can be maintained even if the remaining bowel is as short as 60 cm (Fig. 77.2). The data taken as a whole suggest that it is easier to meet needs for energy and nitrogen by increasing oral intake than the needs for electrolytes and divalent ions. A review of the literature before the availability of PN showed that small bowel resections of up to 33% result in no malnutrition, and resections of up to 50% of normal length can be tolerated without special aids; however, patients with small bowel resection in excess of 75% of normal length require nutritional support to avoid severe malnutrition (19–29).

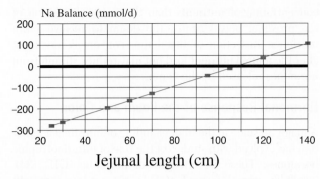

Figure 77.1. Jejunal efflux or absorption of sodium (Na) in relation to length of remaining small bowel. The *dark solid line* is the demarcation at which sodium secretion changes to absorption. (Reprinted with permission from Nightingale JM, Lennard-Jones JE, Walker ER et al. Jejunal efflux in short bowel syndrome. Lancet 1990;336:765–8.)

ADAPTATION OF THE INTESTINE

Following resection, the remaining small bowel hypertrophies and increases in absorptive function (30–33). This process enhances the ability of the remaining bowel to recover the lost function and is thus an important compensatory process. The factors that influence this adaptation are complex and are discussed later, as are the effects of total PN.

Eating exposes the gastrointestinal tract to a unique set of stimuli that do not occur when the bowel is kept constantly empty, a process called bowel rest. The advent of PN resulted in the ability to rest the bowel for short or long periods of time without causing malnutrition, a situation that had not been possible previously. This process nourished the body but excluded the gut from nutrient and hormonal stimuli that occur during the ingestion of an oral diet. The advent of defined formula diets (DFDs) without residue and diets composed of monomers such as glucose instead of polymeric starch modified the stimuli received by the gut when exposed to a normal diet. Because nutrients are absorbed progressively along the length of the bowel, the jejunum is exposed to a higher

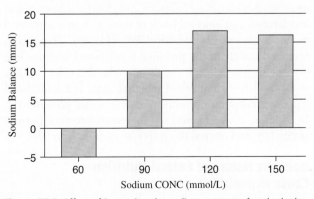

Figure 77.2. Effect of increasing the sodium content of oral rehydration solution on fluid absorption. CONC, concentration. (Reprinted with permission from Lennard-Jones JE. Oral rehydration solutions in short bowel syndrome. Clin Ther 1990;12[Suppl A]:129–38.)

concentration of nutrients than the ileum. Resection of the proximal bowel causes the ileum to receive more nutrients. Resection of the ileum, conversely, does not alter the jejunal nutrient load but may reduce stimuli from hormones released by the ileum.

Hormonal Response of the Ileum and Colon

A major advance in the understanding of intestinal adaptation has evolved with studies of the role of intestinotrophic hormones. These include growth hormone (GH) (34), insulinlike growth factor-I (IGF-I) (35), epidermal growth factor (EGF) (36), transforming growth factor-α (TGF-α) (37), and glucagon-like peptide-2 (GLP-2) (38). In mice, Drucker et al (39) showed that GLP-2 modified to reduce degradation by dipeptidyl peptidase was the most potent intestinotrophic factor. Jeppesen et al (40) showed that in normal individuals, GLP-2 levels in blood rose with a meal. In contrast, there was an absence of such a response in patients with combined ileal and colonic resection. In contrast, patients who had an ileal resection but retained colon had elevated fasting and meal-induced GLP-2 levels (41). These studies show that ileocolonic resection markedly reduces the likelihood of intestinal adaptation and causes patients with a jejunostomy to continue to have severe malabsorption. In contrast, preservation of the colon allows the remaining jejunum to adapt and helps to explain why patients with a remaining colon can often avoid permanent PN. Finally, isolated jejunal resection leaves the hormonal machinery of the ileum and colon intact.

Effect of Excluding Food from the Bowel Lumen

When food is excluded from the lumen, intestinal hypoplasia occurs in experimental animals. At the same time, body composition can be simultaneously maintained by the use of PN. These facts have been extensively documented, and the interested reader is referred to a review by Tappenden (42).

In growing or neonatal animals, PN and bowel rest maintained normal body growth but resulted in reduced bowel length and gastric and pancreatic hypoplasia (43–46). Despite the occurrence of mucosal hypoplasia, the development of disaccharidase enzymes and glucose transport was accelerated, and mucosal levels of these enzymes increased in neonatal animals receiving PN (44, 46). Hypoplasia occurred mainly in the proximal small bowel and was less evident distally (45). In adult animals, the effect of PN and bowel rest diminished mucosal mass but stimulated glucose absorption per milligram of mucosal protein (47). In addition, PN and bowel rest increased intestinal permeability (48) and altered the response to endotoxin (49).

Does the Nature of Enteral Nutrition Cause Hypoplasia?

It is not simply the lack of food but also the nature of the diet that influences mucosal bulk. In neonatal studies, mother's milk was no better than formula (45). However, refined intragastric liquid feeds caused relative hypoplasia as compared with a solid diet (43, 50).

Factors Influencing Bowel Atrophy

In general, it appears that the decreased digestive and absorptive activities of the mucosa during bowel rest are the major reasons for hypoplasia. This concept is supported by the finding that simply increasing the tonicity of the bowel contents results in an increase of the mucosal mass (51). Absorption of amino acids leads to a nonspecific increase of mucosal function and mass (52). Finally, disaccharide hydrolysis followed by absorption stimulates mucosal growth to a greater extent than equivalent monosaccharide absorption (53).

Another factor affecting the mucosa appears to be biliary-pancreatic secretion. Transplantation of the ampulla causes mucosal hypoplasia, whereas infusion of cholecystokinin and secretin stimulates mucosal growth (54, 55). SCFAs were shown to prevent or reduce mucosal atrophy in animals receiving PN and bowel rest, even when SCFAs were given parenterally (56–58). Dietary fiber is the main source of colonic fermentable substrate for SCFA production. Therefore, fiber in the diet aids the maintenance of mucosal mass, and DFD are not quite as good as a solid diet in this regard. Glutamine is a nutrient for the bowel mucosa, and the supplementation of PN with glutamine preserves gastric and colonic mass in solely PN-fed rats but does not preserve small bowel mucosal height (59).

Does Bowel Rest Induce Gut Atrophy in Humans?

In the rat, bowel rest with PN caused atrophy in days (60), but in humans, even after 21 days of bowel rest with PN, there was no change in gut hormone production after a meal (61) or any histologic atrophy (62, 63). In children, bowel rest caused atrophy only when it was prolonged beyond 9 months (63). However, investigators noted a reduction in the size of the microvilli and a fall in brush-border enzyme activity (62).

In summary, animal data suggest that when the bowel is not used, it atrophies. Mucosal atrophy results from a combination of the lack of functional stimulation and the absence of hormonal, biliary, and pancreatic secretion. In addition to food in the lumen in general, the only convincing specific nutrient trophic factors are SCFAs and perhaps glutamine. Finally, the dramatic mucosal atrophy seen in animals on bowel rest while receiving PN does not occur in humans even after a few weeks of bowel rest. Thus, few data suggest that patients receiving PN for short periods need to be fed enteral diets before introduction of a normal diet to avoid malabsorption from bowel mucosal atrophy.

SPECIFIC ASPECTS OF MANAGEMENT

Control of Gastric Hypersecretion and Motility

Reducing acid secretion improves absorption in patients with a short bowel (64). Furthermore, hypersecretion can cause nausea, reflux, and hemorrhage from severe esophageal ulceration; these effects are prevented by proton pump inhibitors (65).

Jejunal Resection with Intact Ileum and Colon

Patients in this category can be fed orally immediately and rarely have any problems.

Ileal Resection of Less than 100 cm with Colon Largely Intact

Patients in this category have so-called bile salt–induced diarrhea, and they are best helped by the administration of 4 g of cholestyramine one to three times a day to bind bile salts. Bile salts are absorbed by the ileum and are recycled. After ileal resection, bile salts remain unabsorbed and enter the colon, where they cause water secretion and diarrhea. Vitamin B_{12} absorption is also impaired in some patients.

Ileal Resection Between 100 and 200 cm with Colon Largely Intact

These patients have little difficulty in maintaining nutrition with an oral diet, but they have almost complete malabsorption of bile salts. In consequence, they have a deficiency of bile salts in the intestinal lumen because bile salt synthesis alone without recycling of bile salts through the ileum is unable to maintain an adequate concentration in the intestinal lumen. These patients have colonic water secretion resulting from entry of bile salt into the colon, as well as malabsorption of fatty acid caused by a low concentration of bile salts in the intestinal lumen. Malabsorbed fatty acids entering the colon increase water secretion. For such patients, fat restriction is mandatory. In patients with a larger resection, the bile salt pool is depleted, and cholestyramine alone is no longer able to prevent diarrhea. Parenteral vitamin B_{12} replacement is required.

Resection in Excess of 200 cm of Small Bowel and Partial Colectomy

Patients in this group require the graduated adaptation program indicated later, in the discussion of general management considerations.

Resection Leaving Less than 60 cm Small Bowel or Only Duodenum: Massive Bowel Resection

Patients in this category need home PN (HPN) indefinitely. However, many patients even in this category may show a surprising degree of adaptation. They may require less PN over time and may benefit from orally absorbed nutrients. In these patients, PN can be reduced when weight gain is excessive, and cautious reduction of HPN does not cause electrolyte imbalance and dehydration.

COMPLICATIONS

Gastric Hypersecretion and Peptic Ulceration

Gastric hypersecretion occurs immediately after intestinal resection and tends to be transient. However, peptic ulceration may occur in some patients. Treatment with histamine (H_2)-blockers and proton pump inhibitors have been found to be successful (65, 66).

Cholelithiasis

After ileal resection, the enterohepatic cycle of bile salts is interrupted. In consequence, bile salt loss occurs in excess of the ability of the liver to increase synthesis, and the bile salt concentration in bile falls. The reduction of the concentration of chenodeoxycholate in the bile increases cholesterol secretion (67). This combination makes the bile lithogenic (68). Clinically, in this situation, an increased incidence of gallstones has been observed. A study in experimental animals has shown an increased incidence of pigment stones (69).

Renal Stones

Hyperoxaluria occurs in patients with short bowel as a result of increased absorption of oxalate by the colon (70). Bile salts in the colon increase oxalate absorption (71). Hyperoxalauria is associated with renal stone formation, and the propensity to form stones is increased by reduced citrate in the urine (72). Treatment involves a low-oxalate diet, cholestyramine to bind bile salts, and use of citrate (e.g., as calcium citrate) to prevent stone formation.

D-Lactic Acidosis

In some patients with a short bowel, a syndrome of slurred speech, ataxia, and altered affect occurs in episodes (73). Superficially, the patient appears "drunk," with slurred speech, impaired gait, and so forth. The cause of this syndrome is microbial fermentation of malabsorbed carbohydrate in the colon to D-xylose with absorption of this metabolite (74). The treatment of this condition involves the use of a low-carbohydrate diet (75).

GENERAL ASPECTS OF MANAGEMENT

Control of Diarrhea

Diarrhea results from a combination of increased secretions, increased motility, and osmotic stimulation of water secretion secondary to malabsorption of luminal contents. Initially after massive bowel resection, diarrhea is controlled by keeping the patient *nil per os* (NPO) to reduce any osmotic component. Gastric hypersecretion can be controlled by the continuous infusion of appropriate doses of proton pump inhibitors. In addition, loperamide can be used to slow gastric and intestinal transit. If loperamide does not work, then codeine or phenoxylate may be tried.

Doses can be escalated as tolerated because many patients appear to have a threshold below which these agents are ineffective. Oral antidiarrheal medications must be taken 20 to 30 minutes before meals to be maximally effective.

Intravenous Fluids

In the immediate postoperative period, all patients with short bowel syndrome require intravenous fluids and electrolytes to replace losses. Sodium and potassium chloride, as well as magnesium, are the most important ions to be replaced; and plasma electrolyte levels should be monitored frequently. Fluid is infused according to measured losses and to maintain an adequate urine output. The infusion is tapered as oral intake is increased.

Strategies to Maintain Fluid and Electrolyte Balance by the Oral Route

The next consideration is to determine the nature of oral feedings. In patients who have more than 100 cm of residual jejunum, refeeding should be progressive, with a view ultimately to feeding a normal oral diet. In patients with less than 100 cm of jejunum as the only small bowel remaining, dietary intake and fluids cause increased fluid loss (18) (see Fig. 77.1). By contrast, in patients who have little small bowel left, the initial target should be small-volume isotonic feedings containing a glucose-electrolyte content similar to the oral rehydration solution (ORS) (Table 77.2). Fluid absorption has been shown to improve with increasing sodium concentration (see Fig. 77.2). In addition, to provide sufficient sodium to absorb dietary carbohydrate, it is necessary to ingest 10 to 15 g of sodium chloride as tablets with meals. Such a regimen avoids osmotic stimulation of secretion and yet stimulates the bowel to absorb (76).

Maintenance of Energy Balance

The absorption of energy is better preserved than is that of fluid and electrolytes and becomes limiting when the bowel is very short (Fig. 77.3). Comparison of Figures 77.1 and 77.3 shows that fluid and electrolyte losses become limiting when 100 cm of jejunum remains, whereas energy absorption becomes limiting when jejunal length is less than 60 to 70 cm. Hyperphagia is the key to meeting energy requirements. In a group of patients with a short bowel, the absorption of carbohydrate and fat

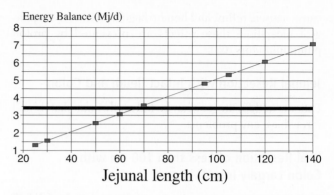

Figure 77.3. The relationship of energy absorption to length of remaining small bowel. The *dark solid line* shows the level at which energy absorption will meet the requirements of an average adult. (Reprinted with permission from Nightingale JM, Lennard-Jones JE, Walker ER et al. Jejunal efflux in short bowel syndrome. Lancet 1990;336:765–8.)

energy was about 60% of intake, whereas protein absorption was about 80% (17). Unpublished data in patients receiving HPN suggest that body weight equilibrates at an absorbed energy intake at about 32 kcal/kg/day. In a 60-kg physiologically normal person, about 1800 kcal/day will be sufficient to maintain weight. If absorption is about 60% of intake, it will be necessary to increase oral energy intake to 3000 to 4000 kcal/day to absorb about 1800 kcal/day.

Progressive feeding should be attempted, as shown in Tables 77.3 and 77.4. The diet should generally be lactose free because lactase levels in such patients are reduced (77).

Carbohydrate Versus Fat Feeding

The ability of the colon to salvage malabsorbed carbohydrate can be used to improve nutrition in patients with a short bowel who have a colon. In these patients, hyperphagia with complex carbohydrates can result in the salvage of as much as 1000 additional kilocalories (78). In contrast, in patients with a jejunostomy and no colon, a high-fat diet was as well absorbed as carbohydrate (79), and it did not result in additional loss of divalent ions. Because of its palatability and high energy density, a high-fat diet is more readily consumed.

Fat restriction has been advocated, especially in patients with a remaining colon, because malabsorbed long-chain

TABLE 77.2	COMPOSITION OF A TYPICAL ORAL REHYDRATION SOLUTION
Glucose	100 mmol/L
Sodium chloride	60 mmol/L
Sodium citrate	60 mmol/L
Magnesium (as gluconate salt)	30 mmol/d
Sodium chloride tablets with food	

TABLE 77.3	MAJOR ISSUES REGARDING ORAL INTAKE IN PATIENTS WITH A SHORT BOWEL

Bowel adaptation requires constant adjustment and individualization of the oral feeding regimen.
Avoid high-fiber, nutrient-poor foods.
Add salt to diet to make the diet "isotonic."
Restrict both hypotonic and hypertonic fluids.
Sip liquids throughout the day.
Avoid specific foods that seem to worsen diarrhea.

TABLE 77.4	ENERGY INTAKE AND THE EFFECTS OF DIETARY FAT AND CARBOHYDRATE

Encourage "hyperphagia" to compensate for malabsorption.
Avoid soluble carbohydrates: sugar and lactose.
Increase both fat and complex carbohydrate intake.
Fat slows intestinal transit time.
Fat allows intake of more energy for the same volume.
Carbohydrate is absorbed by the colon as SCFA after microbial metabolism.
Fat may cause water secretion in colon.
Unabsorbed carbohydrate and excess SCFA can cause osmotic diarrhea.

SCFA, short-chain fatty acid.

fatty acids can cause colonic water secretion and may bind divalent ions such as magnesium and calcium (80). However, in two crossover studies of patients with a short bowel with variable lengths of remaining colon, a high-fat diet was comparable to a high-carbohydrate diet with regard to total fluid, energy, nitrogen, sodium, potassium, and divalent ion absorption (11, 17). Therefore, a low-lactose diet containing high calories from both fat and complex carbohydrate and a high protein intake is recommended in most patients with a short bowel. The objective is to promote hyperphagia by making the diet palatable and acceptable. In adults who require about 30 kcal/kg/day, the aim is to increase intake gradually to about 60 kcal/kg/day to provide sufficient absorbed calories despite malabsorption. The rationale for this approach is discussed by Woolf et al (17).

Micronutrient Supplements

A summary of micronutrients that commonly require supplementation in short bowel syndrome is given in Table 77.5. Vitamin B_{12} levels should be measured, and if they are subnormal, injections of 200 to 1000 μg/month should be instituted (all patients without terminal ileum require vitamin B_{12} supplementation for life). Supplements of potassium, magnesium, and zinc are given as needed to normalized blood levels with serial

TABLE 77.5	MICRONUTRIENT SUPPLEMENTATION IN PATIENTS WITH SHORT BOWL SYNDROME

When zinc and selenium losses are high:
Zinc gluconate	100 mg/d
Selenium	60–100 μg/d

Malabsorption of fat-soluble vitamins:
Vitamin A	10,000 IU/d
Vitamin D	1,25-OH vitamin D 0.25–0.5 μg/d or ergocalciferol 50,000 IU up to several times weekly orally
Vitamin E	1,200 IU/d
Calcium gluconate	1,500 mg/d

Severe osteoporosis
  Alendronate 70 mg orally weekly; consider zoledronate 5 mg intravenously yearly

monitoring. In particular, potassium as gluconate may be added to a concentration of 12 mmol/L in the ORS. In addition, magnesium heptogluconate is especially useful as a supplement to correct hypomagnesemia without causing diarrhea. It is possible to add 30 mmol of magnesium/L of ORS to be sipped over the day.

Enteral Nutrition

Studies by McIntyre et al (79) showed that enteral feedings are not absorbed better than a solid diet in patients with a jejunostomy. However, a more recent study Joly et al (81) showed that even in patients who were studied 3 months after intestinal resection, a tube-fed polymeric diet was better absorbed than an oral diet and, when combined with an oral diet, allowed 7 of 9 patients studied to absorb enough energy and protein to become independent of PN. The difference between an oral diet and a tube-fed diet was better absorption of fat and protein but not carbohydrate, which was well absorbed from an oral diet. Hence, tube feeding or home enteral nutrition (HEN) can potentially be used in many patients to meet energy and protein intake, but it often fails to allow fluid and electrolyte balance. The fluid and electrolyte requirements make the parenteral route essential in many patients. In a large study from northern Alberta where one center provided all HEN therapy (82), only 9 out of 797 patients received HEN for a short bowel. Furthermore, of the patients receiving HEN because of gastrointestinal disorders, 82% of the 89% who survived either went back to an oral diet (77%) or were changed to PN (4.6%). Hence, tube feeding is rarely a long-term option for patients with short bowel syndrome.

Parenteral Nutrition

In patients with less than 100 cm of remaining jejunum and in those with a combined small bowel and colon resection, PN is lifesaving. PN is started in such patients within a few days of the resection, and initially, approximately 32 kcal/kg of a mixed energy substrate and 1 g/kg amino acids are infused with sodium 150 to 200 mM, potassium 60 to 100 mM, calcium 9 to 11 mM, magnesium 7 to 15 mM, and zinc 70 to 100 μmol/day. Among trace elements, zinc is the most important because large losses have been noted in patients with a high endogenous output of intestinal fluids. Oral feedings are simultaneously started, and attempts are made to reduce PN as oral feedings are increased. It will become apparent whether the patient requires PN on a long-term basis. If that is the case, then the patient should be started on a program of HPN. As the bowel adapts over months and even years, the patient requires less PN, and ultimately about 30% of patients who initially required HPN can be weaned off HPN by using up to 2 L of ORS, high-calorie diet, individualized dietary modification, and supplements of potassium, magnesium, calcium, fat-soluble vitamins, and zinc. These individuals are monitored regularly until their body weight is stable, urine output is adequate, and blood electrolytes are in balance.

Hypomagnesemia is a particularly serious problem in these patients. Ingestion of magnesium salts orally may increase diarrhea in many patients, and therefore it often becomes difficult to use magnesium supplements orally. Magnesium heptogluconate has been used successfully for this purpose. This preparation is available as a palatable liquid that is added to the ORS supplement in quantities of 30 mM/day. If this approach is not successful, then magnesium sulfate can be injected intramuscularly in doses of 12 mM one to three times a week or given intravenously to supplement the oral intake.

Vitamin supplementation needs comment. These patients can absorb water-soluble vitamins but have difficulty absorbing fat-soluble vitamins. They may require large doses of vitamin A, D, and E to maintain normal levels. In addition, pills often pass out whole in these patients; hence liquid preparations have to be used. Measurement of these vitamin levels and supplementation with aqueous preparations of vitamin A and E (Aqasol A and E) and 1,25-dihydroxy-vitamin D in doses that normalize the plasma levels are recommended. Normalization may not be possible with oral vitamins in some individuals, especially vitamin E levels. In other patients, an oral diet with intravenous fluid and electrolytes becomes necessary, and in the remainder, full PN may be required for 3 or more days weekly.

In general, patients with short bowel syndrome who require PN are best managed with the assistance of an experienced multidisciplinary nutrition support team.

HORMONE THERAPY

Somatostatin Analog

Long-acting somatostatin analog has become available and can be given subcutaneously. All studies with somatostatin analog showed a reduction in the volume of stool output and an increase in sodium or chloride absorption (83–85). However, the reduction did not seem to be sufficient to avoid PN in patients who required it (84).

Human Growth Hormone

Byrne et al (86, 87), in an observational study and subsequently in a controlled trial, found that a combination of human GH (HGH) and glutamine allowed patients with a short bowel to reduce PN. A systematic review (88) of five controlled clinical trials showed that HGH, with or without glutamine, increased body weight by 1.66 kg (confidence interval [CI], 0.69 to 2.63; $p = .0008$), lean body mass by 1.93 kg (CI, 0.97 to 2.90; $p = .0001$), energy absorption by 4.42 kcal (CI, 0.26 to 8.58; $p = .04$), and nitrogen absorption by 44 g (95% CI, 0.20 to 9.49; $p = .04$). These minor benefits were associated with a 77% incidence of

edema and a 32% incidence of carpel tunnel syndrome. Although all studies showed significant weight gain, only one showed a significant increase in absorption. Hence, HGH seemed to benefit patients mainly by its well-known somatotrophic effect instead of by significantly improving absorption. Furthermore, significant side effects were associated with the use of HGH.

Glucagon-like Peptide-2 Analog

Multicenter, double-blind randomized controlled trials have been completed on the efficacy of daily subcutaneous injections of an analog of GLP-2 that is resistant to enzymatic degradation by enzyme dipeptidyl peptidase IV (89, 90). Results show that this agent appears safe, improves nutrient absorption, and modestly, but significantly, decreases the need for PN in patients with short bowel syndrome who previously required stable PN (89, 90).

ROLE OF INTESTINAL TRANSPLANTATION

HPN is associated with complications that include progressive steatohepatitis resulting in cirrhosis and liver failure (91, 92), catheter-related complications, repeated sepsis, and an inability to cope with the regimen of HPN (91–95). These complications can result in failure of HPN and progressive malnutrition. Under these circumstances, the only alternative is intestinal transplantation (IT). In theory, IT is the ideal solution for the treatment of intestinal failure. The patient who has had an IT can eat and enjoy normal food, does not need complicated machinery to deliver intravenous nutrition, and will avoid the previously mentioned complications of HPN and have an improved quality of life (96). In practice, published data show that the rates of survival at 3 years and at 5 years in PN-dependent patients remain approximately 70% and 63%, respectively, in various series; death is caused by sepsis, rejection, and lymphoma (96–101).

Five-year survival on HPN depends on the primary diagnosis and can be as high as 82% for Crohn disease, a rate that compares unfavorably with 5-year survival for IT (96). Conversely, the rate is about the same as for IT in patients with ischemic bowel and radiation enteritis. However, even in the latter group of patients and in those with pseudo-obstruction, patients receiving HPN who live beyond 3 years (~35% to 40% of the original cohort) have a very long survival over 10 to 15 years of observation (96). Although patient survival at 10 years after IT is about the same (43%), graft survival is much lower, a finding suggesting that HPN in general may still have a better long-term outcome (94). In contrast, although patients who undergo IT do well initially, they have a higher long-term mortality, but the survival rate is continuously improving (96, 101).

When faced with a patient having IT, what should the physician recommend? HPN as primary therapy, IT as primary therapy, or HPN followed by IT if HPN is a failure? The answer to the question is not straightforward because outcome with HPN depends on many factors. These include the primary disease that has resulted in intestinal failure, the age of the patient, the patient's ability to care for the catheter, the length of the surviving bowel, support for the patient, acceptance of HPN by the patient, and narcotic dependence (101). Furthermore, even after years of HPN, many patients can adapt and potentially be weaned off HPN (87). Hence, premature IT may introduce an irreversible procedure in a person who may have recovered spontaneously. The success of IT also depends on pretransplant status, treatment center size, immunosuppressive regimen, and transplant type (isolated intestine, intestine-liver, multivisceral) (96–101).

To give a firm recommendation in an individual patient about HPN or IT, physicians need studies in which all these factors have to be considered in interpreting the outcome or one or the other procedure. At the present time, based on the recommendation by Medicare and Medicaid, the initial therapy for intestinal failure is HPN; and IT is recommended when HPN fails, as defined by the following conditions (101):

1. Impending or overt liver failure secondary to liver injury from PN
2. Thrombosis of two or more central veins
3. Two or more episodes per year of catheter-related systemic sepsis requiring hospitalization
4. A single episode of line-related fungemia, septic shock, or acute respiratory distress syndrome
5. Frequent episodes of severe dehydration despite intravenous fluid in addition to HPN

Other factors to be considered, according to the American Society of Transplantation, include the following:

1. High risk of death attributable to the underlying disease
2. Ultrashort bowel syndrome (gastrostomy, duodenostomy, residual small bowel <10 cm in infants and <20 cm in adults)
3. Intestinal failure with frequent hospitalization, narcotic dependency, or pseudo-obstruction
4. The patient's unwillingness to accept long-term HPN

The contraindications for IT are similar to those in patients eligible for solid organ transplantation. The unanswered question is whether these recommendations promote the best outcome, given that these recommendations were based on retrospective data and expert opinion. In an effort to determine the impact of these recommendations, Pironi et al (102) reported a prospective 5-year study comparing 389 noncandidates for IT and 156 candidates for IT from patients receiving HPN in Europe. Results showed a survival rate of 87% in non-IT candidates, 73% in IT candidates with HPN failure, 84% in those with high-risk underlying disease, 100% in those with high morbidity

intestinal failure, and 54% in IT recipients ($p < .001$). The primary cause of death in patients receiving HPN was the underlying disease in those with HPN duration of 2 years or less and HPN-related conditions in those with an HPN duration of more than 2 years ($p = .006$).

In IT candidates, the death rates were significantly increased in patients with desmoids or liver failure compared with noncandidates (102). In IT candidates who died, the indications for IT were the causes of death in 92% of those with desmoids or liver failure and in 38% of those with other indications ($p = .041$). In IT candidates with catheter-related complications or ultrashort bowel, the survival rate was similar in those who remained on HPN and did not receive IT versus the rate after IT (83% versus 78%; not significant). The authors concluded that (a) HPN is the primary treatment for intestinal failure; (b) desmoid tumors and HPN-related liver failure constitute indications for lifesaving IT; (c) catheter-related complications and ultrashort bowel may be primary indications for IT; and (d) in the early years after initiating HPN, lifesaving IT could be required for some patients at higher risk of death from their underlying disease (102). These observations, taken together, suggest that IT may most likely benefit patients with liver disease and central venous catheter–related thrombosis or sepsis and the small number of patients with desmoid tumors as a cause of intestinal failure.

In summary, the short bowel syndrome is a complex and variable condition that clinically can range from mild, as seen following terminal ileal resection, to a very debilitating condition, following total ileal and colonic resection with an end-jejunostomy. The management varies with the extent and site of resection and the adaptation of the remaining bowel. Complex patients require management by a multidisciplinary team that should include expertise in specialized enteral nutrition and PN support.

REFERENCES

1. O'Keefe SJ, Buchman AL, Fishbein TM. Clin Gastroenterol Hepatol 2006;4:6–10.
2. Malagelada JR. Gastric, pancreatic and biliary response to a meal. In: Johnson JR, ed. Physiology of the Gastrointestinal Tract. New York: Raven Press, 1981.
3. Summers RW, Kent TH, Osborne JW. Gastroenterology 1970; 59:731–9.
4. Ricotta J, Zuidema GD, Gadacz TR et al. Surg Gynecol Obstet 1981;152:310–4.
5. Fordtran JS, Locklear TW. Am J Dig Dis 1966;11:503–21.
6. Powell DW. Intestinal water and electrolyte transport. In: Johnson LR, ed. Physiology of the Gastrointestinal Tract. 2nd ed. New York: Raven Press, 1987.
7. Binder HJ, Mehta P. Gastroenterology 1989;96:989–96.
8. Royall D, Wolever TMS, Jeejeebhoy KN. Am J Gastroenterol 1992;87:751–6.
9. Nylander G. Acta Chir Scand 1967;133:131–8.
10. Reynell PC, Spray GH. Gastroenterology 1956;31:361–8.
11. Woolf GM, Miller C, Kurian R et al. Gastroenterology 1983; 84:823–8.

12. Cummings JH, James WPT, Wiggins HS. Lancet 1973;1: 344–7.

13. Booth CC, Aldis D, Read AE. Gut 1961;2:168–74.

14. Hoffman AF, Poley JR. Gastroenterology 1972;62:918–34.

15. Hylander E, Ladefoged K, Jarnum S. Scand J Gastroenterol 1980;15:853–8.

16. Ladefoged K, Nicolaidou P, Jarnum S. Am J Clin Nutr 1980;33:2137–44.

17. Woolf GM, Miller C, Kurian R et al. Dig Dis Sci 1987;32: 8–15.

18. Nightingale JM, Lennard-Jones JE, Walker ER et al. Lancet 1990;336:765–8.

19. Haymond HE. Surg Gynecol Obstet 1953;61:693–705.

20. McClenahan JE, Fisher B. Am J Surg 1950;79:684–8.

21. Trafford HS. Br J Surg 1956;44:10–13.

22. West ES, Montague JR, Judy FR. Am J Dig Dis 1938;5: 690–2.

23. Pilling GP, Cresson SL. Pediatrics 1957;19:940–8.

24. Martin JR, Patee CJ, Gardner C et al. Can Med Assoc J 1953; 69:429–33.

25. Kinney JM, Goldwyn RM, Barr JS et al. JAMA 1962;179: 529–32.

26. Walker-Smith J. Med J Aust 1967;1:857–60.

27. Clayton BE, Cotton DA. Gut 1961;2:18–22.

28. Anderson CM. Br Med J 1965;5432:419–22.

29. Meyer HW. Surgery 1962;51:755–9.

30. Flint JM. Johns Hopkins Med J 1912;23:127–44.

31. Porus RL. Gastroenterology 1965;48:753–7.

32. Booth CC, Evans KT, Menzies T et al. Br J Surg 1959;46: 403–10.

33. Althausen TL, Doig RK, Uyeyama K et al. Gastroenterology 1950;16:126–39.

34. Yeh KY, Moog F. Dev Biol 1975;472:156–72.

35. Winesett DE, Ulshen MH, Hoyt EC et al. Am J Physiol 1995;268:G631–40.

36. Ulshen MH, Raasch RH. Clin Sci (Lond) 1996;90:427–31.

37. Potten CS, Owen G, Hewitt D et al. Gut 1995;36:864–73.

38. Drucker DJ, Ehrlich P, Asa SL et al. Proc Natl Acad Sci U S A 1996;93:7911–16.

39. Drucker DJ, DeForest L, Brubaker PL. Am J Physiol 1997; 273:G1252–62.

40. Jeppesen PB, Hartmann B, Hansen BS et al. Gut 1999;45: 559–63.

41. Jeppesen PB, Hartmann B, Thulesen J et al. Gut 2000;47: 370–6.

42. Tappenden KA. Gastroenterology 2006;130(Suppl 1):S93–9.

43. Goldstein RM, Hebiguchi T, Luk G et al. J Pediatr Surg 1985; 20:785–91.

44. Shulman RJ. Gastroenterology 1988;95:85–92.

45. Morgan W, Yardley J, Luk G et al. Pediatr Surg 1987;22: 541–5.

46. Gall DG, Chung M, O'Laughlin EV et al. Biol Neonate 1987;51:286–96.

47. Kolter DP, Levine GM, Shiau YF. Am J Physiol 1981;240: 432–36.

48. Purandare S, Offenbartl K, Westrom B et al. Scand J Gastroenterol 1989;24:678–82.

49. Fong YM, Marano MA, Barber A et al. Ann Surg 1989; 210:449–56.

50. Hosoda N, Nishi M, Nakagawa M et al. J Surg Res 1989; 47:129–33.

51. Weser E, Babbitt J, Vandeventer A. Dig Dis Sci 1985;30: 675–81.

52. Levine GM. Gastroenterology 1986;91:49–55.

53. Weser E, Babbit J, Vandeventer A. Gastroenterology 1986; 91:521–7.

54. Hughes CA, Bates T, Dowling RH. Gastroenterology 1978; 75:34–41.

55. Weser E, Bell D, Tawil T. Dig Dis Sci 26:1981;409–16.

56. Koruda MJ, Rolandelli RH, Bliss DZ et al. Am J Clin Nutr 1990;51:685–9.

57. Koruda MJ, Rolandelli RH, Settle RG et al. Gastroenterology 1988;95:715–20.

58. Kripke SA, Fox AD, Berman JM. J Surg Res 1988;44:436–44.

59. Grant JP, Snyder PJ. J Surg Res 1988;44:506–13.

60. Hughes CA, Prince A, Dowling RH. Clin Sci 1980;59:329–36.

61. Greenberg GR, Wolman SL, Cristofides ND et al. Gastroenterology 1981;80:988–93.

62. Guedon C, Schmitz J, Lerebours E et al. Gastroenterology 1986;90:373–78.

63. Rossi TM, Lee PC, Young C et al. Dig Dis Sci 1993;38: 1608–13.

64. Cortot A, Fleming CR, Malagelada JR. N Engl J Med 1979; 300:79–80.

65. Tang SJ, Jose M. Nieto JM et al. J Clin Gastroenterol 2002; 34:62–3.

66. Murphy JP Jr, King DR, Dubois A. N Engl J Med 1979;300: 80–1.

67. Jeejeebhoy KN. Trop Gastroenterol 2010;31:244–8.

68. Roslyn JJ, Pitt HA, Mann LL. Gastroenterology 1983;84: 148–54.

69. Pitt HA, Lewinski MA, Muller EL et al. Surgery 1984;96: 154–62.

70. Dobbins JW, Binder HJ. N Engl J Med 1977;296:298–301.

71. Chadwick VS, Gaginella TS, Carlson GL et al. J Lab Clin Med 1979;94:661–74.

72. Pak CYC, Peterson R, Sakhaee K et al. Am J Med 1985;79: 284–8.

73. Traube M, Bock JL, Boyer JL. Ann Intern Med 1983;98: 171–3.

74. Satoh T, Narisawa K, Konno T et al. Eur J Pediatr 1982;138:324–6.

75. Ramakrishnan T, Stokes P. JPEN J Parenter Enteral Nutr 1985;9:361–3.

76. Griffin GE, Fagan EF, Hodgson AJ. Dig Dis Sci 1982;27: 902–8.

77. Richards AJ, Condon JR, Mallinson CN. Br J Surg 1971;58:493–4.

78. Nordgaard I, Hansen BS, Mortensen PB. Lancet 1994;343: 373–6.

79. McIntyre PB, Fitchew M, Lennard-Jones JE. Gastroenterology 1986;91:25–33.

80. Ovesen L, Chu R, Howard L. Am J Clin Nutr 1983;38: 823–8.

81. Joly F, Dray X, Corcos O et al. Gastroenterology 2009;136: 824–31.

82. Cawsey SI, Soo J, Gramlich LM. Nutr Clin Pract 2010;25: 296–300.

83. Rodrigues CA, Lennard-Jones JE, Thompson DG et al. Aliment Pharmacol Ther 1989;3:159–69.

84. Ladefoged K, Christensen KC, Hegnhoj J et al. Gut 1989;30: 943–9.

85. Dharmsathaphorn K, Gorelick FS, Sherwin RS et al. J Clin Gastroenterol 1982;4:521–4.

86. Byrne TA, Persinger RL, Young LS et al. Ann Surg 1995; 222:243–55.

87. Byrne TA, Wilmore DW, Iyer K et al. Ann Surg 2005;242: 655–61.

88. Wales PW, Nasr A, de Silva N et al. Cochrane Database Syst Rev 2010;(6):CD006321.

89. Jeppesen PB, Gilroy R, Pertkiewicz M et al. Gut 2011;60: 902–14.

90. Vipperla K, O'Keefe SJ. Expert Rev Gastroenterol Hepatol 2011;5:665–78.

91. Bowyer BA, Fleming CR, Ludwig J et al. JPEN J Parenter Enteral Nutr 1985;9:11–17.

92. Cavicchi M, Beau P, Crenn P et al. Ann Intern Med 2000;132:525–32.

93. Howard L. Gastroenterology 2006;130(Suppl 1):S52–9.

94. Messing B, Lemann M, Landais P et al. Gastroenterology 1995;108:1005–10.

95. MacRitchie KJ. Can Psychiatr Assoc J 1978;23:373–9.

96. O'Keefe SJ, Emerling M, Koritsky D et al. Am J Gastroenterol 2007;102:1093–100.

97. Freeman RB, Steffick DE, Guidinger MK et al. Am J Transplant 2008;8:958–76.

98. Jeejeebhoy K, Allard J, Gramlich L. Home parenteral nutrition in Canada. In: Bozetti F, Staun M, Van Gossum A, eds. Home Parenteral Nutrition. Cambridge, MA: CAB International, 2006:36–42.

99. Grant DW, Shah SA. Results of intestinal transplantation. In: Langnas AN, Goulet O, Quigley EMM, Tappenden KA, eds. Intestinal Failure. Malden, MA: Blackwell, 2008: 349–56.

100. DeLegge M, Alsolaiman MM, Barbour E et al. Dig Dis Sci 2007;52:876–92.

101. Fishbein TM. N Engl J Med 2009;361:998–1008.

102. Pironi L, Joly F, Forbes A et al. Gut 2011;60:17–25.

SUGGESTED READINGS

Fishbein TM. Intestinal transplantation. N Engl J Med 2009;361: 998–1008.

Howard L. Home parenteral nutrition: survival, cost, and quality of life. Gastroenterology 2006;130(Suppl 1):S52–9.

Nordgaard I, Hansen BS, Mortensen PB. Colon as a digestive organ in patients with short bowel. Lancet 1994;343:373–6.

O'Keefe SJ, Buchman AL, Fishbein TM et al. Short bowel syndrome and intestinal failure: consensus definitions and overview. Clin Gastroenterol Hepatol 2006;4:6–10.

Woolf GM, Miller C, Kurian R et al. Diet for patients with a short bowel: high fat or high carbohydrate? Gastroenterology 1983;84:823–8.

78 | NUTRITION IN INFLAMMATORY BOWEL DISEASE: IMPLICATIONS FOR ITS ROLE IN THE MANAGEMENT OF CROHN DISEASE AND ULCERATIVE COLITIS[1]

GERALD W. DRYDEN AND DOUGLAS L. SEIDNER

Maintenance of human health requires the continuous ingestion of nutrients coupled with their appropriate digestion and assimilation, both of which require an appropriately functioning digestive tract. Many human diseases interfere with normal digestion. However, disruptions are particularly prominent in inflammatory conditions of the intestinal tract such as Crohn disease (CD) and ulcerative colitis (UC), collectively known as inflammatory bowel disease (IBD). Nutrition plays three roles in IBD: instigator, victim, and healer. This chapter explores ways in which nutritional support benefits patients with IBD; but to understand the crucial role nutrition plays in IBD, the interplay of nutrition with host and environmental factors associated with the development of IBD are examined first.

---

[1]**Abbreviations: AA**, arachidonic acid; **ALA**, α-linoleic acid; **CD**, Crohn disease; **CI**, confidence interval; **DC**, dendritic cell; **DHA**, docosahexaenoic acid; **ECN**, *Escherichia coli* Nissle 1917; **EPA**, eicosapentaenoic acid; **FA**, fatty acid; **FD**, free diet; **GBF**, germinated barley foodstuff; **half-ED**, half-elemental diet; **HLA**, human leukocyte antigen; **IBD**, inflammatory bowel disease; **LA**, linoleic acid; **LTB₄**, leukotriene B$_4$; **OR**, odds ratio; **PEM**, protein-energy malnutrition; **PGE₂**, prostaglandin E$_2$; **PO**, *Plantago ovata*; **RDBPC**, randomized, double-blind, placebo-controlled; **SCFA**, short-chain fatty acid; **TEN**, total enteral nutrition; **TPN**, total parenteral nutrition; **UC**, ulcerative colitis; **WD**, Western diet.

ROLE OF NUTRITION IN THE ETIOLOGY OF INFLAMMATORY BOWEL DISEASE

CD and UC share a common physiologic basis: loss of tolerance to intestinal bacteria. Germ-free animals susceptible to IBD remain inflammation free until exposed to bacteria. However, humans must coexist with their gut flora for many reasons: food digestion, vitamin K production, and pathogen protection, to name a few. Loss of tolerance to one's own flora arises from a triad of factors. First, a genetic mutation encodes susceptibility. More than 70 loci have been identified for CD (1). Second, a trigger is required to initiate inflammation. A breakdown in tolerance against the ever-present intestinal flora ensues. One well-characterized gene involved in CD susceptibility, nucleotide-binding oligomerization domain containing (NOD)-2, encodes for a bacterial defense peptide prominently expressed in ileal mucosa, the site most highly affected in CD (2, 3). However, genetic mutations alone cannot explain the rapid rise in world IBD cases over the past five or six decades (4, 5). Various hypothetical mechanisms listed in Table 78.1 provide potential explanations for the phenomenon of the rapid worldwide expansion of IBD cases (6, 7).

Diet as a Susceptibility Factor

Dietary habits typified as the Western diet (WD) offer one plausible mechanism for transforming IBD into an equal opportunity disease. These food choices, combined with preexisting genetic susceptibilities, could induce rapid proliferation of IBD. For instance, Japan has seen a significant rise in cases of IBD over the past three decades (4). This rise followed large-scale, rapid dietary changes undertaken by the Japanese population. Total calories consumed in the form of fat and animal proteins rose dramatically, displacing rice consumption. Changes in dietary intake have been linked to rising incidence rates for both CD and UC (8, 9).

Univariate analysis in one study implicated rising CD rates with total fat intake, animal fat and protein intake, and a change in the ratio of ω-6 to ω-3 fatty acid (FA) intake, whereas multivariate analysis pointed to increased animal protein intake as the strongest influence associated with new IBD cases (9). Several other studies identified

TABLE 78.1	THEORIES FOR THE RAPID SPREAD OF INFLAMMATORY BOWEL DISEASE

Spread of Western diet
Hygiene hypothesis
Cold-chain hypothesis

individual food choices as risk factors; in particular, refined sugars, fatty foods, and fast food all enhance development of both UC and CD (8, 10), whereas vegetables protect against UC but increase CD risk (8).

As an alternative explanation to an individual's food choices, the cold-chain hypothesis uniquely links systemwide changes in food consumption to the expansion of IBD cases to the rise of commercial refrigeration (11). Post–World War II economic prosperity made the refrigerator widely available. Refrigeration quickly transformed food consumption from a pattern of daily use of perishables to a dependence on long-term refrigerated storage. Support for this theory rests on identification of organisms that thrive at (near)-freezing temperatures. Some psychotropes (*Yersinia* and *Legionella*) are associated with IBD-like infections of the gut (12). These data demonstrate that food choices likely play a role in IBD susceptibility, but elimination of individual food items will not likely alter disease course. However, nutrition still can play a significant therapeutic role in IBD.

Roles of Nutrition

IBD therapy optimally induces rapid disease remission, maintains that remission, and improves quality of life (13). Nutritional therapy can fulfill these goals as a primary IBD intervention. Primary nutrition therapy for IBD traditionally has referred to either total parenteral nutrition (TPN) or total enteral nutrition (TEN). However, the concept of nutritional therapy has broadened to include other tools for an IBD treatment plan, including interventions to alter intestinal epithelial function, enhance enteric flora, or reduce intestinal epithelial inflammation. These options provide clinicians multiple choices for providing therapeutically sound nutritional prescriptions to patients with IBD.

Nutritional Status of Patients with Inflammatory Bowel Disease

Protein-energy malnutrition (PEM)—an imbalance between the body's demand for nutrients, the energy requirements for normal growth and homeostasis, and the available supply of nutrients (14)—is the most common form of malnutrition in patients with IBD, particularly CD (15). Up to 75% of hospitalized CD patients exhibit PEM evidenced by excessive weight loss and hypoalbuminemia (16), whereas up to 50% of outpatient CD patients weigh less than normal, even in remission (17).

TABLE 78.2	MICRONUTRIENTS COMMONLY AFFECTED BY INFLAMMATORY BOWEL DISEASE

	FREQUENCY OF DEFICIENCY		
		ADULT	
MICRONUTRIENT	PEDIATRIC	CD	UC
Water Soluble			
Iron	17%	39%	81%
Zinc	No data	50%	No data
Folate	0%–2%	67%	30%–40%
Vitamin B$_{12}$	0%	48%	5%
Fat Soluble			
Vitamin A	14%	11%	No data
Vitamin D	16%–35%	75%	35%
Vitamin E	6%	No data	No data
Vitamin K	No data	No data	No data

CD, Crohn disease; UC, ulcerative colitis.

Data from Mallon DP, Suskind DL. Nutrition in pediatric inflammatory bowel disease. Nutr Clin Pract 2010;25:335–9; Vagianos K, Bector S, McConnell J et al. Nutrition assessment of patients with inflammatory bowel disease. JPEN J Parenter Enteral Nutr 2007;31:311–9, with permission.

Multiple IBD-related factors contribute to PEM, including mucosal disease–related nutrient malabsorption/loss, systemic cytokine-driven increases in metabolic requirements, and restricted oral intake for controlling diarrhea and abdominal pain related to small bowel strictures. Patients with IBD also exhibit many vitamin and mineral deficiencies (Table 78.2) (16). Although iron deficiency is more commonly found in UC (up to 81%) than in CD, this form of anemia is common in both disease states, affecting at least two thirds of patients. Anemia from folate or vitamin B$_{12}$ deficiencies is more likely in CD (16). Medications used to treat IBD also play a significant role in exacerbating nutrient deficiencies through a variety of mechanisms (Table 78.3). In addition to macronutrient therapy, targeted micronutrient supplementation is often necessary to replete specific deficiencies acquired in the course of IBD (see Table 78.2) (18, 19).

TABLE 78.3	MEDICATION-ASSOCIATED NUTRIENT EFFECTS IN INFLAMMATORY BOWEL DISEASE

DRUG	NUTRIENT AFFECTED	MECHANISM
Sulfasalazine	Folate	Competitive inhibition of jejunal folate conjugation enzyme
Corticosteroids	Calcium	Steroids suppress calcium absorption by small bowel, increase urinary excretion
Cholestyramine	Fat, calcium, fat-soluble vitamins	Impair absorption of fat by bile sequestration
6-Mercaptopurine/ azathioprine	General caloric intake	Can induce nausea, vomiting, dyspepsia

NUTRITION-BASED THERAPY FOR INFLAMMATORY BOWEL DISEASE

Total Parenteral Nutrition

Complete dietary replacement with TPN has the longest history of nutrition therapy for IBD, and likely works by eliminating antigenic stimuli from intact food molecules, altering intestinal bacteria, and removing large, nondigestible food components, which generate obstructive symptoms at intestinal strictures. Introduced as primary or adjunctive therapy for severe cases of IBD in the 1960s (20, 21), early studies were plagued by inconsistent disease activity measurements, clinical end points, and limitations on concomitant steroids (22, 23). Regardless, TPN appeared to induce CD remission effectively (65% to 100%) but rarely maintained it (0% to 33%) (24, 25). In addition, long-term TPN can be complicated by line sepsis, access problems, cholestasis, and high cost. TPN results for UC are less impressive, with lower remission rates (27% to 58%) and abysmal maintenance rates (0% to 15%) (24, 26, 27).

The days heralding TPN as a long-term primary treatment for IBD have passed (23), because poor efficacy, high cost, and frequent side effects prompt evidence-based guidelines currently to not recommend TPN as a primary treatment for IBD (28). There may be a role for supplemental parenteral nutrition or TPN as a short-term adjunctive approach to replete micronutrients and provide macronutrients for anabolism when the patient is hospitalized for an acute IBD flare and otherwise consuming minimal or no enteral nutrients orally or cannot tolerate liquid nutrient formulations, but such a practice is not currently evidence based. These circumstances pertain to the management of patients with short gut, prolonged ileus or obstruction, or postoperative fistulas from anastomotic leaks. In these cases, TPN may help to prevent severe malnutrition, particularly in already malnourished patients who may require elective surgery, including further bowel resection resulting from refractory IBD.

Total Enteral Nutrition

In contrast to the foregoing, over time evidence has mounted for the benefits of TEN for the treatment of active IBD. TEN replaces a patient's caloric and nutrient intake with a processed liquid nutritional supplement administered by mouth or feeding tube. TEN theoretically prevents small bowel mucosal villous atrophy from long-term bowel rest, maintains epithelial integrity, and reduces intestinal immune system activation.

The first randomized, controlled clinical trial demonstrated that TEN could achieve remission as frequently as corticosteroids (29), but several small, follow-on studies produced conflicting results. A well-executed metaanalysis clarified the situation. For induction of clinical remission, the odds ratio (OR) for steroid therapy versus TEN was 0.35 (95% confidence interval [CI], 0.23 to 0.53), indicating short-term superiority of steroid therapy, but not at 1 year (OR, 0.97; 95% CI, 0.31 to 3.00) (30). Unfortunately, poor patient compliance with long-term TEN complicates this form of therapy, at least in adult populations.

Compliance rates vary greatly among adult patients with CD from country to country. Although patients in the United States rarely accept long-term TEN, this approach is an important first-line therapy for both inducing and maintaining CD remission in Japan (31, 32). Similarly, European guidelines promote TEN for adults with active CD complicated by effects of steroids, as supplemental TEN for undernourished children with CD, or as first-line therapy for children with active CD to induce remission (33).

The percentage of calorie intake from TEN influences success. Consumption of greater than or equal to 900 kcal/day of TEN resulted in lower hospitalization rates compared with subjects receiving fewer calories (32). This effect was most noticeable in patients with ileitis. A "half-elemental" diet (half-ED) has also been evaluated for maintaining CD remission (34). Patients in remission by TEN, prednisolone, induction infliximab, or surgery were randomized to half-ED (900 to 1200 kcal) or free diet (FD) and evaluated for relapse over a 2-year follow-up period. Patients in the half-ED group recurred less frequently (35%) than patients in the FD group (64%; CI = 0.16 to 0.98) (34).

When examined in aggregate as a primary therapy, TEN induces remission almost as effectively as corticosteroid therapy, without steroid-related side effects. TEN can be administered via tube or mouth, in elemental or semielemental form, and can be continued on a long-term basis to maintain CD remission induced by all standard methods. In pediatrics, EN improves growth velocity hampered by corticosteroid therapy (35). However, cultural preferences, palatability, feeding tube aversion, and cost hinder widespread use of TEN in the United States.

NUTRITION SUPPLEMENTS FOR INFLAMMATORY BOWEL DISEASE

Probiotics

Basis for Efficacy

Acceptance of unregulated supplements, such as prebiotics and probiotics or other bioactive substances, is high among US patients with IBD. One of the most popular nutritional supplements with patients with IBD today, the use of "beneficial" bacteria for health was first advocated by Elie Metchnikoff in the early twentieth century (36). Given the central role bacteria play in IBD, strategies to enhance anti-inflammatory bacterial populations provide an attractive alternative to pharmacologic therapy. To this point, germ-free human leukocyte antigen (HLA)-B27 transgenic rats exhibit no demonstrable colitis (37). However, animals exposed to single strains or combinations of bacteria develop cecal inflammation.

To evaluate the role of a common probiotic organism in intestinal inflammation, germ-free HLA-B27 rats were monoassociated with *Bacteroides vulgates, Escherichia coli,* or a mixture of bacteria from a CD patient (37). Rats monoassociated with either the bacterial mixture or *B. vulgates* developed cecal inflammation, whereas rats monoassociated with *E. coli* exhibited no significant inflammation. Later, specific pathogen free HLA-B27 transgenic rats were monoassociated with *Bacteroides vulgates* and one of two strains of *Lactobacillus.* Neither *Lactobacilli* species prevented colitis, but when animals received antibiotics after monoassociation, the probiotic *Lactobacillus* GG (LGG) prevented recurrent colitis (38).

These and other studies suggest that probiotics modulate intestinal inflammation via multiple mechanisms. First, they inhibit pathogen growth. This may improve the dysbiosis affecting IBD patients, characterized by deficiencies in favorable bacteria such as *Bacteroides, Bifidobacteria,* and *Lactobacillus* spp., or excessive detrimental bacteria, such as epithelium-associated *E. coli* (39–41). Alternatively, probiotics may impact intestinal flora by releasing antibacterial peptides or displacing toxins or pathogens from intestinal binding sites. One class of antibacterial proteins secreted by Gram-positive bacteria, the lantibiotics, intercalate into the cell wall of pathogenic bacteria by means of a specific lipid component (42). The other class of antibacterial proteins, secreted mainly by *Lactobacilli,* disrupts cell membranes of target bacteria as well as critical intracellular processes (43). Probiotics such as *Lactobacilli* also control pathogenic species by secreting acetic, propionic, and lactic acids (44). These acids decrease pH levels in the local environment, effectively inhibiting pathogenic organisms such as *Salmonella* (45).

Next, probiotics improve mucosal health and integrity. Epithelial barrier integrity is enhanced by *E. coli* Nissle 1917 (ECN) via a bolstering of tight junction complexes (46). Other probiotics reduce intestinal permeability by counteracting the effects of proinflammatory cytokines on epithelial integrity (47–49). Finally, they regulate intestinal immune responses. M-cells lining the intestinal mucosa take up probiotics for processing by dendritic cells (DCs) and subsequent presentation to T and B cells (50, 51). This interaction stimulates secretory IgA production, which in turn enhances the efficacy of the unstirred water layer to repel pathogens (51, 52). Probiotic organisms possess the ability to polarize DCs to express anti-inflammatory cytokines (53, 54). Both *Lactobacillus acidophilus* and *Lactobacillus salivarius* enhance anti-inflammatory regulatory T-cell activity (55), whereas other probiotic organisms actually augment T-helper cell (Th1) immunity against pathogenic organisms. The host immune system can differentiate structural differences between probiotic- and pathogen-derived Toll-like receptor-4 (TLR-4) agonists (56). Unfortunately, despite all the basic science data supporting the use of probiotics for IBD, evidence for a clinical benefit from probiotics has been found lacking.

Probiotic Clinical Trials for Ulcerative Colitis

Reflecting a general enthusiasm for the concept of probiotic therapy for IBD, disproportionately large numbers of review articles have been published on the handful of published probiotic clinical trials. The first clinical trial investigating the role of a probiotic organism in IBD compared ECN (2.5 to 25×10^9 CFU) with 1.5 g mesalamine/day to maintain remission in patients with UC, with no significant difference between relapse rates (56). In another study, patients in remission from mildly, moderately, or severely active colitis were randomized to either oral mesalamine (1.2 g/day) or ECN (5×10^5 viable bacteria twice daily) (57). Similar remission rates were observed for maintenance mesalamine and probiotic (73% and 67%, respectively, $p = .006$) (57).

A much larger maintenance trial comparing ECN with 1.5 g/day mesalamine also documented comparable relapse rates (64% and 67%, respectively, $p = .003$) (58). When 3 different doses of ECN enemas were compared with placebo for induction of remission, the highest dose of 40 mL achieved a 53% remission rate (59). This dose-dependent effect was confirmed in a subsequent study of 90 subjects with mild to moderate UC, with remission rates 52.9% (40 mL), 44.4% (20 mL), 27.3% (10 mL), and 18.2% (placebo) (60).

Another common probiotic agent used in UC trials, VSL#3, also has been used to treat mild-to-moderate UC. An open-label study evaluated VSL#3 (3 g/day) in combination with low-dose balsalazide (2.25 g/day), compared with a moderate dose of balsalazide (4.5 g/day) or mesalazine (2.4 g/day) alone (61). Combination therapy proved to be most effective in inducing 8-week remission, as 85.7% of VSL#3/balsalazide subjects achieved remission versus 80.8% receiving balsalazide or 70% receiving mesalazine alone ($p < .02$). A second open-label study administered VSL#3 twice daily for 6 weeks in 34 patients with mild to moderately active UC, achieving a combined remission/response rate of 77% (62).

A larger, randomized, double-blind, placebo-controlled (RDBPC) evaluation of VSL#3 or placebo administered twice daily to patients with mild-to-moderate UC demonstrated that 32.5% of VSL#3 treated patients attained the primary end point of a decrease of less than 50% from their baseline UC Disease Activity Index score, compared with only 10% of those receiving placebo ($p = .001$) (63). The beneficial effects of VSL#3 also carry over to pediatric patients with UC.

In an RDBPC induction and remission study, either VSL#3 or placebo was added to a standard induction regimen of oral methylprednisolone 1 mg/kg/day plus oral mesalamine 50 mg/kg/day in newly diagnosed patients (64). Subjects receiving VSL3# in combination with standard induction therapy were more likely to achieve remission (92.8%) than subjects receiving standard therapy alone (36.4%) ($p < .001$). A significantly higher percentage of patients treated with mesalamine therapy only

(73.3%) flared within 12 months than those treated with VSL#3 plus mesalamine (21.4%, $p = .014$) (64). In contrast, two studies involving other probiotic organisms were unable to establish an effect on maintenance of remission (65, 66).

Probiotic Clinical Trials for Pouchitis

Studies also have been conducted in the setting of pouchitis. Pouchitis commonly occurs in patients with UC who have undergone total proctocolectomy with ileal pouch anastomosis. When *Lactobacillus* GG (LGG 0.5 to 1×10^{10} CFU/capsule) or placebo was administered as primary therapy for active pouchitis twice daily versus placebo for 3 months, no difference was noted (67). The administration of a fermented milk product containing *Lactobacilli* and *Bifidobacteria* to 41 patients with UC for 4 weeks in open-label fashion produced an endoscopic improvement (68), whereas a second study evaluating this product in 69 patients (51 of whom underwent pouch surgery for UC) only demonstrated improvement in subjects with UC (69). In contrast to the failures as a primary therapy for pouchitis, probiotics have established a more robust record for maintaining remission of medically induced pouchitis. Two RDBPC trials with VSL#3 provided to patients with antibiotic-induced remission demonstrated a highly beneficial outcome (70, 71). Also intriguing is the fact that one sachet of VSL#3 daily, initiated immediately after patients underwent pouch surgery for UC, was significantly better than placebo for preventing a first occurrence of pouchitis (72).

Probiotic Clinical Trials for Crohn Disease

Regarding CD, nine clinical trials were conducted with probiotics before 2011 (73). In contrast to the success seen in UC, only one CD trial has demonstrated an ability to induce remission. The first study conducted in CD, an open-label study of *Lactobacillus* GG in pediatric patients with mild to moderately active CD, demonstrated a large decrease in the baseline CDAI score at week 4 (74). A second small study compared *Lactobacillus* GG with placebo in adult patients with CD with mild to moderate disease activity (75). After equally small numbers of patients in each trial arm were found to be in remission at 6 months, the investigators concluded that there was no benefit from treating with *Lactobacillus* GG.

The effects of probiotics on postoperative recurrence in CD also have been studied. Two studies with *Lactobacillus* GG failed to prevent postoperative recurrence (76, 77), whereas other studies with *Lactobacillus johnsonii* LA1 also proved to be ineffective in preventing postoperative CD (78, 79). Finally, a study evaluating the role of a combination prebiotic/probiotic (Synbiotic 2000) was also unable to prevent postoperative recurrence (80).

Probiotic effects in IBD can be summarized as follows: Certain probiotics can significantly affect the disease course of UC (ECN) or medically induced remission of pouchitis (VSL#3). However, little evidence exists for a beneficial effect of probiotics in CD. Although probiotics exhibit an excellent safety profile, concerns for culture viability and product purity give cause for concern. These concerns, as well as preclinical data documenting significant anti-inflammatory effects in IBD models, have fueled significant interest in developing a class of therapeutic supplements called prebiotics. The term *prebiotic* was coined to describe nondigestible, complex sugars that promote growth of beneficial bacteria (81, 82).

Prebiotics

These substances resist digestion and assimilation in the upper gastrointestinal tract, but are subsequently fermented by beneficial species of bacteria to promote an individual's health. Inulin and oligofructose are naturally occurring prebiotic substances found in plants such as wheat, chicory, leeks, artichokes, asparagus, and garlic (83). Prebiotics potentially diminish intestinal mucosal inflammation by enhancing barrier function, anti-inflammatory effects, and short-chain FA (SCFA) production. Like probiotics, prebiotics possess an attractive safety profile, but they occasionally generate non-serious side effects such as abdominal pain, flatulence, bloating and diarrhea (83).

A prebiotic trial in quiescent UC leveraged knowledge that colonic bacteria fermented the fiber from *Plantago ovata* (PO) seeds into butyrate (84). To test the benefits of PO fiber, 3 groups were compared in open-label fashion: PO seeds 10 g twice daily, mesalamine 500 mg 3 times daily, or a combination. Disease activity flared at similar rates in each group (37% PO, 35% mesalamine, and 23% combination therapy) (84). The benefits of an alternate fiber source produced as a byproduct of brewing beer, germinated barley foodstuff (GBF), was evaluated in 18 patients with mild-to-moderate UC. Treatment with 20 to 30 g GBF for 4 weeks conveyed a significant benefit (85). A subsequent report of 12 months of therapy with GBF revealed a prolonged benefit for GBF-treated subjects, compared with a control group who did not receive GBF (86).

Oat bran, yet another form of dietary fiber that ferments into SCFA, has also shown promise as an IBD treatment through its ability to maintain remission of UC (87). Twenty-three patients with UC received 60 g of oat fiber per day for a total of 12 weeks. No relapses occurred in either groups, but treated patients demonstrated elevated SCFA stool levels.

Purified components of probiotic substances also have benefited IBD patients. A small placebo-controlled, crossover trial in 20 subjects with pouchitis compared 24 g of inulin daily versus placebo. After 3 weeks on therapy, subjects underwent stool collection and pouch endoscopy, followed by a 4-week washout, then crossover to the alternate therapy (88). Although there were no differences in the pouch disease index by treatment, butyrate levels were significantly higher in inulin-treated subjects. Another small, open-label study examining a combination of oligofructose and inulin (15 g/day) in 10 patients with active ileocolonic CD improved disease activity after 3 weeks of treatment (89). Limited positive clinical trial data supporting the use of prebiotics for IBD justifies the need for larger trials. However, blinding subjects to the large volume of ingested prebiotic will be difficult and may adversely contribute to the large placebo effect commonly found in IBD trials.

OMEGA-3 FATTY ACIDS

Omega-3 rich–fish and fish oil make up one final "functional food" therapy that has been of long-standing interest to patients with IBD. Humans produce all but two FAs required for health. These two "essential" FAs consist of linoleic acid (LA; a precursor to the ω-6 series of fatty acids) and α-linolenic acid (ALA; a precursor to the ω-3 fatty acids). Optimal consumption of LA to ALA occurs at a 4:1 ratio (90). However, the heavy plant oil consumption found in the WD has altered this ratio to 15 to 16:1, likely spurring a worldwide increase in inflammatory disorders such as CD and UC (91, 92).

Saturated ω-6 FA precursors of arachidonic acid (AA) accumulate in mammalian cell membranes. Although AA is an important signaling molecule playing a crucial role in regulating inflammation, excessive AA can trigger uncontrolled inflammation. AA is cleaved from membrane phospholipids by the action of phospholipase A2 (93). Downstream products of AA metabolism include

the proinflammatory molecules leukotriene B$_4$ (LTB$_4$) and prostaglandin E$_2$ (PGE$_2$), which are implicated in the activation of inflammatory cells as well as their subsequent vascular adhesion, migration, and chemotaxis (94).

The excessive accumulation of ω-6 FAs in cell membranes induced by WD results in excessive downstream production of LTB$_4$ and PGE$_2$, which have been tied to increasing incidences of several inflammatory disorders (95). On the contrary, consumption of ω-3 FA-rich foods may interfere with the conversion of AA to proinflammatory components, instead shunting metabolism toward the production of less potent molecules such as LTB$_5$ and PGE$_3$ (96, 97).

Although a plausible explanation for the anti-inflammatory properties of ω-3 FAs, research has uncovered an even more convincing mechanism for these effects. Resolution of inflammation was previously attributed to phagocytic depletion of pathogenic antigens and subsequent elimination of chemotactic gradients (98). However, conclusive evidence has established that resolvins and protectins, two classes of molecules derived from ω-3 FA metabolism, actively drive the resolution of inflammation (99, 100). During the initial phases of a host response to pathogens, classic prostaglandins and leukotrienes dominate, generating classic signs of inflammation. At a transition point in the inflammatory process, PGE$_2$ and PGD$_2$ promote the induction of key enzymes involved in the synthesis of lipoxins, resolvins, and protectins, each of which plays a specific role in the reinduction of a state of homeostasis (100). As reviewed in Figure 78.1, resolvins

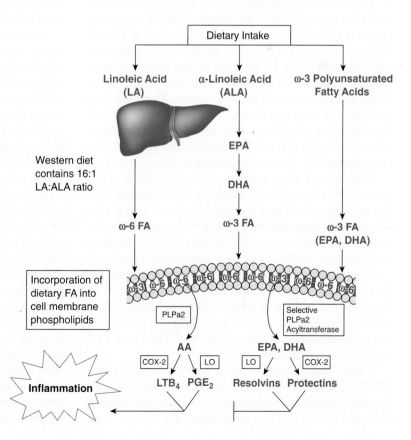

Fig. 78.1. Dietary intake of essential fatty acids and their impact on inflammation. *AA*, arachidonic acid; *COX-2*, cyclooxygenase-2; *DHA*, docosahexaenoic acid; *EPA*, eicosapentaenoic acid; *FA*, fatty acid; *LO*, lipoxygenase; *LTB$_4$*, leukotriene B$_4$; *PGE$_2$*, prostaglandin E$_2$; *PLP*, phospholipase.

and protectins are exclusively derived from the ω-3 fatty acids eicosapentaenoic acid (EPA) and docosahexaenoic acid (DHA) (100).

The elucidation of this mechanism has renewed calls to harness the anti-inflammatory effects of EPA and DHA derived from a diet rich in deep water fish (e.g., salmon, herring, mackerel). Intestinal bacteria from these fish generate copious long-chain ω-3 FA (e.g., EPA and DHA) de novo, which are incorporated into their flesh (90, 101). Ingestion of the fish flesh transfers the EPA and DHA to the consumer.

A more pharmacologic approach using concentrated fish oil has been extensively studied for IBD, with inconclusive results. An initial open-label trial of fish oil in 10 patients with mild to moderately active UC heralded great promise when 7 patients experienced moderate to marked improvement (102). Further supporting the benefits of fish oil, a subsequent crossover trial enrolled 11 patients with mild-to-moderate UC to evaluate fish oil containing 4.2 g ω-3 FA/day. Fifty-six percent of subjects experienced improvement in colitis symptoms while receiving active therapy, whereas only 4% improved while receiving placebo ($p < .05$) (103).

A second small crossover study involving 24 patients with active UC was also conducted using fish oil capsules (104). Subjects experienced disease-related biochemical and histologic improvements while receiving the study drug, but not while receiving placebo. However, a much larger study randomized patients with UC to either fish oil or olive oil and failed to demonstrate a difference between treatment groups (105). Biochemical differences were detected between treatment groups. The lack of clinical differences could be explained by an animal study that used the interleukin-10 knockout mouse model of intestinal inflammation to evaluate the effects of fish oil on colitis and inflammation-induced tumors. This study also used olive oil as a control (106). Olive oil–treated animals developed less inflammation and lower tumor scores than animals receiving fish oil. This suggests that olive oil does not constitute an appropriate placebo to fish oil.

A third small study evaluating fish oil in distal colitis patients did demonstrate efficacy by both a clinical activity index ($p < .05$) and endoscopy ($p = .013$) (107). In an attempt to summarize disparate trial results, a meta-analysis of all comparative trials of fish oil for UC found no overall benefit for fish oil in the maintenance of remission (108). However, a pilot study that explored the impact of dietary salmon in patients with active UC did demonstrate improvement in both a colitis activity index as well as other biochemical parameters, suggesting that food-based interventions aimed at raising intestinal DHA and EPA could be beneficial (109).

A much larger body of evidence has examined fish oil for CD. Several randomized, controlled clinical trials evaluated the role of fish oil in maintaining (generally steroid-induced) remission (110–114), but inconsistent trial designs were hampered by varying forms of fish oil. Early trials demonstrated enhanced remission rates in subjects receiving fish oil (111, 112, 114), whereas the largest trials showed no difference (110, 113). However, when pooled results of studies using enteric coated preparations of fish oil were examined in a metaanalysis, summary data for enteric coated fish oil demonstrated a benefit in maintaining remission at 1 year (relative risk, 0.77; 95% CI, 0.61 to 0.98) (108).

Given the fact that no serious adverse events have been reported to date in fish oil clinical trials, in addition to biochemical evidence that fish oil supplementation alters intestinal mucosal eicosanoid composition in a beneficial way, fish oil supplementation appears to be a safe, if not highly efficacious, nutritional supplement for patients with UC. However, evidence garnered from the EPIC trials (110) reasonably suggests that fish oil does not confer a clinically meaningful benefit in CD. When all the evidence is considered in aggregate, there appears to be no compelling evidence that fish oil supplementation is useful for IBD.

CONCLUSION

In this era of information overload confronting both patients and clinicians, literature regarding nutritional support for IBD is both broad in scope and narrow in conclusive results that can guide practice. Patients with IBD have a profound interest in constructive advice regarding how to best use their daily nutrition intake to positively influence the chronic state of inflammation in their bowels.

Common questions involve how diet is implicated in the onset of IBD, followed by questions regarding whether they can make changes in their diet to make the inflammation go away. The best evidence suggests that a WD may serve as a risk factor. Unfortunately, dietary manipulations to reverse the inflammatory state do not appear to be sufficient in IBD. Profound interventions, such as oral diet elimination combined with replacement enteral formula appear to offer a sound, low-risk therapeutic intervention with possible long-term benefits.

As concluded in a review of nutritional support in IBD, emerging literature (especially in pediatrics) favors the use of such exclusive enteral nutrition in the primary treatment of active CD, but rigorous controlled trials are lacking (115). Additionally, targeted interventions for common deficiencies brought about by the inflammatory disorders of the digestive tract can help avoid and replete micronutrient deficiencies. Beyond that, nutrition support appears to offer no quick and easy "cures" for this notoriously difficult to treat disease process. As summarized by Forbes et al, "Nutrition therapy in adults with IBD is probably both undervalued and underused, but the evidence base needs to be strengthened to confirm its efficacy, determine better those patients most likely to benefit, and optimize the regimens to be employed" (115).

micronutrient deficiencies resulting from this approach, generalized exclusion diets are not recommended for routine use in patients with IBS (1, 43, 45).

Although generalized exclusion diets are not advised, diets specifically avoiding unabsorbed, fermentable short-chain carbohydrates, collectively termed fermentable oligosaccharides, disaccharides, monosaccharides, and polyols (FOD-MAPs), may be of benefit to patients with IBS. FOD-MAPs include fructose and lactose when malabsorbed, poorly absorbed polyols (sorbitol, xylitol), and fructooligosaccharides (fructans) and galactooligosaccharides (raffinose) not cleaved by human hydrolases and thus poorly absorbed (46).

Support for the use of FOD-MAP–restricted diets initially was derived from uncontrolled studies examining restriction of lactose alone (35) or fructose with or without sorbitol (29, 33). A double-blind, randomized, quadruple-arm, placebo-controlled rechallenge trial demonstrated that 70% or more of patients with IBS receiving fructose, fructans, or a combination of both experience inadequate symptom control compared with 14% receiving glucose (46). These findings suggest that the effect of the low FOD-MAP diet resulted from sugar restriction and not from a placebo effect.

Dietary Fiber

Fiber supplementation is a commonly prescribed dietary remedy for IBS. Its use depends on the patient's dominant symptom. Fiber supplementation is most commonly used for patients with constipation and, to a lesser extent, for those with diarrhea. Fiber is believed to alleviate constipation by adding bulk to the stool, which accelerates oral–anal transit and decreases intracolonic pressures (47). For patients with diarrhea, soluble fiber creates a more viscous stool and can improve stool output. When pain, gas, and bloating predominate, use of fiber may actually be counterproductive because fermentation of fiber generates increased gas production.

Evidence supporting the use of fiber in IBS is poor. Most studies were performed between 1976 and 1994, and many were limited by methodologic weaknesses. Several systematic reviews and metaanalyses have been performed to formulate more definitive conclusions (1,48–53). A metaanalysis of the effects of fiber (typically insoluble wheat bran or soluble ispaghula husk) versus placebo in patients with IBS reported that ispaghula husk, but not wheat bran, improved global IBS symptoms over a 6- to 12-week period. However, when only higher quality studies were included, the beneficial effect of ispaghula husk was no longer significant (53). In a randomized study of soluble fiber (psyllium), insoluble fiber (bran), or placebo in patients with IBS over a 12-week period, those treated with soluble fiber had significantly higher relief of abdominal pain compared with the placebo or bran supplementation groups. This study suggests that soluble fiber, but not insoluble fiber, offers symptom relief in a subset of patients with IBS (54).

Based on the available data, the American College of Gastroenterology Task Force on Functional Gastrointestinal Disorders does not endorse fiber as a treatment for IBS, but it does recognize its usefulness for the treatment of constipation (1). In patients with IBS-C, fiber intake should be titrated gradually to minimize the common adverse effects of bloating, abdominal distention, and flatulence.

Probiotics and Prebiotics

The intestinal microbiome may have a pathogenic role in the development of IBS. Manipulation of the gut microflora using prebiotics and probiotics has potential therapeutic value. Probiotics, commonly live *Bifidobacteria* and *Lactobacillus* spp., are available in capsule form or in food items such as yogurts. Prebiotics, commonly nondigestible fructooligosaccharides (oligofructose and inulin) and galactooligosaccharides in food, stimulate the growth and activity of select intestinal bacteria.

A large metaanalysis assessing the efficacy of probiotics versus placebo on global IBS symptoms reported a statistically significant reduction in IBS symptoms across all probiotics used (*Lactobacillus, Bifidobacterium, Streptococcus*, and combinations) compared with placebo (55). These data, however, displayed significant heterogeneity and likely overestimated the treatment effect. In trials that reported IBS symptoms as a continuous variable, probiotic use resulted in a statistically significant improvement in IBS symptoms compared with placebo (55). The optimal probiotic regimen could not be delineated from this review.

Prebiotics have been reported to change stool consistency and improve flatulence and bloating significantly in patients with IBS treated with the prebiotic, *trans*-galactooligosaccharide, when compared with placebo. Concurrent with these effects was an increase in fecal bifidobacterial concentrations, a finding suggesting a potential benefit from the altered microbiota (56).

DIVERTICULAR DISEASE AND DIET

Colonic diverticulosis refers to the development of saclike outpouchings in the colonic wall resulting from herniation of mucosa and submucosa through defects in the muscle layer. Although most patients with diverticulosis remain asymptomatic, up to 25% develop clinically significant disease (57). The spectrum of diverticular disease includes a complex of abdominal pain and altered bowel habits similar to IBS, diverticulitis with or without complications, diverticular hemorrhage, and diverticular colitis (Fig. 80.3).

Diet and Pathophysiology

Fiber deficiency is believed to be central to the development of diverticulosis and diverticular disease. The fiber hypothesis was first proposed by physicians Dennis Burkitt and NS Painter in 1971 while on a medical mission

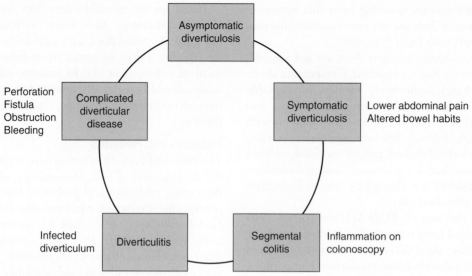

Fig. 80.3. Spectrum of diverticular disease.

in rural Africa. The team noted that diverticular disease, although prevalent in England, was virtually nonexistent in the Ugandan population. This difference was attributed to high fiber consumption among Ugandans and lower fiber intake among the English (58, 59).

The emergence of diverticular disease appeared to parallel a decrease in dietary fiber consumption. Autopsy studies in the early twentieth century detected diverticulosis in 2% to 10% of a Western population, whereas autopsy series in the 1960s revealed prevalence rates of 10% to 66%, depending on the age group studied (59, 60). Over time, diverticular disease increased in developing countries that adopted the Western diet (61). A similar shift was also observed in Japan. In a retrospective study of 1289 barium enemas performed between 1960 and 1970, the prevalence of diverticular disease was 2.6% among Japanese patients who were more than 40 years old, whereas prevalence rates reached 7% to 12% between 1980 and 1990. This rise in diverticular disease followed a reduction in mean daily fiber intake in 1972 to approximately 70% of the 1952 level (58, 62, 63, 64).

A large, prospective study confirmed the inverse relationship between diverticular disease and fiber consumption (65). Unlike the epidemiologic studies, this analysis focused solely on patients with symptomatic diverticular disease. Among an estimated 48,000 men participating in the Health Professionals Follow-Up Study, 385 men with dietary data developed symptomatic diverticular disease over a 4-year period. Patients in the highest quintile of fiber intake had significantly reduced risk of developing diverticular disease compared with patients in the lowest quintile (relative risk [RR], 0.58; 95% confidence interval [CI], 0.41, 0.83; $p = .01$). Conversely, the RR for men on a high-total-fat, low-fiber diet was 2.35 (95% CI, 1.38, 3.98) compared with those on a low-total-fat, high-fiber diet (65). This association was primarily attributable to

consumption of fruit and vegetable fiber rather than cereal fiber (66).

Fiber deficiency is believed to promote diverticula formation by generating low stool mass and reduced luminal size. In this setting, peristaltic forces are transmitted to the colon wall rather than to luminal contents, thus causing mucosa and submucosa to herniate through the weakest points and create sacculations. Less well understood are the variables influencing progression from asymptomatic to symptomatic diverticular disease. One theory is that fiber deficiency alters the gut flora and leads to immunologic changes that stimulate inflammation and diverticulitis (58). Formal studies are needed to understand the relationship between the diet–microbiome and symptomatic diverticular disease more clearly.

Diet in the Management of Diverticular Disease

Prevention of Symptomatic Diverticular Disease

Historically, physicians have advised patients with diverticulosis to avoid consumption of nuts, seeds, popcorn, and other high-fiber foods to prevent symptoms or complications of diverticular disease. This recommendation was based on concerns that large, undigested particles could lodge within a diverticulum, obstruct the neck, or traumatize the mucosa, thus causing inflammation or bleeding. A more recent study, however, suggested that this practice is unnecessary. As part of the Health Professionals Follow-up Study, a cohort of 47,228 men completed periodic medical and dietary questionnaires over an 18-year period (67). During this interval, 801 incident cases of diverticulitis and 383 incident cases of diverticular bleeding were reported. Review of available dietary records failed to establish an association between corn consumption and diverticulitis or between nut, corn, or popcorn consumption and diverticular hemorrhage.

In fact, an inverse relationship was found between nut and popcorn consumption and diverticulitis risk, suggesting a protective effect (67).

Dietary fiber supplementation has been advocated as a means to prevent formation of diverticula and symptomatic diverticular disease (68). At least 6 studies have examined the role of dietary fiber in the management of diverticular disease, including two randomized controlled trials. The first trial randomized 18 patients with diverticulosis to either wheat or bran crisp bread over a 3-month period. Subjects receiving the high-fiber bran product experienced greater improvements in pain and total symptom scores compared with the low-fiber group (69). In contrast, a second randomized trial showed no difference in pain, lower bowel, or total symptom scores in response to a high-fiber diet, although constipation and stool consistency improved (70).

Additional data supporting fiber supplementation in diverticular disease are derived from 4 retrospective, uncontrolled trials, only 1 of which included patients with complicated diverticular disease (i.e., diverticulitis) (68, 71). In this trial, 60 of 100 patients admitted to the hospital with symptomatic diverticular disease had diverticulitis. Seventy-five patients were managed medically whereas 25 required surgery. Following treatment, the medical and surgical groups were started on a high-fiber diet, and 91% remained symptom free after 5 to 7 years of follow up (71).

Diet and Acute Complicated Diverticular Disease

During an acute attack of diverticulitis or diverticular hemorrhage, patients are placed on bowel rest, and their diet is advanced as clinical parameters improve. Although data on dietary advancement are lacking, patients are generally started on a low-fiber diet (10 g/day). As the patient recovers, daily fiber intake can be advanced by 5 g each week until a target intake of 25 to 35 g is achieved (68). As noted, avoidance of nuts and seeds is not necessary.

SUMMARY

IBS is a common clinical disorder with varied presentations, including predominant constipation, predominant diarrhea, or a mixed picture. The pathophysiology of IBS is currently unknown. Significant numbers of patients with IBS consider their gastrointestinal symptoms to be food related and modify their diets. In most instances, reported food intolerances are not substantiated by formal testing for food allergies, malabsorption, or celiac disease. The role of food allergy in the pathogenesis of IBS is controversial. Celiac disease and other problems such as bacterial overgrowth appear to be common comorbidities with IBS symptoms. Individualized dietary counseling may be a helpful adjunct to pharmacologic treatments for IBS. Patients with IBS should eat a balanced diet with few restrictions. Dietary modifications should be based on the dominant gastrointestinal symptoms in individual patients

and may include reductions in specific food items known to exacerbate symptoms or use of increased dietary fiber.

Diverticular disease appears intimately tied to dietary fiber consumption. Epidemiologic data suggest that the emergence of the Western diet and associated decline in fiber intake led to increased rates of diverticular disease. Less well established is the role of fiber deficiency in the progression to symptomatic diverticular disease. Although the American Society of Colorectal Surgeons advocates the use of fiber supplementation to prevent recurrent diverticulitis, the American College of Gastroenterology finds no consistent evidence to support this practice. Despite this contradiction, the National Institute of Health recommends a high-fiber diet in patients with diverticular disease. The low risk of fiber supplementation along with the theoretic benefit lends support to this recommendation.

REFERENCES

1. Brandt LJ, Chey WD, Foxx-Orenstein AE et al. Am J Gastroenterol 2009;104(Suppl):S1–35.
2. Simren M, Mansson A, Langkilde AM et al. Digestion 2001;63:108–15.
3. Monsbakken KW, Vandvik PO, Farup PG. Eur J Clin Nutr 2006;60:667–72.
4. Locke GR 3rd, Zinsmeister AR, Talley NJ et al. Am J Gastroenterol 2000;95:157–65.
5. Young E, Stoneham MD, Petruckevitch A et al. Lancet 1994;343:1127–30.
6. Saito YA, Locke GR 3rd, Weaver AL et al. Am J Gastroenterol 2005;100:2743–8.
7. Boyce JA, Assa'ad A, Burks AW et al. J Allergy Clin Immunol 2010;126:1105–18.
8. Zar S, Kumar D, Benson MJ. Aliment Pharmacol Ther 200; 15:439–49.
9. Bentley SJ, Pearson DJ, Rix KJ. Lancet 1983;2:295–7.
10. Farah DA, Calder I, Benson L et al. Gut 1985;26:164–168.
11. Petitpierre M, Gumowski P, Girard JP. Ann Allergy 1985; 54:538–40.
12. Stefanini GF, Saggioro A, Alvisi V et al. Scand J Gastroenterol 1995;30:535–41.
13. Andre F, Andre C, Colin L et al. Allergy 1995;50:328–33.
14. Bischoff SC, Mayer J, Meier PN et al. Int Arch Allergy Immunol 1997;113:348–51.
15. Carroccio A, Brusca I, Mansueto P et al. Clin Gastroenterol Hepatol 2010;8:254–60.
16. Zar S, Benson MJ, Kumar D et al. Am J Gastroenterol 2005;100:1550–7.
17. Atkinson W, Sheldon TA, Shaath N et al. Gut 2004;53: 1459–64.
18. Zipser RD, Patel S, Yahya KZ et al. Dig Dis Sci 2003;48: 761–4.
19. Fasano A, Berti I, Gerarduzzi T et al. Arch Intern Med 2003;163:286–92.
20. Ford AC, Chey WD, Talley NJ et al. Arch Intern Med 2009; 169:651–8.
21. O'Leary C, Wieneke P, Buckley S et al. Am J Gastroenterol 2002;97:1463–7.
22. O'Leary C, Quigley EM. Am J Gastroenterol 2003;98:720–2.
23. Spiegel BM, DeRosa VP, Gralnek IM et al. Gastroenterology 2004;126:1721–32.

24. Mein SM, Ladabaum U. Aliment Pharmacol Ther 2004; 19:1199–210.

25. Wahnschaffe U, Ullrich R, Riecken EO et al. Gastroenterology 2001;121:1329–38.

26. Wahnschaffe U, Schulzke JD, Zeitz M et al. Clin Gastroenterol Hepatol 2007;5:844–50; quiz 769.

27. Black KE, Murray JA, David CS et al. J Immunol 2002; 169:5595–600.

28. Verdu EF, Huang X, Natividad J et al. Am J Physiol Gastrointest Liver Physiol 2008;294:G217–25.

29. Fernandez-Banares F, Rosinach M, Esteve M et al. Clin Nutr 2006;25:824–31.

30. Corlew-Roath M, Di Palma JA. South Med J 2009;102:1010–2.

31. Bohmer CJ, Tuynman HA. Eur J Gastroenterol Hepatol 2001;13:941–4.

32. Bohmer CJ, Tuynman HA. Eur J Gastroenterol Hepatol 1996; 8:1013–6.

33. Goldstein R, Braverman D, Stankiewicz H. Isr Med Assoc J 2000;2:583–7.

34. Parker TJ, Woolner JT, Prevost AT et al. Eur J Gastroenterol Hepatol 2001;13:219–25.

35. Vernia P, Di Camillo M, Marinaro V et al. Dig Liver Dis 2001;33:234–39.

36. Fernandez-Banares F, Esteve-Pardo M, de Leon R et al. Am J Gastroenterol 1993;88:2044–50.

37. Nelis GF, Vermeeren MA, Jansen W. Gastroenterology 1990;99:1016–20.

38. King TS, Elia M, Hunter JO. Lancet 1998;352:1187–9.

39. Pimentel M, Kong Y, Park S. Am J Gastroenterol 2003; 98:2700–4.

40. Nucera G, Gabrielli M, Lupascu A et al. Aliment Pharmacol Ther 2005;21:1391–5.

41. Evans PR, Piesse C, Bak YT et al. Scand J Gastroenterol 1998;33:1158–63.

42. Lasser RB, Bond JH, Levitt MD. N Engl J Med 1975;293:524–6.

43. Park MI, Camilleri M. Neurogastroenterol Motil 2006;18: 595–607.

44. Jones VA, McLaughlan P, Shorthouse M et al. Lancet 1982; 2:1115–7.

45. Cabre E. Curr Opin Clin Nutr Metab Care 2010;13:581–7.

46. Shepherd SJ, Parker FC, Muir JG et al. Clin Gastroenterol Hepatol 2008;6:765–71.

47. Zuckerman MJ. J Clin Gastroenterol 2006;40:104–8.

48. Akehurst R, Kaltenthaler E. Gut 2001;48:272–82.

49. Bijkerk CJ, Muris JW, Knottnerus JA et al. Aliment Pharmacol Ther 2004;19:245–51.

50. Jailwala J, Imperiale TF, Kroenke K. Ann Intern Med 2000; 133:136–47.

51. Lesbros-Pantoflickova D, Michetti P, Fried M et al. Aliment Pharmacol Ther 2004;20:1253–69.

52. Quartero AO, Meineche-Schmidt V, Muris J et al. Cochrane Database Syst Rev 2005;(2):CD003460.

53. Ford AC, Talley NJ, Spiegel BM et al. BMJ 2008;337:a2313.

54. Bijkerk CJ, de Wit NJ, Muris JW et al. BMJ 2009;339:b3154.

55. Moayyedi P, Ford AC, Talley NJ et al. Gut 2010;59:325–32.

56. Silk DB, Davis A, Vulevic J et al. Aliment Pharmacol Ther 2009;29:508–18.

57. Martel J, Raskin JB. J Clin Gastroenterol 2008;42:1125–7.

58. Korzenik JR. J Clin Gastroenterol 2006;40(Suppl):S112–6.

59. Painter NS, Burkitt DP. Br Med J 1971;2:450–4.

60. Parks TG. Clin Gastroenterol 1975;4:53–69.

61. Segal I, Solomon A, Hunt JA. Gastroenterology 1977;72: 215–9.

62. Nakaji S, Sugawara K, Saito D et al. Eur J Nutr 2002;41: 222–7.

63. Miura S, Kodaira S, Shatari T et al. Dis Colon Rectum 2000;43:1383–9.

64. Nakada I, Ubukata H, Goto Y et al. Dis Colon Rectum 1995;38:755–9.

65. Aldoori WH, Giovannucci EL, Rimm EB et al. Am J Clin Nutr 1994;60:757–64.

66. Aldoori WH, Giovannucci EL, Rockett HR et al. J Nutr 1998;128:714–9.

67. Strate LL, Liu YL, Syngal S et al. JAMA 2008;300:907–14.

68. Tarleton S, DiBaise JK. Nutr Clin Pract 2011;26:137–42.

69. Brodribb AJ. Lancet 1977;1:664–6.

70. Ornstein MH, Littlewood ER, Baird IM et al. Br Med J (Clin Res Ed) 1981;282:1353–6.

71. Hyland JM, Taylor I. Br J Surg 1980;67:77–9.

SUGGESTED READINGS

Brandt LJ, Chey WD, Foxx-Orenstein AE et al. An evidence-based position statement on the management of irritable bowel syndrome. Am J Gastroenterol 2009;104(Suppl):S1–35.

Bijkerk CJ, de Wit NJ, Muris JW et al. Soluble or insoluble fibre in irritable bowel syndrome in primary care? Randomised placebo controlled trial. BMJ 2009;339:b3154.

Boyce JA, Assa'ad A, Burks AW et al. Guidelines for the diagnosis and management of food allergy in the united states: summary of the NIAID-sponsored expert panel report. J Allergy Clin Immunol 2010;126:1105–18.

Strate LL, Liu YL, Syngal S et al. Nut, corn, and popcorn consumption and the incidence of diverticular disease. JAMA 2008;300:907–14.

Tarleton S, DiBaise JK. Low-residue diet in diverticular disease: putting an end to a myth. Nutr Clin Pract 2011;26:137–42.

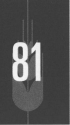

81 NUTRITION IN PANCREATIC DISEASES[1]

AMIT RAINA AND STEPHEN J. D. O'KEEFE

The pancreas, a retroperitoneal glandular organ, serves both endocrine and exocrine functions. The exocrine pancreas secretes at least 10 digestive enzymes, which are essential for the digestion and absorption of nutrients. The endocrine pancreas also secretes several hormones that play a key role in maintaining the metabolic homeostasis of the body. Three major pancreatic disorders discussed in this chapter are acute pancreatitis (AP), chronic pancreatitis (CP), and pancreatic cancer. These diseases, by altering the functioning of the pancreas, can all lead to major derangements in nutritional and metabolic homeostasis, although the underlying pathophysiologic mechanisms are different. This chapter at the outset briefly outlines the role pancreatic enzymes play in the absorption of nutrients and then focuses on pathophysiology, clinical presentation, assessment of nutritional status, and the principles of nutritional therapy in these three major pancreatic diseases.

PHYSIOLOGY OF PANCREATIC SECRETION

Knowledge of the mechanisms of pancreatic secretion is fundamental to the management of patients with pancreatic disease, especially AP. Pancreatic secretion is precisely orchestrated by the release of peptide hormones and neurotransmitters from the gastrointestinal (GI) tract after contact with ingested food. Traditionally, pancreatic stimulation is divided into three phases: the cephalic, gastric, and intestinal phases. The thought of food primes the pancreas to commence the process of zymogen aggregation and secretion. Next, the ingestion and swallowing of food, followed by expansion of the stomach wall, induce vagally mediated pancreatic secretion. Finally, the entry of food into the duodenum induces the most powerful stimulation, associated with acetylcholine and cholecystokinin (CCK) release by the mucosa and propelled by migrating motor complexes. In physiologic studies in healthy volunteers, a liquid formula diet was delivered to different regions of the upper GI tract, and the secretory response was greatest if a polymeric diet was infused into the duodenum (1) (Fig. 81.1). Further, the secretory response could be reduced significantly if the composition was changed to low-fat elemental. Additional studies showed that total parenteral nutrition (TPN) had no stimulatory effect, and that pancreatic rest could be maintained if the enteral feeding was delivered more than 40 cm past the ligament of Treitz (2). Finally, ileal delivery stimulated the ileal brake peptides peptide YY (PYY) and glucagon-like peptide-1 (GLP-1), resulting in inhibition of secretion.

DIGESTION OF NUTRIENTS

Without the pancreas, humans cannot survive because the gland is essential for the digestion of food. The normal pancreas secretes digestive enzymes, together

---

[1]**Abbreviations: AP**, acute pancreatitis; **ARDS**, acute respiratory distress syndrome; **CCK**, cholecystokinin; **CP**, chronic pancreatitis; **CRP**, C-reactive protein; **EN**, enteral nutrition; **GI**, gastrointestinal; **GLP-1**, glucagon-like peptide-1; **ICU**, intensive care unit; **IL**, interleukin; **MAP**, mitogen-activated protein; **MCP-1**, monocyte chemotactic protein-1; **MOFS**, multiorgan failure syndrome; **NG**, nasogastric; **NGJ**, nasogastrojejunal; **PEG**, percutaneous endoscopic gastrostomy; **PN**, parenteral nutrition; **PYY**, peptide YY; **RCT**, randomized controlled trial; **SAP**, severe acute pancreatitis; **SIRS**, systemic inflammatory response; **TNF-α**, tumor necrosis factor-α; **TPN**, total parenteral nutrition.

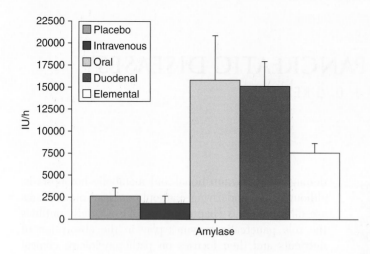

Fig. 81.1. Amylase secretion in response to enteral and parenteral nutrition. Relative amylase secretory responses to enteral and parenteral feeding, illustrating no difference between oral and duodenal feeding of a complex diet, an intermediate response to duodena elemental diet feeding, and no stimulatory effect of intravenous feeding compared with placebo saline.

with water and electrolytes, predominantly bicarbonate, which enhances luminal enzyme function by neutralizing gastric acid. The most active enzymes are lipase, amylase, and trypsin. Amylase (α-amylase) hydrolyzes dietary starch into disaccharides and trisaccharides, which are then broken down by enzymes on the brush border to absorbable forms as glucose and maltose. Pancreatic lipase hydrolyzes fat molecules. Bile salts secreted by the liver aid the digestive action of lipase by coating and emulsifying large fat droplets into smaller droplets, thus increasing the overall surface area for lipase to work. Fat hydrolysis results in formation of monomers (two free fatty acids and one 2-monoacylglycerol), which are then absorbed downstream into the lymphatic system by the lacteals. The main proteolytic enzyme, trypsin, is synthesized in the pancreas in an inactive form, as trypsinogen. Following a meal, when the pancreas is stimulated by CCK and cholinergic reflexes, trypsinogen is released from zymogen stores in the acinar cells and is secreted into the duodenum. Once in the small intestine, the intestinal enzyme enteropeptidase activates it into trypsin by proteolytic cleavage. Trypsins then, by the process of autocatalysis, activate more trypsinogen molecules. Once activated, the trypsin breaks down food proteins and peptides (proteins broken down to peptides in the stomach by pepsin) to amino acids, which are then absorbed by active transport systems.

ACUTE PANCREATITIS

Demographic and Clinical Presentation

AP is an acute inflammatory process of the pancreas that may involve the peripancreatic tissue and even remote organs. In the United States, about 75% to 80% cases of AP are attributed to alcohol abuse or gallstones (3–5). Other factors associated with AP include medications, trauma, infections, and metabolic causes (6). Biliary pancreatitis AP is more common in female patients, and alcoholic AP is more common in male patients (7). Clinical presentation typically consists of severe upper abdominal pain, nausea, and vomiting. Laboratory testing reveals elevated lipase and amylase in the bloodstream.

About 75% of cases of AP in patients admitted to hospitals are mild (edematous and interstitial pancreatitis) and follow a benign, self-limited course, with discharge home by day 4 (8). The remaining 25% cases, called severe AP (SAP), progress with the development of a profound systemic inflammatory response (SIRS), commonly associated with pancreatic gland necrosis, acute peripancreatic fluid collections, and multiorgan failure syndrome (MOFS). All the mortality ($\leq$50%) from the condition is associated with these complications. The inflamed and swollen pancreatic gland may itself or by development of acute fluid collections compress the stomach and duodenum. The result is obstruction to the outflow from the stomach, and patients present clinically with nausea and vomiting. The SIRS is usually associated with ileus and increased mucosal permeability. These critically ill patients often spend weeks in intensive care units (ICUs) and frequently need surgery for pancreatic necrosis and infections. However, early surgery is associated with elevated mortality rates because it is extremely difficult, and every effort should be made to manage patients conservatively for more than 4 weeks with enteral nutrition (EN) until the area of pancreatic necrosis or fluid collection becomes walled off, thus allowing a more definitive approach.

Pathophysiology

Basic understanding of the pathophysiology of AP is essential to comprehend the principles of nutritional therapy in these patients. Figure 81.2 helps illustrate some of what is known to happen in the evolution of the severe disease. AP is initiated by premature activation of trypsinogen within the acinar cells. Once trypsinogen, which normally is stored in zymogens within the acinar cells in an inactive form, is stimulated within the acinar cells, it autoactivates

can help stabilize these patients and improve their functional status, response to therapy, and prognosis. Nutritional evaluation includes generic evaluation parameters such as body mass index, weight change, midarm muscle circumference, triceps skinfold thickness and laboratory measurements such as prealbumin and albumin, although the last two values better reflect disease activity and prognosis.

Nutritional therapy for pancreatic cancer involves pain and nausea control. Megestrol acetate has shown promise in treating these patients by stimulation of appetite and antagonism of the metabolic effects of the catabolic cytokines produced by cancer and immune cells (96). Fish oil can reduce production of proinflammatory cytokines in patients with cancer and may be helpful in reversing the weight loss by modulating the metabolic responses to feeding (97, 98). Clinical studies have yielded mixed findings, however. They probably are helpful, but the optimum dose to maximize weight gain and minimize side effects has not been determined (97–100).

Gordon et al (101) studied use of thalidomide (anti-TNF agent) in patients with advanced pancreatic cancer–related cachexia. Fifty patients with advanced pancreatic cancer who had lost at least 10% of their body weight were randomized to receive thalidomide (200 mg daily) or placebo for 24 weeks in a single-center, double-blind RCT. At 8 weeks, patients taking thalidomide had significantly less weight loss and significantly more arm muscle mass compared with placebo (101).

Another key component in the management of these patients is to recognize and treat pancreatic exocrine insufficiency. Because most of pancreatic cancers are located in the head of the pancreas, the tumor can lead to exocrine glandular insufficiency by blocking the pancreatic duct (102). These patients and those who have undergone pancreaticoduodenectomy benefit from optimum pancreatic enzyme supplementation. Preoperative nutritional support is important to correct fluid, electrolyte, and micronutrient deficiencies, but time should not be wasted trying to correct body mass when the cancer may be at a resectable stage. Postoperative feeding is very important because many patients take time to tolerate normal food after a Whipple procedure. Use of an NGJ feeding system is recommended immediately after surgery because gastric outlet dysfunction nearly always occurs for a variable period.

REFERENCES

1. O'Keefe SJ, Lee RB, Anderson FP et al. Am J Physiol 2003;284:G27–36.
2. Kaushik N, Pietraszewski M, Holst JJ et al. Pancreas 2005;31:353–9.
3. Lankisch PG, Lowenfels AB, Maisonneuve P. Pancreas 2002;25:411–2.
4. Spanier BW, Dijkgraaf MG, Bruno MJ. Best Pract Res 2008;22:45–63.
5. Venneman NG, Buskens E, Besselink MG et al. Am J Gastroenterol 2005;100:2540–50.
6. Walker WA, Goulet O, Kleinman RE et al, eds. Pediatric Gastrointestinal Disease: Pathophysiology, Diagnosis, Management. 4th ed. Hamilton, Ontario, Canada: BC Decker, 2004:1584–97.
7. National Institutes of Health. Drinking in the United States: Main Findings from the 1992 National Longitudinal Alcohol Epidemiologic Survey (NLAES), vol. 6. Bethesda, MD: National Institutes of Health, 1998. NIH publication 99-3519.
8. Abou-Assi S, Craig K, O'Keefe SJ. Am J Gastroenterol 2002;97:2255–62.
9. Gorelick FS, Modlin IM, Leach SD et al. Yale J Biol Med 1992;65:407–20.
10. Leach SD, Modlin IM, Scheele GA et al. J Clin Invest 1991;87:362–6.
11. Aoun E, Chen J, Reighard D et al. Pancreatology 2009;9:777–85.
12. Pezzilli R, Billi P, Miniero R et al. Dig Dis Sci 1995;40:2341–8.
13. Stoelben E, Nagel M, Ockert D et al. Chirurg 1996;67:1231–6.
14. Martin MA, Saracibar E, Santamaria A et al. Rev Esp Enferm Dig 2008;100:768–73 [in Spanish].
15. Ueda T, Takeyama Y, Yasuda T et al. Surgery 2007;142:319–26.
16. Andoh A, Takaya H, Saotome T et al. Gastroenterology 2000;119:211–9.
17. Osman MO, Gesser B, Mortensen JT et al. Cytokine 2002;17:53–9.
18. Shi C, Zhao X, Wang X et al. Scand J Gastroenterol 2005;40:103–8.
19. Makhija R, Kingsnorth AN. J Hepatobiliary Pancreat Surg 2002;9:401–10.
20. Bhatia M, Wong FL, Cao Y et al. Pancreatology 2005;5:132–44.
21. Rahman SH, Ammori BJ, Holmfield J et al. J Gastrointest Surg 2003;7:26–35.
22. Fong YM, Marano MA, Moldawer LL et al. J Clin Invest 1990;85:1896–04.
23. Hegazi R, Raina A, Graham T et al. JPEN J Parenter Enteral Nutr 2011;35:91–6.
24. Shah U, Shenoy-Bhangle AS. N Engl J Med 2011;365:1528–1536.
25. Yadav D, Agarwal N, Pitchumoni CS. Am J Gastroenterol 2002;97:1309–18.
26. Wu BU, Johannes RS, Sun X et al. Gut 2008;57:1698–703.
27. Ranson JH, Rifkind KM, Roses DF et al. Surg Gynecol Obstet 1974;139:69–81.
28. Banks PA, Freeman ML. Am J Gastroenterol 2006;101:2379–400.
29. Mofidi R, Duff MD, Wigmore SJ et al. Br J Surg 2006;93:738–44.
30. Buter A, Imrie CW, Carter CR et al. Br J Surg 2002;89:298–302.
31. Balthazar EJ, Robinson DL, Megibow AJ et al. Radiology 1990;174:331–6.
32. Robert JH, Frossard JL, Mermillod B et al. World J Surg 2002;26:612–9.
33. Muddana V, Whitcomb DC, Khalid A et al. Am J Gastroenterol 2009;104:164–70.
34. Lankisch PG, Weber-Dany B, Maisonneuve P et al. Am J Gastroenterol 2010;105:1196–200.
35. Wu BU, Johannes RS, Sun X et al. Gastroenterology 2009;137:129–35.
36. Teich N, Aghdassi A, Fischer J et al. Pancreas 2010;39:1088–92.
37. Jacobson BC, Vander Vliet MB, Hughes MD et al. Clin Gastroenterol Hepatol 2007;5:946–51.
38. Sathiaraj E, Murthy S, Mansard MJ et al. Aliment Pharmacol Ther 2008;28:777–81.

39. Heyland DK, Dhaliwal R, Drover JW et al. JPEN J Parenter Enteral Nutr 2003;27:355–73.

40. Marik PE, Zaloga GP. Crit Care Med 2001;29:2264–70.

41. Hegazi RA, O'Keefe SJ. Curr Gastroenterol Rep 2007;9:99–106.

42. O'Keefe SJ. Nat Rev Gastroenterol Hepatol 2009;6:207–15.

43. Petrov MS, Kukosh MV, Emelyanov NV. Dig Surg 2006;23:336–44.

44. Petrov MS, van Santvoort HC, Besselink MG et al. Arch Surg 2008;143:1111–7.

45. Ragins H, Levenson SM, Signer R et al. Am J Surg 1973;126:606–14.

46. Vu MK, van der Veek PP, Frolich M et al. Eur J Clin Invest 1999;29:1053–9.

47. O'Keefe SJ. Nat Clin Prac 2007;4:488–9.

48. O'Keefe SJ. Curr Opin Clin Nutr Metab Care 2006;9:622–8.

49. Kumar A, Singh N, Prakash S et al. J Clin Gastroenterol 2006;40:431–4.

50. Eatock FC, Chong P, Menezes N et al. Am J Gastroenterol 2005;100:432–9.

51. O'Keefe SJ, Lee RB, Li J et al. Am J Physiol 2005;289:G181–7.

52. Kalfarentzos F, Kehagias J, Mead N et al. Br J Surg 1997;84:1665–9.

53. O'Keefe SJ, Foody W, Gill S. JPEN J Parenter Enteral Nutr 2003;27:349–54.

54. O'Keefe SJ, Cariem AK, Levy M. J Clin Gastroenterol 2001;32:319–23.

55. Seder CW, Stockdale W, Hale L et al. Crit Care Med 2010;38:797–801.

56. Artinian V, Krayem H, DiGiovine B. Chest 2006;129:960–7.

57. Barr J, Hecht M, Flavin KE et al. Chest 2004;125:1446–57.

58. Martindale RG, McClave SA, Vanek VW et al. Crit Care Med 2009;37:1757–61.

59. Hegazi R, Raina A, Graham T et al. JPEN J Parenter Enteral Nutr 2011;35:91–6.

60. O'Keefe SJ, Ou J, Delany JP et al. World J Gastrointest Pathophysiol 2011;2:138–45.

61. Rolniak S RA, Hegazi R, Centa-Wagner P et al. Gastroenterology 2009;136:A-76.

62. Etemad B, Whitcomb DC. Gastroenterology 2001;120:682–707.

63. Lankisch PG, Lohr-Happe A, Otto J et al. Digestion 1993;54:148–55.

64. Wakasugi H, Funakoshi A, Iguchi H. J Gastroenterol 1998;33:254–9.

65. Manari AP, Preedy VR, Peters TJ. Addict Biol 2003;8:201–10.

66. Duggan S, O'Sullivan M, Feehan S et al. Nutr Clin Pract 2010;25:362–70.

67. Petersen JM, Forsmark CE. Semin Gastrointest Dis 2002;13:191–199.

68. DiMagno EP, Go VL, Summerskill WH. N Engl J Med 1973;288:813–5.

69. Regan PT, Malagelada JR, Dimagno EP et al. Gut 1979;20:249–54.

70. Chowdhury RS, Forsmark CE, Davis RH et al. Pancreas 2003;26:235–8.

71. Hebuterne X, Hastier P, Peroux JL et al. Dig Dis Sci 1996;41:533–9.

72. Giger U, Stanga Z, DeLegge MH. Nutr Clin Pract 2004;19:37–49.

73. Kalvaria I, Labadarios D, Shephard GS et al. Int J Pancreatol 1986;1:119–28.

74. Marotta F, Labadarios D, Frazer L et al. Dig Dis Sci 1994;39:993–8.

75. Nakamura T, Takebe K, Imamura K et al. Acta Gastroenterol Belg 1996;59:10–4.

76. Yokota T, Tsuchiya K, Furukawa T et al. J Neurol 1990;237:103–6.

77. Mann ST, Stracke H, Lange U et al. Metabolism 2003;52:579–85.

78. Glasbrenner B, Malfertheiner P, Buchler M et al. Klin Wochenschr 1991;69:168–72.

79. Marotta F, O'Keefe SJ, Marks IN et al. Dig Dis Sci 1989;34:456–61.

80. Stanga Z, Giger U, Marx A et al. JPEN J Parenter Enteral Nutr 2005;29:12–20.

81. Nordback I, Pelli H, Lappalainen-Lehto R et al. Gastroenterology 2009;136:848–55.

82. Takeyama Y. Clin Gastroenterol Hepatol 2009;7(Suppl):S15–7.

83. Pelli H, Sand J, Laippala P et al. Scand J Gastroenterol 2000;35:552–5.

84. Yadav D, Whitcomb DC. Nat Rev Gastroenterol Hepatol 2010;7:131–45.

85. O'Keefe SJ, Cariem AK, Levy M. J Clin Gastroenterol 2001;32:319–23.

86. Jemal A, Siegel R, Ward E et al. CA Cancer J Clin 2009;59:225–49.

87. Lynch SM, Vrieling A, Lubin JH et al. Am J Epidemiol 2009;170:403–13.

88. Nothlings U, Wilkens LR, Murphy SP et al. J Natl Cancer Inst 2005;97:1458–65.

89. Ghadirian P, Boyle P, Simard A et al. Int J Pancreatol 1991;10:183–96.

90. Stevens RJ, Roddam AW, Beral V. Br J Cancer 2007;96:507–9.

91. Zheng W, Lee SA. Nutr Cancer 2009;61:437–46.

92. Trede M, Schwall G, Saeger HD. Ann Surg 1990;211:447–58.

93. Yeo CJ, Cameron JL, Lillemoe KD et al. Ann Surg 1995;221:721–31.

94. Ryan DP, Grossbard ML. Oncologist 1998;3:178–88.

95. Splinter TA. Ann Oncol 1992;3(Suppl 3):25–7.

96. Berenstein EG, Ortiz Z. Cochrane Database System Rev 2005;(2):CD004310.

97. Fearon KC, Von Meyenfeldt MF, Moses AG et al. Gut 2003;52:1479–86.

98. Brown TT, Zelnik DL, Dobs AS. Int J Gastrointest Cancer 2003;34:143–50.

99. Wigmore SJ, Ross JA, Falconer JS et al. Nutrition 1996;12(Suppl):S27–30.

100. Harle L, Brown T, Laheru D et al. J Altern Complement Med 2005;11:1039–46.

101. Gordon JN, Trebble TM, Ellis RD et al. Gut 2005;54:540–5.

102. Simchuk EJ, Traverso LW, Nukui Y et al. Am J Surg 2000;179:352–5.

SUGGESTED READINGS

Fearon KC, Von Meyenfeldt MF, Moses AG et al. Effect of a protein and energy dense N-3 fatty acid enriched oral supplement on loss of weight and lean tissue in cancer cachexia: a randomised double blind trial. Gut 2003;52:1479–86.

Hegazi R, Raina A, Graham T et al. Early jejunal feeding initiation and clinical outcomes in patients with severe acute pancreatitis. JPEN J Parenter Enteral Nutr 2011;35:91–6.

O'Keefe SJ. A guide to enteral access procedures and enteral nutrition. Nat Rev Gastroenterol Hepatol 2009;6:207–15.

O'Keefe SJ, Anderson FP, Gennings C et al. Physiological effects of enteral and parenteral feeding on pancreaticobiliary secretion in humans. Am J Physiol 2003;284:G27–36.

Stanga Z, Giger U, Marx A et al. Effect of jejunal long-term feeding in chronic pancreatitis. JPEN J Parenter Enteral Nutr 2005;29:12–20.

82

NUTRITION IN LIVER DISORDERS AND THE ROLE OF ALCOHOL[1]

JULIANE I. BEIER, SARAH LANDES, MOHAMMAD MOHAMMAD, AND CRAIG J. MCCLAIN

OVERVIEW OF THE LIVER AND ALCOHOL METABOLISM

The liver is the largest organ in the body, and it has a unique dual blood supply, perfused by both the portal vein (directly exposed to absorbed nutrients) and the hepatic artery. The liver is composed of multiple cell types with differing functions. Hepatocytes make up more than 80% of total liver mass and play a critical role in the metabolism of amino acids and ammonia, lipids, carbohydrates,

vitamins, minerals, hormones, and detoxification of a variety of drugs and xenobiotics. Hepatic stellate cells comprise the major storehouse for vitamin A in the body, and they play a critical role in collagen formation during liver injury and fibrosis. Sinusoidal endothelial cells (SECs) make up approximately half of the nonparenchymal cells of the liver and play an important role in controlling the exchange of materials (including nutrients) between the bloodstream and the liver parenchyma. The SECs express scavenger receptors and act as antigen-presenting cells, to name only a few of the important immune functions of these cells. Hepatic Kupffer cells comprise the largest reservoir of fixed macrophages in the body. They play a protective role against gut-derived toxins that have escaped into the portal circulation, and they are a major producer of cytokines, which can markedly influence nutritional status. Bile duct epithelial cells play a major role in transport (e.g., water, bile), express a variety of transporters, and have important immune functions. All these cell types interact in a coordinated fashion to protect against gut-derived toxins and autoimmune reactions (tolerance), and they modulate hormonal and nutritional status.

The liver is also the main organ for ethanol metabolism. Ethanol is primarily metabolized (~80%) by alcohol dehydrogenase (ADH), oxidizing ethanol to acetaldehyde. However, cytochrome P-450 systems (mainly CYP2E1) and catalase also contribute to the production of acetaldehyde in ethanol metabolism. Whereas ADH transfers electrons from ethanol to the reducing equivalent oxidized nicotinamide adenine dinucleotide phosphate ($NADP^+$), the cytochrome P-450 system transfers the electrons to molecular oxygen (O_2), and catalase reduces hydrogen peroxide (H_2O_2) to water (Fig. 82.1). Ethanol metabolism is considered zero order at physiologically relevant doses, meaning that the oxidation of ethanol is saturated at blood alcohol concentrations (BACs) that cause significant central nervous system (CNS) effects (>0.03%). Whereas the oxidation of ethanol to acetaldehyde is mediated by three distinct enzyme systems, only one enzyme, aldehyde dehydrogenase (ALDH), oxidizes acetaldehyde to acetate (see Fig. 82.1). Analogous to ADH, ALDH uses oxidized nicotinamide adenine dinucleotide (NAD^+) as the electron acceptor for this reaction; however, ALDH is located in the mitochondria of the cell (see Fig. 82.1).

[1]Abbreviations: **ADH**, alcohol dehydrogenase; **AH**, alcoholic hepatitis; **ALD**, alcoholic liver disease; **ALDH**, aldehyde dehydrogenase; **BAC**, blood alcohol concentration; **BCAA**, branched-chain amino acid; **CNS**, central nervous system; **DPI**, diphenyliodonium; **FAEE**, fatty acid ethyl ester; **GSH**, glutathione; **HE**, hepatic encephalopathy; **HIF**, hypoxia-inducible factor; **iNOS**, inducible nitric oxide synthase; **LES**, late evening snack; **LPS**, lipopolysaccharide; **NAD⁺**, oxidized nicotinamide adenine dinucleotide; **NADH**, reduced nicotinamide adenine dinucleotide; **NADP⁺**, oxidized nicotinamide adenine dinucleotide phosphate; **NAFLD**, nonalcoholic fatty liver disease; **NASH**, nonalcoholic steatohepatitis; **PEM**, protein-energy malnutrition; **RNS**, reactive nitrogen species; **ROS**, reactive oxygen species; **RQ**, respiratory quotient; **SAM**, S-adenosylmethionine; **SEC**, sinusoidal endothelial cell; **TLR-4**, Toll-like receptor-4; **TNF**, tumor necrosis factor; **TRIF**, TIR-domain–containing adapter-inducing interferon-β; **VA**, Veterans Affairs; **WKS**, Wernicke–Korsakoff syndrome.

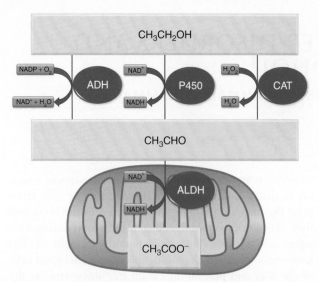

Fig. 82.1. Oxidative metabolism of alcohol by the liver. Alcohol (CH₃CH₂OH) is oxidized to acetaldehyde (CH₃CHO) by three enzyme systems: the microsomal ethanol oxidizing system (MEOS), alcohol dehydrogenase (ADH), and catalase (CAT). Acetaldehyde, in turn, is metabolized to acetate (CH₃COO-) by aldehyde dehydrogenase (ALDH) in the mitochondria. The metabolic and biochemical effects of alcohol metabolism may contribute to ADH. *NAD,* nicotinamide adenine dinucleotide; *NADH,* reduced nicotinamide adenine dinucleotide; *NADP,* nicotinamide adenine dinucleotide phosphate.

This chapter reviews major direct mechanisms of alcohol-induced liver injury, the gut–liver axis, general malnutrition in alcoholic liver disease (ALD), deficiencies of specific nutrients, and nutrition support in ALD. It also highlights how many principles of altered nutrition and nutrition support in ALD apply to other advanced liver diseases (e.g., hepatitis C, nonalcoholic steatohepatitis [NASH]).

DIRECT MECHANISMS OF LIVER INJURY

Ethanol is rapidly removed by the liver as a protective mechanism to prevent CNS depression and injury. However, the toxic metabolic and biochemical processes of ethanol metabolism, including induction of CYP2E1, production of toxic metabolites (e.g., acetaldehyde), and changes of biochemical processes may contribute to the development and progression of ALD.

Induction of CYP2E1

Although the relative contribution of the cytochrome P-450 system to total ethanol metabolism is low, CYP2E1 is strongly induced by alcohol and can contribute to total ethanol metabolism to a far greater extent in alcohol-dependent individuals (1). Inhibitors of CYP2E1 partially blocked hepatic injury caused by ethanol in animal models, a finding supporting this hypothesis (2). It is difficult to determine mechanisms in vivo, and, unfortunately, cultured cells exhibit very low activities of CYP enzymes. Therefore, HepG2 cells that overexpress CYP2E1 have been developed. Research using these cells has supported

the hypothesis that CYP2E1 is involved in hepatocyte damage from alcohol (3).

The exact mechanisms by which CYP2E1 contributes to ALD still need to be elucidated. However, it is proposed that CYP2E1 contributes to oxidative stress caused by alcohol because this enzyme has been shown to be relatively loosely coupled with cytochrome reductase. CYP2E1 can therefore leak electrons to oxygen to form $O_2{}^{\cdot-}$, or it can catalyze lipid peroxidation (4). Furthermore, CYP2E1 can bioactivate hepatotoxic agents (e.g., acetaminophen). The induction of this enzyme by chronic ethanol abuse can therefore increase the risk of liver damage by other agents. This enzyme has also been shown to be induced in Kupffer cells. Macrophages overexpressing CYP2E1 respond more robustly to stimulation in culture (5), and this may contribute to the priming effect of alcohol on these cells. Finally, ALD often correlates with an increase in the formation of autoantibodies, and autoantibodies against oxidatively modified CYP2E1 have been detected in the blood of persons with alcoholism (6).

Production of Toxic Metabolites

Acetaldehyde plays a central role in the toxicity of alcohol. Although acetaldehyde is subsequently oxidized to acetate by ALDHs (see Fig. 82.1), the kinetics of this reaction are relatively slow compared with alcohol oxidation, thus allowing acetaldehyde to accumulate detectably in humans consuming alcohol. Several of the systemic toxic effects of ethanol abuse (e.g., flushing, headaches, and nausea) are mediated, at least in part, by direct or indirect effects of elevated acetaldehyde levels. At the more local level, it is proposed that acetaldehyde also plays an etiologic role in ALD (7). For example, acetaldehyde, which is highly unstable, can form adducts with reactive residues on proteins or small molecules (e.g., cysteines), and these chemical modifications can alter or interfere with normal biologic processes and can be directly toxic to the cell.

Modified biologic molecules may also stimulate the host immune system and cause an autoimmune-like response. Antibodies against such oxidatively modified proteins have been found in both humans and animal models of ALD (8, 9). For example, a hybrid adduct of malondialdehyde and acetaldehyde (MAA), unique to alcohol exposure, has been shown to induce an immune response in both humans with alcoholism and animal models of ALD (10). Furthermore, acetaldehyde promotes enhanced glutathione (GSH) utilization and turnover, which results in significant GSH depletion (11). There are at least five different classes of human ADH isoenzymes, based on differences at the molecular level (12). Single nucleotide polymorphisms (SNPs) in the *ADH* genes that produce functional differences in the kinetic properties of the enzymes and the relative rate of alcohol metabolism have been identified (13). Indeed, correlations between lower ALDH activity and increased risk for ALD have been shown (14).

Other products of ethanol metabolism may also be toxic to the liver. In addition to oxidative metabolism, ethanol can be metabolized via a nonoxidative pathway with fatty acid ethyl esters (FAEEs) as end products (15). These molecules accumulate in the mitochondria and may uncouple oxidative phosphorylation. FAEEs are suspected to contribute to tissue damage in organs that lack oxidative ethanol metabolism (16).

Changes in Biochemical Processes

The concentrations of ethanol in the systemic blood can reach quite high levels; for example a BAC of 0.08% equates to an alcohol concentration of approximately 20 mM in the blood. Because of the first-pass effect of the liver on ethanol, the hepatic concentrations of ethanol are much higher than systemic levels. These high alcohol concentrations, coupled with the impressive rate of metabolism by the liver, stress liver cells biochemically. Indeed, although acetate from ethanol oxidation can enter the citric acid cycle after conversion to acetyl-coenzyme A, the various metabolic and biochemical alterations caused by ethanol exposure result in a negative energy balance (11). It is hypothesized that some of these biochemical changes caused by alcohol metabolism may cause ALD.

Steatosis is one of the earliest hepatic changes caused by alcohol, and it was originally thought to be a pathologically inert histologic change. It is now understood that steatosis may play a critical role not only in the initiation but also in the progression of ALD (17, 18). For example, fatty livers are more sensitive to hepatotoxicity from a second hit, such as endotoxin (17). Furthermore, the degree of fatty infiltration is predictive of the severity of later stages of ALD (i.e., fibrosis and cirrhosis) (19, 20). Because the oxidation of ethanol to acetaldehyde by ADH and the subsequent oxidation to acetate by ALDH use NAD^+ as an electron acceptor, the ratio of reduced nicotinamide adenine dinucleotide (NADH) to NAD^+ is dramatically shifted to a more reduced state. This increase in the reduced state of pyridine nucleotides may also be involved in the accumulation of lipids during alcohol ingestion. Specifically, the shift in the $NADH/NAD^+$ ratio increases the rate of fatty acid synthesis and esterification while simultaneously decreasing mitochondrial β-oxidation of free fatty acids. This change in the redox state can also impair normal carbohydrate metabolism; this has multiple effects, including decreasing the supply of adenosine-5'-triphosphate to the cell (21). Furthermore, investigators have demonstrated that this shift in the pyridine nucleotide redox state can activate the sirtuin family of histone deacetylases (22), which can alter gene expression profiles and thereby indirectly affect the metabolic state of the liver.

Hypoxia

As noted earlier, the oxidation of alcohol by cytochrome P-450 consumes oxygen (see Fig. 82.1). Furthermore, alcohol causes an acute hypermetabolic state in the liver, in which the oxygen consumption rate is doubled (23). This increase in the oxygen extraction rate also increases the intralobular oxygen gradient in the liver (24), thus causing pericentral hypoxia (25, 26). Hypoxia exacerbates the metabolic stress on the liver by further altering the pyridine nucleotide redox state. A decrease in cellular oxygen tension also exacerbates the ethanol-impaired mitochondrial electron flow from decreased delivery of O_2 to the mitochondria. After ethanol levels decrease, subsequent reoxygenation can increase pro-oxidant production via hypoxia or reoxygenation. This effect, in combination with impaired free radical defenses resulting from hypoxia, can contribute to the observed oxidative stress in the liver after alcohol exposure (27, 28).

Oxidative Stress

Reactive oxygen species (ROS) and nitrogen species (RNS) are products of normal cellular metabolism and have beneficial effects (e.g., cytotoxicity against invading bacteria). However, because of the potential of these molecules also to damage normal tissue, the balance between pro-oxidants and antioxidants is critical for the survival and function of aerobic organisms. An imbalance that up-regulates pro-oxidants or down-regulates antioxidants, thus potentially leading to damage, was termed "oxidative stress" by Sies in 1985 (29). There is evidence that oxidative stress causes ALD (30–32). Oxidative stress associated with clinical ALD is most likely not solely the result of increased pro-oxidant formation. Persons with alcoholism replace up to 50% of their total daily calories with ethanol (33); therefore, it is not surprising that they have a high rate of nutritional deficiencies. Alcohol abuse also can lead to malabsorption in the gastrointestinal tract, further exacerbating these deficiencies (34). The net effect is that persons with alcoholism often have lower levels of key dietary antioxidant molecules (21), as well as an overall decreased antioxidant status or capacity. Studies in animal models of ALD established a clear link between oxidative stress and the development of experimental liver damage caused by alcohol, and numerous antioxidants were shown to protect against the damaging effects of ethanol in vitro and in vivo models of ALD (35–37).

The most obvious pathologic changes to the liver during alcohol exposure occur in the hepatocytes. Moreover, the accumulation of products of oxidative stress (e.g., lipid peroxides) is predominantly a hepatocyte event during alcohol administration. This finding indicates that oxidant production by hepatocytes likely plays a key role in alcoholic liver injury. The two major sources of pro-oxidants in hepatocytes are the ethanol-inducible CYP2E1 and mitochondria. The reduction of O_2 to H_2O by the mitochondrion is not complete and proceeds to $O_2^{\cdot-}$ (38). Alcohol exposure even increases the yield of $O_2^{\cdot-}$ from hepatocyte mitochondria (39). Elevated pro-oxidant production by mitochondria not only increases the net yield of pro-oxidants in the hepatocyte but also directly damages mitochondrial proteins and DNA. Direct damage can exacerbate mitochondrial aging and stimulate mitochondrial-mediated apoptotic pathways (40). Moreover, alcohol depletes mitochondrial GSH levels (41), a change that increases the response of hepatocytes to apoptotic stimuli (42). Therefore, it is likely that pro-oxidant production from the mitochondria is critical for the development of severe ALD.

Inflammation is a key factor in the progression of alcohol-induced liver injury. Both resident (e.g., Kupffer cells) and recruited (e.g., neutrophils and lymphocytes) inflammatory cells are involved in this process. ROS production in hepatocytes is predominantly caused passively by electron leakage from biochemical processes, whereas inflammatory cells are active producers of ROS and RNS. The production of these species is critical for host defense, but these species can also cause damage to normal tissue, if they are inappropriately stimulated.

Inappropriate activation of Kupffer cells plays a key role in the initiation of ALD (43, 44). The production of pro-oxidants is increased in activated Kupffer cells. Major sources of pro-oxidants in these cells include NAD(P)H oxidase and the inducible form of nitric oxide synthase (iNOS or NOS2). Studies have shown that the NAD(P)H oxidase inhibitor, diphenyliodonium (DPI), prevents alcohol-induced liver injury in rats fed alcohol enterally (37). However, pharmacologic inhibitors can have nonspecific effects. Indeed, DPI is likely better defined as a flavoprotein inhibitor than a specific NAD(P)H oxidase inhibitor. However, protection against experimental ALD was also observed in mice deficient in NAD(P)H oxidase [p47^{phox} knockout mice (37)]. Together, these results add weight to the hypothesis that $O_2^{\cdot-}$ production from NAD(P)H oxidase plays a key role in the initiation of oxidative stress and experimental ALD. Investigators have demonstrated that iNOS knockout mice (45) and NAD(P)H oxidase–deficient mice (37) are protected against oxidative stress caused by alcohol, a finding indicating that the damaging oxidant in experimental ALD is dependent on the production of $O_2^{\cdot-}$ and NO.

Most research into the role of oxidative stress in alcohol-induced liver injury has focused on Kupffer cells or hepatocytes. However, more recent studies indicate that oxidative stress may play a role in the transformation of stellate cells into myofibroblasts, the critical matrix-deposition cell in the fibrotic liver (46). Indeed, oxidant production within the cell may be involved in its transformation (47). It is unclear at this time how much stellate cells contribute to oxidative stress in the organ as a whole, or whether pro-oxidant production in this cell acts mainly as an autocrine or paracrine signaling event. Because activation of this cell type is key in the progression to fibrosis and cirrhosis in ALD, more research in this area is required.

Oxidative stress can be mediated not only by an increase in ROS and RNS production, but also by a decrease in the antioxidant defenses. For example, alcohol can cause modifications to the cell that may favor oxidative stress. Moreover, persons with alcoholism often have lower antioxidant levels because of nutritional deficiencies. Hypoxia caused by alcohol exposure can impair antioxidant defenses. Additionally, free iron is mobilized by alcohol, and this process can also lead to an increase in transition-metal catalysis to potent oxidants (e.g., the Fenton reaction). Alcohol

exposure also inhibits the 26S proteosome in hepatocytes (2) that is responsible for degrading proteins damaged by ROS and RNS. Thus, when this complex is inhibited, proteins damaged by ROS and RNS accumulate, possibly even in the absence of a real increase in pro-oxidants (48). Finally, many proteins and systems are involved in the antioxidant network. This network does not directly block pro-oxidants, but it serves instead as ancillary reductants and maintains the catalytic activity of antioxidant proteins or small molecules. These reactions are energy dependent. Thus, the biochemical stress caused by alcohol exposure can indirectly impair cellular antioxidant defenses.

GUT–LIVER AXIS

Endotoxin or lipopolysaccharide (LPS) is derived from the cell wall of Gram-negative bacteria. Increased endotoxin levels are observed in patients with ALD and in rodent models of ALD. Increased endotoxin levels are also noted in animal models (high-fat or high-fructose feeding) of nonalcoholic fatty liver disease (NAFLD), and endotoxin/gut-derived toxins have been postulated to play an etiologic role in this disease process. Thus, much of what is described related to the gut–liver axis in ALD likely also applies to NAFLD, NASH, and other forms of liver disease. Elevated endotoxin levels in ALD may originate from gram-negative bacterial overgrowth in the intestine, increased intestinal permeability, or impaired hepatic clearance of endotoxin (49). Endotoxin then stimulates the production of tumor necrosis factor (TNF) and other proinflammatory cytokines through Toll-like receptor (TLR-4) signaling, which plays a critical role in the development and progression of ALD (Fig. 82.2). Other bacteria-derived toxins, such as peptidoglycan and flagellin, may also affect TLR signaling and

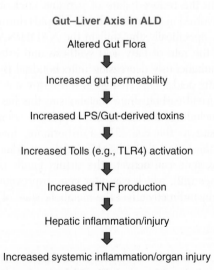

Gut–Liver Axis in ALD

Altered Gut Flora

⬇

Increased gut permeability

⬇

Increased LPS/Gut-derived toxins

⬇

Increased Tolls (e.g., TLR4) activation

⬇

Increased TNF production

⬇

Hepatic inflammation/injury

⬇

Increased systemic inflammation/organ injury

Fig. 82.2. Alterations in gut flora and permeability can lead to activation of hepatic Tolls, subsequent hepatic inflammation or injury, and ultimately systemic inflammation and organ injury. *ALD,* alcoholic liver disease; *LPS,* lipopolysaccharide; *TLR,* Toll-like receptor; *TNF,* tumor necrosis factor.

the United States, and BCAA supplementation is generally not widely used in the United States because of cost and lack of conviction concerning efficacy.

HEPATIC ENCEPHALOPATHY

All the factors involved in the pathophysiology of HE have yet to be elucidated, but the well-known components include increased ammonia levels resulting from decreased detoxification and the increased ratio of aromatic amino acids to BCAAs. The finding that these two processes can be altered by nutritional intervention has led to much new research.

The foremost topic in nutrition and HE has been the long-standing dogma of protein restriction. Given the evidence that cirrhotic patients start catabolism and develop a negative nitrogen balance following a short overnight fast, this concept has since been challenged (87, 88). A study of 30 cirrhotic patients hospitalized for HE showed no difference in the course of the disease between those receiving a normal amount of protein (1.2 g/kg/day) and those initially receiving a low-protein diet (129). Gheorghe et al (130) fed cirrhotic patients with HE a 30 kcal/kg/day and 1.2 g protein/kg/day diet divided into 4 meals including an LES. Of 153 subjects, 122 improved; notably, those with higher grade HE had the most improvement. Subsequently, the European Society for Parenteral and Enteral Nutrition (ESPEN) recommended avoiding protein restriction "at all cost" and for as short a time as possible in cases of severe protein intolerance. For those patients, it is recommended that BCAAs be given at 0.25 g/kg/day until the patient is able to resume normal protein intake (131, 132). This provides amino acids that do not require oxidation by the liver and are available for direct use by other tissues.

BCAAs have been studied in HE, given their role in increasing skeletal muscle and brain glutamine synthesis (thought to aid in breakdown of ammonia) and in increasing the ratio of BCAA to aromatic amino acids, thereby decreasing the amount of aromatic amino acids crossing the blood–brain barrier (133). Data continue to be mixed regarding the direct impact of BCAAs on HE. A 2003 metaanalysis of 11 randomized trials (including a total of 556 patients) demonstrated an overall significant improvement in HE following BCAA supplementation without an impact on survival or on the length of time to effect. However, because of "significant statistical heterogeneity" among these studies, the authors of the metaanalysis concluded that there was no "convincing evidence" of effect (134). As BCAA supplementation continues to be researched and given more recent favorable studies on its impact on disease progression in liver cirrhosis, more consistent data may emerge (see also the previous section on BCAAs).

Supplementation with probiotics, prebiotics, and synbiotics (the combination of probiotics and prebiotics) has been studied because of the potential to alter gut flora and subsequently the pH of the gut lumen. These changes can decrease ammonia production. Most studies involve

mild HE as revealed by psychometric testing, as opposed to overt HE. A study evaluated the use of a probiotic-containing yogurt for patients with nonalcoholic cirrhosis and mild HE and found reversal of symptoms in 12 of 17 study patients and an 88% adherence to the regimen (135). Liu et al (136) studied synbiotics (probiotics plus a fermentable fiber prebiotic) in patients with various forms of liver disease and mild HE (determined by psychometric testing and brainstem auditory evoked potential). These investigators found that patients with cirrhosis and mild HE had fecal overgrowth of *Escherichia coli* and *Staphylococcus* species that decreased after 30 days of synbiotic administration. The groups receiving either synbiotics or the prebiotic were found to have decreased fecal pH, venous ammonia levels, and serum endotoxin levels as compared with placebo. Fifty percent of the subjects in the study groups reversed their mild HE compared with placebo (136). Finally, a metaanalysis reviewed 9 studies involving 349 patients that evaluated synbiotics, probiotics, and lactulose. All studies demonstrated improvement in mild HE compared with placebo; however, limitations noted included short duration of the studies and small numbers of patients (137).

In conclusion, the key nutritional components for patients with HE include avoiding protein restriction, except in patients who are severely intolerant of supplementation. BCAAs may have a role in affecting HE, but further studies are needed; these may be limited, given the acceptance of other treatments including lactulose and rifaximin. Probiotics, prebiotics, and synbiotics appear to have a role in mild HE and can be delivered in something as simple as a yogurt supplement. The impact of other nutritional supplementation in HE, including zinc and L-carnitine, is still being evaluated.

CONCLUSIONS

Malnutrition, both PEM and deficiencies in individual nutrients, is a frequent complication of ALD. Severity of malnutrition correlates with severity of ALD. Malnutrition also occurs in patients with cirrhosis from causes other than alcohol. The mechanisms for malnutrition are multifactorial, and malnutrition frequently worsens in the hospital as a result of fasting for procedures and metabolic complications of liver disease, such as HE. Aggressive nutritional support is indicated in inpatients with ALD, and patients often need to be fed through an enteral feeding tube to achieve protein and calorie goals. Enteral nutritional support clearly improves nutrition status and may improve clinical outcome. Moreover, LESs in outpatients with cirrhosis improve nutritional status and lean body mass. With no Food and Drug Administration–approved therapy for ALD, aggressive nutritional intervention should be considered as front-line therapy, along with discontinuation of alcohol consumption. Many of the observations and therapeutic strategies concerning malnutrition and ALD apply to cirrhosis of other causes, especially hepatitis C.

ACKNOWLEDGMENTS

This work was supported by the National Institutes of Health grants P01 AA017103 (CJM), R01 AA0015970 (CJM), R01 AA018016 (CJM), R01 DK071765 (CJM), R37 AA010762 (CJM), R01 AA018869 (CJM), P30 AA019360 (CJM), and RC2AA019385 (CJM) and the Department of Veterans Affairs (CJM).

REFERENCES

1. Lieber CS. Clin Chim Acta 1997;257:59–84.
2. Bardag-Gorce F, Yuan QX, Li J et al. Biochem Biophys Res Commun 2000;279:23–9.
3. Cederbaum AI, Wu D, Mari M et al. Free Radic Biol Med 2001;31:1539–43.
4. Ekstrom G, Ingelman-Sundberg M. Biochem Pharmacol 1989;38:1313–9.
5. Cao Q, Mak KM, Lieber CS. Am J Physiol Gastrointest Liver Physiol 2005;289:G95–107.
6. Clot P, Albano E, Eliasson E et al. Gastroenterology 1996;111: 206–16.
7. Lieber CS. Biochem Soc Trans 1988;16:241–7.
8. Klassen LW, Tuma D, Sorrell MF. Hepatology 1995;22:355–7.
9. Niemela O. Free Radic Biol Med 2001;31:1533–8.
10. Thiele GM, Worrall S, Tuma DJ et al. Alcohol Clin Exp Res 2001;25:218S–24S.
11. Lieber CS. Clin Chim Acta 1997;257:59–84.
12. Bosron WF, Li TK. Hepatology 1986;6:502–10.
13. Visvanathan K, Crum RM, Strickland PT et al. Alcohol Clin Exp Res 2007;31:467–76.
14. Eriksson CJ. Alcohol Clin Exp Res 2001;25:15S–32S.
15. Laposata M. Prog Lipid Res 1998;37:307–16.
16. Beckemeier ME, Bora PS. J Mol Cell Cardiol 1998;30:2487–94.
17. Yang SQ, Lin HZ, Lane MD et al. Proc Natl Acad Sci U S A 1997;94:2557–62.
18. Day CP, James OF. Hepatology 1998;27:1463–6.
19. Sorensen TI, Orholm M, Bentsen KD et al. Lancet 1984;2:241–4.
20. Teli MR, Day CP, Burt AD et al. Lancet 1995;346:987–90.
21. Lieber CS. Annu Rev Nutr 2000;20:395–430.
22. You M, Cao Q, Liang X et al. J Nutr 2008;138:497–501.
23. Yuki T, Thurman RG. Biochem J 1980;186:119–26.
24. Ji S, Lemasters JJ, Thurman RG. Proc Natl Acad Sci U S A 1982;80:5415–9.
25. Arteel GE, Raleigh JA, Bradford BU et al. Am J Physiol 1996;271:G494–500.
26. Arteel GE, Iimuro Y, Yin M et al. Hepatology 1997;25:920–6.
27. Jones DP. The role of oxygen concentration in oxidative stress: hypoxic and hyperoxic models. In: Sies H, ed. Oxidative Stress. London: Academic Press, 1985:151–95.
28. Shan X, Aw TY, Shapira R et al. Toxicol Appl Pharmacol 1989;101:261–70.
29. Sies H. Oxidative stress: introductory remarks. In: Sies H, ed. Oxidative Stress. London: Academic Press, 1985:1–8.
30. Di Luzio NR. Lab Invest 1966;15:50–63.
31. Arteel GE. Gastroenterology 2003;124:778–90.
32. Shaw S, Jayatilleke E, Ross WA et al. J Lab Clin Med 1981;98:417–24.
33. Patek AJ Jr. Am J Clin Nutr 1979;32:1304–12.
34. Bujanda L. Am J Gastroenterol 2000;95:3374–82.
35. Kono H, Arteel GE, Rusyn I et al. Free Radic Biol Med 2001;30:403–11.
36. Kono H, Rusyn I, Uesugi T et al. Am J Physiol Gastrointest Liver Physiol 2001;280:G1005–12.
37. Kono H, Rusyn I, Yin M et al. J Clin Invest 2000;106:867–72.
38. Boveris A, Chance B. Biochem J 1973;134:707–16.
39. Bailey SM, Pietsch EC, Cunningham CC. Free Radic Biol Med 1999;27:891–900.
40. Cunningham CC, Bailey SM. Biol Signals Recept 2001;10: 271–22.
41. Fernandez-Checa JC, Kaplowitz N, Garcia-Ruiz C et al. Am J Physiol 1997;273:G7–17.
42. Colell A, Garcia-Ruiz C, Miranda M et al. Gastroenterology 1998;115:1541–51.
43. Beier JI, McClain CJ. Biol Chem 2010;391:1249–64.
44. Beier JI, Arteel, GE, McClain CJ. Curr Gastroenterol Rep 2011;13:56–64.
45. McKim SE, Gabele E, Isayama F et al. Gastroenterology 2003;125:1834–44.
46. Poli G. Mol Aspects Med 2000;21:49–98.
47. Kim KY, Rhim T, Choi I et al. J Biol Chem 2001;276:40591–8.
48. Donohue TM Jr. Addict Biol 2002;7:15–28.
49. Purohit V, Bode JC, Bode C et al. Alcohol 2008;42:349–61.
50. Gustot T, Lemmers A, Moreno C et al. Hepatology 2006;43:989–1000.
51. Luckey TD, Reyniers JA, Gyorgy P et al. Ann N Y Acad Sci 1954;57:932–5.
52. Rutenburg AM, Sonnenblick E, Koven I et al. J Exp Med 1957;106:1–14.
53. Broitman SA, Gottlieb LS, Zamcheck N. J Exp Med 1964; 119:633–42.
54. Nolan JP. Yale J Biol Med 1979;52:127–33.
55. Gabuzda GJ. Adv Intern Med 1962;11:11–73.
56. Zieve L. Arch Intern Med 1966;118:211–23.
57. McClain CJ, Zieve L. Portal systemic encephalopathy: recognition and variations. In: Davidson CS, ed. Problems in Liver Diseases. New York: Stratton Intercontinental Medical Book, 1979:162–
58. Adachi Y, Moore LE, Bradford BU et al. Gastroenterology 1995;108:218–24.
59. Keshavarzian A, Choudhary S, Holmes EW et al. J Pharmacol Exp Ther 2001;299:442–8.
60. Nanji AA, Khettry U, Sadrzadeh SM. Proc Soc Exp Biol Med 1994;205:243–7.
61. McClain CJ, Song Z, Barve SS et al. Am J Physiol Gastrointest Liver Physiol 2004;287:G497–502.
62. Iimuro Y, Gallucci RM, Luster MI et al. Hepatology 1997;26:1530–37.
63. Yin M, Wheeler MD, Kono H et al. Gastroenterology 1999; 117:942–52.
64. Honchel R, Ray MB, Marsano L et al. Alcohol Clin Exp Res 1992;16:665–9.
65. Szabo G, Bala S. World J Gastroenterol 2010;16:1321–9.
66. Gao B, Seki E, Brenner DA et al. Am J Physiol Gastrointest Liver Physiol 2011;300:G516–25.
67. McClain CJ, Cohen DA. Hepatology 1989;9:349–51.
68. Khoruts A, Stahnke L, McClain CJ et al. Hepatology 1991;13:267–76.
69. Naveau S, Chollet-Martin S, Dharancy S et al. Hepatology 2004;39:1390–97.
70. Boetticher NC, Peine CJ, Kwo P et al. Gastroenterology 2008;135:1953–60.
71. Wang Y, Kirpich I, Liu Y et al. Am J Pathol 2011;179:2866–75.
72. Kirpich IA, Solovieva NV, Leikhter SN et al. Alcohol 2008;42:675–82.
73. Mendenhall CL, Anderson S, Weesner RE et al. Am J Med 1984;76:211–22.
74. Mendenhall CL, Moritz TE, Roselle GA et al. JPEN J Parenter Enteral Nutr 1995;19:258–65.
75. Mendenhall CL, Roselle GA, Gartside P et al. Alcohol Clin Exp Res 1995;19:635–41.

76. Mendenhall CL, Tosch T, Weesner RE et al. Am J Clin Nutr 1986;43:213–8.

77. Mendenhall CL, Moritz TE, Roselle GA et al. Hepatology 1993;17:564–76.

78. Merli M, Romiti A, Riggio O et al. JPEN J Parenter Enteral Nutr 1987;11:130S–4S.

79. Baker JP, Detsky AS, Wesson DE et al. N Engl J Med 1982;306:969–72.

80. Campillo B. Assessment of nutritional status and diagnosis of malnutrition in patients with liver disease. In: Preedy VR, Lakshman R, Srirajaskanthan R et al, eds. Nutrition, Diet Therapy and the Liver. Boca Raton, FL: CRC Press 2010:22–46.

81. Detsky AS, McLaughlin JR, Baker JP et al. JPEN J Parenter Enteral Nutr 1987;11:8–13.

82. Patek AJ Jr, Post J, et al. J Am Med Assoc 1948;138:543–9.

83. Kearns PJ, Young H, Garcia G et al. Gastroenterology 1992;102:200–5.

84. Cabré E, Rodriguez-Iglesias P, Caballeria J et al. Hepatology 2000;32:36–42.

85. Hirsch S, Bunout D, de la Maza P et al. JPEN J Parenter Enteral Nutr 1993;17:119–24.

86. Hirsch S, de la Maza MP, Gattas V et al. J Am Coll Nutr 1999;18:434–41.

87. Yamanaka H, Genjida K, Yokota K et al. Nutrition 1999;15:749–54.

88. Swart GR, Zillikens MC, van Vuure JK et al. BMJ 1989; 299:1202–3.

89. Plank LD, Gane EJ, Peng S et al. Hepatology 2008;48:557–66.

90. Zhou Z, Wang L, Song Z et al. Am J Pathol 2005;166:1681–90.

91. Zhou Z, Liu J, Song Z et al. Exp Biol Med (Maywood) 2008;233:540–8.

92. Zhong W, McClain CJ, Cave M et al. Am J Physiol Gastrointest Liver Physiol 2010;298:G625–33.

93. McClain CJ, Marsano L, Burk RF et al. Semin Liver Dis 1991;11:321–39.

94. Wells IC Can J Physiol Pharmacol 2008;86:16–24.

95. Rylander R, Megevand Y, Lasserre B et al. Scand J Clin Lab Invest 2001;61:401–5.

96. Guerrero-Romero F, Tamez-Perez HE, Gonzalez-Gonzalez G et al. Diabetes Metab 2004;30:253–8.

97. Poikolainen K, Alho H. Subst Abuse Treat Prev Policy 2008;3:1.

98. Dahle LO, Berg G, Hammar M et al. Am J Obstet Gynecol 1995;173:175–80.

99. Brown KM, Arthur JR. Public Health Nutr 2001;4:593–9.

100. Neve J. Nutr Rev 2000;58:363–9.

101. Czuczejko J, Zachara BA, Staubach-Topczewska E et al. Acta Biochim Pol 2003;50:1147–54.

102. Jablonska-Kaszewska I, Swiatkowska-Stodulska R, Lukasiak J et al. Med Sci Monit 2003;9(Suppl 3):15–8.

103. Gonzalez-Reimers E, Galindo-Martin L, Santolaria-Fernandez F et al. Biol Trace Elem Res 2008;125:22–9.

104. Dworkin BM, Rosenthal WS, Stahl RE et al. Dig Dis Sci 1988;33:1213–7.

105. Bergheim I, Parlesak A, Dierks C et al. Eur J Clin Nutr 2003;57:431–8.

106. Arteel G, Marsano L, Mendez C et al. Best Pract Res Clin Gastroenterol 2003;17:625–47.

107. Evstigneeva RP, Volkov IM, Chudinova VV. Membr Cell Biol 1998;12:151–72.

108. Hill DB, Devalaraja R, Joshi-Barve S et al. Clin Biochem 1999;32:563–70.

109. Lee KS, Buck M, Houglum K et al. J Clin Invest 1995;96:2461–8.

110. de la Maza MP, Petermann M, Bunout D et al. J Am Coll Nutr 1995;14:192–6.

111. Mezey E, Potter JJ, Rennie-Tankersley L et al. J Hepatol 2004;40:40–6.

112. Sanyal AJ, Chalasani N, Kowdley KV et al. N Engl J Med 2010;362:1675–85.

113. Levy S, Herve C, Delacoux E et al. Dig Dis Sci 2002;47:543–8.

114. Hoyumpa AM Jr. Am J Clin Nutr 1980;33:2750–61.

115. Roongpisuthipong C, Sobhonslidsuk A, Nantiruj K et al. Nutrition 2001;17:761–5.

116. Leevy CM, Moroianu SA. Clin Liver Dis 2005;9:67–81.

117. Russell RM. Am J Clin Nutr 1980;33:2741–9.

118. Leo MA, Lieber CS. Am J Clin Nutr 1999;69:1071–85.

119. Malham M, Jorgensen SP, Ott P et al. World J Gastroenterol 2011;17:922–5.

120. Lieber CS, Casini A, DeCarli LM et al. Hepatology 1990;11:165–72.

121. Barak AJ, Beckenhauer HC, Tuma DJ. Alcohol 1994;11:501–3.

122. Song Z, Zhou Z, Chen T et al. J Nutr Biochem 2003;14:591–7.

123. Halsted CH, Villanueva J, Chandler CJ et al. Hepatology 1996;23:497–505.

124. Purohi, V, Abdelmalek MF, Barve S et al. Am J Clin Nutr 2007;86:14–24.

125. Marchesini G, Bianchi G, Merli M et al. Gastroenterology 2003;124:1792–801.

126. Muto Y, Sato S, Watanabe A et al. Clin Gastroenterol Hepatol 2005;3:705–13.

127. Kawamura E, Habu D, Morikawa H et al. Liver Transpl 2009;15:790–7.

128. Kumada H, Okanoue T, Onji M et al. Hepatol Res 2010;40:8–13.

129. Cordoba J, Lopez-Hellin J, Planas M et al. J Hepatol 2004;41:38–43.

130. Gheorghe L, Iacob R, Vadan R et al. Rom J Gastroenterol 2005;14:231–38.

131. Plauth M, Cabre E, Riggio O et al. Clin Nutr 2006;25:285–94.

132. Plauth M, Merli M, Kondrup J et al. Clin Nutr 1997;16:43–55.

133. Holecek M. Nutrition 2010;26:482–90.

134. Als-Nielsen B, Koretz RL, Kjaergard LL et al. Cochrane Database Syst Rev 2003;(2):CD001939.

135. Bajaj JS, Saeian K, Christensen KM et al. Am J Gastroenterol 2008;103:1707–15.

136. Liu Q, Duan ZP, Ha DK et al. Hepatology 2004;39:1441–9.

137. Shukla S, Shukla A, Mehboob S et al. Aliment Pharmacol Ther 2011;33:662–71.

SUGGESTED READINGS

Beier JI, McClain CJ. Mechanisms and cell signaling in alcoholic liver disease. J Biol Chem 2010;391:1249–64.

Muto Y, Sato S, Watanabe A et al. Effects of oral branched-chain amino acid granules on event-free survival in patients with liver cirrhosis. Clin Gastroenterol Hepatol 2005;3:705–13.

Plank LD, Gane EJ, Peng S et al. Nocturnal nutritional supplementation improves total body protein status of patients with liver cirrhosis: a randomized 12-month trial. Hepatology 2008;48:557–66.

Purohit V, Abdelmalek MF, Barve S et al. Role of S-adenosylmethionine, folate, and betaine in the treatment of alcoholic liver disease: summary of a symposium. Am J Clin Nutr 2007;86:14–24.

Sanyal AJ, Chalasani N, Kowdley KV et al. Pioglitazone, vitamin E, or placebo for nonalcoholic steatohepatitis. N Engl J Med 2010;362:1675–85.

83 ENTERAL FEEDING[1]

LAURA E. MATARESE AND MICHELE M. GOTTSCHLICH

Metabolic hallmarks of trauma and surgery include hypermetabolism and erosion of protein stores. Provision of sufficient nutrition to the critically ill patient is vital to optimize conditions that advance recovery. Traditionally, nutrition was regarded as adjunctive care designed to stabilize the patient during repair. More recently, nutrition support has evolved as an emergent medical intervention specifically designed to attenuate the catabolic response to stress, prevent oxidative injury, protect the gastrointestinal (GI) mucosa, modulate the immune response, and promote wound healing. Current clinical practice guidelines strongly recommend enteral nutrition (EN) support for patients who cannot meet their nutrient needs through voluntary oral intake (for purposes of this chapter, EN refers primarily to tube feeding methods). This chapter provides guidelines for the use, implementation time and access substrate characteristics, diseases, specific formulations, and various administration tips that are important to consider during EN support.

---

[1]**Abbreviations: AAA**, aromatic amino acid; **ARDS**, acute respiratory distress syndrome; **BCAA**, branched-chain amino acid; **COPD**, chronic obstructive pulmonary disease; **DM**, diabetes mellitus; **EN**, enteral nutrition; **GI**, gastrointestinal; **HE**, hepatic encephalopathy; **ICU**, intensive care unit; **MUFA**, monounsaturated fatty acid; **PEG**, percutaneous endoscopic gastrostomy; **PN**, parenteral nutrition; **RRT**, renal replacement therapy; **SBS**, short bowel syndrome; **VCO₂**, carbon dioxide production.

ROUTE OF FEEDING: ENTERAL VERSUS INTRAVENOUS

Besides the GI tract's role in digestion, absorption, and secretion, it is now recognized that the gut is a metabolically active organ that performs an important function in nutrient transport as well as immune defense. The deliberation on whether to use EN versus parenteral nutrition (PN) for feeding is largely academic because of the physiologic advantages associated with using normal digestive and absorptive pathways. In practice, if the GI tract is functional, accessible, and safe to use, EN should be given primary consideration with the mindset that intravenously supplied nutrients can be used as adjunctive support. Justification for directing nutrition support to the GI tract includes the fact that enteral nutrients experience first-pass metabolism in the liver, thus maximizing utilization. Furthermore, direct exposure of the small intestine to nutrition stimuli supports the functional integrity of the gut, enhances blood flow, and induces the release of endogenous trophic agents (e.g., cholecystokinin, gastrin, bombesin, and bile salts). Luminal nutrients help maintain normal intestinal pH and gut microbiota, whereas specific enteral nutrients (e.g., glutamine and short-chain fatty acids) provide a source of fuel for the intestine as well as stimulate enterocyte proliferation and growth. From a practical standpoint, enteral formulas mimic oral intake and supply intact nutrients such as fiber, whole proteins, dipeptides, and specialized fatty acids that cannot be delivered parenterally.

The positive effects of EN when compared with PN are well documented (Table 83.1) (1–24). The most consistent beneficial outcome from the use of EN compared with PN is decreased infectious complications (3, 13–17). A decline in mortality has not been clearly demonstrated. EN has also been associated with significant reductions in hyperglycemia (11, 18), hospital length of stay (19–22), and cost of nutrition intervention (11, 22–24).

INDICATIONS AND CONTRAINDICATIONS

EN should be the method of choice for all individuals with adequate digestive and absorptive capacity of the GI tract presenting with clinical conditions in which oral intake is impossible, inadequate, or unsafe to use (25). Determining

TABLE 83.1	POTENTIAL BENEFITS OF USING THE ENTERAL ROUTE FOR NUTRITION SUPPORT

Physiologic
  Maintains GI mucosal integrity
  Preserves gut barrier function
  First-pass metabolism in the liver
  Stimulates release of cholecystokinin
  Promotes digestive and absorptive capabilities of the GI tract
  Augments cellular antioxidant systems
  Decreases incidence of hyperglycemia when compared with PN
  Certain nutrients are not available in PN form (i.e., fiber)
Immunologic
  Decreased bacterial translocation
  Support of gut-associated lymphoid tissue (GALT) and mucosa-associated lymphoid tissue (MALT) for preservation of mucosal immunologic functions
  Lowered risk of infection
  Improved wound healing
Cost benefit
  Shorter length of hospital stay than with PN
  Less expensive than PN
  Simplified procedures and equipment

GI, gastrointestinal; PN, parenteral nutrition.

which patients should receive a feeding tube requires consideration of several factors including the patient's clinical status, diagnosis, prognosis, risk-benefit ratio, discharge plans, quality of life, ethical considerations, and the patient/family wishes. Specific indications for EN are listed in Table 83.2.

Contraindications to enteral feeding relate primarily to the presence and degree of malnutrition, the patient's ability to consume adequate nutrition by mouth, and GI

TABLE 83.2	INDICATIONS AND CONTRAINDICATIONS FOR ENTERAL NUTRITION SUPPORT

INDICATIONS	CONTRAINDICATIONS
Severe dysphagia from obstruction or dysfunction of the oropharynx or esophagus	Inability to gain access to the GI tract
Neurologic impairment, coma, or delirious state	Nonoperative mechanical GI obstruction that cannot be bypassed with a feeding tube
Persistent anorexia	Intractable vomiting or severe GI malabsorption
Psychiatric disorders	Adynamic ileus
Low-output enterocutaneous fistulas	Distal high-output fistulas that cannot be bypassed with a feeding tube
Increased nutritional requirements such as burns or trauma	Severe GI bleeding
Organ system failure	Aggressive nutrition intervention is not consistent with prognosis or patient wishes

GI, gastrointestinal.

integrity and functional capacity. Relative contraindications to enteral intervention include expectation of early resumption of oral intake in a previously well-nourished patient, mechanical intestinal obstruction, intractable severe diarrhea, severe short bowel syndrome (SBS; <100 cm of small intestine), or severe GI bleeding (see Table 83.2). Nevertheless, some of the potential barriers to EN can be circumvented with careful selection of the enteral access device, formula and route of administration.

SPECIAL CONSIDERATIONS

Reperfusion Injury and Low-Flow States

Reperfusion injury and low-flow states in which hypoperfusion of the GI tract is suspected must be considered when initiating enteral feedings. Certain clinical conditions frequently observed in critically ill patients such as hypovolemia, hypotension, and hemorrhagic and septic shock pose a risk for low splanchnic blood flow that can lead to GI dysmotility, increased mucosal permeability, endotoxemia, and multiple system organ failure (26–28). Disproportionate vasoconstriction can occur in response to an insult sustained during critical illness, raising concern that initiation of EN may be poorly tolerated by an underperfused intestine and intestinal ischemia is a potential but rare complication of EN (29–34).

Despite these concerns, evidence indicates that with appropriate patient selection, careful initiation and close monitoring, EN can be used successfully in critically ill patients (30, 32–35). EN may be provided guardedly to patients who are receiving inotropes or pressor agents, while observing for signs of intolerance or gut ischemia (25, 31, 33, 34). EN should be conservative until the patient is stabilized in some situations. For patients requiring significant hemodynamic support (including high-dose vasopressor use, alone or in combination with large volume fluid or blood product resuscitation to maintain cellular perfusion), EN should be withheld or delivered at a very low rate of infusion until the patient is fully resuscitated and stable (24, 34).

Altered Intestinal Anatomy

Patients who have had GI anatomy altered either by surgical resection, reconstruction, or replacement with intestinal transplantation can be fed enterally. The choice of enteral feeding will be largely dependent on the GI anatomy and health of the mucosa. An intact stomach, pancreas, and liver will enhance digestion and absorption. For the patient with SBS, several factors influence tolerance to EN (34, 36–41). In general, adults with more than 100 cm of small bowel ending in stoma or more than 60 cm of small bowel anastomosed to the colon can tolerate EN (via oral food or tube feedings) and achieve adequate nutrition with close monitoring and individualization of the diet. The site and extent of the surgical resection will also impact the patient's ability to tolerate EN. Digestion and absorption of most nutrients occurs in the duodenum and proximal jejunum, whereas the distal 100 cm of ileum is responsible for absorption of vitamin B_{12} and bile salts. Patients with jejunal resections generally tolerate EN unless more than 75% has been resected. The transit time is usually normal and they retain the ability to absorb vitamin B_{12} and bile salts. Resections of the ileum are associated with greater malabsorption. Malabsorption of bile salts can cause fat malabsorption, steatorrhea, and loss of fat-soluble vitamins (42). Since the terminal ileum is the site of vitamin B_{12} absorption, the patient will require supplemental parenteral or nasal vitamin B_{12} for life if the terminal ileum is resected. Patients may also experience rapid intestinal transit and small bowel bacterial overgrowth leading to intolerance of enteral formula. Loss of the ileocecal valve may result in decreased transit time through the proximal gut and loss of fluid and nutrients. Without the ileocecal valve, colonic bacteria can reflux and colonize the small bowel (bacterial overgrowth), which inhibits digestive enzyme activity and worsens chronic diarrhea and GI nutrient loss. For the patient with SBS, bacteria in the colon metabolize undigested carbohydrate and soluble fiber into short-chain fatty acids which provide a source of energy, aid in fluid and electrolyte absorption, and stimulate intestinal adaptation.

A standard, polymeric formula with complex nutrients (intact proteins, typically casein or whey, as well as glucose polymers, and a mixture of long- and medium-chain triglycerides) can be used for most patients with compromised intestinal function. The addition of soluble fiber is especially useful in patients with an intact colon to improve absorptive function and serve as a source of energy via generation of short-chain fatty acids (acetate, propionate, and butyrate) from bacterial metabolism of malabsorbed fiber in the colon (35).

Although the length of the remaining intestine is critical for successful EN in SBS, the health of the intestinal mucosa is also an important consideration. If the mucosa of the remaining bowel is diseased (i.e., Crohn disease, radiation enteritis), absorption will be impaired. For these patients, the use of a predigested EN liquid formula may enhance nutrient absorption and reduce output.

The ability to tolerate EN following surgical resection is also dependent on the amount of adaptation that has occurred (43). Medications (e.g., antidiarrheals, pancreatic enzymes, bile acid sequestrants, antibiotics, and probiotics) can be used during EN therapy to enhance absorption and reduce GI symptoms (44). EN support is also used following intestinal and multivisceral transplantation in those individuals with permanent intestinal failure (45). A jejunostomy tube is placed directly into the allograft at the time of surgery and EN commences within 2 weeks following transplantation (46). As EN is advanced, PN is reduced and oral nutrition is initiated. A standard polymeric formula that is high in protein and low in potassium is used because there are no data to suggest significant malabsorption of the intestinal allograft.

EARLY ENTERAL NUTRITION IN THE INTENSIVE CARE UNIT

The underlying metabolic responses to early enteral feeding and the benefit to clinical outcomes have been well described for the intensive care unit (ICU) patient (47). Secretory IgA, gut-associated lymphoid tissue (GALT), and mucosa-associated lymphoid tissue (MALT) are stimulated by enteral feedings and help fight infection locally in the gut and at distant sites as well (48, 49). An analysis of 12 randomized prospective controlled trials, showed significant reduction in infections and hospital length of stay with the use of immediate postoperative tube feeding or aggressive early oral nutrition versus standard therapy (50). A metaanalysis of 3 high-quality randomized controlled trials in trauma patients (total 126 patients) showed that the provision of early EN was associated with a significant reduction in mortality (odds ratio, 0.20; 95% confidence interval, 0.04 to 0.91) (51). Although GI motility is impaired in critically ill postoperative patients (52), the use of prokinetic agents alone or in combination with opiate antagonists and a multifaceted change in clinical practice (53, 54) aided the delivery of adequate EN support. EN and PN guidelines for critically ill patients have been published by the European Society of Parenteral and Enteral Nutrition (ESPEN) (55, 56) and the American Society for Parenteral and Enteral Nutrition (ASPEN) jointly with the Society of Critical Care Medicine (SCCM) (25). These guidelines make generally well-supported recommendations to initiate normal food intake or enteral feeding early and that EN is the preferred route of nutrition support over PN.

Current clinical practice guidelines suggest that tube feeding should generally be started within 24 hours after surgery for patients undergoing major head and neck surgery or major GI surgery for cancer, if possible (55, 56). In addition, it is recommended that EN should be initiated early in patients with severe trauma and in malnourished surgical patients (25, 55, 56). The presence of bowel sounds is not required to implement enteral feedings (see later). Current clinical practice guidelines (25, 55, 56) and several metaanalyses (50, 57) also favor the early institution of postoperative EN for surgical and acutely ill patients in the ICU setting without, however, uniformity of agreement (58, 59) or a clear definition of "early." Ultimately, the decision to start early enteral intervention must be based not only on the aforementioned recommendations but also individualized based on each patient's condition and special circumstances.

ENTERAL ACCESS

Access to the GI tract can be obtained at the patient's bedside, in the radiology department, the endoscopy suite, or the operating room (52–54). The state of the upper GI tract, the anticipated length of time that enteral feeding will be required and the potential risk of aspiration will determine the type of feeding device needed and its modality of placement. Generally, EN for a period less than 4 weeks can be provided using nasal tubes of variable length (30 to 43 inches) and diameter that are usually made of polyurethane and are 8 to 12 F in diameter. Feedings for longer periods require more permanent tubes such as those placed percutaneously made of silicone and are 18 to 28 F in diameter (gastrostomy tubes) or 8 to 12 F in diameter (jejunostomy tubes) (60–63).

The tip of the feeding tube may be positioned either in the stomach, duodenum or proximal small intestine. Despite several techniques described to correctly place feeding tubes (52–54, 64–69), nasogastric or nasoenteral feeding tube position should be confirmed radiologically before starting tube feeding (70, 71). In the critically ill patient needing temporary enteral feeding, predisposition to aspiration and pneumonia make the use of postpyloric feeding tube placement more clinically rational (72). In addition, postpyloric feeding has been shown to allow for the delivery of more calories and protein with less vomiting compared with nasogastric tube feeding (73). Maintaining nasoenteral tube position without accidental displacement is helped with the use of a nasal bridle and the risk of nasal necrosis is minimized by using umbilical tape instead of a red rubber catheter (68).

Nasogastric tube feeding in the postoperative patient may be risky in case of impaired gastric emptying and high gastric residuals that could lead to vomiting and aspiration. Although poor correlation exists between gastric residual volumes and the risk of aspiration (66), gastric residual volumes greater than 200 to 500 mL should alert the clinician to institute measures to minimize the risk of aspiration such as elevating the head of the bed, avoiding bolus infusion, considering the use of a promotility agent such as erythromycin or a narcotic antagonist such as naloxone and alvimopan, and considering the use of postpyloric feeding (73). In addition, the use of chlorhexidine mouthwash could reduce the risk of ventilator-associated pneumonia (74).

The most common complication related to enteral feeding is diarrhea (75–79), and its cause is multifactorial. It is commonly associated with magnesium or sorbitol-containing medication, antibiotics, infections such as *Clostridium difficile* infections, and formula intolerance. Infectious and inflammatory etiologies, fecal impaction, and medications should be ruled out before starting antidiarrheals. Reducing osmolality or adding soluble fiber or probiotics may be of help (78, 79). If intractable diarrhea persists, the volume of enteral feeding should be reduced until it is tolerated with consideration to addressing the caloric deficit using PN.

When enteral access is required for 4 or more weeks, feeding tubes can be placed endoscopically, laparoscopically, fluoroscopically, or by open abdominal surgery (54). The morbidity and mortality for feeding tubes placed by open surgery as the sole reason for the operation is high, primarily because of the patient's underlying medical conditions. Several techniques for surgical gastrostomies have been described (54, 80–94). At the time of laparotomy for other reasons, the most common approach to gastrostomy tube placement is the Stamm procedure. The introduction of percutaneous endoscopic gastrostomy (PEG) in 1980 (81, 89) revolutionized the technique of obtaining long-term enteral access and remains the most commonly used method for placement of gastrostomy tubes. It has greatly reduced the associated morbidity and mortality in properly selected patients (88–90). Beneficial outcomes with the use of PEGs have been reported for patients with head and neck cancer (85) and with stroke and head trauma (86), whereas its use in patients with dementia is controversial (88).

Many techniques to gain access to the jejunum for EN have been described (90–93). At the time of surgery for other reasons, the Witzel jejunostomy or a modification thereof (94) is commonly used. Gastrojejunal tubes are indicated when gastric decompression is needed, as well as jejunal feeding, as occurs in patients with impaired gastric motility with normal small bowel motility and absorption. These tubes can be placed at the time of surgery or laparoscopically.

ENTERAL FORMULAS

Once a decision has been made to initiate enteral feeding and access has been established, an appropriate formula must be selected. The selection of an enteral formula is based on matching the composition of a formula to the patient's clinical status, GI function, and nutritional requirements. A plethora of enteral formulas is commercially available to the clinician. Although no standard terminology exists, these formulas can be classified according to the composition of the macronutrient sources, and are referred to as polymeric or hydrolyzed. They can be further divided into standard, fiber-supplemented, disease-specific, and immune-modulating categories.

Polymeric Formulas

Polymeric formulas are the most common group of enteral products, and they are typically used for hospitalized, long-term care, and ambulatory patients. These products contain nutrient profiles that mimic a healthy diet so that a daily intake of 1500 to 2000 kcal provides the dietary reference intake for most nutrients. Protein constitutes 12% to 20% of total calories and is supplied as intact protein from eggs, milk, pureed meat, or protein isolates from casein, whey, lactalbumin, soy protein, or egg white. Carbohydrate, an important ingredient because of its energy and protein-sparing actions, originates from corn syrup solids, hydrolyzed cornstarch, or maltodextrin. Fat is included in these formulas as a source of essential fatty acids, carrier of the fat-soluble vitamins, and a calorically dense source of energy. Various oils are used including borage, canola, corn, fish, safflower, soybean, and sunflower oil. Polymeric formulas also contain a full complement of vitamins, minerals, electrolytes, and trace elements in 1 to 2 L. Most formulas are 1.0 Kcal/mL, but high-caloric-density mixtures (1.2, 1.5, or 2.0 Kcal/mL) are useful for those patients requiring fluid restriction.

Concentrated formulas may also be beneficial in terms of reducing volume needs in patients with heightened caloric demands or requirements for bolus, cyclic or nocturnal feedings. Because of the fixed nutrient and synthetic nature of these formulas, products may lack some phytochemicals, micronutrients, and unidentified growth factors that are present in food. Therefore, for those individuals on long-term EN, it may be advisable to consider the use of a commercially available blenderized product derived from whole foods.

Hydrolyzed Formulas

Hydrolyzed formulas, also known as monomeric, oligomeric, predigested, chemically defined, elemental, or semielemental formulas, use crystalline amino acids or hydrolyzed protein from casein, whey, or lactalbumin to provide short-chain peptides and free amino acids. Sources of carbohydrate include hydrolyzed cornstarch, dextrin, and fructose. The content of hydrolyzed formulas usually contributes a smaller percentage of total calories compared with polymeric regimens and is comprised of long- and medium-chain triglycerides. Hydrolyzed formulas were designed for patients with malabsorption and pancreatic insufficiency because these products in theory require less digestion by pancreatic and brush border enzymes. Limited data are available comparing hydrolyzed formulas with standard polymeric feedings. Studies evaluating the use of standard hydrolyzed products in patients with Crohn disease and critical illness (55, 56) found no significant difference in mortality, infections, complications, and diarrhea. However, patients with acute pancreatitis receiving a hydrolyzed formula had a significantly reduced hospital length of stay compared with those patients who received intact nutrients (95). Clinical trials that document the advantages of routine use of hydrolyzed formulas are limited. All hydrolyzed products are expensive and should be limited to those patients with malabsorption who do not tolerate standard polymeric formulas.

Fiber-Supplemented Formulas

Fiber is an important component of the diet and has beneficial metabolic and physiologic effects. Many polymeric formulas have been supplemented with purified fiber to promote bowel regularity, to control diarrhea, or prevent constipation. The fiber content of enteral formulas varies considerably both in amount and type. Functionally, fiber is classified by its solubility in water. Soluble fibers such as pectin and hydrolyzed guar gum are water soluble, have low viscosity, and can easily be added to enteral formulas. They prolong gastric emptying and are rapidly fermented by colonic bacteria to short-chain fatty acids.

Insoluble fibers such as soy polysaccharide and cellulose pass largely unchanged. They increase fecal weight, soften the stool, and shorten transit time. Insoluble fiber is frequently used in the long-term enterally fed patient as a means to prevent constipation. The research evaluating fiber-containing enteral formula in the management of diarrhea has not demonstrated consistent results. A metaanalysis of five randomized controlled trials failed to demonstrate any significant effects of fiber on diarrhea in enterally fed patients (96). The lack of consistent results may be because of differences in the amount and type of fibers used in each of the studies. Some enteral formulas have incorporated blends of soluble and insoluble fibers to promote healthy gut microflora. In a randomized, double blind, crossover trial, the use of a fiber-containing enteral formula resulted in a significant increase in fecal short-chain fatty acids, as well as improved microbiota in patients requiring long-term EN (97).

Disease Specific Formulations

A variety of commercial formulas have been developed for use in disease-specific conditions (98). The macronutrient portion and, in some cases, the micronutrients have been altered to promote improved tolerance and optimize conditions for recovery.

Diabetes and Formulas for Glucose Control

Diet is an important element for metabolic control and reduction of complications in patients with diabetes mellitus (DM). Several enteral formulas for diabetics have been developed for use in acute care with the intent to improve glycemic control and lipid concentrations; as such, the composition of these formulas has decreased carbohydrate, increased fat, and added insoluble fibers. Carbohydrate sources include complex forms such as oligosaccharides, fructose, and soy polysaccharides to prevent the rapid glucose absorption and rise in blood glucose concentration. The fat content is higher in monounsaturated fatty acids (MUFAs) and lower in polyunsaturated and saturated fatty acids. Lipids provide approximately 50% of the calories.

Few randomized controlled trials have been done evaluating the use and outcomes of diabetic formulas in hospitalized patients. Glycemic and lipid control of inpatients with type 2 DM was evaluated using a high-carbohydrate versus a low-carbohydrate, high-monounsaturated fat formula (99). The enteral DM formula with lower carbohydrate and higher MUFAs had a neutral effect on glycemic control and lipid metabolism compared with a high-carbohydrate, lower fat formula. In a randomized, double-blind, controlled, multicenter trial, a low-carbohydrate, high-MUFA DM formula resulted in a reduction in insulin requirements, fasting blood glucose, and hemoglobin A1c (100). Formulas marketed for DM have also been used in critically ill patients. In one study, use of a DM product in hyperglycemic ICU patients resulted in improved glycemic control and decreased insulin requirements but no difference in infectious complications, ICU length of stay, ventilator duration, or mortality (100). Overall, DM formulas can influence blood glucose levels, but the clinical significance of using these formulas remains unclear (101).

Renal Disease Formulas

Renal products have been developed to provide optimal nutrition to patients with a reduced capacity for clearance of various metabolites (102, 103). These formulas are typically lower in total protein but enhanced with essential amino acids and histidine to minimize uremic symptoms. Some of these formulas have increased levels of protein for use during dialysis. They are also calorically dense for fluid management and contain reduced levels of potassium, magnesium, and phosphorus compared with standard formulas. Some products do not contain vitamins or trace elements; others contain reduced amounts or only water-soluble vitamins. No clinical trials have compared the efficacy of enteral renal formulas with standard products, but they may be useful in some clinical situations (55, 102, 103). This will depend on the degree of renal function, the presence or absence of renal replacement therapy (RRT), nutritional status, and nutrient requirements. Patients receiving RRT have increased protein requirements and do not require fluid restriction. In the absence of elevated levels of potassium, magnesium, and phosphorus, patients undergoing dialysis should continue to receive a standard or high-protein formula. However, renal formulas may be useful in those circumstances where RRT is delayed or must be avoided all together. Additionally, with persistent hyperkalemia, hypermagnesemia, or hyperphosphatemia, a specialty renal product may be useful. Despite the lack of controlled clinical trials demonstrating improved outcomes, renal specific nutrition intervention can reduce the degree of protein depletion. For patients intolerant to standard formulas or for those whom dialysis must be delayed, the use of specialty renal formulas will allow provision of nutrients until dialysis can be instituted or renal function improves.

Hepatic Disease Formulas

Patients with liver dysfunction present unique challenges in that they are often malnourished but intolerant to provision of protein because of an imbalance of branched-chain amino acids (BCAAs) and aromatic amino acids (AAAs) resulting in hepatic encephalopathy (HE). The abnormal plasma amino acid patterns are characterized by elevated levels of methionine and AAAs, phenylalanine, tyrosine, free tryptophan, and decreased levels of BCAAs, leucine, isoleucine, and valine. The two groups of amino acid compete for transport across the blood–brain barrier and there is increased uptake of AAAs by the brain. These AAAs act as false neurotransmitters in the central nervous system and contribute to HE (104). Hepatic formulas have increased amounts of BCAAs and decreased amounts of AAAs to normalize the amino acid pattern and improve or reverse HE. In a prospective randomized double-blind trial, the effects of an oral BCAA supplement were compared with an isonitrogenous standard protein or isocaloric carbohydrate supplement in patients with advanced cirrhosis (105). The patients receiving the supplemental BCAAs showed a decrease in death and liver failure and they demonstrated greater improvement in nutritional status. There was no significant difference in incidence of encephalopathy or mortality among the three groups. The initial findings of a Cochrane Review of BCAAs demonstrated an improvement of HE when compared with controls. However, when including only trials with adequate sample sizes and good methodologic quality, no difference in HE, survival, or adverse events was evident (106). Based on the conflicting results in a few studies, the routine use of BCAA-enriched hepatic enteral formulas is not indicated. However, for those patients who are refractory to routine medical therapy for HE and are unable to tolerate standard protein formulas without precipitation of HE, the use of BCAA formulas may be warranted (107).

Pulmonary Disease Formulas

Whereas malnutrition, common in patients with pulmonary disease, can adversely affect respiratory function (108), overfeeding, notably with high-carbohydrate products, can result in added carbon dioxide production (VCO_2) and thus present an added burden to compromised lungs (109, 110). Specialized pulmonary formulas replace carbohydrates with increased amounts of fat to theoretically diminish nutrition-induced metabolic stress in chronic obstructive pulmonary disease (COPD) and acute respiratory distress syndrome (ARDS). Studies comparing the effects of pulmonary products with standard enteral formulas have been conflicting. Angelillo et al demonstrated reduced VCO_2 and respiratory quotient in ambulatory patients with COPD and hypercapnia when these patients were supplied with a high-fat substrate (111). In hospitalized, ventilated patients, VCO_2 and ventilatory time were significantly reduced in patients receiving a high-fat EN compared with a standard enteral formula with higher carbohydrate loads (112–114). However, other studies suggest that differences in VCO_2 and respiratory quotient may be influenced by excessive caloric intake to a greater extent than the composition of the formula. In ambulatory patients with COPD who were receiving a high-fat formula, no significant differences in respiratory quotient were demonstrated with a high-fat formula (113). Talpers et al provided ventilated patients with varying amounts of carbohydrate (40%, 60%, 75%) or total calories (1.0, 1.5, 2.0 times the basal energy expenditure) (114) . There was no significant difference in VCO_2 in the different carbohydrate regimens; however,

VCO_2 increase significantly as the total caloric intake increased. These data question the efficiency of high-fat, low-carbohydrate regimens (110) and suggest that it is more important simply to avoid caloric overfeeding in patients with pulmonary compromise (55).

ARDS, which is characterized by hypoxemia, results from a cascade of events involving free radical proliferation and proinflammatory eicosanoids production. A specialized enteral formula containing borage and fish oils as a source of omega-3 fatty acids (γ-linolenic and eicosapentaenoic acids) along with increased antioxidants (β-carotene and vitamins C and E) has been formulated specifically for use in ARDS and acute lung injury. The metabolism of specialty fatty acids and antioxidants promotes an anti-inflammatory and vasodilatory state, which improves gas exchange. In a multicenter randomized trial, patients receiving an ARDS specialty product showed a significant improvement in oxygenation, fewer days of mechanical ventilation, and reduced ICU stays when compared with the control group receiving a standard formula (115). Similar results have been reported in some additional trials (116–118) as well as in a metaanalysis (119). Results of a study, however, did not show benefits with administration of such EN formulas in ICU patients with lung failure (120). Although the use of enteral pulmonary products for COPD is not strongly supported by the evidence to date, use of anti-inflammatory formulas in ARDS and acute lung injury should probably be considered on an individual basis.

Immune-Enhancing Formulas

So-called immune-enhancing formulas refer to EN products containing varying amounts of specific immune-modulating nutrients such as omega-3 fatty acids, glutamine, arginine, probiotics, and/or antioxidants believed to exert beneficial effects on the immune, inflammatory, and metabolic processes (Table 83.3); however, this remains the subject of controversy and debate (119–123). Numerous studies have been conducted on heterogeneous patient populations using enteral feeding regimens containing a wide spectrum of compositional quantitative differences in nutrients and outcome measures. To evaluate these results and formulate a conclusion, several metaanalyses have been conducted. Beale et al conducted a systematic review of studies including 1557 critically ill patients that demonstrated significant reductions in infection, duration of ventilator support, and hospital stay, without any detrimental effect to mortality in those patients who received immune-enhancing formulas (119). Another metaanalysis of studies involving the use of immunonutrition in critically ill surgical and trauma patients was associated with a significant decrease in the incidence of wound complications and hospital length of stay in patients undergoing GI surgery and in those with critical illness (121). However, there were no differences in mortality or incidence of pneumonia. A systemic review of 24 studies (3013 patients) concluded that EN

TABLE 83.3	SOME CHARACTERISTICS OF COMPONENTS OF IMMUNE-ENHANCING TUBE FEEDINGS

Arginine
  May become conditionally essential in catabolic states
  Necessary for normal T- and B-lymphocyte and macrophage functions
  Role in synthesis of nitric oxide
Glutamine
  May become conditionally essential in catabolic states
  Primary fuel in rapidly proliferating cells such as enterocytes and immune cells
  Protects gut mucosa from injury in animal models
  Improves immune and barrier function of gastrointestinal tract, hence reducing bacterial translocation and sepsis in animal models
Omega-3 fatty acids
  Attenuates inflammatory injury via anti-inflammatory cytokine: ecosanoid network
  Modulates immunity via lymphocyte proliferation and phagocytic activity
  Improves gut barrier function in some animal models
Probiotics and prebiotics
  May prevent or reverse microbiota dysbiosis
  May modulate intestinal immune system
  May enhance gut barrier function
Antioxidants (vitamin A/β-carotene, Vitamin C, Vitamin E, selenium, glutamine)
  Antioxidants may have cytoprotective effects and decrease organ dysfunction
  May negate toxic effects of oxygen free radicals produced during critical illness

supplemented with fish oil improved the outcome of medical ICU patients (with systemic inflammatory response syndrome, sepsis, or ARDS) (124). A metaanalysis of immunonutrition EN in GI surgery patients (21 studies, 2730 patients) concluded that perioperative immunonutrition decreased overall complications, hospital infections, and length of stay without an impact on mortality (125).

Glutamine has been considered a conditionally essential amino acid during catabolic states when endogenous production is insufficient to meet increased requirements (24, 126). Results of several large blinded, randomized trials of enteral glutamine supplementation in ICU patients have been mixed, with some studies showing a decrease in infections (127) and others not (128). Results from ongoing, large, randomized controlled trials incorporating enteral glutamine will be available in the next several years to help determine the utility of this nutrient when added to EN in ICU patients (129).

There has been some concern regarding the use of arginine-enriched products in the subset of patients with sepsis, given the potential to induce hypotension from nitric oxide production (130, 131). However, more recent studies in patients have described no harm from immune products containing arginine (131–133). In spite of extensive preclinical and patient intervention research, a straightforward application of evidence to practice is not presently possible, although some studies identified specific patients in whom immune formulas offer benefits. The currently recommendation is that these specialty products be considered as a nutrition adjunct in patients undergoing major elective surgery and in those with trauma, burns, and head and neck cancer as well as critically ill patients receiving mechanical ventilation (24, 55).

ADMINISTRATION CONSIDERATIONS

EN is not without potential complications and requires proper administration and monitoring (134–136). The choice of method of administration is dictated by the type and site of access. Tube feedings can be administered via bolus, intermittent, or continuous methods. Bolus feedings are administered by gravity or syringe over a short period of time, usually 5 minutes or less. Generally, the patient is fed a volume of 250 to 500 mL of feeding four to six times daily. Feedings provided by this method may result in adverse GI effects because of the sudden delivery of a large, hyperosmolar formula. Intermittent feedings are administered over a longer period of time, generally 20 to 30 minutes, using a feeding container and gravity drip. Because of the longer infusion time, there is generally less GI intolerance than may occur with bolus feedings.

Bolus and intermittent methods are usually reserved for gastric feeding because the stomach can act as a reservoir to handle relative large volumes of formula over a short time. Although the large lumen of gastrostomy tubes allows for easy administration with these techniques, they can also be given through small bore nasogastric tubes. Bolus and intermittent feedings are the most physiologic method of administration because they mimic normal eating and allow the gut to rest between feedings. Additionally, they are the easiest to administer, requiring very little equipment. Feedings can be delivered continuously slowly over 12 to 24 hours, usually with an enteral feeding pump. The use of a pump is more desirable than gravity drip because a constant infusion rate can be sustained and accidental bolus delivery is less likely to occur. In general, continuous administration is usually tolerated best (134) and may be necessary when patients cannot tolerate bolus or intermittent methods. Transpyloric feedings require continuous infusion because the small bowel cannot act as a reservoir for large volumes of feeding delivered within a short time. Enteral formulas are initiated at full strength at 10 to 40 mL/hour and advanced to the goal rate in increments of 10 to 20 mL/hour every 8 to 12 hours as tolerated (136). Tube feedings can be cycled for patients who are transitioning from tube to oral feeding, in an attempt to stimulate appetite, or for those receiving home EN, to allow bowel rest and time off the pump. The feedings may be administered at night and discontinued during the day to afford the patient greater mobility and an opportunity to eat. They also may be infused continuously in an intermittent fashion to accommodate the patient's lifestyle and wishes.

CONCLUSION

EN support is a safe and efficacious way of feeding patients who are unable to eat. It has become not only a food replacement alternative but also through special formulations can optimize metabolic support of the critically ill patient. It is the preferred technique for nourishing patients when a functional intestinal tract can be safely accessed. The use of laparoscopic, endoscopic, radiologic, and bedside feeding tube placement techniques in the intestinal tract makes EN a feasible first choice for nutrition support of virtually any patient.

REFERENCES

1. Windsor AC, Kanwar S, Li AG et al. Gut 1998;42:431–5.
2. Petrov MS, Loveday BPT, Pylypchuk RD et al. Br J Surg 2009;96:1243–52.
3. Kudsk KA, Croce MA, Fabian TC et al. Ann Surg 1992; 215:503–13.
4. Heyland DK, Dhaliwal R, Drover JW et al. JPEN J Parenter Enteral Nutr 2003;27:355–73.
5. Kalfarentzos F, Kehagias J, Mead N et al. Br J Surg 1997; 84:1665–9.
6. Peter JV, Moran JL, Phillips-Hughs J. Crit Care Med 2005; 33:213–20.
7. Bower RH, Talamini MA, Sax HC et al. Arch Surg 1986; 121:1040–5
8. Fukatsu K, Kudsk KA. Surg Clin North Am 2011;91: 805–820.
9. Suchner C, Senftleben U, Eckart T et al. Nutrition 1996; 12:13–22.
10. Simpson F, Doig GS. Intensive Care Med 2005;31:12–23.
11. Gramlich L, Kichian K, Pinilla J et al. Nutrition 2004;20: 843–8.
12. Peng YZ, Yuan ZQ, Xiao GX et al. Burns 2001;27:145–9.
13. Moore FA, Moore EE, Jones TN et al. J Trauma 1989;29: 916–23.
14. Herndon DN, Barrow RE, Stein M et al. J Burn Care Rehabil 1989;10:309–13
15. Miller KR, Kiraly LN, Lowen CC et al. JPEN J Parenter Enteral Nutr 2011;35:643–59.
16. Moore FA, Feliciano DV, Andrassy RJ et al. Ann Surg. 1992; 216:172–83.
17. Kudsk KA, Minard G, Croce MA et al. Ann Surg 1996;224: 531–43.
18. Braunschweig CL, Levy P, Sheean PM, Wang X. Am J Clin Nutr 2001;74:534–42.
19. Taylor S, Fettes S, Jewkes C et al. Crit Care Med 1999; 27:2525–31
20. Neumayer LA, Smout RJ, Horn HG et al. J. Surg Res 2001;95:73–7.
21. Trujillo EB, Young LS, Chertow GM et al. JPEN J Parenter Enteral Nutr 1999;23:109–13.
22. Farber MS, Moses J, Korn M. JPEN J Parenter Enteral Nutr 2005:29:S562–9
23. Braga M, Gianotti L, Gentilini O et al. Crit Care Med 2001; 29:242–8.
24. McClave SA, Martindale RG, Vanek VW et al. JPEN J Parenter Enteral Nutr 2009;33:277–316.
25. Kirton OC, Windsor J, Wedderburn R et al. Chest 1998; 113:1064–9.
26. Flynn MP. Crit Care Med 1991;19:627–41.

27. Matarese LE, Costa G, Bond G et al. Nutr Clin Pract 2007;22:474–81.

28. Schunn CD, Daly JM. J Am Coll Surg 1995;180:410–16.

29. McClave SA, Change WK. Nutr Clin Pract 2003;18:279–84.

30. Melis M, Fichera A, Ferguson MK. Arch Surg 2006;141:701–4.

31. Zaloga GP, Roberts PR, Marik PE. Nutr Clin Pract 2003;18:285–93.

32. Berger MM, Chiolero RL. JPEN J Parenter Enteral Nutr 2009;33:702–9.

33. Metheny NA, Stewart BJ, McClave SA. JPEN J Parenter Enteral Nutr 2011;35:346–55

34. Atia A, Girard-Piper F, Hebuterne X et al. JPEN J Parenter Enteral Nutr 2011;35:229–40.

35. Nordgaard I, Hansen BS, Mortensen PB. Lancet 1994;343:373–6.

36. Nightingale JM, Lennard-Jones JE, Gertner DJ et al. Gut 1992;33:1493–7.

37. Weser E. Clin Gastroenterol 1983;12:443–61.

38. Messing B, Crenn P, Beau P et al. Gastroenterology 1999;117:1043–50.

39. Hoffman AF, Poley Jr. N Engl J Med 1969;281:397–402.

40. Nightingale JM, Kamm MA, van der Sijp JR et al. Gut 1996;39:267–72.

41. Matarese LE, Steiger E. J Clin Gastroenterol 2006;40:S85–93.

42. Abu-Elmagd KM, Costa G, Bond GJ et al. Ann Surg 2009;250:567–81.

43. Matarese LE, Costa G, Bond G et al. Nutr Clin Pract 2007;22:474–81.

44. McClave SA, Heyland DK. Nutr Clin Pract 2009;24:305–15.

45. Colomb V, Goulet O. Curr Opin Clin Nutr Met Care 2009;12:186–90.

46. O'Keefe SJ, Emerling M, Koritsky D et al. Am J Gastroenterol 2007;102:1093–1100.

47. Lewis SJ, Egger M, Sylvester PA, Thomas S. BMJ 2001;323:773–6.

48. Byrnes MC, Reicks P, Irwin E. Am J Surg 2010;199:359–63.

49. Ukleja A. Nutr Clin Pract 2010;25:16–25.

50. Doig GS, Simpson F, Finfer S et al. JAMA 2008;300:2731–41.

51. Doig GS, Heighes PT, Simpson F. Injury 2011;42:50–6.

52. Vanek VW. Nutr Clin Pract 2002;17:275–83.

53. Vanek VW. Nutr Clin Pract 2003;18:50–74.

54. Vanek VW. Nutr Clin Pract 2003;18:201–20.

55. Kreymann KG, Berger MM, Deutz NEP et al. Clin Nutr 2006;25:210–23.

56. Weimann A, Braga M, Harsanyi L et al. Clin Nutr 2006;25:224–44.

57. Doig GS, Heighes PT, Simpson F et al Int Care Med 2009;35:2018–27.

58. Heighes PT, Doig GS, Sweetman EA et al. Anaesth Intensive Care 2010;38:167–74.

59. Bankhead RR, Fang JC. Enteral access devices. In Gottschlich MM, ed. The A.S.P.E.N. Nutrition Support Core Curriculum: A Case Based Approach-The Adult Patient. Silver Spring, MD: American Society for Parenteral and Enteral Nutrition, 2007:233–45.

60. Zaloga GP. Chest 1991;100:1643–6.

61. Baskin WN, Johansen JF. Gastrointest Endosc 1995;42:161–5.

62. Munera-Seeley V, Ochoa JB, Brown N et al. Nutr Clin Pract 2008;23:318–21.

63. Rivera R, Campana J, Hamilton C et al. JPEN J Parenter Enteral Nutr 2011;35:636–42.

64. Rassias AJ, Ball PA, Corwin HL. Crit Care 1998;2:25–8.

65. Marderstein EL, Simmons RL, Ochoa JB. J Am Coll Surg 2004;199:39–47.

66. McClave SA, DeMeo MT, DeLegge MH et al. JPEN J Parenter Enteral Nutr 2002;26:S80–5.

67. Hsu CW, Sun SF, Lin SL et al. Crit Care Med 2009;37:1866–72.

68. Gunn SR, Early BJ, Zenati MS et al. JPEN J Parenter Enteral Nutr 2009;33:50–4.

69. Seder CW, Janczyk R. Nutr Clin Pract 2008;23:651–4.

70. Metheny NA, Schallom L, Oliver DA et al. Am J Crit Care 2008;17:512–19.

71. McClave SA, Lukan JK, Stefater JA et al. Crit Care Med 2005;33:324–30.

72. Fraser RJL, Bryant L. Nutr Clin Pract 2010;25:26–31.

73. Hegazi RA, Wischmeyer PE. Crit Care 2011;15:234.

74. Bellissimo-Rodrigues F, Bellissimo-Rodrigues WT, Viana JM et al. Infect Control Hosp Epidemiol 2009;30:952–8.

75. Wierdsma NJ, Peters JH, Weijs PJ et al. Crit Care 2011;15:R264.

76. Reintam A, Parm P, Kitus R et al. Acta Anaesthesiol Scand 2009;53:318–24.

77. Ferrie S, East V. Aust Crit Care 2007;20:7–13.

78. Fuhrman MP. Nutr Clin Pract 1986;14:83–3.

79. Elia M, Engfer MB, Green CJ et al. Aliment Pharmacol Ther 2008;15:120–45.

80. Gauderer MW, Stellato TA. Curr Prob Surg 1986;23:661–719.

81. Gauderer MWL, Ponsky J, Izant RJ Jr. J Pediatr Surg 1980;15:872–5.

82. Steigman GV, Goff JS, Silas D et al. Gastrointest Endosc 1990;36:1–5.

83. Scott JS, De LaTorre RA, Unger SW. Am Surg 1991;57:338–40.

84. Light VL, Siezak FA, Porter JA. Gastrointest Endosc 1995;42:330–5.

85. Lee JH, Machtay M, Unger LD et al. Arch Otolaryngol Head Neck Surg 1998;124:871–5.

86. Kostadima E, Kaditis AG, Alexopoulos EI et al. Eur Resp J 2005;26:106–11.

87. Murphy LM, Lipman TO. Arch Intern Med 2003;163:1351–3.

88. Garrow D, Pride P, Moran W et al. Clin Gastroenterol Hepatol 2007;1372–8.

89. Torosian MH, Rombeau JL. Surg Gynecol Obstet 1980;150:918–27.

90. Ho CS. Nutr Clin Pract. 1997;12:S17–9.

91. Senkal M, Koch J, Hummel T et al. Surg Endosc 2004;18:307–9.

92. Mack LA, Kaklamanos IG, Livingstone AS et al. Ann Surg 2004;240:845–51.

93. DiSario JA, Baskin WN, Brown RD et al. Gastrointest Endosc 2002;55:901–8.

94. Gerndt SJ, Orringer MB. Surgery 1994;115:164–9.

95. Tiengou LE, Gloro R, Pouzoulet J et al. JPEN J Parenter Enteral Nutr 2006;30:1–5.

96. Yang G, Wu XT, Zhou Y et al. World J Gastroenterol 2005;11:3935–8.

97. Schneider SM, Giarard-Pipau F, Anty R et al. Clin Nutr 2006;25:82–90.

98. Mesejo A, Acosta JA, Ortega C et al. Clin Nutr 2003;295–305

99. Pohl M, Mayr P, Mertl-Roetzer M et al. Eur J Clin Nutr 2005;59:1121–32.

100. Leon-Sanz M, Garcia-Luna PP, Planas M et al. JPEN J Parenter Enteral Nutr 2005;29:21–9.
101. Elia M, Ceriello A, Laube H et al. Diabetes Care 2005; 28:2267–79.
102. Kopple JD. JPEN J Parenter Enteral Nutr 1996;20:3–12.
103. Chiolero R, Berger MM. Contrib Nephrol 2007;156:267–74.
104. Fischer JR. Surgery 1975;78:276–90.
105. Marchesini G, Bianchi G, Merli M et al. Gastroenterology 2003;124:1792–1801.
106. Als-Nielsen B, Koretz RL, Kjaergard LL et al. Cochrane Database Syst Rev 2003;(2):CD001939.
107. Stickel F, Hoehn B, Schuppan D et al. Aliment Pharmacol Ther 2003;18:357–73.
108. Arora NS, Rochester DF: J App Physiol 1982;52:65–70.
109. Covelli HD, Black JW, Olssen MS, Beekman JF. Ann Intern Med 1981;95:579–81.
110. Lochs H, Dejong C, Hammarquvist F et al. Clin Nutr 2006; 25:260–74.
111. Angelillo VA, Bdei S, Durfee D et al. Ann Intern Med 1985; 103:883–5.
112. Al-Saady NM, Blackmore CM, Bennett ED. Intensive Care Med 1989;15:290–5.
113. Akrabawi SS, Mobarhan S, Stoltz R et al. Nutrition 1996; 12:260–5.
114. Talpers SS, Romberger DJ, Bunce SB et al. Chest 1992; 102:551–5.
115. Gadek JE, DeMichele SJ, Karlstad MD et al. Crit Care Med 1999;27:1409–20.
116. Tehila M, Gibstein L, Gordgi D et al. Clin Nutr 2003;22: S1–S20.
117. Singer P, Theilla M, Fisher H et al. Crit Care Med 2006; 34:1033–8.
118. Pontes-Arruda A, Aragao AM, Albuquerque JD. Crit Care Med 2006;34:2325–33.
119. Beale RJ, Bryg DJ, Bihari DJ. Crit Care Med 1999;27: 2799–2805.
120. Heys SD, Walker LG, Smith I et al. Ann Surg 1999;329: 467–77.
121. Heyland DK. Nutr Clin Pract 2002;17:267–72.
122. Cook DJ, Heyland DK. JAMA 2011;306:1599–1600.
123. Wischmeyer P. Curr Opin Anaesthesiol 2011;24:381–8.
124. Marik PE, Zaloga GP. Intensive Care Med 2008;34:1980–90.
125. Cerantola Y, Hübner M, Grass F et al. Br J Surg 2011;98: 37–48.
126. Wernerman J. Ann Intensive Care 2011;1:25.
127. Houdijk AP, Rijnsburger ER, Jansen J et al. Lancet 1998; 352:772–6.
128. Schulman AS, Willcutts KF, Claridge JA et al. Crit Care Med 2005;33:2501–6.
129. Wischmeyer PE, Heyland DK. Crit Care Clin 2010;26: 433–41.
130. Suchner U, Heyland DK, Peter K. Br J Nutr 2002; 87(Suppl 1):S121–32.
131. Martindale RG, McCarthy MS, McClave SA. Minerva Anestesiol 2011;77:463–7.
132. Preiser JC, Luiking Y, Deutz N. Crit Care Med 2011;39: 1569–70.
133. Drover JW, Dhaliwal R, Weitzel L et al. J Am Coll Surg 2011;212:385–99.
134. Plauth M, Cabre E, Riggio O et al. Clin Nutr 2006;25:285–94.
135. Anker SD, John M, Pedersen PV et al. Clin Nutr 2006;25: 311–18.
136. ASPEN Board of Directors. JPEN Parenter Enteral Nutr 2002;26:18A–138SA.

SUGGESTED READINGS

ASPEN Board of Directors. Guidelines for the use of parenteral and enteral nutrition in adult and pediatric patients. JPEN J Parenter Enteral Nutr 2002;26:18A–138SA.

Gramlich L, Kichian K, Pinilla J et al. Does enteral nutrition compared to parenteral nutrition result in better outcomes in critically ill adult patients? A systematic review of the literature. Nutrition 2004;20:843–8.

Kreymann KG, Berger MM, Deutz NEP et al. ESPEN guidelines on enteral nutrition: intensive care. Clin Nutr 2006;25:210–23.

McClave SA, Martindale RG, Vanek VW et al. Guidelines for the provision and assessment of nutrition support therapy in the adult critically ill patient: Society of Critical Care Medicine (SCCM) and American Society for Parenteral and Enteral Nutrition (A.S.P.E.N.). JPEN J Parenter Enteral Nutr 2009;33:277–316.

Weimann A, Braga M, Harsanyi L et al. ESPEN guidelines on enteral nutrition: surgery including organ transplantation. Clin Nutr 2006;25:224–44.

84

PARENTERAL NUTRITION[1]

REX O. BROWN, GAYLE MINARD, AND THOMAS R. ZIEGLER

---

[1]**Abbreviations: AMA**, American Medical Association; **ASPEN**, American Society for Parenteral and Enteral Nutrition; **BSI**, bloodstream infections; **CPN**, central vein parenteral nutrition; **Cr³⁺**, chromium; **EFA**, essential fatty acid; **EN**, enteral nutrition; **ESPEN**, European Society for Parenteral and Enteral Nutrition; **FDA**, Food and Drug Administration; **FFA**, free fatty acid; **GI**, gastrointestinal; **GSHPx**, glutathione peroxidase; **HPN**, home parenteral nutrition; **ICU**, intensive care unit; **LBW**, low birth weight; **LCT**, long-chain triglyceride; **MCT**, medium-chain triglyceride; **Mn²⁺**, manganese; **MVI**, multiple vitamin infusion **PICC**, peripherally inserted central venous catheter; **PN**, parenteral nutrition; **PPN**, peripheral vein parenteral nutrition; **PVC**, polyvinyl chloride; **RCT**, randomized controlled trial; **RES**, reticuloendothelial system; **TNA**, total nutrient admixture.

Malnutrition (e.g., loss of significant lean body mass and/or depletion or frank deficiency of specific essential vitamins, minerals, and trace elements) is common in hospitalized patients and in patients unable to maintain adequate nutrition and hydration by the enteral route. Various factors contribute to protein-energy malnutrition and loss of micronutrients in these settings, including catabolic hormonal and cytokine signals, resistance to anabolic hormones, lack of adequate oral food intake during illness, abnormal nutrient losses (e.g., via drains, renal replacement therapies, wounds, emesis, polyuria), *nil per os* (NPO) status resulting from diagnostic or therapeutic tests and procedures, and increased macronutrient and micronutrient needs during specific illnesses.

Assessment of nutritional status requires comprehensive evaluation and integration of medical and surgical history, current clinical and fluid status, dietary intake patterns, body weight changes, physical examination, and selected biochemical tests. The gastrointestinal (GI; enteral) route should be the first choice for specialized feeding in the hospital setting, with parenteral nutrition (PN) modalities, via peripheral or central vein, reserved for those patients in whom adequate enteral nutrition (EN) is not possible. Thus, a key feature of nutritional assessment is determination of GI signs and symptoms that may preclude use of the enteral route for feeding (e.g., severe, nausea, emesis, diarrhea, partial or complete bowel obstruction, bleeding, fistulas). In such a minority of cases, feeding via the intravenous route by PN support may be indicated.

Current guidelines suggest that goals for caloric intake between 20 and 25 kcal/kg/day and for protein and amino acids between 1.2 and 1.5 g/kg/day are appropriate for most adult hospital patients. These goals can readily be met in most patients with the conventional PN methodologies outlined in the chapter. Adequate vitamins, minerals, electrolytes, essential amino acids, and essential fats must be provided, based on recommended allowances for healthy individuals; although the true requirements for these in subtypes of hospital patients are unknown, conventional PN provides all these substrates, in addition to fluid. Metabolic, infectious, and mechanical complications can occur with PN feeding modalities and can be prevented or diminished with careful monitoring and adherence to current standards of practice. Relatively few

checking proper placement by radiographic study before use, and adequately caring for the insertion site. The use of ultrasound may facilitate central line placement. It reduces the number of failed insertion attempts and overall mechanical complication rates, particularly in the hands of inexperienced personnel, but it does not seem to decrease insertion time significantly (34). In 2011, the US Centers for Disease Control and Prevention published new comprehensive guidelines for the prevention of intravascular catheter-related infection (35).

DELIVERY SYSTEMS

Nutrient solutions for PN are delivered exclusively from plastic bags via electronic pumps. CPN solutions are generally delivered using peristaltic pumps of various types. These have become increasingly sophisticated, automated, and expensive. They ensure even flow rates, overcome the increased resistance of filters of small porosity (especially with continued use), minimize the likelihood of clotting at the catheter tip, and reduce the need for frequent nursing surveillance. Most have an air-in-line alarm system that prevents the occurrence of air embolism.

The use of pliable plastic bags of various sizes eliminates the danger of breakage, simplifies transportation and storage, and reduces storage space requirements before and after filling compared with use of glass or formed-plastic bottles. The usual water solutions of nutrient formulations do not extract measurable amounts of phthalate plasticizer used in the manufacture of polyvinyl chloride (PVC) bags; however, albumin, lipids, and blood take up the plasticizer (36). The amount of plasticizer eluted from PVC administration sets by lipid emulsions is relatively small compared with that from the bags. Plasticizer-free ethylene vinyl acetate tubing and bags have essentially replaced products using PVC.

Dual-chambered plastic bags that allow admixture of macronutrients immediately before infusion of PN are available. These are very convenient for home PN (HPN) use, especially for patients who receive intravenous lipids on a regular basis. Dual-chambered bags are manufactured either empty or with the macronutrients in them (i.e., dextrose in one chamber and amino acids in the other chamber). When lipid is used, the dextrose, amino acids, and electrolytes are added to the bottom chamber of the empty bag and the desired intravenous lipid dose to the upper chamber. Before administration, the plastic divider is removed, and the admixture with lipid is prepared. This increases stability because the total nutrient admixture (TNA) is not prepared until just before infusion.

Filters continue to be recommended during administration of PN formulations (37). In general, filters remove or reduce the infusion of particulate matter, air, and microorganisms into the patient. Particulates are found in large-volume injectables. Particulates have been found to clog pulmonary capillaries and actually cause pulmonary embolus when they exceed 5 μm. Potentially, they could also deposit in other soft tissues such as the brain, spleen, renal medulla, and lung. For those centers that use PPN, in-line filters have been reported to decrease the incidence of phlebitis (5, 6). The two filters used commonly during administration of PN formulations are 0.22- and 1.2-μm filters. The 0.22-μm filter is effective at removing microorganisms, particulates, and air. A 0.22-μm filter with a nylon membrane that has been positively charged has the ability to remove pyrogen (e.g., Gram-negative endotoxin) by electromagnetic forces (5, 6). TNAs should be filtered with 1.2-μm filters because the lipid particles in a stable emulsion are between 0.1 and 1 μm in size. Although lipid particles could be forced through a 0.22-μm filter, it would destabilize the emulsion. The 1.2-μm filter removes organisms such as *Candida albicans* because they are large particles in the range of 3 to 6 μm.

Patients who receive HPN will have several bags of PN stored in a home refrigerator to enhance compatibility before administration. These patients should be taught to remove the PN formulation 2 to 3 hours before administration so the product is closer to room temperature during infusion.

Insulin adsorption to the catheter varies appreciably depending on the binding characteristics of the nutrients present, the type of plastic in the delivery system, the presence of filters, and the concentration of insulin added (5). Insulin adsorption is minimal in TNAs. When insulin is added to PN formulations for diabetic patients, the dosage must be closely monitored until properly adjusted (5, 38, 39).

COMPONENTS AND REQUIREMENTS

Fluid

Fluid requirements for most adult are approximately 30 to 40 mL/kg/day (6). The fluid component of PN plus other intravenous fluids with or without any enteral fluid intake must meet individual requirements as determined by evaluation of the clinical and laboratory data (e.g., physical examination findings relevant to fluid status and plasma sodium and urea concentrations). Consideration of the close interrelationships of water, electrolytes, hormonal factors, and organ function is very important when prescribing a PN formulation. In addition to clinical factors that could cause excessive retention or loss, consideration must be given to fluid intake with medications and "keep-vein-open" infusions, as well as changes in insensible water loss. Meticulous recording of fluid intake and output is necessary. Assessment of volume status by hemodynamic monitoring may be required in some critically ill patients.

Standard PN admixtures can be administered to the patient with increased fluid needs, especially when extra renal losses are involved, with a supplemental intravenous solution to meet needs in the acute care setting. In the home setting, the extra fluid requirements can be added to the PN admixture in one plastic bag or can be given separately. For the patient who is fluid overloaded, the PN prescription should be made as concentrated as possible to minimize intake. Expansion of extracellular fluid is common in hospitalized patients with malnutrition, and this increases body weight and decreases serum concentrations of albumin, prealbumin, and other proteins, independent of nutritional status.

Energy and Macronutrient Requirements

Caloric goals in clinically stable, noncritically ill adult patients are estimated by current clinical practice guidelines at approximately 25 to 30 kcal (6.0 to 7.2 kJ)/kg body weight/day. A ratio of grams of nitrogen to kilocalories (N/kcal) of approximately 1:130 to 150 (1:31 to 36 N/kJ) is a routinely prescribed formula in stable non-ICU patients (5, 6). Shaw et al (40) developed a graphic presentation of the effects of nitrogen and energy intakes on nitrogen and fat balance in depleted patients. The amount of additional protein needed is usually proportionally higher than that of energy; for example, for adult patients acutely stressed by trauma, burns, or infection, the N/kcal ratio is commonly increased (e.g., 1:100). In ICU patients, precise caloric needs for improved clinical outcomes remain unclear, but lower doses (e.g., 20 to 25 kcal/kg/day) are recommended by European and American-Canadian clinical practice guidelines, given the risks associated with higher caloric loads in the ICU setting (see later) (7, 9, 14, 15). The energy goals for infants and children requiring PN are based on age and other factors and are beyond the scope of this chapter, but they have been reviewed in ASPEN guidelines (8, 41).

Currently, several RCTs are in progress to define clinically optimal PN calorie doses in ICU and non-ICU patients more accurately (16). Even though precise energy, protein and amino acid, caloric, fat, and micronutrient needs in the types of patients requiring PN are not well defined by rigorous data, conventional guidelines, based on decades of experience with PN administration, appear to be generally safe and effective for most patients (Table 84.4) (6–16).

Amino Acids

As noted earlier, conventional PN formulations provide all nine essential amino acids and a variety of nonessential amino acids, with the exact amino acid proportion and amount or volume varying as a function of the specific commercial preparation (Table 84.5). Intravenous amino acid solutions have evolved from the original hydrolysates of casein or blood fibrin to formulations of crystalline L-amino acids of different compositions and varying concentrations based in part on the amino acid composition of high-quality dietary proteins. Formulations of crystalline L-amino acids have been developed for specific clinical problems, with varying claims for superiority over more general formulas for use in renal and hepatic failure, in trauma, and for growth of infants (4–8).

TABLE 84.4	GENERAL GUIDELINES FOR MACRONUTRIENT DOSING IN ADULT HOSPITAL PATIENTS
SUBSTRATE	**CALORIE DOSE (g/kg/d)**[a,b,c,d]
Energy dose	Clinically stable: REE × 1–1.3 (or 20–30 kcal/kg/d) ICU: REE × 1–1.2 (or 20–25 kcal/kg/d) Initial PN order with 60%–70% of non–amino acid calories as dextrose and 30%–40% as lipid
Essential + nonessential amino acid dose (g/kg/d)[e]	
Normal renal and hepatic function	1.2–1.5
Hepatic failure (cholestasis)	0.6–1.0 (based on hepatic function)
Encephalopathy	0.6
Acute renal failure, not on renal replacement therapy	0.6–1.0 (based on renal function)
Renal failure, on renal replacement therapy	1.2–1.5

ICU, intensive care unit; PN, parenteral nutrition; REE, resting energy expenditure.

[a]PN amino acids provide 4 kcal/g, dextrose 3.4 kcal/g, and conventional lipid emulsion 10 kcal/g.
[b]Caloric needs can be estimated by indirect calorimetry; these measurements can be inaccurate in mechanically ventilated patients receiving high levels of inspired oxygen or as a result of air leaks or other technical issues with the ventilator.
[c]The Harris-Benedict equation can be used to estimate REE:
Males (kcal/24 hours) = 66.5 + (13.8 × kg body weight) + (5.0 × height in cm) − (6.8 × age in years)
Females (kcal/24 hours) = 655 + (9.6 × kg body weight) + (1.8 × height in cm) − (4.7 × age in years)
[d]In obese subjects, adjusted body weight should be used in the calculation of energy and protein needs by the following equation:

Adjusted body weight = current weight − ideal body weight (from standard tables or equations) × 0.25 + ideal body weight

[e]Some clinical guidelines recommend protein and amino acid doses approaching 2.0 g/kg/day (or higher) in certain subgroups such as with burn injury or renal replacement therapy.

Adapted with permission from Ziegler TR. Parenteral nutrition in the critically ill patient. N Engl J Med 2009;361:1088–97.

Commercial formulations differ among and within manufacturers in amino acid composition and concentrations, depending on clinical purpose; in addition, they may have added electrolytes and/or glucose. Concentrated standard amino acids in a 15% and 20% solution are now available for patients who are fluid overloaded and require PN. Many pharmacies that use automated compounders will stock one strength (usually 15% or 20%) of standard amino acids to make all PN formulations using this component (5, 6).

The typical recommended dose of amino acids for adults is 1.2 to 1.5 g kg/day, but in special circumstances, such as with continuous renal replacement therapy or burn injury (see the chapter on burns and wound healing), higher amino acid doses (approaching 2 g kg/day) have been recommended by some (42, 43). Higher PN amino

TABLE 84.5	COMPOSITION OF COMMERCIAL AMINO ACID PRODUCTS FOR PARENTERAL NUTRITION				
	PROSOL (20%)	AMINOVEN (15%)	TRAVASOL (10%)	TROPH-AMINE (10%)[a]	GLAMIN (13.4%)[b]
Manufacturer	Baxter	Fresenius Kabi	Baxter	B. Braun	Fresenius Kabi
Amino acid (g or mg/ 100 g amino acid)					
EAAS					
Valine	7.20 g	3.66 g	5.80 g	7.80 g	5.45 g
Lysine	6.75 g	7.39 g	5.80 g	8.20 g	6.71 g
Histidine	5.90 g	4.86 g	4.80 g	4.80 g	5.07 g
Isoleucine	5.40 g	3.46 g	6.00 g	8.20 g	4.18 g
Leucine	5.40 g	5.92 g	7.30 g	14.00 g	5.89 g
Phenylalanine	5.00 g	3.66 g	5.60 g	4.80 g	4.36 g
Threonine	4.90 mg	5.73 g	4.20 g	4.20 g	4.18 g
Methionine	3.80 mg	2.53 g	4.00 g	3.40 g	4.18 g
Tryptophan	1.60 mg	1.07 g	1.80 g	2.00 g	1.42 g
EAAs(%)	46%	38%	45%	57%	41%
NEAAS					
Alanine	13.80 g	16.65 g	20.07 g	5.40 g	11.94 g
Glycine	10.30 g	12.32 g	10.30 g	3.60 g	See footnotes
Arginine	9.80 g	13.32 g	11.50 g	12.00 g	8.43 g
Proline	6.70 g	11.32 g	6.80 g	6.80 g	5.07
Glutamic acid	5.10 g	0	0	3.20 g	4.18 g
Serine	5.10 g	6.39 g	5.00 g	3.80 g	3.36
Aspartic acid	3.00 mg	0	0	3.20 g	2.54 g
Tyrosine	250 mg	266 mg	400 mg	2.4 g (as tyrosine and acetyl-L-tyrosine)	See footnotes
Taurine	0	1.33 g	0	250 mg	0
Cysteine	0	0	0	240 mg (as cysteine HCl)	0
Glycyl-glutamine[c]	0	0	0	0	22.58 g
Glycyl-tyrosine[d]					2.57 g
NEAAs (%)	54%	62%	55%	43%	59%

EAAs, essential amino acids; NEAAs, nonessential amino acids; PN, parenteral nutrition.

[a]Designed for infants and young children (including those of low birth weight).
[b]Dipeptide-containing formula.
[c]Glycyl-glutamine dipeptide composition corresponds to 7.66 g glycine and 14.92 g glutamine.
[d]Glycyl-tyrosine dipeptide composition corresponds to 701 mg glycine and 1.70 g tyrosine.

Adapted with permission from Yarandi SS, Zhao VM, Hebbar G et al. Amino acid composition in parenteral nutrition: what is the evidence? Curr Opin Clin Nutr Metab Care 2011;14:75–82.

acid doses are also required for infants and growing children (8). The amino acid load in PN is adjusted downward or upward as a function of the amino acid dosing goal and as a function of the degree of renal and hepatic dysfunction, respectively (6–8, 15). Some guidelines recommend routine addition of glutamine as a conditionally essential amino acid in ICU patients (see the chapter on glutamine) (9). Although it is not questioned that essential and sufficient nonessential amino acids should be provided in PN in amounts needed to sustain adequate protein synthesis and intermediary metabolism, surprisingly, limited data from rigorous, adequately powered RCTs to define optimal doses of total or individual amino acids in PN are available (44, 45). Although some promising data have been published, little rigorous data are available on clinical efficacy of altered doses of specific amino acids in PN, including arginine, branched-chain amino acids, cysteine, or taurine supplementation (45).

Adequate EFAs should be supplied, and conventional intravenous lipid emulsions provide adequate linoleic and α-linolenic fatty acids; generally more than 3% of total kilocalories provided as EFAs are required to prevent EFA deficiency (see later). All essential electrolytes, trace elements, and vitamins are provided in conventional complete PN, but optimal intakes of specific micronutrient intakes to meet individual needs in clinical settings are essentially unknown, and more data are needed. Clinically, a reasonable approach is to maintain specific micronutrients, when measured, within the normal plasma concentration range. Deficiency of an essential nutrient may lead to negative nitrogen balance. For example, single deficiency of potassium, sodium, phosphate, or nitrogen impairs or abolishes retention of other elements, and zinc depletion can itself cause negative nitrogen balance (46, 47).

Carbohydrates

Glucose (dextrose) is the commonly used carbohydrate for caloric contribution in PN and is usually the major source of energy, typically ordered as 60% to 70% of the total

TABLE 84.6	OSMOLALITIES AND ENERGY VALUES OF INTRAVENOUS DEXTROSE PREPARATIONS[a]	
DEXTROSE (%)	OSMOLALITY (mOsm/kg H₂O)	kcal/L
5	278	170
10	523	340
15	896	510
20	1,250	680
25	1,410	850

[a]Dextrose = 3.4 kcal/g.

PN non–amino acid calories (see Table 84.4). Parenteral glucose is in the form of the monohydrate, with 1 g providing approximately 3.4 kcal. It is readily available in various concentrations in liquid form, is relatively inexpensive, and is rapidly metabolized by most patients. Using primarily glucose to meet large energy needs within a tolerable fluid volume requires an extremely hypertonic solution (Table 84.6).

Glucose Metabolism and Hormonal Changes

Infusion of intravenous glucose into humans results in an increase in insulin secretion, thus leading to increased insulin serum concentrations. In stable patients, this adaptive response is often adequate for maintaining normal or nearly normal serum concentrations of glucose. Abrupt cessation of PN can result in rebound hypoglycemia in some patients because the secretion of insulin is not blunted immediately with the withdrawal of the PN infusion. Therefore, clinical practice dictates that intravenous dextrose (usually 5% or 10%) be administered after withdrawal of PN to prevent hypoglycemia, unless the patient is eating some carbohydrate-containing food or is being tube fed (48). Adaptation to increasing loads of parenteral glucose and other nutrients decreased as the duration of infusion was shortened in test subjects, who were relatively stable adults being prepared for or already receiving HPN (49). Because such patients are not uncommon, tolerance to glucose must be checked before large amounts are infused in cyclic fashion. Other studies in adults found that abrupt termination of PN was rarely associated with significant hypoglycemia or its symptoms (50). ASPEN clinical guidelines on preventing hyperglycemia and hypoglycemia in the neonate receiving PN have been published (51). Sudden increases or decreases in glucose infusion can be averted by the use of infusion pumps that can gradually increase infusion of the admixture and taper it automatically, without changing the pump settings.

Glucose metabolism in patients with trauma, injury, burns, and sepsis or advanced cancer that induces weight loss differs markedly from that of physiologically normal persons. The reasonably stable patient can oxidize infused glucose to carbon dioxide (CO_2) efficiently up to approximately 14 mg/kg/minute, whereas the critically ill patient has only about half that capacity: 5 mg/kg/minute in burned patients and 6 to 7 mg/kg/minute in postoperative

patients. Infusion above the limiting rate results in conversion of glucose to fat, with an increase in energy expenditure and an increase above 1 in the respiratory quotient (RQ). Conversion of excess glucose to fat is energy dependent; after oxidation of the resultant fat, the derived energy (as adenosine triphosphate sources) is 30% of that theoretically obtained by direct oxidation of the converted glucose. Altered substrate metabolism in hypercatabolic patients is covered in chapters in the section on nutrition in surgery and trauma.

Control of Blood Glucose Concentrations

Throughout the history of PN, control of hyperglycemia has been an important component of the management of patients receiving this intervention. The administration of PN with a substantial component of dextrose contributes to hyperglycemia; however, it is usually this administration with the combination of an acute disease state (trauma, burns, sepsis), a chronic disease condition (diabetes mellitus), or concomitant pharmacotherapy (corticosteroids, protease inhibitors) that often results in moderate-to-severe hyperglycemia. Critically ill patients are particularly at risk for stress-induced hyperglycemia, which is well known to predispose to infection, possibly by impairing immune functions (6, 52).

A major clinical trial addressing hyperglycemia in critically ill patients was published by Van den Berghe et al in 2001 in which 1548 patients hospitalized in an ICU were randomized to intensive insulin therapy or standard insulin treatment (53). All patients were receiving PN or EN during the study. The intensive insulin therapy group received regular insulin as a continuous infusion to maintain serum glucose concentrations in the normal range of 80 to 110 mg/dL (4.4 to 6.1 mmol/L). The standard insulin treatment group received regular insulin as a continuous infusion when the serum glucose concentration exceeded 215 mg/dL. The goal in this group was to maintain the serum glucose concentrations between 180 and 200 mg/dL (10 and 11.1 mmol/L). The results from this major study demonstrated decreased mortality in the group receiving intensive insulin therapy (53). Several other improvements in hospital morbidity were realized in the group receiving intensive insulin therapy for patients residing in an ICU for more than 5 days: decreased length of ICU stay, decreased time receiving ventilator support, decreased prevalence of acute renal failure, and decreased bacteremia (53).

Both Van den Berghe et al (54) and Finney et al (55) subsequently published data that suggest that the improvements in mortality and clinical outcome result from the control of hyperglycemia and not necessarily the administration of insulin. In a subsequent large ($N = 6104$), multicenter, multinational study of ICU patients by the NICE SUGAR investigators, subjects were randomized within 24 hours after admission to undergo either intensive glucose control, with target blood glucose of 81 to 108 mg/dL (4.5 to 6.0 mmol/L), or conventional glucose control, with a target of 180 mg/dL or less (≤10.0 mmol/L) (56). The two groups had similar clinical characteristics at baseline. Mortality was slightly but significantly higher in the intensive insulin group at 90 days (intensive control 27.5% versus conventional control 24.9%; $p = .02$) (56). The treatment effect did not differ significantly between surgical and medical patients. Severe hypoglycemia (blood glucose level ≤40 mg/dL [2.2 mmol/L]) occurred in 6.8% in the intensive control group and 0.5% in the conventional control group ($p < .001$) (56). There was no other significant clinical outcome difference between the two treatment groups.

Based on this important trial and other studies of tight blood glucose control summarized by Kavanagh and McCowen (57), the current standard of care in ICU patients is to maintain blood glucose between 140 and 180 mg/dL (7.8 and 10.0 mmol/L) via insulin infusion and very close clinical monitoring to prevent hypoglycemia. Clinical practice guidelines by the Endocrine Society recommend a premeal glucose target of less than 140 mg/dL (7.8 mmol/L) and a random blood glucose value of less than 180 mg/dL (10.0 mmol/L) for the majority of hospitalized patients with noncritical illness (58). Studies have not been designed to evaluate tight blood glucose control parameters specifically in patients receiving PN, so these guidelines are currently recommended.

Lipid Emulsions

The clinical use and metabolic or oxidative, immune, and clinical effects of the variety of intravenous lipid emulsions now available for use in PN have been comprehensively reviewed (59–61).

Composition

Parenteral lipid emulsions consist of tiny droplets (≤0.5 μm) with triglyceride as the core and cholesterol derived from egg yolk phosphatides surrounded by a solubilizing and stabilizing surface layer of the emulsifying phospholipids (6). Intravenous lipid emulsions provide both essential linoleic and α-linolenic fatty acids and energy. In the United States, only soybean oil–based or soybean + safflower oil–based emulsions are available, primarily providing omega-6 as the long-chain fatty acid source. These are typically given as separate infusions as a 20% lipid emulsion over 10 to 12 hours/day. When pharmacy PN compounders are used, 20% or 30% lipid emulsions may be mixed with dextrose, amino acids, and micronutrients in the same infusion bag as TNA solutions and are given typically over 24 hours (6–8, 15).

More recently, parenteral lipid emulsions available for use in European and other countries outside of the United States have been formulated with partial substitution of soybean/safflower oil with oils containing MCTs, omega-9 monounsaturated fatty acids, or omega-3 polyunsaturated fatty acids (59, 60). Small studies, most in ICU patients, suggest that larger doses of standard soybean oil–based fat

emulsions may induce proinflammatory and pro-oxidative effects and possibly immune suppression (59–61). These may relate, in part, to arachidonic acid derived from the omega-6 fatty acid component (linoleic fatty acid) and downstream proinflammatory mediators, including leukotriene and other compounds (59–61). In addition, blood lipid peroxidation markers increase and blood α-tocopherol levels decrease in some ICU patients given soybean oil–based lipid emulsion, a finding suggesting that higher doses of vitamin E may be needed (61).

One unblinded small RCT in trauma patients showed that the group receiving soybean oil–based lipid emulsion with PN had a higher hospital infection rate, more days on mechanical ventilation, and a longer length of hospital stay than the control group not receiving lipids with PN (with fewer total calories) (62). Based on this study, and other nonrandomized observational studies, some clinical investigators advocate withholding soybean oil–based lipid emulsion during the first several days of PN in the ICU or in severe sepsis (7). However, rigorous published data on clinical outcome differences among lipid emulsion types remain limited.

Pediatric patients, especially neonates, with intestinal failure (e.g., short gut syndrome) are at particular risk for PN-associated cholestasis and liver dysfunction by mechanisms that remain unclear (63). However, this complication was markedly decreased with administration of fish oil–based PN substituted for soybean oil–based PN in small studies (64–66). Simply reducing the soybean oil–based lipid may be responsible for some or most of these benefits (67).

Several well-powered RCTs are now in progress to assess the clinical efficacy of the newer lipid emulsions compared with soybean oil–based lipids in PN in various clinical conditions in adults, and, with regard to fish oil, in children requiring PN (59–67). For example, in a recent double-blind, parallel group RCT of 100 medical or surgical ICU patients requiring PN, patients receiving an 80% olive oil/20% soybean oil lipid emulsion in PN demonstrated similar clinical outcomes (infections, organ dysfunction, mortality) and plasma inflammatory or oxidative stress indexes and neutrophil functions compared with patients receiving PN with conventional soybean oil–based lipid emulsion (68).

In CPN, a reasonable initial guideline is to provide 30% to 40% of non–amino acid calories as fat emulsion (see Table 84.4). The recommended maximal dose of fat emulsion infusion is approximately 1.0 to 1.3 g/kg/day, with monitoring of blood triglyceride concentrations at baseline and then generally weekly, particularly in patients with known lipid disorders, pancreatitis, or liver or renal disease, to assess triglyceride clearance (15). Triglyceride levels should be maintained at less than 400 to 500 mg/dL to decrease the potential risk of pancreatitis and diminished pulmonary diffusion capacity in patients with severe chronic obstructive lung disease, which may occur with very high triglyceride levels.

Metabolism

After infusion of intravenous fat emulsions into humans, lipoprotein lipase (LPL) acts on the triglyceride portion of this product and converts it to free fatty acids (FFAs). The FFAs can enter the mitochondria via carnitine to be oxidized directly for energy, stored in adipose tissue, or transported to the liver via albumin to be synthesized into complex lipids (69). When the concentration of lipid increases to the level at which binding sites on LPL are saturated, a maximum elimination capacity has been reached. In physiologically normal adults, this maximum rate is about 3.8 g of fat/kg/24 hours, which corresponds to about 35 kcal/kg/24 hours. It increases in starvation (~50%) and even more in trauma (70).

Stability and Safety Factors

The admixture system is potentially unstable. The relevant properties of the phosphatide emulsifiers and various factors influencing stability of the fat emulsions in the presence of various additives in the admixture have been reviewed (71). Driscoll et al (72) found that iron dextran was the most disruptive component of TNAs. These investigators studied the effects of many additives, including amino acids, lipids, dextrose, and monovalent, divalent, and trivalent ions. Based on these results, using more sophisticated analysis, addition of any dose of iron dextran to replete iron stores to a TNA is discouraged. Less microbial growth over 24 hours occurs in TNAs than in intravenous lipid emulsions themselves (71, 72). This finding led the Centers for Disease Control and Prevention to recommend a 12-hour maximal infusion time for intravenous lipid emulsions not in TNAs.

Potential Adverse Effects of Lipid Infusions

Because the ability to metabolize these emulsions is related directly to infant maturity, the risk of lipid accumulation in blood and its sequelae is greatest in the premature infant, the small for gestational age low birth weight (LBW) infant, and the nutritionally depleted older child. Lipid accumulation in the hepatic reticuloendothelial system (RES) with the likelihood of depressed immune responses and its competition with bilirubin and other substances for albumin binding has been described. Cases have been reported, primarily in young children, of bleeding dyscrasia in association with high plasma lipid concentrations and platelets engorged with lipid (6). Reports of altered pulmonary function during acute hyperlipidemia have varied; whereas decreased pulmonary diffusion capacity has been noted by some, other investigators have found no change in lung dynamics but rather have found decreased arterial oxygenation (6, 73, 74).

Patients with acute respiratory distress syndrome who received 500 mL of 20% intravenous lipid emulsion over 8 hours (maximum rate suggested in package inserts) demonstrated a significant decrease in arterial partial pressure of oxygen (PaO_2), fraction of inspired oxygen (FiO_2), and mean pulmonary arterial pressure and a significant increase in pulmonary vascular resistance and pulmonary venous admixture (73, 74). Intravenous lipid emulsions should be administered cautiously over at least 12 hours to patients with acute respiratory distress syndrome. An advantage of TNA PN mixtures, in which lipids are admixed with other PN constituents, is that the lipid component is administered typically over 24 hours in hospital patients. In light of conventional caloric goals in ICU patients (20 to 25 kcal/kg/day maximum), 250 mL of a standard 20% soybean oil–based lipid, which provides 50 g lipid and 500 kcal from fat (10 kcal/g), is a reasonable daily dose. This lipid emulsion dose in PN can be decreased from daily dosing to administration two to three times weekly (or can be temporarily discontinued) if plasma triglycerides rise to more than 400 mg/dL (6, 15).

The increased uptake of long-chain lipids by the RES in patients with hepatosplenomegaly and decreased clearance of lipids led to concern about possible depression of immune responses with such infusions and increased susceptibility to infection. Using clearance of sulfur colloid technetium-99 as a marker of RES function, 3 days of administration of soybean oil–based intravenous fat emulsion resulted in significant impairment in humans receiving PN at a dose of 0.13 g/kg/hour for 10 hours daily. It took 3 days of lipid administration for this measurement of immunologic impairment to occur (75). A follow-up study demonstrated little change from baseline in the clearance of sulfur colloid technetium-99 when a lipid emulsion containing both long-chain triglycerides (LCTs) and MCTs was used (76).

Various immune functions were studied in malnourished patients with cancer who were maintained on either a glucose-based PN formula or one with both glucose and lipid; depressed cell-mediated immunity was noted before starting PN, and no alteration in these parameters was observed with fat infusion (77). Lenssen et al (78) studied 512 patients who underwent either autologous or allogeneic bone marrow transplantation. All patients received PN in the postoperative period, so that oral feeding and PN provided 1.5 times basal energy expenditure. Patients were then stratified by several clinical factors and randomized to either a low dose or a standard dose of intravenous lipid. The low dose was 6% to 8% of total parenteral calories from intravenous lipids, and the standard dose was 25% to 30% of total parenteral calories from intravenous lipids. No significant differences in the incidence in bacteremia and fungemia were noted between the 2 groups of lipid doses. There was still no significant difference between groups when the observation period was extended to 60 days after transplantation. These data strongly suggest that moderate doses of intravenous lipids have no appreciable effect on infection in this immunocompromised patient population.

Although various immune-associated abnormalities of cell-mediated immunity have been shown with infusion of soybean oil–based lipid emulsions, such studies have been small to date, and adequately powered rigorous comparative effectiveness trials in this regard are needed (59, 60). As noted, a double-blind RCT showed no difference in infections or neutrophil immune functions when comparing adult ICU patients receiving an olive oil–based with a soybean oil–based lipid emulsion in PN (68).

Lipids as Pharmacologic Vehicles

Some drugs are now marketed in intravenous soybean oil–based lipid emulsions. One example is propofol, originally marketed for induction of anesthesia, but used commonly for sedation in the critical care setting. It is prepared by the manufacturer in 10% fat emulsion (1.1 kcal/mL), and some patients who require large doses of propofol receive substantial kilocalories per day from this agent (e.g., 20 mL/hour propofol provides 528 kcal/day from the lipid component) (79). In addition, several lipid formulations of amphotericin B have been marketed in the United States; however, the caloric contribution of lipid formulations of amphotericin B is negligible. Clevidipine is an intravenous calcium channel blocker sometimes used to control postoperative hypertension; it is also formulated in a 20% lipid emulsion, providing 2 kcal/mL from fat. Thus, the lipid kilocalories provided from these agents, especially propofol, which is commonly administered for several days or longer in ICU patients, must be taken into account in PN orders to avoid complications from overfeeding calories (see later).

Minerals

Sodium, potassium, calcium, magnesium, phosphate, and chloride are essential nutrients and are all provided in conventional PN on an individual basis (see Table 84.3). Detailed information on electrolyte and mineral depletion and repletion is given in the chapter on electrolytes. Because many patients receiving or needing PN have malabsorption of the alimentary tract or impaired renal reabsorption, or both, often associated with large fluid ionic losses, a continuing concern in the care of such patients is the adequacy of fluid and electrolyte balance (6,7, 80). In general, patients who are critically ill require typically daily monitoring of electrolyte (sodium, potassium, calcium, magnesium, phosphate) concentrations in blood with PN dosing adjustments as needed and close serial monitoring to follow.

The basic daily needs of patients with reasonably normal cardiovascular, intestinal, renal, hormonal, and hydration status are 50 to 60 mEq (mmol) of sodium, 40 mEq (mmol) of chloride and bicarbonate (including those associated with amino acids as acetate), and 40 to 60 mEq (mmol) of potassium. Excessive losses from the intestine or kidney and abnormal retention require appropriate changes, with suitable monitoring as needed. Mineral needs of infants and children have been summarized in the literature (6).

Calcium and phosphorus (as inorganic phosphate) are needed in relatively large amounts by infants; however,

when both are present in relatively large concentrations, solubility in the PN solution becomes a problem. It has been recommended that glycerophosphate or glucose phosphate be given together with calcium gluconate or calcium glycerophosphate as more soluble forms of these nutrients. Reference curves have been developed to estimate calcium and phosphate compatibility in commonly used neonatal PN solutions (81). Recommended pediatric concentrations of calcium, phosphorus, and magnesium per liter of PN solution are given by Greene et al (82). Adults require between 10 and 25 mEq of calcium/day via PN.

Negative calcium balance related to hypercalciuria may occur in adults receiving PN, especially during the infusion period of cyclic PN; supplementation with either sodium or potassium acetate (replacing equimolar amounts of NaCl or KCl) resulted in major decreases in urinary calcium in patients receiving 24-hour and cyclic PN, primarily because of increased renal tubular reabsorption with reduced excretion to near-infusion levels (83). Reports are contradictory concerning whether urinary calcium excretion with 12-hour cyclic PN is greater than that with continuous 24-hour infusion (83). Although this may not be a significant issue for the short-term patient, it may be important for patients receiving prolonged PN because chronic negative calcium balance would result in skeletal calcium loss.

In a case series, six patients receiving long-term PN (mean of 19 years) demonstrated a significantly decreased bone mass when compared with physiologically normal volunteers (84). The patients had higher serum parathyroid hormone concentrations compared with physiologically normal persons, but they had an abnormally low response to sodium acetate infusions, which suggested that they had secondary hyperparathyroidism (84). Metabolic bone diseases, including osteoporosis and osteomalacia, are common in patients receiving PN. Initially considered to be a manifestation of aluminium toxicity from aluminum contamination of PN, metabolic osteopathy during PN is now considered to be a multifactorial syndrome, and exact causes within individual patients may be obscure (85–87).

Hypophosphatemia has multiple causes (see the chapter on phosphorus); however, in patients receiving PN, it is often associated with sudden infusion of glucose, the metabolism of which stimulates transfer of phosphate from plasma to cells (see the later discussion of the refeeding syndrome). Hypophosphatemia can be treated during provision of PN by using a graduated dosing scheme based on the serum phosphorus concentration in patients with normal renal function (88). For serum phosphorus concentrations lower than 1.5 mg/dL, 0.64 mmol/kg was given over 8 hours; doses of 0.32 mmol/kg over 4 to 6 hours and 0.16 mmol/kg over 4 hours were given for serum phosphorus concentrations of 1.6 to 2.2 mg/dL and 2.3 to 3.0 mg/dL, respectively (88). Some data support more aggressive replacement of phosphorus in patients with moderate-to-severe hypophosphatemia (89).

The importance of magnesium and magnesium balance is being appreciated more, especially in the critical care setting, in which serum magnesium concentrations are being assessed with increased frequency, and risk factors for magnesium depletion are now well recognized (see the chapter on magnesium). Although the serum magnesium concentration does not always accurately reflect magnesium status, a low concentration usually indicates magnesium deficiency. Doses for management of moderate to severe deficiency in various clinical situations for various age groups are given in the chapter on magnesium and elsewhere, including in ASPEN guidelines for daily electrolyte and mineral requirements for adults and children (6, 90). Hypermagnesemia may occur with fluctuating or progressively deteriorating renal function or decreasing intestinal or renal magnesium loss; periodic monitoring of blood magnesium concentrations and adjustment in PN are necessary.

Trace Elements

Acceptable direct evidence indicates that iron, iodide, zinc, copper, Cr^{3+}, and selenium are essential human nutrients (6). The biochemical and physiologic roles of these trace elements and the effects of their depletion in humans and other species are reviewed in relevant chapters. Trace element needs of infants and children are summarized in reference 6 and in the chapters on these elements. Table 84.7 summarizes daily trace element recommendations for PN formulations and provides composition of a conventional commercial mixed trace element product. Individual trace elements can also be added to PN solution for repletion.

Mn^{2+} has been found essential for all experimental species studied, but clear evidence of Mn^{2+} deficiency in human beings is lacking. Conversely, Mn^{2+} toxicity in patients receiving PN is well known. In a review, Hardy noted that most PN products contain Mn^{2+} as a contaminant (91). Excessive Mn can lead to hypermanganesemia and reversible Parkinson-like symptoms. Exposure to Mn^{2+} doses at five times the current daily requirements, together with the PN contamination, can lead to neurotoxicity. Whole-blood Mn^{2+} levels are accurate for monitoring and correlate well with Mn^{2+} accumulation in brain by magnetic resonance imaging (91). Current intravenous trace element mixtures contain 500 µg Mn^{2+}, which may be excessive in some patients; thus, periodic blood monitoring is important.

Several generalizations about essential trace elements can be made. The cationic trace elements (iron, zinc, copper, Cr^{3+}, and Mn^{2+}) in their salt forms are highly regulated and tend to be absorbed in small amounts from food by the normal intestine. When in excess in the body, all these elements may be toxic. Giving them intravenously risks excessive retention because intestinal controls are bypassed. Iron particularly is poorly excreted in the urine after PN or blood infusion. Copper, Mn^{2+}, and (to a much smaller extent) molybdate are excreted through the bile into the intestinal tract; hence continued administration of the usual amounts of copper and Mn^{2+} in the presence of excretory liver dysfunction imposes a risk (see later). In contrast, all the anionic forms of trace elements (iodide, selenite, or molybdate) are well absorbed and excreted in the urine; again, excess imposes a risk of toxicity. Many trace elements are present as contaminants in PN components and so contribute variably to the input.

The intravenous iron requirement for the term infant is estimated to be about 100 µg/kg/day; the premature infant probably needs double that amount intravenously. Older children need 1 to 2 mg/day (6). Nonmenstruating women and men whose condition is stable need about 1 mg, and menstruating women need double that amount per day. Iron loss through frequent venipuncture for various tests may be estimated on the basis of 1 mg of iron lost for every 1 mL of packed red cells removed (see the chapter on iron).

When evidence indicates iron depletion, iron may be given intravenously as dilute iron dextran solution in varying amounts after ensuring that the patient has no hypersensitivity to a test dose. Other parenteral iron products include iron sucrose and sodium ferric gluconate. Because neither of the latter two products has been tested in PN formulations, they should be administered separately from the PN formulation. As noted earlier, addition of iron dextran and other iron salts disrupts TNA stability.

Patients who receive chronic PN without iron and who eat very little invariably become iron deficient over time. Iron should be added to the PN solution (preferably a dextrose and amino acid PN solution) to either prevent or treat iron deficiency in this situation. This can be accomplished by adding small daily doses of iron dextran to the PN solution (e.g., 1 to 2 mg/day) or by giving regular doses of therapeutic iron dextran via PN (e.g., 25 to 50 mg/day for 2 to 4 weeks). Patients who have a duodenum and

TABLE 84.7	DAILY TRACE ELEMENT SUPPLEMENTATION RECOMMENDATIONS FOR ADULT PARENTERAL NUTRITION FORMULATIONS	
TRACE ELEMENT	STANDARD DAILY INTAKE DOSAGE RECOMMENDATION	DOSE PROVIDED IN CONVENTIONAL COMMERCIAL PRODUCT[a]
Chromium	10–15 µg	10 µg
Copper	0.3–0.5 mg	1.0 mg
Iron	Not routinely added	None[c]
Manganese	60–100 µg[b]	500 µg
Selenium	20–60 µg	60 µg
Zinc	2.5–5.0 mg	5.0 mg

[a]Multitrace Concentrate (American Regent, Inc., Shirley, NY)
[b]Manganese contamination in various components of parenteral nutrition (PN) can contribute to total intake. Serial blood monitoring of manganese concentrations is indicated with long-term PN use.
[c]Iron dextran can be added to PN formulations that do not contain lipid emulsion.

Adapted with permission from Mirtallo J, Canada T, Johnson D et al. Safe practices for parenteral nutrition. JPEN J Parenter Enteral Nutr 2004;28:S40–70.

proximal jejunum and eat a normal diet during chronic PN usually absorb enough iron to prevent deficiency. These patients may not need supplemental iron via PN. Regular measurement of hemoglobin, serum iron concentration, mean corpuscular volume, and serum ferritin concentration helps in assessing iron stores. During acute stress such as infections, measuring serum iron and ferritin concentrations may not be helpful in the diagnosis of iron deficiency because serum iron concentration decreases, whereas serum ferritin concentration increases.

Serum iodide often remains normal in infants and adults with no added iodide in PN. During 4 or more years of observation in adult patients receiving long-term PN at home without added iodide, the various parameters of thyroid function have remained within normal limits. This is explained by iodide contamination of various mineral additives, by efficient absorption in the upper GI tract of iodides from any ingested diet, and by the use of iodide-containing topical antimicrobial solutions. However, the Centers for Disease Control and Prevention guidelines support the use of chlorhexidine solution for site care dressings of central catheters. This would remove the iodine intake through the skin using previously recommended solutions with this trace element. For the occasional previously depleted adult patient with malabsorption who may have a low serum iodide concentration, 1 μg/kg/day appears adequate during the repletion period. The same amount has been recommended for infants to avoid any risk of deficiency or toxicity.

After the recommendation of an expert committee of the Nutrition Advisory Group of the American Medical Association (AMA) to the Food and Drug Administration (FDA) in 1979 (92), commercial intravenous solutions of zinc, copper, Mn^{2+}, and Cr^{3+} became available, thus ending a period in which such solutions were available only to physicians and pharmacists who personally prepared them. The 2002 and 2004 ASPEN guidelines have suggested decreases in both copper and Mn^{2+} during administration of PN (5, 6). The original zinc recommendations of the AMA committee (92) for stable and for hypermetabolic patients are deemed reasonable, but as noted, much remains to be learned about specific micronutrient needs for optimal biochemical levels and clinical outcomes in hospital patients (15, 93). As in adults, severe diarrhea secondary to infectious disease and the short bowel syndrome in children are associated with increased zinc losses and increased need (93). The 2004 ASPEN clinical practice guidelines for PN are helpful in estimating intestinal losses of zinc, which may approach 12 to 15 mg/L stool (6). In PN, the requirements have been estimated by balance studies to be 3 mg/day in patients without GI losses and a mean of 12 mg/day in patients with diarrhea and fistula losses (94). Periodic checks of serum zinc concentrations in such circumstances are essential. Zinc contamination of PN additives is variable, depending on the specific sources. As a result, total zinc in the formulation may be

as high as 0.3 to 0.4 mg/L (94).

The work of Shike et al (95) showed that, unlike with zinc, increased stool volume is not associated with a major increase in copper excretion, and urinary losses tend to be low; thus, copper accumulates in the body when infused in amounts exceeding those needed for maintenance. On the basis of these and other findings, it is suggested that the range for copper be lowered to 0.3 to 0.5 mg/day for stable patients (see Table 84.7). Caution in copper administration in obstructive jaundice is emphasized because the major excretory route is through bile. Copper deficiency has occurred during PN administration when copper was removed secondary to cholestasis (96). Copper deficiency has also been observed in patients receiving jejunal feeding (which bypasses the duodenum and proximal jejunum where most copper is absorbed), in various malabsorptive conditions, with certain medications, after partial or complete gastric resection, and with roux-en-Y gastric bypass surgery for obesity (97, 98).

The Mn^{2+} content in PN components (99) and the blood concentrations found in PN patients given varying amounts of Mn^{2+} (100) suggested an appreciable reduction in the AMA recommendations. Mn^{2+} contamination of various PN additives produced in the United States may result in an adult receiving 8 to 22 μg/day (see Table 84.7) (100). HPN-treated patients receiving 60 to 120 μg/day (~1.5 to 3 μg/kg/day) of added Mn^{2+} had normal serum concentrations (100). The potential for excessive retention escalates when cholestasis is present (which interferes with Mn^{2+} elimination from the body) and there is continued provision of the amount of Mn^{2+} listed in Table 84.7 in PN.

Even with normal liver function, higher doses in infants and children (101, 102) and in several adults (103, 104) on long-term PN resulted in high blood concentrations associated with high signal intensity in Tl-weighted imaging in the basal ganglia (101–104). Concentrations of plasma (105) or whole blood (100) Mn^{2+} in children showed a significant positive correlation with bilirubin levels. Reducing or omitting supplementary Mn^{2+} resulted in major decreases in blood Mn^{2+} over periods varying from weeks to months (101–105) in children and adults, and the high-intensity signal on magnetic resonance brain imaging disappeared. Neurologic signs were present in one adult on long-term PN containing 1 to 2 mg/day of Mn^{2+}; these signs improved, and serum and urinary Mn^{2+} concentration decreased when Mn^{2+} was omitted from PN. Nine months later, the patient died of a massive GI hemorrhage secondary to her cancer. At autopsy, the Mn^{2+} content of the caudate nucleus and centrum ovale was two to three times that found in some patients not receiving PN (106). In another study, complete withdrawal of Mn^{2+} resulted in a decrease in serum concentrations and brain deposition of Mn^{2+} (107).

As noted in the 1979 AMA report, quantitative data on Cr^{3+} requirements were lacking at that time, and the qualitative suggestions were based on estimates from balance data on healthy persons (92). The current situation is not appreciably clearer, largely because of the difficulty of measuring plasma Cr^{3+} concentrations (normally very low), lack of information on tissue levels of this ion, and lack of controlled studies on very low Cr^{3+} intake. Cr^{3+} appears to function as a regulator of insulin action (93, 108, 109).

The relatively few cases of well-documented symptomatic Cr^{3+} depletion have occurred in adult patients receiving long-term PN with little or no supplementary Cr^{3+} (93). It was associated with sudden occurrence of glucose intolerance, glycosuria, weight loss, and neurologic symptoms, especially peripheral neuropathy. Development of symptoms appeared to be related to prolonged glucose infusions and intestinal fluid losses, both of which increase Cr^{3+} need. The patients responded well to Cr^{3+}, often 250 μg Cr^{3+} infused daily for weeks (108). Cr^{3+} toxicity has not been observed, even with doses greater than 250 μg/day. As noted in a review by Moukarzel, despite published guidelines for routine supplementation of Cr^{3+} in PN, there remain major concerns about the infusion of excess amounts of this trace element (109). Although some patients with malabsorption may become deficient, little information is available on appropriate dosage for use of Cr^{3+} in PN. The data to date suggest that the amounts listed in Table 84.7 may need to be lowered as a general guideline in both adults and children (109).

Recommendations for selenium were not made in the 1979 AMA report. That year saw the first reports in English relating selenium deficiency to Keshan disease in China (see the chapter on selenium) and the report of a case of selenium deficiency in a patient receiving PN (110). Considerable clinical and biochemical information has accrued since then, including selenium deficiency in patients receiving PN, with some deaths associated with cardiomyopathy and reports of muscle tenderness and weakness.

Low plasma concentrations of selenium, to less than 10 μg/mL or less than 0.13 μmol/L, may be present without symptoms. Cohen et al (79) followed up five patients who were receiving HPN without added selenium for an average of 18.6 months. Selenium-dependent glutathione peroxidase (GSHPx) in plasma reached very low levels less than 15% of normal values) in approximately 1 year; GSHPx in red cells reached that level in 1 to 2 years (79). Selenious acid (as selenite salts) is available for intravenous use. Use of 20 to 60 μg/day in PN usually maintains normal plasma concentrations during short-term PN (see Table 84.7). Patients requiring long-term PN or HPN may require higher doses, 100 to 120 μg/day, to maintain normal serum concentrations of selenium (from decreased dietary intake with or without stool loss). Administration of 100 μg/day in the infusate will increase low blood concentrations in most previously depleted, clinically stable patients receiving PN into the normal plasma range (79).

Selenoprotein P concentrations in plasma (measured by radioimmunoassay) correlate well with extracellular GSHPx and selenium as markers for selenium status in deficient patients receiving long-term PN. As noted in a review by Shenkin, critically ill patients or those with severe burns may have higher selenium requirements (111). RCTs suggest that up to 400 μg/day may be beneficial in patients with burn injury, but the evidence is inconclusive regarding benefits of high-dose selenium in sepsis or critical illness. When increased selenium provision is used, or in long-term PN, selenium status should be monitored by measurement of plasma selenium together with a marker of systemic inflammation such as C-reactive protein (111). A double-blind RCT suggested that high-dose selenium (500 μg) if given for 5 days of more as a separate intravenous, was associated with decreased hospital infections in ICU patients receiving mixed PN and EN (112).

The most commonly used commercially available trace element combination products contain four to five individual metals (see Table 84.7). A combination product containing six trace elements (molybdenum plus zinc, copper, Mn^{2+}, Cr^{3+}, and selenium) and one containing seven trace elements (iodine plus the six mentioned earlier) are also commercially available. Use of multiple trace elements in a fixed formula poses the risk of excessive dosage of one or more of the constituents to patients receiving the formula long term and who have metabolic abnormalities that require restriction or omission (6). Furthermore, evidence reviewed in this chapter and recommendations in Table 84.7 suggest that routine needs for some trace elements are appreciably lower than those recommended in the AMA–FDA report (92). A combination of individual trace elements or a decreased volume of a given multitrace element formulation may be necessary when restriction of one or more of the latter is indicated, such as in fulminant liver failure, in which Mn^{2+} can rapidly accumulate.

The issue of toxicity of parenterally administered lead, cadmium, mercury, and aluminum present as contaminants merits consideration because they bypass the normal barriers of the GI tract.

Aluminum is of special concern because its toxicity was well delineated in patients with renal disease who were treated with aluminum-containing phosphate-binding antacids and/or who received aluminum-contaminated water in hemodialysis. Neurologic changes include apraxic motor abnormalities involving speech, myoclonus, seizures, and dementia. Also seen is an osteomalacia refractory to therapy with vitamin D analogs, calcium, or phosphate; bone pain; pathologic fractures; aluminum deposition on bone osteoid front; and microcytic anemia without evidence of iron deficiency (113, 114). Aluminum toxicity has been described in patients of all ages with a variety of therapies, including dialysis, phosphate-binding medications, and PN (115).

Although free amino acid solutions have much smaller amounts of aluminum (e.g., 26 ± 20 μg/L of 10% solution), other PN ingredients may have significant amounts

(63, 140–142). It can progress to portal tract fibrosis and infiltration, liver failure, and death. A large and continuing literature has confirmed PN as a contributing risk factor for hepatobiliary dysfunction of varying degree and incidence (63, 140–142). Reviews of the biochemical, clinical, and histopathologic changes in adults and children have emphasized the multifactorial nature of the problem (63, 140).

In children, degree of prematurity, infection, inability to consume food orally, extent of intestinal dysfunction, number of surgical procedures, duration of PN, and long-term administration of excessive calories are risk factors (63, 141, 142). Immaturity of the hepatic excretory function and the enterohepatic circulation, particularly in the neonate, is one reason for development of cholestasis. Cholestasis has been reported in various series to occur in a significant proportion of infants who are receiving PN, with wide variations among differing populations, criteria, hospital practices, and clinical conditions (63). Use of fish oil in PN to replace soybean oil–based lipid emulsion is described earlier (64, 65). A review of PN-associated liver dysfunction in children concluded that only a few concrete associations and treatment protocols have been established for this condition and that more evidence-based information from rigorous research is needed (63).

In adults, preexisting liver and other diseases, sepsis, preexisting malnutrition, extent of bowel resection and/or damage (such as from radiation), excess nonprotein calories, little or no oral intake, and duration on PN are also associated risk factors for PN-associated liver disease (140–142). Increases may occur in serum transaminase, alkaline phosphatase, γ-glutamyl-transferase, and, less frequently, bilirubin as indicators of hepatic dysfunction.

Adult patients receiving long-term PN (median, 18 months) who were given relative excesses of carbohydrate, fat, and amino acids showed abnormal hepatic function and cholestatic changes. When the amounts of these macronutrients were reduced, jaundice was reversed, and liver function test results and histologic features improved (143). Other investigators noted increasing steatosis with administration of excess calories as carbohydrate or lipid, or both (144). In one study, 43 patients who received PN were randomized to receive either glucose as the sole nonprotein calorie source or a combination of glucose and fat. The dose of nonprotein energy used in this study was moderate compared with that in many of the previous studies. Although the patients were not dramatically overfed (1.5 times calculated basal energy expenditure), alkaline phosphatase and γ-glutamyl-transferase increased significantly in both groups. Aspartate aminotransferase, alanine aminotransferase, and direct bilirubin increased more in the group receiving only glucose as nonprotein calories. It appears that liver enzyme laboratory test results are affected by administration of PN, even when used in moderate doses and when part of the energy dose is given as intravenous lipid emulsion (142, 145).

Various agents have been tested on patients receiving PN who have developed evidence of associated significant hepatic dysfunction and who require continued PN (63, 87). Giving a mixture of MCT and LCT to PN-treated patients as the intravenous lipid source did not cause a change in liver size or grayscale value, whereas LCT infusion increased both (87). On the grounds that metronidazole could depress formation by intestinal bacteria of potentially damaging bile acids, this drug has been tested in patients receiving PN and has been reported by some investigators to reduce abnormalities in liver enzymes compared with untreated control subjects (146, 147). Other antibiotics such as neomycin, gentamicin, and polymyxin B are also being evaluated. It is theorized that the use of enteral antibiotics reduces the bacterial load of the gut, which, in turn, decreases the amount of lipopolysaccharide that crosses into the portal circulation.

Ursodeoxycholic acid, an epimer of chenodeoxycholic acid, has been given with benefit to adults (148) and children (149) receiving long-term PN who developed cholestatic liver disease. Jaundice and enzyme abnormalities regressed, and their clinical condition improved. Cholestyramine, choline, and lecithin have been reported to decrease hepatic steatosis (126, 149).

Gallstones

Sludge in the gallbladder has been observed repeatedly as a PN- and bowel rest–associated risk factor; this situation can progress to gallstone formation as the duration of PN increases (6). Patients who receive long-term PN maintenance because of resection or disease of the terminal ileum usually malabsorb bile salts. Thus, the bile salt pool decreases, and lower levels of bile salts are present in the gallbladder. This situation, in turn, increases the tendency of cholesterol to precipitate in the bile, thus forming the nidus of gallstones (142). There is also an increase in unconjugated bilirubin and calcium, which are present in the stones that form from the accumulated sludge in the gallbladder (150). Impaired gallbladder contraction is important. Ultrasonography indicated development of biliary sludge within 12 days of starting PN in 14 of 23 patients. By 6 weeks, all had sludge; 6 patients developed stones, and 3 required surgery. The sludge disappeared 4 weeks after instituting oral feeding (151).

Gallstones are a significant problem in adults, but even more so in children receiving PN. For example, 9 of 29 children receiving PN developed cholelithiasis; 64% of these with ileal disorders or resections developed stones (152); 6 of 13 children with less than 38 cm of small bowel remaining required a cholecystectomy (153).

These potential problems have led to the following suggestions for management of such patients at risk: nutrition should be provided enterally whenever possible in an effort to decrease biliary stasis, liver function studies should be checked periodically, ultrasound should be used liberally when a cholestatic picture is evident if gallstones are detected, and if laparotomy is to be done for any reason, cholecystectomy should be considered at that time.

Metabolic Bone Disease

Metabolic bone disease is usually a long-term complication of PN administration; however, it is prevalent in several disease states such as short bowel syndrome, inflammatory bowel disease, and cancer (85–87, 154, 155). Patients with these disease states make up a substantial portion of patients receiving HPN, so metabolic bone disease is a multifactorial disorder. Administration of corticosteroids has also been associated with metabolic bone disease because these drugs increase bone resorption and impair osteoblastic activity (155). The work of Pironi et al (156) addressed the prevalence of metabolic bone disease in adult patients receiving long-term PN in Europe. Of 165 patients, 84% had T-scores via dual-energy x-ray absorptiometry that were decreased by more than 1 standard deviation from normal, which meets criteria for osteopenia. Forty-one percent of these patients had T-scores that were decreased by more than 2.5 standard deviations from normal, meeting criteria for osteoporosis (156). Calcium, phosphorus, magnesium, and sodium balance all may be factors in the development of metabolic bone disease, as well as vitamins D and K intake. High doses of protein, especially when given via cyclic PN, increase urinary excretion of calcium and potentially contribute to the development of metabolic bone disease.

Rickets has been described in infants receiving PN. The causative factor appeared to be a need for more calcium and phosphate in the small fluid volume required by the neonate, rather than more vitamin D. Reference has been made earlier to the effects of aluminum contamination on bone.

The histomorphologic features of bone were examined in relation to formula composition in patients receiving long-term HPN who were not subsisting on aluminum-contaminated casein hydrolysate. In a prospective study in Toronto by Shike et al (157), bone biopsies of HPN-treated patients initially showed a hyperkinetic pattern, possibly resulting from initial malnutrition; at 6 to 73 months on HPN, the histologic features changed, with 12 of 16 patients having some degree of osteomalacia. In this study, patients received 500 IU of vitamin D_2 every other day; all other vitamins were supplied except biotin. Because 7 of these patients were hypercalcemic and 6 had elevated 25(OH) vitamin D concentrations, further studies were performed on 11 patients before and after withdrawal of vitamin D_2 (and, by necessity, the accompanying vitamin A) for 6 months (157). Six of 10 patients had less osteoid and increased tetracycline uptake with the vitamin modification, but there was continuing evidence of a high turnover rate. In the 3 symptomatic patients, bone pain subsided, fractures healed, and urinary loss of calcium

and phosphate was decreased. Other investigators have noted improvement in HPN-treated patients with respect to bone fractures and pain after withdrawal of vitamin D from the PN formulations (158).

It has been suggested that PN patients lose a significant amount of bone mass early as a result of hypocalcemia that then stabilizes. Amenorrhea and smoking are also factors. The conclusion is that osteopenia is characteristic of patients receiving long-term PN but that present PN formulations do not necessarily cause deterioration of bone health and may benefit some patients (159). Pironi et al (160) reported impaired bone formation in patients who were receiving PN for more than 1 year. Poor bone formation was positively correlated with low serum osteocalcin concentrations in this population. Substantial data demonstrate that parenteral phosphorus administration via PN in patients receiving HPN decreases hypercalciuria (161, 162). It is likely that phosphorus induces this favorable response by increasing renal tubular calcium absorption (162). Patients receiving HPN should have calcium, phosphorus, and magnesium concentrations monitored regularly. Sufficient acetate should be administered to buffer titratable acids generated by the patient. Vitamin K should be provided daily either as a component of the parenteral vitamin product or as a separate component if it is not contained in the vitamin constituent.

DRUG COMPATIBILITY

The frequency of drug interventions for coexistent illnesses or complications of PN requires ensuring that administering a drug as part of the PN solution or in conjunction with that solution will not produce incompatibility or an adverse reaction. Regular insulin is the most commonly added drug in PN, and it effectively controls blood glucose in most patients, with or without a separate intravenous insulin infusion (6-7, 15). Significant information on PN drug compatibility has been summarized (163–165). Table 84.11 contains compatibility information for PN solutions and many commonly used drugs. Drugs that can or should be administered as continuous infusions and that are compatible with PN solutions are ideal additives, especially in the critical care setting, where fluid intake often must be regulated.

Not all combinations of drugs and different PN solutions have been studied. In addition, some drugs are compatible in traditional dextrose and amino acid PN solutions but not in TNAs (e.g., iron dextran). Still, other drugs are compatible in PN solutions because they are diluted in a large volume of fluid and are incompatible when given during Y-site intravenous administration with the same PN solution. This problem undoubtedly occurs because the drug concentration is high when coinfused with PN through the same tubing. Trissel et al found that 82 of 102 drugs were compatible during Y-site administration with PN solutions (165).

TABLE 84.11	COMPATIBILITIES OF SELECTED DRUGS WITH PARENTERAL NUTRITION SOLUTIONS
Dextrose and amino acids compatible with	Albumin
	Folic acid
	Regular human insulin
	Phytonadione
	Cimetidine
	Heparin
	Iron dextran
	Ranitidine
	Famotidine
	HCl
	Metoclopramide
	Thiamin
Total nutrient admixtures compatible with	Albumin
	Heparin
	Phytonadione
	Cimetidine
	Regular human insulin
	Ranitidine
	Famotidine
	Metoclopramide
	Thiamin
Dextrose and amino acids incompatible with	Amphotericin B
	Phenytoin
	Ampicillin
	Metronidazole
Total nutrient admixtures incompatible with	Amphotericin B
	Methyldopa
	HCl
	Phenytoin
	Iron dextran

HOME PARENTERAL NUTRITION

Since the first patients were discharged from the hospital to home on PN in 1969 and the early 1970s, in the United States and Canada (1, 2, 166), HPN as primary outpatient nutritional support has mushroomed. An HPN registry for the United States and Canada was established at the New York Academy of Medicine during the years 1978 to 1983 to collect and compile the data being accrued by an increasing number of medical centers that discharged patients on HPN. Data were distributed regularly to participants and interested parties. In 1984, this registry became a joint effort of the Oley Foundation and the ASPEN that was originally designated the OASIS Registry and, until recent years, the North American Home Parenteral and Enteral Nutrition Patient Registry (HPEN Registry) produced by the Oley Foundation.

Today, it is very difficult to assess the actual number of patients receiving HPN, but Delegge (167), using Medicare data in 2002, estimated that approximately 40,000 patients received this therapy. Issues related to suitability, training, formulations, and home support have

been extensively identified, and standards on organization, patient selection, and management have been developed (5, 6). ASPEN is currently reestablishing a comprehensive HPN registry.

In 1995, Howard et al (168) published detailed data for 11 diagnoses concerning survival, likelihood of rehabilitation to full and to partial function, and frequency of HPN and non-HPN complications. Annual survival rates of those with GI diseases were 87% or better, with a 50% to 73% likelihood of complete rehabilitation in 1 year, except for patients with radiation enteritis or obstruction with chronic adhesions. In the 3 most common GI diseases (Crohn disease, ischemic bowel disease, and motility disorders), survival rate more than 1 year for patients 18 years or less was about 95%; for those 35 to 55 years old, it was 90%; and for those 65 years old and older, it was about 70%. Howard et al (169) estimated that between 25% and 33% of all patients receiving home nutrition support are more than 65 years of age. Their outcomes are reasonable, so age should not be considered a barrier for offering these means of support. Younger patients were more likely to resume full oral nutrition and have more complete rehabilitation, but they had more septic admissions. The frequency of HPN-related complications was similar in all diagnostic groups: 1 to 2 rehospitalizations per year, one half because of sepsis (169). The newly constituted ASPEN registry will provide sorely needed data on diagnoses and outcomes in patients receiving HPN.

Complications associated with HPN accounted for only 5% of deaths. If earlier experience continues to hold true, a minority of patients account for a majority of rehospitalizations. Howard and Ashley (170) reviewed the management of the common complications associated with HPN.

HPN presents various stresses to the patient and family members (171), including the sudden need to cope with the technical aspects, time demands, and safety issues of HPN after hospital discharge, management of handicaps resulting from primary and secondary illness and their treatments, concerns about meeting costs, patient dependency, and excessive dependence on others. A smooth transition to home care requires adequate predischarge assessment and training of the patient and family in HPN management and close support by the health care team by telephone contact and follow-up at home or in the physician's office to ensure that the patient's condition remains satisfactory.

Dietary intake and other factors at home may require modification of the PN formulation from that deemed satisfactory in the hospital setting. Data from a survey of 178 randomly selected families with a member on HPN for an average of 4.6 years, with 116 follow-up questionnaires (172). Patient and caregiver mean family scores for quality of life, self-esteem, life satisfaction, family cohesion, and quality of patient–caregiver relationship were similar to published norms for other healthy populations and other groups of chronically ill patients. HPN family adaptability and coping scores were higher. There were problems associated with financial strain and mild depression in patients related to increasing duration of PN and being barred from work (although able to) because of their disability classification (172). Additional reports on various quality of life measures in HPN-treated patients have been published (173, 174).

Estimates of the cost of HPN vary from $75,000 to more than $200,000 per patient-year depending on the days of PN/week required (175–178). Many factors enter into the total cost of maintaining a patient on HPN including PN-associated complications and monitoring; such charges vary considerably, depending in part on the method used in their estimations and on differences in the perspectives chosen for the analyses, particularly the matter of estimating benefits gained and/or the effectiveness gained. As summarized by Rhoda et al (179), HPN is a lifesaving treatment for many patients with conditions associated with intestinal failure. Skilled placement and care of the central venous access device reduce the incidence of complications, and careful monitoring of fluid, electrolyte, and macronutrient, and micronutrient status can minimize hyperglycemia, major organ dysfunction, and other metabolic complications. A multidiscipline, integrated nutrition support team can allow patients with intestinal failure who need HPN to live a nearly normal life (179).

FUTURE PERSPECTIVES

As noted earlier, use of PN is a routine component of clinical care worldwide, yet many important areas of uncertainty remain with regard to the optimal use complete PN and parenteral macronutrients and micronutrients in combination with EN (see Table 84.2) (15, 16). However, as noted in several reviews and perspective papers on PN, the future of this therapy looks bright, given the large number of ongoing RCTs in progress, improved knowledge of complications related to PN and how to prevent them, and newer thinking about how to combine PN with EN in clinical settings (180–184). For example, a large RCT from Belgium (4640 patients) was published on the effect of early versus later timing of PN initiation in adult, primarily surgical adult ICU patients who were unable to tolerate adequate amounts of early EN (14). In the early initiation group, supplemental PN to meet the caloric goal of 25 to 30 kcal/kg/day was started on ICU day 2. In the late initiation group, supplemental PN to meet the caloric goal was started on ICU day 7, per 2009 American clinical practice guidelines (7). The early initiation of PN was associated with modestly increased ICU and hospital length of stay, infectious complications, indices of organ dysfunction, and total hospital costs, without a difference in mortality indexes (14). However, most patients in this study were not significantly malnourished at entry, and

those receiving specialized EN or PN on ICU admission were excluded (groups in whom PN use is common in ICU settings). Nonetheless, this important study provides needed evidence that PN initiation in the first few days of an ICU admission to supplement inadequate EN should be used judiciously in adults (14). These results, coupled with those of other ongoing rigorous RCTs studies, will help to define more optimal PN treatment strategies more accurately in the not too distant future (16, 180–184).

REFERENCES

1. Vinnars E, Wilmore D. JPEN J Parenter Enteral Nutr 2003; 27:225–31.
2. Bistrian BR. Nestle Nutr Workshop Ser Clin Perform Programme 2009;12:127–36.
3. Dudrick S, Wilmore DW, Vars HM et al. Surgery 1968;64: 134–42.
4. Anonymous. JPEN J Parenter Enteral Nutr 1993;17:1SA–26SA.
5. Anonymous. JPEN J Parenter Enteral Nutr 2002;26: 1SA–138SA.
6. Mirtallo J, Canada T, Johnson D et al. JPEN J Parenter Enteral Nutr 2004;28:S40–70.
7. McClave SA, Martindale RG, Vanek VW et al. JPEN J Parenter Enteral Nutr 2009;33:277–316.
8. Druyan ME, Compher C, Boullata JI et al. JPEN J Parenter Enteral Nutr 2012;36:77–80.
9. Preiser JC, Schneider SM. Clin Nutr 2011;30:549–52.
10. Cahill NE, Narasimhan S, Dhaliwal R et al. JPEN J Parenter Enteral Nutr 2010;34:685–96.
11. Heyland DK, MacDonald S, Leefe L et al. JAMA 1998; 280:2013–9.
12. Thibault R, Pichard C. Crit Care Clin 2010;26:467–80.
13. Kutsogiannis J, Alberda C, Gramlich L et al. Crit Care Med 2011;39:2691–9.
14. Casaer MP, Mesotten D, Hermans G et al. N Engl J Med 2011;365:506–17.
15. Ziegler TR. N Engl J Med 2009;361:1088–97.
16. Ziegler TR. N Engl J Med 2011;365:562–4.
17. Gura KM. Nutr Clin Pract 2009;24:709–17.
18. Culebras JM, Martin-Peña G, Garcia-de-Lorenzo A et al. Curr Opin Clin Nutr Metab Care 2004;7:303–7.
19. Norwood S, Wilkins HE, Vallina VL et al. Crit Care Med 2000;28:1376–82.
20. Kearns PJ, Coleman S, Wehner JH. JPEN J Parenter Enteral Nutr 1996;20:20–4.
21. Cowl CT, Weinstock JV, Al-Jurf A et al. Clin Nutr 2000;19: 237–43.
22. McGee DC, Gould MK. N Engl J Med 2003;348:1123.
23. Pittiruti M, Hamilton H, Biffi R et al. Clin Nutr 2009;28: 365–77.
24. Fonkalsrud EW, Berquist W, Burke M et al. Am J Surg 1982;143:209–11.
25. Mansfield PF, Hohn DC, Fornage BD et al. N Engl J Med 1994;331:1735–8.
26. Clark-Christoff N, Watters VA, Sparks W et al. JPEN J Parenter Enteral Nutr 1992;16:403–7.
27. Kemp L, Burge J, Choban P et al. JPEN J Parenter Enteral Nutr 1994;18:71–4.
28. Timsit JF, Sebille V, Farkas JC et al. JAMA 1996;276:1416–20.
29. Maki DG, Stolz SM, Wheeler S et al. Ann Intern Med 1997;127:257–66.

30. Timsit JF, Schwebel C, Bouadma L et al. JAMA 2009;301: 1231–41.
31. Camargo LF, Marra AR, Büchele GL et al. J Hosp Infect 2009;72:227–33.
32. Oliveira C, Nasr A, Brindle M et al. Pediatrics 2012;129:318–29.
33. Timsit JF, Dubois Y, Minet C et al. Semin Respir Crit Care Med 2011;32:139–50.
34. Feller-Kopman D. Chest 2007;132:302–9.
35. O'Grady NP, Alexander M, Burns LA et al. Am J Infect Control 2011;39:S1–34.
36. O'Keefe SJ, Burnes JU, Thompson RL. JPEN J Parenter Enteral Nutr 1994;18:256–63.
37. Ball PA. Curr Opin Clin Nutr Metab Care 2003;6:319–25.
38. Alcutt A, Lort D, McCollum N. Br J Surg 1983;70:111.
39. Seres DS. Nutr Clin Pract 1990;5:111–7.
40. Shaw SN, Elwyn DH, Askanazi J et al. Am J Clin Nutr 1983;37:930–40.
41. Mehta NM, Compher C. JPEN J Parenter Enteral Nutr 2009;33:260–76.
42. Rodriguez NA, Jeschke MG, Williams FN et al. JPEN J Parenter Enteral Nutr 2011;35:704–14.
43. Cano NJ, Aparicio M, Brunori G et al. Clin Nutr 2009;28: 401–14.
44. Genton L, Pichard C. Int J Vitam Nutr Res 2011;81:143–52.
45. Yarandi SS, Zhao VM, Hebbar G et al. Curr Opin Clin Nutr Metab Care 2011;14:75–82.
46. Rudman E, Millikan WJ, Richardson TJ et al. J Clin Invest 1975;55:94–104.
47. Starker PM, LaSala PA, Forse A et al. JPEN J Parenter Enteral Nutr 1985;9:300–2.
48. Kauffmann RM, Hayes RM, Jenkins JM et al. JPEN J Parenter Enteral Nutr 2011;35:686–94.
49. Byrne WJ, Lippe BM, Strobel CT et al. Gastroenterology 1981;80:947–56.
50. Krzywda A, Andris DA, Whipple JK et al. JPEN J Parenter Enteral Nutr 1993;17:64–7.
51. Arsenault D, Brenn M, Kim S et al JPEN J Parenter Enteral Nutr 2012;36:81–95.
52. McCowen KC, Malhotra A, Bistrian BR. Crit Care Clin 2001;17:107–24.
53. Van den Berghe G, Wouters P, Weekers F et al. N Engl J Med 2001;345:1359–67.
54. Van den Berghe G, Wouters PJ, Bouillon R et al. Crit Care Med 2003;31:359–66.
55. Finney SJ, Zekveld C, Elia A et al. JAMA 2003;290:2041–7.
56. NICE-SUGAR Study Investigators, Finfer S, Chittock DR et al. N Engl J Med 2009;360:1283–97.
57. Kavanagh BP, McCowen KC. N Engl J Med 2010;363: 2540–6.
58. Umpierrez GE, Hellman R, Korytkowski MT et al. J Clin Endocrinol Metab 2012;97:16–38.
59. Calder PC, Jensen GL, Koletzko BV et al. Intensive Care Med 2010;36:735–49.
60. Mirtallo JM, Dasta JF, Kleinschmidt KC et al. Ann Pharmacother 2010;44:688–700.
61. Wanten GJ, Calder PC. Am J Clin Nutr 2007;85:1171–84.
62. Battistella FD, Widergren JT, Anderson JT et al. J Trauma 1997;43:52–8.
63. Rangel SJ, Calkins CM, Cowles RA et al. J Pediatr Surg 2012;47:225–40.
64. de Meijer VE, Gura KM, Meisel JA et al. Arch Surg 2010;145:547–51.
65. Park KT, Nespor C, Kerner J Jr. J Perinatol 2011;31(Suppl 1): S57–60.
66. Deshpande G, Simmer K. Curr Opin Clin Nutr Metab Care 2011;14:145–50.
67. Cober MP, Killu G, Brattain A et al. J Pediatr 2012;160:421–7.
68. Umpierrez GE, Spiegelman R, Zhao V et al. Crit Care Med 2012;40:1792–8.
69. Kemin Q, Maysoon A, Seo T et al. JPEN J Parenter Enteral Nutr 2003;27:58–64.
70. Adamkin DH, Gelke KN, Andrews BE. JPEN J Parenter Enteral Nutr 1984;8:563–7.
71. Driscoll DF. JPEN J Parenter Enteral Nutr 2003;27:433–8.
72. Driscoll DF, Bhargava HN, Li L et al. Am J Hosp Pharm 1995;52:623–34.
73. Venus B, Smith RA, Patel C et al. Chest 1989;95:1278–81.
74. Suchner U, Katz DP, Fürst P et al. Crit Care Med 2001;29:1569–74.
75. Seidner DL, Mascioli EA, Istfan NW et al. JPEN J Parenter Enteral Nutr 1987;13:614–9.
76. Jensen GL, Mascioli EA, Seidner DL et al. JPEN J Parenter Enteral Nutr 1990;14:467–71.
77. Ota DM, Jessup JM, Babcock GE et al. JPEN J Parenter Enteral Nutr 1985;9:23–7.
78. Lenssen P, Bruemmer BA, Bowden RA et al. Am J Clin Nutr 1998;67:927–33.
79. Cohen HJ, Brown MR, Hamilton D et al. Am J Clin Nutr 1989;49:132–9.
80. Maroulis J, Kalfarentzos F. Clin Nutr 2000;19:295–304.
81. Dunham B, Marcuard S, Khazanie PG et al. JPEN J Parenter Enteral Nutr 1991;15:608–11.
82. Greene HL, Hambidge M, Schanler R et al. Am J Clin Nutr 1988;48:1324–42.
83. Berkelhammer CH, Wood RJ, Sitrin MD. Am J Clin Nutr 1988;48:1482–9.
84. Goodman WG, Misra S, Veldhuis JD et al. Am J Clin Nutr 2000;71:560–8.
85. Acca M, Ragno A, Francucci CM et al. J Endocrinol Invest 2007;30(Suppl):54–9.
86. Diamanti A, Bizzarri C, Basso MS et al. J Bone Miner Metab 2010;28:351–8.
87. Wanten G, Calder PC, Forbes A. BMJ 2011;342:d1447.
88. Clark CL, Sacks GS, Dickerson RN et al. Crit Care Med 1995;23:1504–11.
89. Charon T, Bernard F, Skrobik Y et al. Intensive Care Med 2003;29:1273–8.
90. Sacks GS, Brown RO, Dickerson RN et al. Nutrition 1997;13:303–8.
91. Hardy G. Gastroenterology 2009;137(Suppl):S29–35.
92. Shils ME, Burke AW, Greene HL et al. JAMA 1979;241:2051–4.
93. Btaiche IF, Carver PL, Welch KB. JPEN J Parenter Enteral Nutr 2011;35:736–47.
94. Jeejeebhoy K. Gastroenterology 2009;137(Suppl):S7–12.
95. Shike M, Roulet M, Kurian R et al. Gastroenterology 1981;81:290–7.
96. Spiegel JE, Willenbucher RF. JPEN J Parenter Enteral Nutr 1999;23:169–72.
97. Griffith DP, Liff D, Ziegler TR et al. Obesity 2009;17:827–31.
98. Gletsu-Miller N, Broderius M, Frediani J et al. Int J Obes 2012;36:328–35.
99. Kurkus J, Alcock NW, Shils ME. JPEN J Parenter Enteral Nutr 1984;8:254–7.
100. Shike M, Ritchie ME, Shils ME. Clin Res 1986;34:804A(abst).
101. Fell JME, Reynolds AP, Meadows N et al. Lancet 1996; 347:1218–21.
102. Ono J, Harada K, Kodaka R et al. JPEN J Parenter Enteral Nutr 1995;19:310–2.

103. Ejima A, Imanura T, Nakamura S et al. Lancet 1992;339:426 (letter).

104. Takagi Y, Okada A, Sando K et al. Am J Clin Nutr 2002;75:112–8.

105. Hambidge KM, Sokol RJ, Fidanze SJ et al. JPEN J Parenter Enteral Nutr 1989;13:168–71.

106. Alves G, Thiebot J, Tracqui A et al. JPEN J Parenter Enteral Nutr 1997;21:41–5.

107. Bertinet DB, Tinivella M, Balzola FA et al. JPEN J Parenter Enteral Nutr 2000;24:223–7.

108. Verhage AH, Cheong WK, Jeejeebhoy K. JPEN J Parenter Enteral Nutr 1996;20:123–7.

109. Moukarzel A. Gastroenterology 2009;137(Suppl):S18–28.

110. Van Rijn AM, Thompson CD, McKenzie JM et al. Am J Clin Nutr 1979;43:2076–85.

111. Shenkin A. Gastroenterology 2009;137(Suppl):S61–9.

112. Andrews PJ, Avenell A, Noble DW et al. BMJ 2011;342:d1542.

113. Abumrad NN, Schneider AJ, Steel D et al. Am J Clin Nutr 1981;34:2551–9.

114. Klein GA. Am J Clin Nutr 1995;61:449–56.

115. Wier HA, Kuhn RJ. Ann Pharmacother 2012;46:137–40.

116. Wu WW, Kaplan LA, Horn J et al. JPEN J Parenter Enteral Nutr 1986;10:591–5.

117. Bishop NJ, Morley R, Day JP et al. N Engl J Med 1997;336:1557–61.

118. de Oliveira SR, Bohrer D, Garcia SC et al JPEN J Parenter Enteral Nutr 2010;34:322–8.

119. Mirtallo JM. JPEN J Parenter Enteral Nutr 2010;34:346–7.

120. Vanamee P, Shils ME, Burke AW et al. JPEN J Parenter Enteral Nutr 1979;3:258–62.

121. De Ritter EJ. Pharm Sci 1982;71:1073–96.

122. Kirkemo AK, Burt ME, Brennan M. Am J Clin Nutr 1982;35:1003–9.

123. Thomas MK, Lloyd-Jones DM, Thadhani RI et al. N Engl J Med 1998;338:777–83.

124. Thomson P, Duerksen DR. JPEN J Parenter Enteral Nutr 2011;35:499–504.

125. Anonymous. Nutrition 1999;15:92–6.

126. Buchman AL. Gastroenterology 2009;137(Suppl):S119–28.

127. Buckman AL, Sohel M, Brown M et al. JPEN J Parenter Enteral Nutr 2000;25:30–35.

128. Compher CW, Kinosian BP, Stoner NE et al. JPEN J Parenter Enteral Nutr 2002;26:57–62.

129. Shils ME, Baker H, Frank O. JPEN J Parenter Enteral Nutr 1985;9:179–88.

130. Chen F, Boyce HW, Tripiett L. JPEN J Parenter Enteral Nutr 1983;7:462–4.

131. Steephen AC, Traber MG, Ito Y et al. JPEN J Parenter Enteral Nutr 1991;15:647–52.

132. Lemoyne M, Gossum AV, Kurian R et al. Am J Clin Nutr 1988;48:1310–5.

133. Greene HL, Smith R, Pollack P et al. J Am Coll Nutr 1991;10:281–8.

134. Centers for Disease Control and Prevention. MMWR Morb Mortal Wkly Rep 1997;46:523–8.

135. Zak J, Burns D, Lingenfelser T et al. JPEN J Parenter Enteral Nutr 1991;15:200–1.

136. Ferrie S. Nutr Clin Pract 2012;27:65–8.

137. Palesty JA, Dudrick SJ. Surg Clin North Am 2011;91:653–73.

138. Byrnes MC, Stangenes J. Curr Opin Clin Nutr Metab Care 2011;14:186–92.

139. Zhao VM, Ziegler TR. Crit Care Nurs Clin North Am 2010;22:369–80.

140. Grau T, Bonet A, Rubio M et al. Crit Care 2007;11:R10.

141. Buchman A. JPEN J Parenter Enteral Nutr 2002;26(Suppl):S43–8.

142. Cavicchi M, Beau P, Crenn P et al. Ann Intern Med 2000;132:525–32.

143. Messing B, Colombel JF, Heresbach D et al. Nutrition 1992;8:30–6.

144. Wagner WH, Lowry AC, Silberman H. Am J Gastroenterol 1983;78:199–202.

145. Buchmiller CE, Kleiman-Wexler RL, Ephgrave KS et al. JPEN J Parenter Enteral Nutr 1993;17:301–6.

146. Payne-James JJ, Silk DB. Dig Dis Sci 1991;9:10–24.

147. Lambert JP, Thomas SM. JPEN J Parenter Enteral Nutr 1985;9:501–3.

148. Spagnuolo MM, Iorio R, Vegnente A et al. Gastroenterology 1996;111:716–9.

149. Buchman AL, Dubin M, Venden D et al. Gastroenterology 1992;102:1363–70.

150. Muller EL, Grace FA, Pitt HA. J Surg Res 1986;40:55–62.

151. Messing B, Bories C, Kustlinger F et al. Gastroenterology 1983;84:1012–9.

152. Roslyn JJ, Berquist WE, Pitt HA et al. Pediatrics 1983;71:784–9.

153. Dorney SF, Ament ME, Berquist WE et al. J Pediatr 1985;107:521–5.

154. Seidner DL. JPEN J Parenter Enteral Nutr 2002;26(Suppl):S37–42.

155. Buchman AL, Moukarzel A. Clin Nutr 2000;19:217–31.

156. Pironi L, Morselli AM, Pertkiewicz M et al. Clin Nutr 2002;21:289–96.

157. Shike M, Harrison JE, Sturtridge WC et al. Ann Intern Med 1980;92:343–50.

158. Verhage AH, Cheong WI, Allard JP et al. JPEN J Parenter Enteral Nutr 1995;19:431–6.

159. Saitta JC, Ou SM, Sherrard DJ et al. JPEN J Parenter Enteral Nutr 1993;17:214–9.

160. Pironi L, Zolezzi C, Ruggeri E et al. Nutrition 2000;16:272–7.

161. Wood RJ, Sitrin MD, Rosenberg IH. Am J Clin Nutr 1988;48:632–6.

162. Berkelhammer C, Wood RJ, Sitrin MD. JPEN J Parenter Enteral Nutr 1998;22:142–6.

163. Mühlebach S, Franken C, Stanga Z. Ger Med Sci 2009;7:doc18.

164. Trissel LA, Gilbert DL, Martinez JF et al. Am J Health Syst Pharm 1997;54:1295–300.

165. Trissel LA, Gilbert DL, Martinez JF et al. JPEN J Parenter Enteral Nutr 1999;23:67–74.

166. Shils ME, Wright WL, Turnbull A et al. N Engl J Med 1970;283:341–4.

167. Delegge MH. JPEN J Parenter Enteral Nutr 2002;26(Suppl):S60–2.

168. Howard L, Ament M, Fleming CR et al. Gastroenterology 1995;109:355–65.

169. Howard L, Malone M. Am J Clin Nutr 1997;66:1364–70.

170. Howard L, Ashley C. Gastroenterology 2003;124:1651–61.

171. Gulledge AD, Srp F, Sharp JW et al. Nutr Clin Pract 1987;2:183–94.

172. Smith CE. JPEN J Parenter Enteral Nutr 1993;17:501–506.

173. O'Neill JP, Shaha AR. Surg Clin North Am 2011;91:631–9.

174. Burnette B, Jatoi A. Curr Opin Support Palliat Care 2010;4:272–5.

175. Howard L, Heaphey L, Fleming CR et al. JPEN J Parenter Enteral Nutr 1991;15:384–93.

NTT received their target calories compared to those managed by the primary team.

MANAGEMENT OF THE HOSPITALIZED PATIENT

Malnutrition has a profound impact on patient outcomes and health care costs, which are detailed elsewhere in this textbook. Not surprisingly, the identification of malnutrition in the hospital setting gained attention starting in the 1970s as modern-day treatment options for PN and EN developed and nutrition intervention and therapy became practical realities. Despite these advances, up to 50% of all hospitalized patients have some degree of malnutrition even today (32).

To combat the human and financial costs associated with malnutrition, it is imperative to screen all hospitalized patients for malnourishment or those at risk for malnutrition. Nutrition screening is different from a full nutrition assessment in that the former is meant to be administered quickly and efficiently to identify those who are appropriate for full nutrition assessment by a nutrition expert (33, 34). Various nutrition screening methods are available, which can be conducted by nutrition professionals (e.g., dietetic technicians or registered dietitians), nursing staff, or even completed by the patient (35). Appropriate validated tools include the Malnutrition Universal Screening Tool, Nutritional Risk Screening, Mini Nutrition Assessment, Short Nutritional Assessment Questionnaire, the Malnutrition Screening Tool, and Subjective Global Assessment. The reader is directed to the review by Anthony (35) for a full description of these screening tools.

Instead of using validated screening tools, some institutions have developed their own screening questions based on clinical experience; and others use a laboratory-based screening process, for example, screening based on albumin or prealbumin levels. Although some controversy exists regarding the use of circulating proteins (36), Robinson et al (37) found that a low prealbumin concentration correlated with a dietitian's identification of the presence of malnutrition. No matter what screening method is used, some screening process should be performed.

Once a patient is determined to be at nutritional risk or frankly malnourished, it is typically the dietitian's role to conduct a comprehensive nutrition evaluation. For patients referred to the NTT for management, other team members may conduct the full nutrition assessment in concert with the dietitian (2). The assessment should determine the presence or absence of malnutrition, including micronutrient deficiencies. The assessment should also include the optimal route for feeding the patient. The options include feeding by mouth, or forced feeding with PN or EN.

The nutrition assessment should include optimizing the timing of nutrition intervention. Although timing of nutrition intervention may seem trivial, it can have a large impact on outcome and costs. For example, a metaanalysis of PN treatment in patients with moderate to severe pancreatitis found that initiating PN within 5 days of hospitalization worsens outcome and delays transition to enteral feeding. Thus, it is recommended that one wait 5 days before administering PN to those with acute pancreatitis even if it is clear that PN may ultimately be necessary on hospital admission (38).

Finally, one should assess the risk for refeeding syndrome (39). The refeeding syndrome refers to the phenomenon that occurs when nutrition support is initiated in malnourished patients and is characterized by hypophosphatemia, hypokalemia, hypomagnesemia, thiamin deficiency, hyperglycemia, and fluid intolerance. There have been a number of mortalities associated with the refeeding syndrome. Therefore, it is essential to identify patients at risk before initiating nutrition support, replenish appropriate electrolyte deficiencies, and initiate feeding slowly. In addition to malnourished patients, other at-risk patients include alcoholics and patients receiving prolonged intravenous fluids. The astute NTT will be able to identify patients at risk and initiate and advance nutrition support carefully to avoid complications.

Once the assessment is complete, an appropriate nutrition plan for addressing the identified nutrition problems can be developed. Table 85.3 summarizes the components of a comprehensive nutrition evaluation.

Determining the Route of Nutrition Support

Determining the optimal route of nutrition intervention is one of the most important decisions for patients requiring forced feeding. Ideally, the least invasive method of nutrition is desired, meaning oral administration of a complete diet consisting of healthy foods. For those who cannot get adequate calories and protein from a regular diet, oral nutritional supplements are often the first line of therapy for malnourished patients. For those patients who cannot or will not take adequate nutrition by mouth but have a functional gastrointestinal (GI) tract, enteral feeding that bypasses the mouth is the next line of nutrition intervention. This requires placement of an enteral access device.

TABLE 85.3	**COMPONENTS OF A CLINICAL NUTRITION EVALUATION**

Review and evaluate anthropometric measurements
Review and evaluate biochemical measures
Obtain and evaluate diet history and/or 24-h diet recall and/or food frequency questionnaire
Conduct nutrition-focused physical examination
Calculate energy, protein (and other macronutrients for patients receiving parenteral nutrition), fluid, and micronutrient requirements
Determine optimal route for nutrition support (i.e., oral, enteral, or parenteral)
Develop implementation and monitoring plan

The type of enteral access device depends on the duration of enteral feeding and the function and accessibility of the GI tract. For example, a patient requiring a short-term enteral feeding would be best served by a nasoenteric feeding tube such as a nasogastric or nasojejunal tube. In contrast, a patient requiring long-term enteral support should receive either a gastrostomy or jejunostomy tube if possible. Enteral feeding devices are reviewed elsewhere in this volume and also in reviews by Vanek (40–42).

The success of enteral feeding depends in part on patient factors such as nausea, vomiting, diarrhea, and abdominal pain. Many of these conditions can be managed with the assistance of an NTT. For example, nausea and vomiting may be improved by placing a post-pyloric tube into the duodenum or jejunum, which overcomes issues associated with gastroparesis. Dedicated teams skilled at placement of postpyloric feeding tubes can increase success of tube placement and tolerance of tube feedings (43, 44). Diarrhea can be overcome by selecting an "antidiarrheal" tube feeding regimen. The NTT can help with selecting the most appropriate type of EN formula based on the clinical evaluation and can adjust the formula selection as needed based on patient response.

The success of enteral feeding also depends in part on nursing and physician factors. There is a large debate and comfort level associated with what are "acceptable" gastric residuals when administrating tube feeds. In addition, there are varying tube feeding advancement protocols even if gastric residuals are acceptable. NTTs generally accept higher gastric residuals and advance tube feedings more quickly. NTTs have developed tube feed advancement protocols to assist in this process. This leads to higher success rates with tube feed administration and more rapid achievement of full caloric goals (45–48).

PN is the only option available to feed the patient without a functional GI tract for a prolonged period. A hospitalized patient may be best served by a centrally inserted central catheter designed for short-term use (e.g., 2 to 3 weeks), particularly in the intensive care unit setting. For patients going home on PN for an intermediate period of time (e.g., 6 to 8 weeks), a peripherally inserted central catheter would be a reasonable choice. For a patient requiring long-term PN, a tunneled catheter would be the best choice. For patients requiring PN infusions less than daily, for example, patients with intestinal failure requiring only a few infusions of PN per week to maintain nutritional status, a totally implantable central venous access device (i.e., a totally implantable port) would be an appropriate option. Reviews by Vanek (49, 50) provide an in-depth discussion of central venous access devices.

Proactive Nutrition Intervention

In some cases, it is possible to formulate a nutrition plan preoperatively in anticipation of nutrition needs that a patient may have postoperatively. For example, it is well known in the trauma surgical population that prophylactic

placement of a feeding jejunostomy at the time of exploratory laparotomy allows for early enteral feeding (51). The benefits of early feeding are described elsewhere in this volume.

However, the benefits of prophylactic feeding tube placement are not just limited to trauma patients. Patients undergoing pancreaticoduodenectomy (i.e. the Whipple procedure) have been shown to benefit from this as well. Baradi et al (52) evaluated placement of a jejunal feeding tube at the time of Whipple and compared it with patients who did not receive enteral access. Placement of the feeding tube during the primary procedure reduced the need for PN by 80% and was associated with decreased infection, late complications, and readmission to the hospital. In a similar study in Whipple patients, Mack et al (53) found that the strategy of placing a feeding tube at the time of surgery decreased the incidence of gastroparesis and was associated with decreased length of stay in the hospital and overall costs (Figs. 85.2 and 85.3).

Surgeons often fail to think of placing a feeding tube at the time of complex intra-abdominal surgeries. One important role of the NTT is to recommend placement of a jejunal feeding tube in patients in whom there is a high risk of prolonged gastroparesis. This is especially true if the patient will have postoperative anatomic concerns (e.g., fresh gastric anastomosis) that would preclude safe postoperative feeding tube placement via the nose into the stomach or distally. The goal should be "plan for EN to prevent PN."

Another area in which proactive nutrition intervention is warranted is in severely malnourished patients who are to undergo elective major surgery. The Nutrition Risk

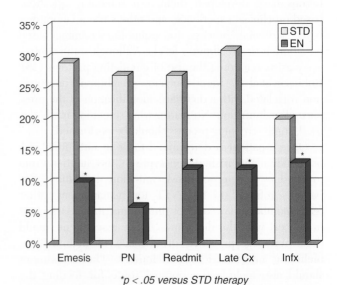

*$p < .05$ versus STD therapy

Fig. 85.2. Benefits of planned enteral access and feeding following pancreaticoduodenectomy. *Cx,* complications; *EN,* enteral nutrition; *Infx,* infection; *PN,* parenteral nutrition; *STD,* standard therapy. (Adapted with permission from Baradi H, Walsh RM, Henderson JM et al. Postoperative jejunal feeding and outcome of pancreaticoduodenectomy. J Gastrointest Surg 2004;8:428–33.)

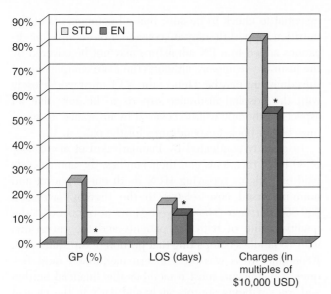

*p < .05 versus STD therapy

Fig. 85.3. Benefits of planned enteral access and feeding following pancreaticoduodenectomy. *EN*, enteral nutrition; *GP*, gastroparesis; *LOS*, length of stay; *STD*, standard therapy; *USD*, United States dollars. (Adapted with permission from Mack LA, Kaklamanos IG, Livingstone AS et al. Gastric decompression and enteral feeding through a double-lumen gastrojejunostomy tube improves outcomes after pancreatico-duodenectomy. Ann Surg 2004;240:845–51.)

Index (NRI) was developed by Buzby et al (54) as part of the protocol for the Veterans Affairs Total Parenteral Nutrition Cooperative Study Group evaluating the effectiveness of perioperative PN in malnourished patients undergoing major abdominal or thoracic surgery (55). The NRI is a scoring system that assesses severity of malnutrition using serum albumin and percent usual body weight (Table 85.4).

Malnourished patients were randomized to receive PN for 7 to 15 days before surgery and 3 days postoperatively or no PN (55). All patients were monitored for major and minor complications for 30 days. Taken as a whole, the patients receiving PN had a higher rate of infectious complications compared with the control. Group subanalyses revealed that those patients who were borderline mal-

nourished or had mild malnutrition based on the NRI had a significantly higher rate of infectious complications and no difference in noninfectious complications compared with those receiving no PN. Of note, and in contrast, the severely malnourished group had a significantly lower rate of noninfectious complications (e.g., anastomotic leak, wound dehiscence, chronic respiratory failure) compared with the control group (5.3% versus 42.9%), whereas infectious complications were comparable. Thus, perioperative PN has a definite role in optimizing the status of severely malnourished patients facing major surgery. The NTT can very easily calculate NRI to help determine which patients are severely malnourished and thus would benefit from 1 to 2 weeks of PN before surgery on an inpatient or outpatient basis.

TRANSITION TO HOME

Home EN (HEN) or home PN (HPN) may be indicated for a number of patients who cannot dependably tolerate oral feedings. The transition to home from the hospital presents several challenges for the patient receiving PN or EN. It is imperative that an inpatient or outpatient NTT be involved in this process to ensure a smooth and successful transition.

Evaluation of the Home Environment

Home nutrition support patients require a safe and supportive home environment to assure a successful transition. This complex therapy requires a patient to have access to clean water, refrigeration, and electricity. The home needs to be clean, free of vermin, and must have a secure storage area for home infusion supplies. In addition, the patient must be able to navigate the home safely, taking into account how the patient will ambulate around the home (including into the bathroom) with an infusion pump and an intravenous pole. The NTT clinicians as well as those involved in coordinating the discharge process can conduct the evaluation of the home environment via patient interview. At times, an in-person home visit is necessary to identify and correct any issues that could preclude safe PN or EN administration (56, 57).

An important aspect of going home on EN or PN is the patient's ability to be independent with the home therapy. In most cases, a clinician will not be able to see the patient at home every day; therefore, the patient or caregiver must learn how to do basic tasks associated with the therapy. For HEN, this may include learning how to decant enteral formula into an enteral feeding bag, priming an enteral feeding pump, learning how to troubleshoot pump problems, and basic care of the enteral access device. For HPN, this would include learning aseptic technique for connecting tubing to a bag of PN, priming the infusion pump, troubleshooting problems with the infusion pump, and appropriate care of the central venous catheter. These tasks can be overwhelming to a patient,

TABLE 85.4	NUTRITION RISK INDEX

NRI: 1.519 × SERUM ALBUMIN (G/L) + 0.417 × (CURRENT WEIGHT/USUAL WEIGHT) × 100	
SCORE	**INTERPRETATION**
>97.5	Borderline malnourished
83.5–97.5	Mildly malnourished
<83.5	Severely malnourished

NRI, Nutrition Risk Index.

Data from Buzby GP, Knox LS, Crosby LO et al. Study protocol: a randomized clinical trial of total parenteral nutrition in malnourished surgical patients. Am J Clin Nutr 1988;47:366–81; and Veterans Affairs Total Parenteral Nutrition Cooperative Study Group. Perioperative total parenteral nutrition in surgical patients. N Engl J Med 1991;325:525–32, with permission.

and the support of a care partner or partners (either family members or a network of friends) is important to promote success in the transition to home. This is especially true for a convalescing patient who may be too weak to care for himself or herself (57, 58).

Patient and Caregiver Education and Support

Education regarding HEN or HPN should start early in the patient's hospital course to ease the transition to home. Once home, the education should continue by clinicians from the home infusion company and/or home nursing agency to assure that the patient and caregivers are proficient in providing the HEN or HPN. Patients and caregivers must be instructed in what to do in an emergency so that they know when to call the home infusion company, when to call the physician, and when to go directly to the local emergency department (56). Various education techniques are available to teach patients and caregivers how to manage the home nutrition therapy. In-person demonstrations, written educational materials, and video resources are all good options to start and then reinforce education to ensure a successful transition to independence (59).

Although NTT health professionals agree on what is necessary to prepare patients adequately for home nutrition therapy, this does not always translate into real preparedness for patients. Silver et al (60) conducted a study of 30 caregivers of patients receiving HEN, including an evaluation of preparedness for caregiving, using the Preparedness for Caregiving Scale. This scale is a validated subset of the Family Caregiving Inventory. Preparedness scores were very low (mean 1.72 on a 5-point scale, with 0 meaning *not prepared at all* and 4 indicating *very well prepared*), and participants noted that they received very little training on HEN before discharge. This finding suggests that patients are often unprepared for receiving home nutrition therapy, particularly EN, a situation that likely contributes to readmission rates to the hospital and unnecessary complications.

Referral to a support organization such as the Oley Foundation may also be beneficial. Smith et al (61) conducted a case-control study evaluating patients who were receiving HPN and who were affiliated with the Oley Foundation and those who were not affiliated. The investigators found that affiliated patients had improved outcomes including improved quality of life, decreased reactive depression scores, and lower incidence of CRBSIs. The Oley Foundation also supported patients receiving HEN, and although this group has not been studied in the same manner as patients receiving HPN, one could expect similar results.

Insurance Coverage

Insurance coverage of nutrition therapy in the home setting is not guaranteed. Although some insurers recognize the importance of in-home coverage, others do not. It is essential to check to be sure that all components of the nutrition support therapy are covered. For example, medications added to a PN admixture may not be covered by the insurance company, although the main components of the admixture may be. Hence, the NTT must work closely with the hospital insurance experts to be sure that all aspects of therapy will be covered by insurance, to minimize out-of-pocket expenditures for the patient.

In a study conducted by Piamjariyakul et al (62, 63) of 80 HPN recipients and their families, the annual costs paid by patients receiving HPN (both out-of-pocket and nonreimbursed cost related to the therapy) averaged $30,866 per year. These investigators also looked at the quality of life of both the patients and the caregivers, with 78 families completing that portion of the study (64). Economic stress was the concern mentioned most frequently. Clinicians must remember this financial burden and refer patients appropriately and early in the clinical course for financial assistance. In addition, it also is a reminder that transition off or reduction of home nutrition should be aggressively pursued for financial as well as clinical reasons. The NTT can also assist in these areas.

Routine Follow-up/Monitoring

Patients receiving home nutrition support require routine monitoring to evaluate the effectiveness of the therapy, assess for complications related to the therapy, and develop a treatment plan as indicated (56). In some hospitals, the inpatient NTT is also responsible for managing outpatients receiving EN or PN. In other hospitals, the primary care physician, primary surgeon, or gastroenterologist may be responsible for managing home nutrition therapy. Ideally, the care of patients receiving in-home nutrition therapy should not be left to the primary care provider alone. Although data comparing management of home nutrition support patients by NTTs versus non-NTT affiliated clinicians are limited, HEN and HPN recipients have well-documented complex medical and nutritional needs (58, 60, 65–68). Given these complexities, a multidisciplinary NTT is best suited to manage these patients and is often recommended as a standard of care (2, 56, 67, 69).

A monitoring plan should be tailored to the individual patient, depending on the type of therapy (i.e., EN or PN), underlying disease, and complexity of the nutrition support regimen (56). Some patients may need to be seen in the clinic only once per year, whereas others may require more frequent follow-up. EN monitoring should follow typical inpatient monitoring guidelines, but it can be conducted less frequently based on patient stability. Good clinical practice dictates at least a yearly follow-up for renewal of the enteral feeding prescription (66, 67). PN monitoring is more intensive than HEN monitoring because of the a higher risk of metabolic and infectious complications with this therapy.

Patients receiving HPN typically receive a weekly in-home visit from a nurse to evaluate the central venous access device, provide routine catheter care, and conduct a general clinical evaluation. As patients become more stable, more time can elapse between clinical and general laboratory monitoring (67, 70). Patients receiving HPN are at particular risk of micronutrient deficiencies; thus, they should have a vitamin and trace element panel checked at least twice per year or more frequently if deficiencies are present and repletion is in progress (71). Metabolic bone disease is a known complication of long-term PN, so a yearly bone density evaluation is also recommended (70, 72).

When patients are transitioning from one mode of nutrition support to another (e.g., transitioning from PN to EN, or PN to an oral diet), frequency of monitoring should increase. Transitional periods put the patient at risk of overfeeding or underfeeding and metabolic complications. In general, patients should participate in their own monitoring by measuring weight daily, conducting a basic assessment of the access device for signs or symptoms of infection or malfunction, and identifying basic clinical problems that require prompt medical evaluation (e.g., central line infection or enteral feeding tube dislodgment), assessing GI tolerance if applicable (e.g., nausea, vomiting, diarrhea, constipation), and contacting the ordering clinician if issues arise.

CONCLUSIONS

Nutrition support therapy is best managed by a dedicated NTT to decrease risks of metabolic and infectious complications, avoid use of inappropriate therapies, and save hospital costs. Nutrition screening is an essential part of hospital care and can identify malnourished patients quickly for evaluation by the NTT. Once EN or PN are initiated, the NTT can assist with transition of the therapy to the home environment as indicated. The team approach to management can continue in the home setting to help prevent complications, achieve or maintain optimal nutritional status for patients, and speed the transition to nutritional autonomy if possible.

REFERENCES

1. Wesley JR. Nutr Clin Pract 1995;10:219–28.
2. DeLegge M, Wooley JA, Guenter P et al. Nutr Clin Pract 2010;25:76–84.
3. Seashore JH, McMahon M, Wolfson M et al. Nutr Clin Pract 2003;18:270–5.
4. Russell M, Stieber M, Brantley S et al. Nutr Clin Pract 2007;22:558–86.
5. DiMaria-Ghalili RA, Bankhead R, Fisher AA et al. Nutr Clin Pract 2007;22:458–65.
6. Rollins C, Durfee SM, Holcombe BJ et al. Nutr Clin Pract 2008;23:189–94.
7. ASPEN Board of Directors. JPEN J Parenter Enteral Nutr 1986;10:441–5.
8. ASPEN Board of Directors. JPEN J Parenter Enteral Nutr 1993;17:1SA–52SA.
9. ASPEN Board of Directors. JPEN J Parenter Enteral Nutr 2002;26:1SA–138SA; errata 2002;26:144.
10. ASPEN Board of Directors. JPEN J Parenter Enteral Nutr 2009;33:255–9.
11. Sitzmann JV, Pitt HA et al. Dig Dis Sci 1989;34:489–96.
12. Trujillo EB, Young LS, Chertow GM et al. JPEN J Parenter Enteral Nutr 1999;23:109–13.
13. Maurer J, Weinbaum F, Turner J et al. JPEN J Parenter Enteral Nutr 1996;20:272–4.
14. DeLegge M, Basel MD, Bannister C et al. Nutr Clin Pract 2007;22:246–9.
15. Martin K, DeLegge M, Nichols M et al. JPEN J Parenter Enteral Nutr 2011;35:122–30.
16. Sriram K, Cyriac T, Fogg LF. Nutrition 2010;26:735–9.
17. Kohli-Seth R, Sinha R, Wilson S et al. Nutr Clin Pract 2009;24:728–32.
18. Kudsk KA, Croche MA, Fabian TC et al. Ann Surg 1992;215:503–11.
19. Matsushima K, Cook A, Tyner T et al. Am J Surg 2010;200:386–90.
20. Nehme AE. JAMA 1980;243:1906–8.
21. Faubion WC, Wesley JR, Khalidi N et al. JPEN J Parenter Enteral Nutr 1986;10:642–5.
22. Goldstein M, Braitman LE, Levine GM. JPEN J Parenter Enteral Nutr 2000;24:323–7.
23. Soufir L, Timsit JF, Mahe C et al. Infect Control Hosp Epidemiol 1999;20:396–401.
24. Berwick DM, Calkins DR, McCannon JC et al. JAMA 2006;295:324–7.
25. Haraden C. What is a Bundle? Available at: http://www.ihi.org/IHI/Topics/CriticalCare/IntensiveCare/ImprovementStories/WhatIsaBundle.htm. 2006. Accessed March 16, 2011.
26. Galpern D, Guerrero A, Tu A et al. Surgery 2008;144:492–5.
27. Koll BS, Straub TA, Jalon HS et al. Jt Comm J Qual Patient Saf 2008;34:713–23.
28. Marra AR, Cal RG, Durao MS et al. Am J Infect Control 2010;38:434–9.
29. Twomey PL, Patching SC. JPEN J Parenter Enteral Nutr 1985;9:3–10.
30. ChrisAnderson D, Heimburger DC, Morgan SL et al. JPEN J Parenter Enteral Nutr 1996;20:206–10.
31. Brown RO, Carlson ST, Cowan GS et al. JPEN J Parenter Enteral Nutr 1987;11:52–6.
32. Norman K, Pichard C, Lochs H et al. Clin Nutr 2008;27:5–15.
33. Charney P. Nutr Clin Pract 2008;23:366–72.
34. Mueller C, Compher C, Druyan ME et al. JPEN J Parenter Enteral Nutr 2011;1:16–24
35. Anthony PS. Nutr Clin Pract 2008;23:373–82.
36. Fuhrman MP, Charney P, Mueller CM. J Am Diet Assoc 2004;104:1258–64.
37. Robinson MK, Trujillo EB, Mogensen KM et al. JPEN J Parenter Enteral Nutr 2003;27:389–95.
38. McClave SA, Chang WK, Dhaliwal R et al. JPEN J Parenter Enteral Nutr. 2006;30:143–56.
39. Solomon SM, Kirby DF. JPEN J Parenter Enteral Nutr 1990;14:90–7.
40. Vanek VW. Nutr Clin Pract 2002;17:275–83.
41. Vanek VW. Nutr Clin Pract 2003;18:50–74.
42. Vanek VW. Nutr Clin Pract 2003;18:201–20.
43. Powers J, Chance R, Bortenschlager L et al. Crit Care Nurse 2003;23:16–24.
44. Marsland C. Nutr Clin Pract 2010;25:270–6.
45. Spain DA, McClave SA, Sexton LK et al. JPEN J Parenter Enteral Nutr 1999;23:288–92.
46. Heyland DK, Cahill NE, Dhaliwal R et al. JPEN J Parenter Enteral Nutr 2010;34:675–84.

47. McClave SA, Snider HL. JPEN J Parenter Enteral Nutr 2002;26:S43–S50.

48. Bankhead R, Boulatta J, Brantley S et al. JPEN J Parenter Enteral Nutr 2009;33:122–67.

49. Vanek VW. Nutr Clin Pract 2002;17:85–98.

50. Vanek VW. Nutr Clin Pract 2002;17:142–55.

51. Jacobs DG, Jacobs DO, Kudsk KA et al. J Trauma 2004;57: 660–79.

52. Baradi H, Walsh RM, Henderson JM et al. J Gastrointest Surg 2004;8:428–33.

53. Mack LA, Kaklamanos IG, Livingstone AS et al. Ann Surg 2004;240:845–51.

54. Buzby GP, Knox LS, Crosby LO et al. Am J Clin Nutr 1988;47:366–81.

55. Veterans Affairs Total Parenteral Nutrition Cooperative Study Group. N Engl J Med 1991;325:525–32.

56. ASPEN Board of Directors. Nutr Clin Pract 2005;20:575–90.

57. Ireton-Jones C, DeLegge MH, Epperson LA et al. Nutr Clin Pract 2003;18:310–17.

58. DiBiase JK, Scolapio JS. Gastroenterol Clin N Am 2007;36: 123–44.

59. Gifford H, DeLegge M, Epperson LA. Nutr Clin Pract 2010;25:443–50.

60. Silver HJ, Wellman NS, Galindo-Ciocon D et al. J Am Diet Assoc 2004;104:43–50.

61. Smith CE, Curtas S, Werkowitch M et al. JPEN J Parenter Enteral Nutr 2002;26:159–63.

62. Piamjariyakul U, Ross VM, Yadrich DM et al. Nurs Econ 2010;28:255–63.

63. Piamjariyakul U, Ross VM, Yadrich DM et al. Nurs Econ 2010;28:323–9.

64. Smith CE, Piamjariyakul U, Yadrich DM et al. Nurs Econ 2010;28:393–9, 414.

65. Howard L. Nutrition 2000;16:625–8.

66. DeLegge MH. JPEN J Parenter Enteral Nutr 2002;28:S4–S7.

67. Rhoda KM, Suryadevara S, Steiger E. Surg Clin North Am 2011; 91: 913–32.

68. Silver HJ, Wellman NS, Arnold DJ et al. JPEN J Parenter Enteral Nutr 2004;28:92–8.

69. Ross VM, Smith CE. Nutr Clin Pract 2011;26:656–64.

70. Seipler J. Nutr Clin Pract 2007;22:340–50.

71. Fuhrman MP. Nutr Clin Pract 2006;21:566–75.

72. Ferrone M, Geraci M. Nutr Clin Pract 2007;22:329–39.

SUGGESTED READINGS

Bankhead R, Boulatta J, Brantley S et al. Enteral nutrition practice recommendations. JPEN J Parenter Enteral Nutr 2009;33:122–67.

DeLegge M, Wooley JA, Guenter P et al. The state of nutrition support teams and update on current models for providing nutrition support therapy to patients. Nutr Clin Pract 2010;25:76–84.

DiBiase JK, Scolapio JS. Home parenteral and enteral nutrition. Gastroenterol Clin North Am 2007;36:123–44.

Mirtallo J, Canada T, Johnson D et al. Safe practices for parenteral nutrition. JPEN J Parenter Enteral Nutr 2004;28:S39–S70.

Trujillo EB, Young LS, Chertow GM et al. Metabolic and monetary costs of avoidable parenteral nutrition use. JPEN J Parenter Enteral Nutr 1999;23:109–13.

86 EPIDEMIOLOGY OF DIET AND CANCER RISK[1]

WALTER C. WILLETT AND EDWARD GIOVANNUCCI

CANCER AS A PUBLIC HEALTH PROBLEM

Following cardiovascular disease, cancer is the second leading cause of death in most affluent countries. It also contributes significantly to mortality rates among adults in developing countries (1, 2). In the United States, about one in three persons will be diagnosed with cancer during their lifetime and about 60% of those diagnosed will die of cancer (3). Because rates of cardiovascular death have been declining rapidly and overall cancer mortality has not substantially changed, cancer will likely become the most important cause of death in the United States (2, 4). Although overall cancer rates among adults vary only modestly around the world, the types of cancers are dramatically different (1, 2). In most affluent countries, cancers of the lung, colon, breast, and prostate contribute most to incidence and mortality. In poorer regions and the Far East, cancers of the stomach, liver, oral cavity, esophagus, and uterine cervix are most important. However, cancer incidence rates are very dynamic; many areas of the world are experiencing a transition from the cancer incidence patterns of poorer to those of affluent areas (1). Rates of breast and colon cancer have been increasing in almost all countries.

Although genetics play an important role in the development of cancer, inherited mutations cannot account for the dramatic differences in cancer rates seen around the world. Populations that move from countries with low rates of specific cancers to areas with high rates, or the reverse, almost invariably achieve the rates characteristic of the new homeland (5–7). The time required to attain the new rate can vary, however, from several decades in the case of colon cancer, to about three generations for breast cancer (7–10). The dramatic changes in cancer rates within a country provide further evidence for the importance of noninherited factors. For example, in Japan rates of colon cancer mortality increased about 2.5-fold between 1950 and 1985 (11).

The dramatic variations in cancer rates around the world and changes over time imply that these malignancies are potentially avoidable if we were able to identify and then avoid the causal factors. For a few cancers, the primary causes are well known, such as smoking in the case of lung cancer; but for most others, the etiologic factors are less well established. However, strong reasons exist to suspect that dietary and nutritional factors may account for many of these variations in cancer rates. First, a role of diet has been suggested by observations that national rates of specific cancers are strongly correlated with aspects of diet such as per capita consumption of fat (12). Also, numerous studies in animals, including a series of detailed experiments conducted during the 1930s (13), clearly demonstrated that dietary manipulations could influence tumorigenesis dramatically.

A multitude of steps in the pathogenesis of cancer have been identified in which dietary factors could plausibly act either to increase or decrease the probability that the clinical cancer will develop. For example, carcinogens in food that can directly damage DNA are discussed elsewhere in this volume, and other dietary factors may block the endogenous synthesis of carcinogens or induce enzymes involved in the activation or deactivation of exogenous carcinogenic substances (14). Oxidative damage to DNA is likely to be an important cause of mutations and potentially can be enhanced by some dietary factors, such as polyunsaturated fats and iron, or reduced by dietary antioxidants or nutrients that are cofactors for antioxidant enzymes, such as selenium or copper (15). Inadequate intake of dietary factors

---

[1]**Abbreviations: EPIC**, European Prospective Investigation into Cancer and Nutrition; **HDL**, high-density lipoprotein; **IGF**, insulinlike growth factor; **RR**, relative risk; **SELECT**, Selenium and Vitamin E Cancer Prevention Trial.

needed for DNA synthesis, repair, and methylation, such as folic acid, also could influence the risk of mutation or gene expression. The rate of cell division influences whether DNA lesions are replicated and is thus likely to influence the probability of cancer developing (15). Thus, energy balance and growth rates, which can be influenced by a variety of essential nutrients, could affect cancer rates. Dietary factors can influence endogenous hormone levels, including estrogens and various growth factors, which can influence cell cycling, and thus potentially cancer incidence. Estrogenic substances found in some plant foods also can interact with estrogen receptors, and thus could either mimic or block the effects of endogenous estrogens (14). Many other aspects of diet can alter cell proliferation or differentiation either by direct hormonal effects, such as by vitamins A or D, or indirectly by influencing inflammatory or irritative processes, such as specific fatty acids that are precursors of prostaglandins or that inhibit their synthesis. Many other examples can be given by which dietary factors could plausibly influence the development of cancer (14, 15).

EPIDEMIOLOGIC INVESTIGATION OF DIET AND CANCER RELATIONSHIPS

The strong suggestions from international comparisons, animal studies, and mechanistic investigations that various aspects of diet may importantly influence risk of cancer raises two critical sets of questions: Which dietary factors are actually important determinants of human cancer? What is the nature of the dose-response relationships? The nature of the dose-response relationships is particularly important because a substance could be carcinogenic to humans, but there could be no important risk within the range of intakes actually consumed by humans. Alternatively, another factor could be critical for protection against cancer, but all persons in a population already may be consuming sufficient amounts to receive the maximal benefit. In either case, no potential exists for reduction in cancer rates by altering current intakes. The important factors to identify are those for which at least some part of the population is either consuming a toxic level or is not eating a sufficient amount for optimal health. Because cancer is a multistage process, the temporal relationship also is critical to identify.

Various epidemiologic approaches can be used to investigate diet and human cancer relationships (Table 86.1). Relationships between diet and nutrition and cancer incidence in epidemiologic studies can be evaluated by collecting data on dietary intake, using biochemical indicators of dietary factors, or measuring body size and composition. Food frequency questionnaires have been used to assess diet in most epidemiologic studies because they provide information on usual diet over an extended

TABLE 86.1	COMPARISON OF TYPES OF STUDIES THAT ADDRESS THE EFFECT OF DIET ON CANCER RISK			
	TYPE OF STUDY			
	Descriptive	Case-Control	Prospective Cohort	Interventional
DESIGN	Cancer rates in populations having different diets are compared by assessing average intake of specific nutrients and determining cancer incidence or mortality.	Earlier diets reported by patients with a particular type of cancer are compared with diets reported by matched controls without cancer.	Incidence of cancer is compared in people whose diets and other potentially relevant factors are determined before follow-up begins.	Incidence of cancer in two groups randomized to specific interventions or to no interventions is compared.
LIMITATIONS	Diet is but one of many variables that distinguish populations. Even crude data on average nutrient intake is difficult to gather. These studies are probably best used to generate hypothesis.	Selection bias may occur if controls do not accurately represent the population from which cases arose. Recall bias can result when patients differ systematically from controls in ability to recall diets. Memory of dietary habits can be faulty among patients and controls.* In rapidly fatal cancers, researchers must often rely on recall of proxy respondents such as spouses.	Selection bias and recall bias should not occur, but thousands or even tens of thousands of people must be enrolled and their health be monitored for many years before statistical power can be achieved.	Adherence to substantial dietary changes is difficult for many people. Participants cannot be easily blinded to their status. Optimal dosages (e.g. of supplemental nutrients) and dose-response relationships can be difficult to ascertain. Duration of intervention required is generally unknown but may be decades.

*Measurements of vitamins in blood are sometimes substituted for dietary recall questionnaires in case-control and cohort studies. However, this strategy is not universally applicable because levels in blood do not always accurately reflect intake. For example, β-carotene blood levels are a good index of dietary intake whereas retinol levels in blood are only weakly related to intake. Blood levels must be interpreted with caution in case-control studies because cancer can change the level of a vitamin in the plasma.

period of time and are sufficiently adequate to be used in large populations. Food frequency questionnaires have been shown to be sufficiently valid to detect important diet–disease relationships in comparisons with more detailed assessments of diet and biochemical indicators (16). Biochemical indicators of diet can be useful in some situations, but for many dietary factors of interest, such as total fat, fiber, and sodium, no useful indicators exist. DNA specimens have been collected from participants in many studies and allow the examination of gene–diet interactions. Until recently, most information on diet and cancer has been obtained from case-control studies. However, many large prospective cohort studies of diet and cancer in various countries are now ongoing and are generating data that are transforming our understanding of nutrition and cancer. Because the number of studies is now becoming large, systematic reviews and metaanalyses that summarize the findings statistically are becoming increasingly important. However, these summaries are limited by the possibility of selective publication of positive results, the difficulty of combining data on diet, which can be expressed in many different ways, and variations in the control of covariates. Analyses that combine the primary data from the original studies, often called pooled analyses, overcome most of these limitations and are a more reliable way to summarize that data, but such analyses are laborious and not always available.

Epidemiologic investigations should be viewed as complementary to animal studies, in vitro investigations, and metabolic studies of diet in relation to intermediate end points, such as hormone levels. Although conditions can be controlled to a much greater degree in laboratory studies than in free-living human populations, the relevance of findings to humans always will be uncertain, particularly in regard to dose-response and temporal relationships. Ultimately, our knowledge is best based on a synthesis of epidemiologic, metabolic, animal, and mechanistic studies.

CURRENT STATE OF KNOWLEDGE FOR SPECIFIC ASPECTS OF DIET

Diet is a complex composite of various nutrients and nonnutritive food constituents, and many types of human cancer exist, each with its own pathogenetic mechanisms. Thus, the combinations of specific dietary factors and cancers are almost limitless. This brief overview focuses primarily on the major cancers of affluent populations and aspects of diet for which strong hypotheses and substantial epidemiologic data exist. Several aspects of diet for which hypothesized preventive roles exist are discussed in further detail in the chapter on chemoprevention.

Energy Balance, Growth Rates, and Body Size

Studies by Tannenbaum and colleagues (13, 17) during the first half of the twentieth century indicated that energy restriction could reduce the development of mammary

tumors in animals profoundly. This finding has been consistently replicated in a wide variety of mammary tumor models and for a wide variety of other tumors (18–22). For example, restriction in energy intake by approximately 30% can reduce mammary tumors by as much as 90% (23). The possibility that this relationship, which is the most consistent and strongest effect of diet in animal studies, also may apply to humans received relatively little attention until recently.

In evaluating the effect of energy restriction on cancer rates in humans, it may be tempting to examine the association between energy intake and incidence of cancer. However, such an approach is likely to be completely misleading because in free-living populations, variation in energy intake is determined largely by energy expenditure in the form of physical activity (24). Thus, for example, energy intake is inversely associated with risk of coronary heart disease owing to the protective effect of exercise against this disease (16). The most sensitive indicators of the balance between energy intake and expenditure are growth rates and body size, which can be measured well in epidemiologic investigations, although they also reflect genetic and other nonnutritional factors. Thus, adult height can provide an indirect indicator of pre-adult nutrition, and adult weight gain and obesity reflect positive energy balance later in life. In populations that were traditionally short, such as the Japanese, rapid gains in height during the last several decades (25) have corresponded with increases in breast and colon cancer rates. Further support for an important role of growth rates comes from epidemiologic studies of age at menarche. An early menarche is a well-established risk factor for breast cancer. The difference in the late age of menarche in China—until recently approximately 17 years (26), compared with 12 and 13 years of age in the United States (27)—contributes importantly to differences in breast cancer rates between these populations. Body mass index, height, and weight have been consistently strong determinants or correlates of age at menstruation (28–30), but the composition of diet appears to have little if any effect. Collectively, these studies provide strong evidence, consistent with animal experiments, that rapid growth rates before puberty play an important role in determining future risk of breast and probably other cancers. Whether the epidemiologic findings result from only restriction of energy intake in relation to requirements for maximal growth, or whether the limitation of other nutrients, such as essential amino acids, may also play a role cannot be determined from available data.

A positive energy balance during adult life and the resultant accumulation of body fat also contributes significantly to several human cancers. The best-established relationships are with cancers of the colon, kidney, pancreas, esophagus (adenocarcinoma), endometrium, and gall bladder (31–38). The relation between body fatness and breast cancer is more complex. Before menopause, women with greater body fat have reduced risk of breast cancer (39, 40), and after menopause a positive but weak association with adiposity is seen. These findings may be the result of anovulatory menstrual cycles in fatter women before menopause (41), which should reduce risk, and the synthesis of endogenous estrogen by adipose tissue in postmenopausal women (42), which is presumed to increase the risk of breast cancer. A complex association between body fat and prostate cancer also may exist (43).

In animal models, reduction in insulinlike growth factor-I (IGF-I) mediates at least part of the effect of energy reduction (44). Insulin is known to be a powerful modulator of bioavailable IGF-I (45). In human studies, increasing evidence exists that high circulating levels of IGF-I and insulin are associated with an increased risk of some cancers that occur in affluent populations, particularly colon cancer (45, 46). In the Physicians' Health Study of male physicians (47), there was 2.5-fold increased risk of colorectal cancer with increasing levels of plasma C-peptide (a marker of insulin secretion) when extreme quintiles (highest versus lowest) were compared. Increasing waist-to-hip ratio is also associated with an increased risk of colon cancer, independently of body mass index (48). In fact, indirect evidence (49) suggests that factors related to energy balance and dietary patterns that stimulate insulin and IGF-I secretion throughout the life span could account largely for the approximately one third of cancers in affluent countries that are believed to be influenced by nutrition (50).

Dietary Fat and Macronutrients

In the landmark 1982 National Academy of Sciences review of diet (51), reduction in fat intake to 30% of calories was the primary recommendation. This objective has been echoed in subsequent dietary recommendations as well (52, 53). Two lines of evidence stimulated this interest in dietary fat as a cause of cancer.

In the first half of the twentieth century, studies by Tannenbaum and colleagues (13, 17) indicated that diets high in fat could promote tumor growth in animal models. A vast literature on dietary fat and cancer in animals has accumulated subsequently (reviewed elsewhere) (22, 51, 54–56). However, although dietary fat has an effect on tumor incidence in most models (57, 58), the influence of fat has not been definitely established to be independent of the effect of energy intake (22, 23, 54, 55, 59). Second, a possible relation of dietary fat intake to cancer incidence also has been hypothesized because the large international differences in rates of cancers of the breast, colon, prostate, and endometrium are strongly correlated with apparent per capita animal fat consumption (12, 60–62).

Fat and Breast Cancer

Although a major rationale for the dietary fat hypothesis has been the international correlation between fat consumption and national breast cancer mortality (12), a study of 65 Chinese counties (63), in which per capita fat intake varied from 6% to 25% of energy, showed only a weak positive association between fat intake and breast cancer mortality. Notably, five counties consumed approximately 25% of energy from fat yet experienced rates of breast cancer far below those of US women with similar fat intake (64), thus providing strong evidence that factors other than fat intake account for the large international differences. Breast cancer incidence rates increased substantially in the United States during the twentieth century, as have the estimates of per capita fat consumption, based on food disappearance data. However, surveys based on reports of individual intake, rather than food disappearance, indicate that consumption of energy from fat, either as absolute intake or as a percentage of energy, actually has declined in the last half of the twentieth century (65, 66), a time during which breast cancer incidence has increased (67).

Many case-control studies have been conducted to investigate the dietary fat effect on breast cancer. In one large study (68), animal fat and total fat intake were not associated with breast cancer. The results from 12 smaller case-control studies were summarized in a metaanalysis by Howe et al (69), which included 4312 cases and 5978 controls. The pooled relative risk (RR) was 1.35 ($p < .0001$) for a 100-g increase in daily total fat intake, although the risk was somewhat stronger for postmenopausal women (RR = 1.48; $p < .001$). This magnitude of association, however, potentially could be compatible with biases resulting from recall of diet or selection of controls (70).

A substantial body of data from cohort studies is now available to assess the relation between dietary fat intake and breast cancer in developed countries. In a pooled analysis of prospective studies that included 4980 incident cases of breast cancer (71), no overall association was seen for overall fat intake over the range of less than 20% to greater than 45% of energy from fat. A similar lack of association was seen among postmenopausal women only and for specific types of fat. Only among the small number of women consuming less than 15% of energy from fat was a significant association seen; breast cancer risk was elevated twofold in this group. The lack of any suggestion of an increase in risk with higher total fat intake was confirmed in an update of the pooled analysis with 7329 incident cases (72, 73) and a more recent large prospective study from Europe with 7119 cases (74). In a large cohort of older American women (3501 cases), a weak and marginally significant positive association was seen with total fat (for highest versus lowest quintile RR 1.11 [95% confidence interval = 1.00 to 1.24]) (75). In the Nurses' Health Study, analyses have been conducted with 14 years of follow-up (2956 cases) (73)—20 years for postmenopausal women (76)—and with up to six assessments of fat intake, which improves the measurement of long-term intake. No indication of an increased risk associated with high fat intake was found.

These studies included mostly postmenopausal women. A study conducted among 90,655 premenopausal women

26 to 46 years of age at baseline found a statistically significant positive association between animal fat, mainly from red meat and high fat dairy sources, and risk of premenopausal breast cancer (77). In the same population, intakes of red meat and total fat (which were not possible to distinguish) during adolescence were associated with greater risk of premenopausal breast cancer (78). Overall, the prospective studies provide strong evidence against any major association between intake of total fat during midlife and breast cancer incidence. The suggestion that intake of animal fat or red meat during adolescence or premenopausal years may increase risk in premenopausal women requires confirmation. It is possible that diet later in life may have little influence on postmenopausal breast cancer, whereas diet earlier in life may impact premenopausal breast cancer. The effect of early life diet on postmenopausal breast cancer also needs to be examined.

The effect of reducing fat intake on risk of breast cancer has been assessed in two large randomized trials. In the Women's Health Initiative trial, 48,000 women were randomized to a low-fat diet that tended to be higher in fruits, vegetables, and whole grains than their usual intake (79). After an average of about 7 years, a nonsignificant 9% lower risk of breast cancer was seen in the intervention group (80). However, no differences in plasma concentrations of triglycerides or high-density lipoprotein (HDL) cholesterol between the groups were seen at any time in the trial. This provides clear evidence that there was little difference in fat intake, because a true difference in fat intake does affect these lipid fractions (81). Even the small and nonsignificant reduction in breast cancer incidence could have been due to the modest difference in weights between groups that is compatible with a nonspecific effect of diet counseling. In the second trial, conducted in Canada among women with higher risk of breast cancer determined by mammograms, a nonsignificant 19% higher risk of breast cancer was seen among those randomized to a low-fat diet (82). In this study, the expected changes in plasma HDL cholesterol and triglycerides were seen, confirming that the hypothesis of fat reduction was actually tested.

Although total fat intake has been unrelated to breast cancer risk in prospective epidemiologic studies, and the results of two randomized trials have not supported a benefit of reducing fat intake in midlife or later, some evidence suggests that the type of fat may be important. In animal mammary tumor models, the tumor-promoting effect of fat intake has been observed primarily for polyunsaturated fats when fed in the presence of diets containing approximately 45% of energy from fat (83, 84). However, in prospective studies, polyunsaturated fat generally has not been associated with higher risk of breast cancer within the much lower range seen in human diets (72, 73). The relatively low rates of breast cancer in southern European countries have suggested that the use of olive oil as the primary fat may reduce risk of breast cancer.

In case-control studies in Spain and Greece, women who used more olive oil had lower risks of breast cancer (85, 86). Furthermore, olive oil has been shown to be protective relative to other sources of fats in some animal studies (54). More evidence should emerge from prospective studies being conducted in southern Europe.

Fat and Colon Cancer

In comparisons among countries, rates of colon cancer are strongly correlated with national per capita disappearance of animal fat and meat, with correlation coefficients ranging between 0.8% and 0.9% (12, 62). Based on these epidemiologic investigations and animal studies, a hypothesis has developed that dietary fat increases excretion of bile acids, which can be converted to carcinogens or promoters (87). However, evidence from many studies that higher body weight increases risk and higher levels of physical activity reduce risk of colon cancer indicates that at least part of the high rates in affluent countries previously attributed to fat intake may result from sedentary lifestyle and excess energy intakes.

With some exceptions (88–91), case-control studies generally have shown an association between risk of colon cancer and intake of fat (92–99) or red meat (100–105). However, in many of these studies, a positive association between total energy intake and risk of colon cancer also has been observed (92–96, 98, 99). A metaanalysis by Howe et al (106) of 13 case-control studies found a significant association between total energy and colon cancer, but saturated, monounsaturated, and polyunsaturated fat were not associated with colon cancer independently of total energy.

The relation between diet and colon cancer has been examined in several large prospective studies. These have not confirmed the positive association with total energy intake in case-control studies (107–111), suggesting that the case-control studies were distorted by reporting bias. Most of the studies did not support an association between fat intake and colon cancer risk independent of energy intake. One exception was the Nurses' Health Study, which showed about a twofold higher risk of colon cancer among women in the highest compared with those in the lowest quintile of animal fat intake (107). However, in a multivariate analysis of these data, which included red meat and animal fat intakes in the same model, red meat intake remained significantly predictive of risk of colon cancer, whereas the association with animal fat was eliminated. A metaanalysis of 13 prospective cohort studies found no appreciable association between total, animal, or plant fat intake and risk of colorectal cancer (112). In a randomized trial of a low-fat dietary pattern, no effect on colorectal cancer incidence was observed (113).

Fat and Prostate Cancer

Associations between fat intake and prostate cancer risk have been seen in many case-control studies (114–124) but sometimes only in subgroups. In a large case-control study among various ethnic groups within the United States (125), consistent associations with prostate cancer risk were seen for saturated fat but not with other types of fat. Some of these studies found stronger associations for fat intake and risk of advanced or fatal disease than for total prostate cancer (121, 125, 126).

The association between fat intake and prostate cancer risk has been assessed in several cohort studies. In a cohort of 8000 Japanese men living in Hawaii, no association was seen between intake of total or unsaturated fat (127). However, diet was assessed with a single 24-hour recall in this study so the lack of association may not be informative. In a study of 14,000 Seventh-Day Adventist men living in California, a positive association between the percentage of calories from animal fat and prostate cancer risk was seen, but this was not statistically significant (128). In the Health Professionals Follow-up Study of 51,000 men, a positive association was seen with intake of red meat, total fat, and animal fat, which was largely limited to aggressive prostate cancers (129). No association was seen with vegetable fats. In another cohort from Hawaii, increased risks of prostate cancer were seen with consumption of beef and animal fat (130). Two small studies of men with prostate cancer suggest that high intake of saturated fat at the time of diagnosis is associated with an increased risk of biochemical failure (131) and prostate cancer–specific death (132). The stronger findings for advanced disease and progression, if confirmed, suggest that dietary fat may influence late stages of carcinogenesis. However, the European Prospective Investigation into Cancer and Nutrition (EPIC) study, a large European cohort study, did not find any association between total, saturated, or monounsaturated fat intake and advanced-stage prostate cancer (133).

A somewhat puzzling observation has been that intake or blood levels of α-linolenic, a fatty acid comprising only about 1% of total energy intake, has been associated with an increased risk of prostate cancer (especially advanced cancers) in two prospective studies (129, 134) and five case-control studies in diverse populations: Uruguay (135), Spain (136), Norway (137), China (138), and the United States (139). However, other studies have not supported this (140–144). Whether or not this association is causal needs to be determined, especially because this fatty acid is beneficial in regard to cardiovascular disease (145, 146). Although further data are desirable, the evidence from international correlations, case-control, and cohort studies is reasonably consistent in support of an association between consumption of fat-containing animal products and prostate cancer incidence, particularly with advanced prostate cancer.

Other Cancers

Rates of other cancers that are common in affluent countries, including those of the endometrium and ovary, are, of course, also correlated with fat intake internationally. Although these have been studied in a small number of

case-control investigations, consistent associations with fat intake have not been seen (147–156). In a prospective study among Iowa women (157), no evidence of relation between fat intake and risk of endometrial cancer was observed. Positive associations have been hypothesized between fat intake and risks of skin (158) and lung cancer, but relevant data in humans are nonsupportive (159, 160). A low-fat dietary pattern intervention suggested that a dietary pattern low in fat may reduce risk of ovarian cancer (161), but this may have been because of chance, as many different cancer sites were examined and the overall association was not statistically significant.

Summary of Fat and Cancer

As the findings from large prospective studies have become available, support for a major relationship between fat intake and breast cancer risk has weakened considerably. For colon cancer, the associations seen with animal fat internationally have been supported in numerous case-control and cohort studies. However, more recent evidence has suggested that this may be explained by factors in red meat other than simply its fat content. Further, the importance of energy balance on colon cancer risk indicates that international correlations probably overstate the contribution of dietary composition to differences in colon cancer incidence. The available evidence most strongly supports an association between animal fat consumption and risk of aggressive or advanced prostate cancer. As with colon cancer, however, the possibility remains that other factors in foods containing animal fat contribute to risk.

Carbohydrates

Coincident with the strong emphasis on lowering dietary fat over the past several decades, grain consumption in the United States increased 50% (162) (http://www.ers.usda.gov/publications/eib33/eib33.pdf). Certain forms of carbohydrate are hypothesized to increase cancer risk, by causing spikes in postprandial blood glucose concentrations and circulating insulin (45). These carbohydrates with a "high glycemic index" (163) are associated with higher postprandial insulin (164) and higher fasting insulin in insulin-resistant states (165). Fasting plasma insulin concentrations, in turn, are inversely correlated with IGF-binding protein-1 (IGFBP-1) and thus increase bioactive IGF-1 concentrations (45). Although associations between high sucrose diets and sucrose-to-fiber ratio have been associated with higher risk of colon cancer in some studies (166), other studies have not observed a significant association between colon cancer and high glycemic load diets (167). In a metaanalysis, a significant increased risk of colorectal cancer was associated with higher glycemic load and index, but there was substantial between study heterogeneity (168). Glycemic index and load were not related to postmenopausal breast cancer in a large prospective cohort (169) but were in some case-control studies (170). However, pancreatic cancer risk was increased by 50% with a high glycemic load diet in a study of women and by 170% among sedentary, overweight women (171). A metaanalysis showed that high glycemic load and index diets were associated with an increased risk of endometrial cancer, a cancer strongly associated with obesity and insulin resistance (168). Although much work is still needed, enough data exist to suggest that abnormal glucose and insulin metabolism, especially in obese, sedentary individuals, is important to consider in carcinogenesis.

Protein

Epidemiologic studies have not found a clear association between high protein intake, at least in adulthood, and risk of cancer. In the vast majority of studies, no evidence exists of deleterious effects of some of the major sources of protein, including fish, poultry, and plant sources. Red meat and dairy products, the other major protein sources, are discussed in the following.

Food Groups

Meat

Red meat intake has been linked with risk of several cancers, most notably of the colon, rectum, and prostate. Meat consumption and colon cancer risk has been the focus of published metaanalyses (172, 173). In a metaanalysis of 13 prospective studies, a 12% to 17% increase in risk with each 100-g increment of red meat intake daily (slightly >3 oz) and a 49% increased risk for each 25-g increment of processed meats daily (about one slice) was observed (172). These findings were largely confirmed in two other metaanalyses (173, 174), but another metaanalysis concluded that the results were not definitive (175). A positive association between red meat intake and colon cancer risk has been observed in many, although, not all, case-control studies, even though meat-related variables, method of assessment, and country of study were quite diverse (176). In the EPIC study population, the absolute risk of developing colorectal cancer within 10 years for a 50-year-old participant was 1.71% for the highest category of red and processed meat intake compared with 1.28% for the lowest category of intake (177). The apparently stronger and more consistent association with red meat compared with fat needs further confirmation, but could result if nonfat components of meat, such as heme iron or carcinogens created by cooking were the primary etiologic factors. This issue has major practical implications because current dietary recommendations (178) support the daily consumption of red meat as long as it is lean.

A review of red meat and prostate cancer determined that 15 of 21 studies found a greater than 30% increased risk associated with higher red meat intake; six of these were statistically significant (179). Six of eight prospective studies found at least a 40% increased risk; three of these were statistically significant. Whether the association is due

to the fat content on meat remains unclear. The evidence for other cancers is less consistent. In a large pooled analysis of eight cohort studies, no association was observed between red meat or total meat intake, and breast cancer risk (180). Other cancers, including those of the bladder, pancreas, and kidney, also may be associated with meat constituents, but not all studies are consistent (181).

Dairy Products

In the United States, dairy products are the major source of dietary calcium and vitamin D and an important source of protein, saturated fat, and minerals. Besides these components, which have been hypothesized to influence cancer risk, dairy products also contain other hypothetically protective (182) and adverse (183) components. Epidemiologic studies of dairy products and colorectal cancer strongly support an inverse association (184). A pooled analysis of 10 cohort studies reported that high milk consumption was associated with a lower risk of colorectal cancer (185). In a more recent metaanalysis of 19 cohort studies, higher intakes of milk and total dairy products (but not cheese) were associated with reduced risk of colon but not rectal cancer (186). For colorectal cancer, the benefit seems largely from calcium and possibly vitamin D. Studies of breast cancer risk (180) have been inconsistent and mostly null, but some studies suggest a possible lower risk of these cancers with higher intakes of low-fat dairy products (187, 188). In a metaanalysis, a decreased risk of breast cancer was observed with higher milk intake, although heterogeneity of results among studies was noted (189). However, one study showed high-fat dairy products associated with an increased risk of premenopausal breast cancer (77).

In contrast with potential benefits for colorectal cancer and possibly breast cancer, high intake of dairy products has been associated with an increased risk of prostate cancer in numerous case-control (190–194) and cohort studies (130, 190, 192, 195–197). Positive associations for prostate cancer have been observed for total dairy intake, as well as specifically for higher intake of milk (192, 197), cheese (198), and yogurt (197). A metaanalysis of 11 cohort studies reported suggestive increases in risk associated with intake of total dairy, milk, and cheese (199). Most (196–198, 200, 201), but not all (202, 203), studies published since this metaanalysis have tended to support an association between higher milk or dairy consumption and prostate cancer risk. Equivocal data also suggest a possible association between higher intake of milk and ovarian cancer (204).

Fruits and Vegetables

Fruits and vegetables have received much interest because they contain numerous substances with potential anticarcinogenic activity. Results from more than 250 epidemiologic studies of fruits and vegetables and cancer have been summarized in several large reviews (181, 205, 206). These reviews concluded that diets high in fruits and vegetables were consistently associated with lower risk of some, but not all, cancers. However, more recent null or weak findings on fruits and vegetables and cancer from large maturing prospective cohort studies have raised doubt about the strength of the association between fruits and vegetable in cancer prevention. For example, prospective studies of stomach cancer and colon or colorectal cancer observe weaker associations for fruits and vegetables than case-control studies (207, 208). An intervention study of fruits and vegetables on recurrence of colorectal adenomas did not find a reduction in risk (209). A large pooled analysis of eight prospective cohort studies found negligible associations between fruits and vegetables and breast cancer (210). Indeed, plant foods probably play a smaller direct role in cancer prevention than previously thought.

Several factors may account for the apparent divergent results from the earlier case-control studies and the more recent prospective studies. First, in some of the case-control studies, recall or selection biases may have occurred. Second, some risk factors for specific cancers have emerged only relatively recently (e.g., tobacco, obesity, physical inactivity for colon cancer), and these were not controlled for in many of the previous analyses. Third, the strength of the results may have been exaggerated in some of the previous reports because several subgroupings of fruits and vegetables (e.g., citrus fruits) may have been considered, but only positive findings were emphasized in the reports. Finally, the source of the potentially protective agents may have changed; for example, in many previous studies the main source of folate was fruits and vegetables, and in the United States multivitamins and fortified foods are associated with higher intakes. A final point is that some types of fruits and vegetables may have potential deleterious effects. For example, potatoes and some fruit juices have a high glycemic index and increase insulin secretion. In the United States 29% of fruit is consumed as fruit juice, and potatoes and potato products make up 27% of total vegetable consumption, whereas broccoli (0.8%) and dark green vegetables (1%) make up a small amount of total vegetables consumed (211).

Although a strong blanket protective role for total fruits and vegetables on total cancer now appears unlikely, fruits and vegetables contain varying levels of potentially protective compounds for specific cancer sites. Combining fruits and vegetables in analyses may obscure potentially strong protective effects of certain phytochemical or botanical subgroups on some cancer sites. From an epidemiologic perspective, some of the promising leads include tomato or lycopene-containing foods and prostate cancer (212); cruciferous vegetables and several cancer sites including prostate, bladder, and lung cancer (208, 213); allium vegetables and stomach cancer (214); folate-rich fruits and vegetables and colon cancer (215); and citrus fruits and lung cancer (216, 217).

Fruits and vegetables contain a myriad of biologically active chemicals, including both recognized nutrients and many more nonnutritive constituents, that potentially could play a role in protection against cancer (14). The identification of the specific protective constituents, or combinations of constituents, is a daunting task and may never be completely possible. Further details on the types and amounts of fruits and vegetables that appear to be particularly protective could provide additional practical guidance for those wanting to select an optimally healthy diet.

Dietary Fiber and Cancer Risk

Interest in dietary fiber is largely the result of Denis Burkitt's observation of low rates of colon cancer in areas of Africa where fiber consumption and stool bulk were high (218). Although fiber was originally seen simply as providing bulk to dilute potential carcinogens and speed their transit through the colon, other hypotheses have suggested that fiber may act by binding carcinogenic substances (219), altering the colonic flora (220–223), reducing the pH (224), or serving as the substrate for the generation of short-chain fatty acids that are the preferred substrate for colonic epithelial cells (225).

A 1992 metaanalysis of case-control studies appeared to support this hypothesis (226), but a later reanalysis of these data, considering study heterogeneity and limited to studies with validated diet assessment instruments, was less supportive (227). Prospective cohort studies of dietary fiber and colon cancer risk, mostly conducted in the 1990s, generally have not supported an association (107, 108, 110, 228, 229). However, more recently published results from a large European study involving 10 countries found a 25% lower risk of colon cancer associated with higher fiber intakes compared with low intakes (230). However, other potentially responsible factors were not included in the analysis (e.g., physical activity, smoking, or other nutrients in high-fiber diets); thus, it is difficult to pinpoint fiber as the responsible factor. In a pooled analysis of 13 prospective studies, dietary fiber was inversely associated with colorectal cancer in age-adjusted analyses but not in the full multivariate model (231). Intervention trials of wheat bran fiber (232), ispaghula husk (psyllium fiber) (233), and a high-fiber/low-fat diet (209) failed to reduce the risk of recurrent adenomatous polyps. Because dietary fiber is complex and heterogeneous, and properties may differ by dietary source, we cannot rule out the possibility that some component at high intakes may not have benefits on colorectal cancer.

Higher intake of fiber also has been hypothesized to reduce risk of breast cancer by interrupting the enterohepatic circulation of estrogens (234). However, in prospective studies, little or no relationship has been observed between fiber intake and risk of breast cancer (64, 235–237).

Alcoholic Beverages

High consumption of alcohol, particularly in combination with cigarette smoking, is a well-established cause of cancer of the oral cavity, larynx, esophagus, and liver

(238). Substantial evidence from case-control and cohort studies indicates that amounts as low as one or two drinks per day increase the risk of breast cancer (239–241). Most evidence indicates that high intake of alcohol increases risk of colorectal cancer (242). A pooled analysis of eight prospective cohort studies confirmed an increased risk at levels of approximately two drinks a day or greater (243). In the upper gastrointestinal tract the carcinogenic effects of alcohol could result from direct contact, and in the liver this could result from toxicity. However, in the large bowel and breast tissue, the mechanisms remain unclear. Nonetheless, an intriguing potential mechanism may involve the well-established antifolate effects of alcohol (244). Evidence from animal and human studies shows that "methyl-poor" diets (high-alcohol, low-methionine, low-folate) are associated with threefold to fourfold increases in risk of both colorectal adenomas and cancer compared with "methyl-rich" diets (low-alcohol, high-methionine, high-folate) (245). These results are quite consistent in men and less so for women, possibly because of their lower alcohol intake (246–248). As with colorectal cancer, folate appears to ameliorate the increased risk of breast cancer associated with alcohol intake (249) in some (246, 247, 250–252), but not all (248), studies. Although the cancer-enhancing effects of alcohol have been established, evidence also indicates that alcohol is associated with a decreased risk of kidney cancer (253–256) and non-Hodgkin lymphoma (257).

Vitamin and Mineral Supplements

Calcium

Calcium has been proposed to reduce risk of colorectal cancer by binding to toxic secondary bile acids and ionized fatty acids to form insoluble soaps in the lumen of the colon (258, 259) or by directly reducing proliferation, stimulating differentiation, and inducing apoptosis in the colonic mucosa (260–262). Large prospective studies have consistently shown a modest and significant inverse association between calcium intake and colorectal cancer risk (263). In an analysis that pooled the results of 10 large, prospective cohort studies, those in the highest quintile of calcium intake had a 22% reduction in risk of colorectal cancer compared with those in the lowest quintile (185). In some data, the risk reduction is achievable by attaining intakes of 700 to 800 mg/day, which suggests a threshold level above which further calcium is not beneficial (188). The findings from observational studies have been confirmed for adenoma (especially advanced adenoma) in randomized, placebo-controlled trials conducted among patients with a history of adenoma (233, 264).

In contrast with colon cancer, higher calcium intake has been associated with an increased risk of total or advanced prostate cancer risk in several case-control (191, 193) and cohort (190, 192, 194, 196, 200, 265) studies. In addition, very high intake of calcium through diet or supplementation was associated with significant excess risks (192, 194,

265). Several studies have suggested that the association is stronger for aggressive forms of prostate cancer, defined by high grade (266) or advanced or lethal prostate cancer (192, 265), although not all studies have confirmed a positive association for calcium (126, 267–269). In studies that simultaneously consider dairy intake and calcium, RR estimates for dairy were attenuated, compared with calcium (192, 196, 198). In an analysis of the EPIC cohort, dairy protein and dairy calcium were both similarly associated with risk of prostate cancer (200).

Few studies on calcium and breast cancer have been reported. One hospital-based case control study reported a statistically significant lower risk (20%) of breast cancer with high versus low calcium intakes (270), whereas results in three others were not significant (270–273). A large prospective study reported a significant inverse association between calcium and breast cancer (187).

Vitamin D

Vitamin D has been of interest based on ecologic studies that populations with greater exposure to ultraviolet light had lower risks of breast (274), colon (275), and prostate cancer (276). The relation between vitamin D status and cancer risk has been investigated using a number of approaches to estimate vitamin D status, including direct measures of circulating 25(OH) vitamin D concentrations, surrogates, or determinants of 25(OH) vitamin D, including region of residence, intake, and sun exposure estimates. Several lines of evidence strongly support a role for vitamin D in lowering risk for colorectal cancer incidence. Studies that have examined circulating 25(OH) D prospectively, in relation to risk of colorectal cancer or adenoma, have generally supported an inverse association (277–288). Although intake is generally not the greatest contributor to vitamin D status, the majority of reported studies found inverse associations between vitamin D intake and either colon or rectal cancer (269, 289–297). This finding was especially evident in studies that took into account supplementary vitamin D and in populations in which milk is fortified with vitamin D.

In contrast with colorectal cancer, for which the evidence has been relatively compelling, the data for other cancers has been less consistent (298–306). Although the data on breast cancer have been not consistent, a meta-analysis of studies on intake of vitamin D suggested a possible modest benefit only in studies in which the intakes exceeded 400 IU/day (307). The evidence also suggests a potential moderate benefit for ovarian cancer risk, especially in overweight women (302, 308–310). To date, most of the epidemiologic studies have examined vitamin D status in relation to incidence of cancer, but emerging evidence suggests that vitamin D may be important for cancer progression and mortality owing to various malignancies (311–316). Further study is needed to establish the role of vitamin D in terms of when in the life span and on what stages of carcinogenesis vitamin D is relevant and the optimal levels required.

Folate

Folate is important for DNA methylation, repair, and synthesis (317–320). Epidemiologic studies have linked low folic acid intake with higher risk of several cancers, most notably colorectal (245), breast (247), and possibly cervical cancer (247). Long-term use of folic acid–containing multivitamin supplements is associated with a 20% to 70% reduction in risk of colon cancer (321–323). One study confirmed a lag of at least 12 to 14 years between low folate intake and increased risk of colorectal cancer (324). Isolated studies in other cancers, including esophageal cancer (325), and leukemia (326), also suggest that inadequate folate intake or metabolism may contribute to carcinogenesis in other sites. Supporting a role of folate is that genotypes for methylenetetrahydrofolate reductase (MTHFR), an enzyme known to be involved in folate metabolism, predicts risk of colon cancer dependent on folate intake or status (245, 327). In contrast with the observational studies, randomized trials for recurrent adenomas in individuals with adenomas tended not to support a benefit of folic acid given at 0.5 mg or 1 mg daily (328, 329). In fact, one trial suggested a possible increased risk of recurrent advanced adenoma or multiple adenomas related to excessive folate (330). These studies indicate that an additional supplement of folic acid is unlikely to be beneficial, and may even be harmful, for those who already have had a colonic neoplasm and have adequate folate intake.

Vitamins C and E

Oxidant byproducts of normal metabolism and smoking cause extensive damage to DNA, protein, and lipids. DNA repair enzymes efficiently repair damage but antioxidant defenses are imperfect (15). Antioxidants may reduce the risk of cancer by neutralizing reactive oxygen species or free radicals that can damage DNA. Vitamin C is the major water-soluble antioxidant, and vitamin E is the major lipid-soluble, membrane-localized antioxidant in humans. However, epidemiologic studies have not consistently supported a role for vitamins C and E in cancer risk (208). Vitamin C can interfere with formation of nitrosamines in the stomach—carcinogens formed endogenously from precursors present in the diet and tobacco smoke. However, chemoprevention trials of stomach cancer in high-risk populations have not conclusively supported a benefit from vitamin C supplements (331), but several antioxidant nutrients were associated with regression of gastric dysplasia (332). In the Alpha-Tocopherol, Beta-Carotene (ATBC) Trial, no association between supplemental α-tocopherol and lung cancer was found, but a 34% lower incidence of prostate cancer among the population of heavy smokers was noted (333). Subsequent prospective analyses of vitamin E supplements (usually as α-tocopherol) in prostate cancer support a possible role limited to smokers (334) but not in nonsmokers (335).

Selenium

Selenium functions through selenoproteins, including selenium-dependent glutathione peroxidases that defend against oxidative stress. The selenium content of food varies depending on the selenium content of soil where plants are grown or animals are raised. Because content can vary more than 10-fold, food composition databases for selenium are unreliable (336). Most epidemiologic evidence on the anticarcinogenic role of selenium stems from biomarker and intervention studies. Selenium has been strongly associated with reduced prostate cancer risk (a secondary end point) in one trial of selenium supplementation and skin cancer (337). Several prospective studies have supported inverse associations between selenium levels in toenails (338–340), a marker of selenium intake over the past year, or in the plasma or serum (341–343). One study (343) suggested that selenium may be important in inhibiting progression of prostate cancers. In contrast with these findings, a prospective study in Finland, a country with low selenium intake during the period of follow-up, showed no relation between serum selenium levels and prostate cancer risk (344). Moreover, beginning in 1984, fertilizers were fortified with selenium in Finland. Despite marked elevations in blood selenium since then, prostate cancer incidence rates continued to rise in Finland, possibly because of enhanced detection, while mortality rates remained relatively stable. The Selenium and Vitamin E Cancer Prevention Trial (SELECT) (345), a large randomized intervention trial with selenium (200 mg) and vitamin E (400 IU), could have addressed the role of selenium definitively, but the trial was ended 4 years early with the investigators reporting no protective effect of selenium on total prostate cancer incidence (346). It will be important to follow up on the men in the SELECT trial for prostate cancer progression, although it is unclear if 4 years of exposure will be adequate.

SUMMARY

Evidence from both animal and epidemiologic studies indicates that, throughout life, excessive energy intake in relation to requirements increases risk of human cancer. Rapid growth rate in childhood leading to greater adult height increases risk of breast, colon, prostate, and other cancers; and accumulation of body fat in adulthood is related to cancers of the colon, kidney, pancreas, and endometrium as well as postmenopausal breast cancer. The overall evidence suggests that the percentage of energy from fat in the diet during midlife and later life is not a major cause of cancers of the breast or colon. Higher intake of meat and dairy products has been associated with greater risk of prostate cancer, which may be related to some component of fat content. Also, red meat consumption has been associated with risk of colon cancer in numerous studies, but this appears to be unrelated to its fat content. Based on prospective studies, a diet high in fruits and vegetables and fiber does not appear to be as protective against cancer as initially believed. Nonetheless, some micronutrients and phytochemicals

262. Lipkin M, Newmark H. N Engl J Med 1985;313:1381–4.

263. Martinez ME, Willett WC. Cancer Epidemiol Biomarkers Prev 1998;7:163–8.

264. Baron JA, Beach M, Mandel JS et al. N Engl J Med 1999;340:101–7.

265. Giovannucci E, Liu Y, Stampfer MJ et al. Cancer Epidemiol Biomarkers Prev 2006;15:203–10.

266. Giovannucci E, Liu Y, Platz EA et al. Int J Cancer 2007; 121:1571–8.

267. Berndt SI, Carter HB, Landis PK et al. Urology 2002;60: 1118–23.

268. Schuurman AG, van den Brandt PA, Dorant E et al. Br J Cancer 1999;80:1107–13.

269. Park SY, Murphy SP, Wilkens LR et al. Am J Epidemiol 2007;166:1259–69.

270. Negri E, La Vecchia C, Franceschi S et al. Int J Cancer 1996;65:140–4.

271. Katsouyanni K, Willett W, Trichopoulos D et al. Cancer 1988;61:181–5.

272. Potischman N, Swanson CA, Coates RJ et al. Int J Cancer 1999;82:315–21.

273. Levi F, Pasche C, Lucchini F et al. Int J Cancer 2001;91: 260–3.

274. Garland FC, Garland CF, Gorham ED et al. Prev Med 1990;19:614–22.

275. Garland CF, Garland FC. Int J Epidemiol 1980;9:227–31.

276. Hanchette CL, Schwartz GG. Cancer 1992;70:2861–9.

277. Garland CF, Comstock GW, Garland FC et al. Lancet 1989;2:1176–8.

278. Tangrea J, Helzlsouer K, Pietinen P et al. Cancer Causes Control 1997;8:615–25.

279. Feskanich D, Ma J, Fuchs CS et al. Cancer Epidemiol Biomarkers Prev 2004;13:1502–8.

280. Levine AJ, Harper JM, Ervin CM et al. Nutr Cancer 2001;39:35–41.

281. Peters U, McGlynn KA, Chatterjee N et al. Cancer Epidemiol Biomarkers Prev 2001;10:1267–74.

282. Platz EA, Hankinson SE, Hollis BW et al. Cancer Epidemiol Biomarkers Prev 2000;9:1059–65.

283. Grau MV, Baron JA, Sandler RS et al. J Natl Cancer Inst 2003;95:1765–71.

284. Braun MM, Helzlsouer KJ, Hollis BW et al. Cancer Causes Control 1995;6:235–9.

285. Wactawski-Wende J, Kotchen JM, Anderson GL et al. N Engl J Med 2006;354:684–96.

286. Otani T, Iwasaki M, Sasazuki S et al. Br J Cancer 2007;97:446–51.

287. Jenab M, Bueno-de-Mesquita HB, Ferrari P et al. BMJ 2010;340:b5500.

288. Woolcott CG, Wilkens LR, Nomura AM et al. Cancer Epidemiol Biomarkers Prev 2010;19:130–4.

289. Garland C, Shekelle RB, Barrett-Conner E et al. Lancet 1985;1:307–9.

290. Kearney J, Giovannucci E, Rimm EB et al. Am J Epidemiol 1996;143:907–17.

291. Bostick RM, Potter JD, Sellers TA et al. Am J Epidemiol 1993;137:1302–17.

292. Martínez ME, Giovannucci EL, Colditz GA et al. J Natl Cancer Inst 1996;88:1375–82.

293. McCullough ML, Robertson AS, Rodriguez C et al. Cancer Causes Control 2003;14:1–12.

294. Benito E, Stiggelbout A, Bosch FX et al. Int J Cancer 1991;49:161–7.

295. Ferraroni M, La Vecchia C, D'Avanzo B et al. Br J Cancer 1994;70:1150–5.

296. Pritchard RS, Gerhardsson de Verdier M. Cancer Epidemiol Biomarkers Prev 1996;5:897–900.

297. Marcus PM, Newcomb PA. Int J Epidemiol 1998;27: 788–93.

298. Gandini S, Boniol M, Haukka J et al. Int J Cancer 2011;128:1414–24.

299. Helzlsouer KJ. Am J Epidemiol 2010;172:4–9.

300. Abnet CC, Chen Y, Chow WH et al. Am J Epidemiol 2010; 172:94–106.

301. Zeleniuch-Jacquotte A, Gallicchio L, Hartmuller V et al. Am J Epidemiol 2010;172:36–46.

302. Gallicchio L, Helzlsouer KJ, Chow WH et al. Am J Epidemiol 2010;172:10–20.

303. Gallicchio L, Moore LE, Stevens VL et al. Am J Epidemiol 2010;172:47–57.

304. Zheng W, Danforth KN, Tworoger SS et al. Am J Epidemiol 2010;172:70–80.

305. Stolzenberg-Solomon RZ, Jacobs EJ, Arslan AA et al. Am J Epidemiol 2010;172:81–93.

306. Purdue MP, Freedman DM, Gapstur SM et al. Am J Epidemiol 2010;172:58–69.

307. Gissel T, Rejnmark L, Mosekilde L et al. J Steroid Biochem Mol Biol 2008;111:195–9.

308. Tworoger SS, Lee IM, Buring JE et al. Cancer Epidemiol Biomarkers Prev 2007;16:783–8.

309. Toriola AT, Surcel HM, Agborsangaya C et al. Eur J Cancer 2010;46:364–9.

310. Toriola AT, Surcel HM, Calypse A et al. Eur J Cancer 2010;46:2799–805.

311. Ng K, Meyerhardt JA, Wu K et al. J Clin Oncol 2008;26: 2984–1991.

312. Zhou W, Heist RS, Liu G et al. J Clin Oncol 2007;25:479–85.

313. Goodwin PJ, Ennis M, Pritchard KI et al. J Clin Oncol 2009;27:3757–63.

314. Newton-Bishop JA, Beswick S, Randerson-Moor J et al. J Clin Oncol 2009;27:5439–44.

315. Ng K, Wolpin BM, Meyerhardt JA et al. Br J Cancer 2009; 101:916–23.

316. Tretli S, Hernes E, Berg JP et al. Br J Cancer 2009;100: 450–4.

317. Duthie SJ, Narayanan S, Blum S et al. Nutr Cancer 2000; 37:245–51.

318. Duthie SJ. Br Med Bull 1999;55:578–92.

319. Wickramasinghe SN, Fida S. Blood 1994;83:1656–61.

320. Blount BC, Mack MM, Wehr CM et al. Proc Natl Acad Sci U S A 1997;94:3290–5.

321. Jacobs EJ, Connell CJ, Patel AV et al. Cancer Causes Control 2001;12:927–34.

322. Giovannucci E, Rimm EB, Ascherio A et al. J Natl Cancer Inst 1995;87:265–73.

323. Giovannucci E, Stampfer MJ, Colditz GA et al. Ann Intern Med 1998;129:517–24.

324. Lee JE, Willett WC, Fuchs CS et al. Am J Clin Nutr 2011; 93:817–25.

325. Prasad MP, Krishna TP, Pasricha S et al. Nutr Cancer 1992; 18:85–93.

326. Thompson JR, Gerald PF, Willoughby ML et al. Lancet 2001;358:1935–40.

327. Chen J, Giovannucci E, Kelsey K et al. Cancer Res 1996; 56:4862–4.

328. Logan RF, Grainge MJ, Shepherd VC et al. Gastroenterology 2008;134:29–38.

329. Wu K, Platz EA, Willett WC et al. Am J Clin Nutr 2009; 90:1623–31.

330. Cole BF, Baron JA, Sandler RS et al. JAMA 2007;297:2351–9.

331. Blot WJ, Li JY, Taylor PR et al. J Natl Cancer Inst 1993; 85:1483–92.

332. Correa P, Fontham ET, Bravo JC et al. J Natl Cancer Inst 2000;92:1881–8.

333. Anonymous. N Engl J Med 1994;330:1029–35.

334. Gann PH, Ma J, Giovannucci E et al. Cancer Res 1999; 59:1225–30.

335. Chan JM, Stampfer MJ, Ma J et al. Cancer Epidemiol Biomarkers Prev 1999;8:893–9.

336. Food and Nutrition Board, Institute of Medicine. Dietary Reference Intakes for Vitamin C, Vitamin E, Selenium, and Carotenoids. Washington, DC: National Academy Press, 2000:529.

337. Clark LC, Combs GF Jr, Turnbull BW et al. JAMA 1996; 276:1957–63.

338. Yoshizawa K, Willett WC, Morris SJ et al. J Natl Cancer Inst 1998;90:1219–24.

339. Vogt TM, Ziegler RG, Graubard BI et al. Int J Cancer 2003; 103:664–70.

340. Helzlsouer KJ, Huang HY, Alberg AJ et al. J Natl Cancer Instit 2000;92:1966–7.

341. Nomura AMY, Lee J, Stemmermann GN et al. Cancer Epidemiol Biomarkers Prev 2000;9:883–7.

342. Brooks JD, Metter EJ, Chan DW et al. J Urol 2001;166:2034–8.

343. Li H, Stampfer MJ, Giovannucci EL et al. J Natl Cancer Inst 2004;96:696–703.

344. Knekt P, Aromaa A, Maatela J et al. J Natl Cancer Inst 1990; 82:864–8.

345. Klein EA, Thompson IM, Lippman SM et al. J Urol 2001; 166:1311–5.

346. Lippman SM, Klein EA, Goodman PJ et al. JAMA 2009; 301:39–51.

SUGGESTED READINGS

Kushi LH, Byers T, Doyle C et al. American Cancer Society guidelines on nutrition and physical activity for cancer prevention: reducing the risk of cancer with healthy food choices and physical activity. CA Cancer J Clin 2006;56:254–81.

Na HK, Oliynyk S. Effects of physical activity on cancer prevention. Ann N Y Acad Sci 2011;1229:176–83.

Ströhle A, Zänker K, Hahn A. Nutrition in oncology: the case of micronutrients. Oncol Rep 2010;24:815–28.

World Cancer Research Fund/American Institute for Cancer Research. Food, Nutrition, Physical Activity, and the Prevention of Cancer: A Global Perspective. Washington, DC: World Cancer Research Fund/American Institute for Cancer Research, 2007.

87 CANCER CACHEXIA[1]

VICKIE E. BARACOS

The presence of a malignant disease is often heralded by a lowered intake of nutrients; however, important distinctions can be made between simple malnutrition and the tumor-bearing state. The pathophysiology of cancer cachexia is characterized by negative protein and energy balance, driven by a variable combination of reduced food intake and concurrent metabolic abnormalities. In addition to the presence of primary anorexia, a legion of nutrition impact symptoms poses barriers to food intake. Superimposed hypermetabolism and hypercatabolism accelerate depletion of physiologic reserves of energy and protein. There is merit in recognizing the onset of cachexia so that nutritional and metabolic interventions to reduce or delay its impact may be implemented. At later stages, cachexia may be clinically refractory because of the presence of rapidly progressive cancer unresponsive to antineoplastic therapy, and the focus of nutrition support shifts away from physiologic and functional outcomes to improvement of food enjoyment and quality of life.

---

[1]**Abbreviations: BMI**, body mass index; **COPD**, chronic obstructive pulmonary disease; **EPCRC**, European Palliative Care Research Collaborative.

CACHEXIA IS DISEASE-ASSOCIATED MALNUTRITION

Multiple definitions and terms for malnutrition and wasting syndromes appear in the literature. International consensus groups have labored to provide clear-cut definitions (1–3). A first important distinction is that cancer is not merely malnutrition or starvation (i.e., defined as a lack of nutrient supply) as the sole cause of depletion of the body reserves. The unqualified term *malnutrition* is relevant in the instance of deficient food supply, as in medical conditions such as anorexia nervosa. Patients with cancer are affected by a more complex pathophysiology driven by a variable combination of reduced food intake and abnormal metabolism, and this superimposed burden of metabolic alteration is regarded as the essential distinction between cachexia and simple malnutrition (Fig. 87.1) (1, 3). Two terms currently found in the literature, disease-associated malnutrition (2) and cachexia (used hereafter in this chapter), can be considered equivalent. *Disease-associated malnutrition* was defined by an international guideline committee constituted to develop a consensus approach to defining the etiology of malnutrition syndromes for adults in the clinical setting (2). These authors defined cancer-associated malnutrition as "a chronic disease or condition that imposes sustained inflammation of a mild to moderate degree." In the view of many researchers and clinical experts, a primary requirement for the development of cachexia is the presence of an inflammatory process (1, 3–6). The presence of a chronic inflammatory state seems to account for seemingly disparate aberrations, including changes in the hypothalamic–pituitary axis, dysautonomia, hypermetabolism, oxidative stress, decreased muscle protein synthesis, and increased ubiquitin-proteosome–mediated muscle protein degradation, together with other metabolic changes such as insulin resistance (7–13). Through its effect on multiple organs and tissues, chronic inflammation leads to the pathophysiologic profile accounting for cachexia.

An international consensus group assembled under the auspices of the European Palliative Care Research Collaborative (EPCRC) developed a conceptual framework for the definition of cancer cachexia (1). This group also underscored the importance of underlying metabolic changes that drive weight loss in the tumor-bearing host.

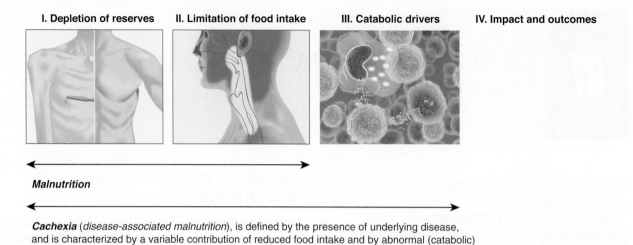

I. Depletion of reserves   **II. Limitation of food intake**   **III. Catabolic drivers**   **IV. Impact and outcomes**

Malnutrition

Cachexia (*disease-associated malnutrition*), is defined by the presence of underlying disease, and is characterized by a variable contribution of reduced food intake and by abnormal (catabolic) metabolism

Fig. 87.1. Conceptual domains of cancer cachexia. Malnutrition is characterized by progressive depletion of body reserves (body weight, adipose tissue, skeletal muscle) when the supply of nutrients is limited. In cachexia, weight loss and depletion of body reserves is greater than would be expected based on the prevailing level of dietary intake, owing to the presence of metabolic abnormalities, which enhance catabolism.

However, although the EPCRC group acknowledged the importance of inflammation, the group also noted that cachexia may exist without overt systemic inflammation. The elevated energy expenditure and capture of substrates by the tumor was identified as a key catabolic driver. Lieffers et al (14) followed the growth of metastatic tumor burden over time in patients with advanced colorectal cancer in a study using serial computed tomography scans. The mean burden of metastatic disease (0.7 kg) and the high specific metabolic rate of tumor marked a quantitatively important contribution of tumor to whole body basal metabolic rate. Endocrine abnormalities such as insulin resistance, high-dose prolonged corticosteroid therapy (which induces Cushing-like muscle atrophy), and hypogonadism are additional endogenous and exogenous changes potentially contributing to catabolism. Finally, Fearon et al (1) underscored the ability of low levels of physical activity to potentiate catabolic stimuli as an exacerbating factor.

Simple malnutrition is reversed by the provision of food, except when malnutrition is severe enough to induce permanent changes (e.g., growth stunting in children). By contrast, cachexia cannot be fully reversed by conventional nutritional support, and this is regarded as one of the defining characteristics of cachexia syndromes (2). Nutrition supplementation alone only partly reverses or prevents negative energy balance and muscle protein loss in active inflammatory states (15). The efficacy of nutritional intervention may be undermined by the presence of catabolic metabolic abnormalities; however, it is a misconception that nutritional support for the patient with cancer cachexia is futile. Inadequate food intake, in any case, aggravates loss of weight and lean tissue, and adequate feeding may help to limit these losses. Food intake is a primary site of intervention, whether by dietetic

counseling, pharmacologic agents intended to stimulate appetite, or artificial nutritional support.

CONTROLS OF ENERGY BALANCE AND METABOLISM IN CANCER CACHEXIA VERSUS HEALTHY INDIVIDUALS

Controls of energy balance and metabolism associated with cancer have many deviations. The involuntary weight loss associated with cancer represents an important failure of the normal control of energy balance. Weight loss is often a presenting symptom and has been long known to predict shortened survival (16). By contrast, energy homeostasis has a high priority in healthy adults, in whom precise metabolic controls help to store food energy optimally or, conversely, to mobilize reserves under appropriate circumstances. A tight coupling of intake with energy expenditure is a mechanism to conserve energy when food supply is limited; in contrast, it also allows for disposing of or storing excess caloric intake. In healthy people, palatable, energy-dense foods retain high incentive value even when immediate energy requirements have been met, and this feature promotes the development of an energy reserve for potential future food shortages. Some individual variation in this response occurs, and the most susceptible individuals exhibit a weak satiety response to fatty meals, a maintained preference for high-fat over low-energy foods in the postingestive satiety period, and a strong hedonic attraction to palatable foods (17).

By contrast to the tight control of energy balance and tendency for energy storage in healthy individuals, patients with cancer lose controls contributing to weight maintenance or gain. Food intake in the patient with cancer may not correlate with degree of weight gain or loss in the usual way (18). Attempts to supplement food intake by either consultation by a dietitian or nutrition supplementation fail to prevent the progressive weight loss (19). Evidence indicates that deliberate ingestion of supplements is counteracted by reduction in food intake at other meals of the day even in patients with cancer whose intake is less than that required to cover the costs of basal metabolism. When Fearon et al (19) provided an energy-dense nutritional supplement to patients with pancreas cancer, these patients consumed 450 kcal/day of this product but had a net increase of total energy intake of only 68 kcal/day because of decreased intake during other meals of the day. Compensating decreases in oral intake at meals mean that supplementation may be completely ineffective in the worst case or merely inefficient in the best case. The hedonic value of food in general, as well as that of palatable high-energy density foods, is also lost to patients with cancer, and spontaneous ideation about food and food enjoyment disappear (20, 21).

Cachexia also differs from malnutrition in the resulting changes in body composition. During simple starvation, all organs lose mass. In the tumor-bearing state, muscle, skin, bone, and adipose tissue are catabolic, whereas organs such as liver and spleen and many parts of the immune system are anabolic and accumulate protein (14). The anabolic state of the liver exceeds the accumulation of liver protein because much of its anabolism is reflected in an increased production of secretory proteins of the acute phase response (22). During starvation, fat stores are mobilized, and most tissues convert to fat-derived fuels (free fatty acids, ketones) to meet metabolic demands. Use of ketones instead of glucose spares protein catabolism and lean body mass. In contrast, glucose production in cancer cachexia is maintained via gluconeogenesis, thus promoting protein catabolism and facilitating muscle wasting and early lean body mass depletion (23). Increased gluconeogenesis during starvation is transient because hepatic glucose production is displaced by β-oxidation of lipid; however, gluconeogenesis and hepatic glucose production are not suppressed in cancer cachexia (24). Finally, during periods when appetite has been stimulated, weight gain in patients with cancer is often transitory and is associated frequently with gain of fat but not protein (25).

Host metabolism is altered in the presence of a tumor, and many of the features are stereotypical responses to infection and injury, as well as cancer (26). These responses of the host organism to cancer appear to be highly organized and conserved (26). Although mobilization of reserves of energy and protein is an important adaptation, high levels of inflammation and catabolism are prognostic of reduced, not increased, survival in patients with cancer (5).

FAILURE OF FOOD INTAKE: ANOREXIA AND NUTRITION IMPACT SYMPTOMS

Dietary intakes of patients with advanced malignant disease have been reported. Individual intakes are quite varied. Mean values of dietary intake are similar to reported basal metabolic rates in the same or similar populations (i.e., 22 to 24 kcal/kg/day) (18, 19, 27). Intake is thus often insufficient to cover even the basal costs of metabolism. Two main elements are considered to contribute to the failure of food intake in cachexia: cancer-associated dysregulation of controls of appetite leading to anorexia and a series of disease- and treatment-related nutrition impact symptoms.

Patients with cancer lack appetite and also experience increased sensations of satiety. These alterations are considered to emanate from the brain, the primary site where food intake is regulated (28). In this organ, specific hypothalamic nuclei integrate cognitive, visual and sensory inputs, and peripheral signals indicating the status of body energy reserves, the activity of the gastrointestinal tract, and nutrient intake. The basic control of feeding behavior is altered in the tumor-bearing state, an effect attributed to proinflammatory cytokines (28).

A second and potentially large dimension to the problem of low dietary intake in patients with cancer is a group of symptoms that pose barriers to food intake above and beyond the presence of anorexia. This component is often termed *secondary cachexia* or, more specifically, secondary nutrition impact symptoms (29–31). The symptoms include, but are not limited to, nausea, vomiting, constipation, diarrhea, defecation after meal (also called dumping syndrome), pain including epigastric and abdominal pain as well as at other sites, dyspnea, fatigue, anxiety, depression, sense of hopelessness, stomatitis, dysgeusia, dental problems, difficulty chewing, dysosmia, xerostomia, thick saliva, and dysphagia. Patients not unusually have two, three, four or more of these symptoms concurrently. Patients with cancers of the head and neck and those with advanced cancers are particularly plagued with a symptom-heavy burden. The symptoms are caused both by the primary disease and the toxic side effects of antineoplastic therapy.

MacDonald et al (8) emphasized that many of the nutrition impact symptoms are potentially treatable causes of poor food intake, and close attention should be paid to their management. Although it is not within the scope of this chapter to address symptom management in detail, clinicians must remember that these symptoms present an obstacle course to the patient attempting to maintain oral intake of normal foods. Pain management is highly important, at whatever site in the body the pain may occur. Cancer evokes many emotional changes, including anxiety, depression, and family and spiritual distress; and the patient and family may experience direct distress around the patient's inability to eat and the family's desire for him or her to do so (20, 21, 32, 33). Numerous problems can be present in the mouth and upper gastrointestinal tract, including deterioration of the condition of teeth and dentures, mouth sores, mucosal breakdown, oral infections, and dry mouth (an especially severe consequence of radiation damage to the salivary glands). Swallowing difficulties may result from tumor involvement or after surgical resection of mouth, tongue, or throat, and food passage may be affected by hypomotility of the gastrointestinal tract. Constipation is a frequent and often severe side effect of the use of opioid analgesics used to treat cancer pain, and meticulous attention also must be paid to bowel care.

Unfortunately, some nutrition impact symptoms that are frequent and severe are poorly understood and thus poorly managed. Chemosensory abnormalities are a good example of such troublesome problems. The changes show a high degree of individual variation, and they may include loss of or distortion of taste and smell, phantom smells, persistent bad tastes, hypersensitivity to odors and tastes, and food aversions with nausea (34–38). These changes limit food intake in proportion with their severity (36, 37) and, not surprisingly, self-perceived quality of life. Taste and smell abnormalities are a direct consequence of cytotoxic cancer therapies, which alter or disrupt the renewal cycle of taste and smell receptors, although these abnormalities are also reported in up to 90% of patients with advanced cancer who are not undergoing active treatment (34, 36, 37). These findings demonstrate that factors other than active therapy are likely to contribute to chemosensory alterations. Empiric proof is lacking for most approaches to the treatment of taste and smell dysfunction in patient populations with cancer. One tactic is to define clearly the clinical features of chemosensory abnormalities, and integrate this knowledge into the development of nutrient-dense foods with features of flavor, odor, texture, and appearance that match the preferences, and thus specifically avoid the aversions experienced by patients with cancer. Some promising results have been obtained with Δ-9 tetra-hydrocannabinol therapy for cancer-associated chemosensory dysfunction (38).

THE THREE STAGES: PRECACHEXIA, CACHEXIA, AND REFRACTORY CACHEXIA

International cachexia consensus groups have attempted to classify the distal ends of the cachexia trajectory. Cachexia begins with initially subtle early manifestations (precachexia), progresses over time, and may culminate in advanced cachexia. The state of a patient wasted unto a state of emaciation is obviously different from that of a patient with limited weight loss. Only recent attention has been paid to these distinct states in the literature. A single publication in 2010 attempted a definition of precachexia (39), and the concept of refractory cachexia was proposed for the first time in 2011 (1).

Onset of Cachexia

The early manifestations of cachexia must be defined to identify individuals at risk and to permit preventive interventions. Nutritional assessments recommended for the evaluation of patients with cancer always begin with the weight loss history, both recent (2 to 4 weeks) and longer

term (3 to 6 months) or in relation to premorbid state. Weight loss of a low grade (2% to 5%) is an initial clue. Because cancer cachexia is characterized by a negative protein and energy balance, assessments usually include some attempt to evaluate the presence of muscle or lean tissue wasting. This evaluation is based on physical examination, blood work, and/or direct and indirect assessments of body composition. The key biologic signs predicting cachexia development remain to be determined exactly and will require validation.

Several important changes in the population demographics of body weight and body composition create an increasingly complex context for the identification of cachexia in its early stages. Specifically, obesity and sarcopenia (severe muscle depletion), conditions described as being of epidemic proportions, increasingly set the point of departure for the cancer trajectory. The normal body weights of adults at the average age of a cancer diagnosis (65 years) have been steadily increasing over the last two decades. This steady upward trend of overall body weight and the well-characterized propensity for obese persons to develop many forms of cancer (40) are reflected in the elevated body mass index (BMI) reported for contemporary patients with cancer at diagnosis, in both early and far-advanced stages of disease (30). Although it would appear obvious that weight loss in persons whose precancer body weight was normal has a different impact and consequence from a loss of similar magnitude in a person who was initially obese, the assumption that weight loss in obese patients with cancer has no consequence or should be encouraged is probably not valid. A significant gap exists in guidelines for the nutritional and metabolic management of the heavier patient with cancer who is losing weight.

Numerous reports are emerging on the prevalence of sarcopenia in patients with cancer (41, 42). Defined sex-specific reference values and standardized measurements are essential to perform assessment of skeletal muscle depletion. Although reference values related to cancer-specific outcomes remain sparse, a generally accepted definition of sarcopenia is absolute muscularity below the 5th percentile. This may be assessed as follows (1):

- Midupper arm muscle area by anthropometry (men, <32 cm^2; women, <18 cm^2)
- Appendicular skeletal muscle index determined by dual-energy x-ray absorptiometry (men, ,7.26 kg/m2; women, <5.45 kg/m^2)
- Lumbar skeletal muscle index determined by computed tomography (men, <55 cm^2/m^2; women, <39 cm^2/m^2)
- Whole body fat free mass index without bone determined by bioelectrical impedance (men, <14.6 kg/m^2; women, <11.4 kg/m^2)

Muscle wasting is not limited to individuals who appear thin or wasted and is often seen in normal weight, overweight, and obese individuals (41, 42). Each patient with cancer presents with a unique weight history and body composition that define the physiologic resources on which he or she is able to draw as the cancer progresses.

Advanced Cachexia

Only half of current cancer diagnoses in Westernized countries end in cure. Cancer spread to organs distant from the site of the primary tumor signifies systemic, progressive, and essentially incurable disease. Advanced cancer may be accompanied by a profound and *refractory cachexia* (1). Cachexia may be clinically refractory because of the presence of rapidly progressive cancer unresponsive to anticancer therapy. Cancer-associated anorexia becomes both total and irreversible at some stage of the disease trajectory. This stage of illness is marked by exponentially increasing rates of loss of muscle and adipose tissue, alongside uncontrolled growth of treatment-resistant metastatic disease (14). The definition of this stage of cachexia is essentially clinical, with an emphasis on unresponsiveness to anticancer therapy and the presence of intense catabolism. Development of more specific diagnostic criteria for this stage of cachexia is awaited; however, refractory cachexia is characterized by a low performance status (World Health Organization score 3 or 4) and a life expectancy of less than 3 months.

The refractory stage delineates cachexia in patients who are entering a phase of their cancer journey in which medical and ethical considerations change the pace and focus of intervention (1). In this stage, patients are unlikely to benefit from interventions aimed at reversing muscle and weight loss (19). These patients should be managed with therapeutic interventions alleviating the consequences and complications of cachexia, such as symptom control (appetite stimulation, nausea) or eating-related distress of patients and families (20, 21, 32, 33).

The psychologic dimensions of the cancer anorexia experience from the perspective of terminally ill patients and their family members are important. Anorexia is not necessarily distressful, but its logical consequence as conceived by the patients and family (i.e., death) certainly is (20, 33). Family members may press the patient to eat, and although this may be done in the sincere belief that it is in the patient's best interest and constitutes a means of empowerment of the patient to control the disease, this may become a considerable source of conflict between the patient and family (33). The ability to provide psychosocial support to patients and families requires that caregivers appreciate the psychologic effect of cancer anorexia and cachexia on these individuals.

The burden and risks of aggressive nutritional support likely outweigh any potential benefit in refractory cachexia. Some appreciation of life expectancy is required for the nutritionist to negotiate comfortably within the span of time leading up to the refractory stage, so that untimely aggressive nutritional strategies may be avoided. Clinical practice guidelines for initiation of parenteral feeding in patients with advanced cancer are explicitly based on an expected survival greater than 2 or 3 months (43, 44). The intent is to provide artificial nutrition only when the patient would be expected to die of starvation before any other consequences of the disease became life-limiting. Instituting parenteral feeding in patients close to death is not desirable because this encumbers them with infusion apparatus and high costs, and exposes them to risks of catheter placement and infection, in a context in which they have little to gain from nutritional support. The nutrition health professional may feel uncomfortable with the clinical prediction of survival, on which the decision to feed parenterally is based. Martin et al (30) provided a nutritional prognostic index for patients with advanced cancer in a palliative setting that may be used to inform the clinical prediction of survival by the care team.

PRINCIPLES OF NUTRITIONAL THERAPY OF CANCER CACHEXIA

The general approach to the management of wasting syndromes is based on an understanding of contributing mechanisms that form the targets for intervention. The most important features of cancer cachexia to take into account when designing therapeutic strategies are its complexity and its individual variation. Evaluations of importance include the following.

Status of Body Reserves

A history of body weight changes and current body composition, including muscle mass, must be taken. The presence of lean tissue wasting is an important consideration for defining the level of protein intake. Nutritional guidelines for the treatment of sarcopenia are available (45).

Assessment of Dietary Intake

Foods, beverages, and nutritional supplements must be reviewed along with a food preferences, dislikes, allergies, and intolerances. Psychosocial factors contributing to food intake, food security, and family relations around food and eating deserve evaluation.

Evaluation of Nutrition Impact Symptoms

Screening and in-depth assessement should be performed when nutrition impact symptoms are present, to develop a symptom treatment plan.

Evaluation of Catabolic Drivers

The presence of inflammation, hypogonadism, basal metabolic rate, and level of physical activity should be quantified to adopt a strategy for metabolic care.

Medical History

A medical history should be taken to identify comorbid conditions that may contribute to wasting (e.g., chronic obstructive pulmonary disease [COPD], chronic heart failure), contribute to metabolic alterations (e.g., diabetes, obesity), or be associated with dietary restrictions (e.g., hypercholesterolemia, diabetes, inflammatory bowel disease). Nutrition planning also must be informed by details of the cancer treatment plan, including radiation, chemotherapy, and surgery, as well as the prognosis, response of cancer to treatment, and expected duration of survival. Details of all medications can help pinpoint medications likely to limit or alter catabolic processes and nutrient use, as well as chemosensory function.

Generally, overall anabolism and muscle anabolism are maximized when nutrients (amino acids for building muscle protein and necessary cofactors and energy fuels) are not limiting. However, the maintenance of an anabolic environment for the use of nutrients is optimized by contractile work (especially resistance-type activity), by the presence of anabolic hormones (insulin and testosterone), and when catabolic factors and inflammation are minimal. An integrated approach of nutrition, resistance exercise, and metabolic or hormonal support has been adopted increasingly in the treatment of wasting both in elderly people (46) and populations with chronic diseases. A central theme of treatment of cachexia in patients with COPD is the trilogy of appetite stimulants or nutritional support, physical activity, and anabolic androgenic steroids, as well as various combinations of these factors (47). Collectively, these data suggest a high degree of reversibility of age-related wasting and show considerable potential for an integrated approach to COPD and other cachexias. These approaches have yet to be fully evaluated in patients with cancer; however, results from other catabolic conditions may share common mechanisms with cancer cachexia and offer insight into important therapeutic principles.

REFERENCES

1. Fearon K, Strasser F, Anker SD et al. Lancet Oncol 2011; 12:489–95.
2. Evans WJ, Morley JE, Argilés J et al. Clin Nutr 2008;27: 793–9.
3. Jensen GL, Mirtallo J, Compher C et al. JPEN J Parenter Enteral Nutr 2010;34:156–9.
4. Penet MF, Winnard PT Jr, Jacobs MA et al. Curr Opin Support Palliat Care 2011;5:327–33.
5. Fearon KC, Voss AC, Hustead DS. Am J Clin Nutr 2006; 83:1345–50.
6. Baracos VE. Annu Rev Nutr 2006;26:435–61.
7. Fearon KC. N Engl J Med 2011;11:365:565–7.
8. MacDonald N, Easson AM, Mazurak VC et al. J Am Coll Surg 2003;197:143–61.
9. Baracos VE. Cytokines and the pathophysiology of skeletal muscle atrophy. In: Anker SD, Hofbauer K, eds. The Pharmacotherapy of Cachexia. Boca Raton, FL: CRC Press, 2005:101–14.
10. de Alvaro C, Teruel T, Hernandez R et al. J Biol Chem 2004; 279:17070–8.
11. Lang CH, Hong-Brown L, Frost RA. Pediatr Nephrol 2005; 20:306–12.
12. Lundholm K, Daneryd P, Korner U et al. Int J Oncol 2004; 24:505–12.
13. Lundholm K, Gelin J, Hyltander A et al. Cancer Res 1994; 54:5602–6.
14. Lieffers JR, Mourtzakis M, Hall KD et al. Am J Clin Nutr 2009;89:1173–9.
15. Zoico E, Roubenoff R. Nutr Rev 2002;60:39–51.
16. Dewys WD, Begg C, Lavin PT et al. Am J Med 1980;69: 491–7.
17. Blundell JE, Stubbs RJ, Golding C et al. Physiol Behav 2005; 86:614–22.
18. Bosaeus I, Daneryd P, Svanberg E et al. Int J Cancer 2001; 93:380–3.
19. Fearon KC, von Meyenfeldt MF, Moses AG et al. Gut 2003;52:1479–86.
20. Shragge JE, Wismer WV, Olson KL et al. Palliat Med 2007; 21:227–33.
21. Hopkinson JB, Fenlon DR, Okamoto I et al. J Pain Symptom Manage 2010;40:684–95.
22. Gabay C, Kushner I. N Engl J Med 1999;340:448–54.
23. Tisdale MJ. Nutrition 1997;13:1–7
24. Tayek JA. J Am Coll Nutr 1992;11:445–56.
25. Loprinzi CL, Schaid DJ, Dose AM et al. J Clin Oncol 1993; 11:152–4.
26. Soeters PB, Grimble RF. Clin Nutr 2009;28:583–96.
27. Hutton JL, Martin L, Field CJ et al. Am J Clin Nutr 2006; 84:1163–70.
28. Guijarro A, Laviano A, Meguid MM. Prog Brain Res 2006;153:367–405.
29. Tong H, Isenring E, Yates P. Supp Care Cancer 2009;17: 83–90.
30. Martin L, Watanabe S, Fainsinger R et al. J Clin Oncol 2010;28:4376–83.
31. Kubrak C, Olson K, Jha N et al. Head Neck 2010;32:290–300.
32. Hopkinson JB. Curr Opin Support Palliat Care 2010;4:254–8.
33. McClement SE, Degner LF, Harlos MS. J Palliat Med 2003;6:737–48.
34. Wismer WV. Curr Opin Support Palliat Care 2008;2:282–7.
35. Brisbois TD, de Kock IH, Watanabe SM et al. J Pain Symptom Manage 2011;41:673–83.
36. Sanchez-Lara K, Sosa-Sanchez R, Green-Renner D et al. Nutr J 2010;9:15.
37. Steinbach S, Hummel T, Böhner C et al. J Clin Oncol 2009; 27:1899–1905.
38. Brisbois TD, de Kock IH, Watanabe SM et al. Ann Oncol 2011; 22:2086–93.
39. Muscaritoli M, Anker SD, Argiles J et al. Clin Nutr 2010; 29:154–9.
40. Renehan AG, Tyson M, Egger M et al. Lancet 2008;371: 569–78.
41. Baracos VE, Reiman T, Mourtzakis M et al. Am J Clin Nutr 2010;91:1133S–7S.
42. Prado CM, Lieffers JR, McCargar LJ et al. Lancet Oncol 2008;9:629–35.
43. Mirhosseini N, Fainsinger RL, Baracos V. J Palliat Med 2005; 8:914–8.
44. Orrevall Y, Tishelman C, Permert J et al. Palliat Med 2009;23:556–64.
45. Morley JE, Argiles JM, Evans WJ et al. J Am Med Dir Assoc 2010;11:391–6.

46. Wolfe RR. J Am Coll Surg 2006;202:176–80.

47. King DA, Cordova F, Scharf SM. Proc Am Thorac Soc 2008; 5:519–23.

SUGGESTED READINGS

Baracos VE. Cancer-associated cachexia and underlying biological mechanisms. Annu Rev Nutr 2006;26:435–61.

Fearon KC. Cancer cachexia and fat-muscle physiology. N Engl J Med 2011;365:565–7.

Fearon K, Strasser F, Anker SD et al. Definition and classification of cancer cachexia: an international consensus. Lancet Oncol 2011;12:489–95.

Muscaritoli M, Anker SD, Argiles J et al. Consensus definition of sarcopenia, cachexia and pre-cachexia: joint document elaborated by Special Interest Groups (SIG) "cachexia-anorexia in chronic wasting diseases" and "nutrition in geriatrics." Clin Nutr 2010;29: 154–9.

Morley JE, Argiles JM, Evans WJ et al. Nutritional recommendations for the management of sarcopenia. J Am Med Dir Assoc 2010;11:391–6.

88

NUTRITIONAL SUPPORT OF THE PATIENT WITH CANCER[1]

DAVID A. AUGUST AND MAUREEN HUHMANN

Cancer is a major public health problem in the United States and worldwide. There were an estimated 1.5 million cases of "serious-minded" (i.e., potentially life threatening) cancer in the United States in 2009, and approximately 560,000 people died from cancer that same year (1). It is projected that by the year 2020, cancer incidence will double worldwide (2). Cancer also has an enormous economic impact. In the United States, medical expenditures directed toward cancer treatment account for more than $200 billion in health care costs and a significant proportion of Medicare spending annually (3). Nutrition and diet play a major role in cancer. Dietary factors are an important component of the identifiable attributable risk of cancer, malnutrition is a cause of some of the significant clinical signs and symptoms that are observed in patients with cancer, and nutrition status is an important prognostic factor in patients with cancer (4). Malnutrition and weight loss often contribute to the death of patients with cancer (1, 4–6). Unfortunately, these issues persist despite decades of basic and clinical research as well as heightened awareness.

PREVALENCE AND SIGNIFICANCE OF MALNUTRITION IN PATIENTS WITH CANCER

Attributable Risk of Nutrition in Cancer

In 1981, Doll and Peto published a widely quoted estimate that 35% of all cancer deaths may be avoided by changes

[1]**Abbreviations: BCM**, body cell mass; **BMI**, body mass index; **CCS**, cancer cachexia syndrome; **cGVHD**, chronic graft versus host disease; **CRF**, corticotropin-releasing factor; **DHA**, docosahexaenoic acid; **ECW**, extracellular water; **EN**, enteral nutrition support; **EPA**, eicosapentaenoic acid; **FFM**, fat-free mass; **GI**, gastrointestinal; **GLN**, glutamine; **GVHD**, graft versus host disease; **HPN**, home parenteral nutrition, **HSCT**, hematopoietic stem cell transplantation; **IFN-γ**, interferon-γ; **IGF-I**, insulinlike growth factor-I; **IL**, interleukin; **LMF**, lipid-mobilizing factor; **α-MSH**, melanocyte-stimulating hormone; **n-3**, omega-3; **NPY**, neuropeptide Y; **PIF**, proteolysis-inducing factor; **PG-SGA**, Patient-Generated Subjective Global Assessment; **PN**, parenteral nutrition; **QOL**, quality of life; **RD**, registered dietitian; **RR**, relative risk; **SGA**, Subjective Global Assessment; **TNF-α**, tumor necrosis factor-α.

content as well as a 30% to 40% loss of body fat (63). Patients with solid tumors can lose as much as 1.34 kg of FFM in 4 weeks (62). These changes in body composition affect surgical outcomes. Patients with cancer with GI malignancies undergoing surgery experience increased rates of severe complications that correlate with decreases in lean body mass (73).

A relationship has been established between weight loss and QOL in oncology patients (74). Increased BCM in head and neck and patients with lung cancer has been associated with improved QOL and Eastern Cooperative Oncology Group performance scores (75). These data suggest opportunities to improve patient outcomes, especially QOL, through nutrition interventions focused on mediating specific changes in the body composition of patients with cancer (in particular, the restoration of lean body mass). Further data are needed to more confidently design specific interventions.

Metabolic Sequelae

The metabolic changes seen in CCS are multiple and variable. They are generally characterized by decoupling of supply and demand, resulting in excessive substrate cycling and turnover (67).

The most striking feature of the energetics of the metabolic response to cancer is its variability. In comparison with control groups, patients with cancer may have reduced, normal, or increased energy expenditure (76–81). The variability is in part caused by the heterogeneity of "cancer," but is also likely owing to differences in host responses to tumor and to the presence of comorbid conditions such as infection. Estimation of energy needs in patients with cancer is problematic because of this heterogeneity in energy expenditure.

Decreased skeletal muscle mass is a hallmark of CCS (29, 67). An apparent failure exists in patients with cancer of the normal mechanism of protein metabolism adaptation seen during simple starvation (82). Despite protein depletion, protein turnover remains normal or is even increased. This appears to result from a combination of decreased synthesis and increased proteolysis. Proteolysis-inducing factor (PIF), detected in the urine of patients with cancer with cachexia, is associated with decreased plasma amino acid levels and decreased protein synthesis (83). PIF activates an RNA-dependent protein kinase, which in turn activates nuclear factor-κB (NF-κB). NF-κB in turn activates the ubiquitin proteasome proteolytic pathway. This NF-κB pathway is proposed as the primary proteolytic pathway in CCS (59).

Depletion of fat stores is a characteristic feature of CCS, accounting for the wasted, "skin-and-bones" appearance of many patients with cancer. Increased turnover of glycerol and fatty acids compared with normal subjects is observed. Glucose infusion fails to suppress lipolysis in patients with cancer (84). Adipose cells from cachectic patients demonstrate increased lipolytic activity (29). TNF-α may play

a role in lipolysis by inhibiting lipoprotein lipase, thereby preventing the ability of adipocytes to extract fatty acids from circulating lipoproteins (i.e., low-density lipoprotein) (59). Lipid-mobilizing factor (LMF) also has been linked with increased lipolysis, increased free fatty acid turnover, and increased serum glycerol. LMF appears to increase lipolysis via increases in hormone sensitive lipase (59). Increased lipid levels in the blood seen in patients with cancer may help the host by fueling the generalized increased substrate turnover characteristic of CCS. Unfortunately, the same lipids also may be used by the tumor to meet essential requirements for polyunsaturated fats such as linoleic and arachidonic acids (85).

Alterations in carbohydrate metabolism are also commonly seen in cancer cachexia. Weight loss in CCS is often associated with glucose intolerance and diminished insulin sensitivity (86, 87). This may be a result of insulin resistance or decreased leptin levels or both (87, 88). Gluconeogenesis may be increased as a result of up-regulated Cori cycle activity in response to tumor production of lactic acid (89, 90). Increased hepatic gluconeogenesis is observed and may result from increased peripheral release of other glucose precursors, especially alanine and glycerol (91, 92). Cytokine mediators of CCS increase glucose demand, which induces gluconeogenic enzymes in the liver, further driving glucose synthesis (89). Host energy depletion can result from increased hepatic gluconeogenesis. Recycling of precursors to produce glucose is an energy-consuming process. The magnitude of this effect may be clinically significant in some patients (82, 93).

Mediators and Mechanisms of Cancer Cachexia Syndrome

A myriad of chemical, metabolic, and clinical factors are implicated in the pathogenesis of CCS. This complexity goes a long way in explaining the historic intractability of CCS to clinical interventions.

Proinflammatory Cytokines and Other Molecular Mediators

Proinflammatory cytokines such as tumor necrosis factor (TNF-α), interferon-γ (IFN-γ), and interleukins 1 and 6 (IL-1 and IL-6) are considered important mediators of CCS. A strong correlation exists between high levels of these factors and the presence of cachexia (59). The tumor appears to be the primary source of these cytokines. IL-6 levels are usually elevated in CCS29. IL-6 induces increased hepatic gluconeogenesis and protein synthesis (94). Increased serum levels of TNF-α have been associated with increases in lipolysis and proteolysis (59). IFN-γ also is associated with increased lipolysis and increased hepatic protein synthesis. IL-1 induces anorexia (95). All of these cytokines may act both peripherally to alter host metabolism and centrally to affect appetite and the host neuroendocrine axis.

Several neuropeptides have been implicated in the pathogenesis of cachexia. Neuropeptide Y (NPY) is orexigenic (appetite stimulating) in the normal state; with decreased production, it causes anorexia. NPY receptors appear resistant to NPY and production of NPY appears to be decreased in cancer cachexia (59). Melanocyte-stimulating hormone (α-MSH) and corticotropin-releasing factor (CRF) are anorexigenic in the normal state. α-MSH and CRF production are stimulated by IL-1, IL-6, and TNF-α, and may be mediators of the effects of these proinflammatory cytokines. Melanocortin signaling also appears to be increased in CCS (59).

Leptin, an adipocytokine crucial for body weight regulation and a modulator of inflammatory and immune responses, controls various processes in both the central nervous system and peripheral tissues. Leptin has been observed to be down-regulated in patients with cancer and cachectic patients (96). This hypoleptinemia may play a role in the increased insulin resistance seen in patients with cancer. However, unlike in healthy individuals, cachectic patients with cancer appear to be resistant to the orexigenic effects of hypoleptinemia (87). The exact impact of hypoleptinemia and its potential as a therapeutic target in cachexia remain to be elucidated.

Impaired Caloric Intake

Although CCS is fundamentally a metabolic syndrome, reduced caloric intake exacerbates the consequences of the underlying metabolic abnormality. Impaired caloric intake is the most significant cause of malnutrition among patients with cancer (97, 98). Changes in taste and appetite, learned food aversions, depression, and disturbances of the GI tract frequently impair adequate calorie intake by patients with cancer. Some of the most common and distressing symptoms in patients with advanced cancers relate to the GI tract. These symptoms may include early satiety, changes in taste, and loss of appetite (99, 100). GI symptoms are often prevalent early in the course of the disease, and may be the first cause of impairment in patients who are otherwise functional. Patients with various malignant diseases and otherwise favorable performance status can experience symptoms of abdominal fullness, pain, taste change, dry mouth, and constipation (32, 101).

Side Effects of Therapy

Unwanted side effects of cancer treatment are an important cause of decreased food intake and malnutrition in some patients with cancer (102).

Surgery induces a stress response characterized by hypermetabolism, tissue wasting, anorexia, and catabolism, all of which contribute to weight loss (102). These effects are often seen in the setting of preexisting nutritional compromise, because patients with cancer commonly are malnourished preoperatively (103). Major surgical resections for cancer may necessitate en bloc removal of adjacent normal tissue with resultant loss of

function. For example, malabsorption can occur after GI, pancreas, and liver resections. It is intuitively evident that the incidence of complications, length of hospitalization, duration of postoperative anorexia, and degree of malnutrition all increase with increasing complexity of the surgical procedure (103, 104).

Chemotherapy and biological therapies for cancer can affect food intake and absorption by inducing GI symptoms such as nausea, vomiting, anorexia, abdominal pain, diarrhea, fever, stomatitis, mucositis, and food aversions (105–107). Symptoms can occur immediately or in a delayed fashion and may last from several hours to days (100). Fatigue and pain induced by chemotherapy also negatively affect nutrition intake (100, 105).

Radiation therapy, especially to the head and neck, abdomen, and pelvis, has the potential to interfere with dietary intake. The effects of radiation therapy to the head and neck may be so severe that it is common to establish enteral access (with a gastrostomy or jejunostomy tube placed endoscopically or surgically) before initiation of therapy to decrease the incidence of malnutrition (108, 109). More than 70% of patients receiving pelvic radiation develop acute inflammatory changes in the small and large intestine, and as many as 50% can go on to develop chronic symptoms (110, 111). Acute, radiation induced injury to GI epithelium is manifested as diarrhea and cramping (111). These can lead to pain, dehydration, and food aversion. Fatigue also may be a prominent side effect of radiation therapy, and can contribute to impaired food intake through a lack of desire to prepare or consume food.

Changes in Taste and Mood

Dysgeusia, or distorted taste, can be a distressing accompaniment of cancer and cancer therapy that interferes with eating. Loss of taste and smell leads to distress and can affect both the psychological and somatic aspects of daily life (106, 107). Dysgeusia is associated with several factors, including direct neurotoxicity to taste buds, xerostomia, and infection. Changes in taste can occur with doses of radiation as low as 200 to 400 centigray (cGy) (112). Dysgeusia probably is related to damage of nerve fibers within the tongue as well as to the outer surface of the taste cells (113). In some cases, taste acuity returns in 2 to 3 months after cessation of treatment; however, in the case of radiation induced dysgeusia, patients may develop permanent hypogeusia (113, 114). The few studies that have investigated it correlate dysgeusia with high levels of perceived symptom distress by patients. This distress is rarely reported to health care providers (106, 107).

Pain and Other Adverse Consequences of Eating

Pain is a common cause of anorexia and/or food aversion. The pain may be a result of the tumor itself or a side effect of anticancer therapy. The experience of pain anywhere in the body can lead to nutritional deterioration (105, 115). Therefore, pain control is a significant element of optimal nutrition care. It is important to note, however, that pain related to eating appears to have the greatest impact on food intake (116, 117). For example, the high cellular turnover rate of oral mucosa makes it susceptible to toxic effects of chemotherapy (118). More than 50% of individuals receiving outpatient chemotherapy may experience stomatitis during treatment (119, 120). The presence of sore mouth during treatment is associated with weight loss and deterioration of nutrition status (121).

The consequences of pain and other symptom distress related to eating may be further exacerbated by development of conditioned food aversions (122). Even a single episode of GI symptom distress associated with chemotherapy treatment and food or beverage consumption can result in eating aversion (123). Occurrence of posttreatment nausea affects subsequent intake of foods consumed within 24 hours after chemotherapy administration or in the first 2 weeks of radiation therapy (123, 124). Fortunately, these aversions appear to be short lived, with most resolving within 2 months (125).

Obstruction, Fistula, and Malabsorption

Mechanical factors related to tumor or complications of therapy may compromise GI tract continuity and normal motility. This effect occurs most commonly as a result of malignant obstruction of the esophagus, stomach, small intestine, colon, or biliary tract, or secondary to tumor-induced changes in gastric wall compliance. Cancer and cancer-related surgery are the most common cause of GI fistulas (126). Symptoms related to mechanical factors may include alterations in taste sensation, early satiety, pain, cramps, vomiting, diarrhea, and constipation (127). Surgery or endoscopic stenting are often the best approaches to dealing with these complications in acceptable risk patients. Unfortunately, before intervention, these symptoms can lead to significant weight loss and malnutrition (128–130). In other circumstances, when patients are poor candidates for invasive procedures or end-of-life issues dominate, palliative care aimed at symptom management is more appropriate (131, 132).

Malabsorption can occur in patients with cancer because of the tumor itself or as a result of surgical treatment. Resection of any significant portion of the small bowel can result in decreased transit time, thereby producing malabsorption. The loss of portions of the small intestine can result in hypergastrinemia and accelerated gastric emptying. An acidic environment in the small bowel lumen deactivates digestive enzymes and deconjugates bile acids, and may result in malabsorption. Significant resection of the lower jejunum and ileum can cause reduced intestinal absorption secondary to the loss of absorptive surface, or short bowel syndrome (133). Resection of the ileocecal valve and significant portions of the colon may lead to diarrhea and bacterial overgrowth (134, 135).

Pancreatic enzymes play an important role in the digestion of starch, protein, and lipid. Pancreatic enzyme deficiency, whether caused by pancreatic duct obstruction, resection, or dysregulation, manifests as malabsorption of fat and steatorrhea. This lack of enzymes can be compensated for, to some extent, by oral administration of pancreatic enzymes, diet modification, and a physiologic shift of the site of digestion to the distal small intestine (136). Pancreaticocibal asynchrony occurs when pancreatic enzyme secretion is mistimed, resulting in malabsorption. This occurs in 16% to 43% of gastrectomy patients (137).

NUTRITION SUPPORT FOR PATIENTS WITH CANCER

Given the deleterious effects of malnutrition on the prognosis of patients with cancer and their QOL, it makes sense to use nutrition support (oral, enteral, or parenteral provision of nutrients) to try to reverse changes in body composition and mass associated with poor outcomes. In fact, given the relationship between nutrition status and poor outcomes, it seems obvious that nutrition support is beneficial in these patients. However, this is not necessarily true. As noted, mere provision of nutrient substrates does not deal with the metabolic consequences of the presence of cancer or CCS. Provision of nutrients does not assure that they will be used effectively. When carefully looked at in clinical settings, it turns out that the use of nutrition support in patients with cancer is most effective when it is limited to special, well-described circumstances. An evidence-based review (138) suggests that nutrition support can be effective in patients with cancer:

1. Who are receiving active anticancer treatment
2. Who are moderately to severely malnourished or are expected to be unable to ingest or absorb adequate nutrients for a "prolonged" period of time (7 to 14 days in perioperative patients and 14 days or longer in nonsurgical patients)

"Routine" use of nutrition support is not indicated to prevent malnutrition in patients undergoing surgery or receiving radiation therapy or chemotherapy who do not meet the listed criteria.

The goal of nutrition intervention in patients with cancer is to support anabolism, body composition, functional status, and QOL (139). In those circumstances in which nutrition support is used, effective and situationally appropriate nutrition care of patients with cancer requires a structured, formal nutrition care process. The process must identify those patients who are at nutritional risk, create a care plan, enact that plan, monitor it, and adjust it as patient and disease factors change. More formally, the nutrition care process should include the following elements: nutrition screening, formal nutrition assessment, formulation of a nutrition care plan, implementation of the plan, patient monitoring, reassessment of the care plan, and then either reformulation of the care plan or termination of therapy (140). This process is iterative and dynamic so that changing patient circumstances are recognized and accommodated. Nutrition care is a multidisciplinary undertaking that is most effective when it includes physicians, nurses, pharmacists, dietitians, psychosocial providers, and physical therapists (141).

Nutrition Screening and Assessment

Early identification of patients at nutrition risk is vital to the prevention of severe malnutrition; however, nutrition status is difficult to quantify. Current weight and weight history (usual body weight, ideal body weight, current weight, and weight loss) are the parameters most commonly used to assess the nutrition status of patients (142). The prevalence of weight loss and malnutrition in oncology patients ranges from 9% to 100% depending on tumor site and stage (11, 143–146). Weight loss is a negative prognostic indicator in patients with cancer (147). Weight loss of greater than 10% has been confirmed to be associated with increased morbidity and mortality regardless of disease process or treatment (147). Although simple, practical, cost effective, and helpful, weight and weight history alone do not capture the extent and full significance of tissue loss in patients with cachexia (148). The purpose of nutrition screening is to identify individuals who are at risk for malnutrition or are currently malnourished. Screening identifies the need for further, in-depth, formal nutrition assessment.

Multiple tools, such as the Mini Nutritional Assessment, the Nutrition Risk Assessment, and the Malnutrition Screening Tool, have been developed to screen for the presence of malnutrition (19, 146, 149–151) (Table 88.4)

TABLE 88.4 **NUTRITION SCREENING AND ASSESSMENT TOOLS FOR PATIENTS WITH CANCER**

Prognostic Nutritional Index[a]: % risk of operative complication = 158 − 16.6 (s. albumin; g/dL) − 0.78 (TSF; mm) − 0.20 (s. transferrin; g/dL) − 5.8 (delayed–type hypersensitivity reaction mm). Validated prospectively.

Nutrition Risk Index[b]: 1.519 (s. albumin; g/dL) + 41.7 (current weight/usual weight); used in Veterans Affairs Total Parenteral Nutrition Cooperative Study Group Trial of perioperative parenteral nutrition to classify patients as well-nourished, or mildly, moderately, or severely malnourished.

Patient Generated Subjective Global Assessment (PG–SGA)[c]: History—Weight change, change in dietary intake, gastrointestinal symptoms, change in functional capacity, diagnosis. Physical examination—Loss of subcutaneous fat, muscle wasting, ankle edema, sacral edema, ascites. Elements are combined to create a numeric score to categorize patients as mildly, moderately, or severely malnourished. Validated prospectively.

TSF, triceps skinfold.

[a]Data from Buzby GP, Mullen JL, Matthews DC et al. Prognostic nutritional index in gastrointestinal surgery. Am J Surg 1980;139:160–7.
[b]Data from The Veterans Affairs Total Parenteral Nutrition Cooperative Study Group. Perioperative total parenteral nutrition in surgical patients. N Engl J Med 1991;325:525–32.
[c]Data from Linn BS, Robinson DS, Klimas NG. Effects of age and nutritional status on surgical outcomes in head and neck cancer. Ann Surg 1988;207:267–73.

(19, 20, 144). Nutrition screening tools should incorporate objective and subjective data. However, a screening tool also should be easy to use, cost effective, valid, reliable, and sensitive. Objective data commonly included in nutrition screening tools include height, weight, weight change, primary diagnosis, disease stage, and the presence of comorbidities (140). No single objective measure is sufficient to determine nutrition risk (152). Because of the incidence and significance of malnutrition in patients with cancer, it is recommended that all patients receive nutrition screening as a component of their initial evaluation (140).

The Patient-Generated Subjective Global Assessment (PG-SGA) (147), a nutrition screening tool commonly used in oncology, is based on a tool developed by Baker et al, the Subjective Global Assessment (SGA) (147, 149, 153). Both the SGA and PG-SGA combine known prognostic indicators such as weight loss, performance status, and nutrition-related symptoms (147). The PG-SGA consists of two sections. The patient-completed section elicits information related to weight history, symptom experience, recent and past food intake, and activity level. The health care professional section includes an evaluation of metabolic demand, disease in relation to nutrition requirements, and findings of the physical examination. The patient and health care provider assessment are combined into a numeric score to categorize patients as mildly, moderately, or severely malnourished and guide potential nutrition interventions and monitoring (154). The PG-SGA may be used serially to assess subtle changes in nutrition status (155).

When patients are identified as malnourished or at nutritional risk by a screening tool such as the PG-SGA, a formal nutrition assessment that includes thorough evaluation of the medical history, dietary history, physical examination, anthropometric measurements, and laboratory data should be performed (152). A review of body composition is integrated with data on disease and clinical status to evaluate effect on metabolism and nutrient requirements. Appraisal of disease and treatment-related symptoms is also necessary to plan nutrition interventions. This process leads to the identification and diagnosis of nutrition issues, which in turn directs the nutrition intervention (156). Planning of the nutrition intervention requires the input of all disciplines involved in patient care. The causes of weight loss or weight gain as well as family situation and socioeconomic issues must be considered (152, 157). Consideration of these factors should be patient focused, with patient preferences helping to guide treatment plans (14). The goals of the intervention must be documented and reevaluated frequently (156). The intervention must be individualized to the patient and consideration should be given to the patient's comfort and wishes (154, 156). Although variable among patients, common nutrition goals include symptom management, weight maintenance, and preservation of functional status

symptoms are present, formal evaluation and intervention by an RD has been shown to be helpful (250). General approaches include the use of antiemetics (ondansetron, chlorpromazine), promotility agents (metoclopramide), antidiarrheals (narcotics, loperamide, atropine), fiber, laxatives, and (when pancreatic insufficiency is suspected) pancreatic enzyme replacement. The National Comprehensive Cancer Network published a thorough set of guidelines for symptom management in patients with cancer that includes management of GI symptoms (251). Several sources also discuss management of GI symptoms from a surgical perspective (252).

HEMATOPOIETIC STEM CELL TRANSPLANTATION

Hematopoietic stem cell transplantation (HSCT) refers to the intravenous infusion of autologous or allogeneic stem cells collected from bone marrow, peripheral blood, or umbilical cord blood to reestablish hematopoietic function. HSCT is used after treatment with high-dose chemotherapy to take advantage of the theoretic benefit of dose dense chemotherapy to improve tumor response. These high doses would otherwise cause irreversible, catastrophic injury to bone marrow function. The ablated bone marrow is reconstituted by the HSCT. When allogeneic HSCT is used, it is accompanied by the use of immunosuppressive drugs to permit engraftment of the allogeneic transplant and prevent potentially fatal graft versus host disease (GVHD). Because of the high doses of chemotherapy used and the prolonged period of associated leukopenia and thrombocytopenia, HSCT may cause considerable physical, social, psychological, and spiritual suffering. Physical symptoms that frequently occur in HSCT include pain, nausea, mucositis, diarrhea, and delirium. Psychological symptoms include depression, anxiety, grief, loss, demoralization, and anger (253).

The incidence of malnutrition before treatment in patients undergoing HSCT is not well described. Malnutrition before HSCT is associated with increased length of stay. Routine nutrition assessment of all patients before HSCT should be undertaken (254).

Chronic GVHD (cGVHD) is a complication of allogeneic HSCT. cGVHD causes oral sensitivity, stomatitis, xerostomia, anorexia, reflux, diarrhea, and dysgeusia, which contribute to suboptimal nutrition status (255). More than 60% of patients undergoing allogeneic HSCT exhibit cGVHD, resulting in weight loss in 28% of patients (255).

Patients commonly require PN during the course of the HSCT because of GI toxicities. PN may be beneficial in patients undergoing HSCT (44, 256–258). Although PN does not appear to reduce toxicity, it may reduce length of stay (44, 259–261) and weight loss in patients undergoing HSCT (258). Furthermore, one study demonstrated a long-term survival advantage in patients who received PN44.

NUTRACEUTICALS

Nutraceuticals are food or dietary supplements believed to provide health benefits (see the chapter on nutraceuticals) (180, 185, 262–287). These are commonly added to the diet through the use of a liquid nutrition supplement fortified with the nutrient(s) of choice.

Arginine

In animal models, arginine influences nitrogen metabolism, wound healing, immunocompetence, and tumor metabolism (267). It is a nonessential amino acid that may become conditionally essential during periods of physiological stress. It is a substrate in the urea cycle and plays a role in protein, creatinine, and polyamine synthesis (268). Parenteral arginine supplementation in patients undergoing colon resection has been shown to enhance immune responsiveness when compared with untreated controls (265). Arginine is not routinely added to PN. Clinical studies of arginine-supplemented EN generally do not demonstrate impact on morbidity or mortality (180, 269, 270). One study of enteral arginine supplementation in patients with head and neck cancer undergoing surgery did suggest improved wound healing and decreased length of stay (271). In one randomized trial of malnourished patients with head and neck cancer, follow-up at 10 years indicated improved survival in those subjects who received supplemental arginine preoperatively (272).

Omega-3 Fatty Acids

n-3 fatty acids, essential in the diet, favor production of prostaglandins in the three series (PGE_3) and leukotrienes in the five series associated with improved immunocompetence and reduced inflammatory responses. n-3 fatty acids also promote reduced levels of the PGE_2 and leukotrienes in the four series known to be immunosuppressive and proinflammatory (273, 274). n-3 fatty acids have been provided in a variety of forms, including enterally as pills and in liquid nutrition supplements, as well as parenterally. Studies of enteral n-3 fatty acid administration in pancreatic patients with cancer indicate that n-3 fatty acid supplementation in the range of 2 to 3 g/day may stabilize body weight (275–277). Parenteral n-3 fatty acid supplementation in patients with colorectal cancer led to improved leukotriene-5 levels and decreased TNF levels (278). Currently, it may be beneficial to provide n-3 fatty acid supplements to patients with pancreas cancer who are losing weight.

Glutamine

GLN, the most abundant amino acid in the human body, is an important substrate for rapidly proliferating cells such as lymphocytes, macrophages, enterocytes, fibroblasts, and renal epithelium (279). GLN is a precursor for the synthesis of purines, pyrimidines, and amino acids and acts as a nitrogen shuttle between tissues (268). Standard PN does not contain GLN because of instability in its free form. When used in PN, GLN is provided as a dipeptide. Common GLN dipeptides stable in an aqueous solution are alanylglutamine and glycylglutamine (280). A meta-analysis of studies that used parenteral GLN postoperatively found parenteral GLN associated with reduced length of stay and decreased incidence of infectious complications (281). One prospective, randomized study of perioperative parenteral GLN in colorectal patients with cancer indicated improved nitrogen balance with GLN supplementation (181). Limited data on the effectiveness of enteral GLN alone exist because it is commonly supplemented in combination with other nutrients. Although in a murine model, enteral GLN supplementation has been shown to decrease intestinal mucosal injury from cisplatin (282), perhaps through up-regulation of GLN transporters by cisplatin, no data in humans exist. Additional studies of GLN efficacy in cancer have been suggested (56).

Immune-Enhancing Enteral Formulas

Multiple studies have investigated the impact of "immunonutrition" or nutritional supplementation with micronutrients or macronutrients with the intent of preserving or improving immune status. The largest clinical trials that have investigated nutritional pharmacologic interventions in perioperative patients with cancer primarily have used a commercially available enteral formula containing supplemental arginine, RNA, and n-3 fatty acids. Several metaanalyses have indicated benefits in surgical patients, including decreased incidence of hospital acquired infections, wound complications, and length of hospital stay with the perioperative use of immune enhancing EN products (283–287). The combination of arginine, n-3 fatty acids, and nucleotides appears to convey the most benefit.

END-OF-LIFE NUTRITION CARE

Despite published guidelines that state that the palliative use of nutrition support is rarely appropriate in patients with cancer, this issue remains controversial (138). However, given the frequency of the use of home PN (HPN) in patients with a cancer diagnosis, it is important to address this issue. Patients' QOL and significant health care resources are at stake (288, 289).

The decision to initiate nutrition support in patients with advanced cancer must include consideration of the patient's and family's wishes, potential risks and benefits, and the patient's estimated survival. The goals of the use of nutrition support in this situation are to improve QOL and prolong life with control of nutrition-related symptoms that cause distress (131). A review cited 5 registry-based studies, 10 retrospective series, 3 prospective studies, and 2 prospective randomized trials relevant to the use of HPN support in terminally ill patients with cancer (132).

Obstruction, malabsorption, fistula, and radiation enteritis were the most frequent indications. The randomized trials are difficult to evaluate because of the failure to use an intention-to-treat analysis in one (290) and the prolonged survival seen in both groups in the other (suggesting they were not imminently terminal) (291). Nevertheless, both suggest some survival benefit. Examples of terminally ill patients with cancer who have demonstrated a favorable response to HPN include patients with a good performance status (e.g., Karnofsky score >50); those with inoperable bowel obstruction; those with minimal symptoms from disease involving major organs such as brain, liver, and lungs; and those with indolent disease progression. American Society for Parenteral and Enteral Nutrition Clinical Guidelines suggest that if patients are to benefit from this complex, intrusive, and expensive therapy, they (a) must be very strongly motivated and physically capable of participating in the their own care; (b) should have an estimated life expectancy of greater than 40 to 60 days; and (c) require strong social and financial support at home, including a dedicated in-home lay care provider (138). Furthermore, they must fail trials of less invasive therapies, including aggressive medical management with antiemetics, narcotics, anticholinergics, and antidepressants. Those patients with a life expectancy of less than 40 days are often well palliated with home intravenous fluid therapy (131). Very few patients evaluated for palliative care with HPN meet these criteria. Frank, compassionate discussions with these patients, their families, and their referring physicians are crucial if optimal decisions are to be made and accepted by all involved.

CLINICAL ALGORITHM FOR THE USE OF NUTRITION SUPPORT IN PATIENTS WITH CANCER

The concepts presented in this chapter suggest an algorithm to guide appropriate use of nutrition support in patients with cancer. A diagnosis of cancer in and of itself identifies the patient as nutritionally at risk. All hospitalized patients with cancer, and many outpatients, should undergo a formal nutrition status assessment to identify those patients who are indeed malnourished. Furthermore, this encounter can be used to counsel patients concerning the nutritional impact of cancer and suggest possible dietary changes to ameliorate the effects of the disease and its treatment.

No indication exists for the *routine* use of specialized nutrition support in patients with cancer. The data are quite clear that adequately nourished patients do not benefit from "adjuvant" nutrition support, and this may actually harm some patients.

For patients undergoing surgery, preoperative nutrition support should be considered in those who are moderately or severely malnourished as determined by the formal nutrition assessment. Oral supplements may be adequate occasionally; most often, either enteral or parenteral support is required to meet nutritional needs and initiate nutritional repletion. At least 7 and preferably 14 days of preoperative support are required to induce the anabolic milieu that best promotes postoperative healing and minimizes nutrition-related complications. For malnourished patients in whom surgery cannot be delayed, or who are recognized postoperatively as unlikely to be able to meet nutritional needs orally within 7 days, early initiation of postoperative nutrition support is important. Preoperative and intraoperative planning that identifies a likely need for postoperative nutrition support can lead to intraoperative establishment of enteral feeding access (a gastrostomy or jejunostomy tube) during an abdominal surgical procedure. The presence of functional GI access can simplify the decision to initiate nutrition support by enteral feedings. In general, enteral feedings are preferred to PN support. However, in those patients without enteral access or in whom the GI tract is not functional, PN should be used. Because of the variable nutrient requirements in patients with cancer, and because perioperative needs are most often dictated by the physiologic status of the patient, protein and calorie requirements must be measured or estimated for each patient. Currently, no proven role exists for nutritional pharmacologic supplements.

In patients receiving chemotherapy or radiation therapy, nutrition support should be reserved for those patients who are moderately to severely malnourished and in whom oral intake is expected to be inadequate for a prolonged period of time ($\geq$14 days).

Patients who are terminally ill and are not receiving active anticancer treatment rarely benefit from EN or PN support. The risk, inconvenience, and discomfort outweigh the potential palliative benefit. Patients who are unable to meet their fluid requirements orally may benefit from intravenous fluid therapy administered intermittently in an ambulatory care setting or at home. On rare occasions, a terminally ill patient not receiving active therapy may derive benefit from HPN if life expectancy is greater than 40 to 60 days, performance status is good, a dedicated and capable care provider is living with the patient, and the costs of the therapy are manageable.

Given the general physiologic and nutritional equivalence of EN and PN in patients with cancer, EN is the preferred method of nutrition whenever possible. EN is simpler, cheaper, and safer if the GI tract is functional and secure enteral access can be established.

REFERENCES

1. Jemal A, Siegel R, Ward E et al. CA Cancer J Clin 2009; 59:225–49.
2. Eaton L. BR MED J 2003;326:728.
3. Meropol NJ, Schulman KA. J Clin Oncol 2007;25:180–6.
4. August D, Huhmann M. Nutritional care of cancer patients. In: Norton J, Barie P, Bollinger R et al, eds. Surgery: Basic Science and Clinical Evidence. 2nd ed. New York: Springer, 2008:2123–49.
5. Warren S. Am J Med Sci 1932;185:610–5.
6. Inagaki J, Rodriguez V, Bodey GP. Cancer 1974;33:568–73.
7. Doll R, Peto R. J Natl Cancer Inst 1981;66:1191–308.
8. Willett WC. Environ Health Perspect 1995;103(Suppl): 165–70.
9. Polednak AP. Cancer Detect Prev 2008;32:190–9.
10. DeWys WD. Cancer 1979;43:2013–9.
11. Dewys WD, Begg C, Lavin PT et al. Am J Med 1980;69: 491–7.
12. Tan BH, Fearon KC. Curr Opin Clin Nutr Metab Care 2008; 11:400–7.
13. McClement S. J Wound Ostomy Continence Nurs 2005; 32:264–8.
14. Ottery FD. Semin Oncol 1995;22:98–111.
15. Puccio M, Nathanson L. Semin Oncol 1997;24:277–87.
16. MacDonald N. J Support Oncol 2003;1:279–86.
17. Studley H. JAMA 1936;106:458–60.
18. Smale BF, Mullen JL, Buzby GP et al. Cancer 1981;47: 2375–81.
19. Buzby GP, Mullen JL, Matthews DC et al. Am J Surg 1980; 139:160–7.
20. The Veterans Affairs Total Parenteral Nutrition Cooperative Study Group. N Engl J Med 1991;325:525–32.
21. Mullen JT, Davenport DL, Hutter MM et al. Ann Surg Oncol 2008;15:2164–72.
22. Calle EE, Rodriguez C, Walker-Thurmond K et al. N Engl J Med 2003;348:1625–38.
23. Friedrich MJ. JAMA 2003;290:2790–1.
24. Fontana L. Eur J Cardiovasc Prev Rehabil 2008;15:3–9.
25. Hunter RJ, Navo MA, Thaker PH et al. Cancer Treat Rev 2009;35:69–78.
26. Wong JR, Gao Z, Merrick S et al. Int J Radiat Oncol Biol Phys 2009;75:49–55.
27. Irwin ML, Mayne ST. Cancer J 2008;14:435–41.
28. Fletcher AL, Marks DL. Curr Opin Support Palliat Care 2007;1:306–11.
29. Tisdale MJ. Curr Opin Gastroenterol 2010;26:146–51.
30. Skipworth RJ, Fearon KC. Eur J Gastroenterol Hepatol 2007; 19:371–7.
31. Penet MF, Winnard PT Jr, Jacobs MA et al. Curr Opin Support Palliat Care 2011;5:327–37.
32. Grosvenor M, Bulcavage L, Chlebowski RT. Cancer 1989; 63:330–4.
33. Warburg O. Science 1956;123:309–14.
34. Warburg O, ed. The Metabolism of Tumours. London: Constable, 1930.
35. Kohlmeier L, Simonsen N, Mottus K. Environ Health Perspect 1995;103(Suppl):177–84.
36. Longo VD, Fontana L. Trends Pharmacol Sci 2010;31:89–98.
37. Roberts DL, Dive C, Renehan AG. Annu Rev Med 2010; 61:301–16.
38. Bozzetti F, Mori V. Clin Nutr 2009;28:226–30.
39. Paz-Filho G, Lim EL, Wong ML et al. Front Biosci 2011; 16:1634–50.
40. Baron PL, Lawrence W Jr, Chan WM et al. Arch Surg 1986; 121:1282–6.
41. Frank JL, Lawrence W Jr, Banks WL et al. Cancer 1992; 69:1858–64.
42. Franchi F, Rossi-Fanelli F, Seminara P et al. J Clin Gastroenterol 1991;13:313–5.
43. Bozzetti F, Gavazzi C, Mariani L et al. Clin Nutr 2004;23: 417–21.
44. Weisdorf SA, Lysne J, Wind D et al. Transplantation 1987; 43:833–8.

45. Hoare M, Young AR, Narita M. Semin Cancer Biol 2011; 21:397–404.

46. Reed JC. J Clin Oncol 1999;17:2941–53.

47. Guenther GG, Edinger AL. Cell Cycle 2009;8:1122–6.

48. Kroemer G, Pouyssegur J. Cancer Cell 2008;13:472–82.

49. Pathania D, Millard M, Neamati N. Adv Drug Deliv Rev 2009;61:1250–75.

50. Kaelin WG Jr, Thompson CB. Nature 2010;465:562–4.

51. DeBerardinis RJ, Cheng T. Oncogene 2010;29:313–24.

52. Enciso JM, Hirschi KK. Curr Cancer Drug Targets 2007; 7:432–7.

53. Kim KC, Friso S, Choi SW. J Nutr Biochem 2009;20:917–26.

54. Cheng WH. Environ Mol Mutagen 2009;50:349–60.

55. Ferguson LR, Philpott M. Curr Cancer Drug Targets 2007; 7:459–64.

56. Kuhn KS, Muscaritoli M, Wischmeyer P et al. Eur J Nutr 2010;49:197–210.

57. Trujillo E, Davis C, Milner J. J Am Diet Assoc 2006;106: 403–13.

58. Davis CD, Milner J. Mutat Res 2004;551:51–64.

59. Fearon K, Strasser F, Anker SD et al. Lancet Oncol 2011; 12:489–95.

60. MacDonald N, Easson AM, Mazurak VC et al. J Am Coll Surg 2003;197:143–61.

61. Muscaritoli M, Anker SD, Argiles J et al. Clin Nutr 2010; 29:154–9.

62. May P, Barber A, D'Olimpio J et al. Am J Surg 2002;183: 471–9.

63. Thibault R, Cano N, Pichard C. Curr Opin Clin Nutr Metab Care 2011;14:261–7.

64. Cohn S, Gartenhaus W, Sawitsky A. Metabolism 1981;30: 222–9.

65. Cohn S, Gartenhaus W, Vartsky D. Am J Clin Nutr 1981;34.

66. Cohn S, Sawitsky A, Vartsky D. Nutr Cancer 1980;2:67–71.

67. Fearon KC. N Engl J Med 2011;11: 365:565–7.

68. Marian M. Support Line 1998;20:3–12.

69. Baker JP, Detsky AS, Wesson DE et al. N Engl J Med 1982; 306:969–72.

70. Giacosa A, Frascio F, Sukkar S et al. Nutr Cancer 1996;12: s20–s3.

71. Shizgal HM. Cancer 1985;55:250–3.

72. Toso S, Gusella M, Menon A et al. Eur J Cancer 1997;33: s58–s9.

73. Fritz T, Hollwarth I, Romaschow M et al. Eur J Surg Oncol 1990;16:326–31.

74. Mariani L, Lo Vullo S, Bozzetti F. Support Care Cancer 2012; 20:301–9.

75. Tchekmedyian S, Fesen M, Price LM et al. Int J Radiat Oncol Biol Phys 2003;57:S283–4.

76. Falconer JS, Fearon KC, Plester CE et al. Ann Surg 1994; 219:325–31.

77. Hansell DT, Davies JW, Burns HJ. Ann Surg 1986;203:240–5.

78. Arbeit JM, Lees DE, Corsey R et al. Ann Surg 1984;199: 292–8.

79. Knox LS, Crosby LO, Feurer ID et al. Ann Surg 1983;197: 152–62.

80. Hyltander A, Drott C, Korner U et al. Eur J Cancer 1991; 27:9–15.

81. Cao DX, Wu GH, Zhang B et al. Clin Nutr 2010;29:72–7.

82. Kern KA, Norton JA. JPEN J Parenter Enteral Nutr 1988;12:286–98.

83. Tisdale MJ. Physiology (Bethesda) 2005;20:340–8.

84. Shaw JH, Wolfe RR. Ann Surg 1987;205:368–76.

85. Hussey HJ, Tisdale MJ. Br J Cancer 1994;70:6–10.

86. Lundholm K, Holm G, Schersten T. Cancer Res 1978;38: 4665–70.

87. Smiechowska J, Utech A, Taffet G et al. J Investig Med 2010;58:554–9.

88. Rofe AM, Bourgeois CS, Coyle P et al. Anticancer Res 1994; 14:647–50.

89. Bongaerts GP, van Halteren HK, Verhagen CA et al. Med Hypotheses 2006;67:1213–22.

90. Lelbach A, Muzes G, Feher J. Med Sci Monit 2007;13: RA168–73.

91. Doyle SL, Donohoe CL, Lysaght J et al. Proc Nutr Soc 2011; 3:1–9.

92. Lundholm K, Edstrom S, Karlberg I et al. Cancer 1982; 50:1142–50.

93. Costa G, Bewley P, Aragon M et al. Cancer Treat Rep 1981;65(Suppl 5):3–7.

94. Argiles JM, Lopez-Soriano FJ. Med Res Rev 1999;19:223–48.

95. Ramos EJ, Suzuki S, Marks D et al. Curr Opin Clin Nutr Metab Care 2004;7:427–34.

96. Diakowska D, Krzystek-Korpacka M, Markocka-Maczka K et al. Cytokine 2010;51:132–7.

97. Fouladiun M, Korner U, Bosaeus I et al. Cancer 2005; 103:2189–98.

98. Ollenschlaeger G, Konkol K, Wickramanayake PD et al. Am J Clin Nutr 1989;50:454–9.

99. Komurcu S, Nelson KA, Walsh D et al. Am J Hosp Palliat Care 2002;19:351–5.

100. Yamagishi A, Morita T, Miyashita M et al. J Pain Symptom Manage 2009;37:823–30.

101. Isenring EA, Bauer JD, Banks M et al. J Hum Nutr Diet 2009;22:545–50.

102. Casey C, Chen LM, Rabow MW. Expert Rev Anticancer Ther 2011; 11:1077–89.

103. Dannhauser A, Van Zyl JM, Nel CJ. J Am Coll Nutr 1995; 14:80–90.

104. Colleoni M, Li S, Gelber RD et al. Lancet 2005;366:1108–10.

105. Tong H, Isenring E, Yates P. Support Care Cancer 2009;17: 83–90.

106. Bernhardson BM, Tishelman C, Rutqvist LE. Eur J Oncol Nurs 2009;13:9–15.

107. Bernhardson BM, Tishelman C, Rutqvist LE. Support Care Cancer 2008;16:275–83.

108. Nugent B, Parker MJ, McIntyre IA. J Hum Nutr Diet 2010; 23:277–84.

109. Paccagnella A, Morello M, Da Mosto MC et al. Support Care Cancer 2010;18:837–45.

110. McGough C, Baldwin C, Frost G et al. Br J Cancer 2004; 90:2278–87.

111. Zimmerer T, Bocker U, Wenz F et al. Z Gastroenterol 2008; 46:441–8.

112. Conger AD. Rad Res 1973;53:338–47.

113. Hovan AJ, Williams PM, Stevenson-Moore P et al. Support Care Cancer 2010;18:1081–87.

114. Chasen MR, Bhargava R. Support Care Cancer 2009;17: 1345–51.

115. Mohan A, Singh P, Kumar S et al. Asian Pac J Cancer Prev 2008;9:557–62.

116. Marin Caro MM, Laviano A et al. Clin Nutr 2007;26: 289–301.

117. Kwang AY, Kandiah M. Am J Hosp Palliat Care 2010;27:117–26.

118. Namukwaya E, Leng M, Downing J et al. Pain Res Treat 2011;2011:393–404.

119. Brown CG, McGuire DB, Peterson DE et al. Cancer Nurs 2009;32:259–70.

120. Brown CG, Beck SL, Peterson DE et al. Support Care Cancer 2009;17:413–28.
121. Murphy BA, Gilbert J, Cmelak A et al. Clin Adv Hematol Oncol 2007;5:807–22.
122. Scalera G. Nutr Neurosci 2002;5:159–88.
123. Schwartz MD, Jacobsen PB, Bovbjerg DH. Physiol Behav 1996;59:659–63.
124. Mattes RD, Curran WJ Jr, Powlis W et al. Physiol Behav 1991;50:1103–9.
125. Mattes RD, Curran WJ Jr, Alavi J et al. Cancer 1992;70:192–200.
126. Falconi M, Pederzoli P. Gut 2001;49(Suppl 4):iv2–10.
127. Nelson KA, Walsh D, Sheehan FA. J Clin Oncol 1994;12:213–25.
128. Lecleire S, Di Fiore F, Antonietti M et al. Gastrointest Endosc 2006;64:479–84.
129. Mourao F, Amado D, Ravasco P et al. Nutr Hosp 2004;19:83–8.
130. Ravasco P, Monteiro-Grillo I, Vidal PM et al. Support Care Cancer 2004;12:246–52.
131. Bachmann P, Marti-Massoud C, Blanc-Vincent MP et al. Br J Cancer 2003;89(Suppl 1):S107–10.
132. Mackenzie ML, Gramlich L. Appl Physiol Nutr Metab 2008;33:1–11.
133. ASPEN Board of Directors. JPEN J Parenter Enteral Nutr 2002;26:1SA–138SA.
134. De Groote MA, Frank DN, Dowell E et al. Pediatr Infect Dis J 2005;24:278–80.
135. Ziegler TR, Evans ME, Fernandez-Estivariz C et al. Annu Rev Nutr 2003;23:229–61.
136. Kahl S, Malfertheiner P. Best Pract Res Clin Gastroenterol 2004;18:947–55.
137. Scholmerich J. Best Pract Res Clin Gastroenterol 2004;18:917–33.
138. August DA, Huhmann MB. JPEN J Parenter Enteral Nutr 2009;33:472–500.
139. Bloch A. Semin Oncol Nurs 2000;16:122–7.
140. Huhmann MB, August DA. Nutr Clin Pract 2009;24:520–6.
141. McMahon K, Brown JK. Semin Oncol Nurs 2000;16:106–12.
142. Bloch A, Charuhas P. Cancer and cancer therapy. In: Gottschlich M, ed. The Science and Practice of Nutrition Support. Dubuque, IA: Kendall Hunt, 2001:148–64.
143. Bozzetti F. Nutrition 2002;18:953–9.
144. Linn BS, Robinson DS, Klimas NG. Ann Surg 1988;207:267–73.
145. Nguyen TV, Yueh B. Cancer 2002;95:553–62.
146. Andreoli A, De Lorenzo A, Cadeddu F et al. Eur Rev Med Pharmacol Sci 2011;15:469–80.
147. Ottery FD. Nutrition 1996;12:S15–9.
148. Wigmore SJ, Plester CE, Richardson RA et al. Br J Cancer 1997;75:106–9.
149. Detsky AS, McLaughlin JR, Baker JP et al. JPEN J Parenter Enteral Nutr 1987;11:8–13.
150. Franch-Arcas G. Clin Nutr 2001;20:265–9.
151. Harvey KB, Moldawer LL, Bistrian BR et al. Am J Clin Nutr 1981;34:2013–22.
152. Committee CoPCQM. J Am Diet Assoc 1994;94:838–9.
153. Isenring E, Bauer J, Capra S. Eur J Clin Nutr 2003;57:305–9.
154. Luthringer S, Kulakowski K. Medical nutrition therapy protocols. In: McCallum P, Polisena C, eds. The Clinical Guide to Oncology Nutrition. Chicago: American Dietetic Association, 2000:24–44.
155. Ferguson M. Oncology 2003;17:13–4; discussion 4–6.
156. Lacey K, Pritchett E. J Am Dietet Assoc 2003;103:1061–72.
157. Ralph JL, Von Ah D, Scheett AJ et al. Clin J Oncol Nurs 2011;15:E114–21.
158. Tripp R. Health Care Food Nutr Focus 2005;22:3–8.
159. Robien K, Levin R, Pritchett E et al. J Am Diet Assoc 2006;106:946–51.
160. Tesauro GM, Rowland JH, Lustig C. Cancer Pract 2002;10:277–83.
161. Isenring E, Bauer J, Capra S. Nutr Dietet 2004;61:46–9.
162. Isenring E, Capra S, Bauer J. J Hum Nutr Diet 2004;17:145–52.
163. Piquet MA, Ozsahin M, Larpin I et al. Support Care Cancer 2002;10:502–4.
164. Ravasco P, Monteiro-Grillo I, Vidal PM et al. J Clin Oncol 2005;23:1431–8.
165. Foschi D, Cavagna G, Callioni F et al. Br J Surg 1986;73:716–9.
166. Meijerink WJ, von Meyenfeldt MF, Rouflart MM et al. Lancet 1992;340:187–8.
167. Muller JM, Brenner U, Dienst C et al. Lancet 1982;1:68–71.
168. Muller JM, Keller HW, Brenner U et al. World J Surg 1986;10:53–63.
169. Bozzetti F, Braga M, Gianotti L et al. Lancet 2001;358:1487–92.
170. Wu GH, Liu ZH, Wu ZH et al. World J Gastroenterol 2006;12:2441–4.
171. Daly JM, Lieberman MD, Goldfine J et al. Surgery 1992;112:56–67.
172. Daly JM, Weintraub FN, Shou J et al. Ann Surg 1995;221:327–38.
173. Di Carlo V, Gianotti L, Balzano G et al. Dig Surg 1999;16:320–6.
174. Braga M, Gianotti L, Vignali A et al. Crit Care Med 1998;26:24–30.
175. Senkal M, Zumtobel V, Bauer KH et al. Arch Surg 1999;134:1309–16.
176. Gianotti L, Braga M, Nespoli L et al. Gastroenterology 2002;122:1763–70.
177. Braga M, Gianotti L, Nespoli L et al. Arch Surg 2002;137:174–80.
178. Farreras N, Artigas V, Cardona D et al. Clin Nutr 2005;24:55–65.
179. Braga M, Gianotti L, Vignali A et al. Surgery 2002;132:805–14.
180. de Luis DA, Izaola O, Cuellar L et al. Eur J Clin Nutr 2004;58:1505–8.
181. Morlion BJ, Stehle P, Wachtler P et al. Ann Surg 1998;227:302–8.
182. Gianotti L, Braga M, Vignali A et al. Arch Surg 1997;132:1222–9; discussion 9–30.
183. Sand J, Luostarinen M, Matikainen M. Eur J Surg 1997;163:761–6.
184. Shirabe K, Matsumata T, Shimada M et al. Hepatogastroenterology 1997;44:205–9.
185. Braga M, Gianotti L, Gentilini O et al. Crit Care Med 2001;29:242–8.
186. Aiko S, Yoshizumi Y, Sugiura Y et al. Surg Today 2001;31:971–8.
187. Jiang XH, Li N, Li JS. World J Gastroenterol 2003;9:1878–80.
188. Hyltander A, Drott C, Unsgaard B et al. Eur J Clin Invest 1991;21:413–20.
189. Aiko S, Yoshizumi Y, Matsuyama T et al. Jpn J Thorac Cardiovasc Surg 2003;51:263–71.
190. Goonetilleke KS, Siriwardena AK. JOP 2006;7:5–13.
191. August D, Huhmann M. Nutritional care of cancer patients. In: Norton J, Barie P, Bollinger R et al, eds. Surgery: Basic Science and Clinical Evidence. 2nd ed. New York: Springer, 2008:2123–50.

192. Braunschweig CL, Levy P, Sheean PM et al. Am J Clin Nutr 2001;74:534–42.
193. Koretz RL, Avenell A, Lipman TO et al. Am J Gastroenterol 2007;102:412–29; quiz 68.
194. Tandon SP, Gupta SC, Sinha SN et al. Indian J Med Res 1984;80:180–8.
195. Bozzetti F, Cozzaglio L, Gavazzi C et al. Tumori 1998;84:681–6.
196. Beer KT, Krause KB, Zuercher T et al. Nutr Cancer 2005;52:29–34.
197. Gavazzi C, Bhoori S, Lovullo S et al. Am J Gastroenterol 2006;101:374–9.
198. Mangar S, Slevin N, Mais K et al. Radiother Oncol 2006;78:152–8.
199. Rabinovitch R, Grant B, Berkey BA et al. Head Neck 2006;28:287–96.
200. Bozzetti F. Clin Nutr 2011;30:714–7.
201. Huckleberry Y. Am J Health Syst Pharm 2004;61:671–82; quiz 83–4.
202. Shike M, Russel DM, Detsky AS et al. Ann Intern Med 1984;101:303–9.
203. Klein S, Kinney J, Jeejeebhoy K et al. JPEN J Parenter Enteral Nutr 1997;21:133–56.
204. Fearon KC, Luff R. Proc Nutr Soc 2003;62:807–11.
205. Klein S, Simes J, Blackburn GL. Cancer 1986;58:1378–86.
206. McGeer AJ, Detsky AS, O'Rourke K. Nutrition 1990;6:233–40.
207. American College of Physicians. Ann Intern Med 1989;110:734–6.
208. Scolapio JS, Picco MF, Tarrosa VB. JPEN J Parenter Enteral Nutr 2002;26:248–50.
209. Sikora SS, Ribeiro U, Kane JM 3rd et al. Support Care Cancer 2009;17:83–90
210. American Gastroenterological Association. Gastroenterology 2001;121:966–9.
211. Popp MB, Wagner SC, Brito OJ. Surgery 1983;94:300–8.
212. Daly J, Thorn A. Neoplastic diseases. In: Kinney J, Jeejeebhoy K, Hill G et al, eds. Nutrition and Metabolism in Patient Care. Philadelphia: Saunders, 1988:567–87.
213. Torosian MH. JPEN J Parenter Enteral Nutr 1992;16:72S–5S.
214. Heys SD, Park KG, McNurlan MA et al. Br J Surg 1991;78:483–7.
215. Pacelli F, Bossola M, Teodori L et al. JPEN J Parenter Enteral Nutr 2007;31:451–5.
216. Andrew IM, Waterfield K, Hildreth AJ et al. Palliat Med 2009;23:680–8.
217. Reid J, McKenna H, Fitzsimons D et al. Int J Nurs Stud 2009;46:606–16.
218. Bartlett DL, Stein TP, Torosian MH. Surgery 1995;117:260–7.
219. Wolf RF, Ng B, Weksler B et al. Ann Surg Oncol 1994;1:314–20.
220. Ng EH, Rock CS, Lazarus DD et al. Am J Physiol 1992;262:R426–31.
221. Tomas FM, Chandler CS, Coyle P, et al. Biochem J 1994;301:769–75.
222. Ottery FD, Walsh D, Strawford A. Semin Oncol 1998;25:35–44.
223. Wren AM, Seal LJ, Cohen MA et al. J Clin Endocrinol Metab 2001;86:5992.
224. Hanada T, Toshinai K, Kajimura N et al. Biochem Biophys Res Commun 2003;301:275–9.
225. DeBoer MD. Nutrition 2008;24:806–14.
226. Lissoni P. Support Care Cancer 2002;10:110–6.
227. Wolf RF, Pearlstone DB, Newman E et al. Ann Surg 1992;216:280–8.
228. Gullett NP, Mazurak VC, Hebbar G et al. Curr Prob Cancer 2011;35:58–90.
229. Loprinzi CL, Michalak JC, Schaid DJ et al. J Clin Oncol 1993;11:762–7.
230. De Conno F, Martini C, Zecca E et al. Eur J Cancer 1998;34:1705–9.
231. Skarlos DV, Fountzilas G, Pavlidis N et al. Acta Oncol 1993;32:37–41.
232. Yeh S, Wu SY, Levine DM et al. J Nutr Health Aging 2000;4:246–51.
233. Mantovani G, Maccio A, Madeddu C et al. Nutrition 2008;24:305–13.
234. Jatoi A, Windschitl HE, Loprinzi CL et al. J Clin Oncol 2002;20:567–73.
235. Moertel CG, Kvols LK, Rubin J. Cancer 1991;67:33–6.
236. Fanelli M, Sarmiento R, Gattuso D et al. Expert Opin Invest Drugs 2003;12:1211–25.
237. Dezube BJ, Sherman ML, Fridovich-Keil JL et al. Cancer Immunol Immunother 1993;36:57–60.
238. Goldberg RM, Loprinzi CL, Mailliard JA et al. J Clin Oncol 1995;13:2856–9.
239. Fearon KC, Barber MD, Moses AG et al. J Clin Oncol 2006;24:3401–7.
240. Mazzotta P, Jeney CM. J Pain Symptom Manage 2009;37:1069–77.
241. Licitra L, Spinazze S, Roila F. Crit Rev Oncol Hematol 2002;43:93–101.
242. Grunberg SM, Deuson RR, Mavros P et al. Cancer 2004;100:2261–8.
243. Fisch M. J Natl Cancer Inst Monogr 2004:105–11.
244. Valente SM, Saunders JM, Cohen MZ. Cancer Pract 1994;2:65–71.
245. Homsi J, Nelson KA, Sarhill N et al. Am J Hosp Palliat Care 2001;18:403–7.
246. Kulkarni SK, Kaur G. Drugs Today (Barc) 2001;37:559–71.
247. Theobald DE, Kirsh KL, Holtsclaw E et al. J Pain Symptom Manage 2002;23:442–7.
248. Fernandez F, Adams F. Head Neck Surg 1986;8:296–300.
249. Abernethy AP, Wheeler JL, Zafar SY. Curr Opin Support Palliat Care 2009;3:41–9.
250. Huhmann MB. The Impact of Medical Nutrition Therapy by a Registered Dietitian on Clinical and Patient Oriented Outcomes in Cancer Patients. Newark, NJ: University of Medicine and Dentistry of New Jersey, 2008.
251. Network NCC. NCCN Clinical Practice Guidelines in Oncology: Palliative Care. In. Fort Washington, PA: National Comprehensive Cancer Network, 2010.
252. Lagman RL, Davis MP, LeGrand SB et al. Surg Clin North Am 2005;85:237–55.
253. Roeland E, Mitchell W, Elia G et al. J Support Oncol 2010;8:100–16.
254. Horsley P, Bauer J, Gallagher B. Bone Marrow Transplant 2005;35:1113–6.
255. Lenssen P, Sherry ME, Cheney CL et al. J Am Dietet Assoc 1990;90:835–42.
256. Charuhas PM, Fosberg KL, Bruemmer B et al. JPEN J Parenter Enteral Nutr 1997;21:157–61.
257. Muscaritoli M, Conversano L, Torelli GF et al. Transplantation 1998;66:610–6.
258. Roberts S, Miller J, Pineiro L et al. Bone Marrow Transplant 2003;32:715–21.

259. Szeluga DJ, Stuart RK, Brookmeyer R et al. Cancer Res 1987;47:3309–16.
260. Ziegler TR, Young LS, Benfell K et al. Ann Intern Med 1992;116:821–8.
261. Schloerb PR, Amare M. JPEN J Parenter Enteral Nutr 1993;17:407–13.
262. Papapietro K, Diaz E, Csendes A et al. Rev Med Chil 2002;130:1125–30.
263. De-Souza DA, Greene LJ. Crit Care Med 2005;33:1125–35.
264. Yao GX, Xue XB, Jiang ZM et al. Clin Nutr 2005;24:510–5.
265. Song JX, Qing SH, Huang XC et al. Di Yi Jun Yi Da Xue Xue Bao 2002;22:545–7.
266. Nakamura K, Kariyazono H, Komokata T et al. Nutrition 2005;21:639–49.
267. Novaes MR, Lima LA, Novaes LC et al. Ann Nutr Metab 2004;48:404–8.
268. Heys SD, Gough DB, Khan L et al. Br J Surg 1996;83:608–19.
269. van Bokhorst-De Van Der Schueren MA, Quak JJ, von Blomberg-van der Flier BM et al. Am J Clin Nutr 2001;73:323–32.
270. De Luis DA, Izaola O, Aller R et al. Ann Nutr Metab 2005;49:95–9.
271. De Luis DA, Izaola O, Cuellar L et al. Eur Rev Med Pharmacol Sci 2009;13:279–83.
272. Buijs N, van Bokhorst-de van der Schueren MA, Langius JA et al. Am J Clin Nutr 2010;92:1151–6.
273. Jho DH, Cole SM, Lee EM, et al. Integr Cancer Ther 2004;3:98–111.
274. Hardman WE. J Nutr 2002;132:3508S–12S.
275. Jatoi A, Rowland K, Loprinzi CL et al. J Clin Oncol 2004;22:2469–76.
276. Fearon K, von Meyenfeldt MF, Moses A et al. Eur J Cancer 2001;37:S27–S8.
277. Moses AW, Slater C, Preston T. Br J Cancer 2004;90:996–1002.
278. Wachtler P, Konig W, Senkal M et al. J Trauma 1997;42:191–8.
279. Savarese DM, Savy G, Vahdat L et al. Cancer Treat Rev 2003;29:501–13.
280. Scheid C, Hermann K, Kremer G et al. Nutrition 2004;20:249–54.
281. Wang Y, Jiang ZM, Nolan MT et al. JPEN J Parenter Enteral Nutr 2010;34:521–9.
282. Nose S, Wasa M, Tazuke Y et al. JPEN J Parenter Enteral Nutr 2010;34:530–7.
283. Marik PE, Zaloga GP. JPEN J Parenter Enteral Nutr 2010;34:378–86.
284. Waitzberg DL, Saito H, Plank LD et al. World J Surg 2006;30:1592–604.
285. Beale RJ, Bryg DJ, Bihari DJ. Crit Care Med 1999;27:2799–805.
286. Cerantola Y, Hubner M, Grass F et al. Br J Surg 2011;98:37–48.
287. Heys SD, Walker LG, Smith I et al. Ann Surg 1999;229:467–77.
288. Howard L. JPEN J Parenter Enteral Nutr 1992;16:93S–9S.
289. Orrevall Y, Tishelman C, Permert J et al. Palliat Med 2009;23:556–64.
290. Lundholm K, Daneryd P, Bosaeus I et al. Cancer 2004;100:1967–77.
291. Shang E, Weiss C, Post S et al. JPEN J Parenter Enteral Nutr 2006;30:222–30.

SUGGESTED READINGS

August DA, Huhmann MB. A.S.P.E.N. clinical guidelines: nutrition support therapy during adult anticancer treatment and in hematopoietic cell transplantation. JPEN J Parenter Enteral Nutr 2009;33:472–500.

Bozzetti F. Nutritional support in oncologic patients: where we are and where we are going. Clin Nutr 2011;30:714–7.

Grosvenor M, Bulcavage L, Chlebowski RT. Symptoms potentially influencing weight loss in a cancer population. Correlations with primary site, nutritional status, and chemotherapy administration. Cancer 1989;63:330–4.

Paccagnella A, Morello M, Da Mosto MC et al. Early nutritional intervention improves treatment tolerance and outcomes in head and neck cancer patients undergoing concurrent chemoradiotherapy. Support Care Cancer 2010;18:837–45.

Tong H, Isenring E, Yates P. The prevalence of nutrition impact symptoms and their relationship to quality of life and clinical outcomes in medical oncology patients. Support Care Cancer 2009;17:83–90.

89 BONE BIOLOGY IN HEALTH AND DISEASE[1]
ROBERT P. HEANEY

---

[1]**Abbreviations: Al**, aluminum; **BMD**, bone mineral density; **[Ca²⁺]**, concentration of calcium ions; **CT**, calcitonin; **DXA**, dual-energy x-ray absorptiometry; **ECF**, extracellular fluid; **OI**, osteogenesis imperfecta; **PTH**, parathyroid hormone; **RANKL**, rank ligand.

BONE COMPOSITION AND STRUCTURE

Bone is a tissue in which cells make up only 2% to 5% of the volume, and nonliving material make up 95% to 98%. It is the nonliving material that gives the bone its basic mechanical properties of hardness, stiffness, and resiliency. This nonliving material consists of a mineral-encrusted protein matrix (also called osteoid), with the mineral comprising about half the volume and the organic matrix the other half. Unlike other connective tissues, virtually no free water is present in the bony material itself. Embedded in this solid material are cells, called osteocytes, residing in lacunae in the matrix and communicating with one another through an extensive network of long cellular processes lying in channels called canaliculi, which ramify throughout the bone. As a consequence of this arrangement, virtually no volume of normal bone is more than a few micrometers from a living cell. Furthermore, even in the dense bone of the shafts of long bones, an extensive network of vascular channels exists, so the most remote osteocyte is typically no more than 90 μm away from a capillary.

Bone Mineral

The mineral of bone is a carbonate-rich, imperfect hydroxyapatite with variable stoichiometry. Calcium comprises 37% to 40%, phosphate 50% to 58%, and carbonate 2% to 8% of this mineral. These values vary somewhat from species to species, and the carbonate component is particularly sensitive to systemic acid–base status (decreasing in acidosis and increasing in alkalosis). In addition, bone mineral contains small amounts of sodium, potassium, magnesium, citrate, and other ions present in the extracellular fluid (ECF) at the time the mineral was deposited, adsorbed onto the crystal surfaces, and trapped there, as the water in the recently deposited matrix is displaced by the growing mineral crystals.

Protein Matrix

The protein matrix of bone, as for tendons, ligaments, and dermis, consists predominantly of collagen, which comprises approximately 90% of the organic matrix. For bone, the collagen is type I. Collagen is a long, fibrous protein, coiled as a triple helix. For the molecules of the protein to coil tightly, no side chains can project from the peptide backbone on the side facing inward. Hence, every third amino acid in the body of the collagen molecule is glycine, which has no side chain. However, projecting outward are the side chains of various other amino acids, such as lysine, which allow the posttranslational formation of tight, covalent bonds between collagen fibers. This cross-linking helps to prevent fibers from sliding along one another when bone is stressed along the axis of the fibers.

Noncollagenous Matrix Proteins

Noncollagenous proteins make up approximately 10% of the organic matrix of bone (1). These proteins include a family of proteins in which glutamic acid residues are carboxylated in the γ position, called gla-proteins, the best studied of which is osteocalcin (or bone gla-protein), which comprises approximately 1.5% of the matrix proteins. Other gla-proteins include osteonectin, fibronectin, matrix gla-protein, osteopontin, and bone sialoprotein. The functions of these many constituents are not entirely clear. Some doubtless serve as chemoattractants for osteoclasts or as points of osteoclast attachment, whereas others stimulate osteoblasts to lay down new bone. Because of these properties of the matrix proteins, bone seems to contain some of the chemical signals for its own remodeling (see later).

The shape and three-dimensional structure of bone are determined by its protein matrix. A bone that has been completely demineralized in the laboratory (by soaking in ethylenediaminetetraacetic or other acid) looks entirely normal; and when sectioned, stained, and examined under a microscope, it reveals all the fine structure of bone. In fact, prior demineralization has been the traditional first step in studying bone histologically (because mineralized bone tends to damage the microtome knives used by histologists to make their sections).

BONE CELLS AND THEIR FUNCTIONS

The four principal bone cells are lining cells, osteoblasts, osteoclasts, and osteocytes. They are responsible both for maintaining the mechanical properties of bone and mediating the calcium homeostatic function of bone.

Lining cells are flat, fibrocyte-like cells covering free surfaces of bone. They are most probably derived from, or closely related to, the osteoblast cell line. They form a membrane that completely covers free bone surfaces and insulates bone from the cells and hormones in the general circulation. They demarcate a virtual compartment between the lining cells on one side and mature bone on the other. This compartment is continuous with the space in canaliculi surrounding osteocyte processes and may well have different ionic composition from that of the ECF located outside, that is, between the lining cells and the capillaries of bone. It is possible that lining cells, by adjusting ion fluxes between the ECF and the

bone compartment, may contribute to the maintenance of calcium ion concentrations in the ECF.

Osteoblasts are derived from marrow stromal cells; they are the cells that lay down bone, first by synthesizing, depositing, and orienting the fibrous proteins of the matrix, and then by initiating changes that render the matrix capable of mineralization. Osteoblasts deposit this matrix between and beneath themselves on a preexisting bone surface, thereby pushing themselves backward as they add new bone.

Bone matrix, when freshly deposited, consists of about half protein and half water and is not immediately mineralizable, just as the similar collagen-based structures, tendon and ligament, do not normally calcify. So the osteoblast still has more work to do after forming and depositing the matrix. The details of the process are not completely clear, but they involve secretion of proteins by the osteoblast into the matrix that it had just previously laid down. These somehow help to create a three-dimensional configuration that allows calcium and phosphate ions in the ECF to arrange themselves in the apatite crystal habitus. Osteoblasts also secrete an enzyme called alkaline phosphatase that hydrolyzes various phosphate compounds in the local environment, thereby increasing phosphate ion concentration at the mineralizing site and at the same time removing natural crystal inhibitors (e.g., pyrophosphate). Finally, as mineral is deposited, it displaces the water of the original matrix. The apatite crystals that form are spindle shaped and are oriented parallel to and between the collagen fibers.

Osteoclasts are derived from the monocyte–macrophage line of cells, are usually multinucleated, and are the cells that resorb bone. They do this first by attaching firmly to a microscopic bony surface and then walling off a small region of that surface. The attachment involves linkage between proteins called integrins in the cell membrane of the osteoclast with proteins in the bone matrix, such as osteopontin, that exhibit a particular amino acid sequence (RGD, i.e., arginine-glycine-asparagine). Once firmly attached, osteoclasts secrete acid and proteolytic enzymes into this confined space. These dissolve the mineral and digest the matrix. The osteoclasts then release the breakdown products into the ECF around the resorption site, whence they are carried away by the circulating blood. After working for a short period of time (measured in days), the osteoclasts undergo programmed cell death (apoptosis), leaving their excavation to be refilled by osteoblasts. The calcium they dissolve from bone mineral seems to trigger or augment this apoptotic process, as osteoclasts blocked from producing acid accumulate on bone surfaces and have longer life spans. When examined histologically in sections of bone, these processes necessarily appear localized. However, the activity is more typically a "project," moving along a bony surface, with osteoclastic work preceding and the osteoblastic formation filling in behind.

The calcium and phosphorus released into the bloodstream at a resorption site will usually be used to mineralize remodeling sites elsewhere in the skeleton, currently in their formation phase. However, the protein fragments are metabolized or excreted. Some of the amino acids released in collagen degradation reenter the body's amino acid pool and can be reused for protein synthesis elsewhere. However, those that have undergone posttranslational modification (e.g., proline to hydroxyproline and the amino acids involved in collagen cross-linking) cannot be reused. For this reason, bone remodeling requires a continuing supply of fresh dietary protein.

Osteocytes are osteoblasts that have stopped matrix synthesis and have become embedded in bone as the other bone-forming cells around them continue to add new layers of matrix. Osteocytes are responsible for monitoring the amount of strain (bending) that occurs in their domains when bone is mechanically loaded and for reporting that information to lining cells on nearby anatomic bone surfaces, which may then initiate local bone remodeling projects. One of the ways they do this is by secreting a hormone, sclerostin, that reduces osteoblast activity (see below). The full extent of their function is not known, but it is clear that bone with dead osteocytes (from whatever cause) is often excessively fragile.

The activity of these bone cells is influenced by a large number of both systemic and local hormonal agents. Additionally, the cells influence the activity of one another. Table 89.1 lists a few of the many agents influencing osteoblasts and osteoclasts (see the later section on revision of bony material). This is a rapidly developing field of investigation, and much is still to be learned. The osteoblasts, or cells of the osteoblast lineage, occupy a central position, not only in forming bone but also in processing systemic signals to the bone remodeling apparatus (see the later section on revision of bony material). Thus, although parathyroid hormone (PTH) is responsible for stimulating bone resorption, no PTH receptors are present on the osteoclast. Rather, they are found on osteoblasts (and related cells) that, in response to PTH binding, release or express on their surfaces agents (e.g., RANK ligand [RANKL]) that stimulate osteoclast activity. By contrast, the osteoclasts do possess

calcitonin (CT) receptors and are thus able to respond very rapidly to the antiresorptive signal provided by secreted CT.

BONE ARCHITECTURE

Bone consists of a dense outer shell, or cortex, and an internal, chambered system of interconnected plates, rods, and spicules called cancellous or trabecular bone (Fig. 89.1). In the shafts of the long bones, the cortical component predominates, creating a hollow tube, whereas nearer the joints, the cortex becomes thinner and the interior is made up of an extensive latticework of cancellous bone. Bones such as the vertebrae, pelvis, sternum, and shoulder blades possess a thin outer rind of cortex and a more or less even distribution of cancellous bone on the inside. The internal, three-dimensional architecture of cancellous bone is arranged along the lines of force that a particular bone experiences and hence provides maximum structural strength with minimum material.

The proportions both of mineral and matrix and of calcium and phosphorus are essentially identical in cortical and cancellous bone. Sometimes the issue has been confused in the literature because of the difficulty of removing adherent marrow elements from cancellous bone samples before chemical analysis. Fundamentally, however, bone is bone. On the other hand, cancellous bone turns over (remodels) much more rapidly than cortical bone. This is partly because of the much greater surface area of cancellous bone. (Remodeling always starts from a microanatomic bone surface and burrows into the bony material. See the later section on revision of bony material.) It is also partly the result of the generally greater contact with hemopoietic marrow in cancellous bone.

TABLE 89.1	HUMORAL FACTORS ACTING ON BONE CELLS
OSTEOBLASTS	**OSTEOCLASTS**
Parathyroid hormone	Calcitonin
1,25(OH)$_2$ vitamin D	Bisphosphonate drugs
Glucocorticoids	Interleukin-1
Insulinlike growth factors (IGFs)	Colony-stimulating factor-1 (CSF-1)
Transforming growth factor-β (TGF-β)	TGF-α
Interleukin-6	TGF-β
	RANK ligand
Parathyroid hormone–related peptide (PTHrP)	Gallium nitrate
Osteoprotegerin	
Bone morphogenetic protein (BMP)	
Sclerostin	

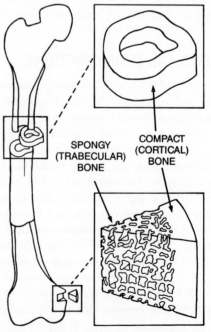

Fig. 89.1. Gross and microarchitecture of a typical long bone. (Copyright Robert P. Heaney, 1996.)

of bone contains more calcium than the entire circulating blood volume in an adult. Thus, in comparison with other nutrients, the calcium reserve is huge. Although low-calcium diets usually deplete the bony reserves, they do so slowly. Thus, whereas the *population-level* risk of fracture rises immediately, it will take many years for bone strength to be sufficiently reduced to lead to a perceptible increase in an *individual person's* risk of fracture (see earlier). The slow expression of the effect of calcium deficiency led many nutritional scientists in the past to the erroneous (and seemingly nonsensical) conclusion that calcium was not important for adult bone strength. Nevertheless, a nutritional deficiency that develops over 30 years is just as truly a deficiency as one that develops over 30 days.

Low intakes of calcium and phosphorus can both limit bone acquisition during growth and cause bone loss after maturity. Calcium intake operates most directly through modulation of remodeling, as described earlier. In the antler example previously cited, if summer foliage were not calcium rich, each cycle of antler formation would deplete the skeleton, bony replacement would fail to occur, and bone mass would fall progressively over the animal's adult life. Because human calcium requirements rise with age (3), and because calcium intakes tend to fall in elderly persons, precisely such depletion occurs in most human populations as they age.

Inadequate phosphorus availability also affects bone, but in a different way. The osteoblast environment is one of continuous mineralization, with the matrix extracting phosphate (as well as calcium) from the fluid bathing the bone-forming cells. Although calcium makes up approximately 40% of the bone mineral, phosphate (PO_4^{3-}) accounts for nearly 60%. Thus, phosphorus is fully as important for bone building as is calcium. Rapid growth is not possible without a high blood phosphate concentration, a fact that explains the substantially higher blood phosphate values in children. When phosphate concentrations in the blood entering bone are low, mineralization extracts as much phosphate from the blood as it can, but in so doing, it creates a local environment severely depleted of phosphate. Osteoblasts, like all cells, need phosphate for their own metabolism. The result is serious interference with osteoblast function: matrix deposition is slowed, and osteoblast initiation of mineralization is reduced even more. These abnormalities produce the typical histologic pattern of rickets and osteomalacia in bone (see later).

Vitamin D

Vitamin D has many bony effects, such as facilitating the development of osteoclast precursors at an activated remodeling locus and augmenting osteoclast response to resorptive stimuli. The vitamin also stimulates synthesis and release of osteocalcin by osteoblasts (see earlier). However, its major importance for bone is its facilitation of intestinal absorption of calcium (and to some extent phosphorus) from the diet. Severe vitamin D deficiency causes rickets and osteomalacia (see later). Milder shortages of the vitamin reduce calcium availability to the body and produce a situation of calcium deficiency, resulting in osteoporosis. Because of the traditional (if simplistic) identification of vitamin D deficiency with rickets and osteomalacia, it has been customary to refer to less extreme degrees of vitamin D shortage as *insufficiency*. This distinction is no longer useful. All degrees of vitamin D inadequacy that produce disease should be termed *deficiency*.

Vitamin K

Vitamin K functions in the γ-carboxylation of the glutamic acid residues of several bone gla-proteins, the best studied of which is osteocalcin. Vitamin K deficiency results both in undercarboxylation of osteocalcin and in reduced osteocalcin synthesis. The net effect of these changes on bone strength or integrity is not certain. However, low vitamin K status is associated in epidemiologic studies with low bone mass, increased hip fracture risk, and increased cardiovascular mortality (4).

Micronutrients

Vitamin C and certain trace minerals (notably copper, zinc, and manganese) are important cofactors for the synthesis or cross-linking of matrix proteins. Copper and vitamin C are perhaps the best studied in this regard. Copper is the cofactor for lysyl oxidase, the enzyme responsible for cross-linking collagen fibrils. Interference with cross-linking results in structurally weak bone. Ascorbic acid is also a required cofactor for the cross-linking of collagen fibrils; and in its absence, bone strength is impaired. In the presence of deficiencies of these micronutrients during growth, severe bone abnormalities can result. These abnormalities include stunting of growth, deformity of bones, and epiphyseal dysplasia. Whether adults can develop sufficient deficiencies of these nutrients to interfere significantly with bone integrity remains unknown.

SKELETAL DISORDERS AND THEIR NUTRITIONAL CORRELATES

Osteoporosis

Osteoporosis is a multifactorial condition of the skeleton in which skeletal strength is reduced sufficiently so that fractures occur on minor trauma. Generally, osteoporosis exhibits reduced bone mass (i.e., both matrix and mineral) as well as various microstructural disturbances of bony architecture (5). A simple decrease in quantity of bone is sometimes called osteopenia (literally, "shortage of bone"). By current World Health Organization standards, bone mass is measured by x-ray absorptiometry as an areal density, termed *bone mineral density* (BMD, sometimes aBMD). Osteopenia is characterized by a BMD value at hip or spine between 1 and 2.5 standard deviations below the young normal adult mean. BMD values more than 2.5 standard deviations below young adult normal are now called osteoporosis, whether or not a fracture is present. BMD is, unfortunately, a poor way to represent bone structural strength, because it explicitly eliminates the important influence of bone size. A larger bone with a lower density is usually stronger—less likely to fracture—than a smaller, denser bone.

A common feature of most cases of osteoporosis is elevated bone remodeling, particularly in postmenopausal women (6). Remodeling activity, although designed to repair weakened bone, actually makes it temporarily weaker during the remodeling process; and when remodeling is in excess of mechanical need, it causes only weakness. Estrogen deficiency, low calcium intake, and vitamin D deficiency all contribute to a harmful postmenopausal rise in bone remodeling.

Lack of exercise and alcohol abuse also contribute to the development of this disorder. Given diets typical of the elderly persons in Europe and North America, it can be estimated that inadequate calcium intake and low vitamin D status are responsible for one third to two thirds of all osteoporotic fractures. (For this reason, the US Food and Drug Administration allows an osteoporosis health claim on the labels of certain calcium-rich foods.)

Rickets and Osteomalacia

Rickets is a disorder of the growth apparatus of bone (see earlier) in which the growth cartilage fails to mature and mineralize normally (7). Growth is stunted, and various deformities about the growth plates occur. Osteomalacia is the corresponding disorder in adults, in whom newly deposited bone matrix fails to mineralize adequately. New matrix formation is slowed in both conditions, but mineralization is retarded even more; thus, unmineralized matrix accumulates on microscopic bone surfaces. For this reason, the proportion of mineral to matrix drops. In severe cases, unmineralized bone may constitute so large a proportion of the skeleton that individual bones lose their stiffness and become severely deformed (bowed legs and misshapen pelves).

The stereotypical forms of rickets and osteomalacia are those associated with vitamin D deficiency. The principal pathogenesis of these common forms follows from insufficient intestinal absorption mainly of calcium (and to some extent phosphorus) from the diet. In attempting to keep blood calcium concentrations close to normal values, the body raises PTH secretion. Because one of the effects of PTH is to increase renal clearance of phosphate, this adaptive response drives the already reduced blood phosphate concentrations down to concentrations such that severe phosphate deficiency develops, first locally in the vicinity of the osteoblasts and chondrocytes and then in other tissues as well (producing, e.g., muscle weakness, tenderness, and pain).

Rickets and osteomalacia also develop for reasons other than vitamin D deficiency, including extreme calcium deficiency, fluoride toxicity, and cadmium poisoning, as well as in association with certain rare vascular malignant diseases. The toxins or products of tumor metabolism, such as fibroblast growth factor-23 (FGF-23), interfere with normal osteoblast function or, alternatively, lower the renal phosphorus threshold. Typical of the latter mechanism is a group of heritable abnormalities of renal phosphate transport, the most common of which is X-linked hypophosphatemia (8). These conditions have in common the inability to maintain the blood phosphate concentrations required for growth. Such forms of rickets, just like that owing to vitamin D deficiency, produce their bony effects primarily because of severe hypophosphatemia. This group of disorders in the past was called vitamin D–resistant rickets. These disorders do not respond to usual doses of vitamin D (hence their name). Therapy is directed at elevating serum phosphate.

Paget's Disease of Bone

Paget's disease is a local but often multifocal disorder of the bone remodeling process of uncertain etiology. Resorption proceeds erratically, with formation filling in with new bone behind it. Bone architecture and even external bone shape are disordered. During the early resorptive phase, the bone is excessively fragile and may fracture readily. The high level of bone remodeling is usually accompanied by high concentrations of remodeling markers (see later), particularly serum alkaline phosphatase. When the process involves the skull, bony growths may constrict the cranial nerve passages and may lead to deafness, for example. No nutritional correlates of this disorder are known.

Parathyroid Dysfunction

Because PTH is the principal determinant of the amount of remodeling activity in the skeleton, one could expect significant skeletal manifestations of parathyroid functional disorders. However, the reality is complicated. Patients with hypoparathyroidism have reduced remodeling, slightly greater than average bone mass, and probably fewer fractures. By contrast, patients with severe, long-standing hyperparathyroidism may have reduced bone mass; subperiosteal bone loss; widespread, very active bone remodeling; and even cysts in bone filled with osteoclast-like cells. Cases of this extreme type are rare today, and generally patients with primary hyperparathyroidism have no abnormalities of the skeleton detectable by ordinary x-ray studies. However, untreated mild primary hyperparathyroidism is now known to result in increased fracture risk, not for reasons of decreased bone mass but because of increased PTH-mediated bone remodeling. When PTH hypersecretion is pulsatile, and the peaks are short lived, PTH is actually trophic for bone and can produce quite large increases in spine bone density. For that reason, PTH 1-34 is now an approved therapy for osteoporosis.

Osteogenesis Imperfecta

Osteogenesis imperfecta (OI) is a group of heritable disorders in which one of several mutations may occur in the genes encoding for the collagen molecules that comprise the bulk of bone matrix (9). Patients with OI have fragile skeletons with reduced bone mass. In one of the common forms of OI, long bones typically have narrow shafts as well as reduced mass. Patients with OI commonly suffer many fractures throughout life, often starting in utero. When some other amino acid replaces glycine in the collagen molecule, the triple helix will not coil properly, collagen synthesis is reduced, and the matrix is abnormal. The severity of the defect depends on the position of the substitution in the chain of the collagen molecule. Fractures heal normally. Other collagen-based connective tissues are also affected in certain forms of the disease, including dentin, ligaments and tendons, and sclerae. Despite the manifest abnormality of the bone matrix, the reason for the reduction in bone mass is unclear.

Bony Manifestations of Diseases of Nonskeletal Systems

Patients with chronic liver disease, but especially with biliary cirrhosis, commonly have a bone disease that is basically osteoporosis (10). Patients who are to undergo liver transplantation often have severe osteoporosis, attributable to a combination of the underlying disease, the immobilization that inevitably accompanies the severe disability of these very sick patients, and the treatments they have received.

Patients with end stage renal disease often have a complex bone disease consisting of a varying mixture of osteosclerosis, osteomalacia, and hyperparathyroid bone disease (11). Exact expression of these varied abnormalities depends on the medical regimens the patients receive, specifically the way in which these regimens manage calcium, phosphorus, and vitamin D metabolism for the patient.

Patients with a variety of disorders of the small intestine, but especially those with gluten-sensitive enteropathy, malabsorb fat-soluble vitamins and hypersecrete calcium and magnesium into the digestive juices. As a result, these patients are commonly deficient in vitamin D, calcium, and magnesium. They often have severe osteoporosis and may have osteomalacia as well.

Patients who have had organ transplants commonly have osteoporosis (12), in part because they present for organ transplantation with already reduced bone mass and in part because the immunosuppressive therapy used to sustain the transplant itself causes bone loss.

Aluminum and Bone

Aluminum (Al) is not strictly speaking a nutrient, but it is extremely common in the environment, is a major component of antacids, and is widely used as cookware. Only a small fraction of ingested Al is absorbed, and absorbed Al is promptly excreted in the urine in healthy persons. However, in patients with severely compromised renal function, particularly in those treated with large doses of Al-containing antacids to block phosphorus absorption, Al accumulates at the mineralizing sites of the bone remodeling process. It was thought at one time to be responsible for the unique bony pathologic features of end-stage renal disease, but it is now considered only a minor contributor to renal osteopathy. Experimentally, Al has shown an ability to increase trabecular bone density in animals, particularly in combination with fluoride. The ultimate significance of this finding remains uncertain.

SKELETAL MANIFESTATIONS OF SYSTEMIC NUTRIENT DEFICIENCIES

Protein-Calorie Malnutrition

As noted, the cells of bone are as dependent on total nutrition as are other cells, and bone suffers in starvation just as do other tissues. However, bone strength is not immediately affected in acute malnutrition, especially in adults. The bony effects of protein-calorie malnutrition are most obvious in two situations: one is during growth, when both growth rates and bone mass accumulation are retarded by malnutrition; and the other is in the repair of fractures, especially in elderly persons. Protein-calorie malnutrition is common among elderly persons, and when they break a bone, such as the hip, serious complications and even death may ensue. Protein supplementation has been shown to reduce these complications substantially, and it is an important and necessary component of the treatment of most patients with hip fractures (13). The reason for the trophic effect of protein on bone is partly that dietary protein helps to sustain normal insulinlike growth factor-I (IGF-1) concentrations, needed for bone growth and repair (14), and partly that, as discussed, bone formation requires fresh dietary protein.

Magnesium Deficiency

Magnesium deficiency occurs in severe intestinal malabsorption (e.g., gluten-sensitive enteropathy, fistulas, or ileal resection, especially with high-fat diets) or with urinary losses from renal tubular defects. Initially, magnesium deficiency impairs bony responsiveness to PTH and thus leads to hypocalcemia despite a rising PTH level. As deficiency progresses, parathyroid response falters, and PTH secretion falls. The hypocalcemia of magnesium deficiency is thus the result of impairment of the calcium regulatory system and is unresponsive to calcium supplementation (15). Less severe degrees of magnesium deficiency in these same syndromes are associated with reduced bone mass, also unresponsive to calcium supplementation. In addition to other needed treatments (e.g., calcium), magnesium supplements are necessary in these patients. Finally, silent magnesium deficiency often accompanies low vitamin D status. The mechanism is uncertain. The deficiency manifests itself as a failure to elevate PTH secretion in response to the poor calcium absorption of vitamin D deficiency.

INVESTIGATION OF NUTRIENT EFFECTS ON THE SKELETON

As noted, the effects of nutrient deficiencies on the skeleton express themselves slowly in adults. For this same reason, nutrient effects on the skeleton of any kind are difficult to detect and easy to misinterpret.

Change in Bone Mass

As noted, bone is a composite of mineral and matrix, and bone mass refers to the quantity of such bone present in the whole organism (or in a particular body region). Technically, changes in bone mass itself cannot be measured in vivo, because no way of detecting the organic component of the composite is known. However, in conditions of health, and in fact in most bone diseases, the proportion of mineral and matrix is about the same (50:50, by volume). In addition, quite good methods are available for measuring bone mineral. Mineral content can be measured either for the whole skeleton or for various regions of interest by x-ray absorptiometric methods (see later). *Change* in bone mass is measured either by classic metabolic balance methods or serial absorptiometry.

The classic nutritional approach to nutrient status is the measurement of a metabolic balance, in this case calcium (or phosphorus) balance. Because more than 99% of body calcium is in the skeleton, total body calcium balance reflects predominantly bone balance. Moreover, because calcium is essentially never removed from or added to preformed bone tissue (rather, units of tissue itself are removed or added), it follows that body calcium balance is a direct measure of bone tissue balance. The balance method is theoretically the ideal way of assessing change in bone mass, but it is expensive, and balance studies are difficult to perform accurately. The principal source of this difficulty, for poorly absorbed nutrients such as calcium, is that most of the ingested calcium ends up in the feces. Accurate timing of fecal excretion is nearly impossible. Moreover, the lag time between ingestion and fecal excretion averages several days in healthy adults, and failure to take that lag time into account leads to serious misinterpretation of calcium balance results (16). Colored dye markers demarcating treatment periods are not adequate safeguards. Rather, continuous intake markers (e.g., polyethylene glycol [PEG 3350]) are required, and fecal output must be adjusted both for its polyethylene glycol content and the time lag.

A newer approach, and one ideally suited to measurement of the quantity of bone present, is the direct measurement of bone mineral (17), either in a specific region or in the skeleton as a whole, by the technique of dual-energy x-ray absorptiometry (DXA). A tightly col-

limated beam of x-rays is passed back and forth across the body (or one of its regions), and absorption of its photons is measured by a detector on the side opposite the x-ray source. Absorption is a function of the amount of mineral present in the path of the beam. This method measures, for example, spine mineral content in as little as 2 to 5 minutes and has a reproducibility on the order of 1% to 2% in healthy young adults.

Because total body calcium in an adult is in the range of 900 to 1500 g, and because change in bone mass (in other words, positive or negative calcium balance) is rarely more than approximately 100 mg/day (and usually much less), it follows that closely spaced, repeat measurements by DXA will produce results within the reproducibility error of the method. For that reason, measurements in persons must usually be separated by 12 to 24 months. (Less time will not allow for measurable change to occur.) Thus, although DXA permits rapid and accurate measurement of bone *mass*, it is not very sensitive to the sorts of *change in mass* that have physiologic or nutritional significance.

The Remodeling Transient

Any intervention, nutritional or otherwise, that alters bone remodeling activity will produce a transient change (18) in calcium balance (or bone mass), which results from the asynchrony of the remodeling cycle (see earlier). Because of the temporal separation of resorption and formation at each remodeling site, suppression of remodeling will produce a prompt but temporary increase in bone mass (Fig. 89.7). If this follows, for example, the administration of supplemental calcium, phosphorus, or vitamin D, the retention of bone mineral should not be interpreted to

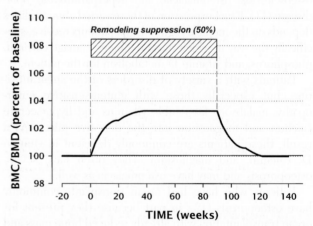

Fig. 89.7. Positive bone remodeling transient in a healthy person who is not calcium deficient, in response first to a large increase in calcium intake (sufficient to suppress remodeling by 50%) and then to its later withdrawal. The vertical axis is bone mass (i.e., either bone mineral content [BMC] or bone mineral density [BMD]), expressed as a percentage of the baseline value. The initial rise in bone mass does not continue past one remodeling cycle (40 weeks in this illustration), and the bone gained by remodeling suppression is lost once again when remodeling returns to its previous level. (Copyright Robert P. Heaney, 1996.)

mean that the patient has a preexisting deficiency. (Such a deficiency may be present, of course, but positive balance will occur whether or not deficiency is present, simply because initially the resorptive component of remodeling is reduced more than the formative component.) Because the remodeling cycle lasts at least 3 months in healthy young adults, bone mass and calcium balance continue to change under the influence of this asynchronous remodeling for at least that long. The process may actually take a year or more in elderly persons for formation and resorption once again to come into equilibrium. Response to nutritional interventions can be interpreted only *after* the transient is complete. If balance is more positive at that time (or bone mass by DXA is still increasing), only then can one safely conclude that the subjects needed more of the nutrient than they had previously been receiving. Because these constraints are rarely followed, much of the calcium literature is contradictory and confusing.

Bone Histomorphometry

The term *histomorphometry* means the measurement of shapes on histologic specimens of bone (19). As noted, many substances attach to bone crystals as they are forming and then become trapped as more bone is laid down on top of them. Some of those substances, like the tetracycline antibiotics, fluoresce brilliantly when they are illuminated by ultraviolet light. Histomorphometry takes advantage of that property by giving patients paired, timed doses of tetracycline several days before obtaining a bone biopsy (typically from the iliac crest). Specimens are sectioned on special microtomes without first removing the mineral and are then examined with an ultraviolet microscope. Figure 89.4 presents a typical photomicrograph from such a labeled biopsy. Because the distance between fluorescent lines can be measured with a calibrated eyepiece or by shape-sensing software, and because the times of administration are known, one can derive a direct and reasonably precise estimate of the rate at which the remodeling cells are working and how active the remodeling process may be. Among other histologic features, measurements are made not only of the distance between labels but also of the extent of bone surface covered with a label. This method is very useful for studying bone biology and disease, but it has limited applicability to the study of nutritional problems affecting bone.

Biochemical Markers of Bone Remodeling

In the synthesis of bone collagen, the ends of the collagen molecules are clipped off as the triple helix is assembled, the proline molecules in the peptide chain are converted to hydroxyproline, and cross-links are developed between the side chains of adjacent collagen fibrils, involving particularly lysine and hydroxylysine protruding from the backbone of the peptide chain. Additionally, both alkaline phosphatase and the noncollagenous proteins are secreted

TABLE 89.2	BIOCHEMICAL MARKERS OF BONE REMODELING
FORMATION	**RESORPTION**
Serum alkaline phosphatase	Urine hydroxyproline
Bone specific	Urine pyridinium cross-links
Total	Pyridinoline
Serum osteocalcin	Deoxypyridinoline
Serum procollagen type I	Peptide cross-links
propeptide	Urine amino terminal
Carboxyterminal	cross-links (NTx)
propeptide (P1CP)	Urine carboxyterminal
	cross-links (CTx)
Amino terminal	Serum carboxyterminal
propeptide (P1NP)	cross-links (CTx)

into the matrix; in this process, some of these substances leak into the bloodstream, where they can be measured. Later, when bone is broken down, the hydroxyproline residues and the cross-links, because they cannot be recycled, are metabolized or excreted. All these activities leave residues or produce effects that can be measured in serum or urine. Collectively, these circulating or excreted substances are called biochemical biomarkers of bone remodeling (20). They reflect in a general way the level of bone remodeling activity. Table 89.2 summarizes the principal markers currently in use together with the component of remodeling they are thought to reflect most directly. In this connection, when remodeling activity changes, ultimately, both resorption and formation generally change, almost always in the same direction, and often to very nearly the same extent. Under steady-state conditions, therefore, a marker for either formation or resorption may be used as an index of remodeling activity.

Although measurements of bone biomarkers can be a relatively inexpensive way of assessing bone remodeling activity under differing nutritional conditions, they are at most only semiquantitative. In other words, a 50% drop in a resorption marker does not mean a 50% reduction in the amount of bone resorbed. In addition, the markers exhibit important discrepancies among themselves. For example, serum alkaline phosphatase is high in nutritional rickets despite a generally low level of new bone apposition, and $1,25(OH)_2$ vitamin D elevates serum osteocalcin apparently without altering actual bone-forming activity (21).

The effects of nutritional deficiencies on the relationship between marker concentration or excretion and the process it reflects have not been studied. Nevertheless, to the extent that a nutritional deficiency alters bone remodeling, one can expect to find corresponding changes in remodeling markers. Thus, the accelerated bone loss of the aged that results from calcium deficiency is associated with elevated excretion of deoxypyridinoline and hydroxyproline. Calcium supplementation both stops or slows the bone loss and reduces urinary excretion of these resorption markers.

REFERENCES

1. Gokhale JA, Robey PG, Boskey AL. The biochemistry of bone. In: Marcus R, Feldman Kelsey J, eds. Osteoporosis, vol 1. 2nd ed. San Diego: Academic Press, 2001:107–88.
2. Kannus P, Haapasalo H, Sievanen H et al. Bone 1994;15:279–84.
3. NIH Consensus Conference. JAMA 1994;272:1942–8.
4. Vermeer C. Vitamin K and bone health. In: Burckhardt P, Dawson-Hughes B, Heaney RP, eds. Nutritional Aspects of Osteoporosis. 2nd ed. San Diego: Elsevier Academic Press, 2004:79–92.
5. Marcus R, Majumder S. The nature of osteoporosis. In: Marcus R, Feldman D, Kelsey J, eds. Osteoporosis, vol 2. 2nd ed. San Diego: Academic Press, 2001:3–17.
6. Heaney RP. Bone 2003;33:457–65.
7. Pettifor JM. Nutritional and drug-induced rickets and osteomalacia. In: Favus MJ, ed. Primer on the Metabolic Bone Diseases and Disorders of Mineral Metabolism. 5th ed. Washington, DC: American Society for Bone and Mineral Research, 2003:399–407.
8. Glorieux FH. Hypophosphatemic vitamin D resistant rickets. In: Favus MJ, ed. Primer on the Metabolic Bone Diseases and Disorders of Mineral Metabolism. 5th ed. Washington, DC: American Society for Bone and Mineral Research, 2003:414–7.
9. Shapiro JR. Osteogenesis imperfecta and other defects of bone development as occasional causes of adult osteoporosis. In: Marcus R, Feldman D, Kelsey J, eds. Osteoporosis, vol 2. 2nd ed. San Diego: Academic Press, 2001:271–301.
10. Herlong HF, Recker RR, Maddrey WC. Gastroenterology 1982;83:103–8.
11. Goodman WG, Coburn JW, Ramirez JA et al. Renal osteodystrophy in adults and children. In: Favus MJ, ed. Primer on the Metabolic Bone Diseases and Disorders of Mineral Metabolism. 5th ed. Washington, DC: American Society for Bone and Mineral Research, 2003:430–47.
12. Epstein S. J Bone Miner Res 1996;11:1–7.
13. Delmi M, Rapin CH, Bengoa JM et al. Lancet 1990;335:1013–6.
14. Wüster C, Rosen C. Growth hormone, insulin-like growth factors: potential applications and limitations in the management of osteoporosis. In: Marcus R, Feldman D, Kelsey J, eds. Osteoporosis, vol 2. 2nd ed. San Diego: Academic Press, 2001:47–67.
15. Rude RK. Magnesium depletion and hypermagnesemia. In: Favus MJ, ed. Primer on the Metabolic Bone Diseases and Disorders of Mineral Metabolism. 5th ed. Washington, DC: American Society for Bone and Mineral Research, 2003:292–5.
16. Heaney RP. Bone Miner 1986;1:99–114.
17. Faulkner KG. Clinical use of bone densitometry. In: Marcus R, Feldman D, Kelsey J, eds. Osteoporosis, vol 2. 2nd ed. San Diego: Academic Press, 2001:433–58.
18. Heaney RP. J Bone Miner Res 1994;9:1515–23.
19. Recker RR, Barger-Lux MJ. Transilial bone biopsy. In: Bilezikian JP, Raisz L, Rodan GA, eds. Principles of Bone Biology. 2nd ed. San Diego: Academic Press, 2002:1595–664.
20. Garnero P, Delmas PD. Biochemical markers of bone turnover in osteoporosis. In: Marcus R, Feldman D, Kelsey J, eds. Osteoporosis, vol 2. 2nd ed. San Diego: Academic Press, 2001:459–77.
21. Feldman D, Malloy PJ, Gross C. Vitamin D: biology, action, and clinical implications. In: Marcus R, Feldman D, Kelsey J, eds. Osteoporosis, vol 1. 2nd ed. San Diego: Academic Press, 2001:257–303.

SUGGESTED READINGS

Gokhale JA, Robey PG, Boskey AL. The biochemistry of bone. In: Marcus R, Feldman D, Kelsey J, eds. Osteoporosis, vol. 1. 2nd ed. San Diego: Academic Press, 2001;108–88.

Heaney RP. Nutrition and risk for osteoporosis. In: Marcus R, Feldman D, Nelson D et al., eds. Osteoporosis. 3rd ed. San Diego: Elsevier, 2008:799–836.

Favus MJ, ed. Primer on the Metabolic Bone Diseases and Disorders of Mineral Metabolism. Washington, DC: American Society for Bone and Mineral Research.

90 PREVENTION AND MANAGEMENT OF OSTEOPOROSIS[1]

KATHERINE L. TUCKER AND CLIFFORD J. ROSEN

Osteoporosis is a progressive deterioration in bone microarchitecture associated with loss of bone mineral density (BMD), leading to increasing risk of fracture with time. The prevalence of this condition in the United States exceeds 12 million adults 50 years old or older, with more than 40 million additional older adults at higher risk of developing osteoporosis because of low BMD. Total incident fractures for the US population 50 years old or older were estimated at more than 2 million in 2005, with 71% of these in women (1). Extrapolating to 2025, approximately 4 of every 10 women more than 50 years old in the United States are expected to experience a fracture. Black adults tend to have a lower prevalence of osteoporosis and fracture than white adults (2). A few studies have shown bone density and fracture risk in Hispanics as between that of non-Hispanic whites and blacks. However, data

---

[1]**Abbreviations: BMD**, bone mineral density; **DASH**, Dietary Approaches to Stop Hypertension; **DXA**, dual energy x-ray absorptiometry; **FOS**, Framingham Osteoporosis Study; **FRAX**, Fracture Risk Assessment Tool; **IGF-I**, insulinlike growth factor-I; **IOM**, Institute of Medicine; **NHANES**, National Health and Nutrition Examination Survey; **NHS**, Nurses' Health Study; **OPG**, osteoprotegerin; **PTH**, parathyroid hormone; **RANKL**, receptor activator of nuclear factor B ligand; **RDA**, recommended dietary allowance; **WHI**, Women's Health Initiative; **WHO**, World Health Organization.

from the National Health and Nutrition Examination Survey (NHANES) III (1988 to 1994) and the NHANES 2005 to 2008 suggest that prevalence of low BMD may be decreasing in non-Hispanic whites but increasing in Hispanics (3, 4).

In the United States, the burden of osteoporosis resulting in hip fractures was estimated at 17 to 20 billion dollars annually, including acute and rehabilitative care (5). Medical costs aside, the effect of a hip fracture can be devastating for the individual. Large percentages of older hip fracture patients do not regain the ability to walk unassisted, approximately one third are admitted into long-term care, and excess mortality ranges from 10% to 20% during the following year (6).

BONE MINERAL DENSITY AND OSTEOPOROSIS

Osteoporosis is characterized by low BMD and compromised bone strength, leading to increasing risk of fracture. Osteoporotic bone tissue shows deterioration of microarchitecture, with thinner trabeculae, reduced mineralization, and thinning of cortical surfaces associated with increased cortical porosity (7). Total BMD is the result of a delicate balance between bone resorption by osteoclasts and bone formation by osteoblasts during continuous remodeling. During childhood, bone growth requires a balance in favor of bone acquisition and peak bone mass, whereas in young adults, BMD tends to be relatively stable. With aging, osteoclast activity begins to exceed that of osteoblasts and loss of bone occurs (8). After the onset of menopause in women, bone loss accelerates to two to six times premenopausal rates, and then gradually slows to about 1% annually by 10 years after menopause (9, 10). In contrast, longitudinal studies in older men suggest consistent albeit slow bone loss (i.e., ~1% per year) (10).

Individually, changes in bone mass also reflect numerous exposures that affect the remodeling balance. Therefore, osteoporosis prevention depends on optimizing peak bone mass, minimizing exposures that lead to bone loss, and optimizing nutritional exposures for bone maintenance throughout life. For more discussion of bone biology and composition, see the chapter on bone and joint biology. An overview of associated factors, discussed in more detail later, can be found in Table 90.1.

TABLE 90.1	KEY MESSAGES FOR BONE HEALTH

Risk statistics:
  More than 12 million adults, 50 years and older, have osteoporosis in the United States.
  An estimated 4 out of 10 women more than 50 years old may experience a fracture.
  A large percentage of older patients with hip fracture do not regain the ability to walk unassisted and are admitted into long-term care.
  Excess mortality ranges from 10% to 20% during the year after a hip fracture.
General risk factors:
  Aging increases risk because of declining muscle strength, loss of balance, gait difficulties, arthritis, poor vision, and use of medications.
  The WHO FRAX (fracture risk assessment tool) includes older age, female sex, low BMI, prior fracture, parental hip fracture, current smoking, long-term use of glucocorticoids, rheumatoid arthritis, conditions leading to secondary osteoporosis (type 1 diabetes, osteogenesis imperfecta, untreated hyperthyroidism, hypogonadism or premature menopause, chronic malnutrition or malabsorption, chronic liver disease), and consumption of three or more alcoholic drinks per day in calculating fracture risk.
Nutrients and bone health:
  Clearly protective nutrients include calcium, magnesium, potassium, vitamin D, and vitamin K.
  Likely protective nutrients include silicon, strontium, vitamin C, vitamin E, vitamin B_{12}, vitamin B_6, folate, carotenoids, and protein.
  Possible negative effects may be seen with high intakes of sodium, phosphorus, iron, fluoride, and vitamin A.
Caffeine and alcohol:
  Excessive caffeine is a risk factor, but may be offset with calcium intake.
  Moderate alcohol intake appears protective, but heavy alcohol intake poses a significant risk.
Body weight and composition:
  Low body mass index and weight loss are risk factors for low bone mineral density and fracture.
  For any given weight, however, abdominal fat mass may contribute to risk.
Physical activity:
  Weight-bearing physical activity and resistance exercises are protective of bone mineral density.
  Strength and balance exercises improve muscle function and reduce falls.
  Aerobic exercise is important during weight reduction to protect against bone loss with weight loss.
Genetics:
  Family history of fracture and identification of bone-sensitive gene polymorphisms show that genetic risk factors are important. However, this risk may be mitigated with optimal diet, physical activity, restriction to moderate alcohol consumption, and avoidance of smoking.

Measuring Bone Mineral Density

In the last three decades, measurements of BMD have improved significantly. The most widely used method is dual energy x-ray absorptiometry (DXA), which captures the energy absorbed as x-rays pass through the bone from an energy source on one side to a detector on the other. Single x-ray absorptiometry also has been widely used, but is appropriate only for areas without much overlying tissue, such as the wrist or heel. Newer techniques include quantitative computed tomography, to measure metabolically active trabecular bone, and ultrasound, which captures the modulation of sound waves as they pass through the tissue.

DXA provides measures of BMD at specific locations of the hip and spine, in g/cm^2. These measures are compared with population standards to provide a T-score, used by physicians in defining osteoporosis or osteopenia. Scores indicate the extent to which an individual is above or below the mean optimal density using standard deviation units. A score higher than −1 is considered normal; between −1 and −2.5 is considered osteopenia (low bone mass); and lower than −2.5 is osteoporosis. The World Health Organization (WHO) international reference standard for the description of osteoporosis in postmenopausal women and in men 50 years old or older, uses DXA measures of the femoral neck from non-Hispanic white women, 20 to 29 years old, in the NHANES III (11). Z-scores, which relate bone density to healthy individuals of the same age and sex, are often used in younger individuals. With the exception of the NHANES, few studies have been conducted in racial and ethnic minorities and, although practitioners discuss whether different racial and ethnic groups should have different reference standards, the WHO currently recommends use of a single standard for optimal comparison across groups.

Bone Mineral Density and Risk of Fracture

Measuring BMD to define osteoporosis is important because an inverse relationship exists with risk of fracture in older adults. A metaanalysis of 12 cohorts in diverse populations showed that DXA femoral neck BMD was a strong predictor of subsequent fracture risk for both men and women (12). Although hip fracture is the most serious, other fractures may also have important effects on health and independence. Vertebral compression factures, which shift vertebrae into a wedge shape leading to kyphosis, or curved spine, can cause chronic pain and disability and are more common in women than men (13).

Risk of fracture increases with age because of changes in bone quality, declining bone density, and falls, which increase with aging because of declining muscle strength, loss of balance, gait difficulties, arthritis, poor vision, and use of medications (14). In the Framingham Osteoporosis Study (FOS) of older adults, important risk factors associated with bone loss over time in women included age, lower weight, and weight loss, whereas estrogen use was protective; in men, bone loss was associated with smoking. Surprisingly, no association was seen in either men or women between bone loss and physical activity, caffeine intake, calcium intake, or serum 25-OH vitamin D concentration (15). In the Rotterdam Study of older adults, bone loss was associated with lower weight and smoking in both men and women, whereas calcium intake was protective in men but not women (16). A large study of 9516 older US women found that risk of fracture was associated with previous fracture, greater height, fair or poor self-rated health, hyperthyroidism, treatment with benzodiazepines or anticonvulsants, greater caffeine intake, and spending up to 4 hours/day standing (17).

To better assess risk, the WHO developed the Fracture Risk Assessment Tool (FRAX) (18). This tool calculates the 10-year risk of fracture with weighted scores for age, sex, BMI, prior fragility fracture, parental hip fracture, current smoking, long-term use of glucocorticoids, rheumatoid arthritis, conditions leading to secondary osteoporosis (e.g., type 1 diabetes, osteogenesis imperfecta, untreated hyperthyroidism, hypogonadism, premature menopause [<45 years], chronic malnutrition or malabsorption, or chronic liver disease), consumption of three or more alcoholic drinks per day and, BMD if available (19). Although helpful and widely used, this tool is constantly being updated and adapted as more information becomes available (20). The FRAX tool does not consider nutritional determinants of risk. However, it provides a useful base from which to investigate the effects of nutritional variables, after other contributors to risk are taken into account.

NUTRITIONAL DETERMINANTS OF BONE DENSITY AND FRACTURE RISK

As living tissue, with constant resorption and rebuilding, bone appears to be responsive to a wide range of nutrients. Some of these have only recently been understood and others continue to be actively investigated. Food sources of the minerals and vitamins most clearly associated with bone status are provided in Table 90.2.

Minerals

Although calcium and vitamin D have long been known to be important for long-term fracture risk, more recent research has shown that bone mass is, in fact, sensitive to a wide variety of nutritional exposures. Dietary intake is a centrally important modifiable factor in the development of peak bone mass and in the protection against bone loss with aging. Because bone undergoes continuous remodeling, an adequate supply of nutrients is required to support

TABLE 90.2	GOOD DIETARY SOURCES OF KEY NUTRIENTS FOR BONE HEALTH	
	DAILY VALUE[a]	FOODS
Calcium	1,000 mg	Milk, yogurt, and cheese
		Small or canned fish with edible bones (sardines, salmon)
		Calcium set tofu
		Fortified soy milk
Magnesium	400 mg	Whole grains and whole grain cereals (wheat bran, wheat germ, brown rice, quinoa, oatmeal, raisin bran, shredded wheat)
		Nuts (almonds, cashews, peanuts, peanut butter)
		Mature beans and peas (soybeans, pinto beans, kidney beans, black-eyed peas, lentils)
		Dark green leafy vegetables (spinach, collards, kale, swiss chard)
		Fish (halibut, pollock, tuna, haddock)
		Dark chocolate, cocoa
Potassium	3,500 mg	Baked potato, sweet potato
		Tomato paste, tomato sauce
		Mature beans (kidney beans, white beans, soy beans, lima beans, lentils)
		Yogurt, milk
		Fish (halibut, rockfish, cod, trout)
		Winter squash
		Orange juice
		Banana
Vitamin D	400 IU (10 μg)	Fatty fish (herring, salmon, sardines, swordfish)
		Fortified milk and yogurt
		Fortified breakfast cereals
Vitamin K	80 μg	Dark green leafy vegetables (kale, swiss chard, collard greens, spinach)
		Dark salad greens (leaf lettuce, watercress, raw spinach)
		Cruciferous vegetables (broccoli, brussels sprouts)
		Vegetable oils (soybean oil, canola oil)

[a]The daily value is the suggested intake for a 2,000-kcal (8.374 MJ) diet, and is the amount used on food labels. Individual requirements vary.

bone formation and retention. The bone matrix is composed of calcium, phosphorus, protein, and trace minerals, including magnesium, and these are of primary importance. However, additional dietary components affect the remodeling balance through effects on calcium regulation, inflammation, DNA methylation, and other regulatory processes that stimulate bone resorption or formation. Understanding these relationships is important, because it points to dietary quality as a critical factor in bone status, as opposed to an earlier focus mainly on calcium supplementation for prevention of bone loss (21, 22).

Calcium

Calcium is the major mineral component of bone mass, and nearly 99% of the calcium in the adult human body is contained in bones in the form of hydroxyapatite. Children need relatively large amounts of calcium to lay down new bone with rapid growth. The 1997 Food and Nutrition Board set adequate intakes at 1300 mg (32.5 mmol) per day for children 9 to 18 years old, for maximizing peak bone mass to protect against osteoporosis later in life (23). However, supplementation studies in children have shown mixed results. A 2000 review of calcium supplementation and bone concluded that calcium contributed to higher BMD primarily at cortical bone sites, was most effective in populations with low baseline calcium intake, and was more effective in pubertal than prepubertal children (24). A more recent review of 19 calcium supplementation trials in 2859 children found that calcium supplementation had a small effect on upper limb BMD but no effect on femoral neck or lumbar spine (25). No evidence was found for effect modification by sex, baseline calcium intake, pubertal stage, ethnicity, or level of physical activity; and it was concluded that calcium supplementation in children is unlikely to reduce the risk of fracture either in childhood or later adulthood.

A broader review of calcium trials, including adults, found that all but 2 of 52 trials showed better bone balance with calcium intervention, greater bone gain during growth, reduced bone loss with aging, or reduced fracture (26). In contrast, a more recent metaanalysis of 4 clinical trials, with 6504 subjects and 139 hip fractures, calculated a pooled RR between calcium and placebo of 1.64 (95% confidence interval, 1.02, 2.64), indicating higher, not lower, risk (27). A follow-up after completion of a large, 3-year, placebo-controlled trial of calcium and vitamin D supplementation in older men and women showed that most of the BMD benefits accrued during the trial were lost 2 years after supplementation ended (28). A lack of efficacy of calcium supplements was also seen in the Women's Health Initiative (WHI), in which 36,282 postmenopausal women 50 to 79 years of age were randomly assigned to 1000 mg calcium and 400 IU (10 μg) vitamin D_3 daily, versus placebo, and followed for 7 years. Although the calcium–vitamin D supplementation resulted in small improvements in hip BMD, it did not reduce hip fracture risk in all healthy postmenopausal women. However,

subgroup analyses showed that supplemented women more than 60 years old, but not younger women, did have a lower risk of hip fractures (29). Together, these studies question the conventional wisdom that calcium supplementation has major protective effects against fracture risk. However, few studies have considered baseline status. It seems likely that those with inadequate calcium intake would benefit more from supplements than those with adequate intakes.

It is also likely that dietary sources of calcium may be more effective than calcium supplements. An NHANES III follow-up analysis found that low recalled milk intake during childhood and adolescence was associated with significantly lower hip BMD and a doubling of fracture risk among women 50 years of age and older (30). A large 5-year study of British adults found that fracture risk was 75% higher among women with baseline calcium intakes less than 525 versus 1200 mg or more per day, and the association was stronger for women less than 50 years of age than for older women (31). However, in the Nurses' Health Study (NHS), women who reported drinking two or more glasses of milk per day versus up to one per week did not differ significantly in hip fracture incidence (32).

Intervention studies with calcium-rich foods have shown beneficial effects on bone. In one, spinal bone loss was significantly lower in premenopausal women who used dairy foods to raise calcium intake from 900 to 1500 mg (22.5 to 37.5 mmol) per day, relative to controls (33). In another, three additional servings of yogurt per day led to significant reduction in urinary excretion of bone turnover markers in older women (34). Calcium in foods like milk and yogurt may be used more effectively than supplements because it comes packaged with other important nutrients that work together, including vitamin D, protein, potassium, and magnesium.

Phosphorus

Phosphorus is essential for bone, but too much phosphorus in combination with low calcium intake can lead to reduced calcium bioavailability and potential bone loss. Although uncommon, phosphorus deficiency can lead to reduced mineralization and bone resorption. Deficiency has been seen in older adults with malnutrition, intestinal malabsorption, or long-term use of medications that bind phosphorus, including antacids (35). In the general population, excess phosphorus is more of a concern than deficiency. The US diet tends to be high in phosphorus relative to calcium. Mean intakes of phosphorus in the NHANES 2007 to 2008 study were 1123 and 1550 mg/day, for women and men, relative to a recommended dietary allowance (RDA) of 700 mg; whereas mean intakes of calcium were 833 and 1038 mg for women and men relative to an RDA of 1000 to 1200 mg (36, 37).

Excess phosphate form complexes with calcium that interfere with calcium absorption, which may in turn lower serum calcium and lead to secretion of parathyroid hormone (PTH), lower $1,25(OH)_2D$ production, lower intestinal calcium absorption and, consequently, bone resorption to release calcium from bone (38). Short-term metabolic studies have documented some of these mechanisms (39, 40).

One major source of excess phosphorus in the US diet is phosphoric acid from cola drinks. Two studies in teenage girls found that cola consumption significantly increased the odds of fracture (41). In the FOS, women consuming cola daily had significantly lower hip BMD than those who consumed cola less than once per week (42). In contrast, a short-term metabolic study, showed negligible effects of phosphoric acid–containing beverages on urinary calcium excretion, and concluded that the effects seen in observational studies may be caused by milk displacement (43). However, milk displacement did not explain the significant negative effects seen for cola in the FOS, and there was no effect of other soft drinks. It is likely that regular exposure to phosphoric acid may cause small BMD losses, which accumulate to measurable losses over time.

Magnesium

Magnesium is important to the formation of pure hydroxyapatite and may enhance bone strength through its role in crystallization (44). It also is known to regulate active intestinal calcium transport. In animal studies, experimental magnesium deficiency decreased bone volume and trabecular thickness, bone mass, PTH, $1,25(OH)_2$ vitamin D concentration, and osteoprotegerin (OPG), whereas it increased receptor activator of nuclear factor B ligand (RANKL) and osteoclastogenesis (45–48).

Magnesium concentrations were significantly lower in women with osteoporosis than those with normal bone mass (49). In observational studies, magnesium intake was significantly positively associated with BMD, and protective against bone loss (50–52). This is important because magnesium intakes tend to be consistently low; daily median intakes from NHANES data ranged from 177 mg among African-American women to 326 mg among non-Hispanic white men, relative to recommendations of 320 and 420 mg for women and men, respectively (53). Some intervention studies with magnesium have shown benefit on bone mass in adolescent girls (54), in suppressing bone turnover markers in young men (55), and protecting against bone loss in osteoporotic women (56), findings suggesting that this important mineral may be underappreciated for its important role in bone health. However, too few randomized controlled trials with magnesium exist to support widespread use of magnesium supplementation to prevent osteoporosis.

Potassium

Potassium promotes renal calcium retention and is also important in neutralizing the acid load of most diets, which may protect against calcium loss from the bones. Potassium administration increased serum osteocalcin concentration and decreased urinary hydroxyproline excretion (57). Several population-based studies have demonstrated protective associations between potassium intake and bone status. In premenopausal women, a difference of 8% in femoral neck BMD between the highest and lowest quartiles of potassium intake was seen (58). In perimenopausal and early postmenopausal women, dietary potassium was associated with lower bone resorption and greater BMD (57). In older adults in the FOS, potassium showed protective associations with BMD in men and women at baseline, and with lower BMD loss over time in men (50). In another study of elderly women, higher urinary potassium excretion at baseline was associated with 4% greater total body BMD and 11% greater trabecular BMD at 5 years (59). One author noted that relative to preagricultural humans, the modern human diet is deficient in potassium (2500 mg versus 7000 mg/day) and contains excess sodium (~4000 mg versus 600 mg/day) (60). This combination may have particularly negative effects on bone.

Sodium

Sodium intake in the United States is considerably higher than recommended. NHANES 2007 to 2008 data showed that in contrast to recommendations of approximately 1500 mg, mean daily sodium intakes in US adults were 4043 mg for men and 2884 mg for women (36, 61). This likely contributes to renal calcium excretion. Studies have shown that each 1000 mg of additional sodium was associated with a 20-mg increase in urinary calcium loss—the amount likely to be absorbed from 80 mg of dietary calcium (62), and consequently with lower BMD. The optimal intake balance for protecting bone was approximately 1000 mg calcium and less than 2000 mg sodium per day.

The effect of sodium also may depend on potassium exposure. A metabolic study found that postmenopausal women given 5175 mg of sodium per day had increases in urinary calcium and N-telopeptide, whereas those given sodium plus potassium citrate had decreases in urinary calcium and no increase in N-telopeptide (63). In the Dietary Approaches to Stop Hypertension (DASH) sodium trial, a diet high in fruit, vegetables, low-fat dairy, and thus high in potassium, was randomly assigned, versus a control diet, for 30 days. The DASH diet significantly reduced serum markers of bone turnover and additionally reducing sodium led to further reduction in serum osteocalcin decreased PTH in the control group, and lowered urinary calcium in both (64). In another study of postmenopausal women who reduced sodium intake to less than 2000 mg/day for 6 months, urinary calcium excretion and bone turnover markers were reduced (65). However, other studies have been less clear about the effects of sodium on bone (66, 67); and one study showed no adverse effect on BMD of 3000 mg of sodium, compared with 1500 mg/day, when participants were supplemented to ensure adequate calcium and vitamin D intakes (68).

Fluoride

Fluoride has long been known to prevent tooth decay and has been added to most water supplies in the United States. Fluoride substitutes for the hydroxyl group in hydroxyapatite, forming fluorapatite. Fluoride has been shown to result in bone with larger crystals and higher BMD, but lower elasticity (69). The effect of fluoride on fracture has been controversial, with both protective effects (70) and increased risk (71, 72) being reported. In the largest randomized, placebo-controlled trial of sodium fluoride in postmenopausal women with osteoporosis, spine BMD increased, but so did vertebral fracture risk (71). A metaanalysis of 25 studies showed that fluoride treatment increased spine and hip BMD, but with no effect on fracture risk. However, the protective effect was seen with low doses (≤20 mg/day of fluoride equivalents) (73). A more recent comparison of bone tissue from individuals in municipalities with and without fluoridated water, showed no differences in the physical characteristics of bone (74). Fluoride supplementation, either in short- or long-acting forms, is not approved by the US Food and Drug Administration for the prevention or treatment of osteoporosis.

Iron

Iron is an important cofactor for hydroxylases in collagen formation. Both low iron intake and iron overload have been negatively associated with bone. Iron overload has been associated with low BMD in patients with genetic hemochromatosis and with African hemosiderosis (75, 76). However, low iron is more of a concern in the general population. Rats fed iron-deficient diets showed compromised bone morphology, strength and density, and decreased serum osteocalcin (77, 78). Studies in postmenopausal women have reported that higher iron intake was associated with greater baseline BMD (79) and, prospectively, with lower loss of BMD in a subset of women using hormone replacement therapy and taking 800 mg calcium per day (80). In contrast, however, another study showed no association between iron status and BMD in women (81).

Silicon

Silicon is important for collagen and glycosaminoglycan formation in bone and cartilage, influencing the formation of the organic matrix. Silicon is also a major ion of osteogenic cells. Orthosilicic acid, the form of silicon absorbed in the diet, appears to be associated with bone formation through increased synthesis of collagen type I and stimulation of osteoblasts (82, 83). Chicks fed a silicon-deficient diet developed abnormally shaped bones (84), whereas the addition of silicon to the diet of depleted rats resulted in fewer osteoclasts, increased bone formation, decreased bone turnover, and increased BMD (85, 86).

Few studies have been conducted in humans, but those studies have shown protective effects. In the FOS, dietary silicon was positively associated with BMD at hip sites for men and premenopausal women but not postmenopausal women (87). French patients with osteoporosis showed significant improvements in trabecular bone volume with silicon treatment (88), and femoral BMD increased in female osteoporosis patients given intramuscular silicon, compared with others given fluoride, oral magnesium, or controls (89). These results suggest that higher silicon intake may be protective of BMD, but more studies are needed to confirm this.

Other Minerals

Copper is a cofactor for lysyl oxidase, which catalyses cross-linking of lysine and hydroxyproline in collagen. Animals with induced copper deficiency have reduced bone strength (90) and greater bone loss with aging (91). In women, plasma copper concentration was correlated with lumbar spine BMD (92), and lower copper status has been noted in elderly patients with fracture, relative to matched controls (93). A controlled feeding study in men showed increased activity of bone resorption markers when moved from a high (6 mg/day) to low (0.7 mg) copper diet, and this was reversed by returning to the high copper diet (94). However, another study did not replicate this effect (95).

Zinc may affect bone through its role in nucleic acid and protein metabolism (96). Lower serum and bone zinc and higher urinary zinc have been noted in patients with osteoporosis (97). In animals, zinc increased alkaline phosphatase and DNA synthesis, which may stimulate bone formation (98). Supplementation with zinc gluconate has been shown to increase alkaline phosphatase activity (99). In one study, postmenopausal women were randomized to treatment with calcium plus copper and zinc versus calcium plus corn starch. After 2 years, women with usual daily zinc intakes less than 8.0 mg benefited from the copper and zinc supplements, but women consuming adequate amounts of dietary zinc actually lost more BMD than control women (100).

Boron intake may protect bone by decreasing urinary calcium, phosphorus, and magnesium losses and increasing serum estradiol (101). In rats, boron deprivation altered trabecular bone and reduced the force needed to break the femur, confirming the importance of boron to cortical bone strength and trabecular bone microarchitecture (102). The systemic administration of boric acid reduced alveolar bone loss in periodontal disease in rats (103). However, no randomized trials of boron supplementation to prevent bone loss or prevent fractures exist.

Strontium has similarities to calcium, and it has received increasing interest as a treatment for osteoporosis. Doses of 1 to 2 g/day of strontium ranelate for 2 years or longer increased BMD in postmenopausal women by 2% to 3%, relative to placebo (104), and reduced both vertebral and nonvertebral fracture risk (105, 106). The increase in BMD is predictable and occurs in all treated individuals because of the ability of strontium to incorporate within the hydroxyapatite crystal. However, fracture risk cannot

and have been associated with lower bone loss induced by periodontitis in animal models (223–225).

Several animal studies support a protective association between n-3 fatty acids or higher n-3 to n-6 ratio and bone health. Few studies have been conducted in humans. Increasing ratios of n-6 to n-3 fatty acid intakes were associated with lower hip BMD in the Rancho Bernardo Study (226), and intake of fish containing n-3 fatty acids was associated with less BMD loss in astronauts (227). In the FOS, three or more, versus fewer, servings of fatty fish per week was associated with protection against 4-year loss of femoral neck BMD, although interactions between n-3 fatty acids with arachidonic acid were seen. Women with relatively high EPA + DHA intakes had higher baseline BMD when arachidonic acid intakes were also high; whereas men with the lowest EPA + DHA intakes in combination with high arachidonic acid intakes lost more BMD over time than did those with low arachidonic acid, suggesting that both types of fatty acids must be adequate for optimal protection of bone (228). It may be that in the presence of high n-3 intakes, production of prostaglandin E2 is suppressed, thus allowing other positive effects of arachidonic acid. Arachidonic acid can be synthesized from linoleic acid, which itself has been hypothesized to have negative effects on bone in high amounts, because of activation of NF-$\kappa\beta$ (229, 230).

Few studies of fatty acid intakes and fracture exist, and those that do have reported contradictory findings (231–234). Protective effects with supplementation with fish oil or n-3 fatty acids on BMD have been reported in postmenopausal women (235, 236), but another study saw no effect on BMD or bone turnover markers in women given fish oil and calcium versus calcium alone for 12 months (237). Adults randomly assigned to a diet high in α-linolenic acid versus an average US diet had significantly lower serum N-telopeptide concentration (238). The complexity of these relationships suggest that the effect of specific types of fatty acids on bone status and fracture risk may be dependent on other factors, and more complex analyses in larger studies may be needed to clarify these associations.

Other Food Constituents and Dietary Patterns

Caffeine

Some evidence shows that caffeine has a negative effect on bone, although study results vary. BMD was significantly lower in growing rats supplemented with 0.2% caffeine for 20 weeks, compared with controls, and osteoclastogenesis of bone marrow cells isolated from caffeine-treated rats was enhanced (239). The viability of bone marrow–derived mesenchymal stem cells from rats decreased in a concentration-dependent manner with higher caffeine, with negative effects on osteoblastogenesis (240). In human osteoblast cells, increasing caffeine incrementally decreased $1,25(OH)_2D_3$–induced VDR expression and alkaline phosphatase activity, affecting osteoblastic function (241).

In humans, caffeine is known to increase short-term urinary calcium excretion (242). However, a 2002 review concluded that caffeine had no effect on total 24-hour urinary calcium excretion, and the negative effect of caffeine on calcium absorption may be offset by "as little as 1 to 2 tablespoons of milk" (243). Consistently, observational studies of postmenopausal women found that consumption of 2 or more cups of coffee per day was associated with lower BMD only in those who did not regularly drink milk (244), and that bone loss was higher with 2 or more cups of coffee per day only when calcium intakes were less than 800 mg/day (242). Similarly, in a cohort of 31,527 Swedish women, intake of 4 or more cups of coffee daily was associated modestly with increased fracture risk, but mainly in women with low calcium intake (245). In Framingham, caffeine intake was associated with risk of hip fracture in elderly women but not in men (246). In contrast, however, elderly Swedish men, but not women, consuming 4 or more cups of coffee per day had significantly lower hip BMD. This association was modified by genotypes for cytochrome P-450 1A2 (CYP1A2), associated with metabolism of caffeine, but not with calcium intake (247).

Alcohol

Osteoporosis is commonly seen in chronic alcoholism (248). Heavy use of alcohol is associated with multiple nutritional deficiencies which, as described throughout this chapter, are likely to have their own negative effects on bone. In addition, ethanol itself appears to have direct effects on bone remodeling, affecting both BMD and bone strength. Long-term administration (3 months) of alcohol at a dose roughly equivalent to 1 L of wine per day in male adult rats showed a 10% reduction in bone density and a 12% reduction of mechanical strength of the femur (249). A review in 2012 concluded that the decrease in bone mass and strength seen with heavy alcohol consumption is mainly owing to a decrease in bone formation, with evidence of osteocyte apoptosis, oxidative stress, and Wnt signaling pathway modulation (250).

In contrast, moderate alcohol use has been associated with higher BMD in several studies of older adults (251, 252) and with lower bone loss over time (253). In the FOS, hip BMD was 3% to 5% greater in men consuming one to two drinks per day of total alcohol or beer, and hip and spine BMD were 5% to 8% greater in postmenopausal women consuming more than two drinks per day of total alcohol or wine. However, in men, more than two drinks per day of distilled liquor were associated with significantly lower BMD. The tendency toward stronger associations between BMD and beer or wine, relative to liquor, suggests that constituents other than ethanol may contribute to bone health (254). Together, the evidence is strong to support beneficial effects of moderate alcohol consumption but harmful effects of heavy alcohol consumption on bone status. Mechanisms for protective effects could include the estrogenic effects of ethanol, which stimulates the conversion of androstenedione to estrone. Additional compounds, such as silicon or polyphenols specifically in beer and wine, may offer additional benefit.

Although beneficial for BMD, less is known about moderate alcohol use and fracture. A metaanalysis of three cohort studies from Canada, Australia, and the Netherlands found that alcohol intake of more than two drinks per day versus less was associated with almost 70% greater hip fracture risk (255). Another study found a U-shaped association, in which hip fracture was lowest among drinkers consuming up to two drinks per day relative to either abstainers or heavier drinkers (256).

Dietary Patterns

It is increasingly clear that bone is sensitive to a wide variety of nutrients and exposures. Although studies usually have examined nutrients one at a time to understand associations and mechanisms, the final effect depends on many together. Therefore, it is useful to look at the total dietary pattern to see if combinations of these nutrients in the diet has an effect that may be greater than that of any single nutrient. Because so many food constituents are likely to affect bone, including an array of phytonutrients not yet fully explored, it may be expected that healthy diets may provide better overall support for bone growth, repair, and maintenance than any single nutrient or even food product.

In the FOS, individuals were divided into dietary pattern groups using cluster analysis (257). Men consuming a diet high in fruits, vegetables, and breakfast cereals had significantly greater hip BMD than all other diet pattern groups, whereas those consuming the most candy had significantly lower BMD. Women consuming the candy pattern also had the lowest BMD, whereas an alcohol pattern, in addition to the fruit and vegetable pattern, had the highest BMD. Dairy and meat groups tended to have intermediate BMD. Consistent with the evidence for individual nutrients, the fruit and vegetable group had the highest intakes of magnesium, potassium, vitamin C, and vitamin K. Similarly, in Scottish women 50 to 59 years old, a "healthy" pattern was associated with lower bone resorption, whereas a pattern characterized by snack foods was associated with lower femoral neck BMD (258). A UK study of postmenopausal twin pairs also showed a positive association between hip BMD and a pattern containing wine but a negative association with a traditional twentieth-century English diet (fried fish, fried potatoes, baked beans, red and processed meats, savory pies, and cruciferous vegetables) (259). Another UK study found significant associations between a pattern high in fruit intake and spine BMC in adolescents and older women and femoral neck BMC in adolescent boys (260). In Australian women 18 to 65 years old, a dietary pattern consisting of refined cereals, soft drinks, fried potatoes, sausages and processed meat, vegetable oils, beer, and takeout foods was significantly associated with lower total body BMC relative to other patterns. In contrast, a pattern

consisting of legumes, seafood, seeds, nuts, wine, rice and rice dishes, other vegetables, and vegetable dishes was positively associated with BMD at the hip and spine and with total body BMC (261). Most recently, an analysis of the NHANES 1999 to 2002 data found no association between the 2005 Healthy Eating Index score and bone turnover markers. However, milk intake was significantly negatively associated with urinary N-telopeptide-to-creatinine ratio and women with the highest added sugars intake had the highest serum bone–specific alkaline phosphatase associated with bone formation, but also with higher bone turnover (262).

A Canadian cohort study showed that a baseline dietary pattern characterized by fruits, vegetables, and whole grains was associated with 14% lower risk of fracture in women, with a similar pattern that did not reach significance in men (263). Dietary pattern intervention also has been shown to be effective. The DASH diet (high in fruit, vegetables, and low-fat dairy products) was shown to significantly reduced bone turnover. The addition of low sodium intake reduced calcium excretion in both the DASH and usual diet groups and further reduced serum osteocalcin in the DASH group (64). Another study compared the effects on bone turnover with 14 weeks of a low-sodium DASH-type diet versus a high-carbohydrate low-fat diet (both with >800 mg of calcium per day). The DASH group showed significant decreases in urinary sodium and calcium, an increase in urinary potassium, and lower bone turnover markers relative to the high-carbohydrate low-fat diet group (264).

Together, the evidence supports the role of an overall healthy diet, beyond adequate calcium intake, for optimal bone health. Pattern analysis is consistent with nutrient analyses showing that diets rich in fruits, vegetables, and low-fat dairy products; moderate in alcohol; and low in sodium appear to be important.

OTHER RISK FACTORS FOR OSTEOPOROTIC FRACTURE

Body Weight and Body Composition

Numerous studies show that higher total body weight is directly associated with greater BMD and lower risk of fracture. Further, weight loss is associated with loss in BMD. One review suggested that each 10% weight loss may lead to 1% to 2% bone loss (265). However, total weight consists of fat-free mass and fat tissue, and it is likely that these components may have differing effects on bone. With the recognition of fat as an endocrine organ, the effect of fat mass on bone may extend beyond its mechanical load on the skeleton.

Abdominal fat mass is more metabolically active, and produces hormones, chemokines, and cytokines that may contribute to inflammation (266) and insulin resistance (267), both of which may negatively affect bone and increase risk of fracture (268, 269). A few studies

(270, 271) have shown that when the mechanical loading effect of body weight was statistically removed, fat mass was negatively associated with bone. In Dutch men and women, most initial relationships between measures of fat distribution and BMD were positive but became negative after BMI adjustment. However, insulin or adiponectin concentrations did not explain either the positive or negative associations (272). Other studies noted that visceral, but not subcutaneous, fat had negative associations with femur strength in young women, hip and spine BMD in obese adolescent girls, and BMD in Korean men and women (273–276). In Puerto Rican adults in Boston, the likelihood of osteopenia or osteoporosis at the hip increased by 10% to 16% for every 100 g increase in body weight–adjusted abdominal fat mass (277). Although total body weight improves BMD, central obesity may have negative effects on bone status.

Physical Activity

In addition to the gravitational effect of body weight, a clear association exists between weight-bearing exercise and BMD (278). Improvements in bone mass also have been shown with resistance exercise (279). Strength and balance exercises improve muscle function and reduce falls, further reducing the risk of fracture (280). Increased aerobic exercise during weight loss is important to mitigate the bone loss otherwise seen with weight reduction (281). A genetically controlled study with twins showed that long-term physical activity during adulthood led to thicker cortices in long bone shafts, higher bending strength, and higher trabecular density and compressive strength in distal bones (282). One review concluded that high force (weight lifting) or high-impact (jumping) exercises have the greatest effect on bone, whereas non–weight-bearing exercises, such as swimming, do not affect bone (278).

Genetics

Although it is clear that bone responds to many environmental exposures, investigators have estimated that approximately 80% of the variance in peak bone mass, and a smaller proportion of the variance in bone loss with aging, may result from heritability (283). The identification of important genetic variants and gene–environment interactions is an active area of research. A family history of hip fracture may be predictive of a twofold increased risk of fracture (284). Studies of candidate gene polymorphisms and genome-wide association studies have identified genes associated with BMD or fragility fracture, including genes coding for the low-density lipoprotein receptor–related protein 5 (LRP5), estrogen receptor alpha (ESR1), and OPG (284). A large quantitative trait analysis resulted in confirmation for 74 SNPs at 32 loci in replication sets of Icelandic, Danish, and Australian adults, with 3 regions near genes previously identified: the *RANKL* gene, OPG, and ESR1, and 2 additional

regions. Several loci were also associated with osteoporotic fractures, including loci close to the *RANK* gene (285). A review noted that most of the known genes involved in osteoporosis encode components of pathways involved in bone synthesis or resorption, but that only a small proportion of the total genetic variation involved in osteoporosis has been identified (286).

One of the earliest genetic markers examined in relation to a dietary interaction was that for the vitamin D receptor, which has been associated with BMD in several populations (287). Women with the low BMD vitamin D receptor genotype had more rapid bone loss and failed to increase calcium absorption in response to lower calcium intake (288, 289). In another example, Greek postmenopausal carriers of the A allele versus the GG homozygotes of the rs4988321 polymorphism in the LRP5 had lower spine BMD only when calcium intake was less than 680 mg/day, a finding suggesting that adequate calcium intake may eliminate the negative effect of this polymorphism on BMD (290). Other reported gene–diet interactions affecting bone include observations that a high-fat diet may be detrimental or beneficial to bone mass depending on the presence of specific allelic variants in the *PPARG* gene, as shown in both mice and humans (291); evidence that $Alox5^{-/-}$ mice placed on a high-fat diet gain more fat mass and lose more bone mass, relative to wild-type controls (292); and evidence that high saturated fat intake in women with the APOE −219T/T and +113C/C genotypes is detrimental to bone status (293). The understanding of genetic determinants and gene–environment interactions remains at an early stage of investigation, and progress in this area is expected to accelerate in the near future.

STRATEGIES FOR THE PREVENTION AND MANAGEMENT OF OSTEOPOROSIS

An extensive body of research has identified numerous modifiable risk factors for osteoporosis and fracture. It is now clear that many aspects of diet and nutrition are important for bone health, including not only adequate intake of calcium and vitamin D but also of magnesium, potassium, other trace minerals, vitamin K, B vitamins, carotenoids, vitamins C and E, protein, and essential fatty acids. At the same time, it is important to avoid excess intakes of phosphorus, vitamin A, and sodium, and to maintain moderate alcohol intake. Although osteoporosis is one area in which BMI has been shown to be protective, we now understand that abdominal adiposity can have negative effects on bone through the release of certain cytokines. Weight-bearing physical activity is protective and is particularly important during weight loss, which may otherwise lead to bone loss as well. Muscle-strengthening exercises also can help to protect against weight loss–associated bone loss and help to strengthen muscles to reduce the risk of falling. Increased muscle mass also may contribute to greater bone strength among individuals across all age groups. Finally, we are in the early stages of understanding gene–nutrition interactions and expect that in the future, more personalized advice may be given based on genetic profiles for osteoporosis prevention.

With respect to management of osteoporosis, particularly for individuals who continue to be at high risk based on family history, age, previous fractures, or low bone mass, dietary recommendations for calcium and vitamin D remain an important cornerstone of the treatment approach, which often includes pharmacologic agents such as bisphosphonates. Most societies and advocacy groups recommend a minimum of 1200 mg of calcium per day either from the diet or with supplements, and at least 600 to 800 IU of vitamin D per day, both of which are in line with the IOM recommendations for the general population (2, 36, 294–296).

Dietary calcium is the preferred form for obtaining required calcium, because data from WHI suggest that excess calcium (i.e., >2000 mg/day) from supplements can be associated with a greater risk of nephrolithiasis (297). Serum 25(OH)D concentrations in osteoporotic patients should be maintained at or higher than 20 ng/mL (50 nmol/L). This usually can be achieved by adequate sunlight exposure and careful attention to diet, but frequently requires addition of a supplement containing 200 to 400 IU of vitamin D_3. In patients with malabsorption, gluten enteropathy, liver disease, gastric or intestinal bypass, or patients taking long-term antiseizure medications, 1000 to 2000 IU/day or more of vitamin D is often required to maintain blood concentrations higher than 20 ng/mL. Some practitioners prescribe 50,000 units of vitamin D_2 once weekly to improve compliance and maintain serum 25(OH)D concentrations at or higher than 20 ng/mL (50 nmol/L). In summary, calcium and vitamin D are essential components of any treatment regimen for osteoporosis. However, research suggests that many aspects of the diet and numerous nutrients contribute to bone health, emphasizing the importance of focusing on overall dietary quality in addition to medical approaches. Combining supplementation of vitamin D and calcium, as needed, with lifestyle changes and in some cases, drugs, to prevent further bone loss can reduce the risk of devastating osteoporotic fractures.

ACKNOWLEDGMENTS

The chapter was informed by an earlier version written by Bess Dawson-Hughes. We have no disclosures to report.

REFERENCES

1. Burge R, Dawson-Hughes B, Solomon DH et al. J Bone Miner Res 2007;22:465–75.
2. US Department of Health and Human Services. Bone Health and Osteoporosis: A Report of the Surgeon General. Office of the Surgeon General. Rockville, MD, 2004.
3. Looker AC, Melton LJ 3rd, Borrud LG et al. Osteoporos Int 2012;23:771–80.
4. Looker AC, Melton LJ 3rd, Borrud LG et al. Osteoporos Int 2012;23:1351–60.
5. Becker DJ, Kilgore ML, Morrisey MA. Curr Rheumatol Rep 2010;12:186–91.
6. Dempster DW. Am J Manag Care 2011;17(Suppl):S164–9.
7. Dempster DW, Shane E, Horbert W et al. J Bone Miner Res 1986;1:15–21.
8. Heaney RP, Abrams S, Dawson-Hughes B et al. Osteoporos Int 2000;11:985–1009.
9. Ensrud KE, Palermo L, Black DM et al. J Bone Miner Res 1995;10:1778–87.
10. Jones G, Nguyen T, Sambrook P et al. BMJ 1994;309:691–5.
11. World Health Organization. WHO Scientific Group on the Assessment of Osteoporosis at Primary Health Care Level. Geneva: World Health Organization, 2007.
12. Johnell O, Kanis JA, Oden A et al. J Bone Miner Res 2005;20:1185–94.
13. Cooper C, Atkinson EJ, O'Fallon WM et al. J Bone Miner Res 1992;7:221–7.
14. Grisso JA, Kelsey JL, Strom BL et al. N Engl J Med 1991;324:1326–31.
15. Hannan MT, Felson DT, Dawson-Hughes B et al. J Bone Miner Res 2000;15:710–20.
16. Burger H, de Laet CE, van Daele PL et al. Am J Epidemiol 1998;147:871–9.
17. Cummings SR, Nevitt MC, Browner WS et al. N Engl J Med 1995;332:767–73.
18. World Health Organization. Fracture Risk Assessment Tool (FRAX). World Health Organization Collaborating Centre for Metabolic Bone Diseases, University of Sheffield, UK. Available at: http://www.shef.ac.uk/FRAX/index.jsp. Accessed February 5, 2012.
19. Kanis JA, McCloskey EV, Johansson H et al. Osteoporos Int 2010;21(Suppl):S407–13.
20. Kanis JA, Hans D, Cooper C et al. Osteoporos Int 2011;22:2395–411.
21. Tucker KL, Bhupathiraju SN. Micronutrients and bone. Chapter 18 in: Cho KH, Michel JP, Buldau J et al, eds. Textbook of Geriatric Medicine, International. Seoul, Korea: Argos, 2010.
22. Tucker KL. Curr Osteoporos Rep 2009;7:111–7.
23. Food and Nutrition Board, Institute of Medicine. Dietary Reference Intakes for Calcium, Phosphorus, Magnesium, Vitamin D, and Fluoride. Washington, DC: National Academy Press, 1997.
24. Wosje KS, Specker BL. Nutr Rev 2000;58:253–68.
25. Winzenberg T, Shaw K, Fryer J et al. BMJ 2006;333:775.
26. Heaney RP. J Am Coll Nutr 2000;19:83S–99S.
27. Bischoff-Ferrari HA, Dawson-Hughes B, Baron JA et al. Am J Clin Nutr 2007;86:1780–90.
28. Dawson-Hughes B, Harris SS, Krall EA et al. Am J Clin Nutr 2000;72:745–50.
29. Jackson RD, LaCroix AZ, Gass M et al. N Engl J Med 2006;354:669–83.
30. Kalkwarf HJ, Khoury JC, Lanphear BP. Am J Clin Nutr 2003;77:257–65.
31. Key TJ, Appleby PN, Spencer EA et al. Public Health Nutr 2007;10:1314–20.
32. Feskanich D, Willett WC, Colditz GA. Am J Clin Nutr 2003;77:504–11.
33. Baran D, Sorensen A, Grimes J et al. J Clin Endocrinol Metab 1990;70:264–70.

34. Heaney RP, Rafferty K, Dowell MS. J Am Diet Assoc 2002;102:1672–4.

35. Lotz M, Zisman E, Bartter FC. N Engl J Med 1968;278:409–15.

36. US Department of Agriculture. What We Eat in America, NHANES 2007–2008. Nutrient Intakes from Food: Mean Amounts Consumed per Individual by Race/Ethnicity and Age, in the United States, 2007–2008. Available at: http://www.ars.usda.gov/ba/bhnrc/fsrg. 2010. Accessed February 12, 2012.

37. Food and Nutrition Board, Institute of Medicine. Dietary References Intakes for Calcium and Vitamin D. Washington, DC: National Academies Press, 2011.

38. Clark I. Am J Physiol 1969;217:865–70.

39. Kemi VE, Karkkainen MU, Karp HJ et al. Br J Nutr 2008; 99:832–9.

40. Kemi VE, Karkkainen MU, Rita HJ et al. Br J Nutr 2010; 103:561–8.

41. Wyshak G, Frisch RE. J Adolesc Health 1994;15:210–5.

42. Tucker KL, Morita K, Qiao N et al. Am J Clin Nutr 2006;84:936–42.

43. Heaney RP, Rafferty K. Am J Clin Nutr 2001;74:343–7.

44. Li M, Hasegawa T, Masuki H et al. J Oral Biosci 2010;52:94–9.

45. Creedon A, Flynn A, Cashman K. Br J Nutr 1999;82:63–71.

46. Rude RK, Kirchen ME, Gruber HE et al. Miner Electrolyte Metab 1998;24:314–20.

47. Rude RK, Gruber HE, Wei LY et al. Nutr Metab 2005;2:24.

48. Rude RK, Gruber HE, Norton HJ et al. Bone 2005;37:211–9.

49. Mutlu M, Argun M, Kilic E et al. J Int Med Res 2007;35: 692–5.

50. Tucker KL, Hannan MT, Chen H et al. Am J Clin Nutr 1999;69:727–36.

51. Ryder KM, Shorr RI, Bush AJ et al. J Am Geriatr Soc 2005;53:1875–80.

52. New SA, Robins SP, Campbell MK et al. Am J Clin Nutr 2000;71:142–51.

53. Ford ES, Mokdad AH. J Nutr 2003;133:2879–82.

54. Carpenter TO, DeLucia MC, Zhang JH et al. J Clin Endocrinol Metab 2006;91:4866–72.

55. Dimai HP, Porta S, Wirnsberger G et al. J Clin Endocrinol Metab 1998;83:2742–8.

56. Stendig-Lindberg G, Tepper R, Leichter I. Magnes Res 1993;6:155–63.

57. Sebastian A, Harris ST, Ottaway JH et al. N Engl J Med 1994;330:1776–81.

58. Macdonald HM, New SA, Fraser WD et al. Am J Clin Nutr 2005;81:923–33.

59. Zhu K, Devine A, Prince RL. Osteoporos Int 2008;20:335–40.

60. Lanham-New SA. J Nutr 2008;138:172S–7S.

61. Institute of Medicine. Strategies to Reduce Sodium Intake in the United States. Washington DC: National Academies Press, 2010.

62. Devine A, Criddle RA, Dick IM et al. Am J Clin Nutr 1995;62:740–5.

63. Sellmeyer DE, Schloetter M, Sebastian A. J Clin Endocrinol Metab 2002;87:2008–12.

64. Lin PH, Ginty F, Appel LJ et al. J Nutr 2003;133:3130–6.

65. Carbone LD, Barrow KD, Bush AJ et al. J Bone Miner Metab 2005;23:506–13.

66. Greendale GA, Barrett-Connor E, Edelstein S et al. J Am Geriatr Soc 1994;42:1050–5.

67. Carbone LD, Bush AJ, Barrow KD et al. J Bone Miner Metab 2003;21:415–20.

68. Ilich JZ, Brownbill RA, Coster DC. Eur J Appl Physiol 2010; 109:745–55.

69. Grynpas MD, Chachra D, Limeback H. The action of fluoride on bone. Chapter 23 in: Henderson JE, Goltzman D, eds. The Osteoporosis Primer. New York: Cambridge University Press, 2000.

70. Pak CY, Sakhaee K, Adams-Huet B et al. Ann Intern Med 1995;123:401–8.

71. Riggs BL, Hodgson SF, O'Fallon WM et al. N Engl J Med 1990;322:802–9.

72. Kleerekoper M, Peterson EL, Nelson DA et al. Osteoporos Int 1991;1:155–61.

73. Vestergaard P, Jorgensen NR, Schwarz P et al. Osteoporos Int 2008;19:257–68.

74. Chachra D, Limeback H, Willett TL et al. J Dent Res 2010;89:1219–23.

75. Guggenbuhl P, Deugnier Y, Boisdet JF et al. Osteoporos Int 2005;16:1809–14.

76. Schnitzler CM, Macphail AP, Shires R et al. J Bone Miner Res 1994;9:1865–73.

77. Medeiros DM, Plattner A, Jennings D et al. J Nutr 2002;132: 3135–41.

78. Katsumata S, Tsuboi R, Uehara M et al. Biosci Biotechnol Biochem 2006;70:2547–50.

79. Harris MM, Houtkooper LB, Stanford VA et al. J Nutr 2003;133:3598–602.

80. Maurer J, Harris MM, Stanford VA et al. J Nutr 2005;135:863–9.

81. Unfer TC, Muller EI, de Moraes Flores EM et al. Clin Chim Acta 2007;384:113–7.

82. Reffitt DM, Ogston N, Jugdaohsingh R et al. Bone 2003;32: 127–35.

83. Jugdaohsingh R. J Nutr Health Aging 2007;11:99–110.

84. Carlisle EM. Ciba Found Symp 1986;121:123–39.

85. Hott M, de Pollak C, Modrowski D et al. Calcif Tissue Int 1993;53:174–9.

86. Rico H, Gallego-Lago JL, Hernandez ER et al. Calcif Tissue Int 2000;66:53–5.

87. Jugdaohsingh R, Tucker KL, Qiao N et al. J Bone Miner Res 2004;19:297–307.

88. Schiano A, Eisinger F, Detolle P et al. Rev Rhum Mal Osteoartic 1979;46:483–6.

89. Eisinger J, Clairet D. Magnes Res 1993;6:247–9.

90. Jonas J, Burns J, Abel EW et al. Ann Nutr Metab 1993;37:245–52.

91. Rico H, Roca-Botran C, Hernandez ER et al. Menopause 2000;7:413–6.

92. Chaudhri MA, Kemmler W, Harsch I et al. Biol Trace Elem Res 2009;129:94–8.

93. Conlan D, Korula R, Tallentire D. Age Ageing 1990;19:212–4.

94. Baker A, Harvey L, Majask-Newman G et al. Eur J Clin Nutr 1999;53:408–12.

95. Cashman KD, Baker A, Ginty F et al. Eur J Clin Nutr 2001;55:525–31.

96. Beattie J, Avenell A. Nutr Res Rev 1992;5:167–88.

97. Atik OS. J Am Geriatr Soc 1983;31:790–1.

98. Yamaguchi M, Yamaguchi R. Biochem Pharmacol 1986;35: 773–7.

99. Peretz A, Papadopoulos T, Willems D et al. J Trace Elem Med Biol 2001;15:175–8.

100. Nielsen FH, Lukaski HC, Johnson LK et al. Br J Nutr 2011;106:1872–9.

101. Nielsen FH, Hunt CD, Mullen LM et al. FASEB J 1987;1:394–7.

102. Nielsen FH, Stoecker BJ. J Trace Elem Med Biol 2009; 23:195–203.

103. Demirer S, Kara MI, Erciyas K et al. Arch Oral Biol 2012;57:60–5.

104. Reginster JY, Bruyere O, Sawicki A et al. Bone 2009;45:1059–64.

105. Meunier PJ, Roux C, Ortolani S et al. Osteoporos Int 2009;20:1663–73.
106. Seeman E, Boonen S, Borgstrom F et al. Bone 2010;46:1038–42.
107. Kanis JA, Johansson H, Oden A et al. Osteoporos Int 2011;22:2347–55.
108. Roschger P, Manjubala I, Zoeger N et al. J Bone Miner Res 2010;25:891–900.
109. Bae YJ, Kim MH. Biol Trace Elem Res 2008;124:28–34.
110. Strause L, Saltman P, Smith KT et al. J Nutr 1994;124:1060–4.
111. Mithal A, Wahl DA, Bonjour JP et al. Osteoporos Int 2009;20:1807–20.
112. Cranney A, Horsley T, O'Donnell S et al. Evid Rep Technol Assess (Full Rep) 2007:1–235.
113. Moschonis G, Katsaroli I, Lyritis GP et al. Br J Nutr 2010;104:100–7.
114. Cummings SR, Browner WS, Bauer D et al. N Engl J Med 1998;339:733–8.
115. van Schoor NM, Visser M, Pluijm SM et al. Bone 2008;42:260–6.
116. Looker AC, Mussolino ME. J Bone Miner Res 2008;23:143–50.
117. Garnero P, Munoz F, Sornay-Rendu E et al. Bone 2007;40:716–22.
118. Dawson–Hughes B, Harris SS, Krall EA et al. N Engl J Med 1997;337:670–6.
119. Chapuy MC, Pamphile R, Paris E et al. Osteoporos Int 2002;13:257–64.
120. Trivedi DP, Doll R, Khaw KT. BMJ 2003;326:469.
121. Heikinheimo RJ, Inkovaara JA, Harju EJ et al. Calcif Tissue Int 1992;51:105–10.
122. Lips P, Graafmans WC, Ooms ME et al. Ann Intern Med 1996;124:400–6.
123. Meyer HE, Smedshaug GB, Kvaavik E et al. J Bone Miner Res 2002;17:709–15.
124. Komulainen MH, Kroger H, Tuppurainen MT et al. Maturitas 1998;31:45–54.
125. Grant AM, Avenell A, Campbell MK et al. Lancet 2005;365:1621–8.
126. Porthouse J, Cockayne S, King C et al. BMJ 2005;330:1003.
127. Lyons RA, Johansen A, Brophy S et al. Osteoporos Int 2007;18:811–8.
128. Law M, Withers H, Morris J et al. Age Ageing 2006;35:482–6.
129. Zhu K, Bruce D, Austin N et al. J Bone Miner Res 2008;23:1343–8.
130. Bischoff–Ferrari HA, Willett WC, Wong JB et al. Arch Intern Med 2009;169:551–61.
131. Winzenberg T, Powell S, Shaw KA et al. BMJ 2011;342:c7254.
132. Sanders KM, Stuart AL, Williamson EJ et al. JAMA 2010;303:1815–22.
133. Bugel S. Vitam Horm 2008;78:393–416.
134. Sokoll LJ, Sadowski JA. Am J Clin Nutr 1996;63:566–73.
135. Booth SL, Broe KE, Gagnon DR et al. Am J Clin Nutr 2003;77:512–6.
136. Feskanich D, Weber P, Willett WC et al. Am J Clin Nutr 1999;69:74–9.
137. Szulc P, Chapuy MC, Meunier PJ et al. Bone 1996;18:487–8.
138. Luukinen H, Kakonen SM, Pettersson K et al. J Bone Miner Res 2000;15:2473–8.
139. Cashman KD, O'Connor E. Nutr Rev 2008;66:532–8.
140. Emaus N, Gjesdal CG, Almas B et al. Osteoporos Int 2010;21:1731–40.
141. Shiraki M, Shiraki Y, Aoki C et al. J Bone Miner Res 2000;15:515–21.
142. Peterkofsky B. Am J Clin Nutr 1991;54:1135S–40S.
143. Kipp DE, McElvain M, Kimmel DB et al. Bone 1996;18:281–8.
144. Sahni S, Hannan MT, Gagnon D et al. Osteoporos Int 2009;20:1853–61.
145. Melhus H, Michaelsson K, Holmberg L et al. J Bone Miner Res 1999;14:129–35.
146. Zhang J, Munger RG, West NA et al. Am J Epidemiol 2006;163:9–17.
147. Raisz LG. J Bone Miner Res 1993;8(Suppl):S457–65.
148. Wu D, Mura C, Beharka AA et al. Am J Physiol 1998;275:C661–8.
149. Arjmandi B, Juma S, Beharka A et al. J Nutr Biochem 2002;13:543.
150. Norazlina M, Ima-Nirwana S, Gapor MT et al. Exp Clin Endocrinol Diabetes 2000;108:305–10.
151. Pasco JA, Henry MJ, Wilkinson LK et al. J Womens Health (Larchmt) 2006;15:295–300.
152. Wolf RL, Cauley JA, Pettinger M et al. Am J Clin Nutr 2005;82:581–8.
153. Lucock M. Mol Genet Metab 2000;71:121–38.
154. Eastell R, Vieira NE, Yergey AL et al. Clin Sci (Lond) 1992;82:681–5.
155. Carmel R. Arch Intern Med 1988;148:1712–4.
156. Kim GS, Kim CH, Park JY et al. Metabolism 1996;45:1443–6.
157. Herrmann M, Schmidt J, Umanskaya N et al. Bone 2007;41:584–91.
158. Cagnacci A, Baldassari F, Rivolta G et al. Bone 2003;33:956–9.
159. Rejnmark L, Vestergaard P, Hermann AP et al. Calcif Tissue Int 2008;82:1–11.
160. Bozkurt N, Erdem M, Yilmaz E et al. Arch Gynecol Obstet 2009;280:381–7.
161. Gjesdal CG, Vollset SE, Ueland PM et al. J Bone Miner Res 2007;22:747–56.
162. Ravaglia G, Forti P, Maioli F et al. J Gerontol A Biol Sci Med Sci 2005;60:1458–62.
163. Yazdanpanah N, Zillikens MC, Rivadeneira F et al. Bone 2007;41:987–94.
164. Morris MS, Jacques PF, Selhub J. Bone 2005;37:234–42.
165. Tucker KL, Hannan MT, Qiao N et al. J Bone Miner Res 2005;20:152–8.
166. Dhonukshe-Rutten RA, Lips M, de Jong N et al. J Nutr 2003;133:801–7.
167. Stone KL, Bauer DC, Sellmeyer D et al. J Clin Endocrinol Metab 2004;89:1217–21.
168. Macdonald HM, McGuigan FE, Fraser WD et al. Bone 2004;35:957–64.
169. McLean RR, Jacques PF, Selhub J et al. J Clin Endocrinol Metab 2008;93:2206–12.
170. Saito M, Fujii K, Marumo K. Calcif Tissue Int 2006;79:160–8.
171. Lubec B, Fang-Kircher S, Lubec T et al. Biochim Biophys Acta 1996;1315:159–62.
172. Elshorbagy AK, Gjesdal CG, Nurk E et al. Bone 2009;44:954–8.
173. Zhu K, Beilby J, Dick IM et al. Osteoporos Int 2009;20:1183–91.
174. Leboff MS, Narweker R, LaCroix A et al. J Clin Endocrinol Metab 2009;94:1207–13.
175. Perier MA, Gineyts E, Munoz F et al. Osteoporos Int 2007;18:1329–36.
176. Sato Y, Honda Y, Iwamoto J et al. JAMA 2005;293:1082–8.
177. Herrmann M, Umanskaya N, Traber L et al. Clin Chem Lab Med 2007;45:1785–92.
178. Green TJ, McMahon JA, Skeaff CM et al. Am J Clin Nutr 2007;85:460–4.

had gout in the previous year, and that 6.1 million adults in the United States had previously had gout (40). The prevalence of gout is increasing in the United States and around the world (34, 36, 41, 42). Gout is much more frequent in men than in women; however, because of greater longevity, gout will become an increasing problem in women (36, 39, 42, 43).

Mechanisms of Hyperuricemia

Uric acid is the end product of purine catabolism in humans. Xanthine oxidase catalyzes the oxidation of hypoxanthine to xanthine and ultimately to uric acid. Hyperuricemia is defined as a serum uric acid concentration greater than 7.0 mg/dL in men or greater than 6.0 mg/dL in women and is a common feature in all types of gout. Although hyperuricemia is a risk factor for gouty arthritis, the majority of individuals with hyperuricemia will not develop gout (36, 44). Overt manifestations of gout are more likely when the serum urate is greater than 9.0 mg/dL and the urinary uric acid excretion is greater than 800 mg/day (45).

The basic mechanisms of hyperuricemia are overproduction (~10% of patients) and underexcretion (~90% of patients) of uric acid. Overproduction could result from myeloproliferative disorders, malignant diseases, or hemolytic anemias. Metabolic inborn errors that cause increased purine and urate production include hypoxanthine-guanine phosphoribosyltransferase deficiency, phosphoribosylpyrophosphate synthetase overactivity, and glucose-6-phosphatase deficiency. Inhibitors of xanthine oxidase are frequently used when individuals overproduce uric acid. Impaired urate clearance may result from renal failure, dehydration, diabetic ketoacidosis, ethanol intake, diuretics, or use of specific medications (see later) (46). Uricosuric agents may be considered for the treatment of impaired urate excretion.

Gout may be classified as primary or secondary (36). Primary gout is related to an inborn error or an acquired metabolic defect. Examples of secondary gout include the use of drugs that increase serum urate concentrations (diuretics, tacrolimus, methoxyflurane, cyclosporine, ethambutol, pyrazinamide, cytotoxic chemotherapies, ethanol, low-dose salicylates, levodopa, ribavirin, interferon, or teriparatide) (36). Other drugs and nutrients are known to lower serum urate concentrations (ascorbic acid, benzbromarone, calcitonin, citrate, estrogen, fenofibrate, losartan, probenecid, high-dose salicylates, and sulfinpyrazone) (47).

Metabolic and Lifestyle Profiles of Individuals with Hyperuricemia and Gout

The classic profile of an individual with gout is an obese, hypertensive, middle-aged man who eats rich foods and drinks alcohol (39).

Metabolic Syndrome and Gout

Strong correlations exist among obesity, insulin resistance, and serum uric acid concentrations and between renal uric acid clearance and degree of insulin resistance (48). Choi et al (49) determined the relationship between metabolic syndrome, defined as ≥3 of the following criteria: abdominal obesity (waist circumference >102 cm in men or >88 cm in women), hypertriglyceridemia (≥150 mg/dL), low high-density lipoprotein cholesterol (<40 mg/dL in men or <50 mg/dL in women), hypertension (>130/85 mg Hg), and high fasting glucose (≥110 mg/dL) (50) and gout prevalence. The prevalence of metabolic syndrome was 62.8% (95% confidence interval [CI], 51.8% to 73.6%) in patients with gout and 25.4% (23.5% to 27.3%) in patients without gout. In addition, a history of gout was shown to be an independent risk factor for the development of type 2 diabetes (51).

Dietary Correlates of Hyperuricemia and Gout

Dietary purines can contribute up to one third of the uric acid in the body (52). However, subjects with gout receiving a purine-free diet had little change in plasma uric acid compared with those receiving a regular diet (53). A variety of foods have been reported to increase serum uric acid and to increase gouty attacks, including meats, seafood, yeast, yeast extracts, peas, beans, lentils, asparagus, spinach, mushrooms, and beer and alcoholic drinks (54). Data from the NHANES III survey showed that, after adjusting for age, uric acid concentrations in adults differed between extreme quintiles by 0.48 mg/dL for total meat intake (95% CI, 0.34 to 0.61; p for trend <.001), 0.16 mg/dL for seafood (95% CI, 0.06 to 0.27; p for trend .005), and inversely by 21 mg/dL for total dairy food intake (95% CI, 0.37 to 0.04; p for trend = .02), indicating that higher meat and seafood consumption, but not total protein, may be related to hyperuricemia (42, 55). In the Health Professionals Follow-up Study, men in the highest quintiles of meat and seafood intakes had 41% and 51% increased risk of gout, respectively, although the consumption of purine-rich vegetables was not associated with risk (42, 56). Individuals consuming a serving of milk one or more times per day had lower serum uric acid than those consuming no milk (55). Yogurt consumption at least every other day was also associated with lower serum uric acid compared with individuals not consuming yogurt (55). Data from the NHANES III also showed that the adjusted odds ratio for hyperuricemia in individuals consuming 6 cups or more of coffee per day, compared with no coffee consumption, was 0.57 (95% CI, 0.35 to 0.94; p for trend .001) (57). Tea consumption was not associated with hyperuricemia, and the authors suggested that the inverse association with coffee intake may be mediated by components other than caffeine. Another study using NHANES III data found that consumption of soft drinks containing fructose, but not artificially sweetened soft drinks, was associated with higher serum uric acid concentrations (58). The metabolism of fructose has been shown to generate uric acid more than other sugars (59). Data from the Health Professionals Follow-up Study showed that greater vitamin C intake was associated with lower uric acid (60). At intake higher than 400 to 500 mg/day of vitamin C, serum uric acid concentrations plateaued (54, 61). The risk of gout was prospectively evaluated over a 23-year period in 47,150 men who had no history of gout at baseline (56). Increased risk of gout was positively associated with higher consumption of meat and inversely associated with higher intake of dairy products. There were no relationships with intakes of total protein or purine-rich vegetables.

Alcohol and Hyperuricemia and Gout

Various mechanisms linking hyperuricemia and gout to alcohol consumption have been postulated. These include (a) production of temporary lactic acidosis; (b) stimulation of purine production by accelerated degradation of adenosine triphosphate to adenosine monophosphate by conversion of acetate to acetyl-coenzyme A during alcohol metabolism; (c) high purine content in beer, particularly guanosine; and (d) consumption of lead-contaminated alcohol causing a reduction in renal urate excretion and subsequent hyperuricemia (54). NHANES III data showed that intake of beer and liquor, after adjustment for other risk factors, predicted elevated uric acid concentrations (62). Data from the Health Professionals Follow-up

Study suggested a positive dose-response relation between total alcohol intake and gout (63). The relative risk for hyperuricemia with beer or liquor consumption was greater than for wine intake. Analyses from the Nutrition and Health Survey in Taiwan found that increasing beer intake was independently associated with hyperuricemia (serum uric acid greater than 6.6 mg/dL for women or 7.7 mg/dL for men) in men, but not women (61).

Dietary Therapy

Pharmacologic therapy with allopurinol or febuxostat, which decreases oxidation of purines to uric acid, and uricosuric agents, such as probenecid and sulfinpyrazone, have changed gout therapy. Dietary therapies may have additive benefits to pharmacologic therapy, although they rarely lower serum urate concentrations by more than 1 mg/dL, even with severe purine restriction (39, 53, 64, 65). Dietary management of gout is particularly useful during a gouty flare (66–68). Figure 91.2 displays the impact of dietary components on gout risk. The American Dietetic Association Nutrition Care Manual (69) recommends that during an acute gouty attack, the patient should do the following: (a) consume 8 to 16 cups

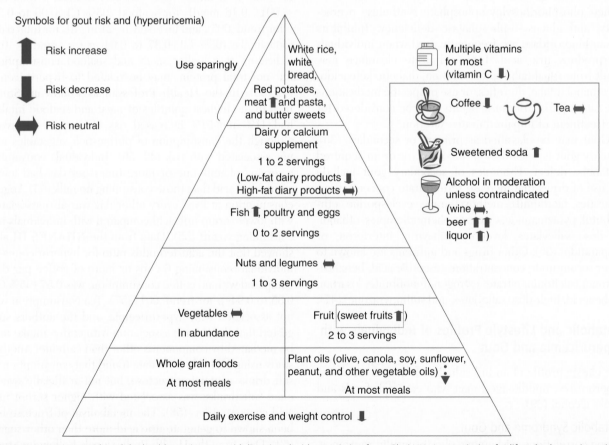

Fig. 91.2. Dietary gout risk and the healthy eating pyramid. (Reprinted with permission from Choi HK. A prescription for lifestyle change in patients with hyperuricemia and gout. Curr Op in Rheumatol 2010;22:165–72.)

of fluid/day, at least half as water; (b) abstain from alcohol; (c) limit animal foods; (d) eat a moderate amount of protein with recommended sources as low-fat or nonfat dairy, tofu, eggs, and nut butters; and (e) limit meat, fish, and poultry to 4 to 6 ounces/day. During remission from a gout flare, the recommendations are as follows: (a) consume 8 to 16 cups of fluid/day, at least half as water; (b) abstain from alcohol; (c) follow a well-balanced eating plan following the Dietary Guidelines for Americans and, as tolerated, consume animal foods and continue to eat a moderate amount of protein; and (d) maintain a desirable body weight and avoid fasting or high-protein diets for weight loss (69). Choi (67) recommend the following guidelines for patients with gout: (a) exercise daily and reduce weight; (b) limit red meat intake; (c) tailor seafood intake to individual risk for cardiovascular disease and consider omega-3 fatty acid supplements; (d) drink skim milk or consume other low-fat dairy products daily up to 2 servings per day; (e) consume vegetable protein, nuts, legumes, and purine-rich vegetables; (f) reduce alcoholic beverages to less than 1 or 2 drinks per day for men or 1 drink for women; (g) limit sugar-sweetened softdrinks and other beverages containing high-fructose corn syrup; (h) allow coffee drinking if already drinking coffee; and (i) consider taking vitamin C supplements.

Summary

Unfortunately the actual dietary practices of individuals with gout appear to be inconsistent with current recommended diet therapy recommendations (70). New goals for gout management include a major emphasis on diet therapy to reduce insulin resistance and produce weight loss in overweight patients.

OSTEOARTHRITIS

Definition

OA, also known as degenerative joint disease, is a progressive disorder of the joints caused by gradual loss of cartilage, resulting in the development of bony spurs and cysts at the margins of the joints (71).

Epidemiology

Estimates from the NHANES III and the NHIS estimate that 27 million adults in the United States have OA (40). The most commonly affected joints are knees, hips, and hands with individuals 50 years or older; and women more often affected than men (40). The prevalence of radiographic knee arthritis in US adults without and with symptoms was estimated as 37.4% and 12.1%, respectively, from NHANES III (72). Demographic characteristics associated with radiographic knee arthritis included body mass index (BMI) of 30 or greater, advancing age, non-Hispanic black race, and men doing manual labor.

Nutrient Intakes of Patients with Osteoarthritis

In a series of 12 patients with OA, more than 50% consumed diets with less than 67% of the recommended dietary allowances (RDAs) for iron, zinc, vitamin E, folate, and vitamin B_6 (73). Of 82 older ambulatory patients, 80% had BMI of 27 or greater (74). Seventy-nine percent of 77 patients participating in a multidisciplinary program for the management of OA were obese, and the degree of obesity was related to the pain of arthritis. Dietary intakes of vitamin D, folate, pyridoxine, and zinc averaged less than 80% of the RDA (75). In another study, patients with OA were, on average, 15 lbs (6.8 kg) overweight, whereas patients with RA averaged 10 lbs (4.5 kg) underweight (76).

Two studies evaluated the relationship of vitamin K status with OA. Radiographs in 672 Framingham Offspring Study participants showed that the mean number of knee joints with osteophytes decreased with greater phylloquinone concentration (77). The prevalence ratio of OA, osteophytes, joint space narrowing, and number of joints with all three features in the hand were also inversely associated with phylloquinone. A Japanese study with 719 individuals aged 60 years or older analyzed radiographs of the knee with Kellgren/Lawrence grading (0 = *normal* to 4 = *severe*) and found that 70.8% had a score of 2 or higher. Age, BMI, and female gender predicted the presence of OA (78, 79). The only dietary factor inversely associated with radiographic knee arthritis was vitamin K. Vitamin K status could be important in the gamma carboxylation of vitamin K–dependent proteins, such as matrix Gla protein. However, in a clinical trial, vitamin K supplementation was not associated with greater bone mineral density (BMD) or lower bone turnover compared with placebo (80).

Nutritional Correlates

The Chingford Study (81) of 1003 adult women found radiographic evidence of knee OA in 118. Elevated blood glucose and moderately elevated serum cholesterol were significantly related to radiographic unilateral knee OA. Bilateral knee OA was significantly associated with hypertension, and elevated cholesterol. In contrast, the Baltimore Longitudinal Study of Aging (82) found that no metabolic factors (blood pressure, fasting lipids, or 2-hour glucose tolerance test) were related to knee radiograph OA after adjusting for age and obesity in 464 men and 275 women aged greater than 40 years.

Obesity

Numerous studies have shown a positive relationship between obesity, elevated BMI, and knee OA (83–96). Body fat distribution does not seem to affect the risk of development of knee OA; however, emerging data suggest that elevated fat mass is associated with increased concentrations of inflammatory mediators and adipokines that affect cartilage and joints (96).

In the Framingham cohort, Felson noted that weight loss of 5.1 kg over 10 years decreased the odds of incident knee OA by 50% (86). In 142 obese patients with radiographic evidence of knee OA and reported disability related to the arthritis (97), each kilogram of weight loss was associated with an approximate 4-unit reduction of knee joint forces including compressive force, resultant force, abduction moment, and medial rotation moment. Each pound of weight loss was associated with an approximately fourfold reduction in load on the knee. The 18-month Arthritis, Diet and Activity Promotion Trial of 316 community-dwelling individuals 60 years of age or older (98) showed that a diet plus exercise intervention improved Western Ontario and McMaster Universities Osteoarthritis Index (WOMAC) scores significantly relative to exercise only, diet only, or control groups. Both the diet-only and the diet-plus-exercise groups had significant weight loss, but only the diet-plus-exercise group had significant reduction in self-reported pain ($p \leq .05$) with a 30.3% decrease in pain over the 18-month intervention. There was no difference in radiographic progression across intervention groups. The same study found that serum biomarkers (cartilage oligomeric protein, hyaluronan, antigenic keratin sulfate, and transforming growth factor-β1) were relatively stable over 18 months; however, higher serum hyaluronan was correlated with worse radiographic classification, lending support for the idea that OA is a metabolically active disease (99).

Another clinical trial of obese patients with OA with a mean age of 62.5 years, compared a very low energy diet (415 kcal/day) to a low energy diet (810 kcal/day) for 16 weeks (100). After 8 weeks, both groups were shifted to a 1200 kcal/day diet of normal foods and meal replacements. There was no significant difference between diets in pain response, and both groups had significant improvement in symptoms.

The Action for Health in Diabetes trial prospectively evaluated 2203 obese subjects with baseline knee pain, randomized to an intensive lifestyle intervention (ILI) program (with support for behavioral change in diet and physical activity) versus an education group (general education about healthy eating and physical activity) (101). The ILI group had greater weight loss (−9.02 versus −0.78 kg; $p < .001$) and more improvement in WOMAC score ($p < .001$) and in physical function, relative to the education group.

Bariatric surgical procedures are increasingly being used to assist weight loss (102). Hooper et al followed 47 obese women and 1 man (mean age 44 ± 9 years, mean BMI = 51 ± 8 kg/m^2) who had an open or laparoscopic roux-en-Y gastric bypass for 12 months (103). The mean weight loss in the women was 41 ± 15 kg. They reported a 51% reduction in WOMAC pain score, a 64% decrease in stiffness, and a 74% improvement in function. Another study followed 53 patients who underwent laparoscopic gastric banding for 2 years and reported significant weight loss and substantial improvement in OA (104).

In summary, a strong relationship exists between obesity and OA. The relationships between obesity and OA are likely related to mechanical factors, but also metabolic factors. Strategies to reduce weight have been shown to decrease both the onset and progression of OA in weight-bearing joints.

Vitamin D

Because of the importance of vitamin D in collagen and bone metabolism, there has been an interest in the effect of vitamin D status on OA incidence and progression. Participants in the Framingham Heart Study with low dietary intakes of vitamin D and low 25-hydroxy vitamin D (25-OH vitamin D) (less than 30 ng/mL) were more likely to have progression of established OA, but these factors did not affect the risk for development of OA (105). The authors hypothesized that low vitamin D status may hinder the response of bone to cartilage damage (105). Data from the Study for Osteoporotic Fractures Research Group found that elderly women in the lowest tertile of serum 25-OH vitamin D were 3 times more likely to develop hip joint space narrowing than women with levels in the highest tertile (106). Data from both the Framingham Osteoarthritis Study and the Boston Osteoarthritis of the Knee Study (BOKS) showed no association between 25-OH vitamin D level and radiographic worsening of arthritis (107). Additionally, in the BOKS trial, there was no relationship of 25-OH vitamin D to cartilage loss, as measured by magnetic resonance imaging. In 880 subjects from the Tasmanian Older Adult Cohort Study, with a mean age of 61 years, sunlight exposure and serum 25-OH vitamin D concentration were associated with medial and lateral tibial cartilage loss in women and in individuals with knee pain, but not in men or individuals without OA on knee radiographs or knee pain (108).

In 1248 subjects from the Rotterdam Study of the elderly, (baseline 1991 to 1993 and follow-up 1997 to 1999), the adjusted odds ratio for progression of knee OA was 7.7 (95% CI, 1.3 to 43.5) for individuals in the lowest versus highest tertile of vitamin D intake (109). Individuals with low BMD were more likely to have incident knee OA ($p = .03$), and poor vitamin D status particularly influenced the progression of knee OA in individuals with low BMD. In the Osteoporotic Fractures in Men Study (110), individuals with radiographic hip arthritis at follow-up (4.6 years) had more hip pain and higher prevalence of vitamin D insufficiency and vitamin D deficiency at baseline, compared with controls. The authors concluded that men with vitamin D deficiency were twice as likely to have prevalent radiographic hip OA, and suggested that vitamin D supplementation is warranted.

Although there is a suggestion that low vitamin D status is cross-sectionally related to hip and knee OA incidence and progression, not all studies have confirmed this relationship. Double-blind, placebo-controlled supplementation trials will be necessary to determine if there is a causal relationship.

Glucosamine and Chondroitin Sulfate as Therapy

The use of glucosamine sulfate and chondroitin sulfate nutritional supplements for the relief of pain in OA is based on their bioavailability, anabolic effects such as increased chondrocyte proliferation, increased extracellular matrix biosynthesis, increased sulfate intake, and reduction in catabolic effects mediated by proteinases, cytokines, and other catabolic mediators. Several trials using radiolabeled compounds have demonstrated that blood concentrations increase following an oral dose in concert with an increase in synovial concentrations. Although numerous in vitro studies support these effects, there is a lack of evidence for them in humans, with the exception of the increase in sulfate intake (111).

The clinical efficacy of these compounds is controversial. A double-blind, placebo-controlled trial of glucosamine sulfate (1500 mg/day) in patients with lumbar osteoarthritis concluded that there was no relief of lower back pain at 6 or 12 months of therapy compared with placebo (112). A larger double-blind, placebo-controlled 2-year study of 662 patients with knee OA using glucosamine sulfate (1500 mg/day), chondroitin sulfate (1200 mg/day), or both, found that none of the treatments significantly reduced the WOMAC index relative to placebo (113). The same group found no radiographic evidence of these treatments in reducing the progression of knee OA (114).

A non–placebo-controlled study demonstrated that glucosamine sulfate plus omega-3 fatty acids was superior to glucosamine alone in reducing the WOMAC index in patients with hip or knee OA (115). Another non–placebo-controlled study tested a combination of glucosamine, chondroitin, and quercetin in patients with OA and in patients with RA and reported both clinical and biochemical beneficial effects (in synovial fluid) only in patients with OA (116). The lack of a placebo group and the combination therapy make it difficult to make conclusions about the effects of glucosamine and/or chondroitin alone.

In 2009, a large systematic review of the glucosamine and chondroitin trials concluded that there was only modest reduction of joint space loss with glucosamine, and that the possibility that sulfate was the active substance should be tested (111). Glucosamine sulfate, up to 2000 mg/day, and chondroitin sulfate, up to 1200 mg/day, are apparently safe with no reported adverse effects at these oral dosing levels (117).

Medical Foods

A relatively new therapeutic approach to OA is the use of medical foods, which came into existence in 1988 (118). As shown in Table 91.2, they are a class of substances between a dietary supplement and a drug. Important distinctions from dietary supplements include a sound, scientific rationale for their use, and like drugs, medical foods require a prescription and physician supervision. They are naturally existing substances that help to restore normal homeostatic physiologic and metabolic processes in a patient with a disease, but that cannot be obtained from a normal diet in sufficient quantities. An example would be digestive enzymes used to treat cystic fibrosis patients with exocrine pancreatic insufficiency (118).

Morgan et al tested the safety of a medical food, flavocoxid (a proprietary blend of free B ring flavonoids

TABLE 91.2	DIFFERENCES AMONG MEDICAL FOODS, DIETARY SUPPLEMENTS, AND DRUGS		
PRODUCT CLASS ATTRIBUTE	DIETARY SUPPLEMENT	MEDICAL FOOD	DRUG
Governing regulation	DSHEA	Orphan Drug Act (amendments, 1988)	Federal Food, Drug, and Cosmetic Act (1938, as amended by FDA Modernization Act of 1997)
Intended population	Healthy	Diseased	Diseased
Ingredients	Nutritional	Nutritional, not in ordinary diet	Mostly synthetic; can be nutritional
Product basis	"General expectation" of desired product performance	Dietary need (metabolic imbalance can be restored by special ingredients)	Safe and effective for disease and patient population
Safety standard	"General expectation" of safety (ingredients on market before DSHEA)	GRAS (safe for public use)	Approved by NDA or ANDA or used as DESI ("grandfathered")
Scientific requirements	None	Recognized science (follows good scientific practices, accepted in clinical practice or peer review)	Preclinical and phases I, II, and III
Physician supervision	None	Required	Required if prescription drug
Dosing	Oral	Oral or enteral	Any
Distribution	Health food stores, mass market	Hospitals, retail pharmacies	Hospitals, retail pharmacies

ANDA, abbreviated new drug application; DESI, Drug Efficacy Study Implementation; DSHEA, Dietary Supplements Health and Education Act of 1994; FDA, Food and Drug Administration; GRAS generally recognized as safe; NDA, new drug application.

Adapted with permission from Morgan SL, Baggott JE. Medical foods: products for the management of chronic diseases. Nutr Rev 2006;64:495–501.

and flavans from the root of *Scutellaria baicalensis* and from the bark of *Acacia catechu*) for the management of knee OA (119). The rationale was that pain and inflammation mediated by excess arachidonic acid metabolites could be reduced by flavocoxid inhibition of cyclooxygenase and lipoxygenase enzymes, which are essential for the biosynthesis of arachidonic acid metabolites (e.g., prostaglandins, thromboxanes, prostacyclin, leukotrienes). Thus, the OA patient has excessive arachidonic acid release and metabolism (disease and dyshomeostasis), which can, in part, be corrected by flavocoxid (120).

Human trials of flavocoxid showed that it did block arachidonic acid metabolism both systemically (serum) and locally (synovial fluid) and, possibly as a consequence, reduced free radical production in synovial fluid (121). However, flavocoxid did not substantially inhibit production of thromboxanes, platelet aggregation, or increase bleeding time in healthy subjects (122).

The safety of flavocoxid was established in a 12-week, double-blind, placebo-controlled study (119). No differences in adverse effects of flavocoxid compared with placebo were reported using a 250 mg twice daily dose. A shorter trial reported that flavocoxid (500 mg twice daily) was as effective as naproxen (500 mg twice daily) in reducing the signs and symptoms of OA (123). The use of medical foods provides the clinician with alternative therapies, which may have a safer adverse event profile than pharmacologic agents.

Summary

Obesity and metabolic syndrome with OA strongly overlap. The efficacy of nutritional supplements such as glucosamine and chondroitin sulfate is controversial. Medical foods may be useful in knee OA.

RHEUMATOID ARTHRITIS

Definition

RA is an inflammatory disease of the synovial lining of the joint and results in pain, stiffness, swelling, joint damage, and loss of function. Inflammation most often affects joints of the hands and feet and tends to be symmetrical. This symmetry helps distinguish RA from other forms of the disease (124). Approximately 1% of the US population (approximately 2.1 million people) has RA (125). Patients with RA may have excess death, radiographic deterioration of joints, and reduced functional status, despite disease-modifying antirheumatic drug (DMARD) treatment (126–128).

Mechanisms Affecting Nutritional Status

RA can affect nutritional status through several mechanisms (129–131). Joint swelling and tenderness can impair the ability to prepare food, involvement of the temporomandibular joint can impair chewing, and general joint involvement can impair self-feeding. In addition, patients may have xerostomia that can impair food intake. Many of the pharmacologic therapies used to treat RA also have side effects that further impair food intake, such as nausea with MTX or proteolysis with corticosteroid therapy (132, 133). The catabolic and inflammatory aspects of the disease also affect nutritional status. Table 91.3 displays mechanisms by which RA may affect nutritional status.

Nutrient Intakes and Vitamin Concentrations in Patients with Rheumatoid Arthritis

In 1943, 31 patients with RA were evaluated to determine their dietary history for the year before onset (134). Although their dietary intakes were not substantially different from those of a cross-section of families in the North Atlantic States, more than two-thirds of patients had diets that were low in calcium, thiamine, and riboflavin, and approximately 50% had low intake of vitamin C. In 1996, Kremer (135) found that patients with RA had diets that were high in total fat, low in fiber, and deficient in micronutrients. Among 41 patients with active RA, diets were low in pyridoxine, zinc, magnesium, folate, and copper.

Morgan et al (131, 136) evaluated the nutrient intake and status of 32 MTX-treated adults with RA (131).

TABLE 91.3	ADVERSE EFFECTS OF RHEUMATOID ARTHRITIS ON NUTRITIONAL STATUS

Increased nutrient requirements
  Increased metabolism and nitrogen losses increase protein requirements.
  Inflammation increases micronutrient requirements (i.e., antioxidant vitamins).
Diminished intake
  Articular disease diminishes the ability to self-feed, shop, and prepare foods.
  Morning stiffness may decrease morning appetite.
  Temporomandibular joint disease may impair the ability to chew.
  Depression from chronic disease may impair food intake.
  Sjögren syndrome and xerostomia may impair food intake.
Diminished absorption
  Abnormalities of the small bowel, liver, and pancreas may decrease absorption of nutrients.
  Drug therapy (e.g., salicylazosulfapyridine) may inhibit nutrient absorption.
Inadequate utilization
  Drug therapy (e.g., methotrexate, salicylazosulfapyridine, and nonsteroidal anti-inflammatory drugs) may inhibit enzymes of intermediary metabolism.
  Vitamin B_{12} deficiency can reduce folate uptake and retention by the cells.
Increased excretion
  Urinary excretion of nutrients may be increased in the catabolic state of active disease and by some drug treatments (e.g., prednisone).
  Chronic blood loss from nonsteroidal anti-inflammatory agents may increase the need for hematopoietic precursors (e.g., iron).

Intakes of pyridoxine, calcium, magnesium, and zinc were less than 33% of the 1989 RDA. Thirty percent had deficient plasma folate, and 23% had deficient erythrocyte folate before starting MTX therapy. In a subsequent study, 79 patients (mean age, 53 years; mean disease duration, 9 years) were followed for 1 year after starting MTX therapy (136). Based on the average of five 24-hour dietary recalls, the patients consumed less than 67% of the recommended dietary intake for folate, vitamin B_{12}, vitamin E, calcium, iron, magnesium, copper, and zinc. Before the start of MTX therapy, 47% of patients had deficient plasma folate and 11% had deficient erythrocyte folate concentrations.

Nutritional Status of Patients with Rheumatoid Arthritis and Juvenile Rheumatoid Arthritis and Body Composition

Comorbidities of RA include loss of lean body mass, termed *rheumatoid cachexia*, which is the end product of the hypermetabolism associated with this disease (137–141). Sir James Paget first described rheumatoid cachexia in 1873 (142). In patients with rheumatoid cachexia, there may be an increase in fat mass with coexisting loss of lean body mass called cachectic obesity (141).

In 1984, Helliwell et al (143) evaluated 50 patients with RA and 50 normal controls, using anthropometric and biochemical measurements, including serum albumin, transferrin, retinol-binding protein, thyroxine-binding prealbumin, zinc, and folic acid concentrations. Patients were classified as being malnourished if they had a reduction in one anthropometric measurement with two or more biochemical abnormalities. The upper arm muscle circumference was low in 14% of patients and most of the biochemical measures (serum albumin, transferrin, retinol-binding protein, thyroxine-binding prealbumin, zinc, and folic acid) were low in the patients. Thirteen out of 50 patients (26%) met the criteria for malnutrition (low anthropometry plus two or more biochemical measures), versus none of the controls (143).

Collins et al (144) studied 38 hospitalized patients with RA (144). A likelihood of malnutrition index was calculated for 38 hospitalized patients with RA that included serum folate and vitamin C levels, triceps skin fold or a BMI calculation, arm muscle area corrected for bone area, a total lymphocyte count, serum albumin and a hematocrit. Twenty-seven of 38 patients (71%) had a high likelihood of malnutrition, based on this index.

Mody et al (145) assessed the nutritional status of 220 patients with RA using triceps skinfold, upper arm muscle circumference, BMI, percentage ideal body weight, and serum albumin. Forty-five of 220 patients (20%) had a low value in one or more anthropometric measures, and 6 (3%) had low albumin. Obesity, defined as a BMI greater than 30, was found in 10% of this population. In contrast, Kalla et al (146) compared 65 patients with RA with 71 matched controls using anthropometric

measurements and serum protein concentrations. Lean body mass was similar in the controls and patients, and corticosteroid therapy had no effect on anthropometric measurements.

Hernandez-Beriain et al (147) evaluated 75 outpatients with RA having variable functional class, radiologic stage, rheumatoid factor seropositivity status, presence of extraarticular disease, and disease duration. Nutritional status was evaluated by measurements of weight, height, midupper arm circumference, and triceps skinfold, and calculation of midarm muscle area and midarm fat area. Lean body mass, as evaluated by midupper arm circumference, was lower in patients with lower RA functional class; 24% of 75 RA outpatients had anthropometric measurements below the 10th percentile, and 14% were below the 5th percentile. The authors concluded that patients with poorer functional class, more severe radiographic disease, or with extraarticular disease had worse nutritional status and loss of lean body mass than patients with less severe disease.

Munro and Capell (148) evaluated BMI, upper arm fat mass (an estimate of body fat mass), and upper arm muscle area (an estimate of body somatic muscle mass) by anthropometric measurements. Similarly, greater than half of patients with RA had values in the lowest 10th percentile for upper arm muscle area; reflecting a loss in somatic muscle stores and the catabolic nature of the disease. In addition, in female patients, there was a correlation between low fat mass and elevated erythrocyte sedimentation rates and C-reactive protein levels. The wasted patients were also more limited in their ability to perform activities of daily living as assessed by the Health Assessment Questionnaire (HAQ) which measures functional status.

Roubenoff et al (137) found that in 24 patients, 67% were cachectic, and their lean body mass was inversely associated with numbers of swollen joints. This suggested that protein catabolism and gluconeogenesis may be required to maintain a high level of disease activity. Chronic caloric deficits were apparently not a cause of lower lean body mass. Elevated tumor necrosis factor (TNF)-α was found in 3 out of 5 patients with flaring joints. TNF-α was not elevated in patients with less active disease. A later study showed that lean body mass was 13% lower in patients considered to be in control (without change in medication over the past year) than in matched controls, indicating that there was a loss of approximately one third of mobilizable muscle cell mass (149). Cytokine production from peripheral blood mononuclear cells was also increased in these patients, and higher interleukin (IL)-1β and TNF-α production was associated with increased resting energy expenditure.

Morgan et al (136) measured BMI in 79 patients starting MTX for RA. Sixty percent had BMI less than 25, and 4% were severely underweight (BMI less than 18); but 40% were overweight or obese. Roubenoff et al (150) found that low physical activity by women with RA results in lower total energy expenditure. Although patients with RA are at risk for cachexia, poor food choices and inactivity may also put them at risk for obesity (151, 152).

A more recent study (153) evaluated body composition by dual-energy x-ray absorptiometry (DXA) in 60 patients hospitalized for RA. The mean BMI for women and men, respectively, were 24.4 and 26.9. However, by calculation of the fat-free mass index (fat-free mass/kg/m^2), 52% of the women and 30% of the men were malnourished. They also evaluated the Subjective Global Assessment (SGA) (154–156) and Mini Nutritional Assessment (MNA) (157, 158) malnutrition screening tools. The MNA had poor specificity and good sensitivity, whereas the SGA had good specificity and poor sensitivity to detect malnutrition. The authors suggested that the MNA be used as a screening tool, followed by body composition analysis determined by DXA. In another study of 80 outpatients with RA, the same investigators (159) completed DXA, bioelectrical impedance analysis (BIA), BMI, the MNA, and waist circumference. Twenty-six percent of women and 21% of men had low fat-free mass index and, in this cohort, the MNA and waist circumference were poor predictors of rheumatoid cachexia. DXA and BIA had good general agreement, but because limits of agreement were wide, they concluded that BIA may be of limited usefulness in clinical practice.

Other investigations have generally confirmed the relationship between chronic inflammation and rheumatoid cachexia/cachectic obesity (141). A cross-sectional study of 14 patients with RA and 14 patients with noninflammatory arthritis (160), using measured resting energy expenditure (REE), joint counts for tenderness and swelling; and the modified Stanford HAQ (m-HAQ) (161, 162) found that REE, adjusted for fat-free mass, was significantly higher in the patients with RA compared with patients with noninflammatory arthritis (1498 ± 162 kcal versus 1330 ± 206 kcal; $p < .031$). In addition, REE and IL-6 concentrations were higher, and fat-free mass lower, in patients with active arthritis, suggesting that hypermetabolism and loss of fat-free mass are associated with active inflammatory disease.

Giles et al matched 189 men and women with RA to non-RA controls and used DXA to determine body composition (163). Women, but not men, with RA, had higher likelihood of sarcopenia, obesity, and sarcopenic obesity than those without RA. Abnormal body composition was associated with higher self-reported disability scores (m-HAQ), higher C-reactive protein, greater joint deformity, rheumatoid factor seropositivity, and lack of current treatment with a DMARD. In another investigation in 197 subjects (164), higher disability scores by m-HAQ were predicted by increasing fat mass and lower lean body mass. The m-HAQ score was 0.52 units higher for individuals in the highest versus lowest quartile of fat mass ($p < .001$) and 0.81 units higher for subjects in the lowest versus highest quartile of lean body mass ($p < .001$). Various inflammatory mediators have been associated with disability and cachexia including low

IGF-1/IGFBP-1 ratio (165) (insulinlike growth factor-I and its regulating binding protein insulinlike growth factor-binding protein-I).

Toms et al evaluated 400 patients with RA for metabolic syndrome (166). Older age and high HAQ score were associated with higher prevalence of metabolic syndrome, whereas MTX therapy was associated with reduced likelihood of metabolic syndrome. In contrast, Stavropoulos-Kalinoglou correlated physical activity, dietary intake from a 3-day food diary, and inflammatory status (IL-6, IL-1, TNF-α levels) with BMI and body fat determined by bioelectrical impedance (167). They found no relationship between inflammatory markers and BMI or body fat. Instead, higher levels of activity had the highest association with lower body fat and low BMI.

Several strategies have been used to try to alter the detrimental effects of chronic stress of RA on body composition (168, 169). Progressive resistance exercise has been shown to increase strength, but was not accompanied by changes in body composition (168, 169). Rall et al (170) showed that treatment with MTX normalized leucine kinetics, probably as a result of a reduction in protein catabolism. In a study of obese patients with RA, a weight reduction program which emphasized caloric restriction, protein supplements and physical exercise for 12 weeks was demonstrated to maintain lean body cell mass and maintain physical functioning (171).

One intervention study used β-hydroxybutyric acid, glutamine, and arginine versus a placebo mixture of alanine, glutamic acid, glycine, and serine for 12 weeks to treat the hypermetabolism in RA (172) similar to the nutrition support of stressed hospitalized patients. The β-hydroxybutyric acid, glutamine, and arginine were not more effective than the placebo mixture in reversing cachexia in patients with RA.

Diet Therapy

Complementary and Alternative Nutritional Therapies
The use of complementary/alternative diet approaches for treatment of RA is common. In a sample of 296 patients, 60.5% admitted to the use of some sort of alternative therapy such as herbs/algae or cartilage components (173). Various compounds have been studied for their efficacy in RA (174); although many have preliminary data, stronger human studies are necessary for most of them. Probiotic supplements have not been found to improve symptoms in RA (175).

Effects of Specific Foods on Rheumatic Symptoms
In a study of 742 patients with RA, juvenile RA, ankylosing spondylitis, psoriatic arthropathy, primary fibromyalgia, and OA, one-third of patients with RA reported a worsening of symptoms with specific foods (176). Forty-three percent of patients with juvenile RA reported an exacerbation of symptoms with specific foods. The foods that were most frequently cited in worsening joint symptoms were meat, wine, alcohol, coffee, sweets, sugar, chocolate, apples, and citrus fruits (177).

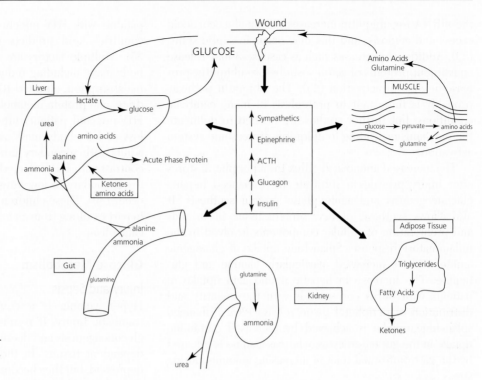

Fig. 92.2. Neuroendocrine and metabolic consequences of injury. *ACTH,* adrenocorticotropic hormone.

secondary infections may cause even further elevations in the REE. A few patients with AIDS exhibit metabolic rates similar to that seen in starvation (17).

Protein Metabolism

Injury and Sepsis

The large reserve of protein in skeletal muscle are rapidly mobilized in response to the increased energy demands after injury or acute inflammatory illnesses, and the extent of urinary nitrogen loss correlates with this activity. The

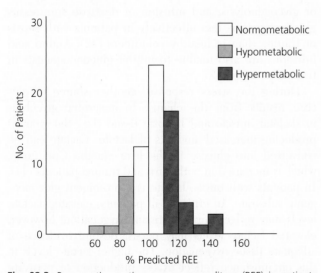

Fig. 92.3. Preoperative resting energy expenditure (REE) in patients with cancer. (Adapted with permission from Luketich JD, Mullen JL, Fuerer ID et al. Ablation of abnormal energy expenditure by curative tumor resection. Arch Surg 1990;125:337–41.)

accelerated rate of protein catabolism generally parallels the increase in oxygen consumption and represents a constant fraction of total oxidation after injury (3).

If allowed to proceed unabated, the net protein catabolism leads to loss of lean muscle mass and, in turn, may contribute to organ dysfunction or failure. Muscle myofibrillar protein is a prominent source of protein mobilization and reduced protein synthesis and inhibition of amino acid uptake by muscle is demonstrable (19). In animal models, important mediators of muscle catabolism include glucocorticoids, as well as certain cytokines, particularly tumor necrosis factor (TNF) and interleukin-1 (IL-1) (20). These and other inflammatory mediators that affect muscle protein metabolism can be produced by the myocyte or by nonmyocyte cells (i.e., macrophages), either locally at the site of injury or from a distance (21).

The cellular mechanisms involved in tissue protein breakdown in catabolic illness are not clearly defined. Animal studies indicate that under some catabolic conditions (e.g., sepsis), nonlysosomal, energy-dependent proteolysis may occur (22). This involves activation of the ubiquitin-proteasome–dependent pathway that increases mRNAs encoding ubiquitin and proteasomes in muscle. In this pathway, proteins destined for degradation are ligated to the polypeptide ubiquitin and then degraded by a protease that acts on ubiquinated proteins (23). The ubiquitination of proteins destined to undergo proteolysis by the proteasome is regulated by ubiquitin ligases as well as other enzymes. Ubiquitin ligases also appear to be involved in increased breakdown of proteins in atrophying muscle (24). Other studies indicated that the mRNA for ubiquitin increases during glucocorticoid excess and acidosis, and this may occur in septic states (23). Additional proteases such as caspase-3 may release constituent proteins of actomyosin before ubiquitin-proteasome system activation (25). The ubiquitin pathway probably is important in proteolysis in many catabolic conditions, but further studies are needed to delineate the mechanisms leading to ubiquitin-proteasome system activation.

The increased amino acid efflux from peripheral stores after injury provides a substrate for enhanced hepatic gluconeogenesis and acute phase protein synthesis. It also allows synthesis of new protein tissue in wounds and proliferation of cellular components involved in the inflammatory response. Splanchnic uptake of glucogenic amino acids is increased, particularly alanine and glutamine. The increase in hepatic amino acid uptake in patients with burns corresponds with the quantity and distribution of peripheral tissue release (26). Enhanced splanchnic uptake is achieved by increased glutamine uptake in the gut enterocytes, whereas alanine is released by the gastrointestinal tract in increasing amounts during stress (27).

During the postinjury response, alanine and glutamine are also preferentially released from muscle stores. Although these amino acids make up approximately 6% of protein in muscle stores, they constitute 60% to 80% of the free amino acids released in response to insult (28, 29). Glutamine availability may become limited during catabolic illness, and mortality in critically ill patients has been associated with low glutamine levels (30).

Cancer

Patients with cancer and significant weight loss exhibit protein kinetics qualitatively similar to that observed in traumatized or infected patients. Whole body protein turnover rates are increased in some patients, with increases in protein synthesis as well as catabolism (31, 32). Attempts have been made to correlate the increase in protein turnover rates with changes in REE or weight loss. Isotope infusion studies suggest a significant increase in whole body protein catabolism in patients with cancer and cachexia compared with noncachectic patients with cancer or patients with benign disease (33). Although the whole body protein turnover rate is increased in other studies, it does not appear to correlate with energy expenditure or weight loss in most patients with cancer (8).

Human Immunodeficiency Virus Infection

In contrast with other patient populations, those infected with HIV in general show an elevated REE with decreased protein synthesis and catabolism in the absence of secondary infection. Preliminary data indicate that protein catabolism and a negative nitrogen balance occur when a patient with AIDS becomes secondarily infected (15). Despite effective antiretroviral therapy, the loss of lean body mass continues to be a common finding in patients with HIV infection, particularly in low-resource countries, and predicts morbidity and mortality (34, 35). Multiple factors are implicated in the loss of lean body mass, including reduced nutritional intake, nutrient malabsorption, elevated REE, and altered lipid, carbohydrate, and protein metabolism (17, 36, 37). Asymptomatic HIV-infected patients often do not exhibit a significant loss of lean body mass as compared with HIV-infected adults with secondary infections (38). This finding is in contrast with HIV-infected children, in whom growth failure secondary to low rates of lean tissue deposition may occur (39). These children have reduced protein balance, in part resulting from an inability to down-regulate protein catabolism.

Glucose Metabolism

Injury and Sepsis

Hyperglycemia is a common response to septic or traumatic injury. It results from both increased hepatic gluconeogenesis and decreased glucose uptake by insulin-dependent tissues. In the ebb phase, insulin levels are depressed, but they become normal to elevated during the flow phase, although remaining depressed in relation to the degree of hyperglycemia. The persistent hyperglycemia suggests injury-induced insulin resistance (3). In addition, studies using hepatic vein cannulations in thermally injured patients show increased uptake of gluconeogenic amino acids by the splanchnic tissues (26).

Stress-induced alterations in glucose metabolism result in decreased skeletal muscle uptake of glucose and decreased glucose incorporation into fatty acids by adipocytes (3). The decreased uptake by skeletal muscle is the result of peripheral insulin resistance, which may be mediated in part by excess cortisol and catecholamines (40, 41). In these stressed patients, hyperglycemia fails to suppress hepatic gluconeogenesis or glycogenolysis; and infusion of dextrose suppresses gluconeogenesis less effectively in patients with sepsis or trauma than in healthy volunteers (42). Amino acid infusions are also unable to inhibit gluconeogenesis in trauma patients (43).

During the stress response, another source of glucose results from the change to anaerobic glycolysis in skeletal muscle and hypoxic tissue (i.e., the wound) producing increased amounts of lactate. Lactate can be converted into glucose in the liver via the Cori cycle, which is increased in both burn and trauma patients (44). In patients with burns, lactate is a prominent gluconeogenic substrate. In critically ill patients, elevated lactate levels may reflect impaired tissue oxygenation; however, elevated lactate levels may persist despite evidence of adequate tissue oxygenation. The higher lactate levels in this circumstance reflect excess production of pyruvate as a consequence of accelerated glycolysis resulting from increased glucose uptake and glycogen breakdown rather than tissue hypoxia (45).

The efficiency of glucose oxidation is altered by trauma (46), surgical stress (45), and burn injury (47). Maximum glucose oxidative capacity appears to be inversely related to the severity of the injury. The decrease in oxidation may be the result of reduced activity of intracellular enzymatic metabolic pathways, such as pyruvate dehydrogenase (48).

Cancer

Glucose intolerance is often observed in association with malignant disease, and glucose intolerance has been documented in diverse cancer populations with advanced disease (49–51). This glucose intolerance may be related, in part, to other influences of cancer, such as weight loss, because glucose intolerance also occurs in response to weight loss attributable to calorie deprivation in benign disease (31).

Numerous reports note increased endogenous glucose production in patients with cancer (49, 52, 53), with an observed increase in glucose turnover rate affected by tumor stage (52, 54) and histology (50, 52). Studies comparing patients with early or advanced gastrointestinal malignant diseases indicated that rates of glucose turnover were significantly higher in patients with advanced lesions (50, 52, 54). Tumor histology may also influence glucose turnover rates. Patients with sarcoma (55) and leukemia (50) exhibit glucose turnover rates two to three times normal, whereas patients with lymphoma have a glucose turnover rate similar to that of normal subjects (50). Other studies indicate that the increased glucose turnover is related specifically to the cancer. The increase in glucose turnover rate is significantly higher in patients with cancer and weight loss than in the cancer-free population with comparable weight loss (31). Another study demonstrated that patients with cancer and progressive weight loss had markedly elevated rates of glucose turnover, whereas weight-stable patients with cancer had glucose turnover rates similar to those in normal volunteers (56). These findings contrast with the decreased glucose turnover rates in patients with weight loss attributable to uncomplicated undernutrition (54).

Regulation of hepatic glucose production is also altered in patients with cancer. Although infusion of glucose in normal subjects suppresses hepatic gluconeogenesis, glucose infusion reduces glucose production by only 70% in patients with early or advanced gastric cancer (52). In patients with sarcoma or leukemia, hepatic glucose production was decreased by less than one third (50, 57).

Increased gluconeogenesis via the Cori cycle represents a substantial proportion of the observed increase in glucose turnover rate in patients with cancer. During this cycle, lactate released from anaerobic glycolysis in peripheral tissue is recycled to glucose in the liver in an energy-requiring reaction. Increased Cori cycle activity occurs in patients with cancer, particularly those with weight loss (56). The increase in Cori cycle activity seems to be a specific response to the neoplasm and not directly related to weight loss. The source of the lactate molecules

remains a matter of debate. Other studies indicate that the tumor itself may exert distal effects on host carbohydrate metabolism; the rates of glucose uptake and lactate release from forearm tissue of patients with cancer were significantly higher than from the tissues of physiologically normal subjects (31). Taken together, it seems probable that increased glycolysis in both the tumor and host tissues contributes to the increased lactate production. Increased glucose oxidation is also observed in patients with cancer and weight loss (56).

Human Immunodeficiency Virus Infection

Hyperglycemia does not appear to be a prevalent finding in patients who are HIV positive. Abnormalities of glucose homeostasis (insulin resistance) and related metabolic abnormalities such as hypertriglyceridemia, low high-density lipoprotein levels, or development of an atherogenic profile are frequently associated with body composition changes in HIV-infected patients receiving antiretroviral therapy (58, 59). Impaired glucose tolerance is a common result with standard oral glucose tolerance testing in HIV-infected patients with lipodystrophy. A 50% reduction in insulin sensitivity was documented in HIV-infected patients with lipodystrophy as compared with HIV-infected patients who had not experienced fat redistribution (60). Duration and modality of antiretroviral therapy appear to contribute to insulin resistance (61).

Lipid Metabolism

Injury and Sepsis

As a major source of endogenous fuel representing 80% of potential energy reserves, lipid stores represent the most effective energy source to be used during the early flow phase after injury. Immediately after insult, enhanced lipolysis mediated by sympathetic stimulation of adipose tissue and activation of tissue-specific lipases by norepinephrine and glucagon occurs (3). Leptin, a hormone that stimulates fatty acid oxidation and is expressed by adipocytes, is now considered a stress-related hormone. Leptin suppresses adrenal synthetic activity and may be responsible for the functional adrenal insufficiency frequently observed in severe injury and stress conditions (62). Insulin, insulinlike growth factor-I (IGF-I), thyroid hormones, somatotropin release–inhibiting factor, glucocorticoids, and β-adrenergic agonists are known to enhance leptin production.

A decreased respiratory quotient is also seen in patients with worsening sepsis, and isotopic studies have corroborated increased fat oxidation in these patients (63). Other studies have demonstrated that with increased severity of sepsis, oxidation and clearance of lipids from the bloodstream decrease, a finding suggesting utilization inefficiency that may account for the feeding-resistant protein wasting in concert with preservation of fat stores observed during critical illness (64).

Cancer

A large body of evidence indicates that much of the weight loss seen in cancer cachexia is the result of depletion of body fat (54, 65, 66). Whole body lipolysis rates in patients with cancer have been reported to be both increased and normal (67, 68). Several possible mechanisms have been proposed for increased lipolysis in patients with cancer including increased lipolysis resulting from decreased food intake and malnutrition; stimulation of lipolysis caused by the stress response with adrenal medullary stimulation, increased circulating catecholamines, and insulin resistance; and the release of lipolytic factors produced by the tumor or by myeloid tissue cells (69). Consistent with enhanced rates of lipolysis, increased fat oxidation has been reported in many patient populations with cancer (31, 68).

Human Immunodeficiency Virus Infection

In contrast to the response to injury and malignant disease, adipose tissue is often conserved in patients with AIDS at the expense of body cell mass (34). Various direct and indirect lipid metabolic changes have been described in HIV-infected patients with lipodystrophy, including insulin resistance, hypertriglyceridemia, and low high-density lipoprotein levels (61). The role of protease inhibitors in lipodystrophy associated with HIV remains largely uncharacterized; however, studies indicate impaired differentiation of preadipocytes, apoptosis of subcutaneous adipocytes, and reduced mRNA levels of key transcriptional factors involved in adipogenesis, such as sterol regulatory element–binding protein 1c and peroxisome-proliferator-activated receptor γ (70–72). Grunfeld and Feingold, in their review of metabolic disturbances in HIV, described decreased triglyceride clearance attributable to decreased lipoprotein lipase activity, with a resultant marked triglyceridemia (15). Hepatic synthesis of fatty acids increases (73), and the levels of circulating free fatty acids are elevated (74). No correlation appears to exist between the alterations in triglyceride metabolism and wasting in AIDS.

MEDIATORS OF THE HYPERCATABOLIC RESPONSE

A characteristic neuroendocrine response is usually evident during the ebb and flow phases after injury, including increases in catecholamines and glucocorticoids levels (3, 75). Investigations of the short-term influences of these hormones in healthy subjects, however, have not reproduced the extent of net protein catabolism observed after severe injury (28). Hence, acute increases in counter-regulatory hormones cannot fully account for much of the observed metabolic response to severe stress and injury. Attention has been directed to other inducible mechanisms of hypercatabolic stress, including alterations of autonomic nervous system function and inflammatory

cytokines that can integrate and transfer information from the injury site and influence systemic host responses. The next section focuses on the role of these mediators in the postinjury response.

Neuroimmunoendocrine Response

The neuroendocrine and immune systems are interrelated by sharing chemical mediators (hormones, cytokines, steroids, neuropeptides, and neurotransmitters) and their associated receptors. These shared chemical mediators and receptors in turn promote an integrated molecular response of the neuroimmunoendocrine system to stress, inflammation, and infection. Sensory afferent and postganglionic sympathetic neurons also influence inflammation by secreting proinflammatory or anti-inflammatory neuropeptides, such as substance P and somatostatin, into the site of inflammation.

Intact afferent neural pathways are essential for mediating the early response to injury as demonstrated by the classic studies of Hume and Egdahl who used sectioning of peripheral nerves, cervical spinal cord, or medulla oblongata, and the blockage of the adrenocorticoid response to burn injury (76). Clinical studies show lower adrenocorticotropic hormone (ACTH) or growth hormone (GH) release in response to minor tissue injury (herniorrhaphy) in patients receiving spinal anesthesia than in those receiving general anesthesia (77). The CNS also appears to be instrumental in the hypermetabolic response to injury. One study demonstrated that administration of inert gas anesthesia to hypermetabolic patients with burns lowered their core temperatures and metabolic rates (78).

Afferent signals from the site of injury, baroreceptors sensing hypovolemia, and infection can each elicit hypothalamic mechanisms to stimulate the anterior pituitary to secrete prolactin, ACTH, antidiuretic hormone, and GH (79). The vagal afferent fiber is an important sensory pathway for intraperitoneal stimuli (80, 81). ACTH release stimulates an increase in adrenal glucocorticoid secretion. Evidence of increased ACTH secretion has been observed after elective operations, extensive trauma (82), thermal injury (83), and infection (84). Cortisol appears unaffected and remains high from the outset of the flow phase whereas patients experiencing a more inflammatory stress may also demonstrate diminished ultradian and circadian secretion of pituitary hormones (85). Whether this loss of variability contributes to the diminished efficiency of nutritional support often observed in such patients is unknown (79).

Thyroid-stimulating hormone levels do not appear to be greatly affected during the early postinjury phase. However, a characteristic pattern of normal thyroxine (T_4), elevated triiodothyronine receptor (rT_3), and depressed triiodothyronine (T_3) during prolonged periods of stress also occurs (86). In patients with this euthyroid sick syndrome, proposed mechanisms include impaired responsiveness of the thyroid to thyroid-stimulating hormone, reduced serum binding of thyroid hormones, and reduced peripheral conversion of T_4 to T_3. Glucocorticoids inhibit the enzymatic conversion of T_4 to T_3. Proinflammatory cytokines appear not to inhibit this glucocorticoid-mediated inhibition of the conversion of T_4 to T_3 (87).

Catecholamines

The production of catecholamines rapidly increases in response to any serious injury. Postinjury levels of catecholamines correlate to some extent with the severity of initial injury. These elevated levels are most pronounced during the early postinjury period (48 hours) and decrease during recovery (75, 88). The net metabolic influence of catecholamines is to increase energy expenditure, hepatic glycogenolysis, glycolysis, and lipolysis with resultant increase in free fatty acid concentration. Catecholamine excess also acutely decreases the efflux of amino acids from peripheral tissue while increasing lactate release from skeletal muscle. This was confirmed by epinephrine infusion into healthy subjects (28, 89). Although the precise effect of adrenergic stimulation on protein kinetics is controversial, studies indicate that β stimulation promotes gluconeogenesis and may limit skeletal muscle nitrogen loss, whereas α-adrenergic stimulation leads to protein catabolism (90, 91). A study of β-blockade in pediatric patients with severe burns demonstrated attenuation of hypermetabolism and reversal of muscle-protein catabolism. (92).

Cortisol

Glucocorticoid excess promotes negative nitrogen balance (89) but shows little influence on overall energy expenditure (93). Cortisol causes a slight increase in free fatty acid concentration, promotes hepatic gluconeogenesis, and increases peripheral tissue amino acid efflux. In normal subjects, cortisol infusion alone produces the same net body and peripheral tissue nitrogen loss as that produced by combined cortisol, epinephrine, norepinephrine, and glucagon infusion (89). Glucocorticoids mediate muscle catabolic activity in part via the ubiquitin-proteasome pathway and calcium-dependent protein degradation (23). During sepsis and other catabolic conditions, glutamine use increases with increased glutamine synthetase expression and activity in skeletal muscle and lung. Overall, glutamine levels are reduced in muscle during critical illness and are proposed to be an important mechanism of stimulated muscle breakdown and inhibited protein synthesis (94). Glucocorticoids appear to regulate the expression and activity of glutamine synthetase in skeletal muscle, thus possibly playing a role in glutamine-mediated muscle breakdown (95).

Insulin

Insulin levels are initially decreased during the ebb phase after injury, but are mildly to markedly increased during the early flow phase. Hyperglycemia and hyperinsulinemia are characteristic of the early stress response. As noted earlier, insulin resistance is often evident in adipocytes and skeletal myocytes (40). The role of the characteristic hyperinsulinemia observed after injury remains unclear because critical organs, the CNS, hematogenous cells, wounds, and the kidney incorporate glucose in an insulin-independent manner. Nevertheless, continuous infusion of glucose and insulin results in decreased urine urea nitrogen excretion as well as decreased amino acid efflux and decreased 3-methylhistidine excretion (a marker of protein catabolism) (96). Major studies have examined the relationship between insulin, blood glucose, and clinical outcomes in critically ill patients and show decreased morbidity and mortality with tighter regulation of glucose levels via insulin infusions (97, 98); however, the overall guidelines for intensive insulin therapy and the upper blood glucose control targets among seriously ill patients remains somewhat controversial, given the risk for hypoglycemia with very tight blood glucose control (98, 99).

Glucagon

Circulating glucagon levels increase during the hypermetabolic postinjury phase and correlate roughly with the severity of injury (82, 100). Glucagon appears to exert little independent influence on peripheral tissue metabolism (101), but is a potent stimulant of the hepatic cyclic adenosine monophosphate system, facilitating hepatic uptake of amino acids (102) and gluconeogenesis (103).

Cytokines

Proinflammatory Cytokines

Many proinflammatory cytokines were originally characterized by their effect on immunologic function but were also noted to have important influences on hemodynamic and metabolic responses (104). During early postinjury or infectious conditions, the initial cytokine response to such insults likely mediates beneficial protective signaling of the immune system (105). Nevertheless, excessive acute production of some cytokines, such as TNF-α, may promote a shock-like state (106). Prolonged production of cytokines within tissues may also sustain some metabolic effects of the hypercatabolic state (21).

Diverse cell types of both myeloid and nonmyeloid origin produce proinflammatory cytokine peptides. These proteins may function by autocrine (acting on the same cell), paracrine (acting on cells in the immediate area), or systemic mechanisms of action. They produce local tissue responses by cell-to-cell interaction at very low concentrations, but also may exert systemic effects in higher concentrations. Although many cytokines are now well characterized, those showing the more prominent proinflammatory activities, including TNF-α, IL-1, IL-6, and interferon-γ (IFN-γ), have been more widely studied from a metabolic perspective (Table 92.2).

TABLE 92.2	MAJOR CYTOKINES INVOLVED IN THE HYPERMETABOLIC RESPONSE	
CYTOKINE	CELL SOURCE	METABOLIC EFFECTS
Tumor necrosis factor-α	Monocytes or macrophages, lymphocytes, Kupffer cells, glial cells, endothelial cells, natural killer cells, mast cells	Decrease free fatty acid synthesis Increased lipolysis Increased peripheral amino acid loss Increased hepatic amino acid uptake Fever
Interleukin-1	Monocytes or macrophages, neutrophils, lymphocytes, keratinocytes, Kupffer cells	Increased adrenocorticotropic hormone Increased hepatic acute phase protein synthesis Fever
Interleukin-6	Monocytes or macrophages, keratinocytes, endothelial cells, fibroblasts, T cells, epithelial cells	Increased acute phase protein synthesis Fever
Interferon-γ	Lymphocytes, pulmonary macrophages	Increased monocyte respiratory burst

Reprinted with permission from Matarese G, La Cava A. The intricate interface between immune system and metabolism. Trends Immunol 2004;25:195–6.

Tumor Necrosis Factor

TNF has been implicated as the initiating signal for a variety of cellular and metabolic events seen in seriously ill patients. TNF administration to healthy subjects elicits a systemic response resembling that observed during septicemia (106), including increased stress hormone release, temperature elevation, and increased acute phase protein synthesis (107). The systemic effects of bacterial liposaccharide (endotoxin) are replicated, if not largely mediated, by the initial effects of TNF activity. TNF may circulate predominately as a complex with its soluble receptors, making detection of the bioactive ligand more difficult, and increased levels of these soluble TNF receptor complexes are seen in response to diverse inflammatory stimuli, including sepsis, cancer, and AIDS. Nevertheless, elevated levels of bioactive TNF are detected in many disease states, including bacterial infection, thermal injury, tumor-bearing states, and AIDS (108). The metabolic effects of TNF and perhaps in concert with other proinflammatory cytokines are to promote the redistribution of body protein and lipid stores (106).

Interleukin-1

IL-1 is produced by macrophages or monocytes, neutrophils, lymphocytes, and keratinocytes (105); and it exerts multiple immunologic and metabolic effects, including stimulation of ACTH, induction of fever, hepatic acute phase protein synthesis, alteration of energy metabolism, inhibition of fatty acid synthesis, and adipocyte differentiation (109, 110). Like TNF activity, IL-1 activity is regulated by shedding of soluble receptors as well as by unique, naturally occurring receptor antagonist (IL-1ra) (111). IL-1ra binds to the IL-1 receptor without an agonist influence. IL-1ra–deficient mice exhibit growth retardation, resistance to high-fat diet–induced obesity, and reduced activity of lipoprotein lipase, and have low insulin levels (110).

Interleukin-6

Elevated levels of IL-6 are frequently detected in patients with acute infection (112), injury, and tumor-bearing states (113), as well as after elective surgical procedures (114). The biologic actions of this protein include regulation of acute phase protein synthesis after injury and differentiation of lymphocytes. In one study, administration of IL-6 to humans induced modest changes in the kinetics of glucose and protein (115). IL-6 is produced in large part by adipose tissue, and circulating levels correlate with body mass index, insulin sensitivity, and glucose.

Interferon-γ

IFN-γ is secreted from lymphocytes and macrophages and exerts antiviral effects as well as protection against bacteria, fungi, and parasites. It enhances TNF production in response to endotoxin and increases the cytotoxicity of monocytes, possibly by enhancing respiratory burst activity (116). A direct role for IFN-γ in directing altered metabolic processes has not been defined in humans, although its administration does induce cachexia and loss of protein and lipid stores in animals (117).

Anti-inflammatory Cytokines

Regulation of the various cytokines produced in response to injury or disease is complex and involves counterregulation by anti-inflammatory cytokines such as IL-10, which down-regulates secretion of proinflammatory cytokines (i.e., TNF and IL-1) as well as suppresses macrophage and T-cell functions. Counterregulatory mechanisms likely are important in maintaining a counterbalance to unopposed systemic inflammation and hypercatabolism and may play a role in restoration of metabolic homeostasis and anabolism (104).

Neuroendocrine Response and Cytokines

The response to injury, infection, and ischemia/reperfusion is associated with concurrent activation of the hypothalamic-pituitary-adrenal axis (HPA). Glucocorticoid secretion, mediated by ACTH and indirectly through cytokines, is a potent anti-inflammatory mechanism. The α-glucocorticoid receptor binds the steroid hormone, translocates to the nucleus, and binds to the glucocorticoid-responsive elements. Some glucocorticoid-responsive elements down-regulate the transcription of other genes (e.g., most cytokines) and prevent transcription initiated by transcriptional factors such as nuclear factor-κB (118). Glucocorticoids can inhibit production of TNF or IL-6, and cortisol infusion attenuates the endogenous TNF response to endotoxin administration (93). Catecholamine infusion also inhibits endotoxin-induced TNF production while simultaneously increasing release of IL-10 (119). Proinflammatory cytokines such as TNF and IL-1 initiate a cascade of inflammatory responses by activating nuclear factor-κB, which, in turn, stimulates proinflammatory genes. Glucocorticoids bound to glucocorticoid receptor interact with nuclear factor-κB in the nucleus and alter its ability to promote transcription of cytokine-responsive genes (120).

Hence, the neuroimmunoendocrine milieu elicited by injury, infection, or other hypermetabolic conditions may serve to alter cytokine mediator activities in a complex manner. It remains to be determined exactly to what extent these parallel signaling pathways direct the human metabolic response.

Autonomically Mediated Anti-inflammatory Pathways

It is now recognized that CNS derived vagal efferent signals may also exert anti-inflammatory influences on peripheral immune systems (121). This mechanism, commonly termed the "cholinergic anti-inflammatory pathway," was originally discovered to activate nicotinic α7 receptors on tissue macrophages, although it is now evident that some projections act via terminal catecholaminergic signals. Although the anti-inflammatory influence of vagally mediated signals has documented only reduced TNF-α levels during vagal stimulation, other proinflammatory cytokine levels are diminished as a result of this effect (122).

Although the anti-inflammatory influence of efferent vagal signaling in animal models is well established, currently no evidence indicates that this influences the catabolic consequences of injury or other illnesses in animals. Further, evidence suggesting that efferent vagal signaling correlates to inflammatory responses in seriously ill humans is conflicting (123, 124). Another largely overlooked aspect of efferent vagal activity is the diurnal pattern of such signaling. Under healthy, free-living conditions, humans exhibit circadian patterns of both sympathetic and parasympathetic (vagal) signals (125). During severe inflammatory conditions, this circadian pattern of autonomic signaling may be attenuated (126) and the implications for both immune and metabolic competence are largely unknown. Although it is known that more prolonged inflammatory conditions may also eventuate in limited amplitude variation and rhythmicity of neuroendocrine activity (85), the implications of this

loss of variability on peripherally dependent immune and metabolic processes that normally respond to circadian and ultradian dynamics are also unknown (127, 128).

SYSTEMIC AND ORGAN REACTIONS

The concept that patients subjected to inflammatory stress for extended periods should receive nutritional supplementation during their hospital course has been the subject of several metaanalyses and clinical guidelines that are discussed elsewhere. Several classic studies of nutritional support in injured patients are instructive for the interested reader (129–131).

A fundamental objective of nutrition support for the hypermetabolic patient is the provision of sufficient nonprotein energy sources and protein substrate to alleviate, or significantly attenuate, the net catabolism of endogenous energy and protein sources. Both enteral and parenteral nutrition support in mildly stressed, depleted patients demonstrably improves nitrogen balance during the recovery phase after injury (132). Current thinking clearly emphasizes a preference for enteral nutrient provision wherever feasible. The most effective composition of such feedings and the minimal level of enteral nutrient intake that may serve to optimize intestinal barrier function remain to be determined. At present, it appears that nutrient requirements should be provided enterally whenever possible to achieve these intestinal function benefits. Trials are currently under way to determine whether early supplementation of enteral feedings will benefit the hypermetabolic, critically ill patient population.

Studies suggest a potential mechanism underlying the clinical benefits of enteral feeding during severe inflammatory conditions. Animal models of induced inflammation demonstrate that intraluminal administration of lipid activates intestinal cholecystokinin receptors and enhances afferent vagal signals. Given the requirement for intact afferent and efferent vagal circuits to regulate systemic inflammatory mediator production, these observations lend support to the clinical perception that enteral feedings are beneficial (Fig. 92.4) (133).

NUTRITIONAL SUPPORT IN PROLONGED STRESS

The hypermetabolic patient who responds to appropriate therapeutic interventions will proceed to an anabolic stage of recovery and eventually to positive nitrogen balance. However, some patients continue to be hypermetabolic and may develop multiorgan system failure. The pathogenesis of organ system failure remains to be clarified, but is it doubtless multifactorial. As noted earlier, however, considerable evidence indicates that this condition is often associated with diminished variation in systemic autonomic and endocrine signaling. Whether these disrupted rhythms are responsive to nutritional interventions during prolonged stressful conditions remains to be determined (128, 134).

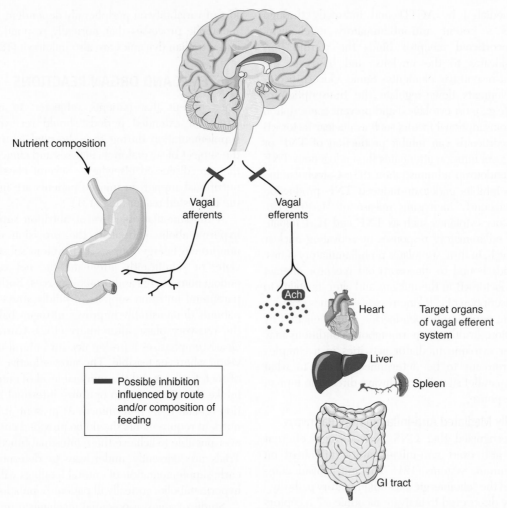

Fig. 92.4. The vagal afferent signals induced by luminal nutrients (e.g., lipids) maintain the activity of efferent vagal signals that can influence peripheral tissue immune function. A disruption or attenuation of either signaling pathway *(blue bars)* may adversely affect the systemic host response and/or solid organ function. *Ach,* acetylcholine; *GI,* gastrointestinal. (Adapted with permission from Lowry SF. A new model of nutrition influenced inflammatory risk. J Am Coll Surg 2007;205[Suppl 4]:S65–68).

ACKNOWLEDGMENTS AND DISCLOSURE

We were supported, in part, by grant R01 GM34695 from the United States Public Health Service. There are no conflicts of interest with respect to the presented materials.

REFERENCES

1. Cuthbertson DP, Stewart CP. Br Med J 1945;2:815.
2. Moore FD. Metabolic Care of the Surgical Patient. Philadelphia: WB Saunders, 1959.
3. Balija TM, Lowry SF. Curr Opin Infect Dis 2011;24:248–53.
4. Matzinger P. Annu Rev Immunol 1994;12:991–1045.
5. Rock KL, Latz E, Ontiveros F et al. Annu Rev Immunol 2010;28:321–42.
6. Medzhitov R. Nature 2007;449:819–26.
7. Bozzetti F, Pagnoni AM, Del Vecchio M. Surg Gynecol Obstet 1980;150:229–34.
8. Skipworth RJ, Stewart GD, Dejong CH et al. Clin Nutr 2007;26:667–76.
9. Knox LS, Crosby LO, Feurer ID et al. Ann Surg 1983;197:152–62.
10. Luketich JD, Mullen JL, Feurer ID et al. Arch Surg 1990;125:337–41.
11. Hursting SD, Berger NA. J Clin Oncol 2010;28:4058–65.
12. Falconer JS, Fearon KC, Plester CE et al. Ann Surg 1994;219:325–31.
13. Fredrix EW, Soeters PB, Wouters EF et al. Cancer Res 1991;51:6138–41.
14. Drott C, Persson H, Lundholm K. Clin Physiol 1989;9:427–39.
15. Grunfeld C, Feingold KR. N Engl J Med 1992;327:329–37.
16. Hommes MJ, Romijn JA, Godfried MH et al. Metabolism 1990;39:1186–90.
17. Melchior JC, Salmon D, Rigaud D et al. Am J Clin Nutr 1991;53:437–41.
18. Hommes MJ, Romijn JA, Endert E et al. Am J Clin Nutr 1991;54:311–15.
19. Zamir O, Hasselgren PO, Higashiguchi T et al. Mediat Inflamm 1992;1:247–50.
20. Aversa Z, Alamdari N, Hasselgren PO. Crit Rev Clin Lab Sci 2011;48:71–86.
21. Pedersen BK. J Appl Physiol 2009;107:1006–14.

22. Tiao G, Fagan JM, Samuels N et al. J Clin Invest 1994;94:2255–64.

23. Franch HA, Price SR. Curr Opin Clin Nutr Metab Care 2005;8:271–5.

24. Sacheck JM, Hyatt JP, Raffaello A et al. FASEB J 2007;21:140–55.

25. Du J, Wang X, Miereles C et al. J Clin Invest 2004;113:115–23.

26. Wilmore DW, Goodwin CW, Aulick LH et al. Ann Surg 1980;192:491–504.

27. Souba WW, Wilmore DW. Surgery 1983;94:342–50.

28. Fong YM, Albert JD, Tracey K et al. J Trauma 1991;31:1467–76.

29. Fong YM, Tracey KJ, Hesse DG et al. Surgery 1990;107:321–6.

30. Oudemans-van Straaten HM, Bosman RJ et al. Intensive Care Med 2001; 27:84–90.

31. Eden E, Edstrom S, Bennegard K et al. Cancer Res 1984;44:1718–24.

32. Heber D, Chlebowski RT, Ishibashi DE et al. Cancer Res 1982;42:4815–9.

33. Shaw JH, Humberstone DA, Douglas RG et al. Surgery 1991;109:37–50.

34. Kotler DP, Tierney AR, Wang J et al. Am J Clin Nutr 1989;50:444–7.

35. Suttajit M. Asia Pac J Clin Nutr 2007;16(Suppl):318–22.

36. Selberg O, Suttmann U, Melzer A et al. Metabolism 1995;44:1159–65.

37. Yarasheski KE, Zachwieja JJ, Gischler J et al. Am J Physiol 1998;275:E577–83.

38. Macallan DC, McNurlan MA, Milne E et al. Am J Clin Nutr 1995;61:818–26.

39. Jahoor F, Abramson S, Heird WC. Am J Clin Nutr 2003;78:182–9.

40. Deibert DC, DeFronzo RA. J Clin Invest 1980;65:717–21.

41. Diethelm AG. Ann Surg 1977;185:251–63.

42. Nelson KM, Long CL, Bailey R et al. Metabolism 1992;41:68–75.

43. Long CL, Nelson KM, Geiger JW et al. J Trauma 1996;40:335–41.

44. Wolfe RR, Herndon DN, Jahoor F et al. N Engl J Med 1987;317:403–8.

45. Wolfe RR, Martini WZ. World J Surg 2000;24:639–47.

46. Vanhorebeek I, Langouche L, Van den Berghe G. Crit Care Med 2007;35(Suppl):S496–502.

47. Burke JF, Wolfe RR, Mullany CJ et al. Ann Surg 1979;190:274–85.

48. Vary TC, Siegel JH, Nakatani T et al. Am J Physiol 1986;250:E634–40.

49. Holroyde CP, Skutches CL, Boden G et al. Cancer Res 1984;44:5910–13.

50. Humberstone DA, Shaw JH. Cancer 1988;62:1619–24.

51. Lundholm K, Edstrom S, Karlberg I et al. Cancer 1982;50:1142–50.

52. Shaw JH, Wolfe RR. Surgery 1987;101:181–91.

53. Bozzetti F, Arends J, Lundholm K et al. Clin Nutr 2009;28:445–54.

54. Kokal WA, McCulloch A, Wright PD et al. Ann Surg 1983;198:601–4.

55. Shaw JH, Humberstone DM, Wolfe RR. Ann Surg 1988;207:283–9.

56. Holroyde CP, Gabuzda TG, Putnam RC et al. Cancer Res 1975;35:3710–4.

57. Waterhouse C. Ann N Y Acad Sci 1974;230:86–93.

58. Carr A, Samaras K, Burton S et al. AIDS 1998;12:F51–8.

59. Hadigan C, Meigs JB, Corcoran C et al. Clin Infect Dis 2001;32:130–9.

60. Andersen O, Haugaard SB, Andersen UB et al. Metabolism 2003;52:1343–53.

61. Leung VL, Glesby MJ. Curr Opin Infect Dis 2011;24:43–9.

62. Bornstein SR, Uhlmann K, Haidan A et al. Diabetes 1997;46:1235–8.

63. Stoner HB, Little RA, Frayn KN et al. Br J Surg 1983;70:32–5.

64. Tissot S, Normand S, Khalfallah Y et al. Am J Physiol 1995;269:E753–8.

65. Coss CC, Bohl CE, Dalton JT. Curr Opin Clin Nutr Metab Care 2011; 14:268–73.

66. Blum D, Omlin A, Baracos VE et al. Crit Rev Oncol Hematol 2011;80:114–44.

67. Eden E, Edstrom S, Bennegard K et al. Surgery 1985;97:176–84.

68. Legaspi A, Jeevanandam M, Starnes HF Jr et al. Metabolism 1987;36:958–63.

69. Klein S, Wolfe RR. J Clin Invest 1990;86:1403–8.

70. Bastard JP, Caron M, Vidal H et al. Lancet 2002;359:1026–31.

71. Domingo P, Matias-Guiu X, Pujol RM et al. AIDS 1999;13:2261–7.

72. Dowell P, Flexner C, Kwiterovich PO et al. J Biol Chem 2000;275:41325–32.

73. Hellerstein MK, Grunfeld C, Wu K et al. J Clin Endocrinol Metab 1993;76:559–65.

74. Grunfeld C, Kotler DP, Hamadeh R et al. Am J Med 1989;86:27–31.

75. Vanhorebeek I, Langouche L, Van den Berghe G. Nat Clin Pract Endocrinol Metab 2006;2:20–31.

76. Hume DM, Egdahl RH. Ann Surg 1959;150:697–712.

77. Newsome HH, Rose JC. J Clin Endocrinol Metab 1971;33:481–7.

78. Taylor JW, Hander EW, Skreen R et al. J Surg Res 1976;20:313–20.

79. Lowry SF. Surg Clin North Am 2009;89:311–26.

80. Goehler LE, Gaykema RP, Hansen MK et al. Auton Neurosci 2000;85:49–59.

81. Maier SF, Goehler LE, Fleshner M et al. Ann N Y Acad Sci 1998;840:289–300.

82. Meguid MM, Brennan MF, Aoki TT et al. Arch Surg 1974;109:776–83.

83. Popp MB, Srivastava LS, Knowles HC Jr et al. Surg Gynecol Obstet 1977;145:517–24.

84. Beisel WR. Am J Clin Nutr 1977;30:1236–s47.

85. Van den Berghe G, de Zegher F, Bouillon RJ. Clin Endocrinol Metab 1998;83:1827–34.

86. van der Poll T, Van Zee KJ, Endert E et al. J Clin Endocrinol Metab 1995;80:1341–6.

87. Mebis L, Van den Berghe G. Best Pract Res Clin Endocrinol Metab 2011;25:745–57.

88. Jaattela A, Alho A, Avikainen V et al. Br J Surg 1975;62:177–81.

89. Gelfand RA, Matthews DE, Bier DM et al. J Clin Invest 1984;74:2238–48.

90. Kraenzlin ME, Keller U, Keller A et al. J Clin Invest 1989;84:388–93.

91. Shaw JH, Holdaway CM, Humberstone DA. Surgery 1988;103:520–5.

92. Herndon DN, Hart DW, Wolf SE et al. N Engl J Med 2001;345:1223–9.

93. Barber AE, Coyle SM, Marano MA et al. J Immunol 1993;150:1999–2006.

94. MacLennan PA, Brown RA, Rennie MJ. FEBS Lett 1987;215:187–91.

95. Lukaszewicz GC, Souba WW, Abcouwer SF. Shock 1997; 7:332–8.

96. Inculet RI, Finley RJ, Duff JH et al. Surgery 1986;99:752–8.

97. van den Berghe G, Wouters P, Weekers F et al. N Engl J Med 2001;345:1359–67.

98. NICE-SUGAR Study Investigators, Finfer S, Chittock DR. N Engl J Med 2009;360:1283–97.

99. Kavanagh BP, McCowen KC. N Engl J Med 2010;363: 2540–6.

100. Alberti KG, Batstone GF, Foster KJ et al. JPEN J Parenter Enteral Nutr 1980;4:141–6.

101. Pozefsky T, Tancredi RG, Moxley RT et al. Diabetes 1976; 25:128–35.

102. Warren RS, Donner DB, Starnes HF Jr et al. Proc Natl Acad Sci U S A 1987;84:8619–22.

103. Felig P, Wahren J, Hendler R. J Clin Invest 1976;58:761–5.

104. Fong Y, Moldawer LL, Shires GT et al. Surg Gynecol Obstet 1990;170:363–78.

105. Dinarello CA. Annu Rev Immunol 2009;27:519–50.

106. van der Poll T, Lowry SF. Shock 1995;3:1–12.

107. Michie HR, Spriggs DR, Manogue KR et al. Surgery 1988;104:280–6.

108. Lahdevirta J, Maury CP, Teppo AM et al. Am J Med 1988; 85:289–91.

109. Haddad JJ, Saade NE, Safieh-Garabedian B. J Neuroimmunol 2002;133:1–19.

110. Matsuki T, Horai R, Sudo K et al. J Exp Med 2003;198:877–88.

111. Fischer E, Van Zee KJ, Marano MA et al. Blood 1992;79: 2196–2200.

112. Helfgott DC, Tatter SB, Santhanam U et al. J Immunol 1989; 142:948–53.

113. Gelin J, Moldawer LL, Lonnroth C et al. Biochem Biophys Res Commun 1988;157:575–9.

114. Shenkin A, Fraser WD, Series J et al. Lymphokine Res 1989;8:123–7.

115. Stouthard JM, Romijn JA, Van der Poll T et al. Am J Physiol 1995;268:E813–9.

116. Nathan CF, Murray HW, Wiebe ME et al. J Exp Med 1983;158:670–89.

117. Matthys P, Dijkmans R, Proost P et al. Int J Cancer 1991;49:77–82.

118. Scheinman RI, Gualberto A, Jewell CM et al. Mol Cell Biol 1995;15:943–53.

119. van der Poll T, Coyle SM, Barbosa K et al. J Clin Invest 1996;97:713–9.

120. Webster JC, Oakley RH, Jewell CM et al. Proc Natl Acad Sci U S A 2001;98:6865–70.

121. Tracey KJ. Nature 2002;420:853–9.

122. van Westerloo DJ, Giebelen IA, Florquin S et al. Gastroenterology 2006;130:1822–30.

123. Huston JM, Tracey KJ. J Intern Med 2011;269:45–53.

124. Jan BU, Coyle SM, Macor MA et al. Shock 2010;33:363–8.

125. Bonnemeier H, Richardt G, Potratz J et al. J Cardiovasc Electrophysiol 2003;14:791–9.

126. Norris PR, Ozdas A, Cao H et al. Ann Surg 2006;243:804–12.

127. Haimovich B, Calvano J, Haimovich AD et al. Crit Care Med 2010;38:751–8.

128. Lowry SF, Calvano SE. J Leukoc Biol 2008;83:553–7.

129. Buzby GP, Williford WO, Peterson OL et al. Am J Clin Nutr 1988;47:357–65.

130. Moore FA, Moore EE, Jones TN et al. J Trauma 1989;29: 916–22; discussion 922–3.

131. Muller JM, Brenner U, Dienst C et al. Lancet 1982;1:68–71.

132. Shenkin A, Neuhauser M, Bergstrom J et al. Am J Clin Nutr 1980;33:2119–27.

133. Lowry SF. J Am Coll Surg 2007;205:S65–8.

134. Schibler U, Ripperger J, Brown SA. J Biol Rhythms 2003; 18:250–60.

93

NUTRITION SUPPORT FOR THE PATIENT WITH SURGERY, TRAUMA, OR SEPSIS[1]

KENNETH A. KUDSK

Specialized nutrition support plays an integral role in the preoperative and postoperative management of patients undergoing major surgical procedures or after severe injuries when the patients are unable to take adequate oral intake. Both parenteral and enteral support reduce

major wound dehiscence and anastomotic leaks in select populations undergoing major general surgical procedures (see elsewhere in this volume). When provided enterally, nutrition also reduces septic complications, especially in severely injured trauma patients. Nutrition does not play an essential role in the treatment of sepsis itself but rather in the prevention of sepsis; and the role of nutrition in sepsis is not well defined. The key issue is appropriate use of nutrition and choosing the appropriate patients to use this sophisticated therapy because specialized nutrition support can potentially cause injury as well as provide benefit. When the therapy is used in patients not at risk of nutrition-related complications, only the complications of therapy are seen. However, when delivered to patients at risk of wound or septic complications, nutrition can reduce these complications.

HISTORY OF NUTRITION SUPPORT

Techniques for intragastric feeding have existed for hundreds of years (1), but parenteral nutrition (PN) is a relatively new, highly technical field, which rapidly advanced during the 1970s (2–6). The goals of nutrition support are to prevent further deterioration of nutritional status, replenish host defenses and lean tissue, improve clinical outcome, and support adjunctive therapies, which otherwise would be impossible in a catabolic, malnourished patient. Patients with total or near total intestinal loss, malnourished patients with chronic inflammatory mucosal disease interfering with normal absorption, or those with fistulas precluding ingestion of adequate oral nutrition could not survive their illness without nutritional support. Indications are less clear when no preexisting malnutrition exists or patients quickly resume oral intake. However, preemptive nutritional therapy reduces the risk of subsequent complications in specific patient populations. Despite limited evidence for use in some patients, nutrition support is commonly prescribed because of the recognized relationships among severe malnutrition, morbidity, and mortality; the high incidence of protein malnutrition in hospitalized patients; the recognition that prolonged starvation impairs healing; and a generalization of data from clinical trials demonstrating benefit in at-risk patients. Fortunately, the risks from nutrition therapy are minimized and benefits increased when experienced

---

[1]**Abbreviations: AAG**, α-1-acid glycoprotein; **ALB**, albumin; **ARDS**, acute respiratory distress syndrome; **ATI**, Abdominal Trauma Index; **BEE**, basal energy expenditure; **CRP**, C-reactive protein; **DH**, delayed hypersensitivity; **FDA**, Food and Drug Administration; **GCS**, Glasgow Coma Scale; **GI**, gastrointestinal; **hGH**, human growth hormone; **ICU**, intensive care unit; **IgA**, immunoglobulin A; **IGF-I**, insulinlike growth factor-I; **IL**, interleukin; **ISS**, Injury Severity Score; **IV**, intravenous; **IVLE**, intravenous lipid emulsion; **LBM**, lean body mass; **LCFA**, long-chain fatty acid; **LCT**, long-chain triglyceride; **LOS**, length of stay; **MAdCAM-1**, mucosal addressin cellular adhesion molecule; **MCT**, medium-chain triglyceride; **MODS**, multiple organ dysfunction syndrome; **NCJ**, needle catheter jejunostomy; **PN**, parenteral nutrition; **PNI**, Prognostic Nutritional Index; **PUFA**, polyunsaturated fatty acid; **RDI**, recommended dietary intake; **RQ**, respiratory quotient; **SGA**, Subjective Global Assessment; **SIADH**, syndrome of inappropriate antidiuretic hormone; **ST**, structured triglyceride; **TFN**, transferrin; **TNF**, tumor necrosis factor; **TPN**, total parenteral nutrition.

professionals deliver this complex technical therapy to appropriate patient populations.

IDENTIFICATION OF THE AT-RISK SURGICAL PATIENT

Identifying the at-risk patient is limited by the tools available. Several scoring systems can quantify the risk of complications—particularly septic complications—following blunt or penetrating trauma. In multiple trials, enteral nutrition improves outcome by reducing sepsis compared with starvation or parenteral feeding (7–12). Trauma patients are not traditionally considered nutritionally at risk because most are young and well nourished, although alcohol and drug abuse are common. General surgical patients with preexisting nutritional deficits have been harder to stratify because specialized scoring systems do not exist, although several principles apply. Preoperative albumin (ALB) is the single best indicator of postoperative complications and mortality following major surgery (13), but low ALB may reflect liver disease, fluid resuscitation, or inflammation, rather than nutritional status.

The Trauma Patient

In most studies, the Injury Severity Score (ISS) (14), Abdominal Trauma Index (ATI) (15), or both have stratified patients to complication risk. The ISS scores the three most severely injured body regions of the six, which include head and neck, musculoskeletal, soft tissue, abdominal, thoracic, or head. The ISS correlates with mortality and morbidity. In randomized prospective studies, early enteral feeding improves the outcome of patients with an ISS greater than 18 to 20 compared with intravenous (IV) feeding or fasting (15).

The ISS underestimates risk when severe injuries are isolated to a single body area. The ATI identifies risk for infection in patients with intra-abdominal injuries (Table 93.1) (15). Each intra-abdominal organ has a risk factor that when multiplied by the magnitude of that organ's injury, correlates with risk of sepsis from that injury. Injuries to the pancreas, colon, major vascular structures, duodenum, and liver pose the highest risk. The ATI can be calculated during surgery by summing the scores of each injured organ. An ATI greater than or equal to 20 to 25 poses the greatest risk for sepsis. Sepsis rates are also high with ATI values less than 20 if injuries such as severe pulmonary and chest wall injury, severe closed head injury, spinal cord injury, major soft tissue injuries, or multiple lower extremity fractures exist. These patients have an ISS greater than 20. With ATI greater than 20 to 25 or ISS greater than or equal to 18 to 20, enteral nutrition is usually tolerated and reduces septic complications (9, 12).

General Surgical Patients

Severely malnourished patients are susceptible to wound dehiscence, infections, anastomotic leaks, and so on.

With no gold standard to determine nutritional status, a complete history and physical examination, determination of body weight changes, and the use of select serum tests help identify risk for nutrition-related complications.

The simplest screen is a history and physical with identification of unintentional weight loss because a strong correlation exists between impaired protein status and postoperative complications (16). Unintentional weight loss greater than 10% occurring over 6 months with increased metabolic requirements indicates nutritional risk. Two calculations are commonly used (17):

$$\% \text{ Body weight loss} = \frac{usual\ weight - current\ weight}{usual\ weight} \times 100$$

or

$$\% \text{ Usual body weight} = \frac{current\ body\ weight}{usual\ body\ weight} \times 100$$

Symptoms of abdominal pain, chronic diarrhea, anorexia, or lethargy often accompany weight change. Anthropometric measurements, creatinine–height index, and delayed cutaneous hypersensitivity to a battery of antigens are rarely used in practice currently (18–20). Assessment of lymphocyte count or lymphocyte transformation also is not specific. Protein-calorie malnutrition decreases ALB synthesis, but a decrease in protein degradation can maintain serum levels. This occurs with marasmus when protein and calorie intake are severely restricted. Lower levels of constitutive transport proteins such as ALB ($t_{1/2} = 21$ days), transferrin (TFN; $t_{1/2} = 8$ days), or thyroxin-binding prealbumin ($t_{1/2} = 2$–3 days) may reflect the degree of malnutrition (21). However, inflammatory conditions (e.g., trauma, sepsis, peritonitis) increase serum interleukin-6 (IL-6), which stimulates the acute phase protein response (22) to increase C-reactive protein (CRP) and α-1-acid glycoprotein (AAG) and reduce constitutive protein production. Therefore, initial protein assessment should include CRP with ALB or prealbumin. Low constitutive proteins with a low CRP more likely indicate preexisting malnutrition. Elevated CRP with depressed constitutive proteins may reflect inflammation, protein-calorie malnutrition, or both.

Combinations of these parameters have been used in predictive models to quantify risk. The Prognostic Nutritional Index (PNI) (23) is calculated as follows:

$$\text{PNI (\%)} = 158 - 16.6\ (\text{ALB}) - 0.78\ (\text{TSF}) - 0.20\ (\text{TFN}) - 5.8\ (\text{DH})$$

where PNI is the percentage of risk of complication, ALB is serum ALB in g/dL, TSF is the triceps skinfold thickness in millimeters, TFN is the serum TFN in mg/dL, and DH is delayed hypersensitivity reactive to one of three recall antigens. With DH, 0 = nonreactive; 1 = less than 5 mm induration; and 2 = greater than 5 mm induration. Because DH is rarely used, an alternative applies a lymphocyte score of 0 to 2, where

TABLE 93.1	CALCULATED RISK OF SEPSIS BY THE ABDOMINAL TRAUMA INDEX[a]

ORGAN INJURED	RISK FACTOR	SCORING	ORGAN INJURED	RISK FACTOR	SCORING
High risk			**Low risk**		
Pancreas	(5)	1. Tangential 2. Through-and-through (duct intact) 3. Major debridement or distal duct injury 4. Proximal duct injury 5. Pancreaticoduodenectomy	Kidney	(2)	1. Nonbleeding 2. Minor debridement or suturing 3. Major debridement 4. Pedicle or major calyceal injury 5. Nephrectomy
Large intestine	(5)	1. Serosal injury 2. Single wall injury 3. ≤25% wall injury 4. >25% wall injury 5. Colon wall and blood supply	Ureter	(2)	1. Contusion 2. Laceration 3. Minor debridement 4. Segmental resection 5. Reconstruction
Major vascular	(5)	1. ≤25% wall 2. >25% wall 3. Complete transection 4. Interposition grafting or bypass 5. Ligation	Bladder	(1)	1. Single wall 2. Through-and-through 3. Debridement 4. Wedge resection 5. Reconstruction
Moderately high risk					
Duodenum	(4)	1. Single wall 2. ≤25% wall 3. >25% wall 4. Duodenal wall and blood supply 5. Pancreaticoduodenectomy	Extrahepatic biliary	(1)	1. Contusion 2. Cholecystectomy 3. ≤25% wall 4. >25% wall 5. Biliary enteric reconstruction
Liver	(4)	1. Nonbleeding, peripheral 2. Bleeding, central, of minor debridement 3. Major debridement 4. Lobectomy 5. Lobectomy with caval repair or extensive bipolar débridement	Bone	(1)	1. Periosteum 2. Cortex 3. Through-and-through 4. Intra-articular 5. Major bone loss
Moderate risk					
Stomach	(3)	1. Single wall 2. Through-and-through 3. Minor debridement 4. Wedge resection 5. >35% resection	Small bowel	(1)	1. Single wall 2. Through-and-through 3. ≤25% wall 4. >25% wall 5. Wall and blood supply or >5 injuries
Spleen	(3)	1. Nonbleeding 2. Cautery or hemostatic agent 3. Minor debridement or suturing 4. Partial resection 5. Splenectomy	Minor vascular	(1)	1. Nonbleeding small hematoma 2. Nonbleeding large hematoma 3. Suturing 4. Ligation of isolated vessels 5. Ligation of named vessels

[a]The Abdominal Trauma Index is calculated by multiplying the risk of sepsis (column 2) by the severity of injury (column 3) for each individual organ injured and summing the individual scores for all injuries.

Data from references 8, 15, and 57, with permission.

0 = less than 1000 total lymphocytes/mm^3; 1 = 1000 to 2000/mm^3 and 2 = greater than 2000/mm^3. ALB drives the results, rendering it susceptible to nonnutritional factors such as inflammation, preexisting liver disease, and edema. The PNI predicts complications better than ALB alone (24).

The Prognostic Inflammatory and Nutrition Index (PINI) (23–25) correlates recovery with acute phase and constitutive proteins as follows:

$$PINI = \frac{CRP \times AAG}{PA \times ALB}$$

CRP, AAG, and prealbumin are measured in mg/dL, whereas ALB is measured in g/dL. Because the AAG elevation and ALB depression are prolonged and slow to recover, CRP and PA drive the equation, although sensitivity and specificity are lost when AAG and ALB are not included.

The Subjective Global Assessment (SGA) (26, 27) examines changes in organ function and body composition, the disease process, and the restriction of nutrient intake to predict nutrition status. The SGA is more valuable than anthropometry, which suffers from interobserver variability, hydration state, and age.

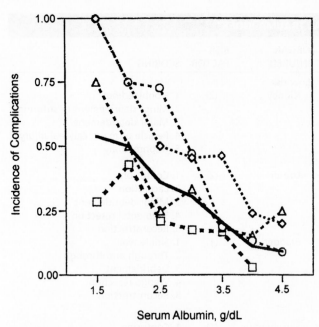

Fig. 93.1. Complications increase as albumin levels drop in patient surgical populations *(solid line)*. Complication rates, however, vary by surgical procedure. Patients undergoing esophageal *(squares* connected by *dots)* and pancreatic *(circles* connected by *dots)* procedures have developed complications at a higher rate at the same albumin level compared with patients undergoing gastric *(triangles* connected by *dashed lines),* or colon *(squares* connected by *dashed lines).* (Reprinted from Kudsk KA, Tolley EA, DeWitt C et al. Preoperative albumin and surgical site identifies surgical risk of major post–operative complications. JPEN J Parenter Enteral Nutr 203;27:1–9, with permission from the American Society for Parenteral and Enteral Nutrition [ASPEN]. ASPEN does not endorse the use of this material of any form other than its entirety.)

The most stressful gastrointestinal (GI) operations are esophagectomy and pancreatic surgery. Complications increase as preoperative ALB levels drop in elective surgery on these organs (Fig. 93.1) (28). Patients undergoing esophagectomy with ALB less than 3.5 g/dL or pancreatic or gastric operations with ALB less than 3.25 g/dL have increased risk for major postoperative complications; risk increases as ALB drops.

THE PHYSIOLOGIC RESPONSE TO SURGERY AND INJURY

The metabolic, physiologic, inflammatory, and cytokine responses to surgery and injury have been well described (29–58). These are also covered in detail elsewhere in this volume.

NUTRITIONAL REQUIREMENTS

Estimating Total Caloric Requirements

The nutrient prescription should meet the metabolic demands of the patient. Overfeeding increases oxygen consumption, generates hepatic lipogenesis, produces immunosuppression (secondary to hyperglycemia or lipid

deposition), and increases CO_2 production, and should be avoided.

The most common way to determine basal energy expenditure (BEE) is the Harris-Benedict formula:

$$\text{In men: BEE} = 66.5 + (13.8 \times \text{body weight in kg}) + (5.0 \times \text{height in cm}) - (6.8 \times \text{age in years})$$

$$\text{In women: } 665 + (9.6 \times \text{body weight in kg}) + (1.8 \times \text{height in cm}) - (4.7 \times \text{age in years})$$

In earlier decades, these values were multiplied by stress and activity factors, but indirect calorimetry shows that stress and activity factors often result in overfeeding when they are used (59, 60).

Indirect calorimetry measures expired CO_2 and O_2 consumption via expired gas to determine the overall resting energy expenditure via the Weir equation. Measurements under controlled conditions approximate the Harris-Benedict equation within 5% to 10% demonstrating that large stress factors are unnecessary. The respiratory quotient (RQ) ratio analyzes the substrate used by the patient because each fuel has a characteristic RQ during metabolism (carbohydrate RQ = 1.0; protein RQ = 0.8; fat RQ = 0.7). Lipogenesis has an RQ value of approximately 8, and a calculated RQ greater than 1 is diagnostic of overfeeding. Unfortunately, small errors in measurement of inspired or expired $\dot{V}O_2$ because of chest tube losses or leaks at a tracheostomy in patients administered a high O_2 concentration can produce a 100% error (61). Thus, the patients who could benefit most from these measurements—the most critically ill, ventilated patients—are those most likely to have tainted values. The technique is labor intensive and requires defined protocols. Because critically ill surgical patients rarely have needs greater than or equal to 15% above the calculated BEE, providing 20 to 30 kcal/kg/day results in 90% of patients receiving adequate nutrition with overfeeding in only 10% to 20% (59, 60). Total requirements are met by administering fat (10 kcal/g IV or 9.1 kcal/g enteral), carbohydrate (4.0 kcal/g enteral and 3.4 kcal/g hydrated glucose), and protein (4 kcal/g) (59).

A modest caloric intake may yield better clinical outcomes in some critically ill patients. Medical intensive care unit (ICU) patients receiving between approximately 9 and 18 kcal/kg/day through enteral and/or parenteral feedings achieved spontaneous ventilation before ICU discharge and had greater survival to hospital discharge than patients receiving 18 to 28 kcal/kg/day (62). The modest caloric intake is also improved outcome compared with patients given a caloric intake of 0 to 9 kcal/kg/day. A specific range for caloric intake may exist for which calories exceeding or failing to meet this intake can have a negative impact on patient outcome. Trauma studies have demonstrated that patients receiving only 40% of goal enteral nutrition intake exhibited significantly fewer infectious complications compared with PN patients receiving greater than 50% of the goal calories (9). Whether these results are because of avoiding overfeeding or some other mechanism is unknown, but providing less than 100% of calculated needs may be beneficial.

Evidence suggests that obesity is an independent risk factor for ICU death (63, 64), and "permissive underfeeding" has been used in obese postoperative patients requiring PN. A hypocaloric, high-protein regimen promotes use of endogenous fat in stressed obese patients while maintaining lean tissue mass. One study showed that hypocaloric, high-protein PN administered to obese patients produced an average weight loss of 2.3 kg/week over 48 days while maintaining positive nitrogen balance with complete healing of wound dehiscence, abscesses, and fistulae (65). Typical hypocaloric PN formulations provide total 22 kcal/kg/day and 2 g protein/kg/day based on ideal body weight for patients with BMI between 30 and 40 and 25 kcal/kg/day and 2.5 g protein/kg/day for patients with a BMI greater than 40. More research on caloric dosing in catabolic patients is clearly needed because of the relative lack of rigorous controlled clinical trials in this area (66).

Glucose Requirements

Hepatic gluconeogenesis produces hyperglycemia as glucose production increases from 2 to 2.5 mg/kg/minute normally to 4 to 5 mg/kg/minute during stress (56, 67). Maximal rate of glucose oxidation is 5 mg/kg/minute (7.2 g/kg/day), which is easily exceeded (68). In a 70-kg person, 2 L of 25% dextrose contains 500 g of glucose, which reaches this maximal level. Traditional recommendations have been to maintain blood glucose values lower than 200 mg/dL because of effects on neutrophils, but data suggest that even tighter control (80 to 120 mg/dL) with insulin improves clinical outcome (53). Mortality dropped in a large group of ICU patients (primarily cardiac surgery patients). It was unclear whether insulin had the primary effect on the cardiac response or through other effects because general surgical patients in that study (including trauma, vascular, and other intra-abdominal procedures) showed no significant improvement with the aggressive insulin treatment. Further work is necessary, but current recommendations are that glucose should be maintained much lower than 180 mg/dL and ideally 140 to 180 mg/dL (and possibly <150 mg/dL in surgical ICU patients) via insulin infusion and very close clinical monitoring to prevent hypoglycemia (56, 69).

Protein Requirements

Adult patients without renal dysfunction should generally receive 1.2 to 1.5 g/kg/day of protein (or amino acids), although this recommendation is not based on rigorous clinical trial data (59). Higher amounts of protein may be indicated in certain conditions (e.g., renal failure patients receiving renal replacement therapy, burn injury). Children also require higher levels of protein per kilogram to account for growth needs (59). If blood urea nitrogen

TABLE 93.2	GENERAL GUIDELINES FOR PROTEIN REQUIREMENTS BASED ON STRESS OR CHANGES IN ORGAN DYSFUNCTION
CLINICAL SITUATION	**RECOMMENDED PROTEIN INTAKES**
Maintenance	1.0 g/kg/d actual BW
Stress or repletion	1.3–2.0 g/kg/d actual BW
Renal failure/before dialysis	0.8–1.0 g/kg/d dry BW
Renal failure/hemodialysis	1.2–1.5 g/kg/d dry BW
Renal failure/peritoneal/CVVHD	1.5–2.0 g/kg/d dry BW
Burn injury	2.0–2.5 g g/kg/d dry BW
Hepatic failure	0.6–1.2 g/kg/d dry BW
Liver transplant	1–1.5 g/kg/d dry BW
Bone marrow transplant	1.5–2.0 g/kg/d dry BW

BW, body weight; CVVHD, continuous venovenous hemodialysis.

exceeds 100 mg/dL, protein should be decreased (e.g., to 1.0 to 1.3 g/kg/day). With hemodialysis or renal supportive techniques such as continuous arterial venous hemodialysis or continuous venovenous hemodialysis, protein requirements actually increase to 1.5 to 2.0 g/kg/day because of protein losses across the dialysis membranes. Burn patients typically require 2.0 to 2.5 g/kg/day owing to urinary and wound losses (59). Table 93.2 summarizes European and US clinical practice guidelines for protein and amino acid needs in catabolic patients (70, 71).

Fat Requirements

Glucose should provide approximately 50% to 60% of total calories (approximately 70% to 80% of nonprotein calories) (59, 70, 71). The balance of nonprotein calories should be given as 1 to 1.5 g/kg/day of fat with triglyceride levels less than 300 mg/dL (70, 71). Hyperlipidemia with triglycerides greater than 500 mg/dL mandates withholding IV lipid emulsion (IVLE) in PN until triglyceride levels decrease to a safer range. The maximum recommended dose of IV lipid is 2.5 g/kg/day in the adult, but this should be used rarely (70, 71). Fat calories can be increased to 50% of requirements in select patients with severe hyperglycemia or high CO_2 production, but with risks of hyperlipidemia, cholestasis, immunosuppression, and increased infection (59, 70, 71). Suspected overfeeding with increased CO_2 should be treated by reduction in total calories (59, 70, 71).

Vitamin Requirements

In April 2000, the Food and Drug Administration (FDA) modified requirements for adult parenteral multivitamins recommending changes to the earlier 12-vitamin formulation (73). Changes included higher dosages of vitamins B_1 (thiamin), vitamin B_6 (pyridoxine), vitamin C (ascorbic acid), and folic acid, and the addition of vitamin K (phylloquinone) (Table 93.3). The vitamin content of the original formula was based on the known nutritional needs of healthy individuals to prevent nutrient deficiency. Clinicians suggested that

TABLE 93.3 OLD VERSUS NEW FDA RECOMMENDATIONS FOR ADULT PARENTERAL MULTIVITAMIN FORMULATIONS

VITAMIN	OLD RECOMMENDATIONS[a]	NEW RECOMMENDATIONS[b]
Vitamin A	3,300 IU (1 mg retinol)	3,300 IU (1 mg retinol)
Vitamin D_2	200 IU (5 μg cholecalciferol)	200 IU (5 μg cholecalciferol)
Vitamin E	10 mg (α-tocopherol)	10 mg (α-tocopherol)
Vitamin K	None	150 μg
Thiamin (B_1)	3 mg	6 mg
Riboflavin (B_2)	3.6 mg	3.6 mg
Pyridoxine (B_6)	4 mg	6 mg
Niacin	40 mg	40 mg
Pantothenate	15 mg	15 mg
Biotin	60 μg	60 μg
Folate	400 μg	600 μg
Cyanocobalamin (B_{12})	5 μg	5 μg
Ascorbic acid (C)	100 mg	200 mg

[a]Data from American Medical Association Department of Foods and Nutrition. Multivitamin preparations for parenteral use. A statement by the Nutrition Advisory Group. JPEN J Parenter Enteral Nutr 1979;3:258–62, with permission.
[b]Data from Food and Drug Administration. Parenteral multivitamin products: drugs for human use; Drug efficacy study implementation, Amendment. Fed Reg 2000;65:21200–1.

requirements may be greater in seriously ill patients requiring specialized nutrition (74). Higher dosages of vitamin C or vitamin E may play a critical role in antioxidant defense. Patients undergoing abdominal aortic aneurysm surgery (75) received 600 IU of oral vitamin E daily for 8 days before surgery. The vitamin E reduced ischemic-reperfusion tissue injury on muscle biopsies compared with patients without supplementation. Patients following trauma or emergency surgery were randomized to vitamins C and E (α-tocopherol 1000 IU every 8 hours orally and ascorbic acid 1000 mg every 8 hours IV during an ICU stay up to 28 days) or nothing (76). No difference in pneumonia or acute respiratory distress syndrome (ARDS) was detected but multiple organ dysfunction syndrome (MODS) was significantly lower with vitamin treatment, although the incidence of MODS occurring in both groups was low. Although micronutrient requirements for critically ill patients are unknown, additional studies suggest that higher dose for a variety of vitamins, such as vitamins A, C and D, are likely higher than as recommended currently in Table 93.3 (59, 71, 74, 77).

The effect of the acute-phase response on fluid distribution and measured vitamin concentrations has been studied after orthopedic surgical procedures (78). Plasma vitamin A, vitamin E, and pyridoxal-5'-phosphate drop in association with a CRP increase over a 7-day period. Vitamin concentrations returned to baseline as the acute-phase response resolved. Reductions in vitamin concentrations should be interpreted with care during the acute-phase response. Supplemental vitamins may be indicated when low vitamin concentrations persist during the absence of an acute-phase response.

Acute injury or illness occurs with progressive vitamin deficiencies during convalescence. Children with greater than or equal to 40% of the total body surface area burns remain deficient in vitamin D up to 7 years after the burn (79). Low levels of circulating 25-hydroxyvitamin D correlate with bone mineral density Z-scores, a finding

suggesting that vitamin D depletion after burn injury could contribute factor to bone loss. Newer evidence suggests a defect in the skin production of cholecalciferol, vitamin D_3, is responsible for low serum vitamin D (80). A fivefold reduction was observed in the conversion of 7-dehydrocholesterol to previtamin D_3 in burn scar skin compared with unburned skin. This implies that survivors of large burns should be assessed for hypovitaminosis D, bone disease, and other consequences of vitamin D deficiency and replete with vitamin D based on blood 25-hydroxyvitamin D levels.

Trace Element Requirements

Trace elements should be added to PN formulations daily, but as noted for vitamins, exact needs for specific trace elements in catabolic patients are unknown. Standard trace element solutions contain selenium, chromium, zinc, copper, and manganese, which are essential in numerous metabolic pathways. Biochemical and functional alterations develop during severe deficiency states. Acute zinc deficiency results in diarrhea, mood changes, dermatitis that starts in the nasolabial folds and spreads to the groin, subsequent alopecia, and increased infections. Zinc concentrations are high in small bowel fluid and should be supplemented with small bowel fistulas and high ileostomy outputs. Low copper produces neutropenia (but neutrocytosis does occur during infection) and a picture of iron deficiency anemia because the iron is not transported to the bone marrow from sites of red blood cell destruction. Chromium deficiency is associated with glucose intolerance resulting from low levels of glucose tolerance factor. Low plasma selenium is associated with more ventilator-associated pneumonia, organ failure, and mortality in critically ill patients, and a few studies show efficacy with high-dose selenium administration in critically ill patients (81, 82). High urinary and cutaneous losses of selenium, zinc, and copper occur after burn and trauma (83). Supplementation of these trace elements improved immune responsiveness, reduced pulmonary infectious episodes, and lowered ICU stay after burns compared with patients receiving standard doses (83). Chromium and zinc are excreted via the kidney, whereas copper and manganese are excreted through the biliary tract. If serum bilirubin levels exceed 10 m/dL during hepatic failure, trace element solutions should be withheld and only selenium, chromium, and zinc should be provided. Clearly more data are needed to define biochemically and clinically optimal doses of trace elements in hospital patients, including those after trauma, operation and infection (59, 84).

ROUTE OF NUTRITION SUPPORT

Enteral versus Parenteral Nutrition

In general, the enteral route is preferable to parenteral feeding if access to and function of the GI allows enteral feeding (70, 71). Although gastroparesis occurs during critical illness or after injury, access directly into the small intestine allows adequate nutrition to meet nutrient needs. Experimentally, parenteral feeding decreases brush border enzyme activity, probably increases mucosal permeability, reduces villous height, and generates inhibitory effects on gut mucosal immunity (85–88). Each factor is benefited by enteral feeding.

Substantial clinical data support the use of enteral nutrition. Many studies were performed in trauma patients (6–12), in whom small bowel cannulation during celiotomy allowed randomization to early enteral feeding, parenteral feeding or no specialized nutrition. Almost uniformly, studies showed significant reductions in pneumonia and intra-abdominal abscesses (if at risk of intra-abdominal abscess) with enteral feeding. In particular, patients with an ATI greater than or equal to 20 or an ISS greater than or equal to 18 to 20—patients most at risk for infectious complications—benefited the most (9). Gastroparesis usually resolves within 3 to 4 hours after isolated closed head injury, unless the patient is in a barbiturate coma, and enteral feeding should be instituted as gastroparesis resolves. Earlier feeding via small bowel tubes placed endoscopically provides no additional benefit (89). If gastroparesis persists, a tube should be advanced with electromagnetic tracking or with endoscopy or fluoroscopy into the distal duodenum/proximal small intestine. Because airway placement occurs in 1.5% to 2% of patients with blind placement often with lethal results, this technique is not advised.

Similar results occur in general surgical patients. In a number of trials, early enteral nutrition improved postoperative infections, immunologic parameters, and GI tract function (10, 90–92). However, no benefit of early enteral feeding occurred in studies that primarily enrolled well-nourished patients undergoing major surgical procedures where uncomplicated postoperative course is usual

(93, 94). However, studies that recruited significant numbers of malnourished patients showed improved outcome with enteral and parenteral feeding (91, 92, 95, 96). Early postoperative nutrition precludes further loss in lean body mass (LBM) owing to starvation and should be delivered enterally rather than parenterally when possible. Enteral and parenteral feeding has been studied in inflammatory bowel disease (97, 98), following transplantation (99, 100), and in patients with a mild-to-moderate pancreatitis (101). Uniformly, reports show beneficial effects with the use of enteral feeding when clinically tolerated. A large European trial in greater than 4500 critically ill adult patients showed that the addition of PN concomitant with early enteral feeding (within the first 2 days) was not beneficial compared with waiting on the initiation of PN until after 7 days (102). Patients in both groups received identical IV micronutrients (vitamins, minerals, and trace elements) at entry, whereas the early use of PN was associated with more infections and organ dysfunction and a longer length of hospital stay than the subjects who received only early enteral tube feeds and IV micronutrients, without a difference in mortality between groups (84, 102).

Perioperative Nutrition Support

Preoperative and postoperative nutrition support studies have provided conflicting results. A critical issue in the interpretation of these data is patient selection because many studies recruited patients who were not at risk of nutrition-related complications. Particularly when a PN arm was included, the results often demonstrated an increase in septic complications with parenteral feeding in patients who could otherwise have had no complications. An example is the Veterans Administration Cooperative Study (95), which randomized preoperative surgical patients to parenteral feeding for 7 to 15 days preoperatively or to a control group with ad libitum access to a diet. The amount of parenteral feeding in that study exceeded current recommendations, which may have aggravated the negative effects, including via hyperglycemia (53, 56). Overall, there was a trend toward a reduction in healing complications (wound dehiscence, anastomotic dehiscence, fistula formation) with parenteral feeding, but with an increased rate of infectious complications, particularly pneumonia. After stratification by preexisting malnutrition, severely malnourished patients clearly benefited from parenteral feeding with fewer healing complications and no increase (and some decrease) in infections. In trials of perioperative nutrition, almost all trials with negative results or a negative effect of nutrition recruited mostly well-nourished patients (93–95). Trials that included mostly malnourished patients demonstrated significant benefit with perioperative nutrition (91, 92, 95). One can conclude that well-nourished patients—identified after a careful nutritional history and physical—are unlikely to benefit from specialized nutrition, whereas patients with preexisting nutritional deficits will benefit.

One exception exists. A metaanalysis showed that patients undergoing elective GI procedures who received enteral diet supplemented with arginine, omega-3 fatty acids, and nucleotides in the perioperative period had significant improvement in their postoperative course, with fewer infectious and other complications, but without a change in mortality versus patients who received conventional enteral feedings (103).

ROLE OF THE GUT IN HOST DEFENSE

General consensus exists from numerous randomized prospective clinical trials in trauma patients and general surgical patients (7–12, 89–92) that GI feeding is more beneficial that PN when the GI tract is functional. Experimentally, parenteral feeding results in very rapid atrophy of intestinal villi (85). These changes also occur within humans, but not to a lesser degree (104). Injury, hemorrhagic shock, ischemia, and sepsis alter gut permeability to macromolecules and also produce a release of virulence factors in bacteria that increases their toxicity (86, 105). Gut permeability increases in trauma patients, but it normalizes quite quickly (106, 107). Unidentified GI factors released into the thoracic duct have been implicated in multiple organ dysfunctions in animal models of ischemia reperfusion (108,109). It is also unclear whether starvation potentiates the release of this factor in animal models.

The gut plays a pivotal role in mucosal immunity (110–117). Bacteria are kept in check with peristalsis, competing bacterial populations, mucin, immunoglobulin A (IgA), and other factors. Experimentally, lack of enteral feeding reduces T and B cells within lamina propria, Peyer patches, and intraepithelial space (110) leading to reduced IgA stimulating cytokines IL-4 and IL-10 and a decrease in lung and intestinal IgA (111). The entry site for T and B cells destined for the mucosal immune system are the Peyer patches, which express mucosal addressin cellular adhesion molecule (MAdCAM-1) on the high endothelial venules to attract the T and B cells (112, 113). MAdCAM-1 expression decreases when the GI tract is not fed (114). After cells are sensitized in the Peyer patches to antigens absorbed from the intestinal lumen, they are distributed to intestinal and extraintestinal sites such as the lung, genitourinary tract, and lactating mammary gland (115). As MAdCAM-1 levels drop and fewer cells enter the mucosal immune system, T and B cells drop in the GI and respiratory tracts of parenterally fed mice resulting in loss of antibacterial and antiviral defenses (116, 117). Immunologic memory is intact because the reinstitution of enteral feeding reverses these defects.

Systemic and intraperitoneal protection also is affected by route of feeding. Enteral feeding reduces the lethality of intraperitoneal bacteria compared with parenteral feeding. PN blunts before bacterial peritonitis suppresses release of intraperitoneal tumor necrosis factor (TNF), which inhibit bacterial proliferation (118) resulting in a higher systemic TNF response to intraperitoneal sepsis. This has been confirmed in human subjects (119).

Types of Feeding

Enteral Diet

Gastroparesis complicates the course of most critically ill patients, which precludes early intragastric feeding. One exception is burned patients who have less gastroparesis when tube fed within 8 to 12 hours of injury (120). When gastroparesis occurs, enteral access beyond the ligament of Treitz allows enteral feeding. Chemically defined "elemental" diets usually are not necessary (86, 121) and should be reserved for patients with mucosal disease or significant GI intolerance. In most critically ill patients, an isotonic diet containing soluble fiber can be given (70, 71). The fiber limits diarrhea, which is usually caused by antibiotics, bacterial overgrowth, *Clostridium difficile* infection, gastric motility agents, or sorbitol-rich elixirs rather than the enteral formula (122–124). Isotonic diets containing 1 kcal/mL can be administered through nasojejunal tubes, 5F and 7F needle catheter jejunostomies (NCJs), or size 14, 16, or 18 catheters. Diets administered into the small bowel should be started in hemodynamically stable patients at a rate of 15 to 25 mL/hour and advanced every 12 to 24 hours as tolerated. Intragastric feedings start at a faster rate—usually 50 mL/hour—to test for gastroparesis. If residuals are not elevated (>200 to 250 mL 4 hours after starting) diets can be advanced to the goal rate (120–122).

Specific Substrates

Specific substrates may benefit certain critically ill or injured patients. Glutamine, arginine, omega-3 fatty acids, and nucleotides have been combined in formulas commonly referred to as pharmaconutrition or "immune-enhancing diets" (70, 103). Production of glutamine, the most abundant free amino acid in the body, increases during stress and sepsis. However, serum and intracellular levels drop as this amino acid becomes "conditionally essential" during times of high metabolic rate (125, 126). It provides substrate for enterocytes, rapidly proliferating cells, and T lymphocytes. Both enteral and parenteral feedings supplemented with glutamine have been shown to be effective (12, 125, 126). Unfortunately, glutamine is difficult to solubilize and degrades into ammonia and pyroglutamate, two toxic products during heat sterilization that have limited its use with IV feeding (see elsewhere in this volume). Arginine is a precursor of nitric oxide, nitrites, and nitrates and promotes proliferation of stimulated T cells. It plays a role in cellular immunity and fibroblast proliferation and serves as a secretagogue for growth hormone, prolactin, glucagon, and insulin production (127). Arginine administration has long been studied in nutritional support (see elsewhere in this volume).

Polyunsaturated fatty acids (PUFAs) contain double bonds at several positions. Omega-6 fatty acids are found in vegetable oils, whereas omega-3 fatty acids are found in fish oil and canola oil (rapeseed oil). Humans cannot synthesize these PUFAs, but can rapidly incorporate them into cell membranes. Omega-6 fatty acids are incorporated as arachidonic acid and subsequently metabolized with phospholipases to produce prostaglandin E_2, thromboxane A_2, and leukotriene B_4. These prostanoids and leukotrienes are immunosuppressive and proinflammatory. They inhibit killer cell activity, impair antibody formation, and blunt cell-mediated immunity. Omega-3 PUFAs are metabolized to prostanoids of the three and five series, including prostaglandin PGI_3, thromboxane A_3, and leukotriene B_5 via the lipoxygenase pathway. These products are neither immunosuppressive nor proinflammatory. More research on enteral products enriched with these lipids is needed (70, 71, 84, 103). Nucleotides provide RNA for cell proliferation, DNA and RNA synthesis, and immunocyte function (70). Formulas supplemented with these nutrients have shown clinical effects. Severely injured trauma patients or those undergo upper GI resection for malignancies significantly benefited with reduced infectious complications, hospital stay, and total complications (12, 91, 92, 128). No benefit occurs when they are used in well-nourished elective general surgical patients unlikely to have postoperative complications (93, 94), with the exception of two studies that preoperatively provided patients with a liter of the diets before colorectal surgery (96). Under those circumstances, well-nourished patients appeared to benefit.

The use of arginine-supplemented tube feedings in frankly septic patients has been questioned, and although the issue is still controversial, investigators have speculated that arginine may have adverse effects in some septic patients (70, 129). More recent data demonstrate that it may be more generalizable to a wider range of septic patients (130). Fortunately, most septic patients do tolerate enteral feeding, but clinicians should be circumspect in administering arginine-enriched diets to frankly septic patients (129). Trauma increases cellular arginase, which rapidly metabolizes arginine (127). In this condition, supplemental arginine may benefit by normalizing serum levels. In frank sepsis, however, arginase levels are depressed and more arginine may be metabolized to nitric oxide, which may increase vasodilatation rendering it toxic. However, given emerging safety and efficacy data, it has been advocated that rigorous trials on administration of arginine in ICU patients may be justified now (130).

Access for Enteral Feeding

Most enteral feeding is delivered into the stomach when surgical access was not obtained or celiotomy not performed (70, 131, 132). Small-bore tubes should be used because large nasogastric tubes increase reflux and may cause pressure necrosis at the nasal site with ulcers or strictures along the path. A stylet in tubes eases their passage but carries a risk of airway placement in 1.5% to 2% of patients with pneumothorax in 30% to 40% of

misplaced tubes, which can be fatal. Position must be confirmed by either aspiration of gastric juice or confirmation by radiography. Simple air insufflation will not distinguish between placement in the left lower lobe or within the stomach. Data show that electromagnetic tracking of the tube eliminated all airway complications. During intragastric feeding, the bed should be kept elevated at least 30 to 35 degrees because the gastroesophageal junction is dependent in supine patients (132).

More distal tube placement is necessary when gastric residuals are high ($\geq$330 to 350 mL) or evidence exists of aspiration or reflux of tube feedings into the throat. If celiotomy is not indicated, small-bore tubes can be advanced via electromagnetic tracking, fluoroscopy, or endoscopy. Blind placement is discouraged. Although no strong evidence exists that placing the tube beyond the stomach precludes gastric reflux and aspiration, advancement of the tube into the distal duodenum or proximal small intestine may provide some protection because direct small bowel feedings rarely reflux into the stomach. Intragastric feeding is not recommended in severely neurologically impaired patients or those with recurrent pneumonia secondary to reflux. A major drawback to nasojejunal is frequent dislodgement (132).

If celiotomy is necessary, access is part of the preoperative and intraoperative plan. Recurrent aspiration pneumonia, severe gastroesophageal reflux, or expected prolonged gastroparesis can be bypassed with direct small bowel access using a large-bore (14F, 16F, or 18F) tube, a 5F or 7F NCJ, or a transgastric jejunostomy. NCJs can function for 3 to 4 weeks if cared for properly. Medications should not be administered via NCJ because elixirs coagulate tube feedings, causing tube occlusion. NCJs tolerate commercially prepared fiber-containing diets without problems. The advantage of 4F, 16F, or 18F tubes, however, is that they can be removed and replaced with a tube of similar diameter if they become dislodged or clog. They also tolerate administration of medications better if irrigated with 20 to 30 mL of water before and after their administration. NCJ tubes cannot be replaced. Important points in the creation of any jejunostomy are as follows: (a) A tube should be located far enough distal to the ligament of Treitz at a site where an adequate mesentery precludes it being pulled off the anterior abdominal wall if the patient becomes distended. (b) Witzel Tunnel construction eliminates potential tube dislodgement into the peritoneal cavity. (c) It should be sutured to the anterior abdominal wall for approximately 4 cm to preclude volvulus at the attachment point. (d) The tube should be sutured to the abdominal wall at the lateral edge of the rectus sheath or more lateral to reduce chance of small bowel herniation over the jejunostomy site. (e) The external portion of the catheter should be kept short to prevent dislodgement by confused patients (70, 132).

Tube feedings can be administered into the small intestine in hemodynamically stable patients who are off vasopressors for hemodynamic stability and after resuscitation is complete. Adequate urinary output is evidence of good splanchnic perfusion. Isotonic solutions are preferable to hypertonic solutions to minimize diarrhea. In addition, use of diet with soluble fiber reduce diarrhea because the fiber is metabolized by bacteria to produce short-chain fatty acids (e.g., acetoacetate, butyrate, propionate) that are substrates for colonocyte metabolism to preserve water absorption. Formulas with medium-chain triglycerides (MCTs) may be better tolerated than long-chain triglycerides (LCTs) because they are more easily digested. However, LCTs must be administered because MCTs have no essential fatty acids. Abdominal distention, emesis, diarrhea, tube dislodgement, and electrolyte abnormalities are the most common complications associated with enteral feeding. Aspiration is most likely with intragastric feeding and can be minimized by administration of prokinetic agents, elevation of the head of the bed to at least 30 degrees, frequent residuals checks, and discontinuation of feedings or advancement of the tube beyond the ligament of Treitz if residuals are high or gastric reflux exists (70).

Diarrhea usually results from the sorbitol in elixirs used to administer medications, antibiotic usage with bacterial overgrowth, *C. difficile*, or failure to stop motility agents. In addition, magnesium-containing antacids may cause diarrhea. In patients with diarrhea, *C. difficile* toxin should be checked; diets converted to a fiber-containing isotonic diet; and all enterally administered medications discontinued. In addition, the need for antibiotic therapy should be reviewed and discontinued if possible.

Tube dislodgement usually occurs during nursing care through movement or turning of the patient. With surgically placed small-bore feeding tubes, the external portion should be kept short and well fixed with a suture at the skin level.

Electrolyte abnormalities are common with both enteral parenteral feeding. Refeeding syndrome with hypokalemia, hypophosphatemia, or hypomagnesemia occurs in malnourished patients and warrants supplementation with the specific electrolytes. In addition, most enteral products have 30 to 40 mEq of sodium; therefore, hyponatremia occurs, especially if IV fluids (particularly piggybacks) are D5W. Hypernatremia occurs with concentrated formula, and 1 mL of water should be administered for each calorie to maintain hydration. Rare complications include small bowel necrosis or pneumatosis intestinalis. Although the etiology for this pathology is unknown, it has been associated with small bowel feedings in patients who are on pressors, are hemodynamically unstable, or are unresuscitated. It also appears as a motility disorder in patients received tube feedings with fiber after 5 to 7 days, resulting in fecalization of the distal small bowel. Intragastric feedings are safe even in unstable patients on pressors because small intestinal intolerance is manifested

by high residuals, which protect the small intestine. If residuals remain low, it is a sign that small bowel tolerance is adequate and they can be advanced toward the goal rate (70).

Parenteral Feeding

Glucose

Monohydrated glucose is used in PN to provide carbohydrate and meet increased energy requirements. Glucose control in critically ill patients has received considerable attention. One study in surgical ICU patients showed reduced mortality and infections using an aggressive insulin protocol, maintaining serum glucose levels between 80 and 108 mg/dL (53). The improvement occurred only after cardiac surgery with no benefit after trauma, vascular, transplant, or general surgical procedures. In a second trial by the same authors, no benefit was found in a population of critically ill medical patients (56). A third trial of both medical and surgical patients (the NICE-SUGAR trial) failed to find any benefit with tight glucose control (69). Potentially important differences among the trials exist. Patients treated with insulin in the single surgical ICU trial received 19 to 20 kcal/kg/day (parenteral and/or enteral) with approximately 70 U insulin/day in an insulin protocol adjusted by dedicated research nurses (53, 56). In the NICE-SUGAR trial, patients in several ICUs received approximately 10 kcal/kg/day of enteral feeding with 50 U insulin/day administered by ICU nurses. Despite promising results in the surgical ICU study, these design differences render it difficult to reach a conclusion regarding the role of intense glucose control (69). Most agree that blood glucose levels should be controlled at levels less than 180 mg/dL and possibly less than or equal to 130 to 150 mg/dL in surgical ICU patients (56).

Amino Acids

During parenteral feeding, standard amino acid solutions appear comparable in nutrient value. Specialty formulas for stress, sepsis, hepatic failure, or renal failure are commercially available, but benefits from their use are unclear (70, 71, 84). Several studies examined the use of supplemental glutamine (125). Glutamine is not available in commercial amino acid products in the United States because of its limited stability in solution and breakdown during heat sterilization to dangerous metabolic byproducts, pyroglutamic acid, and ammonia. For safe administration of glutamine, a cold sterilization and filtration process ensures the purity and stability of IV glutamine prepared from glutamine powder. In several clinical trials, glutamine supplementation had a beneficial effect on lymphocytes (133, 134) and reduced infections in bone marrow transplant patients (135), but this was not duplicated in patients with solid organ malignancies. Studies in critically ill patients are limited but seem to show reduced hospital stay and better survival in some patient subgroups, as summarized elsewhere in this volume.

Intravenous Lipid Emulsions

In the United States, all IVLEs available for parenteral feeding are derived from soybean or soybean and safflower oil combinations. These vegetable oils are long-chain fatty acids (LCFAs) and deliver the essential fatty acids, linoleic acid (omega-6) and α-linolenic acid (omega-3) (70, 71, 136). Linoleic acid is the major fatty acid in IVLEs, ranging from 44% to 65%, with α-linolenic acid present in concentrations of 4% to 11%. Alterations in immune function occur with large infusions of IVLEs over short periods of time because of products of omega-6 fatty acid metabolism that are proinflammatory and immunosuppressive. When infusions of IVLEs exceed 0.12 g/kg/hour, there appears to be impairment of neutrophil or monocyte/macrophage function (136). Studies of IVLEs on cellular immunity show inconsistent results, and no studies show any effect on humoral immunity.

IVLE infusion can affect pulmonary function. Elevated mean pulmonary artery pressure and pulmonary venous admixture with declines in arterial oxygen levels to fractional inspired oxygen ratio (PaO_2/FIO_2) were noted when IVLE infusion rates were greater than 0.12 g/kg/hour in patients with ARDS who did (137) and did not have sepsis (138, 139). Trauma patients receiving no IVLE with PN during the first 10 days of hospitalization experienced almost a 2-week reduction in mechanical ventilator days compared with patients randomized to receive PN with IVLE. Unfortunately, these improvements cannot be solely attributed to withholding IVLEs and may be related to the fact that they also received fewer calories (70, 71, 140).

To circumvent the problems with LCFA-based IVLEs, alternative lipid sources such as MCTs have been studied (136). MCTs possess metabolic advantages over LCFAs. MCTs are cleared more rapidly, independent of carnitine for transport into mitochondria, and less likely to be deposited in the liver or adipose tissue. Work with MCTs in mechanically ventilated patients shows that MCTs are tolerated, but they may increase oxygen consumption. Pure MCT formulations lack the essential fatty acids, linoleic acid, and α-linolenic acid, and always must be combined with LCFAs. MCFAs are ketogenic and must be used with caution in diabetic patients. They are contraindicated if ketosis or acidosis exists. MCFAs and LCFAs have been combined into lipid emulsions to minimize any adverse effects of MCFA alone. Combinations exist in two forms: physical mixtures of MCFAs and LCFAs or structured triglycerides (STs). STs are formed by hydrolysis and reesterification of MCFAs and LCFAs on the same glycerol backbone. STs provide both essential fatty acids and MCFAs, which are rapidly cleared from the serum. STs produce a more positive nitrogen balance and significant weight gain with enhanced lipid clearance in

catabolic patients when compared with physical mixtures of MCFAs/LCFAs (141). Combination IVLE products are not currently marketed in the United States for use in clinical practice.

Electrolytes

Surgery and injury often create fluid and electrolyte imbalances requiring adjustments in the PN formula (18, 59, 70). (Please also see details in other chapters.)

Sodium. Sodium is the principal extracellular cation, and the amount required in PN is based on clinical need. The amount of sodium chosen is usually similar to 0.45% saline with 70 to 80 mEq/L added to the PN. Congestive heart failure, edema, cirrhosis, or nephrotic syndrome cause fluid overload manifested as hypervolemic hyponatremia resulting from excess total body sodium with an even greater excess in total body water. Severe sodium restriction is required with sodium withheld from the PN (18).

Syndrome of inappropriate antidiuretic hormone secretion (SIADH) is a less common cause of hyponatremia in critically ill patients. Central nervous system pathology resulting from head injury, meningitis, or subarachnoid hemorrhage is associated with this clinical state. Pharmacologic agents, including carbamazepine, chlorpropamide, tricyclic antidepressants, clonidine, and cyclophosphamide, also may be responsible. SIADH is diagnosed by a combination of low serum sodium (in the absence of fluid overload), low serum osmolality, elevated urine osmolality relative to serum osmolality, and urine sodium greater than 40 mEq/L (18). Antidiuretic hormone stimulates water absorption without sodium in the kidney so that urine sodium and tonicity are high relative to serum. The appropriate therapy is water restriction.

Patients with large nasogastric losses, high ileostomy or pancreatic fistula outputs, or large bowel losses often require substantial quantities of sodium. Hypernatremia develops if the sodium and fluid losses are not replaced. If serum sodium exceeds 150 mEq/L, no more than 40 mEq/day of sodium should be added to the PN. Medication records should be reviewed for "hidden" sodium contained in ALB, medications in 0.9% saline, and sodium-containing antibiotics. Other medications, such as lactulose, produce dehydration from volume depletion by causing excessive diarrhea.

Potassium. Potassium is principally an intracellular cation, and inclusion in PN is dictated by clinical need. With normal renal function, 40 mEq/L of potassium usually is sufficient to maintain homeostasis (18). Potassium needs are influenced by acid–base status. During metabolic acidosis (pH <7.2), excess hydrogen ions is present in serum exchanges with intracellular potassium, causing hyperkalemia. Conversely, hypokalemia occurs with metabolic alkalosis.

Renal insufficiency (creatinine clearance <30 mL/minute) also is associated with impaired potassium clearance and hyperkalemia. In general, hyperkalemia in acute renal failure warrants potassium removal from PN until levels are less than 4.0 mEq/L, when potassium can be added in modest doses (e.g., 10 mEq/L). Many medications alter serum potassium levels. Hyperkalemia can occur with potassium-sparing medications such as angiotensin-converting enzyme inhibitors, spironolactone, triamterene, and amiloride. Heparin is an aldosterone antagonist causing sodium wasting and potassium retention. Both systemic and low-dose heparin may cause this problem, especially in patients with diabetes or chronic renal failure. Trimethoprim in trimethoprim/sulfamethoxazole, used frequently for Gram-negative systemic infections, is a weak diuretic with potassium-sparing activities. Reducing potassium in PN is warranted when patients receive these medications, even those with normal renal function. If serum potassium concentrations exceed 5.1 mEq/L, no more than 20 mEq/day of potassium should be included in the PN formulation (18).

Hypokalemia occurs with potassium-wasting medications, such as amphotericin B, aminoglycosides, antipseudomonal penicillins (i.e., ticarcillin), loop/thiazide diuretics, glucocorticoids, insulin, and inhaled beta agonists (i.e., albuterol).

Calcium. Calcium gluconate is used in PN because it is more stable and less likely to precipitate with phosphorus than chloride salt. Up to 98% of total body calcium is in bone and is readily mobilized, as needed under the influence of parathyroid hormone. The recommended dietary intake (RDI) for parenteral calcium is approximately 10 mEq or 200 mg/day. Patients with high losses, such as those with severe short bowel syndrome or massive blood transfusions, may require substantially more calcium in PN. Dosage increases of 5 mEq daily for acute care are reasonable, but simultaneous monitoring of serum phosphorus is recommended. Calcium is highly protein bound (especially to ALB). The following formula allows adjustment of serum calcium for low ALB concentrations:

$$\text{Corrected calcium} = [(4\text{-ALB}) \times 0.8] + \text{Measured calcium}$$

Lower amounts of calcium may be required for patients with hyperphosphatemia, metastatic cancer, or hyperparathyroidism. Usually 10 mEq/day is a sufficient amount in PN (18).

Magnesium. Magnesium is closely linked to calcium metabolism. The parenteral RDI for magnesium is approximately 10 mEq or 120 mg/day (18). Patients with short bowel syndrome, chronic alcoholism, or burns may require larger doses for homeostasis and can be advanced incrementally by 50% of the parenteral RDI. Medications associated with magnesium wasting include amphotericin B, aminoglycosides, cyclosporin A, cisplatin, loop and thiazide diuretics, and piperacillin (18). Dysrhythmias, hypocalcemia (a common problem after trauma), and irritability are avoided with magnesium monitoring and appropriate treatment. IV magnesium therapy usually is necessary when moderate-to-severe magnesium deficiency

TABLE 93.4	GRADUATED DOSING SCHEME FOR MAGNESIUM REPLACEMENT THERAPY
SERUM MAGNESIUM CONCENTRATION (mg/dL)^a	**MAGNESIUM DOSE/ INFUSION PERIOD^b**
1.5–1.8	0.5 mEq/kg/12 h
1.1–1.4	1.0 mEq/kg/24 h
≤1	1.5 mEq/kg/24 h

^{a}The normal serum magnesium concentration is 1.7 to 2.3 mg/dL.
^{b}Use 50% of the recommended doses when creatinine clearance is less than 30 mL/min.

is caused by poor absorption of oral magnesium salts. Magnesium has a renal tubular threshold similar to glucose; therefore, rapid administration over a short period of time (<4 hours) invariably results in high urinary losses and no change is serum values. A weight-based regimen for magnesium deficiency with a slow IV infusion over 12 to 24 hours facilitates magnesium retention (Table 93.4). Magnesium status should be considered in a hypokalemic patient because magnesium is a cofactor for the Na-K ATPase pump. Magnesium replacement should be considered for low-normal serum magnesium concentrations in the presence of hypokalemia because magnesium is an intracellular cation and serum concentrations may not reflect intracellular status accurately. Generally, 12 mEq/L is appropriate in total parenteral nutrition (TPN), depending on the prevailing blood level, dextrose dose, and renal function. Hypermagnesemia usually occurs with renal failure requiring removal of magnesium in the PN until the serum levels return to the normal (18, 59).

Phosphorus. Phosphorus influences multiple organ systems including respiration, myocardial function, platelet, and red and white blood cell function. The parenteral RDI of phosphorus is approximately 30 mmol or 1000 mg/day. If omitted from TPN formulations, potentially life-threatening hypophosphatemia may develop within a week of TPN therapy if phosphate is not added to PN, especially in patients who are malnourished (18, 59). Hypophosphatemia commonly occurs in approximately 30% of critically ill patients receiving PN. Patients with a history of alcohol abuse, poor nutritional status preinjury, or long-term use of antacids or sucralfate are at a greater risk for developing phosphorus deficiency. Drug-induced hypophosphatemia results from intracellular shift of phosphorus or urinary wasting. Such drugs include antacids, sucralfate, diuretics, theophylline, and insulin. Generally, PN should contain approximately 15 to 30 mmol/day of phosphorus, depending on the prevailing blood level, dextrose dose, and renal function. Treatment of hypophosphatemia is dictated by severity, usually by IV replacement (18). If both potassium and phosphate are required, add potassium phosphate (usually 15 to 22.5 mmol/L) to the PN. A graduated scheme for phosphorus replacement based on the serum phosphorus concentration is shown in Table 93.5.

TABLE 93.5	GRADUATED DOSING SCHEME FOR PHOSPHORUS REPLACEMENT THERAPY
SERUM PHOSPHORUS CONCENTRATION (mg/dL)[a]	PHOSPHORUS DOSE/ INFUSION PERIOD[b]
2.3–3.0	0.16 mmol/kg/4 h
1.6–2.2	0.32 mmol/kg/4–6 h
≤1.5	0.64 mmol/kg/8 h

[a]The normal serum phosphorus concentration is 2.5 to 4.5 mg/dL.
[b]Use 50% of the recommended dose when creatinine clearance is less than 30 mL/minute.

Hyperphosphatemia is less common than hypophosphatemia and usually occurs with renal compromise. Medications that increase serum phosphorus levels include IVLEs and phosphorus-containing enemas in renal failure. If renal dysfunction exists, 3 to 5 mmol/L of phosphorus in PN are appropriate.

Chloride and acetate salts in PN depend on the acid–base status of the patient. In cases of metabolic alkalosis, only use chloride salts of either sodium or potassium. Conversely, during acidosis, use sodium or potassium acetate salts. Under no circumstances should calcium chloride or sodium bicarbonate be used in PN, because they result in insoluble precipitates that can cause fatal respiratory failure.

MONITORING NUTRITION SUPPORT THERAPY

Fluid status should be evaluated daily (18, 70–72). PN should be concentrated and sodium reduced if patients gain 1 to 2 kg over a 24-hour period. Levels of glucose, sodium, potassium, acid–base status, and renal function should be performed daily with calcium, phosphorus, and magnesium measured at least three times a week. Triglycerides, liver function tests, complete blood count with differential, prothrombin time, and thromboplastin time should be assessed weekly during the acute phase of injury (18, 59).

A nitrogen balance can be calculated using a 24-hour urine collection for volume and urea nitrogen to determine severity of catabolism, with the caveat that intake and output measures must be strictly accurate (142). Nitrogen balance is defined as the difference between nitrogen intake from diet and nitrogen excretion from stool and urine.

Serum protein concentrations can monitor nutritional status because certain protein increases reflect protein anabolism. Serum ALB concentration is the most common protein used to assess nutritional status although its use is limited in critically ill patients because of redistribution from the intravascular to the interstitial space, dilution with IV fluids, its long half-life (~21 days), and reduced production during the acute phase response (59, 70). During recovery, prealbumin and TFN are more sensitive to nutrition support because of shorter half-lives of 2 and 7 days, respectively. Serum CRP, a positive acute phase protein, increases during inflammation and stress and decreases rapidly during recovery. An acutely elevated CRP together with acute drops in serum prealbumin likely indicates an underlying inflammatory condition rather than deteriorating nutritional status. However, a low prealbumin with a low CRP likely reflects inadequate calories and/or protein. These basic principles assist the clinician in appropriately adjusting a nutrition regimen.

ANABOLIC AGENTS

Limited data support use of growth hormone, insulin-like growth factor-I (IGF-I), or anabolic steroids in critically ill patients, with most work performed in burned and trauma patients. Burned patients receiving human growth hormone (hGH) have reduced mortality compared with control patients (11% versus 37%, $p < .03$) (143). Pediatric burn victims receiving 0.2 mg/kg/day of hGH had a significant decrease in donor-site healing times at first (9.1 ± 0.4 versus 7.4 ± 0.6, $p < .05$, respectively) and second harvest (9.0 ± 0.7 versus 5.7 ± 0.3, $p < .05$, respectively) compared with placebo treatment. Length of hospital stay (LOS/percent total body surface area) also was shortened significantly with recombinant growth hormone treatment (144).

These encouraging results were tempered by the FDA, which released a drug warning in 1997 reporting a higher mortality rate in critically ill patients receiving hGH following two studies conducted in Finland and Europe. A multicenter, double-blind, randomized, placebo-controlled trial involved 532 ICU patients in four separate groups: cardiac surgery, abdominal surgery, multiple trauma, and acute respiratory failure (145). Patients received either 0.10 ± 0.02 mg/kg of hGH daily or placebo until discharge from the ICU or a maximum of 21 days. The hGH group experienced mortality caused by multiple organ failure, hyperglycemia, uncontrolled infection, and septic shock of 39% versus 20% with placebo in the Finnish trial and 44% versus 18% in the European trial ($p < .001$). The relative risk of dying with hGH was 1.9 (95% confidence interval, 1.3 to 2.9) in the Finnish study and 2.4 (95% confidence interval, 1.6 to 3.5) in the European study. Increased mortality persisted after accounting for diagnostic group, Acute Physiology and Chronic Health Evaluation II (APACHE II) score, and age. Most deaths in the European study occurred in the first 10 days, whereas 50% of deaths in the Finnish study occurred during the first 10 days of treatment and the remainder occurred after 3 weeks.

The causes of increased mortality in this study are unclear. Takala et al (145) theorized that hGH caused a modulation in immune function. Human growth factor can augment or inhibit production of reactive oxygen species and proinflammatory cytokines and reduce or increase susceptibility to endotoxin or bacterial in animals. hGH could be beneficial or detrimental depending on the clinical condition (146). Hyperglycemia has been attributed to defective nonoxidative glucose disposal, an increase in splanchnic glucose release, and increased peripheral resistance (147). In addition, insulin resistance induced by hGH could deprive cells of glucose, leading to an energy deficit.

IGF-I administration has been studied in critical care patients to diminish or block the catabolic process. Kudsk et al (148) studied recombinant IGF-I at 0.01 mg/kg/hour with aggressive PN on CD4/CD8 rations in head-injured patients with a Glasgow Coma Scale score (GCS) of 4 to 10. IGF-I administration increased CD4:CD8 ratios and elevated IGF-I levels.

In a second study of head injury patients given PN, IGF-I–treated patients demonstrated weight gain despite a significantly higher measured energy expenditure and lower calorie intake ($p = .02$), decreased nitrogen excretion, and improved nitrogen balances. Improvements in GCS scores also were noted in those patients receiving IGF-I (149).

Nutrition support with anabolic steroids has been used to preserve LBM after surgery and trauma. Early studies using of nandrolone and stanozolol reported improved nitrogen balance with decreases in nitrogen excretion (150–153). Gervasio et al (153) investigated oxandrolone administered 10 mg twice daily in multiple trauma patients in a prospective, double-blind, placebo-controlled study with early enteral nutrition. Both groups were highly catabolic at baseline. Nitrogen balance remained negative throughout the study and no differences in serum prealbumin over time, hospital LOS, ICU stay, or episodes of pneumonia or sepsis were noted in the study. The use of anabolic agents in ICU and post-ICU patients clearly requires further study. Nascent use of newer pharmacologic modulators of the hypercatabolic response to critical illness have emerged, including studies on the use of metformin, glucagon-like peptide-1 and peroxisome proliferator-activated receptor agonists (154).

REFERENCES

1. Dudrick SJ, Palesty JA. Surg Clin North Am 2011;91:945–64.
2. Wilmore DW. JPEN J Parenter Enteral Nutr 2000;24:1–4.
3. Dudrick SJ, Wilmore DW, Vars HM et al. Surgery 1968; 64:134–6.
4. Rhoads JE, Dudrick SJ. History of intravenous nutrition. In: Rombeau JL, ed. Clinical Nutrition: Parenteral Nutrition. 2nd ed. Philadelphia: Saunders, 1993:1–10.
5. Kudsk KA, Carpenter G, Petersen S et al. J Surg Res 1981; 31:105–10.
6. Kudsk KA, Stone JM, Carpenter G et al. J Trauma 1983; 23:605–9.
7. Moore EE, Jones TN. J Trauma 1986;26:874–879.
8. Moore FA, Moore EE, Jones TN et al. J Trauma 1989;29:916–23.
9. Kudsk KA, Croce MA, Fabian TC et al. Ann Surg 1992; 215:503–11.
10. Doig GS, Heighes PT, Simpson F et al. Injury 2011;42:50–56.
11. Moore FA, Feliciano DV, Andrassy RJ et al. Ann Surg 1992;216:172–83.
12. Kudsk KA, Minard G, Croce MA. Ann Surg 1996;224:531–40.
13. Khuri SF, Daley J, Henderson W et al. J Am Coll Surg 1997;185:315–27.
14. Baker SP, O'Neill B. J Trauma 1976;16:822–85.
15. Borlase BC, Moore EE, Moore FA. J Trauma 1990;30:1340–4.
16. Winsor JA, Hill GL. Ann Surg 1988;208:209–14.
17. Blackburn GL, Bistrian BR, Maini BS et al. JPEN J Parenter Enteral Nutr 1977;1:11–22.
18. ASPEN Board of Directors and Clinical Guidelines Task Force. JPEN J Parenter Enteral Nutr 2002;26(Suppl): 1SA–138SA.
19. Hall JC, O'Quigley J, Giles GR et al. Am J Clin Nutr 1980; 33:1846–51.
20. Jensen GL, Wheeler D. Curr Opin Crit Care 2012;18:206–11.
21. Kudsk KA, Jacobs DO. Perioperative management. In: Norton JA, Bollinger RR, Chang AE et al, eds. Surgery: Scientific Basis and Current Practice. New York: Springer, 2000:123–50.
22. Kudsk KA, Minard G, Wojtysiak SL et al. Surgery 1994; 116:516–23.
23. Buzby GP, Mullen JL, Mathews DC et al. Am J Surg 1980;139:160–7.
24. Kyle UG, Pirlich M, Schuetz T et al. JPEN J Parenter Enteral Nutr 2004;28:99–104.
25. Dessi M, Noce A, Agnoli A et al. Nutr Metab Cardiovasc Dis 2009;19:811–15.
26. Detsky AS, McLaughlin JR, Baker JP et al. JPEN J Parenter Enteral Nutr 1987;11:8–13.
27. Gupta D, Vashi PG, Lammersfeld CA et al. Ann Nutr Metab 2011;59:96–106.
28. Kudsk KA, Tolley EA, DeWitt RC et al. JPEN J Parenter Enteral Nutr 2003;27:1–9.
29. Hassan-Smith Z, Cooper MS. Best Pract Res Clin Endocrinol Metab 2011;25:705–17.
30. Hermans G, Vanhorebeek I, Derde S et al. Crit Care Med 2009;37:S391–7.
31. Robinson K, Prins J, Venkatesh B. Crit Care 2011;15:221.
32. Cuthbertson DP. JPEN J Parenter Enteral Nutr 1979;3:108–29.
33. Deitrick JE, Whedon GD, Shorr E. Am J Med 1948;4:3–13.
34. Cerra FB. Nutrition in the care of the patient with surgery. In: Mattox KL, Feliciano DV, Moore EE, eds. Trauma. 3rd ed. Stamford, CT: Appleton & Lange 1996:1155–76.
35. Shaw-Delanty SN, Elwyn DH, Askanazi J et al. Clin Nutr 1990;9:305–10.
36. Shaw JHF, Wolfe RR. Ann Surg 1989;207:63–72.
37. Shaw JHF, Klein S, Wolfe RR. Surgery 1985;97:557–68.
38. Threlfall CJ, Maxwell AR, Stoner HB. J Trauma 1984;24:516–23.
39. Wilmore DW, Smith RJ, O'Dwyer ST et al. Surgery 1988; 104:917–23.
40. Souba WW. Annu Rev Nutr 1991;11:285–308.
41. Balija TM, Lowry SF. Curr Opin Infect Dis 2011;24:248–53.
42. Lowry SF. Surg Clin North Am 2009;89:311–26.
43. Long CL, Kinney JM, Geiger JW. Metabolism 1976;25:193–201.
44. Ohzato H, Yoshizaki, K, Nishimoto N et al. Surgery 1992;111:201–9.
45. Stoner HB, Frayn KN, Barton RN et al. Clin Sci 1979;56: 563–573.
46. Nanni G, Siegel JH, Coleman B et al. J Trauma 1984;24: 14–30.
47. Kenler AS, Swails WS, Driscoll DF et al. Ann Surg 1996; 223:316–33.
48. Vogel TR, Dombrovskij VY, Carlson JL et al. Ann Surg 2010; 252: 1065–71.
49. Wolfe R, O'Donnell T, Stone M et al. Metabolism 1980; 29:892–900.
50. McHoney M, Eaton S, Pierro A. Eur J Pediatr Surg 2009; 19:275–85.

51.   van Hall G. Curr Opin Clin Nutr Metab Care 2012;15:85–91.
52.   Blackburn GL. Surg Clin North Am 2011;91:467–80.
53.   van den Berghe G, Wouters P, Weekers F et al. N Engl J Med 2001;345:1359–67.
54.   Tracey KJ, Beutler B, Lowry SF et al. Science 1986;234:470–4.
55.   Besedovsky H, Del Rey A, Sorkin E et al. Science 1986;233:652–4.
56.   Kavanagh BP, McCowen KC. N Engl J Med 2010;363:2540–6.
57.   Kudsk K, Brown R. Acute care surgery: principles and practice. In: Moore EE, Feliciano DV, Mattox KI eds. Trauma. 4th ed. New York: McGraw-Hill, 2000:1369–1405.
58.   Vanhorebeek I, Gubnst J, Derde S et al. J Clin Endocrinol Metab 2012;97:E59–64.
59.   Ziegler TR. N Engl J Med 2009;361:1088–97.
60.   Hwang TL, Hwang SL, Chen MF. J Trauma 1993;34:247–51.
61.   Campbell SM, Kudsk KA. JPEN J Parenter Enteral Nutr 1988;12:610–12.
62.   Krishnan JA, Parce PB, Martinez A et al. Chest 2003;124:297–305.
63.   Goulenok C, Monchi M, Chicke JD et al. Chest 2004;125:1441–5.
64.   Bercault N, Boulain T, Kuteifan K et al. Crit Care Med 2004;32:998–1003.
65.   Dickerson RN, Rosato EF, Mullen JL. Am J Clin Nutr 1986;44:747–55.
66.   Heyland DK, Dhaliwal R, Jiang X et al. Crit Care 2011;15:R268.
67.   Long CL, Schaffel N, Geiger JW et al. JPEN J Parenter Enteral Nutr 1979;3:452–56.
68.   Wolfe R, Allsop J, Burke J. Metabolism 1979;28:210–20.
69.   NICE-SUGAR Study Investigators, Finfer S, Chittock DR et al. N Engl J Med 2009;1283–97.
70.   McClave SA, Martindale RG, Vanek VW et al. JPEN J Parenter Enteral Nutr 2009; 33:277–316.
71.   Singer P, Berger MM, Van den Burghe G et al. Clin Nutr 2009;28:387–400.
72.   Talpers SS, Romberger DJ, Dunce SB et al. Chest 1992;102:551–55.
73.   Food and Drug Administration. Fed Reg 2000;65:20.
74.   Luo M, Fernandez-Estivariz C, Jones DP et al. Nutrition 2008;24:37–44.
75.   Novelli GP, Adembri C, Gandini E et al. Am J Surg 1997;173:206–9.
76.   Nathens AB, Neff MJ, Jurkovich GJ et al. Ann Surg 2002;236:814–22.
77.   Fukushima R, Yamazaki E. Curr Opin Clin Nutr Metab Care 2010;13:662–8.
78.   Louw JA, Werbeck A, Louw ME et al. Crit Care Med 1992;20:934–41.
79.   Klein GL, Langman CB, Herndon DN. J Trauma 2002;52:346–50.
80.   Klein GL, Chen TC, Holick MF et al. Lancet 2004;363:291–92.
81.   Andrews PJ, Avenell A, Noble DW et al. BMJ 2011;343:d1542
82.   Manzanares W, Biestro A, Torre MH et al. Intensive Care Med 2011;37:1120–7.
83.   Berger MM, Spertini FS, Shenkin A et al. Am J Clin Nutr 1998;68:365–71.
84.   Ziegler TR. N Engl J Med 2011;365:562–4.
85.   Levine GM, Derin JJ, Steiger E et al. Gastroenterology 1974;67:975–82.
86.   Hegazi RA, Wischmeyer PE. Crit Care 2011;15:234.
87.   Kudsk KA. Amer J Surg 2002;183:370–98.
88.   van der Meij BS, van Bokhorst-de van der Schueren MA, Langius JA et al. Am J Clin Nutr 2011;94:1248–65.
89.   Minard G, Kudsk KA, Melton S et al. JPEN J Parenter Enteral Nutr 2000;24:145–9.
90.   Fan St, Lo CM, Lai EC et al. N Engl J Med 1994;331:1547–52.
91.   Daly JM, Liebernab MD, Goldfine J et al. Surgery 1992;112:56–67.
92.   Daly JM, Weintraub FN, Shou J et al. Ann Surg 1995;221:327–38.
93.   Brennan MF, Pisters PWT, Posner M et al. Ann Surg 1994;220:436–44.
94.   Heslin MJ, Latkany L, Leung D et al. Ann Surg 1997;226:567–77.
95.   The Veteran Affairs Total Parenteral Nutrition Cooperative Study Group. N Engl J Med 1991;325:525–32.
96.   Braga M, Gianotti L, Nespoli L et al. Arch Surg 2002;137:174–80.
97.   Ginzalez-Huix F, Fernandez-Banares F, Esteve-Comas M et al. Am J Gastroenterol 1993;88:227–32.
98.   Gonzalez-Huix F, de Leon R, Fernandez-Banares F et al. Gut 1993;34:778–82.
99.   Wicks C, Somasundaram S, Bjarnason I et al. Lancet 1994;344:837–40.
100. Hasse JM, Blue LS, Liepa GU et al. JPEN J Parenter Enteral Nutr 1995;19:437–43.
101. McClave SA, Greene LM, Snider HL et al. JPEN J Parenter Enteral Nutr 1997;21:14–20.
102. Casaer MP, Mesotten D, Hermans G et al. N Engl J Med 2011;365:506–17.
103. Cerantola Y, Hubner M, Grass F et al. Br J Surg 2011;98:37–48.
104. van der Hulst RRWJ, von Meyenfeldt MF, van Kreel BK et al. Lancet 1993;341:1363–15.
105. Deitch EA. Perspect Crit Care 1988;1:1–13.
106. Janu P, Li J, Minard G et al. Surg Forum 1996;47:7–9.
107. Moore FA, Moore EE, Poggetti R et al. J Trauma 1991;31:629–36.
108. Deitch EA, Shi HP, Lu Q et al. Crit Care Med 2004;32:533–8.
109. Adams CA Jr, Hauser CJ, Adams JM et al. Shock 2002;18:513–7.
110. Li J, Gocinski B, Henken B et al. J Trauma 1995;39:44.
111. Wu Y, Kudsk KA, DeWitt RC et al. Ann Surg 1999;229:662–8.
112. Gomez EE, Lan J, Kang W et al. JPEN J Parenter Enteral Nutr 2007;31:47–52.
113. Ikeda S, Kudsk KA, Fukatsu K et al. Ann Surg 2003;237:677–85.
114. Zarzaur BL, Fukatsu K, Johnson CJ et al. Surg Forum 2001;52:194–6.
115. Fukatsu K, Kudsk KA. Surg Clin North Am 2011;91:755–70.
116. Kudsk KA, Li J, Renegar KB. Ann Surg 1996;223:629.
117. King BK, Kudsk KA, Li J et al. Ann Surg 1999;229:272–8.
118. Lin MT, Saito H, Fukushima R et al. Ann Surg 1996;223:84–93.
119. Fong Y, Marano MA, Barber E et al. Ann Surg 1989;210:449–56.
120. McDonald WS, Sharp CW Jr, Deitch EA. Ann Surg 1991;213:177–83.
121. Collier P, Kudsk KA, Glezer J et al. Nutr Clin Pract 1994;9:101–3.
122. Yuan Y, Ren J, Gu G et al. Nutr Clin Prac 2011;26:688–94.
123. Eisenberg PG. Nutr Clin Pract 1993;8:119–23.
124. Guenter PA, Settle RG, Permutter S et al. JPEN J Parenter Enteral Nutr 1991;15:277–80.
125. Yarandi SS, Zhao VM, Hebbar G et al. Curr Opinion Clin Nutr Metab Care 2011;14:75–82.
126. Griffiths RD, Jones C, Palmer TE. Nutrition 1997;13:295–302.
127. Kirk SJ, Barbul A. JPEN J Parenter Enteral Nutr 1990;14:226S–9S.

128. Moore FA, Moore EE, Kudsk KA et al. J Trauma 1994;37: 607–15.

129. Heyland DK, Novak F, Drover J et al. JAMA 2001;286: 944–53.

130. Manzanares W, Heyland DK. Crit Care Med 2012;40:350–2.

131. Bertolini G, Iapchino G, Radrizzani D et al. Intensive Care Med 2003;29:834–40.

132. Vanek VW. Nutr Clin Prac 2003;18:201–20.

133. Chang WK, Yang KD, Shaio MF. Clin Immunol 1999;93: 294–301.

134. Wilmore DW, Shabert JK. Nutrition 1998;14:618–26.

135. Ziegler TR, Young LS, Benfell K et al. Ann Intern Med 1992;116:821–8.

136. Wanten GL, Calder PC. Am J Clin Nutr 2007;13:180–6.

137. Smirniotis V, Kostopanagiotou G, Vassiliou J et al. Intensive Care Med 1998;24:1029–33.

138. Hwang TL, Huang SL, Chen MF. Chest 1990;97:934–8.

139. Venus B, Smith RA, Patel C et al. Chest 1989;95:1278–81.

140. Battistella FD, Widergren JT, Anderson JT et al. J Trauma 1997;43:52–60.

141. Kruimel JW, Naber TH, van der Vliet JA et al. JPEN J Parenter Enteral Nutr 2001;25:237–44.

142. Miller SJ. Hosp Pharm 1990;25:61–5, 70.

143. Knox J, Demling R, Wilmore D et al. J Trauma 1995;39: 526–32.

144. Herndon DN, Barrow RE, Kunkel KR et al. Ann Surg 1990; 212:424–73.

145. Takala J, Ruokonen E, Webster NR et al. N Engl J Med 1999;341:785–92.

146. Taylor BE, Buchman TG. Curr Opin Crit Care 2008;14:438–44.

147. Jeevanandam M, Holaday NJ, Peterson SR. Metabolism 1996;45:450–6.

148. Kudsk KA, Mowatt-Larssen C, Bukar J et al. Arch Surg 1994;129:66–70.

149. Hatton J, Rapp RP, Kudsk KA et al. J Neurosurg 1997;86: 779–86.

150. Debroy MA, Wolf SE, Zhang XJ et al. J Trauma 1999;47: 904–10.

151. Hausmann DF, Nutz V, Rommelsheim K et al. JPEN J Parenter Enteral Nutr 1990;14:111–14.

152. Hansell DT, Davies JW, Shenkin A et al. JPEN J Parenter Enteral Nutr 1989;13:349–58.

153. Gervasio JM, Dickerson RN, Swearingen J et al. Pharmacotherapy 2000;20:1328–31.

154. Gauglitz GG, Williams FN, Herndon DN et al. Curr Opin Clin Nutr Metab Care 2011;14:176–81.

SUGGESTED READINGS

ASPEN Board of Directors and Clinical Guidelines Task Force. Guidelines for the use of parenteral and enteral nutrition in adult and pediatric patients. JPEN J Parenter Enteral Nutr 2002; 26(Suppl):1SA–138SA.

Casaer MP, Mesotten D, Hermans G et al. Early versus late parenteral nutrition in critically ill adults. N Engl J Med 2011;365:506–17.

Dudrick SJ, Palesty JA. Historical highlights of the development of enteral nutrition. Surg Clin North Am 2011;91:945–64.

Fukatsu K, Kudsk KA. Nutrition and gut immunity. Surg Clin North Am 2011;91:755–70.

McClave SA, Martindale RG, Vanek VW et al. Guidelines for the Provision and Assessment of Nutrition Support Therapy in the Adult Critically Ill Patient: Society of Critical Care Medicine (SCCM) and American Society for Parenteral and Enteral Nutrition (ASPEN). JPEN J Parenter Enteral Nutr 2009;33:277–316.

with compromised hepatic or renal function (i.e., lactate elimination diminished). Moreover, metformin must be used cautiously in the subacute period after burn injury.

Novel Therapeutic Options

Other approaches to treat hyperglycemia after burn injury are currently being investigated in trials. These include different combinations of diabetes drugs, glucagon-like peptide-1 (an insulin incretin), and agonists of peroxisome proliferator-activated receptor-γ (PPAR-γ). PPAR-γ agonists, which include pioglitazone and fenofibrate, heighten insulin sensitivity in diabetic individuals. A blind, controlled, randomized trial showed that fenofibrate increased mitochondrial oxidation of glucose and improved insulin sensitivity, thus serving to reduce plasma glucose levels (131). Moreover, a comparison of muscle tissue from placebo- and fenofibrate-treated patients revealed that after hyperinsulinemic (euglycemic) clamp, fenofibrate-treated patients had better insulin receptor signaling, as seen by greater tyrosine phosphorylation of the insulin receptor and insulin receptor substrate-1 (131). Active investigation of these agents is ongoing and will define their potential utility in the near future.

CONCLUSION

Severely burned patients have unique and profound nutritional requirements because of the prolonged postburn hypermetabolic, hypercatabolic response. EN support should be initiated early to optimize overall burn care; it has contributed greatly to the significant inhibition of LBM loss normally observed in severely catabolic patients (20). Furthermore, neither nonpharmacologic nor pharmacologic strategies are sufficient to fully block the responses triggered by severe burns. Rather, all these therapeutic approaches have helped decrease morbidity and mortality. Modulation of the hypermetabolic response and adequate feeding are important aspects of burn care; they are paramount to restoring structure and function.

REFERENCES

1. Hart DW, Wolf SE, Mlcak R et al. Surgery 2000;128:312–9.
2. Reiss E, Pearson E, Artz CP. J Clin Invest 1956;35:62–77.
3. Rutan RL, Herndon DN. Arch Surg 1990;125:392–5.
4. Wilmore DW, Mason AD Jr, Pruitt BA Jr. Ann Surg 1976;183:314–20.
5. Yu YM, Tompkins RG, Ryan CM et al. JPEN J Parenter Enteral Nutr 1999;23:160–8.
6. Cuthbertson D. Lancet 1942;1:433–6.
7. Goldstein DS, Kopin IJ. Stress 2007;10:109–20.
8. Selye H. Br Med J 1950;1:1383–92.
9. Selye H. Nature 1951;168:149–50.
10. Selye H, Fortier C. Psychosom Med 1950;12:149–57.
11. Herndon DNEA. J Trauma 1981;21:701–5.
12. Lee JO, Herndon DN. Nestle Nutr Workshop Ser Clin Perform Programme 2003;8:39–49; discussion 56.
13. Newsome TW, Mason AD Jr, Pruitt BA Jr. Ann Surg 1973;178:215–7.
14. Barrow RE, Hawkins HK, Aarsland A et al. Shock 2005;24:523–8.
15. Barrow RE, Wolfe RR, Dasu MR et al. Ann Surg 2006;243:115–20.
16. Herndon DN, Hart DW, Wolf SE et al. N Engl J Med 2001;345:1223–9.
17. Wolfe RR, Herndon DN, Peters EJ et al. Ann Surg 1987;206:214–21.
18. Chang DW, DeSanti L, Demling RH. Shock 1998;10:155–60.
19. Wilmore DW, Long JM, Mason AD Jr et al Ann Surg 1974;180:653–69.
20. Jeschke MG, Chinkes DL, Finnerty CC et al. Ann Surg 2008;248:387–401.
21. Wilmore DW, Aulick LH. Surg Clin North Am 1978;58:1173–87.
22. Jeschke MG, Gauglitz GG, Kulp GA et al. PLoS One 2011;6:e21245.
23. Hart DW, Wolf SE, Chinkes DL et al. Ann Surg 2000;232:455–65.
24. Bessey PQ, Jiang ZM, Johnson DJ et al. World J Surg 1989;13:465–70; discussion 71.
25. Jahoor F, Desai M, Herndon DN, Wolfe RR. Metabolism 1988;37:330–7.
26. Herndon DN, Tompkins RG. Lancet 2004;363:1895–902.
27. Kinney JM, Long CL, Gump FE et al. Ann Surg 1968;168:459–74.
28. Wilmore DW, Aulick LH, Mason AD et al. Ann Surg 1977;186:444–58.
29. Carter EA, Tompkins RG, Babich JW et al. Metabolism 1996;45:1161–7.
30. Gauglitz GG, Herndon DN, Kulp GA et al. J Clin Endocrinol Metab 2009;94:1656–64.
31. Long CL, Spencer JL, Kinney JM et al. J Appl Physiol 1971;31:110–6.
32. Wolfe RR, Durkot MJ, Allsop JR et al. Metabolism 1979;28:1031–9.
33. Tappy L, Schwarz JM, Schneiter F et al. Crit Care Med 1998;26:860–7.
34. van den Berghe G, Wouters P, Weekers F et al. N Engl J Med 2001;345:1359–67.
35. Jahoor F, Shangraw RE, Miyoshi H et al. Am J Physiol 1989;257:E323–31.
36. Shaw JH, Wolfe RR. Ann Surg 1989;209:63–72.
37. Wolfe RR, Herndon DN, Jahoor F et al. N Engl J Med 1987;317:403–8.
38. Greenhalgh DG, Saffle JR, Holmes JHT et al. J Burn Care Res 2007;28:776–90.
39. Murray CK, Loo FL, Hospenthal DR et al. Burns 2008;34:1108–12.
40. Pruitt BA Jr, McManus AT, Kim SH et al. World J Surg 1998;22:135–45.
41. Im MJ, Hoopes JE. J Surg Res 1970;10:459–64.
42. Falcone PA, Caldwell MD. Clin Plast Surg 1990;17:443–56.
43. Mochizuki H, Trocki O, Dominioni L et al. Ann Surg 1984;200:297–310.
44. Dominioni L, Trocki O, Fang CH et al. JPEN J Parenter Enteral Nutr 1985;9:269–79.
45. Saffle JR. Nutritional support of the burned patient. In: Herndon DN, ed. Total Burn Care. 3rd ed. Philadelphia: WB Saunders, 2007:398–419.
46. Wolf SE, Rose JK, Desai MH et al. Ann Surg 1997;225:554–65; discussion 65–9.
47. Deitch EA. Surgery 1990;107:411–6.
48. van Elburg RM, Uil JJ, de Monchy JG et al. Scand J Gastroenterol Suppl 1992;194:19–24.

49. Hart DW, Wolf SE, Chinkes DL et al. J Trauma 2003;54: 755–61; discussion 61–4.

50. Mochizuki H, Trocki O, Dominioni L et al. Curr Surg 1985;42:121–5.

51. McDonald WS, Sharp CW Jr, Deitch EA. Ann Surg 1991;213:177–83.

52. Tinckler LF. Br J Surg 1965;52:140–50.

53. Raff T, Hartmann B, Germann G. Burns 1997;23:19–25.

54. Gore DC, Rutan RL, Hildreth M et al. J Burn Care Rehabil 1990;11:400–4.

55. Smith LC, Mullen JL. Surg Clin North Am 1991;71:449–57.

56. Suman OE, Mlcak RP, Chinkes DL et al. Burns 2006;32: 335–42.

57. Goran MI, Peters EJ, Herndon DN et al. Am J Physiol 1990; 259:E576–85.

58. Hart DW, Wolf SE, Herndon DN et al. Ann Surg 2002; 235:152–61.

59. Wolfe RR, Allsop JR, Burke JF. Metabolism 1979;28: 210–20.

60. Sheridan R, Choucair R, Donelan M et al. J Burn Care Rehabil 1998;19:528–30.

61. Wolfe RR. JPEN J Parenter Enteral Nutr 1998;22:190.

62. Demling RH, Seigne P. World J Surg 2000;24:673–80.

63. Mochizuki H, Trocki O, Dominioni L et al. JPEN J Parenter Enteral Nutr 1984;8:638–46.

64. Alexander JW, Saito H, Trocki O et al. Ann Surg 1986; 204:1–8.

65. Huschak G, Zur Nieden K, Hoell T et al. Intensive Care Med 2005;31:1202–8.

66. Mayes T, Gottschlich MM, Kagan RJ. J Burn Care Res 2008; 29:82–8.

67. Wolfe RR, Goodenough RD, Burke JF et al. Ann Surg 1983; 197:163–71.

68. Yu YM, Ryan CM, Burke JF et al. Am J Clin Nutr 1995;62: 960–8.

69. Melville S, McNurlan MA, McHardy KC et al. Metabolism 1989;38:248–55.

70. Hoerr RA, Matthews DE, Bier DM et al. Am J Physiol 1993; 264:E567–75.

71. Yu YM, Young VR, Castillo L et al. Metabolism 1995;44: 659–66.

72. Matthews DE, Marano MA, Campbell RG. Am J Physiol 1993;264:E109–18.

73. Norbury WB. Modulation of the hypermetabolic response after burn injury. In: Herndon DN, ed. Total Burn Care. 3rd ed. Philadelphia: WB Saunders 2007:420–33.

74. Patterson BW, Nguyen T, Pierre E et al. Metabolism 1997;46:573–8.

75. Soeters PB, van de Poll MC, van Gemert WG et al. J Nutr 2004;134:1575S–82S.

76. De Souza DA, Greene LJ. Crit Care Med 2005;33:1125–35.

77. Souba WW. Annu Rev Nutr 1991;11:285–308.

78. Gore DC, Jahoor F. Arch Surg 1994;129:1318–23.

79. Garrel D. JPEN J Parenter Enteral Nutr 2004;28:123.

80. Wischmeyer PE, Lynch J, Liedel J et al. Crit Care Med 2001;29:2075–80.

81. Zhou YP, Jiang ZM, Sun YH et al. JPEN J Parenter Enteral Nutr 2003;27:241–5.

82. Cerra FB, Mazuski JE, Chute E et al. Ann Surg 1984;199: 286–91.

83. Gamliel Z, DeBiasse MA, Demling RH. J Burn Care Rehabil 1996;17:264–72.

84. Gottschlich MM, Mayes T, Khoury J et al. J Am Diet Assoc 2004;104:931–41; quiz 1031.

85. Mayes T, Gottschlich MM, Warden GD. J Burn Care Rehabil 1997;18:365–8; discussion 4.

86. Rock CL, Dechert RE, Khilnani R et al. J Burn Care Rehabil 1997;18:269–78; discussion 8.

87. Berger MM, Shenkin A. J Trace Elem Med Biol 2007;21: 44–8.

88. Berger MM, Spertini F, Shenkin A et al. Am J Clin Nutr 1998;68:365–71.

89. Selmanpakoglu AN, Cetin C, Sayal A et al. Burns 1994;20: 99–103.

90. Hunt DR, Lane HW, Beesinger D et al. JPEN J Parenter Enteral Nutr 1984;8:695–9.

91. Cunningham JJ, Leffell M, Harmatz P. Nutrition 1993;9: 329–32.

92. Gosling P, Rothe HM, Sheehan TM et al. J Burn Care Rehabil 1995;16:481–6.

93. Shakespeare PG. Burns Incl Therm Inj 1982;8:358–64.

94. Voruganti VS, Klein GL, Lu HX et al. Burns 2005;31:711–6.

95. Berger MM, Baines M, Raffoul W et al. J Clin Nutr 2007; 85:1293–300.

96. Berger MM, Binnert C, Chiolero RL et al. Am J Clin Nutr 2007;85:1301–6.

97. Berger MM, Eggimann P, Heyland DK et al. Crit Care 2006;10:R153.

98. Battistella FD, Widergren JT, Anderson JT et al. J Trauma 1997;43:52–8; discussion 8–60.

99. Fong YM, Marano MA, Barber A et al. Ann Surg 1989; 210:449–56; discussion 56–7.

100. Herndon DN, Barrow RE, Stein M et al. J Burn Care Rehabil 1989;10:309–13.

101. Herndon DN, Stein MD, Rutan TC et al. J Trauma 1987; 27:195–204.

102. Klein GL, Wolf SE, Langman CB et al. J Clin Endocrinol Metab 1998;83:21–4.

103. Takala J, Ruokonen E, Webster NR et al. N Engl J Med 1999; 341:785–92.

104. Demling RH. Burns 1999;25:215–21.

105. Gore DC, Honeycutt D, Jahoor F et al. J Surg Res 1991; 51:518–23.

106. Ramirez RJ, Wolf SE, Barrow RE et al. Ann Surg 1998; 228:439–48.

107. Branski LK, Herndon DN, Barrow RE et al. Ann Surg 2009; 250:514–23.

108. Herndon DN, Ramzy PI, DebRoy MA et al. Ann Surg 1999; 229:713–20; discussion 20–2.

109. Spies M, Wolf SE, Barrow RE et al. Crit Care Med 2002; 30:83–8.

110. Jeschke MG, Herndon DN, Barrow RE. Ann Surg 2000;231: 408–16.

111. Cioffi WG, Gore DC, Rue LW 3rd et al. Ann Surg 1994;220: 310–6; discussion 6–9.

112. Demling RH, Orgill DP. J Crit Care 2000;15:12–7.

113. Wolf SE, Edelman LS, Kemalyan N et al. J Burn Care Res 2006;27:131–41.

114. Jeschke MG, Finnerty CC, Suman OE et al. Ann Surg 2007;246:351–62.

115. Murphy KD, Thomas S, Mlcak RP et al. Surgery 2004;136: 219–24.

116. Suman OE, Thomas SJ, Wilkins JP et al. J Appl Physiol 2003; 94:2273–81.

117. Baron PW, Barrow RE, Pierre EJ et al. J Burn Care Rehabil 1997; 18:223–7.

118. Gore DC, Honeycutt D, Jahoor F et al. Ann Surg 1991; 213:568–73; discussion 73–4.

119. Pereira CT, Jeschke MG, Herndon DN. Novartis Found Symp 2007;280:238–48; discussion 48–51.

120. Gauglitz GG, Herndon DN, Jeschke MG. J Burn Care Res 2008;29:683–94.

121. Dandona P, Chaudhuri A, Mohanty P et al. Curr Opin Clin Nutr Metab Care 2007;10:511–7.

122. Van den Berghe G, Wilmer A, Hermans G et al. N Engl J Med 2006;354:449–61.

123. Ellger B, Debaveye Y, Vanhorebeek I et al. Diabetes 2006; 55:1096–105.

124. Ingels C, Debaveye Y, Milants I et al. Eur Heart J 2006; 27:2716–24.

125. Brunkhorst FM, Engel C, Bloos F et al. N Engl J Med 2008; 358:125–39.

126. Langouche L, Vanhorebeek I, Van den Berghe G. Nat Clin Pract 2007;3:270–8.

127. Finney SJ, Zekveld C, Elia A et al. JAMA 2003;290:2041–7.

128. Dellinger RP, Levy MM, Carlet JM et al. Crit Care Med 2008;36:296–327.

129. Gore DC, Wolf SE, Herndon DN et al. J Trauma 2003;54: 555–61.

130. Gore DC, Herndon DN, Wolfe RR. J Trauma 2005;59: 316–22; discussion 22–3.

131. Cree MG, Zwetsloot JJ, Herndon DN et al. Ann Surg 2007;245:214–21.

SUGGESTED READINGS

Branski LK, Herndon DN, Barrow RE et al. Randomized controlled trial to determine the efficacy of long-term growth hormone treatment in severely burned children. Ann Surg 2009;250:514–23.

Gauglitz GG, Williams FN, Herndon DN et al. Burns: where are we standing with propranolol, oxandrolone, recombinant human growth hormone, and the new incretin analogs? Curr Opin Clin Nutr Metab Care 2011;14:176–81.

Herndon DN, Tompkins RG. Support of the metabolic response to burn injury. Lancet 2004;363:1895–902.

Jeschke MG, Chinkes DL, Finnerty CC et al. Pathophysiologic response to severe burn injury. Ann Surg 2008;248:387–401.

Williams FN, Branski LK, Jeschke MG et al. What, how, and how much should patients with burns be fed? Surg Clin North Am 2011;91:609–29.

95 NUTRITIONAL DISORDERS OF THE NERVOUS SYSTEM[1]

GUSTAVO C. ROMÁN

[1]**Abbreviations: ALA**, α-linolenic acid; **ATP**, adenosine triphosphate; **CNS**; central nervous system; **CoA**, coenzyme A; **CSF**, cerebrospinal fluid; **FAO**, Food and Agriculture Organization; **GABA**, γ-aminobutyric acid; **HIV**, human immunodeficiency virus; **IDD**, iodine deficiency disorder; **IF**, intrinsic factor; **LDL**, low-density lipoprotein; **5MH₄F**, 5-methyltetrahydrofolate; **MMA**, methylmalonic acid; **MS**, multiple sclerosis; **NAD**, nicotinamide adenine dinucleotide; **NADP**, nicotinamide adenine dinucleotide phosphate; **1,25(OH)₂D**, 1,25-dihydroxyvitamin D; **POWs**, prisoners of war; **SAM**, S-adenosyl methionine; **SCD**, subacute combined degeneration; **TPN**, total parenteral nutrition; **T₃**, triiodothyronine; **T₄**, thyroxine; **TSH**, thyroid-stimulating hormone; **WKS**, Wernicke-Korsakoff syndrome.

Brain function is unavoidably dependent on a constant dietary supply of appropriate nutrients. Regrettably, large segments of the world population have limited access to basic foodstuffs. Despite increases in agricultural production, hunger remains a widespread worldwide problem as a result of poverty, war, population displacement, and social unrest. Hunger creates a vicious cycle of poor health, lack of energy, and mental impairment that reduces people's ability to work thereby increasing poverty.

According to the United Nations Food and Agriculture Organization (FAO), nearly 30% of the world population, some 777 million people worldwide, are malnourished (1). This represents more than 35% of tropical Africa's population, about 25% of the people in India, and 5% to 20% of Latin America and Caribbean populations. Of them, 150 million children worldwide are underweight, and 182 million are physically and cognitively stunted. Moreover, protein-energy malnutrition contributes to 5 million child deaths per year.

Less recognized, however, are the effects of malnutrition on the nervous system. These may range from isolated involvement of the peripheral nervous system that produces blindness, deafness, paralysis, or sensory deficits to complex lesions of the spinal cord and central nervous system (CNS) that lead to mental retardation, cognitive dysfunction, and gait limitations. Nutritional deficiencies affecting the nervous system are not restricted to developing nations, however. Selected groups in the developed world also suffer from the neurologic consequences of nutritional deficiencies as a result of meager diets. Populations at risk include the poor, the homeless, people addicted to alcohol and substance abusers, some patients with chronic psychiatric conditions, and demented elderly persons. Also affected are persons with restrictive dietary habits such as strict vegans or those suffering from eating disorders such as bulimia and anorexia nervosa, as well as patients with impaired absorption of nutrients from intestinal malabsorption syndromes.

A rampant form of malnutrition peculiar to developed nations is obesity, frequently accompanied by metabolic syndrome, hypertension, and diabetes that may manifest with secondary neurologic signs and symptoms as a result of stroke, obstructive sleep apnea, and peripheral neuropathy. According to the FAO, obesity is also beginning to affect developing nations, a situation resulting in the coexistence in the same population of undernutrition and obesity. This problem is called "the double burden of malnutrition" (1).

NUTRITION AND COGNITIVE FUNCTION

A constant dietary supply of appropriate nutrients including glucose, amino acids, fatty acids, vitamins, and minerals is required for normal brain function (2). Food is also needed to maintain the integrity of cellular membranes in the brain and the production of neurotransmitters (3). Although the brain represents only 2% of the body mass, it consumes 20% of the energy provided by the diet and 20% of the oxygen inhaled. Children consume twice more glucose than adults do, and the newborn brain requires 60% of the energy provided by the diet. Therefore, the effects of prolonged hypoglycemia can be devastating for newborns and children, given that the brain is totally dependent on dietary glucose, and glycogen reserves are limited. Many of the fatalities and permanent sequelae resulting from cerebral malaria in children are caused by the severe hypoglycemia induced by the malarial infection and quinine treatment (4), in addition to the direct damage induced by the parasite (5). In elderly persons, decreased cognitive performance occurs with relatively mild hypoglycemia (6). Similarly, cognitive dysfunction worsens the outcome of treatment in patients with type 2 diabetes (7).

Appropriate dietary supply of amino acids is needed to synthesize proteins and neurotransmitters in the nervous system. The quality of dietary proteins influences brain protein formation. Tryptophan, a precursor of serotonin (5-hydroxytryptamine)—the neurotransmitter involved in appetite and satiety, sleep, blood pressure, pain sensitivity, and mood—is particularly important because 5-hydroxytryptamine cannot cross the blood–brain barrier. Metabolically active brain sites such as hippocampus, basal ganglia, and hypothalamus are particularly sensitive to the effects of malnutrition, loss of energy, and amino acid supply.

Studies in experimental animals and in humans have demonstrated the importance of appropriate nutrition during crucial—and relatively brief—periods of brain growth (8–12). Neurons and glia are formed and begin migration by 22 weeks of gestation; and by late pregnancy, marked axonal and neural proliferation result in substantial brain growth. Brain weight at birth is about 350 g, increasing during the first year of life to about 1100 g or 70% of the adult brain weight. In 1969, Winick and Rosso (13, 14) demonstrated that early malnutrition stunts brain growth and development. Children dying of severe malnutrition during pregnancy and from marasmic malnutrition in early life had smaller head circumferences, decreased brain weight, and lower brain content of total protein, DNA and RNA compared with normal controls. Early malnutrition also affects processes involved in brain maturation such

as neurogenesis, neuronal and glial migration, number of synapses, and degree of myelination.

These changes are largely irreversible and cause permanent cognitive deficiencies (11, 15, 16). The extent of the cognitive and neurologic damage depends on factors such as severity and duration of the nutritional deficiency, the stage of brain development, and associated diseases such as diarrhea from *Giardia lamblia* (17) and other causes, as well as familial, social, cultural, and economic factors. Nonetheless, substantial evidence indicates that reduced breast-feeding, low birth weight, iron and iodine deficiency, and protein-energy malnutrition are associated with long-term deficits in psychomotor brain function (12). Follow-up studies of perinatal malnutrition showed, 15 and 20 years later, residual deficits in brain size, cognition, and psychosocial achievements (6, 11). Ivanovic et al (18) and Leiva et al (19) demonstrated, among high school students in Chile, residual effects of early malnutrition manifested by smaller head circumferences and brain volumes determined by magnetic resonance imaging. Lower IQ and more severe learning difficulties resulted in worse school performance, higher school desertion, and lower enrollment in higher education institutions in those with history of early malnutrition, compared with classmates from a common socioeconomic background who had a normal nutritional history.

Similar, although less severe, problems also occur in premature and low birth weight infants (20). In clinical trials comparing breast milk with preterm formula alone or as a supplement to maternal milk, in preterm infants weighing less than 1200 g, children fed banked breast milk took longer to reach 2000 g than did infants fed a preterm formula. Lucas et al (21) found that IQs, short-term memory, and attention at 8 years of age were better in children fed maternal milk than in controls, even after adjustment for maternal education and social class. Breast milk lowers low-density lipoprotein (LDL) cholesterol and C-reactive protein, findings indicating decreased risk of atherosclerosis late in life (22).

Maternal milk contains certain factors, particularly lipids, that promote brain maturation in periods of rapid growth. The brain is 60% structural lipid and depends on dietary lipids. Lack of both linoleic acid and α-linolenic acid (ALA) is incompatible with life. Of major dietary importance are ω-3 fatty acids of the ALA family (2). Arachidonic acid and docosahexaenoic acid (DHA) are large contributors to nonmyelin membranes and must be provided by the diet. Differentiation and functioning of cultured brain cells, oligodendrocytes, and astrocytes require ALA and ω-3 fatty acids. Brain, retina, and visual development are affected by diets with insufficient amounts of essential fatty acids, such as those found in soy oil–based formula products (20).

In adults, decreased dietary levels of ω-3 fatty acids (particularly from fish consumption) increase the risk of cardiovascular disease and stroke (23), depression (24), in particular postpartum depression, as well as cognitive decline and dementia (25, 26). An appropriate dietary provision of ω-3 fatty acids during aging may prevent abnormal phospholipid metabolism, thus ensuring membrane maintenance and preventing cognitive decline (27, 28).

MICRONUTRIENT DEFICIENCIES AND COGNITIVE FUNCTION

From the public health viewpoint, iodine is the most important micronutrient for the prevention of brain disorders causing lower intellectual functioning, psychomotor delay, and mental retardation (29). Universal salt iodization may solve the worldwide problem of iodine deficiency disorders (IDDs). The World Health Organization considers that 50 million people have some degree of mental impairment caused by IDDs (30, 31).

Also of major public health importance is the deficiency of other micronutrients capable of affecting the nervous system; these include deficiencies of iron, copper, zinc, and selenium, as well as vitamin B_{12}, folate, and vitamin A. The magnitude of these problems is staggering (31): for example, 2 billion people—more than 30% of the world's population—suffer from iron deficiency anemia, most often in developing countries in association with malaria and hookworm infections. Anemia contributes to 20% of all maternal deaths of pregnant women. Between 100 and 140 million children have vitamin A deficiency, and of these, 250,000 to 500,000 become blind every year, and half of them die prematurely. Multinutrient food fortification appears to be a cost-effective treatment (32).

Iodine Deficiency Disorders

IDDs occur in areas of the earth where iodine was leached from the soil by the effects of rain, glaciations, and flooding waters. These areas typically include flood plains and mountainous regions such as the Alps, the Balkans, the Andes, the Himalayas, and the New Guinea Highlands (33). The populations of these regions suffer from high prevalence of endemic cretinism, goiter, short stature, and deafness. The neurologic importance of IDDs resides in the definite risk of fetal brain damage resulting from thyroid hormone deficiency during critical periods of brain development, both in utero and in the early postpartum period (34, 35).

Normal pregnancy causes a progressive increase of serum thyroid-stimulating hormone (TSH) along with a corresponding rise of serum thyroglobulin. In areas with moderate dietary iodine deficiency, a steady decrease of free thyroxine (T_4) occurs during gestation; TSH increases, resulting in a 20% to 30% enlargement of the thyroid volume that leads to goiter (35). Serum TSH and thyroglobulin values are even higher in neonates born to mothers with iodine deficiency. These changes in neonatal TSH frequently occur with levels of maternal iodine deficiency that would not affect the thyroid function in nonpregnant adults.

In areas with moderate iodine deficiency (iodine ingestion = 20 to 49 µg/day), clinically euthyroid children and adults often have definite abnormalities of psychomotor and intellectual development including lower IQ, slower visual-motor performance, loss of fine-motor skill, deficits in perceptual and neuromotor abilities, apathy, and low developmental quotients (35). A metaanalysis of 19 studies from 8 countries included 2676 subjects ranging in age from 2 to 30 years who were living in iodine-deficient regions. Iodine deficiency resulted in a mean loss of 13.5 IQ points at global population level; that is, 82% of children with normal iodine intake scored better than iodine-deficient children (36). Loss of intellectual capacity and deafness from IDDs constitute public health problems with a major impact on socioeconomic development.

Endemic Cretinism and Other Forms of Iodine Deficiency Disorders

Endemic cretinism is a congenital disorder of the CNS manifested by deaf-mutism, mental retardation, spastic diplegia, squint, and signs of bulbar damage (37). Partial manifestations include isolated deafness or deaf-mutism and mental retardation without pyramidal tract signs. In some endemic places (New Guinea, Thailand, Indonesia, the Andes), the usual signs of childhood myxedema—coarse puffy skin, macroglossia, umbilical hernia, short stature, and skeletal disproportion—occur rarely, whereas these signs predominate in other endemic areas (China, Congo). Therefore, two forms of the syndrome of endemic cretinism are recognized: neurologic and myxedematous.

Endemic cretinism is different from congenital hypothyroidism, which occurs in 1 in 3500 newborns (38). Congenital hypothyroidism results from deficient thyroid function in the fetus and the newborn, resulting from endocrine factors unrelated to dietary iodine deficiency.

Halpern et al (39) studied the neurologic features associated with both types of endemic cretinism in 104 persons with myxedematous cretinism from China and in 35 persons from central Java (Indonesia), who had the predominantly neurologic form. Both types of endemic cretinism had a similar pattern of neurologic involvement with mental retardation, proximal pyramidal and extrapyramidal signs, squint, deafness, primitive reflexes, and typical gait with laxity and deformities of joints. Those with serious hypothyroidism had calcification of basal ganglia on cerebral computed tomography. Therefore, both forms of endemic cretinism represent the most severe degree of brain damage from in utero maternal and fetal hypothyroidism, resulting from dietary iodine deficiency. The myxedematous type is explained by continuing postnatal thyroid hormone deficiency with impaired growth, skeletal retardation, and sexual immaturity. Thiocyanate toxicity from cassava consumption plays a role in myxedematous endemic cretinism. The combined effect of iodine and selenium deficiency is also relevant.

Thiocyanate Toxicity. Numerous staple foods in the tropics contain large amounts of cyanogenic glycosides. These include cassava (*Manihot esculenta* Crantz: *yuca* in Spanish, *manioc* in French), yam, sweet potato, corn, millet (*Sorghum* sp.), bamboo shoots, and beans such as *Phaseolus vulgaris* (40). Tobacco smoke (*Nicotiana tabacum*) also contains considerable amounts of cyanide (150 to 300 μg per cigarette). Hydrolysis of plant glycosides releases cyanide as hydrocyanic acid. Acute intoxication occurs by rapid cyanide absorption through the gastrointestinal tract or the lungs. Detoxification is mainly to thiocyanate in a reaction mediated by a sulfurtransferase (rhodanase) converting thiosulfate into thiocyanate and sulfite. The sulfur-containing essential amino acids—cystine, cysteine, and methionine—provide the sulfur for these detoxification reactions. Also important is vitamin B_{12} with conversion of hydroxocobalamin to cyanocobalamin.

Thiocyanate from cassava is goitrogenic (41); it inhibits thyroid peroxidase and prevents the incorporation of iodine into thyroglobulin (42). Thiocyanate may also form thiourea. These mechanisms explain the damaging neurologic effects of cyanide, diets poor in sulfur-containing amino acids, and low dietary iodine intake.

Selenium. In 1990, Vanderpas et al (43) found combined iodine and selenium deficiency associated with cretinism in northern Congo. Selenium is present in high concentrations in the normal thyroid (34) and in glutathione peroxidase and superoxide dismutase, the enzymes for detoxification of toxic oxygen radicals. It is also present in deiodinase, the enzyme for peripheral conversion of T_4 to triiodothyronine (T_3). Selenium deficiency decreases T_4 catabolism and allows excessive production of peroxide (H_2O_2), with thyroid cell destruction, fibrosis, and thyroid failure (34).

Pathogenesis of Brain Lesions Induced by Iodine Deficiency

Thyroid hormones affect neuronal differentiation, migration, neural networking, and synaptogenesis through binding of T_3 to nuclear receptors regulating gene expression in different brain regions (44). Thyroid hormone receptors are present in the human fetus by 8 weeks of gestation and increase about 10-fold between 10 and 18 weeks of gestation. Kester et al (45) found that T_3 is required by the human cerebral cortex before midgestation. T_4 from the mother is the only source and correlates with deiodinase (D_2) activity in the cortex. For these reasons, even moderately low T_4 maternal levels may be damaging to the fetus. Haddow et al (46) found, in mothers with increased TSH during the second trimester of pregnancy, that the strongest predictor of infant mental development was the mothers' free T_4 levels at 12 weeks of gestation. Furthermore, low levels of free T_4 at both 12 and 32 weeks of gestation resulted in worse infant cognitive outcome.

Lavado-Autric et al (47) and Ausó et al (48) produced in the rat an experimental model of transient maternal hypothyroxinemia—low T_4 but normal T_3—demonstrating that transient and mild thyroid function deficits in the mother during early gestation produced permanent abnormalities in cortical cytoarchitecture, with presence of heterotopic neuronal migration in hippocampus and somatosensory cortex. Migration of cortical neurons along the scaffolding provided by radial glia is regulated by the *reelin-dab* signaling system. Reelin is an extracellular protein secreted by Cajal-Retzius neurons that binds to membrane receptors on migrating neurons, phosphorylating the disabled homolog 1 (Dab1) to guide cells to their destination. Hypothyroidism reduces reelin expression and enhances Dab1 expression and could explain these migratory abnormalities (49, 50). Based on the foregoing mechanisms, Román (51) proposed that early maternal hypothyroxinemia could induce autism.

Treatment and Prevention

The results of salt iodination programs in Switzerland offer important evidence of their beneficial effects at population levels (52). Before 1922, the prevalence of cretinism in some Swiss cantons was 0.5%, and 100% of the schoolchildren had goiter; 30% of young men were unfit for military service because of large goiters. Salt iodination began in 1922 at low levels; by 1930, no cases of cretinism occurred, and goiter disappeared rapidly among schoolchildren. Some cantons that allowed salt iodination only in 1952 lagged behind in these achievements. The incidence of isolated deafness, mental deficiency, and short stature also decreased after implementation of salt iodination.

In 1971, Pharoah et al (53) demonstrated, in a case-control trial in the Jimi Valley of New Guinea, the effects of iodine in the prevention of congenital cretinism. Each alternate family received intramuscular injections of iodine in oil, whereas controls received saline injections. Of the women who received placebo, 534 children were born, and 26 of these children had endemic cretinism; whereas among 498 children of treated women, 7 children had endemic cretinism, but 6 of these women were already pregnant when they received the iodine injections. In 1994, Cao et al (54) studied an area of severe iodine deficiency in Xinjiang, China. Oral iodine was provided to 689 children from birth to 3 years of age and to 295 women at each trimester of pregnancy. Neurologic abnormalities occurred in 2% of children born to mothers treated early versus 9% among those treated in the third trimester. Microcephaly decreased from 27% in the untreated group to 11% of the treated children, and developmental quotients at 2 years of age also increased. Treatment in the third trimester of pregnancy or after delivery did not improve neurologic status, but head growth and developmental quotients improved slightly. Treatment during the first trimester improved neurologic outcome. In conclusion, based on these and other controlled clinical trials, treatment with iodized oil or iodized salt before or during early pregnancy prevents endemic cretinism and brain damage. Provision of iodized salt is the most cost-effective strategy (55).

Cognitive Effects of Iron Deficiency

Iron is an essential cofactor for numerous proteins involved in neuronal function. Both iron deficiency anemia and excessive iron accumulation in the brain are associated with neurologic disturbances. The brain has limited access to plasma iron because of the blood–brain barrier (56). Apathy and poverty of movement have been observed in iron-deficient children. A review by Grantham-McGregor and Ani (57) showed that anemic children usually have poor cognition and lower school achievement than non-anemic children. With treatment, most but not all of them tend to improve; however, school achievement generally remains lower in children with prior iron deficiency anemia than in nonanemic controls. Lozoff and Brittenham (58) showed that severe and chronic iron deficiency in infancy continues to cause developmental and behavioral delay more than 10 years after iron treatment. Iron deficiency causes lower cognitive, motor, attentional, and developmental scores, including failure to respond to test stimuli, short attention span, unhappiness, increased fearfulness, withdrawal, and increased body tension. In adults, anemia limits maximal physical performance, endurance, and spontaneous activity.

With aging, there is accumulation of iron-containing molecules in the brain, particularly in Alzheimer and Parkinson diseases, perhaps caused by enhanced generation of reactive oxygen species (ROS) and higher neuronal vulnerability. Iron accumulation also occurs in other neurologic diseases, such as congenital aceruloplasminemia, Friedreich ataxia, Hallervorden-Spatz disease, neuroferritinopathy, neurodegeneration with brain iron accumulation, and restless legs syndrome (56).

Cognitive Effects of Zinc Deficiency

Dietary zinc deficiency is a common nutritional disorder around the world (29). Zinc treatment of deficient children improves growth, immunity, and motor development in infants and toddlers. Zinc deprivation during periods of rapid growth impairs brain and sexual development. There are few studies in children on the cognitive, motor, and behavioral changes associated with zinc deficiency and supplementation (59, 60).

Neurologic Effects of Copper Deficiency

Copper is an essential cofactor for numerous enzymes such as copper-zinc superoxide dismutase, ceruloplasmin ferroxidase, and cytochrome oxidase. Menkes disease and Wilson disease are congenital metabolic copper abnormalities resulting from mutations of two related genes, *MNK* and *WND*, which encode proteins belonging to P-type adenosine triphosphatase (ATPase) cation transporters (61). Menkes disease is caused by mutations of the *ATP7A* gene resulting in abnormally low intestinal absorption of copper, low ceruloplasmin, and secondary deficiency in copper-dependent mitochondrial enzymes in brain, skin, hair ("kinky hair"), blood vessels, and other organs. In contrast, Wilson disease (hepatolenticular degeneration) results from mutations of the *ATP7B* gene with decreased plasma ceruloplasmin and excessive copper in blood and urine, as well as excessive copper deposition in brain, liver, eyes, and other organs. Treatment includes low-copper diet and use of chelating agents (penicillamine, trientine) or inhibitors of intestinal absorption (zinc acetate).

Copper deficiency may result also from total parenteral nutrition (TPN), prior vitamin B_{12} deficiency, intestinal malabsorption from gastric resection or bariatric surgery (62), and zinc overload, particularly with use of zinc-containing adhesive denture creams (63). Copper deficiency may mimic cobalamin deficiency manifesting with anemia from myelodysplasia (64), spinal cord involvement with subacute combined degeneration (SCD) (65), peripheral neuropathy, optic neuropathy, and periventricular white matter lesions (66). Oral copper supplementation improves functional activities of daily living in patients with copper deficiency (67).

NUTRITIONAL NEUROPATHIES AND MYELONEUROPATHIES

The polyneuropathies observed in association with alcoholism are usually considered nutritional, although a specific vitamin cannot be identified as causal. Alcohol may play a secondary neurotoxic role, but it also displaces food in the diet, increases the metabolic demands for B-group vitamins, and decreases absorption of thiamin, folic acid, and liposoluble vitamins because of impaired pancreatic function. Symptoms vary from weakness, dysesthesias, and pain to the asymptomatic patient with absent ankle reflexes. Sensory and motor deficits predominate distally and symmetrically in the legs; the face and trunk are not involved. Sensitivity to pressure palsies is often present. On neuropathologic examination, the nutritional neuropathies show predominantly sensory axonal degeneration.

It appears pointless to incriminate one particular factor as the cause of polyneuropathy seen in conditions of severe dietary restriction, alcoholism, or widespread malabsorption. Nevertheless, B-group vitamin deficiencies have long been thought to be the main cause of nutritional disorders, particularly when they are associated with alcoholism.

Neurologic signs occur relatively late during malnutrition. Symptoms appear when a combination of factors finally leads to a deficiency of essential nutrients that is severe enough to injure the nervous system or when protective nutrients—such as sulfur-containing amino acids and antioxidant carotenoids such as lycopene—become unavailable. The most sensitive elements are highly active metabolic neurons, such as dorsal root ganglia, large myelinated distal axons, bipolar retinal neurons, and cochlear neurons. These are the first to suffer damage

after ingestion of the African silkworm *Anaphe venata*, is probably the result of a heat-resistant thiaminase that induces thiamin deficiency (97).

Nutritional Amblyopia. Nutritional amblyopia is also known as tobacco-alcohol amblyopia, deficiency amblyopia, nutritional optic neuropathy, and tropical amblyopia (Mádan, 1898). The pathologic lesion appears to be confined to the maculopapillary bundle, with resulting central or cecocentral scotomata, loss of color vision, and pallor of the temporal side of the optic disc. Nutritional amblyopia was also observed among POWs in the Far East between 1942 and 1945 (71, 98–104). Cruickshank (71) described *camp blindness*, as follows:

> On examination there was lowered visual acuity of one or both eyes with difficulty in reading. Central or paracentral scotomata just above or below the point of fixation were constant findings. They varied in size but were usually larger for red than for black or white. Ophthalmoscopy in the early stages usually revealed a normal fundus. In patients with symptoms of long duration, pallor of the temporal side of the disc developed, frequently corresponding with the maculopapillary bundle.

The specific deficit responsible for nutritional amblyopia has not been established. A combination of deficits of thiamin, vitamin B_{12}, folate, and perhaps riboflavin has been invoked. In patients with Cuban optic neuropathy, Sadun (105, 106) postulated an acquired mitochondrial energy failure of macular neurons resulting from a combination of dietary deficiency of folic acid and ingestion of low doses of methanol, manifested by elevation of formate in serum and cerebrospinal fluid (CSF). Retinal mitochondria can be impaired genetically (Leber hereditary optic neuropathy) by nutritional deficit of folate and vitamin B_{12} or by toxic factors (methanol, ethambutol or cyanide). These metabolic optic neuropathies are characterized by bilaterally symmetric visual impairment with loss of central visual acuity, dyschromatopsia, cecocentral visual field defects, temporal optic disc atrophy, and specific loss of nerve fiber layer in the maculopapillary bundle. The resulting mitochondrial derangement would lead to ATP depletion that compromises axonal transport.

Burning Feet. According to Bruyn and Poser (107), "burning feet" was first described in 1826 by J. Grierson, a British medical officer in the Indian Army. This complex symptom was also commonly found in POW camps in tropical regions, where it was called "the happy feet," probably because pain kept patients walking at night. Cruickshank (108), who studied 500 cases, described the following symptoms appearing among POWs about 3 months after imprisonment:

> The suffering men were unable to sleep because of the severe burning pain in the soles of the feet. The earliest sign was a dull throbbing in the balls of the feet appearing in the evening at the end of the work day. The pains were always worst at night, keeping the patient awake. The patients became worn out from pain and loss of sleep; rapid loss of weight occurred and the appetite often became poor. Tightly gripping and massaging the feet gave some relief and men adopted a characteristic attitude in bed, sitting forward, cross-legged, gripping

their feet. On examination the patient's face wears an expression of chronic distress with dark shadows under the eyes. The constant pain and the loss of sleep produce an exhausted, red-eyed, irritable patient. Some are almost tearful from the pain. The only abnormal findings in the feet were hyperesthesia to pin prick and light touch in the majority and excessive sweating in some of the severe cases, sensory deficits in a stocking and glove distribution, and depressed or absent ankle reflexes, without severe paresis.

In Cruickshank's experience, thiamin and riboflavin deficiencies were not likely cause of burning feet among POWs. He used nicotinic acid (niacin) with good results in 68% of 500 cases, but pellagra or niacin deficiency alone is not a probable cause of this syndrome. Pantothenic acid was useful in some patients, and experimental deficiency of pantothenic acid in pigs produced dorsal myelopathy and sensory neuropathy. Folic acid deficiency itself has been associated with cases of myelopathy and sensory neuropathy in humans. The treatment of burning feet remains symptomatic.

More recently, the condition known as burning feet is a symptom of patients with distal sensory neuropathy from human immunodeficiency virus (HIV) infection (109). Patients with HIV infection and burning feet show a dying back axonal degeneration of long axons in distal regions, loss of unmyelinated fibers, and variable degree of macrophage infiltration in peripheral nerves and dorsal root ganglia. Skin biopsies (109) show reduction in nerve fiber density, increased frequency of fiber varicosities, and fragmentation of cutaneous nerve fibers.

Vitamin B_2 (Riboflavin) Deficiency

Ariboflavinosis is associated with nonspecific signs such as angular cheilosis, glossitis (beefy-red tongue), scaling dermatitis, normochromic normocytic anemia, and superficial interstitial keratitis. Recommended treatment is with vitamin B complex that usually contains a mixture of riboflavin, thiamin, niacin, folic acid, vitamin B_{12}, pantothenic acid, and biotin. In the presence of a deficiency syndrome with interstitial keratitis, vitamin A is also recommended.

Niacin Deficiency (Pellagra)

Since the 1600s, pellagra (Italian *pelle*, skin; and *agra*, rough) was epidemic in Mediterranean Europe and north Africa. In the southeastern United States from 1910 until 1935, the incidence reached 170,000 cases per year. Pellagra continues to occur among patients with alcoholism, malabsorption syndromes, and chronic diseases, as well as in malnourished populations that consume corn (maize) as staple food. Niacin, as nicotinamide, is an essential component of nicotinamide adenine dinucleotide (NAD) and NAD phosphate (NADP), two coenzymes crucial in oxidation-reduction reactions. Nicotinic acid is used for the treatment of hyperlipidemia, particularly in type 2 diabetes (110).

Humans obtain niacin from the diet or from tryptophan. Dietary leucine, found in millet in Asia and Africa, blocks the conversion of tryptophan to niacin. The traditional Central and South American treatment of corn with alkaline lime before baking the tortillas increases niacin content. Pellagra may occur in carcinoid syndrome as a result of conversion of tryptophan to serotonin by the tumor, as well as in Hartnup disease, caused by defective intestinal absorption of several amino acids.

The three Ds—dermatitis, diarrhea, and dementia—characterize the clinical manifestations of pellagra. The dermatitis typically occurs in areas exposed to sunlight, including the neck (Casal collar, 1762). The dermatitis of acute pellagra begins as an erythema that resembles sunburn with slow tanning and exacerbation by sunlight. Oral scalding, burning sensations of the tongue, glossitis, anorexia, abdominal pain, and recurrent bouts of diarrhea also occur. The dementia is preceded by insomnia, fatigue, nervousness, irritability, and depression. Suicide by drowning was said to be a common occurrence. The cognitive deficits include confusion, mental dullness, apathy, and memory impairment. Typical neuropathologic lesions of pellagra affect Betz cells in the motor cortex, smaller pyramidal cortical neurons, large neurons of basal ganglia and motor cranial nuclei, dentate nucleus, and anterior horn cells. Affected neurons appear swollen, rounded, with eccentric nuclei and loss of Nissl particles. Some alcoholic patients have similar brain lesions in the absence of overt pellagra. Pellagra neuropathy is indistinguishable from beriberi neuropathy, but it fails to respond to niacin treatment alone, and B-complex vitamin treatment is recommended.

Diagnosis and Treatment

No definitive laboratory tests exist for pellagra. The diagnosis is supported by low levels of serum niacin, tryptophan, NAD, and NADP. A combined excretion of N-methylnicotinamide and pyridone of less than 1.5 mg/24 hours indicates severe niacin deficiency. Treatment is with niacin (nicotinic acid) or with nicotinamide, which does not cause the flushing caused by niacin. The adult dose for acute pellagra is nicotinamide, 100 mg orally every 6 hours for several days or until resolution of major acute symptoms, followed by oral administration of 50 mg every 8 to 12 hours until all skin lesions heal. In severe cases with neurologic involvement, 1 g three to four times daily should be provided, initially by the parenteral route. The dose for children is 10 to 50 mg orally every 6 hours until resolution of the symptoms and signs of pellagra. Therapy should also include other B vitamins, zinc, copper and magnesium, as well as a diet rich in calories. Some data support the use of niacin in HIV-infected patients because HIV induces niacin depletion.

Vitamin B$_6$ (Pyridoxine)

Vitamin B$_6$ exists in three natural forms, pyridoxol, pyridoxal, and pyridoxamine. Ingested pyridoxol is phosphorylated and then oxidized to pyridoxal phosphate, an important coenzyme in the metabolism of amino acids, including the conversion of α-ketoglutarate to glutamate and of glutamate to GABA. Vitamin B$_6$ deficiency may cause niacin deficiency as a result of impaired tryptophan metabolism. Increased homocysteine responds to pyridoxine, vitamin B$_{12}$, or folate, depending on the type of depletion.

Vitamin B$_6$ Deficiency

Pyridoxine is found in virtually all foods, thus making dietary deficiency unlikely, although increased requirements occur in pregnancy and lactation, estrogen use, hyperthyroidism, high-protein diets, and elderly persons. Faulty preparation may destroy pyridoxine in baby formula, with resulting infantile seizures. Infants of mothers deficient in vitamin B$_6$ may also suffer neonatal seizures. The latter two mechanisms of seizure causation are different from pyridoxine dependency, a rare autosomal recessive disorder causing intractable seizures in neonates and infants.

The clinical manifestations of pyridoxine deficiency resulting from use of the antagonist desoxypyridoxine include seborrheic dermatitis, angular cheilosis, glossitis, peripheral neuropathy, and convulsions. Pyridoxine deficiency is common in patients with alcoholism because of displacement of pyridoxal phosphate by acetaldehyde. Isoniazid and penicillamine combine with pyridoxal phosphate to inactivate it. Long-term treatment of tuberculosis with isoniazid may result in distal, symmetric neuropathy that may progress to sensory ataxia and limb weakness. Pathologic examination reveals axonal degeneration and regeneration of both myelinated and unmyelinated fibers. Isoniazid acetylation by N-acetyltransferase is a genetically determined polymorphism; the acetylated drug is more easily excreted by the kidney. In Western populations, half are slow acetylators with an increased risk of developing neuropathy (and hepatotoxicity) with standard doses. Isoniazid neuropathy is reversible by discontinuation of the drug, or vitamin B$_6$ supplementation. Acute isoniazid overdose is characterized by the clinical triad of repetitive seizures that are unresponsive to anticonvulsants, metabolic acidosis with a high anion gap, and coma. The recommended therapy for isoniazid intoxication is pyridoxine. Prevention of neuropathy in patients taking isoniazid is with oral pyridoxine 50 to 100 mg/day for the duration of the isoniazid treatment.

Vitamin B$_6$ Intoxication

Megadoses of pyridoxine greater than 200 mg/day have been associated with sensory neuropathy and severe ataxia, but without weakness (111). In experimental animals (112), histologic examination revealed widespread neuronal degeneration in the dorsal root ganglia and gasserian ganglia, as well as degeneration of sensory nerve fibers in peripheral nerves, the dorsal columns of the spinal cord, and the descending spinal tract of the trigeminal nerve. The mechanism of action of megadoses of pyridoxine

responses, and the Babinski sign. In a large series of patients with pernicious anemia (136), common symptoms included loss of cutaneous sensation, weakness, urinary or fecal incontinence, and orthostatic hypotension. About one in four patients had no evidence of anemia. The final stage in untreated cases is an ataxic paraplegia, with spasticity and contractures; flaccid paraplegia may occur in some patients with severe peripheral nerve involvement. Response to treatment was inversely related to duration and severity of the neurologic symptoms and the anemia before diagnosis.

Early pathologic changes involve separation of myelin lamellae, vacuolization, and axonal damage with minimal gliosis, involving first the dorsal columns of the cervical and upper thoracic cord. Late lesions are scattered irregularly in posterior and lateral funiculi and disclose a typical honeycomb appearance. Vacuolar myelopathy, pathologically identical to SCD, occurs in patients with acquired immunodeficiency syndrome (137). Based on a postulated abnormality of cobalamin-dependent transmethylation leading to reductions of SAM, a clinical trial with L-methionine was completed; unfortunately, the results were negative (138). As mentioned earlier, low copper levels may mimic the clinical manifestations of pernicious anemia and SCD resulting from cobalamin deficiency.

Optic Neuropathy. Visual symptoms secondary to involvement of the optic nerves were commonly seen in untreated pernicious anemia. Clinically, patients have loss of visual acuity and color vision, with cecocentral scotomata, similar to those of other nutritional optic neuropathies described earlier. At autopsy, spongy degeneration of the optic nerves is usually found. In a model of dietary vitamin B_{12} deficiency in monkeys (139), neuropathologic examination revealed loss of ganglion cells in the macula with early involvement of the maculopapillary bundles, extending to the retrobulbar portion of the optic nerves. CNS changes in the monkeys occurred after 33 to 45 months of deficiency, similar to the time required to produce vitamin B_{12} deficiency in humans. A more readily animal model is obtained in a fruit bat exposed to inhaled nitrous oxide (140).

Peripheral Neuropathy. A mild form of sensory peripheral neuropathy probably occurs in vitamin B_{12} deficiency, with typical stocking-and-glove distribution, but most of the sensory symptoms result from dorsal column involvement. A review of clinical electrophysiologic studies in SCD (141) showed posterior column dysfunction and damage to the central motor pathway. A few patients had axonal neuropathy and, more rarely, demyelinating neuropathy. Motor evoked potentials and median somatosensory evoked potentials became normal with cobalamin treatment, but tibial somatosensory evoked potentials remained abnormal in most patients.

Other Forms of Presentation. Unusual forms of presentation of vitamin B_{12} deficiency (142) include cranial neuropathies with hoarseness from vocal cord paralysis, disturbances of taste and smell, tinnitus, nocturnal tabetic-type pains, upward or lateral gaze limitation, cerebellar dysfunction, and movement disorders occurring in addition to more typical manifestations of SCD.

Neuropsychiatric Symptoms. Mental symptoms are frequent in pernicious anemia and range from confusional episodes and maniac behavior to depression and progressive decline of memory, orientation, and cognition leading to dementia. Cerebral white matter lesions typical of vitamin B_{12} deficiency are the probable neuropathologic substrate. Neuropsychiatric symptoms have been correlated with reduced CSF levels of SAM (143, 144).

Diagnosis and Treatment. The diagnosis of vitamin B_{12} deficiency from pernicious anemia is usually made in the presence of positive anti-IF antibodies, low levels of vitamin B_{12}, and increased levels of MMA and homocysteine. Macrocytic anemia and neutrophil polysegmentation may not be present.

The neurologic complications of vitamin B_{12} deficiency usually respond to intramuscular injections of 1000 μg of vitamin B_{12} daily for 5 days to replenish the stores, followed by monthly injections of 500 to 1000 μg indefinitely. A sublingual form of vitamin B_{12} is also available. For preventive treatment, oral preparations of vitamin B_{12} appear to be adequate.

Folic Acid

After intestinal absorption, mainly 5-methyltetrahydrofolate ($5MH_4F$) enters the circulation; folate reserves are limited, and deficits may occur after a few months of negative balance. Tetrahydrofolates act as acceptors of one-carbon fragments for the synthesis of purines, methionine, and deoxythymidine monophosphate for the synthesis of DNA. Decreased absorption is present in patients with alcoholism, in malabsorption, as well as with ingestion of phenytoin and oral contraceptives. There are increased requirements for folic acid in pregnancy and lactation, in infants and adolescents, and in patients with active hematopoiesis and cancer.

Neurologic Manifestations of Folate Deficiency

Folate deficiency produces megaloblastic anemia identical to that of vitamin B_{12} deficiency, but isolated folic acid deficiency rarely produces SCD and peripheral neuropathy. Folic acid deficiency may produce isolated increase of homocysteine.

Ramaekers and Blau (145) described a neurologic syndrome called idiopathic cerebral folate deficiency in children with low CSF levels of $5MH_4F$ but with normal folate metabolism outside the nervous system. Onset is at about 4 months of age, with restlessness, irritability, and altered sleep, followed by psychomotor retardation, cerebellar ataxia, spastic paraplegia, dyskinesias, and visual and hearing loss; one third of the children have seizures. Periventricular demyelination and cerebral atrophy are seen. The syndrome is caused by nonfunctional CSF receptor-mediated folate receptor protein 1 (FR1). Patients usually respond to oral folate supplementation. Secondary forms of cerebral folate deficiency include long-term use of antifolate and anticonvulsant drugs, Rett syndrome, Aicardi-Goutieres syndrome, 3-phosphoglycerate dehydrogenase deficiency, dihydropteridine reductase deficiency, aromatic amino acid decarboxylase deficiency, and Kearns-Sayre syndrome.

Congenital errors of folate metabolism include (146) methylenetetrahydrofolate reductase deficiency, characterized by mental retardation, seizures, schizophrenia, or vascular disease, without hematologic abnormalities. This is the most common congenital error of folate metabolism. Laboratory tests show low folate in serum, red blood cells, and CSF, associated with homocystinuria. Methionine synthase deficiency causes megaloblastic anemia associated with mental retardation. Glutamate formiminotransferase cyclodeaminase deficiency manifests with severe mental retardation. Rarely, dihydrofolate reductase deficiency manifests with folate-responsive neonatal megaloblastic anemia.

Neural Tube Defects and Folate. One of the most common malformations of the CNS is spina bifida, resulting from fusion failure of the caudal neural tube. Up to 70% of spina bifida cases can be prevented by maternal folic acid supplementation (147). Other causes include chromosome abnormalities, single gene disorders, and teratogenic exposure. The mechanism of protection is unknown, but it may include genes that regulate folate transport and metabolism. Maternal risk factors include low dietary intake of iron, magnesium, and niacin (148), as well as maternal use of antiepileptic drugs that increase the risk for neural tube defects (149). Tea drinking during pregnancy may increase the risk because of tea catechins that inhibit the activity of the enzyme dihydrofolate reductase (150).

Genetic susceptibility to folate deficiency occurs in subjects with gene mutations of the enzyme 5,10-methylenetetrahydrofolate reductase (MH_4FR). A common gene mutation (C677T) results in decreased activity of this enzyme (151) and increased homocysteine levels. The effects are probably worsened by low folate levels and possibly also low riboflavin levels; this mutation may increase the risk of depression in elderly persons as a result of the dysfunction of methylation metabolic pathways critical to the synthesis of norepinephrine and serotonin (151).

Treatment of Folate Deficiency

Folate deficiency readily responds to dietary modification and oral folic acid supplements. Oral doses of 1 mg folic acid per day are considered safe. However, before instituting folic acid treatment, it is mandatory to exclude concurrent cobalamin deficiency because in the presence of combined deficiencies of folate and cobalamin, folate therapy alone may result in hematologic improvement with simultaneous—and sometimes irreversible—neurologic deterioration.

Pantothenic Acid

Pantothenate is bound to CoA, a critical component of carbohydrate and fatty acids metabolism, and it acts against apoptosis and cell damage by quenching oxygen free radicals. The Hallervorden-Spatz syndrome was linked with the gene *PANK2* on chromosome 20, which encodes pantothenate kinase, an essential step for the synthesis of CoA from pantothenate (152), thus causing abnormalities of fatty acid synthesis and energy metabolism, as well as increasing concentration of cysteine-iron deposits in basal ganglia. The Hallervorden-Spatz syndrome is characterized pathologically by iron deposits and axonal spheroids in basal ganglia.

Vitamin E (α-Tocopherol)

This lipid-soluble vitamin was initially identified as an indispensable nutrient for fertility in animals; however, α-tocopherol is also a potent antioxidant that prevents cell membrane injury from lipid peroxidation. Tocopherol is absorbed into chylomicrons in the small intestine and is transported bound to α-tocopherol transfer protein.

Vitamin E deficiency occurs with poor diets, malabsorption (153), short bowel and blind-loop syndromes (154), cystic fibrosis (155), celiac disease, and chronic cholestatic liver disease, as well as in abetalipoproteinemia and in isolated genetic defects of the α-tocopherol transfer protein. The Italian form of ataxia with vitamin E deficiency (156) is a rare autosomal recessive disorder caused by mutations in the α-tocopherol transfer protein gene on chromosome 8q13. Affected patients have a progressive spinocerebellar syndrome and low plasma levels of vitamin E (156). Vitamin E deficiency has also been described in patients with tropical myeloneuropathies, probably associated with dietary deficiency and tropical malabsorption (157).

There is a rare syndrome of isolated vitamin E deficiency with neurologic manifestations with onset in childhood, without fat malabsorption (158). Symptoms include tremor, tremulous dysarthric speech, gait ataxia from loss of vibratory sensation and proprioception, and global areflexia. Cerebellar deficits include dysmetria, slowed finger movements, and postural tremor. The gait is wide based, with prominent lordosis and genu recurvatum with pseudodystonic extension of the knees and inversion of the feet. Ophthalmoplegia, retinitis pigmentosa, dysarthria, generalized muscle weakness, and extensor plantar responses are present in some cases. The symptoms progress from hyporeflexia, ataxia, limitations in upward gaze, and strabismus to long-tract defects, weakness, and visual field constriction. Patients with severe, prolonged deficiency may develop complete blindness, dementia, and cardiac arrhythmias (158).

76. Cuba Neuropathy Field Investigation Team. N Engl J Med 1995;333:1176–82.

77. Román GC. Neurology. 1994;44:1784–6.

78. Diniz A da S, Pacheco Santos LM. J Pediatr (Rio J) 2000;76 (Suppl):S311–22.

79. Biesalski HK, Nohr D. J Nutr 2004;134 (Suppl):3453S–7S.

80. Smith J, Steinemann TL. Int Ophthalmol Clin 2000;40: 83–91.

81. Beaton GH, Martorell R, L'Abbé KA et al. Bol Sanit Panam 1994;117:506–18.

82. D'Souza RM, D'Souza R. J Trop Pediatr 2002;48:323–7.

83. Collins MD, Mao GE. Annu Rev Pharmacol Toxicol 1999; 39:399–430.

84. Singleton CK, Martin PR. Curr Mol Med 2001;1:197–207.

85. Galvin R, Bråthen G, Ivashynka A et al. Eur J Neurol 2010; 17:1408–18.

86. Silverman B, Franklin GM, Bolin R et al. MMWR Morb Mortal Wkly Rep 1997;46:523–8.

87. Smith SW. J Emerg Med 1998;16:587–91.

88. Martínez M, Román GC, de la Hoz F et al. Biomédica (Colombia)1996;16:41–51.

89. Spillane JD. Nutritional Disorders of the Nervous System. Edinburgh: E & S Livingstone, 1947.

90. Cruickshank EK. Proc Nutr Soc 1946;5:121–7.

91. Aguiar AC, Costa VM, Ragazzo PC et al. Arq Neuropsiquiatr 2004;62:733–6.

92. Koike H, Iijima M, Mori K et al. Nutrition 2004;20:961–6.

93. Victor M, Adams RD, Collins GH. The Wernicke-Korsakoff Syndrome: A Clinical and Pathological Study of 245 Patients, 82 with Post-Mortem Examinations. Philadelphia: FA Davis, 1971.

94. Blass JP, Gibson GE. N Engl J Med 1977;297:1367–70.

95. Jung EH, Sheu KF, Blass JP. J Neurol Sci 1993;114:123–7.

96. Brokate B, Hildebrandt H, Eling P et al. Neuropsychology 2003;17:420–8.

97. Adamolekun B, McCandless DW, Butterworth RF. Metab Brain Dis 1997;12:251–8.

98. Fisher CM. Can Serv Med J 1955;11:157–99.

99. Denny-Brown D. Medicine (Baltimore) 1947;26:41–113.

100. Wilkinson PB, King A. Lancet 1944;1:528–31.

101. Spillane JD, Scott GI. Lancet 1945;2:261–4.

102. Clarke CA, Sneddon IB. Lancet 1946;1:734–7.

103. Hobbs HE, Forbes FA. Lancet 1946;2:149–53.

104. Smith DA. Brain 1946;69:209–22.

105. Sadun A. Trans Am Ophthalmol Soc 1998;96:881–923.

106. Sadun A. Semin Ophthalmol 2002;17:29–32.

107. Bruyn GW, Poser CM. The History of Tropical Neurology: Nutritional Disorders. Canton, MA: Science History Publications, 2003:19–28.

108. Cruickshank EK. Lancet 1946:2:369–71.

109. Pardo CA, McArthur JC, Griffin JW. J Peripher Nerv Syst 2001;6:21–7.

110. Grundy SM, Vega GL, McGovern ME et al. Arch Intern Med 2002;162:1568–76.

111. Schaumburg H, Kaplan J, Windebank A et al. N Engl J Med 1983;309:445–8.

112. Krinke G, Schaumburg HH, Spencer PS et al. Neurotoxicology 1981;2:13–24.

113. Andrès E, Goichot B, Schlienger JL. Arch Intern Med 2000; 160:2061–2.

114. Russell-Jones GJ, Alpers DH. Pharm Biotechnol 1999;12: 493–520.

115. Hathout L, El-Saden L. J Neurol Sci 2011:301:1–8.

116. Andrès E, Goichot B, Perrin AE et al. Rheumatology (Oxford) 2001;40:1196–7.

117. Andrès E, Noel E, Ben Abdelghani M. Ann Pharmacother 2003;37:1730.

118. Andrès E, Noel E, Goichot B. Arch Intern Med 2002;162: 2251–2.

119. Selzer RR, Rosenblatt DS, Laxova R et al. N Engl J Med 2003;349:45–50.

120. Stabler SP, Allen RH. Annu Rev Nutr 2004;24:299–326.

121. Rogers LM, Boy E, Miller JW et al. Am J Clin Nutr 2003;77:433–40.

122. Andrès E, Loukili NH, Noel, E et al. CMAJ 2004;171: 251–9.

123. Wolters M, Strohle A, Hahn A. Prev Med 2004;39:1256–66.

124. Carmel R. Clin Chem 2003;49:1367–74.

125. van Asselt DZ, Thomas CM, Segers MF et al. Ann Clin Biochem 2003;40:65–9.

126. Gailus S, Höhne W, Gasnier B et al. J Mol Med 2010;88: 459–66.

127. Humphrey LL, Fu R, Rogers K et al. Mayo Clin Proc 2008; 83:1203–12.

128. Dufouil C, Alperovitch A, Ducros V et al. Ann Neurol 2003; 53:214–21.

129. Vermeer SE, Van Dijk EJ, Koudstaal PJ et al. Ann Neurol 2002;51:285–9.

130. Garcia A, Zanibbi K. CMAJ 2004;171:897–904.

131. Seshadri S, Beiser A, Selhub J et al. N Engl J Med 2002; 346:476–83.

132. Garcia A, Haron Y, Evans L et al. J Am Geriatr Soc 2004; 52:66–71.

133. Homocysteine Studies Collaboration. JAMA 2002;288: 2015–22.

134. Smith D, Smith SM, de Jager CA et al. PLoS 2010;5:e12244.

135. Scalabrino G, Buccellato FR, Veber D et al. Clin Chem Lab Med 2003;41:1435–7.

136. Healton EB, Savage DG, Brust JC et al. Medicine (Baltimore) 1991;70:229–45.

137. Petito CK, Navia BA, Cho ES et al. N Engl J Med 1985; 312:874–9.

138. Di Rocco A, Werner P, Bottiglieri T et al. Neurology 2004; 63:1270–5.

139. Chester EM, Agamanolis DP, Harris JW et al. Acta Neurol Scand 1980;61:9–26.

140. van der Westhuyzen J, Fernandes-Costa F, Metz J. Life Sci 1982;31:2001–10.

141. Hemmer B, Glocker FX, Schumacher M et al. J Neurol Neurosurg Psychiatry 1998;65:822–7.

142. Ahn TB, Cho JW, Jeon BS. Eur J Neurol 2004;11:339–41.

143. Bottiglieri T, Hyland K. Acta Neurol Scand 1994;154 (Suppl):19–26.

144. Stanger O, Fowler B, Pietrzik K et al. Expert Rev Neurother 2009;9:1393–412.

145. Ramaekers VT, Blau N. Dev Med Child Neurol 2004;46: 843–51.

146. Zittoun J. Baillieres Clin Haematol 1995;8:603–16.

147. Mitchell LE, Adzick NS, Melchionne J et al. Lancet 2004; 364:1885–95.

148. Groenen PM, van Rooij IA, Peer PG et al. J Nutr 2004;134: 1516–22.

149. Frey L, Hauser WA. Epilepsia 2003;44(Suppl):4–13.

150. Ye R, Ren A, Zhang L et al. Epidemiology 2011;22:491–6.

151. Almeida OP, Flicker L, Lautenschlager NT et al. Neurobiol Aging 2005;26:251–7.

152. Gordon N. Eur J Paediatr Neurol 2002;6:243–7.

153. Harding AE, Muller DPR, Thomas PK et al. Ann Neurol 1982;12:419–24.

154. Brin MF, Fetell MR, Green PH. Neurology 1985;35:338–42.

155. Sitrin MD, Lieberman F, Jensen WE et al. Ann Intern Med 1987;107:51–4.

156. Mariotti C, Gellera C, Rimoldi M et al. Neurol Sci 2004; 25:130–7.

157. Tranchant D, Darracq R, Ticolat R. Presse Med 1986;15: 1729–30.

158. Tanyel MC, Mancano LD. Am Fam Physician 1997;55: 197–201.

159. Berman K, Brodaty H. CNS Drugs 2004;18:807–25.

160. Jialal I, Devaraj S. J Nutr 2005;135:348–53.

161. Holick MF. J Cell Biochem 2003;88:296–307.

162. Cantorna MT, Mahon BD. Exp Biol Med 2004;229: 1136–42.

163. Munger KL, Zhang SM, O'Reilly E et al. Neurology 2004; 62:60–5.

164. VanAmerongen BM, Dijkstra CD, Lips P et al. Eur J Clin Nutr 2004;58:1095–109.

165. Dumas M, Jauberteau-Marchan MO. Med Hypotheses 2000;55:517–20.

166. McMichael AJ, Hall AJ. Neuroepidemiology 2001;20:165–7.

167. Jansen SC, van Dusseldorp M, Bottema KC et al. Ann Allergy Asthma Immunol 2003;91:233–40.

168. Matalas AL, Zampelas A, Stavrinos V et al, eds. The Mediterranean Diet: Constituents and Health Promotion. CRC Press Modern Nutrition Series. Boca Raton, FL: CRC Press, 2001.

169. Trichopoulou A, Tina Costacou T, Trichopoulos D. N Engl J Med 2003;348:2599–608.

170. Serra-Majem L, Román B, Estruch R. Nutr Rev 2006;64: S27–47.

171. Estruch R, Martinez-Gonzalez MA, Corella D et al. Ann Intern Med 2006;145:1–11.

172. Scarmeas N, Stern Y, Tang MX et al. Ann Neurol 2006;59: 912–21.

173. Lambert M. Am Fam Physician 2011;83:993–1001.

174. Ard JD, Coffman CJ, Lin PH et al. Am J Hypertens 2004;17:1156–62.

175. Shawcross D, Jalan R. Lancet 2005;365:431–3.

176. Kircheis G, Wettstein M, Dahl S et al. Metab Brain Dis 2002;17:453–62.

177. Freeman JM, Kelly MT, Freeman JB. The Epilepsy Diet Treatment: An Introduction to the Ketogenic Diet. New York: Demo Publications, 1994.

178. Vaisleib II, Buchhalter JR, Zupanc ML. Pediatr Neurol 2004; 31:198–202.

96

BEHAVIORAL DISORDERS AFFECTING FOOD INTAKE: EATING DISORDERS AND OTHER PSYCHIATRIC CONDITIONS[1]

JANELLE W. COUGHLIN, MARGARET SEIDE, AND ANGELA S. GUARDA

Eating disorders are driven behavioral disorders resulting in significant functional impairment and, in extreme cases, death. They occur along a spectrum, so that diagnostic boundaries are often blurred. The fourth edition of the *Diagnostic and Statistical Manual of Mental Disorders* (*DSM-IV*) (1) distinguishes three major categories of eating disorders: anorexia nervosa (AN), bulimia nervosa (BN), and eating disorder not otherwise specified (EDNOS).

Binge-eating disorder (BED) is usually accompanied by obesity and is subsumed under the EDNOS category. BED is currently under consideration as a distinct eating disorder in DSM-V and has become the focus of significant clinical and scientific attention.

Unlike BED, AN and BN are perhaps better thought of as "dieting disorders" (2). Both are characterized by an overvalued fear of fatness that drives a set of disturbed behaviors, including restricting food intake, binge eating, excessive exercise, self-induced vomiting, and abuse of laxatives, diuretics, and diet pills. Engagement in these behaviors, coupled with the physiologic consequences of starvation and/or the binge-purge-restrict cycle, sustains and heightens food preoccupation and body image disturbance. This chapter reviews the diagnosis, epidemiology, etiology, complications, and treatment of eating disorders and concludes with a summary of other psychiatric conditions and frequently prescribed psychotropic medications that may affect food intake. Although obesity is often the consequence of repetitive overeating or binge eating, it is primarily a medical condition and is addressed in chapters reserved solely for this topic.

OVERVIEW OF EATING DISORDERS

Anorexia Nervosa

AN is a syndrome of self-starvation characterized by weight loss to a level below 85% of expected body weight. Weight loss is accompanied by fear of fatness and, in girls and women, amenorrhea or the absence of three or more consecutive menstrual cycles. AN is further subdivided into a restricting (AN-R) or a binge-eating/purging (AN-P) subtype. Individuals with AN-R restrict food intake and often excessively exercise and fidget in the service of weight loss but do not binge or engage in purging behaviors. By contrast, AN-P includes regular binge-eating and/or purging behaviors (e.g., self-induced vomiting and abuse of laxatives, diuretics, and enemas).

Bulimia Nervosa

BN is a dieting disorder characterized by episodes of binge eating followed by compensatory behaviors aimed at preventing weight gain. Binge eating is defined as consumption of an amount of food definitely larger than

[1]**Abbreviations: AN**, anorexia nervosa; **ADHD**, attention deficit hyperactivity disorder; **BED**, binge-eating disorder; **BMI**, body mass index; **BN**, bulimia nervosa; **CBT**, cognitive-behavioral treatment; **DSM**, *Diagnostic and Statistical Manual of Mental Disorders*; **EDNOS**, eating disorder not otherwise specified; **IPT**, interpersonal psychotherapy; **TPN**, total parenteral nutrition.

most people would eat in a similar period, under similar circumstances, and is associated with a sense of loss of control over eating. Typical binge foods are high-fat, high-calorie, "forbidden" foods, and amounts consumed are 1000 to 2000 calories or more per binge (3). Between binges, bulimic individuals typically restrict intake and only consume "safe," low-calorie, low-fat foods. Other compensatory behaviors following a binge can include purging, vomiting, abuse of laxatives or diuretics, or excessive exercise. As in AN, dieting and preoccupation with thinness develop into a consuming passion that is difficult to interrupt and impairs psychologic and social function. The distinction between AN-P and BN is primarily one of weight. Individuals who binge and purge but are less than 85% of ideal body weight or a body mass index (BMI) of about 17.5 and are amenorrheic are given the diagnosis of AN-P, whereas those who are less underweight, or are normal weight or overweight, are given the diagnosis of BN. The two subtypes of BN are purging (BN-P) and nonpurging (BN-NP). Individuals with BN-NP do not self-induce vomiting or abuse laxatives or diuretics; rather, they alternate episodes of binge eating with fasting or excessive exercise to avoid weight gain.

Eating Disorder Not Otherwise Specified

EDNOS is a heterogeneous diagnostic category. It includes partial-syndrome cases of AN and BN, BED, and atypical eating disorders. For partial-syndrome AN or BN, the diagnosis of EDNOS does not imply minor clinical significance. Indeed, these cases may be associated with morbidity equal to or greater than full-syndrome cases of AN or BN (4). An example would be an individual whose baseline weight was obese and who developed intense fear of fatness and extreme dieting behaviors, rapidly losing more than 40% of his or her body weight yet failing to meet the underweight criterion for AN or the binge frequency criterion for BN.

BED is defined as regular binge eating, twice a week or more, associated with a subjective sense of loss of control over eating but lacking the compensatory behaviors typical of BN. BED differs from BN in several additional ways. Individuals with BN restrict their food choices and calorie intake when not bingeing yet often are more impulsive and consume more calories during binges than do individuals with BED. Patients with BED overeat more consistently throughout the day than do patients with BN (5) and are more likely to be overweight or obese.

Examples of atypical eating disorders include globus hystericus, or fear of swallowing, resulting in severe weight loss and functional impairment, and psychogenic vomiting syndromes. In some cases, these may be factitious disorders, conditions in which the behavior persists in part because the sick role has become rewarding to the affected individual.

EPIDEMIOLOGY

Epidemiologic data on eating disorders is limited for several reasons. Both AN and BN have relatively low prevalence in the general population. Furthermore, most patients are ambivalent about seeking treatment and minimize their symptoms. A minority of cases reaches clinical attention, so research on clinical samples inevitably underestimates the true incidence of these psychiatric conditions (6).

The prevalence of AN among young women is approximately 0.3%, with girls and women 10 times more likely to develop AN than boys and men (6). The age- and sex-adjusted incidence in the general population is approximately 8 cases per 100,000 population per year. Across the life span, AN is most likely to have its onset among girls and women ages 15 to 19 years, who comprise an estimated 40% of documented new cases. In one epidemiologic sample, incidence rates in this age group increased steadily from 1935 to 1989 (7). It is unclear how much this increase reflects better detection and increased care seeking as awareness of the diagnosis among both clinicians and the general public has increased.

Incidence rates of BN are consistently higher than those reported for AN across studies, approximating 12 cases per 100,000 population per year (6). These are likely to be underestimates because of the more secretive nature of this disorder and because affected individuals lack the starved habitus that makes AN easier to detect. The higher incidence and prevalence of BN are also partly explained by research suggesting that as many as 40% of patients with AN progress to BN over time as a result of the challenges of maintaining a low body weight through primarily restrictive behaviors (8). In comparison with AN, the age of onset in BN is later, with 20- to 24-year-old women being at greatest risk. Prevalence estimates for BN are 1% for girls and women and 0.1% for boys and men, the same gender distribution found in AN (6).

EDNOS is a phenomenologically heterogeneous group, and epidemiologic information on it is scant at best, although the prevalence of partial-syndrome eating disorders is at least twice that of full-syndrome eating disorders (9). Only three population studies of the prevalence of BED have been completed, and these reveal a prevalence of 2% to 3%, a more equal female-to-male distribution (approximately 2:1), and a later age of onset than that of AN or BN of 30 to 50 years (10). Rates of BED are much higher, on the order of approximately 25%, in clinical samples of obese individuals seeking weight-loss treatment (11).

ETIOLOGY: RISK AND SUSCEPTIBILITY FACTORS

Although knowledge of the pathogenesis of eating disorders remains limited, it is clear that the etiology of these conditions is multifactorial and in most cases includes the interaction of both genetic and environmental predisposing factors. These interactions and how they contribute to risk remain largely unexplored and are believed to vary significantly among individuals.

Genetics

Family, twin, and molecular studies suggest that eating disorders are genetically influenced. Cross-transmission of AN, BN, and EDNOS within families suggests a shared familial liability (12). Prevalence of eating disorders in relatives of eating-disordered probands is 7 to 12 times that of controls, and monozygotic twins have significantly higher concordance rates of AN and BN than their dizygotic counterparts (13); however, eating disorders do not necessarily breed true (i.e., relatives of probands with AN have increased rates of AN or BN, not increased rates of AN specifically). Twin studies have found heritability estimates of 58% to 76% for AN, 54% to 76% for BN, 38% to 61% for BED, and 32% to 72% for attitudes commonly associated with eating disorders (e.g., body dissatisfaction and weight preoccupation) (13, 14). Attempts to identify biologic markers for AN and BN have led some researchers to investigate polymorphisms in serotonin- and dopamine-related genes. Other studies have targeted leptin and estrogen receptors, genes involved in weight regulation, feeding, and energy expenditure (15). Although promising, research on these biologic markers has produced inconsistent findings and therefore awaits further investigation.

Personality

Research has identified several personality traits associated with eating disorders including elevated harm avoidance (15), neurotic personality features, and low self-esteem (16). Perfectionism, conscientiousness, persistence, and obsessive qualities are often discriminating features of AN, whereas elevated impulsivity, novelty seeking, negative emotionality, stress reactivity, and personality traits associated with antisocial, borderline, histrionic, and narcissistic personality disorders are more commonly associated with BN (15, 17). Family studies have found increased levels of some of these traits in first-degree relatives of individuals with eating disorders, a finding suggesting that the heritability of AN and BN may be related in part to the heritability of these personality characteristics (17).

Developmental Factors

Eating disorders are significantly more prevalent in menstruating girls and women than in prepubertal girls, a finding implicating a role for ovarian hormones and sexual development in the activation of disordered eating (18). Perception of being overweight prepubertally (19) and early-onset menarche (20) have emerged as specific aspects of puberty that may increase eating disorder vulnerability. Early-maturing girls have higher adiposity before menarche, are more dissatisfied with their bodies, and are more likely to engage in weight-loss efforts than girls who go through puberty on time or later in life (20). Environmental changes associated with the transition to college, including high levels of stress, performance and achievement demands, and role and identity changes, are factors significantly related to disordered eating (21) and may make this developmental milestone one that places late adolescents at risk of developing eating disorders. Past trauma, namely, childhood sexual abuse, may heighten the risk of developing eating disorders; however, early sexual abuse has been associated with other psychiatric conditions, thus making it difficult to determine whether a direct link between eating disorders and childhood sexual abuse exists or whether early sexual abuse and mental health are more broadly linked (22).

Sociocultural Factors

The sociocultural model of eating disorders posits that eating disorders and body image disturbances are the result of pervasive societal pressures on girls and women to be thin. According to this model, messages idealizing thinness are transmitted to members of society through the mass media, peers, and families. Although this model explains why eating disorders are more common in Western cultures that value thinness, only a small minority of the population develops eating disorders; therefore, sociocultural factors alone are not a sufficient explanation for the development of an eating disorder. However, pressures to be thin starting around the age of puberty may trigger the onset of dieting behavior in otherwise vulnerable individuals.

Mass Media

Slender female models and images (e.g., cartoons, computer graphics) saturate the Western mass media. Internalization, or acceptance, of these societal standards of thinness may lead to low self-esteem, negative affect, dieting, and/or eating disorders in girls and women (23). Experimental studies have consistently shown that girls and women exposed to media images of thinness experience greater body dissatisfaction in comparison with those exposed to heavier or neutral images (24). The negative effect of these images is heightened when girls and women viewing slender images have already internalized thin beauty ideals or have high baseline levels of body image disturbance.

Peers

Pressure to be thin from peers (25) and past history of weight-related teasing (26) may impact body dissatisfaction among girls and women and may increase the risk of disordered eating behaviors; however, at least one study reported that weight-related teasing does not predict body dissatisfaction in adolescent girls (27). Because most studies of teasing are retrospective, they are also affected by recall bias, which may be stronger in individuals with body dissatisfaction who are at risk of eating disorders.

Similarly, although members of adolescent female cliques often have comparable levels of body image disturbance, it is unclear whether body image is directly influenced by peers or whether adolescents simply seek homogeneous peer groups. Among college sorority sisters, bingeing and purging behaviors are passed from one individual to another, much like the spreading of a disease (a contagion effect), a finding suggesting a direct social influence of peers on disordered eating (28).

Family

Parents are the most dominant sociocultural factor affecting young children, and parents' direct comments about their child's weight, particularly comments of mothers, have been identified as the most consistent factor associated with children's concerns and behaviors related to weight and shape (29, 30). Familial dynamics are also important predisposing factors in eating disorders. Girls who eat alone, who have parents who are not married (31), or who perceive their family communication, parental caring, and parental expectations as low (32) are at increased risk of disordered eating. Indeed, investigators have suggested that low perceived social support from family, coupled with low self-esteem, high body concern, and use of escape-avoidance coping, places women at high risk of developing eating disorders (33).

CONSEQUENCES AND COMPLICATIONS

Social and Developmental Complications

Eating is a highly social activity, and eating disorders inevitably impair interpersonal function. Affected individuals become socially isolated in an attempt to hide or avoid confrontation regarding their food choices or amounts eaten and spend increasing time engaged in eating rituals and exercise routines that take precedence over age-appropriate social engagements. Formation of intimate relationships and sexual function are often impaired by starvation's effect on libido and heightened body image concerns. Because they primarily affect young women and girls, AN and BN often result in the interruption of normal developmental tasks including separation-individuation from parents, identity formation, and the development of meaningful peer relationships.

Psychologic Complications

Individuals with eating disorders describe a consuming and constant preoccupation with food and weight that occupies much of their waking time and worsens with starvation. Furthermore, starvation results in a syndrome characterized by low mood, apathy, anhedonia, and decreased concentration and energy that is indistinguishable from major depression but reverses within days or weeks of refeeding (34). Besides starvation-related increases in obsessional preoccupation with food and weight and depressive symptoms, family studies have confirmed increased rates of affective disorders, alcohol abuse, and anxiety disorders in first-degree relatives of individuals with AN and BN (17). This finding suggests that comorbid psychiatric conditions are common and may complicate the treatment course unless they are addressed in parallel with the eating disorder. Finally, demoralization and loss of self-esteem often accompany patients' attempts to control their behaviors and the realization that these behaviors have impaired their functioning.

Physical Complications and Signs

Physical complications arise as a consequence of starvation and/or purging behaviors. Therefore, the diagnostic group at highest risk is AN-P—underweight starved patients who employ purging techniques in the service of weight loss. Besides complications of the eating disorder itself, treatment and refeeding are associated with potential medical risks.

Starvation-Related Complications

Malnutrition and starvation in AN are associated with numerous physical signs and symptoms. Patients often appear emaciated, with muscle wasting and weakness on examination, and may develop lanugo, the growth of fine, diffuse body hair. Physiologic responses to self-starvation are aimed at conserving energy and include bradycardia, hypotension, hypothermia, and interruption of the hypothalamic-pituitary-ovarian axis. Estrogen, follicle-stimulating hormone, and luteinizing hormone revert to prepubertal levels, as a result of disturbances in gonadotropin-releasing hormone pulsatility, resulting in amenorrhea and infertility. In prepubertal patients, normal secondary sexual characteristics, such as breast development and height, may be halted by malnutrition (35). Patients frequently complain of cold intolerance, fatigue, and gastrointestinal symptoms, including bloating, early satiety, and constipation. Starvation also results in delayed gastric emptying, delayed gastrointestinal transit times, and constipation (36). Anemia is common, and pancytopenia and bone marrow suppression can occur in severely malnourished patients (37). Osteoporosis is a largely irreversible consequence of AN, occurring relatively early in the course of the disorder; most affected girls and women develop significant decreases in bone density within a year of onset, and osteoporosis also can be a complication for boys and men with AN (38). Osteoporosis results in elevated fracture risk, and patients with chronic AN are at risk of debilitating hip fractures and spinal compression fractures. Unlike in menopausal osteoporosis, little evidence suggests a protective role for estrogen in preventing bone loss, and weight restoration is the only intervention known to stop bone mineral loss (39). Finally, hypoglycemia is common in starvation; and depleted glycogen stores in AN complicate serum glucose regulation. Chronic hypoglycemia also may underlie some of the neuroendocrine disruptions observed in this condition. Disturbances in glucose counter regulatory hormones in AN include alterations in growth hormone, cortisol, and catecholamines. These changes may in turn contribute to the maintenance of anorectic behaviors and cognitions (40).

Purging-Related Complications

Patients who vomit may present with visible bilateral parotid and salivary gland hypertrophy and with Russell sign—calluses on the dorsum of the hand resulting from reflexive biting during manual stimulation of the gag reflex to induce vomiting. Dental caries and enamel erosion of the lingual surface of the teeth are also common. Recurrent vomiting can lead to esophagitis and reflux, and some patients ruminate or chew and spit food as part of their disorder (41). Ipecac abuse is especially dangerous because its active ingredient, emetine, is cardiotoxic and has a long half-life, accumulating in cardiac muscle and increasing the risk of life-threatening cardiomyopathy.

Laxative abusers often use large quantities of laxatives daily and may develop laxative dependence and rebound constipation. Besides acute dehydration and presyncopal or syncopal symptoms, chronic laxative and diuretic abuse can lead to renal damage and nephrocalcinosis. Both vomiting and laxative abuse can result in electrolyte and acid–base imbalances as well as dehydration. The most common serious electrolyte imbalance is hypokalemia, which increases the risk of potentially lethal cardiac arrhythmias.

Refeeding Syndrome

Refeeding syndrome is the term used to describe the constellation of severe metabolic abnormalities that may arise in AN as a result of rapid weight restoration (42). These complications are more likely to occur with parenteral and enteral refeeding than with oral refeeding but are risks in any severely malnourished patient. In severely starved patients with a BMI (measured as weight in kilograms divided by the square of the height in meters) of 14 or lower, refeeding should be initiated gradually, starting with 1200 to 1500 kcal/day and advancing to 3500 kcal/day in increments no larger than 500 calories every 2 to 3 days (43). The initial diet should be low in salt, lactose, and fat to minimize malabsorption and edema.

Severe hypophosphatemia, a serious potential complication of refeeding and a hallmark of the refeeding syndrome, results from the intracellular shift of serum phosphate needed for the regeneration of adenosine triphosphate, 2,3-diphosphoglycerate, and glycerol-3-phosphate involved in cellular anabolic processes. Hypophosphatemia is associated with cardiac and neuromuscular dysfunction and with hematologic red and white blood cell dysfunction. Intracellular shifts in potassium and magnesium leading to low serum levels of these two electrolytes contribute to an increased risk of cardiac arrhythmia, as well as to gastrointestinal and neuromuscular complications. Rapid extracellular fluid expansion resulting in peripheral edema is common in malnourished patients during early refeeding; and in extreme cases, congestive heart failure is a risk. Abrupt cessation of laxative or diuretic abuse and vomiting behavior can contribute to fluid retention. Patients who purge using these techniques tend to have chronically elevated aldosterone levels from metabolic alkalosis induced by volume depletion, which may take several weeks to normalize (44). Finally, severely underweight patients are at risk of Wernicke encephalopathy related to thiamin deficiency. Thiamin supplementation intramuscularly or intravenously before refeeding in severely starved patients is recommended (45).

TREATMENT

AN and BN are behavioral disorders and, like addictions, once established, tend to take on a life of their own. Although certain stressors and risk factors are associated with their onset, disordered eating patterns eventually sustain themselves. Initial treatment goals include normalizing eating patterns and restoring weight in underweight patients by using behavioral psychotherapeutic interventions. Starvation perpetuates a preoccupation with food (34), and weight restoration is well established as necessary, if not sufficient, for recovery from AN (46). Similarly, in BN, repeated engagement in the restrict-binge-purge cycle exacerbates symptomatic preoccupations with weight and shape and the drive to diet. Psychotherapy aimed at elucidating underlying individual vulnerabilities to these disorders may provide a meaningful narrative to patients to help them understand the development of their disorder, but it is unlikely to bring about behavioral change. Therefore, primarily insight-oriented approaches are best reserved for a later stage in treatment once eating behavior has been normalized.

Patients with AN or BN tend to be ambivalent about treatment because they experience their dieting behaviors as rewarding and do not want to stop them. Successful treatment can be seen as requiring a cognitive shift or conversion, from viewing dieting as a solution to seeing it as the primary impairment to healthy function. Treating clinicians often find themselves in a battle of wills with patients who deny or minimize the severity of their problems. Motivating patients with AN or BN to change their behavior requires significant role induction and the building of a strong therapeutic alliance between clinician and patient. The clinician is faced with the task of repeatedly confronting the patient about the self-destructive consequences of his or her behavior in the presence of the patient's resistance to change.

Evidence-Based Treatment

To date, the most comprehensive practice guidelines for the treatment of eating disorders are those of the American Psychiatric Association (46) and the National Institute for Clinical Excellence (47). Decisions about the appropriate setting for treatment and the introduction of pharmacotherapy should be made by professionals familiar with these guidelines who are able to assess psychiatric, behavioral, and medical factors associated with eating disorders. Treatment often requires collaboration and close communication within a multidisciplinary team, which may include psychiatrists, general practitioners, psychologists, social workers, professional counselors, nutritionists, nurses, and/or occupational therapists.

Outpatient Treatment

Randomized clinical trials provide strong empirical evidence in support of cognitive behavioral treatment (CBT) of eating disorders, particularly for BN and BED (47) with early response to treatment being the best predictor of good outcome at 1 year (48). CBT involves several components: (a) normalization of eating behavior, (b) self-monitoring and maintaining of food records, (c) correcting cognitive distortions that sustain disordered eating habits, and (d) relapse-prevention techniques. Interpersonal psychotherapy (IPT), a treatment that focuses on maladaptive interpersonal patterns and relationships, is an effective alternative to CBT for treatment of both BN and BED; however, IPT is typically of longer duration and has fewer studies supporting its efficacy in comparison with CBT.

In contrast with BN and BED, a paucity of controlled research addresses the outpatient treatment of AN. One exception is adolescent AN of short duration. This subset of patients has been found to respond best to outpatient family therapy that instructs parents to take control of their child's food intake (49). Family therapy is equally effective whether the patient is treated separately from his or her parents or conjointly as a family, although parent training and separated family therapy techniques are easier to learn and disseminate among clinicians than conjoint family therapy (50, 51). In the case of adult AN, evidence-based trials of outpatient interventions are scant and are plagued by methodologic problems such as high dropout rates. Furthermore, outpatient trials have been ineffective at achieving weight restoration in this population. A double-blind controlled trial of CBT for relapse prevention in AN, however, suggests that once weight is restored in an inpatient setting, follow-up outpatient CBT is more effective than nutritional counseling in preventing relapse at 1-year follow-up (52).

Inpatient Treatment and Partial Hospitalization

The presence of comorbid psychiatric problems, dangerously low BMI, metabolic complications or abnormalities, suicidality, pregnancy, type 1 diabetes, or self-injurious behaviors often warrant inpatient hospitalization in patients with eating disorders (46). Most patients admitted to inpatient specialty units for eating disorders have AN, because uncomplicated BN is usually treatable in an outpatient setting. Only those patients with BN who are treatment resistant or who have serious medical or psychiatric comorbidity are likely to be admitted as inpatients. Although few randomized clinical trials exist, naturalistic studies have yielded certain conclusions about the efficacy

of acute inpatient treatment for AN. Behavioral units are well established in achieving rapid weight restoration in severely underweight patients on the order of 2 to 4 lb/week (~1 to 2 kg/week) (43, 46). The less structured partial hospital setting also can be effective for weight restoration; however, rates of weight gain are slower, averaging 0.5 to 2 lb/week, and some patients may not be treatable in this setting because of compliance problems. Partial hospital treatment also can be useful when applied in a stepdown sequence as a transitional level of care between inpatient and weekly outpatient treatment. In this model, inpatient treatment is used to block eating disorder behaviors and establish healthy eating patterns, and patients are then given increasing levels of independence over eating as they make the transition to a less restrictive setting.

Medications

The role of pharmacotherapy in the treatment of eating disorders is limited. Most randomized controlled trials are of short duration, and many lack adequate follow-up data. Although several agents have been found useful, especially for the treatment of BN and BED, no agent to date has been conclusively shown to assist patients with AN to gain weight outside the setting of a structured inpatient behavioral refeeding program. Preliminary open-label and uncontrolled studies suggest that the atypical antipsychotics, olanzapine in particular, may hold promise in acutely underweight patients with AN (53). Very few medication trials have assessed the utility of medication for relapse prevention following inpatient behavioral weight restoration. One small randomized, controlled study suggested that fluoxetine may be helpful in preventing relapse in weight-restored patients with AN (54); however, a larger multisite study failed to replicate this finding (55).

In the case of BN, several controlled studies have found that antidepressants are helpful in decreasing urges to binge and purge, although their effect is usually smaller than that of CBT. The best studied antidepressant in BN is fluoxetine, which, at high doses of 60 to 80 mg/day, was found superior to placebo in decreasing bulimic behaviors (56). Lower doses are ineffective, however, and few patients achieve abstinence with medication alone. Importantly, it appears that the antibulimic effect of fluoxetine is independent of its antidepressant effects.

In the case of BED, the anticonvulsant topiramate was found to be effective in decreasing both binge frequency and weight in patients with BED (57). However, this agent is poorly tolerated and has frequent, uncomfortable side effects, including paresthesias and mental confusion as well as a risk of metabolic acidosis and oligohidrosis.

Role of the Nutritionist

In the case of both AN and BN, education about normal eating should include instruction on scheduling three regular meals a day, eating normal portion sizes, expanding food repertoire (which is often very narrow), and avoiding diet foods. Patients should be encouraged to consume all foods in moderation and in normal combinations and to avoid fat-free or sugar-free diet products. An exception to the latter may be the case for patients with BED or BN who are overweight. These patients are likely to benefit from additional guidance on eating fewer high-calorie, high-fat foods; introducing more fruits, vegetables, and whole-grain unprocessed foods; increasing the water density of foods consumed; and engaging in a regular exercise program as well as decreasing sedentary activities, such as watching television. Vegetarianism that develops after the onset of dieting behavior is common in both AN and BN and should be discouraged because it is often used to disguise dieting. Careful questioning usually reveals that preferred vegetarian foods are limited to those low in calories.

Instruction in the diabetic exchange system as a method of estimating portion sizes is easily adapted to the treatment of eating disorders, and this system is useful in teaching portion sizes without focus on calorie counting. Patients with BN or BED should be instructed to eat approximately 2000 kcal/day with an initial goal of weight maintenance. Although most patients with BN are dissatisfied with their body shape and want to lose weight, it is important to stress that interrupting bulimic behavior and weight maintenance are the initial goals of treatment. Restricting intake in the service of weight loss is likely to exacerbate bingeing behavior unless the bulimia is in remission for 6 months or more. In the case of BED, many clinicians believe that behavioral weight loss management strategies can exacerbate bingeing unless they are introduced after a normal eating pattern is established. Data on very-low-calorie diets and behavioral weight loss strategies in BED currently are mixed, although some studies suggest that the combination of CBT and behavioral weight loss strategies may prove effective when instituted in a complementary fashion.

Patients with AN who need to gain weight should be instructed to consume the same normal, healthy, 2000-cal diet plus three high-calorie liquid supplements between meals, totaling an additional 1000 to 1500 kcal/day to gain weight. These supplements should be thought of as "prescribed medication." On a diet of 3000 to 3500 kcal/day, patients should be able to gain 1 to 4 lb/week. While on this weight-gain diet, patients should stop all exercise, or they will be unlikely to gain weight. For severely underweight persons with a BMI of 14.5 or lower, calories may need to be titrated more slowly to minimize the risk of refeeding edema (see the earlier section on refeeding complications). Compulsive weighing should be discouraged, and patients should be instructed to limit weighing to weekly sessions with a nutritionist or therapist. This allows the patient the opportunity to discuss and process her reactions to any change in her weight with her clinician. The treating clinician should instruct patients on how to keep a food log and should review food diaries weekly because self-monitoring is one of the most effective tools in achieving behavioral change. In the case

of both AN and BN, patients are strongly motivated to restrict their intake to low–calorie density foods and are fearful of gaining weight.

Persistent encouragement, persuasion, and guidance to change dietary patterns usually are necessary to achieve behavior change in this population. Gastrointestinal symptoms and complaints of nausea, heartburn, abdominal pain, gas, and constipation are common during the early stages of refeeding (58). These symptoms are believed to be secondary to the delayed gastric emptying and gastric transit times or gastroesophageal reflux disease that are common consequences of purging and starvation in eating disorders. Education and reassurance that these symptoms will resolve over several weeks of refeeding is critical to improving patient compliance with the prescribed diet.

The outpatient treatment of eating disorders often requires a multidisciplinary approach and initially may involve weekly meetings with a nutritionist, an eating disorder therapist, and a physician. Excellent communication among clinicians is essential to this team approach, and clinicians must be alert to the potential for "splitting" in the service of the eating disorder. This occurs when patients distort the recommendations of one clinician in their report to another member of the team.

Enteral and Parenteral Feeding

AN is characterized by refusal to eat rather than by inability to eat or a nonfunctional gastrointestinal tract. Therefore, oral feeding is the safest method of weight restoration from both a physiologic standpoint and because this disorder is marked by narrowing of the food repertoire and conditioned avoidance of high-calorie density foods. The variety of foods consumed at discharge from inpatient specialty treatment was shown to be related to outcome (59). These data, together with clinical experience, suggest that repeat exposure to diverse foods of differing calorie density and normalization of eating patterns are important components of treatment. Although supplemental nocturnal nasogastric feeding has been advocated by some to boost weight gains achieved by oral feeding in a behavioral inpatient program (60), it has not been shown to result in rates of weight gain that match those of expert behavioral oral refeeding programs (61, 62). When access to a specialized behavioral inpatient eating disorders program is limited, however, an attempt at enteral feeding for severely underweight individuals who fail to gain weight with oral feeding may be warranted. The use of total parenteral nutrition (TPN) has been described as a means of supplementation for AN patients who are refusing oral or nasogastric feeding. However, TPN should be reserved for patients with severe gastrointestinal complications that preclude the normal functioning of the gastrointestinal tract, because severely cachectic patients are immunocompromised and at elevated risk of sepsis or opportunistic infections, such as candidiasis, with TPN (63). TPN has further been shown to impair gastric emptying and gut motility, which are often already disrupted in this population (63), and it is associated with gut atrophy (64). Finally, both TPN and enteral feeding incur greater risk of refeeding syndrome than oral feeding and both fail to address the restricted eating repertoire and avoidance of high-calorie foods that are hallmarks of anorectic eating behavior. Therefore, the use of TPN or enteral feeds should be considered only as a temporary measure to achieve a medically stable weight before transfer into a specialized behavioral treatment program.

Prognosis and Outcomes

Outcome studies of AN and BN suggest that approximately 50% of patients with eating disorders recover fully, 25% to 30% improve significantly, and 15% to 20% continue to have unrelenting eating disorders following treatment, with mortality rates ranging from 1% to 13% in AN and 0% to 3% in BN (65, 66). Naturalistic studies reveal that the risk of relapse in these disorders is substantial, and recovery is characterized by a fluctuating course with frequent readmissions and exacerbations (67). Less is known about the long-term outcomes of BED treatment; however, the disorder appears to be unstable, waxing and waning with and without treatment and responding well to placebo and wait-list conditions (68).

OTHER PSYCHIATRIC CONDITIONS AFFECTING FOOD INTAKE

Mood Disorders

Although significant changes in body weight are commonly associated with eating disorders, it is not uncommon for individuals who are clinically depressed to lose or gain weight. Major depression is characterized by depressed mood and diminished interest in pleasurable activities accompanied by changes in sleep patterns, difficulty concentrating, loss of libido, lack of energy, feelings of worthlessness or guilt, thoughts of death or suicide, and a disturbance in appetite (1). Children who are depressed often present as irritable, instead of sad and tearful, and may fail to gain weight as expected.

In contrast to eating disorders, changes in appetite that occur during depressive episodes are not driven by fear of fatness and obsession with dieting and food. Rather, depressed individuals frequently report that they have lost interest in eating and tend to identify their weight loss as a problem. These individuals are less likely to become distressed over the thought or reality of resuming normal eating and may even express a desire to do so. Furthermore, their eating pattern does not reflect the restriction of fats, sweets, and high-calorie foods that is typical of AN. Rather, they just eat less and describe losing a taste for food. Eating patterns in this population also may reflect decreased consumption of fish, fruits, and vegetables possibly because of decreased motivation to cook or prepare foods (69).

Not all depressed individuals report decreased appetite, and some display a marked increase in appetite and cravings and complain that they find themselves coping with sadness by overeating and indulging in high-calorie foods. A past history of food deprivation or self-imposed caloric restriction has been found to moderate the likelihood of overeating during an acute episode of a mood disorder (70, 71) and there appears to be a complicated bidirectional association between obesity and depression. Both longitudinal and cross-sectional data link depression to increased lifetime risk of obesity in women; however, the reverse is also true, with obesity being predictive of a future depressive episode (72).

Besides depression, adjustment disorders in response to acute stressors and grief reactions also can be characterized by transient anorexia or loss of appetite accompanied by weight loss.

Schizophrenia

Schizophrenia is a psychotic disorder often characterized by delusions, hallucinations, disorganized speech and behaviors, and affective flattening (1). Individuals frequently become paranoid in response to delusional thoughts, which are erroneous, often bizarre, perceptions of reality that are strongly held, even in the presence of clear contradictory evidence. Although the content of delusions may include a variety of themes, they sometimes involve food or eating. An example of a delusion involving food or eating includes a person's belief that his or her food is contaminated or that he or she is being watched while eating. Such paranoid thinking often results in refusal to eat and, in turn, significant weight loss. Psychiatric management, which includes antipsychotic medication, supportive psychotherapy, and family-based interventions, is commonly recommended for individuals exhibiting delusional and other psychotic symptoms. Cessation of delusional thinking is often necessary for behaviors, such as eating and self-care, to improve.

Substance Use Disorders

Substance use disorders also can affect weight and eating. The effect of different substances on food intake varies depending on substance class and level of use. Substance dependence is characterized by tolerance, withdrawal, extensive and persistent use, functional impairment, and continued use in the presence of physical and psychologic consequences (1). Substance abuse lacks the tolerance and withdrawal that characterize substance dependence, but includes significant adverse and harmful substance–related consequences, such as legal problems or failure to meet social obligations. Substance intoxication is a more acute reversible psychologic and behavioral reaction to a substance and does not necessarily imply frequent and persistent use.

Marijuana use is associated with increased appetite and food intake, and symptoms of cannabis withdrawal include increased irritability, depression, and decreased food intake (73). Alcoholism is associated with abnormal consummatory behaviors and susceptibility to overweight, obesity, and eating disorders (74). Patients with severe alcoholism may eat sporadically and obtain most of their caloric intake from alcohol, resulting in nutritional deficiencies, including risk of Wernicke-Korsakoff syndrome from inadequate thiamin intake. Whereas obesity is prevalent among individuals with a history of significant alcohol consumption, overweight is uncommon in the advanced stages of alcoholism, during which multiple, often irreversible, organ dysfunction is accompanied by severe illness, weight loss, and malnutrition. Cocaine and other amphetamines stimulate the central nervous system and usually decrease appetite and food intake, resulting in weight loss, which can be severe at times. Occasionally, individuals with an eating disorder may abuse these substances to lose weight.

Drug-induced disturbances in food intake are unlikely to be reversed without significant changes in substance use. Therefore, treatment of substance-induced effects on appetite is secondary to treatment of substance dependence, abuse, and intoxication.

Attention Deficit Hyperactivity Disorder

With a prevalence of 2% to 18%, attention deficit hyperactivity disorder (ADHD) is one of the most common psychiatric conditions seen in childhood (75, 76). The cause of ADHD is presumed to be multifactorial, with contributions from both genes and environment (77). One environmental factor that may play a role in the onset or maintenance of ADHD is diet. The popular notion that high-sugar diets worsen or precipitate ADHD was first proposed in 1922 (78). However, a review of double-blind, placebo-controlled studies evaluating the effects of sugar intake on child behavior does not support this hypothesis (79). Another popular view, first introduced by Ben Feingold in the 1970s, concerns the putative effect of food additives, including artificial food colorings on child behavior (80). Unlike with sugar intake, evidence linking artificial food colorings to worsening of ADHD symptoms in children is growing. A 2005 metaanalysis of double-blind, placebo-controlled trials suggested that, for children with ADHD, artificial food colorings worsen ADHD symptoms (81). The mechanism by which this could occur is uncertain. Azo dyes promote urticaria in some individuals, and the effect of histamine release on the central nervous system has been postulated as a mediator for symptomatic worsening in children with ADHD (77). Others have suggested that the orange food dye tartrazine increases urinary zinc excretion resulting in zinc deficiency. Because zinc is an essential cofactor for more than 100 enzymes, zinc deficiency interferes with cell processes relevant to healthy brain function, including serotonin and dopamine metabolism and essential fatty acid conversion pathways (76). A cross-sectional epidemiologic study found an increased odds ratio for ADHD in 14-year-old adolescents who consumed a Western dietary pattern versus a healthier pattern. The Western diet was high in processed foods containing saturated fats, refined sugars, and sodium, and low in omega-3 free fatty acids, fiber, and folate (82). This Western diet also was presumed to be higher in food additives, including artificial food colorings and preservatives, although this was not directly assessed in the study. In 2004, Jim Stevenson of the University of Southampton, United Kingdom showed that children exhibited increased hyperactivity, as assessed by parents, teachers, and trained observers, following administration of preservatives and artificial dyes. The Southampton study resulted in the British Food Standards Agency advising parents to eliminate food colorings from the diets of children who exhibit hyperactive behaviors and urging food manufacturers to remove artificial colorings from foods marketed to children. By contrast, the Food and Drug Administration never issued a similar warning regulating food colorings in foods marketed to children in the United States. A second study by Stevenson's group examined the effect of food additives on hyperactive behavior in a community sample of 3- and 8- to 9-year-old children. The study employed a randomized, double-blinded, placebo-controlled crossover trial of a food challenge containing a mix of food colorings and the commonly used preservative sodium benzoate (83). Results replicated the group's previous study supporting a role for food additives in exacerbating hyperactive behaviors (inattention, impulsivity, and overactivity) in a nonclinical community sample of young children.

Increased consumption of processed food may worsen ADHD symptoms in some children not only because of the increased intake of food additives but also because of associated nutritional deficiencies associated with a Western diet high in processed foods. Several studies have found omega-3 deficiencies in children with ADHD. Imaging studies have documented reduced blood flow to the frontal lobes in children with ADHD (84); and as optimal blood flow to the brain depends on several nutrients including omega-3 fatty acids, thiamin, pyridoxine, and folic acid, deficiencies in these compounds may account for worsening of ADHD symptoms (75). These data have raised interest in interventions employing essential fatty acid supplements (76, 85). To date however, randomized controlled trials have not convincingly demonstrated behavioral treatment effects for essential fatty acid supplementation (86). Dietary supplementation studies examining one or more micronutrients have similarly failed to yield consistent data supporting behavioral improvements in patients with ADHD (87).

Psychotropic Medications: Effects on Food Intake

Many psychopharmacologic agents used in the treatment of psychiatric disorders have effects on appetite and food intake (88). Regularly weighing patients who are taking psychotropic medications is crucial to the recognition of weight-related side effects early in treatment. If these problems arise, switching to a different agent that is weight neutral or lowering the dose can be helpful interventions and can increase patient compliance with medication. Several antidepressants, mood stabilizers, and antipsychotics are associated with weight gain and increased appetite, whereas stimulant drugs used in the treatment of ADHD tend to reduce appetite and may result in weight loss.

Among the antidepressants, the older tricyclic drugs, especially amitriptyline and imipramine, as well as the newer agent mirtazapine, are associated with the largest weight gains. The monoamine oxidase inhibitors phenelzine and tranylcypromine are less likely to be associated with weight changes but require adherence to a strict low-tyramine diet to avoid the risk of a hypertensive crisis. For this reason, the latter agents are poor choices in patients unlikely to follow a prescribed diet. The two most frequently used mood stabilizers, lithium and valproate, can both result in weight gain. Lithium also can cause fluid retention and edema in some patients. In contrast, the newer mood stabilizer, topiramate, has been associated with significant weight loss and appetite suppression, with average weight loss of 3 to 10 kg (~7 to 22 lb) over several weeks.

Several antipsychotic agents are associated with weight gain. Of the conventional neuroleptics, chlorpromazine and thioridazine have the highest rates of weight gain. Although the newer atypical neuroleptics—clozapine, olanzapine, and quetiapine—have a more favorable side effect profile in other respects compared with conventional agents, they often result in significant weight gain and can affect glucose and lipid metabolism, resulting in new-onset type 2 diabetes or hyperlipidemia. Careful baseline screening and follow-up of weight, waist circumference, fasting plasma glucose and fasting lipid profile is recommended when using these agents to monitor risk of metabolic syndrome (89).

Psychostimulant drugs used in the treatment of ADHD, including dextroamphetamine, pemoline, and methylphenidate, decrease appetite and often result in weight loss, although only a minority of patients are likely to complain of this side effect to their prescribing physician (90). Stimulants also may suppress growth and result in stunting of height when administered to children long term. All children treated with psychostimulants should be monitored regularly using developmental growth charts and periodic weight and height measurements, and a careful review of systems should be performed at each visit. Weight loss typically occurs during the first few months of treatment followed by attenuation, whereas the effects on height take at least 1 year to become fully apparent (91).

In 2002, the Food and Drug Administration approved a nonstimulant agent for the treatment of ADHD,

atomoxetine. Despite not being a stimulant, similar rates of weight loss are observed in users of this medication, although weight loss with atomoxetine may be more closely linked to gastrointestinal side effects of nausea, vomiting, and dyspepsia than to the loss of appetite itself seen with stimulants (91).

REFERENCES

1. American Psychiatric Association. Diagnostic and Statistical Manual of Eating Disorders. 4th ed. Washington, DC: American Psychiatric Association, 2000:583–95.
2. Beumont PJV, Touyz SW. Eur Child Adolesc Psychiatry 2003;12(Suppl):120S–4S.
3. Fairburn CG, Harrison PJ. Lancet 2003;361:407–16.
4. Watson TL, Andersen AE. Acta Psychiatr Scand 2003;108:175–82.
5. Walsh BT, Boudreau G. Int J Eat Disord 2003;34(Suppl):30S–8S.
6. Hoek HW, van Hoeken D. Int J Eat Disord 2003;34:383–96.
7. Lucas AR, Crowson CS, O'Fallon WM et al. Int J Eat Disord 1999;148:397–405.
8. Eckert ED, Halmi KA, Marchi P et al. Psychol Med 1995;25:143–56.
9. Shisslak CM, Crago M, Estes LS. Int J Eat Disord 1995;18:209–19.
10. Dingemans AE, Bruna MJ, van Furth EF. Int J Obes 2003;26:299–307.
11. Yanovski SZ. Int J Eat Disorders 2003;34(Suppl):117S–20S.
12. Strober M, Freeman R, Lampert C et al. Am J Psychiatry 2000;157:393–401.
13. Klump KL, Kaye WH, Strober M. Psychiatr Clin North Am 2001;24:215–25.
14. Bulik CM, Sullivan, PF, Kendler KS. Int J Eat Disord 2003;33:293–8.
15. Klien DA, Walsh BT. Int J Psychiatry 2003;15:205–16.
16. Cervera S, Lahortiga F, Martinez-Gonzalez MA et al. Int J Eat Disord 2003;33:271–80.
17. Lilenfeld LR, Kaye WH, Greeno CG et al. Arch Gen Psychiatry 1998;55:603–10.
18. Klump KL, McGue M, Iacono WG. Int J Eat Disord 2003;33:287–92.
19. Ackard DM, Peterson CB. Int J Eat Disord 2001;29:187–94.
20. Striegel-Moore RH, McMahon RP, Biro FM et al. Int J Eat Disord 2001;30:421–33.
21. Rosen JC, Compas BE, Tacy B. Int J Eat Disord 2001;29:280–8.
22. Everill JT, Waller G. Int J Eat Disord 1995;53:1–11.
23. Thompson JK, Stice E. Curr Directions Psychol Sci 2001;10:181–3.
24. Groesz LM, Levine MP, Murnen SK. Int J Eat Disord 2002;31:1–16.
25. Stice E, Maxfield J, Wells T. Int J Eat Disord 2003;34:108–17.
26. Lunner K, Werthem EH, Thompson JK et al. Int J Eat Disord 2000;28:430–5.
27. Stice E, Whitenton K. Dev Psychol 2002;38:669–78.
28. Crandall CS. J Pers Soc Psychol 1988;55:588–98.
29. Thelen MH, Cormier JF. Behav Ther 1995;26:85–99.
30. Smolak L, Levine MP, Schermer F. Int J Eat Disord 1999;25:263–71.
31. Martinez-Gonzalez MA, Gual P, Lahortiga F et al. Pediatrics 2003;111:315–20.
32. Neumark-Sztainer D, Story M, Hannan PJ et al. Int J Eat Disord 2000;28:249–58.

33. Ghaderi A. Eat Behav 2003;3:387–96.
34. Keys A, Brozek J, Henschel A et al. The Biology of Human Starvation 2. Minneapolis: University of Minnesota Press, 1950.
35. Russell GF. J Psychiatr Res 1985;19:363–9.
36. Hadley SJ, Walsh BT. Curr Drug Targets CNS Neurol Disord 2003;2:1–9.
37. Devuyst O, Lambert M, Rodhain J et al. Q J Med 1993;86:791–9.
38. Bachrach LK, Guido D, Katzman DK et al. Pediatrics 1990; 86:440.
39. Mehler PS. Int J Eat Disord. 2003;33:113–26.
40. Mattingly D, Bhanji S. J R Soc Med 1995;88:191–5.
41. Guarda AS, Coughlin JW, Cummings M et al. Eat Behav 2004;5:231–9.
42. Solomon SM, Kirby DF. JPEN J Parenter Enteral Nutr 1990; 14:90–7.
43. Guarda AS, Heinberg LJ. Inpatient and partial hospital approaches to the treatment of eating disorders. In: Thompson JK, ed. Handbook of Eating Disorders and Obesity. New York: John Wiley and Sons, 2003:297–322.
44. Schulte M, Mehler P. Metabolic abnormalities in eating disorders. In: Mehler PS, Andersen AE, eds. Eating Disorders: A Guide to Medical Care and Complications. Baltimore: Johns Hopkins University Press, 1999:76–86.
45. Winston AP, Jamieson CP, Madira W et al. Int J Eat Disord 2000;28:451–4.
46. American Psychiatric Association. Am J Psychiatry 2000; 157(Suppl):1S–39S.
47. National Institute for Clinical Excellence. Eating Disorders: Core Interventions in the Treatment and Management of Anorexia Nervosa, Bulimia Nervosa and Related Eating Disorders. Clinical Guideline 9. London: National Collaborating Center for Mental Health, 2004:1–35.
48. Fairburn CG, Agras WS, Walsh BT et al. Am J Psychiatry 2004;161:2322–4.
49. Lock J, Le Grange D, Agras WS et al. Arch Gen Psychiatry 2010;67:1025–32.
50. Eisler I, Dare C, Hodes M et al. J Child Psychiatry Psychol 2000;41:727–36.
51. Lock J, Le Grange D, Agras WS et al. Treatment Manual for Anorexia Nervosa: A Family-Based Approach. New York: Guilford Press, 2001.
52. Pike KM, Walsh BT, Vitousek K et al. Am J Psychiatry 2003; 160:2046–9.
53. Bissada H, Tasca GA, Barbar AM et al. Am J Psychiatry 2008; 165:1281–8.
54. Kaye WH, Nagata T, Weltzin TE et al. Biol Psychiatry 2001; 49: 644–52.
55. Walsh BT, Kaplan AS, Attia E et al. JAMA 2006;295:2605–12.
56. Romano S, Halmi K, Sarkar NP et al. Am J Psychiatry 2002; 159:96–102.
57. McElroy SL, Arnold LM, Shapira NA et al. Am J Psychiatry 2003;160:255–61.
58. Rigaud D, Bedig G, Merrouche M et al. Dig Dis Sci 1988; 33:919–25.
59. Schebendach JE, Mayer LE, Devlin MJ et al. Am J Clin Nutr 2008;87:810–6.
60. Robb AS, Silber TJ, Orrell-Valente JK et al. Am J Psychiatry 2002;159:1347–53.

61. Guarda AS. Physiol Behav 2008;94:113–20.
62. Attia E, Walsh BT. N Engl J Med 2009;360:500–6.
63. Melchior JC, Corcos M. J Adolesc Health 2008;44:410–11.
64. Zaloga GP. Lancet 2006;367:1101–11.
65. Agras WS, Brandt HA, Bulik CM et al. Int J Eat Disord 2004;35: 509–21.
66. Keel PK, Mitchell JE. Am J Psychiatry 1997;154:313–21.
67. Strober M, Freeman R, Morrell W. Int J Eat Disord 1997;22:339–60.
68. Stunkard AJ, Allison KC. Int J Eat Disord 2003;34(Suppl): 107S–16S.
69. Tanskanen A, Hibbeln JR, Hintikka J et al. Arch Gen Psychiatry 2001;58:512–3.
70. Van Strien T. Int J Eat Disord 1996;19:83–92.
71. Ouwens MA, van Strien T, van Leeuwe JF. Appetite 2009; 53:245–8.
72. Simon GE, Von Korff M, Saunders K et al. Arch Gen Psychiatry 2006;63:824–30.
73. Haney M. J Clin Pharmacol 2002;42(Suppl):34S–40S.
74. Thiele T, Navarro M, Sparta DR et al. Neuropeptides 2003;37:321–37.
75. Cruz NV, Bahna SL. Pediatr Ann 2006;35:744–5,748–54.
76. Sinn N. Nutr Rev 2008;66:558–68.
77. Stevenson J, Sonuga-Barke E, McCann D et al. Am J Psychiatry 2010;169:1108–15.
78. Shannon WR. Am J Dis Child 1922;24:89–94.
79. Wolraich ML, Wilson DB, White JW. JAMA 1995;274: 1617–21.
80. Feingold MJ. Am J Nurs 1975;75:797–803.
81. Schab DW, Trinh NHT. J Dev Behav Pediatr 2004;25:423–34.
82. Howard AL, Robinson M, Smith GJ et al. J Atten Disord 2011;15:403–11.
83. McCann D, Barrett A, Cooper A et al. Lancet 2007;370: 1560–67.
84. Bradley JD, Golden CJ. Clin Psychol Rev 2001;21:907–29.
85. Curtis LT, Patel K. J Altern Complement Med 2008;14: 79–85.
86. Raz R, Gabis L. Dev Med Child Neurol 2009;51:580–92.
87. Sinn N, Bryan J. J Dev Behav Pediatr 2007;28:82–91.
88. Vanina Y, Podolskaya A, Sedky K et al. Psychiatr Serv 2002;53:842–7.
89. Marder SR, Essock SM, Miller AL et al. Am J Psychiatr 2004; 161:1334–49.
90. Cascade E, Kalali AH, Wigal SB. Psychiatry (Edgmont) 2010; 7:13–5.
91. Vitiello B. Child Adolesc Psychiatr Clin North Am 2008;17: 459–74, xi.

SUGGESTED READINGS

American Dietetic Association. Nutrition intervention in the treatment of anorexia nervosa, bulimia nervosa, and eating disorders not otherwise specified (EDNOS). J Am Diet Assoc 2001;101:810–9.

American Psychiatric Association Work Group on Eating Disorders. Practice guidelines for the treatment of patients with eating disorders (revision). Am J Psychiatry 2000;157(Suppl):1–39.

Keys A, Brozek J, Henschel A et al. The Biology of Human Starvation. Minneapolis: University of Minnesota Press, 1950.

97 NUTRITION, DIET, AND THE KIDNEY[1]

JOEL D. KOPPLE

[1]Abbreviations: **aBW**, actual body weight; **ACE**, angiotensin-converting enzyme; **ACEI**, angiotensin-converting enzyme inhibitor; **AKI**, acute kidney injury; **Apo**, apolipoprotein; **ARB**, angiotensin receptor blocker; **BMI**, body mass index; **CKD**, chronic kidney disease; **CPD**, chronic peritoneal dialysis; **CRF**, chronic renal failure; **CRP**, C-reactive protein; **CVVH**, continuous venovenous hemofiltration; **CVVHD**, continuous venovenous hemofiltration with concurrent hemodialysis; **DRI**, dietary reference intake; **ESRD**, end stage renal disease; **GFR**, glomerular filtration rate; **GH**, growth hormone; **HDL**, high-density lipoprotein; **ICU**, intensive care unit; **IDL**, intermediate-density lipototein; **IGF-I**, insulinlike growth factor-I; **IL**, interleukin; **KDOQI**, Kidney Disease Outcome Quality Initiative; **LDL**, low-density lipoprotein; **Lp(a)**, lipoprotein (a); **LPD**, low-protein diet; **MD**, maintenance dialysis; **MDRD**, Modification of Diet in Renal Disease; **MHD**, maintenance hemodialysis; **NKF**, National Kidney Foundation; **nPNA**, protein equivalent of total nitrogen appearance; **PEM**, protein-energy malnutrition; **PEW**, protein-energy wasting; **PTH**, parathyroid hormone; **RDA**, recommended dietary allowance; **SUN**, serum urea nitrogen; **TGF-β**, transforming growth factor-β; **TLC**, Therapeutic Lifestyle Changes; **TNF-α**, tumor necrosis factor-α; **TPN**, total parenteral nutrition; **UNA**, urea nitrogen appearance; **VLDL**, very-low-density lipoprotein;.

KIDNEY FUNCTION

The kidney has three primary functions: excretory, endocrine, and metabolic. All three functions may be impaired in renal disease and may affect the patient's nutritional status and management. When injury, necrosis, and scarring of the renal parenchyma cause a loss of renal function, the quantity of the substances that are filtered by the kidney falls. However, many aspects of renal function undergo adaptive changes that preserve homeostasis and minimize the derangements in plasma and tissue concentrations of substances that normally are excreted by the kidney. Prominent among these adaptions are nephron hypertrophy and an increase in blood flow and glomerular filtration rate (GFR) in those nephrons that are still functional. Chronic kidney disease (CKD) has been classified into five stages, as shown in Table 97.1 (1).

Water and many organic compounds and minerals accumulate in renal failure (2). Low-protein diets (LPDs), various minerals, and other compounds reduce accumulation of many of these substances. Eventually, renal failure may become so severe that the aforementioned adaptive mechanisms are no longer adequate to maintain homeostasis,

failure in animals and humans, particularly, but not only, in diabetic patients (83–87). ACEIs and ARBs reduce urinary protein excretion in patients with kidney disease and reduce or abolish microalbuminuria in diabetic and nondiabetic patients (88, 89). Aldosterone increases activity of enzymes in the kidney as well as other organs. These changes engender activation of some cytokines that promote renal fibrosis and collagen matrix formation (90).

Medications that block binding of aldosterone to aldosterone receptors reduce proteinuria in rats and people with CKD and slow progression of CKD in rats (91, 92). The effects of these blockers on progression of CKD in humans are not well established; patients receiving aldosterone receptor blockers must be monitored for hyperkalemia induced by these blockers (91, 92). Antihypertensive medicines also slow progression of CKD by reducing blood pressure.

Human Studies on the Effect of Dietary Therapy on Progression of Chronic Renal Failure

To what extent are the animal data applicable to patients? From the mid-1970s to the present, many, but not all, dietary studies in humans with renal insufficiency have indicated that a low intake of dietary protein and phosphorus will retard the rate of progression of renal failure (93–104). Some evidence indicates that a low protein and phosphorus intake may each act separately to slow progressive renal failure (61). The earlier studies of this question in humans suffered from one or more major defects in experimental design. Later studies, in general, were better designed. Diet studies generally evaluated low-protein, low-phosphorus diets that provide about 0.40 to 0.60 g protein/kg body weight/day or a very LPD containing about 0.28 g/kg/day (e.g., ~16 to 25 g protein/day). This latter diet was supplemented with 10 to 20 g/day of the nine essential amino acids or of mixtures of several essential amino acids and ketoacid or hydroxyacid analogs of the other essential amino acids (93, 95–98, 100, 103). These diets were compared with either a more liberal diet containing approximately 1.0 g or more of protein/kg/day and more phosphorus or to an ad libitum diet.

The ketoacid or hydroxyacid analog is structurally identical to its corresponding essential amino acid, except that the amino (NH_2) group attached to the second (α) carbon of the amino acid is replaced with a keto group or hydroxy group, respectively. The ketoacid and hydroxyacid analogs can be transaminated in the body to the respective amino acids, although a proportion of the analogs are degraded rather than transaminated. Because the ketoacids and hydroxyacids lack the nitrogen containing amino group on the α carbon, these compounds provide the patient with a lesser nitrogen load. Because they are degraded in the body, they should engender fewer waste products that normally accumulate in renal failure. Ketoacid analogs of the branched-chain amino acids, especially of leucine, may be

somewhat more likely to promote protein anabolism, possibly by decreasing protein degradation (105, 106).

The largest and most intensive examination of whether low-protein, low-phosphorus diets retard the rate of progression of renal disease was the National Institutes of Health–funded Modification of Diet in Renal Disease (MDRD) Study (103, 104). This project investigated, in an intention-to-treat analysis, the effects of 3 levels of dietary protein and phosphorus intakes and 2 blood pressure management goals on the progression of CKD. A total of 840 adults with various types of renal disease, but excluding diabetes mellitus, were divided into 2 study groups according to their GFR.

In Study A, 585 patients with a GFR, measured by iodine-148 iothalamate clearances, of 25 to 55 mL/1.73m^2/ minute were examined. Patients were randomly assigned to either a usual-protein, usual-phosphorus diet (1.3 g/kg standard body weight/day of protein and 16 to 20 mg/kg/ day of phosphorus) or to a low-protein, low-phosphorus diet (0.58 g/kg/day of protein and 5 to 10 mg/kg/day of phosphorus) and also to either a moderate or strict blood pressure goal: mean arterial blood pressure 107 mm Hg (113 mm Hg for those ≥61 years of age) or 92 mm Hg (98 mm Hg for those ≥61 years of age). Study B included 255 patients with a baseline GFR of 13 to 24 mL/1.73 m^2/ minute. Patients were randomly assigned to the low-protein, low-phosphorus diet or to the very-low-protein, very-low-phosphorus diet (0.28 g/kg/day of protein and 4 to 9 mg/kg/day of phosphorus) with a ketoacid-amino acid supplement (0.28 g/kg/day). They were also randomly assigned to either the moderate or strict blood pressure control groups, as in Study A. The adherence to the dietary protein prescription in the different diet groups was good (103).

Among participants in Study A, those prescribed the LPD had significantly faster declines in GFR during the first 4 months than those assigned to the usual-protein diet. Thereafter, the rate of decline of the GFR in the low-protein, low-phosphorus group was significantly slower than in the group fed the usual-protein, usual-phosphorus diet. Over the course of the entire treatment period, there was no difference in the overall rate of progression of renal failure in the two diet groups. However, it is likely that the initial greater fall in GFR in the patients prescribed the LPD may reflect a hemodynamic response to the reduction in protein intake rather than a greater rate of progression of the parenchymal renal disease. This response could in fact be beneficial, reflecting a reduction of intrarenal hyperfiltration and intrarenal hypertension. If this explanation is correct (and it is not proven that it is correct), the subsequently slower rate of progression of disease after the first 4 months of dietary treatment is consistent with a beneficial effect of this intervention on the renal disease. In Study B, the very LPD group had a marginally slower decline of GFR than the LPD group; the average rate of decline did not differ significantly between the two groups ($p = .066$).

In the MDRD Study, the very-low-protein ketoacid-amino acid supplemented–diet was not compared with the usual protein intake. Moreover, it is possible that the lack of significant effect of the LPD on the progression of renal failure could reflect the rather short mean duration of treatment in the MDRD study—2.2 years. Indeed, if the trend toward slower progression of renal failure in the LPD groups that was present at the termination of the MDRD study had persisted during a longer follow-up period, a statistically significantly slower progression would have been observed with the 0.60 g/kg protein diet in Study A and the very-low-protein, ketoacid-amino acid–supplemented diet in Study B. Several other characteristics of the patient population and study design of the MDRD may have led to the lack of a statistically significant difference in progression of renal failure between the diet groups (107).

It is also reported that vegetarian LPDs providing soy protein may retard progression of CRF more effectively than diets of similar protein content that contain animal protein (52, 108, 109). The mechanisms of such an effect is not known, but it may be related to the total content and different composition of fats in the vegetarian diet. The vegetarian diet is reported to improve the serum lipid profile in patients with CKD and the nephrotic syndrome (109, 110).

Several published metaanalyses have evaluated clinical trials of the effects of LPDs on the rate of progression of kidney failure. In general, the LPDs were also low in phosphorus. These metaanalyses each evaluated a somewhat different series of clinical trials, only some of which included the MDRD study (111–114). Three of the metaanalyses used, as the key outcome, the onset of end stage renal disease (ESRD) as determined by the patient with CRF who is starting treatment with MHD or CPD or receiving a kidney transplant (111, 112, 114). These metaanalyses reported statistically significant reductions in the relative risk of a patient with CRF assigned to the LPDs reaching this end point to 0.54, about 0.67, and 0.61, respectively. One metaanalysis used the rate of decrease in GFR as the key outcome (113). This last study described a slowing in the progression of renal failure of only 6% which, although statistically significant, was of questionable clinical significance.

The discrepancy between these two sets of findings may be explained in part by the fact that ingestion of LPDs leads to a reduction in the generation of metabolic products of protein and amino acids, and that some of these metabolic products are toxic. Indeed, patients ingesting LPDs are reported to be started on MHD or CPD at lower GFRs than are individuals with higher protein intakes. The fact that LPDs may ameliorate uremic symptoms and delay the need to inaugurate dialysis treatment or renal transplantation can be considered to be an advantage in itself to these LPDs, even if the degree of delay in the rate of progression of CKD is not very large. In this regard, in another study, elderly patients with GFRs of 5 to 7 mL/minute/1.73 m^2 were randomly assigned to treatment with MD or with a very-low-protein ketoacid-amino acid diet. The latter patients were treated with the ketoacid diet for 1.0 to 58.1 months (median, 10.7) (115). The patients who were assigned to the ketoacid diet appeared to fare as well clinically and nutritionally as did those who were assigned initially to MD.

The foregoing metaanalyses also examined clinical trials that used an intention-to-treat type of analysis, whereby the data from individuals assigned to a given dietary intake were included in the results, whether or not they adhered to the dietary prescription or even were available for follow-up testing. Thus, these studies do not rule out the possibility that people who adhere closely to these LPDs may not have a significant delay in the rate of progression of their CKD.

Another metaanalysis analyzed the results of five prospective clinical trials of the effects of LPDs on progression of renal failure in patients with insulin-dependent diabetes mellitus (112). This analysis indicated that LPDs also retard progression in these individuals. However, the results were much less definitive because smaller numbers of patients were analyzed; two of the trials had no randomized, concurrent control group, and the key end points were less definitive.

In a secondary analysis of Study B, in which the decrease in GFR was correlated with the actual quantity of protein ingested, there was no effect of ingesting the LPD versus the very LPD supplemented with ketoacids and amino acids on the progression of renal failure (104). However, in Study A, when the data from the two groups were combined and then analyzed, there was a significant inverse relationship between the protein intake actually ingested, as determined from the urea nitrogen appearance (UNA) (see later), and the rate of decline in GFR (104). The actual dietary protein intake associated with the lowest rate of decline in GFR was about 0.62 g/kg/day. More recently, at least one other small-scale randomized controlled study compared treatment with a very-low-protein, ketoacid-amino acid–supplemented diet to a 0.6 g/day protein diet in patients with CKD. The results indicated that the ketoacid diet was more effective at slowing progression of CKD (116).

The mechanism of action by which ketoacid diets retard progression of renal failure is unclear. Studies suggest that alkalinization of the urine can retard the progression of renal failure (117–119). Because ketoacids in the dietary supplements are present as alkaline salts, perhaps it is the alkali in these supplements that actually retards progression of renal failure, if the rate of progression is indeed slowed.

A 12-year follow-up analysis was conducted in the Study A MDRD patients concerning the hazard ratio, adjusted for baseline characteristics, of developing ESRD or a combination of either ESRD or all-cause mortality (120). ESRD was defined as commencing MD therapy or receiving a kidney transplant. This study indicated that during the first 6 years after the onset of the dietary protein prescription, there was a statistically significant adjusted lower hazard ratio of incurring ESRD, or the combination of either ESRD or mortality in those assigned to the 0.60 g protein/kg/day diet versus those assigned to the 1.3 g protein/kg/day diet (120). This difference tended to reverse itself in the second 6-year period of follow-up.

In Study B patients, those assigned to the ketoacid supplemented diet had a significantly greater hazard ratio, adjusted for baseline factors, for death after they developed ESRD during the 12 years after assignment to their diet prescription (121). These data are particularly intriguing because patients were treated in the study, on average, only for the first 2.2 years of follow-up and were then referred back to their usual physicians. Moreover, with few exceptions, ketoacid mixtures were not available to patients in the United States after the MDRD Study ended. Thus, the Study B patients could not have taken ketoacids during most of this 12-year observation period. A rather large, retrospective study from France did not confirm any difference in long-term mortality rate in patients with CKD who are prescribed ketoacid diets (122). However, this study compared survival of these former patients with survival data from the French dialysis registry and with patients who underwent transplant procedures in Bordeaux. It is possible that the patients who agreed to take the ketoacid diets were a more motivated, capable, disciplined, and healthier group of individuals; and one could imagine that, all else equal, their survival rate should be greater than that of the average French dialysis patient.

The Nurses' Health Study compared spontaneous protein intakes of individuals with different levels of GFR, determined from their serum creatinine concentrations (123). In this study, 1624 women, aged 42 to 68 years, had their protein intake measured in 1990 and again in 1994 using a semiquantitative food frequency questionnaire. Those women with mildly reduced baseline estimated GFR levels that were greater than 55 mL/minute/1.73 m^2 but less than 80 mL/minute/1.73 m^2 showed a fall in GFR of -1.69 mL/minute/1.73 m^2 per 10-g increase in protein intake. However, after adjustment for measurement of error, the change in estimated GFR was -7.72 mL/minute/1.73 m^2 per 10-g increase in protein intake. This association was of borderline statistical significance. A high intake of nondairy animal protein in people with mild renal insufficiency was associated with a significantly greater fall in estimated GFR (-1.21 mL/minute/1.73 m^2 per 10-g increase in nondairy animal protein intakes). A retrospective study in renal transplant recipients indicated that those recipients who spontaneously ingested higher protein diets experienced greater losses of GFR (124).

Taken together, the post hoc analysis of the MDRD Study data, the results of the approximately 12 years of follow-up to the MDRD Study, the Nurses' Health Study, the study in renal transplant recipients, the four metaanalyses, and the newer randomized ketoacid studies all point to the probability that LPDs will retard the rate of progression of renal failure in individuals with CKD. Moreover, because these LPDs often engender sufficiently lower uremic toxicity for a given level of reduced renal function, patients fed these diets may be able to avoid MHD, CPD, or renal transplantation at GFR levels that would require individuals ingesting higher protein intakes to commence such therapy.

An interesting question is whether LPDs may prevent or retard the development of renal failure in individuals with no underlying renal disease. At the present time, there are no clear answers to this question.

Another unresolved issue is whether LPDs will retard progression of renal failure in patients receiving ACEIs and/or ARBs. Because dietary protein restriction exerts many of the same hemodynamic and other physiologic effects on the kidney as do ACEIs and ARBs (44, 45, 125), it is possible that the renal-protective effects of LPDs, when combined with ACEIs and ARBs, are replicative, rather than additive. In a rather small study, 82 patients with type 1 diabetes mellitus were randomly assigned to an LPD (0.60 g protein/kg/day) or a more usual-protein diet (126); most of the patients were receiving ACEIs. In this 4-year trial, the low-protein group experienced a 10% incidence of death or ESRD as compared with 27% in the patients eating the usual-protein diet ($p < .042$). There was no difference in the rate of decline in GFR in the 2 groups (126).

Because proteinuria is associated with greater progression of renal failure and increased risk of cardiovascular disease, and because ACEIs and ARBs, even in combination, and blood pressure lowering may reduce proteinuria but not eradicate it, there may be a role for LPDs at least in persistently proteinuric patients. More research in this area is clearly needed.

NUTRITIONAL ALTERATIONS IN THE NEPHROTIC SYNDROME

The nephrotic syndrome is a kidney disorder characterized by losses of large quantities of protein in the urine ($\geq$3.0 g/day), low serum albumin concentrations, high serum levels of cholesterol and other fats, and accumulation of excess body water to form edema (127). This condition is caused by diseases that affect the glomerulus and increase glomerular permeability to protein. Because patients with the nephrotic syndrome have large urinary protein losses and their appetite is frequently poor, they often develop protein wasting and debility. Certain vitamins and most trace elements are protein bound in plasma, and these patients are therefore also at risk for developing deficiencies of these nutrients when these proteins are lost in the urine. Excessive urinary iron, copper, and vitamin D losses and vitamin D deficiency have been reported in patients with the nephrotic syndrome (127, 128). Malnutrition may occur in nephrotic patients even when they do not have advanced kidney failure. For a given type of renal disease, heavy proteinuria is associated with more rapid progression of renal failure, possibly because of the incorporation of proteins into the glomerular mesangium that may cause sclerosis or inflammatory responses (129). Many growth factors and other bioactive substances are also bound to proteins that are filtered by the leaky glomerulus in patients with the nephrotic syndrome. It is postulated that some of these bioactive compounds, when filtered and exposed to the renal tubular lumen or renal interstitium, may promote progressive renal damage (130). As indicated earlier, protein-restricted diets, ACEIs, ARBs, and aldosterone receptor antagonists may each reduce renal losses of protein (131–134). Using these medicines in nephrotic patients to reduce proteinuria while maintaining a sufficiently high protein intake to increase both albumin and total body protein mass may be desirable.

NUTRITIONAL AND METABOLIC CONSEQUENCES OF CHRONIC RENAL FAILURE

CRF causes pervasive nutritional and metabolic disorders that may affect virtually every organ system. These abnormalities are reviewed briefly.

Clinical, Nutritional, and Metabolic Disorders

Advanced CRF is a complex disorder caused by a marked reduction in the excretory, endocrine, and metabolic functions of the kidney. Patients with CRF eventually develop uremia, which refers to the accumulation of nitrogenous metabolites in the blood in combination with the clinical signs and symptoms of advanced renal failure. Most of these compounds are products of amino acid and protein metabolism. Quantitatively, the most prominent are urea, creatinine, other guanidine compounds and uric acid (Fig. 97.1). It is generally believed that some of these compounds are toxic in high concentrations.

The many signs and symptoms of uremia include weakness, a feeling of ill health, insomnia, fatigue, loss of appetite, nausea, vomiting, weight loss, diarrhea, itching, muscle cramps, hiccups, twitching or jerking of the extremities, fasciculations, tremors, emotional irritability, and decreased mental concentration and comprehension. A characteristic fetid breath, caused at least partly by exhalation of methylamines, is often present.

Altered serum concentrations of other electrolytes and acidemia (excessive accumulation of hydrogen ion in the blood) can occur and can have profound and life-threatening effects on the physiologic processes and metabolism of the body (see Fig. 97.1). Abnormalities in water and electrolyte balance and acidemia are caused by impaired ability of the failing kidney to regulate, by excretion, the content of water, salts, and acids in the body. The sodium and water disturbances associated with renal

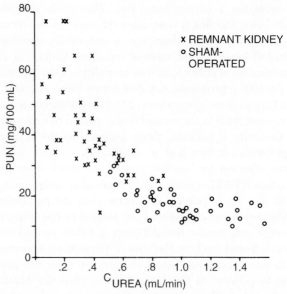

Fig. 97.1. Relationship between plasma urea nitrogen (PUN) and the glomerular filtration rate as indicated by urea clearance in Sprague-Dawley rats with chronic renal insufficiency and sham-operated controls. Chronic renal failure was produced by ligation of two thirds to three fourths of the arterial supply to the left kidney and contralateral nephrectomy. (Reprinted with permission from Kopple JD. Nutrition and the kidney. In: Alfin-Slater BB, Kritchevsky D, eds. Human Nutrition: A Comprehensive Treatise. Vol 4. New York: Plenum Publishing, 1979:409–57.)

failure can lead to congestive heart failure and hypertension or, if excessive sodium depletion occurs, reduction in extracellular fluid volume and a fall in blood pressure. When renal failure is not in the end stage or nearly so, most of these clinical and metabolic disorders can be ameliorated or prevented with dietary and medicinal therapy. Untreated uremia can lead to lethargy, loss of consciousness, coma, convulsions, and death.

Advanced CRF causes pervasive alterations in the absorption, excretion, or metabolism of many nutrients. These disorders include the following: accumulation of chemical products of protein metabolism (2), a decreased ability of the kidney either to excrete a large sodium load or to conserve sodium rigorously when dietary sodium is restricted (135); impaired renal ability to excrete water, potassium, calcium, magnesium, phosphorus, trace elements, acids, and other compounds; a tendency to retain phosphorus (136–140); decreased intestinal absorption of calcium (137) and possibly iron (140); and a high risk for developing certain vitamin deficiencies, particularly vitamin B_6, vitamin C, folic acid, and the most potent known form of vitamin D, 1,25-dihydroxycholecalciferol (138, 141). The patient with CRF is also likely to accumulate certain potentially toxic chemicals, such as aluminum, that normally are ingested in small amounts and excreted in the urine (140).

Uremia is also a polyendocrinopathy, and many of the metabolic and clinical manifestations of uremia are caused by the endocrine disorders. Many hormone concentrations are elevated in renal failure, particularly those of the peptide hormones, because of the impaired ability of the kidney to degrade peptides. These elevated peptide hormones include PTH, leptin, glucagon, insulin, growth hormone (GH), prolactin, luteinizing hormone, often follicle-stimulating hormone (FSH), and gastrin (137, 142–150). Increased secretion of some hormones, such as PTH and insulin, may contribute to elevated plasma levels. Patients with CRF have altered thyroid hormone levels that are similar to the euthyroid sick syndrome, but hypothyroidism is not common (151). Of the hormones elaborated by the kidney, plasma erythropoietin and 1,25-dihydroxycholecalciferol are reduced (5–8, 138); and plasma renin activity may be increased, normal, or decreased.

Serum GH is elevated, and IGF-I levels are usually normal in renal failure, but there is resistance to the activity of both GH and IGF-I (152, 153). Sensitivity to glucagon is reversed by hemodialysis, although hyperglucagonemia persists (143). Resistance to the peripheral action of insulin occurs (154). These effects on insulin and glucagon contribute to the mild glucose intolerance usually present in nondiabetic patients with CRF (144). Obesity, which is common in patients with CKD, may contribute to glucose intolerance. Impaired actions of hormones in uremia may result from circulating inhibitors in serum, down-regulation of receptor number, or postreceptor defects in the signal transduction system. Cytosolic calcium participates in certain cell signaling systems. Elevated basal cytosolic calcium, induced by hyperparathyroidism, appears to be one of the postreceptor signal transduction disorders induced by CRF (155).

Most of the products of metabolism that accumulate in renal failure do so as the result of decreased excretion. The ability of the failing kidney to synthesize or metabolize many compounds, including amino acids, is also impaired. In CRF, the kidney displays reduced catabolism of glutamine, impaired synthesis of alanine, and decreased conversion of glycine to serine and citrulline to urea (156, 157). Serum and tissue taurine levels are often low.

Quantitatively, the most important end product of nitrogen metabolism is urea (158). In a clinically stable patient with CRF who eats at least 40 g of protein per day, the net quantity of urea produced each day contains an amount of nitrogen equal to about 80% to 90% of the daily nitrogen intake. Guanidines are the next most abundant end product of nitrogen metabolism. Guanidino compounds include creatinine, creatine, and guanidinosuccinic acid (2, 158). Many polypeptides and small proteins also accumulate in CRF (158). Most certainly, many compounds contribute to uremic toxicity. Prime suspects for uremic toxins include urea, guanidine compounds, phenolic acids, proinflammatory cytokines, carbonyl compounds, oxidants (see later), and some of the hormones elevated in uremic plasma, especially PTH and possibly glucagon (2, 143, 155, 158–160).

Altered gastrointestinal function may affect nitrogen metabolism in patients with CRF. The gastrointestinal tract metabolizes urea, uric acid, creatinine, and choline and synthesizes or releases from larger molecules dimethylamine, trimethylamine, ammonia, sarcosine, methylamine, and methylguanidine and certain tryptophan metabolites (158). The gut metabolism or synthesis of many of these compounds is increased in CRF, possibly because of the rise in the quantity of intestinal bacterial flora (161).

Some of the metabolic alterations in uremia are adaptive homeostatic responses that offer both benefits and disadvantages to the patient (159). Hyperparathyroidism is an example. As the kidneys fail, impaired excretion of phosphorus leads to phosphorus retention. Concomitantly, the diseased and scarred renal parenchyma is less able to convert 25-hydroxycholecalciferol to the most potent metabolite of vitamin D, 1,25-dihydroxycholecalciferol, a powerful suppressor of PTH secretion (138). Low plasma concentrations of 1,25-dihydroxycholecalciferol lead to an increase in PTH secretion.

In addition, deficiency of 1,25-dihydroxycholecalciferol both impairs intestinal calcium absorption and causes resistance to the actions of PTH in bone (137, 138). These alterations also promote hypocalcemia and contribute to the development of hyperparathyroidism. Elevated serum PTH reduces renal tubular reabsorption of phosphorus (enhancing urine phosphorus excretion), lowers serum phosphorus, promotes renal synthesis of 1,25-dihydroxycholecalciferol, mobilizes calcium from bone, and increases intestinal calcium absorption, although intestinal calcium absorption usually remains low or, in mild renal insufficiency, normal. The benefits derived from these homeostatic actions are that more normal concentrations of plasma phosphorus and calcium are maintained in patients with mild to more advanced renal insufficiency. The trade-off is the development of hyperparathyroidism (159, 160). PTH has been implicated as a pervasive uremic toxin that adversely affects many organs and tissues and contributes to the uremic syndrome (160). Fibroblast growth factor-23 (FGF23) is another hormone that regulates phosphorus homeostasis by reducing renal tubular phosphorus reabsorption and promoting urinary phosphorus excretion (139). Anemia, which usually is primarily, but not exclusively, the result of impaired erythropoiesis caused by deficiency of erythropoietin, can be treated effectively with this hormone (8). To reduce the risks of adverse events, including possibly higher mortality, and the high costs of therapy, sufficient erythropoietin is usually given to raise the hemoglobin levels only to the currently recommended levels of about 11 to 12 g/dL (162, 163). Large doses of iron are usually given intravenously to patients undergoing MD and orally or intravenously to patients with CKD, to attain a higher serum total iron binding saturation. Erythropoietin and other erythropoiesis-stimulating agents are expensive and, in large doses, possibly hazardous medications, and these higher serum iron levels will often decrease the amount of these medications needed to maintain target hemoglobin levels (164).

When kidney failure is a complication of an underlying systemic disease, such as diabetes mellitus, hypertension, or lupus erythematosus, other manifestations of these underlying diseases may also adversely affect the patient and may be progressive. All of these problems do not seriously affect every patient, and many patients with CRF or who are undergoing dialysis lead full and productive lives.

With the institution of dietary therapy or treatment with MHD or CPD, blood levels of many metabolic products that accumulate in uremic plasma decrease, and the patient may experience clinical improvement. MHD or CPD enables patients to live for many years with essentially no renal function. Despite such improvement, however, many clinical and metabolic disorders may persist or even progress. These include the following: oxidative and carbonyl stress; an inflammatory state; type IV hyperlipidemia and other disorders of lipid metabolism (165, 166); a high incidence of cardiovascular, cerebrovascular, and peripheral vascular disease (167); osteodystrophy with disordered bone architecture, osteoporosis, or osteomalacia (aluminum toxicity often contributes to the osteomalacia) (137, 168); anemia (6–8); impaired immune function and decreased resistance to infection; mildly impaired peripheral and central nervous system function; muscle weakness and atrophy; frequent occurrence of viral hepatitis (169); sexual impotence and infertility; generalized protein-energy wasting (PEW) (170–178); a general feeling of ill health or emotional depression; and poor rehabilitation (179). Most of these complications can be aggravated by poor nutritional intake or improved with good nutrition.

The foregoing considerations indicate that the intestinal absorption, excretion, and/or metabolism of virtually every nutrient may be altered in CRF. In addition, the decreased intake of food and excessive intake of certain minerals, such as phosphorus, sodium, or potassium, may alter clinical or nutritional status. Moreover, medicinal therapy may adversely affect nutrient metabolism in renal failure. For example, anticonvulsant medications may cause deficiencies of vitamin D and folic acid; hydralazine, isoniazid, and other medications may cause vitamin B_6 deficiency (180). Part of the challenge of dietary therapy for such patients is to provide for the altered requirements and tolerance of many nutrients that occur in CRF.

Protein-Energy Wasting

Patients with CRF, and particularly in those undergoing MHD or CPD, frequently show evidence of wasting and particularly PEW (see Table 97.2). The term PEW is used because not all causes of PEW are the result of inadequate nutrient intake (170–178, 181, 182).

Evidence for PEW includes decreased relative body weight (i.e., the patient's body weight divided by the weight of physiologically normal people of the same age, height, sex, and skeletal frame size); body mass index (BMI);

skinfold thickness (an estimate of total body fat); arm muscle mass; total body nitrogen and potassium; subjective global nutritional assessment (SGA); low growth rates in children; decreased serum concentrations of many proteins including albumin, transthyretin (prealbumin), and transferrin; and low muscle alkali-soluble protein. The plasma amino acid pattern, which is pathognomonic for renal failure, also has similarities to that found in malnutrition.

The findings of PEW are sometimes observed in nondialyzed patients with CRF, but they are more prevalent in patients undergoing MHD or CPD. Not every dialysis-treated patient has evidence for these disorders; however, virtually every survey of patients undergoing MD indicates that these patients have an increased prevalence of PEW (170–178, 181). PEW is only mild to moderate in most dialyzed patients with this condition. About 6% to 8% of dialysis-treated patients have severe wasting. In addition to PEW, patients with CRF are at higher risk for malnutrition of iron, zinc, and certain vitamins, including vitamin B_6, vitamin C, folic acid, 1,25-dihydroxycholecalciferol, and possibly carnitine and often other nutrients (183–188).

There are many causes of wasting in CRF (Table 97.3) (171). First, dietary intake is often inadequate, particularly for energy requirements (170, 175, 189, 190). The low dietary intake is mainly the result of anorexia. This is caused by uremic toxicity, a CRF-related inflammatory state, the anorexigenic effects of acute or chronic superimposed illnesses, and emotional depression. Associated illnesses may also impair the patient's physical ability to procure, ingest, or digest foods or to receive or use tube feeding. In addition, the dietary prescription in renal failure, which is low in protein and other nutrients and may be difficult to prepare or be unpalatable, can lead to low nutrient intakes.

Second, the superimposed illnesses that patients with CRF frequently sustain often induce a catabolic state (191–193). Third, the dialysis procedure itself may induce wasting. Hemodialysis and peritoneal dialysis removes free amino acids, peptides or bound amino acids (194–197), water-soluble vitamins (141), proteins (with peritoneal dialysis and, to a much lesser extent, with hemodialysis) (195, 198), glucose (during hemodialysis with glucose-free dialysate) (199), and probably other bioactive compounds. Hemodialysis also increases net protein breakdown, especially by activating the complement cascade system and inducing release of catabolic cytokines (see later) (200, 201). Fourth, excessive accumulation of acid in blood (acidemia) engenders protein catabolism (202). Fifth, patients with CRF sustain blood losses. Because blood is a rich source of protein, these losses may contribute to protein depletion. The blood losses are caused by frequent blood drawing for laboratory testing, the common occurrence of occult gastrointestinal bleeding, and sequestration of blood in the hemodialyzer and blood tubing (203).

Other possible, but not well established, causes of wasting include the following: altered endocrine activity, particularly resistance to insulin (154), GH, and IGF-I (152, 153); hyperglucagonemia (143), hyperparathyroidism (137, 155, 159,

TABLE 97.3	EVIDENCE FOR PROTEIN-ENERGY WASTING IN PATIENTS WITH ADVANCED CHRONIC KIDNEY FAILURE[a]

Decreased
  Body weight
  Height (children)
  Growth (children)
  Body fat (skinfold thickness)
  Fat free solids
  Intracellular water
  Muscle mass (midarm muscle circumference)
  Total body potassium (nondialyzed patients)
  Total body nitrogen (patients receiving chronic peritoneal dialysis)
  Total albumin mass, synthesis, and catabolism
  Valine pools (nondialyzed patients)
  Serum
    Total protein
    Albumin
    Transferrin
    Prealbumin
    C3
    C3 activator
    Cholinesterase
  Plasma
    Leucine
    Isoleucine
    Total tryptophan
    Valine
    Tyrosine
    Valine/glycine ratio
    Essential/nonessential ratio
  Muscle
    Alkali-soluble protein
    RNA/DNA ratio
    Valine
    Tyrosine
Normal to increased
  Plasma
  Glycine

[a]Patients with chronic renal failure may have normal values for these parameters, but statistical comparisons indicate that the levels are often abnormal in these individuals.

160), and possibly deficiency of 1,25-dihydroxycholecalciferol (137); endogenous uremic toxins; exogenous uremic toxins, such as aluminum; and loss of metabolic functions of the kidney. Because the kidney is a metabolic organ that synthesizes or degrades many biologically valuable compounds, including amino acids (156, 157), the loss of these activities in kidney failure could possibly disrupt the body's metabolism and promote wasting.

Inflammation and Oxidant and Carbonyl Stress in Chronic Renal Failure and Patients Undergoing Maintenance Dialysis

Patients with CRF and those undergoing MD frequently show evidence of inflammation. This evidence includes increased serum levels of such acute phase proteins as C-reactive protein (CRP), serum amyloid A, and ceruloplasmin. Serum levels of negative acute phase proteins,

including albumin, transferrin, transthyretin (prealbumin), and cholesterol-carrying lipoproteins may decrease not only as a result of PEW but also as a direct result of inflammation (190, 204–210). Most surveys suggest that serum CRP levels are increased in about 30% to 50% of US and European MHD-treated patients and perhaps lower in Asian MHD-treated patients (207). Serum proinflammatory cytokines, including tumor necrosis factor-α (TNF-α), interleukin-1 (IL-1), and IL-6, are commonly elevated in patients with advanced CRF (207). In patients with advanced CRF and those receiving MD, there is also an accumulation in serum of compounds that cause oxidant or carbonyl stress (207, 211, 212). Oxidant stress refers to cellular injury caused by exposure of the cell to compounds that oxidize chemicals in the cell (211). Carbonyl stress refers to cellular injury caused by carbon-containing compounds that react with compounds in the cell (212). Homocysteine is such a carbonyl-reactive compound that is increased in serum in patients with CRF and MD treatment and that, when elevated, exerts several adverse effects on the vascular endothelium (213–217).

Causes of inflammation in individuals with CRF include comorbid illnesses, CRF (which itself leads to an increase in serum levels of several oxidants, reactive carbonyl compounds, and proinflammatory cytokines), oxidant and carbonyl stress, chronic low-grade infections (e.g., by chlamydia), and reaction to the vascular access prostheses that are necessary to perform hemodialysis, the hemodialyzer itself, the peritoneal dialysis catheter (for CPD-treated patients) and (for MHD- or CPD-treated patients) dialyzer tubing or impure dialysate (205, 206, 210, 218)

Why Are Protein-Energy Wasting and Inflammation of Great Concern to Nephrologists?

The current high interest in PEW and inflammation stems from the fact that measures of either of these two conditions are epidemiologically linked to increased risk of morbidity and mortality in patients undergoing MD (19, 209–211, 219). Markers of inflammation have been particularly linked to atherosclerosis and cardiovascular morbidity and mortality (206–208, 217). Moreover, laboratory research indicates that certain acute phase proteins, oxidants, reactive carbonyl compounds, and proinflammatory cytokines can be directly toxic to the endothelium. These compounds may cause inflammation, cellular proliferation, and increased matrix deposition in the endothelium with the formation of inflamed atherosclerotic plaques that are likely to rupture and increase the likelihood of myocardial infarction or stroke. The increased risk of morbidity and mortality in patients undergoing MD who have PEW and/or inflammation is of particular importance because the adjusted mortality rate for MD-treated patients in the United States is very high, approximately 21% to 22% per year (193). Hence, in a population that is already at high risk for morbidity and mortality, the identification of clinical characteristics that demonstrate the presence of a subgroup of these individuals who are at even greater risk for these adverse outcomes is a cause for alarm. At the same time, it affords a potential opportunity to develop interventions that may improve such poor prognoses.

There is an overlap between the manifestations of protein-energy malnutrition (PEM) and inflammation. Thus, both PEM and inflammation display reduced serum levels of such negative acute phase proteins as albumin, transferrin, transthyretin, and cholesterol-carrying lipoproteins (204, 206, 209, 210, 218, 220). The lowest serum levels of these proteins are generally found with inflammation rather than PEM. Inflammation may cause PEM by inducing anorexia (e.g., TNF-α and IL-6 are anorexigens) and also by engendering a hypercatabolic state (206, 220–222). Whether PEM may predispose to inflammation, for example, by increasing the risk of infection or enhancing the inflammatory response to other stimuli, is not certain.

The relative contributions of PEM and inflammation to the high morbidity and mortality of patients with CRF are controversial, especially because the syndrome of PEM shares many clinical manifestations with inflammation. Because inflammatory processes may cause endothelial injury and/or predispose to atherosclerosis and vascular thrombosis, it is easy to perceive why there would be a causal connection between inflammation and morbidity and mortality from vascular disease.

These considerations have led some investigators to question whether PEM by itself is hazardous or whether it is only an important risk factor for morbidity and mortality when it occurs in association with inflammation (223). Intuitively, it seems that a nutrient intake that is inadequate to maintain a healthy quantity of body protein mass or that does not provide adequate energy must eventually place the patient at risk for increased morbidity and mortality. PEM may, among its other adverse consequences, predispose to inflammation and vascular disease. This is a question that demands further investigation. PEM and inflammation occur together so commonly in patients with ESRD that some investigators have described them as components of a single syndrome referred to as the malnutrition-inflammation complex syndrome (224).

Numerous researchers have pointed out that relationships between traditional risk factors and mortality are markedly altered or even reversed in patients undergoing MD as compared with the public at large. These altered risk factor patterns have been observed for body BMI or weight for a given height, predialysis serum total cholesterol, LDL cholesterol, and predialysis creatinine, serum urea nitrogen (SUN), UNA (net urea production; see later), blood pressure, magnitude of acidosis, and possibly serum homocysteine and PTH levels (209, 210, 219, 225–234).

Although several explanations have been advanced to explain these phenomena, the most likely mechanism is related to the malnutrition-inflammation complex syndrome (225, 227, 231, 232). Patients undergoing MD who eat inadequately, who have major comorbid conditions, or who have evidence for systemic inflammation are more likely to have low BMI, serum cholesterol, and homocysteine and also be at greater risk for mortality. Individuals who are healthier are more likely to have a greater appetite and to have a higher body weight, a greater protein intake, and hence a higher UNA and serum urea, greater metabolic acid production and metabolic acidosis, and possibly higher serum homocysteine. Serum total cholesterol and LDL cholesterol tend to be higher in healthy people who are less likely to be inflamed and also have greater food intakes. Because of their greater muscle mass and appetite, these individuals tend to have higher predialysis serum creatinine concentrations. They are less likely to suffer from cardiac pump failure and to have low blood pressures. Also, because they are healthier, they are more likely to live longer.

Survival bias may also account for some of the paradoxic risk factors (i.e., those individuals with abnormal levels of the normal risk factors may be more likely to die earlier, before they start MD therapy). These explanations cannot completely account for the altered risk factor patterns in MD-treated patients because it turns out that markedly obese individuals (those with BMI of ≥45 kg/m^2) have greater unadjusted 2-year mortality rates than those patients who are overweight or mildly obese (228, 235). Clearly, further research is needed in this area.

DIETARY MANAGEMENT OF CHRONIC RENAL DISEASE AND CHRONIC RENAL FAILURE

A recommended plan for nutrient intake is given in Table 97.4 for patients with CRF who are not undergoing dialysis therapy as well as for patients undergoing MHD or CPD. This section explains this approach to the dietary management of these patients.

General Principles of Dietary Therapy

The widespread metabolic disorders, frequent occurrence of PEW, obesity and diabetes, cardiovascular, cerebrovascular, and peripheral vascular disease, and evidence that nutrient intake may retard the progression of renal failure indicate that nutritional management is a critical aspect of the treatment of CKD. The five goals of dietary therapy are to prevent or correct PEW, to prevent or treat obesity and diabetes mellitus, to prevent or minimize uremic toxicity and the metabolic derangements of renal failure, to reduce risk of adverse cardiac and vascular events, and to retard or to stop the rate of progression of renal failure.

Adherence to specialized diets is difficult and stressful for most patients and their families. Generally, it requires patients to undergo a major change in their behavior patterns and to forsake many of their traditional sources of daily pleasure. The patient must procure special foods, prepare special recipes, usually forgo or severely limit intake of many favorite foods, and often eat foods that are not desirable. Demands are made on the time, effort, and

TABLE 97.4	RECOMMENDED NUTRIENT INTAKE FOR NONDIALYZED PATIENTS WITH CHRONIC RENAL FAILURE AND PATIENTS UNDERGOING MAINTENANCE HEMODIALYSIS OR CHRONIC PERITONEAL DIALYSIS

	CHRONIC RENAL FAILURE[a]	MAINTENANCE HEMODIALYSIS OR CHRONIC PERITONEAL DIALYSIS[b]
Protein	Low-protein diet: 0.60–0.75 g/kg/d $\geq$0.35 g/kg/d of high-biologic-value protein Where ketoacid/essential amino acid supplements are available, about 0.28 g/kg/d of these supplements may be prescribed with a very low protein diet (0.3 g/kg/d of protein of any biological quality)	Hemodialysis[b] 1.1–1.2 g/kg/d $\geq$50% high-biologic-value protein CPD 1.2–1.3 g/kg/d $\geq$50% high-biologic-value protein; Protein-energy wasted CPD patients may be given up to 1.5 g/kg/d
Energy[c]	$\geq$35 kcal/kg/d unless patient's relative body weight is >120% or patient gains unwanted weight	
Fat (% of total energy intake)[d,e]	30–40	30–40
Polyunsaturated/saturated fatty acid ratio[e]	1.0:1.0	1.0:1.0
Carbohydrates[f]	Rest of nonprotein calories	
Total fiber intake[e]	20–25 g	20–25 g
Minerals	Range of intake	
Sodium	1,000–3,000 mg/d[g]	750–1,000 mg/d[g]
Potassium	40–70 mEq/d	40–70 mEq/d
Phosphorus	5–10 mg/kg/d[h,j,k]	8–17 mg/kg/d[h,k]
Calcium	800 mg/d[i]	800 mg/d[i]
Magnesium	200–300 mg/d	200–300 mg/d
Iron	$\geq$10–18 mg/d[j]	See text
Zinc	15 mg/d	15 mg/d
Water	$\leq$3,000 mL/d usually as tolerated[g]	750–1,500 mL/d[g]
Vitamins	Diets to be supplemented with these quantities	
Thiamin	1.5 mg/d	1.5 mg/d
Riboflavin	1.8 mg/d	1.8 mg/d
Panthothenic acid	5 mg/d	5 mg/d
Niacin	20 mg/d	20 mg/d
Pyridoxine HCl	5 mg/d	10 mg/d or 5 mg/d
Vitamin B$_{12}$	3 µg/d	3 µg/d
Vitamin C	70 mg/d	70 mg/d
Folic acid	about 1 mg/d	1 mg/d
Vitamin A	No addition	No addition
Vitamin D	See text	See text
Vitamin E	15 IU/d	15 IU/d
Vitamin K	None[k]	None[k]

CPD, chronic peritoneal dialysis.

[a]GFR greater than 4 to 5 mL/1.73 m^2/minute and about 75 mL/1.73 m^2 or lower (see text).

[b]Protein intake for maintenance hemodialysis (MHD)–treated patients generally should be at or near 1.2 g/kg/day; for CPD-treated patients who are not malnourished, it should be about 1.2 to 1.3 g/kg/day.

[c]This includes energy intake from dialysate in CPD-treated patients.

[d]Refers to percentage of total energy intake (diet plus dialysate); if triglyceride levels are markedly elevated, the percentage of fat in the diet may be increased to about 40% of total calories; otherwise, 30% of total calories is preferable.

[e]These dietary recommendations are considered less crucial than the others, unless hypercholesterolemia is present (see text).

[f]Should be primarily complex carbohydrates, if tolerated by the patient.

[g]Can be higher in CPD-treated patients or in those nondialyzed patients with chronic renal failure and in hemodialysis-treated patients who have greater urinary losses.

[h]Phosphate binders are often needed as well.

[i]Dietary calcium needs vary according the patient's clinical condition and other components of the treatment regimen (see text).

[j]10 mg/day for male patients and nonmenstruating female patients; at least 18 mg/day for menstruating female patients; may be increased with erythropoietin therapy.

[k]Vitamin K supplements may be needed for patients who are not eating and who are receiving antibiotics.

emotional support system of the family or close associates. Therefore, it is incumbent on the physician not to prescribe radical changes in dietary intake without a clear indication that such changes may be beneficial to the patient. To ensure successful dietary therapy, patients with CKD must undergo extensive training in the principles of nutritional therapy and the design and preparation of diets, and they need continuous encouragement regarding dietary adherence. When nutritional intake is not carefully monitored, patients tend to adhere poorly to dietary prescriptions. They may eat too little of certain nutrients rather than too much.

TABLE 97.5   **RECOMMENDED MEASURES FOR MONITORING NUTRITIONAL STATUS OF MAINTENANCE DIALYSIS PATIENTS**

CATEGORY	MEASURE	MINIMUM FREQUENCY OF MEASUREMENT
I. Measurements that should be routinely performed in all patients	Predialysis or stabilized serum albumin	Monthly
	% of usual postdialysis (MHD) or postdrain (CPD) body weight	Monthly
	% of standard (NHANES II) body weight	Every 4 mo
	Subjective global assessment (SGA)	Every 6 mo
	Dietary interview and/or diary	Every 6 mo
	nPNA	Monthly MHD; every 3–4 mo CPD
II. Measure that can be useful to confirm or extend the data obtained from the measures in category I	Predialysis or stabilized serum prealbumin	As needed
	Skinfold thickness	As needed
	Midarm muscle area, circumference, or diameter	As needed
	Dual-energy x-ray absorptiometry	As needed
III. Clinically useful measures that, if low, may suggest the need for a more rigorous examination of protein-energy nutritional status	Predialysis or stabilized serum Creatinine	As needed
	Urea nitrogen	As needed
	Cholesterol	As needed
	Creatinine index	

CPD, chronic peritoneal dialysis; MHD, maintenance hemodialysis; NHANES, National Health and Nutrition Examination Survery; nPNA, net protein quivalent of total nitrogen appearance.

National Kidney Foundation/DOQI guidelines reproduced with permission from the editor of the American Journal of Kidney Diseases from National Kidney Foundation DOQI Clinical Practice Guidelines for Nutrition in Chronic Renal Failure. Am J Kidney Dis 35:(Suppl. 2), S1–S140, 2000.

A team approach to dietary management may improve adherence to the special diet. The team should include the physician, dietitian, close family members, nursing staff, and, where available, psychologists or social workers. Diet plans should be designed specifically for the individual tastes of the patient. A problem-oriented approach to dietary compliance can be very effective (207). At each visit, the physician should monitor dietary intake and should discuss the results with the patient. The physician must strongly support the dietitian's efforts to train and counsel the patient and to obtain dietary compliance. The patient's family and close associates can provide moral support to the patient and assist with acquisition and preparation of foods. To promote adherence to the diet, the entire medical team should assume an energetic, positive, and sympathetic approach. Research indicates that the foregoing techniques can enable many patients to attain acceptable levels of dietary compliance (236).

Patients with advanced renal failure are at particular risk for inadequate energy intake. Because the prescribed diets are often marginally low in some nutrients, such as protein, and high in others, such as energy fuels, and PEW is not infrequent, it is important periodically to evaluate the adequacy of the diet and the patient's nutritional status. Such evaluation should include assessment of protein-energy nutritional status, mineral and bone metabolism, parathyroid status and bone densitometry, risk factors for cardiovascular disease (e.g., high serum phosphorus and CRP levels), and urine albumin excretion including the presence of microalbuminuria. The National Kidney Foundation (NKF) Kidney Disease Outcome Quality Initiative (KDOQI) Clinical Practice Guidelines for Nutrition in Chronic Renal Failure recommendations for evaluation of protein-energy nutritional status in patients undergoing MD are shown in Table 97.5.

The dietitian is often best qualified to perform anthropometry. To maintain good dietary compliance and to monitor fluid and electrolyte disorders and clinical and nutritional status, it is often preferable for the physician and dietitian to see the patient with stage 3 to 5 CKD frequently, often monthly. Patients with slowly progressive mild or moderate renal insufficiency may be able to see the physician and dietitian less frequently.

Cross-sectional studies indicate that dietary protein and energy intake begin to fall and that protein-energy nutritional status begins to deteriorate when the GFR decreases to roughly one-half normal (~50 to 55 mL/minute) (237). The decline in nutritional status is gradual and usually mild to moderate until the GFR falls rather severely, to less than 10 mL/minute, and when the patient is commencing MD therapy (170, 189, 237, 238). Although nutritional status may improve during the first few months of dialysis therapy (239), the protein-energy nutritional status at the onset of chronic dialysis treatment appears to be a good predictor of both nutritional status 2 to 3 years later and of longevity (170, 240). Hence, particular effort should be made to prevent malnutrition when the patient approaches the time when dialysis should be instituted and during the first few weeks of chronic dialysis therapy. Such effort should be directed toward maintaining good nutritional intake during this period, rapidly instituting therapy for supervening illnesses, and maintaining good nutritional intake during such illnesses.

Urea Nitrogen Appearance and the Ratio of Serum Urea Nitrogen to Serum Creatinine

The control of protein intake is pivotal to the nutritional management of patients with acute renal failure or CRF. Hence, one must accurately monitor nitrogen intake. Fortunately, this is possible for most patients. Those who are in nitrogen balance should have a total nitrogen output (appearance) equal to nitrogen intake minus about 0.5 g nitrogen per day for unmeasured losses from growth of skin, hair, and nails and from sweat, respiration, flatus, and blood drawing (241). For clinical purposes, a slightly positive or negative balance does not substantially alter the use of the nitrogen output to estimate intake. If patients are in very positive or negative balance, such as from pregnancy or severe infection, nitrogen output may not reflect intake. However, it is usually readily apparent to the clinician whether the patient is in very positive or negative balance and whether the nitrogen output will reflect intake.

The measurement of total nitrogen output or appearance is too laborious and expensive to be widely applied for clinical uses. However, because urea is the major nitrogenous product of protein and amino acid degradation, the UNA can be used to estimate total nitrogen output and hence nitrogen intake (242–244). UNA refers to the amount of urea that appears or accumulates in body fluids and all outputs, such as urine, dialysate, and fistula drainage. The term UNA is used rather than urea production or generation because some urea is degraded in the gastrointestinal tract; the ammonia released from urea is largely transported to the liver and is converted back to urea (245, 246). Thus, the enterohepatic urea cycle has little effect on urea or total nitrogen economy, and this cycle can be ignored without compromising the ability of the UNA to estimate total nitrogen output or intake accurately. Moreover, the recycling of urea cannot be measured without costly and time consuming isotope studies. UNA is calculated as follows:

Equation 1:

$$\text{UNA (g per day)} = \text{urinary urea nitrogen (g per day)}$$
$$+ \text{ dialysate urea nitrogen (g per day)}$$
$$+ \text{ change in body urea nitrogen (g per day)}$$

Equation 2:

$$\text{Change in body urea nitrogen (g per day)} =$$
$$(\text{SUN}_f - \text{SUN}_i, \text{g/L per day}) \times \text{BW}_i(\text{kg}) \times (0.60 \text{ L/kg})$$
$$+ (\text{BW}_f - \text{BW}_i, \text{kg per day}) \times \text{SUN}_f(\text{g/L}) \times (1.0 \text{ L/kg})$$

where i and f are the initial and final values for the period of measurement, SUN is serum urea nitrogen (grams per liter), BW is body weight (kilograms), 0.60 is an estimate of the fraction of body weight that is water, and 1.0 is the fractional distribution of urea in the weight that is gained or lost (i.e., 100%).

The estimated proportion of body weight that is water may be increased in patients who are edematous or lean and decreased in individuals who are obese or very young. Changes in body weight during the 1- to 3-day period of measurement of UNA are assumed to results entirely from changes in body water. In patients undergoing hemodialysis, the urea concentration in dialysate is low and difficult to measure accurately, and UNA can be calculated during the interdialytic interval and then normalized to 24 hours. Because many patients undergoing dialysis have little or no urinary excretion, the equation for calculating their UNA during the interdialytic interval often can be simplified to Equation 2.

In our metabolic studies, the relationship between UNA and total nitrogen appearance (output) in chronically uremic patients not undergoing dialysis is as follows (244):

Equation 3:

$$\text{Total nitrogen appearance (g per day)} =$$
$$1.19 \text{ UNA (g per day)} + 1.27$$

If the individual is more or less in neutral nitrogen balance, the UNA also will correlate closely with nitrogen intake. Equation 4 describes observed relationships between UNA and dietary nitrogen intake in clinically stable nondialyzed, largely patients with stage 5 CRF who are in neutral protein balance.

Equation 4:

$$\text{Dietary nitrogen intake (g per day)} =$$
$$1.20 \text{ UNA (g per day)} + 1.74$$

Multiplication of equation 3 by 6.25 will convert total nitrogen output to net protein degradation (grams per day), that is, the difference between the absolute rates of body protein degradation and protein synthesis. Multiplication of equation 4 by 6.25 will convert dietary nitrogen intake to dietary protein intake (grams per day). When both nitrogen intake and UNA are known, nitrogen balance can be estimated from the difference between nitrogen intake and total nitrogen appearance estimated from the UNA. If the patient is markedly anabolic, such as from pregnancy, particularly in its later stages, equation 4 will underestimate nitrogen intake. For patients who have large protein losses, such as from nephrotic syndrome or peritoneal dialysis, or who are acidemic and have sufficient kidney function to excrete large quantities of ammonium, equations 3 and 4 will underestimate both nitrogen appearance and nitrogen intake. In most circumstances, however, these conditions are not present, and the UNA provides a powerful tool for monitoring nitrogen output and intake or estimating balance. Maroni et al and other researchers described similar techniques for monitoring these parameters (241, 243).

The relationships among the UNA, total nitrogen appearance, and dietary nitrogen intake in patients undergoing continuous ambulatory peritoneal dialysis are shown in equations 5 and 6 (244). Other researchers have described rather similar equations (247). Because protein losses in peritoneal dialysate are variable, in some equations, an independent term is added for the daily nitrogen losses from protein in peritoneal dialysate. As indicated previously, multiplication of these terms by 6.25 can convert the equations to net protein output (grams per day) or, in clinically stable patients who are in approximately neutral protein balance, to dietary protein intake (grams per day).

Equation 5:

$$\text{Total nitrogen appearance (g per day)} = 0.94 \text{ UNA} + 5.54$$

Equation 6:

$$\text{Dietary nitrogen intake (g per day)} = 0.97 \text{ UNA} + 6.80$$

The UNA (also called Gu) can be calculated in hemodialysis patients by urea kinetic modeling (242, 248). This technique essentially involves the predialysis and postdialysis SUN and body weight, the urea clearance characteristics of the dialysis, and the blood flow, dialysate flow, and duration of the dialysis therapy.

The relationships among UNA, net protein degradation, and dietary protein intake in MHD-treated patients have been described in other studies (244, 248). Net protein degradation in dialyzed patients, normalized to body weight, usually referred to as the nPNA (normalized protein equivalent of total nitrogen appearance) or nPNA (normalized protein catabolic rate) (249). A critique of the precision and reproducibility of these calculations is presented elsewhere (244, 248). The nPNA or nPCR often reported refers to net total body protein degradation, which underestimates total protein intake (compare equations 3 and 4 with equations 5 and 6).

The ratio of SUN to serum creatinine also correlates closely with dietary protein or amino acid intake in patients with CRF who are not undergoing dialysis treatment. This relationship can be used to estimate the recent daily intake of such patients. Although this ratio is not as precise as the UNA and can be influenced by certain clinical factors (250), it is easy and inexpensive to measure.

Dietary Prescription

For purposes of nutritional prescription, the body weights in this chapter refer to the standard (normal) body weights from the National Health and Nutrition Examination Survey (NHANES) data (251). An exception are individuals who are obese (e.g., >115% of standard body weight) or very underweight (e.g., <90% of standard body weight). For these patients, their adjusted actual body weight (aBW) may be used for the body weight term (252). The adjusted aBW appears to be gaining in popularity but has not yet been validated by experimental data. The aBW,

modified from an American Dietetic Association report (252), is calculated as follows:

$$\text{Adjusted aBW} = \text{standard (normal) BW} + ([\text{edema-free aBW} - \text{standard (normal) BW}] \times 0.25)$$

Protein Intake

Glomerular Filtration Rate Higher Than 70 mL/ 1.73 m^2 per Minute. Virtually no data exist concerning the optimal dietary protein and phosphorus intakes for patients with CKD and mild impairment in renal function. At present, we do not routinely restrict protein for patients with a GFR higher than 70 mL/1.73 m^2/minute except perhaps to 0.80 to 1.0 g/kg body weight/day, unless renal function is clearly declining. In the latter case, the patient is treated as indicated in the next paragraph.

Glomerular Filtration Rate 25 to 70 mL/1.73 m^2 per Minute. The studies, including the metaanalyses (see earlier), indicating that low-protein, low-phosphorus diets may retard the need for chronic dialysis, dialysis, or renal transplantation must be qualified because it is not yet certain that these diets will add additional benefits to patients receiving ACEIs and/or ARBs. On the other hand, followed properly, a high-energy diet providing 0.60 g protein/kg body weight per day is safe. This should be explained to the patient, but regardless of whether or not protein is restricted, there are many other aspects of dietary therapy that cannot be ignored. If the patient agrees to dietary therapy, a diet is offered providing 0.60 g protein/kg/day, of which at least 35 g/kg/day is high biologic value protein, to ensure a sufficient intake of the essential amino acids. This quantity of protein should maintain neutral or positive nitrogen balance (243, 244, 253, 254), and, for many patients, it should not be excessively burdensome. If this diet is too difficult to adhere to or if the patient cannot maintain an adequate energy intake with this diet, the protein intake may be increased up to 0.75 or 0.80 g/kg/day. An alternative approach is to prescribe a diet providing about 7 to 10 g/day of the nine essential amino acids and 0.50 to 0.73 g protein of miscellaneous quality/kg/day. The greater amount of low-quality protein that can be ingested with this latter diet may improve its palatability and facilitate the patient's ability to ingest sufficient energy.

Glomerular Filtration Rate Lower than 25 mL/ 1.73 m^2 per Minute without Dialysis. At this level of renal failure, the potential advantages to using a low-protein, low-phosphorus diet become more compelling. First, at this degree of renal insufficiency, potentially toxic products of nitrogen metabolism begin to accumulate in larger quantities. The LPD will generate fewer potentially toxic nitrogenous metabolites. Second, because the LPD generally contains less phosphorus and potassium, the intake of these minerals can be reduced more readily with this diet (see later sections on recommended phosphorus and potassium intakes). As a result of these first two factors, the patient may be less uremic for a given low level of GFR and may be able to delay the onset of dialysis treatments safely. As indicated earlier, these diets may also retard the progression of CKD. Third, some patients with CRF eat too little protein rather than too much. Specific training and encouragement to follow a prescribed diet may increase the likelihood that the patient will not ingest too little protein. Patients should be prescribed a protein intake as described in the previous paragraph (see Table 97.4).

Although there is a lack of evidence from the MDRD Study that the ketoacid-amino acid–supplemented very LPDs retard the rate of progression of renal failure, because such diets may not be safe (see earlier) (121), and because ketoacid-essential amino acid supplements are not currently available in the United States, they are not recommended. As indicated earlier, more recent studies suggested that the ketoacid-amino acid–supplemented very LPDs may retard progression of CKD (116). There is insufficient research experience to evaluate the potential for very LPDs providing about 0.30 g protein/kg/day supplemented with about 15 to 20 g of essential amino acids to retard progression, and these diets are therefore not currently recommended.

When the GFR falls to less than about 5 mL/1.73 m^2/minute, there is no evidence that patients fare as well with LPDs as with regular dialysis and higher protein intakes. Because patients with these low GFR levels may be at high risk for PEW and long-term sequelae of uremic toxicity (170, 189, 237, 238), it is recommended that MD treatment or renal transplantation be inaugurated at this time. Support for an alternative approach may be found in the study indicating that elderly patients with GFRs of 5 to 7 mL/minute/1.73 m^2 appear to fare as well clinically when they are fed very LPDs supplemented with a ketoacid-amino acid mix as when they are started on MD therapy with higher protein intakes (115). If patients cannot maintain a sufficiently high energy intake to maintain their body weight and there is no other identifiable cause for weight loss, chronic dialysis therapy should be considered (255). This is especially important because PEW at the commencement of MD therapy is a predictor for higher mortality.

Nephrotic Syndrome. Evidence indicates that a rather LPD (e.g., 0.80 g protein/kg/day) may slow progression of renal failure, cause a decrease in urine protein excretion, and maintain or actually slightly increase serum albumin levels (132, 133, 256). This evidence has led to recommendations for a reduction in dietary protein prescription for nephrotic patients. A vegetarian, soy-based, LPD also decreases proteinuria and serum lipid levels in nephrotic patients (108–110). Until more information is available, it is recommended that patients with the nephrotic syndrome be prescribed a diet containing about 0.70 g protein/kg/day and an additional 1.0 g/day of high biologic value protein for each gram of urinary protein lost each day above 5.0 g/day. ACEIs and ARBs reduce proteinuria

(131), lower blood pressure, retard progression of renal failure, and may protect against atherosclerotic disease and therefore should be given preference in the treatment of hypertension in these patients (84–87). LPDs, when added to ACEIs and ARBs, may further reduce proteinuria. Aldosterone receptor antagonists may also reduce proteinuria (81), but serum potassium must be carefully monitored with ACEIs, ARBs, and aldosterone receptor antagonists because these three drugs may each reduce urinary potassium excretion and cause dangerous hyperkalemia. Patients with the nephrotic syndrome should be given multivitamins, including vitamin D supplements, and must be monitored for depletion of protein and protein-bound nutrients including vitamin D analogs and trace elements.

Maintenance Dialysis Therapy. Few studies of dietary protein requirements have been conducted in patients undergoing MHD (257, 258). It seems clear that these patients have greater protein needs because of the removal of amino acids and peptides by dialysis procedures (194–196), probably as a result of inflammation and catabolic stimuli from the hemodialysis procedure, including activation of complement, and other metabolic disorders such as acidemia (201, 256). Based on available evidence from nitrogen balance studies and clinical monitoring of outpatients, the NKF KDOQI Clinical Practice Guidelines recommend that MHD patients receive 1.1 to 1.2 g protein/kg/day (see Table 97.4) (255). Our studies confirm that most clinically stable MHD patients will maintain protein balance with a diet providing an adequate energy intake and 1.0 g protein/kg/day, but a safe intake that will maintain balance in most patients probably requires about 1.15 g protein/kg/day. CPD-treated patients lose each day into dialysate about 9 g protein, a small amount of peptides, and about 2.5 to 4.0 g/day of amino acids, and they are also subjected to inflammatory and other catabolic stimuli (196, 198). Also based on nitrogen balance studies, the NKF KDOQI guidelines recommend that CPD-treated patients should be prescribed 1.2 to 1.3 g protein/kg/day (255, 259). Patients undergoing CPD who are protein depleted may be prescribed up to 1.5 g protein/kg/day. At least 50% of the daily protein intake of all patients undergoing MD should be of high biologic value.

Some physicians suggest that MHD or CPD patients may maintain their body protein mass with lower dietary protein intakes (e.g., ~0.9 g protein/kg/day). The foregoing recommendations, although based on relatively small numbers of studies, are designed to maintain good protein nutrition for most (i.e., ~97%) of patients undergoing MD. This reasoning is consistent with the deliberations used by the World Health Organization to determine the recommended dietary protein intakes for normal adults (260). Hence, although some patients may maintain good protein nutrition with lower daily protein intakes, there is no demonstrated method for identifying which individuals can maintain nitrogen balance with these lower protein diets.

Because of the high incidence of protein malnutrition in these patients (169–178, 181, 207), the higher protein intakes recommended in this chapter should be prescribed.

Consistent with the foregoing recommendations, the European Best Practice Guidelines (EBPG) Guideline on Nutrition recommends at least 1.1 g protein/kg ideal body weight/day for MHD-treated patients (261), and the Australian and New Zealand evidence based practice guidelines for the nutritional management of chronic kidney disease recommend 1.2 to 1.4 g protein/kg ideal body weight/day for clinically stable MHD patients and at least 1.2 g protein/kg ideal body weight/day for clinically stable CPD patients with at least 50% of the protein of high biologic value (262).

Energy

Studies in nondialyzed patients with CRF and those undergoing MHD indicate that energy expenditure is normal or nearly normal when patients are lying in bed, sitting, following ingestion of a standard meal, and during defined exercise (263–265). Nitrogen balance studies in nondialyzed patients with stages 4 and 5 CKD who were ingesting diets providing 0.55 to 0.60 g protein/kg/day and 15, 25, 35, or 45 kcal/kg/day indicate that the energy intake necessary to ensure neutral or positive nitrogen balance is approximately 35 kcal/kg/day (263). Similar findings were obtained in nitrogen balance studies of MHD-treated patients who were ingesting 1.1 g protein per kg per day and 25, 35, or 45 kcal/kg/day (266). However, virtually every survey of energy intake in nondialyzed patients with stage 4 or 5 CKD and in patients undergoing MHD or CPD indicates that, on average, the dietary intake is lower than this level and is usually substantially lower than 30 kcal/kg daily (267–271). In nondialyzed patients with CRF and in patients undergoing MHD, the finding that—unless they were obese before developing CRF—decreased body fat is one of the more prominent alterations in nutritional status supports the contention that these patients require more energy than they usually ingest (267, 269–271). In contrast, CPD-treated patients not uncommonly gain fat, probably because of the additional energy intake from glucose absorbed from the dialysate in the peritoneal cavity and the subsequent increase in circulating insulin levels.

The NKD KDOQI Guidelines recommend that patients up to 60 years old who are undergoing MHD and CPD should ingest at least 35 kcal/kg/day, and those who are 60 years or older should ingest 30 kcal/kg/day (255). The same energy intakes, adjusted for age, are recommended for individuals with GFR levels lower than 50 kcal/kg/day. Patients who are obese with an edema-free body weight greater than 120% of desirable body weight may be treated with lower calorie intakes. Some patients, particularly those with mild renal insufficiency and young or middle-aged women, may become obese on this energy intake or may refuse to ingest the recommended calories out of fear of obesity. These individuals may require a lower energy prescription.

Many commercially available high-calorie foodstuffs are low in protein, phosphorus, sodium, and potassium. A nephrology dietitian can recommend these foodstuffs, as well as other low-protein, high-calorie foods that can be prepared readily at home.

Lipids

Patients with stage 4 and 5 CKD and patients undergoing MHD and CPD have a high incidence of increased serum triglyceride levels, intermediate-density lipoprotein (IDL), and very-LDL (VLDL), as well as serum lipoprotein (a) Lp(a); serum high-density lipoprotein (HDL) cholesterol is often low in patients with CRF and those undergoing MHD (165, 272–276). Patients receiving CPD often have higher serum total cholesterol, triglycerides, LDL cholesterol, and apolipoprotein-B (Apo-B) levels than do patients undergoing MHD (277, 278). Qualitative changes in the apolipoprotein concentrations also occur; among these is an increase in small dense LDL (sd LDL) (279).

A major metabolic abnormality in patients with CRF and those undergoing MD is a decreased degradation rate for triglyceride-rich lipoproteins. This reduced catabolic rate leads to increased quantities of Apo-B–containing triglyceride-rich lipoproteins in IDL and VLDL and reduced concentrations of HDL. The key alteration in the apolipoprotein levels appears to be a decreased ratio of Apo-AI to Apo-CIII (280).

In addition, because diets for patients with CKD are usually restricted in protein, sodium, potassium, and water, it may be difficult for many patients to take in sufficient energy without ingesting large amounts of purified sugars that may increase triglyceride production. Activities of plasma and hepatic lipoprotein lipase and lecithin:cholesterol acyltransferase (LCAT) are decreased in CRF (281). Moreover, the actions of carnitine may sometimes be impaired (282, 283).

Patients with the nephrotic syndrome usually have hypertriglyceridemia with increased serum total cholesterol and LDL cholesterol. LDL, IDL, VLDL, and Lp(a) are increased (258), and serum HDL tends to be low. Serum, phospholipids, and Apo-B, Apo-CII, Apo-CIII, and Apo-E are increased, whereas Apo-AI and Apo-AII are normal (284). Elevated serum cholesterol is caused by increased hepatic synthesis of lipoproteins and cholesterol and reduction in LDL receptor activity, which plays an important role in the clearance of IDLs. These changes are stimulated by urinary albumin losses. Decreased activity of lipoprotein lipase contributes to the elevated serum triglyceride levels. Patients have elevated plasma cholesterol ester transfer protein (CETP) and decreased catabolism of LDL apolipoprotein, at least by the more typical receptor pathway.

Renal transplant recipients may have type IIb hyperlipidemia with high serum total cholesterol and LDL cholesterol. LDL and IDL lipoproteins are increased. Type IIa and type IV hyperlipidemia also is often present

receiving $1,25(OH)_2$ vitamin D. Another medication for treatment of secondary hyperparathyroidism in patients with stages 4 and 5 CKD and in those undergoing dialysis is cinacalcet. This medication increases the sensitivity of the calcium receptor parathyroid gland so that lower levels of serum calcium suppress PTH secretion. Cinacalcet suppresses hyperparathyroidism in patients with CRF and reduces serum calcium and phosphorus levels and the serum calcium-phosphorus product (339).

The US National Institute of Medicine proposed that the recommended dietary allowance (RDA) of vitamin D (cholecalciferol) for physiologically normal males and females from age 1 through 70 years is 600 IU/day (340). For men and women 71 years old or older, an RDA of 800 IU/day of vitamin D is proposed. These recommendations are based on the amount of dietary vitamin D, estimated from the scientific literature, to promote bone growth and maintenance in healthy people (340). Because vitamin D may have other beneficial effects, it is possible that an adequate vitamin D intake to attain these other benefits may require higher doses. This is clearly an area in need of further research.

At present, a supplement of vitamin D_3 (cholecalciferol), 800 IU/day, is recommended for patients with stage 3 to 5 CKD. Some patients do not maintain normal serum 25-hydroxycholecalciferol levels at this dose. As an alternative, one may measure serum 25-hydroxycholecalciferol levels. If they are less than 30 ng/mL (20 ng/mL to cover the needs of ≥97.5% of the general population according to the National Institute of Medicine [340]), larger doses of cholecalciferol may be prescribed, up to 1200 or even 2000 IU/day, if necessary. Some physicians prescribe vitamin D_2 (ergocalciferol) instead of cholecalciferol. Patients with stage 3 to 5 ckd may also be tested for serum 1,25-dihydroxycholecalciferol (calcitriol) levels. If low, one of the activated vitamin D sterols (calcitriol, alphacalcidol, paricalcitol, or doxercalciferol) may also be prescribed. However, these blood tests are not inexpensive. For patients with stage 5D CKD, therapy with an activated vitamin D sterol should be provided. Whether such patients with stage 5D CKD also need supplemental vitamin D_2 or D_3 is not known.

Treatment of nondialyzed patients with stage 3 to 5 CKD with calcitriol or other vitamin D sterols usually is started at 0.25 to 0.50 μg/day. The serum calcium must be monitored carefully, and if it is low and does not rise by at least 0.5 mg/dL with any particular dosage, the dose may be increased by 0.25 to 0.50 μg/day every 4 to 6 weeks. Hypercalcemia is treated by temporary withdrawal of calcitriol. Ultimately, the best criterion for effective treatment with 1,25-dihydroxycholecalciferol is improvement in bone anatomy as determined by bone histology, radiographs, and densitometry, although such monitoring is usually not necessary. Improvement in muscle function or abolition of severe hypocalcemia also may indicate appropriate dosage of calcitriol. With time, the requirements for

1,25-dihydroxycholecalciferol and the tolerance for this vitamin may decrease, and the maintenance dosage may have to be reduced. This change may occur after there has been sufficient bone healing so that the skeleton no longer serves as a sink for calcium and phosphorus.

Calcitriol should not be started if serum calcium is elevated (normal range, ~8.4 to 9.5 mg/dL), serum phosphorus is not more than slightly increased, and the calcium-phosphorus product is less than 55 mg^2/dL^2. Indications for other vitamin D sterols are described earlier. As indicated previously, serum calcium and phosphorus should be monitored during therapy to ensure that the concentrations are normal. In renal failure, many of the beneficial effects of 1,25-dihydroxycholecalciferol (calcitriol) can be reproduced by administration of other vitamin D sterols, often with less risk of hypercalcemia (see earlier).

A syndrome called aplastic or hypoplastic bone disease has been described in patients receiving chronic dialysis (137, 341–343). It is characterized by relatively low serum PTH concentrations, decreased bone osteoblasts, and marked reduction in bone turnover. The syndrome can be caused by aluminum toxicity (137, 341, 342). It is postulated that treatment with large doses of calcium binders of phosphate or vitamin D analogs with consequent suppression of PTH is a cause of this disorder (137, 341, 343).

Magnesium

People with stage 5 CRF have net absorption of approximately 50% of ingested magnesium from the intestinal tract (net absorption is the difference between dietary intake and fecal excretion) (341). The absorbed magnesium is excreted primarily by the kidney. Hence, hypermagnesemia may occur in CRF (344). Because the restricted diets of patients with CRF are low in magnesium (usually ~100 to 300 mg/day for a 40-g protein diet), serum magnesium levels are usually normal or only slightly elevated unless the patient ingests substances that are high in magnesium content, such as magnesium-containing antacids and laxatives (298, 344). Nondialyzed patients with CRF need to ingest about 200 mg/day of magnesium to maintain neutral balance (298). The optimal dietary magnesium allowance for the patient undergoing chronic dialysis has not been well defined. It is influenced by the level of magnesium in the dialysate; at current dialysate magnesium concentrations, the optimal dietary magnesium allowance is probably about 200 to 250 mg/day.

Sodium and Water

Sodium is freely filterable by the glomerulus. In the normal kidney, the renal tubules usually reabsorb well over 99% of the filtered sodium. As renal insufficiency progresses and the GFR decreases, the fractional renal tubular reabsorption of sodium also falls progressively. Thus, many patients with renal failure are able to maintain sodium balance with a normal salt intake. Normally, only about 1 to 3 mEq/day of sodium will be excreted in the feces, and in the nonsweating individual, only a few milliequivalents per day of sodium are lost through the skin. Despite an adaptive reduction in the renal tubular reabsorption of sodium, when ESRD supervenes, patients may be unable to excrete the quantity of sodium ingested, and they may develop edema, hypertension, or congestive heart failure. This syndrome is particularly likely to occur when the GFR is lower than 4 to 10 mL/minute. When renal insufficiency is complicated by congestive heart failure, the nephrotic syndrome, or advanced liver disease, the propensity for sodium retention is increased. With decreased ability to excrete sodium, restriction of sodium and water intake and the use of diuretic medications may be necessary. In renal failure, hypertension often is more easily controlled with sodium restriction and may be accentuated with increased sodium intake at least partly because of expansion of the extracellular fluid volume (345).

In addition, nondialyzed patients with stage 4 to 5 CKD often have an inability to conserve sodium normally (135, 136). A low sodium intake may not be sufficient to replace urinary and extrarenal sodium losses, and the patient may develop sodium depletion, a decrease in extracellular fluid volume, blood volume, and renal blood flow and a further reduction in GFR. Volume depletion may be difficult to recognize. An unexplained weight loss or decrease in blood pressure may be a sign of this condition. Nondialyzed patients with CRF who do not have evidence for fluid overload, hypertension, or heart failure may be cautiously given a greater sodium intake to determine whether their GFR can be improved slightly by extracellular volume expansion.

In general, when sodium balance is well controlled, thirst will regulate water balance adequately. However, when the GFR falls to less than 2 to 5 mL/minute, there is a particular risk of overhydration. In diabetic patients, hyperglycemia may also increase thirst and enhance positive water balance. For patients with far-advanced renal failure whose total body water is at the desired level (as indicated by normal or nearly normal blood pressure, absence of edema, and normal serum sodium), urine volume may be a good guide to water intake. The daily water intake should equal the urine output plus approximately 500 mL to replace insensible losses.

In most nondialyzed patients with advanced renal failure, a daily intake of 1000 to 3000 mg (40 to 130 mEq) of sodium and 1500 to 3000 mL of fluid will maintain sodium and water balance. The requirement for sodium and water varies markedly, and each patient must be managed individually. Patients undergoing MHD or CPD usually become oliguric or anuric after several weeks to 1 or 2 years of treatment. For MHD-treated patients, sodium and total fluid intake generally should be restricted to about 1000 to 1500 mg/day and 750 to 1500 mL/day,

respectively. Patients undergoing CPD usually tolerate a greater sodium and water intake because salt and water can be easily removed each day by using hypertonic dialysate, which increases the flow of water from the body into the peritoneal cavity where it can be drained. Maintaining a large dietary sodium and water intake allows the quantity of fluid removed from the CPD patient and hence the daily dialysate volume to be increased. This increase may be advantageous because the daily clearance of small molecules with CPD is directly related to the volume of dialysate outflow. In nondialyzed patients with CRF or in those undergoing MD who are not anuric and who gain excessive sodium or water despite attempts at dietary restriction, a potent loop diuretic, such as furosemide or bumetanide, may be tried to increase urinary sodium and water excretion.

Potassium

Normally, the kidney provides the major route for potassium excretion. In CRF, potassium retention may occur and may lead quickly to fatal hyperkalemia. Two factors act to mitigate this process in renal failure. First, as long as urine output remains at approximately 1000 mL/day or greater, tubular secretion of potassium in the remaining functioning nephrons tends to be increased, and therefore the renal potassium clearance does not fall as markedly as the GFR. Second, fecal excretion of potassium is increased owing to enhanced large intestinal secretion (253). Thus, patients with CRF usually do not become hyperkalemic except in the following circumstances: excessive intake of potassium; acidemia, oliguria, or hypoaldosteronism (e.g., secondary to decreased renin secretion by the diseased kidney or renal tubular resistance to the actions of aldosterone); or catabolic stress. Patients with stage 4 or 5 CKD (GFR <29 mL/minute) including those undergoing MHD, in general, should receive no more than 70 mEq of potassium per day. Some patients, particularly those with less advanced CRF, may tolerate higher potassium intakes; they may be identified by liberalizing their dietary potassium and carefully monitoring serum potassium levels. The common use of ACEIs, ARBs, and/or aldosterone receptor blockers increases the risk of hyperkalemia by reducing the secretion or actions of aldosterone. Even individuals with normal kidney function may need to restrict their potassium intake if they take these medications and develop hyperkalemia.

Trace Elements

Several factors tend to either increase or decrease the body burden of certain trace elements in patients with renal failure (346–348). Many trace elements are excreted primarily in the urine, and they may accumulate with renal failure (347, 349). Elements such as iron, zinc, and copper, which are protein bound, may be lost in excessive quantities when there are large urinary protein losses, such as in the nephrotic syndrome (349). Occupational exposure or pica may increase the burden of some trace elements. The effect of the excessive or deficient dietary intake in the patient with kidney failure on body pools of trace elements is not well understood (348). Because many trace elements bind avidly to serum proteins, when present even in small quantities in dialysate, they may be taken up into blood and cause toxicity. It is therefore recommended that, as a routine practice, dialysate should be purified of trace elements before use. In certain circumstances, therapeutic doses of trace elements may be administered through dialysis, as has been done for zinc (350). Assessment of the trace element pools in patients with renal failure is difficult because the serum binding protein concentrations or affinities for trace elements may be altered, and red cell levels of trace elements may not reflect concentrations in other tissues.

Dietary requirements for trace elements have not been well defined in uremic patients (Table 97.5). Trace element supplementation should be undertaken with caution because impaired urinary excretion of trace elements increases the risk of overdosage.

Oral iron supplements are often given to patients who are iron deficient or, as a routine treatment, for patients who have a propensity to develop iron deficiency (e.g., individuals who frequently have marginal or low serum iron, reduced percent saturation of the iron binding capacity, or decreased ferritin levels). Iron requirements increase when erythropoietin therapy is started and hemoglobin synthesis rises. Ferrous sulfate, 300 mg up to three times per day, one-half hour after meals, may be used. Some patients develop anorexia, nausea, constipation, or abdominal pain with ferrous sulfate and may tolerate other iron compounds better, such as ferrous fumarate, gluconate, or lactate. For most patients undergoing MD who are receiving erythropoietin or other erythropoiesis-stimulating agents, oral iron therapy will not maintain adequate serum iron levels; these patients may be treated with intramuscular or, more usually, intravenous iron (351, 352). The need for larger intravenous iron doses is particularly common, because somewhat more elevated serum iron concentrations reduce the doses of erythropoiesis-stimulating agents needed to maintain the same blood hemoglobin levels. As previously mentioned, ferric citrate, which has been proposed as an intestinal phosphate binder, may possibly also raise serum iron levels modestly and could supplant the need for intravenous iron in some patients with CKD (329).

The zinc content of most tissues is normal in renal failure (348), although serum and hair zinc is often low and red cell zinc is usually increased (347, 350, 353, 354). In nondialyzed patients with CRF, the fractional urinary excretion of zinc is increased; however, because the GFR is reduced, total urinary excretion of zinc tends to be normal or reduced (346). Fecal zinc is increased (353), and a dietary zinc intake greater than the dietary reference intakes (DRIs) (355) may be necessary to maintain normal body zinc pools. Further studies are needed to confirm this. Some reports indicate that dysgeusia, poor food intake, and impaired sexual function, which are common problems of patients undergoing MD, may be improved by giving patients zinc supplements (350, 353, 356, 357). Other studies have not confirmed this (303).

As previously indicated, in nondialyzed patients with CRF and in those receiving MD, increased body burden of aluminum has been implicated as a cause of a progressive dementia syndrome (particularly in patients receiving MHD), osteomalacia, weakness of the muscles of the proximal limbs, and anemia (137, 323, 324, 341, 342). Although contamination of dialysate with aluminum was previously the major source of aluminum toxicity in many dialysis centers, current methods of water treatment have removed virtually all aluminum from dialysate. At present, ingestion of aluminum binders of phosphate is probably the major cause of the excess body burden of aluminum (323, 324). Many nephrologists now use aluminum binders sparingly if at all, and rely more on low-phosphorus diets and nonaluminum phosphate binders (see earlier) to control serum phosphorus levels (330–333). Aluminum toxicity, which is no longer a common serious problem, may be treated by reduction of aluminum intake and by intravenous infusions of desferrioxamine, a chelator of aluminum (357). This chelator can be removed from the body by hemodialysis or peritoneal dialysis.

Vitamins (Other Than Vitamin D)

Patients with more advanced CKD (i.e., stages 3 to 5) are prone to deficiencies of water-soluble vitamins unless supplements are given (141). Vitamin deficiencies occur for the several reasons. First, vitamin intake is often low because of anorexia and poor food intake and also because many foods that are high in water-soluble vitamins are often restricted owing to the elevated potassium content. The typical diet for nondialyzed CRF and MD patients frequently contains less than the DRI for certain water-soluble vitamins (358, 359). Second, the metabolism of certain water-soluble vitamins tends to be altered in CRF (360, 361). Third, many medications interfere with the intestinal absorption, metabolism, or actions of vitamins (180, 200). Fourth, dialysis treatment removes water-soluble vitamins.

Vitamin B_6, vitamin C, and folic acid are the water-soluble vitamins most likely to be deficient in nondialyzed patients with CRF and in patients undergoing MD. Vitamin B_{12} deficiency is uncommon in CRF because the daily requirement is small (2.4 μg/day for nonpregnant, nonlactating adults) (359), the body can store relatively large quantities of this vitamin, and vitamin B_{12} is protein bound in plasma and hence is poorly dialyzed.

Some studies indicate that many MHD-treated patients may subsist for months with no vitamin supplementation and without developing deficiencies of water-soluble vitamins (362). However, these latter studies have not demonstrated that, without vitamin supplements, a small but substantial proportion of patients will not develop water-soluble vitamin deficiencies, particularly after 1 or more years of dialysis treatment. Because water-soluble vitamin deficiencies are caused by several different mechanisms in these patients, because vitamin deficiency may develop gradually, after months or years of dialysis treatment, and because water-soluble vitamin supplements are safe, it would seem prudent to continue to use them routinely.

Daily supplements for most vitamins are not well defined in renal failure (141). Evidence indicates that, in addition to vitamin intake from foods, the following daily supplements of vitamins will prevent or correct vitamin deficiency (see Table 97.4): pyridoxine hydrochloride, 5 mg in nondialyzed patients with CRF and 10 mg in patients undergoing MHD or CPD (363); folic acid, 1 mg; and the RDAs for physiologically normal individuals for the other water-soluble vitamins (358, 359). Patients with CRF probably require less than 1.0 mg/day of folic acid; however, because this vitamin is safe and some evidence suggests that there may be competitive interference with its actions (360, 364), it may be advisable to prescribe this dose of folic acid until more definitive studies of the requirements are carried out. A supplement of 3 μg/day of vitamin B_{12} is recommended, because this intake of vitamin B_{12} is considered safe for normal individuals and for patients with renal failure, and the RDA for vitamin B_{12} of 2.4 μg/day is therefore rounded upward.

A supplement of only 70 mg/day of vitamin C is advised. This is less than the RDA for vitamin C of 90 mg/day for men and 75 mg/day for nonpregnant, nonlactating women (358). This amount of supplemental vitamin C is recommended because ascorbic acid can be metabolized to oxalate. Large doses of ascorbic acid have been associated with increased plasma oxalate levels in patients with renal failure (365, 366). Oxalate is highly insoluble, and there is concern that high plasma oxalate concentrations may lead to its precipitation in soft tissues. In the nondialyzed patient with stage 3 to 5 CKD, it is possible that oxalate deposition in the kidney may cause further impairment in renal function. Moreover, this is the recommendation for a vitamin C supplement; patients are expected to ingest additional vitamin C with their foods.

Because serum retinol-binding protein and vitamin A are elevated in uremia (367), the routine use of supplemental vitamin A is not recommended, particularly given that even relatively small doses of vitamin A (i.e., 7500 to 15000 IU/day) may cause bone toxicity (368). Additional vitamin E and vitamin K are probably not necessary. However, patients who receive antibiotics for extended periods and who do not ingest foods containing vitamin K may need vitamin K supplements (369). The vitamin needs for people with stage 2 to 4 CKD have been reviewed (370). Unfortunately, less is known about the vitamin requirements of these individuals than of people with ESRD or who are receiving MD.

Acidosis and Alkali

Metabolic acidosis occurs frequently in nondialyzed patients with CRF because the ability of the kidney to excrete acidic metabolites is impaired. Particularly in the earlier stages of CRF or with primary tubular disorders in the kidney, metabolic acidosis can also be caused by excessive renal losses of bicarbonate. Acidosis refers to a process or processes that promote the accumulation of acid (protons) in the body; acidemia indicates an excess of protons in the blood. The rate of acid production is probably normal or lower than normal in stable patients with advanced CRF. Acidemia can cause many adverse effects (Table 97.6), including increased protein degradation, enhanced bone reabsorption and reduced bone mass, more rapid progression of renal failure, and symptoms of lethargy and weakness (117–119, 371–376)..

The NKF KDOQI Clinical Practice Guidelines both on nutrition in renal disease and on bone and mineral metabolism in renal disorder both recommend that serum bicarbonate be maintained at 22 mEq/L or higher (1, 255). However, more recent studies suggested that to prevent increased body protein losses and to retard progression of renal failure, an arterial blood pH higher than 7.36 to 7.38 and possibly as high as 7.43 to 7.45 or a serum bicarbonate of about 24 to 25 mEq/L is necessary (376).

Ingestion of low-nitrogen diets may prevent or reduce the severity of the acidosis by decreasing the endogenous generation of acidic products of protein metabolism. Alkali supplements are often necessary for preventing or treating the acidosis of CRF. Sodium bicarbonate tablets or citrate solutions such as Bicitra or Shohl solution may be taken orally in divided daily doses. In general, alkali salts containing potassium should be avoided, to prevent hyperkalemia. The dose of alkali required is not well defined. A dose of sodium citrate providing the equivalent of 1.0 mEq of bicarbonate/kg body weight/day in three divided doses was used in one study (118). In the other study, an average of about 22 mmol/day of sodium bicarbonate was given in three divided doses (119). Estimated GFR for inclusion in the first study was 20 mL/minute or more but less than 60 mL/minute; in the second study, renal function for inclusion was CKD stage 4 and 5.

TABLE 97.6	**ADVERSE CONSEQUENCES OF METABOLIC ACIDEMIA**

1. Increased protein catabolism and reduced body protein
2. Bone disease and bone loss
3. More rapid progression of kidney failure
4. Multiple endocrine disorders
5. Increased serum levels of some pro-inflammatory cytokines
6. Systemic inflammation
7. Increased β_2-microglobulin
8. Hypertriglyceridemia
9. Hypotension (with severe acidemia)
10. Malaise and weakness (with severe acidemia)

patients are receiving amino acid infusions as compared with when they are not (399, 400).

Patients with AKI who receive nutritional support may also receive hemodialysis treatment for several hours daily as often as every day rather than three times weekly, which is the usual treatment for clinically stable patients receiving MHD. If AKI persists for more than 2 to 3 weeks, patients undergoing regular dialysis treatment are often treated as are patients who are undergoing MHD, with about 1.0 to 1.2 g/kg/day of protein or amino acids for hemodialysis-treated patients or 1.2 to 1.5 g/kg/day for peritoneal dialysis–treated patients.

Other Nutritional Techniques to Reduce Hypercatabolism

Some investigators have proposed adding amino acids and additional glucose to the dialysate of patients undergoing CPD or MHD (401, 402). The nutrients diffuse into the body during dialysis. At present, these techniques may provide supplemental nutrition but cannot be used for total nutritional support.

Because the metabolic status of patients with AKI often facilitates the catabolism of protein, amino acids, and other energy substrates (384–389, 395), there may be advantages to administering agents that promote anabolic processes or reduce catabolic pathways. As mentioned previously, the nitrogen intake appears to be used more efficiently if a greater proportion of the administered amino acids is essential (387, 389, 396). This hypothesis has not yet been tested clinically. In addition, studies in catabolic patients without renal failure suggest that intravenous infusions in which a large proportion of the amino acids are composed of branched-chain amino acids (i.e., isoleucine, leucine, and valine) may have a specific anabolic effect (403, 404). Not all studies confirm these findings. Ketoacid analogs of the branched-chain amino acids have also been shown to promote anabolism both when studied in in vitro preparations and when given to nonuremic individuals who are not hypercatabolic (105, 106). The intravenous infusion of the salt complex of α-ketoglutarate and ornithine in postoperative patients receiving TPN is reported to reduce UNA and to increase nitrogen balance (405). Severely stressed patients without renal failure display a rapid fall in intracellular muscle glutamine (406). Administration of glutamine improves protein balance in these patients (406, 407). Arginine also may increase nitrogen balance (408).

Anabolic steroidal compounds, many of which are androgenic and resemble testosterone, have been used in patients with AKI (409, 410). These agents can reduce UNA and increase nitrogen balance; they also have been reported to decrease the need for dialysis treatments. In vitro studies of skeletal muscle from rats with AKI indicate that insulin may increase synthesis and reduce degradation of protein (385). Studies in catabolic patients who do not have renal failure indicate that insulin may decrease the UNA (411, 412). Insulin infusions combined with

tight glucose control in intensive care unit (ICU) patients are reported to reduce mortality (413–416). It is not clear whether this reduced mortality results from the greater amounts of glucose infused rather than from the insulin infusions and/or the tight control of blood glucose levels (414). By contrast, wider variations in blood glucose levels and more frequent episodes of hypoglycemia during insulin and glucose infusions are associated with increased mortality in ICU patients who are receiving insulin infusions with tight glucose control (413–415).

Thus, the results of randomized prospective trials on intensive insulin therapy have not been consistent, and many of the trials suggest that intensive insulin treatment (i.e., to attain a maintenance of blood glucose between 80 and 110 mg/dL) does not improve survival and may increase the risk of mortality, possibly by engendering hypoglycemia or wider variations in blood glucose. More recent guidelines suggest that for ICU patients who become hyperglycemic, blood glucose should be maintained at higher concentrations; some experts suggest blood glucose levels between 140 and 180 mg/dL (416). Algorithms are available for the employment of insulin and glucose infusions (416). Blood glucose must be monitored closely in these patients. Computerized insulin infusion algorithms may be particularly helpful (416).

Recombinant DNA–synthesized human GH has been used to improve nitrogen balance in postoperative, acutely stressed patients without renal failure, and the results have been encouraging (417, 418). This hormone has also improved nitrogen balance in stable, malnourished patients undergoing MD (419). However, individuals who are acutely stressed from infection or physical trauma or who receive low quantities of nutrients sometimes become refractory to GH, possibly because of down-regulation of GH receptors with reduced ability to express IGF-I (420). Moreover, in very ill ICU patients, the use of GH has been associated with increased mortality (421), possibly because of increased blood glucose levels engendered by the GH injections. Therefore, for the present, GH should not be given to patients who are very ill.

In rats with ischemic- or toxin-induced AKI, IGF-I may enhance recovery of renal function (422, 423). However, studies in sick ICU patients with AKI suggest that IGF-I therapy does not enhance the rate of recovery of renal function, reduce the need for dialysis treatment, or improve survival (424). Because IGF-I appears to stimulate growth of dedifferentiated cells, neither GH nor IGF-I should be given to patients with active malignant disease.

Several other growth factors—epidermal growth factor (425), hepatocyte growth factor (426), hormones (thyroxin [427], atrial natriuretic peptide) (428), or adenine nucleotides (429)—are reported to enhance recovery of renal function in experimental animals or in preliminary studies in humans. None of these agents have yet been shown to improve renal function in well-controlled clinical trials in humans with AKI.

Energy

Patients with AKI appear to have the same energy expenditure and needs as do individuals with similar types and severities of coexistent illnesses but who do not have renal failure. The exception to this is the patient with AKI who is receiving small amounts of amino acids or protein in an attempt to decrease the generation of uremic toxins and thereby reduce or avoid altogether the need for dialysis treatment (see the previous section). Studies suggest, but have not definitively demonstrated, that when small amounts of amino acids or protein are taken, higher energy intakes may enhance the efficiency of utilization of these nutrients and reduce protein wasting (383, 387, 388, 395).

In two studies of patients with AKI who were not randomized for energy intake, those who died were found to have a higher energy expenditure and more negative energy balance (383) or lower energy intake (383, 387) than those who survived. As a result of these findings, we usually administer about 30 kcal/kg standard (normal) weight per day (see Table 97.4) (251, 430), except in patients who are substantially obese (e.g., $>\sim 125\%$ standard body weight, BMI $\geq \sim 32$ kg/m^2) (222).

Higher intakes (i.e., about 35 kcal/kg/day) may be used for the patients who are treated with small amounts of amino acids or protein in an effort to avoid dialysis treatment or CVVHD three times weekly or more or who have a high energy need as estimated by the following techniques. The patient's energy needs may be estimated by multiplying the Harris-Benedict equation (431) or the World Health Organization equations (432) for calculating the daily energy requirements of normal individuals by a stress factor to adjust for the patient's illness (433) and by 1.25. This latter term (1.25) is included to ensure that a surfeit of energy is provided to promote anabolism or to diminish the rate of catabolism of the patient; the value of this term has not been clearly demonstrated. Energy expenditure, measured by indirect calorimetry, can also be multiplied by 1.25 to estimate the daily energy requirement. Some authorities recommend lower energy intakes for AKI patients, closer to 20–30 kcal/kg per day (434) although, again, large clinical trials have not tested the value of such lower intakes.

As indicated earlier, with the almost routine use of CVVHD or dialysis frequencies exceeding three times weekly to treat the hypercatabolic patient with AKI who, for example, has a systemic inflammatory response syndrome (SIRS), the amino acid or protein intakes are commonly increased to about 1.5 to 2.5 g/kg/day intakes. At this level of amino acid and protein intake, the need for an increased energy intake (e.g., determined by multiplying calculated energy needs by 1.25) may not be necessary. Unfortunately, prospective studies to test this hypothesis are not available.

Larger energy intakes are not used because there appears to be little nutritional advantage to administering more calories to catabolic patients. Indeed, because high energy intakes generate more carbon dioxide from the infused carbohydrate and fat, they can promote hypercapnia if pulmonary function is impaired (435). Carbon dioxide retention is particularly likely to occur with very high carbohydrate loads. In addition, high energy intakes may cause obesity and fatty liver (436), and they may increase the water load to the patient.

Because most patients with AKI do not tolerate large water intakes, glucose is usually administered in a 70% solution. Again, the common exception to this is the patient receiving CVVH or CVVHD or frequent hemodialysis or peritoneal dialysis. The glucose and amino acid solutions are mixed, so the amino acids and energy are provided simultaneously (see Table 97.6). Lipid emulsions should also be given. At the least, patients receiving TPN for more than 5 days should receive lipids. Patients require about 25 g/day of lipids to prevent essential fatty acid deficiency. Some investigators have recommended giving up 30% to 40% calories as lipids to provide sufficient fatty acids to organs that normally use lipids as their main energy source and to more closely approximate the normal US dietary intake. However, some researchers have reported that infusions of large amounts of fat emulsions, such as 50 g over 8 to 12 hours, may impair the function of the reticuloendothelial system (437); they have questioned whether infusion of lipid emulsions could lower host resistance. A prudent approach may be to infuse lipid emulsions over at least 12 hours, if not 24 hours, to prevent marked increases in plasma lipids. For patients who are septic or at high risk of severe sepsis, probably no more than 10% to 20% of total calories should be provided from fat. For patients who are not septic and not at high risk of infection, about 20% to 30% of calories may be given as lipid emulsions. Intravenous lipid emulsions are available in 10% (1.1 kcal/mL) and 20% (2.0 kcal/mL) solutions. With careful attention to aseptic control, the lipid emulsions may be mixed with glucose and amino acids (438).

Minerals

A mineral prescription for parenteral nutrition in acute renal failure is shown in Table 97.7. Any recommended intake of minerals is tentative and must be adjusted according to the clinical status of the patient. If the serum concentration of an electrolyte is increased, it may be advisable to reduce the quantity infused or to not administer it at the onset of parenteral nutrition. The patient must be monitored closely, because the hormonal and metabolic changes that often occur with initiation of parenteral nutrition may cause the serum electrolytes to fall rapidly. This occurrence is particularly likely for serum potassium and phosphorus. On the other hand, a low concentration of a mineral may indicate a need for greater than usual intake of that element. Again, metabolic changes and the impaired GFR can lead to a rapid rise in the serum concentrations during repletion.

Trace elements are probably not necessary in parenteral nutrition solutions given to catabolic patients with AKI unless this is the sole source of nutritional support for at least 2 to 3 weeks or the patients are known to have depletion of certain trace elements. The nutritional requirements for trace elements have not been established for AKI or CRF patients receiving TPN.

Vitamins

Vitamin requirements have not been well defined for patients with AKI. Tentative recommendations for vitamin intake for patients receiving parenteral nutrition are shown in Table 97.7. Much of the recommended intake is based on information obtained from studies in patients with CRF, physiologically normal individuals, or acutely ill patients without CRF. Vitamin A is probably best avoided for the first several days of nutritional support, because in CRF, serum vitamin A levels are elevated and small doses of vitamin A have been reported to cause toxicity in patients undergoing MD (367, 378). After the first several days of nutritional therapy, a dose of vitamin A that is between one half and the complete RDA for vitamin A (355) for normal individuals may be given daily.

Vitamin D is fat soluble, and vitamin stores should not become depleted during the few days to weeks that most patients with AKI receive parenteral nutrition. However, many normal individuals, and particularly elderly persons, have been shown to have insufficiency (15 to <30 nM) or deficiency (<15 nM) of serum 25-hydroxycholecalciferol. It may be helpful to check serum levels for this hormone in patients with AKI and give cholecalciferol or ergocalciferol supplements if serum levels are low. The turnover of the active metabolite, 1,25-dihydroxycholecalciferol (calcitriol), is much faster than 25-hydroxycholecalciferol. Hence, calcitriol may be needed in patients with AKF (336).

Although vitamin K is fat soluble, vitamin K deficiency has been reported in patients without CRF who are not eating and are receiving antibiotics (369). Vitamin K therefore should be given routinely to patients receiving parenteral nutrition (see Table 97.7). Ten milligrams per day of pyridoxine hydrochloride (8.2 mg/day of pyridoxine) is recommended because studies in clinically stable or sick patients undergoing MHD indicate that this quantity may be necessary to prevent or correct vitamin B_6 deficiency (363). Patients should probably not receive more than about 60 mg of ascorbic acid per day because of the risk of increased oxalate production (365, 366).

The nutrient intake of patients with AKI must be carefully reevaluated each day and sometimes more frequently. This reevaluation is particularly important in patients with AKI because they may undergo rapid changes in their clinical and metabolic condition.

Peripheral Parenteral Nutrition

Parenteral nutrition through a peripheral vein avoids the risks of inserting a catheter into a great vein, including the superior vena cava. If a peripheral vein is used, the osmolality of the infusate must be restricted to reduce the risk of thrombophlebitis. Thus, it is necessary to use a larger volume of fluid and/or a lower intake of nutrients. Both approaches may have undesirable consequences for patients with AKI. It has been argued that the financial cost of TPN administered through a peripheral vein is about the same as or greater than the cost of administration through a central vein because of the large quantities of isotonic lipid emulsions used to provide the energy needs when peripheral veins are used.

Peripheral partial parenteral nutrition may be advantageous for patients with AKI who are able to ingest or be tube fed only part of their daily nutritional requirements. The peripheral infusions may enable these patients to receive adequate nutrition without resorting to TPN through a large flow vein. In these patients, it is often most practical to infuse an 8.5% to 10% amino acid solution or a 20% lipid emulsion into a peripheral vein and to administer as much as possible of the other essential nutrients, including carbohydrates, through the enteral tract.

The peripheral vascular access used for hemodialysis can also be used for parenteral nutrition. Because there is a high blood flow through the vascular access used for hemodialysis, hypertonic solutions can be used, and the water load to the patient can be reduced. This technique probably increases the risk of infection or thrombosis in the vascular access, however, and it should not be used in patients who will need hemodialysis access for extended periods.

Supplemental or Intradialytic Parenteral Nutrition

Infusion of amino acids and glucose and/or lipids may be given as a nutritional supplement to patients with AKI or CRF who eat poorly. Supplemental amino acids, glucose, and/or lipids can be infused conveniently during the hemodialysis procedure. Because most patients in need of nutritional supplements have decreased intake of both amino acids and energy, the recommended approach is to infuse 40 to 42 g of essential and nonessential amino acids and 200 g of D-glucose (150 g of D-glucose if the hemodialysate contains glucose). This preparation is infused throughout the hemodialysis procedure at a constant rate into the blood leaving the dialyzer. Such a technique minimizes the normal fall in amino acid and glucose pools that occurs as a result of dialysis losses of these nutrients. Most of the infused glucose and amino acids are retained; the amino acid losses into dialysate increase by only about 4 to 5 g (194). Lipid infusions can be substituted for some of the infused glucose but are more expensive and possibly pose some risk of reducing host resistance to infection (437). Patients who have low serum phosphorus or potassium concentrations at the onset of dialysis treatment may require supplements of these electrolytes during the amino acid and glucose supplementation. To prevent reactive hypoglycemia, the infusion should not be stopped until the end of hemodialysis; and, ideally, the patient should eat a carbohydrate source 20 to 30 minutes before the end of the infusion.

It is controversial whether intravenous supplements with amino acids, glucose, and/or lipids thrice weekly for about 3 to 4 hours during hemodialysis are beneficial to patients who are undergoing MHD and who eat poorly (439). Two retrospective analyses suggest that in malnourished MHD-treated patients, intradialytic parenteral nutrition may reduce the mortality rate (440, 441). One study indicated that this benefit was observed only when the serum albumin was 3.3 g/dL or lower (441). Intradialytic parenteral nutrition should be used only in patients who cannot increase their intake of foods or take oral or enteral supplements. The intravenous supplements should be continued only if nutritional or clinical assessment indicates that these nourishments are beneficial to the patient. This is clearly an area that requires further investigation.

Amino Acids That May Predispose to Acute Kidney Injury

Several studies in rats suggest that amino acid or protein intake may increase the susceptibility to AKI caused by ischemia or aminoglycoside nephrotoxicity (442–445). The nutrients seem to increase both the incidence and the severity of AKI induced by these agents. Although some studies have demonstrated this effect with large doses of intravenous amino acids or dietary protein (442–445), the quantities of amino acids and protein that may be prescribed for patients, on a per body weight basis, can also predispose to AKI in animal studies (443, 444). D-Serine, DL-ethionine, and L-lysine appear to be particularly nephrotoxic (443, 445). It is not known whether amino acid or protein intake will predispose to AKI in humans. If either one does, then patients who receive nephrotoxic medicines or who are at high risk for renal ischemia may possibly benefit from low amino acid or protein intakes during those periods of time when they are at high risk. On the other hand, in vitro studies also indicate that some amino acids, particularly L-glycine and L-alanine, may protect renal tubular cells from ischemic or nephrotoxic injury (446). This is also an area in need of more research.

REFERENCES

1. National Kidney Foundation. Am J Kidney Dis 2003;42(Suppl 3):S1–201.
2. Lindholm B, Heimbürger O, Stenvinkel P et al. Uremic toxicity. In: Kopple JD, Massry SG, eds. Nutritional Management of Renal Disease. 2nd ed. Philadelphia: Lippincott Williams & Wilkins, 2003:63–98.
3. Takeda M, Endou H. Renal cell metabolism. In: Massry SG, Glassock RJ, eds. Massry & Glassock's Textbook of Nephrology, vol 1. 4th ed. Philadelphia: Lippincott Williams & Wilkins, 2001:110–21.
4. Hausmann MJ, Rabkin R, Dahl DC. Role of kidney in hormone metabolism. In: Massry SG, Glassock RJ, eds. Massry & Glassock's Textbook of Nephrology, vol 1. 4th ed. Philadelphia: Lippincott Williams & Wilkins, 2001:141–50.
5. Don BR, Schambelan M, Lo JC. Endocrine hypertension: effects of hormones on renal function. In: Greenspan FS, Gardner DG, eds. Basic and Clinical Endocrinology. 7th ed. New York: McGraw-Hill, 2004:414–38.
6. Hausmann MJ, Rabkin R. Kidney and endocrine system. In: Massry SG, Glassock RJ, eds. Massry & Glassock's Textbook of Nephrology, vol 1. 4th ed. Philadelphia: Lippincott Williams & Wilkins, 2001:139–230.
7. Jean G, Terrat JC, Vanel T et al. Nephrol Dial Transplant 2008;23:3670–6.
8. Wolf M, Betancourt J, Chang Y et al. J Am Soc Nephrol 2008;19:1379–88.
9. St Peter WL, Li S, Liu J et al. Pharmacotherapy 2009;29:154–64.
10. Palmer SC, McGregor DO, Craig JC et al. Cochrane Database Syst Rev 2009;(4):CD008175.
11. Palmer SC, McGregor DO, Craig JC et al. Cochrane Database Syst Rev 2009;(4):CD005633.
12. Kokko KE, Montero A, Lakkis FG et al. Hormones and the kidney. In: Schrier RW, ed. Diseases of the Kidney, vol 1. 7th ed. Philadelphia: Lippincott Williams & Wilkins, 2001:265–313.
13. Eschbach JW, Kelly MR, Haley R et al. N Engl J Med 1989;321:158–62.
14. Rabkin R, Landau, D. Effect of nutritional status and changes in protein intake on renal function. In: Kopple JD, Massry SG, Kalantar-Zadeh K, eds. Nutritional Management of Renal Disease. 3rd ed. New York: Academic Press, 2013.
15. Klahr S, Tripathy K. Arch Intern Med 1966;118:322–5.
16. Klahr S, Tripathy K, Garcia FT et al. Am J Med 1967;43:84–96.
17. Klahr S, Tripathy K, Lotero H. Am J Med 1970;48:325–31.
18. Ibrahim HN, Weber ML. Curr Opin Nephrol Hypertens 2010;19:534–8.
19. Ichikawa I, Purkerson ML, Klahr S et al. J Clin Invest 1980;65:982–8.
20. Hirschberg R, Kopple JD, Blantz RC et al. J Clin Invest 1991;87:1200–6.
21. Hirschberg R, Kopple JD. J Am Soc Nephrol 1991;1:1034–40.
22. Owen OE, Felig P, Morgan AP. J Clin Invest 1969;48:574–83.
23. Gutman AB, Yu TF. Am J Med 1968;45:756–79.
24. Bosch JP, Lew S, Glabman S et al. Am J Med 1986;81:809–15.
25. Smoyer WE, Brouhard BH, Rassin DK et al. J Lab Clin Med 1991;118:166–75.
26. Castellino P, Hunt W, DeFronzo RA. Kidney Int 1987;32(Suppl 22):S15–20.
27. Hirschberg R, Kopple JD. Kidney Int 1987;32:382–7.
28. Mitch WE, Walser M, Buffington GA et al. Lancet 1976;2:1326–28.
29. Rutherford WE, Blondin J, Miller JP et al. Kidney Int 1977;11:62–70.
30. Barsotti G, Guiducci A, Ciardella F et al. Nephron 1981;27:13–117.
31. Cotran R. Kidney Int 1982;21:528.
32. McCormack LJ, Beland JE, Schnekloth RE et al. Am J Pathol 1958;34:1011–22.
33. Kleinknecht C, Grunfeld JP, Gomez PC et al. Kidney Int 1973;4:390–400.
34. Rodriguez-Iturbe B, Garcia R, Rubio L et al. Clin Nephrol 1976;5:198–206.
35. Torres VE, Velosa JA, Holley KE et al. Ann Intern Med 1980;92:776–84.
36. Deen WM, Maddox DA, Robertson CR et al. Am J Physiol 1974;227:556–62.
37. Hostetter TH, Olson JL, Rennke HG et al. Am J Physiol 1981;241:F85–93.
38. Hostetter TH, Troy JL, Brenner BM. Kidney Int 1981;19:410–5.
39. Olson JL, Hostetter TH, Rennke HG et al. Proceedings of the American Society of Nephrology. Thorofare, NJ: Charles B. Slack, 1979:87A.

40. Olson JL, Hostetter TH, Rennke HG et al. Kidney Int 1982;22:112–26.
41. Farr LE, Smadel JE. J Exp Med 1939;70:615–27.
42. Addis T. Glomerular Nephritis: Diagnosis and Treatment. New York: Macmillan, 1948.
43. Kirsch R, Frith L, Black E et al. Nature 1968;217:578–9.
44. Brenner BM, Meyer TW, Hostetter TH. N Engl J Med 1982;307:652–9.
45. Meyer TW, Lawrence WE, Brenner BM. Kidney Int 1983;24(Suppl 16):S243–7.
46. Schrier RW, Harris DCH, Chan L et al. Am J Kidney Dis 1988;12:243–9.
47. Nath KA, Hostetter MK, Hostetter TH. J Clin Invest 1985;76:667–75.
48. Paller MS, Hostetter TH. Am J Physiol 1986;251:F34–9.
49. Williams M, Young JB, Rosa RM et al. J Clin Invest 1986;78:1687–93.
50. Wang S, Hirschberg R. J Biol Chem 2004;279:23200–6.
51. Wang S, Wilkes MC, Leof EB et al. FASEB J 1005;19:1–11.
52. Walls J, Williams SJ. Contr Nephrol 1988;60:179–87.
53. Mauer S, Steffes MW, Azar S et al. Kidney Int 1989;35:48–59.
54. Mogensen CE. Diabetes 1976;25:872–9.
55. Mogensen CE, Steffes MW, Deckert T et al. Diabetologia 1981;21:89–93.
56. Mogensen CE, Christensen CK, Vittinghus E. Diabetes 1983;32(Suppl 2):64–78.
57. Niwa T, Nagoya J. Med Sci 2010;72:1–11.
58. Niwa T. J Ren Nutr 2010;20(Suppl):S2–6.
59. Niwa T. Ther Apher Dial 2011;15:120–4.
60. Ibels LS, Alfrey AC, Haut L et al. N Engl J Med 1978;298:122–6.
61. Barsotti G, Giannoni A, Morelli E et al. Clin Nephrol 1984;21:4–59.
62. Lumlertgul D, Burke TJ, Gillum OM et al. Kidney Int 1986;29:658–66.
63. Gimenez LF, Solez K, Walker GW. Kidney Int 1987;31:93–9.
64. Harris DCH, Hammond WS, Burke TJ et al. Kidney Int 1987;31:41–6.
65. Kopple JD, Feroze U. J Ren Nutr 2011;21:66–71.
66. French SW, Yamanaka W, Ostwald R. Arch Pathol 1967;83:204–10.
67. Kasiske BL, O'Donnell MP, Schmitz PG et al. Kidney Int 1990;37:880–91.
68. Wellmann K, Wolk BW. Lab Invest 1970;22:144–5.
69. Keane WF, O'Donnell MP, Kasiske BL et al. J Am Soc Nephrol 1990;1:S69–74.
70. Kasiske BL, O'Donnell MP, Cleary MP et al. Kidney Int 1988;33:667–72.
71. Campese VM, Park J. Clin J Am Soc Nephrol 2007;2:1100–3.
72. Barcelli UO, Weiss M, Pollack VE. J Lab Clin Med 1982;100:786–97.
73. Susuki S, Shapiro R, Mulrow PJ et al. Prostaglandins Med 1980;4:377–82.
74. Knecht A, Fine LG, Kleinman KS et al. Am J Physiol 1991;261:F292–9.
75. Komers R, Meyer TW, Anderson S. Pathophysiology and nephron adaptation in chronic renal failure. In: Schrier RW, ed. Diseases of the Kidney, vol 3. 7th ed. Philadelphia: Lippincott Williams & Wilkins, 2001:2689–718.
76. Zurier RB, Damjanov O, Sayadoff DM et al. Arthritis Rheum 1977;20:1449–56.
77. Kelley VE, Winkelstein A, Izui S. Lab Invest 1979;41:531–7.
78. McLeish KR, Gohara AF, Cunning WT III. J Lab Clin Med 1980;96:470–9.
79. Rahman MA, Nakazawa M, Emancipator SN et al. Kidney Int 1986;29:343 (abstr).
80. Badr KF, Brenner BM, Wasserman M et al. Kidney Int 1986;29:328 (abstr).
81. Don BR, Blake S, Hutchison FN et al. Am J Physiol 1989;256:F711–8.
82. Anderson S, Meyer TW, Rennke HG et al. J Clin Invest 1985;76:612–9.
83. Tolins JP, Raij L. Hypertension 1990;16:452–61.
84. Ruggenenti P, Perna A, Benini R et al. J Am Soc Nephrol 1999;10:997–1006.
85. Brenner BM, Cooper ME, de Zeeuw D et al. N Engl J Med 2001;345:861–9.
86. Lewis EJ, Hunsicker LG, Clarke WR et al. N Engl J Med 2001;345:851–60.
87. Ruggenenti P, Perna A, Gherardi G et al. J Kidney Dis 2000;35:1155–65.
88. Lewis EJ, Hunsicker LG, Bain RP et al. N Engl J Med 1993;329:1456–62.
89. Viberti G, Mogensen CE, Groop LC et al. JAMA 1994;271:275–9.
90. Blasi ER, Rocha R, Rudolph AE et al. Kidney Int 2003;63:1791–800.
91. Campese VM, Park J. J Hypertens 2006;24:2157–9.
92. Ku E, Campese VM. Pediatr Nephrol 2009;24:2301–7.
93. Walser M. Clin Nephrol 1975;3:180–6.
94. Maschio G, Oldrizzi L, Tessitore N et al. Kidney Int 1982;22:371–6.
95. Alvestrand A, Ahlberg M, Bergstrom J. Kidney Int 1983;24(Suppl 16):S268–72.
96. Barsotti G, Morelli E, Giannoni A et al. Kidney Int 1983;24(Suppl 16):S278–84.
97. Gretz N, Korb E, Strauch M. Kidney Int 1983;24(Suppl 16):S263–7.
98. Mitch WE, Walser M, Steinman TI et al. N Engl J Med 1984;311:623–9.
99. Rosman JB, Meijer S, Sluiter WJ et al. Lancet 1984;2:1291–5.
100. Walser J, LaFrance ND, Ward L et al. Kidney Int 1987;32:123–8.
101. Ihle BU, Becker GJ, Whitworth JA et al. N Engl J Med 1989;321:1773–7.
102. Zeller J, Whittaker E, Sullivan L et al. N Engl J Med 1991;324:78–84.
103. Klahr S, Levey AS, Beck GJ et al. N Engl J Med 1994;330:877–84.
104. Levey AS, Adler S, Caggiula AW et al. Am J Kidney Dis 1996;27:652–63.
105. Mitch WE, Walser M, Sapir DG. J Clin Invest 1981;67:553–62.
106. Tischler ME, Desautels M, Goldberg AL. J Biol Chem 1982;257:1613–21.
107. Kopple, JD. Nutritional management of nondialyzed patients with chronic renal failure. In: Kopple JD, Massry SG eds. Nutritional Management of Renal Disease. 2nd ed. Philadelphia: Lippincott Williams and Wilkins, 2004:379–432.
108. Williams AJ, Baker F, Walls J. Nephron 1987;46:83–90.
109. D'Amico G, Gentile MG, Manna G et al. Lancet 1992;339:1131–4.
110. D'Amico G, Remuzzi G, Maschio G et al. Clin Nephrol 1991;35:237–42.
111. Fouque D, Laville M, Boissel JP et al. BMJ 1992;304:216–20.
112. Pedrini MT, Levey AS, Lau J et al. Ann Intern Med 1996;124:627–32.

113. Kasiske BL, Lakatua JD, Ma JZ et al. Am J Kidney Dis 1998;31:954–61.

114. Fouque D, Wang P, Laville M et al. Nephrol Dial Transplant 2000;12:1986–92.

115. Brunori G, Viola BF, Parrinello G et al. Am J Kidney Dis 2007;49:569–80.

116. Mircescu G, Gârneata L, Stancu SH et al. J Ren Nutr 2007; 17:179–88.

117. Shah SN, Abramowitz M, Hostetter TH et al. Am J Kidney Dis 2009;54:270–77.

118. de Brito-Ashurst I, Varagunam M, Raftery MJ et al. J Am Soc Nephrol 2009;20:2075–84.

119. Phisitkull S, Khannal A, Simon J et al. Kidney Int 2010;77: 617–23.

120. Levey AS, Greene T, Sarnak MJ et al. Am J Kidney Dis 2006; 48:879–88.

121. Menon V, Kopple JD, Wang X et al. Am J Kidney Dis 2009;53:208–17.

122. Chauveau P, Couzi L, Vendrely B et al. Am J Clin Nutr 2009;90:969–74.

123. Knight EL, Stampfer MJ, Hankinson SE et al. Ann Intern Med 2003;138:460–7.

124. Bernardi A, Biasia F, Pati T et al. Am J Kid Dis 2003;41:S146–52.

125. Hostetter TH, Rosenberg ME. J Am Soc Nephrol 1990;1:S55–8.

126. Hansen HP, Tauber-Lassen E, Jensen BR et al. Kidney Int 2002;62:220–8.

127. Schnaper HW, Robson AM. Nephrotic syndrome: minimal change disease, focal glomerulosclerosis, and related disorders. In: Schrier RW, ed. Diseases of the Kidney, vol 2. 7th ed. Philadelphia: Lippincott Williams & Wilkins, 2001:1773–831.

128. Kaysen GA. Nutritional and non-nutrtional management of the nephrotic syndrome. In: Kopple JD, Massry SG, Kalantar-Zadeh K, eds. Nutritional Management of Renal Disease. 3rd ed. New York: Academic Press, 2013.

129. Ibels LS, Gyory AZ. Medicine 1994;73:79.

130. Hirschberg R, Wange S. Curr Opin Nephrol Hypertens 2005;14:43–52.

131. Taguma Y, Kitamoto Y, Futaki G et al. N Engl J Med 1985; 313:1617–20.

132. Kaysen GA, Gambertoglio J, Jimenez I et al. Kidney Int 1986; 29:572–7.

133. Zeller KR, Raskin P, Rosenstock J et al. Kidney Int 1986; 29:209.

134. Kaysen GA, Davies RW. J Am Soc Nephrol 1990;1:S75–9.

135. Gonick HC, Maxwell MH, Rubini ME et al. Nephron 1966;3:137–52.

136. Hebert LA, Haddad N, Shim RL. Nutritional management of water, sodium, potassium, chloride and magnesium in renal disease. In: Kopple JD, Massry SG, Kalantar-Zadeh K, eds. Nutritional Management of Renal Disease. 3rd ed. New York: Academic Press, 2013.

137. Martin K. Calcium, parathyroid hormone and bone disease in kidney disease and chronic kidney failure. In: Kopple JD, Massry SG, Kalantar-Zadeh K, eds. Nutritional Management of Renal Disease. 3rd ed. New York: Academic Press, 2013.

138. Thadhani RI, Christov M. Vitamin D in kidney disease. In: Kopple JD, Massry SG, Kalantar-Zadeh K, eds. Nutritional Management of Renal Disease. 3rd ed. New York: Academic Press, 2013.

139. Houston J, Isakova T, Wolf F. Phosphorus and FGF23 in chronic kidney disease. In: Kopple JD, Massry SG, Kalantar-Zadeh K, eds. Nutritional Management of Renal Disease. 3rd ed. New York: Academic Press, 2013.

140. Swaminathan S. Trace element metabolism in kidney disease. In: Kopple JD, Massry SG, Kalantar-Zadeh K, eds. Nutritional Management of Renal Disease. 3rd ed. New York: Academic Press, 2013.

141. Chazot C, Kopple JD. Vitamin metabolism and requirements in kidney disease and kidney failure. In: Kopple JD, Massry SG, Kalantar-Zadeh K, eds. Nutritional Management of Renal Disease. 3rd ed. New York: Academic Press, 2013.

142. Rabkin R, Simon NM, Steiner S et al. N Engl J Med 1970;282:182–7.

143. Sherwin RS, Bastl C, Finkelstein FO et al. J Clin Invest 1976; 57:722–31.

144. Vajda FJE, Martin TJ, Melick RA. Endocrinology 1969;84: 162–4.

145. Cuttelod S, Lemarchand-Beraud T, Magnenat P et al. Metabolism 1974;23:101–3.

146. Davidson WD, Moore TC, Shippey W et al. Gastroenterology 1974;66:522–5.

147. Samaan N, Freeman RM. Metabolism 1970;19:102–13.

148. Nagel TC, Frenkel N, Bell RH et al. J Clin Endocrinol Metab 1973;36:428–32.

149. Lim VS, Fang VS. Am J Med 1975;58:655–62.

150. Tourkantonis A, Spiliopoulos A, Pharmakioltis A et al. Nephron 1981;27:271–2.

151. Hershman JM, Krugman LG, Kopple JD et al. Metabolism 1979;27:755–9.

152. Fouque D, Peng SC, Kopple JD. Kidney Int 1995;47:876–83.

153. Ding H, Gao CL, Hirschberg R et al. J Clin Invest 1996; 97:1064–75.

154. McCaleb ML, Wish JB, Lockwood DH. Endocrinol Res 1985;11:113–25.

155. Fadda GZ, Hajjar SM, Perna AF et al. J Clin Invest 1991; 87:255–61.

156. Kopple JD, Fukuda S. Am J Clin Nutr 1980;33:1363–72.

157. Tizianello A, De Ferrari G, Garibotto B et al. J Clin Invest 1980;65:1162–73.

158. Kopple JD. Products of nitrogen metabolism and their toxicity. In: Massry SG, Glassock RJ, eds. Massry & Glassock's Textbook of Nephrology, vol 2. 4th ed. Philadelphia: Lippincott Williams & Wilkins, 2001:1262–78.

159. Bricker NS. N Engl J Med 1972;286:1093–9.

160. Massry SG, Smogorzewski M. Semin Nephrol 1994;14:219–31.

161. Simenoff ML, Burke JF, Saukkonen JJ et al. Lancet 1976;2:818–21.

162. Locatelli F, Aljama P, Canaud B et al. Nephrol Dial Transplant 2010;25:2846–50.

163. Clement FM, Klarenbach S, Tonelli M et al. Arch Intern Med 2009;169:1104–12.

164. Besarab A, Coyne DW. Nat Rev Nephrol 2010;6:699–710.

165. Krol E, Rutkowski B, Wroblewska M et al. Miner Electrolyte Metab 1996;22:13–5.

166. Attmann PO, Alaupovic P. Nephron 1991;57:401–10.

167. Lindner A, Charra B, Sherrard D et al. N Engl J Med 1974;290:697–701.

168. Malluche HH, Faugere MC. Kidney Int 1990;38:193–211.

169. Briggs WA, Lazarus JM, Birtch AG et al. Arch Intern Med 1973;132:21–8.

170. Kopple JD. Nutrition in renal failure: causes of catabolism and wasting in acute or chronic renal failure. In: Robinson RR, ed. Nephrology, vol 2. Proceedings of the IXth International Congress of Nephrology. New York: Springer, 1984: 1498–515.

171. Cianciaruso B, Brunori G, Kopple JD et al. Am J Kidney Dis 1995;26:475–86.

172. Canada-USA Peritoneal Dialysis Study Group. J Am Soc Nephrol 1996;7:198–207.

173. Woodrow G, Oldroyd B, Turney JH et al. Nephrol Dial Transplant 1996;11:1613–8.

174. Palop L, Martinez JA. Am J Clin Nutr 1997;66:498S–503S.

175. Dwyer JT, Cunniff PJ, Maroni BJ et al. J Renal Nutr 1998;8:11–20.

176. Aparicio M, Cano N, Chauveau P et al. Nephprol Dial Transplant 1999;14:1679–86.

177. Chung S, Na MH, Lee SH et al. Perit Dial Int 1999;19:S517–22.

178. Williams AJ, McArley A. J Ren Nutr 1999;9:157–62.

179. Carlson DM, Duncan DA, Naessens JM et al. Mayo Clin Proc 1984;59:769–75.

180. Hirschberg R. Drug-nutrient interactions in renal failure. In: Kopple JD, Massry SG, Kalantar-Zadeh K, eds. Nutritional Management of Renal Disease. 3rd ed. New York: Academic Press, 2013.

181. Lowrie EG, Lew NL. Am J Kidney Dis 1990;15:458.

182. Fouque D, Kalantar-Zadeh K, Kopple J et al. Kidney Int 2008;73:391–8 (erratum in Kidney Int 2008;74:393).

183. Delano BG, Manis JG, Manis T. Nephron 1977;19:26.

184. Lawson DH, Boddy K, King PC et al. Clin Sci 1971;41: 345–51.

185. Mahajan SK, Prasad AS, Lambujon J et al. Am J Clin Nutr 1980;33:1517–21.

186. Kopple JD, Mercurio K, Blumenkrantz MJ et al. Kidney Int 1981;19:694–704.

187. Sprenger KBG, Bundschu D, Lewis K et al. Kidney Int 1983;24(Suppl 16):S315–8.

188. Bellinghieri G, Savica V, Mallamace A et al. Am J Clin Nutr 1983;38:523–31.

189. Kopple JD, Berg R, Houser H et al. Kidney Int 1989;36(Suppl 27):S184–94.

190. Velasquez M, Mehrotra M, Wing M, Raj D. Causes of protein-energy wasting in chronic kidney failure. In: Kopple JD, Massry SG, Kalantar-Zadeh K, eds. Nutritional Management of Renal Disease. 3rd ed. New York: Academic Press, 2013.

191. Grodstein GP, Blumenkrantz MJ, Kopple JD. Am J Clin Nutr 1980;33:1411–6.

192. Keane WF, Collins AJ. Am J Kidney Dis 1994;24:1010–8.

193. US Renal Data System. Am J Kidney Dis 2005;45(Suppl 1): S1–280.

194. Wolfson M, Jones MR, Kopple JD. Kidney Int 1982;21: 500–6.

195. Ikizler TA, Flakoll PJ, Parker RA et al. Kidney Int 1994;46:830–7.

196. Kopple JD, Blumenkrantz MJ, Jones MR et al. Am J Clin Nutr 1982;36:395–402.

197. Chazot C, Shahmir E, Matias B et al. Kidney Int 1997;52: 1663–70.

198. Blumenkrantz MJ, Gahl GM, Kopple JD et al. Kidney Int 1981;19:593–602.

199. Wathen RL, Keshaviah P, Hommeyer P et al. Am J Clin Nutr 1978;31:1870–5.

200. Gutierrez A, Alvestrand A, Wahren J et al. Kidney Int 1990; 38:487–94.

201. Gutierrez A, Bergström J, Alvestrand A. Clin Nephrol 1992; 38:20.

202. Mehrotra R, Kopple JD, Wolfson M. Kidney Int Suppl 2003;88:S13–25.

203. Linton AL, Clark WF, Driedger AA et al. Nephron 1977;19:95–8.

204. Kopple JD. Dietary considerations in patients with chronic renal failure, acute renal failure, and transplantation. In: Schrier RW, ed. Diseases of the Kidney. 7th ed. Philadelphia: Lippincott Williams & Wilkins, 2001:3085–138.

205. Kopple JD, Coburn JW. Medicine 1973;52:597–607.

206. Carrero JJ, Stenvinkel P. Inflammation. In: Kopple JD, Massry SG, Kalantar-Zadeh K, eds. Nutritional Management of Renal Disease. 3rd ed. New York: Academic Press, 2013.

207. Kalantar-Zadeh K, Stenvinkel P, Pillon L et al. Adv Ren Replace Ther 2003;10:155–59.

208. Kalantar-Zadeh K, Kopple JD, Kamranpour N et al. Kidney Int 2007;72:1149–56.

209. Rambod M, Kovesdy CP, Bross R et al. Am J Clin Nutr 2008;88:1485–94.

210. Rambod M, Bross R, Zitterkoph J et al. Am J Kidney Dis 2009;53:298–309.

211. Shah S. Oxidative stress. In: Kopple JD, Massry SG, Kalantar-Zadeh K, eds. Nutritional Management of Renal Disease. 3rd ed. New York: Academic Press, 2013.

212. Miyata T. Carbonyl stress in kidney disease and kidney failure. In: Kopple JD, Massry SG, Kalantar-Zadeh K, eds. Nutritional Management of Renal Disease. 3rd ed. New York: Academic Press, 2013.

213. Bachmann J, Tepel M, Raidt H et al. J Am Soc Nephrol 1995;6:121–5.

214. Robinson K, Gupta A, Dennis V et al. Circulation 1996;94:2743–8.

215. Kalantar-Zadeh K, Block G, Humphreys MH et al. J Am Soc Nephrol 2004;15:442–53.

216. Welch GN, Loscalzo J. N Engl J Med 1998;338:1042–50.

217. Kopple JD. Am Soc Artificial Int Organs J 1997;43:246–50.

218. Kalantar-Zadeh K, Kopple JD. Nutritional management of patients undergoing maintenance hemodialysis. In: Kopple JD, Massry SG, Kalantar-Zadeh K, eds. Nutritional Management of Renal Disease. 3rd ed. New York: Academic Press, 2013.

219. Noori N, Kovesdy CP, Dukkipati R et al. Am J Clin Nutr 2010;92:1060–70.

220. Bologa RM, Levine DM, Parker TS et al. Am J Kidney Dis 1998;32:107–14.

221. Garcia-Martinez C, Llovera M, Agell N et al. Biochem Biophys Res Commun 1994;201:682–6.

222. Sarraf P, Frederich RC, Turner EM et al. J Exp Med 1997;185:171–5.

223. Stenvinkel P, Heimburger O, Lindholm B et al. Nephrol Dial Transpl 2000;15:953–60.

224. Kalantar-Zadeh K, Kopple JD. Am J Kidney Dis 2001;38: 1343–50.

225. Kopple JD, Zhu X, Lew NL et al. Kidney Int 1999;56:1136–48.

226. Port FK, Ashby VB, Dhingra RK et al. J Am Soc Nephrol 2002;13:1061–6.

227. Kalantar-Zadeh K, Block G, Humphreys MH et al. Kidney Int 2003;63:793–808.

228. Liu Y, Coresh J, Eustace JA et al. JAMA 2004;291:451–9.

229. Kalantar-Zadeh K, Block G, Humphreys MH et al. J Am Soc Nephrol 2004;15:442–53.

230. Kalantar-Zadeh K, Kopple JD, Humphreys MH et al. Nephrol Dialysis Transplant 2004;19:1507–19.

231. Johansen KL, Young B, Kaysen GA et al. Am J Clin Nutr 2004;80:324–32.

232. Leavey SF, McCullough K, Hecking E et al. Nephrol Dial Transplant 2001;16:2386–94.

233. Kalantar-Zadeh K, Kilpatrick RD, McAllister CJ et al. 2004 (submitted).

234. Kalantar-Zadeh K, Kilpatrick RD, McAllister CJ et al. J Am Soc Nephrol 2004;15:126A.

235. Kopple JD. Am J Clin Nutr 2005;81:1257–66.

236. Martino S, Chwastiak L, Finkelstein F. Motivating the kidney disease patient to dietary adherence and other healthy lifestyle activities. In: Kopple JD, Massry SG, Kalantar-Zadeh K, eds. Nutritional Management of Renal Disease. 3rd ed. New York: Academic Press, 2013.

237. Kopple JD, Greene T, Chumlea WC et al. Kidney Int 2000;57:1688–703.

238. Ikizler TA, Greene JH, Wingard RL et al. J Am Soc Nephrol 1995;6:1386–91.

239. Mehrotra R, Berman N, Alistwani A et al. Am J Kidney Dis 2002;40:133–42.

240. Salusky I, Fine RN, Nelson P et al. Proceedings of the American Society of Nephrology 15th Annual Meeting [abstract]. December 1982:66A.

241. Calloway DH, Odell ACF, Margen SJ. Nutr 1971;101: 775–86.

242. Sargent JA, Gotch FA. J Am Diet Assoc 1979;75:547–51.

243. Maroni BJ, Steinman TI, Mitch WE. Kidney Int 1985;27: 58–65.

244. Kopple JD, Gao XL, Qing DP. Kidney Int 1997;52:486–94.

245. Varcoe R, Halliday D, Carson ER et al. Clin Sci Mol Med 1975;43:379–90.

246. Walser M. J Clin Invest 1974;53:1385–92.

247. Bergström J, Fürst P, Alvestrand A et al. Kidney Int 1993;44:1048–57.

248. Blake P, Daugirdas J. Quantification and prescription: general principles. In: Jacobs C, Kjellstrand CM, Koch KM et al. eds. Replacement of Renal Function by Dialysis. 4th rev ed. Dordrecht, Kluwer Academic Publishers, 1996:619–56.

249. Kopple JD, Jones MR, Keshaviah PR et al. Am J Kidney Dis 1995;26:963–81.

250. Kopple JD, Coburn JW. JAMA 1974;227:41–4.

251. Frisancho AR. Am J Clin Nutr 1984;40:808.

252. American Dietetic Association. Manual of Clinical Dietetics. Chicago: American Dietetic Association, 1988:623.

253. Kopple JD, Coburn JW. Medicine 1973;52:583–95.

254. Kopple JD. Treatment with low protein and amino acid diets in chronic renal failure. In: Barcelo R, Bergeron M, Carriere S, eds. Proceedings of the VIIIth International Congress of Nephrology. Basel, S. Karger, 1978:497–507.

255. National Kidney Foundation. Am J Kidney Dis 2000;35(Suppl 2):S1–140.

256. Kaysen GA, Al-Bander H. Am J Nephrol 1990;10:36.

257. Borah MF, Schoenfeld PY, Gotch FA et al. Kidney Int 1978;14:491–500.

258. Kopple JD, Shinaberger JH, Coburn JW et al. Trans Am Soc Artif Intern Organs 1969;15:302–8.

259. Blumenkrantz MJ, Kopple JD, Moran JK et al. Kidney Int 1982;21:849–61.

260. World Health Organization. Energy and Protein Requirements. Report of a Joint FAO/WHO/UNU Expert Consultation. Geneva: World Health Organization, 1985:1–206. Technical Report series No. 724.

261. Fouque D, Vennegoor M, Ter Wee P et al. Nephrol Dial Transplant 2007;22(Suppl 2):ii45–87.

262. Australia and New Zealand Renal Guidelines Taskforce. Evidence based practice guidelines for the nutritional management of chronic kidney disease. Nutrition & Dietetics 2006;63(Suppl. 2):S35–S45.

263. Kopple JD, Monteon FJ, Shaib JK. Kidney Int 1986;29: 734–42.

264. Monteon FJ, Laidlaw SA, Shaib JK et al. Kidney Int 1986; 30:741–7.

265. Schneeweiss B, Graninger W, Stockenhuber F et al. Am J Clin Nutr 1990;52:596–601.

266. Slomowitz LA, Monteon FJ, Grosvenor M et al. Kidney Int 1989;35:704–11.

267. Wolfson M, Strong CJ, Minturn D et al. Am J Clin Nutr 1984; 39:547–55.

268. Marckmann P. Clin Nephrol 1988;29:75–8.

269. Kopple JD. Kidney Int 1978;14:340–8.

270. Kluthe R, Luttgen FM, Capetianu T et al. Am J Clin Nutr 1978;31:1812–20.

271. Blumenkrantz MJ, Kopple JD, Gutman RA et al. Am J Clin Nutr 1980;33:1567–85.

272. Appel G. Kidney Int 1991;39:169–83.

273. Attman PO. Nephrol Dial Transplant 1993;8:294.

274. Cocchi R, Viglino G, Cancarini G et al. Miner Electrolyte Metab 1996;22:22–5.

275. Wanner C, Bartens W, Nauck M et al. Miner Electrolyte Metab 1996;22:26–30.

276. Vaziri, ND. Altered lipid metabolism and serum lipids in kidney disease and kidney failure. In: Kopple JD, Massry SG, Kalantar-Zadeh K, eds. Nutritional Management of Renal Disease. 3rd ed. New York: Academic Press, 2013.

277. Roncari DAK, Breckenridge WC, Khanna R et al. Perit Dial Bull 1988;1:136–41.

278. Boeschoten EW, Zuyderhoudt FMJ, Krediet RT et al. Perit Dial Bull 1988;19:8–13.

279. Deighan CJ, Caslake MJ, McConnell M et al. Am J Lidney Dis 2000;35:852–62.

280. Samuelsson O, Attmann PO, Knight-Gibson C et al. Nephrol Dial Transplant 1991;9:1580–5.

281. Chan MK, Varghese Z, Moorhead JF. Kidney Int 1981;19: 625–37.

282. Ciman M, Rizzoli V, Moracchiello M et al. Am J Clin Nutr 1980;33:1489–92.

283. Bellinghieri G, Savica V, Mallamace A et al. Am J Clin Nutr 1983;38:523–31.

284. Joven J, Villabona C, Vilella E et al. N Engl J Med 1990; 323:579–84.

285. Ibels LS, Alfrey AC, Weil R III. Am J Med 1978;64:634.

286. Nelson J, Beauregard H, Gélinas M et al. Transplant Proc 1988;20:1264–70.

287. Dimény E, Fellström B, Larsson E et al. Transplant Proc 1992;24:366.

288. Expert Panel on Detection, Evaluation, and Treatment of High Blood Cholesterol in Adults. JAMA 2001;285:2486–97.

289. Thomas ME, Harris KPG, Ramaswamy C et al. Kidney Int 1993;44:1124–9.

290. Wanner C, Krane V, Marz W et al. N Engl J Med 2005;353: 238–48 (erratum in N Engl J Med 2005;353:1640).

291. Fellstrom BC, Jardine AG, Schmieder RE et al. N Engl J Med 2009;360:1395–407.

292. Liu Y, Coresh J, Eustace JA et al. 2004;291:451–9.

293. Kovesdy CP, Anderson JE, Kalantar-Zadeh K. J Am Soc Nephrol 2007;18:304–11.

294. Kilpatrick RD, McAllister CJ, Kovesdy CP et al. J Am Soc Nephrol 2007;18:293–303.

295. Tonelli M, Moyé L, Sacks FM et al. J Am Soc Nephrol 2003;14:1605–13.

296. Ciman M, Rizzoli V, Moracchiello M et al. Am J Clin Nutr 1980;33:1489–92.

297. Bellinghieri G, Savica V, Mallamace A et al. Am J Clin Nutr 1983;38:523–31.

298. Guarnieri G, Toigo G, Crapesi L et al. Kidney Int 1987; 32(Suppl 22):S116–27.

299. Wanner C, Horl WH. Nephron 1988;50:89.

300. Pierides AM, Alvarez-Ude F, Kerr DNS et al. Lancet 1979; 2:1279–82.

301. Leaf A, Weber PC. N Engl J Med 1988;318:549.

302. Donadio JV Jr, Bergstralh EJ, Offord KP et al. N Engl J Med 1994;331:1194–9.

303. Manis T, Deutsch J, Finestein EI et al. Am J Clin Nutr 1980;33:1485–8.

304. Hamazaki T, Nakazawa R, Tateno S et al. Kidney Int 1984;26:1–84.

305. Bremer J. Physiol Rev 1983;63:1420.

306. Vacha GM, Corsi M, Giorcelli G et al. Curr Ther Res 1985;37:505.

307. Hiatt WR, Koziol BJ, Shapiro JI et al. Kidney Int 1992; 41:1613–9.

308. Golper TA, Wolfson M, Ahmad S et al. Kidney Int 1990; 38:904–11.

309. Ahmad S, Robertson HT, Gloper TA et al. Kidney Int 1990; 38:912–8.

310. van Es A, Henny FC, Kooistra MP et al. Contrib Nephrol 1992;98:28–35.

311. Golper TA, Ahmad S. Semin Dial 1992;5:94–98.

312. Labonia WD. Am J Kidney Dis 1995;26:757–64.

313. Symposium on Role Dietary Fiber in Health. Am J Clin Nutr 1978;31:S1–S291.

314. Parillo M, Riccardi G, Pacioni D et al. Diabetes Care 1985;8:620.

315. Anderson JW, Zettwoch N, Feldman T et al. Arch Intern Med 1988;148:292.

316. Anderson JW, Chen WL. Am J Clin Nutr 1979;32:346.

317. Rampton DS, Cohen SL, Crammond V De B et al. Clin Nephrol 1984;21:159–63.

318. Noori N, Kalantar-Zadeh K, Kovesdy CP et al. Clin J Am Soc Nephrol 2010;5:683–92.

319. Kovesdy CP, Kuchmak O, Lu JL et al. Am J Kidney Dis. 2010;56:842–51. (comment in: Am J Kidney Dis 2010;56: 813–6).

320. Kidney Disease: Improving Global Outcomes (KDIGO) CKD-MBD Work Group. Kidney Int 2009;76(Suppl 113):S1–130.

321. Kalantar-Zadeh K, Gutekunst L, Mehrotra R et al. Clin J Am Soc Nephrol 2010;5:519–30.

322. Noori N, Sims JJ, Kopple JD et al. Iran J Kidney Dis 2010;4:89–100.

323. Cannata JB, Briggs JD, Junor BJR. BMJ 1983;286:1937–8.

324. Sedman AB, Miller NL, Warady BA et al. Kidney Int 1984;26:201–4.

325. Chertow GM, Burke SK, Raggi P. Kidney Int 2002;62: 245–52.

326. Chertow GM. J Am Soc Nephrol 2003;14:S310–4.

327. Al-Baaj F, Speake M, Hutchison AJ. Nephrol Dial Transplant 2005;20:775–82.

328. Lacour B, Lucas A, Auchere D et al. Kidney Int 2005;67: 1062–9.

329. Geisser P, Philipp E. Clin Nephrology 2010;74:4–11.

330. Nolan CR, Califano JR, Butzin CA. Kidney Int 1990;38:937–41.

331. Schaefer K, Scheer J, Asmus G et al. Nephrol Dial Transplant 1991;6:170–5.

332. Mai ML, Emmett M, Sheikh MS et al. Kidney Int 1989; 36:690–5.

333. Pflanz S, Henderson IS, McElduff N et al. Nephrol Dial Transplant 1994;9:1121.

334. Boudville N, Inderjeeth C, Elder GJ et al. Clin Endocrinol 2010;73:299–304.

335. Kopple JD, Massry SG. Am J Nephrol 1988;8:437–48.

336. Reichel H, Koeffler HP, Norman AW. N Engl J Med 1989;320:980–91.

337. Boudville N, Inderjeeth C, Elder GJ et al. Clin Endocrinol 2010;73:299–304.

338. Teng M, Wolf M, Ofsthun MN et al. J Am Soc Nephrol 2005;16:1115–25.

339. Drüeke TB, Ritz E. Clin J Am Soc Nephrol 2009;4:234–41.

340. Food and Nutrition Board, Institute of Medicine. Dietary Reference Intakes for Calcium and Vitamin D. Washington, DC: National Academies Press, 2011.

341. Sherrard DJ, Hercz G, Pei Y et al. Kidney Int 1993;43: 436–42.

342. Faugere MC, Malluche HH. Kidney Int 1986;30:717–22.

343. Hercz G, Pei Y, Greenwood C et al. Kidney Int 1993;44: 860–6.

344. Randall RE Jr, Cohen MD, Spray CC Jr et al. Ann Intern Med 1964;61:73–8.

345. Koomans HA, Roos JC, Boer P et al. Hypertension 1982; 4:190–7.

346. Lawson DH, Boddy K, King PC et al. Clin Sci 1971;41: 345–51.

347. Chen SM. J Formosan Med Assoc 1990;89:220.

348. Rudolph H, Alfrey AC, Smythe WR. Trans Am Soc Artif Intern Organs 1973;19:456–65.

349. Cartwright GE, Gubler CJ, Wintrobe MM. J Clin Invest 1954;33:685.

350. Sprenger KBG, Bundschu D, Lewis K et al. Kidney Int 1983;24(Suppl 16):S315–8.

351. Taylor JE, Peat N, Porter C et al. Nephrol Dial Transplant 1996;11:1079–83.

352. Ahsan N. J Am Soc Nephrol 1998;9:664–8.

353. Mahajan SK, Bowersox EM, Rye DL et al. Kidney Int 1989;27:S269–73.

354. Mansouri K, Halsted JA, Gombos EA. Arch Intern Med 1970;125:88–93.

355. Food and Nutrition Board, Institute of Medicine. Dietary Reference Intakes for Vitamin A, Vitamin K, Arsenic, Boron, Chromium, Copper, Iodine, Iron, Manganese, Molybdenum, Nickel, Silicon, Vanadium, and Zinc. Washington, DC: National Academy Press, 2002.

356. Mahajan SK, Abraham J, Hessburg T et al. Kidney Int 1983;24(Suppl 16):S310–4.

357. Antoniou LD, Shalhoub RJ, Sudhakar T et al. Lancet 1977;2:895–8.

358. Food and Nutrition Board, Institute of Medicine. Dietary Reference Intakes for Vitamin C, Vitamin E, Selenium, and Carotenoids. Washington, DC: National Academy Press, 2000.

359. Food and Nutrition Board, Institute of Medicine. Dietary Reference Intakes for Thiamin, Riboflavin, Vitamin B_6, Vitamin B_{12}, Pantothenic Acid, Biotin, and Choline. Washington, DC: National Academy Press, 1998.

360. Jennette JC, Goldman ID. J Lab Clin Med 1975;86:834–43.

361. Spannuth CL Jr, Warnock LG, Wagner C et al. J Lab Clin Med 1977;90:632–7.

362. Descombes E, Hanck AB, Fellay G. Kidney Int 1993;43: 1319–28.

363. Kopple JD, Mercurio K, Blumenkrantz MJ et al. Kidney Int 1981;19:694–704.

364. Kopple JD, Swendseid ME. Kidney Int 1975;7(Suppl 2): S79–84.

365. Balcke P, Schmidt P, Zazgornik J et al. Ann Intern Med 1984;101:344–5.

366. Pru C, Eaton J, Kjellstrand C. Nephron 1985;39:112–6.

367. Smith FR, Goodman DS. J Clin Invest 1971;50:2426–36.

368. Yatzidis H, Digenis P, Fountas P. Br Med J 1975;2:352–3.

369. Udall JA. J Am Med Assoc 1965;194:127.

370. Steiber AL, Kopple JD. J Ren Nutr 2011;21:355–68.

371. May RC, Kelly RA, Mitch WE. J Clin Invest 1987;79: 1099–103.

372. Reaich D, Channon SM, Scrimgeour CM et al. Am J Physiol 1992;263:E735–9.

373. Mehrotra R, Kopple JD, Wolfson M. Kidney Int 2003;88(Suppl):S13–25.

374. Ballmer PE, McNurlan MA, Hulter HN et al. J Clin Invest 1995;95:39–45

375. Sonikian M, Gogusev J, Zingraff J et al. J Am Soc Nephrol 1996;7:350–6.

376. Mehrotra R, Bross R, Wang H et al. Am J Clin Nutr 2009;90:1532–40.

377. Savica V, Bellinghieri G, Kopple JD. Annu Rev Nutr 2010;30:365–401.

378. US Renal Data System. 2005 Annual Data Report. Available at: http://www.usrds.org. Accessed June 22, 2012.

379. Kalantar-Zadeh K, Kopple JD, Kilpatrick RD et al. Am J Kidney Dis 2005;46:489–500.

380. Kalantar-Zadeh K, Kuwae N, Wu DY et al. Am J Clin Nutr 2006;83:202–10.

381. Kovesdy CP, Kalantar-Zadeh K. Semin Nephrol 2009;29:3–14.

382. Dornfeld LP, Maxwell MH, Waks A et al. Kidney Int 1987;22:S254–58.

383. Mault JR, Bartlett RH, Dechert RE et al. Trans Am Soc Artif Intern Organs 1983;29:390–4.

384. Flugel-Link RM, Salusky IB, Jones MR et al. Am J Physiol 1983;244:E615–23.

385. Clark AS, Mitch WE. J Clin Invest 1983;72:836–45.

386. Frohlich J, Scholmerich J, Hoppe-Seyler G et al. Eur J Clin Invest 1974;4:453–8.

387. Feinstein EI, Blumenkrantz MJ, Healy H et al. Medicine 1981;60:124–37.

388. Feinstein EI, Kopple JD, Silberman H. Kidney Int 1983;26(Suppl 16):S319–23.

389. Kopple JD. JPEN J Parenter Enteral Nutr 1996;20:3–12.

390. Abel RM, Abbott WM, Beck CH Jr et al. Am J Surg 1974;128:317–23.

391. Abel RM, Shih VE, Abbott WM et al. Ann Surg 1974;180: 350–5.

392. Abel RM, Beck CH Jr, Abbott WM et al. N Engl J Med 1973;288:695–9.

393. Baek SM, Makabali GG, Bryan-Brown CW et al. Surg Gynecol Obstet 1975;141:405–8.

394. McMurray SD, Luft FC, Maxwell DR et al. Arch Intern Med 1978;138:950–5.

395. Leonard CD, Luke RG, Siegel RR. Urology 1975;6:154–7.

396. Kopple JD, Swendseid ME. Am J Clin Nutr 1974;27: 806–12.

397. Nakasaki H, Katayama T, Yokoyama S et al. JPEN J Parenter Enteral Nutr 1993;17:86–90.

398. Mehta RL. Semin Nephrol 1994;14:64–82.

399. Davenport A, Roberts NB. Crit Care Med 1989;17:1010.

400. Davies SP, Reaveley DA, Brown EA et al. Crit Care Med 1991;19:1510.

401. Feinstein EI, Collins JF, Blumenkrantz MJ et al. Prog Artif Organs 1984;1:421–6.

402. Kopple JD, Bernard D, Messana J et al. Kidney Int 1995;47:1148–57.

403. Cerra FB, Upson D, Angelico R et al. Surgery 1982;92: 192–200.

404. Daly M, Mihranian MH, Kehoe JI et al. Surgery 1983;94: 151–9.

405. Leander U, Fürst P, Vesterberg K et al. Clin Nutr 1985;4: 43–51.

406. Hammarqvist F, Wernerman J, Ruston A et al. Ann Surg 1989;209:455–61.

407. Stehle P, Zander J, Mertes N et al. Lancet 1989;1:231–3.

408. Daly JM, Reynolds J, Thom A et al. Ann Surg 1988;208: 512–23.

409. McCracken BH, Parsons FM. Lancet 1958;2:885–6.

410. Gjorup S, Thaysen JH. Acta Med Scand 1960;167:227–38.

411. Hinton P, Allison SP, Littlejohn S et al. Lancet 1971;1: 767–9.

412. Woolfson AMJ, Healtley RV, Allison SP. N Engl J Med 1979;300:14–7.

413. Meyfroidt G, Keenan DM, Wang X et al. Crit Care Med 2010;38:1021–9.

414. Marik PE, Preiser JC. Chest 2010;137:544–51.

415. Hermanides J, Bosman RJ, Vriesendorp TM et al. Crit Care Med 2010;38:1430–4.

416. Kavanagh BP, McCowen KC. N Engl J Med 2010;363: 2540–6.

417. Ponting GA, Halliday D, Teale JD et al. Lancet 1988;1:438–40.

418. Wilmore DW. N Engl J Med 1991;325:695.

419. Kopple JD, Brunori G, Leiserowitz M et al. Nephrol Dial Transpl 2005;20:952–8.

420. Dahn MS, Lange P, Jacobs LA. Arch Surg 1988;123:1409.

421. Takala J, Ruokonen E, Webster NR et al. N Engl J Med 1999;341:785–92.

422. Miller SB, Martin DR, Kissane J et al. Proc Natl Acad Sci U S A 1992;89:11876–80.

423. Ding H, Kopple JD, Cohen A et al. J Clin Invest 1993;91: 2281–7.

424. Hirschberg R, Kopple JD, Lipsett P et al. Kidney Int 1999;55:2423–32.

425. Humes HD, Cieslinski DA, Coimbra TM et al. J Clin Invest 1989;84:1757–61.

426. Miller SB, Martin DR, Kissane J et al. Am J Physiol 1994;266:F129–34.

427. Siegel NJ, Gaudio KM, Katz LA et al. Kidney Int 1984;25: 906–11.

428. Rahman SN, Kim GE, Mathew AS et al. Kidney Int 1994;45:1731–8.

429. Siegel NJ, Glazier WB, Chaudry IH et al. Kidney Int 1980;17:338–49.

430. Kopple JD, Jones MR, Keshaviah PR et al. Am J Kidney Dis 1995;26:963–81.

431. Harris JA, Benedict FG. A Biometric Study of Basal Metabolism in Man. Publication no. 279. Washington, DC: Carnegie Institute, 1919.

432. Garrel DR, Jobin N, de Jonge LHM. Nutr Clin Pract 1996;11:99–103.

433. Wilmore DW. The Metabolic Management of the Critically Ill. New York: Plenum Press, 1977:314.

434. Druml W. Nutritional management of acute kidney injury. In: Kopple JD, Massry SG, Kalantar-Zadeh K, eds. Nutritional Management of Renal Disease. 3rd ed. New York: Academic Press, 2013.

435. Askanazi J, Elwyn DH, Silverberg BS et al. Surgery 1980;87:596–8.

436. Jeejeebhoy KN, Langer B, Tsallas G et al. Gastroenterology 1976;71:943–53.

437. Seidner DL, Mascioli EA, Istfan NW et al. JPEN J Parenter Enteral Nutr 1989;13:614–9.

438. Driscoll DF, Baptista BJ, Bistrian BR et al. Am J Hosp Pharm 1986;43:416–9.

439. Dukkipati R, Kalantar-Zadeh K, Kopple JD. Am J Kidney Dis 2010;55:352–64.

440. Capelli JP, Kushner H, Camiscioli TC et al. Am J Kidney Dis 1994;23:808–16.

441. Chertow GM, Ling J, Lew NL et al. Am J Kidney Dis 1994;24:912–20.

442. Zager RA, Johannes G, Tuttle SE et al. J Lab Clin Med 1983;101:130–40.

443. Zager RA, Venkatachalam MA. Kidney Int 1983;24:620–5.

444. Malis CD, Racusen C, Solez K et al. J Lab Clin Med 1984;103:660–76.

445. Andrews PM, Bates SB. Kidney Int 1987;32(Suppl 22): S76–80.

446. Weinberg JM. Semin Nephrol 1990;10:491–500.

98 HEMATOLOGIC ASPECTS OF IRON DEFICIENCY AND LESS COMMON NUTRITIONAL ANEMIAS[1]

CHRISTOPHER R. CHITAMBAR AND ASOK C. ANTONY

---

[1]**Abbreviations: HIV**, human immunodeficiency virus; **MCV**, mean corpuscular volume; **RBC**, red blood cell; **sTfR**, soluble transferrin receptor; **WHO**, World Health Organization; **ZPP**, zinc protoporphyrin.

Iron deficiency is the most common and widespread nutritional disorder in the world. As well as affecting a large number of children and women in developing countries, it is the only nutrient deficiency which is also significantly prevalent in industrialized countries. The numbers are staggering: 2 billion people—over 30% of the world's population—are anaemic, many due to iron deficiency, and in resource-poor areas, this is frequently exacerbated by infectious diseases. Malaria, HIV/AIDS, hookworm infestation, schistosomiasis, and other infections such as tuberculosis are particularly important factors contributing to the high prevalence of anaemia in some areas.

Iron deficiency affects more people than any other condition, constituting a public health condition of epidemic proportions. More subtle in its manifestations than, for example, protein-energy malnutrition, iron deficiency exacts its heaviest overall toll in terms of ill-health, premature death and lost earnings.

Iron deficiency and anaemia reduce the work capacity of individuals and entire populations, bringing serious economic consequences and obstacles to national development. Overall, it is the most vulnerable, the poorest and the least educated who are disproportionately affected by iron deficiency, and it is they who stand to gain the most by its reduction.

—World Health Organization (WHO) Report on Iron-deficiency Anemia (1)

GENERAL CONCEPTS

Iron deficiency looms largest among the factors that contribute to the global burden of anemia, which affects one third of the world's population and has serious consequences for maternal and perinatal health and child development (2). In many developing countries, more than half of specific groups of individuals are affected. Even in developed countries, the problem of iron deficiency is significant (Table 98.1). The WHO quotation cited above encapsulates the fundamental problem that this chapter aims to highlight. Coincident with the diagnosis of iron deficiency is the imperative for identification of all underlying root causes, which must be addressed to prevent a recurrence of iron deficiency after iron replacement.

From the public health point of view, the main hematopoietic nutrients are iron, folate, and vitamin B_{12}. These nutrients are discussed in separate chapters. Whereas other trace metals and vitamins contribute to normal hematopoiesis, their clinical role independent of the three major nutrients is of lesser public health importance. Nevertheless, when patients continue to have anemia despite repletion with iron, folate, and vitamin B_{12}, and other causes for anemia have been ruled out, the additional

TABLE 98.1	PREVALENCE OF IRON DEFICIENCY FROM THE UNITED STATES NATIONAL HEALTH AND NUTRITION EXAMINATION SURVEYS, 1988 TO 1994 AND 1999 TO 2000[a]			

SEX AND AGE GROUPS (y)	1988–1994		1999–2000	
	%	(95% CI)[a]	%	(95% CI)
Both sexes				
1–2	9	(6–11)	7	(3–11)
3–5	3	(2–4)	5	(2–7)
6–11	2	(1–3)	4	(1–7)
Males				
12–15	1	(0.1–2.0)	5	(2–8)
16–69	1	(0.6–1.0)	2	(1–3)
≥70	4	(2–3)	3	(2–7)
Females (nonpregnant)				
12–15	9	(6–12)	9	(5–12)
16–19	11	(7–14)	16	(10–22)
20–49	11	(10–13)	12	(10–16)
White, non-Hispanic	8	(7–9)	10	(7–13)
African-American, non-Hispanic	15	(13–17)	19	(14 –24)
Mexican-American	19	(17–21)	22	(17–27)
50–69	5	(4–7)	9	(5–12)
≥70	7	(5–8)	6	(4–9)

CI, confidence interval.

[a]All racial and ethnic groups, except where noted.

Adapted with permission from Centers for Disease Control and Prevention. Iron deficiency: United States, 1999–2000. MMWR Morb Mortal Wkly Rep 2002;51:897–9.

role of other trace metals and vitamins should be sought. Anemia is defined as a low concentration of hemoglobin in the blood. Optimum hemoglobin values at different ages are presented in Table 98.2.

Iron and Hematopoiesis

Of a total of 4 to 5 g of iron in the body, about 3 g of iron is in hemoglobin—which is the oxygen carrier in erythrocytes (red blood cells [RBCs])—whereas some iron is in myoglobin, the remainder is in various heme and nonheme enzymes, including cytochromes that are necessary for oxidative reactions producing energy. Iron is also critical for cell proliferation because ribonucleotide reductase, an iron-dependent enzyme, is required for DNA synthesis. Because the major requirement for iron in the body is for hemoglobin in RBCs, an early manifestation of iron deficiency is anemia.

The formation of blood cells (hematopoiesis) occurs in the bone marrow medullary cavity of virtually all bones in the newborn, but in adults, active blood formation is confined to the central skeleton (skull, vertebral column, ribs, and pelvis) and upper ends of the humerus and femur. All hematopoietic cells arise from a very small population of self-renewing stem cells that, under the influence of a range of growth factors, give rise to RBCs, white blood cells (polymorphonuclear neutrophils, eosinophils, basophils, monocytes, lymphocytes), and platelets. Because the turnover of blood cells is normally greater

TABLE 98.2	HEMOGLOBIN CUTOFFS USED TO DEFINE ANEMIA AT SEA LEVEL[a]

AGE OR SEX GROUP	HEMOGLOBIN LOWER THAN THE VALUES (g/dL) DEFINES ANEMIA
Men	13.0
Nonpregnant women	12.0
Pregnant women	11.0
Children (6 mo–5 y)	11.0
Children (5–11 y)	11.5
Children (12–13 y)	12.0

[a]The optimal hemoglobin value should be higher than these values for various ages and sex. The hematocrit is usually three times the hemoglobin value. Individuals living at an altitude of 4000 ft or more have higher normal blood values; the hemoglobin should be approximately 1 g/dL higher for people residing at approximately 6500 to 7000 ft altitude.

Data from Gleason G, Scrimshaw N. An overview of the functional significance of iron deficiency. In: Kraeme K, Zimmerman MB, eds. Nutritional Anemia. Basel: Sight and Life Press, 2007:45–58; and Biesalki HK, Erhardt J. Diagnosis of nutritional anemia: laboratory assessment of iron status. In: Kraeme K, Zimmerman MB, eds. Nutritional Anemia. Basel: Sight and Life Press, 2007:37–43, with permission.

than that of other tissues in the body, deficiency of any of the three important nutrients—iron, vitamin B_{12} (cobalamin), and folate (folic acid, pteroylglutamic acid)—can become limiting for hematopoiesis. The bone marrow, with its prodigious production of RBCs (2×10^{11} RBCs/day/adult), can further augment erythropoiesis in response to blood loss or hemolysis by sixfold by using stored iron from ferritin and hemosiderin in the liver, spleen, and bone marrow. Iron is incorporated into hemoglobin-synthesizing immature erythroid cells in the marrow via transferrin receptor–mediated endocytosis of transferrin-bound iron. Transferrin receptor expression is greatest in the early stages of erythroid development when hemoglobin synthesis occurs and is lost as these cells mature into RBCs that are released to the circulation (3).

IRON DEFICIENCY AND ITS CLINICAL CONSEQUENCES

Physiologic Adaptation to Iron Deficiency

Impairment of normal RBC production results in a fall in the hemoglobin concentration (anemia), RBC count, and packed red cell volume (hematocrit) below the levels shown in Table 98.2. The decrease in hemoglobin leads to a reduction in the oxygen-carrying capacity of the blood and impairment of oxygen delivery to tissues. Three separate physiologic responses are called into play to compensate for the development of anemia: First, there is a change in the binding of hemoglobin to oxygen so that oxygen is more efficiently unloaded from RBCs to tissues. Second, the cardiac output of blood increases so that more blood (and oxygen) is delivered to the rest of the body. Third, an increase in the level of the erythropoiesis-stimulating hormone, erythropoietin, stimulates RBC production in the bone marrow.

When anemia develops over a prolonged period of time, these compensatory mechanisms allow a patient to continue normal activity with minimal or no symptoms. Indeed, the severity of the anemia is often disproportionate to the symptoms. Most patients, however, become symptomatic when the hemoglobin drops to less than 7 to 8 g/dL. Other factors such as a patient's age, physiologic conditioning, and the presence of other medical problems will often determine whether symptoms develop at a particular hemoglobin level. For example, patients with underlying cardiac dysfunction may develop symptoms related to anemia when the hemoglobin falls to less than 10 g/dL.

Causes of Iron Deficiency

As in most micronutrient mineral deficiencies, the major causes of iron deficiency involve reduced dietary intake, malabsorption, increased loss, or increased requirement (and, less important for public health, defects in iron utilization). And more often the rule rather than the exception, several causes may be found in the same individual.

The primary factors contributing to widespread iron deficiency in developing countries include diets low in bioavailable iron that are superimposed on increased demands for iron that cannot be met during pregnancy and growth, menorrhagia in women of childbearing age, and gastrointestinal blood loss. The latter two conditions are the main causes of iron deficiency in adults in developed countries.

Malabsorption of iron may occur following resection of the stomach (total or partial gastrectomy) or surgical bypass of the duodenum, gastric achlorhydria, and tropical or nontropical (celiac) sprue.

Common causes of gastrointestinal tract blood loss include peptic ulcer disease, gastric erosions resulting from chronic use of nonsteroidal anti-inflammatory drugs (NSAIDs, including aspirin) or steroids, gastroesophageal hiatal hernia, colonic diverticulosis or polyps, gastrointestinal mucosal angiodysplasia, malignant disease, and parasitism.

Urinary iron losses can result from lesions within the genitourinary tract (including stones) and intravascular RBC hemolysis (especially from malaria).

Polyparasitism and Parasite-Related Blood Loss

In many developing countries, gastrointestinal blood loss from hookworm infestation with *Ancylostoma duodenale* or *Necator americanus* is a major cause of iron-deficiency anemia. Approximately 740 million people worldwide are infected with hookworm. Each worm attaches itself to the duodenum and jejunum of the gastrointestinal tract and sucks blood and serum protein, with resulting iron deficiency and malnutrition. With light infestation by hookworm, the blood loss is 2 mL/day, but with heavy infestation it can be approximately 100 mL/day. *N. americanus* consumes 0.03 mL blood/worm/day, whereas *A. duodenale*

consumes much more, at 0.15 to 0.23 mL blood/worm/day. Hemoglobin values of less than 11 g/dL can be seen with infestation by 40 to 160 worms. The number of hookworm eggs in the stool can serve as an indirect measure of hookworm burden. With approximately 1000 eggs/g of feces, the patient may have a blood loss equivalent to 1 mg iron lost/day. Even *Trichuris trichiura* (whipworm) roundworm infestation can lead to a loss of 0.005 mL blood/worm/day. Schistosomiasis (*Schistosoma hematobium*) of the bladder can also lead to significant blood loss in the urine that causes iron deficiency (4).

Infection and infestation with multiple parasites are the norm in the tropics and subtropics and are likely to have a major impact generally on nutrition and more particularly on anemia (5). More than half of children studied in various geographic regions harbor high worm burdens of *Ascaris, Trichuris,* and hookworm (6, 7), as well as amebiasis and, in endemic areas, schistosomiasis. Young women are also common victims of polyparasitism, and approximately 44 million pregnant women are infected with hookworm worldwide, with 7.5 million in sub-Saharan Africa alone (8).

A successful large-scale universal program that was built into an existing public health structure addressed the problem of anemia among 52,000 Vietnamese women of reproductive age (9, 10). The key was improving the hemoglobin and iron status of these women before they became pregnant by giving them weekly iron and folic acid supplementation combined with a regular deworming program (9). This type of innovative approach is applicable to thousands of women of reproductive age in Southeast Asia and Africa, nearly half of whom have, primarily, iron deficiency that is often accompanied by folate and vitamin B_{12} deficiency.

CLINICAL PRESENTATIONS OF IRON DEFICIENCY

In early stages of iron deficiency, individuals can be entirely asymptomatic; and the discovery of iron-deficiency anemia may be made only as a result of a routine blood count. Eventually, however, patients with iron deficiency will develop symptoms ascribed to anemia. An initial complaint of most patients with significant anemia is that they feel tired or tire easily with exertion. Pica (eating of materials such as ice, clay, paper, dirt) may be seen, particularly in children. Obsessive eating of ice (pagophagia) may be specific to iron deficiency and disappears within 1 to 2 weeks of iron treatment; eating of ice was noted in approximately 8% of 553 African-American women with iron deficiency in pregnancy (11). Patients with iron deficiency may also complain of a sensation of pins and needles (paresthesia) in the hands and feet. Palpitations (awareness of their own heartbeat), tinnitus (ringing or whistling noise in the ears or head), headache, irritability, dizziness, and generalized weakness may be present. Anemia may produce shortness of breath on exertion accompanied by a rapid heartbeat.

In older individuals with severe anemia, cardiac pain (angina) and cardiac failure may develop. Additional symptoms related to iron deficiency include cracks at the angles of the mouth (angular stomatitis) (Fig. 98.1), difficulty in swallowing, and a sensation of a lump in the throat (dysphagia). Some patients complain of soreness of the mouth and tongue (from impaired squamous cell regeneration from iron deficiency) that may be aggravated by hot drinks or spicy foods (Fig. 98.2).

Physical examination of individuals with iron-deficiency anemia reveals pallor of the conjunctiva and skin, pale blue sclera, and misshapen nails that break easily and may be spoon shaped (koilonychia) (Fig. 98.3). The heart and pulse rate may be rapid, and a systolic heart murmur may be detected on cardiac auscultation. Heart failure characterized by pulmonary edema, a congested liver, and edema of the lower extremities may develop. In patients with long-standing severe anemia, the spleen may be enlarged, with the spleen tip palpable under the left costal margin. Radiographic evaluation of patients for dysphagia may reveal the cause as a postcricoid web in the esophagus (Fig. 98.4); these patients are at increased risk for developing esophageal cancer.

Patients with iron-deficiency anemia may have additional clinical complaints and findings that are not the result of anemia itself but are related to the underlying cause of iron deficiency. For example, tarry-colored or bright red stools suggest iron loss from gastrointestinal bleeding, whereas bloody or Coca-Cola—colored urine suggests urinary iron loss from genitourinary bleeding or intravascular hemolysis, respectively.

Signs and Symptoms of Iron Deficiency among Special Groups

Children can present with cognitive impairment, decreased physical capacity, and reduced immunity. The motor and social development of children (and young adults) with iron deficiency is generally poor. These children are less responsive, show less activity on the playground, have increased fatigue (and other nonspecific symptoms related to increased worm burden), and anorexia.

There is also a clear relationship between increased susceptibility to infections among children with iron deficiency (12). Such children are more frequently absent (because of frequent infections) and are less likely to attend school; and when they do attend school, their overall poor school performance may be poor. Improving school children's performance by iron supplements led to substantial improvement in 3 months (13); anemic Thai children had lower scores in Thai language, mathematics, and other subjects compared with iron-replete children. This finding has obvious implications for developing countries if iron-deficient children are not treated. Another feature of severe iron deficiency among children is their inability to maintain body temperature in cold climates (they need protective clothing).

Iron deficiency leads to defective information processing and impaired cognitive development in adult women, and there is improvement in verbal learning and memory with administration of iron (14). These young women should be targeted for optimization of their iron status; such interventions can improve their physical endurance and changes in mood and ability to concentrate even when they do not have frank anemia.

Even among adults working in the field (as rubber tappers, workers in tea plantations, and rice fields) in Indonesia and Sri Lanka, iron replenishment led to an overall improvement in productivity that led to increased wages (12) and therefore a greater capacity for earning a steady income. Even when a financial incentive was removed, the overall performance was better among those adults treated with iron.

Nonhematologic Effects of Iron Deficiency

Development and Work Performance

Iron deficiency in pregnancy is accompanied by increased maternal morbidity, including premature labor and low birth weight infants (15). Human and animal studies have shown that tissue iron deficiency produces a decrease in work performance even when the hemoglobin is within a normal range, and work performance improves with iron supplementation (12). Even athletes with chronic iron deficiency may experience symptoms of decreased endurance without the presence of anemia.

Neurologic Effects

Iron is present in large quantities in certain parts of the brain and is required for the activity of enzymes that are components of neurotransmitter metabolism, which is critical for normal cognition. The iron content of parts of the brain is comparable to that of liver and continues to increase until the third decade of life. In children, impaired mental development was found when hemoglobin levels were less than 10 g/dL at 5 years (16). Iron-deficient children showed reduced attention and poor learning performance. This was manifested in lower scores in mental and motor function that returned to normal when tests were repeated after iron therapy.

Immunity

Cell-mediated (T-lymphocyte) immunity and neutrophil killing of phagocytosed bacteria may be impaired in iron-deficient patients (6). Neutrophils ingest and kill organisms by the production of reactive oxygen species, a process referred to as the oxidative burst, which depends on the activity of iron-containing enzymes. Conversely, because microorganisms require iron for their growth, parenteral iron treatment can precipitate latent infection (17). Several studies have shown an increase in malarial attacks in children following treatment of iron deficiency without simultaneous antimalarial prophylaxis (18).

LIFE STAGE–SPECIFIC ISSUES IN IRON DEFICIENCY

Neonates and Infants

A normal newborn has approximately 75 mg iron/kg body weight, of which two thirds is in hemoglobin. Premature (low birth weight) infants have much less iron stores and need dietary iron at an earlier age than full-term infants. Infants born of women with iron-deficiency anemia are at increased risk for neonatal death from premature birth and low birth weight. About 50% of the iron for a normal 6-month-old infant can be obtained from breast milk. However, by 6 months, the iron stores received at birth are used up for normal growth; so if the mother is anemic, the child will also be depleted of iron earlier. Intramuscular iron dextran given to the premature infant can benefit overall iron stores (19); however, it is also recognized that oral iron would be safer if the child could be followed in the long term. As of now, any parenteral iron given to infants should be under the aegis of a controlled clinical trial.

Human breast milk contains about 0.5 mg iron/L. The bioavailability is high, with 50% iron absorbed. This contrasts with cow's milk formulas or unfortified cow's milk, in which only 10% to 20% of the iron is available for absorption. Hence, cow's milk formulas are usually fortified with iron to supply 6 to 12 mg/L. Breast milk supplies sufficient iron to full-term infants to meet their needs for the first 4 to 5 months of life. Because weaning foods often consist of cereals with iron of low bioavailability, many of these cereals contain added iron and ascorbate. Such foods are a major source of iron in the first 1 or 2 years of life.

During infancy, the most iron is required between 6 and 18 months. This is the period of highest risk, when nutritional iron deficiency can manifest in serious and potentially permanent intellectual impairment with cognitive defects and poor social development (20). Even infants in the United States with borderline iron deficiency who did not have frank anemia responded to supplemental iron with a significant increase in mental development index scores (+21.6 points) as measured by the Bayley Scales of Mental Development (21).

Delayed cord clamping for a full 120 seconds, measured from the time of delivery of the infant's shoulders, has now been shown to have a beneficial effect on the infant's iron stores from between 27 and 47 mg when measured at 6 months (22). This procedure had the impact of a higher RBC, mean corpuscular volume (MCV), ferritin, and total body iron. A confirmatory study that also delayed cord clamping showed raised mean venous hematocrit immediately after birth (23). Thus, this is a simple, efficient way to increase the net iron stores for the baby at birth.

Children

The question whether iron supplements can increase the risk of infections has been answered. A systematic review of 22 randomized controlled trials, involving more than 7000 children, concluded that iron supplementation (via oral or parenteral iron) or fortified formula milk or cereals has *no* apparent harmful effect on the overall incidence of infectious illnesses in children, except for a small risk of diarrhea, which was deemed unlikely to have an impact on public health (24). In addition, all children found to have iron-deficiency anemia in areas of high malaria prevalence should be given supplementary iron as a component of a proactive intervention that also includes provision of treated bed nets and antimalarial drugs (12).

Adolescents

The next growth spurt that occurs in adolescence and at menarche marks the other phase when iron requirement peaks. This is the period when a woman is at risk for additional complications if she becomes pregnant, a not uncommon occurrence, especially in the developing world. A cross-sectional study among adolescents in Sri Lanka revealed that 50% of boys and nearly 60% of girls had anemia predominantly from iron deficiency (25).

Women and Pregnancy

Anemia with hemoglobin less than 7 g/dL places pregnant women at serious risk for increased maternal mortality (cardiac failure during labor from anemia, poor tolerance of hemorrhagic blood loss during labor, slower wound-healing time, and also increased risk for infection). Indeed, because intravenous iron given during this time can significantly increase the risk for infections, prophylactic oral iron administered well before labor is best (26).

Menstruating women need 2.8 mg/day (whereas men need 0.9 mg/day). Women need 0.8 mg/day in the first trimester of pregnancy, 4 to 5 mg/day in the second trimester, and more than 6 mg/day in the third trimester. Thus, women require an extra 1000 mg iron to meet the needs of a normal pregnancy (220 mg iron during pregnancy going to term), to expand their RBC mass (500 mg), and to provide iron for the placenta and developing fetus. The full-term fetus has approximately 290 mg iron, and the placenta has approximately 25 mg iron. During lactation, women need 2.4 mg/day (27). All this has to be set against the total body iron of 2500 mg present in an adult woman with normal iron absorption of 1 to 2 mg/day. This amount of iron is more than can be provided by a good diet, so serum iron and ferritin levels both fall steadily throughout pregnancy. Thus, iron deficiency in pregnancy results from increased demands for iron that cannot be met from stores and diet. The problem facing women with preexisting anemia is that when they become pregnant, there is an increased risk of maternal death, preterm delivery, impaired fetal growth, low birth weight infants, and increased neonatal mortality. Moreover, because maternal iron deficiency predicts iron deficiency in the fetus, there may be additional cognitive

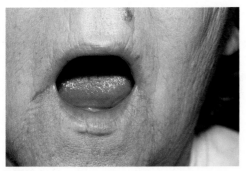

Fig. 98.1. Angular stomatitis (fissures at the angles of the mouth) in iron deficiency.

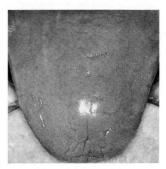

Fig. 98.2. Glossitis.

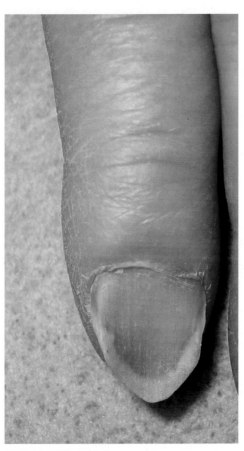

Fig. 98.3. Koilonychia.

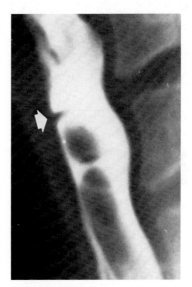

Fig. 98.4. Esophageal web in iron deficiency.

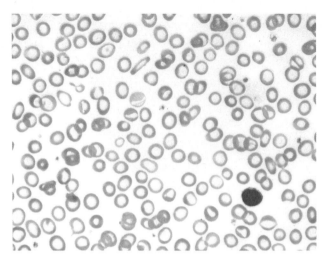

Fig. 98.5. Iron-deficiency anemia: red blood cells.

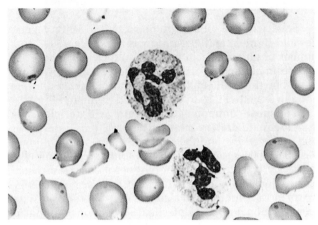

Fig. 98.6. Blood smear in vitamin B$_{12}$ deficiency showing hypersegmentation (more than five lobes in the nuclei) of the neutrophils.

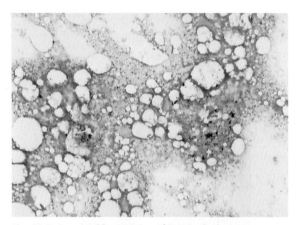

Fig. 98.7. Prussian blue staining of iron in the bone marrow.

and adverse developmental issues in the newborn. Hence, prophylactic oral iron supplement is invariably required during pregnancy and is the best approach (26).

A double-blind, cluster-randomized controlled trial from rural Western China demonstrated a longer gestation and a reduction in risk of early neonatal mortality by 54% in women who took iron and folic acid compared with those taking folic acid alone (28). Similar findings in the United States among women who were not anemic demonstrated a lower incidence of low birth weight and preterm deliveries in women taking iron supplements (29, 30).

Elderly Persons

Whereas an adult man has approximately 500 to 1000 mg of storage iron and older men have even more, the iron stores in women seldom reach 500 mg. In elderly persons, anemia resulting in a reduction of oxygen-carrying capacity of the blood leads to fatigue, cardiovascular complications (including heart failure) and poor physical capacity arising from reduced muscle strength (31), increased disability with decreased performance, and increased all-cause mortality among nursing home residents (32). For those persons with iron deficiency and mild or moderate heart failure with ventricular systolic dysfunction, the efficacy of intravenous iron infusion in improving symptoms and measurable quality of life benefits was demonstrated; within 4 weeks of initiation of therapy, these persons were able to increase their distance in the 6-minute walk test by more than 30 m (33).

DIAGNOSIS OF IRON DEFICIENCY

Laboratory Tests

The development of iron-deficiency anemia with its characteristic morphologic changes in RBCs is preceded by stages of iron depletion and iron-deficient erythropoiesis. In the early stages of *iron depletion*, a decrease in iron stores in the bone marrow reticuloendothelial cells occurs, with a decrease in plasma ferritin levels to approximately 20 μg/mL. A marked change in serum iron levels is generally not seen at this early stage. However, a decrease in the percentage of transferrin saturated with iron (transferrin saturation) and an increase in the iron-binding capacity of transferrin are noted. An increase in iron absorption also occurs at this stage.

With progression to *iron-deficient erythropoiesis*, iron stores in reticuloendothelial cells are depleted, and ferritin and plasma iron levels decrease to below normal values. (The normal range for ferritin is 30 to 400 ng/mL for men and 13 to 150 ng/mL for women. The normal range for iron is 65 to 175 μg/dL for men and 50 to 170 μg/dL for women). In addition, transferrin saturation decreases to less than 15% (normal = 16% to 50%), and RBC zinc protoporphyrin (ZPP) is increased to more than 30 μg/dL.

At this stage, a mild decrease in hemoglobin is seen, but the RBCs appear normal in size and appearance (referred to as normocytic and normochromic).

With the appearance of frank *iron-deficiency anemia*, there is a further decrease in hemoglobin (see Table 98.2) with a decrease in plasma ferritin to less than 10 μg/mL and MCV to less than 80 femtoliters/cell. These smaller RBCs (referred to as microcytes) contain less hemoglobin than normal RBCs, so the mean corpuscular hemoglobin concentration is also reduced. A further decrease in serum iron and transferrin saturation to less than 10% with an increase in transferrin iron-binding capacity and RBC protoporphyrin is also seen at this stage.

Although the development of microcytic and hypochromic RBCs is characteristic of iron-deficiency anemia, the decrease in hemoglobin generally precedes the appearance of microcytosis. Hence, in early iron-deficiency anemia, the MCV is normal, and the population of smaller RBCs in the circulation may be fully hemoglobinized and not hypochromic. However, later on, the peripheral blood smear shows RBCs with reduced hemoglobin content that is manifested as a reduced area of central pallor (hypochromia) in the RBC that becomes more prominent with worsening anemia. (Normochromic RBCs have central pallor that occupies one third of the cell). In severe iron-deficiency anemia, RBC morphology may become significantly altered, with RBCs appearing as thin rings with bizarre shapes (Fig. 98.5).

When iron-deficiency anemia coexists with either vitamin B_{12} deficiency or folate deficiency (megaloblastic anemia), the peripheral blood smear shows an increase in nuclear segmentation in neutrophils (hypersegmentation) (Fig. 98.6), which is a hallmark of megaloblastic anemia. In contrast to iron-deficiency anemia, which produces RBC microcytosis, megaloblastic anemia is associated with an increase in MCV (macrocytosis); both types of cells may be observed on the peripheral smear. Hence, with combined iron and vitamin B_{12} or folate deficiency, the average MCV of microcytes and macrocytes—when measured by an automated counter—is usually in the normal range (masked megaloblastosis) (34). Iron-deficiency anemia is not associated with changes in white blood cell number; however, an increase in the platelet count is often seen.

Although the diagnosis of iron deficiency as the cause of anemia can usually be established by measurements of serum iron, transferrin, and serum iron-binding capacity and a review of the peripheral blood smear, in certain conditions these measurements may not be reliable indicators of iron deficiency. For example, chronic inflammatory conditions (e.g., tuberculosis, arthritis, hepatitis, enteritis) may be associated with mild microcytic anemia suggestive of iron deficiency. However, in these situations, the plasma ferritin level may be elevated as an acute phase reactant and thus is not a reliable marker of iron status. An analysis of the bone marrow to demonstrate the *absence* of stainable iron in the marrow has long been considered the "gold standard" for establishing iron deficiency. Figure 98.7 shows normal staining of iron in the marrow.

Although not widely used in clinical medicine, other tests to detect early iron deficiency have been shown to be of value. ZPP is normally present in trace amounts in RBCs during hemoglobin synthesis. With failure of iron delivery for hemoglobin synthesis, the level of ZPP accumulates in RBCs, thus resulting in an increase in the RBC ZPP/heme ratio. Studies in pediatric populations have shown that an increased ZPP/heme ratio is a reliable indicator of iron-deficient erythropoiesis (35–37). However, concerns about the use of ZPP as a marker of iron deficiency exist; the test is sensitive to interference by drug and plasma components, and a significant number of RBCs being analyzed must be new RBCs synthesized in the iron-deficient state (38).

Another marker, the soluble transferrin receptor (sTfR), has been shown to be present in increased levels in the circulation in iron deficiency. Measurement of serum sTfR level and calculation of the ratio of sTfR/log ferritin (i.e., logarithmic transformation of the serum ferritin level) is of value in estimating body iron stores, especially when serum iron and transferrin levels are not reliable as a result of the clinical conditions described earlier, and analysis of the marrow is not feasible. The sTfR/log ferritin ratio is increased in iron deficiency. A present obstacle to the routine use of sTfR measurements for determining iron deficiency appears to be lack of standardization among the available assays (39).

Clinical Considerations in Diagnosis and Treatment

An important factor that aggravates iron deficiency is an increased need for iron in individuals with preexisting marginal iron stores. This can occur in several clinical circumstances: when individuals contract malaria or have blood losses from high worm burdens; when women are in the last trimester of pregnancy, are lactating, or are weaning their infants; and in adolescents during their growth spurt.

In developing countries, multiple micronutrient deficiencies often coexist in a single individual, so it is often impossible to distinguish the etiopathologic factors that led to anemia. It is estimated that iron deficiency—resulting from inadequate iron intake that often coexists with infection-related hemolysis of RBCs (malaria) and excess blood loss from parasitic infestation of the intestine (hookworm, whipworm) or bladder (schistosomiasis)—is primarily responsible for one half of the cases of anemia in these populations (40).

Deficiency of other micronutrients (e.g., vitamin B_{12}, folate, riboflavin, and vitamin A, individually or in combination) or infectious diseases (e.g., malaria, human immunodeficiency virus [HIV] infection, or tuberculosis, individually or in combination), and hemoglobinopathies

that protect against malaria (sickle cell disease, thalassemias, glucose-6-phosphate dehydrogenase deficiency) are the cause of the remainder. Vitamin A and zinc deficiency result in increased susceptibility to respiratory and diarrheal illness (41, 42) that further contributes a component of chronic disease anemia. A good example of the plethora of etiologic factors contributing to anemia in children was reported from Malawi (43). Therefore, treatment must be individualized, with all coexisting factors that perpetuate the anemia addressed together with supplementation of the deficient minerals and micronutrients.

Differential Diagnosis

Whereas microcytic hypochromic anemia is the hallmark finding of iron-deficiency anemia, similar RBC morphology can be seen in a few other conditions that must be differentiated from iron deficiency to avoid inappropriate diagnostic testing and treatment. For example, the decrease in globin synthesis that occurs in thalassemic syndromes also produces mild to moderate microcytic hypochromic anemia in individuals with a thalassemia trait. The diagnosis of thalassemias can be excluded by hemoglobin electrophoresis and more specialized tests.

Anemia of chronic disease may resemble iron deficiency because both have small RBCs and a low serum iron level; however, the serum iron-binding capacity is normal or low in the anemia of chronic disorders, whereas in iron deficiency it is raised. Because ferritin is an acute phase reactant, its levels may be elevated in the anemia secondary to chronic disease. The sTfR concentration is not elevated in chronic disease (in contrast to ferritin), and therefore, measurement of the sTfR/log ferritin ratio has been suggested as a means to discriminate between iron-deficiency anemia and anemia of chronic disease. Distinguishing iron deficiency from anemia of chronic disease may still require direct examination of the marrow for iron stores. Measurement of markers of inflammation such as C-reactive protein may also be useful in establishing the presence of inflammation as a cause of anemia (39).

PREVENTION AND TREATMENT OF IRON DEFICIENCY

Iron Supplementation and Iron Fortification of Foods

Food fortification and dietary supplementation are the traditional methods for replenishing specific vulnerable groups deficient in one or more micronutrients. Whereas dietary supplements can provide a sufficient quantity of micronutrients in specific amounts, the number of individuals who benefit is far smaller than with food fortification, which covers entire populations at far lower cost, provided the vehicle used for fortification actually reaches the entire target population (44). Various traditionally eaten staple foods that have been used as vehicle

99 NUTRITION IN RESPIRATORY DISEASES[1]

NEAL M. PATEL AND MARGARET M. JOHNSON

Cellular respiration is essential for the functioning of all tissues. Food substrate is converted to usable energy by the formation of high-energy phosphate bonds. Oxygen (O_2) fuels this process, and carbon dioxide (CO_2) is produced as a byproduct. The respiratory system supplies the necessary O_2 and eliminates the CO_2 produced. Adequate nutrition is essential for development, growth, and function of the respiratory system. This chapter summarizes the normal structure and function of the respiratory system, the changes encountered with common diseases, and the impact of nutritional status on the epidemiology and pathophysiology of pulmonary disease.

[1]**Abbreviations: ARDS**, acute respiratory distress syndrome; **BMI**, body mass index; **CF**, cystic fibrosis; **CO_2**, carbon dioxide; **COPD**, chronic obstructive pulmonary disease; **ICU**, intensive care unit; **MIP**, maximum inspiratory pressure **O_2**, oxygen; **REE**, resting energy expenditure; **V_A**, alveolar minute ventilation; **V_E**, total minute ventilation; **V_T**, tidal volume.

STRUCTURE AND FUNCTION OF THE RESPIRATORY SYSTEM

Control of Breathing

Afferent signals arising from pontomedullary portion of the brainstem control resting rhythmic breathing patterns. Voluntary and involuntary input from higher cerebral centers, and changes in pH and partial pressure of arterial O_2 (PaO_2) and CO_2 ($PaCO_2$), can override these rhythmic impulses and alter respiratory patterns as needed to meet the changing metabolic demands of the organism.

Respiratory Muscles

Inspiration is achieved when a negative intrathoracic pressure is generated by the active contraction of the inspiratory muscles, creating a pressure gradient between the mouth, and the distal air spaces, the alveoli. Moving down this pressure gradient, air fills the lungs until the alveoli and atmospheric pressure equilibrate. Relaxation of the inspiratory muscles returns the thoracic cage to its resting position, thus reversing the pressure gradient and leading to exhalation.

The diaphragm, the primary muscle of respiration, is dome shaped at rest. With contraction, it flattens and descends, increasing both the vertical and anterior-posterior dimensions of the thoracic cage. The diaphragm does not have intrinsic automaticity properties such as cardiac muscle, and thus can fatigue when demand exceeds supply. Both fatigue (1), a reversible inability of a muscle to generate a prior attainable force, and weakness, the chronic inability to attain adequate force, may cause inadequate ventilation.

Diseases directly affecting the respiratory muscles are uncommon, but the respiratory muscles are an important compensatory mechanism in lung disease. In increased demand states such as exercise, or in the presence of muscle dysfunction from malnutrition, the compensatory capacity is overwhelmed leading to diminished functional capabilities.

Lung Parenchyma

The lungs are composed of the conducting airways, the alveoli, and the capillary beds, which form the gas-exchanging units, the supporting interstitial structures, the pulmonary vasculature, and immune effector cells.

Tracheobronchial Tree (Conducting Airways)

The conducting airways are a series of progressively, dichotomously branching tubular structures extending from the trachea. The trachea and proximal main airways, the bronchi, offer structural support to the airways but do not participate in gas exchange. Gas exchange occurs at the level of the distal respiratory bronchioles and the alveoli. The tracheobronchial tree is lined with ciliated columnar bronchial epithelial cells and submucosal glands that humidify, warm, and filter the inspired air and contribute to the bronchial mucus layer (2).

Smooth muscle, innervated by the parasympathetic and the nonadrenergic, noncholinergic nervous pathways, lines the tracheobronchial tree. Muscle contraction imparts rigidity to the airways and reduces the caliber of the airway lumen resulting in increased resistance to bulk gas flow. Additionally, airway edema, inflammation, and excessive mucus also narrow the airway (2), diminishing gas flow.

Terminal Respiratory Units

The terminal respiratory unit, consisting of respiratory bronchioles, alveolar ducts, and alveoli, is the gas-exchanging unit. Gas exchange occurs at the alveolar–capillary membrane, which consists of the alveolar epithelium and capillary endothelium, their basement membranes, and the contiguous interstitial space (2). Surfactant, a complex phospholipid and protein mixture that lines the alveolus, reduces its surface tension decreasing its tendency to collapse at low lung volumes.

Pulmonary Physiology

The ultimate purpose of the respiratory system is to transfer O_2 from the inspired air to the bloodstream and CO_2 from the bloodstream to the exhaled air. The respiratory and cardiac systems work in conjunction to provide a continuous supply of oxygenated blood to the peripheral tissues. After circulating to the periphery where O_2 is extracted, blood is returned to the right side of the heart and is pumped through the pulmonary arteries to the pulmonary capillaries. At the alveolar-capillary interface, O_2 diffuses down a concentration gradient from the O_2-rich alveolar gas to the pulmonary capillary blood. Most of the transferred O_2 binds to hemoglobin in the red blood cells; a small percentage is dissolved in the plasma. Simultaneously, CO_2 diffuses down a concentration gradient from the capillary blood to the alveolus.

O_2-enriched gas is continuously replenished at the alveolar level through inspiration. Approximately 30% of each inspired breath remains in the conducting airways and thus does not participate in gas exchange; this is anatomic dead space. A small fraction of each inspired breath reaches alveoli that are not perfused, and thus, do not allow gas transfer. This volume of gas is physiologic dead space. Effective alveolar minute ventilation (VA) is the difference between the total minute ventilation (VE) and the sum of anatomic and physiologic dead space ventilation (Table 99.1).

Efficient gas exchange is contingent on the delivery of gas to perfused alveoli and adequate capillary blood flow. Inadequate gas flow causes perfused alveoli not to be ventilated. The complete absence of ventilation to perfused alveoli is called shunt. Supplying inspired air to nonperfused alveoli increases physiologic dead space, thereby decreasing the effective tidal volume (VT). This is commonly seen in emphysema as a result of capillary bed obliteration.

Increased VE initially can compensate for mismatched gas and blood flow. Ultimately, however, if metabolic demands exceed these compensatory mechanisms, gas exchange abnormalities will develop.

Additional Respiratory System Functions

In addition to gas exchange functions, the lung acts as a "filter" for the blood and also has extensive metabolic functions. The lung synthesizes surfactant and other substances, including histamine and arachidonic acid. The effects of nutrition on these functions are largely unknown.

COMMON PULMONARY PATHOPHYSIOLOGY

Various diseases can affect the respiratory system and ultimately compromise gas exchange. Bulk gas flow can be diminished by airway obstruction or restriction. In obstructive disease, the airway lumen is narrowed, creating increased resistance to flow. Prototypical obstructive diseases include asthma, emphysema, and chronic bronchitis. Decreased compliance of the respiratory system leads to restrictive disease. The loss of compliance can be result from abnormalities in the lung parenchyma, respiratory muscles, or chest wall. Pulmonary fibrosis, the prototypical restrictive disease, is characterized by a loss of compliance of the lung parenchyma as a result of interstitial fibrosis. Other diseases, such as pneumonia and pulmonary edema, decrease the lung compliance by filling the alveolar spaces. Decreased compliance increases the work required to maintain adequate bulk gas flow.

Pulmonary function tests measure exhaled gas volumes and flow rates. Abnormalities in respiratory muscle function decrease the maximum pressures attainable with inspiration and expiration. Arterial blood gas determinations, which measure the arterial pH, $PaCO_2$, and PaO_2, can evaluate the efficiency of gas exchange. Other tests, including timed walk tests or cardiopulmonary exercise tests, can more comprehensively assess the interaction of the respiratory and cardiac systems with the peripheral muscles. These tests allow one to measure the impact of various nutritional interventions on lung function.

EFFECTS OF MALNUTRITION ON DEVELOPMENT, STRUCTURE, AND FUNCTION OF THE RESPIRATORY SYSTEM

Development

Both animal and human investigations demonstrate that inadequate nutrition during fetal development is deleterious. In animal models, fetal malnutrition results in pulmonary hypoplasia (3, 4). Inadequate protein during development diminishes collagen and elastin synthesis and causes pathologic changes similar to those in emphysema (5). The timing of nutrition insults affects their manifestations: Early malnutrition leads to small but normally proportioned animals, whereas later insults result in lung size disproportionately small for body size (6). In humans, a direct correlation exists between low birth weight and subsequent decreases in pulmonary function (7, 8).

Respiratory Muscles

Diaphragm weight correlates with body weight in animal models and both healthy and emphysematous humans (9–11). Poorly nourished patients have diminished maximal respiratory muscle strength as measured by maximum inspiratory pressure (MIP) and maximum expiratory pressure (MEP) (11). The extent of muscle strength loss exceeds the loss of muscle mass, a finding suggesting coexistent myopathy of the remaining muscle (11).

The diaphragm is composed of both type I and type II fibers, and malnutrition affects these fibers differently. In grossly underfed and protein-malnourished animals, the cross-sectional area of both types of fibers is greatly reduced, but the fast-twitch fibers (type II) are quantitatively more affected (12–14). These observations suggest that malnutrition should diminish peak pressure generation but have a more limited impact on endurance.

Ventilatory Drive

The impact of nutrition on respiratory drive is incompletely understood. Caloric and nutrient restrictions decrease the hypoxic respiratory drive in normal subjects (15, 16). Severe anorexia nervosa decreases V_E, which may reverse on refeeding (17).

Host Defenses

Malnutrition increases general susceptibility to infections, but it specifically alters pulmonary defense mechanisms. Animal models of severe malnourishment have demonstrated decreased alveolar macrophage counts (18), phagocytosis, and microbial killing (19). In patients with tracheostomies, nutritional status inversely correlates with lower respiratory tract bacterial colonization (20). Malnourished patients also are predisposed to pulmonary infections because of inadequate clearance of respiratory secretions resulting from ineffective cough from muscle weakness and a greater propensity for alveolar collapse.

PROTOTYPICAL LUNG DISEASES: RELATION TO NUTRITIONAL STATUS

Critical Illness and Acute Respiratory Failure

Critically ill patients often have multisystem organ failure, commonly including the respiratory system. Respiratory dysfunction is often the result of acute respiratory distress syndrome (ARDS), a syndrome characterized by hypoxemic respiratory failure in the setting of a severe systemic critical illness or isolated pulmonary disease. This section reviews nutritional supplementation in the critically ill patient, with specific attention to ARDS.

Nutrition in Critical Illness: Metabolic Requirements

The nutritional milieu of critical illness is characterized by hypermetabolism, protein catabolism, and insulin resistance leading to impaired glucose use and hyperglycemia. Because of the inherent complications of both underfeeding and overfeeding, proper estimation of caloric requirements is an essential but challenging task. Energy requirements can be estimated using standard population-based regression formulas, such as the Harris-Benedict equation (21). However, predictive formulas were derived from physiologically normal subjects at rest and do not address the stress and hypercatabolism of critical illness. "Correction stress factors," ranging from 1.2 to 1.5 times the calculated resting energy expenditure (REE) are suggested, but their correlation with indirect calorimetry measurements is often suboptimal (22, 23).

O_2 consumption ($\dot{V}O_2$), which can be used as an estimate of caloric needs, can be calculated by the Fick equation

$$\dot{V}O_2 = CO \div (Ca_{O_2} - Cv_{O_2})$$

where CO is the cardiac output and Ca_{O_2} and Cv_{O_2} are the O_2 content of arterial and mixed venous blood, respectively. This approach requires invasive monitoring with a pulmonary artery catheter, and a relatively stable patient.

Alternatively, $\dot{V}O_2$ can be assessed with a metabolic cart that measures exhaled gases directly. This technique is not universally available, and it requires expensive equipment, technical expertise, and a stable fraction of inspired O_2. Despite these limitations, this technique offers the advantage of continuous measurements rather than intermittent snapshots of one's caloric needs.

The $\dot{V}O_2$ (mL/minute) obtained by either the Fick equation or by the gas exchange method is converted to kilocalories/day by using the caloric value of O_2 (4.69 to 5.05 kcal/L of O_2 consumed) or the modified Weir equation if V_{CO_2} (CO_2 production) is also known (24).

Substrate Supplementation: Implications for Ventilatory Requirements

Patients with acute respiratory failure typically are in a hypercatabolic state and rely in part on proteolysis of protein stores to meet their immediate metabolic needs. Nutritional supplementation may spare consumption of endogenous protein, although the amount of glucose required differs from that needed in normal fasting adults (25). Intravenous fat emulsions, if administered with a minimum of 500 kcal/day of carbohydrate (26), and exogenous protein supplementation also can limit proteolysis (26).

The appropriate mix of carbohydrate, fat, and protein calories must be individualized. Carbohydrates produce more CO_2 during oxidation than fat or protein. For every molecule of glucose completely oxidized, six molecules of CO_2 are produced, giving a respiratory quotient of 1 (Table 99.1), whereas the oxidation of fat and protein produces less CO_2, with a respiratory quotient of 0.7 and 0.8, respectively. V_A must be increased when CO_2 production increases to maintain a normal partial pressure of arterial Pa_{CO_2}. In the presence of underlying lung disease, the ability to increase V_A may be limited.

TABLE 99.1	DEFINITION OF RESPIRATORY PHYSIOLOGY TERMS AND ABBREVIATIONS
TERM	**DEFINITION**
Tidal volume (V_T)	Volume of gas moved during a single respiration
Minute ventilation (V_E)	Amount of air moved in and out of the lungs in 1 minute; $V_E = V_T \times$ respiratory rate (RR) per minute
Dead-space ventilation (V_D)	Amount of inspired gas that does not participate in gas exchange; ventilation of nonperfused alveoli
V_D/V_T	Fraction of each tidal volume that is dead space
Alveolar minute ventilation (V_A)	Amount of inspired air able to participate in gas exchange; alveolar ventilation is the difference between total minute ventilation and dead-space ventilation
Forced vital capacity (FVC)	Volume of gas that can be forcibly exhaled after a maximal inhalation
Forced expiratory volume in 1 second (FEV_1)	Volume of gas expired in the first second of a forced expiration
Stroke volume (SV)	Amount of blood pumped by the heart in a single beat
Cardiac output (CO)	Volume of blood pumped by the heart in 1 minute (heart rate [HR] $\times$ SV)
Pa_{O_2}	Partial pressure of oxygen in the arterial blood
Pa_{CO_2}	Partial pressure of carbon dioxide in the arterial blood
$\dot{V}_{O_2}$	Oxygen consumption (mL/min)
$\dot{V}_{CO_2}$	Carbon dioxide production (mL/min)
Compliance	Change in volume per unit change of pressure
Respiratory quotient (RQ)	Molecules of oxygen used/molecule of carbon dioxide produced
Mixed venous blood	Deoxygenated blood returned to the heart; samples for measurements are obtained from a catheter in the pulmonary artery

Timing and Route of Nutritional Support

Malnutrition at the onset of critical illness is associated with poor outcomes, and improved clinical outcomes are associated with nutritional support (27). However, the optimal composition and timing of the initiation of feedings remains uncertain (28).

Enteral Feeding and Pulmonary Issues. Enteral feeding is most commonly accomplished through a nasogastric tube or nasoduodenal tube. Potential mechanical risks are associated with enteric feeding tubes, including misplacement in the tracheobronchial tree or pleural space; thus, radiographic confirmation of proper placement is mandatory before initiation of feeding. It is uncertain if the risk of aspiration differs between gastric and duodenal feedings (29, 30). Postpyloric feedings should be considered in those with significant gastroesophageal reflux disease, high risk for aspiration, on high doses of sedatives/paralytics, or intolerance to gastric feeding. Maintaining patients in a semirecumbent position, rather than supine, decreases the risk of aspiration (31).

Parenteral Nutrition and Pulmonary Issues. Parenteral nutrition is delivered through a central or peripheral vein. Central vein infusions allow for the delivery of more concentrated solutions; thus, it minimizes obligate fluid requirements. In patients with ARDS, limited fluid intake shortens the duration of mechanical ventilation (32). The addition of heparin (33), sterile line placement, and restriction of catheter use exclusively to alimentation (34) may limit catheter-associated complications such as thrombosis and infection. Infusion of lipid emulsions decrease diffusing capacity and oxygen saturation by causing ventilation and perfusion mismatch; thus, its use is typically avoided if possible.

Acute Respiratory Distress Syndrome and Acute Lung Injury

Optimal nutritional support in ARDS has been investigated. Patients with ARDS have lower levels of dietary antioxidants, including vitamin E, vitamin C, retinol, and β-carotene, than healthy controls (35). Decreased plasma concentrations of tocopherol and vitamin E and elevated lipoperoxides indicative of oxidative damage commonly are seen in patients with ARDS (36); findings prompting speculation that antioxidant supplementation may be beneficial. Although a prospective randomized trial examining the efficacy of supplementation with α-tocopherol and vitamin C did not decrease pulmonary mortality or the development of ARDS, the intervention group did have a significantly lower incidence of multisystem organ failure, shorter duration of intensive care unit (ICU) stay, and mechanical ventilation (37).

The specific dietary lipid alters the profile of eicosanoids produced by inflammatory cells, which may have clinical relevance. Linoleic acid, an n-6 fatty acid, is converted to arachidonic acid, which is the precursor of many proinflammatory prostaglandins and leukotrienes (38). Alternatively, linolenic acid, an n-3 fatty acid, is converted to eicosapentaenoic acid, which produces eicosanoids with much less inflammatory potential (38).

Gadek et al prospectively assessed the effects of enteral feedings enriched with eicosapentaenoic acid (and fish oil), γ-linolenic acid, and antioxidants in 98 patients with ARDS. Compared with controls, the treatment group had more ventilator-free and ICU-free days, earlier improvements in oxygenation, less new organ failure development, and a nonsignificant trend toward decreased mortality (16% versus 25%; $p = .31$) (39).

Currently, the ARDS network is performing a prospective, randomized trial of initial trophic enteral feeding followed by advancement to full-calorie enteral feeding versus early advancement to full-calorie enteral feeding. This trial will be conducted simultaneously with a one comparing omega-3 fatty acid, γ-linolenic acid, and antioxidant supplementation with a comparator.

Chronic Lung Diseases

Chronic lung disease generally is classified as obstructive or restrictive, based on the primary physiologic abnormality, as discussed. Obstructive lung diseases include asthma, chronic bronchitis, emphysema, cystic fibrosis (CF), and bronchiectasis. Emphysema and chronic bronchitis are most commonly the result of tobacco abuse and are collectively labeled chronic obstructive pulmonary disease (COPD).

Restrictive diseases include infiltrative or fibrotic diseases of the lung parenchyma as well as extrapulmonary processes such as muscular weakness, thoracic cage abnormalities, and neurologic diseases that result in similar physiologic impairments. Investigations of the interrelationships between nutrition and chronic pulmonary disease have focused on COPD, asthma, and CF.

Obstructive Lung Disease

COPD causes substantial and increasing morbidity and mortality in the United States and worldwide. An imbalance of proteases and antiproteases resulting in destruction of the elastin and collagen lung matrix causes emphysema. Tobacco use greatly contributes to this imbalance. Tobacco smoke causes neutrophils to migrate into the lung and release elastase and other proteases. Oxidants inhaled from tobacco smoke and released from activated inflammatory cells recruited into the airways impair endogenous antiproteases.

Several naturally occurring antioxidants are present in the lower respiratory tract to counter inhaled oxidants. The extent to which dietary supplementation with antioxidants may protect against tobacco or other environmentally induced pulmonary damage is not established. Concerns exist about deleterious effects of β-carotene supplementation (see the section on lung cancer).

Approximately 25% of chronic smokers develop clinically relevant COPD (40), and the amount of tobacco exposure does not fully account for disease development.

Therefore, it is hypothesized that one's diet may serve either a predisposing or protective role in COPD development. Supporting this hypothesis is the observation of pathologic changes similar to emphysema in patients with anorexia nervosa (41).

Dietary antioxidants intake and pulmonary function appear to be inversely related (42–45). Serum levels of β-carotene and retinol correlated with maintenance of ventilatory function in the Beta-Carotene and Retinol Efficacy Trial (46). These findings mirrored those of an earlier trial (47). However, baseline data from participants in the Atherosclerosis Risk in Communities study failed to demonstrate this relationship (48).

Because the type of ingested dietary fat may affect systemic inflammation, the Atherosclerosis Risk in Communities study investigated the relationship between dietary intake of n-3 fatty acids and the subsequent development of COPD in 8960 current or former smokers. There was a quantity-dependent inverse relationship between the two after controlling for the intensity of tobacco use (49). Sharp et al and Schwartz et al demonstrated similar results in 6346 and 2526 subjects, respectively (44, 50).

Mechanisms of Malnutrition

Malnutrition affects up to 60% of patients with COPD (51–53), and it is associated with poor outcomes (54–56). Persons who are less than 90% of ideal body weight have greater 5-year mortality after correction for the severity of lung disease (51). In a cohort of 4088 patients, 5-year survival was 24% in those with a body mass index (BMI) lower than 20% and 59% for those with a BMI greater than 30 (Fig. 99.1) (54). Patients who are underweight and have poor nutritional intake have been shown to have increased incidence of COPD exacerbations (57). Inadequate nutrition may be a modifiable identifier for

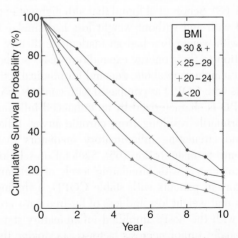

Fig. 99.1. Prognostic influence of body mass index in patients with chronic obstructive pulmonary disease. *BMI*, body mass index. (Reprinted with permission from Chailleux E, Laaban JP, Veale D. Prognostic value of nutritional depletion in patients with COPD treated by long-term oxygen therapy: data from the ANTADIR observatory. Chest 2003;123:1463.)

| TABLE 99.2 | RANDOMIZED CONTROLLED TRIALS EVALUATING NUTRITIONAL SUPPORT IN CHRONIC OBSTRUCTIVE PULMONARY DISEASE | | | |

AUTHOR (y)	NO.	DURATION (wk)	WEIGHT GAIN?	OTHER OUTCOMES
Wilson (1986)	6	3	Yes	Improved MIP
Lewis (1987)	10	8	No	No change in MIP
Knowles (1988)	25	8	No	No change in MIP
Efthimiou (1988)	7	12	Yes	Improved MIP
Otte (1989)	28	13	Yes	No change in pulmonary function
Fuenzalida (1990)	9	21	Yes	Improved immune response
Whittaker (1990)	6	2.3	Yes	MIP improved
Rogers (1992)	15	4	Yes	Improved MIP
Schols (1995)	135	8	Yes	Improved MIP
Creutzberg (2003)	64	8	Yes	Improved MIP, handgrip strength, peak workload, symptoms
Cai (2003)	60	3	Yes	Increased FEV_1

FEV_1, forced expiratory volume in 1 second; MIP, maximum inspiratory pressure.

deleterious outcomes in COPD, with intervention improving survival and functional status (58).

Malnutrition and weight loss in association with advanced lung disease, the pulmonary cachexia syndrome, results from both inadequate intake caused by hyperinflation-induced early satiety and chronic systemic inflammation (59). Patients with COPD generally are hypermetabolic. Measured REE exceeds the predicted REE by the Harris-Benedict equation in patients with COPD with and without weight loss (11, 60, 61). The increased work of breathing and greater energy expenditure for respiratory muscle activity account for the bulk of the increase in REE. Additionally, diet-induced thermogenesis and the O_2 cost associated with eating limit the ability to consume adequate calories to effect weight gain.

Investigations examining the adequacy of caloric intake are challenging. Most rely on patient food recall that is inherently inaccurate (62). Commonly, intake is adequate to meet energy requirements at rest but insufficient for metabolic demands of activity or for intercurrent illness (58, 62, 63). Schols et al found that although patients with COPD with and without weight loss had similar REEs, those with weight loss had an inadequate dietary intake in relation to their energy expenditure (64). Studies also suggest a higher metabolic demand for physical activity in patients with COPD as compared with controls (65).

COPD is characterized by an enhanced inflammatory state primarily resulting from chronic airway inflammation and circulating inflammatory mediators that may contribute to malnutrition (66). Skeletal muscle loss has been correlated with circulating levels of inflammatory mediators in patients with stable COPD, a finding suggesting that weight loss and loss of fat-free mass are associated with the host's amplified inflammatory state (59). Additionally, tumor necrosis factor-α, a cytokine that can induce cachexia, is elevated in weight-losing patients with COPD even in the absence of an acute infection (67). Nutritional supplementation combined with low-intensity exercise not only produced an improvement in weight, exercise capacity, and quality of life but also significantly reduces various proinflammatory markers (68).

Nutritional Supplementation

Numerous investigators have prospectively studied the effects of prolonged (>2 weeks) nutritional supplementation on patients with COPD (Table 99.2). Most of these studies are small, thus limiting their conclusions. Although the heterogeneity in study design limits the utility of meta-analysis, a review of the available data suggested no significant benefit in lung function, anthropometric measures, or exercise capacity in patients with stable COPD (69).

Recognizing individual variability and tailoring dietary interventions based on specific needs is likely to result in the most appropriate interventions. Slinde et al demonstrated significant anthropometric and functional improvements with a 1-year individualized dietary intervention in patients undergoing rehabilitation (70). Advanced age, anorexia, and an elevated systemic inflammatory response characterize patients who are unable to gain weight (71).

Anabolic Steroid or Growth Hormone and Appetite Stimulant Administration

Administration of supplemental growth hormone and anabolic steroids has been studied as adjuvant therapy to improve nutritional status in patients with COPD. Various investigators have shown improvements in nitrogen balance (72), body weight, lean body mass (73, 74), and maximum inspiratory pressures with growth hormone use (75). Rudman et al showed that growth hormone supplementation could increase lean body mass and a decrease in adipose tissue mass (76). Burdet et al demonstrated an increase in lean body mass with growth hormone but no effect on inspiratory or peripheral muscle strength (74). The use of exogenous growth hormone may allow protein synthesis while minimizing the thermogenic effect of nutritional replacement by reducing the total number of calories needed for anabolism. Schols et al compared the effects of nutritional supplementation with or without anabolic steroids with placebo in patients with COPD enrolled in a rehabilitation program. Nutritional support in combination with anabolic steroids increased fat-free body mass and MIP in subjects who were depleted at baseline (77). In 23 malnourished patients with COPD who had reduced respiratory muscle strength, synthetically derived testosterone improved BMI, weight, and lean body mass but did not affect exercise capacity (78). In two similarly designed studies, supplementation with growth hormone increased lean body mass but did not improve functional capabilities (73, 74, 79). Recognizing that body weight is an independent predictor of survival, supplements that increase weight may improve outcomes, but data validating this assumption are lacking. In a single study, the appetite stimulant megestrol acetate led to weight gain in patients with COPD but no improvement in respiratory muscle function or exercise tolerance (80).

Nutrient Composition and Administration

As described, the oxidation of carbohydrates produces more CO_2 for each mole of O_2 consumed than fats. Therefore, it has been suggested that a high-fat diet would be superior to a high-carbohydrate diet in patients with limited ventilatory reserve. Angelillo et al randomized patients with COPD with hypercarbia to a high-carbohydrate (74% carbohydrate calories) or a low-carbohydrate (28% carbohydrate calories) diet (81). The low-carbohydrate diet resulted in lower CO_2 production and arterial $PaCO_2$ and higher PaO_2. Kwan and Mir documented similar findings in patients fed a low-carbohydrate diet. The clinical impact of these findings is unclear. Brown et al showed a reduction in 12-minute walk distance after a large-carbohydrate meal in patients with COPD (82). In normal subjects, however, altering dietary fat and carbohydrate proportions did not change exercise gas exchange or mean V_E (83).

Electrolyte deficiencies, including hypokalemia, hypocalcemia, and hypophosphatemia, can adversely affect respiratory muscle function (see elsewhere in this volume). Diaphragmatic contractility improves after phosphorus replacement in hypophosphatemic patients (84). This observation is particularly relevant to patients with COPD who require mechanical ventilation because intracellular shifts of phosphorus follow correction of respiratory acidosis with ventilatory support. The clinical manifestations of hypophosphatemia result from intracellular phosphorus depletion resulting from chronic hypophosphatemia. Aubier et al reported that acute lowering of the serum calcium reduces maximum diaphragmatic contractility (85). Restoring normal intracellular concentrations of these ions may improve respiratory muscle strength.

Despite the paucity of proven beneficial effects of nutritional supplementation in malnourished patients with COPD, it is recommended that interventions be undertaken to restore or maintain a normal BMI. Such supplementation should be instituted in conjunction with a regular exercise program and routine reassessment of the patient's progress and nutritional status.

Asthma

Prostanoids released from inflammatory cells contribute greatly to the pathophysiologic changes of asthma, and dietary fat composition may alter prostanoid production. Epidemiologic studies from the 1960s and 1970s demonstrated a low incidence of asthma in populations whose diets were rich in fish oil that was rich in eicosapentaenoic acid (85). Clinical investigations of fish oil supplementation show changes in inflammatory cells but variable effects on clinical markers of disease (86, 87). A review of randomized trials failed to substantiate a therapeutic role for either dietary or supplemental eicosapentaenoic acid (88).

Both inhaled and intravenous magnesium supplements have been suggested to augment standard β-agonist therapy in acute asthma. Although the efficacy of magnesium therapy has been more fully established in pediatric populations than in adults (89), a study of 55 adults assessed the impact of oral supplementation magnesium in asthmatic patients aged 21 to 55 years. The study group showed improvement in objective measures of bronchial reactivity to methacholine, peak expiratory flow measurments, and subjective measures of asthma control and quality of life (90).

Antioxidant supplementation has been suggested as a means to modulate effects of airway injury in patients with asthma who are exposed to ozone and other air pollutants. Children with asthma in Mexico City were randomized to receive either a combined vitamin E and C supplement or placebo. Supplementation attenuated the loss of small airway function in those children with moderate-to-severe disease (91).

Lung Cancer

Lung cancer is the leading cause of cancer deaths. Most cases are attributable to tobacco abuse, with a direct relationship between exposure intensity and cancer incidence. However, only approximately 10% to 20% of heavy smokers develop lung cancer, a finding suggesting a role for either genetic or environmental predispositions.

Retinol, Carotenoids, and α-Tocopherol

Epidemiologic studies suggested that reduced intake and serum levels of carotenoids or retinoids correlated with increased incidence of lung cancer. The National Cancer Institute in Milan prospectively examined the use of retinoids in the prevention of secondary tumors in patients with lung cancer (92). Patients with localized disease were randomized to retinyl palmitate treatment or a control group. A greater disease-free interval and fewer new malignancies related to tobacco use were seen in the treatment group, but there was no improvement in overall survival. Subsequently, the Alpha-Tocopherol, Beta-Carotene Cancer Prevention Group randomized 29,133 male smokers to α-tocopherol, β-carotene, both agents, or placebo (93). Supplementation with α-tocopherol or β-carotene did not decrease the incidence of lung cancer.

However, total mortality was 8% higher in those participants who received β-carotene than in those who did not, primarily from an increase in mortality from lung cancer and ischemic heart disease. In the Beta-Carotene and Retinol Efficacy Trial, former smokers, current smokers, and asbestos workers were randomized to receive β-carotene and vitamin A or placebo. The intervention group had a 1.28 greater relative risk for lung cancer development (94). These troubling results raised still unresolved concerns regarding prooncogenic effects of β-carotene and prompted early termination of the trial.

Alternatively, the Physicians Health Study randomized 22,000 male physicians to β-carotene (50 mg) supplementation or placebo every other day for an average of 12 years. No difference in the rates of overall malignancy or any specific type of malignancy was seen (95). Finally, 1024 asbestos workers were studied in South Africa in a nonblinded fashion, with a comparison made between supplemental β-carotene (30 mg) and retinol (25,000 IU). The incidence of malignant mesothelioma was significantly lower in the retinol group compared with the β-carotene group but overall lung cancer incidence was the same (96). Currently, β-carotene, α-tocopherol supplementation, or other studied supplements such as flavonoids, N-acetylcysteine, or isotretinoin cannot be recommended for lung cancer chemoprevention.

Fruits and Vegetables

Diets rich in fruits and vegetables may decrease the incidence of lung cancer. More than 10 studies have demonstrated an inverse relationship between fruit and vegetable intake and the incidence of lung malignancy irrespective of tobacco history (97–99). Special attention has been paid to intake of carrots in particular. Consumption of five or more carrots a week in women was associated with a decreased risk of lung cancer (100, 101).

Dietary Fat

Epidemiologic data in the 1980s serendipitously uncovered a potential relationship between dietary intake of saturated fat and lung cancer (102). Subsequent case-control studies demonstrated a positive association between saturated fat intake and lung cancer incidence (103–105) and attributable mortality. In a multicountry study including more than 12,000 participants, lung cancer mortality correlated with saturated fat consumption (106).

Cystic Fibrosis

CF is an autosomal recessive disorder characterized by impaired chloride transport in various organs. Clinical manifestations include bronchiectasis, recurrent respiratory infections, and pancreatic dysfunction resulting in fat-soluble vitamin deficiency. Malnutrition is exceedingly common in CF, and inadequate weight gain is often the dominant finding in children at presentation. Nutritional status has been directly correlated with mortality and morbidity (107), and maintenance of adequate nutrition is a vital goal of therapy.

Numerous factors lead to malnutrition in CF. Malabsorption resulting from pancreatic dysfunction is the major contributing factor. Moreover, similar to patients with COPD, REE is 25% to 80% greater in patients with CF (108), primarily because of the increased work of breathing (109).

Abnormal cellular mitochondrial function also contributes to increased $\dot{V}O_2$ (110). Although the mechanism is incompletely delineated, it is likely that the CF gene abnormalities alter cellular aerobic respiration.

Because of chronic infection, circulating inflammatory cytokines, catecholamines, and cortisol are elevated in CF, with concomitant increases in REE (111). Antimicrobial treatment of pulmonary infections can reduce REE and promote weight gain (109), but the chronicity and recurrence of infection make it difficult to achieve sustained improvements.

Nutritional assessment should be undertaken at the time of the diagnosis and periodically thereafter to ensure adequate nutrient intake. Generally it is recommended that a patient with CF consume 120% to 150% of the recommended caloric intake of age- and sex-matched controls (112).

Pancreatic insufficiency decreases the absorption of fat-soluble nutrients such as β-carotene and vitamins K, A, D, and E. β-Carotene deficiency is common in patients with CF, and supplementation is recommended (113). Vitamin K deficiency typically occurs only in conjunction with antibiotic use, and thus supplementation is recommended at those times (114).

Up to 50% of patients have vitamin A deficiency, leading to visual defects in up to 18% (115). Low vitamin A levels correlate with poor lung function and offer prognostic value (116). Serum measurements of vitamin A or retinol-binding protein should be obtained when the patient is in a noninfected state because levels vary widely in the presence of with inflammation.

Osteoporosis is a persistent problem in CF that is frequently accompanied by vitamin D deficiency. Malabsorption, inadequate exposure to sunlight, and poor hepatic function all contribute to this deficiency. Supplementation of both calcium and vitamin D is recommended to ensure bone health.

Vitamin E is highly fat soluble and correlates well with fat malabsorption. Severely deficient states are characterized by hemolytic anemia, neuromuscular degeneration, and cognitive deficits. Annual assessment of vitamin E levels and supplementation, when deficient, are recommended.

Iron and zinc deficiency are common in CF. Iron supplements are indicated in the presence of iron deficiency anemia. Zinc supplementation is suggested in children who have failed to meet developmental landmarks (112). Supplementation with n-3 fatty acids may be beneficial, but confirmatory research is necessary (117).

Despite advances in our understanding of the genetic defect of CF, treatment is still largely supportive. A high-calorie, high-protein diet with supplemental pancreatic enzymes and multivitamins is recommended. Aggressive nutritional intervention, even using enteral feedings when indicated, may aid in weight maintenance and improve lung function (118).

Lung Transplantation

Lung transplantation is a therapeutic option for patients with end stage lung disease resulting from a variety of illnesses. Both malnutrition and obesity are commonly recognized problems before and after lung transplantation, and they have a direct impact on a patient's clinical course.

Malnutrition is encountered in up to 60% of patients seeking evaluation for lung transplantation (119). A BMI less than 17 kg/m^2 is associated with an increased risk of mortality (120). It is unclear whether improving malnutrition perioperatively improves outcomes (121, 122) and delaying lung transplantation to improve nutritional status may adversely affect the outcome (123).

Lung transplantation may reverse malnutrition. In 37 patients followed after lung transplantation, total weight and fat-free mass increased 16.6% and 14.0%, respectively, in the first year after the transplant (124). Greater weight gain following transplantation is associated with improved survival (125).

Pretransplant obesity is associated with increased mortality (120, 126) and weight loss is often recommended before listing for transplant. Weight reduction alone may improve function sufficiently to delay or obviate the need for transplantation (127).

Other Clinical Considerations

Compromised nutritional status may exacerbate or be worsened by respiratory illness. For example, protein malnutrition causing hypoalbuminemia alters the threshold for transudation of fluid into the lung parenchyma and pleural space and results in pulmonary edema and pleural effusions.

Specific respiratory diseases impose particular nutritional demands. Patients with malignant disease metastatic to the pleura may drain large amounts of protein into the pleural space. Repeated thoracentesis to drain this fluid results in severe protein wasting. Patients with chylothorax caused by disruption of the thoracic duct may lose massive amounts of protein, fat, and electrolytes into the pleural space. Parenteral alimentation or oral medium-chain triglycerides are often beneficial in replacing the lost nutrients.

Systemic corticosteroids, which are used in a variety of pulmonary diseases, have numerous potential deleterious side effects, including fluid retention and weight gain, with resultant increases in work of breathing. In animal models, steroids are associated with increased atrophy of type II fibers in the diaphragm (128). In 64 nutritionally depleted patients with COPD, the beneficial effects of nutritional supplementation were attenuated in those receiving systemic steroids (129). Dietary suppressants, including aminorex and fenfluramine (Redux), have been associated with the development of pulmonary hypertension (130).

Although this chapter focuses on the adverse respiratory effects of malnutrition and low body weight, obesity also profoundly affects respiratory function. Excessive weight on the chest and elevation of the hemidiaphragm because of increased abdominal pressure may cause restrictive ventilatory impairment. In extreme cases, these mechanical changes interact with abnormalities of the respiratory center (decreased sensitivity to hypoxemia and hypercarbia) and culminate in the obesity–hypoventilation syndrome. Moreover, increased body weight is a major risk factor for obstructive sleep apnea, which may lead to the development of pulmonary hypertension. Weight loss is the primary treatment for both these conditions.

REFERENCES

1. Roussos C, Macklem PT. N Engl J Med 1982;307:786–97.
2. Murray JF. The Normal Lung: The Basis for Diagnosis and Treatment of Pulmonary Disease. 2nd ed. Philadelphia: WB Saunders, 1986.
3. Lechner AJ, Winston DC, Bauman JE. J Appl Physiol 1986;60:1610–4.
4. Fariday EE. J Appl Physiol 1975;39:535–40.
5. Kalenga M, Shaheen S, Barker DJ. Thorax 1994;49:533–6.
6. Eeckhout Y. Pediatr Res 1989;26:125–7.
7. Shaheen S, Barker DJ. Thorax 1994;49:533–6.
8. Chan KN, Noble-Jamieson CM, Elliman A et al. Arch Dis Child 1989;64:1284–93.
9. Barker DJ, Godfrey KM, Fall C et al. BMJ 1991;303:671–5.
10. Rochester DF, Pradel-Guena M. J Appl Physiol 1973;34:68–74.
11. Goldberg AL, Odessey R. Am J Physiol 1972;223:1384–91.
12. Lewis MI, Sieck GC, Fournier M et al. J Appl Physiol 1986;60: 596–603.
13. Goldspink G, Ward PS. J Physiol (Lond) 1979;296:453–69.
14. Oldfors A, Mair WG, Sourander P. J Neurol Sci 1983;59:291–302.
15. Doekel RC Jr, Zwillich CW, Scoggin CH et al. N Engl J Med 1976;295:358–61.
16. Baier H, Somani P. Chest 1984;85:222–5.
17. Ryan CF, Whittaker JS, Road JD. Chest 1992;102:1286–8.
18. Moriguchi S, Sone S, Kishino Y. J Nutr 1983;113:40–6.
19. Shennib H, Chiu RC, Mulder DS et al. Surg Gynecol Obstet 1984;158:535–40.
20. Niederman MS, Merrill WW, Ferranti RD et al. Ann Intern Med 1984;100:795–800.
21. Harris JA, Benedict FG. Standard Basal Metabolism Constants for Physiologists and Clinicians: A Biometric Study of Basal Metabolism in Man. Philadelphia: JB Lippincott, 1919:223.
22. Weissman C, Kemper M, Askanazi J et al. Anesthesiology 1986;64:673–9.
23. Liggett SB, Renfro AD. Chest 1990;98:682–6.
24. Damask MC, Schwarz Y, Weissman C. Crit Care Clin 1987;3:71–96.

25. Elwyn DH, Kinney JM, Jeevanandam M et al. Ann Surg 1979;190:117–27.

26. Edens NK, Gil KM, Elwyn DH. Clin Chest Med 1986;7:3–17.

27. Alberda C, Gramlich L et al. Int Care Med 2009;35:1728–37.

28. Heighes PT, Doig GS, Simpson F et al. Anaesth Int Care 2010;38:167–74.

29. Zaloga GP. Chest 1991;100:1643–6.

30. Strong RM, Condon SC, Solinger MR et al. JPEN J Parenter Enteral Nutr 1992;16:59–63.

31. Torres A, Serra-Batlles J, Ros E et al. Ann Intern Med 1992; 116:540–3.

32. Wiedemann HP, Wheeler AP et al. N Engl J Med 2006; 354:2564–75.

33. Imperial J, Bistrian BR, Bothe A Jr et al. J Am Coll Nutr 1983;2:63–73.

34. Kruse JA, Shah NJ. Nutr Clin Pract 1993;8:163–70.

35. Metnitz PG, Bartens C, Fischer M et al. Int Care Med 1999; 25:180–5.

36. Richard C, Lemonnier F, Thibault M et al. Crit Care Med 1990;18:4–9.

37. Nathens AB, Neff MJ, Jurkovich GJ et al. Ann Surg 2002; 236:814–22.

38. Zaloga GP. Nutrition and prevention of systemic infection. In: Taylor RW, Shoemaker WC, eds. Critical Care State of the Art. Fullerton, CA: Society of Critical Care Medicine, 1991:31–80.

39. Gadek JE, DeMichele SJ, Karlstad MD et al. Crit Care Med 1999;27:1409–20.

40. Lokke A, Lange P et al. Thorax 2006;61:935–9.

41. Chan IH, Birmingham CL, Mayo JR. In: 89th Scientific Assembly and Annual Meeting of the Radiological Society of North America. Chicago: Radiological Society of North America, 2003.

42. Britton JR, Pavord ID, Richards KA et al. Am J Respir Crit Care Med 1995;151:1383–7.

43. Strachan DP, Cox BD, Erzinclioglu SW et al. Thorax 1991; 46:624–9.

44. Schwartz J, Weiss ST. Am J Clin Nutr 1994;59:110–4.

45. Schwartz J, Weiss ST. Am J Epidemiol 1990;132:67–76.

46. Chuwers P, Barnhart S, Blanc P et al. Am J Respir Crit Care Med 1997;155:1066–71.

47. Morabia A, Menkes MJ, Comstock GW et al. Am J Epidemiol 1990;132:77–82.

48. Shahar E, Folsom AR, Melnick SL et al. Am J Respir Crit Care Med 1994;150:978–82.

49. Shahar E, Folsom AR, Melnick SL et al. N Engl J Med 1994;331:228–33.

50. Sharp DS, Rodriguez BL, Shahar E et al. Am J Respir Crit Care Med 1994;150:983–7.

51. Wilson DO, Rogers RM, Wright EC et al. Am Rev Respir Dis 1989;139:1435–8.

52. Sahebjami H, Doers JT, Render ML et al. Am J Med 1993; 94:469–74.

53. Schols AM, Soeters PB, Dingemans AM et al. Am Rev Respir Dis 1993;147:1151–6.

54. Chailleux E, Laaban JP, Veale D. Chest 2003;123:1460–6.

55. Gray-Donald K, Gibbons L, Shapiro SH et al. Am J Respir Crit Care Med 1996;153:961–6.

56. Thomas DR. Clin Geriatr Med 2002;18:835–9.

57. Hallin R, Janson C et al. Respir Med. 2006;100:561–7.

58. Schols AM, Slangen J, Volovics L et al. Am J Respir Crit Care Med 1998;157:1791–7.

59. Eid AA, Ionescu AA, Nixon LS et al. Am J Respir Crit Care Med 2001;164:1414–8.

60. Goldstein SA, Thomashow BM, Kvetan V et al. Am Rev Respir Dis 1988;138:636–44.

61. Donahoe M, Rogers RM, Wilson DO et al. Am Rev Respir Dis 1989;140:385–91.

62. Ryan CF, Road JD, Buckley PA et al. Chest 1993;103:1038–44.

63. Wilson DO, Rogers RM, Sanders MH et al. Am Rev Respir Dis 1986;134:672–7.

64. Schols AM, Soeters PB, Mostert R et al. Am Rev Respir Dis 1991;143:1248–52.

65. Baarends EM, Schols AM, Pannemans DL et al. Am J Respir Crit Care Med 1997;155:549–54.

66. Vernooy JH, Kucukaycan M, Jacobs JA et al. Am J Respir Crit Care Med 2002;166:1218–24.

67. Di Francia M, Barbier D, Mege JL et al. Am J Respir Crit Care Med 1994;150:1453–5.

68. Sugawara K, Takahashi H. Respir Med 2010;102:970–7.

69. King DA, Cordova F, Scharf SM. Proc Am Thorac Soc 2008;5:519–23.

70. Slinde F, Gronberg AM, Engstrom CR et al. Respir Med 2002;96:330–6.

71. Creutzberg EC, Schols AM, Weling-Scheepers CA et al. Am J Respir Crit Care Med 2000;161:745–52.

72. Suchner U, Rothkopf MM, Stanislaus G et al. Arch Intern Med 1990;150:1225–30.

73. Casaburi R, Porszasz J, Burns MR et al. Am J Respir Crit Care Med 1997;155:1541–51.

74. Burdet L, de Muralt B, Schutz Y et al. Am J Respir Crit Care Med 1997;156:1800–6.

75. Pape GS, Friedman M, Underwood LE et al. Chest 1991;99:1495–500.

76. Rudman D, Fellor AG, Angraj HS. N Engl J Med 1991; 323:1–6.

77. Schols AM, Soeters PB, Mostert R et al. Am J Respir Crit Care Med 1995;152:1268–74.

78. Ferreira IM, Verreschi IT, Nery LE et al. Chest 1998;114: 19–28.

79. Sharma S, Arneja A et al. Chron Respir Dis 2008;5:169–76.

80. Weisberg J, Wanger J et al. Chest 2002;121:1070–8.

81. Angelillo VA, Bedi S, Durfee D et al. Ann Intern Med 1985;103:883–5.

82. Brown SE, Nagendran RC, McHugh JW et al. Am Rev Respir Dis 1985;132:960–2.

83. Sue CY, Chung MM, Grosvenor M et al. Am Rev Respir Dis 1989;139:1430–4.

84. Aubier M, Murciano D, Lecocguic Y et al. N Engl J Med 1985;313:420–4.

85. Horrobin DF. Med Hypoth 1987;22:421–8.

86. Arm JP, Horton CE, Spur BW et al. Am Rev Respir Dis 1989;139:1395–400.

87. Thien FC, Mencia-Huerta JM, Lee TH. Am Rev Respir Dis 1993;147:1138–43.

88. Woods RK, Thien FC, Abramson MJ. Cochrane Database Syst Rev 2002:CD001283.

89. Ciarallo L, Sauer AH, Shannon MW. J Pediatr 1996;129: 809–14.

90. Kazaks AG, Uriu-Adams JY et al. J Asthma 2010;47:83–92.

91. Romieu I, Sienra-Monge JJ, Ramirez-Aguilar M et al. Am J Respir Crit Care Med 2002;166:703–9.

92. Pastorino U, Infante M, Maioli M et al. J Clin Oncol 1993; 11:1216–22.

93. Alpha-Tocopherol, Beta-Carotene Cancer Prevention Study Group. N Engl J Med 1994;330:1029–35.

94. Omenn GS, Goodman GE, Thornquist MD et al. N Engl J Med 1996;334:1150–5.

95. Hennekens CH, Buring JE, Manson JE et al. N Engl J Med 1996;334:1145–9.

96. de Klerk NH, Musk AW, Ambrosini GL et al. Int J Cancer 1998;75:362–7.

97. Brennan P, Fortes C, Butler J et al. Cancer Causes Control 2000;11:49–58.

98. Jansen MC, Bueno-de-Mesquita HB, Rasanen L et al. Int J Cancer 2001;92:913–8.

99. Voorrips LE, Goldbohm RA, Verhoeven DT et al. Cancer Causes Control 2000;11:101–5.

100. Speizer FE, Colditz GA, Hunter DJ et al. Cancer Causes Control 1999;10:475–82.

101. Rachtan J. Acta Oncol 2002;41:389–94.

102. Byers TE, Graham S, Haughey BP et al. Am J Epidemiol 1987;125:351–63.

103. Hinds MW, Kolonel LN, Lee J et al. Am J Clin Nutr 1983; 37:192–3.

104. Jain M, Burch JD, Howe GR et al. Int J Cancer 1990;45: 287–93.

105. Stefani ED, Boffetta P, Deneo-Pellegrini H et al. Nutr Cancer 1999;34:100–10.

106. Mulder I, Jansen MC, Smit HA et al. Int J Cancer 2000;88:665–71.

107. Corey M, McLaughlin FJ, Williams M et al. J Clin Epidemiol 1988;41:583–91.

108. Pencharz P, Hill R, Archibald E et al. J Pediatr Gastroenterol Nutr 1984;3(Suppl):147S–53S.

109. Bell SC, Saunders MJ, Elborn JS et al. Thorax 1996;51:126–31.

110. Feigal RJ, Shapiro BL. Nature 1979;278:276–7.

111. Elborn JS, Cordon SM, Western PJ et al. Clin Sci (Lond) 1993; 85:563–8.

112. Borowitz D, Baker RD, Stallings V. J Pediatr Gastroenterol Nutr 2002;35:246–59.

113. Renner S, Rath R, Rust P et al. Thorax 2001;56:48–52.

114. Beker LT, Ahrens RA, Fink RJ et al. J Pediatr Gastroenterol Nutr 1997;24:512–7.

115. Rayner RJ, Tyrrell JC, Hiller EJ et al. Arch Dis Child 1989; 64:1151–6.

116. Duggan C, Colin AA, Agil A et al. Am J Clin Nutr 1996;64: 635–9.

117. Innis SM, Davidson AG. Annu Rev Nutr 2008;28:55–72.

118. Steinkamp G, von der Hardt H. J Pediatr 1994;124:244–7.

119. Calanas-Continente AJ, Cervero Pluvins C, Munoz Gomariz E et al. Nutr Hosp 2002;17:197–203.

120. Madill J, Gutierrez C, Grossman J et al. J Heart Lung Transplant 2001;20:288–96.

121. Forli L, Bjortuft O, Vatn M et al. Ann Nutr Metab 2001; 45:159–68.

122. Forli L, Pedersen JI, Bjortuft O et al. Respiration 2001;68: 51–7.

123. Snell GI, Bennetts K, Bartolo J et al. J Heart Lung Transplant 1998;17:1097–103.

124. Kyle UG, Nicod L, Romand JA et al. Transplantation 2003; 75:821–8.

125. Singer LG, Brazelton TR, Doyle RL et al. J Heart Lung Transplant 2003;22:894–902.

126. Kanasky WF Jr, Anton SD, Rodrigue JR et al. Chest 2002; 121:401–6.

127. Forsythe J, Cooley K, Greaver B. Prog Transplant 2000; 10:234–8.

128. Lewis MI, Monn SA, Sieck GC. J Appl Physiol 1992;72: 293–301.

129. Creutzberg EC, Wouters EF, Mostert R et al. Nutrition 2003; 19:120–7.

130. Abenhaim L, Moride Y, Brenot F et al. N Engl J Med 1996; 335:609–16.

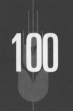

100 NUTRITION AND INFECTIOUS DISEASES[1]

ALICE M. TANG, ELLEN SMIT, AND RICHARD D. SEMBA

HISTORICAL OVERVIEW

The relationship between nutrition and infectious diseases was largely characterized in the twentieth century. In the early part of the century, the idea of certain "substances," "accessory food factors," or "vitamines" essential for health emerged (1–3); and knowledge of vitamins and deficiency diseases grew rapidly in the period following 1912 (4). The study of nutrition and infectious diseases was facilitated by developments in immunology, such as the description of humoral antibodies, serologic tests for the diagnosis of infectious diseases, and assays for measurements of immunologic protection (5). By the late 1930s and early 1940s, it became generally accepted that some dietary deficiencies could increase the risk of infectious diseases (6–8). With fortification of foods, improvement in diet, and a general increase in the standard of living, micronutrient deficiencies declined and became less of a public health problem in developed countries.

In 1968, a World Health Organization (WHO) expert committee reviewed the interactions between nutrition and infection (9) and concluded the following:

> Infections are likely to have more serious consequences among persons with clinical or subclinical malnutrition, and infectious dis-

eases have the capacity to turn borderline nutritional deficiencies into severe malnutrition. In this way, malnutrition and infection can be mutually aggravating and produce more serious consequences for the patient than would be expected from a summation of the independent effects of the two.

This work provided the foundation for research on nutrition and infection that has followed to the present, much of which has taken place in developing countries, where micronutrient deficiencies are more prevalent.

GENERAL PRINCIPLES

Infection with a pathogen usually triggers a series of responses; these vary depending on the infectious agent. Response to bacterial infection commences with the release of microbial products such as lipopolysaccharides and peptidoglycans from bacterial cell walls, bacterial DNA, and exotoxins; viral infections start with the release of viral double-stranded RNA and viral glycoproteins. Depending on the type of pathogen and its ability to evade the immune response, the location of the infection, host immune status, and other factors, a localized response with influx of polymorphonuclear leukocytes, macrophages, and natural killer cells may occur. Polymorphonuclear cells release inflammatory mediators from granules, including reactive oxygen intermediates such as hydroxyl radicals, hydrogen peroxide, reactive nitrogen, and superoxide anion, and antimicrobial enzymes such as lysozyme, proteases, collagenases, and phospholipases. Macrophages may phagocytize antigens and express cytokines such as interleukin (IL)-1 that attract T lymphocytes to the site of inflammation. The complement system may be activated. If the pathogen is not contained, these localized events may amplify and lead to a larger systemic condition—the acute phase response—which is characterized by fever, somnolence, anorexia, and cachexia and is accompanied by metabolic alterations such as loss of muscle and negative nitrogen balance, fat catabolism, and impaired gluconeogenesis. The acute phase response also can be triggered by other factors, including trauma, burns, surgery, tissue infarction, exposure to chemicals or radiation, and advanced cancer.

During the acute phase response, changes occur in many plasma proteins, or acute phase proteins, which have been defined as proteins whose plasma concentrations

---

[1]**Abbreviations: AIDS**, acquired immunodeficiency syndrome; **ARI**, acute respiratory infection; **DALY**, disability-adjusted life year; **HAART**, highly active antiretroviral therapy; **HIV**, human immunodeficiency virus; **IFN**, interferon; **IL,** interleukin; **MHC**, major histocompatibility complex; **NF-κB**, nuclear factor-κB; **TB**, tuberculosis; **TNF**, tumor necrosis factor; **UNICEF**, United Nations Children's Fund; **VDR**, vitamin D receptor; **WHO**, World Health Organization.

increase (positive acute phase proteins) or decrease (negative acute phase proteins) by at least one fourth during inflammatory disorders (10, 11). The liver is the main site of synthesis of most acute phase proteins. C-reactive protein (10), α-1-acid glycoprotein (12), and serum amyloid A (13) are among the best characterized positive acute phase proteins. Other positive acute phase proteins include ferritin, haptoglobin, and ceruloplasmin, and negative acute phase proteins include albumin and transthyretin.

Cytokines play an important role in the acute phase response as inducers of acute phase proteins and hormones, as modulators of inflammation, and as activators and inhibitors of central nervous system functions related to appetite and metabolism (14). Cytokines that have been implicated in the anorexia that occurs during infection include IL-1β, IL-6, and tumor necrosis factor-α (TNF-α) (14). IL-1β and TNF-α are produced primarily by macrophages and can be triggered by stimuli such as bacterial wall products, lipopolysaccharide, viruses, parasites, and microbial superantigens. IL-6 is produced by monocytes, T lymphocytes, endothelial cells, and fibroblasts and is a major stimulator of the production of acute phase proteins in the liver. These cytokines may have a direct effect on hypothalamic neurons involved in appetite and other neural mediators such as serotonin, corticotropin-releasing factor, and β-melanocyte–stimulating hormone, and decreases in dopamine and neuropeptide Y. There may be increased cytokines in the circulation as well as the brain that modulate appetite during the acute phase response (15).

MALNUTRITION AND SPECIFIC INFECTIOUS DISEASES

The nutritional consequences of infection, no matter which microorganism is causing it, tend to be predictable. Any infection, whether symptomatic or asymptomatic, is accompanied by losses of some nutrients from the body and redistribution of other nutrients. The magnitude of these changes depends on the severity and duration of the infection. Metabolic and nutritional responses that are specific to certain organisms occur when the infection becomes localized within a single organ system. For example, diarrheal infections cause sizeable losses of fluid and electrolytes, whereas paralytic forms of infection result in wasting of bone and muscle. If the infection can be cured or eliminated naturally by the host immune system, lost body nutrients can then be replenished over a period of weeks to months. If the infectious process is not eliminated and becomes chronic, however, body composition can become markedly altered, and a new equilibrium of body nutrient balances is reached at a cachectic, or extremely wasted, level.

The impact of malnutrition on the severity of infection has been investigated most extensively in children with measles, diarrheal disease, respiratory infections, and malaria and in children and adults with tuberculosis (TB) and human immunodeficiency virus (HIV) infection.

Measles

Measles is a highly contagious disease caused by a virus. An estimated 278,358 cases of measles and 164,000 measles-related deaths were reported during 2008 (16, 17). The number of deaths in 2008 reflects a decrease of 78% since 2000 after the launch of the Measles Initiative, a vaccination campaign in high-risk countries jointly led by the American Red Cross, United Nations Foundation, US Centers for Disease Control and Prevention, United Nations Children's Fund (UNICEF), and WHO. Most measles deaths continue to occur in the Southeast Asia region, as defined by the WHO (16). Deaths from measles are largely the result of an increased susceptibility to secondary bacterial and viral infections, and the underlying mechanism includes immune suppression related to malnutrition, especially vitamin A deficiency (18). Complications may occur in 10% to 30% of cases and include pneumonia, diarrhea, malnutrition, otitis media, mouth ulcers, corneal epithelial keratitis, corneal ulceration, and blindness.

Measles virus is an enveloped RNA virus in the genus *Morbillivirus* of the family paramyxoviridae. One known serotype and eight clades (A to H) of measles exists. Measles is spread when a susceptible person inhales aerosolized droplets containing measles virus. Viral replication occurs initially in macrophages in the lymphoid tissue of the nasopharynx, respiratory mucosa, and lungs (19). The measles virus enters human cells through a cell surface receptor known as signaling lymphocyte activation molecule (20). Viremia allows measles virus to spread to multiple organs, including the skin, liver, and conjunctiva, and a prodrome of fever, cough, and conjunctivitis occurs approximately 14 days after infection.

The immune response to measles is thought to be consistent with T-helper type 2–like immune responses in which antibody responses predominate and are driven by IL-4, IL-6, and IL-10. Antibody responses against measles virus proteins are detectable at the onset of the rash. Immune suppression often accompanies measles infection and increases the susceptibility to secondary infections. Delayed-type hypersensitivity skin test responses and in vitro proliferation of lymphocytes to viral antigens are often minimal or absent in measles infection (19). Infants are protected against measles virus infection by passively acquired maternal antibody to measles.

Although most people recover from measles, those with malnutrition or coinfections are at increased risk of complications (21–24). In the classic early investigation of a measles outbreak in the Faroe Islands by Peter Panum and August Manicus in 1846, the most severe diarrheal disease and highest mortality were described among those patients with greatest poverty and poor diet (25). Malnourished children have more severe disease and higher mortality (26, 27). More persistent measles infection and viral shedding also have (23) been reported in malnourished children (21). A close synergism exists between measles and vitamin A deficiency. One study in Zaire demonstrated that severely vitamin A–deficient children were three times more likely to die of measles than were children with better vitamin A status before infection (28). Children with measles who are vitamin A deficient also have a much higher risk of xerophthalmia, corneal ulceration, keratomalacia, and subsequent blindness (29).

Vitamin A supplementation has shown to reduce the morbidity and mortality of measles among preschool children (30–34). Vitamin A supplementation appears to reduce the infectious complications associated with measles immune suppression, such as pneumonia and diarrheal disease, and these effects have been associated with modulation of immune responses by vitamin A (35, 36). In a randomized controlled trial in South Africa, children with severe measles who received vitamin A supplementation recovered more quickly from complications and were hospitalized for significantly fewer days. Their risk of death or a major complication was half that of their untreated counterparts (32). A metaanalysis of studies in the United Kingdom, South Africa, and Tanzania showed that vitamin A therapy for measles reduced mortality by 67% (37). Another metaanalysis of five randomized controlled clinical trials found that at least two doses of 200,000 IU of vitamin A on consecutive days were needed for significant reduction in measles mortality. Although one dose did not have a significant effect, two doses resulted in a 62% reduction in mortality (38). High-dose vitamin A therapy is now accepted as part of standard recommended treatment of measles infection in developing countries. Improving vitamin A status and immunization coverage are also cornerstones of current measles prevention efforts.

Malaria

Malaria is caused by a parasitic infection with protozoan organisms of the genus *Plasmodium*. In 2008, an estimated 247 million cases of malaria and approximately 1 million deaths from malaria occurred worldwide; more than 85% of malaria cases were in Africa (39). Of the four *Plasmodium* species that infect humans (*Plasmodium falciparum*, *Plasmodium vivax*, *Plasmodium malariae*, and *Plasmodium ovale*), the most serious morbidity and mortality are caused by *P. falciparum* (40). Malarial infection begins when a female *Anopheles* mosquito bites a human and releases sporozoites from the salivary gland into the circulating blood of the host. Sporozoites then enter hepatocytes, and in the preerythrocytic cycle, sporozoites grow and develop in the liver into thousands of merozoites. The hepatocytes then release merozoites, which invade

erythrocytes. In the asexual erythrocytic cycle, merozoites develop into schizonts, and erythrocytes rupture, releasing more merozoites that can invade erythrocytes. In the sexual stage, some merozoites develop into gametocytes that are taken up in a blood meal by a mosquito, and within the mosquito, these gametocytes develop in microgametes and macrogametes.

In addition to the type of parasite, the extent of transmission and illness depends on the species of the *Anopheles* vector, human immunity, and climate. Specifically, vector species that have a long life span and species that prefer to bite humans over animals increase the chances of human transmission. Adults can develop some, but not complete, immunity to malaria after years of exposure, and transmission is highest in higher temperature and humid conditions (39). Transmission can be significantly reduced by insecticide-treated mosquito nets and indoor spraying with insecticides.

Malaria symptoms include fever, chills, and flu-like illness; and, if left untreated, malaria can progress to severe illness and death. Treatment generally includes antimalarial drugs, although regimens depend on the country and region where the infection occurs. Natural history studies suggest that the severity of malaria may be related to nutritional status. Some studies in the older literature have reported that malnutrition, and specifically protein-energy malnutrition, is protective against malaria. In particular, refeeding after famine appeared to increase the risk of malaria, especially among persons who are carriers of the disease (41, 42). Nevertheless, comprehensive reviews on protein-energy malnutrition showed that persons with better nutritional status have less severe malaria and a lower risk of death (40, 43–45).

Specific nutrients have been shown to affect malaria morbidity. Vitamin A, in particular, influences the incidence as well as the morbidity related to malaria (46–48). A randomized, placebo-controlled clinical trial was conducted in Papua New Guinea to examine the effects of vitamin A supplementation (60 mg retinol equivalents every 3 months) on malarial morbidity in preschool children (49). Children between 6 and 60 months of age were randomly allocated to receive vitamin A or placebo every 3 months. A weekly morbidity surveillance and clinic-based surveillance were established for monitoring acute malaria, and children were followed up for 1 year. Vitamin A significantly reduced the incidence of malaria attacks by about 20% to 50% for all except those with extremely high levels of parasitemia. Similarly, vitamin A supplementation reduced clinic-based malaria attacks, which consisted of self-solicited visits to the clinic by mothers who thought that their children should be seen because of fever. Vitamin A supplementation had little impact in children less than 12 months of age and the greatest effect among children 13 to 36 months old.

Studies of the benefits of zinc on malaria incidence and morbidity have shown conflicting results. Several studies

AIDS (167). The risk of progression to AIDS was higher in those persons with vitamin B$_{12}$ deficiency (153). Low serum zinc levels were associated with reduced secretory function of the thymus (168) and HIV disease progression (164, 169). Low serum or plasma selenium concentrations were associated with an increased risk of progression to AIDS and higher mortality (170–172).

In 2003, the report issued by the WHO also included recommended micronutrient requirements for people living with HIV infection (141). At the time, little scientific evidence existed in the form of randomized controlled clinical trials to recommend micronutrient intakes higher than the recommended dietary allowance. Since then, data from several clinical trials of multiple micronutrient supplementation in HIV-infected adults have been published (173–180). The earliest and largest of these, a trial of HIV-infected pregnant women in Tanzania, showed that multivitamin supplementation compared with placebo had several beneficial outcomes in HIV-infected pregnant women, including greater increases in T-cell counts during and after pregnancy, as well as better birth outcomes (reduced fetal deaths and low birth weight) (181) and improved weight gain during pregnancy (182). Further follow-up of the same women over several years demonstrated continued benefits of multiple micronutrients on T-cell counts, lower viral loads, slower HIV progression, and improved overall survival (173). Additional analyses of these trial participants showed a beneficial effect of micronutrients on maternal wasting (183), maternal and child hemoglobin status (184), as well as maternal depression and quality of life (185).

The other clinical trials published since 2003 were much smaller and were conducted in different geographic regions (Southeast Asia, Africa, United States) with differing population characteristics (including differing levels of micronutrient deficiency at baseline) and using different mixes and doses of multiple micronutrients, thus making it difficult to draw any generalizable conclusions. Some of these studies were conducted among pregnant women (179), others among people coinfected with TB (176, 177), and only one in a population treated with antiretroviral therapy (180). Therefore, it is not surprising that the results of these trials were mixed. Two trials demonstrated the benefit of multiple micronutrient supplementation on improving CD4 counts (175, 180). Three trials showed a reduction in mortality (174, 176, 178), although this reduction was only in specific subgroups of the population for two of these studies (174, 176). Because the duration of follow-up for most these trials was less than 1 year, the long-term effects of micronutrient supplementation are still unknown.

In conclusion, some evidence from clinical trials indicates that multiple micronutrient supplementation may benefit some subgroups of people living with HIV infection. However, these trials were largely conducted at a time when HIV-infected populations had little or no access to antiretroviral therapy. Currently, people living with HIV infection in many resource-poor countries are beginning to gain access to antiretroviral therapy, so the effects of micronutrient supplementation on HIV outcomes need to be reassessed in light of this change. In addition, although most of these trials used high doses of multiple micronutrients and did not measure underlying micronutrient status in the participants, it is still unclear what the minimal and most effective doses would be to improve HIV-related outcomes in different circumstances.

SUMMARY

The causes of malnutrition are complex and involve food, society, health, and caring practices. The theoretic framework for the causes of malnutrition used by UNICEF classifies the causes as immediate (individual level), underlying (household or family level), and basic (societal level) (186). A malnourished child has reduced immunity to infection and can have more severe and frequent episodes of illness. Illnesses such as diarrheal disease can reduce appetite, increase malabsorption of nutrients, hasten losses of nutrients, and thus can further perpetuate a cycle of malnutrition and infection. On the level of the household, problems may exist with food security (i.e., access to safe food of sufficient quality and quantity to ensure adequate health for all family members). The quality and quantity of food should meet the requirements for protein, energy, and micronutrients. Access to food can depend on financial, social, and physical factors. Given the close relationship between malnutrition and infection, factors that affect hygiene on the household level, such as clean water and sanitation, affect malnutrition. Inadequate maternal and child care practices are also underlying household causes of malnutrition. Lack of or early cessation of breast-feeding, the lack of safe, high-quality complementary foods, withholding of food and liquids to a child with diarrhea, inadequate practices of food sharing at the table, poor knowledge of personal hygiene, and lack of immunizations are some specific examples of practices at the household level that are underlying causes of malnutrition (186). On the societal level, low status of women, inadequate health services, lack of jobs, and poverty are causes that underlie malnutrition.

The theoretic framework of UNICEF for the causes of malnutrition suggests multiple levels for interventions to reduce morbidity and mortality from infectious diseases. It also suggests that such strategies range from improved roads and sanitation, maternal education, and immunizations to food fortification and micronutrient supplementation.

REFERENCES

1. Grijns G. Geneeskundig Tijdschrift Nederl Indië 1901;41:3.
2. Hopkins FG. Analyst 1906;31:385–404.
3. Funk C. J State Med 1912;20:341–68.
4. Carpenter KJ. J Nutr 2003;133:3023–32.
5. Silverstein AM. A History of Immunology. San Diego: Academic Press, 1989.

6. Heilbron IM, Jones WE, Bacharach AL. Vitam Horm 1944;2: 155–213.

7. Robertson EC. Medicine 1934;13:123–206.

8. Clausen SW. Physiol Rev 1934;14:309–50.

9. Scrimshaw NS, Taylor CE, Gordon JE. Interactions of Nutrition and Infection. Geneva: World Health Organization, 1968.

10. Gabay C, Kushner I. N Engl J Med 1999;340:448–54.

11. Gitlin JD, Colten HR. Molecular biology of acute phase plasma proteins. In: Pick E, Landy M, eds. Lymphokines, vol 14. San Diego: Academic Press, 1987:123–53.

12. Fournier T, Medjoubi N, Porquet D. Biochim Biophys Acta 2000;1482:157–71.

13. Uhlar CM, Whitehead AS. Eur J Biochem 1999;265:501–23.

14. Langhans W. Nutrition 2000;16:996–1005.

15. Plata-Salaman CR. Int J Obes Relat Metab Disord 2001;25: S48–S52.

16. Ebrahim GJ. J Trop Pediatr 2010;56:219–20.

17. Centers for Disease Control and Prevention. MMWR Morb Mortal Wkly Rep 2009;58:1321–6.

18. Perry RT, Halsey NA. J Infect Dis 2004;189:S4–S16.

19. Griffin DE. Curr Top Microbiol Immunol 1995;191:117–34.

20. Tatsuo H, Ono N, Tanaka K et al. Nature 2000;406:893–7.

21. Dossetor J, Whittle HC, Greenwood BM. Br Med J 1977;1: 1633–5.

22. Chen LC, Rahman M, Sarder AM. Int J Epidemiol 1980;9: 25–33.

23. Koster FT, Curlin GC, Aziz KM et al. Bull World Health Org 1981;59:901–8.

24. World Health Organization. WHO Vaccine Preventable Diseases: Monitoring System, 2004 Global Summary. Geneva: World Health Organization, 2004.

25. Manicus A. Ugeskrift Laeger 1847;6:189–210.

26. Smedman L, Lindeberg A, Jeppsson O et al. Ann Trop Paediatr 1983;3:169–76.

27. Alwar AJ. East Afr Med J 1992;69:415–8.

28. Markowitz LE, Nzilambi N, Driskell WJ et al. J Trop Pediatr 1989;35:109–12.

29. Semba RD, Bloem MW. Surv Ophthalmol 2004;49:243–55.

30. Ellison JB. Br Med J 1932;2:708–11.

31. Barclay AJ, Foster A, Sommer A. Br Med J (Clin Res Ed) 1987;294:294–6.

32. Hussey GD, Klein M. N Engl J Med 1990;323:160–4.

33. Coutsoudis A, Broughton M, Coovadia HM. Am J Clin Nutr 1991;54:890–5.

34. Ogaro FO, Orinda VA, Onyango FE et al. Trop Geogr Med 1993;45:283–6.

35. Coutsoudis A, Kiepiela P, Coovadia HM et al. Pediatr Infect Dis J 1992;11:203–9.

36. Benn CS, Balde A, George E et al. Lancet 2002;359:1313–4.

37. Glasziou PP, Mackerras DE. BMJ 1993;306:366–70.

38. Sudfeld CR, Navar AM, Halsey NA. Int J Epidemiol 2010;39(Suppl 1):i48–i55.

39. World Health Organization. Malaria. Fact sheet no. 94. Geneva: World Health Organization, 2010.

40. Shankar AH. Malaria. In: Semba RD, Bloem MW, eds. Nutrition and Health in Developing Countries. Totowa, NJ: Humana Press, 2001:177–207.

41. Murray J, Murray A. Perspect Biol Med 1977;20:471–83.

42. Murray MJ, Murray AB, Murray NJ et al. Am J Clin Nutr 1978;31:57–61.

43. Caulfield LE, Richard SA, Black RE. Am J Trop Med Hyg 2004;71:55–63.

44. Murray MJ, Murray AB, Murray MB et al. Lancet 1976;1: 1283–5.

45. Famine Inquiry Commission: Report on Bengal. New Delhi: Government of India, 1945.

46. Stürchler D, Tanner M, Hanck A et al. Acta Trop 1987;44:213–27.

47. Galan P, Samba C, Luzeau R et al. Int J Vitam Nutr Res 1990; 60:224–8.

48. Friis H, Mwaniki D, Omondi B et al. Am J Clin Nutr 1997; 66:665–71.

49. Shankar AH, Genton B, Semba RD et al. Lancet 1999;354: 203–9.

50. Bates CJ, Evans PH, Dardenne M et al. Br J Nutr 1993; 69:243–55.

51. Shankar AH, Genton B, Baisor M et al. Am J Trop Med Hyg 2000;62:663–9.

52. Sazawal S, Black RE, Ramsan M et al. Lancet 2007;369:927–34.

53. Richard SA, Zavaleta N, Caulfield LE et al. Am J Trop Med Hyg 2006;75:126–32.

54. Shankar AH. J Infect Dis 2000;182(Suppl):S37–S53.

55. Müller O, Becher H, van Zweeden AB et al. BMJ 2001; 322:1567.

56. Zinc Against Plasmodium Study Group. Am J Clin Nutr 2002; 76:805–12.

57. International Nutritional Anemia Consultative Group. Safety of Iron Supplementation Programs in Malaria-Endemic Regions. Washington, DC: International Life Science Institute, 2000.

58. Ojukwu JU, Okebe JU, Yahav D et al. Cochrane Database Syst Rev 2009;CD006589.

59. World Health Organization. Diarrheal Disease. Fact sheet number 330.2009.

60. Lanata CF, Black RE. Diarrheal diseases. In: Semba RD, Bloem MW, eds. Nutrition and Health in Developing Countries. 2nd ed. Totowa, NJ: Humana Press, 2008:139–78.

61. Black RE, Brown KH, Becker S. Am J Clin Nutr 1984;39: 87–94.

62. Chen LC, Huq E, Huffman SL. Am J Epidemiol 1981;114: 284–92.

63. Gartner LM, Morton J, Lawrence RA et al. Pediatrics 2005;115:496–506.

64. Sazawal S, Black RE, Bhan MK et al. N Engl J Med 1995; 333:839–44.

65. Bhutta ZA, Bird SM, Black RE et al. Am J Clin Nutr 2000; 72:1516–22.

66. United Nations Children's Fund/World Health Organization. Clinical Management of Acute Diarrhoea: Joint statement. 2004:1–13.

67. McLaren DS, Shirajian E, Tchalian M et al. Am J Clin Nutr 1965;17:117–30.

68. Cohen N, Rahman H, Sprague J et al. World Health Stat Q 1985;38:317–30.

69. Khatry SK, West KP Jr, Katz J et al. Arch Ophthalmol 1995; 113:425–9.

70. Schaumberg DA, O'Connor J, Semba RD. Eur J Clin Nutr 1996;50:761–4.

71. Doesschate JT. Causes of Blindness in and Around Surabaja, East Java, Indonesia. Doctoral Thesis. University of Jakarta, Indonesia, 1968.

72. Sommer A. Nutritional Blindness: Xerophthalmia and Keratomalacia. New York: Oxford University Press, 1982.

73. Beaton GH, Martorell R, L'Abbe KA et al. Effectiveness of Vitamin A Supplementation in the Control of Young Child Morbidity and Mortality in Developing Countries. ACC/SCN state-of-the-art nutrition policy discussion paper no. 13. New York: United Nations, 1993.

74. World Health Organization. Initiative for Vaccine Research: Acute Respiratory Infections. 2009. Available at: http://

www.who.int/vaccine_research/diseases/ari/en/index.html. Accessed September 13, 2012.

75. Lanata CF, Black RE. Acute lower-respiratory infections. In: Semba RD, Bloem MW, eds. Nutrition and Health in Developing Countries. 2nd ed. Totowa, NJ: Humana Press, 2008:179–214.

76. Brown KH, Peerson JM, Baker SK et al. Food Nutr Bull 2009; 30:S12–S40.

77. Ninh NX, Thissen JP, Collette L et al. Am J Clin Nutr 1996; 63:514–9.

78. Sazawal S, Black RE, Bhan MK et al. Am J Clin Nutr 1997; 66:413–8.

79. Sazawal S, Black RE, Jalla S et al. Pediatrics 1998;102:1–5.

80. Meeks GJ, Witter MM, Ramdath DD. Eur J Clin Nutr 1998;52:34–9.

81. Penny ME, Peerson JM, Marin RM et al. J Pediatr 1999; 135:208–17.

82. Bhandari N, Bahl R, Taneja S et al. BMJ 2002;324:1358–60.

83. Bhutta ZA, Black RE, Brown KH et al. J Pediatr 1999;135: 689–97.

84. Roth DE, Caulfield LE, Ezzati M et al. Bull World Health Org 2008;86:356–64.

85. Vitamin A and Pneumonia Working Group. Bull WHO 1995; 73:609–19.

86. Mahalanabis D, Lahiri M, Paul D et al. Am J Clin Nutr 2004; 79:430–6.

87. Brooks WA, Yunus M, Santosham M et al. Lancet 2004; 363:1683–8.

88. Marshall I. Cochrane Database Syst Rev 2000;CD001364.

89. Hulisz D. J Am Pharm Assoc 2004;44:594–603.

90. Beaton GH, Martorell R, L'Abbe KA et al. Effectiveness of Vitamin A Supplementation in the Control of Young Child Morbidity and Mortality in Developing Countries. ACC/SCN state-of-the-art nutrition policy discussion paper no. 13. New York: United Nations, 1993.

91. World Health Organization. Initiative for Vaccine Research: Parasitic Disease. 2011. Available at: http://www.who.int/vaccine_research/diseases/soa_parasitic/en/index2.html. Accessed September 13, 2012.

92. Pawlowski ZS, Schad GA, Stott GJ. Hookworm Infection and Anemia: Approaches to Prevention and Control. Geneva: World Health Organization, 1991.

93. Loukas A, Prociv P. Clin Microbiol Rev 2001;14:689–703.

94. Hotez PJ, Brooker S, Bethony JM et al. N Engl J Med 2004;351:799–807.

95. Smillie WG, Augustine DL. Am J Dis Child 1926;31:151–68.

96. Smillie WG, Augustine DL. South Med J 1926;19:19–28.

97. Smillie WG, Spencer CR. J Educ Psychol 1926;17:314–21.

98. Waite JH, Neilson IL. J Am Med Assoc 1919;73:1877–9.

99. Strong EK. Effects of Hookworm Disease on the Mental and Physical Development of Children. New York: Rockefeller Foundation, 1916. International Health Commission Publication No. 3.

100. Semba RD. Nutrition: epidemiology and public health overview. In: Ward JW, Warren C, eds. Safer and Healthier America: The Advancement of Public Health in the 20th Century. New York: Oxford University Press, 2005.

101. Stoltzfus RJ, Albonico M, Chwaya HM et al. Am J Clin Nutr 1998;68:179–86.

102. Stephenson LS, Latham MC, Kurz KM et al. Am J Trop Med Hyg 1989;41:78–87.

103. Boivin MJ, Giordani B. J Pediatr Psychol 1993;18:249–64.

104. Dossa RA, Ategbo EA, de Koning FL et al. Eur J Clin Nutr 2001;55:223–8.

105. Christian P, Khatry SK, West KP Jr. Lancet 2004;364:981–3.

106. World Health Organization. Global Tuberculosis Control: A Short Update to the 2009 Report. Geneva: World Health Organization, 2009.

107. Atun R, Raviglione M, Marais B et al. Lancet 2010;376:940–1.

108. USAID Africa's Health in 2010 project. Nutrition and Tuberculosis: A Review of the Literature and Considerations for TB Control Programs. Washington, DC: US Agency for International Development, 2008.

109. Chocano-Bedoya P, Ronnenberg AG. Nutr Rev 2009;67:289–93.

110. Houben EN, Nguyen L, Pieters J. Curr Opin Microbiol 2006;9:76–85.

111. Takashima T, Ueta C, Tsuyuguchi I et al. Infect Immun 1990; 58:3286–92.

112. Wallis RS, Vjecha M, mir-Tahmasseb M et al. J Infect Dis 1993; 167:43–8.

113. Ogawa T, Uchida H, Kusumoto Y et al. Infect Immunol 1991; 59:3021–5.

114. Macallan DC. Diagn Microbiol Infect Dis 1999;34:153–7.

115. van Lettow M, Whalen C. Tuberculosis. In: Semba RD, Bloem MW, eds. Nutrition and Health in Developing Countries. 2nd ed. Totowa, NJ: Humana Press, 2008:275–306.

116. Gupta KB, Gupta R, Atreja A et al. Lung India 2009;26:9–16.

117. van LM, Fawzi WW, Semba RD. Nutr Rev 2003;61:81–90.

118. Munro WT, Leitch I. Proc Nutr Soc 1945;3:155–64.

119. Getz HR, Long ER, Henderson HJ. Am Rev Tuberc 1951;64:381–93.

120. Thorn PA, Brookes VS, Waterhouse JA. Br Med J 1956;1:603–8.

121. Downes J. Milbank Mem Fund Q 1950;28:127–59.

122. Cegielski JP, McMurray DN. Int J Tuberc Lung Dis 2004; 8:286–98.

123. Blumenthal A, Isovski F, Rhee KY. Transl Res 2009;154:7–14.

124. Liu PT, Stenger S, Li H et al. Science 2006;311:1770–3.

125. Abba K, Sudarsanam TD, Grobler L et al. Cochrane Database Syst Rev 2008;(4):CD006086.

126. Villamor E, Mugusi F, Urassa W et al. J Infect Dis 2008;197: 1499–505.

127. Range N, Andersen AB, Magnussen P et al. Trop Med Int Health 2005;10:826–32.

128. Joint United Nations Programme on HIV/AIDS. Global Report: UNAIDS Report on the Global AIDS Epidemic 2010. Geneva: Joint United Nations Programme on HIV/AIDS, 2010.

129. Semba RD, Tang AM. Br J Nutr 1999;81:181–9.

130. Castetbon K, Kadio A, Bondurand A et al. Eur J Clin Nutr 1997;51:81–6.

131. McCorkindale C, Dybevik K, Coulston AM et al. J Am Diet Assoc 1990;90:1236–41.

132. Tang AM, Graham NMH, Kirby AJ et al. Am J Epidemiol 1993;138:937–51.

133. Baum M, Cassetti L, Bonvehi P et al. Nutrition 1994;10: 16–20.

134. Baum MK, Shor-Posner G, Bonvehi P et al. Ann N Y Acad Sci 1992;669:165–74.

135. Sharpstone D, Gazzard B. Lancet 1996;348:379–83.

136. Kotler DP, Goetz H, Lange M et al. Ann Intern Med 1984; 101:421–8.

137. Keating J, Bjarnason I, Somasundaram S et al. Gut 1995; 37:623–9.

138. Sandler NG, Wand H, Roque A et al. J Infect Dis 2011; 203:780–90.

139. Brenchley JM, Douek DC. Curr Opin HIV AIDS 2008;3: 356–61.

140. Stockmann M, Fromm M, Schmitz H et al. AIDS 1998; 12:43–51.

141. WHO. Nutrient Requirements for People Living with HIV/AIDS: Report of a Technical Consultation, 13–15 May 2003. Geneva: World Health Organization, 2004.

142. Crenn P, Rakotoanbinina B, Raynaud JJ et al. J Nutr 2004; 134:2301–6.

143. Ware LJ, Jackson AG, Wootton SA et al. Br J Nutr 2009; 102:1038–46.

144. Shevitz AH, Knox TA, Spiegelman D et al. AIDS 1999;13: 1351–7.

145. Fitch KV, Guggina LM, Keough HM et al. Metabolism 2009; 58:608–15.

146. Kosmiski LA, Kuritzkes DR, Lichtenstein KA et al. AIDS 2001;15:1993–2000.

147. Kosmiski LA, Kuritzkes DR, Sharp TA et al. Metabolism 2003; 52:620–5.

148. Semba RD, Miotti PG, Chiphangwi JD et al. Lancet 1994; 343:1593–7.

149. Phuapradit W, Chaturachinda K, Taneepanichskul S et al. Obstet Gynecol 1996;87:564–7.

150. Semba RD, Ndugwa C, Perry RT et al. Nutrition 2005; 21:25–31.

151. Tang AM, Smit E. Vitamins C and E, and HIV infection. In: Friis H, ed. Micronutrients and HIV Infection. Boca Raton, FL: CRC Press, 2001:111–34.

152. Beach RS, Mantero-Atienza E, Shor-Posner G et al. AIDS 1992;6:701–8.

153. Tang AM, Graham NMH, Chandra RK et al. J Nutr 1997; 127:345–51.

154. Paltiel O, Falutz J, Veilleux M et al. Am J Hematol 1995;49: 318–22.

155. Boudes P, Zittoun J, Sobel A. Lancet 1990;335:1401–2.

156. Semba RD, Kumwenda N, Hoover DR et al. Eur J Clin Nutr 2000;54:872–7.

157. Semba RD, Shah N, Strathdee SA et al. J Acquir Immune Defic Syndr 2002;29:142–4.

158. Mueller BU, Tannenbaum S, Pizzo PA. J Pediatr Hematol Oncol 1996;18:266–71.

159. Totin D, Ndugwa C, Mmiro F et al. J Nutr 2002;132:423–9.

160. Koch J, Neal EA, Schlott MJ et al. Nutrition 1996;12:515–8.

161. Mantero-Atienza E, Sotomayor MG, Shor-Posner G et al. Nutr Res 1991;11:1237–50.

162. Semba RD. Nutr Rev 1998;56:S38–S48.

163. Shankar AH, Prasad AS. Am J Clin Nutr 1998;68:447S–63S.

164. Baum MK, Shor-Posner G, Lu Y et al. AIDS 1995;9:1051–6.

165. Semba RD, Graham NMH, Caiaffa WT et al. Arch Intern Med 1993;153:2149–54.

166. Semba RD, Miotti P, Chiphangwi JD et al. J Acquir Immune Defic Syndr Hum Retrovirol 1997;14:219–22.

167. Tang AM, Graham NMH, Semba RD et al. AIDS 1997;11: 613–20.

168. Falutz J, Tsoukas C, Gold P. J Am Med Assoc 1988;259: 2850–1.

169. Graham NMH, Sorenson D, Odaka N et al. J Acquir Immune Defic Syndr 1991;4:976–80.

170. Baum MK, Shor-Posner G, Lai S et al. J Acquir Immune Defic Syndr Hum Retrovirol 1997;15:370–4.

171. Campa A, Shor-Posner G, Indacochea F et al. J Acquir Immune Defic Syndr Hum Retrovirol 1999;20:508–13.

172. Kupka R, Msamanga GI, Spiegelman D et al. J Nutr 2004; 134:2556–60.

173. Fawzi WW, Msamanga GI, Spiegelman D et al. N Engl J Med 2004;351:23–32.

174. Jiamton S, Pepin J, Suttent R et al. AIDS 2003;17:2461–9.

175. McClelland RS, Baeten JM, Overbaugh J et al. J Acquir Immune Defic Syndr 2004;37:1657–63.

176. Range N, Changalucha J, Krarup H et al. Br J Nutr 2006; 95:762–70.

177. Semba RD, Kumwenda J, Zijlstra E et al. Int J Tuberc Lung Dis 2007;11:854–9.

178. Kelly P, Katubulushi M, Todd J et al. Am J Clin Nutr 2008; 88:1010–7.

179. Kawai K, Kupka R, Mugusi F et al. Am J Clin Nutr 2010; 91:391–7.

180. Kaiser JD, Campa AM, Ondercin JP et al. J Acquir Immune Defic Syndr 2006;42:523–8.

181. Fawzi WW, Msamanga GI, Spiegelman D et al. Lancet 1998; 351:1477–82.

182. Villamor E, Msamanga G, Spiegelman D et al. Am J Clin Nutr 2002;76:1082–90.

183. Villamor E, Saathoff E, Manji K et al. Am J Clin Nutr 2005; 82:857–65.

184. Fawzi WW, Msamanga GI, Kupka R et al. Am J Clin Nutr 2007;85:1335–43.

185. Smith Fawzi MC, Kaaya SF, Mbwambo J et al. HIV Med 2007; 8:203–12.

186. UNICEF. The State of the World's Children. New York: Oxford University Press, 1998.

SUGGESTED READINGS

Beaton GH, Martorell R, L'Abbe KA et al. Effectiveness of Vitamin A Supplementation in the Control of Young Child Morbidity and Mortality in Developing Countries. ACC/SCN state-of-the-art nutrition policy discussion paper no. 13. New York: United Nations, 1993.

Beisel WR. Nutrition and infection. In: Linder MC, ed. Nutritional Biochemistry and Metabolism, with Clinical Applications. New York: Elsevier, 1985:369–94.

Scrimshaw NS, Taylor CE, Gordon JE. Interactions of Nutrition and Infection. Geneva: World Health Organization, 1968.

Semba RD, Bloem MW, eds. Nutrition and Health in Developing Countries. Totowa, NJ: Humana Press, 2001:177–207.

World Health Organization. Nutrient Requirements for People Living with HIV/AIDS: Report of a Technical Consultation, 13–15 May 2003. Geneva: World Health Organization, 2004.

developed because of neuromuscular weakness and progressed to pulmonary hypertension and thromboembolic phenomena. The scleroderma-like symptoms included Raynaud phenomenon, sicca syndrome, dysphagia, and contractures caused by thickening skin collagen. Vascular lesions were noted in all organs, apparently resulting from endothelial proliferation and thrombosis. All patients in the late group had antinuclear antibody and many had antibodies against smooth muscle and skeletal muscle (17). These pathologic and clinical features are consistent with an autoimmune mechanism for the illness. Because the precise causative agent and its mechanism have not been delineated, this serious epidemic might occur again if similar circumstances exist. Also, it is unknown whether the toxin might be present in small amounts in other foods, and thus might be producing or aggravating other clinical conditions.

Melamine

Melamine (2,4,6-triamino-1,3,5-triazine [Fig. 101.1]) is an industrial chemical used for manufacturing of plastics, adhesive, fabrics, and flame retardants. Several years ago, melamine was intentionally added to pet foods and dairy products including infant formula in China to increase the "apparent" protein content of these products (18, 19). Melamine gives a strong positive result in the Kjedahl and Dumas methods for nitrogen determination, which often are used to assess the protein content of foods. In 2007, wheat gluten from China was adulterated with melamine and that wheat gluten was subsequently used to manufacture pet foods. Many pets in North America suffered renal toxicity as a result of consuming the pet food contaminated with melamine and the related substance, cyanuric acid (18). When melamine and cyanuric acid are consumed together, crystals of melamine cyanurate form readily in the kidney tubules leading to acute renal failure. An unknown number of pet cats and dogs died as a result of kidney failure. Subsequently, in 2008, infant formula and other milk products in China were found to be adulterated with melamine; cyanuric acid was not detected in this episode. As many as 294,000 infants and young children in China were affected by the contaminated foods (19) leading to 50,000 hospitalizations and at least 6 fatalities. As in the pet food episode, renal toxicity was the primary manifestation. Apparently, melamine alone under some conditions can lead also to the formation of crystals in the renal tubules leading to nephrolithiasis.

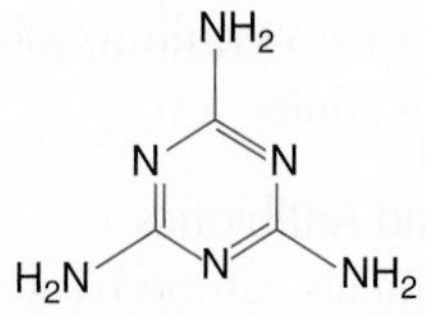

Fig. 101.1. Structure of melamine.

FOOD CONTAMINANTS

Potentially hazardous chemicals may contaminate foods from a variety of sources, including natural contaminants, agricultural chemicals, industrial contaminants, and processing-induced contaminants. The natural contaminants can include mycotoxins from molds, phycotoxins from marine algae, and bacterial toxins. Other contaminants are manufactured and have useful purposes although not intended to occur in foods.

Agricultural Chemicals

Many different chemicals are used in modern agricultural practices. Residues of these agrichemicals can occur in raw and processed foods. Federal regulatory agencies evaluate the safety of such chemicals and regulate and monitor their use on plant food products and in food-producing animals (2). The major categories of agricultural chemicals include insecticides, herbicides, fungicides, fertilizers, and veterinary drugs including antibiotics.

Insecticides

Insecticides are added to foods to control insect pests. Insecticides fall into several major categories including organochlorine compounds (dichlorodiphenyltrichloroethane [DDT], chlordane, and others, many of which are now banned), organophosphate compounds (e.g., parathion and malathion), carbamate compounds (e.g., carbaryl and aldicarb), botanical compounds (e.g., nicotine and pyrethrum), and inorganic compounds (e.g., arsenicals).

Insecticide residues in foods are not particularly hazardous, especially on an acute basis, because of the exceedingly low residue levels of insecticides found in most foods. Certainly, large doses of insecticides can be toxic to humans. Some are neurotoxins such as the organophosphates and carbamates, which are cholinesterase inhibitors and act by blocking synaptic nerve transmission. Insecticide residues in foods pose a low degree of hazard for several reasons: (a) the level of exposure is very low; (b) some insecticides are not very toxic to humans; (c) some insecticides decompose rapidly in the environment; and (d) many different insecticides are used, which limits exposure to any one particular insecticide (1).

Acute food poisoning incidents attributable to the proper use of insecticides on foods are exceedingly rare. Most episodes of pesticide intoxications have resulted from the misuse of pesticides, including contamination of foods during storage and transport, the use of pesticides in food preparation because of their mistaken identity as common food ingredients such as sugar and salt, and their misuse in agricultural practice on crops for which they are not intended to be used (20).

Aldicarb poisonings are one of the best examples of acute food poisoning episodes associated with pesticides. In one noteworthy episode, an outbreak of aldicarb intoxication from watermelons occurred on the West Coast in 1985 (21). The use of aldicarb on watermelons is illegal because excessive levels of aldicarb become concentrated in the edible portion of the melon. In this incident, several farmers used aldicarb illegally, resulting in consumer illnesses and the recall and destruction of thousands of watermelons. The outbreak involved a total of 1373 illness reports with 78% classified as probable or possible aldicarb poisoning cases (21, 22). Thus, this episode is the largest known outbreak of pesticide poisoning in North America (21, 22). Aldicarb has also been involved in several other food poisoning outbreaks. These incidents were associated with ingestion of hydroponically grown cucumbers (22, 23). The symptoms of aldicarb intoxication include nausea, vomiting, diarrhea, and mild neurologic manifestations such as dizziness, headache, blurred vision, and loss of balance (21–23).

Chronic intoxications resulting from pesticide residues in foods have been a long-standing concern (24). For example, DDT is a known animal carcinogen. Because of these concerns for human health and additional concerns resulting from their potential for accumulation in the environment, many organochlorine pesticides have been banned or allowed only under very restricted use conditions. Despite the concerns, the evidence that the low residual amounts of insecticides on foods present a carcinogenic risk to human consumers is not particularly strong.

Several important crops including corn and potatoes have been genetically engineered for insecticide resistance. These genetically engineered, insect-resistant crops contain a novel gene that produces a naturally occurring insecticidal protein toxin from *Bacillus thuringiensis* (Bt). Bt toxins have been used for decades in organic agriculture. The Bt proteins produced by the genetically engineered crops have been thoroughly examined and appear to be quite safe for human consumption (25).

Herbicides

Herbicides are applied to agricultural crops to control the growth of weeds. Several classes of herbicides include chlorophenoxy compounds (e.g., 2,4-D), dinitrophenols (e.g., dinitroorthocresol), bipyridyl compounds (e.g., paraquat), substituted ureas (e.g., monuron), carbamates (e.g., propham), and triazines (e.g., simazine).

In most circumstances, herbicide residues in foods do not present any hazard to consumers. Food poisoning incidents have never resulted from the proper use of herbicides on food crops. The lack of hazard from herbicide residues is associated with the low level of exposure, their low degree of toxicity to humans and selective toxicity toward plants, and the use of many different herbicides, which limits exposure to any particular herbicide (2). Most herbicides pose little hazard to humans simply because they are selectively toxic to plants. The bipyridyl compounds are an exception. These herbicides, including diquat and paraquat, are nonselective and are toxic to humans, with effects on the lung (26). However, no food poisoning incidents have ever been attributed to inappropriate use of the bipyridyl compounds.

Fungicides

Fungicides are used to curtail the growth of molds on food crops. Important fungicide categories include captan, folpet, dithiocarbamates, pentachlorophenol, and the mercurials. The hazards from foodborne fungicides are miniscule because exposure is quite low, most fungicides do not accumulate in the environment, and fungicides typically are not very toxic (2). Several exceptions exist, including the mercurial compounds and hexachlorobenzene. Mercurial fungicides often are used to treat seed grains to prevent mold growth during storage. These seed grains are typically colored pink and are intended for planting rather than consumption. However, especially in times of famine, consumers are tempted to eat the seed grain. On several occasions, consumers have eaten these treated seed grains and developed mercury poisoning (20). Deaths have resulted in several severe episodes. More commonly, mild cases occur. Mild cases of mercury intoxication can be manifested in gastrointestinal symptoms such as abdominal cramps, nausea, vomiting, and diarrhea and dermal symptoms such as acrodynia and itching (20).

Hexachlorobenzene caused one of the most massive outbreaks of pesticide poisoning in recorded history. More than 3000 individuals were affected in this incident in Turkey from 1955 through 1959 in which seed grain was consumed rather than planted (27). Hexachlorobenzene had been used to treat the seed grain. The symptoms were severe with a 10% mortality rate, porphyria cutanea tarda, ulcerated skin lesions, alopecia, porphyrinuria, hepatomegaly, and thyroid enlargement (27).

Fertilizers

Fertilizers are typically combinations of nitrogen and phosphorus compounds. Nitrogen fertilizers are oxidized to nitrate and nitrite in the soil. Both nitrate and nitrite are hazardous to humans if ingested in large amounts (2). Infants are particularly susceptible to nitrate and nitrite intoxication (2). Fertilizers present little, if any, risk to consumers in most typical situations. However, some plants, such as spinach, can accumulate nitrate to hazardous levels if allowed to grow on overly fertilized fields (28, 29). Because nitrite is more toxic than nitrate, the situation can be worsened if nitrate-reducing bacteria are allowed to proliferate on these foods. As another example, improper storage of carrot juice has allowed the proliferation of nitrate-reducing bacteria, resulting in the accumulation of hazardous levels of nitrite in the product (30). After ingestion of low doses, the symptoms include flushing of the face and extremities, gastrointestinal discomfort, and headache; in larger doses, cyanosis, methemoglobinemia, nausea, vomiting, abdominal pain, collapse, and death can occur (26). The lethal dose of nitrite is estimated at approximately 1 g in adults (28).

Veterinary Drugs and Antibiotics

Food-producing animals can be treated with a variety of veterinary drugs especially antibiotics. If properly used, residues in foods are typically quite low. Acute food poisoning incidents have not occurred as a result of properly used veterinary drugs and antibiotics (2). Concerns have arisen from the use of veterinary drugs. One of the best examples is penicillin, a common antibiotic used in animal as well as human health. Some consumers are allergic to penicillin primarily as a result of its use in human medicine. Questions exist regarding the potential for allergic reactions to penicillin residues resulting from its use in food-producing animals. However, the likelihood of allergic reactions to the very low levels of penicillin residues found in foods is quite remote (31).

Chemicals Migrating from Packaging Materials and Containers

Foods often are packaged for convenience, shelf stability, and protection from microbial agents. These packages and containers also contain chemicals, and under certain circumstances chemicals can migrate from the packaging material into the edible portion of the foods. Chemicals migrating from packaging materials into foods and beverages typically do not present a significant hazard. A variety of chemicals, including plastics monomers, plasticizers, stabilizers, printing inks, and others, do migrate at extremely low levels into foods. Concerns have arisen about the potential chronic toxicity of bisphenol A (BPA) migrating from packaging materials into foods (32). In addition to BPA, the migration of lead, zinc, tin, and other heavy metal residues from packaging materials or storage containers into foods are long-standing concerns (33). The storage of acidic foods in certain packages or containers can result in the leaching of these toxic heavy metals into the food.

Bisphenol A

BPA is a monomer used in the manufacture of plastics including the production of polycarbonate resins used to make baby bottles and water bottles and in the epoxy resins used as the internal linings of cans for soft drinks and beer. Residues of BPA can migrate into foods and beverages stored in containers containing BPA (33). The National Toxicology Program (NTP) has indicated that some concerns exist for adverse effects on the brain, behavior, and prostate glands in fetuses, infants and children at current exposure levels (32). Considerable debate exists relative to the magnitude of the risk associated with these levels of exposure and little concern exists for any risk to exposed adults. Despite the debate, efforts are being made to lessen the extent of exposure to BPA.

Lead

Environmental exposure to lead is a significant public health concern. However, exposure to lead via foods has always been a comparatively moderate contributor to overall environmental lead exposure. The migration of lead from lead-soldered cans was once a source of some concern. However, lead-soldered cans have been successfully phased out of use totally in the United States.

Now, the main issue with lead contamination results from the occasional use of lead-based glazes on pottery or paint on glassware that may come in contact with acidic foods or beverages. Lead is a well-known toxicant that can affect the nervous system, the kidney, and the bone.

Tin

Metal cans for food storage are typically constructed using tin plate. These cans have inner surfaces that are lined with a lacquer material when cans are used for acidic foods or beverages. The inappropriate use of unlacquered cans for acidic food products such as tomato juice or fruit cocktail has resulted in cases of acute tin intoxication (34). Because tin is poorly absorbed, the primary symptoms are bloating, nausea, abdominal cramps, vomiting, diarrhea, and headache occurring 30 minutes to 2 hours after consumption of the acidic product (34).

Zinc

The inappropriate storage of acidic foods or beverages in galvanized containers can result in acute zinc intoxication (33, 35). Episodes have involved fruit punch and tomato juice (33). Zinc is a potent emetic. The symptoms of zinc intoxication include irritation of the mouth, throat, and abdomen; nausea; vomiting; dizziness; and collapse (2).

Industrial Chemicals

Industrial and environmental pollutants have the potential to migrate into foods on occasion. In most circumstances, rather small and inconsequential (from a health perspective) residual amounts are found. On rare occasions, hazardous levels of such chemicals enter the food supply often with devastating consequences from both a health and economic perspective. A few prominent examples will illustrate the potential magnitude of this issue.

Polychlorinated Biphenyls and Polybrominated Biphenyls

Food contamination with polychlorinated biphenyls (PCBs) and polybrominated biphenyls (PBBs) has occurred on several occasions (2). PCBs and PBBs are persistent in the environment. These compounds are fat soluble so they tend to accumulate in the fat depots of various organisms; concentrations often magnify upward along the food chain. PCBs and PBBs are considered to be toxic pollutants from industrial practices. PBBs are commonly used as fire retardants, whereas PCBs are frequently used in transformer fluid. PCBs and PBBs are not particularly worrisome as acute toxicants in foods. However, because they are lipid soluble, elimination from the body is slow and the chronic effects of exposure to these contaminants in foods are of concern. PBBs were involved in one of the most infamous industrial contamination incidents ever in the United States involving the accidental contamination of dairy feed in Michigan (36). This incident resulted in the destruction of many cows and their milk. Although the health consequences of this incident remain uncertain, the economic impact was considerable. PCBs were responsible for cases of human illness associated with contaminated rice bran oil in Japan in one of the most infamous international episodes of industrial contamination of foods (37). The PCBs leaked from a heat exchanger used to deodorize the oil. The resulting syndrome was called *yusho* (meaning "oil disease") by the Japanese. *Yusho* was characterized by chloracne, weakness, numbness of limbs, swelling of eyelids, discharges from the eyes, dark skin pigmentation, and liver damage (37, 38). Acute symptoms were evident at exposure doses as low as 0.5 g. The toxic effects were chronic in many of the victims, persisting for 8 years or more after exposure. Prolonged symptoms included chloracne, menstrual disturbances, fatigue, headache, fever, cough, digestive disturbances, and numbness of the extremities (37, 38). Such incidents continue to occur periodically although fortunately without the human toll experienced in the *yusho* episode. Leaking transformers have contributed to the contamination of feeds with PCBs, which led to the destruction of chickens, eggs, and egg-containing food products (2).

Mercury

Minamata disease, caused by mercury intoxication, is another classic example of food contamination by industrial pollutants. The episode occurred over a number of years and resulted from an industrial firm located on the shores of Minamata Bay in Japan that dumped mercury-containing wastes into the bay from 1953 until the early 1960s. In the bay, bacteria in the sediment converted the inorganic mercury into highly toxic methylmercury. Although elemental mercury is poorly absorbed from the gastrointestinal tract, organomercury compounds including methylmercury are much more efficiently absorbed and are thus more toxic as food contaminants. Fish in the bay became contaminated with the methylmercury, and consumers became ill from eating this fish. More than 1200 cases of mercury intoxication occurred among consumers of Minamata Bay fish (39). The symptoms included tremors and other neurotoxic effects and kidney failure.

Gulf of Mexico Oil Spill

In 2010, a massive oil spill occurred in the Gulf of Mexico from a ruptured oil well. The Gulf of Mexico is a very rich source of seafood. Seafood harvests were temporarily halted because of concerns over the possibility of petrochemical residues affecting the seafood. Although no illnesses were documented, this environmental catastrophe prompted consumer worry and economic hardships. Thus, even the threat of food contamination with industrial pollutants can be disruptive. Many challenges exist for assessment of the risk/safety of seafood after an oil spill (40).

Natural Contaminants

Contaminants can also enter the food supply through various natural means. Bacterial toxins, mycotoxins from molds, and phycotoxins from marine algae are relevant examples.

Bacterial Toxins

Pathogenic bacteria typically cause foodborne disease by the infectious route. The pathogenesis mechanism involves invasion of cells and tissues, multiplication, and symptom causation as a result of cellular injury, inflammation, and/or disturbance of key physiologic processes. Although infectious bacteria are properly viewed as contaminants of food, this chapter is focused on chemical contaminants. The infectious pathogens are living microorganisms and thus will not be considered further.

A few bacteria are toxigenic and produce exogenous toxins in foods before they are eaten. For these bacteria, the ingestion of the toxins initiates the disease process even if the bacteria are destroyed in processing or preparation. The best examples of bacterial intoxication are the staphylococcal enterotoxins and botulinal toxins.

The staphylococcal enterotoxins can be produced in foods by certain strains of *Staphylococcus aureus* (41). The *S. aureus* grows on foods under certain conditions such as temperatures between 10° and 45°C and produces the enterotoxin during growth. When ingested, these protein enterotoxins cause nausea and vomiting with a rapid onset time of 1 to 6 hours. Staphylococcal food poisoning is one of the most common forms of foodborne disease in the United States. Low microgram levels of the staphylococcal enterotoxins are sufficient to elicit symptoms (41). Nine distinct (but structurally related) enterotoxins have been identified as being produced by various strains of *S. aureus* (41). The enterotoxins are small proteins with molecular weights of 25,000 to 29,000 Da. The enterotoxins bind to some as-yet unidentified site in the small intestine and transmit a signal to the vomiting center in the brain. The enterotoxins are more stable to digestion than most proteins and are quite heat resistant. For this reason, staphylococcal food poisoning is often associated with cooked foods that have been cooked after improper storage that allowed the proliferation of *S. aureus*.

The botulinal toxins are potent neurotoxins produced in foods under anaerobic conditions by *Clostridium botulinum* (42). Toxin formation can occur in canned foods that have been improperly processed. The commercial canning process is predicated on the destruction of this organism and its spores so that the spores will not germinate, grow, and produce toxin on storage of the canned product. Seven toxin types have been identified as being produced by various strains of *C. botulinum*, although types A, B, and E are most commonly associated with foodborne illness (42). The botulinal toxins are proteins with a molecular mass of approximately 150 kDa (42). The neurotoxin inhibits the release of acetylcholine at the synapses and thus affects the peripheral nervous system. Botulinal toxins are among the most potent toxins known to humans. Clinical symptoms begin to develop 12 to 48 hours after exposure to the toxin, with weakness, dizziness, and mouth dryness occasionally accompanied by nausea and vomiting. Neurologic symptoms follow, including blurred vision, inability to swallow, aphasia, and weakness of the skeletal muscles. Symptoms can ultimately progress to respiratory paralysis and death. The vegetative cell of *C. botulinum* and the botulinal toxins are easily destroyed by heat, but the spores of *C. botulinum* are heat resistant. Thus, spores can survive improper thermal processing and will germinate and grow under suitable anaerobic conditions (42). Infant botulism is a related illness. In infant botulism, the spores enter the gastrointestinal system early in life before competitive microflora are in place to resist their germination and growth (42). The growth of *C. botulinum* ensues in the intestinal tract where toxin production occurs and causes severe illness. Honey is one of the more frequent sources of the spores in the infant diet (42).

Several other examples exist of toxins produced by bacteria growing on foods including (a) histamine associated primarily with scombroid fish poisoning (43) and (b) the diarrheic and emetic syndromes caused by *Bacillus cereus*, another spore-forming microorganism that can occasionally provoke foodborne disease (44).

Mycotoxins

Mycotoxins are produced by a wide variety of molds that can grow on many different foods (45). The first recognition of mycotoxins emanated from the observation of domestic animals fed moldy animal feeds. Although their effects on humans are not so clearly established, many of the mycotoxins are potentially hazardous to humans as well. The aflatoxins and fumonisins will be discussed as the primary examples.

Aspergillus molds are known to produce several types of mycotoxins, but the aflatoxins are the most notable examples (45). The aflatoxins are produced primarily by *Aspergillus flavus* and *Aspergillus parasiticus*, molds that often contaminate peanuts and corn. Several types of aflatoxins have been identified in legumes and cereals including aflatoxins B and G. Dairy cows fed aflatoxin-contaminated grains or oilseeds are known to release a related form of aflatoxin, aflatoxin M, into their milk. The aflatoxins are potent carcinogens, especially affecting the liver (45). The role of aflatoxins in human carcinogenesis remains uncertain but they are among the most potent animal carcinogens known.

Fusarium molds produce a number of different mycotoxins, including the trichothecenes, fumonisins, and zearalenone (45), but only the fumonisins will be discussed as an example. Fumonisins are produced primarily by *Fusarium verticillioides* and several other *Fusarium* species (45). These molds contaminate various grains and soybeans but are a particular problem with corn. The fumonisins have been implicated in equine leukoencephalomalacia, a fatal neurotoxic syndrome in horses, characterized by extensive necrosis of the white matter in the brain (45). Fumonisins are known rodent carcinogens (46). Although their effects on humans remain unknown, low-level contamination of grains with fumonisins seems to be fairly common.

Algal Toxins

Marine algae are capable of producing a number of potentially hazardous substances; it is estimated that 60 to 80 species out of approximately 4000 known marine phytoplankton are capable of producing potentially toxic algal blooms (47). These toxins are ingested by shellfish and fish, resulting in the development of potentially hazardous seafoods. These algal toxins pass through the food chain from smaller organisms to larger ones; the largest ones are often the most toxic. However, in all cases, the fish and shellfish are only toxic in circumstances where they have the opportunity to feed on toxic marine algae. Several acute illnesses are associated with such seafood, and ciguatera poisoning, paralytic shellfish poisoning, amnesic shellfish poisoning, and tetrodotoxin poisoning will be discussed as examples (48–50).

Ciguatera Poisoning

Ciguatera poisoning results from the ingestion of fish that have fed on toxic dinoflagellate algae. Ciguatera poisoning is probably the most common cause of foodborne disease of chemical etiology on a worldwide basis. This foodborne illness is common throughout the Caribbean and much of the Pacific but is now encountered around the world because of the improved distribution of fish (49, 50). In the United States, the illness occurs most frequently in Florida, Hawaii, and the Virgin Islands (49). Fish that inhabit reef and shore areas in temperate regions, such as grouper, red snapper, barracuda, amberjack, kingfish, Spanish mackerel, mahi-mahi, sea bass, surgeon fish, and eels are the most commonly implicated species, although many different fish species can likely be involved (49). These fish acquire the toxic agent(s) by feeding on smaller fishes that acquire the toxin from the poisonous planktonic algae (49). Several species of dinoflagellate algae appear able to produce toxins of the type associated with ciguatera poisoning; *Gambierdiscus toxicus* is one of the most prominent (49, 50).

Several toxins may be involved in ciguatera poisoning, but the major toxin is a lipid-soluble, polyether compound with a molecular weight of 1112, known as ciguatoxin (50). Ciguatoxin has ionophoric properties (50). Although the toxins accumulate in the liver and viscera of the fish, enough can enter the muscle tissues to result in ciguatera poisoning among humans ingesting these fish (49). The toxins are heat-stable and thus unaffected by processing or cooking practices (49).

The symptoms of ciguatera poisoning are variable. This may be because of the role of several different dinoflagellate algae and several different toxins in this syndrome (49). Gastrointestinal and neurologic manifestations are the predominant symptoms (49, 51), although in some cases, the gastrointestinal symptoms predominate, whereas in other cases, the neurologic symptoms predominate (51). The gastrointestinal complaints include nausea, vomiting, diarrhea, and abdominal cramps. The neurologic symptoms include dysesthesia, paresthesia especially in the perioral region and extremities, pruritus, vertigo, muscle weakness, malaise, headache, and myalgia. A peculiar reversal of hot and cold sensations occurs in about 65% of all patients (51). In severe cases, the neurologic manifestations can progress to delirium, pruritus, dyspnea, prostration, brachycardia, and coma (51). Many patients recover within a few days or weeks. However, treatment can be difficult, and some deaths from cardiovascular collapse have been encountered (49, 51).

Paralytic Shellfish Poisoning

Paralytic shellfish poisoning occurs as the result of ingesting molluscan shellfish, such as clams, mussels, cockles, and scallops, which have become poisonous by feeding on toxic dinoflagellate algae (49, 52). Paralytic shellfish poisoning occurs worldwide with an estimated 2000 human cases occurring each year (52). Toxic dinoflagellate algae belonging to three genera—*Alexandrium, Gymnodinium,* and *Pyrodinium*—have been implicated (52). Because the blooms of the toxic dinoflagellates are quite sporadic, most shellfish will be hazardous only during the times of the blooms (49). In most shellfish species, the toxins are cleared from their system within a few weeks after the end of the dinoflagellate bloom (49). However, a few species, such as the Alaskan butter clam, seem to retain the toxin for long periods (49). Saxitoxins are the causative agents involved in paralytic shellfish poisoning (49, 53). Saxitoxins bind to and block the sodium channels in nerve membranes (49, 53). Processing and cooking have no effect on the toxicity of the heat-stable saxitoxins in the shellfish (49). Because the saxitoxins can block nerve transmission, they are potent neurotoxins. The symptoms of paralytic shellfish poisoning include a tingling sensation and numbness of the lips, tongue, and fingertips followed by numbness in the legs, arms, and neck; ataxia; giddiness; staggering; drowsiness; incoherent speech progressing to aphasia; rash; fever; and respiratory and muscular paralysis (49). Death from respiratory failure does occur with some frequency, usually within 2 to 12 hours depending on the dose ingested (49). No antidotes are known, although prognosis is good if the victim survives the first 24 hours of the illness (49).

Amnesic Shellfish Poisoning

Amnesic shellfish poisoning was first recognized in 1987 as the result of an outbreak in Canada (54). This outbreak involving ingestion of mussels from Prince Edward Island was associated with more than 100 cases and at least 4 deaths (54, 55). A planktonic alga, now identified as a *Pseudo-nitzschia* species, which was blooming in an isolated area of Prince Edward Island at the time of the outbreak, was implicated as the source of the toxin (56). Domoic acid, a neuroexcitatory amino acid, was identified as the toxin (57). Amnesic shellfish poisoning is characterized by gastrointestinal symptoms and unusual neurologic abnormalities (54). The gastrointestinal symptoms include vomiting, abdominal cramps, and diarrhea usually occurring in the first 24 hours after onset of the illness. The neurologic symptoms, which had onset

within 48 hours, were severe incapacitating headaches, confusion, loss of short-term memory, and, in a few cases, seizures and coma. Severely affected patients who did not die experienced prolonged neurologic sequelae including memory deficits and motor or sensorimotor neuronopathy or axonopathy (55).

Tetrodotoxin or Pufferfish Poisoning

Tetrodotoxin poisoning is also a seafood-related illness. However, the tetrodotoxins are likely bacterially produced, rather than produced by marine algae. Pufferfish poisoning occurs primarily in Japan and China, because those are the primary areas of the world where pufferfish are frequently consumed (58). More than 30 species of pufferfish are found worldwide, although most species are not considered to be toxic (49). The most hazardous pufferfish belong to the genus *Fugu*, which are considered in Japan and China to be delicacies (58). Pufferfish are also sometimes referred to as blowfish. The toxin in pufferfish is a potent neurotoxin called tetrodotoxin (49). For many years, the toxins were thought to be produced by the fish. More recently, new evidence suggests that marine bacteria may be the original source of the toxins (59). Tetrodotoxins are heat stable and, like the saxitoxins, act by blocking the sodium channels in nerve cell membranes (49). The symptoms of tetrodotoxin poisoning usually begin with a tingling sensation of the fingers, toes, lips, and tongue, followed by nausea, vomiting, diarrhea, and epigastric pain (60). Twitching, tremors, ataxia, paralysis, and death often ensue (60). A fatality rate of about 60% occurs in untreated cases (60). The tetrodotoxins accumulate in the liver, viscera, and roe of the pufferfish. Careful cleaning of the fish before ingestion of the edible muscle is required to safeguard against tetrodotoxin intoxication (49). Although tetrodotoxin was once thought to be a single chemical entity (49), it is now recognized that various bacteria belonging to species such as *Alteromonas, Vibrio,* and others can produce different but related forms of tetrodotoxin that vary in potency (58). Although tetrodotoxin poisoning is primarily associated with *Fugu* fishes, similar, if not identical, toxins occur in newts, frogs, marine snails, octopuses, crabs, starfishes, and other marine species (61).

PROCESSING-INDUCED TOXICANTS

Processing-induced toxicants form under certain processing conditions, especially heat treatments. As processing treatments prolong the shelf life of foods and guard against microbial hazards, the development of processing-induced toxicants is a classic risk versus benefit puzzle. Several examples of processed-induced toxicants, such as heterocyclic aromatic amines, hydroxymethylfurfural, advanced glycation end products, nitrosamines, and acrylamide, form as a result of food processing and preservation commonly used in the food industry as well as in the home. Acrylamide formation during heat processing of foods containing high levels of carbohydrates and asparagine residues has been extensively studied, and this serves as a good example of processing-induced toxicants.

Acrylamide

Acrylamide (2-propenamide) is a colorless and odorless crystalline solid used in making polyacrylamide and acrylamide copolymers that are used in the paper and textile industries, as flocculants in wastewater treatment, as soil conditioning agents, and as grouting agents for construction of dam foundations, tunnels, and sewers (62, 63). The association of acrylamide in foods was made when researchers were investigating the occurrence of dead fish, paralyzed cattle, and neurotoxic symptoms in railway tunnel makers in Sweden in the late 1990s. Acrylamide polymer was used as a sealant in the tunnel, and some of this sealant entered a nearby stream leading to the contamination of the local water. Researchers found high levels of acrylamide-hemoglobin adducts in tunnel workers, fish, and cattle in the immediate area but also found higher background levels of these adducts in humans that were not exposed to the contaminated water as compared to background levels found in fish and cattle that were not exposed to the water (63). This led researchers to question whether cooked foods could be the source of acrylamide exposure in humans. The first animal study conducted to examine this question found that rats fed fried feed had higher levels of the acrylamide-hemoglobin adducts than rats fed a standard diet (64). Since this study, several world regulatory agencies as well as independent researchers have analyzed and reported levels of acrylamide in foods. French fries, potato chips, breakfast cereals, cookies, brewed coffee, breads and toasts, and pies and cakes are the foods in the US diet that contained the highest levels of acrylamide (65).

Acrylamide forms in foods during the Maillard reaction, which leads to desirable color, flavor, and aroma development in cooked foods. Acrylamide will form due to a reaction between the amino acid, asparagine, and reducing sugars such as glucose and fructose under elevated temperatures (higher than 120°C) and in low-moisture conditions. The highest levels of acrylamide are found in fried, baked, and broiled foods, whereas acrylamide does not form in foods that are boiled or microwaved (66). Acrylamide is rapidly absorbed from the gastrointestinal tract and is distributed throughout the body where it is metabolized to form glycidamide, which is a reactive epoxide that is thought to be responsible for the genotoxic effects of acrylamide exposure (63). Acrylamide has also been shown to be neurotoxic and carcinogenic in animal models, which lead the International Agency for Research on Cancer (IARC) to classify acrylamide as a category 2A carcinogen (probably carcinogenic to humans). Several epidemiologic studies have investigated the association between oral exposure to acrylamide from food sources and the incidence of several types of cancer in humans; however, none of these studies were able to establish a cause-and-effect relationship (63).

NATURAL TOXICANTS

In addition to the naturally occurring contaminants, natural constituents of foods may be hazardous under some circumstances of exposure. Fungi, plants, and occasionally, animals can contain hazardous levels of various naturally occurring toxicants. Of course, such fungi, plants, and animals should not be consumed as food but are accidentally or intentionally consumed on occasion, resulting in foodborne illness. Beyond the poisonous species, many other plants and animals contain levels of naturally occurring toxicants that are probably not hazardous to humans ingesting typical amounts of these foods. However, the ingestion of abnormally large quantities of such foods and their naturally occurring toxicants is potentially hazardous. The naturally occurring toxicants in some plants are inactivated or removed during processing or preparation of foods prior to consumption, but the failure to adhere to such processing and preparation practices can result in foodborne illness.

Poisonous Animals

Acute intoxications occur with very few animal species, although several species of poisonous fish and other marine animals are known to exist (67). Pufferfish is the most often cited example, although it now appears that the toxin in pufferfish may actually emanate from bacteria (58). Animal tissues and products are not generally hazardous unless ingested in abnormally large quantities, at least not on an acute basis. Of course, this statement does not take into account the nutritional concerns with cholesterol and saturated fats. Although overconsumption of cholesterol and saturated fat on a chronic basis may be considered as potentially deleterious to health, these substances generally are not regarded as toxicants. In fact, animal tissues and products contain very few naturally occurring toxicants. The best example is vitamin A (2, 10) as previously discussed. Milk can occasionally contain hazardous substances but these are typically contaminants that are secreted into the milk after the cow has eaten a poisonous plant (68). Ovomucoid, a protein in egg whites, is a trypsin inhibitor, but this activity is diminished by cooking (69). Molluscan shellfish may contain arsenical compounds but typically at levels that are not considered to be hazardous (70). Additional examples are difficult to find.

Poisonous Plants

In contrast, a very large number of poisonous plants exist in nature (71). Classically, plants such as water hemlock and nightshade were used to poison one's enemies. Consumers purchasing foods from commercial sources usually avoid the ingestion of poisonous plants. However, intoxications occur each year among individuals who have harvested their own foods in the wild (72). For example, an elderly couple died after preparing herbal tea from materials they had gathered in the forest surrounding their home. They mistook foxglove for comfrey; foxglove contains digitalis, a potent cardiotoxic substance (73). In another example, a team member in a desert survival course died after eating a salad prepared in part from jimsonweed (72). Jimsonweed contains tropane alkaloids including atropine. Atropine has potent anticholinergic properties, and individuals ingesting jimsonweed and other plants containing tropane alkaloids suffer neurotoxic effects. Although digitalis and atropine are both useful pharmaceutical agents, their ingestion from natural sources in uncontrolled doses can be fatal. Many more such examples could be cited.

Plant food products purchased from commercial sources rarely cause acute intoxications. However, occasional exceptions do exist. In one well-investigated episode, a commercial herbal tea sold to the Mexican-American population in Arizona was contaminated with *Senecio longilobus*, a well-known poisonous plant (74). The herbal tea was called gordolobo yerba, and it was promoted as a cure for colic, viral infections, and nasal congestion in infants. The number of infants and others who ingested the hazardous tea is not known, but six infants died. This tea contained 1.5% of dry weight of pyrrolizidine alkaloids, and one of the deceased infants was estimated to have consumed 66 mg of the alkaloids over a 4-day period. *Senecio* plants contain a group of chemicals known as pyrrolizidine alkaloids that can cause both acute and chronic symptoms (75). Chronic low doses produce liver cancer and cirrhosis (75). The acute symptoms associated with the contaminated herbal tea included ascites, hepatomegaly, venoocclusive liver disease, abdominal pain, nausea, vomiting, headache, and diarrhea (74). The infants who died experienced liver failure.

Although the herbal tea episode involved acute intoxication, pyrrolizidine alkaloids can also cause chronic intoxications if ingested in smaller quantities over more extended periods of time (75, 76). With such long-term, low-level intake, the effects on the liver are cumulative, with irreversible liver damage occurring in small increments over months or even years. Eventually, cirrhosis and liver cancer are the principal manifestations of chronic intoxication with pyrrolizidine alkaloids. Several of the pyrrolizidine alkaloids are well-documented carcinogens in laboratory animals. The lifelong ingestion of herbal products containing low levels of potentially carcinogenic pyrrolizidine alkaloids presents unknown carcinogenic risks. For example, many herbal teas commonly contain lower levels of pyrrolizidine alkaloids that are not typically hazardous on an acute basis. For example, comfrey (*Symphytum officinale*) typically contains a total alkaloid level of 0.003% to 0.02% including a pyrrolizidine alkaloid, symphytine, which is apparently insufficient to elicit acute illness. It is unknown whether long-term intake of comfrey tea would significantly increase the risk of development of liver cancer. Thousands of alkaloids with varying degrees of toxicity are known to occur in plant tissues (76, 77). Some, like the pyrrolizidine alkaloids in *Senecio*, are very hazardous, whereas others are much less hazardous. Some commonly consumed plant foods contain alkaloids at levels that are not considered to be acutely toxic at typical levels of consumption. Comfrey tea would be one example.

In some cases, plant-derived foods contain naturally occurring toxicants at doses that are not acutely toxic at typical levels of consumption but that can be toxic when large quantities of the food are eaten. Examples would include solanine and chaconine in potatoes, oxalates in spinach and rhubarb, furan compounds in mold-damaged sweet potatoes, and cyanogenic glycosides in lima beans, cassava, and many fruit pits (76). Because so many possible examples exist, the cyanogenic glycosides serve as an illustrative example (78). Cyanogenic glycosides can release cyanide from enzymatic action occurring during the storage and processing of the foods or on contact with stomach acid. Although wild varieties of lima beans can contain high and potentially hazardous levels of cyanogenic glycosides, the commercial varieties of lima beans contain minimal amounts of these cyanogenic glycosides having a hydrocyanic acid (HCN) yield of 10 mg/100 g of lima beans (wet weight). Because the lethal oral dose of cyanide for humans is 0.5 mg/kg, a 70-kg adult would have to ingest 35 mg of cyanide, an amount that would require the ingestion of at least 350 g of lima beans. Such levels of consumption are quite unlikely, and human illnesses from cyanide intoxication from ingestion of commercially harvested lima beans have not been reported. Wild varieties of lima beans contain much higher levels of the cyanogenic glycosides (up to 300 mg HCN/100 g). Other plant sources of cyanogenic glycosides also exist. In Africa and South America, cyanide intoxications have occurred from the consumption of cassava (78, 79). Cassava is sometimes ingested in large quantities in these areas because of a lack of other foods. Acute cyanide intoxication has also occurred from the ingestion of fruit pits (80) including the grinding of pits with the fruit in food processors during the preparation of jams and wines. The symptoms of cyanide intoxication include a rapid onset of peripheral numbness and dizziness, mental confusion, stupor, cyanosis, twitching, convulsions, coma, and death (78).

In some cases, plant foods would be hazardous if eaten raw, but processing and preparation ensure the safety of these foods. In these situations, the toxic constituents of plants are inactivated or removed during processing and preparation. For example, raw soybeans contain trypsin inhibitors, lectins, amylase inhibitors, saponins, and various antivitamins (81). Fortunately, these toxicants are inactivated during the heating and fermentation processes used with soybeans. If these toxicants are not removed or inactivated, foodborne illness can occur. For example, raw kidney beans contain lectins, which are typically inactivated during cooking. In the United Kingdom, immigrants who did not appreciate the importance of thorough cooking of kidney beans have ingested undercooked kidney beans leading to the onset of nausea, vomiting, abdominal pain, and bloody diarrhea from the lectins (82).

Poisonous Mushrooms

Mushrooms are often poisonous, so the harvesting of mushrooms in the wild can be a hazardous practice.

Incidents of mushroom poisoning occur each year around the world (83). Poisonous mushrooms contain various naturally occurring toxicants, which can be classified into groups I to VI (84).

The group I toxins are the most hazardous. Group I toxins include amatoxin and phallotoxin. Amatoxin is characteristically produced by *Amanita phalloides*, the death cap mushroom. Acute amatoxin intoxication occurs in three stages. In the first stage, abdominal pain, nausea, vomiting, diarrhea, and hyperglycemia begin to develop 6 to 24 hours after ingestion of the mushrooms. A short period of remission then occurs. In the third and often fatal stage, severe liver and kidney dysfunction leads to hypoglycemia, convulsions, coma, and death. Death resulting from hypoglycemic shock occurs 4 to 7 days after the onset of symptoms. The group II toxins are hydrazines. Gyromitrin, produced by *Gyromitra esculenta* or false morel mushrooms, is the best known example. The symptoms elicited by ingestion of false morel mushrooms include a bloated feeling, nausea, vomiting, watery or bloody diarrhea, abdominal pain, muscle cramps, faintness, and ataxia occurring with a 6 to 12 hour onset time. Muscarine is the most characteristic of the group III toxins that affect the autonomic nervous system. Muscarine occurs in fly agaric (*Amanita muscarina*), sometimes in association with the group I toxins. Symptoms include perspiration, salivation, lacrimation with blurred vision, abdominal cramps, watery diarrhea, constriction of the pupils, hypotension, and a slowed pulse occurring rapidly following the ingestion of the poisonous mushrooms.

Coprine is a group IV toxin that causes symptoms only when ingested with alcoholic beverages. Coprine is produced by *Coprinus atramentarius*. Symptoms include flushing of the neck and face, distension of the veins in the neck, swelling and tingling of the hands, metallic taste, tachycardia, and hypotension progressing to nausea and vomiting. Symptoms begin within 30 minutes of ingestion of the mushrooms but only if alcoholic beverages are also consumed simultaneously. Symptoms can persist for up to 5 days.

The groups V and VI toxins are hallucinogenic, ostensibly exerting their actions on the central nervous system causing hallucinations. The group V toxins include ibotenic acid and muscimol. The group V toxins cause dizziness, drowsiness followed by hyperkinetic activity, confusion, delirium, incoordination, staggering, muscular spasms, partial amnesia, a comalike sleep, and hallucinations beginning 30 minutes to 2 hours after ingestion. Fly agaric is a good source of the group V toxins. The group VI toxins include psilocybin and psilocin. The symptoms of the group VI toxins include pleasant or aggressive mood, anxiety, unmotivated laughter and hilarity, compulsive movements, muscle weakness, drowsiness, hallucinations, and sleep. Mexican mushrooms, *Psilocybe mexicana*, contain the group VI toxins. Symptoms usually begin within 30 to 60 minutes after ingestion of the mushrooms, and recovery is often spontaneous in 5 to 10 hours. When the

dose of the group VI toxins is high, prolonged and severe sequelae, even death, can occur.

REFERENCES

1. Taylor SL. Food toxicology. In: Metcalfe DD, Sampson HA, Simon RA, eds. Food Allergy: Adverse Reactions to Foods and Food Additives. 3rd ed. Elmsford, NY: Blackwell, 2003:475–86.
2. Taylor SL. Chemical intoxications. In: Cliver DO, Riemann HP, eds. Foodborne Diseases. 2nd ed. San Diego: Academic Press, 2002:305–16.
3. Taylor SL, Byron B. J Food Prot 1984;47:249.
4. Lockey S. Ann Allergy 1959;17:719–25.
5. Bush RK, Taylor SL, Hefle SL. Adverse reactions to food and drug additives. In: Adkinson NF, Yunginger JW, Busse WW et al, eds. Middleton's Allergy Principles and Practice. 6th ed. St. Louis: Mosby, 2003:1645–63.
6. Stevenson DD. Tartrazine, azo, and non-azo dyes. In: Metcalfe DD, Sampson HA, Simon RA, eds. Food Allergy: Adverse Reactions to Foods and Food Additives. 3rd ed. Elmsford, NY: Blackwell, 2003:351–9.
7. Cheskin LJ, Miday R, Zorich N et al. JAMA 1998;279:150–2.
8. Food and Nutrition Board, Institute of Medicine. Dietary Reference Intakes: A Risk Assessment Model for Establishing Upper Intake Levels for Nutrients. Washington, DC: National Academy Press, 1998.
9. Munro IC. In: Taylor SL, Scanlan RA, eds. Food Toxicology: A Perspective on the Relative Risks. New York: Marcel Dekker, 1989:151–67.
10. DiPalma JR, Ritchie DM. Annu Rev Pharmacol Toxicol 1977;17:133–48.
11. Press E, Yeager L. Am J Public Health 1962;52:1720–8.
12. Campana L, Redmond S, Nitzkin JL et al. JAMA 1983;250:160.
13. Burkhalter J, Shore M, Wollstadt L et al. MMWR Morb Mortal Wkly Rep 1981;30:11–2.
14. Kilbourne EM, Rigau-Perez JG, Heath CW Jr et al. N Engl J Med 1983; 309:1408–14.
15. de la Paz MP, Philen RM, Borda IA et al. Food Chem Toxicol 1996;34:251–7.
16. World Health Organization. Toxic Oil Syndrome: Current Knowledge and Future Perspectives. Copenhagen: WHO Regional Publications, European series no. 42, 1992.
17. Rodriguez M, Nogura AE, Del Villaras S et al. Arthritis Rheum 1982;25:1477–80.
18. Dobson RLM, Motlagh S, Quijano M et al. Toxicol Sci 2008; 106:251–62.
19. Ingelfinger JR. N Engl J Med 2008;359:2745–8.
20. Ferrer A, Cabral R. Food Addit Contam 1991;8:755–76.
21. Green MA, Heumann MA, Wehr HM et al. Am J Public Health 1987;77:1431–4.
22. Goldman LR, Beller M, Jackson RL. Arch Environ Health 1990;45:141–7.
23. Goes EA, Savage EP, Gibbons G et al. Am J Epidemiol 1980;111:254–60.
24. Concon JM. Food Toxicology: Part B, Contaminants and Additives. New York: Marcel Dekker, 1988.
25. Sanders PR, Lee TC, Groth ME et al. Safety assessment of insect-protected corn. In: Thomas JA, ed. Biotechnology and Safety Assessment. 2nd ed. London: Taylor & Francis, 1998:241–56.
26. Taylor SL, Nordlee JA, Kapels LM. Pediatr Allergy Immunol 1992;3:180–7.
27. Schmid R. N Engl J Med 1960;268:397–8.

28. Fassett DW. Nitrates and nitrites. In: Committee on Food Protection. Toxicants Occurring Naturally in Foods. 2nd ed. Washington, DC: National Academy of Sciences, 1973:7–25.

29. Spinios A. Munchen Med Wochenschr 1964;106:1180–2.

30. Keating JP, Lell ME, Straus AW et al. N Engl J Med 1973; 288:825–6.

31. Dewdney JM, Edwards RG. J R Soc Med 1984;77:866–77.

32. NTP-CERHR. Monograph on the Potential Health Reproductive and Developmental Effects of Bisphenol A. Bethesda, MD, National Institutes of Health, 2008. NIH publication 08-5994.

33. Hughes JM, Horwitz MA, Merson MH et al. Am J Epidemiol 1977;105:233–44.

34. Barker WH Jr, Runte V. Am J Epidemiol 1972;96:219–26.

35. Brown MA, Thom JV, Orth GL et al. Arch Environ Health 1964;8:657–60.

36. Hecht A. FDA Consum 1976 Dec-1977 Jan:21–5.

37. Kuratsune M, Yoshimura T, Matsuzaka J et al. Environ Health Perspect 1972;1:119–28.

38. Higuchi K, ed. PCB Poisoning and Pollution. New York: Academic Press, 1976.

39. Kurland LT, Faro SN, Siedler H. World Neurol 1960;1: 370–95.

40. Gilroy DJ. J Toxicol Environ Health A 2000;60:317–29.

41. Balaban N, Rasooly A. Int J Food Microbiol 2000;61:1–10.

42. Parkinson NG, Ito K. Botulism. In: Cliver DO, Riemann HP, eds. Foodborne Diseases. 2nd ed. San Diego: Academic Press, 2002:249–59.

43. Hungerford JM. Toxicon 2010;56:231–43.

44. Griffiths MW, Schraft H. *Bacillus cereus* food poisoning. In: Cliver DO, Riemann HP, eds. Foodborne Diseases. 2nd ed. San Diego: Academic Press, 2002:261–70.

45. Richard JL. Int J Food Microbiol 2007;119:3–10.

46. Howard PC, Eppley RM, Stack ME et al. Environ Health Perspect 2001;109(Suppl 2):277–82.

47. Smayda TJ. Limnol Oceanogr 1997;42:1137–53.

48. James KJ, Carey B, O'Halloran J et al. Epidemiol Infect 2010;138:927–40.

49. Taylor SL. Food Technol 1988;42:94–8.

50. Dickey RW, Plakas SM. Toxicon 2010;56:123–136.

51. Farstad DJ, Chow T. Wilderness Environ Med 2001;12: 263–9.

52. Van Dolah FM. Environ Health Perspect 2000;108(Suppl 1): 133-41.

53. Shimizu Y. The chemistry of paralytic shellfish toxins. In: Tu AT, ed. Handbook of Natural Toxins, vol. 3. Marine Toxins and Venoms. New York: Marcel Dekker, 1988:63–85.

54. Perl TM, Bedard L, Kosatsky T et al. N Engl J Med 1990; 322:1775–80.

55. Teitelbaum JS, Zatorre RJ, Carpenter S et al. N Engl J Med 1990;322:1781–7.

56. Bates SS, Bird CJ, DeFreitas ASW et al. Can J Fish Aquatic Sci 1989;46:1203–15.

57. Wright JLC, Boyd RK, DeFreitas ASW et al. Can J Chem 1989;67:481–90.

58. Hwang DF, Noguchi T. Adv Food Nutr Res 2007;52: 142–236.

59. Yasumoto T, Yasumura D, Yotsu M et al. Agric Biol Chem 1986;50:793–5.

60. Mines D, Stahmer S, Shepherd SM. Emerg Med Clin North Am 1997;15:157–77.

61. Wakely JF, Fuhrman GJ, Fuhrman FA et al. Toxicon 1966; 3:195–203.

62. Zhang YU, Zhang Y. Crit Rev Food Sci Nutr 2007:521–42.

63. Mills C, Mottram DS, Wedzicha BL. Acrylamide. In: Stadler RH, Lineback DR, eds. Process-Induced Food Toxicants: Occurrence, Formation, Mitigation, and Health Risks. Hoboken, NJ: John Wiley, 2009:23–50.

64. Tareke E, Rydberg P, Karlsson P et al. Chem Res Toxicol 2000;13:517–22.

65. Roach JAG, Andrzejewski ML, Gay D et al. J Agric Food Chem 2003;51:7547–54.

66. Tareke E, Rydberg P, Karlsson P et al. J Agric Food Chem 2002;50:4998–5006.

67. Halstead BW. Other poisonous marine animals. In: Hui YH, Gorham JR, Murrell KD et al, eds. Foodborne Disease Handbook: Diseases Caused by Hazardous Substances, vol 3. New York: Marcel Dekker, 1994:497–528.

68. Beier RC, Nigg HN. Toxicology of naturally occurring chemicals in foods. In: Hui YH, Gorham JR, Murrell KD et al, eds. Foodborne Disease Handbook: Diseases Caused by Hazardous Substances, vol 3. New York: Marcel Dekker, 1994:1–186.

69. Doell BH, Ebden CJ, Smith CA. Qual Plant Foods Hum Nutr 1981;31:139– 44.

70. Whanger PD. Factors affecting the metabolism of nonessential metals in foods. In: Hathcock JN, ed. Nutritional Toxicology, vol. I. New York: Academic Press, 1982:163–208.

71. Smith RA. Poisonous plants. In: Hui YH, Gorham JR, Murrell KD et al, eds. Foodborne Disease Handbook: Diseases Caused by Hazardous Substances, vol 3. New York: Marcel Dekker, 1994:187–226.

72. Huxtable RJ. Perspect Biol Med 1980;24:1–14.

73. Cooper L, Grunenfelder G, Blackmon J et al. MMWR Morb Mortal Wkly Rep 1977;26:257–9.

74. Stillman AE, Huxtable R, Consroe P et al. Gastroenterology 1977;73:349–53.

75. Coulombe RA. Adv Food Nutr Res 2003;45:61–99.

76. Sinden SL, Deahl KL. Alkaloids. In: Hui YH, Gorham JR, Murrell KD, Cliver DO, eds. Foodborne Disease Handbook: Diseases Caused by Hazardous Substances, vol 3. New York: Marcel Dekker, 1994:227–59.

77. Rietjens IM, Martena MJ, Boersma MG et al. Mol Nutr Food Res 2005;49:131–58.

78. Vetter J. Toxicon 2000;38:11–36.

79. Cliff J, Muquingue H, Nhassico D et al. Food Chem Toxicol 2011;49:631–5.

80. Morse DL, Harrington JM, Heath CW. N Engl J Med 1976;295:1264.

81. Liener IE. Crit Rev Food Sci Nutr 1994;34:31–67.

82. Rodhouse JC, Haugh CA, Roberts D et al. Epidemiol Infect 1990;105:485–91.

83. Diaz J. Crit Care Med 2005;33:419–26.

84. Spoerke DG Jr. Mushrooms: epidemiology and medical management. In: Hui YH, Gorham JR, Murrell KD et al, eds. Foodborne Disease Handbook: Diseases Caused by Hazardous Substances, vol 3. New York: Marcel Dekker, 1994:433–62.

SUGGESTED READINGS

Botana LM, ed. Phycotoxins: Chemistry and Biochemistry. Ames, IA: Blackwell, 2007.

Reddy CS, Hayes AW. Foodborne toxicants. In: Principles and Methods of Toxicology. 5th ed. New York: Informa Healthcare, 2007:633–92.

Riemann HP, Cliver DO, eds. Foodborne Infections and Intoxications. Amsterdam: Elsevier/Academic Press, 2006.

Stadler RH, Lineback DR, eds. Process-Induced Food Toxicants: Occurrence, Formation, Mitigation, and Health Risks. Hoboken, NJ: John Wiley, 2009.

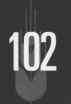

102   FOOD ALLERGIES AND INTOLERANCES

STEVE L. TAYLOR AND JOSEPH L. BAUMERT

Centuries ago, the Roman philosopher Lucretius stated, "What is food to one is bitter poison to another." Food allergies and related illnesses can be collectively referred to as *individualistic* adverse reactions to foods." These illnesses affect certain individuals within the population but not others. Although these individualistic adverse reactions to foods are often grouped together under the general heading of "food allergy," in fact a variety of different types of illnesses are involved. Several different types of individualistic adverse reactions to foods occur that have different symptoms, severity, prevalence, and causative factors. This fact is not widely recognized by physicians and consumers.

When properly diagnosed by medical professionals, food allergies and related diseases can be treated successfully; and symptoms can be avoided by following specific avoidance diets. Nutritional advice is often desirable in the construction of safe and effective avoidance diets. However, consumers sometimes do not seek medical attention for these conditions, relying instead on self-diagnosis or parental diagnosis of the conditions experienced by infants and young children. Consumers perceive that food allergies are quite common (1), whereas in fact many self-diagnosed cases of food allergy incorrectly associate foods with a particular malady or ascribe various mild forms of postprandial eating discomfort to this category of illness. As a result, some consumers mistakenly attempt to avoid certain foods. Although the result of such needless avoidance diets is harmless in many cases, nutritional problems can occur, especially when attempts are made to avoid many foods.

DEFINITION AND CLASSIFICATION

Most consumers and some physicians improperly classify any abnormal response to ingestion of food as a food allergy.

---

[1]**Abbreviations: CAP**, ImmunoCAP test; **DBPCFC**, double-blind, placebo-controlled food challenge; **ELISA**, enzyme-linked immunosorbent assay; **FAO**, Food and Agriculture Organization; **G6PD**, glucose-6-phosphate dehydrogenase; **GSH**, glutathione; **IgE**, immunoglobulin E; **NADPH**, nicotinamide adenine dinucleotide phosphate; **OAS**, oral allergy syndrome; **SPT**, skin prick test.

TABLE 102.1	CLASSIFICATION OF INDIVIDUALISTIC ADVERSE REACTIONS TO FOODS

True food allergies
  Antibody-mediated food allergies
    Immunoglobulin E–mediated food allergies (e.g., peanut, cows' milk), including oral allergy syndrome
    Exercise-associated food allergies
  Cell-mediated food allergies
    Celiac disease
    Food protein–induced enterocolitis
    Food protein–induced enteropathy
    Food protein–induced proctitis
    Other types of delayed hypersensitivity
  Either antibody-mediated or cell-mediated
    Allergic eosinophilic gastroenteritis
    Allergic eosinophilic esophagitis
Food intolerances
  Anaphylactoid reactions
  Metabolic food disorders
    Lactose intolerance
    Favism
  Idiosyncratic reactions
  Sulfite-induced asthma

In fact, several different types of individualistic adverse reactions are known to occur, and only certain types of reactions can be correctly classified as true food allergies.

A classification scheme for the different types of individualistic adverse reactions to foods or food sensitivities that occur in association with food ingestion is provided in Table 102.1. Two major groups of food sensitivity are known: true food allergies and food intolerances (2). Although true food allergies involve abnormal immunologic mechanisms, food intolerances do not. The differences between *immunologic* food allergies and *nonimmunologic* food intolerances are significant for the affected individual. Food intolerances usually can be managed by limiting the amount of the food or food ingredient that is eaten; total avoidance usually is not necessary. In contrast, *total avoidance* of the offending food typically is necessary with true food allergies. In addition, allergy-like intoxication can occur with certain foods (3). Although this form of food poisoning sometimes is clinically confused with food allergy, it is distinctly different because all consumers are potentially susceptible.

Food allergies are abnormal immunologic responses to a particular food or food component, usually a naturally occurring protein (4, 5). Immediate hypersensitivity reactions and delayed hypersensitivity reactions are well-documented types of immunologic responses that can occur in certain individuals on ingestion of specific foods. Immediate hypersensitivity reactions are immunoglobulin E (IgE) mediated, with symptoms ensuing within minutes of ingesting the offending food. Delayed hypersensitivity reactions are cell mediated, with symptoms developing 48 to 72 hours after ingesting the offending food. The role of cell-mediated reactions in food allergies is far less well established, with the exception of celiac

disease, which is the only type of delayed hypersensitivity discussed in this chapter.

In contrast, *food intolerances* do not involve abnormal responses of the immune system (6). Three mechanistically distinct forms of food intolerances are recognized: anaphylactoid reactions, metabolic food disorders, and idiosyncratic reactions.

As the name implies, *allergy-like intoxications* often are confused with true food allergies because the symptoms are identical (3). Histamine poisoning is the primary example of an allergy-like intoxication.

IMMUNOGLOBULIN E–MEDIATED FOOD ALLERGIES

IgE-mediated food allergies are arguably the most important class of food sensitivities. Although the number of affected individuals is relatively small, the reactions in some individuals in this group can be life threatening, especially if a significant quantity of the offending food is ingested inadvertently. Also, the degree of tolerance for the offending food is small, making the implementation of safe and effective avoidance diets more difficult.

Mechanism

IgE-mediated or immediate hypersensitivity reactions are associated with the rapid onset of symptoms, usually within minutes to a few hours, after the ingestion of the offending food. Immediate hypersensitivity reactions are mediated by an allergen-specific IgE antibody, as depicted in Figure 102.1 (4). Food allergens are typically naturally occurring proteins in foods (7). In IgE-mediated food allergies, exposure to the allergen stimulates the production of allergen-specific IgE antibodies in susceptible individuals (5, 6). The allergen-specific IgE attaches itself to the surface of mast cells in various tissues and basophils in the blood. This process is known as sensitization.

During the sensitization phase, the susceptible individual may form allergen-specific IgE antibodies on exposure to a specific food protein. However, even among susceptible individuals, exposure to food proteins does not usually result in the formation of IgE antibodies. In normal individuals, exposure to a food protein in the gastrointestinal tract results in oral tolerance through either the formation of protein-specific IgG, IgM, or IgA antibodies or no immunologic response whatsoever (clonal anergy) (8, 9). Heredity and other physiologic factors are important in predisposing individuals to the development of IgE-mediated allergies, including food allergies (10). Monozygotic and dizygotic twins demonstrate that genetics is an extremely important parameter, and identical twins may inherit the likelihood of responding to the same allergenic food, such as peanuts (11, 12). Approximately 65% of patients with clinically documented allergy have first-degree relatives with allergic disease (10). Conditions that

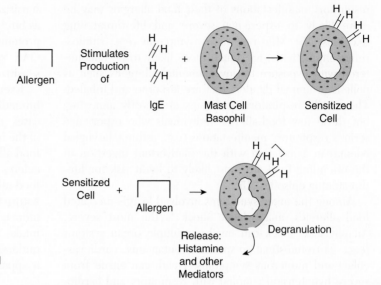

Fig. 102.1. Mechanism of immunoglobulin E–mediated food allergy.

increase the permeability of the small intestinal mucosa to proteins such as viral gastroenteritis, premature birth, and cystic fibrosis also seem to increase the risk of development of food allergy.

Although no symptoms occur during the sensitization process, the affected individual is now primed for an allergic reaction. On subsequent exposure to the allergenic food, the allergen cross-links IgE molecules on the surface of the mast cell or basophil membrane, causing these cells to release various mediators of the allergic reaction into the bloodstream and tissues. Dozens of physiologically active mediators of the allergic reaction have been identified (13). Histamine is one of the most important mediators of the immediate hypersensitivity reaction and can elicit inflammation, pruritus, and contraction of the smooth muscles in the blood vessels, gastrointestinal tract, and respiratory tract (6). Other important mediators include various leukotrienes and prostaglandins (6, 13). The released mediators interact with receptors in various tissues, eliciting a wide range of physiologic responses. Because the mediators are released into the bloodstream, systemic reactions involving multiple tissues and organs can ensue.

Allergies to pollens, mold spores, animal danders, dust mites, certain drugs (e.g., penicillin), and bee venom also occur through this same IgE-mediated mechanism. Susceptible individuals may form allergen-specific IgE to one or several substances, including food allergens. Occupational food allergies are also known to occur where individuals are affected by contact with or inhalation of the offending food rather than its ingestion (14).

Symptoms

Numerous symptoms can be associated with IgE-mediated food allergies, ranging from mild and annoying to severe and life threatening (Table 102.2) (2). Only a few of

these symptoms will occur in each allergic individual. The nature of the symptoms and their severity depend on several factors, including the individual, the amount of the offending food ingested, the tissue receptors that are affected, and the length of time since the last previous exposure.

As noted in Table 102.2, the symptoms of IgE-mediated reactions can involve the gastrointestinal tract, skin, or respiratory tract. Gastrointestinal and cutaneous symptoms are among the more common manifestations. Although respiratory symptoms are much less commonly encountered in food-allergic reactions, individuals with

TABLE 102.2	SYMPTOMS ASSOCIATED WITH IMMUNOGLOBULIN E–MEDIATED FOOD ALLERGY

Gastrointestinal
  Nausea
  Vomiting
  Diarrhea
  Abdominal cramping
  Oral allergy syndrome
Cutaneous
  Urticaria
  Dermatitis or eczema
  Angioedema
  Pruritus
Respiratory
  Rhinitis
  Rhinoconjunctivitis
  Asthma
  Laryngeal edema
  Heiner syndrome
Generalized
  Anaphylactic shock

For additional information see Sellge G, Bischoff SC. The immunological basis of IgE-mediated reactions. In: Metcalfe DD, Sampson HA, Simon RA, eds. Food Allergy: Adverse Reactions to Foods and Food Additives. 4th ed. Malden, MA: Blackwell Science, 2008:15–28.

respiratory manifestations of their food allergies may be more likely to experience severe and life-threatening reactions (15). Mild respiratory symptoms (e.g., rhinitis, rhinoconjunctivitis) are much more likely to be encountered with exposure to environmental allergens such as pollens or animal danders that are airborne and inhaled. These mild respiratory symptoms are mostly annoying, but those few food-allergic individuals who experience serious respiratory manifestations (e.g., asthma, laryngeal edema) in association with the inadvertent ingestion of the offending food are most likely to be at risk for life-threatening episodes (15).

Among the many symptoms involved in IgE-mediated food allergies, anaphylactic shock is the most severe. Anaphylactic shock can involve multiple organ systems (e.g., gastrointestinal, respiratory, cutaneous, cardiovascular) and numerous symptoms. Death can ensue from severe hypotension coupled with respiratory and cardiovascular complications. Comparatively few individuals are susceptible to suffering such severe reactions on food ingestion. The severity of an allergic reaction depends on the degree of sensitivity of the individual and the amount of the offending food that is ingested (2). The inadvertent ingestion of allergenic foods has resulted in deaths (15–18). Anaphylactic shock is a common cause of death in these fatalities. Deaths have occurred with most of the common allergenic foods, although peanuts, tree nuts, and crustacea seem to be more frequently implicated in severe food allergies than some of the other commonly allergenic foods. The prevalence of severe allergic reactions to foods is uncertain. Although the number of deaths occurring from IgE-mediated food allergies is not recorded in most countries, approximately 100 deaths are thought to occur in the United States each year (2, 17).

Although severe and potentially fatal allergic reactions such as anaphylactic shock are obviously a focus of much concern, mild symptoms are much more likely to occur with IgE-mediated food allergies. Perhaps the most common and possibly the mildest form of IgE-mediated food allergy is the so-called oral allergy syndrome (OAS) (19). OAS symptoms are confined to the oropharyngeal area, including pruritus, urticaria, and angioedema. OAS is most frequently associated with the ingestion of various fresh fruits and vegetables (19). OAS is an IgE-mediated reaction to specific proteins present in fresh fruits and vegetables (19). Most of the fruit and vegetable allergens involved in OAS are apparently quite susceptible to digestive proteases in the gastrointestinal tract (19), thus systemic reactions are rarely encountered to these foods. These fruit and vegetable allergens are also apparently heat labile (19), as the heat-processed versions of these foods are not typically involved in initiation of OAS. A more stable allergen called lipid transfer protein has been implicated in allergic reactions to certain fruits, and these reactions are more likely to be systemic and severe (19). With OAS, affected individuals are initially sensitized to one or more pollens in the environment, such as birch or mugwort pollens, that cross-react with related proteins found in fresh fruits and vegetables (19). With OAS, sensitization to pollen increases the likelihood of sensitization to specific foods.

Exercise-induced food allergies are a subset of the immediate hypersensitivity reactions to foods. In these cases, exercise must be done coincident with ingestion of the food for symptoms to occur (20). Exercise-induced food allergies have been associated with shellfish, wheat, celery, and peach. The symptoms of exercise-induced food allergies are individualistic, variable, and similar in nature to those involved in other food allergies. Exercise-induced allergies can also exist without any role for food intake (20). The mechanism of this illness is not well understood, although the involvement of IgE antibodies is apparent.

Sources

The Food and Agriculture Organization (FAO) of the United Nations has established that peanuts, soybeans, fish, crustacea, milk, eggs, tree nuts, and wheat are the most common allergenic foods on a worldwide basis (21). Perhaps 90% of all IgE-mediated food allergies are caused by these eight foods or food groups, sometimes referred to as the big eight. The big eight actually involves many more than eight foods because several food groups are included. Fish refers to all species of finfish, although some species of fish such as cod and salmon are more commonly allergenic than others (22, 23). Shrimp, prawns, crab, lobster, and crayfish are included in the category of crustacea; most individuals with crustacean allergy are sensitive to all species (24). Egg-allergic individuals are allergic to the eggs of all avian species (25). Furthermore, both egg white and egg yolk contain allergens (26), although egg white is considered to be the more potent sensitizing fraction. Milk-allergic individuals are primarily sensitized to cows' milk, but typically are also reactive to the milk of other species, including goat and sheep (27). The commonly allergenic tree nuts include almonds, walnuts, pecans, cashews, Brazil nuts, macadamias, pistachios, hazelnuts (filberts), hickory nuts, chestnuts, and pine (pinyon) nuts (2). Although sometimes included in the tree nut category, coconuts, kola nuts, and shea nuts are rarely, if ever, allergenic. Cross-reactions do not inevitably occur with closely related foods. Although there are several hundred species of edible legumes, peanuts and soybeans account for the vast majority of legume-related food allergies. However, several other legumes, including lentils, beans, and garbanzo beans (chickpeas), occasionally have caused serious allergic reactions (28, 29).

Although the eight most commonly allergenic foods and food groups account for more than 90% of all IgE-mediated food allergies on a global basis, more than

TABLE 102.3	PRIORITY ALLERGENIC FOODS BY REGION			
FOOD	UNITED STATES	CANADA	EUROPEAN UNION	AUSTRALIA/NEW ZEALAND
Peanut	X	X	X	X
Tree nuts	X	X	X	X
Soybean	X	X	X	X
Wheat[a]	X	X	X	X
Milk	X	X	X	X
Eggs	X	X	X	X
Fish	X	X	X	X
Crustacea	X	X	X	X
Molluscs		X	X	
Sesame seed		X	X	X
Mustard		X	X	
Celery			X	
Lupine			X	

[a]Or cereals containing gluten, which include wheat.

160 other foods have been documented in the medical literature on one or more occasions to elicit food allergies (30). Any food that contains protein has the potential to elicit allergic sensitization. Generally, foods that are major sources of protein and that are frequently consumed in the diet are most likely to cause allergic reactions. However, certain foods that are considered to be good sources of protein, such as beef, pork, chicken, and turkey, are rarely allergenic (30).

Although the FAO list of the eight most commonly allergenic foods or food groups is reasonably well accepted, various regulatory jurisdictions have established their own list of commonly allergenic foods (Table 102.3). These lists are used for food labeling regulations in these areas. The lists partially reflect the fact that unique cultural dietary patterns may affect the comparative prevalence of specific allergenic foods. For example, lists in Canada, the European Union, and Australia/New Zealand include sesame seed, a common allergenic food among certain Asian and Middle Eastern cultures (31). By contrast, sesame seed allergy appears to be comparatively uncommon in the United States. Although the earliest European lists included sesame seed, mustard, and celery (uniquely allergenic in central Europe, where celeriac is a more common food ingredient), the development of a scientific approach to construction of such lists in Europe (32) led to a decision to add molluscan shellfish and an emerging allergenic food, lupine (33), to the European Union list. Molluscan shellfish are also on the list in Canada. Mustard is on the list of commonly allergenic foods in the European Union and Canada, even though the prevalence of mustard allergy is not very well established; mustard allergy has principally been reported in France and Spain for unexplained reasons (34). Buckwheat is included on the list of commonly allergenic foods in Japan and Korea and appears to be a commonly allergenic food in those countries, probably because of frequent exposure to soba noodles (35).

Food Allergens

Virtually all of the allergens in foods are naturally occurring proteins (7). However, foods contain millions of proteins and relatively few are known to be allergens. Allergenicity does not appear to be an inherent property of proteins, although all proteins are capable of provoking immune reactions under selected circumstances. Some commonly allergenic foods, including peanuts, eggs, milk, and soybeans, contain multiple allergens (7). Other commonly allergenic foods appear to contain only a single major allergen, including cod and Brazil nut (7). Major allergens are generally defined as proteins for which 50% or more of the allergic patients have specific IgE (7). Plant food allergens tend to fall into certain functional categories, such as some of the pathogenesis-related proteins or certain classes of storage proteins (36). For example, the 2S albumins, storage proteins rich in sulfur-containing amino acids, are major allergens in peanuts, Brazil nuts, sesame seeds, walnuts, sunflower seeds, and mustard (37). Similarly, several pan-allergens appear to exist in allergenic animal species, such as the parvalbumin in fish (38) and tropomyosin in crustaceans (39).

Prevalence

Allergic diseases are estimated to affect 10% to 25% of the general population (4). The prevalence of IgE-mediated food allergies in the United States can be estimated at 3.5% to 4.0% of the population, based on surveys indicating that the prevalence of shrimp, peanut, tree nut, and fish allergies as 1.9%, 0.76%, 0.62%, and 0.4% of the overall population (40, 41). IgE-mediated food allergies are more common among infants and young children than among adults; the prevalence in children under the age of 3 is in the range of 5% to 8% (42). Although food allergies develop most commonly in early childhood, they can develop later in life. For example, crustacea are among the most common allergenic foods among adults (41), but that food allergy is rarely seen among young children, probably because of their infrequent ingestion of crustacea.

The prevalence of IgE-mediated food allergies to specific foods has been evaluated primarily on the basis of random digit-dial telephone surveys (40, 41). For certain types of food allergies, including immediate hypersensitivity reactions associated with noteworthy symptoms, these telephone surveys are arguably reasonably accurate. However, clinical confirmation of these estimates has not been obtained, making prevalence estimates uncertain (43). A large effort is being completed in Europe, through a project called EuroPrevall, to prepare a more reliable estimate of prevalence based on clinical confirmation. As noted, there is general agreement that eight foods or food groups comprise the majority of IgE-mediated food allergies (21). This is based primarily on comparative prevalence studies conducted in allergy clinics with groups of patients (44).

Fewer studies have attempted to determine the prevalence of specific food allergies among the general population. The prevalence of adverse reactions to foods, as confirmed by double blind, placebo-controlled food challenge (DBPCFC) during the first 3 years of life among 480 consecutively born infants in a community in Colorado, was 8% (45). Of these children, 25 (5.2%) were suspected to be allergic to cows' milk, but DBPCFC confirmed sensitivity to cows' milk in only 11 (2.3%) (45). In a prospective study of 1,749 newborns in a single hospital in Denmark during 1985, 39 (2.2%) were found to have adverse reactions to cows' milk (46). Similarly, Jakobsson and Lindberg (47) followed a cohort of 1079 Swedish newborns and found that 1.9% developed sensitivity to cows' milk. A prevalence rate of 2.8% was observed in challenge studies conducted on a group of Dutch infants (48). The overall prevalence of food allergies among a birth cohort in Australia was estimated at about 8.5%, with 3.2% for egg, 2.0% for milk, 1.9% for peanut, and 0.42% for sesame seed (49).

Persistence

Many young children outgrow their food allergies within a few months to several years after the onset of the hypersensitivity (6, 50). As many as 80% to 87% of children identified with food allergies are able to tolerate the offending food by 3 years of age (50). Allergies to certain foods, such as cows' milk, are more commonly outgrown than are allergies to other foods, such as peanut (50). Exceptions do exist, as perhaps 20% of peanut-allergic individuals ultimately become tolerant (51), and a subpopulation of milk-allergic children fail to achieve tolerance over time (50). The mechanisms involved in the loss of sensitivity to specific foods are not precisely known, but the development of immunologic tolerance is definitely involved (9). The emergence of tolerance has been examined closely in children with milk and egg allergy, showing that those milk- and egg-allergic children who are destined to achieve tolerance first are able to tolerate these foods in baked form (52, 53). Presumably these patients are reactive to conformational epitopes on the milk and egg proteins that are more likely to be disrupted by the high temperature conditions of baking. In contrast, the children who fail to reach tolerance tend to be reactive to linear sequences of amino acids on the milk and egg allergens that would be unaffected by food processing.

Prevention

The prevention of allergic sensitization and the development of IgE-mediated food allergies require early identification of high-risk infants. IgE-mediated food allergies are most likely to develop in infants born to parents with histories of allergic disease of any type (e.g., pollens, mold spores, animal danders, bee venoms, food). Several strategies have been advocated for the prevention of allergic sensitization in high-risk infants, although agreement on the optimal approach has not been achieved. Strategies include exclusion of commonly allergenic foods such as cows' milk, eggs, and peanuts from the infant diet; breast-feeding for an extended period; possible use of hypoallergenic infant formulae; and the exclusion of commonly allergenic foods from the diet of the nursing mother (54, 55). Maternal dietary restriction during pregnancy (excluding commonly allergenic foods such as peanuts) did not prevent the development of food allergy in infants in several studies (54, 55), which suggests that sensitization does not occur in utero. Nevertheless, avoidance of peanuts during pregnancy has been advocated by some clinicians (56). Although exclusion of commonly allergenic foods from the environment of high-risk infants seems logical, this approach is not based on clinical evidence of its efficacy. In fact, evidence suggests that the early introduction of peanuts into the diets of young infants may lower the likelihood of sensitization to peanuts (57). For some decades, breast-feeding for an extended period has been advocated for high-risk infants. However, the evidence actually suggests that exclusive breast-feeding for extended periods of time delays, but may not prevent, the development of IgE-mediated food allergies (58).

The observation has been made that infants on occasion can be sensitized to allergenic foods through exposure to the allergens in breast milk (59, 60). Apparently, certain allergenic food proteins are resistant to maternal digestion, are absorbed at least to a small extent from the small intestine, and are secreted in breast milk leading to sensitization. Maternal dietary avoidance of certain commonly allergenic foods, such as peanuts, during the lactation period is advocated because it will help to prevent sensitization through breast milk. However, the elimination of certain other commonly allergenic foods, such as milk and eggs, is not recommended for nursing mothers because these foods are usually considered to be too important nutritionally.

TABLE 102.4	CEREAL SOURCES OF GLUTEN
Wheat	
Rye	
Barley	
Spelt	
Kamut	
Triticale	
Durum wheat or semolina	
Club wheat	
Emmer	
Einkorn	
Farro	

inflammatory reaction results in a so-called flat lesion in the gut. The cell-mediated immunologic reaction in the gut is characterized by this villous atrophy along with crypt hyperplasia, lymphoid infiltration of the epithelium, edema of the lamina propria, and impaired absorptive function of the epithelium, including increased fluid secretion and enhanced permeability (124). This inflammatory process damages the absorptive epithelium of the small intestine, resulting in a decreased number of epithelial cells that are critical to digestion and absorption. The mucosal enzymes necessary for digestion and absorption are also altered in the damaged cells. Thus, the absorptive cells are functionally compromised, leading to nutrient malabsorption (6). It appears as though a defect in mucosal processing of gliadin in celiac patients provokes the generation of toxic peptides that contribute to the abnormal immunologic response and the subsequent inflammatory reaction (125).

Symptoms and Sequelae

The inflammatory process occurring in celiac disease results in a severe malabsorption syndrome characterized by diarrhea, bloating, weight loss, anemia, bone pain, chronic fatigue, weakness, various nutritional deficiencies, muscle cramps, and, in children, failure to thrive (124, 126). Although the risk of death is quite low (127), untreated celiac disease is associated with considerable discomfort. Individuals suffering from celiac disease for long periods are also at increased risk for development of T-cell lymphomas (124, 128), and are more likely than others to have various other diseases, particularly those of an autoimmune nature (126). Examples include dermatitis herpetiformis, thyroid diseases, Addison disease, pernicious anemia, autoimmune thrombocytopenia, sarcoidosis, insulin-dependent diabetes mellitus, IgA nephropathy, and Down syndrome (126).

Sources

Celiac disease is associated with the ingestion of wheat, rye, barley, or related grains (22, 129). Although oats were once thought to be a causative factor, the role of oats has now been discounted (130). However, oats are often

contaminated with wheat in commerce, so caution may still be necessary (6). Spelt, Kamut, einkorn, emmer, and club wheat are varieties of wheat that are also thought to trigger celiac disease in susceptible individuals (6). Triticale, a cross between wheat and rye, also must be avoided.

Causative Factor

The prolamin fractions of wheat, rye, and barley are implicated in the causation of celiac disease. Because the prolamin fraction of wheat is known as gluten, celiac disease is sometimes referred to as gluten-sensitive enteropathy. In wheat, the gliadin or alcohol-soluble fraction is the component of the gluten fraction involved in the elicitation of celiac disease, although the glutenin, or alcohol-insoluble fraction, is also likely involved (125, 131). Because the prolamins are the major storage proteins in these grains, all varieties of wheat, rye, and barley are considered hazardous for celiac sufferers.

Prevalence and Persistence

The prevalence of celiac disease remains a subject of intense scrutiny. The diagnosis of celiac disease can be difficult. Celiac disease appears to be latent or subclinical in some individuals, with symptoms only appearing occasionally (132, 133). The prevalence of celiac disease appears highest in certain European populations and in Australia (126, 134), although this may relate to more thorough diagnostic approaches. Celiac disease may occur in as many as 1 in every 250 people in some European groups (126). In the United States, the prevalence of celiac disease generally is perceived to be much lower. However, improved diagnosis has led to an increased estimate of prevalence in the United States to 1 in every 133 people (135), although many of these individuals have latent celiac disease. Considerable variability is observed in the prevalence of celiac disease among various European populations (126, 134, 136). Celiac disease is a lifelong condition. Although celiac disease may occur in a latent phase in some affected individuals, oral tolerance for gluten proteins does not seem to occur.

Management and Minimal Eliciting Dose

Like IgE-mediated food allergies, celiac disease is treated with an avoidance diet (137). Those with celiac disease attempt to avoid all sources of wheat, rye, barley, and related grains, including a wide variety of common food ingredients derived from these grains (137). The need to avoid ingredients that do not contain protein from the implicated grains is debatable but widely practiced (6). Most of these individuals also avoid oats, because of the frequent contamination of oats with wheat from shared farms, harvesting equipment, and storage facilities (6). Gluten-free foods are available commercially. The definition of gluten-free in most countries is less than 20 ppm gluten. The United States has no definition for gluten free but is considering a limit of 20 ppm. The minimal eliciting dose for wheat, rye, barley, and related grains among celiac sufferers is unknown. Many individuals with celiac disease go to great lengths to avoid all sources of wheat, rye, barley, and triticale. Although this has not been conclusively proved, a few studies have concluded that up to 10 mg of gliadin per day can be tolerated by most patients with celiac disease (138).

Detection

An ELISA has been developed for the detection of gluten and related proteins from wheat, rye, and barley (139). Current ELISA kits on the market allow the detection of gluten at levels of 5 ppm or above. This assay is used to assure that gluten-free products are properly labeled.

FOOD INTOLERANCES

As noted, food intolerances are the other major category of food-associated adverse reactions that affect only certain individuals. Food intolerances include all of those individualistic adverse reactions to foods in which the immune system is not directly involved in the pathogenesis. The major categories include anaphylactoid reactions, metabolic food disorders, and idiosyncratic reactions. Anaphylactoid reactions are associated with the release of histamine and other mediators of allergic disease from mast cells without the intervention of IgE (6). Some foods may contain substances that destabilize mast cell membranes, causing the spontaneous release of histamine. However, no such substances have ever been identified in foods, so this remains controversial.

Metabolic food disorders result from a genetically inherited defect in the ability to metabolize a food component or a genetically inherited sensitivity to a food component that affects some critical metabolic process. Examples of metabolic food disorders are lactose intolerance and favism. Lactose intolerance results from an inherited deficiency of the enzyme β-galactosidase in the intestinal mucosa (140). In favism, an inherited deficiency in the enzyme glucose-6-phosphate dehydrogenase in erythrocytes results in a heightened sensitivity to naturally occurring oxidant compounds in fava beans (141).

Idiosyncratic reactions are adverse reactions to foods that occur through unknown mechanisms (6). Many different mechanisms theoretically could be involved, and a range of symptoms could occur. However, the role of foods in many of these reactions has not been well established. Sulfite-induced asthma is discussed as an example, because the cause-and-effect relationship has been well established in this case.

LACTOSE INTOLERANCE

Lactose intolerance is a metabolic food disorder associated with a deficiency of the enzyme β-galactosidase or lactase in the intestinal mucosa (140). As a result, lactose, the primary sugar in milk and milk products, cannot be metabolized into its component monosaccharides, galactose and glucose. In contrast to the monosaccharides, undigested lactose cannot be absorbed across the small intestinal mucosa and passes into the colon, where resident bacteria metabolize it into CO_2, H_2, and H_2O. The characteristic symptoms of lactose intolerance are bloating, flatulence, abdominal cramping, and frothy diarrhea (6, 140).

Sources, Properties, and Occurrence in Foods

Lactose, the principal sugar in milk and milk products, is a disaccharide, 4'-(β-D-galactopyranoside)-D-glucopyranose. This disaccharide is unique and is found exclusively in milk and milk products, including milk, ice cream, cottage cheese, and yogurt. Hard cheeses contain only small amounts of lactose. The usual treatment for lactose intolerance is the avoidance of dairy products containing lactose. Individuals with lactose intolerance appear to tolerate yogurt and acidophilus milk better than other dairy products, despite the fact that these products contain appreciable amounts of lactose (142, 143). Apparently, these fermented products have inherent lactase activity, which is partially able to survive digestive processes and assist with the metabolism of lactose in the small intestine (140).

Prevalence

Lactose intolerance affects many people worldwide. It occurs with high frequency among black Americans, Native Americans, Hispanics, Asians, Jews, and Arabs, and has been reported to affect as many as 60% to 90% of individuals in such groups (144). The prevalence among North American non-Hispanic whites is about 6% to 12% (145). β-Galactosidase levels are high in virtually all infants at birth (140). However, after infancy, many individuals in the ethnic groups mentioned lose up to 90% of intestinal β-galactosidase activity (146, 147). This normal pattern of loss of β-galactosidase activity is transmitted by a recessive gene and should be considered a normal physiologic event (140). The levels of β-galactosidase found in infants tend to persist into adulthood in a few ethnic populations, such as non-Hispanic whites, presumably as an adaptation to the widespread historical use of dairy products in these cultures (140). β-Galactosidase persistence is inherited as an autosomal dominant characteristic (148). Although genuine lactose intolerance affects many individuals, 15% to 30% of self-diagnosed, lactose-intolerant individuals in the United States have satisfactory levels of β-galactosidase and thus should not display the symptoms of lactose intolerance on the ingestion of dairy products (149).

Minimal Eliciting Dose and Management

In contrast to IgE-mediated food allergies, lactose-intolerant individuals can tolerate some amount of lactose in their diets (2). In the majority of lactose-intolerant individuals, symptoms following the consumption of 12 g of lactose, an amount equivalent to one cup of milk, are trivial (149). The frequency and severity of symptoms increase as the lactose dose exceeds 12 g (148, 150). Lactose-intolerant individuals display variability in their individual tolerances for lactose (140). Lactose ingested with a meal containing high amounts of solids or fat is better tolerated than a similar amount of lactose in fluid milk (140), and lactose in yogurt and acidophilus milk is better tolerated than lactose from other dairy products (142, 143). Most adults consume less than 25 g of lactose per day, whereas infants commonly consume greater than 50 g per day (140).

Lactose intolerance is not a severe illness. Symptoms are confined to the gastrointestinal tract and are usually mild (6). Symptom severity can vary, dependent on β-galactosidase activity, gastrointestinal transit time, lactose load, and colonic fermentation (140, 147). The symptoms can be avoided by the implementation of a dairy product avoidance diet (6). However, because dairy products provide 75% of the calcium intake in US diets, the implementation of dairy product avoidance diets from childhood can place individuals at increased risk for postmenopausal osteoporosis (140). The emergence of lactose-hydrolyzed dairy products in the marketplace provides lactose-intolerant individuals with another means to control their reactions. Although lactose intolerance may affect more individuals, the symptoms are mild in general, and the tolerance for lactose in the diet equates to fewer problems in the implementation of a safe and effective avoidance diet.

FAVISM

Favism results from intolerance to the consumption of fava beans or the inhalation of pollen from the *Vicia faba* plant. Sensitive individuals suffer from acute hemolytic anemia on exposure (141). The characteristic symptoms of favism include pallor, fatigue, dyspnea, nausea, abdominal and/or back pain, fever, and chills. Rarely, hemoglobinuria, jaundice, and renal failure occur. The onset time is quite rapid, usually occurring 5 to 24 hours after ingestion. Recovery is prompt and spontaneous assuming no further exposure occurs. Favism occurs most frequently in areas in which the plant grows and the crop is harvested and sold in local markets, and is most prevalent when the *Vicia faba* plant is in bloom, causing elevated levels of airborne pollen, and when the beans are available in the market.

Individuals susceptible to favism are those with an inherited deficiency of erythrocyte glucose-6-phosphate dehydrogenase (G6PD) (140). G6PD is a critical enzyme in erythrocytes, in which it is essential to maintain levels of the reduced form of glutathione (GSH) and nicotinamide adenine dinucleotide phosphate (NADPH); GSH and NADPH prevent oxidative damage to the cells. Thus, the red blood cells of individuals with G6PD deficiency are more susceptible to oxidative damage. Fava beans contain several naturally occurring oxidants, including vicine and convicine, which are able to damage the erythrocytes of G6PD-deficient individuals. G6PD deficiency is the most common inherited enzymatic defect in humans on a worldwide basis, affecting 100 million people (140). G6PD deficiency occurs with the highest frequency among Eastern Jewish communities in Israel, Sardinians, Cypriot Greeks, African-Americans, and certain African populations. The trait is virtually nonexistent in northern European nations, North American Indians, and Eskimos. Favism occurs primarily in the Mediterranean area, the Middle East, China, and Bulgaria, where fava beans are frequently consumed. The diagnosis of G6PD deficiency is made through an assay for enzymatic activity of G6PD in isolated red blood cells. Susceptible individuals can avoid the effects of favism by avoiding the ingestion of fava beans and/or the inhalation of the plant pollen.

SULFITE-INDUCED ASTHMA

Sulfite sensitivity is an idiosyncratic reaction of undefined mechanism, associated with the ingestion of sulfites in foods and medications (151). Although scattered reports exist of other manifestations of sulfite sensitivity, including anaphylaxis (151, 152), asthma is the only symptom that has been clearly linked to sulfite ingestion in multiple subjects as the result of carefully controlled clinical challenge studies (151, 153).

Sources, Properties, and Occurrence in Foods

Sulfites are used as food additives in a variety of foods (154). Sulfites exist in several forms: sulfur dioxide, sodium metabisulfite, potassium metabisulfite, sodium bisulfite, potassium bisulfite, and sodium sulfite, although all of these ingredients have similar chemistries in foods, dependent on pH (154). Sulfites also occur naturally in foods, especially fermented foods, as the result of formation by yeast (154). The residual levels of sulfites in foods range from less than 10 ppm in many food products to greater than 2000 ppm in certain dried fruits (154). Naturally occurring levels of sulfites are typically quite low. Sulfites are added to foods for a variety of purposes, including the control of enzymatic and nonenzymatic browning (e.g., potatoes), the prevention of undesirable bacterial growth (e.g., corn wet milling and wine making), the conditioning of dough (e.g., some frozen dough products), the prevention of oxidation, and the bleaching of selected products (e.g., maraschino cherries and hominy). When added to foods, the fate of sulfites is complex (154). In acidic foods, sulfites can be released into the surrounding atmosphere as SO_2 gas. Sulfites can also react with numerous food components, including carbohydrates, proteins, and others. These reactions can be either reversible or irreversible depending on the nature of the reaction. Very little free, unbound sulfite remains in most sulfited foods, with a few exceptions such as lettuce (155).

Prevalence and Severity

Although asthma is the most prominent symptom involved in sulfite sensitivity, only a small percentage of asthmatics are sulfite sensitive (156). Challenge studies indicate that severe or steroid-dependent asthmatics, about 20% of the overall asthmatic population, are primarily at risk, although only about 5% of them are sulfite sensitive (156). Extrapolating from challenge study results, perhaps 150,000 sulfite-sensitive asthmatics exist in the US population. Despite the small size of the at-risk population, sulfites are capable of causing severe reactions in sensitive individuals. The provocation of asthma can be life threatening, and deaths have occurred from the ingestion of sulfites by sulfite-sensitive asthmatics (151, 157). Anaphylaxis appears to be another rare but severe manifestation of sulfite sensitivity (152). However, it should be emphasized that only a few such cases have been described in the medical literature.

Management

Sulfite-sensitive asthmatics must avoid the ingestion of sulfites in their diets (154). Fortunately the presence of sulfites must be declared on the ingredient labels of packaged foods when residual levels exceed 10 ppm (2). Sulfite use is banned from many fresh food products such as lettuce, in which high residual levels were associated with provocation of particularly severe reactions (158). However, sulfite-sensitive asthmatics can tolerate the ingestion of small quantities of sulfites (153, 156). Challenge results support the hypothesis that sulfite-sensitive asthmatics are more tolerant of sulfites in foods than they are of inorganic sulfites in capsules or other common challenge vehicles (151, 158). Apparently the reaction of sulfites with food components removes some of the sulfite from having the capability to trigger asthmatic reactions in sensitive individuals (158). The tolerance for sulfited foods appears to vary with the nature of the food, suggesting that the form of bound sulfite is likely important (158). Because of the release of SO_2 vapor from acidic beverages, sulfite-sensitive asthmatics may be more sensitive to sulfited beverages than to other forms of sulfite in foods (158, 159). They also appear to be more sensitive to residues of unbound sulfites in foods such as lettuce (158) than to sulfited foods that contain bound sulfites such as shrimp and potatoes (158). Sulfite-sensitive asthmatics can tolerate some sulfite in the diets, but the thresholds are low in some individuals.

ALLERGY-LIKE INTOXICATIONS (HISTAMINE POISONING)

Histamine poisoning is the most commonly encountered allergy-like intoxication (3). Outbreaks of histamine intoxication are often referred to as scombroid fish poisoning and occur with some frequency in the United States, Europe, Japan, and other countries.

Symptoms and Features

As noted, histamine is one of the primary mediators released from mast cells in IgE-mediated food allergies. Thus, similar symptoms occur in histamine intoxication and IgE-mediated food allergy. The symptoms are variable and not particularly definitive, although the illness is typically rather mild (160). Gastrointestinal symptoms such as nausea, vomiting, diarrhea, and abdominal cramps are common. Tingling, itching, and burning sensations often occur in the mouth. Cutaneous symptoms include flushing, urticaria, angioedema, and other itchy rashes. Hypotension is common, as are headache and palpitations. In the study of a large series of outbreaks in the United Kingdom, the most common symptoms were rash, diarrhea, flushing and sweating, and headache (161). Because such symptoms are not definitive, there is frequent misdiagnosis of histamine intoxication. Although histamine intoxication is usually mild, serious cardiac and respiratory complications can occur on rare occasions (3, 162).

Symptoms of histamine poisoning typically appear within minutes to a few hours after ingestion of the offending food (3). Histamine intoxication is a self-limited illness and symptoms usually subside within a few hours. However, when untreated, symptoms can persist for as long as 24 to 48 hours (3). The dose of exposure and/or the susceptibility of the affected individual affect symptom duration. Effective treatment (see the following) leads to a prompt resolution of the symptoms.

Diagnosis and Treatment

The diagnosis of histamine poisoning is often contingent on associating the ingestion of one of the more commonly implicated foods with the rapid onset of symptoms (3). A beneficial response to antihistamines further strengthens the diagnosis (3). The diagnosis can be confirmed only by analysis of the suspect food and detection of unusually high levels of histamine (3). Samples of the incriminated food should be sought immediately whenever histamine intoxication is suspected. The accepted procedure for the analysis of histamine in food involves extraction, clean-up, and fluorometric analysis (163). When the food sample is not available, vomitus and/or stomach contents could be analyzed for histamine, but baseline data on histamine levels in these materials are not readily available (3).

Because of similarities in symptoms and the beneficial effects of antihistamines, histamine poisoning is often misdiagnosed as an allergic reaction to food. However, histamine intoxication can be readily distinguished from IgE-mediated food allergies (3). With histamine intoxication, the patient typically has no prior history of allergic reactions to the implicated food. By contrast, the patient usually is well aware of existing IgE-mediated food allergies. In addition, SPTs with commercial extracts of the food will be negative if no IgE-mediated allergy exists in the patient. However, if an extract is made of the actual incriminated food, the SPT can be positive owing to the presence of histamine in the extract (3). In many situations, the presence of symptoms in dining companions offers another clue. With histamine intoxication, the attack rates in group outbreaks are often 50% to 100%. Meanwhile, with IgE-mediated food allergies, it is rare to encounter two individuals sharing the same meal who experience the same food allergy. Finally, histamine intoxication can be distinguished from IgE-mediated food allergy by analysis of the incriminated food and detection of abnormally high levels of histamine.

Antihistamines are the most effective treatment for histamine intoxication. Both H1 and H2 antagonists are effective (164, 165). Even without treatment, the symptoms of histamine intoxication usually subside within a few hours (3).

Sources and Formation

The most common cause of histamine poisoning is certain types of spoiled fish (3). This illness is sometimes referred to as scombroid fish poisoning because of its frequent association with fish from the families *Scomberesocidae* and *Scombridae*, such as tuna, skipjack, mackerel, and bonito. Scombroid fish poisoning is a bit of a misnomer however because certain types of nonscombroid fish are also commonly involved, including mahi-mahi, bluefish, jack mackerel, sardines, yellowtail, anchovies, and herring. In the United States, mahi-mahi has become one of the most frequent offending foods in cases of histamine intoxication (3). These species of fish do not elicit histamine poisoning unless they contain elevated levels of histamine; the Food and Drug Administration considers 50 mg of histamine per 100 g of fish to be hazardous for tuna based on the investigation of numerous outbreaks (166).

Outbreaks of histamine poisoning from cheese occur with far less frequency than from fish (3). Swiss cheese has been implicated in several outbreaks in the United States (3, 167). Typically, the histamine contents of cheeses are quite low. Histamine may be a cause of wine intolerance (168), although few clinical studies have been conducted to confirm this possibility. In a challenge study with 125 mL of red wine containing 50 μg of histamine, 22 of 28 patients experienced a significant rise in plasma histamine within 30 minutes along with some symptoms consistent with histamine intoxication (168).

Histamine formation in foods is associated with the growth of bacteria possessing the enzyme histidine decarboxylase, which converts the amino acid histidine into histamine. Few bacterial species are capable of the prolific histamine formation necessary to develop hazardous levels food products. In fish, *Morganella morganii* and *Klebsiella pneumoniae* are two species with such capabilities (3, 169). When fish with high levels of free histidine in their edible tissues are contaminated with such histamine-producing bacteria (and most are not), the bacteria can convert large amounts of histidine to histamine in a relatively short

period of time, when the fish are held at elevated temperatures. Such fish will not necessarily appear to be spoiled even though they contain hazardous levels of histamine. In cheese, certain species of lactobacilli are probably responsible for histamine formation, although this is an unusual trait among lactobacilli (3). Several factors may contribute to histamine formation in cheese, including higher ripening temperatures, excessive proteolysis, high pH, and low salt concentrations (170). The Swiss cheese–making process is especially conducive to histamine formation, and levels of histamine in Swiss cheese appear to be dependent primarily on the number of histamine-producing bacteria in the raw milk supply (170).

Toxicology

Histamine is much less potent when taken orally than it is when released or administered intravenously (171). Humans can tolerate milligram levels of histamine orally without untoward effects (172). The lack of toxicity of orally administered histamine is not surprising, because humans have several enzymes in the intestinal mucosa—diamine oxidase and histamine-N-methyltransferase—which are capable of detoxifying histamine (171).

In fact, the role of histamine in scombroid fish poisoning has been questioned (173, 174). No correlation was observed between the dose of histamine and the likelihood of an adverse reaction when human subjects consumed mackerel samples that had been implicated in outbreaks of scombroid fish poisoning (173, 174). However, the antihistamine chlorpheniramine abolished the adverse effects observed in some individuals with specific samples of spoiled mackerel (174). Thus, Ijomah et al (174) postulated that spoiled fish may contain an as-yet-unidentified substance that induces release of endogenous histamine from mast cells, so that scombroid fish poisoning is the result of the release of endogenous histamine rather than the ingestion of exogenous histamine. Thus, histamine poisoning could be an anaphylactoid reaction, as described earlier. In contrast, Morrow et al (175) asserted that exogenous histamine was the likely causative agent in scombroid fish poisoning because high levels of histamine and one of its metabolites, N-methylhistamine, were found in the urine of three individuals experiencing scombroid fish poisoning from marlin. They were unable to find elevated urinary levels of the prostaglandin D_2 metabolite, 9α,11β-dihydroxy-15-oxo-2,3,18,19-tetranorprost-5-ene-1,20-dioic acid, suggesting that mast cell degranulation had not occurred (175). The use of tryptase as a measure of mast cell degranulation would have been preferable, but to our knowledge has never been tried.

Some individual variability in susceptibility to histamine poisoning is likely (3). Considerable variability was observed in individual susceptibility to ingestion of mackerel fillets that had been implicated in a scombroid fish poisoning outbreak (173). Some individuals are likely compromised in their ability to detoxify and excrete histamine (3). Several drugs including isoniazid can inhibit the detoxification of histamine and are likely to potentiate its toxicity. Isoniazid has been implicated as a contributing factor in several outbreaks of histamine poisoning (176, 177). Alternatively, individuals taking antihistamines for various reasons may be protected to some extent from the effects of histamine (3).

Preventive Measures

Although the role of exogenous histamine remains controversial, the bulk of the scientific evidence suggests that histamine plays a central role in scombroid fish poisoning. The key to the prevention of histamine intoxication is to prevent spoilage and histamine formation (3). Although efforts have focused on preventing the formation of histamine, the histamine-releasing factor, if present, also must be formed during spoilage because freshly caught and/or properly refrigerated/frozen fish do not cause illness (3). Holding fish at temperatures below 5°C, after catching, prevents histamine formation (171). Most histamine-producing bacteria in fish are enteric bacteria; therefore, human handling of the fish after catching may be the source of contamination, and good hygienic practices during distribution, storage, handling, processing, and preparation could prevent contamination of the fish. With cheese, histamine formation can be controlled by reducing the number of histamine-producing bacteria in the raw milk (170). Thus, the risk should be small in cheese made from pasteurized milk (3).

CONCLUSIONS

Food allergies and other individualistic adverse reactions to foods affect only a small percentage of the population. However, the reactions can be very severe and even life threatening in some cases of IgE-mediated food allergy and sulfite-induced asthma. The primary management strategies for these illnesses are the avoidance of the offending food or food ingredient. However, the avoidance of a specific food or food ingredient can be a daunting daily task, and complete success is unlikely.

IgE-mediated food allergies are well understood and relatively easy to diagnose. The prevalence of IgE-mediated food allergies appears to be increasing in the United States, and awareness of the consequences of IgE-mediated food allergies is increasing around the world. Much progress has been made in the identification and characterization of the allergenic proteins in foods, methods for the detection of allergenic residues in foods, and food industry practices to control allergenic residues. However, many unresolved issues remain, such as clear establishment of minimal eliciting doses allowing the development of safe and effective regulatory guidelines, the allergenicity of food ingredients derived from allergenic sources, the prediction of the allergenicity of novel proteins contained in genetically engineered foods, methods for preventing allergic sensitization in infants, and improved treatment modalities for those with food allergies.

The role of delayed hypersensitivity reactions in food allergies is much less clear. Certainly, celiac disease may be more common than previously appreciated and severe consequences, such as an increased prevalence of lymphoma, may accompany celiac disease. A better understanding of the role of other foods in delayed hypersensitivity reactions would be helpful in the treatment of affected individuals. The role of certain food ingredients in food intolerances such as lactose intolerance and sulfite-induced asthma is well established. However, the role of foods or food additives in these illnesses is much less clear. Here, research should be focused on establishment of clear cause-and-effect relationships. Histamine poisoning can be confused diagnostically with food allergy, but histamine poisoning can be distinguished readily in many circumstances by the presence of multiple cases among individuals sharing the same meal. Histamine poisoning is not an individualistic adverse reaction to food and can be controlled by limiting bacterial histamine formation in foods.

REFERENCES

1. Sloan AE, Powers ME. J Allergy Clin Immunol 1986;78: 127–33.
2. Taylor SL, Hefle SL. Food Technol 2001;55(9):68–83.
3. Taylor SL, Hefle SL. Allergylike intoxications from foods. In: Frieri M, Kettelhut B, eds. Food Hypersensitivity and Adverse Reactions: A Practical Guide for Diagnosis and Management. New York: Marcel Dekker, 1999:141–53.
4. Sellge G, Bischoff SC. The immunological basis of IgE-mediated reactions. In: Metcalfe DD, Sampson HA, Simon RA, eds. Food Allergy: Adverse Reactions to Foods and Food Additives. 4th ed. Malden, MA: Blackwell Science, 2008:15–28.
5. Rubio-Tapia A, Murray J. Gluten-sensitive enteropathy. In: Metcalfe DD, Sampson HA, Simon RA, eds. Food Allergy: Adverse Reactions to Foods and Food Additives. 4th ed. Malden, MA: Blackwell Science, 2008:211–22.
6. Taylor SL, Hefle SL. Allergic reactions and food intolerances. In: Kotsonis FN, Mackey MA, eds. Nutritional Toxicology. 2nd ed. New York: Taylor & Francis, 2002:93–121.
7. Breiteneder H, Mills ENC. Food allergens: molecular and immunological characteristics. In: Metcalfe DD, Sampson HA, Simon RA, eds. Food Allergy: Adverse Reactions to Foods and Food Additives. 4th ed. Malden, MA: Blackwell Science, 2008:43–61.
8. Sicherer SH, Sampson HA. Clin Exp Allergy 1999;29:507–12.
9. Bjorksten B. Development of immunological tolerance to food antigens. In: Metcalfe DD, Sampson HA, Simon RA, eds. Food Allergy: Adverse Reactions to Foods and Food Additives. 4th ed. Malden, MA: Blackwell Science, 2008:90–8.
10. Chandra RK. Food allergy: setting the theme. In: Chandra RK, ed. Food Allergy. St. John's, Newfoundland, Canada: Nutrition Research Education Foundation, 1987;3–5.
11. Lack G, Fox DES, Golding J. J Allergy Clin Immunol 1999;103:S95.

12. Sicherer SH, Furlong TJ, Maes HH et al. J Allergy Clin Immunol 2000;106:53–6.

13. Hsu ID, Boyce JA. Biology of mast cells and their mediators. In: Adkinson NF Jr, Holgate ST, Bochner BS et al, eds. Middleton's Allergy: Principles and Practice. 7th ed. St. Louis: Mosby Elsevier, 2009;311–28.

14. Sikora M, Cartier A, Aresery M et al. Occupational reactions to food allergens. In: Metcalfe DD, Sampson HA, Simon RA, eds. Food Allergy: Adverse Reactions to Foods and Food Additives. 4th ed. Malden, MA: Blackwell Science, 2008:223–50.

15. Sampson HA, Mendelson L, Rosen J. N Engl J Med 1992; 327:380–4.

16. Yunginger JW, Sweeney KG, Sturner WQ et al. JAMA 1988; 260:1450–2.

17. Bock SA, Munoz-Furlong A, Sampson HA. J Allergy Clin Immunol 2007;119:1016–8.

18. Pumphrey RSH, Gowland MH. J Allergy Clin Immunol 2007;119:1018–9.

19. Wang J. Oral allergy syndrome. In: Metcalfe DD, Sampson HA, Simon RA, eds. Food Allergy: Adverse Reactions to Foods and Food Additives. 4th ed. Malden, MA: Blackwell Science, 2008:133–43.

20. Williams AN, Simon RA. Food-dependent exercise- and pressure-induced syndromes. In: Metcalfe DD, Sampson HA, Simon RA, eds. Food Allergy: Adverse Reactions to Foods and Food Additives. 4th ed. Malden, MA: Blackwell Science, 2008:584–95.

21. Food and Agriculture Organization. Report of the FAO Technical Consultation on Food Allergies, Rome, Italy, November 13–14. Food and Agricultural Organization of the United Nations, 1995.

22. Bernhisel-Broadbent J, Scanlon SM, Sampson HA. J Allergy Clin Immunol 1992;89:730–7.

23. Hansen TK, Bindslev-Jensen C. Allergy 1992;47:610–7.

24. O'Neill CE, Lehrer SB. Food Technol 1995;49:103–16.

25. Langeland T. Allergy 1983;39:399–412.

26. Anet J, Back JF, Baker RS et al. Int Arch Allergy Appl Immunol 1985;77:364–71.

27. Dean TP, Adler BR, Ruge F et al. Clin Exp Allergy 1993; 23:205–10.

28. Lopez-Torrejon G, Salcedo G, Martin-Esteban et al. J Allergy Clin Immunol 2003;112:1208–15.

29. Martinez San Ireneo M, Ibanez MD, Fernandes-Caldes E et al. Int Arch Allergy Immunol 2008;147:222–30.

30. Hefle SL, Nordlee JA, Taylor SL. Crit Rev Food Sci Nutr 1996;36S:69–89.

31. Taylor SL, Hefle SL, Soylemez G et al. Food Allergy Intolerance 2002;3:115–22.

32. Bjorksten B, Crevel R, Hischenhuber C et al. Reg Toxicol Pharmacol 2008;51:42–52.

33. European Commission. Official J Eur Union L 2007;310:11–14.

34. Rance F, Dutau G, Abbal M. Allergy 2000;55:496–500.

35. Imai T, Akasawa A, Iikura Y. Int Arch Allergy Immunol 2001;124:312–4.

36. Breiteneder H, Ebner C. J Allergy Clin Immunol 2000;106: 27–36.

37. Pastorello EA, Pravettoni V, Calamari M et al. Allergy 2002; 57(Suppl 72):106–10.

38. Bugajska-Schretter A, Elfman L, Fuchs T. J Allergy Clin Immunol 1998;101:67–74.

39. Reese G, Ayuso R, Lehrer SB. Int Arch Allergy Immunol 1999;119:247–58.

40. Sicherer SH, Munoz-Furlong A, Godbold JH et al. J Allergy Clin Immunol 2010;125:1322–6.

41. Sicherer SH, Munoz-Furlong A, Sampson HA. J Allergy Clin Immunol 2004;114:159–65.

42. Sampson HA. Curr Opinion Immunol 1990;2:542–7.

43. Rona RJ, Keil T, Summers C et al. J Allergy Clin Immunol 2007;120:638–46.

44. Sampson HA, McCaskill CC. J Pediatr 1985;107:669–75.

45. Bock SA. Pediatrics 1987;79:683–8.

46. Host A, Halken S. Allergy 1990;45:587–96.

47. Jakobsson I, Lindberg T. Acta Pediatr Scand 1979;68:853–9.

48. Schrander JJP, van den Bogart JPH, Forget PP et al. Eur J Pediatr 1993;152:640–4.

49. Hill DJ, Hosking CS, Zhie CY et al. Environ Toxicol Pathol 1997;4:101–10.

50. Wood RA. Natural history of food allergy. In: Metcalfe DD, Sampson HA, Simon RA, eds. Food Allergy: Adverse Reactions to Foods and Food Additives. 4th ed. Malden, MA: Blackwell Scientific, 2008:461–9.

51. Skolnick HS, Conover-Walker MK, Koerner CB et al. J Allergy Clin Immunol 2001;107:367–74.

52. Lemon-Mule H, Sampson HA, Sicherer SH et al. J Allergy Clin Immunol 2008;122:977–83.

53. Nowak-Wegrzyn A, Bloom KA, Sicherer SH et al. J Allergy Clin Immunol 2008;122:342–7.

54. Zeiger RS, Heller S, Mellon MH et al. J Allergy Clin Immunol 1989;84:72–89.

55. Muraro A, Dreborg S, Halken S et al. Pediatr Allergy Immunol 2004;15:291–307.

56. Warner JO, Jones CA, Kilburn SA et al. Pediatr Allergy Immunol 2000;13S:6–8.

57. du Toit G, Katz Y, Susieni P et al. J Allergy Clin Immunol 2008;122:984–91.

58. Zeiger RS, Heller S. J Allergy Clin Immunol 1995;95: 1179–90.

59. Van Asperen PP, Kemp AS, Mellis CM. Arch Dis Child 1983;58:253–256.

60. Gerrard JW. Ann Allergy 1979;42:69–72.

61. Isolauri E, Rautava S, Kalliomaki M. Curr Opinion Allergy Clin Immunol 2002;2:263–71.

62. Lee J, Seto D, Bielory L. J Allergy Clin Immunol 2008; 121:116–21.

63. Businco L, Dreborg S, Einarsson R et al. Pediatr Allergy Immunol 1993;4:101–11.

64. von Berg A, Filipiak-Pittroff B, Kramer U et al. J Allergy Clin Immunol 2008;121:1442–7.

65. Vandenplas Y, Hauser B, Van den Borre C et al. Eur J Pediatr 1995;154:488–94.

66. Nowak-Wegrzyn A, Sampson HA. Med Clin North Am 2006;90:97–127.

67. Bock SA, Sampson HA, Atkins FM et al. J Allergy Clin Immunol 1988;82:986–97.

68. Taylor SL, Moneret-Vautrin DA, Crevel RWR et al. Food Chem Toxicol 2010;48:814–9.

69. Metcalfe DD. Nutr Rev 1984;42:92–7.

70. Sampson HA, Ho DG. J Allergy Clin Immunol 1997;100: 444–51.

71. Simons FER, Akdis CA. Histamine and H_1 antihistamines. In: Adkinson NF Jr, Holgate ST, Bochner BS et al, eds. Middleton's Allergy: Principles and Practice. 7th ed. St. Louis: Mosby Elsevier, 2009:1517–47.

72. Kemp SF, Lemanske RF Jr, Simons FER. Allergy 2008;63: 1061–70.

73. Taylor SL, Bush RK, Busse WW. N Engl Reg Allergy Proc 1986;7:527–32.

74. Cordle CT. J Nutr 2004;134:1213S–19S.

75. Zeiger RS, Sampson HA, Bock SA et al. J Pediatr 1999; 134:614–22.

76. Kleinman RE, Bahna S, Powell GF, Sampson HA. Pediatr Allergy Immunol 1991;4:146–55.

77. Saylor JD, Bahna SL. J Pediatr 1991;118:71–4.

78. Rosenthal E, Schlesinger Y, Birnbaum Y et al. Acta Paediatr Scand 1991;80:958–60.

79. Hefle SL, Taylor SL. Food Technol 1999;53:62–70.

80. Teuber SS, Brown RL, Haapanen LAD. J Allergy Clin Immunol 1997;99:502–7.

81. Kanny G, de Hauteclocque C, Moneret-Vautrin DA. Allergy 1996;51:952–7.

82. Hoffman DR, Collins-Williams C. J Allergy Clin Immunol 1994;93:801–2.

83. Businco L, Cantani A, Longhi M et al. Ann Allergy 1989; 62:333–5.

84. Muller U, Weber W, Hoffmann A et al. Z Lebensm Unter Forsch 1998;207:341–51.

85. Gu X, Beardslee T, Zeece M et al. Int Arch Allergy Immunol 2001;126:218–25.

86. Taylor SL, Dormedy ES. Adv Food Nutr Res 1998;42:1–44.

87. Gern JE, Yang E, Evrard HM et al. N Engl J Med 1991; 324:976–9.

88. McKenna C, Klontz KC. Ann Allergy Asthma Immunol 1997; 79:234–6.

89. Hansen TK, Poulsen LK, Stahl Skov P et al. Food Chem Toxicol 2004;42:2037–44.

90. Andre F, Cavagna S, Andre C. Int Arch Allergy Immunol 2003;130:17–24.

91. Taylor SL, Kabourek JL, Hefle SL. J Food Sci 2004;69:R175–80.

92. Hamada Y, Nagashima Y, Shiomi K. Biosci Biotechnol Biochem 2001;65:285–91.

93. Taylor SL, Hefle SL. Curr Allergy Clin Immunol 2001;14:12–18.

94. Taylor SL, Hefle SL. Can J Allergy 2000;5:106–10.

95. Herian AM, Taylor SL, Bush RK. J Food Sci 1993;58:385–88.

96. Bernhisel-Broadbent J, Scanlon SM, Sampson HA. J Allergy Clin Immunol 1992;89:730–7.

97. Herian AM, Taylor SL, Bush RK. Int Arch Allergy Appl Immunol 1990;92:193–8.

98. Moneret-Vautrin D, Guerin L, Kanny G et al. J Allergy Clin Immunol 1999;104:883–8.

99. Bernhisel-Broadbent J, Sampson HA. J Allergy Clin Immunol 1989;83:435–40.

100. Sicherer SH. Hidden and cross-reacting food allergens. In: Metcalfe DD, Sampson HA, Simon RA, eds. Food Allergy: Adverse Reactions to Foods and Food Additives. 4th ed. Malden, MA: Blackwell Science, 2008:310–22.

101. Taylor SL, Hefle SL, Bindslev-Jensen C et al. J Allergy Clin Immunol 2002;109:24–30.

102. Taylor SL, Baumert JL. Curr Allergy Asthma Rep 2010; 10:265–70.

103. Yuninger JW, Gauerke MB, Jones RT et al. J Food Prot 1983; 46:625–8.

104. Laoprasert N, Wallen ND, Jones RT et al. J Food Prot 1998; 61:1522–4.

105. Hefle SL, Furlong TJ, Niemann L et al. J Allergy Clin Immunol 2007;120:171–6.

106. Taylor SL, Hefle SL, Bindslev-Jensen C et al. Clin Exp Allergy 2004;34:689–94.

107. Taylor SL, Hourihane JO'B. Food allergen thresholds of reactivity. In: Metcalfe DD, Sampson HA, Simon RA, eds. Food Allergy: Adverse Reactions to Foods and Food Additives. 4th ed. Malden, MA: Blackwell Science, 2008:82–9.

108. Threshold Working Group. J Food Prot 2008;71:1043–88.

109. Vierk K, Falci K, Wolyniak C, Klontz KC. J Allergy Clin Immunol 2002;109:1022–6.

110. Taylor SL, Nordlee JA. Food Technol 1996;50:231–4, 238.

111. Poms R, Klein CL, Anklam E. Food Addit Contam 2004; 21:1–31.

112. Niemann L, Taylor SL, Hefle SL. J Food Sci 2009;74:T51–7.

113. Lee PW, Hefle SL, Taylor SL. J Food Sci 2008;73:T62–8.

114. Taylor SL, Lehrer SB. Crit Rev Food Sci Nutr 1996;36:S91–118.

115. Sicherer SH, Noone SA, Barnes-Koerner C et al. J Pediatr 2001;138:688–93.

116. Jankiewicz A, Baltes W, Bogl K et al. J Sci Food Agric 1997;75:357–70.

117. Bernhisel-Broadbent J, Strause D, Sampson HA. J Allergy Clin Immunol 1992;90:622–9.

118. Astwood JD, Leach JN, Fuchs RL. Nature Biotechnol 1996;14:1269–73.

119. Codex Alimentarius Commission. Alinorm 03/34: Joint FAO/WHO Food Standard Programme, Codex Alimentarius Commission, Twenty-Fifth Session, Rome, 30 June–5 July, 2003. Appendix III: Guideline for the Conduct of Food Safety Assessment of Foods Derived from Recombinant-DNA Plants; and Appendix IV: Annex on the Assessment of Possible Allergenicity, 2003:47–60.

120. Goodman RE, Vieths S, Sampson HA et al. Nature Biotechnol 2008;26:73–81.

121. Nordlee J, Taylor SL, Townsend JA et al. N Engl J Med 1996; 334:688–92.

122. Taylor SL, Goodman RE. Cereal Foods World 2007;52:174–8.

123. Strober W. J Allergy Clin Immunol 1986;78:202–11.

124. Marsh MN. 1992. Gastroenterology 1992;102:330–54.

125. Cornell HJ. Amino Acids 1996;10:1–19.

126. Troncone R, Greco L, Auricchio S. Pediatr Clin North Am 1996;43:355–73.

127. Logan RFA, Rifkind EA, Turner ID et al. Gastroenterology 1989;97:265–71.

128. O'Mahoney S, Ferguson A. Gluten-sensitive enteropathy (celiac disease). In: Metcalfe DD, Sampson HA, Simon RA, eds. Food Allergy: Adverse Reactions to Foods and Food Additives. Boston: Blackwell Scientific, 1991:186–98.

129. Anand BS, Piris J, Truelove SC. Q J Med 1978;47:101–10.

130. Janatuinen EK, Pikkarainen PH, Kemppainen TA et al. N Engl J Med 1995;333:1033–7.

131. Wieser H. Acta Pediatr Suppl 1996;412:3–9.

132. Duggan JM. Med J Aust 1997;166:312–5.

133. Troncone R. Acta Pediatr 1995;34:1252–7.

134. Logan RFA. Descriptive epidemiology of celiac disease. In: Branski, D, Rozen,P, Kagnoff MF, eds. Gluten-Sensitive Enteropathy, Frontiers Gastrointestinal Research, vol 19. Basel: Karger, 1992:1–14.

135. Fasano A, Berti I, Gerarduzzi T et al. Arch Intern Med 2003;163:286–92.

136. George EK, Mearin ML, van der Velde EA et al. Pediatr Res 1995;37:213–8.

137. Hartsook EI. Cereal Foods World 1984;29:157–8.

138. Hekkens WTJM, van Twist de Graaf M. Nahrung 1990;34: 483–7.

139. Skerritt JH, Hill AS. J Assoc Off Anal Chem 1991;74: 257–64.

140. Suarez FL, Savaiano DA. 1997. Food Technol. 1997;51:74–6.

141. Mager J, Chevion M, Glaser G. Favism. In: Liener IE, ed. Toxic Constituents of Plant Foodstuffs. 2nd ed. New York: Academic Press, 1980:265–94.

142. Gallagher CR, Molleson AL, Caldwell JH. Cult Dairy Prod J 12977;10:22–4.

143. Kolars JC, Levitt MD, Aouji M et al. N Engl J Med 1984; 310:1–3.

144. Kocian J. Int J Biochem 1988;20:1–5.

145. Sandine WE, Daly M. J Food Prot 1979;42:435–7.

146. Gilat T, Russo S, Gelman-Malachi E et al. Gastroenterology 1972;62:1125–7.

147. Scrimshaw NS, Murray EB. Am J Clin Nutr 1988;48: 1083–159.

148. Johnson AO, Semenya JG, Buchowski MS. Am J Clin Nutr 1993;57:399–401.

149. Suarez FL, Savaiano DA, Levitt MD. N Engl J Med 1995; 333:1–4.

150. Reasoner J, Maculan TP, Rand AG et al. Am J Clin Nutr 1981; 34:54–60.

151. Bush RK, Taylor SL. Adverse reactions to food and drug additives. In: Adkinson ND Jr, Holgate ST, Bochner BS et al, eds. Middleton's Allergy Principles and Practices. 7th ed. St. Louis: Mosby Elsevier, 2008:1169–87.

152. Prenner BM, Stevens JJ. Ann Allergy 1976;37:180–82.

153. Stevenson DD, Simon RA. J Allergy Clin Immunol 1981; 68:26–32.

154. Taylor SL, Higley NA, Bush RK. Adv Food Res 1986;30:1–76.

155. Martin LB, Nordlee JA, Taylor SL. J Food Prot 1986;49:126–9.

156. Bush RK, Taylor SL, Holden K et al. Am J Med 1986;81: 816–21.

157. Yang WH, Purchase ECR, Rivington RN. J Allergy Clin Immunol 1986;78:443–9.

158. Taylor SL, Bush RK, Selner JC et al. J Allergy Clin Immunol 1988;81:1159–67.

159. Delohery J, Simmul R, Castle WD et al. Am Rev Respir Dis 1984;130:1027–32.

160. Taylor SL, Stratton JE, Nordlee JA. Clin Toxicol 1989;27: 225–40.

161. Bartholomew BA, Berry PR, Rodhouse JC et al. Epidemiol Infect 1987;99:775–782.

162. Borysiewicz L, Krikler D. Br Med J 1981;282:1434.

163. Anonymous. Histamine in seafood: fluorometric method. In: Helrich K, ed. Official Methods of Analysis of the Association of Analytical Chemists, 15th ed. Arlington, VA: Association of Official Analytical Chemists, 1990:876–7.

164. Dickinson G. Ann Emerg Med 1982;11:487–9.

165. Blakesley ML. Ann Emerg Med 1983;12:104–6.

166. Food and Drug Administration. Decomposition and histamine: raw, frozen tuna and mahi-mahi; canned tuna; and related species. Compliance Policy Guide 7108.24. Washington, DC: US Government Printing Office, 1995.

167. Taylor SL, Keefe TJ, Windham ES et al. J Food Prot 1982; 45:455–7.

168. Wantke F, Gotz M, Jarisch R. N Engl Reg Allergy Proc 1994;15:27–32.

169. Halasz A, Barath A, Simon-Sarkadi L et al. Trends Food Sci Technol 1994;5:42–9.

170. Sumner SS, Roche F, Taylor SL. J Dairy Sci 1990;73:3050–8.

171. Taylor SL. CRC Crit Rev Toxicol 1986;17:91–128.

172. Weiss S, Robb GP, Ellis LB. Arch Intern Med 1932;49:360–2.

173. Clifford MN, Walker R, Ijomah P et al. Food Addit Contam 1991;8:641–52.

174. Ijomah P, Clifford MN, Walker R et al. Food Addit Contam 1991;8:531–42.

175. Morrow JD, Margolies GR, Rowland J et al. N Engl J Med 1991;324:716–20.

176. Uragoda CG, Kottegoda SR. Tubercle 1977;58:83–9.

177. Senanayake N, Vyravanathan S. Toxicon 1981;19:184–5.

SUGGESTED READINGS

Adkinson NF Jr, Holgate ST, Bochner BS et al, eds. Middleton's Allergy: Principles and Practice. 7th ed. St. Louis: Mosby Elsevier, 2009.

Bulush A, Poole S, Deeth C et al. Biogenic amines in fish: roles in intoxication, spoilage and nitrosamine formation: a review. Crit Rev Food Sci Nutr 2009;49:369–77.

Freeman HJ, Chopra A, Clandinin MT et al. Recent advances in celiac disease. World J Gastroenterol 2011;17:2259–72.

Metcalfe DD, Sampson HA, Simon RA, eds. Food Allergy: Adverse Reactions to Foods and Food Additives. 4th ed. Malden, MA: Blackwell Science, 2008.

103 DRUG–NUTRIENT INTERACTIONS[1]

LINGTAK-NEANDER CHAN

A drug–nutrient interaction is defined as the result of a physical, chemical, physiologic, or pathophysiologic relationship between a drug and nutrient status, a nutrient, multiple nutrients, or food in general (1). The causes of most clinically significant drug–nutrient interactions are usually multifactorial. Failure to identify and properly manage drug–nutrient interactions can lead to very serious consequences (2). In the case of treating an infection, for instance, some drug–nutrient interactions can result in reduced absorption of certain oral antibiotics and lead to suboptimal antibiotic concentrations at the site of infection (2, 3). This predisposes the patient to treatment failure and antibiotic resistance in the future. A drug–nutrient interaction also may become a burden on health care costs if its associated complications, such as treatment failure or adverse events, result in increased length of hospital stay and overall resource utilization. In some instances, the impacts of unrecognized and unmanaged drug–nutrient interactions may take years to surface. Metabolic bone disease secondary to vitamin D deficiency in transplant recipients or patients with epilepsy usually takes months to years to progress (4–8). Without proper monitoring of mineral and vitamin status and early intervention, accelerated bone loss or bone fracture may occur.

PREDICTORS

Research has shown that the main predictors for having a drug–nutrient interaction in a given patient are increased age, presence of multiple chronic illnesses, and the concurrent use of multiple medications and supplements (9). Critically ill patients—especially those who receive continuous enteral feeding—may also be at risk for developing drug–nutrient interactions (10, 11). The presence of polypharmacy (i.e., using multiple drugs to manage different disease states) further increases patients' risk for problematic drug–nutrient interactions (12). Elderly patients, patients who have underlying malnutrition, or obese patients are more likely to experience more severe adverse events from a drug–nutrient interaction because of the changes in body composition and physiologic reserves (13–18). Patients with multiple chronic diseases are also more prone to having adverse events. Genetics can be an important factor in determining the appropriate dose and clinical response to a particular drug or nutrient. Polymorphism of the methylenetetrahydrofolate reductase gene (*MTHFR*) may affect the amount of pyridoxine, cobalamin, folic acid, and riboflavin requirement, which may play a role in determining the threshold intake in preventing certain drug–nutrient interactions (19–21). Although the clinical significance has not been well documented, it is possible that some genetic polymorphisms also may have a protective effect against experiencing clinically significant drug–nutrient interactions.

CLASSIFICATION

A drug–nutrient interaction may result in an alteration of the *kinetic* or *dynamic* profile of a drug or a nutrient (22). The magnitude of change determines whether the

---

[1]**Abbreviations: ATP**, adenosine triphosphate; **AUC**, area-under-the-concentration-time curve; **CYP**, cytochrome P-450; **GI**, gastrointestinal; **GLP1**, type 1 glucagon-like peptide; **MAO**, monoamine oxidase; **MAOI**, monoamine oxidase inhibitor; *MTHFR*, methylenetetrahydrofolate reductase gene; **P-gp**, P-glycoprotein; **t_max**, time to reach maximal detectable concentration; **TPGS**, D-α-tocopheryl-polyethylene-glycol-1000 succinate.

interaction is clinically significant and requires intervention. *Pharmacokinetics* refers to the quantitative description of drug disposition, which includes absorption, distribution, metabolism, and excretion of the compound. Pharmacokinetic parameters such as half-life, bioavailability, time to reach maximal detectable concentration (t_{max}), and area-under-the-concentration-time curve (AUC) often are used to provide quantitative comparisons. Half-life refers to the time it takes for the drug concentration (usually in the plasma) to reduce by one-half. It is used commonly to reflect the rate of removal or clearance of the drug from the body. Bioavailability refers to the fraction of the drug administered that becomes available in the body. By definition, intravenous administration provides 100% bioavailability. Oral administration, in many cases, produces lower bioavailability because of incomplete absorption or loss of the active component from presystemic effect. Oral bioavailability is usually the most significant parameter affected by drug–nutrient interactions, although the rate of absorption, metabolic clearance, and tissue distribution of compounds may also be altered. The parameter t_{max} is used to determine the time to achieve peak plasma concentration of a particular compound. If the drug or nutrient is administered orally, t_{max} reflects the rate of oral absorption. Age, underlying medical conditions, types of diet consumed, surgical interventions to the gastrointestinal tract, and concurrent medications can all affect t_{max}. The parameter AUC is used to reflect the overall exposure of a drug by the patient. It is affected by oral bioavailability, clearance and, in some cases, the rate of absorption. The disposition and kinetics of a nutrient (i.e., nutrikinetics) can also be described by these mathematical parameters. For instance, one can estimate the effect of a drug on the disposition of vitamin D by comparing the bioavailability, distribution, and elimination rate of calcidiol and calcitriol before and after the introduction of the drug.

Pharmacodynamics refers to the clinical or physiologic effects of the drug. For example, coadministration of folic acid to a patient taking the antiepileptic agent phenytoin may lead to a reduction in serum phenytoin concentration (pharmacokinetic effect). If the reduction in phenytoin concentration is clinically significant, the patient may experience increased frequency or duration of seizure activities (pharmacodynamic effect).

The four types of drug–nutrient interactions are categorized based on the nature and the mechanisms of the interactions (22). Each type is described briefly in the following paragraphs, and the terms "object agent" and "precipitant agent" are used. An *object agent* refers to the drug or the nutritional element that is affected by the interaction. A *precipitant agent* refers to the drug or the nutritional element that causes the interaction.

Type I: Ex vivo bioinactivations, which refers to the interaction between the drug and the nutritional element or formulation through biochemical or physical reactions. Some of the examples of this type of interaction involve hydrolysis, oxidation, neutralization, precipitation, and complexation. These reactions usually take place when the interacting agents are in direct physical contact and occur usually before the nutrients or drugs enter the body. In other words, these interactions usually occur in the delivery device.

Type II: Interactions affecting absorption, which affect drugs and nutrients delivered only by mouth or via enteral delivery devices. These interactions cause either an increase or decrease of oral bioavailability of the object agent. The precipitant agents may modify the function of an *enzyme* (*type A* interaction) or a *transport mechanism* (*type B* interaction) that is responsible for the biotransformation or transport of the object agent before reaching systemic circulation. In some cases, *complexation, binding, or other deactivating processes* occur in the gastrointestinal (GI) tract (*type C interaction*) and impair the object agent from being absorbed.

Type III: Interactions affecting systemic/physiologic disposition, which occur after the drug or the nutritional element has been absorbed from the gastrointestinal tract and entered into the systemic circulation. The mechanisms involve changing the cellular or tissue distribution, systemic metabolism or transport, or penetration to specific organ/tissues of the object compound. In some cases, the interaction between the precipitant agent and the object agent may involve changing the function of other cofactors (e.g., clotting factors) or hormones.

Type IV: Interactions affecting the elimination or clearance of drugs or nutrients, which may involve the modulation, antagonism, or impairment of renal or enterohepatic elimination.

FACTORS AFFECTING DRUG–NUTRIENT INTERACTIONS

The two factors that play the most significant role in the occurrence of drug–nutrient interactions are the host and the drug (or nutrient) itself (Fig. 103.1). The host factor refers to the individual's response to a drug or nutrient. Age, sex, body size, body composition, lifestyle, underlying diseases and medical conditions, and genetics can affect the response (Table 103.1). The drug or nutrient factor is always affected by the amount, time, and route of administration. For instance, type II drug–nutrient interaction occurs exclusively when both the nutrient and the drug are administered orally or via enteral route and can essentially be eliminated by administration via the intravenous route. Many type IIC interactions (complexation in the GI tract) can be avoided by simply spacing out the administration time. Type I interactions are far more common with drugs and nutrients administered intravenously.

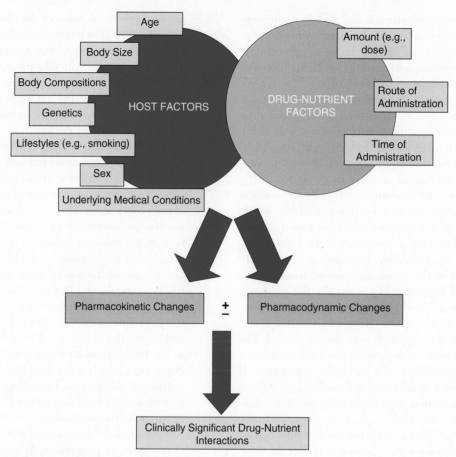

Fig. 103.1. Factors contributing to drug–nutrient interactions. Not all pharmacokinetic or pharmacodynamic changes may lead to clinically significant interactions.

The potential for drug–nutrient interactions increases exponentially with the addition of every drug or dietary supplement (23).

MECHANISM

Ex Vivo Bioinactivations

Before reaching the GI tract or the venous blood (as in the case of intravenous administration), drugs and

TABLE 103.1	PATIENT POPULATIONS WITH SIGNIFICANTLY HIGHER RISK OF EXPERIENCING ADVERSE EVENTS FROM DRUG–NUTRIENT INTERACTIONS

Patients with acquired immunodeficiency syndrome
Patients with cancer
Elderly patients
Malnourished patients
Patients with gastrointestinal tract dysfunctions or surgery (e.g., bariatric surgery, Crohn disease)
Patients receiving enteral nutrition
Pregnant women
Transplant recipients

nutrients are sometimes mixed in the delivery system, where physicobiochemical reactions may occur ex vivo between drugs and nutrients in a delivery vehicle or tubing, in which the active ingredients can be deactivated before being absorbed. The resultant biophysical change as the result of the interaction is described as physical incompatibility. This commonly happens with parenteral products, because physical incompatibility is often associated with the formation of precipitates in a solution. Some of the physical incompatibility can even be visually detected. Precipitation from calcium and phosphate salts is a classic example of physical incompatibility resulting in the formation of the insoluble particles. Nevertheless, visual inspection is not the most accurate approach to rule out the presence of physical incompatibility because some of the precipitants formed may be too small to be visible by naked eyes (24). Intravenous lipid products, conversely, are formulated as opaque emulsions (oil mixed in water). Therefore, physical incompatibility cannot be determined by visual inspection. As a general rule, practitioners should not rely on visual inspection to determine the presence of type I interactions (Table 103.2).

REFERENCES

1. Santos CA, Boullata JI. Pharmacotherapy 2004;25:1789–1800.
2. Radandt JM, Marchbanks CR, Dudley MN. Clin Infect Dis 1992;14:272–84.
3. Neuvonen PJ. Drugs 1976;11:45–54.
4. Offermann G, Pinto V, Kruse R. Epilepsia 1979;20:3–15.
5. Farhat G, Yamout B, Mikati MA et al. Neurology 2002;58: 1348–53.
6. Mikati M, Wakim RH, Fayad M. J Med Liban 2003;51: 71–3.
7. Drezner MK. Epilepsy Behav 2004;5(Suppl 2):S41–7.
8. Fitzpatrick LA. Epilepsy Behav 2004;5(Suppl 2):S3–15.
9. Lewis CW, Frongillo EA Jr, Roe DA. J Am Diet Assoc 1995;95:309–15.
10. Btaiche IF, Chan LN, Pleva M et al. Nutr Clin Pract 2010; 25:32–49.
11. Magnuson BL, Clifford TM, Hoskin LA et al. Nutr Clin Pract 2005;20:618–24.
12. Salazar JA, Poon I, Nair M. Expert Opin Drug Saf 2007;6: 695–704.
13. Akamine D, Filho MK, Peres CM. Curr Opin Clin Nutr Metab Care 2007;10:304–10.
14. MacDonald L, Foster BC, Akhtar H. J Pharm Pharm Sci 2009;12:367–77.
15. Noble RE. Metabolism 2003;52(Suppl 2):27–30.
16. Cheymol G. Clin Pharmacokinet 2000;39:215–31.
17. Murry DJ, Riva L, Poplack DG. Int J Cancer Suppl 1998; 11:48–51.
18. Krishnaswamy K. Clin Pharmacokinet 1989;17(Suppl 1):68–88.
19. Varela-Moreiras G. Biomed Pharmacother 2001;55:448–53.
20. Bailey LB, Gregory JF III. J Nutr 1999;129:919–22.
21. Carmel R, Green R, Rosenblatt DS et al. Hematology (Am Soc Hematol Educ Program) 2003:62–81.
22. Chan LN. Curr Opin Clin Nutr Metab Care 2002;5:327–32.
23. Hansten PD. Sci Med 1998;Jan/Feb:16–25.
24. Mirtallo JM. J Infus Nurs 2004;27:19–24.
25. Fleisher D, Li C, Zhou Y. Clin Pharmacokinet 1999;36: 233–54.
26. Singh BN. Clin Pharmacokinet 1999;37:213–55.
27. Schmidt LE, Dalhoff K. Drugs 2002;62:1481–502.
28. Pedrazzoni M, Ciotti G, Davoli L et al. J Endocrinol Invest 1989;12:409–12.
29. Borovicka J, Schwizer W, Mettraux C et al. Am J Physiol 1997;273:G374–80.
30. Costarelli V, Sanders TA. Br J Nutr 2001;86:471–7.
31. Konturek JW, Thor P, Maczka M et al. Scand J Gastroenterol 1994;29:583–90.
32. Ogunbona FA, Smith IF, Olawoye OS. J Pharm Pharmacol 1985;37:283–4.
33. Lange H, Eggers R, Bircher J. Eur J Clin Pharmacol 1988; 34:315–7.
34. Conway EL, Phillips PA, Drummer OH et al. J Pharm Sci 1990;79:228–31.
35. Hoon TJ, McCollam PL, Beckman KJ et al. Am J Cardiol 1992;70:1072–6.
36. Hashiguchi M, Ogata H, Maeda A et al. J Clin Pharmacol 1996;36:1022–8.
37. Waldman SA, Morganroth J. J Clin Pharmacol 1995;35:163–9.
38. Gill KS, Wood MJ. Clin Pharmacokinet 1996;31:1–8.
39. Oguey D, Kolliker F, Gerber NJ et al. Arthritis Rheum 1992;35:611–4.
40. Kozloski GD, DeVito JM, Kisicki JC et al. Arthritis Rheum 1992;35:761–4.
41. Hamilton RA, Kremer JM. J Rheumatol 1995;22:630–2.
42. Dupuis LL, Koren G, Silverman ED et al. J Rheumatol 1995;22:1570–3.
43. Patsalos PN. Clin Pharmacokinet 2004;43:707–24.
44. Crevoisier C, Zerr P, Calvi-Gries F et al. Eur J Pharm Biopharm 2003;55:71–6.
45. Wiley J, Tatum D, Keinath R et al. Gastroenterology 1988;94: 1144–9.
46. Kaneko H, Sakakibara M, Mitsuma T et al. Am J Gastroenterol 1995;90:603–9.
47. Brundin T, Wahren J. Am J Physiol 1991;260:E232–7.
48. Dauzat M, Lafortune M, Patriquin H et al. Eur J Appl Physiol Occup Physiol 1994;68:373–80.
49. Szinnai C, Mottet C, Gutzwiller JP et al. Scand J Gastroenterol 2001;36:540–4.
50. Ramchandani VA, Kwo PY, Li TK. J Clin Pharmacol 2001;41: 1345–50.
51. Gao L, Ramzan I, Baker AB. Anaesth Intensive Care 2000; 28:375–85.
52. Janssen P, Vanden Berghe P, Verschueren S et al. Aliment Pharmacol Ther 2011;33:880–94.
53. Soffer EE, Thongsawat S, Hoodwerf BJ et al. Dig Dis Sci 1999;44:50–5.
54. Schirra J, Katschinski M, Weidmann C et al. J Clin Invest 1996;97:92–103.
55. Levanon D, Zhang M, Orr WC et al. Am J Physiol 1998;274: G430–4.
56. Chey WY, Chang TM. J Gastroenterol 2003;38:1025–35.
57. Rezek M, Novin D. J Nutr 1976;106:812–20.
58. Moran TH, Ladenheim EE, Schwartz GJ. Int J Obes Relat Metab Disord 2001;25(Suppl 5):S39–41.
59. Herzlich B, Herbert V. Am J Gastroenterol 1986;81:678–80.
60. Neal G. Gut 1990;31:59–63.
61. Howden CW. J Clin Gastroenterol 2000;30:29–33.
62. Ruscin JM, Page RL II, Valuck RJ. Ann Pharmacother 2002;36:812–6.
63. Sagar M, Janczewska I, Ljungdahl A et al. Aliment Pharmacol Ther 1999;13:453–8.
64. Hall SD, Thummel KE, Watkins PB. Drug Metab Dispos 1999;27;161–6.
65. Ito K, Kusuhara H, Sugiyama Y. Pharm Res 1999;16:225–31.
66. Lee SL, Wang MF, Lee AI et al. FEBS Lett 2003;544:143–7.
67. Wacher VJ, Salphati L, Benet LZ. Adv Drug Deliv Rev 2001;46:89–102.
68. van Waterschoot RA, Schinkel AH. Pharmacol Rev 2011;63: 390–410.
69. Benet LZ, Cummins CL, Wu CY. Int J Pharm 2004;277:3–9
70. Dresser GK, Spence JD, Bailey DG. Clin Pharmacokinet 2000;38:41–57.
71. Huang SM, Hall SD, Watkins P et al. Clin Pharmacol Ther 2004;75:1–12.
72. Lown KS, Bailey DG, Fontana RJ et al. J Clin Invest 1997; 99:2545–53.
73. Zhou S, Gao Y, Jiang W et al. Drug Metab Rev 2003;35: 35–98.
74. Henderson L, Yue QY, Bergquist C et al. Br J Clin Pharmacol 2002;54:349–56.
75. Mannel M. Drug Saf 2004;27:773–97.
76. Mucksavage JJ, Chan LN. Dietary supplement interactions with medications. In: Boullata JI, Armenti VT, Malone M, eds. Handbook of Drug-Nutrient Interactions. Totowa, NJ: Humana Press, 2004:217–33.
77. Mai I, Bauer S, Perloff ES et al. Clin Pharmacol Ther 2004;76:330–40.
78. Bauer S, Stormer E, Johne A et al. Br J Clin Pharmacol 2003;55:203–11.

79. Frye RF, Fitzgerald SM, Lagattuta TF et al. Clin Pharmacol Ther 2004;76:323–9.

80. Smith P. Pharmacotherapy 2004;24:1508–14.

81. Mueller SC, Uehleke B, Woehling H et al. Clin Pharmacol Ther 2004;75:546–57.

82. Tannergren C, Engman H, Knutson L et al. Clin Pharmacol Ther 2004;75:298–309.

83. Morimoto T, Kotegawa T, Tsutsumi K et al. J Clin Pharmacol 2004;44:95–101.

84. Hebert MF, Park JM, Chen YL et al. J Clin Pharmacol 2004;44:89–94.

85. Hall SD, Wang Z, Huang SM et al. Clin Pharmacol Ther 2003;74:525–35.

86. Pfrunder A, Schiesser M, Gerber S et al. Br J Clin Pharmacol 2003;56:683–90

87. Markowitz JS, Donovan JL, DeVane CL et al. JAMA 2003;290:1500–4.

88. Dintaman JM, Silverman JA. Pharm Res 1999;16:1550–6.

89. Johnson BM, Charman WN, Porter CJ. AAPS PharmSci 2002;4:E40.

90. Chan L, Humma LM, Schriever CA et al. Clin Pharmacol Ther 2004;75:P95.

91. Hennessy M, Kelleher D, Spiers JP et al. Br J Clin Pharmacol 2002;53:75–82.

92. Bauer LA. Neurology 1982;32:570–2.

93. Au Yeung SC, Ensom MH. Ann Pharmacother 2000;34:896–905.

94. Guengerich FR. Am J Clin Nutr 1995;61:651S–8S.

95. Ioannides C. Xenobiotica 1999;29:109–54.

96. Cashman JR, Lattard V, Lin J. Drug Metab Dispos 2004;32:222–9.

97. Dickerson RN, Charland SL. Pharmacotherapy 2002;22:1084–90.

98. Earl-Salotti GI, Charland SL. J Parenter Enteral Nutr 1994;18:458–65.

99. Wilmana PF, Brodie MJ, Muclow JC et al. Br J Clin Pharmacol 1979;8:523–8.

100. Brodie MJ, Boobis AR, Toverud EL et al. Br J Clin Pharmacol 1980;9:523–5.

101. Gandhi M, Aweeka F, Greenblatt RM et al. Annu Rev Pharmacol Toxicol 2004;44:499–523.

102. Evans WE, McLeod HL. N Engl J Med 2003;348:538–49.

103. Mizutani T. Drug Metab Rev 2003;35:99–106.

104. Evans WE, Relling MV. Nature 2004;429:464–8.

105. Nebert DW, Russell DW. Lancet 2002;360:1155–62.

106. Paoloni-Giacobino A, Grimble R, Pichard C. Clin Nutr 2003;22:429–35.

107. Loktionov A. J Nutr Biochem 2003;14:426–51.

108. Booth SL, Centurelli MA. Nutr Rev 1999;57:288–96.

109. Khan T, Wynne H, Wood P et al. Br J Haematol 2004;124:348–54.

110. Volz HP, Gleiter CH. Drugs Aging 1998;13:341–55.

111. Youdim MB, Weinstock M. Neurotoxicology 2004;25:243–50.

112. Suzzi G, Gardini F. Int J Food Microbiol 2003;88:41–54.

113. Brown C, Taniguchi G, Yip K. J Clin Pharmacol 1989;29:529–32.

114. Yamada M, Yasuhara H. Neurotoxicology 2004;25:215–21.

115. Tein I. J Inherit Metab Dis 2003;26:147–69.

116. Dietary Supplement Health and Education Act of 1994. Pub L No. 103–417 (October 25 1994). Codified at 42 USC 287C–11.

117. Dickerson RN, Garmon WM, Kuhl DA et al. Pharmacotherapy 2008;28:308–13.

118. Dickerson RN. Nutrition 2008;24:1048–52.

119. Dickerson RN, Maish GO 3rd, Minard G et al. Nutr Clin Pract 2010;25:646–52.

120. Ehrenpreis ED, Guerriero S, Nogueras JJ et al. Ann Pharmacother 1994;28:1239–40.

121. Healy DP, Brodbeck MC, Clendening CE. Antimicrob Agents Chemother 1996;40:6–10.

122. Rodman DP, Stevenson TL, Ray TR. Pharmacotherapy 1995;15:801–5.

123. Hasegawa T, Nara K, Kimura T et al. Pediatr Transplant 2001;5:204–9.

124. Madigan SM, Courtney DE, Macauley D. Clin Nutr 2002;21:531–2.

SUGGESTED READINGS

Bailey DG. Fruit juice inhibition of uptake transport: a new type of food-drug interaction. Br J Clin Pharmacol 2010;70:645–55.

MacDonald L, Foster BC, Akhtar H. Food and therapeutic product interactions: a therapeutic perspective. J Pharm Pharm Sci 2009;12:367–77.

Santos CA, Boullata JI. An approach to evaluating drug-nutrient interactions. Pharmacotherapy 2005;25:1789–800.

Seden K, Dickinson L, Khoo S et al. Grapefruit-drug interactions. Drugs 2010;70:2373–407.

Wohlt PD, Zheng L, Gunderson S et al. Recommendations for the use of medications with continuous enteral nutrition. Am J Health Syst Pharm 2009;66:1458–67.

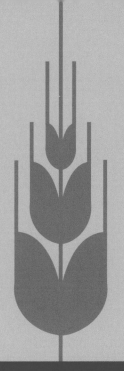

PART V

NUTRITION OF POPULATIONS

A. NUTRITION IN A CHANGING WORLD

104 FOUNDATIONS OF A HEALTHY DIET[1]

WALTER C. WILLETT AND MEIR J. STAMPFER

Nutritional science has provided a wealth of data ranging from detailed molecular descriptions of nutrients and their actions to epidemiologic findings from large prospective studies and controlled randomized studies on selected population groups. Integrating this vast literature into a description of a healthy diet is a challenging yet essential step to provide the public and those responsible for food programs with the best information regarding their food choices. Efforts to develop descriptions of a healthy diet include the US Dietary Guidelines for Americans (1), a synthesis by the Institute of Medicine (IOM) (2) and the World Health Organization (WHO) (3). Because information on diet and health is accruing rapidly, these syntheses of dietary information require frequent updating, which is recognized by the requirement that the US Dietary

Guidelines be reviewed every 5 years. This chapter discusses considerations for developing the definition of a healthy diet and briefly reviews some of the main issues, recognizing that they are addressed in detail elsewhere in this text. Finally, several alternative representations of a healthy diet are described.

Until recently, a primary focus of human nutrition was the prevention of nutrient deficiency, and achieving the recommended dietary allowances (RDAs) (4) for essential nutrients was the central objective. This approach led to the development of the seven food groups during World War II and later the "basic four" (meat, dairy, grains, and fruits and vegetables) as the definition of a healthy diet to be conveyed to the public (5). This effort, together with selective fortification and greater availability of a variety of foods, successfully eliminated clinically evident nutrient deficiencies from the United States and Europe. In the last several decades, the definition of a healthy diet has been expanded to include the optimization of long-term health. An underlying motivation for this expansion in scope has been epidemiologic evidence that coronary heart disease (CHD) and cancer have become the major causes of death in Western countries. Thus, considerations regarding a healthy diet have come to include macronutrient composition, qualitative aspects of macronutrients such as the glycemic index, food constituents not considered to be nutrients such as fiber and carotenoids, and possible benefits of essential nutrients at intakes above those known to prevent overt deficiency.

In describing a healthy diet, an immediate issue is whether this should be expressed as foods or nutrients. Using foods is attractive because this provides an easy form of communication that is recognizable by all. Although this is desirable in principle, those attempting to describe an optimal diet only in terms of foods find this challenging. The main reason is that the same foods can be made in many ways. For example, a cracker can be made with lard, partially hydrogenated vegetable oil, or nonhydrogenated corn oil; and vegetables served at a restaurant can be prepared in butter, margarine of unknown composition, or olive oil. The implications for health vary greatly. This issue is becoming increasingly important as the proportion of the food supply that is already processed or is eaten away from home increases. Most groups that have grappled with these issues have developed guidelines

---

[1]**Abbreviations: CHD**, coronary heart disease; **FDA**, Food and Drug Administration; **HDL**, high-density lipoprotein; **HEI**, healthy eating index; **HIV**, human immunodeficiency virus; **IOM**, Institute of Medicine; **LDL**, low-density lipoprotein; **MTHFR**, methylenetetrahydrofolate reductase; **PKU**, phenylketonuria; **RDA**, recommended dietary allowance; **USDA**, United States Department of Agriculture; **WHO**, World Health Organization.

that are hybrids, using a combination of food and nutrient criteria. For example, many written guidelines include both a quantitative description of fat intake and suggestions about servings of fruits and vegetables. However, when translating dietary guidance into graphic form (e.g., a food guide pyramid), this is often done by only using foods, which may fail to convey essential information.

QUANTITY VERSUS QUALITY OF DIET

Excessive body fat caused by an imbalance between energy intake and expenditure is currently the most important nutritional problem in developed countries and is rapidly becoming a global epidemic. A definition of a healthy diet that fails to address this would be deficient. Some well-intended guidelines are highly prescriptive in terms of energy intake or servings per day of each food group. A fundamental problem is that even the healthiest combination of foods consumed in slight excess, by only a few percent, over an extended period of time, will lead to overweight. Even with the best of methods, our assessments of intake are not sufficiently precise to measure these fine differences, and our assessments of energy expenditure are at least as imperfect. This problem is further compounded by the imprecise estimation of intake of quantities of foods by individuals and even by differences in definitions of serving sizes among branches of government (e.g., the US Food and Drug Administration [FDA] and US Department of Agriculture [USDA]). For these reasons, attempts to address overweight by detailed definitions of energy intake in dietary guidelines will not be successful. Weight itself, however, is well measured and represents a sensitive indicator of the long-term balance between energy intake and expenditure. For this reason, a definition of a healthy diet needs to be closely linked with the importance of maintaining a healthy weight and the need to make adjustments in intake or physical activity if an imbalance exists. Whether the qualitative aspects of diet may help facilitate weight control is discussed later in this chapter.

DOES DIETARY GUIDANCE NEED TO BE INDIVIDUALIZED?

For many years nutritionists have recognized that individuals differ in their response to nutrient intakes (e.g., in the response of serum cholesterol to dietary cholesterol [6], or the response of blood pressure to sodium intake [7]). In extreme cases of inborn genetic defects (e.g., phenylketonuria [PKU]), standard diets can be lethal. The elucidation of the human genome and rapid identification of polymorphisms in almost all genes is creating new opportunities to individualize dietary guidance. For example, a homozygous polymorphism in the methylenetetrahydrofolate reductase (MTHFR) gene, present in about 10% of the population, increases the amount of dietary folic acid needed to minimize blood concentrations of homocysteine (8). Does this mean that special dietary guidance needs to be given to those persons? Although we could now easily screen for MTHFR polymorphisms and individualize dietary advice, this is still probably not a logical strategy, and having different dietary advice for folic acid for different persons would create considerable complexity within populations and even within families. Because these variations probably exist for almost every nutrient, the possible combinations are almost infinite and would mean that each person would have a unique dietary recommendation. An alternative is to define healthy diets that would be sufficiently high in folic acid to meet the needs of this subset of the population. This has been the general approach in setting RDAs, whereby a margin of error has been added above average requirements to include individual variations in nutrient needs. This is an appropriate approach when variation in requirements is known to exist and we have no practical way of identifying individuals with different requirements or the reason for these differences, and often it is still a reasonable strategy even though we have the potential to identify individual differences in requirements.

The ability to identify individuals with different requirements allows more detailed studies to be sure that their needs are being met. Also, for some carefully selected genetic variants, different dietary approaches may be appropriate (e.g., PKU, as mentioned). Also, it may well be that diets to address specific abnormalities, such as elevated cholesterol, will be prescribed based on genetic information.

Genetic variation is only one of several factors that can influence nutritional requirements, and may not even be the most important. Age, body size, activity level, and pregnancy have long been recognized as factors to be considered, and requirements often are specific for these groups. However, as Hegsted pointed out (9), if requirements are expressed in terms of dietary quality (e.g., as nutrient densities), many of the differences in requirements diminish. One fundamentally important influence on the response to diet is the underlying degree of insulin resistance. This was described by Jeppesen et al (10, 11), who noted that the adverse effects of high carbohydrate intake on metabolic markers of the insulin resistance syndrome were strongly correlated with baseline insulin resistance. This relation has been confirmed in population studies showing a much stronger relation between the dietary glycemic load and blood triglyceride concentrations (12) and risk of CHD (13) among persons with a greater body mass index, which is a major determinant of insulin resistance. The implication is that a person who is lean and active can better tolerate a high-carbohydrate diet than someone who is less active and overweight. This also has important implications on a population basis because of strong evidence that most Asian groups have a higher prevalence of insulin resistance, possibly because of genetic reasons, compared with European populations (14). Neel (15) described this as the "thrifty gene." Until recently, these populations generally were highly active and lean, and thus protected from the adverse effects of this genetic predisposition. However, with the reductions in activity and gains in body weight that typically accompany a modern lifestyle, the ability to tolerate a diet high in refined carbohydrates diminishes. Nevertheless, this does not necessarily require different dietary recommendations if diets with low amounts of refined carbohydrate, even if not as critical, would be desirable for other populations as well.

SPECIFIC CONSIDERATIONS IN FORMULATING A HEALTHY DIET

Traditionally, animal experiments and small human metabolic studies provided the data underlying the basis of dietary recommendations, based on short-term or extreme effects, such as overt deficiency. Inevitably, the study of chronic disease in humans has required epidemiologic approaches. Until recently, these largely consisted of international comparisons and case-control studies, which examined dietary factors retrospectively in relation to cancer and other diseases. Now, large prospective studies of many thousands of persons are providing data, based on both biochemical indicators of diet and dietary questionnaires, which have been rigorously validated (16). Ideally, each potential relationship between diet and a health outcome would be evaluated in a randomized trial (17), but this is often not feasible because of practical constraints. The best available evidence usually is based on a synthesis of epidemiologic, metabolic, animal, and mechanistic studies. Major aspects of diet are discussed briefly here.

Dietary Fat and Specific Fatty Acids

Until recently, reviews on diet and health consistently recommended reducing total fat intake, usually to 30% of energy or less (17–19), to decrease CHD and cancer. The classical diet–heart hypothesis has rested heavily on observations that total serum cholesterol concentrations predict CHD risk; serum cholesterol has thus functioned as a surrogate marker of risk in hundreds of metabolic studies. These studies, summarized as equations by Keys (20) and Hegsted (21), indicated that, compared with carbohydrates, saturated fats and dietary cholesterol increase and polyunsaturated fat decreases serum cholesterol, whereas monounsaturated fat has no influence. These widely used equations, although valid for total cholesterol, have become less relevant with the recognition that the high-density lipoprotein (HDL) cholesterol fraction is strongly and inversely related to CHD risk, and the ratio of total cholesterol to HDL is a better predictor (22–25). Substitution of carbohydrate for saturated fat (the basis of most dietary recommendations until recently) tends to reduce HDL as well as total and low-density lipoprotein (LDL) cholesterol; thus, the ratio does not change appreciably (26). In contrast, substituting monounsaturated fat for saturated fat reduces LDL without affecting HDL, thus providing an improved ratio (26). In addition, monounsaturated fats, compared with carbohydrate, reduce blood sugar and triglycerides in those with type 2 diabetes (27).

Although different saturated fats vary in their influence on LDL concentration (28), this finding probably has limited practical importance because intakes of the various saturated fats are strongly correlated with each other in usual diets, and there is no direct evidence that stearic acid is a lesser risk factor for CHD than other saturated fatty acids (29).

Uncertainty about Optimal Polyunsaturated Fat Intake

The metabolic studies predicting total serum cholesterol (20, 21) suggested that polyunsaturated fat intake should be maximized, and the American Heart Association has recommended intakes of up to 10% of energy (compared with US averages of approximately 3% in the 1950s and 6% at present). Concerns have arisen from animal studies in which omega-6 polyunsaturated fat (typically as corn oil) has promoted tumor growth (30), and the possibility that high intakes of omega-6 relative to omega-3 fatty acids might be proinflammatory and promote coronary thrombosis. However, as described in the following, available evidence from human studies has not supported these concerns at levels of omega-6 fatty acid intakes at least up to 10% of calories.

Dietary Fat and Incidence of CHD

In Keys' pioneering ecologic study of diets and CHD in seven countries (31, 32), total fat intake had little association with population rates of CHD; indeed, the lowest rate was in Crete, which had the highest fat intake because of the large consumption of olive oil. Saturated fat intake, however, was positively related to CHD. In contrast to international comparisons, which are potentially confounded by many different factors, little relationship has been seen with saturated fat intake in prospective studies of individuals when compared with the same percentage of energy from carbohydrate (33, 34). However, polyunsaturated fat, mainly linoleic acid, has been inversely associated with risk of CHD in these prospective studies, especially when compared with saturated fat intake. Similarly, dietary intervention trials generally have shown little effect on CHD incidence when carbohydrate replaces saturated fat, but replacing saturated fat with polyunsaturated fat has reduced incidence of CHD (35). At intakes within the dietary range, the benefits of omega-3 fatty acids appear to be primarily in prevention of fatal arrhythmias that can complicate CHD rather than in prevention of infarction (36, 37). The amount of long-chain (marine) omega-3 fatty acids needed to prevent arrhythmia is remarkably small—on the order of 250 mg/day—and fish consumption twice a week appears to provide most of the potential reduction of sudden death (38). The 18-carbon omega-3 fatty acid, α-linolenic acid, also appears to reduce risk of coronary heart disease (39, 40) and may be particularly important when fish intake is low. Based on theoretic concerns about competition in the elongation and desaturation pathways, some have hypothesized that dietary omega-6 fatty acids, mainly linoleic acid, are proinflammatory and counteract the benefits of omega-3 fatty acids; thus some have proposed that the ratio of omega-6 to omega-3 fatty acids is especially important in the prediction of heart disease (41). However, linoleic acid appears to have anti-inflammatory effects mediated by other pathways and does not increase inflammatory markers in humans (42). Also, because both omega-3 and omega-6 fatty acids are essential and reduce the risk of heart disease, their ratio has been unrelated to risk (43); consuming adequate amounts of both are important (44). The optimal amount of linoleic acid in the diet is not yet clear; in the US population, the benefits for heart disease appear to increase monotonically with greater intakes, but few individuals consume more than 10% of energy.

Trans-Fatty Acids

Trans-fatty acids are formed by the partial hydrogenation of liquid vegetable oils in the production of margarine and vegetable shortening and can account for as much as 40% of these products. *Trans*-fatty acids increase LDL and decrease HDL (45); raise the proportion of small, dense, and atherogenic LDL particles (46); raise lipoprotein(a) (47, 48) and increase inflammatory markers that have been related to CHD risk (49, 50). In the most detailed prospective study to date, *trans*-fatty acid intake was strongly associated with risk of CHD (33) and, as predicted by metabolic studies, this association was stronger than for saturated fat. The association between *trans*-fatty acid intake and risk of CHD has been confirmed in other prospective studies (51). Since 2006, the FDA has required food labels to include the *trans*-fat content of foods, which has resulted in major decreases in the amounts used (52); and banning of *trans*-fat in restaurants in New York and elsewhere has led most national restaurant chains to eliminate them from their products.

Relation between Dietary Fat and Risk of Type 2 Diabetes. The relation between dietary fat and risk of type 2 diabetes appears to be similar to that for CHD (53). The overall percentage of fat does not appear to be related to risk. However, polyunsaturated fat is inversely associated with risk, consistent with its effect on insulin resistance, and *trans*-fat has been positively associated with risk (53, 54), consistent with evidence of its effects on inflammatory markers noted in the preceding discussion. Consumption of red meat, particularly processed red meat, has associated with greater risk (55, 56).

Dietary Fat and Cancer. One justification for low-fat diets has been the belief that these would reduce the incidence of cancers of the breast, colon and rectum, and prostate (18, 57). The primary evidence has been that countries with low-fat intake (also the less affluent areas) have had low rates of these cancers (57, 58). These correlations have been primarily with animal fat and meat intake rather than with vegetable fat consumption.

The hypothesis that fat intake increases breast cancer risk has been supported by most animal models (59, 60), although no association was seen in a large study that did not use an inducing agent (61). Moreover, much of the effect of dietary fat in the animal studies appears to be caused by an increase in total energy intake, and energy restriction profoundly decreases incidence (30, 59, 61). Data from many large prospective studies, including approximately 8000 cases in more than 300,000 women, have been published (62). In none of these studies was the risk of breast cancer significantly elevated among those with the highest fat intake, and the summary relative risk for the highest versus lowest category of dietary fat composition was 1.03 (62). In a pooled analysis, no reduction in risk was seen, even in those with less than 20% of energy from fat (63). In two large randomized trials, interventions to reduce intake of total fat did not significantly influence risk of breast cancer (64, 65). Thus, over the range of fat intake consumed by middle-aged women, total dietary fat does not appear to increase breast cancer risk. During adolescence and early adulthood, higher intake of animal fat, particularly from dairy products and red meat, has been associated with greater risk of premenopausal breast cancer (66–68). Vegetable fat was not associated with risk of breast cancer in this study, suggesting that some components of animal foods rather than fat itself may increase risk.

Although associations between dietary fat and risk of colorectal cancer had been seen in earlier retrospective case-control studies, little relation has been seen in prospective studies (69). However, associations between red meat consumption, particularly processed meats, and colorectal cancer risk have been seen in both case-control and cohort studies (69), suggesting that components other than fat, such as heat-induced carcinogens (70) or the high content of readily available iron, may be responsible (71). Like breast and colon cancer, prostate cancer rates are much higher in affluent compared with poor and Eastern countries (58). More detailed epidemiologic studies are limited, but intake of total fat generally has not been associated with this type of cancer (69). A positive association has been seen with intake of α-linolenic acid in some studies, but the overall evidence is unclear at this time (72).

Overweight is an important cause of morbidity and mortality, and short-term studies have suggested that reducing the fat content of the diet induces weight loss (73). However, in randomized studies lasting a year or longer, reductions in fat to 20% to 25% of energy had minimal effects on overall long-term body weight (74).

In summary, there is little evidence that dietary fat itself is associated with risk of CHD. Metabolic and epidemiologic data are consistent in suggesting that intake of partially hydrogenated vegetable fats should be minimized. Metabolic studies, epidemiologic studies, and randomized trials indicate that replacement of saturated fat by polyunsaturated fat reduces the risk of coronary heart disease, but the benefits are minimal if carbohydrate rather than unsaturated fat replaces the saturated fat. Although the evidence is more limited, controlled feeding studies of blood lipids as well as the experience of southern European populations suggest that consuming a substantial proportion of energy as monounsaturated fat in the form of olive oil is associated with low rates of coronary heart disease. Available evidence also suggests that total fat reduction has little effect on breast cancer risk, although reducing red meat intake likely decreases the incidence of coronary heart disease, diabetes, colon cancer, and possibly premenopausal breast cancer.

Carbohydrates

Because protein varies only modestly across a wide range of human diets, higher carbohydrate consumption, in practice, is the reciprocal of a low-fat diet. For reasons discussed under the topic of fat, a high-carbohydrate diet can have adverse metabolic consequences. In particular, such diets are associated with an increase in triglycerides and a reduction in HDL cholesterol (25), and these adverse responses are aggravated in the context of insulin resistance (10, 75, 76).

Complex Carbohydrates

The traditional distinction between simple and complex carbohydrates is not useful in dietary recommendations because some forms of complex carbohydrates, such as starch in potatoes, are very rapidly metabolized to glucose. Instead, emphasis is better placed on whole grain and other less-refined complex carbohydrates as opposed to the highly refined products and sugar generally consumed in the United States. Adverse consequences of highly refined grains appear to result from both the rapid digestion and absorption of these foods, as well as the loss of fiber and micronutrients in the milling process. The glycemic response after carbohydrate intake, which has been characterized by the glycemic index, is greater with highly refined foods as compared with less-refined whole grains (77). The greater glycemic response caused by highly refined carbohydrates is accompanied by increased plasma insulin concentrations and augments the other adverse metabolic changes caused by carbohydrate consumption, noted in the preceding section, to a greater degree than with less-refined foods (12). Higher intakes of refined starches and sugar, particularly when associated with low fiber intake (78), are associated with increased risk of type 2 diabetes (79, 80) and CHD (13, 78). In contrast, higher intake of fiber from grain products has been associated consistently with lower risks of CHD and diabetes

(53, 81). Whether these benefits are mediated by only fiber itself, or in part by the accompanying micronutrients is not clear, but for practical reasons this distinction is not essential. Anticipated reductions in colon cancer risk by diets high in grain fiber have not been supported in most prospective studies (82). However, reduced constipation and risk of colonic diverticular disease (83) are clear benefits of such diets.

The importance of micronutrients in the prevention of many chronic conditions has reemphasized the problem of "empty calories" associated with diets high in sugar and highly refined carbohydrates. In the standard milling of white flour, as much as 60% to 90% of vitamins B_6 and E, folate, and other nutrients are lost (84); this may be nutritionally critical for persons with otherwise marginal intakes. Thiamin, riboflavin, folate, and niacin currently are replaced by fortification, but other nutrients remain substantially reduced.

Protein

Average protein consumption in the United States exceeds conventional requirements (18), and adequate intake can be maintained on most reasonable diets. Optimal protein intake has been widely debated, and high intakes are advocated in many popular diets, but long-term data are limited. Substituting protein or monounsaturated fat for carbohydrate reduces blood pressure and improves blood lipids (85) and has been associated with lower risk of CHD (86).

Protein Sources

The specific sources of dietary protein have important implications for long-term health, probably more related to the other constituents of these foods than to the protein itself. As noted, fish consumption is related to lower risk of sudden cardiac death, probably because of its content of omega-3 fatty acids. Also, regular consumption of nuts has been related to lower risk of CHD in multiple studies (87) and type 2 diabetes (88), likely because of their high content of unsaturated fatty acids and possibly also their high content of micronutrients and other phytochemicals. Soy products are high in polyunsaturated fatty acids and presumably are beneficial with regard to CHD risk—but little direct evidence is available, and the same applies to other legumes. Poultry fat is relatively unsaturated compared with that of red meat, which is the primary contributor to saturated fat intake in the US diet. Not surprisingly, higher consumption of red meat compared with the same number of servings of fish, poultry, or nuts has been positively related to risk of CHD (89). As noted, consumption of red meat, particularly processed meats, also has been related to risks of several cancers and type 2 diabetes. This extensive body of evidence supports the replacement of red meat with a combination of nuts, fish, poultry, and legumes as protein sources for overall long-term health.

Vegetables and Fruits

Advice to eat a generous amount of vegetables and fruits (18) has been justified largely by anticipated reductions in cancer and cardiovascular disease. However, more recent cohort studies have tended to show much weaker— or no—relation between overall fruit and vegetable consumption and risks of common cancers (90–92). However, inverse relationships have been seen for renal cell (93) and estrogen receptor–negative breast cancer (94). The possibility remains for a small overall benefit, or benefits, only of specific fruits or vegetables against specific cancers. For example, considerable evidence suggests that lycopene, mainly from tomato products, reduces the risk of prostate cancer, but overall consumption of fruits is unrelated to risk (69, 95).

In contrast to the data for cancer, the epidemiologic evidence quite consistently supports a benefit of higher intake of fruit and vegetable consumption for the prevention of cardiovascular disease (96). Evidence that elevated blood homocysteine is an independent risk factor for coronary heart and cerebrovascular disease (97, 98), and that concentrations can be reduced by increasing folic acid intake (99), suggest one mechanism. High intake of vegetables reduces blood pressure (100); the active factors remain unclear, but potassium is a likely contributor (101). Other benefits of higher fruit and vegetable intake are likely to include lower risk of neural tube defects, the most common severe birth defect (102), resulting from higher folate intake. Intake of the carotenoids lutein and zeaxanthin, which are high in green leafy vegetables, has been inversely related to risk of cataracts (103, 104).

Calcium and Dairy Products

Recommendations to consume large amounts of dairy products, at least three servings (1) on a daily basis, derive primarily from the importance of calcium in maintaining bone strength. Calcium supplements in conjunction with vitamin D have reduced fracture incidence in some studies (104, 105), but benefits of calcium cannot be distinguished from those of vitamin D. The optimal calcium intake remains uncertain. Intakes of 1200 mg/day or higher are recommended for women greater than 50 years old and men greater than 70 years old in the United States. However, the basis of the recommended levels, balance studies lasting less than 2 weeks (106), is fundamentally flawed because these very short-term studies are likely to reflect transient movements of calcium into and out of bone. A review of calcium requirements in the United Kingdom concluded that 700 mg/day was adequate (107) and the WHO determined that 500 mg/day was sufficient (3). Many populations have low fracture rates despite minimal dairy product consumption and low overall calcium intake by adults (108, 109).

In large prospective studies, higher consumption of calcium (110) or milk (111) as an adult has consistently not been associated with lower overall fracture incidence. Although randomized trials of calcium without vitamin D have been small, no significant reduction in overall fracture risk has been found (110), and risk of hip fracture was increased. At best, the benefits of high calcium intake are minor compared with those from regular physical activity (112, 113) or vitamin D supplements (114).

Inverse associations have been reported between calcium intake and blood pressure in some studies (115), but in a review of trials of supplementation, little overall effect was seen (116). In a metaanalysis of randomized trials of calcium without vitamin D, higher risk of cardiovascular disease was seen (117). Low calcium and low dairy product consumption is associated with a modestly elevated risk of colon cancer (118), but most benefits appear to be achieved with calcium intake of about 800 mg/day. Evidence from a randomized trial that calcium supplementation modestly reduces colon adenoma recurrence adds important evidence of causality to the epidemiologic studies (119).

Although recommended calcium intakes can be achieved by a high consumption of greens and certain other vegetables, greatly increased intakes would be required for most adults to achieve the calcium intakes recommended in the United States by diet without high consumption of milk and other dairy products. However, these recommended intakes of calcium appear to be substantially more than needed. The WHO and the United Kingdom recommended that adequate intakes for adults can be achieved by a reasonable diet with one serving of dairy per day. Alternatively, a modest calcium supplement (e.g., 500 mg/day) with vitamin D (see the following) would achieve these intakes without any calories or saturated fat; thus, dairy product consumption can be considered an optional rather than a necessary dietary component. Enthusiasm regarding high dairy consumption also should be tempered by the suggestion in many studies that this is associated with increased risks of advanced or fatal prostate cancer (69, 120). Whether an increased risk is caused by calcium, endogenous hormones, or other factors in milk remains unclear.

Salt and Processed Meats

Reduction of salt (sodium chloride) intake from an average of approximately 8 to 10 g/day to less than 6 g/day will decrease blood pressure to a modest degree on average. Law et al (121) concluded that a 3-g/day reduction would reduce the incidence of stroke by 22% and CHD by 16%. Although the decrease in risk of cardiovascular disease achieved by reducing salt consumption is modest for most individuals, the overall number of cardiovascular deaths potentially avoided is large, an estimated 50,000 to 90,000 per year in the United States (122), supporting policies to reduce salt consumption, particularly in processed foods and by institutions. In many case-control studies, the consumption of salty and pickled foods has been associated with stomach cancer (69). However, because this cancer is relatively rare in the United States, further benefit from reducing salt intake would be small.

Alcohol

Many adverse influences of heavy alcohol consumption are well recognized, but moderate consumption has both beneficial and harmful effects, greatly complicating decisions for individuals. Overwhelming epidemiologic data indicate that moderate consumption (one to two drinks per day) reduces the risk of myocardial infarction (123, 124) by approximately 30% to 40%. Although this effect has been hypothesized to be the result of antioxidants in red wine, similar protective effects for equivalent amounts of alcohol have been seen for all types of alcoholic beverages (125, 126). In contrast, modest positive associations with risk of breast cancer incidence have been observed in more than 30 studies (127) for similar levels of alcohol intake, possibly because alcohol appears to increase endogenous estrogen levels (128, 129). The overall effect of alcohol, as represented by total mortality, appears beneficial for up to about two drinks per day in men (130). Overall, a similar relation with total mortality is seen among women, but no net benefit was observed among those at low risk of CHD because of younger age or lack of coronary risk factors (131). Several studies suggest that the adverse effects of alcohol on cancer risk may be mitigated by adequate intake of folate, but the evidence is inconsistent.

Vitamin Supplements

The role of vitamin supplements and food fortification has been debated on both a philosophic and scientific level. Some nutritionists have believed as a matter of principle that nutritional needs should be met by diet alone. However, often, this is not possible (e.g., when iodine levels are low in the soil), and iodine fortification has been a great public health advance. Also, a large percentage of the US population appears to have suboptimal blood concentrations of vitamin D, largely because of limited solar exposure at northern latitudes during the winter. In addition, low incomes and limited access can be serious barriers to optimal food intakes; to achieve the recommended 400 μg/day of folate from natural foods alone can be expensive. Many of these shortcomings can be remedied efficiently and effectively by some combination of fortification and supplementation.

The most firmly established benefit of vitamin supplementation against the background of a Western diet is that folic acid supplements, in the amounts contained in typical multiple vitamins, can reduce the risk of neural tube defects by approximately 70% (132). This is probably an indicator of more widespread consequences of suboptimal folate intakes. For example, higher folate intake and long-

term use of multiple vitamins have been associated with lower risk of colonic neoplasias (133, 134). Low folate intake, along with suboptimal status of vitamins B_6 and B_{12}, contribute to elevated blood homocysteine concentrations and, potentially, the risk of cardiovascular disease (98, 135). In randomized trials among patients with advanced heart disease and stroke, folate supplementation has had little effect (136), but among healthy persons with lower folate intakes, supplements may contribute to the prevention of cardiovascular disease, especially stroke (137). Since 1998, grain products in the United States have been fortified with folic acid, which is likely to have reduced the value of additional supplemental folic acid, but many US residents still have intakes below the RDA of 400 μg/day.

Many elderly persons have suboptimal vitamin B_{12} status, mainly resulting from loss of stomach acid, which is needed to liberate vitamin B_{12} from food sources. In contrast, vitamin B_{12} in supplements or from fortified foods is readily absorbed without stomach acid. The health consequences of marginal status of vitamin B_{12} remain unclear, but interactions with folate intake may be important in cognitive function (138).

Vitamin D has established roles in bone health and potentially in reducing risks of some cancers, cardiovascular disease, diabetes, infectious diseases, and other conditions. In a 2010 report, an IOM panel concluded that only the data for bone health were sufficient for making recommendations, that a blood concentration of 50 nmol/L (20 ng/mL) was adequate for 97% of the US adult population, the RDA was 600 to 800 IU/day for adults (106), and the upper limit should be 4000 IU/day. Even though approximately 33% of adults have blood concentrations less than 50 nmol/mL and very few adults obtain the RDA from their diets (139), the panel did not recommend use of supplements or screening for low vitamin D blood concentrations. This report has been unusually controversial because the conclusions appear illogical, and blood concentrations greater than 75 nmol/L have been associated with lower risks of falls (140), colorectal cancer (141), bone mineral density (142), and other health outcomes, although these relationships have been established by randomized trials only for falls. This well illustrates the frequent situation in which ideal data do not exist. The IOM panel took a position at one end of a spectrum, that randomized trials with clinical end points are required to make recommendations for higher intakes. However, decisions must be made with the best available evidence; and a reasonable alternative position, given current data, is to use a supplement of 1000 to 2000 IU/day, which will bring most people to 75 nmol/L (although some persons need more, especially those with darker skin and little sun exposure). Even reaching the current RDA is very difficult to do using food alone, because natural sources of vitamin D are few (mainly fish), and recommendations to increase sun exposure could lead to elevations in skin cancer. More data are needed to refine recommendations, but it may not be possible to exclude benefits for some end points such as cancer risk using randomized trials because the necessary duration of supplementation is unclear and adherence in trials typically decreases with time.

Many US adults, especially women, take calcium supplements primarily to reduce the risk of osteoporosis and fractures. However, as noted, the evidence for the current high recommendations for calcium intake are based on short-term balance studies that may be misleading, and findings from randomized trials and prospective studies do not support a reduction in fracture risk with higher intakes. In contrast, in a metaanalysis of randomized trials of calcium supplements without vitamin D, those receiving the supplements experienced a twofold higher risk of hip fracture compared with placebo (140). Also, calcium supplements may increase the risk of kidney stones (143) and myocardial infarction (117, 144). Thus, the current evidence suggests that persons who consume at least one serving of milk or other dairy food per day and who achieves the WHO adequate intake of 500 mg/day, should not take a calcium supplement. For those not consuming dairy products daily, a supplement of 500 mg/day might be considered, but the evidence is not clear that this will be beneficial in the context of an overall healthy diet.

The prevalence of iron deficiency in the United States, determined by the use of three plasma biomarkers, is 9% to 12% among adolescent and adult females aged 12 to 49 years (145). Among non-Hispanic black and Mexican-American women, the prevalence is 19% to 22%. These rates are much higher than in men or older women (approximately 5%) and primarily result from menstrual losses rather than deficient diets. The current US Dietary Guidelines recommend increases in lean red meat by premenopausal women to address iron deficiency (1). However, heme iron continues to be absorbed and to accumulate even if iron stores are adequate, and higher intakes of red meat and heme iron have been associated with an increased risk of coronary heart disease (89) and type 2 diabetes (146, 147), probably at least in part because of excessive iron stores. Thus, the inclusion of an RDA amount of inorganic iron—the absorption of which will be better regulated—in a multiple vitamin/mineral used by premenopausal women appears to be a better solution. In contrast to red meat, this has no saturated fat, cholesterol, or excessive energy and costs much less.

Few long-term trials of multivitamins have been completed. In a randomized trial conducted in a region of China with low consumption of fruits and vegetables, a supplement containing β-carotene, vitamin E, and selenium reduced incidence of stomach cancer (148). In a study conducted among Tanzanian women infected with human immunodeficiency virus (HIV), a multiple vitamin containing B vitamins, vitamin E, and vitamin C reduced progression of the disease and HIV-related mortality (149). The French Su.Vi.Max trial of a combination of zinc and low-dose antioxidants yielded a significant 31% reduction in cancer incidence and lower overall mortality

in men, but results were not significant among women, who had a better nutritional status at baseline (150). Whether these benefits would be seen in the background of dietary intakes in the United States is not clear.

Any recommendation for use of nutritional supplements should carefully consider possible adverse effects. One of the few adverse effects of vitamin supplement use at the RDA level appears to be an increase in risk of hip fractures caused by vitamin A when consumed at 5000 IU/day in the form of retinol. Higher intake of preformed vitamin A (retinol) has been associated with excess risk of hip fracture in prospective studies (151, 152), and elevated risks were seen for both use of multiple vitamins and specific supplements of vitamin A. Also, serum retinol concentrations have been associated with future risk of fractures (153). These effects may be caused by competition at the vitamin D receptor (154) and might not have occurred if vitamin D concentrations were adequate. The amount of retinol in most multiple vitamins has been reduced.

Because intakes of many micronutrients appear marginal for many Americans (155, 156), and very few meet all the current dietary guidelines (157), the risks of using an RDA-level multiple vitamin appear minimal; the use of a daily multiple vitamin with 1000 to 2000 IU of vitamin D appears rational for many Americans. The cost of this is low, especially compared with consumption of fresh fruits and vegetables. Any suggestion about supplements should not replace efforts to improve diets, but major dietary improvements are challenging for many and some deficiencies are not simply caused by poor diets (e.g., iron in premenopausal women, vitamin B_{12} in older persons, and vitamin D in people who work indoors or have darker skin).

SUMMARY

Any description of a healthy diet must be made with the recognition that information is currently incomplete and conclusions are subject to change with new data. Most of the major diseases contributing to morbidity and mortality in the United States develop over many decades, and large-scale nutritional epidemiologic studies have only begun in the last 25 years; thus, a full picture of the relation between diet and disease will require additional decades of careful investigation. Nevertheless, in combining available metabolic, clinical, and epidemiologic evidence, several general conclusions that are unlikely to change substantially can be drawn.

1. Staying lean and active throughout life has major health benefits. Because most people in developed countries work at sedentary jobs, weight control usually requires conscious daily physical activity as well as some effort to avoid overconsumption of calories.

2. Dietary fats should be primarily in the form of non-hydrogenated plant oils. Butter, lard, and fat from red meat should be used sparingly, and *trans*-fatty acids

from partially hydrogenated vegetable oils should be avoided.

3. Grains should be consumed primarily in a minimally refined, high-fiber form, and intakes of refined starches and simple sugars should be low. Sugar-sweetened beverages should be consumed only occasionally if at all.

4. Vegetables and fruits should be consumed in abundance (five servings per day is minimal) and should include green leafy and orange vegetables daily. Fruit juice should be limited to not more than about one small glass per day.

5. Red meat should be consumed only occasionally and in low amounts if at all; nuts, legumes, poultry, and fish in moderation, are healthy alternatives.

6. The optimal consumption of dairy products and calcium intake is not known, but dairy products are not essential. High consumption of milk (e.g., more than two servings per day) does not appear to be beneficial and may increase risk of prostate cancer. Calcium needs are higher for growing children, adolescents, and lactating women; supplements (including vitamin D) should be considered if dietary sources are low.

7. For most people, taking a daily RDA-level (Daily Value) multiple vitamin containing 1000 to 2000 IU of vitamin D provides a sensible nutritional safety net. Because menstrual losses of iron may not be replaced adequately by iron intake on the low-energy diets of women in a sedentary society and iron deficiency is common before menopause, it is reasonable for most premenopausal women to use a multiple vitamin that also contains iron.

8. Salt intake should be kept low; the American Heart Association target of 1500 mg/day is reasonable for most people (158).

REPRESENTATION OF AN OVERALL HEALTHY DIET AND VALIDATION

To inform the public and provide guidance for food programs and services, many summary representations of a healthy diet have been developed. The approaches include written guidelines, graphic displays, and dietary indices or scores.

Guidelines and Pyramids

Examples of dietary guidelines include the Dietary Guidelines for Americans (1) that are updated every 5 years, the Population Nutrient Intake Goals created by the WHO (3), and those developed by the professional organizations such the American Heart Association and American Cancer Society (Table 104.1). Usually, these are created by committees of experts, ideally using the

TABLE 104.1	**EXAMPLES OF DIETARY GUIDELINES**			
FACTOR	US DIETARY GUIDELINES[a]	WHO DIETARY GOALS[b]	AMERICAN HEART ASSOCIATION EATING PLAN FOR HEALTHY AMERICANS[c]	AMERICAN CANCER SOCIETY GUIDELINES ON NUTRITION AND PHYSICAL ACTIVITY[d]
Weight control	BMI <25	BMI <25	Adjust calories to maintain healthy weight	Maintain healthful weight throughout life; strive for BMI <25
Fat	<10% E saturated, minimize trans	15%–30% of E	<30% E, <10% polyunsaturated, <15% monounsaturated	
Protein	choose a variety	10%–15% of E	—	Emphasize plant sources
Carbohydrates	at least half of all grains as whole grains	55%–75% of E	6+ servings grains, starchy vegetables	Chose whole grains
Fruits and vegetables	half your plate	400 g/day	5+ servings/day	5+ servings/day
Dairy	fat-free or low fat milk	—	2–4 servings/day	
Alcohol	0–1 servings/day, women	—	0–1 servings/day, women	0–1 servings/day, women
	0–2 servings/day, men		0–2 servings/day, men	0–2 servings/day, men
Sugar, sweets	drink water instead of sugary drinks	Free sugars <10% of E		
Physical activity	activity to maintain caloric balance	30 min most days	30 min/day	30–45 min, 5+ times/wk
Other	<1500 mg sodium for most <300 mg cholesterol		<2,400 mg sodium, 300 mg cholesterol/day	Red meat

BMI, body mass index; E, energy.

[a]US Department of Agriculture, US Department of Health and Human Services. Nutrition and Your Health: Dietary Guidelines for Americans 2010. 7th edition. Washington, DC: US Government Printing Office, 2010.
[b]World Health Organization, Food and Agriculture Organization. Diet, Nutrition and the Prevention of Chronic Diseases: Report of a Joint WHO/FAO Expert Consultation. Geneva: World Health Organization, 2003. Technical Report Series No. 916.
[c]Krauss RM, Eckel RH, Howard B et al. AHA Dietary Guidelines: revision 2000: A statement for healthcare professionals from the Nutrition Committee of the American Heart Association. Stroke 2000;31:2751–66.
[d]Byers T, Nestle M, McTiernan A et al. American Cancer Society guidelines on nutrition and physical activity for cancer prevention: Reducing the risk of cancer with healthy food choices and physical activity. CA Cancer J Clin 2002;52:92–119.

best available evidence. However, in reality, consistency with earlier versions of the same guideline and with other guidelines is often given high priority, even when the other guidelines were based on little evidence. Thus, these processes are inherently slow to evolve and may lag considerably.

Graphic depictions of a healthy diet often are used to convey information to the public in a way that is intended to be friendly and effective. Examples of this include the original US Food Guide Pyramid (159), the 2010 dish-based icon (160) (http://www.choosemyplate.gov/), figures meant to be based on the Guidelines for Americans, and the Healthy Eating Pyramid developed at Harvard School of Public Health (161) (Fig. 104.1). Many other countries and organizations have developed similar graphics and there is no consensus on the ideal shape or method of conveying information. Condensing the massive literature on diet and health into a simple figure is challenging and requires that only the most important information be addressed. Whether these figures should represent volume, energy, or frequency of consumption also is unclear.

Indices

Dietary indices or scores have been created to represent a healthy diet. These are usually based on a priori information from many sources and have been used to assess diets of individuals or food programs (Table 104.2). One example is the Healthy Eating Index (HEI) (162), which was designed to be a quantitative measure of adherence to the US Dietary Guidelines and Food Guide Pyramid. Conceptually, this has been an important advance because

it provides a method for determining the degree to which federal food programs are consistent with the guidelines; an updated version has been created to represent the 2005 Dietary Guidelines (163). Other indices include those designed to summarize the important dietary factors in predicting risk of CHD (164) and the Mediterranean diet (165). An alternative approach to creating a dietary score is to use stepwise regression or other multivariate techniques to create a prediction score based on a health outcome in a specific population. This has been used to develop a prediction score for colon cancer (166).

Validation of Dietary Indices

The value of any dietary index or score depends on whether greater adherence is related to better health. If the index emphasizes irrelevant aspects of diet or fails to make important distinctions, its usefulness is impaired. A direct assessment of the validity of an index is to determine whether individuals with higher scores have better long-term health outcomes, taking into account other risk factors. As an example, the HEI was widely used to evaluate individual diets and food programs, but without examining the validity of the index. To address this, in parallel studies of 67,272 women and 38,622 men, McCullough et al (167, 168) examined whether higher scores on the HEI predicted future risk of major chronic disease, defined as any cancer, myocardial infarction, stroke, or death excluding those resulting from trauma. Although clear inverse relations were seen in age-adjusted analyses, after accounting for smoking, physical activity, and other risk factors, those with the highest HEI scores did not fare appreciably better than those with low scores (Fig. 104.2), indicating that

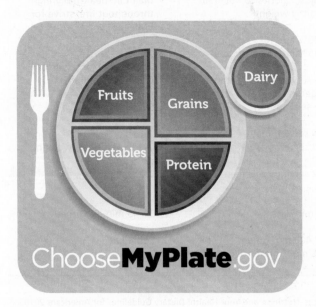

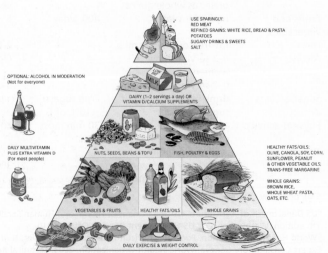

Fig. 104.1. Examples of graphical representations of a healthy diet: the US Department of Agriculture (USDA) Food Guide Pyramid, the USDA Choose MyPlate, and the Healthy Eating Pyramid (HEP). (HEP is reproduced with permission from Harvard School of Public Health. Healthy Eating Pyramid. 2000. Available at: http://www.hsph.harvard.edu/nutritionsource/.)

TABLE 104.2	PRESENTATION OF A HEALTHY DIET BY INDICES		
HEALTHY EATING INDEX[a]	**REVISED HEALTHY EATING INDEX**[b]	**CORONARY HEART DISEASE DIETARY INDEX**[c]	**MEDITERRANEAN DIET SCORE**[d]
Grains (servings/day)	Vegetables (servings/day)	Low *trans*-fat	Vegetables (g/day)
Vegetables (servings/day)	Fruits (servings/day)	High ratio of polyunsaturated to saturated fat	Legumes (g/day)
Fruits (servings/day)	Nuts and soy protein (servings/day)	High cereal fiber	Fruits and nuts (g/day)
Milk (servings/day)	Ratio of white to red meat	High marine omega-3 fatty acids	Cereals (g/day)
Meat (servings/day)	Cereal fiber (g/day)	High folate	Fish (g/day)
Total fat (% of E)	*Trans*-fat (% of E)	Low glycemic load	Red meat, poultry (g/day)
Saturated fat (% of E)	Polyunsaturated to saturated fat ratio		Dairy products (g/day)
Cholesterol (mg/day)	Duration of multivitamin use		Alcohol
Sodium (mg/day)	Alcohol (servings/day)		Monounsaturated to saturated fat ratio
Variety			
Each item scored 0–10	Each item scored 1–10, except	Each item scored	Each item scored 0–1
Total score range = 0–100	multivitamin use 2.5–7.5	1–5 (quintiles)	by adherence. For items
	Score range = 2.5–87.5	Score range = 6–30	1–5 at or above median
			intake scores 1. For items
			6–9 at or above median
			intake scores 0.
			Score range = 0–9

E, energy.

[a]US Department of Agriculture. The Healthy Eating Index. Washington, DC: US Government Printing Office, 1995.
[b]McCullough ML, Feskanich D, Stampfer MJ et al. Diet quality and major chronic disease risk in men and women: moving toward improved dietary guidance. Am J Clin Nutr 2002;76:1261–71.
[c]Stampfer MJ, Hu FB, Manson JE et al. Primary prevention of coronary heart disease in women through diet and lifestyle. N Engl J Med 2000;343:16–22.
[d]Trichopoulou A, Costacou T, Bamia C et al. Adherence to a Mediterranean diet and survival in a Greek population. N Engl J Med 2003;348:2599–608.

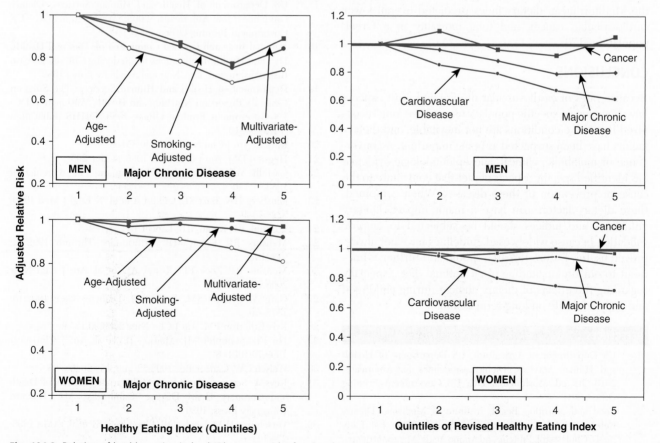

Fig. 104.2. Relation of healthy eating index (HEI) score to risk of major chronic disease. (Data from references 167 to 169.)

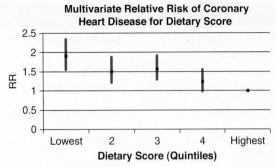

Fig. 104.3. Multivariate relative risk of coronary heart disease for dietary score. The score is based on intake of *trans* fat, ratio of polyunsaturated to saturated fat, long-chain n-3 fatty acids, cereal fiber, and glycemic load. (Data from Stampfer MJ, Hu FB, Manson JE et al. N Engl J Med 2000;343:16–22.)

the overall index had little value. A revised HEI, reflecting modified guidelines that took into account the type of fat, form of carbohydrate, and sources of protein, did significantly predict lower rates of major chronic disease, especially cardiovascular disease, in both men and women (169). In evaluations of other indices, a five-variable dietary score developed by Stampfer strongly predicted lower risk of CHD (164) (Fig. 104.3). When combined with not smoking, regular physical activity, avoidance of overweight, and moderate alcohol consumption, these findings indicate that greater than 80% of CHD is avoidable by diet and lifestyle changes. In another analysis, the Mediterranean dietary index predicted overall lower cardiovascular, cancer, and total mortality in a Greek population (170).

CONCLUSIONS

Because rates of cardiovascular disease and most cancers have been low in specific populations, we have long recognized that these conditions are not inevitable, and dietary factors have been suspected as being important. A convergence of metabolic, clinical, and epidemiologic evidence has identified specific aspects of diet that contribute to the cause or prevention of these diseases. When combined, these dietary factors can have a major impact. Dietary guidelines and indices should be subjected to empiric validation because widely used guidelines have not always proved useful. Future research should add further refinement to our understanding of an optimal diet, especially regarding the effects of dietary choices during childhood and early adult life on long-term health.

REFERENCES

1. US Department of Agriculture, US Department of Health and Human Services. Dietary Guidelines for Americans, 2010. 7th ed. Washington, DC: US Government Printing Office, 2010.
2. Food and Nutrition Board, Institute of Medicine. Dietary Reference Intakes for Energy, Carbohydrate, Fiber, Fat, Fatty Acids, Cholesterol, Protein, and Amino Acids (Macronutrients).

Washington, DC: National Academy of Sciences, 2002. Available at: http://www.nap.edu/catalog/10490.html. Accessed September 14, 2012.
3. World Health Organization, Food and Agriculture Organization. Diet, Nutrition and the Prevention of Chronic Diseases: Report of a Joint WHO/FAO Expert Consultation. Geneva: World Health Organization, 2003. Technical Report Series No. 916.
4. Food and Nutrition Board. Recommended Dietary Allowances. 10th rev ed. Washington, DC: National Academy Press, 1989.
5. Hayes O, Trulson MF, Stare FJ. J Am Diet Assoc 1955; 31:1103–7.
6. Katan MB, Beynen AC, de Vries JH et al. Am J Epidemiol 1986;123:221–34.
7. Beeks E, Kessels AG, Kroon AA et al. J Hypertens 2004; 22:1243–9.
8. Bailey LB, Gregory JF 3rd. J Nutr 1999;129:919–22.
9. Hegsted DM. Clin Nutr 1985;4:159–63.
10. Jeppesen J, Chen YDI, Zhou MY et al. Am J Clin Nutr 1995; 61:787–91.
11. Jeppesen J, Chen YD, Zhou MY et al. Am J Clin Nutr 1995; 62:1201–5.
12. Liu S, Manson JE, Stampfer MJ et al. Am J Clin Nutr 2001; 73:560–6.
13. Liu S, Willett WC, Stampfer MJ et al. Am J Clin Nutr 2000; 71:1455–61.
14. Dickinson S, Colagiuri S, Faramus E et al. J Nutr 2002; 132:2574–9.
15. Neel J. Am J Human Genet 1962;14:353–62.
16. Willett WC. Nutritional Epidemiology. 2nd ed. New York: Oxford University Press, 1998.
17. US Department of Health and Human Services. Dietary Guidelines for Americans, 2005. Washington, DC: US Government Printing Office, 2005.
18. National Research Council Committee on Diet and Health. Diet and Health. Implications for Reducing Chronic Disease Risk. Washington, DC: National Academy Press, 1989.
19. Department of Health and Human Services. The Surgeon General's Report on Nutrition and Health. Washington, DC: US Government Printing Office, 1988. DHHS publication (PHS) 50210.
20. Keys A. Am J Clin Nutr 1984;40:351–9.
21. Hegsted DM. Am J Clin Nutr 1986;44:299–305.
22. Castelli WP, Abbott RD, McNamara PM. Circulation 1983;67:730–4.
23. Ginsberg HN, Barr SL, Gilbert A et al. N Engl J Med 1990; 322:574–9.
24. Mensink RP, Katan MB. Lancet 1987;1:122–5.
25. Mensink RP, Katan MB. Arterioscler Thromb 1992;12: 911–19.
26. Mensink RP, Zock PL, Kester AD et al. Am J Clin Nutr 2003;77:1146–55.
27. Garg A, Grundy SM, Koffler M. Diabetes Care 1992;15: 1572–80.
28. Kris-Etherton PM. Am J Clin Nutr 2009;90:13–4.
29. Hu FB, Stampfer MJ, Manson JE et al. Am J Clin Nutr 1999;70:1001–8.
30. Welsch CW. Cancer Res 1992;52(Suppl 7):2040S–8S.
31. Keys A. Seven Countries: A Multivariate Analysis of Death and Coronary Heart Disease. Cambridge, MA: Harvard University Press, 1980.
32. Verschuren WM, Jacobs DR, Bloemberg BP et al. JAMA 1995; 274:131–6.

33. Hu F, Stampfer MJ, Manson JE et al. N Engl J Med 1997; 337:1491–9.
34. Jakobsen MU, O'Reilly EJ, Heitmann BL et al. Am J Clin Nutr 2009;89:1425–32.
35. Sacks F. J Cardiovasc Risk 1994;1:3–8.
36. GISSI-Prevention Investigators. Lancet 1999;354:447–55.
37. Albert CM, Campos H, Stampfer MJ et al. N Engl J Med 2002;346:1113–8.
38. Albert CM, Hennekens CH, O'Donnell CJ et al. JAMA 1998;279:23–8.
39. de Lorgeril M, Renaud S, Mamelle N et al. [Erratum in: Lancet 1995;345:738]. Lancet 1994;343:1454–9.
40. Campos H, Baylin A, Willett WC. Circulation 2008;118: 339–45.
41. Simopoulos AP, Leaf A, Salem N Jr. Prostaglandins Leukot Essent Fatty Acids 2000;63:119–21.
42. Willett WC. J Cardiovasc Med (Hagerstown) 2007;8(Suppl 1): S42–5.
43. Hu FB, Stampfer MJ, Manson JE et al. Am J Clin Nutr 1999; 69:890–7.
44. Goyens PL, Spilker ME, Zock PL et al. Am J Clin Nutr 2006; 84:44–53.
45. Ascherio A, Katan MB, Zock PL et al. N Engl J Med 1999; 340:1994–8.
46. Lichtenstein AH, Ausman LM, Jalbert SM et al. N Engl J Med 1999;340:1933–40.
47. Nestel P, Noakes M, Belling B. J Lipid Res 1992;33:1029–36.
48. Mensink RP, Zock PL, Katan MB et al. J Lipid Res 1992;33:1493–1501.
49. Mozaffarian D, Pischon T, Hankinson SE et al. Am J Clin Nutr 2004;79:606–12.
50. Baer DJ, Judd JT, Clevidence BA et al. Am J Clin Nutr 2004;79:969–73.
51. Mozaffarian D, Katan MB, Ascherio A et al. N Engl J Med 2006;354:1601–13.
52. Mozaffarian D, Jacobson MF, Greenstein JS. N Engl J Med 2010;362:2037–9.
53. Hu FB, van Dam RM, Liu S. Diabetologia 2001;44:805–17.
54. Riserus U, Willett WC, Hu FB. Prog Lipid Res 2009;48: 44–51.
55. van Dam RM, Willett WC, Rimm EB et al. Diabetes Care 2002;25:417–24.
56. Fung TT, Schulze MB, Manson JE et al. Arch Intern Med 2004;164:2235–40.
57. Prentice RL, Sheppard L. Cancer Causes Control 1990;1: 81–97.
58. Armstrong B, Doll R. Int J Cancer 1975;15:617–631.
59. Ip C. Quantitative assessment of fat and calorie as risk factors in mammary carcinogenesis in an experimental model. In: Mettlin CJ, Aoki K, eds. Recent Progress in Research on Nutrition and Cancer: Proceedings of a Workshop Sponsored by the International Union Against Cancer, Held in Nagoya, Japan, November 1–3, 1989. New York: Wiley-Liss, 1990: 107–17.
60. Freedman LS, Clifford C, Messina M. Cancer Res 1990; 50:5710–19.
61. Appleton BS, Landers RE. Adv Exp Med Biol 1986;206: 99–104.
62. Smith-Warner SA, Spiegelman D, Adami HO et al. Int J Cancer 2001;92:767–74.
63. Hunter DJ, Spiegelman D, Adami HO et al. N Engl J Med 1996;334:356–61.
64. Prentice RL, Caan B, Chlebowski RT et al. JAMA 2006; 295:629–42.
65. Martin LJ, Li Q, Melnichouk O et al. Cancer Res 2011;71: 123–33.
66. Cho E, Spiegelman D, Hunter DJ et al. J Natl Cancer Inst 2003;95:1079–85.
67. Linos E, Willett WC, Cho E et al. Cancer Epidemiol Biomarkers Prev 2008;17:2146–51.
68. Cho E, Chen WY, Hunter DJ et al. Arch Intern Med 2006;166:2253–9.
69. World Cancer Research Fund/American Institute for Cancer Research. Second Expert Report: Food, Nutrition, Physical Activity, and the Prevention of Cancer: A Global Perspective. London: WCRF, 2007.
70. Gerhardsson de Verdier M, Hagman U, Peters RK et al. Int J Cancer 1991;49:520–5.
71. Babbs CF. Free Radic Biol Med 1990;8:191–200.
72. Carayol M, Grosclaude P, Delpierre C. Cancer Causes Control 2010;21:347–55.
73. Bray GA, Popkin BM. Am J Clin Nutr 1998;68:1157–73.
74. Willett WC, Leibel RL. Am J Med 2002;113(Suppl 9B): 47S–59S.
75. Jeppesen J, Hollenbeck CB, Zhou MY et al. Arterioscler Thromb Vasc Biol 1995;15:320–4.
76. Willett WC, Stampfer M, Chu N et al. Am J Epidemiol 2001;154:1107–12.
77. Jenkins DJ, Wolever TM, Taylor RH et al. Am J Clin Nutr 1981;34:362–6.
78. Barclay AW, Petocz P, McMillan-Price J et al. Am J Clin Nutr 2008;87:627–37.
79. Salmeron J, Manson JE, Stampfer MJ et al. JAMA 1997; 277:472–7.
80. Salmeron J, Ascherio A, Rimm EB et al. Diabetes Care 1997;20:545–50.
81. Hu FB, Willett WC. JAMA 2002;288:2569–78.
82. Park Y, Hunter DJ, Spiegelman D et al. JAMA 2005;294: 2849–57.
83. Aldoori WH, Giovannucci EL, Rockett HR et al. J Nutr 1998;128:714–9.
84. Schroeder HA. Am J Clin Nutr 1971;24:562–73.
85. Appel LJ, Sacks FM, Carey VJ et al. JAMA 2005;294: 2455–64.
86. Hu FB, Stampfer MJ, Manson JE et al. Am J Clin Nutr 1999;70:221–7.
87. Hu FB, Stampfer MJ. Curr Atheroscler Reports 1999;1:204–9.
88. Jiang R, Manson JE, Stampfer MJ et al. JAMA 2002;288: 2554–60.
89. Bernstein AM, Sun Q, Hu FB et al. Circulation 2010; 122(9):876–83.
90. Koushik A, Hunter DJ, Spiegelman D et al. J Natl Cancer Inst 2007;99:1471–83.
91. Smith-Warner SA, Spiegelman D, Yaun SS et al. JAMA 2001;285:769–76.
92. Smith-Warner SA, Spiegelman D, Yaun SS et al. Int J Cancer 2003;107(6):1001–11.
93. Lee JE, Giovannucci E, Smith-Warner SA et al. Cancer Epidemiol Biomarkers Prev 2006;15:2445–52.
94. Fung TT, Hu FB, Holmes MD et al. Int J Cancer 2005; 116:116–21.
95. Giovannucci E. J Natl Cancer Inst 1999;91:317–31.
96. Hung HC, Joshipura K, Jiang R et al. J Natl Cancer Inst 2004;21:1577–84.
97. Stampfer MJ, Malinow MR, Willett WC et al. JAMA 1992; 268:877–81.
98. Selhub J, Jacques PF, Bostom AG et al. N Engl J Med 1995; 332:286–91.

99. Tucker KL, Olson B, Bakun P et al. Am J Clin Nutr 2004; 79:805–11.

100. Sacks FM, Svetkey LP, Vollmer WM et al. N Engl J Med 2001;344:3–10.

101. Sacks FM, Willett WC, Smith A et al. Hypertension 1998; 31:131–8.

102. Werler MM, Shapiro S, Mitchell AA. JAMA 1993;269: 1257–61.

103. Chasan-Taber L, Willett WC, Seddon JM et al. Am J Clin Nutr 1999;70:509–16.

104. Brown L, Rimm EB, Seddon JM et al. Am J Clin Nutr 1999;70:517–24.

105. Chapuy MC, Arlot ME, Duboeuf F et al. N Engl J Med 1992;327:1637–42.

106. Institute of Medicine. Dietary Reference Intakes for Calcium and Vitamin D. Washington, DC: National Academy of Sciences, 2010.

107. Scientific Advisory Committee on Nutrition (SACN). Key Dietary Recommendations. London: SACN, 2002.

108. Nordin BEC. Clin Orthop 1966;45:17–20.

109. Hegsted DM. J Nutr 1986;116:2316–19.

110. Bischoff-Ferrari HA, Dawson-Hughes B, Baron JA et al. Am J Clin Nutr 2007;86:1780–90.

111. Bischoff-Ferrari HA, Dawson-Hughes B, Baron JA et al. J Bone Miner Res 2010; 21: 1121–32.

112. Feskanich D, Willett W, Colditz G. JAMA 2002;288:2300–6.

113. Wickham CAC, Walsh K, Cooper C et al. BMJ 1989;299: 889–92.

114. Bischoff-Ferrari HA, Willett WC, Wong JB et al. Arch Intern Med 2009;169:551–61.

115. McCarron DA, Morris CD, Henry HJ et al. Science 1984; 224:1392–8.

116. Cutler JA, Brittain E. Am J Hypertens 1990;3:137S–146S.

117. Bolland MJ, Avenell A, Baron JA et al. BMJ 2010;341:c3691.

118. Cho E, Smith-Warner S, Spiegelman D et al. J Natl Cancer Inst 2004;96:1015–22.

119. Baron JA, Beach M, Mandel JS et al. N Engl J Med 1999; 340:101–7.

120. Giovannucci E. Nutritional and environmental epidemiology of prostate cancer. In: Kantoff PW, Carroll PR, D'Amico AV, eds. Prostate Cancer: Principles and Practice. Philadelphia: Lippincott Williams & Wilkins, 2002:117–39.

121. Law MR, Frost CD, Wald NJ. BMJ 1991;302:819–24.

122. Bibbins-Domingo K, Chertow GM, Coxson PG et al. N Engl J Med 2010;362:590–9.

123. Klatsky AL, Armstrong MA, Friedman GD. Am J Cardiol 1990;66:1237–42.

124. Hines LM, Stampfer MJ, Ma J et al. N Engl J Med 2001; 344:549–55.

125. Hines LM, Rimm EB. Postgrad Med J 2001;77:747–52.

126. Mukamal KJ, Conigrave KM, Mittleman MA et al. N Engl J Med 2003;348:109–18.

127. Smith-Warner SA, Spiegelman D, Yaun SS et al. JAMA 1998;279:535–40.

128. Reichman ME, Judd JT, Longcope C et al. J Natl Cancer Inst 1993;85:722–27.

129. Hankinson SE, Willett WC, Manson JE et al. J Natl Cancer Inst 1995;87:1297–1302.

130. Boffetta P, Garfinkel L. Epidemiology 1990;1:342–8.

131. Fuchs CS, Stampfer MJ, Colditz GA et al. N Engl J Med 1995;332:1245–50.

132. MRC Vitamin Study Research Group. Lancet 1991;338:131–7.

133. Lee JE, Willett WC, Fuchs CS et al. Am J Clin Nutr 2011;93:817–25.

134. Kim DH, Smith-Warner SA, Spiegelman D et al. Cancer Causes Control 2010;21:1919–30.

135. Rimm EB, Willett WC, Hu FB et al. JAMA 1998;279:359–64.

136. Clarke R, Halsey J, Lewington S et al. Arch Intern Med 2010;170:1622–31.

137. Wang X, Qin X, Demirtas H et al. Lancet 2007;369:1876–82.

138. Selhub J, Morris MS, Jacques PF et al. Am J Clin Nutr 2009;89:702S–6S.

139. Looker AC, Johnson CL, Lacher DA et al. Vitamin D status: United States, 2001–2006. NCHS Data Brief 2011:1–8.

140. Bischoff-Ferrari HA, Dawson-Hughes B, Staehelin HB et al. BMJ 2009;339:b3692.

141. Lee JE, Li H, Chan AT et al. Cancer Prev Res (Phila) 2011; 4:735–43.

142. Bischoff-Ferrari HA, Dietrich T, Orav EJ et al. Am J Med 2004;116:634–9.

143. Jackson RD, LaCroix AZ, Gass M et al. N Engl J Med 2006; 354:669–83.

144. Bolland MJ, Grey A, Avenell A et al. BMJ 2011;342:d2040.

145. Centers for Disease Control. MMWR Morb Mortal Wkly Rep 2002;51:897–9.

146. Rajpathak S, Ma J, Manson J et al. Diabetes Care 2006; 29:1370–6.

147. Qi L, Meigs J, Manson JE et al. Diabetes 2005;54:3567–72.

148. Blot WJ, Li JY, Taylor PR et al. J Natl Cancer Inst 1993; 85:1483–92.

149. Fawzi WW, Msamanga GI, Spiegelman D et al. N Engl J Med 2004;351:23–32.

150. Hercberg S, Galan P, Preziosi P et al. Arch Intern Med 2004;164:2335–42.

151. Feskanich D, Singh V, Willett WC et al. JAMA 2002;287:47–54.

152. Melhus H, Michaelsson K, Kindmark A et al. Ann Intern Med 1998;129:770–78.

153. Michaelsson K, Lithell H, Vessby B et al. N Engl J Med 2003;348:287–94.

154. Johansson S, Melhus H. J Bone Miner Res 2001;16:1899–905.

155. Block G, Patterson B, Subar A. Nutr Cancer 1992;18:1–29.

156. Block G, Abrams B. Ann N Y Acad Sci 1993;678:244–54.

157. Krebs-Smith SM, Guenther PM, Subar AF et al. J Nutr 2010;140:1832–8.

158. Appel LJ, Frohlich ED, Hall JE et al. Circulation 2011; 123:1138–43.

159. US Department of Agriculture. The food guide pyramid. Home and Garden Bulletin No. 252. Washington, DC: GPO, 1992:30.

160. US Department of Agriculture. ChooseMyPlate, 2011. Available at: http://www.choosemyplate.gov. Accessed March 26, 2012.

161. Harvard School of Public Health. Healthy Eating Pyramid. 2000. Available at: http://www.hsph.harvard.edu/nutritionsource/. Accessed September 14, 2012.

162. Kennedy ET, Ohls J, Carlson S et al. J Am Diet Assoc 1995; 95:1103–8.

163. Guenther PM, Reedy J, Krebs-Smith SM et al. Development and Evaluation of the Healthy Eating Index 2005: Technical Report. Washington, DC: US Department of Agriculture, Center for Nutrition Policy and Promotion, 2007.

164. Stampfer MJ, Hu FB, Manson JE et al. N Engl J Med 2000; 343:16–22.

165. Trichopoulou A, Lagiou P, Kuper H et al. Cancer Epidemiol Biomarkers Prev 2000;9:869–73.

166. McCullough ML, Robertson AS, Rodriguez C et al. Cancer Causes Control 2003;14:1–12.

167. McCullough ML, Feskanich D, Stampfer MJ et al. Am J Clin Nutr 2000;72:1214–22.

heart disease and stroke in US women (48), and with lower incidence of type 2 diabetes in US adults. In the Insulin Resistance Atherosclerosis Study (IRAS), adults in the highest, versus the lowest, tertile of DASH adherence score were 69% less likely to develop incident diabetes over 5 years (49). However, one cohort study using a DASH score did not find associations with hypertension or cardiovascular mortality in a large cohort of US women; the investigators noted that adherence to the score may have been too low to see an effect (50).

DASH diet scores have also been examined in youth. An intervention with adolescents with prehypertension or hypertension who were randomly assigned to standard of care or to a DASH diet intervention showed that those in the DASH group had greater declines in systolic blood pressure (51). Among youth 10 to 22 years of age with type 1 diabetes, those in the highest DASH diet score tertile had significantly lower blood pressure (52), lower LDL/HDL cholesterol ratios, and lower glycosylated hemoglobin than those in the lowest tertile (53). Prospectively, adolescent girls in the Prospective National Growth and Health Study had lower gains in BMI over 10 years, when in the highest, versus the lowest, quintile of DASH diet score (54).

Together, the evidence for the DASH diet in chronic disease prevention is strong. Although designed specifically for lowering blood pressure, this diet has been shown to have beneficial effects on other metabolic indicators, a finding suggesting that it is likely a beneficial behavior for health in most individuals. Given the general success of the DASH diet, it has been promoted for general population use by the National Heart, Lung, and Blood Institute (55), the Mayo Clinic (56), the American Heart Association (57), and in a popular book (58).

Dietary Patterns from Observed Healthy Populations: The Mediterranean Diet Score

The DASH diet is not the only approach to healthy eating, however. The AHEI, described earlier, was a modification of the original HEI to include additional evidence on diet and health, particularly aspects of an observed dietary pattern that has been associated with lower chronic disease risk relative to other regional patterns: the Mediterranean diet. This diet was first highlighted in 1970 by Ancel Keys in his seven-country study (59). CHD was noted to be lower in the Mediterranean region than other parts of the world, although total fat intake—in the form mainly of olive oil—was not low. In 1995, a Mediterranean diet pyramid was introduced, following an expert conference sponsored by Oldways Preservation & Exchange Trust (http://www.oldwayspt.org/mediterraneandiet) and the World Health Organization/Food and Agriculture Organization Collaborating Center in nutritional epidemiology at the Harvard School of Public Health in Boston (60). This pyramid was based on the food patterns of Crete, other parts of Greece, and southern Italy in the 1960s (61). The 1960s

Mediterranean diet was characterized by high intakes of fruit, vegetables, breads and cereals, potatoes, beans, and nuts and seeds, with olive oil as the principal source of fat; low to moderate amounts of cheese and yogurt, fish, poultry, and eggs; moderate amounts of wine, consumed mainly with meals; and low intakes of red meat. This diet is low in saturated fat (≤8% of energy), with total fat from 25% to more than 35%.

A score specifically to describe adherence to the traditional Mediterranean diet was first developed in Greece and included 1 point each for being above the sex-specific median for 6 items (ratio of monounsaturated to saturated fat; alcohol consumption; intake of legumes; intake of cereals, bread, and potatoes; intake of fruit; intake of vegetables) and for being below the median for 2 items (intake of meat and meat products and intake of milk and dairy products) (62). In a relatively small sample of elderly adults followed for 4 to 5 years, each additional point in the score was associated with 17% lower risk of mortality. The association of the total score with mortality was considerably stronger than for any of the individual components. This analysis was then scaled up to a large Greek population (almost 26,000 adults), followed for a mean of 3.7 years, with adaptations to the score to limit alcohol to 10 to 50 g/day for men or 5 to 25 g/day for women and to add high fish intake, thus bringing the new score to 9 possible points (63). Again, the investigators found that higher adherence to the Mediterranean diet was associated with a 25% reduction in total mortality with 2 score points, with hazard ratios of 0.76 (95% confidence interval, 0.59 to 0.98) for cancer mortality and 0.67 (0.47 to 0.94) for CHD.

Since then, this score, or an adapted version of it, has been used in numerous studies, with results showing protection against CHD and cancer mortality in in several countries, including large studies in the United States. (64). Among others, studies have shown that higher Mediterranean diet scores were associated with lower risk for several cancers (65), hypertension (66), obesity (67), abdominal obesity (68), and diabetes (69). In addition, adherence to a Mediterranean-type diet has been associated with lower risk of Alzheimer disease (70) and of Parkinson disease (71), as well as improved fertility (72) and better birth outcomes (73). Interventions using this diet have also shown success in management of the metabolic syndrome (when supplemented with nuts) (74), with weight loss (relative to a low-fat diet) (75), and to improved control of arthritis symptoms (76).

Empiric Dietary Patterns: Principal Components and Cluster Analyses

The patterns described previously have been well tested, and results support the importance of a total diet approach to health. However, it is likely that multiple combinations of dietary constituents may be beneficial, and it is important to continue to understand how people choose to eat and how this relates to health outcomes. From this perspective, there has been growing interest in extracting dietary pattern behavior from within existing population groups. This is important for continued improvement in understanding the types of diets that may be beneficial to diverse groups of individuals as well as for understanding existing behavior as a baseline for change.

The methods most commonly used to derive patterns from data include principal components analysis (PCA), which identifies factors within the correlation matrix, and cluster analysis, which maximally separates individuals into groups with similar versus differing food intake patterns (77). Both approaches require initial definition of food group variables from the dietary data. Because of the empiric nature of the methods, there is no clearly accepted list of food groups, and many different assumptions have been used. These assumptions range from the use of individual food codes (78) (which does not tend to perform well because of multiple zeros and collinearity of some items that may be overweighted in the overall pattern as recipes, such as salad items) to a small number of major food groups (79), which may mask important differences in actual pattern and their associations with other foods (e.g., grouping all dairy products together rather than identifying selection of low-fat products).

Food groups may be included in the analysis in several forms. The two most common forms are percentage of contribution to total calories, which allows a pattern to emerge relative to requirement or intake, and the number of servings of food groups, which is useful when total energy intake is not available.

Early analyses tended to use grams of food intake, which can be problematic when creating food groups because of variations in weight from water content. Over time, the field has tended to settle in on similar food groups of intermediate size ranging, for the most part, from about 30 to about 50 groups, as a balance that minimizes zeros and distorted collinearity in the data but that preserves separation of behaviors within traditional food groups (77).

Principal Components Analysis

PCA identifies dimensions of correlations in the data to create factors that explain variance in the correlation or covariance matrix. Although there are variations in approaches to PCA, the standard approach that has been used most frequently in nutritional epidemiologic studies is to define the factors within the correlation matrix of food group intakes. This results in weighted linear combinations of food groups that are intercorrelated and therefore describe an eating pattern in the population with continuous degrees of adherence (Table 105.2). Because factors continue to be generated, with decreasing variance explained sequentially up to the number of variables entered, it is necessary to select the number of meaningful factors to retain. This is generally done based on eigenvalues (percentage of variance explained), scree

TABLE 105.2   EXAMPLE OF DIETARY PATTERNS DETERMINED BY PRINCIPAL COMPONENTS ANALYSIS[a]

FOOD GROUP	PRUDENT PATTERN	WESTERN PATTERN
Other vegetables	0.75	
Green leafy vegetables	0.64	
Dark yellow vegetables	0.63	
Cruciferous vegetables	0.63	
Legumes	0.61	
Fruit	0.57	
Tomatoes	0.56	
Fish	0.51	
Garlic	0.42	
Poultry	0.36	
Whole grains	0.35	
Red meat		0.63
Processed meat		0.59
Refined grains		0.49
Sweets and desserts		0.47
French fries		0.46
High-fat dairy		0.45
Eggs		0.39
High-sugar drinks		0.38
Snacks		0.37
Condiments		0.36
Margarine		0.34
Potatoes		0.33
Butter		0.31

[a]Absolute values <0.030 not listed.

Adapted with permission from Hu FB, Rimm EB, Stampfer MJ et al. Prospective study of major dietary patterns and risk of coronary heart disease in men. Am J Clin Nutr 2000;72:912–21. Data are from the Health Professionals Follow-Up Study.

plots (visual plots of sequential variance explained), and interpretability.

Once the factors retained are identified, these are then rotated, usually with a varimax rotation procedure, to improve clarity and to remove overlapping variance. Because there can be considerable subjectivity based not only on the food group definitions but also in analysis decisions, early use of PCA raised concerns about whether it would provide replicable solutions. However, as best practices have evolved in the field, and results and patterns have been identified as generally replicable when expected to be, this method has gained acceptance and is now used regularly (80).

Once the rotated factors are extracted, each individual is given a factor score for each derived factor. The score is calculated as the sum of the factor loadings for each food group within the factor, which is the correlation of the food group to the overall intercorrelation of the factor (ranging from −1.0 to +1.0), multiplied by the actual intake of the respective food group by the individual. This sum creates unique individual scores, expressed in standardized Z-score form (81). The result is a set of continuous factor score variables that may then be used in subsequent analyses on health measures. Using the method described earlier results in orthogonal variables, so that all the retained factors may be put into the same model as linear variables, without influencing the others. In practice, many studies divide the factors into quintiles or other quantiles to associate intakes with health outcomes.

Pioneering work on deriving dietary patterns using factor analysis was done by Schwerin et al (79, 82) using data from the 10-state survey and National Health and Nutrition Examination Survey I (NHANES I). These investigators used gram weights of 15 food groups as the input variables and retained 7 patterns. They noted that certain eating patterns were significantly associated with better health, measured as absence of biochemical deficiencies and clinical symptoms, and emphasized that understanding existing dietary patterns is important because ". . . the findings offer knowledge of how people actually eat, rather than of what they should eat" (82). They further noted that this is important for behavior change because "educational and communications experience alike teach that change is more successfully engineered from the base of individual's existing behavior and attitudes, than from the goal one seeks to reach" (82).

Using this method in a case control study of colon cancer in several US sites, Slattery et al (83) were the first to label two major patterns as "prudent," characterized by high factor loadings on fresh fruit, cruciferous vegetables, carrots and tomatoes, legumes, salad, and other vegetables; and "Western," characterized by high loadings on processed meat, red meat, eggs, refined grains, and added sugars. These investigators found that greater adherence to the Western pattern was associated with significantly greater risk of colon cancer in both men and women, whereas adherence to the prudent pattern was associated with lower risk. Subsequently, Hu et al (84, 85) identified similar patterns in the Male Health Professionals Study and showed that they were predictive of CHD. The prudent pattern of Hu et al was characterized by higher intake of vegetables, fruit, legumes, whole grains, fish, and poultry; and the Western pattern was characterized by higher intake of red meat, processed meat, refined grains, sweets and desserts, french fries, and high-fat dairy products. After adjustment for age and CHD risk factors, those in the highest (versus lowest) quintile of the prudent pattern score were 30% less likely to have incident CHD (nonfatal myocardial infarction or fatal CHD) over 8 years of follow-up, whereas those in the highest (versus lowest) quintile of the Western pattern score were 64% more likely to have incident CHD. Since then, studies have shown protective associations with the prudent pattern and risk associations with the Western pattern with numerous health outcomes in varying populations.

A 2004 review identified 58 studies that used factor analysis to derive dietary patterns (86). At that time, some type of prudent or healthy diet was identified by most studies, and some type of Western or high-meat diet was identified by many. Although this terminology has been widely adopted, with generally "healthy" patterns labeled as prudent and high meat, refined grains patterns as Western, there is usually some, and sometimes considerable,

variation in specific foods loading on each factor across studies (77). Other patterns reported frequently have included "desserts and sweets" or "alcoholic beverages."

Patterns across many diverse studies have been significantly associated with measures of CVD, CHD, obesity, cancers, metabolic syndrome, hypertension, hyperlipidemia, diabetes, and all-cause mortality. More recent studies include a review and metaanalysis that showed an estimated 11% decreased risk of breast cancer in the highest (versus lowest) categories of prudent and healthy dietary patterns ($p = .02$) in pooled cohort studies and a 21% increased risk for the highest (versus lowest) categories of alcohol intake dietary patterns ($p = .01$) (87). Another study, in middle-aged participants, found that a processed food dietary pattern was associated with depressive symptoms 5 years later, whereas a whole foods pattern was protective (88).

PCA dietary patterns have been applied also to maternal and child health. In the Norwegian Mother and Child Cohort Study (MoBa), 23,423 nulliparous pregnant women completed a food frequency questionnaire at gestational weeks 17 to 22. PCA identified dietary patterns labeled vegetables, processed food, potato and fish, and cakes and sweets. Women in the highest (versus lowest) tertile of the PCA pattern characterized by vegetables, plant foods, and vegetable oils were 28% less likely to develop preeclampsia, whereas women in the highest (versus lowest) tertile of the pattern characterized by processed meat, salty snacks, and sweet drinks were 21% more likely to develop this condition (89). Another study found no association between maternal dietary pattern and child asthma at 3 years (90).

Cluster Analysis

Cluster analysis is a popular alternative to PCA for extracting a posteriori dietary patterns. Rather than linking correlated variables in linear combinations that result in individual scores, cluster analysis groups individuals into mutually exclusive categories based on the similarity of their eating behaviors. In this method, the algorithm examines the similarity of variables within individuals and then groups individuals with similar patterns in multidimensional space by minimizing differences within groups and maximizing differences among groups (91). Most of the studies using cluster analysis use a K-means approach to grouping, which is efficient with large samples and has been shown to have good reproducibility with dietary patterns (92). One study compared different approaches and confirmed that the K-means produced the most reproducible dietary clusters (92).

This method is iterative and creates clusters based on the mean intakes, or centroids, of the input variables. Once preliminary groups are defined, all individuals are reassigned to the nearest cluster center (by Euclidian distance) until no more reassignment occurs, thus maximizing separation. This method has the advantage of directly describing mean intakes of subgroups, thereby providing quantitative information on subgroup diets

TABLE 105.3	EXAMPLE OF DIETARY PATTERNS FROM CLUSTER ANALYSIS[a]				
	STARCHY VEGETABLES (*n* = 174)	SWEETS AND STARCHY GRAINS (*n* = 173)	RICE, BEANS, AND OIL (*n* = 170)	HEALTHY (*n* = 170)	WHOLE MILK (*n* = 138)
Starchy vegetables	**9.9 ± 7.6**	0.7 ± 1.8	4.6 ± 4.7	1.5 ± 2.4	3.6 ± 3.9
Poultry	**8.0 ± 5.5**	4.0 ± 3.5	**8.0 ± 5.4**	5.7 ± 4.2	5.7 ± 4.9
Sweet baked goods	1.6 ± 2.7	**10.4 ± 9.4**	1.0 ± 1.9	2.3 ± 3.0	2.5 ± 3.9
Bread	5.6 ± 4.5	**9.0 ± 6.6**	4.4 ± 3.9	6.9 ± 4.7	5.2 ± 4.4
Pasta	1.5 ± 2.0	**4.6 ± 5.7**	1.9 ± 3.2	3.4 ± 4.1	1.6 ± 2.3
Candy and sugars	1.8 ± 3.1	**3.9 ± 6.1**	1.7 ± 4.0	1.9 ± 3.1	2.2 ± 2.9
Meat	4.6 ± 3.7	**6.2 ± 4.4**	4.5 ± 3.8	3.6 ± 3.1	3.6 ± 3.0
Dairy desserts	3.4 ± 3.0	**4.8 ± 4.9**	2.2 ± 2.1	3.3 ± 3.2	3.0 ± 2.6
Rice	12.2 ± 4.0	2.7 ± 3.8	**22.7 ± 4.8**	5.0 ± 4.7	10.1 ± 6.0
Beans and legumes	4.9 ± 3.3	2.1 ± 3.3	**6.7 ± 4.2**	2.4 ± 2.3	3.4 ± 2.8
Added oil and fats	8.2 ± 3.4	6.2 ± 4.4	**12.4 ± 2.9**	5.3 ± 3.6	7.1 ± 3.2
Breakfast cereal	4.3 ± 4.3	4.8 ± 4.7	2.4 ± 3.5	**12.9 ± 8.1**	5.8 ± 5.2
Low-fat milk	2.2 ± 3.8	2.2 ± 3.1	2.0 ± 4.0	**7.7 ± 9.6**	0.2 ± 0.7
Citrus fruit	4.1 ± 4.0	3.0 ± 3.0	2.4 ± 3.4	**5.0 ± 6.2**	3.2 ± 3.3
Other fruit	6.7 ± 5.7	4.4 ± 4.6	3.3 ± 3.2	**7.3 ± 5.2**	3.7 ± 3.2
Whole milk	3.7 ± 3.9	3.9 ± 4.7	5.6 ± 5.7	4.1 ± 4.2	**20.3 ± 7.5**
Soft drinks	2.2 ± 3.5	3.0 ± 4.9	2.8 ± 3.8	1.5 ± 3.5	**3.8 ± 5.1**

[a]Values are percentage of total energy from each food group. Food groups contributing less than 3.5% of energy to any cluster group are omitted here for simplicity. Numbers in boldface boldface identify the pattern (column) with the greatest intake of that food group, relative to the other patterns.

Adapted with permission from Lin H, Bermudez OI, Tucker KL. Dietary patterns of Hispanic elders are associated with acculturation and obesity. J Nutr 2003;133:3651–7. Data are from the Massachusetts Hispanic Elders Study.

and their risk with associated variables (Table 105.3). Although more intuitive than factor scores, grouping in this way results in a loss of statistical power, relative to the continuous factor measures described earlier. Therefore, it is most useful with large samples. The clustering method requires that the number of clusters be prespecified, and this introduces some subjectivity into the final selection, not unlike that with PCA. Most investigators run several sets of clusters and make a final decision based on distribution of individuals and on interpretability of patterns.

An early example of cluster analysis identified four patterns among older adults in the Boston area (93). Four major patterns were identified, with relatively high consumption of alcohol; milk, cereals, and fruits; bread and poultry; or meat and potatoes. The milk, breakfast cereals, and fruits group had the highest micronutrient intakes and plasma concentrations; the high meat and potato group had the lowest micronutrient intakes and plasma folate and vitamin B_6; the high alcohol had the lowest plasma riboflavin and vitamin B_{12} but the highest HDL cholesterol; and the bread and poultry group had the highest mean BMI. These findings confirmed expected patterns and reinforced the idea that overall dietary pattern can capture nutritional status. Healthy dietary patterns identified by cluster analysis have been associated with lower measures of subclinical heart disease (94, 95), lower gains in BMI or waist circumference over time (96), lower plasma triglycerides (97), greater insulin sensitivity and lower systemic inflammation in older adults (98), higher bone mineral density (99), more years of healthy life (100), lower incidence of diabetes and coronary events (101), and lower risk of adenocarcinoma of the esophagus and stomach (102).

Most recently, the Coronary Artery Risk Development in Young Adults (CARDIA) study identified the same prudent (higher intakes of fruit, whole grains, milk, and nuts and seeds) and Western (higher intakes of fast food, meat and poultry, pizza, and snacks) patterns often identified with PCA (103). In a 20-year follow-up, these investigators examined the interaction of diet soft drink consumption with these patterns on risk of metabolic syndrome. Prudent nonconsumers of nondiet soft drinks had the lowest risk of high waist circumference, high triglycerides, and the metabolic syndrome compared with Western consumers.

Results with more specific clusters include the observation that, although a meat and potatoes cluster showed the expected highest gains in BMI over time, a cluster high in refined grains showed the greatest gains in waist circumference over 4 years in older adults (96). The Health ABC study found that older adults in a high-fat dairy products cluster or a sweets and baked products cluster had 40% greater risk of mortality, relative to a healthy cluster, over years of follow-up (104).

Comparison of Principal Components Analysis with Cluster Analysis

Comparison of PCA with cluster analysis has shown good general replicability of patterns. In the Baltimore Longitudinal Study of Aging (97), similar patterns were identified by both methods. Both identified a healthy pattern, and both of these were associated with lower plasma triglycerides than other patterns. Further, alcohol patterns identified by both methods were associated with higher total cholesterol. A large UK study of children found that both PCA and cluster analysis identified three

- Identification of tolerable upper levels of intake, given changes in the food supply, including increased use of dietary supplements
- Greater consideration of chronic disease end points as well as more traditional endpoints in determining nutrient adequacy or adverse health effects

Additionally, the original vitamins, minerals, proteins, and calories specified in 1941 expanded over time to include a range of nutrient substances, including food constituents, such as total fiber and water. Table 106.1 shows the increasing number of nutritional substances for which reference values have been developed.

The DRIs now serve as a science standard for federal nutrition guidance and are either the statutory or de facto standard for virtually all national nutrition assistance programs. Over time, they have been applied in everyday life—such as by bankruptcy courts to determine income for food expenses—and they have increasingly been used by dietetic practitioners in settings very different from those imagined in the 1940s, when the concern was an adequate food supply and military preparedness. They are now also used as a basis for nutritional standards in a number of other countries.

KEY COMPONENTS

In the 1990s, the DRIs were envisioned as a set of values that would include more than an RDA; specifically, additions were outlined that became known as the estimated average requirement (EAR) and the tolerable upper intake level (UL). Activities in 1997 and beyond added other types of nutrient reference values to the DRIs. The types of values that comprise the DRIs at this time are shown in Table 106.2 and are discussed in the next section.

DRIs, along with descriptive text, are contained in six volumes published by NAS between 1997 and 2004 (http://www.iom.edu/dris). These publications represent the first generation of DRIs. To help users understand the application of the DRIs, two publications were created to provide general guidance. One is focused on applications related to dietary assessment (8) and the other on applications for dietary planning (9). In 2006, NAS issued *Dietary Reference Intakes: The Essential Guide to Nutrient Requirements* (10), which is also available in French. It provides an overall summary of the DRIs through 2004. After a 2007 workshop that focused on lessons learned during the development of the initial set of DRIs (11), a new report initiated the second generation of DRIs. Specifically, in 2009 to 2010, the DRIs for calcium and vitamin D were reviewed and updated, and a report was published in 2011 (12). Tables containing all the current DRI values can be viewed at the website http://www.iom.edu/dris. A range of US and Canadian government agencies have provided support for DRI development.

The current life stage groups associated with the DRIs were determined at the same time the DRIs were

TABLE 106.1	NUTRIENTS WITH ESTABLISHED REFERENCE VALUES: 1941–2010	
1941	**1989**[a]	**1997–2004/2010**[b]
Protein	Protein	Protein
Calcium	Calcium	Calcium
Iron	Iron	Iron
Vitamin A	Vitamin A	Vitamin A
Thiamin	Thiamin	Thiamin
Vitamin C	Vitamin C	Vitamin C
Riboflavin	Riboflavin	Riboflavin
Nicotinic acid	Nicotinic acid	Niacin
Vitamin D	Vitamin D	Vitamin D
Calories	Energy	Energy and physical activity
	Vitamin K	Vitamin K
	Vitamin B_6	Vitamin B_6
	Folate	Folate
	Vitamin B_{12}	Vitamin B_{12}
	Vitamin E	Vitamin E
	Magnesium	Magnesium
	Phosphorus	Phosphorus
	Iodine	Iodine
	Selenium	Selenium
	Zinc	Zinc
	Chromium	Chromium
	Copper	Copper
	Fluoride	Fluoride
	Pantothenic acid	Pantothenic acid
	Biotin	Biotin
	Manganese	Manganese
	Molybdenum	Molybdenum
	Potassium	Potassium
	Sodium	Sodium
	Chloride	Chloride
	Total water	Total water
	Choline	Choline
	Carbohydrate	Carbohydrate
	Total fiber	Total Fiber
	Linoleic acid (n-6)	Linoleic acid (n-6)
	α-Linolenic acid (n-3)	α-Linolenic acid (n-3)
		Arsenic
		Boron
		Nickel
		Silicon
		Vanadium
		Amino acids

[a]Values for chromium, copper, fluoride, pantothenic acid, biotin manganese, and molybdenum were expressed in 1989 as estimated safe and adequate daily dietary intakes. Potassium was expressed as an estimated minimum requirement.
[b]Vitamin D and calcium were reviewed in 1997 and again in 2010. All other nutrients were reviewed once during the 1997–2004 time period. Carotenoids were reviewed, but no dietary reference intake (DRI) established.

Adapted with permission from Yates AA. Dietary reference intakes: rationale and application. In: Shils ME, Shike M, Ross AC et al. Modern Nutrition in Health and Disease. 10th ed. Baltimore: Lippincott Williams & Wilkins, 2006:1672–7.

developed, using the new 1994 approach for nutrient reference values. The life stage groupings took into account developmental and gender differences as well as additional factors such as the age at which young children enter institutional feeding settings, the onset of menarche,

TABLE 106.2	NUTRIENT REFERENCE VALUES THAT COMPRISE DIETARY REFERENCE INTAKES[a]
NUTRIENT REFERENCE VALUE	**DESCRIPTION**
Estimated average requirement (EAR)	Reflects the estimated median daily requirement and is particularly appropriate for applications related to planning and assessing intakes for groups of persons
Recommended dietary allowance (RDA)	Derived from the EAR and intended to cover the requirements for 97%–98% of the population
Tolerable upper intake level (UL)	Highest average daily intake that is likely to pose no risk
Adequate intake (AI)	*Used when an EAR/RDA cannot be developed; average recommended daily intake level based on observed or experimental intakes*
Acceptable macronutrient distribution range (AMDR)	*An intake range for an energy source associated with reduced risk of chronic disease*
Estimated energy requirement (EER)	*Average daily dietary energy intake predicted to maintain energy balance in a healthy adult of defined age, gender, weight, height, and level of physical activity that is consistent with good health*

[a]Italics denote DRI reference values developed after the initial DRI plan.

Adapted with permission from Food and Nutrition Board, Institute of Medicine. How Should the RDAs Be Revised? Washington, DC: National Academy Press, 1994.

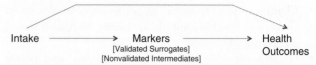

Fig. 106.1. Effect of nutrient intake on health outcome: direct versus indirect measurement.

and detailed. Data are often limited for key topic areas and for some life stage groups, and scientific judgment is required.

The health outcomes of interest for DRIs—sometimes referred to as the "indicators" or "end points"—are considered in relation to the direct effect of intake on the health outcome, as shown by the upper line in Figure 106.1. More commonly, the indicator used relates to an indirect effect. That is, the effect of intake on a marker for the health outcome (bottom line in Fig. 106.1) is considered rather than a measure of the outcome itself. For example, the number and type of polyps is measured rather than the onset of a cancer.

The challenge is to ensure that the marker is a valid reflection of the health outcome of interest. With few exceptions, the approach to identifying and validating such markers is not as well developed for nutrients as for other substances such as pharmaceuticals and toxins. There is often confusion and inadvertent overlap regarding markers of intake and markers of effect, and guiding principles for ensuring the appropriateness of nutrient-related markers are not well articulated. Further, studies often fail to examine a range of intakes—that is, they are not designed to identify a dose-response—but instead use a single intake/dose level. As described in the following, the ability to identify a dose-response relationship is critical to DRI development. There are often calls for more studies on dose-response relationships and on the relationship between a marker of a health outcome and the outcome it purports to reflect (11, 14).

The selection of health outcomes for DRI development usually relates to the following:

- Evidence demonstrates a causal relationship
- Selection of health outcome supports protection of public health
  - Adequacy: Preference for outcome with relatively high intake—not necessarily outcome with most data or even strongest data
  - Upper level: Preference for outcome with relatively low intake—not necessarily outcome that is most "severe"
- Selection may differ by life stage group

Some examples of indicators (i.e., the health outcomes and markers) used for DRI development for adequate intakes are shown in Table 106.3. Indicators can be described and labeled in various ways, for example, as "clinical," "biochemical," and "functional" measures. Factorial models and balance studies also are used.

and the age at which retirement generally occurs, which potentially affect energy requirements (13). Additionally, these life stage differences mean that the outcomes of interest in setting a nutrient requirement or an upper intake level differ for different life stage groups. The specific life stage groups for the DRIs can be viewed by accessing the website containing the DRI tables.

FRAMEWORK FOR DEVELOPMENT

The basic task for developing DRIs appears simple: Identify the health outcome that the nutrient affects, and then determine how much of the nutrient causes that effect, so that a requirement for the nutrient can be specified. In the case of tolerable upper levels, the adverse effect must be identified and likewise the level that causes such an effect must be determined. For example, the question may be how much nutrient X ensures healthy bones or how much nutrient Y reduces the risk of coronary heart disease. In practice, the process is complicated

TABLE 106.3	EXAMPLES OF INDICATORS (OUTCOMES AND MARKERS) USED FOR DIETARY REFERENCE INTAKE DEVELOPMENT FOR ADEQUACY REFERENCE VALUES		
NUTRIENT	**VALUE**	**INDICATOR**	**TYPE OF INDICATOR**
Thiamin	EAR	Urinary thiamin excretion	Biochemical
Vitamin C	EAR	Antioxidant functions in leukocytes	Functional
Vitamin A	EAR	Amount of dietary vitamin A required to maintain a given body-pool size in well-nourished adults	Factorial model
Magnesium	EAR	Magnesium balance studies	Nutrient balance
Fluoride	AI	Prevention of dental caries	Clinical
Pantothenic acid	AI	Pantothenic acid intakes	(direct estimation)

AI, adequate intake; EAR, estimated average requirement.

Adapted with permission from a background paper developed by Dr. Margaret Cheney for a 2007 workshop. Food and Nutrition Board, Institute of Medicine. The Development of DRIs 1994–2004: Lessons Learned and New Challenges: Workshop Summary. Washington, DC: National Academies Press, 2008.

Principles of a Distribution

The foundation of DRI development, and hence the rationale for the types of DRI values, is the specification of a distribution—an arrangement of data values showing the frequency of occurrence throughout the range of various possible values (10). The specific distribution of interest is the amount of a nutrient that affects the health outcome, as shown in Figure 106.2 (given the assumption that requirements for nutrients are normally distributed). The y axis on the left of the figure demarcates the frequency with which the intake level meets the required need, or more precisely affects the health outcome. Under conditions of normality, the highest frequency is that of the median, mean, and mode of the distribution, in this case reflecting the amount consumed to affect the outcome.

Those asked to develop DRIs must examine the available data to develop the frequency distribution of requirements.

In turn, the distribution is the basis for determining the EAR and RDA. As illustrated in Figure 106.2, the task is statistically based: The EAR is the median (as well as the mean) of the identified distribution, and the RDA is that level at the far end of the distribution that is greater than the needs of almost the entire population (97.5%). In short, the EAR is the point at which one half of the population has requirements that are lower than the value and one half has requirements that are higher. The RDA is calculated by using the principle that two standard deviations above that median/mean value reflects an intake level that is greater than the requirements of almost 98% of the group.

A key question is, Why are these two values specified in the DRI reports? After all, for many years before the 1990s, only a single value (the RDA) was established. The scientific discussions surrounding the applications of the DRI values (8, 9) determined that, in planning and assessing

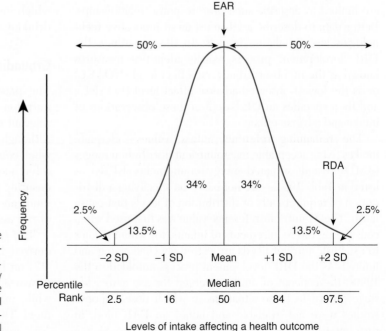

Fig. 106.2. Generic frequency distribution for intake required to affect a health outcome. *EAR,* estimated average requirement; *RDA,* recommended dietary allowance. (Reprinted with permission from the National Academy of Sciences from Food and Nutrition Board, Institute of Medicine. Dietary Reference Intakes: The Essential Guide to Nutrient Requirements. Washington, DC: National Academies Press, 2006. Courtesy of the National Academies Press, Washington, DC.)

diets, different types of nutrient reference values should be used depending upon their application and whether the interest is in a group of persons or an individual (see the section on applications). From a utility perspective, especially on an international basis, the EAR is the "foundation" reference value (11, 14). It is a scientifically derived estimate of human nutrient requirements. The RDA, conversely, is a recommended intake to cover the needs of 97.5% of the population, and is viewed as an application of the EAR estimate. Indeed, the cut-point used for a recommended intake could vary from situation to situation or country to country. That is, some may choose to establish a population-based recommended intake that would cover a different percentage of their population. Variance around the EAR may be another factor that would affect the establishment of a recommended intake (11, 14).

At times it can be challenging for those new to the DRIs to embrace the relevance and importance of specifying requirement distributions as opposed to identifying a single level of intake that is known to have benefit. This is understandable, in that many scientists are well versed in what might be referred to as the "clinical" or "medical" model in which the goal is to address the needs of a specific individual presenting to the clinician and requiring specific advice about treatment. In contrast, the DRIs relate to a "public health" model, in which the goal is to describe the requirements on a population basis and apply these understandings to a range of applications.

In principle, the development of the UL would also seek to describe a distribution—that is of intakes that cause the adverse event to occur when high levels of intake are consumed. However, given that studying levels of intake that cause harm is precluded by ethical considerations in all but the most careful of clinical situations or through case reports on accidental overdoses, data are limited to describe such dose-response relationships. Better data to describe a UL must await innovative technologies and simulation models. In the meantime, the DRI development process usually identifies measures known as the no-observed-adverse-effect level (NOAEL) or as the lowest-observed-adverse-effect level (LOAEL), and then specifies an UL based on these observations of intake and adverse effects.

The remaining reference intake values—adequate intakes (AIs), acceptable macronutrient distribution ranges (AMDRs), and estimated energy requirements (EERs), as listed in Table 106.2—are not based on specifying a distribution of requirements or distribution of levels that cause harm. The AI nutrient reference value was first used when considering the requirements of infants, for whom studies to establish nutrient needs are extremely challenging and limited. As the DRI development process unfolded in the 1990s, the concept of an AI emerged for use across life stage groups in those situations in which dose-response studies were not available and hence an EAR (and, in turn, an RDA) could not be specified (13). The AI is a recommended average daily intake—but not labeled as an

RDA because they are developed differently—based on observed or experimentally determined approximations of intakes that appear to be consistent with an apparently healthy population (10, 13). AIs have been identified as problematic for at least some users of the DRIs because, although they are useful as a guide for recommending an intake to an individual, they cannot readily be used in the statistical approaches for planning and assessing diets of groups of persons (11, 14), as described in the section on applications.

The AMDR reflects a range of intakes of an energy source (i.e., macronutrients [protein, amino acids, carbohydrates, fat, and fatty acids]) associated with the risk of chronic disease. The ranges take into account the need to ensure adequate intakes of the essential nutrients contained in such energy sources (10, 15). Questions have been posed as to whether such values can be more systematically developed in the future and how such values should be used (11, 14).

The EER is defined as the average dietary energy intake that is predicted to maintain energy balance in a healthy adult of a defined age, gender, weight, height, and a level of physical activity consistent with good health (10, 15). The EER is based on prediction equations for normal-weight individuals; however, the EER does not represent the exact dietary energy intake needed to maintain energy balance for a specific individual. Rather, the EER reflects the average needs for those with the specified characteristics, for example weight, height, age, and gender (10).

Finally, reference values for water intake were established in 2005 as AIs (16). They are based on median total water intakes from US survey data and represent intake considered to prevent effects of dehydration (10, 16). They are specified as intake levels of *total* water, which includes water contained in food, beverages, and drinking water.

Grounding in Risk Assessment Approaches

The practice of risk assessment, as developed in non-nutrition fields, has been acknowledged as a useful and relevant organizing structure for DRI development (11). Although the term "risk" may give nutritionists pause when considering the effects of a nutrient, in fact nutrient reference values address the question of nutritional risk by ensuring that the risk of too little as well as the risk of too much are avoided. Figure 106.3 shows comparative levels of risk associated with the nutrient reference values.

The conceptual underpinnings of risk assessment are derived from a 1983 National Research Council report (17) on how scientific deliberations should be organized to assess risk in a manner that meets the users' needs while maintaining the scientific integrity of the assessment. The framework is based on the assumption that the "risk assessors" (in this case, the DRI committees) evaluate the science and identify the reference values, whereas

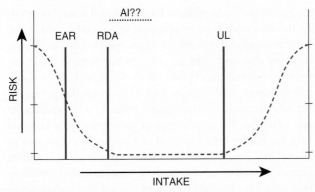

Fig. 106.3. Level of risk of adequacy associated with estimated average requirement (EAR) and recommended dietary allowance (RDA) and of adverse events associated with the tolerable upper intake level (UL). Risk for the adequate intake (AI) is approximately that of the RDA, although unknowns surrounding risk are associated with this reference value.

the "risk managers" (in this case, DRI users ranging from government officials to individual practitioners) determine whether and how they apply and integrate DRIs into health policy development, regulations, health programs, and related uses. The importance of separating the activities of evaluating the science and determining public health policy has been described in an international report issued by two agencies of the United Nations (18). Examples of these different activities are provided in this report.

The risk assessment approach is predicated on the need to (a) make the scientific evaluation transparent and well documented, and (b) be structured so that uncertainties can be taken into account and appropriate scientific judgment employed and outlined. In the field of public health protection—which is often the end point of risk assessment—scientific judgment in the face of limited data is preferable to the alternative of providing no guidance because data are limited. In the absence of scientific conclusions from risk assessors (even if only scientific opinion), risk managers lack any basis upon which to proceed with public health protection on the one hand and research protocols on the other.

The organizing scheme that risk assessment provides for DRI development constitutes a four-step process (the steps may be iterative):

1. Outcome identification: Conduct and describe a literature review to identify potential health outcomes of interest as the basis for a nutrient reference value.
2. Dose-response specification: Evaluate and describe the data, determining the outcome that will provide public health protection. Outline the dose-response relationship based on the available data. Establish reference values.
3. Intake assessment: Carry out a comparison between the established reference values and real-world intake in order to identify potential public health concerns or other issues that would be important for risk managers or other users to know in applying the DRI values.

4. Implications/risk characterization: Characterize the overall risk assessment, highlighting key challenges and uncertainties, caveats for use of the values, special populations at risk, and next steps for improved assessments in the future.

Challenge of Literature Review and Evaluation

The amount of data that a DRI committee must review has grown over the years and can be considerable, depending upon the nutrient. Studies must first be arrayed in a summary fashion and rated on the quality of the design, and then integrated so that a clear picture of the totality of the evidence can emerge. The most recent DRI report on calcium and vitamin D used a variety of data presentation techniques including evidence maps and forest plots (12). Next, committees must delve into key studies in detail, at times checking or reanalyzing the data provided in the reports. When such reanalyses cause the committee to come to different conclusions than the publication authors, the reanalysis is documented and explained in the DRI report.

To assist DRI committees in arraying and summarizing data, specific use of systematic evidence-based reviews (SEBRs) has been advocated (11, 19, 20). Certainly, evidence has long been evaluated and used for DRI development, but there is a newer interest in assisting committees by providing independent systematic compilations developed by groups such as the Agency for Healthcare Research and Quality (http://www.ahrq.gov). For SEBRs, scientists trained in summarizing health-related studies independently create comprehensive and documented data arrays. The appropriateness and relevance of such summaries for DRI work are dependent upon ensuring that such activities incorporate an advisory panel or other expert guidance that outlines the questions and criteria for the data analyzers to ensure its relevance for the end use, for example, DRI development (19). Moreover, SEBR inclusion in DRI work does not "make decisions" for the committee or eliminate the extensive evaluation and integration needed on the part of the committee. Nonetheless, concern has been voiced that such summaries may be overly controlled by methodologists ignorant of the key questions, or that SEBRs usurp committee decision making (11). However, the inclusion of SEBRs for DRI development and other scientific reports from the FNB has met with apparent success (12, 21). Well-conducted SEBRs are expensive and complicated to conduct, so their role in future DRI development may be judicious and dependent upon the size of the available data base.

Institute of Medicine Committee Process

The development of a DRI report and other consensus reports issued by NAS and the Institute of Medicine (IOM), the health arm of NAS that houses FNB, follow a process that ensures the outcome is independent, objective and, nonpartisan (http://www.nationalacademies.org/study process/index.html). Committee members are selected in order to provide an appropriate range of expertise for the study question as well as a balance of perspectives. Committee members are screened for conflicts of interest. All volunteer their time, serve as individual experts—not as representatives of organizations or interest groups—and each member is asked to contribute to the work on the basis of his or her own expertise and scientific judgment of the evidence.

Consensus committees of the type used to develop DRIs operate under certain requirements, laid out in Section 15 of the Federal Advisory Committee Act (http://www.nationalacademies.org/coi/bi-coi_form-0.pdf), which relates to reports for government use that are developed under the auspices of NAS. If the Section 15 stipulations are followed in convening committees and developing reports, the government can readily use the advice and recommendations provided by Academy reports. Typically, the committee process involves following:

- Creating websites to post provisional committee biosketches for comment and to accept information and data
- Meeting as a committee in closed deliberations, intended to allow frank debate among committee members, all of whom can make different scientific judgments and therefore must work to find ways for consensus conclusions
- Holding public information-gathering workshops and designating meeting sessions open to the public.

After data evaluation and detailed committee discussion, an initial report is developed. Under the academy process, this version of the report is then reviewed by a separate group of experts. Written comments from these reviewers are compiled. The committee's response, and the changes made as a result of the reviewers' comments, are overseen by the report's monitor and coordinator, who are appointed by NAS and IOM. The review process provides additional perspectives on the topic and ensures that the reasoning for the committee's conclusions are well presented, clearly justified, and can stand up to the expected scrutiny.

When the reviewers' input has been addressed to the satisfaction of the monitor and coordinator, the report is publicly released by the IOM and hard copy publication follows. The committee does not know the identities of the reviewers during the review process. Once the report is finalized, the names of reviewers are listed in the published report.

APPLICATIONS: GROUPS AND INDIVIDUALS

DRIs provide standards for good nutrition and serve as a yardstick by which to measure progress toward that goal (10). They are applicable to the general population (sometimes referred to as a normal, healthy population) and are not intended to address the needs of diseased persons. In the absence of more appropriate guidance and if not contraindicated, DRIs are, at times, used to plan and assess diets for diseased persons (11). As mentioned, DRIs are tools for assessing and planning diets. As such, their application is wide and diverse, and it draws on the principles for distributions—distributions related to requirements and to intake. The application of these principles, coupled with the earlier establishment of a probability approach to assess prevalence of nutrient inadequacy in groups, and its proxy EAR cut-point approach (22), necessitated specification for users on how DRIs are to be applied in real-world settings to plan and assess nutrient intake. Two reports developed by DRI subcommittees (8, 9) provide guidance for user application, including appropriate application of DRIs for assessment and planning for specific purposes and inappropriate applications; appropriate assumptions about intake and requirement distributions; adjustments needed to minimize potential error in dietary intake data; and appropriate use of DRI values of specific nutrients.

The DRI value to be used—notably, EAR versus RDA—depends on the type of activity being carried out. Applications are categorized by whether they are intended to assess or plan diets and whether they focus on a group or an individual. For example, the goal of *assessing* nutrient intake of groups is to determine the prevalence of inadequacy (or excessive nutrient intakes) within a particular group of people; and the goal of *planning* nutrient intakes for groups is to achieve usual intakes that meet the requirements of most individuals, but that are not excessive (10).

The concept of planning and assessing for groups versus individuals has been represented as a "two-by-two table," as shown in Table 106.4. As a general matter, EARs relate to considerations for groups, whereas RDAs relate to considerations for individuals. When AIs must be used because an EAR and RDA are lacking, there is a greater level of uncertainty. Table 106.2 includes brief summaries of the stipulated applications, which are further outlined in the 2006 summary publication (10), but a full reading of the guidance documents (8, 9) is recommended for users of the DRIs.

To illustrate real-world application of this paradigm on a national basis, Table 106.5 identifies US government use of the components of the two-by-two table. Applications in Canada are often similar to those in the United States. As shown in the table, some activities are classified as simultaneously assessment and planning. Although recognized as an important advance in DRI applications, questions about how the two-by-two approach works conceptually and during the implementation process have been discussed (11). Some have asked whether there are special issues if a program fits within more than one box of the table. Further, although DRIs are specified for individual nutrients, their application occurs in the context of the total diet, creating some challenges for users. Others have noted that the emerging world of statistical methods and its relevant guidance for application of the

TABLE 106.4	TWO-BY-TWO TABLE FOR DIETARY REFERENCE INTAKE APPLICATION

ASSESSING GROUPS	PLANNING FOR GROUPS
Goal is to determine the prevalence of inadequate or excessive nutrient intakes within a group on individuals.	Goal is low prevalence of inadequate intakes; required definition of acceptable low prevalence
Intakes should be adjusted to represent usual intakes	Considers entire distribution of usual nutrient intakes
Use of EAR, probability approach, and short-cut EAR method	RDA should not be used.
ASSESSING INDIVIDUALS	**PLANNING FOR INDIVIDUALS**
Goal is to determine if intake is meeting his or her nutrient requirement	Goal is to achieve low probability of inadequacy while not exceeding UL for each nutrient
Qualitative and quantitative considerations RDA should not be used	RDA often used as a guide

EAR, estimated average requirement; RDA, recommended dietary allowance; UL, tolerable upper intake level.

For additional detail, see Food and Nutrition Board, Institute of Medicine. Dietary Reference Intakes: The Essential Guide to Nutrient Requirements. Washington, DC: National Academies Press, 2006, from which this table is abstracted.

TABLE 106.5	EXAMPLES OF US GOVERNMENT DIETARY ASSESSING AND PLANNING ACTIVITIES USING DIETARY REFERENCE INTAKES

ACTIVITY	FOCUS	GOVERNMENT PROGRAM
Assessing	Groups	Healthy People 2010 Initiative US National Food Supply Food Additives Review
	Individuals	MyPyramid Tracker
	Groups and individuals	Healthy Eating Index
Planning	Individuals	Thrifty Food Plan MyPyramid Food Guidance System
	Groups and individuals	Nutrition Education
Assessing and planning	Groups	Human Nutrition Research Programs
	Groups and individuals	Dietary Guidelines for Americans Child and Adult Care Food Program Summer Food Service Program National School Lunch and School Breakfast Programs Women, Infants, and Children's Supplemental Nutrition Program

Adapted with permission from background paper developed by the US Federal DRI Steering Committee for a 2007 workshop in Food and Nutrition Board, Institute of Medicine. The Development of DRIs 1994–2004: Lessons Learned and New Challenges: Workshop Summary. Washington, DC: National Academies Press, 2008.

DRIs (particularly for those working with individuals) requires more research. Additionally, the question of whether it is possible to simplify the application of DRIs for "everyday practitioners" has also been raised (11). Application of the approach to develop nutrition standards for groups can be found in three IOM reports: food packages for women, infants, and children (http://www.iom.edu/Reports/2005/WIC-Food-Packages-Time-for-a-Change.aspx); school meal standards (http://www.iom.edu/Reports/2009/School-Meals-Building-Blocks-for-Healthy-Children.aspx); and guidance for child and adult care food programs (http://www.iom.edu/Reports/2010/Child-and-Adult-Care-Food-Program-Aligning-Dietary-Guidance-for-All.aspx).

EMERGING ISSUES

Incorporation of Chronic Disease Outcomes

The interest in incorporating chronic disease outcomes (e.g., cancers, heart disease, or macular degeneration) into the spectrum of health outcomes relevant to DRIs has engendered focused discussion. On the one hand, there is agreement that use of chronic disease indicators to set nutrient reference values does not signal that data of lesser quality than that for nonchronic disease outcomes is acceptable. Rather, concern about ensuring that a causal relationship is established and the ability to sort through the confounding factors associated with measurement of chronic disease remains paramount. On the other

hand, there is a need to determine whether and in what ways the development of DRIs may need to be adapted when the outcome of interest is chronic disease. In July 2009, the IOM organized an informal planning meeting to discuss approaches that may be used to elucidate and resolve challenges for the inclusion of chronic disease indicators into DRI development. The meeting was cochaired by Stephanie Atkinson and Elizabeth Yetley, and the points included here are from the discussions of that meeting. Several issues may warrant exploration:

- The current model based on establishing a threshold effect of benefit for all persons in the group may not be applicable to chronic disease outcomes.
- A chronic disease "model" may require obtaining a distribution for effect (both benefit and harm) by examining intake distributions relative to multiple indicators, as opposed to selecting just one indicator, as is central to the EAR threshold model.
- If multiple (or a composite of) chronic disease outcomes are used, criteria are needed to practically

determine how many diseases can be meaningfully considered or how to prioritize disease outcomes if they yield quite different intake-response curves.

- Developing reference values based on chronic disease outcomes likely requires accuracy in quantifying the intakes associated with health outcomes as compared with the relative differences often reported in research studies.

In addition, in the case of the use of associational studies, the ramifications of the likelihood that the dose-response relationship for chronic disease risk may not be linear have been pointed out (11). This topic was discussed by Susan Mayne during a 2007 workshop on lessons learned in DRI development (11); the text included is based on her workshop remarks. Different statistical approaches are used to analyze nutrients in relation to chronic disease risk. In the single-study approach, one examines nutrient intake or status in relation to a chronic disease outcome. The typical approach is to express the intake or status data in quantiles, then examine the relationships across these quantiles and statistically test for linear trends. Nutrient intake or status can also be examined as a continuous variable (11). The relationship between intake or status of nutrient X and disease Y can be modeled using regression. Both of these approaches typically assume a linear relationship, which may or may not be a valid assumption.

As shown in Figure 106.4, a hypothetical example using folate status and breast cancer risk is illustrative. Although some studies find protective effects with higher folate status, other studies identify suggestions of adverse effects or at least no benefit. The disparate findings may be because the relationship between folate and breast cancer risk is nonlinear (23). The linearity of the relationship depends in the part of the dose-response curve in which it lies (see Fig. 106.4). Thus, another aspect of addressing chronic disease outcomes in DRI development is awareness that dose-response associations for nutrients and chronic disease may be nonlinear and thus considerable care in describing the dose-response relationship is an important concern.

Approach to Updating Dietary Reference Intakes

In the past, nutrient reference values were regularly reviewed and the efforts were carried out for all nutrients simultaneously. Comprehensive reviews in six related groupings were undertaken with the advent of the DRI approach for developing nutrient reference values (13):

- Calcium, vitamin D, phosphorus, magnesium, and fluoride
- Folate, vitamin B_{12}, B vitamins, and choline
- Vitamins C and E, selenium, β-carotene, and other carotenoids
- Vitamins A and K, arsenic, boron, chromium, copper, iron, iodine, manganese, molybdenum, nickel, silicon, vanadium, and zinc
- Energy, carbohydrate, fiber, fat, fatty acids, cholesterol, protein, and amino acids
- Water, sodium, potassium, chloride, and sulfate

The reports were issued during the time span of 1997 to 2004 and, as shown in Table 106.1, they addressed more than 30 nutrient substances. Once the initial reviews were completed, the experience was examined and the mode for future updates considered (11). It now seems that comprehensive routine review of all nutrient reference values is neither practical nor necessary. Data that would warrant changes to DRI values do not necessarily emerge for all nutrients during any given time span, yet some nutrients may experience a large or unexpected spurt in research interest and relevant findings. In other words, updating of nutrient reference value has gravitated to an "as-needed" basis. Therefore, as discussed during the 2007 workshop on lessons learned in DRI development (11), the new challenge is in identifying the factors that "trigger" an update.

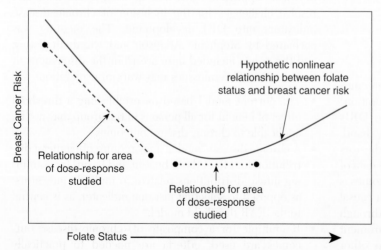

Fig. 106.4. Hypothetic nonlinear relationship between folate status and breast cancer risk as compared with relationships for different areas of the dose-response curve. (Modified with permission by the American Society for Nutrition from Ulrich CM. Folate and cancer prevention: a closer look at a complex picture. Am J Clin Nutr 2007:86:271–3.)

The US and Canadian governments initiated a trigger-like effort relevant to the DRIs for vitamin D (24). A working group of US and Canadian government scientists outlined an approach and rationale in deciding whether a review of the 1997 vitamin DRIs was warranted. They considered that the need for a new nutrient review should be evaluated against criteria set a priori. After selecting the criterion of significant new and relevant research, the working group used results from a systematic review and two conferences on vitamin D and health to evaluate whether significant new and relevant scientific evidence had become available (24). This effort was carefully defined so as not to prejudge whether the new evidence would in fact change the existing DRI values, but only to consider if additional and relevant data had become available. The decisions as to whether and in what ways the DRIs reference values for the nutrient might be revised were specifically left for the IOM committee to consider. Currently, the government sponsors and the IOM are drawing on the calcium and vitamin D experience and exploring approaches for identifying other nutrients in need of review.

DISCLOSURE

The responsibility for the content of this chapter rests with us and does not necessarily represent the views of the Institute of Medicine (IOM) or its committees.

REFERENCES

1. US Department of Agriculture, US Department Health and Human Services. Dietary Guidelines for Americans, 2010. 7th ed. Washington, DC: US Government Printing Office, 2010.
2. Health Canada. Eating Well with Canada's Food Guide. Ottawa, ON: Health Promotion and Programs Branch, Minister of Public Works and Government Services Canada, 2007.
3. Dupont JL, Harper AE. Nutr Rev 2002;60:342–8.
4. National Research Council. Recommended Dietary Allowances: Protein, calcium, iron, vitamin A, vitamin B (thiamin), vitamin C (ascorbic acid), riboflavin, nicotinic acid, vitamin D. Washington, DC. 1941.
5. Food and Nutrition Board, Institute of Medicine. How Should the RDAs Be Revised? Washington, DC: National Academy Press, 1994.
6. Roberts LJ. N Y State J Med 1944;44:59–65.
7. Yates AA. Dietary reference intakes: rationale and applications. In: Shils ME, Shike M, Ross AC et al. Modern Nutrition in Health and Disease. 10th ed. Baltimore: Lippincott Williams & Wilkins, 2006:1672–7.
8. Food and Nutrition Board, Institute of Medicine. Dietary Reference Intakes: Applications in Dietary Assessment. Washington, DC: National Academy Press, 2000.
9. Food and Nutrition Board, Institute of Medicine. Dietary Reference Intakes: Applications in Dietary Planning. Washington, DC: National Academy Press, 2003.
10. Food and Nutrition Board, Institute of Medicine. Dietary Reference Intakes: The Essential Guide to Nutrient Requirements. Washington, DC: National Academies Press, 2006.
11. Food and Nutrition Board, Institute of Medicine. The Development of DRIs 1994–2004: Lessons Learned and New Challenges: Workshop Summary. Washington, DC: National Academies Press, 2008.
12. Food and Nutrition Board, Institute of Medicine. Dietary Reference Intakes for Calcium and Vitamin D. Washington, DC: National Academies Press, 2011.
13. Food and Nutrition Board, Institute of Medicine. Dietary Reference Intakes for Calcium, Phosphorus, Magnesium, Vitamin D, and Fluoride. Washington, DC: National Academy Press, 1997:1–432.
14. Taylor CL. Framework for DRI Development: Components "Known" and Components "To Be Explored." Washington, DC: National Academies Press, 2008. Available at: http://www.iom.edu/dris. Accessed September 15, 2012.
15. Food and Nutrition Board, Institute of Medicine. Dietary Reference Intakes for Energy, Carbohydrate, Fiber, Fat, Fatty Acids, Cholesterol, Protein, and Amino Acids. Washington, DC: National Academy Press, 2002.
16. Food and Nutrition Board, Institute of Medicine. Dietary Reference Intakes for Water, Potassium, Sodium, Chloride and Sulfate. Washington, DC: National Academy Press, 2004.
17. National Research Council. Risk Assessment in the Federal Government: Managing the Process. Washington, DC, National Academy Press, 1983.
18. World Health Organization. A Model for Establishing Upper Levels of Intake for Nutrients and Related Substances: A Report of a Joint FAO/WHO Technical Workshop on Food Nutrient Risk Assessment. Geneva: World Health Organization, 2006.
19. Russell R, Chung M, Balk EM et al. Am J Clin Nutr 2009; 89:728–33.
20. Chung M, Balk EM, Ip S et al. Am J Clin Nutr 2010;92:273–6.
21. Institute of Medicine and National Research Council. Weight Gain During Pregnancy: Reexamining the Guidelines. Washington, DC: The National Academies Press, 2009.
22. National Research Council. Nutrient Adequacy: Assessment Using Food Consumption Surveys. Washington, DC: National Academy Press, 1986.
23. Ulrich CM. Am J Clin Nutr 2007:86:271–3.
24. Yetley EA, Brule D, Cheney MC et al. Am J Clin Nutr 89:719–27.

SUGGESTED READINGS

Beaton GH. When is an individual an individual versus a member of a group? Nutr Rev 2006;1:211–5.

Murphy SP, Barr SI, Yates AA. The recommended dietary allowance (RDA) should not be abandoned: an individual is both an individual and a member of a group. Nutr Rev 2006;1:313–8.

107 FOOD LABELING[1]

F. EDWARD SCARBROUGH

In the United States, several federal agencies share responsibility for regulating foods. The Centers for Disease Control and Prevention (CDCP), the Environmental Protection Agency (EPA), the Federal Trade Commission (FTC), the National Oceanic and Atmospheric Administration (NOAA), and the Alcohol and Tobacco Tax and Trade Bureau (TTB) all have a role in regulating food. However, when discussing labeling related to health and nutrition, we need focus only on the Food and Drug

---

[1]**Abbreviations: CDCP**, Centers for Disease Control and Prevention; **Codex**, Codex Alimentarius Commission; **CSPI**, Center for Science in the Public Interest; **DRI**, dietary reference intake; **DRV**, daily reference value; **DSHEA**, Dietary Supplement Health and Education Act; **DV**, daily value; **EC**, European Commission; **EPA**, Environmental Protection Agency; **FAO**, Food and Agriculture Organization; **FDA**, Food and Drug Administration; **FD&C Act**, Food, Drug and Cosmetic Act of 1938; **FDAMA**, Food and Drug Administration Modernization Act; **FMIA**, Federal Meat Inspection Act; **FNB**, Food and Nutrition Board; **FPLA**, Fair Packaging and Labeling Act; **FSIS**, Food Safety and Inspection Service; **FTC**, Federal Trade Commission; **IOM**, Institute of Medicine; **NAS**, National Academies of Science; **NLEA**, Nutrition Labeling and Education Act; **NOAA**, National Oceanic and Atmospheric Administration; **OWG**, Obesity Working Group; **PDCAAS**, Protein Digestibility–Corrected Amino Acid Score; **PER,** protein efficiency ratio; **PPIA**, Poultry Products Inspection Act; **RACC**, reference amount commonly consumed; **RDA**, recommended dietary allowance; **RDI**, reference daily intake; **RNI**, recommended nutrient intake; **TTB**, Alcohol and Tobacco Tax and Trade Bureau; **USDA**, United States Department of Agriculture; **WHO**, World Health Organization; **WTO**, World Trade Organization

Administration (FDA) and the Food Safety and Inspection Service (FSIS). The FDA is responsible for the labeling of all foods except meat, poultry, and egg products, which is the responsibility of the FSIS.

THE LEGAL BASIS FOR FOOD LABELING IN THE UNITED STATES

In 1906, partially in response to the public uproar caused by the publication of *The Jungle* by Upton Sinclair (1), which graphically detailed the horrendous sanitary and working conditions in the meat-packing industry, Congress passed the Federal Food and Drugs Act (2) and the Federal Meat Inspection Act (3), authorizing the federal government to regulate the safety and quality of food. Both acts prohibited misbranded (i.e., mislabeled) foods from moving in interstate commerce.

In 1938, the Federal Food and Drugs Act was replaced by the Federal Food, Drug, and Cosmetic Act (FD&C Act), which is still the basic law in the United States (4). This law, and subsequent interpretations through regulations and court decisions, has proved to be a valuable tool for FDA control of food labeling.

The FD&C Act was strengthened in 1967 through passage of the Fair Packaging and Labeling Act (FPLA). Among other things, the FPLA requires that the labels of processed packaged foods bear the name of the food, the net contents, and the contact information for the manufacturer or distributor.

NUTRITION LABELING

History in the United States

In 1969, the White House Conference on Food, Nutrition, and Health was convened to address deficiencies in the US diet (5). The conference recommended that the FDA consider the development of a system for identifying the nutritional qualities of food (6).

Largely in response to the White House Conference's recommendation, in 1971, the FDA proposed regulations on labeling of foods with information on cholesterol, fat, and fatty acid composition (7) and in 1972, proposed regulations on nutrition labeling (8). Final rules were published in 1973 (9) and went into effect in 1975. An essential feature of these regulations was that nutrition labeling was required only when a nutrient was added to the food or a claim was made on the label or in advertising about the food's nutritional properties. In 1984, the regulations were expanded when the FDA added sodium to the list of nutrients required on nutrition labeling. Potassium also was added as an optional nutrient (10).

In the 1980s, with continuing interest in the role of diet in disease and health, several major studies were initiated. Notable among these was the 1988 release of *The Surgeon General's Report on Nutrition and Health* (11). This report represents the federal government's first formal recognition of the role of diet in certain chronic diseases. In 1989, the National Academy of Sciences (NAS) issued *Diet and Health: Implications for Reducing Chronic Disease Risk* (12), which presented additional evidence of the growing acceptance of diet as a factor in the development of chronic diseases, such as coronary heart disease and cancer. Also, the NAS' Food and Nutrition Board, under contract to the FDA and the USDA's FSIS, convened a committee to consider how food labels could be improved to help consumers adopt or adhere to healthy diets. The committee's report, *Nutrition Labeling: Issues and Directions for the 1990s* (13), presented a number of recommendations to the government.

In response, Secretary of Health and Human Services Louis Sullivan announced that reform of the food label was a major priority for the FDA (14), and the FDA along with the FSIS held a series of public meetings around the country (15). In 1990, the FDA proposed extensive food labeling changes, including mandatory nutrition labeling for most foods (16). However, before the FDA could publish its final regulations, Congress, which had been discussing food labeling, passed the Nutrition Labeling and Education Act (NLEA) on November 8, 1990 (17). In many aspects, the requirements of the NLEA mirror those in the FDA's proposed regulations of 1990. Perhaps the NLEA's most important aspect is that the new law gave the FDA explicit authority to require nutrition labeling and control nutrient claims and health messages on food labeling. One notable section of the NLEA, the so-called hammer provision (18), required the FDA to publish proposed regulations within 1 year of the passage of the Act (or the law became the final regulations without regulatory interpretation) and to publish final regulations within 2 years (or the proposed regulations became the final regulations). In 1991, the FDA issued more than 20 proposals to implement the NLEA (19). In addition, the agency issued a final rule on *voluntary* point-of-purchase nutrition information for raw produce and fish. In 1992, the FDA issued final regulations, which became effective in 1993 (20). Even though the United States Department of Agriculture (USDA) was not subject to the NLEA, the FSIS, in coordination with the FDA, simultaneously issued proposals and final rules for mandatory nutrition labeling of processed meat and poultry, and *voluntary* point-of-purchase nutrition information for raw meat and poultry. In 2003, the FDA amended the nutrition

labeling regulations to require that *trans*-fatty acids be declared on the nutrition label (21).

Requirements

The Food and Drug Administration

General. Nutrition labeling is required on all foods regulated by the FDA, with certain exceptions, as shown in Table 107.1.

When food is not in a packaged form, nutrition information may be given with a counter card, sign, tag, or in a loose-leaf binder.

Serving Size. FDA regulations require that nutrition information be given on the basis of a "serving size." In many other countries, as discussed later, nutrition information is expressed on the basis of a specific weight or volume, such as 100 g or 100 mL. The FDA and many consumer advocates have argued, however, that 100 g, for example, is not relevant because many foods are consumed in quantities of more or less than 100 g or 100 mL. The counterargument is that not all consumers eat the same amount of a food in a serving, and the specific weight or volume allows much easier comparison among different foods.

Before 1990, the only requirement was that food manufacturers chose a "reasonable" serving size. In the years leading up to passage of the NLEA, many consumers were of the opinion that manufacturers were manipulating serving sizes, declaring smaller serving sizes to make

TABLE 107.1	FOODS EXEMPT FROM NUTRITION LABELING

Food manufactured by small businesses (*annual gross sale of food less than $50,000*)

Food served in restaurants, and so forth or delivered to homes ready for immediate consumption

Delicatessen-type food, bakery products and confections that are sold directly to consumers from the location where prepared

Foods that provide no significant nutrition (*Examples include instant coffee [plain, unsweetened] and most spices.*)

Infant and junior foods (other than infant formula) for children up to 4 years of age (*These categories have modified, age-appropriate label provisions.*)

Dietary supplements (*Different regulations apply.*)

Medical foods[a]

Bulk foods shipped for further processing or packaging before retail sale

Fresh produce and seafood (*A voluntary nutrition labeling program covers these foods through the use of the appropriate means such as shelf labels, signs, and posters.*)

Donated food that is given free (not sold) to the consumer.

Custom-processed fish and game meats

[a]Section 5(b) of the Orphan Drug Act: "[A medical food is] a food which is formulated to be consumed or administered enterally under the supervision of a physician and which is intended for the specific dietary management of a disease or condition for which distinctive nutritional requirements, based on recognized scientific principles, are established by medical evaluation."

the content for nutrients that consumers were seeking to minimize appear more favorable, or larger serving sizes, to overemphasize more positive nutrients.

An important feature of the NLEA is that the FDA was required to "establish regulations defining serving size or other unit of measure." This section of the law proved to be one of the more difficult to implement because of the vast number of food products, the facts that new foods were constantly being introduced and consumption patterns were changing, and that the amount of a particular food consumed varies significantly from person to person. The FDA approached this task by consulting nationwide food consumption surveys (primarily the 1977 to 1978 and 1987 to 1988 Nationwide Food Consumption Surveys conducted by the USDA) (22), and considered three statistical estimates, that is, the mean (average), the median (50th percentile), and the mode (most frequent value), for each product category. Using this procedure, the FDA established reference amounts commonly consumed (RACC), expressed in grams or milliliters, for approximately 150 different food categories, and provided a process for manufacturers to derive serving sizes from the RACC.

Given their complexity, there has been continued concern about serving sizes declared on food packages, particularly in what constitutes a single serving. For example, the Center for Science in the Public Interest (CSPI) filed a petition (23) with the FDA in 2004, requesting that the definition for a single serving be increased for three categories of food: soft drinks/beverages, muffins, and snack foods. The CSPI also suggested that the FDA should consider whether cutoff levels for other categories of oversized "single-serve" foods, such as candy bars, dried soups, frozen entrees, pizza crusts, and fruit cups, should be raised. For example, a serving of soft drink is defined as 8 oz, and 16-oz, 20-oz, and 24-oz bottles are labeled as containing multiple servings.

Another area of concern has been the increase in portion sizes typically consumed by Americans (24–26). Many nutritionists consider these increased portion sizes a major contributor to the critical obesity problem in the United States (27). In 2003, the FDA created an Obesity Working Group (OWG), charged with developing an action plan to help consumers lead healthier lives through better nutrition. A principal charge to the OWG was to "develop an approach for enhancing and improving the food label to assist consumers in preventing weight gain and reducing obesity." In its final report, the OWG recommended that the FDA re-examine regulations on serving sizes, specifically, (a) whether to require that food packages that can reasonably be consumed at one eating occasion declare the whole package as a single serving; (b) which, if any, RACC of food categories need to be updated; and (c) whether to provide for comparative calorie claims for smaller portions of identical foods (28).

In 2005, to address the issues being raised about serving sizes, the FDA published an advance notice of proposed rulemaking, requesting comments on serving sizes (29).

Nutrients in the Nutrition Facts Panel. The following nutrients are either required to be on the Nutrition Facts panel or may be included voluntarily:

- Calories (may also be expressed as total calories): The caloric content per serving is declared in 5-calorie increments up to 50 calories and 10-calorie increments above 50 calories. Energy content may also be expressed as kilojoules in parentheses. FDA regulations provide several methods for determining caloric content, including (a) Atwater factors (30); (b) general factors 4, 4, and 9, for protein, carbohydrate, and fat, respectively, or the same general factors but with insoluble fiber subtracted from total carbohydrate; (c) specific factors approved by the FDA; or (d) bomb calorimetry. The term "energy" may be added in parentheses following "Total Calories."
- Calories from fat: Calories from fat are declared in the same manner and increments as calories. If a serving contains less than 0.5 g of fat, calories from fat may be omitted and the statement, "Not a significant source of calories from fat" is placed at the bottom of the table of nutrient values.
- Calories from saturated fat: Calories from saturated fat may be *voluntarily* declared.
- Fat (total fat): Fat is defined as total lipid fatty acids. Amounts are rounded to the nearest 0.5-g increment below 5 g and to the nearest gram increment above 5 g, and can be stated as zero if the serving contains less than 0.5 g.
- Saturated fat (or saturated): Saturated fat is required to be listed, with the same increments and rounding rules as fat.
- *Trans*-fat (or *trans*): *Trans*-fat is defined as the sum of all unsaturated fatty acids that contain one or more isolated (i.e., nonconjugated) double bonds in a *trans*-configuration and must be declared with the same increments and rounding rules as fat.
- Polyunsaturated fat (or polyunsaturated): Polyunsaturated fat is defined as *cis*-, *cis*-methylene-interrupted polyunsaturated fatty acids, and may be declared voluntarily. The declaration is indented under the declaration for total fat.
- Monounsaturated fat (or monounsaturated): Monounsaturated fat is defined as *cis*-monounsaturated fatty acids and may be declared *voluntarily* except when polyunsaturated fat is declared or a claim about fatty acids or cholesterol is made.
- Cholesterol: Cholesterol is expressed in milligrams per serving to the nearest 5-mg increment, and may be declared as zero if a serving contains less than 2 mg and the product makes no claim about fat, fatty acids, or cholesterol content. If cholesterol is not required to be declared, the statement "Not a significant source of cholesterol" is placed at the bottom of the table of nutrient values.

- Sodium: Sodium, in milligrams per serving, must be declared to the nearest 5-mg increment when the serving contains 5 to 140 mg of sodium, and to the nearest 10-mg increment when the serving contains greater than 140 mg. Sodium may be declared as zero for servings containing less than 5 mg.
- Potassium: Potassium may be voluntarily declared, using the same units and criteria as for sodium.
- Total carbohydrate: The Nutrition Facts panel must contain a statement of carbohydrate content, expressed in grams. If a serving contains less than 1 g carbohydrate, the label may contain a statement, "less than 1 gram." Servings containing less than 0.5 g of carbohydrate may be declared as zero carbohydrate. Carbohydrate content is determined by difference, that is, the subtraction of the sum of the crude protein, total fat, moisture, and ash from the total weight of the food (31).
- Dietary fiber: Dietary fiber content must be declared, using the same criteria as for total carbohydrate.
- Soluble fiber and insoluble fiber: The content per serving of either or both soluble and insoluble fiber may be voluntarily declared, using the same criteria as for dietary fiber.
- Sugars: Sugars, defined as the sum of all free monosaccharides and disaccharides (e.g., glucose, fructose, lactose, sucrose), are declared in gram units, again using the same criteria as for total carbohydrate.
- Sugar alcohol: When sugar alcohols are present in a food, the sugar alcohol content of a serving must be declared in the Nutrition Facts panel, in gram units. Sugar alcohols are defined as the sum of saccharide derivatives in which a hydroxyl group replaces a ketone or aldehyde group and whose use in the food has been approved by the FDA (e.g., mannitol, xylitol, sorbitol).
- Other carbohydrate: Other carbohydrate is defined as the difference between total carbohydrate and the sum of dietary fiber, sugars, and sugar alcohol, and the content per serving may be declared voluntarily.
- Protein: Protein is declared in gram units for servings containing more than 1 g of protein. Protein content is calculated by multiplying the nitrogen content of a serving by a factor of 6.25 (unless other factors are required for specific foods) (32). The FDA also includes a number of protein quality criteria. Protein quality is determined by the protein digestibility–corrected amino acid score (PDCAAS) (33). Except in the case of a food marketed to children less than 4 years old, the protein quality must be at least 20%; otherwise, the label must state that the food is not a significant source of protein. For foods marketed to children less than 4 years old, the PDCAAS must be at least 40% for the food to qualify as a significant source of protein. For foods marketed to infants, the older protein efficiency ratio (PER; which is a biologic assay of the quality of a particular protein, measured as the gain in weight of an animal per gram of the protein eaten) is still cited as the measure of protein quality, and the PER must be at least 40% of the reference standard, casein, for the food to be considered a source of protein.
- Vitamins and minerals: Vitamins and minerals are expressed as a percentage of the daily value (DV). Vitamin A, vitamin C, calcium, and iron, in that order, are required to be listed. Any other vitamin or mineral listed in Table 107.2 may be declared, unless the nutrient is added to the food or a claim is made about the nutrient, in which case the percent DV must be declared. Exceptions are made for nutrients in standardized foods (e.g., thiamin, riboflavin, niacin in enriched flour) *and* when the standardized food is used as an ingredient in another food. Exemptions are also made for nutrients added to food strictly for technologic purposes (e.g., ascorbic acid added as an antioxidant). The percentages for vitamins and minerals are expressed to the nearest 2% increment, up to and including the 10% level, the nearest 5% increment above 10%, and up to the 50% level, and the nearest 10% increment above the 50% level. Amounts of vitamins and minerals present at less than 2% of the reference daily intake (RDI) may be declared as zero.

RDA, DRV, RDI, DV, RNI, and DRI. This veritable alphabet soup of acronyms has an interesting and ongoing history. The recommended dietary allowance (RDA) was developed during World War II by a committee of the NAS Food and Nutrition Board, at the request of the US military, to investigate nutritional issues that

TABLE 107.2	REFERENCE DAILY INTAKES
NUTRIENT	REFERENCE DAILY INTAKES (RDI)
Vitamin A	5,000 IU
Vitamin C	60 mg
Calcium	1,000 mg
Iron	18 mg
Vitamin D	400 IU
Vitamin E	30 IU
Vitamin K	80 μg
Thiamin	1.5 mg
Riboflavin	1.7 mg
Niacin	20 mg
Vitamin B$_6$	2 mg
Folate	400 μg
Vitamin B$_{12}$	6 μg
Biotin	300 μg
Pantothenic acid	10 mg
Phosphorus	1,000 mg
Iodine	150 μg
Magnesium	400 mg
Zinc	15 mg
Selenium	70 μg
Copper	2.0 mg
Manganese	2.0 mg
Chromium	120 μg
Molybdenum	75 μg
Chloride	3,400 mg

might affect national defense. The committee created a set of recommendations for standard daily allowances for each nutrient, which would be used for nutrition recommendations for military personnel, civilians, and food relief overseas. The final set of guidelines, RDA, was accepted in 1941. The Food and Nutrition Board has periodically reviewed the RDAs and revised them as necessary. More recently, in a project jointly with the governments of Canada and the United States, the Food and Nutrition Board replaced the RDAs (United States) and the recommended nutrient intakes (RNIs) (Canada) with dietary reference intakes (DRIs) and is in the process of issuing a series of reports to establish RDI. For example, a report on energy and the macronutrients carbohydrate, fiber, fat, fatty acids, cholesterol, protein, and amino acids was published in 2005 (34). Another report in this series, on calcium and vitamin D, was also released. A listing of the DRIs for various nutrients and population groups can be found on the NAS IOM website (35).

In its mandatory nutrition labeling proposal of 1990, the FDA replaced the US RDA (label reference values based on the RDA) with two sets of reference values, RDIs for vitamins and minerals and daily reference values (DRVs) for macronutrients and sodium and potassium. Although the FDA considered it necessary to distinguish between RDIs and DRVs for regulatory purposes, the agency did not consider the distinction to be important for consumers' understanding of the nutrition information presented on the food label. On its own, the FDA arrived at the single term daily value (DV) to use on the label. The agency had determined through studies that many consumers interpreted RDA, DRV, and DRI to be requirements rather than recommendations. Also, some DRV are used for dietary planning to limit the intake of certain nutrients (e.g., fat), whereas others represent targets for adequate intake (e.g., fiber). In 2007, the FDA published an advance notice of proposed rulemaking to request comments on establishing new reference values (i.e., RDI and DRV) (36).

The current DRVs, shown in Table 107.3, are based on a reference caloric intake of 2000 calories per day.

Format. A significant feature of the FDA regulations implementing the NLEA was the creation of the Nutrition Facts label, now seen on almost all packaged food in the

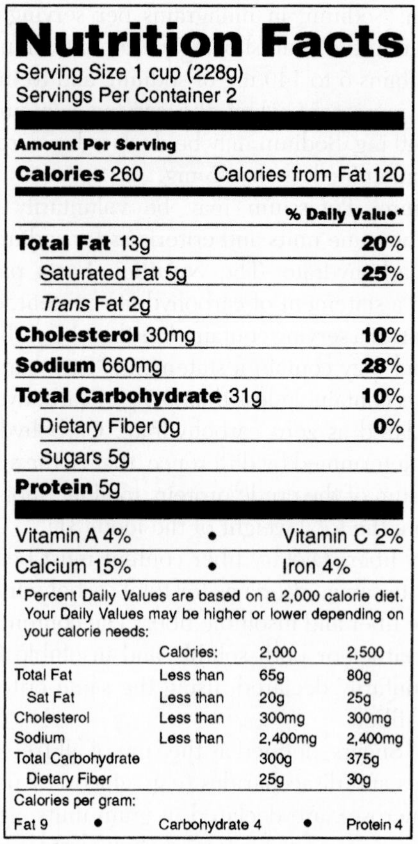

Fig. 107.1. Example of basic Nutrition Facts label.

United States. Kessler et al described the process that the FDA followed in developing the Nutrition Facts label (37). The regulations are quite specific in specifying type sizes, colors, letter separation, and mandatory graphic elements (38). An example of the basic label format is given in Figure 107.1.

The regulations allow for other formats for specific conditions. If insufficient space exists on the label for the basic format, for example, a vertical format is permitted on small packages. For packages containing two or more separate foods, an aggregate format is presented. Labeling in other languages is permitted, provided the first language is English. Nutrition information is given on the product *as packaged*, but additional information may be provided on the nutrient content as prepared (e.g., a cake mix may show the nutrient content of the mix and of the cake when baked according to directions). A simplified format is permitted if the product contains insignificant amounts of eight or more of the following nutrients: calories, total fat, saturated fat, *trans*-fat, cholesterol, sodium, total carbohydrate, dietary fiber, sugars, protein, vitamin A, vitamin C, calcium, and iron.

Compliance. FDA regulations specify the analytic methods the agency uses to check the accuracy of nutrition information. Manufacturers are free to use any analytic method to determine nutrient values, but the agency's designated method is used in case of a dispute. The FDA has

TABLE 107.3	DAILY REFERENCE VALUES	
FOOD COMPONENT	**UNIT OF MEASUREMENT**	**DAILY REFERENCE VALUES (DRV)**
Fat	grams (g)	65
Saturated fatty acids	grams (g)	20
Cholesterol	milligrams (mg)	300
Total carbohydrate	grams (g)	300
Fiber	grams (g)	25
Sodium	milligrams (mg)	2,400
Potassium	milligrams (mg)	3,500
Protein	grams (g)	50

defined two classes of nutrients for purposes of compliance: *class I* (added nutrients in fortified or fabricated foods), and *class II* (naturally occurring [indigenous] nutrients). For *class I*—vitamin, mineral, protein, dietary fiber, or potassium—the nutrient content must be at least equal to the value for that nutrient declared on the label. For *class II*—vitamin, mineral, protein, total carbohydrate, dietary fiber, other carbohydrate, polyunsaturated or monounsaturated fat, or potassium—the nutrient content must be at least equal to 80% of the value declared on the label. Foods are considered misbranded if the declaration of calories, sugars, total fat, saturated fat, *trans*-fat, cholesterol, or sodium is less than 80% of the amount found in the food. Reasonable excesses of vitamins, minerals, protein, total carbohydrate, dietary fiber, other carbohydrate, polyunsaturated fat, monounsaturated fat, or potassium greater than labeled amounts are acceptable. Reasonable deficiencies of calories, sugars, total fat, saturated fat, *trans*-fat, cholesterol, or sodium less than labeled amounts are acceptable. The FDA also has provided guidance on the creation of databases for determining nutrient values (39).

The United States Department of Agriculture

FSIS has responsibility for the regulation of labeling for meat and poultry products under the Federal Meat Inspection Act (FMIA) and the Poultry Products Inspection Act (PPIA) (40) and is also authorized to regulate food labeling for exotic species of animals under the Agricultural Marketing Act of 1946 (41). Therefore, because the NLEA amended the Federal Food, Drug, and Cosmetic Act only, the USDA was not mandated to adopt mandatory nutrition labeling for products under its jurisdiction. However, in coordination with the FDA, the USDA voluntarily adopted sweeping new regulations mandating that most foods bear nutrition labeling. Nutrition labeling is now required for all meat and poultry products intended for human consumption and offered for sale, except single-ingredient, raw products and other exempt products (42). The requirements for meat and poultry products are virtually identical to those for foods regulated by the FDA.

Restaurant Labeling

Previously, the FDA provided guidance on nutrition labeling of restaurant food (43). In Code of Federal Regulations §101.10, the agency said that nutrient information must be provided, on request, for any restaurant food or meal for which a nutrient content or health claim is made. The regulation requires that information on the nutrient amounts that are the basis of the claim is provided. For example, a claim that a meal or food is low in fat must provide the total grams of fat in the food or meal. Nutrient amounts may be determined from recipes, cookbooks, databases, and so on, and no specific format was mandated. Several jurisdictions, such as New York City, Philadelphia, Massachusetts, California, and several major counties, have mandated nutrition labeling on restaurant foods (44).

On March 23, 2010, President Obama signed the health care reform bill (45). Section 4205 of the new law expanded provisions of the NLEA, establishing new nutrition labeling requirements for standard menu items offered for sale in a "restaurant or similar retail food establishment that is part of a chain with 20 or more locations doing business under the same name (regardless of the type of ownership of the locations) and offering for sale substantially the same menu items." Establishments subject to the new requirements must disclose, in a clear and conspicuous manner, the following:

- The number of calories contained in the standard menu item
- A succinct statement concerning suggested daily caloric intake

In addition, restaurants also must provide certain additional nutrition information, such as fat content and information on other nutrients to consumers on request. The additional information must be in writing and available on the premises of the restaurant or retail service establishment. Some foods are exempt from the requirements, such as items that are not listed on a menu or menu board (e.g., condiments, daily specials) or temporary menu items that appear on the menu for fewer than 60 days per calendar year.

In March 21, 2011, the FDA issued proposed regulations to implement the new requirements. The regulations address standardization of recipes and methods of preparation, reasonable variation in serving size and formulation of menu items, space on menus and menu boards, inadvertent human error, training of food service workers, variations in ingredients, and the format and manner of the nutrient content disclosure requirements. The FDA also established regulations for determining and disclosing the nutrient content for standard menu items available in different flavors, varieties, or combinations, but that are listed as single menu items (e.g., soft drinks, ice cream, pizza, doughnuts, children's combination meals).

Vending machines are also subject to the new requirements, with certain exceptions. Calorie content must be provided by the vending machine operator when an article of food sold from a vending machine does not permit the purchaser to examine the product's Nutrition Facts panel before purchasing the article or does not otherwise provide visible nutrition information at the point of purchase.

On July 7, 2010, FDA announced that the agency was seeking public comments and information to help the agency implement the new federal law (46). The Health Care Reform Act preempts state and local laws that require nutrient disclosures. The new labeling requirements create a national standard that supersedes existing state and local requirements.

Dietary Supplement Labeling

The labeling of dietary supplements is governed by the Dietary Supplement Health and Education Act of 1994 (DSHEA) (47), which differs somewhat from the provisions of the NLEA. Under the DSHEA, the FDA has established regulations that govern the following:

- Nutrition labeling, statement of identity, and ingredient labeling (48)
- Nutrient content and health claims, comparative percentage claims, and mandatory structure/function claim disclaimer (49)
- Requirements to use the nutrient content claims "high potency" and "antioxidants" (50)
- Defining structure/function claims that can be used for dietary supplements (51)
- Mandatory warning statement for iron-containing supplements and special packaging requirements for high-potency iron supplements (52)

Dietary supplements, including their labeling, are covered in another chapter.

International Nutrition Labeling

Codex

The Codex Alimentarius Commission (Codex), a body of the United Nations, cosponsored by the Food and Agriculture Organization (FAO) of the United Nations and the World Health Organization (WHO), was established in 1963 to develop internationally agreed upon food standards that would protect the health of consumers and ensure fair practices in food trade (53). Codex is recognized by the World Trade Organization (WTO) as the benchmark for settling trade disputes involving food safety (54). Codex has developed guidelines for nutrition labeling that call for mandatory nutrient declaration for foods for which nutrition claims are made, but voluntary for all other foods (55). When nutrition labeling is applied, the amount of energy, protein, available carbohydrate (excluding dietary fiber), fat, and any other nutrient for which a claim is made must be declared. When a claim is made regarding the type or amount of carbohydrate, the amount of total sugars must be listed. When a claim is made regarding the amount and/or type of fatty acids or the amount of cholesterol, the amounts of saturated fatty acids, monounsaturated fatty acids, and polyunsaturated fatty acids and cholesterol should be declared. Many countries have followed Codex guidelines in establishing their nutrition labeling regulations (56).

Other Countries

As of January 2012, approximately 63 countries have some form of nutrition labeling requirements (57). Many require nutrition labeling when a nutritional claim is made and for foods for special dietary uses (e.g., the European Union [EC], Ecuador, Hungary, Indonesia, Japan, Singapore, South Africa, Thailand, and Vietnam). Others require nutrition labeling on certain foods for special dietary uses and other specified categories of foods (e.g., Gulf Cooperation Council member countries [Bahrain, Kuwait, Oman, Qatar, Saudi Arabia, and United Arab Emirates], Costa Rica, Croatia, Mauritius, Morocco, Nigeria, Peru, Philippines, and Venezuela). Nutrition labeling is required on most prepackaged foods in other countries, including the United States, Canada, Australia, New Zealand, Argentina, Brazil, Paraguay, Uruguay, Israel, Malaysia, and India. A number of individual countries are briefly discussed in the following sections.

China, Hong Kong, and Chinese Taipei (Taiwan). On April 21, 2010, China notified the WTO of the National Food Safety Standard for Nutrition Labeling of Prepackaged Foods as TBT/N/CHN/734. This measure "prescribes the basic principles and requirements for the nutrition labeling and claims on prepackaged foods directly offered to consumers." The Chinese regulations take effect on January 1, 2013 (57). On May 28, 2008, Hong Kong's Legislative Council passed a nutrition labeling regulation that took effect on July 1, 2010. The new labeling regulation required all prepackaged food sold in Hong Kong to include energy plus seven nutrients, including protein, carbohydrate, fat, saturated fat, trans-fat, sodium, and sugars. Taiwan has provided notification of intent to require nutrition labeling on all products manufactured after January 1, 2008. The required labeling elements will include energy, protein, fat (saturated and trans-), carbohydrate, sodium, and any other nutrients for which a claim is made. The labeling shall be expressed in units of 100 g or grams per serving. Number of servings per package shall also be declared.

Mexico. Mexico has proposed that a nutritional declaration on the label will be mandatory instead of voluntary.

Canada. Canada requires nutrition labeling on most prepackaged foods, using a Nutrition Facts label similar to that of the United States, with the obvious difference of bilingual (French and English) requirements. The regulations governing nutrition labeling in Canada were issued in 2003 (58) with subsequent amendments in 2005 (59). The Canadian regulations tightly control the format of the nutrition label, with a decision tree used to select among almost 30 main formats, along with a number of subformats for each main format. For example, vertical formats must be considered before horizontal or linear formats.

Australia and New Zealand. Foods sold in Australia and New Zealand are regulated by a binational agency, Food Standards Australia New Zealand. Packaged food sold in the two countries, with certain specified exceptions, must contain a Nutrition Information panel. Declaration of percent DV is optional. The regulations governing nutrition labeling in Australia and New Zealand can be found in the Australian standards (60).

Argentina, Brazil, Paraguay, and Uruguay. Mandatory nutritional food labeling has been applied in these countries since August 2006 for packaged food, except for some specifically chosen foods. In 2006, Mercosur established that all food labels must include information on *trans*-fatty acid content (61). Nutrition information is given per serving, with the mandatory nutrients (energy, carbohydrate, protein, total fat, saturated fat, *trans*-fat, dietary fiber, and sodium). The percent coverage of DVs also must be declared, according to FAO/WHO advice, except for *trans*-fat, which has no recommended value. For sodium, instead of a DV, a goal value of 2400 mg was used. The addition of some optional nutrients, such as specific carbohydrates (sugars, polyalcohols, starch), other fat components (cholesterol, monounsaturated and polyunsaturated fatty acids), and soluble and insoluble fiber is permitted. Vitamins and minerals may be included only if their amount per serving is higher than 5% of the RDI established by the FAO/WHO.

Israel. Israel is noteworthy for introducing mandatory nutrition labeling for the four major nutrients (energy, fat, protein, carbohydrate) on prepackaged foods in 1993. The nutrients are declared "per 100g/100ml" (with "per serving" as a voluntary addition).

Malaysia and Southeast Asian Countries. The Ministry of Health, Malaysia, amended the Food Regulations on September 29, 2005 to make nutrition labeling mandatory for certain foods, as well as to regulate health and nutrition claims. The Malaysian regulations closely follow the Codex guidelines on nutrition labeling in terms of format, components to be included, and mode of expression. In other Southeast Asian countries—notably Indonesia, the Philippines, Singapore, and Thailand—nutrition labeling is voluntary, unless the food is fortified or claims are made. Thailand also requires nutrition labeling on some snack foods, such as potato chips, popcorn, extruded snacks, cookies, crackers, and filled wafers. Thailand and the Philippines have drafted regulations very similar to those of the NLEA requirements in the United States (62).

India. Since 2008, packaged foods sold in India must declare nutritional information on the label (63). The label must also contain a mark of one of three organizations (the International Organization for Standardization, the Food Products Order regulated by the Ministry of Food Processing Industries, or the Agricultural Information Network under the Ministry of Agriculture) responsible for checking the information.

European Union. Nutrition labeling is harmonized throughout the EU. Nutrition labeling is subject to Council Directive 90/496/EEC (64), issued in 1990, but subsequently amended, perhaps most significantly by Council Directive 2008/100/EC of October 28, 2008 regarding recommended daily allowance definitions (65). Nutrition labeling is scheduled to become mandatory for all foods sold in the EU after January 1, 2014 (66). Claims are allowed only for energy, protein, carbohydrate, fat, dietary fiber, sodium, and vitamins and minerals.

The information that must be provided includes energy, protein, carbohydrate, and fat, unless a claim referring to sugars, saturated fatty acids, dietary fiber, or sodium exists, in which case the amount of sugar, saturated fat, fiber, and sodium also must be included. The amounts of monounsaturated fatty acids, polyunsaturated fatty acids, cholesterol, and vitamins and minerals also may be given. Nutrient amounts are declared per 100 g or per 100 mL, but also may be given per serving or per package. Information on vitamins and minerals is expressed as percentage of the recommended daily allowance (RDA).

CLAIMS

Nutrient Content Claims

United States

As another significant feature of the NLEA, the FDA was required to develop, by regulation, standard definitions for nutrient content claims. Such claims describe the level of a nutrient or dietary substance (e.g., fiber) in the product, using terms such as free, high, or low, or they compare the level of a nutrient in a food to that of another food, using terms such as more, reduced, or lite. The FDA and USDA defined a number of core claims (e.g., free, low, lean, extra lean, high, good source, reduced, less, light, fewer) as well as a number of synonyms. For example, synonyms for "free" include zero, no, without, trivial source of, negligible source of, and insignificant source of. Synonyms for "low" include little (few for calories), contains a small amount of, and low source of. The use of nutrient content claims on conventional foods is limited to nutrients for which a DV exists, based on the nutrient intake recommendations of the US dietary guidelines, or the NAS. Information on the criteria for the use of nutrient content claims can be found on the FDA website (67).

A few things should be noted, because there continues to be consumer confusion about certain terms. First, "free" does not mean zero. Rather, because absolute zero is difficult to measure and assure, "free" denotes an insignificant amount of a nutrient in terms of the daily diet. Second, foods that are naturally "free" or "low" in a nutrient without further processing must indicate this fact when making a claim. Required statements such as "broccoli, a fat-free food" or "celery, a low-calorie food" are intended to help consumers understand that this broccoli or celery is not different from other broccoli or celery.

In one of the more recent additions to the nutrient content regulations, the FDA and USDA defined "healthy" to be an implied nutrient content claim that characterizes a food that has "healthy" levels of total fat, saturated fat, cholesterol, and sodium (68).

International Considerations

Nutrient content claims are permitted in several countries. The Codex also has established guidelines for nutrient content claims. Under Codex guidelines, the only nutrient content claims permitted are those relating to energy, protein, carbohydrate, fat and its components (e.g., saturated fat or *trans*-fat), fiber, sodium, and vitamins and minerals, for which Codex has adopted Nutrient Reference Values. Unlike the regulations in the United States, the Codex claims are based on 100 g for solid foods and 100 mL for liquids. For example, "low" fat may be claimed for foods with 3 g or less fat per 100 g for solid foods or 1.5 g or less for liquids. Further information about the Codex guidelines for nutrient content claims may be found in the Codex publication, Food Labelling (69), available on the Codex website (70).

Health Claims

United States

A "health claim" describes a relationship between a food or food component and reduced risk of a disease- or health-related condition. A health claim has two essential components: a substance (food or food component), and a disease- or health-related condition. A statement lacking either one of these components does not meet the regulatory definition of a health claim. For example, statements that address a role of dietary patterns or general categories of foods (e.g., fruit and vegetables) in health are considered to be dietary guidance rather than health claims. Dietary guidance statements used on food labels must be truthful and non-misleading. Statements that address a role of a specific substance in maintaining normal healthy structures or functions of the body (e.g., calcium builds strong bones) are considered to be structure–function claims. Unlike health claims, dietary guidance statements and structure–function claims are not subject to FDA review and authorization.

Three ways by which the FDA exercises oversight of health claims are (a) NLEA authorized health claims; (b) health claims based on authoritative statements; and (c) qualified health claims.

1. NLEA Authorized Health Claims: NLEA provides for food label health claims that characterize a relationship between a food, food component, or dietary ingredient and the risk of a disease (e.g., "diets high in calcium may reduce the risk of osteoporosis"), provided the claims are authorized by an FDA regulation. The FDA authorizes these types of health claims based on an extensive review of the scientific literature, generally as a result of the submission of a health claim petition, using a *significant scientific agreement* standard to determine that the nutrient–disease relationship is well established. Claims that have been authorized by NLEA regulations include: calcium and osteoporosis (71); sodium and hypertension (72); fat and cancer (73); saturated fat and cholesterol and coronary heart disease (74); fiber-containing grain products, fruits, and vegetables and cancer (75); fruits, vegetables, and grain products that contain fiber, particularly soluble fiber,

and coronary heart disease (76); fruits and vegetables and cancer (77); folate and neural tube defects (78); noncariogenic carbohydrate sweeteners and dental caries (79); soluble fiber from certain foods and coronary heart disease (80); soy protein and coronary heart disease (81); and plant sterol–stanol esters and coronary heart disease (82).

2. Health Claims Based on Authoritative Statements. The Food and Drug Administration Modernization Act of 1997 (FDAMA) (83) provided a second way for the use of a health claim on foods. The FDAMA permits, after notification to FDA, health claims based on an "authoritative statement" from a scientific body of the US Government or the NAS. FDAMA-notified claims include whole grain foods and heart disease and certain cancers ("Diets rich in whole grain foods and other plant foods and low in total fat, saturated fat, and cholesterol may reduce the risk of heart disease and some cancers."); potassium and high blood pressure and stroke ("Diets containing foods that are a good source of potassium and that are low in sodium may reduce the risk of high blood pressure and stroke."); fluoridated water and dental carries ("Drinking fluoridated water may reduce the risk of [dental caries or tooth decay]."); and saturated fat, cholesterol, and *trans*-fat, and heart disease ("Diets low in saturated fat and cholesterol, and as low as possible in *trans* fat, may reduce the risk of heart disease.").

3. Qualified Health Claims. The FDA's 2003 Consumer Health Information for Better Nutrition Initiative provided for the use of qualified health claims when emerging evidence exists for a relationship between a food or food component and reduced risk of a disease or health-related condition (84). In this case, the evidence is not well established enough to meet the significant scientific agreement standard required for the FDA to issue an authorizing regulation. Examples of such claims for which the FDA has found insufficient evidence to establish a regulation include tomatoes and/or tomato sauce and prostate, ovarian, gastric, and pancreatic cancers; calcium and colon/rectal cancer and calcium and recurrent colon/rectal polyps; green tea and cancer; nuts and heart disease; monounsaturated fatty acids from olive oil and coronary heart disease; unsaturated fatty acids from canola oil and coronary heart disease; corn oil and heart disease; phosphatidylserine and cognitive dysfunction and dementia; chromium picolinate and diabetes; and calcium and hypertension, pregnancy-induced hypertension, and preeclampsia .

Qualifying language is included as part of the preceding claims to indicate that the evidence supporting them is limited. Examples of qualifying statements include "Although there is scientific evidence supporting the claim, the evidence is not conclusive," "Some scientific evidence suggests... however, FDA has determined that this evidence is limited and not conclusive," and "Very limited and preliminary scientific research suggests... FDA concludes that there is little scientific evidence supporting this claim."

International

Codex. Codex has developed very general guidelines on health claims, which state,

> Health claims must be based on current relevant scientific substantiation and the level of proof must be sufficient to substantiate the type of claimed effect and the relationship to health as recognized by generally accepted scientific review of the data and the scientific substantiation should be reviewed as new knowledge becomes available. The health claim must consist of two parts:
>
> 1. Information on the physiological role of the nutrient or on an accepted diet–health relationship; followed by
> 2. Information on the composition of the product relevant to the physiological role of the nutrient or the accepted diet–health relationship unless the relationship is based on a whole food or foods, whereby the research does not link to specific constituents of the food.

Any health claim must be accepted by or be acceptable to the competent authorities of the country where the product is sold.

European Union. Internationally, one of the more interesting developments has been the European Union's attempt to reign in health claims on food labels. In December 2006, the European Council and Parliament adopted a regulation on nutrition and health claims made on foods (85). This regulation lays down harmonized rules across the European Union for the use of health claims such as "reducing blood cholesterol." The European Food Safety Authority is required to validate claims based on scientific studies submitted by manufacturers. The agency is looking at more than 4000 health claims and has rejected more than 80% so far. An example of a rejected claim is that green tea is good for blood pressure, cholesterol levels, bones, and teeth, or that it works as an antioxidant, reducing the effects of aging (86).

Front-of-the-Package Issues

The use of symbols, logos, and icons on the front to communicate nutritional information of food labels has become prevalent throughout the marketplace in many countries (e.g., United Kingdom, Sweden, Australia, and the United States). Different systems use different criteria for permitting front-of-the-package displays, and some systems are proprietary. This has raised concerns that the meaning of different rating systems may be confusing to consumers. The FDA, along with the CDCP, asked the NAS to conduct a review of front-of-the-package nutrition rating systems and symbols. The committee considered the potential benefits of a single, standardized front-of-the-package food guidance system, regulated by the FDA. The Committee also developed conclusions about which system(s) are most effective in promoting health and how

to maximize the use and effectiveness of the system(s) (87). The FDA also announced that it was undertaking two quantitative consumer research studies on the relative effectiveness of existing and alternative labeling schemes in helping US consumers make better dietary decisions (88).

An excellent review of the various nutrition rating systems in a number of countries can be found on the website of the National Policy and Legal Analysis Network to Prevent Childhood Obesity of the Public Health Law Center of William Mitchell College of Law (89).

OTHER PUBLIC HEALTH LABELING

Ingredient Labeling

Requirements

FDA regulations require that ingredients be listed on the label in descending order of predominance by weight (90). Two ingredients, not nutrients, namely salt and sugar, have attracted considerable public health interest.

Issues

Added Salt. The majority of sodium intake by individuals comes from salt added to processed foods and prepared meals by food manufacturers, restaurants, and food service establishments. Concern about high sodium intakes prompted Congress in 2008 to request that the NAS develop a report on strategies on sodium intake. The report, sponsored by the FDA, CDC, and the National Heart, Lung, and Blood Institute and released in 2010, presented the FDA with several recommendations (91). It recommended that the FDA should set standards for salt added to processed foods and prepared meals, and that it should gradually step down the maximum amount of salt that can be added to foods, through a series of incremental reductions. The committee also recommended that the DV for sodium be changed from the current 2400 mg per day to 1500.

Added Sugar. Another ingredient that continues to create significant controversy is added sugar. Current nutrition labeling regulations require that, when the amount of sugar in a food is declared, all sugars, including naturally occurring sugar (e.g., lactose in milk) are included. Primarily because of the national obesity epidemic, many groups have called on the FDA to focus on added sugars as a healthy concern. In the most recent *Dietary Guidelines for Americans*, the Dietary Guidelines Advisory Committee recommended that added sugar be limited to 25% of total calorie consumption (92). The FDA is looking at this issue.

REFERENCES

1. Sinclair U. The Jungle. New York: Doubleday, Jabber & Company, 1906.
2. Federal Food and Drugs Act of 1906. Pub L No. 59-384, 34 Stat 768 (1906), 21 USC § 1-15 (1934). Repealed in 1938 by 21 USC § 329(a)

3. Federal Meat Inspection Act of 1906, 34 Stat 674. Amended by Pub L No. 59-242, 34 Stat 1260 (1967). Codified at 21 USC §§ 601 et seq.

4. Federal Food, Drug, and Cosmetic Act, 21 USC §341-350f.

5. White House Conference on Food, Nutrition and Health. J Nutr 1969;99:257–60.

6. White House Conference on Food, Nutrition and Health: Final Report. Washington, DC: US Government Printing Office, 1969.

7. Fed Regist 1971;33:11521–2.

8. Fed Regist 1972;34:6493–7.

9. Fed Regist 1973;38:2125–32.

10. Fed Regist 1984;49:15510–35.

11. US Department of Health and Human Services, Public Health Service. Aging. In: The Surgeon General's Report on Nutrition and Health. Washington, DC: US Government Printing Office, 1988. DHHS (PHS) publication 88-50210.

12. National Research Council, Diet and Health. Implications for Reducing Chronic Disease Risk. Washington, DC: National Academy Press, 1989.

13. National Academy of Sciences. Nutrition Labeling: Issues and Directions for the 1990s. Washington, DC: National Academy Press, 1990.

14. Hilts PJ. New York Times, March 8, 1990.

15. Fed Regist 1989;54:32610.

16. Fed Regist 1990;55:29476–533.

17. NLEA, Public Law 101-585, Nov. 8, 1990.

18. Magill ME. Food Drug Law J 1995;50:149–90.

19. Fed Regist 1991;56:6036–878.

20. Fed Regist 1993;58:2066–941.

21. Fed Regist 2003;68:41433–506.

22. Fed Regist 1993;58:2236–7.

23. Center for Science in the Public Interest. Petition for Rulemaking on Nutrition Labeling for Food and Beverages Sold in Single-Serving Containers, 2004.

24. US Department of Health and Human Services, National Institutes of Health, National Heart, Lung, and Blood Institute. Portion Distortion! Do You Know How Food Portions Have Changed in 20 Years? Available at: http://hin.nhlbi.nih.gov/portion/index.htm. Accessed September 15, 2012.

25. Smiciklas-Wright H, Mitchell DC, Mickle SJ et al. J Am Diet Assoc 2003;103:41–7.

26. Nielsen SJ, Popkin BM. JAMA 2003;289:450–3.

27. Young LR, Nestle M. J Am Diet Assoc 2003;103:231–4.

28. Working Group on Obesity. Calories Count. 2004. Available at: http://www.fda.gov/Food/LabelingNutrition/ReportsResearch/ucm081696.htm. Accessed September 15, 2012.

29. Fed Regist 2005;70:17010–14.

30. Atwater WO. US Farmers' Bull 1910;142:48.

31. Merrill AL, Watt BK. USDA Handbook. Washington, DC: US Government Printing Office, 1973.

32. Official Methods of Analysis of the AOAC International. 15th ed. Arlington, VA: The Association of Official Analytical Chemists, 1990.

33. Food and Agriculture Organization/World Health Organization. Report of the Joint FAO/WHO Expert Consultation on Protein Quality Evaluation. Rome: Food and Agriculture Organization, 1991.

34. Food and Nutrition Board, Institute of Medicine. Dietary Reference Intakes for Energy, Carbohydrate, Fiber, Fat, Fatty Acids, Cholesterol, Protein, and Amino Acids. Washington, DC: National Academies Press, 2005.

35. Dietary Reference Intakes. Available at: http://www.iom.edu/Reports/2006/Dietary-Reference-Intakes-Essential-Guide-Nutrient-Requirements.aspx. Accessed September 15, 2012.

36. Fed Regist 2007;72:62149–75.

37. Kessler DA, Mande JR, Scarbrough FE et al. Harvard Health Policy Review 2003;4(2):13–24.

38. 21 Code of Federal Regulations 101.9(d).

39. Bender MM, Scarbrough FE. The World of Ingredients 1995:54-6.

40. Poultry Products Inspection Act of 1957. Public Law 85-172, as amended.

41. Agricultural Marketing Act of 1946. As Amended Through Public Law 110–246.

42. 9 Code of Federal Regulations 317.400 (meat); 9 Code of Federal Regulations 381.500 (poultry)

43. 21 Code of Federal Regulations 101.10.

44. State and local laws/bills/regulations: 2009–2010. Available at: http://www.cspinet.org/new/pdf/ml_bill_summaries_09.pdf.

45. Patient Protection and Affordable Care Act of 2010. Pub L No. 111-148.

46. Fed Regist 2010;75:39026–8.

47. Dietary Supplement Health and Education Act of 1994. Pub L 103-417.

48. Fed Regist 1997;62:49825–58.

49. Fed Regist 1997;62:49859–68.

50. Fed Regist 1997;62:49868–81.

51. Fed Regist 2000;65:999–1050.

52. Fed Regist 1997;62:2217–50.

53. Codex Alimentarius Commission. Procedural Manual, 20th ed. Available at: ftp://ftp.fao.org/codex/Publications/ProcManuals/Manual_20e.pdf. Accessed September 15, 2012

54. World Trade Organization. Available at: http://www.wto.org/english/thewto_e/coher_e/wto_codex_e.htm. Accessed September 15, 2012.

55. Guidelines on Nutrition Labelling, CAC/GL 2-1985. Available at: http://www.codexalimentarius.org/standards/list-of-standards/en/. Accessed September 15, 2012

56. Lewis CJ, Randell A, Scarbrough FE. Food Control 1996;7: 285–293.

57. European Food Information Council. Global Update on Nutrition Labelling, 2012, Executive Summary. Available at: http://www.eufic.org/upl/1/default/doc/GlobalUpdateExecSumJan2012_PUBLIC_Final.pdf. Accessed September 15, 2012.

58. Canada Gazette. Part II. 2003;1:154–403.

59. Canada Gazette. Part I. 2005;1:1570–1620.

60. Food Standards Australia New Zealand. Available at: http://www.foodstandards.gov.au/foodstandards/foodstandardscode.cfm. Accessed September 15, 2012

61. Mercosul Technical Regulation for Nutritional Labeling of Packaged Foods 12/12/2003 [English translation] Montevideo: Mercosul, 2003. Available at: http://www.anvisa.gov.br/alimentos/informacao_nutricional_alegacoes_saude_cenaario_global_regulamentacoes.pdf. Accessed September 15, 2012.

62. E-Siong Tee, Tamin S, Ilyas R et al. J Clin Nutr 2002;11: S80–6.

63. Prevention of Food Adulteration. Available at: http://www.pfndai.com/Gazette%20pdfs/002_664_2008.pdf. Accessed September 15, 2012.

64. European Parliament and Council. Nutrition Labelling Rules of Foodstuffs. Council Directive 90/496/EEC, 1990.

65. European Parliament and Council. Recommended Daily Allowances Definitions. 2008 Council Directive. Available at: http://eur-lex.europa.eu/LexUriServ/LexUriServ.do?ur=OJ:L:2008:285:0009:0012:EN:PDF.

66. Regulation EU No 1169/2011 of the European Parliament and the Council of 25 October 2011 on the provision of food information to consumers. Available at http://eur-lex

.europa.eu/LexUriServ/LexUriServ.do?uri=OJ:L:2011:304:0018:0063:EN:PDF. Accessed September 15, 2012

67. Criteria for the Use of Nutrient Content Claims. Available at: http://www.fda.gov/Food/GuidanceComplianceRegulatory Information/default.htm. Accessed September 15, 2012.

68. 21 Code of Federal Regulations §101.65.

69. FAO/WHO. Food Labelling. 5th ed. Rome: Food and Agriculture Organization, 2007.

70. Codex Alimentarius, Thematic Compilations. Available at: ftp://ftp.fao.org/codex/Publications/Booklets/Labelling/Labelling_2007_EN.pdf. Accessed September 15, 2012.

71. 21 Code of Federal Regulations 101.72.

72. 21 Code of Federal Regulations 101.74.

73. 21 Code of Federal Regulations 101.73.

74. 21 Code of Federal Regulations 101.75.

75. 21 Code of Federal Regulations 101.76.

76. 21 Code of Federal Regulations 101.77.

77. 21 Code of Federal Regulations 101.78.

78. 21 Code of Federal Regulations 101.79.

79. 21 Code of Federal Regulations 101.80.

80. 21 Code of Federal Regulations 101.81.

81. 21 Code of Federal Regulations 101.82.

82. 21 Code of Federal Regulations 101.83.

83. The Food and Drug Administration Modernization Act of 1997. Pub L 105-115.

84. Consumer Health Information for Better Nutrition Initiative: Task Force Final Report. Available at: http://www.fda.gov/Food/LabelingNutrition/LabelClaims/QualifiedHealthClaims/QualifiedHealthClaimsPetitions/ucm096010.htm. Accessed September 15, 2012

85. European Parliament and Council. Nutrition and Health Claims Made on Foods. Regulation (EC) No 1924/2006, 2006.

86. European Food Safety Authority. Available at: http://www.efsa.europa.eu/en.

87. Institute of Medicine, Front-of-Package Nutrition Rating Systems and Symbols: Promoting Healthier Choices, Washington DC, National Academies Press, 2012

88. Fed Regist 2009;74:62786–92.

89. Armstrong K. 2010. Stumped at the Supermarket; Making sense of nutrition rating systems. Available at http://changelab solutions.org/publications/stumped-supermarket. Accessed September 15, 2012.

90. 21 Code of Federal Regulations §101.4

91. Henney JE, Taylor CL, Boon CS, eds. Strategies to Reduce Sodium Intake in the United States. Washington, DC: National Academies Press, 2010.

92. Fed Regist 2010;75:33759–60.

SUGGESTED READINGS

Armstrong K. Childhood Obesity. St. Paul, MN: Public Health Law Center, William Mitchell College of Law, 2010. Available at: http://nplan.org.

FDA Consumer Information. How to Understand and Use the Nutrition Facts Label. Available at: http://www.fda.gov/Food/ResourcesForYou/Consumers/NFLPM/ucm274593.htm.

FDA Consumer Information. Make Your Calories Count: Use the Nutrition Facts Label for Healthy Weight Management. Available at: http://www.fda.gov/Food/ResourcesForYou/Consumers/NFLPM/ucm275438.htm.

FDA Consumer Information. Spot the Block Using the Nutrition Facts Label to Make Healthy Food Choices: A Program for Tweens. Available at: http://www.fda.gov/Food/ResourcesForYou/Consumers/KidsTeens/ucm115810.htm.

Taylor C, Wilkening V. J Am Diet Assoc 2008;(Part 1)107:437–42; (Part 2)107:618–23.

World Health Organization. Nutrition labels and health claims: the global regulatory environment. Available at: http://whqlibdoc.who.int/publications/2004/9241591714.pdf.

108 FOOD ASSISTANCE PROGRAMS[1]
CRAIG GUNDERSEN

Low-income families in the United States face numerous challenges. One central challenge is limitations in the ability to acquire enough food for their families. In 2010, for example, 14.5% of Americans were food insecure (i.e., they were uncertain of having, or unable to acquire, enough food for all their members because they had insufficient money or other resources) (1). These proportions were substantially higher among certain subgroups of the population, including children and low-income households.

---

[1]**Abbreviations: ABAWDs**, able-bodied adults without dependents; **CACFP**, Child and Adult Care Food Program; **CCFP**, Child Care Food Program; **EBT**, electronic benefit transfer; **NSLP**, National School Lunch Program; **SBP**, School Breakfast Program; **SNAP**, Supplemental Nutrition Assistance Program; **SSI**, Supplemental Security Income; **TANF**, Temporary Assistance for Needy Families; **TEFAP**, Emergency Food Assistance Program; **USDA**, US Department of Agriculture; **WIC**, Special Supplemental Nutrition Program for Women, Infants, and Children.

That millions of persons in the United States go without sufficient food is a serious issue and policy concern. Moreover, a well-established set of consequences exists associated with food insecurity. Research has shown that children in households suffering from food insecurity are more likely to have fair or poor general health (2–9), psychosocial problems (8, 10–13), frequent stomachaches and headaches (10), increased odds of being hospitalized (3), greater propensities to have seen a psychologist (10), behavior problems (14, 15), lower intakes of important nutrients (16–18), worse developmental outcomes (19–21), more chronic illnesses (8), impaired functioning (13), impaired mental proficiency (22), and higher levels of iron deficiency with anemia (23, 24) than are children in food-secure households. Food-insecure adults have been shown to have lower intakes of a variety of nutrients (25–28), a broad set of physical health problems (29–33), mental health challenges (31, 34), and chronic diseases (35, 36), including type 2 diabetes (29, 35, 37). Among senior adults in particular, the negative health consequences of food insecurity include lower intakes of a variety of nutrients (38, 39), lower skinfold thickness (38), greater likelihood of reporting fair or poor health (38–40), higher levels of depression (39–41), poorer quality of life (41), and lower levels of physical performance (41).

Although research on food insecurity and its consequences is relatively recent, the US government has long recognized that millions of Americans face serious nutritional challenges. In response, the United States has established a food assistance safety net composed of several distinct programs. The largest food assistance program in the United States is the Supplemental Nutrition Assistance Program (SNAP). Three additional programs directed toward children are the Special Supplemental Nutrition Program for Women, Infants, and Children (WIC); the National School Lunch Program (NSLP); and the School Breakfast Program (SBP). Smaller, but important, programs include The Emergency Food Assistance Program (TEFAP) and the Child and Adult Care Food Program (CACFP).

SUPPLEMENTAL NUTRITION ASSISTANCE PROGRAM

The SNAP (formerly known as the Food Stamp Program) is by far the largest US food assistance program, serving approximately 46 million individuals in 2011, with an annual benefit distribution of $75.7 billion. Participants receive benefits for the purchase of food in authorized retail food outlets. Benefits are distributed through an electronic benefit transfer (EBT) card, which is operationally similar to an automated teller machine (ATM) card. The level of benefits received by a household is determined by income level and family size. In 2010, the average monthly benefit was $288/month for a family of four, with the maximum benefit for a family of four being $668. The central goal of SNAP is to be a core component of the safety net against hunger (42).

History

A form of SNAP (food stamps) began in 1939, when low-income persons were allowed to buy orange stamps equal to their normal food expenditures and to then receive supplemental blue stamps that were valued at 50% of the household's normal food expenditures. Although orange stamps could be used to buy any food, blue stamps could only be used to buy food that the US Department of Agriculture (USDA) determined to be surplus. In 1961, a pilot program retained the purchased food stamps, but eliminated stamps specifically for surplus foods. In 1964, The Food Stamp Act was passed in which, among other things, each state developed the eligibility standards to use within its borders. Recipients purchased their food stamps, paying an amount corresponding with their normal food expenditures, and then received a predetermined amount of food stamps, based on that considered necessary, to obtain a low-cost, nutritionally adequate diet (the purchase requirement). All food items except alcoholic beverages and imported foods were deemed suitable for purchase with food stamps.

The Food Stamp Act of 1977 made a major change by eliminating the so-called purchase requirement, because it was thought to discourage participation. With the elimination of the purchase requirement on January 1, 1979, there was a 1.5 million participant increase compared with the preceding month. In the 1980s, the recognition of hunger as a serious issue in the United States led to further improvements in the Food Stamp Program, such as elimination of sales taxes on food stamp purchases, the reinstatement of categoric eligibility (discussed later), and an increased resource limit.

In the past two decades, other changes to the program have been made. The 1993 Mickey Leland Childhood Hunger Relief Act allowed households with children to more easily gain access to needed SNAP benefits by raising the cap on the dependent care deduction and simplifying the household definition. The Personal Responsibility and Work Opportunities Reconciliation Act of 1996 (PRWORA) enacted other major changes, including restrictions on eligibility for most legal immigrants, time limits on food stamp receipt for healthy adults with no dependent children, and requirements for states to implement the EBT system.

In 2002, the Food Security and Rural Investment Act re-established eligibility to qualified legal immigrants, modified the standard deduction to vary by household size and inflation; and provided incentives to encourage states to maintain high standards within the administration of the program.

The American Recovery and Reinvestment Act Plan of 2009 lead to some temporary changes in SNAP. In particular, it provided an increase in the monthly benefits of SNAP participants, expanded eligibility for jobless adults, and added federal dollars to support the administration of the program.

Eligibility Criteria

Eligibility for SNAP is defined at the household level. More specifically, a household is defined as one containing people who live together and purchase and prepare meals together. To be eligible for SNAP, households have to first meet a monthly gross income test. Under this criterion, a household's income (before any deductions) has to be less than 130% of the poverty line. As an example, in 2010, a SNAP household with three persons and a monthly income less than $1984 would be gross income eligible. The gross income test does not apply to all households, however; households with at least one elderly member or one disabled member do not have to meet this test.

Households with an elderly or disabled member and most other households have to pass the net income criteria, wherein net income is defined as gross income minus certain deductions. The allowable deductions include (a) a standard deduction for all households; (b) a 20% earned income deduction; (c) a dependent care deduction when care is necessary for work, training, or education; (d) a legally owed child support payments deduction; (e) a medical costs deduction for elderly and disabled people; and (f) an excess shelter cost deduction. To be eligible, this net income must be less than the poverty line. As an example, in 2010, a SNAP household with net income of less than $1526/month would be net income eligible. Households in which all members receive Supplemental Security Income (SSI) or Temporary Assistance for Needy Families (TANF) are considered to be automatically eligible for SNAP, and do not have to pass either the gross or the net income tests.

The final test for SNAP eligibility is the asset test. For most households, the total assets of a household must be less than $2000. When determining eligibility with respect to assets, some resources are not counted, such as one's home and up to $4650 of the fair market value of one car per adult household member. Similarly, one car per teenaged household member may be deducted if the teenager is using it for work, and a vehicle's value is not counted if it is needed to transport a disabled household member. Exceptions to these rules apply: Households with an elderly or disabled person have an asset limit of $3000; those where everyone received SSI or TANF do not have an asset test. Many states have the ability to waive the asset test.

Able-bodied adults without dependents (ABAWDs), between the ages of 18 and 50 years, must be employed to receive SNAP. If they are not employed, they can lose their SNAP benefits. In areas with particularly high unemployment rates or limited employment opportunities, this so-called ABAWD requirement is waived.

Research Evaluations

Determinants of Participation

A high proportion of households eligible for SNAP do not participate. This is ascribed to three main factors. First, there may be stigma associated with receiving SNAP. Stigma encompasses a wide variety of sources, from a person's own distaste for receiving SNAP, to the fear of disapproval from others when redeeming SNAP, to the possible negative reaction of caseworkers (43, 44). Second, transaction costs can diminish the attractiveness of participation. Examples of such costs include travel time to, and time spent in, a SNAP office; the burden of transporting children to the office or paying for child care services; and the direct costs of paying for transportation. A household faces these costs on a repeated basis, because it must recertify its eligibility. Third, the benefit level can be quite small— for some families, as low as $10 per month.

Because the Government Performance and Results Act of 1993 calls for policy makers to assess the effects of federal programs, the extent of nonparticipation by eligible households is closely followed. To this end, national SNAP participation, defined as the percentage of eligible people who actually participate in food stamps, has been used to assess performance for nearly 25 years. In 2008, a 2-year performance target of 68% of the eligible population was set.

The most recently calculated food stamp participation data show that approximately 67% of eligible people in the United States received food stamp benefits in 2008 (45). However, participation varied greatly from state to state. Missouri, Tennessee, Oregon, Maine, West Virginia, Michigan, Louisiana, and Kentucky had significantly higher participation rates than two thirds of the remaining states, whereas Wyoming, Nevada, California, and Utah had significantly lower rates. In 2007, among the eligible working poor—those who work but are still in need—56% received food stamps. As for all eligible people, participation by the working poor varied widely across states. Reasons for this variation across states include, among other factors, differences in macroeconomic conditions and social policies (46).

Impacts on Health Outcomes

Given the large number of people reached by SNAP and the total cost of SNAP benefits, policymakers and program administrators are very interested in the success of SNAP in improving the health and well-being of recipients. The central goal of SNAP is the alleviation of food insecurity.

Comparisons between eligible households that do and do not participate in SNAP show that the prevalence of food insecurity is substantially higher among participants.

For example, using data from the Current Population Survey from 2003, food insecurity was 52% higher among participants (47). This difference, which holds even after controlling for other factors, is perplexing to policymakers because it suggests that SNAP is not successful in achieving its central goal. However, the reality is more complex.

Researchers have addressed this paradoxical result in two main ways. First, the higher rates of food insecurity could be the result of adverse selection, because households more likely to be food insufficient are also more likely to be in SNAP, and encouraging those who are most at risk of food insecurity to join the program is a central goal (48). After controlling for this, researchers have found that SNAP recipients either have the same probability of food insecurity as nonrecipients or are less likely to be food insecure (49, 50). Another possible issue is measurement error with respect to SNAP participation. SNAP participation is misreported in major surveys, with errors of omission (i.e., saying that one does not receive SNAP when one really does) being substantially more likely than errors of commission (51, 52) This systematic misreporting can lead to incorrect conclusions about the relationship between SNAP and food insecurity. One study found that even with low levels of misreporting, the usual positive association between SNAP and food insecurity disappears (47).

SPECIAL SUPPLEMENTAL NUTRITION PROGRAM FOR WOMEN, INFANTS, AND CHILDREN

The goal of the WIC in the US social safety net is to "provide supplemental nutritious food as an adjunct to good health during such critical times of growth and development [during pregnancy, the postpartum period, infancy, and early childhood] to prevent the occurrence of health problems" (P.L. 94–105). To meet this goal, WIC provides nutritious foods, nutrition education, and referrals to health and other social services to participants. WIC is designed for low-income, nutritionally at-risk, pregnant, postpartum, and breast-feeding women, and infants and children up to age 5 years. WIC is not an entitlement program, meaning that Congress does not set aside funds to allow every eligible individual to participate in the program. Instead, WIC is a federal grant program, for which Congress authorizes a specific amount of funding each year. The USDA Food and Nutrition Service (FNS) provides these funds to state agencies, such as state health departments, to pay for WIC foods, nutrition education, and administrative costs. WIC operates through 2000 local agencies, 10,000 clinic sites, 50 state health departments, 34 Indian Tribal Organizations, the District of Columbia, and 5 territories.

History

WIC was launched as a pilot program in 1972 and made permanent in 1974. Formerly known as the WIC. WIC's name was changed to emphasize its role as a nutrition

3.   Cook J, Frank D, Berkowitz C et al. J Nutr 2004;134: 1348–1432.
4.   Cook J, Frank D, Levenson S et al. J Nutr 2006;136:1073–6.
5.   Dunifon R, Kowaleski-Jones L. Soc Serv Rev 2003;77:72–92.
6.   Gundersen C, Kreider B. J Health Econ 2009;28:971–83.
7.   Kirkpatrick S, McIntyre L, Potestio M. Arch Pediatr Adolesc Med 2010;164:754–62.
8.   Weinreb L, Wehler C, Perloff J et al. Pediatrics 2002;110:e41.
9.   Yoo J, Slack K, Hall J. Am J Public Health 2009;99:829–836.
10. Alaimo K, Olson C, Frongillo E. Pediatrics 2001;108:44–53.
11. Alaimo K, Olson C, Frongillo E. J Nutr 2002;132:719–25.
12. Kleinman R, Murphy J, Little M et al. Pediatrics 1998;101:e3.
13. Murphy J, Wehler C, Pagano M et al. J Am Acad Child Adolesc Psychiatry 1998;37:163–70.
14. Slack K, Yoo J. Soc Serv Rev 2005;79:511–36.
15. Whitaker R, Phillips S, Orzol S. Pediatrics 2006;118:e859–e68.
16. Kaiser L, Melgar-Quinonez H, Lamp C et al. J Am Diet Assoc 2002;102:924–9.
17. Kaiser L, Melgar-Quinonez H, Townsend M et al. J Nutr Educ Behav 2003;35:148–53.
18. Matheson D, Varady J, Varady A et al. Am J Clin Nutr 2002;76:210–17.
19. Hernandez D, Jacknowitz A. J Nutr 2009;139:1517–24.
20. Jyoti D, Frongillo E, Jones S. J Nutr 2005;135:2831–9.
21. Rose-Jacobs R, Black M, Casey P et al. Pediatrics 2008;121: 65–72.
22. Zaslow M, Bronte-Tinkew J, Capps R et al. Matern Child Health J 2009;13:66–80.
23. Eicher-Miller H, Mason A, Weaver C et al. Am J Clin Nutr 2009;90:1358–71.
24. Skalicky A, Meyers A, Adams W et al. Matern Child Health J 2006;10:177–85.
25. Bhattacharya J, Currie J, Haider S. J Health Econ 2004;23: 839–62.
26. Dixon L, Winkelby M, Radimer K. J Nutr 2001;131:1232–46.
27. McIntyre L, Glanville T, Raine K et al. Can Med Assoc J 2003;168:686–91.
28. Olson C. Top Clin Nutr 2005;20:321–8.
29. Nelson K, Cunningham W, Andersen R et al. J Gen Intern Med 2001;16:404–11.
30. Pheley A, Holben D, Graham A et al. J Rural Health 2002;18: 447–54.
31. Siefert K, Heflin C, Corcoran M et al. Women Heath 2001;32:159–77.
32. Stuff J, Casey P, Szeto K et al. J Nutr 2004;134:2330–5.
33. Vozoris N, Tarasuk V. J Nutr 2003;133:1200–6.
34. Huddleston-Casas C, Charnigo R, Simmon L. Public Health Nutr 2009;12:1133–40.
35. Biros M, Hoffman P, Resch K. Acad Emerg Med 2005; 12:310–17.
36. Sullivan A, Clark S, Pallin D et al. J Emerg Med 2010;38:524–8.
37. Seligman H, Bindman A, Vittinghoff E et al. Soc Gen Intern Med 2007;22:1018–23.
38. Lee J, E. Frongillo J. Nutr 2001;131:1503–9.
39. Ziliak J, Gundersen C, Haist M. The Causes, Consequences, and Future of Senior Hunger in America. Special report by the University of Kentucky Center for Poverty Research for the Meals on Wheels Association of America Foundation. Lexington, KY: University of Kentucky Center for Poverty Research, 2008.
40. Holben D, Barnett M, Holcomb J. J Hunger Environ Nutr 2006;1:89–99.
41. Klesges L, Pahor M, Shorr R et al. Am J Public Health 2001;91:68–75.
42. US Department of Agriculture Food and Nutrition Service. Annual Historical Review: Fiscal Year 1997. Washington, DC: US Department of Agriculture, 1999.
43. Ranney C, Kushman J. South Econ J 1987;53:1011–27.
44. Moffitt R. Am Econ Rev 1983;73:1023–35.
45. US Department of Agriculture Food and Nutrition Service. Current Perspective on SNAP Participation. Washington, DC: US Department of Agriculture, 2009.
46. Ziliak J, Gundersen C, Figlio D. South Econ J 2003;69:903–19.
47. Gundersen C, Kreider B. J Hum Resour 2008;43:352–82.
48. Gundersen C, Jolliffe D, Tiehen L. Food Policy 2009;34:367–76.
49. Gundersen C, Oliveira V. Am J Ag Econ 2001;84:875–87.
50. DePolt R, Moffitt R, Ribar D. Pacific Econ Rev 2009;14: 445–73.
51. Bollinger C, David M. J Am Stat Assoc 1997;92:827–35.
52. Bollinger C, David M. J Bus Econ Stat 2001;19:129–41.
53. Bitler M, Currie J, Scholz J. J Hum Resour 2003;38:1139–79.
54. Gundersen C. Child Youth Serv Rev 2005;27:99–114.
55. Bitler M, Gundersen C, Marquis G. Rev Ag Econ 2005;27(3): 433–8.
56. Arcia G, Crouch L, Kulka R. Am J Agric Econ 1990;72:218–26.
57. Basiotis P, Kramer-LeBlanc C, Kennedy E. Fam Econ Nutr Rev 1998;11:4–16.
58. Oliveira V, Gundersen C. US Department of Agriculture Economic Research Service: Food Assistance and Nutrition Research Report 5. Washington, DC: US Department of Agriculture, 2000.
59. Siega-Riz A, Kranz S, Blanchette D et al. J Pediatrics 2004; 144:229–34.
60. Swensen A, Harnack J, Ross J. J Am Diet Assoc 2001;101:903–8.
61. Ahluwalia I, Hogan V, Grummer-Strawn et al. Am J Public Health 1998;88:1374–7.
62. Brown H, Watkins K, Hiett A. Am J Obstet Gynecol 1996; 174:1279–83.
63. Gueorguieva R, Morse S, Roth J. Matern Child Health J 2009; 13:479–88.
64. Moss N, Carver K. Am J Public Health 1998;88:1354–61.
65. Black M, Cutts D, Frank D et al. Pediatrics 2004;114:169–76.
66. Devaney B, Bilheimer L, Schore J. J Policy Anal Manag 1992;11:573–92.
67. Figlio D, Hamersma S, Roth J. J Pub Econ 2009;93:235–45.
68. Kowaleski-Jones L, Duncan G. Am J Public Health 2002;92: 799–804.
69. Kim I, Hungerford D, Kuester S et al. MMWR 1992;41: 26–42.
70. Yip R, Pravanta I, Scanlon K et al. MMWR 1992;41:1–24.
71. El-Bastawissi A, Peters R, Sassen K et al. Matern Child Health J 2007;11:611–21.
72. Altucher K, Rasmussen K, Barden E et al. J Am Diet Assoc 2005;105:709–15.
73. Carlson A, Senauer B. Am J Agric Econ 2003;85:479–91.
74. Buescher P, Horton S, Devaney B et al. Am J Public Health 2003;93:145–150.
75. Lee B, Mackey-Bilaver L. Child Youth Serv Rev 2007;29: 501–17.
76. Jacknowitz A, Novillo D, Tiehen L. Pediatrics 2007;119: 281–89.
77. Bitler M, Currie J. J Policy Anal Manag 2005;24:73–93.
78. Jiang M, Foster M, Gibson-Davis C. Child Youth Serv Rev 2010;32:264–73.
79. Joyce T, Gibson D, Colman S. J Policy Anal Manag 2005;24: 661–85.
80. Joyce T, Racine A, Yunzal-Butler C. J Policy Anal Manag 2008;27:277–303.

81.   Beal A, Kuhlthau K, Perrin J. Public Health Rep 2003;118: 368–76.
82.   Chatterji P, Brooks-Gunn J. Am J Public Health 2004;94:1324–7.
83.   Houghton M, Graybeal T. J Am Diet Assoc 2001;101:245–7.
84.   McCann M, Baydar N, Williams R. J Hum Lact 2007;23: 314–24.
85.   Ryan A, Zhou W. Pediatrics 2005;117:1136–46.
86.   Gleason P, Suitor C. Am J Agric Econ 2003;85:1047–61.
87.   Akin J, Guilkey D, Popkin B. Am J Agric Econ 1983;65:477–85.
88.   Grainger C, Senauer B, Runge C. J Cons Affairs 2007;41: 265–84.
89.   Millimet D, Tchernis R, Husain M. J Hum Resour 2010;45: 640–54.
90.   Gundersen C, Kreider B, Pepper J. J Econometrics 2012;166: 79–91.
91.   Nord M, Romig K. J Children Poverty 2006;12:141–58.
92.   Devaney B, Fraker T. Am J Agric Econ 1989;71:932–48.
93.   Sampson A, Dixit S, Meyers A et al. Ambulatory Child Health 1995;1:14–22.
94.   Bartfeld J, Ahn H. J Nutr 2011;141:470–5.

SUGGESTED READINGS

Gundersen C, Kreider B, Pepper J. The Economics of Food Insecurity in the United States. Applied Economic Perspectives and Policy, 2011;33(3):281–303.

Jolliffe D, Ziliak J, eds. Income Volatility and Food Assistance in the United States. Kalamazoo, MI: WE Upjohn Institute for Employment Research, 2008.

Institute of Medicine. Planning a WIC Research Agenda: Workshop Summary. Washington, DC: National Academies Press, 2011.

Institute of Medicine. School Meals: Building Blocks for Healthy Children. Washington, DC: National Academies Press, 2010.

Nord M, Coleman-Jensen A, Andrews M et al. Household Food Security in the United States, 2009. Economic Research Report 108. Washington, DC: US Department of Agriculture Economic Research Service, 2009.

Oliveira V. Informing Food and Nutrition Assistance Policy: 10 Years of Research at ERS. Miscellaneous publication 1598. Washington, DC: U.S. Department of Agriculture Economic Research Service, 2007.

109 THE NUTRITION TRANSITION: GLOBAL TRENDS IN DIET, LIFESTYLE, AND NONCOMMUNICABLE DISEASES[1]

BENJAMIN CABALLERO

Food has been a critical factor for the survival of the human species since the beginning of time. For centuries, humans have struggled to secure enough food for survival, and to achieve a body size that optimized chances of survival, productivity, and reproduction. In the past century, the dramatic increase in access to dietary energy by millions of people in the developing world and the relative reduction in infectious disease burden, for the first time in history, have led to an increase in the body size of the human species that exceeds the desirable limits. Around the year 2002, a sort of milestone was reached: The number of overweight people on the planet exceeded the number of underweight people (1). Today, we confront a global epidemic of overweight and obesity, which is leading inevitably to a dramatic increase in diabetes, cardiovascular diseases, and other conditions associated with excess body mass. Furthermore, in many countries, undernutrition (underweight) coexists with overnutrition (overweight), even within the same household (2, 3). About 1 billion adults are overweight, and more than 300 million are clinically obese.

[1]**Abbreviations: BMI**, body mass index; **GDP**, gross domestic product; **GNP**, gross national product; **LMICs**, low- and middle-income countries; **QSR**, quick service restaurant; **SES**, socioeconomic status; **UN**, United Nations; **WHO**, World Health Organization.

THE PERSISTENT PROBLEM OF UNDERNUTRITION

Approximately 20 million children in the world are severely undernourished, and half of them will die every year—more than 1000 per hour. The World Health Organization (WHO) estimated that more than two thirds of those deaths are preventable by simple relatively low-cost interventions (4), because the leading causes of death—diarrhea, pneumonia, and malaria—are treatable or preventable. Poverty continues to be a major underlying factor in the persistent burden of undernutrition and preventable diseases in children. Approximately half the world population lives on less than $2 per day, and 20% of these on less than $1 per day. Poverty level correlates strongly with the prevalence of underweight. The role of socioeconomic status (SES) on the nutrition transition is further discussed later.

THE GLOBAL EPIDEMIC OF OBESITY

Overweight/obesity is an important risk factor for death. It ranks fifth among leading mortality risks, and is responsible for 7% to 8% of deaths globally. Overweight has been a longstanding public health concern in developed countries, but the focus on developing countries is relatively recent. The WHO Technical Report No. 894, one of the first devoted to the "global epidemic" of obesity, was published in 2000 (5). Since then, the focus and research on global obesity, as well as on related chronic, noncommunicable disorders associated with excess weight, have expanded considerably (6).

The global obesity epidemic continues its upward trend in most countries and regions. An analysis by Finucane et al (7) provided evidence of this continuing progression. Between the period evaluated, 1980 to 2008, body mass index (BMI) increased in all but eight of the 199 countries studied. Flat trends were observed in some Eastern European countries in women and in Central Africa and South Asia in men. The data also showed a wide range of mean BMI in different populations, from 19.9 in men from Congo to 35 in women from Nauru. The authors estimated that, as of 2008, there were 1.46 billion individuals in the world with excess body weight (BMI $\geq$25), of whom about 35% were obese (BMI >30). The data showed a moderate excess of obesity in women relative to men, but with wide

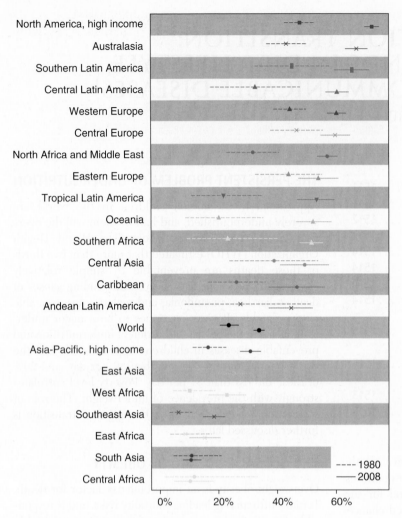

Fig. 109.1. Global prevalence of obesity, men. Changes in prevalence between 1980 and 2008 in selected countries. (Reproduced with permission from Finucane MM, Stevens GA, Cowan MJ et al. National, regional, and global trends in body-mass index since 1980: systematic analysis of health examination surveys and epidemiological studies with 960 country-years and 9.1 million participants. Lancet 2011;377:557–67.)

country and regional variations. Figures 109.1 and 109.2 depict the changes in prevalence of obesity between 1980 and 2008. Well-recognized caveats in interpreting combined datasets from different countries exist, particularly with the use of a single cutoff point to define overweight and obesity across regions. Nevertheless, these data provide an important assessment of trends in the obesity epidemic since 1980.

Obesity prevalence is also on the rise in young children (0 to 5 years of age). Estimates indicate that the global prevalence of overweight and obesity in this age group has increased from 4.2% in 1990 to 6.7% in 2010 (8). This is equivalent to 43 million overweight or obese children, of whom 35 million are in developing countries. This same report projected that by the year 2020 the prevalence will reach 9.1%, or approximately 60 million children.

THE NUTRITION TRANSITION

The term "transition" has been used to describe the epidemiologic transition (9), and it was applied by Popkin and others to describe trends associated with diet, food consumption, and chronic diseases that are occurring in the developing world (10, 11). This nutrition transition can be seen as part of the changes that shaped human

health during the last half of the twentieth century, namely, the demographic, economic, and technologic changes that developing countries experienced during that period (12, 13). The nutrition transition has been driven by three major factors: changes in global food availability and dietary intake, urbanization, and a lifestyle characterized by low levels of physical activity. Technical advances in communications also have played an important role by facilitating the rapid and extensive dissemination of cultural preferences and lifestyle trends.

DIETARY TRENDS

Since the 1980s and 1990s, major shifts in diet quantity and composition have occurred across the world. Per capita energy availability increased markedly. In the developing world (excluding sub-Saharan Africa), this increase averaged approximately 600 kcal/day, but was as much as 1000 kcal/day in China (14). Overall, low- and middle-income countries (LMIC) have seen modest declines in consumption of cereals and pulses and an increase in animal food sources, whereas a low consumption of fruit and vegetables continues to be a concern.

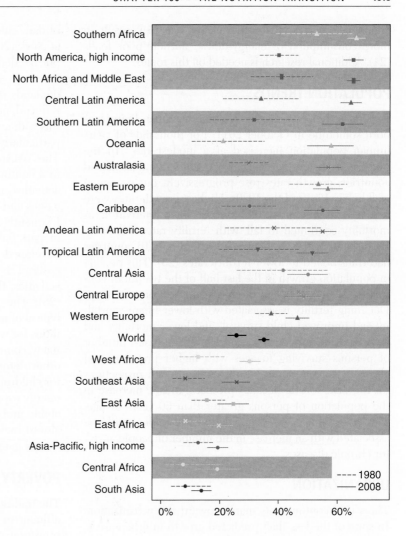

Fig. 109.2. Global prevalence of obesity, women. Changes in prevalence between 1980 and 2008 in selected countries. (Reproduced with permission from Finucane MM, Stevens GA, Cowan MJ et al. National, regional, and global trends in body-mass index since 1980: systematic analysis of health examination surveys and epidemiological studies with 960 country-years and 9.1 million participants. Lancet 2011;377:557–67.)

Major contributors to the increase in total dietary energy intake are vegetable oils and refined carbohydrates (sugars). Projections indicate that fat and sugar consumption will continue to be the main factors driving the increased dietary energy availability (15).

The previous relationship between income and diet in poor countries led to the traditional concept that a low per capita gross national product (GNP) is associated with a heavily plant-based diet, of low energy density; this diet profile has been progressively altered by global trends in food production and marketing. Food balance sheets and other research data from developing countries (16, 17) have shown that current diets in LMIC have increasing proportions of calories derived from fat (primarily vegetable oils) and refined carbohydrates. A number of factors may explain these changes in diet composition. First, there has been an increase in worldwide availability of relatively cheap vegetable oil (18, 19). Second, cultural perceptions of diet quality, influenced by commercial advertisement, have led to the consumption of more processed food products, many containing refined sugars. A quest for variety and convenience (i.e., prepared foods) also has been cited as an important factor (20). In a model

to assess the impact of urbanization, Drewnowski and Popkin predicted a substantial increase in consumption of caloric sweeteners as urbanization increases (21). The continuing expansion of the fast food market in LMICs is also of concern. More than half the revenues of the US fast food industry are obtained outside of the United States, mostly by the rapid growth of minimum service food stands (quick service restaurants [QSRs]) in LMICs (22). Another important factor determining food access and quality in developing countries is the dramatic expansion of retail food chains (supermarkets). In many LMICs, almost half the daily calories are now obtained from supermarkets, and this trend continues to grow.

In the United States, supermarkets appear to have a favorable effect on food quality, in part because they may provide more variety and quantity of produce and healthier options of processed foods (23). Thus, the concern in developed countries centers on "food deserts," areas with no supermarkets, in which individuals purchase food in convenience stores in gas stations, or small corner stores with limited offerings. Although data from LMICs on this topic are still scarce, some evidence points to an opposite effect of supermarkets in developing countries. Data from

Guatemala suggest that supermarket use may result in more consumption of energy-dense, nutrient-poor foods (24). Additional research is needed on this topic.

POPULATION TRENDS

Experts estimated that the 7 billionth human being was born sometime in October 2011. For thousands of years human population increased at a modest rate. In the mid-1800s, as mortality began to decline in industrialized countries, growth rates rose progressively, but remained well below 1% until the 1920s. Highest growth rates were reached in the mid-1900s, but declined thereafter, as mortality continued to fall, with fertility rates following. By the end of the twentieth century, all but 16 countries had transitioned to lower fertility rates (25). This decline in population growth in the last half of the twentieth century is a key element in the modern nutrition transition. Declining fertility is associated with lower infant mortality and improved child survival, and lower mortality and increased life expectancy result in an increased number of persons surviving to ages with higher prevalence of chronic, noncommunicable diseases. Growth projections for the next several decades predict a drastic increase in the population of persons greater than 60 years of age. This aging of the world population will undoubtedly be associated with an increase in the number of people at risk for chronic diseases.

URBANIZATION

The world continues its march toward full urbanization. In spite of the less-than-predicted growth in urban areas, the percentage of individuals living in an urban environment continues to increase. In some regions, such as Latin America, approximately 80% of the population is already urbanized. Predictions suggest that most people added to the world population in the next 20 years will reside in urban areas (25). Urban dwelling has several characteristics that greatly affect dietary intake and energy balance. First, the energy cost of basic survival activities (e.g., securing water and food) tends to be substantially lower. Second, labor energy demands are also reduced relative to those of typical rural work. Similarly, food availability differs in quantity and composition, usually with an increase in total dietary energy and a higher proportion of fats and refined sugars (17). These factors combine to facilitate a positive energy balance and consequent excess weight gain. Other factors characteristic of urban dwelling, such as television viewing, street violence, and the lack of open spaces, also facilitate an indoor, sedentary lifestyle and thus a further decline in energy expenditure.

SEDENTARY LIFESTYLE

The energy demands of daily living are important contributors to total energy needs in rural populations. Securing food, water, and firewood consumes a significant portion of daily caloric allowance, in addition to the energy spent at work (26). In the urban environment, the energy output needed for survival activities is sharply reduced, and the most common types of jobs are also lower in energy demands relative to rural work. As energy expenditure is reduced, persons find it more and more difficult to match this with an equivalent reduction in dietary energy intake, particularly when energy-dense foods are widely available. The "Westernization" of lifestyle in LMICs has resulted in a continuing increase in sedentary, low-energy output activities, including television viewing and use of video games and computers. In many LMICs, economic growth frequently involves creation of jobs in the service sector, in part fueled by outsourcing of service activities from developed countries that are searching for lower labor costs (27). These type of jobs usually involve sedentary activities, thus further reducing daily energy expenditure (28). The design of zoned, car-centered communities, typical of many industrialized countries, restricts opportunities for walking and cycling as part of daily activities. In many communities, public safety and street violence are other deterrents to outdoor physical activity, particularly for children. The end result is a chronic reduction in daily energy expenditure, which coupled with the ample availability and the consumption of energy-dense foods leads almost inevitably to a positive energy balance and excess weight gain.

POVERTY AND THE NUTRITION TRANSITION

The traditional view that obesity primarily affects the most affluent in society has been challenged by the nutrition transition. An analysis of data from 37 developing countries (29) suggests that although low-income countries (gross domestic product [GDP] ~$800/year) generally have a low prevalence of obesity, this prevalence increases rapidly in developing countries with an intermediate-level GNP (~$2000/year). A good example of this association between obesity and SES trends is Brazil, a country in rapid socioeconomic transition. In the 1980s, undernutrition was more prevalent and overweight less prevalent in lower socioeconomic groups. Ten years later, the prevalence of both undernutrition and overnutrition was higher among the poor (29). Data from China also suggest that income growth may have a negative effect on the diet of the urban poor (30). Although the causes of these shifts are complex, it is likely that in lower income populations, food availability is a limiting factor for energy intake; and frequent infections associated with a contaminated environment further increase energy requirements. As income increases, access to energy-dense foods—albeit of poor nutritional value—may increase, allowing for higher total energy intake.

Urbanization, frequently associated with economic development, does not necessarily improve socioeconomic status among the poor. Using data from the World Bank, Haddad et al reported an overall increase in urban poverty in less developed countries in the last 20 years of the twentieth century (31). In 11 of the 14 countries examined, the prevalence of underweight children in urban areas also increased. The same data show that doubling the per capita GNP produced only a 10% reduction in the prevalence of underweight in children. Furthermore, some health indicators show a wider gap between the richest and the poorest in urban compared with rural populations (32, 33).

Poverty also may have more negative consequences in urban than in rural areas. In the urban environment of LMICs, families usually depend on their income to buy food, and therefore are highly vulnerable to market manipulations, advertisements, and food prices (34). When families need to spend 50% or more of their income on food, as is the case in many LDCs, food price becomes a powerful factor driving food choice. The association between economic development (measured by gains in per capita GDP) and obesity is highly variable, in part conditioned by the stage of transition in diet, lifestyle, and income of each country. One evaluation of cross-sectional data on women from 54 countries (35) found a modest positive correlation between BMI and per capita GDP.

THE DOUBLE BURDEN OF DISEASE AMONG THE POOR

The increasing prevalence of obesity in LMICs results in the coexistence of undernutrition and overnutrition in the same population, even in the same family (3, 36, 37). By some estimates, as many as 60% of households in Southeast Asia may have at least one underweight and one overweight member, frequently an underweight child–overweight mother pair (38). This "dual burden" poses a major challenge to the development of integrated prevention programs.

EARLY UNDERNUTRITION AND ADULT DISEASES

The relationship between nutritional status early in life and adult disease was brought to the forefront by a series of epidemiologic observations describing the association between low birth weight and diabetes, cardiovascular

diseases, and respiratory disorders in adult life (39–42). Other studies extended these associations to extrauterine growth faltering, and the subsequent phase of accelerated ("catch-up") growth as important determinants of later obesity in older children and adults (43–46). Using medical records from Dutch populations who suffered severe nutritional deprivation during World War II, Susser and Stein (47) identified similar associations between impaired fetal growth and subsequent risk of adult diseases. Overall, these data point to critical early periods of structural and functional differentiation, during which altered nutritional conditions may produce long-lasting effects (48–51). The implications of this phenomenon for developing countries is significant because of their high prevalence of impaired fetal and postnatal growth, which would result in an additional risk burden for adult populations now facing the nutrition transition. Experts recognize that a narrow window of opportunity exists early in life to restore normal growth in vulnerable children, before such efforts carry with them the adverse long-term consequences described in the preceding (52). It is also clear that fetal and early life undernutrition, important risk factors for adult diseases, can and should be addressed within the traditional health policy programs focused on maternal and child health.

THE EMERGENCE OF CHRONIC, NONCOMMUNICABLE DISEASES

The global trends in diet and lifestyle are also fostering an alarming increase in related conditions, some of them mediated by excess weight gain. According to the WHO (53), the most prevalent disease risk factors globally are high blood pressure (13% of deaths), tobacco use (9%), high blood glucose (6%), physical inactivity (6%), and overweight/obesity (5%). These factors, along with low consumption of fruit and vegetables, are responsible for more than 50% of deaths from cardiovascular disease, which is the leading cause of death globally (Table 109.1). Therefore, it is not surprising that worldwide, overweight/obesity cause

TABLE 109.1	LEADING CAUSES OF ATTRIBUTABLE MORTALITY AND BURDEN OF DISEASE WORLDWIDE		
ATTRIBUTABLE MORTALITY (%)		**ATTRIBUTABLE DALYs (%)**	
1. High blood pressure	12.8	1. Childhood underweight	5.9
2. Tobacco use	8.7	2. Unsafe sex	4.6
3. High blood glucose	5.8	3. Alcohol use	4.5
4. Physical inactivity	5.5	4. Unsafe water, sanitation, hygiene	4.2
5. Overweight and obesity	4.8	5. High blood pressure	3.7
6. High blood cholesterol	4.5	6. Tobacco use	3.7
7. Unsafe sex	4.0	7. Suboptimal breastfeeding	2.9
8. Alcohol use	3.8	8. High blood glucose	2.7
9. Childhood underweight	3.8	9. Indoor smoke from solid fuels	2.7
10. Indoor smoke from solid fuels	3.3	10. Overweight and obesity	2.3
59 million total deaths in 2004		1.5 billion total DALYs in 2004	

DALYs, disability-adjusted life years.

Adapted with permission from World Health Organization. Global Health Risks: Mortality and Burden of Disease Attributable to Selected Major Risks. Geneva: World Health Organization, 2009.

more deaths than underweight, and that the burden of disease associated with diet and physical inactivity in LMIC is equivalent to that of human immunodeficiency virus infection/acquired immunodeficiency syndrome and tuberculosis combined (53).

The obesity epidemic also constitutes the main factor responsible for another epidemic, that of type 2 diabetes. The number of people with diabetes has increased from 153 million in 1980 to 347 million in 2008 (54). Similarly, the number of persons with high fasting plasma glucose (an antecedent of type 2 diabetes) has also increased, most notably in North America, Oceania, and Saudi Arabia. Of the top 10 countries with the highest diabetes prevalence, 6 are in the developing world, led by India and China (55). It is predicted that in the next 10 years the number of individuals with diabetes in India will reach 60 million.

POLICY IMPLICATIONS

The evidence supporting the significant adverse health impact of the nutrition transition in developing countries has been accumulating steadily for several decades. Today, a few chronic diseases associated with diet and lifestyle are responsible for more than half of the world's deaths. Ample consensus exists that three key modifiable risk factors are tobacco use, unhealthy diet, and physical inactivity. In the past few years, international organizations such as the WHO have defined an operational framework for global tobacco control (56) and a strategy for diet, physical activity, and health (14). In addition, the enormous economic implications of chronic diseases for health care costs and productivity in developing countries are also becoming clear. Nevertheless, support and funding for a vigorous response to the problem have been limited so far, and only a few countries have included well-defined strategies to prevent noncommunicable diseases in their public health programs. The fact that many of these risk factors are the result of profound changes in global food production and commerce, cultural influences, and adoption of certain models of economic development is undoubtedly a major challenge. These are not factors that can be modified overnight, but they are certainly modifiable. Initiatives in Brazil, China, and several other countries provide hope that the much-needed political will is emerging.

The Millenium Development Goals (57) provide a unifying template for efforts to eliminate poverty and disease from the developing world. One key goal is to reduce undernutrition, which would result in an important reduction in chronic disease risk associated with early growth faltering, as discussed. The goal of improving maternal health also would have a positive effect on gestational performance and fetal growth, another factor associated with obesity and chronic diseases later in life. Therefore, it is clear that fetal and early life undernutrition, important risk factors for adult diseases, can and should be addressed within the traditional health policy programs focused on maternal and child health.

Improving the food environment by making healthy foods available and affordable and restricting the marketing of unhealthy foods, particularly to children, is another ongoing challenge. As noted earlier, because of the high price elasticity of food in developing countries, eating patterns are difficult to change without some form of market regulation and control, which may run counter to the free market principles demanded by many international lenders. Furthermore, many governments do not have the clout to overcome financial and political pressures opposing regulation, usually under the banner of freedom of commerce. Nevertheless, a broad range of initiatives are taking shape at the national, multinational, and local levels. A large majority of governments pledged to implement the WHO Diet and Physical Activity strategy as well as the Tobacco Control Framework. The increasing concern of governments culminated in the United Nations (UN) Summit on Chronic Diseases in September 2011, only the second time in the history of the UN system that heads of state met exclusively to focus on a health topic (58). On the nongovernment front, grassroots efforts to create activity-friendly communities and healthy and sustainable living environments are emerging across the world (59, 60).

REFERENCES

1. Gardner G, Halweil B. Overfed and Underfed: The Global Epidemic of Malnutrition. Washington, DC: Worldwatch Institute, 2000.
2. Doak CM, Adair LS, Monteiro C et al. J Nutr 2000;130:2965–71.
3. Caballero B. 2005. N Engl J Med 352:1514–6.
4. World Health Organization. World Health Report. Geneva: World Health Organization, 2010.
5. World Health Organization. Report of a WHO Consultation. Geneva: World Health Organization, 2000.
6. Caballero B. Epidemiol Rev 2007;29:1–5.
7. Finucane MM, Stevens GA, Cowan MJ et al. Lancet 2011; 377:557–67.
8. de Onis M, Blossner M, Borghi E. Am J Clin Nutr 2010; 92:1257–64.
9. Omran AR. Milbank Mem Fund Q 1971;49:509–38.
10. Popkin BM. Nutr Revs 1994;52:285–98.
11. Caballero B, Popkin BM. The Nutrition Transition: Diet and Disease in the Developing World. London: Academic Press, 2002:1–8.
12. Popkin BM. World Dev 1999;27:1905–16.
13. Popkin BM. Am J Clin Nutr 2006;84:289–98.
14. World Health Organization, Food and Agriculture Organization. Report of a Joint WHO/FAO Expert Consultation. Geneva: World Health Organization, 2002.
15. Food and Agriculture Organization. World Agriculture: Towards 2015/2030. Rome: Food and Agriculture Organization, 2002.
16. Food and Agriculture Organization. Food Production. 2011. Available at: http://www.fao.org/docrep/014/i2280e/i2280e00. htm. Accessed September 20, 2012.
17. Popkin BM. Proc Nutr Soc 2011;70:82–91.
18. Popkin BM, Gordon-Larsen P. Int J Obes Relat Metab Disord 2004;28:S2–S9.
19. Caballero B, Popkin BM, eds. The Nutrition Transition: Diet and Disease in the Developing World. London: Academic Press, 2002:109–128.

20. US Department of Agriculture Economic Research Service. Changing Structure of Global Food Consumption and Trade. Washington, DC: US Department of Agriculture Economic Research Service, 2001.

21. Drewnowski A, Popkin BM. Nutr Revs 1997;55:31–43.

22. Fast Food: Global Industry Guide. Limassol, Cyprus: Market Publishers, 2010.

23. Franco M, Diez-Roux AV, Nettleton JA et al. Am J Clin Nutr 2009;89:897–904.

24. Asfaw A. Dev Policy Rev 2008;26:16.

25. Caballero B, Popkin BM, eds. The Nutrition Transition: Diet and Disease in the Developing World. London: Academic Press, 2002:147–164.

26. Immink MD, Blake CC, Viteri FE et al. Arch Latinoam Nutr 1986;36:247–59.

27. Worth RF. In New York Tickets, Ghana Sees Orderly City. The New York Times. October 19, 2002.

28. Weng X, Caballero B. Obesity and Related Diseases in China: The Impact of the Nutrition Transition in Urban and Rural Adults. New York: Cambria Press, 2007.

29. Monteiro CA, Conde WL, Lu B et al. Int J Obes Relat Metab Disord 2004;28(Suppl 3):S2–S9.

30. Du S, Mroz TA, Zhai F et al. Soc Sci Med 2004;59:1505–15.

31. Haddad L, Ruel MT, Garrett JL. World Dev 1999;27:1891–904.

32. Menon P, Ruel M, Morris SS. Socioeconomic Differentials in Child Stunting Are Consistently Larger in Urban Than in Rural Areas. 2000. Available at: http://www.ifpri.org/publication/socio-economic-differentials-child-stunting-are-consistently-larger-urban-rural-areas-0. Accessed September 20, 2012.

33. Gwatkin DR, Guillot M, Heuveline P. Lancet 1999;354:586–9.

34. Regmi A, Deepak MS, Seale JL et al. Cross-Country Analysis of Food Consumption Patterns. Washington, DC: US Department of Agriculture Economic Research Service, 2001.

35. Subramanian SV, Perkins JM, Ozaltin E et al. Am J Clin Nutr 2011;93:413–21.

36. Doak CM, Adair LS, Bentley M et al. Int J Obes (Lond) 2005;29:129–36.

37. Garrett JL, Ruel MT. Food Nutr Bull 2005;26:209–21.

38. Popkin BM, Horton SH, Kim S. Food Nutr Bull 2001;22:3–57.

39. Cheung YB, Low L, Osmond C et al. Hypertension 2000;36:795–800.

40. Eriksson JG, Forsen T, Tuomilehto J et al. Diabetes 1999;48:A72-A.

41. Eriksson JG, Forsen T, Tuomilehto J et al. Br Med J 2001;322:949–53.

42. Martorell R, Stein AD, Schroeder DG. J Nutr 2001;131:874S–80S.

43. Ong KK, Loos RJ. Acta Paediatrica 2006;95:904–8.

44. Ibanez L, Ong K, Dunger DB et al. J Clin Endocrinol Metab 2006;91:2153–8.

45. Ibanez L, Suarez L, Lopez-Bermejo A et al. J Clin Endocrinol Metab 2008;93:925–8.

46. Ong KK, Ahmed ML, Emmett PM et al. BMJ 2000;320:967–71.

47. Susser M, Stein Z. Nutr Revs 1994;52:84–94.

48. Symonds ME, Gardner DS. Curr Opin Clin Nutr Metab Care 2006;9:278–83.

49. Caballero B. J Pediatr 2006;149:S97–S9.

50. Morrison JL. Clin Exp Pharmacol Physiol 2008;35:730–43.

51. Kawamura M, Itoh H, Yura S et al. Endocrinology 2007;148:1218–25.

52. Victora CG, de Onis M, Hallal PC et al. Pediatrics 2010;125:e473–80.

53. World Health Organization. Global Health Risks: Mortality and Burden of Disease Attributable to Selected Major Risks. Geneva: World Health Organization, 2009.

54. Danaei G, Finucane MM, Lu Y et al. Lancet 2011;378:31–40.

55. Wild S, Roglic G, Green A et al. Diabetes Care 2004;27:1047–53.

56. World Health Organization. Framework Convention for Tobacco Control. 2005. Available at: http://www.who.int/fctc/en/index.html. Accessed September 20, 2012.

57. United Nations. Millenium Development Goals. 2011. Available at: http://www.un.org/millenniumgoals/. Accessed September 20, 2012.

58. United Nations. High-Level Meeting on Noncommunicable Disease Prevention and Control. 2011. Available at: http://www.who.int/nmh/events/un_ncd_summit2011/en/. Accessed September 20, 2012.

59. Cicliovias Recreativas. Available at: http://www.ciclovias recreativas.org/. Accessed September 20, 2012.

60. 8-80 Cities. Available at: http://www.8-80cities.org. Accessed September 20, 2012.

SUGGESTED READINGS

Ahsan Karar Z, Alam N, Streatfield PK. Epidemiological transition in rural Bangladesh, 1986–2006. Global Health Action 2009;2.

Caballero B, Popkin BM. The Nutrition Transition: Diet and Disease in the Developing World. London: Academic Press, 2002.

Prentice A, Webb F. Obesity amidst poverty. Int J Epidemiol 2006;35:24–30.

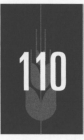

110

FOOD-BASED DIETARY GUIDELINES FOR HEALTHIER POPULATIONS: INTERNATIONAL CONSIDERATIONS[1]

RICARDO UAUY, SOPHIE HAWKESWORTH, AND ALAN D. DANGOUR

The modern approach toward defining the nutritional adequacy of diets has progressed over the past two centuries in parallel with scientific understanding of the biochemical and physiologic basis of human nutritional requirements in health and disease. The definition of essential nutrients and nutrient requirements has provided the scientific underpinnings for nutrient-based dietary recommendations, which now exist for virtually every essential nutrient known (1–6). However, obvious limitations exist to the reductionist nutrient-based approach because people consume foods and not nutrients. Moreover, the effect of specific foods and of dietary patterns on health goes well beyond the combination of essential nutrients the food may contain.

[1]**Abbreviations: Apo-E**, apolipoprotein-E; **DRI**, dietary reference intake; **EAR**, estimated average requirement; **FAO**, Food and Agriculture Organization; **FBDG**, food-based dietary guideline; **IDD**, iodine deficiency disorders; **LDL**, low-density lipoprotein; **RNI**, recommended nutrient intake; **RUTF**, ready-to-use therapeutic food; **SNP**, single nucleotide polymorphism; **WHO**, World Health Organization.

Given our present understanding of food–health relationships, it seems likely that a large variety of foods can be combined in varying amounts to provide a healthy diet. Thus, it is difficult to determine a precise indispensable intake of individual foods that can, when combined with other foods, provide a nutritionally adequate diet under all conditions. The prevailing view is that a large set of food combinations are compatible with nutritional adequacy, but that no given set of foods can be extrapolated as absolutely required or sufficient across different ecologic settings. Trends in the globalization of food supply provide clear evidence that dietary patterns and even traditionally local foods can move across geographic niches.

Recommended nutrient intakes (RNIs) are customarily defined as the intake of energy and specific nutrients necessary to satisfy the requirements of a group of healthy individuals. These are discussed further in the chapter on dietary reference intakes (DRIs). This nutrient-based approach has served well to advance science but has not always fostered the establishment of nutritional and dietary priorities consistent with broad public health interests at national and international levels. For example, the emphasis on protein quality of single food sources placed a premium on the development of animal foods and failed to include amino acid complementarities, which increase the quality of mixed vegetable protein sources. We now know that human protein needs can also be met with predominantly plant-based protein sources. In contrast to this nutrient-based approach, food-based dietary guidelines (FBDGs) address health concerns related to dietary insufficiency, excess, or imbalance with a broader perspective, considering the totality of the effects of a given dietary pattern (7). They are more closely linked to the diet–health relationships of relevance to the particular country or region of interest (8). In addition, they take into account the customary dietary pattern, the foods available, and the factors that determine the consumption of foods. They consider the ecologic setting, the socioeconomic and cultural factors, and the biologic and physical environment that affects the health and nutrition of a given population or community. Finally, they are easy to understand and accessible for all members of a population.

In this chapter we examine the steps required to develop FBDGs, strategies which can be employed to

has been tested and used by various countries with necessary local adaptations to ensure better implementation.

The initial step is the establishment of a working group that includes all relevant stakeholders. Membership should be broad, representing private and government institutions, agricultural and food industries, communication and anthropology specialists, nutrition scientists, consumer organizations, public health, and medical nutritionists. There should be thorough discussion of the relevant nutrition problems of the region of interest based on up-to-date survey information, ideally representing different regions and population groups. Information will be required on the prevailing nutrition-related disease issues of the population in question as well as on habitual diet patterns and food availability data. Once identified, the dietary component of the public health nutritional problem should be defined further. Dietary factors (nutrient excess, deficit or imbalance) should be examined beyond mean population intakes because there may be overconsumption or underconsumption in specific population groups. For example, there may be a shift in the overall population intake or a distinct subpopulation that does not consume the given nutrient. These problems should be addressed differently, in the first case increasing the nutrient intake for the complete population and in the latter case acting to increase the intake of the specific population subgroup of underconsumers. This can represent a practical problem, because in some cases it may be virtually impossible to identify such a subgroup and implementation strategies may be difficult to target at a particular group alone.

The working group should discuss and prioritize the set of major public nutrition problems that will be addressed by the FBDGs and explore the foods available to improve the nutritional problem. There may be a need to explore whether it is possible to change the pattern of agricultural production and food distribution. There also may be a need to modify food subsidies, apparent or hidden, or other government policies that affect food consumption. The economic constraints in implementing food-based approaches should be considered, as well as the possible solutions. This will clearly be different for urban societies who depend on an industrialized food supply, and self-sufficient farmers who consume what they produce.

The working group should then define a set of FBDGs that will address the nutrient intake/food patterns that require modification, considering the social, cultural, and economic factors that exist. A statement discussed and approved by all working group members should support each guideline technically. This may include circulating the draft and receiving input from technical parties not present in the working group. All iterations necessary to bring about technical consensus should be explored. The final draft of this step, including the messages that will reach consumers, should then be pilot tested with consumer groups and modified to secure understanding by the target group. The results of the pilot tests should be used in establishing the revised guidelines.

The final set of guidelines and supporting technical statements should then be released for ample critical public review by all relevant groups. The support of international technical experts and relevant UN agencies may be helpful at this stage. Experience suggests that the Internet can be used to enhance input from consumer groups. Subsequent to final modifications resulting from the public consultation process, the FBDGs will be ready for final approval, publication in various formats, dissemination, and implementation for general use. The lower portion of Figure 110.2 provides a summary of potential end-users of the FBDGs.

The impact of FBDGs in modifying food intake patterns and the relevant public nutrition problems should be periodically assessed. Measures to enhance their applicability such as mass media and educational campaigns, incorporation into school curricula, and inclusion in other health promotion programs should be implemented. Based on periodic assessment, the guidelines should be reexamined and/or revised within a set period, normally every 5 to 10 years, to ensure that they remain current and scientifically valid.

Effectiveness and National Variation

Experience with FBDGs over the past decade suggests that they offer a feasible, effective, and sustainable approach to promote healthy eating of the population in general and to address nutrition problems in vulnerable groups. They foster a practical, consumer-oriented approach to reach specific nutritional goals for a given population. A focus on foods and food groups helps in the development of clear, easy-to-understand, behavioral messages suitable for the target audience. FBDGs often go beyond the remit of "foods"; for example they may promote a healthy weight, encourage physical activity, and provide advice about water and food safety. Guidelines are often further simplified into schematic representations of the agreed dietary advice such as the UK Eatwell Plate (18) and the USDA health pyramid (19) to provide greater clarity to consumers.

Importantly, FBDGs must facilitate choices for consumers that are consistent with their preferences, food culture, and economic resources. Typically, such guidelines recommend a minimum number of servings from each of four to seven basic food groups. FBDGs also commonly suggest the need to limit intake of certain food components, such as saturated and *trans*-fatty acids, added sugars, and salt. For example, one of the key recommendations of the US Dietary Guidelines is to "consume a variety of nutrient-dense foods and beverages within and among the basic food groups while choosing foods that limit the intake of saturated and *trans*-fats, cholesterol, added sugars, salt, and alcohol" (20). FBDGs must also take into account the needs of population subgroups, especially those at particular risk, and will often specify guidelines for these groups such as older people or women of childbearing age.

Food-based strategies offer many benefits that go beyond the prevention and control of nutrient deficiencies. For example, FBDGs

- Help prevent and control both macro- and micronutrient deficiencies by addressing underlying causes
- Support health promotion and preventive medicine
- Should be cost effective and sustainable
- Can be adapted to different cultural and dietary traditions and to strategies that are feasible at the local level
- Address multiple nutrition problems simultaneously
- Minimize the risk of toxicity and adverse nutrient interactions because the amounts of nutrients consumed are within usual physiologic levels
- Support the role of breast-feeding and the special diet and care needs of infants and young children
- Can foster the development of sustainable, environmentally sound, food production systems
- May serve to alert agricultural planners to the need to protect the micronutrient content of soils and crops
- Build partnerships among governments, consumer groups, the food industry, and other organizations to achieve the shared goals of overcoming nutrition-related health problems
- Empower people to become more self-reliant using local resources
- Provide opportunities for social interaction and enjoyment

Many nations have developed FBDGs for their populations and we have provided an example from each world region in Table 110.1. The FAO is compiling these as part of an online resource (21). Dietary guidelines from different countries tend to be similar in their purposes and uses, but the process of development can be distinct depending on the stakeholders involved. They are intended for use not only by health professionals but also by members of the general population and thus are mostly worded in simple, concrete terms. The similarity among national guidelines is striking: they all place an emphasis on balance, moderation (especially with regard to fat, sugar, salt, and alcohol), and variety and they all highlight the importance of consuming sufficient portions of fruits, vegetables, and grains. However, they also vary quite considerably, both in the wording used and the level of detail provided to the consumer.

Once FBDGs have been developed, they must be put into practice to be effective; that is, the general public must be aware of the guidelines and encouraged to follow them. A number of important barriers exist to the effectiveness of FBDGs at a national level (22). These range from the time-consuming and cumbersome consultation process initially required to develop the guidelines to the lack of consumer involvement in the development, so that their needs are not understood or placed at the center of the process. FBDGs can be ineffective because of a lack of understanding and/or misunderstanding by the consumers or the influence of other, often more powerful, factors

on food choice (22). A review of the implementation of FBDGs in four countries (Chile, Germany, New Zealand, and South Africa) found that they were often not included in wider health promotion strategies and their effectiveness was often not evaluated sufficiently. The investigators suggested several recommendations for improving FBDG implementation at a national level (22):

- National governments should undertake monitoring of FBDG implementation regularly, with intermediate indicators, and identify barriers to success.
- National governments should endorse the FBDG and lead its implementation, ensuring its value is also understood by nonhealth professionals and is used as a basis for the national catering industry.
- Promotion of FBDGs should be conducted through various mass media.
- FBDGs should be used to align wider agriculture, food, and nutrition policies and should underpin national health strategies.

STRATEGIES TO IMPROVE DIET QUALITY IN INTERNATIONAL PUBLIC HEALTH NUTRITION

Within the remit of public health nutrition, recommended nutrient intakes can be applied to assess the adequacy of diets and FBDGs used to improve diet quality and thus health. With our increasingly sophisticated understanding of the role of nutrition in the development and prevention of disease, the necessity of ensuring individuals are consuming a diet of adequate quantity and quality becomes ever more apparent. A diet consisting of a diverse range of foodstuffs as outlined by national FBDGs should be sufficient to meet the nutritional needs of the population and to ensure optimal intakes for a healthy life. In practice, many diets are not meeting these guidelines and alternative strategies to improve nutrient intake must be considered. FBDGs may be just one of many steps aimed at improving health by improving diet quality and in the next section we explore some other strategies available for improving nutritional status, particularly in lower income country settings.

Food Security

Populations in lower income countries often consume a monotonous diet out of need rather than choice, because access to different foods can be curtailed by economic factors. The percentage increase in the demand of a food item when income increases by 1% is called the elasticity of demand of the given food item. Most staple foods such as rice, wheat, and corn have low income elasticity; that is, even if income increases greatly, the increase in the amount of staple foods eaten will be small. However, meat and animal food products have high income elasticity; that is, there is a large effect of income on consumption patterns. This can clearly be seen in the fact that the amount of animal protein foods consumed by

TABLE 110.1	DIVERSITY OF NATIONAL FOOD-BASED DIETARY GUIDELINES
COUNTRY	**FOOD-BASED DIETARY GUIDELINES**
South Africa, 2004 (57)	For adults and children more than 7 years old: • Enjoy a variety of foods. • Be active. • Make starchy foods the basis of most meals. • Eat dry beans, split peas, lentils, and soya regularly. • Chicken, fish, milk, meat, or eggs can be eaten daily. • Drink lots of clean, safe water. • Eat plenty of vegetables and fruits every day. • Eat fats sparingly. • Use salt sparingly. • Use food and drinks containing sugar sparingly and not between meals. • If you drink alcohol, drink sensibly.
India, 1998 (58)	• A nutritionally adequate diet should be consumed through a variety of foods. • Additional food and extra care are required during pregnancy and lactation. • Exclusive breast-feeding should be practiced for 4–6 mo. Breast-feeding can be continued up to 2 years. • Food supplements should be introduced to infants by 4–6 mo. • An adequate and appropriate diet should be followed by children and adolescents, both in health and disease. • Plenty of green leafy vegetables, other vegetables, and fruits should be used. • Cooking oils and animal foods should be used in moderation, and vanaspati/ghee/butter should be used only sparingly. • Overeating should be avoided to prevent overweight and obesity. Proper physical activity is essential to maintain desirable body weight. • Salt should be used in moderation. • Foods consumed should be safe and clean. • Healthy and positive food concepts and cooking practices should be adopted. • Water should be taken in adequate amounts and beverages should be consumed in moderation. • Processed and ready-to-eat foods should be used judiciously. • Sugar should be used sparingly. • The elderly should eat a nutrient-rich diet to keep fit and active.
United Kingdom, 2006 (59)	The Health Ministry recommends that all healthy individuals should consume a diet that contains • Plenty of starchy foods such as rice, bread, pasta, and potatoes (choosing whole grain varieties whenever possible) • Plenty of fruit and vegetables; at least five portions of a variety of fruits and vegetables a day • Moderate amounts of protein-rich foods such as meat, fish, eggs, and alternatives such as nuts and pulses • Moderate amounts of milk and dairy, choosing reduced-fat versions or eating smaller amounts of full fat versions or eating them less often • Less saturated fat, salt, and sugar
Chile, 2005 (60)	• Consume dairy foods three times a day (milk, yogurt, soft cheeses) prefer low-fat or nonfat dairy. • Eat at least two vegetables and three fruits per day (select different color fruits and vegetables). • Eat beans, chick peas, lentils, or green peas at least twice a week; these can replace meats. • Eat fish, at least twice a week, cooked, steamed, or grilled. • Prefer foods with low saturated fats and cholesterol. • Reduce your consumption of sugar and salt. • Drink six to eight glasses of water per day.
Oman, 2009 (61)	• Vary your diet, making it healthy and balanced. • Choose whole grains and cereals, and consume potatoes, with their skin. • Consume three to five servings of vegetables daily. • Consume two to four servings of fruits daily. • Consume fish, poultry, eggs, or lean meat. • Consume one serving of legumes daily. • Consume milk or dairy products daily. • Limit your fat intake and choose your snacks wisely. • Follow the five keys to safer food. • Be active, exercise regularly, and drink plenty of water.

(continued)

TABLE 110.1	DIVERSITY OF NATIONAL FOOD-BASED DIETARY GUIDELINES *(Continued)*
Canada, 2007 (62)	• Eat at least one dark-green and one orange vegetable every day. • Enjoy vegetables and fruit prepared with little or no added fat, sugar, or salt. • Have vegetables and fruits more often than juice. • Select whole grains for at least half of one's grain products. • Choose grains products that are low in fat, sugar, and salt. • Drink skim, 1% or 2% milk each day. • Consume meat alternatives such as beans, lentils, and tofu often. • Eat at least two servings of fish each week. • Select lean meat and alternatives prepared with little or no added fat or salt. • Include a small amount of unsaturated fat each day. • Satisfy thirst with water. • Limit foods and beverages high in calories, fat, sugar, or salt. • Be active every day.

the wealthiest 20% of the world's population is four times larger than that consumed by the poorest 20%.

If access to food was not dependent on income but on need, the food available globally would be sufficient to meet the needs of humankind. A corollary to this conditional statement is that unless economic constraints in food consumption are overcome, dietary diversification will fail. The prevention of malnutrition of women and children through dietary means in economically deprived population groups will not work unless people have access to foods that are adequate in both quantity and quality. This is part of the human rights–based approach: the right to food (23). Food security cannot be determined based on the availability of food energy alone; nutritional security requires that all essential micronutrients are covered by the food supply. In the absence of major changes in income distribution in certain lower income countries, and/or major accelerations in economic growth, other possible alternatives to achieve adequate dietary intake must be sought. Some of the most common strategies are discussed in the following sections.

Improving Dietary Diversity

Micronutrient deficiencies are widespread in low- and middle-income countries and within certain population groups in high-income countries. Although accurate prevalence figures are hard to calculate, deficiencies in key micronutrients are estimated to underpin a substantial proportion of the global burden of disease (24). Public health strategies to improve micronutrient intake range from food-based approaches focused on dietary diversity to supplementation programs.

Increasing dietary diversity among the poor to achieve the complementation of cereal/tuber-based diets with micronutrient-rich foods is believed to be the most sustainable option for improving nutritional intake in the long term. Achieving this diversity, however, can take longer to implement than alternative strategies, not least because initiatives often require family incomes to reach a sufficient level to provide adequate high quality, nutrient-dense diets (25). The following strategies have

been used to promote dietary diversification in different settings.

Small-Scale Community Vegetable and Fruit Gardens

These projects have the potential to increase the production and consumption of micronutrient-rich foods at the community or household level. The success of such projects requires a good knowledge and understanding of local conditions, as well as the involvement of women and overall community participation. These are key elements to support, achieve, and sustain the beneficial nutritional change at the household level. In addition, land availability and water supply are common constrains that often require local government intervention or support.

Household Production of Poultry, Fish, and Other Small Animals

These are excellent sources of highly bioavailable essential micronutrients, such as vitamin A, iron, and zinc. The production of animal foods at the local level may permit communities to access foods that otherwise are not available because of their high costs. These types of projects also need support to overcome the cost constraints of implementation and training of producers.

Implementation of Large-Scale Commercial Vegetable and Fruit Production

This initiative has the objective of providing micronutrient-rich foods at reasonable prices, through effective and competitive markets that lower consumer costs without reducing producers' prices.

Reduction of Postharvest Losses and Nutritional Value of Micronutrient-Rich Foods

Improvement of storage and food preservation facilities of fruits and vegetables significantly reduces postharvest losses. At the household level, the promotion of effective cooking methods (minimal cooking of vegetables) and practical ways of preserving foods (solar drying of seasonal micronutrient-rich foods, like grapes, mangoes, peaches and apricots), may significantly increase the access to bioavailable micronutrient-rich foods. At the commercial level, grading, packing, transport, and marketing practices can reduce losses and optimize income generation.

Fortification of Plant and Animal Foods

Food fortification can be a very cost-effective public health intervention, provided it is used as part of a food-based approach in which diets are known to be failing. Fortification should not be seen as a replacement to dietary diversification programs but can be a complementary part of wider prevention strategies and is often used as a strategy to combat micronutrient deficiencies (25). Three essential conditions must be met in any fortification program: (a) the fortificant should be effective, bioavailable, acceptable, and affordable; (b) the selected food vehicle should be easily accessible and eaten in regular amounts by all sectors of society; and (c) detailed production instructions and monitoring procedures should be in place and enforced by law.

Biofortification

Biofortification refers to the addition of nutritional value to agricultural products during production. Advances in technology such as the improvement of soils and enhanced plant micronutrient content via classical plant breeding or genetic modification have become a promising area for future research into the most effect method of improving nutritional intakes. Developments in genetic modification, for example, may hold the potential of achieving micronutrient sufficiency from staple foods. One of the best-known examples is the genetically modified "golden rice" that provides β-carotene to increase vitamin A intake (26) and that could have important public health impacts if widely adopted (27). The elimination of antinutritional factors that affect bioavailability of minerals either through traditional breeding or genetic modifications may also enhance the utilization of iron and zinc in regular plant foods.

The nutritional quality of animal foods can also be affected by production practices; for example the type and quantity of fats present in monogastric animals may be determined by the feed provided. Thus if chicken are free-range fed, they will have lower total fat and more n-3 fatty acids than if they are given a maize-based feed and constrained in their movements. Eggs can be enriched in long chain n-3 fatty acids if animals are provided fish meal or flax seed in their feed. Pork fat can be improved in nutritional quality if animals are fed meals high in polyunsaturated fatty acids (e.g., soy oil) (28). Milk and meat from ruminants are more difficult to alter through diet because microbial fermentation in the rumen modifies ingested nutrients significantly. However, new techniques of microencapsulation do permit the delivery of nutrients beyond the rumen. Cattle living in constrained environments and given cereal-based diets have a higher total fat than their pasture-fed counterparts. Genetic modification also allows drastic changes in fatty acid composition of animal tissues; the introduction of an n-3 desaturase gene from a worm (the nematode *Caenorhabditis elegans*) into mice produced a dramatic increase in the DHA content of milk and muscle from these mammals (29).

Novel methods such as these potentially provide a way to enhance the nutritional quality of diets without having to drastically modify consumption patterns. These approaches may prove acceptable to food producers who are reluctant to change their traditional food productions systems, and will allow consumers to maintain their customary diet and still achieve the desired nutrient intake goals. However, many of these techniques remain controversial and will require evidence of effectiveness and safety before they can be widely implemented.

Fortification of Agricultural Products

Traditionally, fortification refers to the processing end of the food chain, encompassing the addition of nutrients (usually micronutrients) to processed foods. Fortification can be single, with only one nutrient (fortificant) added, or multiple, to include two or more nutrients. Food fortification programs in high-income countries are well-established, with cereal products, margarine, and milk often fortified with common micronutrients. Increasingly, fortification is being considered as a cost-effective option to combat micronutrient deficiencies in lower-income countries. Some examples are outlined here.

Iron.   Iron deficiency is the most common form of micronutrient deficiency, with more than 2 billion people estimated to be anemic worldwide (30). Iron fortification of various foodstuffs has been implemented in many countries, but data on the effectiveness of these interventions are lacking. Iron fortification of infant formula in the United States and of wheat and maize flours in Venezuela has been associated with a reduction in anemia among children (31, 32).

The choice of a suitable iron compound is a key feature of any successful fortification strategy, because those with the highest relative bioavailability often can cause unpalatable changes to the chosen food vehicle (25). The effect of fortification on micronutrient bioavailability is illustrated in Figure 110.3 using iron fortification of wheat and maize as examples (33). The presence of inhibitors in the maize renders iron less bioavailable than in wheat, and this demands the use of iron compounds that can be better absorbed. At the same time, these compounds react with the food matrix, limiting the amount that can be used without affecting the sensory properties or the shelf-life of the food products made from the staple. Thus, both iron compound and compatibility of the food matrix are crucial in determining the amount of iron that can be included and effectively absorbed from the food (34).

Iodine.   Iodine deficiency is the second most widespread micronutrient deficiency worldwide, with profound impacts on health and development (35). Iodine is sparsely distributed on the earth surface, and foods produced in soils poor or lacking in iodine do not supply adequate amounts of this micronutrient in the diet. Only foods of marine origin are naturally rich sources of iodine and as a result, iodine deficiency disorders (IDDs) are widespread. Salt iodization has been shown to be an

% Fe absorption based on fortificant and food matrix

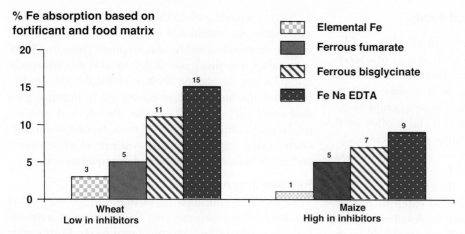

**Compatibility with food matrix
Max Fe load (mg/kg)**

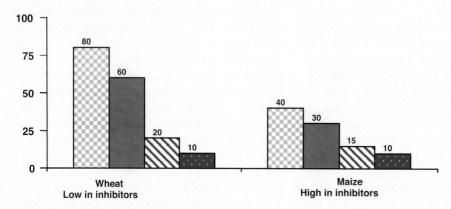

**Biologic impact
Fe absorbed mg per 100 g of product**

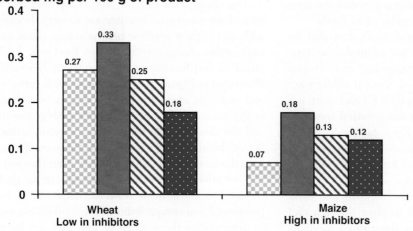

Fig. 110.3. The biologic impact of iron (Fe) fortification depends on the interaction of the iron fortificant and the food matrix, which determine percent absorption, maximal iron load compatible with the food, and the resulting absorbed iron from the consumption of 100 g of the fortified food. Refined wheat flour represents a matrix with a low amount of inhibitors, whereas industrially produced maize dough for tortilla manufacturing is an example of a matrix with a high content of inhibitors [phytates, $Ca(OH)_2$]. Numbers on top of bars correspond to respective value. Biologic impact is the product of the percentage of absorbed iron and maximal iron load depending on fortificant used and food matrix; a small amount of iron derived from the matrix has been included in the final calculation. Na EDTA, sodium ethylenediaminetetraacetic acid. (Modified with permission from Uauy R, Hertrampf E, Reddy M. Iron fortification of foods: overcoming technical and practical barriers. J Nutr 2002;132[Suppl]:849S–52S.)

effective means of controlling IDDs in countries where it has been adopted (25), and the WHO recommends universal salt iodization (the iodization of all salt for human consumption) as a strategy to control IDDs (36). The target of eradication of IDDs by 2000 has not yet been met, however, because of issues of implementation and sustainability that often pose a challenge to even the most effective fortification programs (37).

Folic Acid Fortification. The process of milling cereal crops removes much of their micronutrient content, particularly B vitamins such as folic acid. In response, cereal products such as flour are often fortified with these micronutrients. Mandatory fortification of grain products with folic acid was introduced in the United States in 1998, and many countries have now also adopted this practice. Effectiveness studies have suggested that mandatory fortification in the United States has reduced the rate of neural tube defects by 26% (38), whereas reductions of up to 50% have been reported in Chile (39). Despite these clear beneficial effects, some countries have made the decision not to adopt mandatory fortification out of concern that high intakes may have adverse effects on neurologic function in people with low vitamin B_{12} intakes, particularly the elderly (40).

Ready-to-Use Therapeutic Foods. Milk powder fortified with appropriate micronutrient compositions has long been used to treat acute malnutrition in children; a humanitarian disaster that continues to affect more than 20 million children younger than 5 years old (41). Lipid-based products with similar consistency have been developed and shown to be effective at treating malnutrition in the community (42). A major advantage of the ready-to-use therapeutic foods (RUTFs) is that they do not require mixing with water and are stable in storage, thus making them suitable for use in the community. The WHO now recommends RUTFs for the community-based management of severe acute malnutrition without complications (42). There also has been considerable interest in the potential for RUTFs to be used for prevention of undernutrition, but this is not without controversy and at present lacks a strong evidence base (43).

Nutritional Supplementation

It was established at the International Conference on Nutrition in 1992 (44) that supplementation should be restricted to vulnerable groups that cannot meet their nutrient needs through food. These include the following: women of childbearing age, infants and young children, elderly people, those with low socioeconomic status, displaced people, refugees, and those in other emergency situations. Supplementation is often the fastest and most effective way to control nutrient deficiencies quickly in a population but programs can suffer from high costs, a lack of effective distribution system, and the need for compliance (25). Supplements may be in the form of pills, capsules, or gels containing single or multiple micronutrients. Supplementation programs are now an established method of combating micronutrient deficiencies; two of the most common are described here.

Iron and Folate Supplementation for Pregnant Women
Much of the world has a low dietary intake of bioavailable iron, and as a result, iron deficiency is prevalent. Anemia in pregnancy is an important risk factor for maternal mortality and for adverse birth outcomes (24). Combined iron and folate supplements to pregnant women are now recommended in most countries in the world and have been shown to be effective at increasing hemoglobin levels (45). It has been suggested that weekly iron and folic acid supplementation in women of reproductive age may be even more effective at improving health because of the targeting of vulnerable women before pregnancy (46).

Vitamin A Supplementation for Infants and Children
The provision of vitamin A supplements to infants and children up to age 6 has been shown to be an effective method of reducing mortality in the Asian contexts in which these interventions have been studied (45). Vitamin A deficiency is also a leading cause of blindness in young children and is thought to affect more than 250 million children worldwide. The WHO currently recommends regular high-dose vitamin A supplementation between 6 months and 6 years as a simple and cost-effective method for improving child health in regions where intake is low. The neonatal period is now also a key area of research to investigate the effectiveness of vitamin A supplements at this earlier time (47).

FUTURE CONSIDERATIONS FOR FOOD-BASED DIETARY GUIDELINES

Genetic Polymorphisms and the Role of Nutrigenetics

Present knowledge of genetics indicates that close to 30,000 genes encode the biologic basis of what makes us *Homo sapiens*, and approximately 3000 of these are key for most organic functions. Mutations in these 3000 genes occur infrequently (1 to 0.01 per 1000 births), but some will result in changed requirements to meet individual nutritional needs. Some examples include individuals who are not able to metabolize phenylalanine and require a nearly phenylalanine free diet, others who cannot absorb zinc efficiently and thus require an intake several times the normal recommendation, and still others who find the population average copper intake to be toxic as in the case of Wilson' disease (48). However, because these mutations are rare and occur similarly across different regions of the world, we need not establish specific recommendations for different populations (49–51).

More recently, we have begun to unravel the significance of changes in a given base pair of the DNA strand, so-called single nucleotide polymorphisms (SNPs). These occur approximately once per 1000 base pairs; and although in most cases SNPs are silent, they can affect the expression of one or more genes and thus may have major consequences for nutrient metabolism. The concept of biochemical individuality coined by Garrod (52) acquires new meaning with the understanding of the intricate nature of gene expression and the interaction between genes and SNPs. At present, most investigators agree that close to 15 million distinct SNPs exist, and they make us truly unique.

At this stage, we are just beginning to discover the implications of genetic and epigenetic influences on the nutritional needs of individuals and population groups. Whether biochemical/genomic individuality leads to nutritional individuality remains to be seen, and if this is the case, we may need to redefine the approach used to establish dietary recommendations. Table 110.2 summarizes

TABLE 110.2	HUMAN GENETIC POLYMORPHISMS THAT AFFECT RECOMMENDED NUTRIENT INTAKES

NUTRIENT	GENE	POLYMORPHIC ALLELE (REFERENCE)
Vitamins		
Folate	*MTHFR*	A222V (63)
	CBS	844ins68 (64)
	GCPII	H475Y (65–67)
Vitamin B12	*MTR*	N919G (64)
	MTRR	122M (64)
Vitamin D	*VDR*	Multiple (68)
Minerals		
Iron	*HFE*	C282Y (69, 70)
Copper	*pATPase7-B*	Multiple (71, 72)
Zinc	*SLC39A4*	Several (73)
Lipids		
	FABP-2	Multiple (74)
	Apo B	Multiple (75, 76)
	Apo C3	Multiple (77)
	Apo E	E2, E3, E4 (78)
Alcohol	*ADH1B*	ADH2*2 (79–81)
	ADH3	ADH3*1 (82)
	ALDH2	ALDH2*2 (82)
Carbohydrate		
Lactose	*LD*	Promoter (83)

gene polymorphisms that define specific nutritional needs based on current knowledge, and the example of apolipoprotein E-(Apo-E) is discussed further below. For now, unless the genetic factor defines a special nutritional need that establishes a strong susceptibility for a given health disorder, we do not consider it in defining nutritional recommendations. This may change as we increase our ability to detect these genetic conditions and to do something about them, such as changing lifelong exposure to given levels of nutrients.

Apolipoprotein E Polymorphism and Fat Intake

The Apo-E gene locus is highly polymorphic and has been extensively studied with regard to cardiovascular disease risk. The best-characterized polymorphism is the epsilon missense mutation that results in a different configuration of the protein known as E2, E3, or E4, depending on the isoform resulting from the mutation (53). Numerous studies have investigated the association between these isoforms and an individual's responsiveness to dietary fat content (54, 55). Although findings are inconsistent, some evidence suggests that individuals with the Apo-E4 isoform tend to show the greatest low-density lipoprotein (LDL) cholesterol response to dietary fat interventions (54). Studies have shown that individuals can vary in the LDL cholesterol response to increased fish intake, with some individuals showing lowered LDL but some having raised levels. It has been suggested that one explanation of these different responses could be an individual's Apo-E polymorphism.

This example demonstrates the potential importance of nutrition–genotype interactions for explaining disease risk profiles and for informing dietary advice as part of a cohesive public health strategy.

Global Food-Based Dietary Guidelines: Are They Possible, Desirable, and Achievable?

FBDGs have the potential to be an effective method of improving the health of the population. As nutrition-related disease patterns move away from those caused by the lack of a single nutrient to more complex interactions of deficiency and excess, it has become even more important to focus on foods rather than nutrients when defining dietary advice. Although FBDGs have been an accepted method of addressing these issues, nutrient requirements still form the basis of many food labels and consumer advice. Some investigators have argued that the concept of RNIs when applied to macronutrients in particular is misleading and counterproductive (56). Thus it will be important to refocus nutritional guidelines on foods rather than nutrients. Effective, well-implemented FBDGs will be the cornerstone of this approach, and a pertinent question is whether global FBDGs are possible and desirable?

The possibility of defining one set of dietary guidelines is indeed attractive, considering the need for uniformity in the global village. Why should the optimal diet be different from one population to the next? Cultural and/or ethnic differences may result in the selection of population-specific foods to meet human nutritional needs, but they do not necessarily imply different dietary guidelines. The only justification for this would be if there was a solid genetic basis for nutritional individuality.

However, universal guidelines present new problems and novel challenges. A single unified set of guidelines will fail to address cultural diversity and the complex social, economic, and political interactions between humans and their food supply. The user needs of FBDGs have changed and it is no longer sufficient to prevent disease of mind and body, we now want to extend our healthy life years and minimize the loss of function associated with ageing. The bottom panel of the scheme presented in Figure 110.1 serves to exemplify the different uses of dietary guidelines and also the expectations that may be associated to these different groups.

Are unified guidelines achievable? The answer to this is that for some guidelines this is certainly possible, although a one-size-fits-all approach should not be applied. Guidelines most likely can be harmonized following a unified approach to defining them, but there must be room to accommodate nutritional individuality. Global guidelines will fail unless they provide the necessary options for individuals and societies to select the foods they prefer and combine them in the way that best suits their tastes and other sensory requirements. Most consumers will agree that food is far too important to be left solely in the hands of the experts.

REFERENCES

1. Food and Agriculture Organization/World Health Organization. Calcium Requirements. Geneva: World Health Organization, 1962. WHO Technical Report Series No. 230.

2. Food and Agriculture Organization/World Health Organization. Requirements of Vitamin A, Thiamine, Riboflavin and Niacin. Geneva: World Health Organization, 1962. WHO Technical Report Series No. 326.

3. Food and Agriculture Organization/World Health Organization. Requirements of Ascorbic Acid, Vitamin D, Vitamin B12, Folate and Iron. Geneva: World Health Organization, 1970. WHO Technical Report Series No. 452.

4. Food and Agriculture Organization/World Health Organization. Human Vitamin and Mineral Requirements: Report of a Joint FAO/WHO Expert Consultation. Rome: Food and Agriculture Organization, 2002.

5. Food and Agriculture Organization/World Health Organization/United Nations University. Human Energy Requirements: Report of a Joint FAO/WHO/UNU Expert Consultation. Geneva: World Health Organization, 2004.

6. Food and Agriculture Organization/World Health Organization/UNU. Protein and Amino Acid Requirements in Human Nutrition. Geneva: World Health Organization, 2007. WHO Technical Report Series No. 935.

7. Uauy R, Hertrampf E. Food-based dietary recommendations: possibilities and limitations. In: Bowman B, Russell R, eds. Present Knowledge in Nutrition. 8th ed. Washington, DC: ILSI Press, 2001:636–49.

8. Food and Agriculture Organization/World Health Organization. Preparation and Use of Food-Based Dietary Guidelines: Report of a Joint FAO/WHO Expert Consultation. Geneva: World Health Organization, 1996.

9. US Department of Agriculture. Dietary Guidelines for Americans. 5th ed. Washington DC: US Departments of Agriculture and of Health and Human Services, 2000.

10. Young VR. J Nutr 2002;132:621–9.

11. Viteri FE. Prevention of iron deficiency. In: Howson CP, Kennedy ET, Horwitz A, eds. Prevention of Micronutrient Deficiencies: Tools for Policymakers and Public Health Workers. Washington, DC: National Academy Press, 1998:45–102.

12. Food and Agriculture Organization/World Health Organization/IAEA. Zinc. In: Trace Elements in Human Nutrition and Health. Geneva: World Health Organization, 1996.

13. Hawkesworth S, Dangour A, Johnston D et al. Philos Trans R Soc 2010;365:3083–97.

14. Messer E. Soc Sci Med 1997;44:1675–84.

15. Food and Nutrition Board, National Academy of Medicine. Dietary Reference Intakes: Applications in Dietary Assessment. Washington DC: National Academy Press, 2001.

16. Lutter CK, Dewey KG. J Nutr 2003;133:3011S–20S.

17. Nestel P, Briend A, de Benoist B et al. J Pediatr Gastroenterol Nutr 2003;36:316–28.

18. UK Food Standards Agency. The Eatwell Plate. Available at: http://www.eatwell.gov.uk. Accessed August 18, 2010.

19. US Department of Agriculture. My Pyramid. Available at: http://www.mypyramid.gov. Accessed August 18, 2010.

20. US Department of Health and Human Services and U.S. Department of Agriculture. Dietary Guidelines for Americans. 6th ed. Washington, DC: U.S. Government Printing Office, 2005.

21. Food and Agriculture Organization. Food-Based Dietary Guidelines. Available at: http://www.fao.org/ag/humannutrition/nutritioneducation/fbdg. Accessed August 18, 2010.

22. Keller I, Lang T. Public Health Nutr 2008;11:867–74.

23. Food and Agriculture Organization. Rome Declaration on World Food Security and World Food Summit Plan of Action. Rome: Food and Agriculture Organization, 1996.

24. Black RE, Allen LH, Bhutta ZA et al. Lancet 2008;371:243–60.

25. Allen L, de Benoist B, Dary O et al. Guidelines on Food Fortification with Micronutrients. Geneva: World Health Organization and Food and Agriculture Organization of the United Nations, 2006.

26. Paine JA, Shipton CA, Chaggar S et al. Nat Biotechnol 2005;23:482–7.

27. Stein AJ, Sachdev HP, Qaim M. Nat Biotechnol 2006;24:1200–1.

28. Stewart JW, Kaplan ML, Beitz DC. Am J Clin Nutr 2001;74179–87.

29. Kang JX, Wang J, Wu L et al. Nature 2004;427:504.

30. World Health Organization. Iron Deficiency Anaemia: Assessment, Prevention and Control. A Guide for Programme Managers. Geneva: World Health Organization, 2001.

31. Yip R, Walsh KM, Goldfarb MG et al. Pediatrics 1987;80:330–4.

32. Layrisse M, Chaves JF, Mendez C et al. Am J Clin Nutr 1996;64:903–7.

33. Oyarzun MT, Uauy R, Olivares S. Arch Latinoam Nutr 2001;51(1):7–18.

34. Uauy R, Hertrampf E, Reddy M. J Nutr 2002;132(Suppl):849S–52S.

35. de Benoist B, Andersson M, Egli I et al. Iodine Status Worldwide: WHO Global Database on Iodine Deficiency. Geneva: World Health Organization, 2004.

36. World Health Organization. Progress Towards the Elimination of Iodine Deficiency Disorders (IDD). Geneva: World Health Organization, 1999.

37. Hetzel BS. Bull World Health Organ 2002;80:410–3; discussion 3–7.

38. Williams LJ, Mai CT, Edmonds LD et al. Teratology 2002;66:33–9.

39. Hertrampf E, Cortes F. Nutr Rev 2004;62:S44–S48; discussion S49.

40. Scientific Advisory Committee on Nutrition. Folate and Disease Prevention. London: The Stationary Office, 2006.

41. United Nations Children's fund. Tracking Progress on Child and Maternal Nutrition: A Survival and Development Priority. New York: United Nations Children's Fund, 2009.

42. World Health Organization/World Food Programme/United Nations University. Community-Based Management of Severe Acute Malnutrition. A Joint Statement by WHO, WFP, and the UN. Geneva: World Health Organization, 2007.

43. Hendricks KM. Nutr Rev 2010;68:429–35.

44. Food and Agriculture Organization, World Health Organization. International Conference on Nutrition: World Declaration and Plan of Action for Nutrition Rome: Food and Agriculture Organization, 1992.

45. Bhutta ZA, Ahmed T, Black RE et al. Lancet 2008;371:417–40.

46. World Health Organization. Weekly Iron–Folic Acid Supplementation (WIFS) in Women of Reproductive Age: Its Role in Promoting Optimal Maternal and Child Health. Position Statement. Geneva: World Health Organization, 2009.

47. World Health Organization. Technical Consultation on Neonatal Vitamin A Supplementation Research Priorities: Meeting Report. Geneva: World Health Organization, 2009.

48. Uauy R, Maass A, Araya M. Am J Clin Nutr 2008;88:867S–71S.

49. Risch NJ. Nature 2000;405:847–56.
50. Davey Smith G, Ebrahim S. Int J Epidemiol 2003;32:1–22.
51. Stover PJ. Physiol Genomics 2004;16:161–5.
52. Garrod A. Lancet 1902;2:1616–20.
53. Rall SC Jr, Weisgraber KH, Mahley RW. J Biol Chem 1982;257:4171–8.
54. Masson LF, McNeill G, Avenell A. Am J Clin Nutr 2003;77:1098–111.
55. Masson LF, McNeill G. Curr Opin Lipidol 2005;16:61–7.
56. Mozaffarian D, Ludwig DS. JAMA 2010;304:681–2.
57. Department of Health. South African Guidelines for Healthy Eating. Pretoria, South Africa: Nutrition Directorate, 2004.
58. National Institute of Nutrition. Dietary Guidelines for Indians: A Manual. Hyderabad, India: Indian Council of Medical Research, 1998.
59. Food Standards Agency. FSA Nutrient and Food Based Guidelines for UK Institutions. London: Food Standards Agency, 2006.
60. Ministry of Health Chile. Guidelines for a Healthy Life: Food, Physical Activity and Tobacco. Santiago, Chile: Ministry of Health, 2005. Available at: http://www.minsal.cl.
61. Ministry of Health Oman. The Omani Guide to Healthy Eating. Oman: Ministry of Health, 2009.
62. Health Canada. Eating Well with Canada's Food Guide. Ottawa: Health Canada, 2007.
63. Bailey LB. J Nutr 2003;133(Suppl 1):3748S–53S.
64. Jacques PF, Bostom AG, Selhub J et al. Atherosclerosis 2003;166:49–55.
65. Devlin AM, Ling EH, Peerson JM et al. Hum Mol Genet 2000;9:2837–44.
66. Ordovas JM. Biochem Soc Trans 2002;30:68–73.
67. Afman LA, Trijbels FJ, Blom HJ. J Nutr 2003;133:75–7.
68. Uitterlinden AG, Fang Y, Bergink AP et al. Mol Cell Endocrinol 2002;197:15–21.
69. Griffiths W, Cox T. Hum Mol Genet 2000;9:2377–82.
70. Lee P, Gelbart T, West C et al. Blood Cells Mol Dis 2002;29:471–87.
71. Bull PC, Thomas GR, Rommens JM et al. Nat Genet 1993;5:327–37.
72. Hsi G, Cullen LM, Moira Glerum D et al. Genomics 2004;83:473–81.
73. Dufner-Beattie J, Wang F, Kuo YM et al. J Biol Chem 2003;278:33474–81.
74. Weiss EP, Brown MD, Shuldiner AR et al. Physiol Genomics 2002;10:145–57.
75. Hubacek JA, Pistulkova H, Skodova Z et al. Ann Clin Biochem 2001;38:399–400.
76. Bentzen J, Jorgensen T, Fenger M. Clin Genet 2002;61:126–34.
77. Brown S, Ordovas JM, Campos H. Atherosclerosis 2003;170:307–13.
78. Fullerton SM, Clark AG, Weiss KM et al. Am J Hum Genet 2000;67:881–900.
79. Bosron WF, Li TK. Hepatology 1986;6:502–10.
80. Ferguson RA, Goldberg DM. Clin Chim Acta 1997;257:199–250.
81. McCarver DG. Drug Metab Dispos 2001;29:562–5.
82. Loew M, Boeing H, Sturmer T et al. Alcohol 2003;29:131–5.
83. Poulter M, Hollox E, Harvey CB et al. Ann Hum Genet 2003;67:298–311.

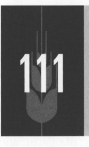

111 APPROACHES TO PREVENTING MICRONUTRIENT DEFICIENCIES[1]

LINDSAY H. ALLEN

HISTORICAL PERSPECTIVE

Since the 1930s, there has been a major evolution in our understanding concerning appropriate nutritional interventions for populations that are undernourished. The term "undernourished" includes signs of protein-energy malnutrition as well as growth stunting and evidence of specific nutrient deficiencies. In the 1930s, the main global nutrition problem was perceived to be lack of protein. Opinion then changed gradually in the 1960s to the general assumption that protein-energy malnutrition was the underlying problem and in the 1970s to the recognition that, except in cases or situations of a severe lack of food (famine and hunger) or where staple foods are low in protein (e.g., cassava), protein deficiency is not the problem. In the late 1970s, the focus shifted to preventing undernutrition by promoting breast-feeding and improving complementary feeding by adding foods such as legumes. Lack of energy (from lack of food) was investigated in the 1980s as the possible cause of chronic undernutrition in the Nutrition Collaborative Research Support Program, but that research revealed that poor dietary quality and lack of specific micronutrients were the strongest predictors of growth stunting, delays in child development, and many other adverse outcomes (1, 2).

In the 1980s, the need and opportunity for micronutrient interventions started to receive major attention. It had certainly been known for decades that severe deficiencies of vitamin A, iron, iodine, and other micronutrients increased mortality and morbidity and impaired child development, but there was little awareness before 1980 that marginal deficiencies of micronutrients could adversely affect human function and that many more functions were affected than evident from the clinical symptoms of severe deficiency. Once this reality was recognized, along with the widespread prevalence of multiple micronutrient deficiencies that result from poor-quality diets, the scientific community, agencies, governments, and others involved with improving nutrition tested and developed a wide range of interventions including the following: single and, later, multiple, nutrient supplements; fortification with single or multiple micronutrients; and food-based improvements.

This chapter describes options for delivering the micronutrients of most importance to public health. More detail on micronutrient assessment and function is available in the chapters on specific nutrients.

VITAMIN A

The World Health Organization (WHO) estimates that 5.2 million preschoolers and 7 million pregnant women suffer from clinical signs of vitamin A deficiency (most commonly night blindness), and 190 million have deficiency without clinical symptoms. Most of these people live in South and Southeast Asia and sub-Saharan Africa.

The need for large-scale interventions to prevent vitamin A deficiency was recognized in the mid-1980s, when preschooler mortality in Sumatra—where deficiency was prevalent—was reduced by 34% with high-dose (200,000 IU) capsules 6 months apart (3). This was later confirmed by a metaanalysis of additional studies (4). Currently, more than 70% of children 6 to 59 months old receive the recommended twice-yearly high-dose supplements (100,000 IU for those 6 to 11 months old and 200,000 IU for those 12 to 59 months old). Effective distribution of the supplements is often supported by public health campaigns promoting "vitamin A days" or combined vaccination and vitamin A promotions.

[1]**Abbreviations: HFP**, homestead food production; **LNS**, lipid-based nutrient supplement; **NaFeEDTA**, sodium iron ethylenediaminetetraacetic acid; **NTD**, neural tube defect; **UL**, tolerable upper intake limit; **USI**, universal salt iodization; **WHO**, World Health Organization.

A metaanalysis of 21 studies showed that neonatal high-dose supplementation reduced all-cause mortality by 12%, but it had no effect during the first 6 months of age (5). In children 6 to 59 months old, mortality was reduced by 25% and diarrhea by 30%. There was no significant effect on deaths from measles or meningitis, although the reduction in deaths from these conditions was almost 30%.

The benefits of giving lower doses of vitamin A to women starting in the periconceptional period were investigated in two studies adequately powered to determine the effect on maternal and infant mortality. The supplements provided the daily recommended intake in a single weekly dose. The first study, in rural Nepal, showed a 40% reduction in pregnancy-related mortality with retinol as the supplement and a 49% reduction with β-carotene (6). However, when the study was replicated in rural Bangladesh, these supplements had no effect on pregnancy-related mortality, which the investigators suggested was the result of the lower mortality rates (better delivery care) and vitamin A status in the Bangladeshi women (7). Providing high-dose supplements to infants within a few days of birth has produced inconsistent effects on infant mortality (8). Additional trials of this question are ongoing in India, Ghana, and Tanzania.

For women of reproductive age, supplementation with high-dose preformed vitamin A (200,000 IU) is restricted to the first 6 weeks postpartum when there is a low risk of their becoming pregnant. This mitigates concern that a high dose could have teratogenic effects on the embryo; the tolerable upper intake limit (UL) for vitamin A is 3000 IU (µg retinol equivalent [RE]) daily for women of reproductive age based on this concern. β-Carotene does not present this risk. Supplementing breast-feeding mothers during early lactation increases the secretion of retinol in breast milk and improves infant vitamin A status. In fact, breast milk vitamin A concentration is a good indicator of the effectiveness of vitamin A intervention programs for women and infants (9). After the first 6 weeks postpartum, when high-dose supplements can no longer be used, maternal intake can be increased through low-dose supplements or foods rich in preformed vitamin A or β-carotene.

Food sources are highly variable in their content of vitamin A and its precursor carotenoids. Animal source foods including milk, eggs, and liver are a good source of retinol. Some fruits and vegetables contain β-carotene and other carotenoids that can be converted to vitamin A and improve vitamin A status (10). One of the most concentrated natural sources of carotenoids is red palm oil, in which carotenoids are present as precursor carotenoids if these are not removed by processing (11). Biofortification for improving vitamin A status can be achieved effectively with orange-fleshed sweet potatoes and golden rice. For example, in Mozambique, Helen Keller's Reaching Agents of Change Project is providing orange-fleshed sweet potatoes to 600,000 households. Vitamin A–rich cassava is also being investigated.

IRON

Iron is often cited as being the most common nutrient deficiency in the world. It is certainly prevalent, especially in menstruating women and in infants and children, although "neglected" nutrients such as riboflavin and vitamin B_{12} may in fact be more common. Pending more definitive data, the WHO states that approximately 50% of anemia worldwide is the result of iron deficiency. Causes of the remainder are incompletely understood but include malaria, thalassemias, vitamin A deficiency, and parasitic infections such as hookworm and schistosomiasis. No strategy to control iron deficiency can be complete unless infections that cause iron deficiency are controlled.

Interventions to prevent and treat iron deficiency are justified because iron deficiency increases the risk of anemia, reduces work capacity and performance, increases the risk of depression, and impairs the cognitive development of children (12). Iron deficiency anemia in infancy may affect major dopamine pathways, leading to persistently poor inhibitory control and executive function later in childhood and adult life (13).

Iron can be provided as ferrous sulfate or other iron salts in tablets or in syrup for infants and young children. These can treat anemia within about 2 to 3 months or can prevent the development of iron deficiency in young children and pregnant women. The recommended daily dose is 3 mg/kg for children up to 5 years and 60 mg for adults; 60 mg is the recommended UL because of the risk of intestinal distress at higher levels. Higher doses are often given in the mistaken assumption that they will be more effective for increasing hemoglobin, but iron absorption is down-regulated as intakes increase, and in some trials, 20 mg/day was as effective as 60 mg for pregnant women.

Iron supplements do not have to be consumed every day to be effective, and taking a supplement once per week can reduce the risk of iron deficiency anemia. The WHO recommends once-weekly iron (60 mg of elemental iron as 300 mg ferrous sulfate, 180 mg ferrous fumarate, or 500 mg ferrous gluconate) and folic acid (2800 µg) supplementation for menstruating adolescent girls and adult women living in areas where the prevalence of anemia in this group is 20% or higher (14). Supplementation can be stopped for 3 months and restarted for another 3 months. Efficacy for treating anemia depends predominantly on the total amount of iron delivered and not on the frequency of delivery; in Bangladesh, most of the hemoglobin response to 60 mg/day supplements occurred with the first 20 tablets, and response plateaued after 40 tablets (15). In pregnant women, the demands for iron are particularly high, so daily, rather than weekly, supplementation is recommended (60 mg/day with 400 µg folic acid) (14). In areas where the prevalence of anemia is higher than 40%, the supplements should be continued for 3 months postpartum.

It is possible that supplemental iron exacerbates the adverse effects of malaria in infants and young children, especially in those who are not iron deficient initially and in areas where malaria prophylaxis and health care are poor (16). Research is ongoing to determine the underlying mechanisms and whether adverse effects may be avoided by providing the iron with meals or in fortified foods.

Iron fortification of food is a common strategy for the prevention of iron deficiency. This approach avoids problems frequent in supplementation programs such as lack of pill distribution and poor participant compliance. One review discussed the reasons that iron deficiency anemia continues to be so prevalent even though the first flour fortification programs (in Canada, the United States, and the United Kingdom) started in the 1940s (17). These issues include concerns about the safety of supplementation and fortification, technical constraints to the addition of iron to foods, the complexities of assessing iron status, and lack of knowledge about the adverse consequences of iron deficiency.

One review of the effectiveness of iron fortification of wheat flour concluded that only 7 out of 78 countries evaluated were likely to detect a positive effect even if the program was implemented effectively (18). The main reason for this is that millers have used less bioavailable iron compounds such as atomized or hydrogen-reduced iron powders because they cost less and do not cause adverse taste and color reactions with food; however, these substances are absorbed poorly. Less reactive yet bioavailable forms of iron such as ferrous fumarate, sodium iron ethylenediaminetetraacetic acid (NaFeEDTA), and micronized ferric pyrophosphate are being used increasingly in flours, condiments (salt, curry, fish sauce, soy sauce), and complementary foods for infants. Where 150 to 300 mg wheat flour is consumed daily, the recommendation is to add 20 ppm iron as NaFeEDTA or 30 ppm as dried ferrous fumarate or ferrous sulfate (18). If sensory problems occur or to reduce cost, 60 ppm of electrolytic iron can be used. Only NaFeEDTA is recommended for high-extraction wheat flour.

In general, food-based strategies to improve iron status have been less effective than supplementation or fortification. Meat and meat products are often expensive, and even feeding 70 g daily for 9 months did not improve the iron status of young Guatemalan children (Allen et al, unpublished data). Increasing intake of food high in ascorbic acid did not improve iron status of Mexican women, even though their diet was high in poorly available iron (19). In many plant-based diets, iron bioavailability is poor because of the high content of phytates and/or tannins. Although absorption from such foods can be improved by soaking or pretreatment with phytases, this is not a common or popular practice.

Biofortification of staple foods shows some promise for improving the iron status of populations. For example, rice with a high content of iron (which only added 1.4 mg/day to the usual dietary intake) did slightly improve iron stores in Filipina women (20). Biofortified beans and pearl millet are being explored by Harvest Plus.

IODINE

In large areas of the world, iodine deficiency is endemic because of the low amount of iodine in water, soil, and plants and animals raised in the region. Two billion people are affected by this deficiency. Iodine deficiency disorders occur over the range of severe to mild deficiency. Consequences include cretinism (as a result of maternal deficiency during pregnancy, and often irreversible) and goiter with severe deficiency, low birth weight and growth stunting, lethargy, and a loss of up to 13 IQ points. The primary intervention is iodization of salt and universal salt iodization (USI), one of the earliest examples of large-scale fortification to prevent micronutrient deficiency. Today, approximately 70% of households in the developing world consume adequately iodized salt; small amounts of iodine are added to table salt as sodium iodide, potassium iodide, and/or potassium iodate, to achieve a concentration of more than 15 ppm iodine. Iodine salts can also be added to other foods, such as flour, water, and milk. The iodine status of a population and the adequacy (or excess) of USI should be monitored by measuring urinary iodine in school-age children. About one third of school-age children still have insufficient iodine intake, although the situation has improved over recent years.

Iodine deficiency is also a problem in many industrialized countries (21), and in some countries, it is reappearing because of less use of iodophors by the dairy industry, which used to increase the iodine content of milk. The best solution in at-risk wealthier countries is to ensure that food manufacturers use iodized salt because about 90% of salt is consumed in processed foods. In such countries, there is often concern about using salt as a fortification vehicle because of its health risks, but it is still possible to add enough iodine in up to 5 g salt per day. Where iodized salt is not adequately consumed, iodized oil can be provided in capsules, although this is more expensive per capita. For the many pregnant women in European countries with low iodine status, a daily 150-μg supplement is recommended to prevent abnormal thyroid function in the mother and infant and adverse effects on mental development of the children (22). Breast-feeding infants may also be at risk because iodine levels are low in the milk of iodine-depleted women, and infants consume low amounts of salt (23). Such infants need adequately iodized complementary foods.

FOLIC ACID AND VITAMIN B$_{12}$

Folic acid supplementation and fortification programs are widely implemented with the primary goal of preventing neural tube defect (NTD) births. In women at high risk of an NTD delivery, poor folate status interacts with genetic and environmental risk factors to produce an infant with an NTD. The condition is not caused by folate deficiency alone.

At least 52 countries mandate folic acid fortification of flour. This has reduced the incidence of NTDs from 19% to 40% where impact has been monitored (24). The level of reduction is greater in populations with a higher prevalence of NTD and poorer folate status before fortification. The global prevalence of folate deficiency is uncertain, and this deficiency is possibly more common in industrialized than developing countries. Legumes are a good source of folate, as are many fruits and vegetables, but refined flour and other cereals are not (25).

The prevalence of NTD ranges from 5 to 8 per 10,000 in countries with effective folic acid fortification programs, most of which aim to supply 400 μg/day, to 40 per 10,000 population. The number of NTDs prevented per year is very small compared with the population exposed to additional folic acid; in the United Kingdom, where fortification has not been implemented, it has been estimated that if flour were to be fortified with 300 μg folic acid/100 g, 77 to 162 birth defects would be prevented, whereas 370,000 to 780,000 people would be exposed to excess folic acid (26). Thus, unnecessary or excessive fortification and supplementation should be avoided. Concerns about the safety of folic acid fortification include possible proliferation of preexisting colorectal tumors (although it may protect against their initiation), adverse effects on immune function, and exacerbation of the functional effects of vitamin B_{12} deficiency. For example, in vitamin B_{12}–deficient US elderly persons, those with the highest serum folate concentration had a greater risk of anemia and cognitive impairment and evidence of altered vitamin B_{12} metabolism, although higher serum folate protected against cognitive impairment in those with adequate vitamin B_{12} status (27). It is likely that people with the highest serum folate consumed supplements in addition to folic acid–fortified products.

The WHO recommends that iron supplements for pregnant women should contain 400 μg folic acid. This has been long-standing advice because evidence at the time suggested that additional folic acid would prevent megaloblastic anemia in pregnancy in some populations, although this condition is now rare. The recommendation continued after it was proven that folic acid could prevent NTDs. However, supplements are effective for preventing NTDs only if they are taken before conception through the first 4 to 6 weeks after conception. Because folic acid supplements often lower plasma homocysteine, a risk factor for poor pregnancy outcomes, and may prevent other birth defects, the recommendation to include folic acid with iron is not likely to change. It has not been investigated whether folic acid supplementation in pregnancy is beneficial where flour is fortified with the vitamin, and because folic acid intakes would be high in this situation, the potential for exacerbation of vitamin B_{12} deficiency should be studied.

Vitamin B_{12} deficiency and depletion are very common in populations whose intake of animal-source foods is low (28). Contrary to popular belief, it is not necessary to be a strict vegetarian to develop this deficiency. Vitamin B_{12} fortification of flour at 2 μg/100 g is recommended for such populations (28), although its efficacy in mandatory fortification programs has yet to be evaluated. Dual fortification with folic acid and vitamin B_{12} would reduce concern about potential adverse effects of folic acid fortification on vitamin B_{12} status, and vitamin B_{12} may also contribute to lowering the prevalence of NTDs. Elderly people worldwide are at risk of vitamin B_{12} deficiency because of low gastric acid secretion, which impairs the release of the vitamin from food. It is recommended that they obtain a substantial proportion of their daily requirement as the synthetic vitamin in supplements or fortified foods, which would be more readily absorbed.

ZINC

Zinc deficiency occurs in populations that consume low intakes of bioavailable zinc because their staple diets are low in animal-source foods and high in phytate, which inhibits zinc absorption. Major losses of zinc occur in diarrheal diseases and especially in chronic diarrhea, contributing to growth stunting. One estimate of the global prevalence of zinc deficiency is 30%, and it is most prevalent in children less than 5 years of age. This may be an overestimate because biomarkers of zinc status are poor, and deficiency prevalence is estimated from the prevalence of growth stunting (which is multicausal) and diets low in bioavailable zinc.

There is reasonable consensus that zinc, when supplemented alone, benefits linear growth, with a 0.37 ($\pm$0.25) cm higher gain in children less than 5 years when 10 mg/day is given for 24 weeks (29). It is unlikely, however, that zinc alone would be given as a supplement except for the treatment of diarrhea, and when zinc is combined with iron in a supplement, it seems to be less effective for increasing growth (29). Zinc losses are much increased during diarrhea, and giving supplements during an episode reduces the duration and severity of the event as well as diarrhea incidence in the subsequent 2 to 3 months. The recommendation is to start zinc supplements early in a diarrheal episode, 10 mg/day for 14 days for children less than 6 months of age and 20 mg for older infants and children (30).

In randomized, placebo-controlled zinc supplementation trials, supplements (usually 10 mg zinc) reduced child mortality and morbidity related to gastrointestinal and respiratory infections (31), as well as malarial morbidity. The most recent metaanalysis revealed that supplements reduce all-cause mortality by 9%, diarrhea-specific mortality by 13%, and pneumonia-specific mortality by 19%, but none of these effects are statistically significant. No effect on malaria-specific mortality was noted (32).

Fortification of flour or other cereals with zinc has not been shown to be very effective for improving zinc status, although the zinc appears to be absorbed. Nevertheless, there are no reasons not to include zinc as a flour fortificant when possible. The amount to be added depends on the type of flour and the populations and subgroups targeted (33). Food-based approaches include soaking and fermentation to enable endogenous phytases to release zinc from phytate (34). Biofortified rice is being tested in Bangladesh and India and in wheat in India and Pakistan.

VITAMIN D

Vitamin D deficiency is widespread in populations with limited skin synthesis of the vitamin, which requires ultraviolet radiation. These populations include persons in more northern and southern latitudes, groups with more pigmented skin, groups whose clothing covers almost all the body, and individuals who are rarely exposed to sunlight or who use heavy sunscreen. Few foods can provide sufficient vitamin D in such situations, exceptions being fatty fish, fish liver, and eggs. Cow's milk is fortified with the vitamin in many countries; in the United States (100 IU/cup) and Canada (35 to 40 IU/100 mL), this fortification has reduced the incidence of rickets in young children and has improved the status of the rest of the population since the 1930s. Margarine and breakfast cereals are often fortified with the vitamin.

Breast-fed infants are at higher risk of vitamin D deficiency because breast milk is low in the vitamin, and it is recommended that exclusively and partially breast-fed infants should be supplemented with 400 IU/day until they are weaned and consuming at least 1000 IU/day in formulas or fortified milk.

Elderly persons are at higher risk of vitamin D deficiency because of their propensity to spend less time outdoors and the substantially reduced ability of their skin to synthesize the precursor form of the vitamin. Supplements are often recommended for this age group and have prevented bone loss and hip fractures.

MULTIPLE MICRONUTRIENT INTERVENTIONS

Dietary quality is often inadequate in poor populations, predominantly because of a low intake of animal source foods. Such foods are good sources of preformed vitamin A, riboflavin, bioavailable iron and zinc, choline, vitamin D, and calcium, among other nutrients, and the only source of vitamin B_{12}. Thus, such populations are typically deficient in multiple micronutrients, and it is often more efficient, as well as necessary, to design interventions to address them all simultaneously.

Infants and Children

Exclusive breast-feeding is recommended for the first 6 months of life, after which nutrient-dense complementary foods should be introduced. In many circumstances, it is difficult to supply young children with complementary foods that are adequate to supply the micronutrients they need in addition to breast milk (35); the child must like and be able to consume the foods. This can be a difficulty with meat, for example, and the food must be affordable and available. The role of caregivers, who make decisions about what is feasible, healthy, and affordable, is critical in all micronutrient delivery interventions for young children (36).

An increasingly popular approach to preventing multiple deficiencies in this age group is the use of micronutrient powders. These preparations have the advantage that they can be added to usual family foods, their bioavailability is good, and compliance can be better than with supplements. They are especially useful for adding to cereals and family foods used as complementary foods for infants and young children. Anemia was reduced even when caretakers used the powders "flexibly" over the course of 4 months (37). A review of micronutrient powder use in large-scale programs that included social marketing concluded that there were improvements in anemia in some subgroups but not others, a reduction in stunting in Nepal and Kenya but not in Bangladesh, and an increase in diarrhea in Nepali children (38). The main challenge is to achieve adequate and sustainable use by the beneficiaries.

Another strategy for delivering multiple micronutrients to this age group is with lipid-based nutrient supplements (LNSs). LNSs were developed to support the recovery of children with severe malnutrition, and they are now being investigated for their efficacy and effectiveness for preventing growth stunting. LNSs are usually made from a legume base such as peanuts, with or without dry milk, and consumed from sachets or a container, either alone or mixed with infant cereals or family foods. Advantages include the stability of the micronutrients in the lipid matrix, the ability to adjust the dose with age, and the ready consumption by children. It has been suggested that the fatty acid, and especially omega-3, content of LNSs may promote growth and development, and trials examining this question are ongoing. LNSs tend to be more expensive than tablets (or micronutrient powders), so caretakers must have the resources to buy them, or the LNSs need to be subsidized or donated. LNSs can also be used by pregnant or lactating women.

Fortification of special complementary foods for infants and young children is another popular strategy for preventing multiple micronutrient deficiencies. It is most often realized through centralized fortification and commercial products. A public-private partnership in China provides a useful example of how to develop and market successfully a fortified complementary food made from local products (full-fat soy powder) (39). A metaanalysis of randomized controlled trials showed that providing multiple micronutrients in fortified foods is as effective as supplementation for improving linear growth of young children (40). Special attention must be given to the formulation of these foods and the forms of fortificants.

Pregnant and Lactating Women

Recognizing that multiple micronutrient deficiencies are common and that there is relatively little cost increase when supplements for pregnant women provide multiple micronutrients rather than iron or iron plus folic acid alone, the benefits of these two strategies were compared in a series of studies that mostly used the United Nations International Multiple Micronutrient Preparation (UNIMMAP) supplement containing the daily recommended intake of 14 micronutrients. Although the trials were conducted rather independently over the course of some years, a metaanalysis was conducted that enabled conclusions to be drawn from all the available data. Compared with iron plus folic acid supplements alone (no trials had a placebo control), multiple micronutrients significantly reduced low birth weight (by 11%) and small for gestational age births (by 10%), but they had no other clear impacts (41). A more recent metaanalysis included newer trials for a total of 17 studies and also concluded that multiple micronutrients had no additional effect over iron plus folic acid for reducing anemia in the third trimester, and that small for gestational age births were reduced by 9% in women with a body mass index of at least 22 kg/m^2 (42). For women delivering at home, there was a 47% higher risk that the infant would die soon after birth, but not where more than 60% of births occurred in health facilities. Overall, neonatal mortality was not increased, but concerns about increased mortality risk remain to be resolved before multiple micronutrient supplements are recommended over iron plus folic acid supplements. Another unresolved issue is whether increasing the dose of micronutrients or supplying them in fortified food is more effective than recommended daily amounts of micronutrients alone (43).

There are few clear recommendations for micronutrient interventions targeted to lactating women. This is surprising because maternal nutrient requirements are substantially higher in lactation than they are in pregnancy, and the amount of many nutrients secreted in breast milk depends on maternal intake and status. These include all the B vitamins except folic acid; vitamins A, C, and D; selenium; and iodine (44). Research is in progress to determine the extent to which breast milk concentrations of these nutrients can be increased by maternal supplementation and subsequently improve infant status.

AGRICULTURAL INTERVENTIONS

Using agriculture as a platform to prevent micronutrient deficiencies has several potential advantages. Homestead food production (HFP) is a particularly attractive intervention that is generating much interest. HFP can increase micronutrient intake with micronutrient-rich crops, especially fruits and vegetables, and biofortified cereals and other crop staples. The latter has been successful for vitamin A (carotenoids) and is being developed for iron and zinc. Animal source food production needs to be increased to improve intakes of those nutrients found only in such foods (e.g., vitamin B$_{12}$) or that are much more bioavailable from those foods (e.g., iron and zinc, vitamin A). Successful examples of increased animal source food production have included education and support with small loans, resulting in higher income from sales that can benefit women in particular (see http://www.partnership-africa.org/content/hidden-hunger-story-enam-project-ghana-and-child-nutrition). Although most such programs have been relatively small in scale and inadequately evaluated (45), Helen Keller International scaled up HFP in Bangladesh that has improved food security for 5 million people. Improving micronutrient intake through agriculture can benefit the entire household, whereas supplementation programs are often targeted to pregnant women and young children.

STRENGTHS AND WEAKNESSES OF DIFFERENT APPROACHES

Olney et al (45) reviewed different programs (supplementation, fortification, and dietary modification) and platforms (health-based, agriculture-based, and market-based approaches and social protection programs) that can deliver micronutrients based on seven performance criteria: targeting, efficacy, quality of implementation, utilization, impact, coverage, and sustainability. Micronutrient delivery often occurs through existing health programs or centers, usually targeted as supplements or micronutrient powders to pregnant women and children and as fortified complementary foods. Such strategies are supported by the WHO's Integrated Management of Childhood Illness (IMCI) program, for example. When these strategies are delivered with appropriate education concerning their importance, acceptance and coverage are generally good. Obvious caveats are that the micronutrient supply must be dependable, clients must use the health care services on a regular basis, and staff must be trained to deliver the education information.

The investigators concluded that all the foregoing programs and platforms can be effective if key program elements are in place. These elements include the following: the need to educate consumers and programs about the importance of micronutrients and how they should be used; ensuring that the supply of products and quality of interventions is adequate, including access to well-trained staff; rigorous evaluations of the effectiveness, delivery, and impact of the interventions to support the goal of scaling up to reach larger populations; and timely dissemination of the results of such evaluations to policymakers and program implementers.

The program and platforms should not be an "either-or" choice because the diversification of approaches can mean better coverage. However, care needs to be taken

actin) results in more myosin crossbridge binding to actin filaments and thereby creates more tension within the muscle. The amount of calcium ion released from the sarcoplasmic reticulum is related to how frequently the motor neuron stimulates the muscle. Thus, increased activation of a motor neuron results in increased force developed in that motor neuron's motor unit (motor neuron and muscle fibers it innervates). Peak force for a motor unit is normally achieved at a neural action potential frequency of approximately 50 Hz (lower frequency for slow motor units and higher frequency for fast motor units). In addition, more force is generated when more motor units are activated.

A larger muscle cross-sectional area increases the number of myosin crossbridge heads available to bind with actin filaments and the potential for maximum force production. Anatomic structure can also influence force production. Maximal force is measured at the end of a lever system (e.g., the hand during an arm curl). The ratio of the length of levers and attachment point of the tendon to bone (e.g., forearm length to elbow's axis of rotation in relation to distance of attachment of the biceps brachii to the axis of rotation) affects force applied at the end of the lever system.

Other factors affect maximal force production, including angle of muscle pennation (pennate muscle fibers extend at an angle from the tendon as the barbs do from a feather). A more acute pennation angle increases force. Fiber type also influences strength and power production. Type II muscle fibers have greater strength and power potential than do type I muscle fibers. Because creatine kinase activity and myokinase activity are related to strength independent of muscle size, and because both seem to be increased in strength-trained individuals, high-energy phosphate availability in the myofibril probably can be limiting to expression of maximal force [17].

CARDIORESPIRATORY FITNESS (AEROBIC FITNESS)

Mode of exercise, heredity, state of training, gender, and age all affect an individual's $\dot{V}O_{2max}$. $\dot{V}O_{2max}$ is generally evaluated during a progressive exercise task requiring large muscle groups. Treadmill walking or running results in the highest $\dot{V}O_{2max}$ for most individuals. Because slightly lower peak values of oxygen uptake are normally found for other activities such as bicycling, $\dot{V}O_{2max}$ should be defined as peak oxygen uptake, if it is likely that a higher value could have been obtained with another modality.

$\dot{V}O_{2max}$ is normally reported relative to body mass (mL O_2/kg body weight/minute) when cardiorespiratory fitness is used to evaluate the ability of an individual to move his or her body mass (i.e., during walking or running). Estimates of physiologic capacity are confounded by variations in fat mass when adjustments are made with body mass, however, because fat mass increases body mass but does not contribute markedly to $\dot{V}O_2$ during exercise. An adjustment for fat-free mass (mL O_2/kg fat-free mass/minute) is made when $\dot{V}O_{2max}$ relative to physiologically active fat-free mass is important.

Efforts have been made to determine the proportion of $\dot{V}O_{2max}$ that is related to hereditary or training [2]. Training can increase $\dot{V}O_{2max}$ much more in some individuals than in others, and the genetic effect of aerobic fitness is probably approximately 40% [2]. An appropriate aerobic endurance training program increases $\dot{V}O_{2max}$ approximately 20% over 12 to 16 weeks in an untrained person, but some individuals improve less than 10% and others improve up to 50%. Aerobic capacity in women is typically 10% to 30% lower than in men, even among trained athletes. Table 112.2 illustrates typical $\dot{V}O_{2max}$ values for various groups.

Genetic factors probably account for significant amounts of the variation in fat distribution as well aerobic capacity. Untrained rats that have high aerobic fitness have lower visceral fat contents and reduced metabolic risk compared with untrained rats with low fitness [18]. Independent of AEE and total body fat, women who have relatively high aerobic fitness have relatively low visceral fat [19]. Taken together, these two studies suggest a genetic link between high aerobic fitness and a more favorable fat distribution.

AGING

After the age of approximately 30 years, both cardiorespiratory and strength fitness decline at approximately 1% per year [2, 17]. The rate of decline in fitness can be decreased but not stopped despite continuing high activity levels. The decline in cardiorespiratory fitness is related to reduced central and peripheral function [20]. Maximum heart rate declines at approximately one beat/year and is the main contributor to reduced maximum cardiac output. Losses of muscle mass, peripheral blood flow capacity, and capacity of skeletal muscle to generate ATP from oxidative processes also occur.

TABLE 112.2	TYPICAL MAXIMUM OXYGEN UPTAKE VALUES IN HEALTHY INDIVIDUALS (IN mL O_2/kg BODY WEIGHT/min)		
	UNTRAINED	TRAINED	ELITE ENDURANCE ATHLETE
Young man (20–30 y)	40–45	57–62	75–85
Older man (50–60 y)	33–38	47–53	58–64
Young woman (20–30 y)	32–36	45–52	63–70
Older woman (50–60 y)	25–30	36–42	45–52

The primary cause of the decline in strength fitness with age is atrophy of skeletal muscle, defined as sarcopenia. Skeletal muscle sarcopenia is characterized by atrophy of both type I and type II muscle fibers, although sarcopenia occurs more rapidly in type II muscle fibers. Muscle fiber necrosis and increased intramuscular content of adipose and connective tissues also occur with aging (17, 21), and they probably contribute to a decrease in muscle quality (strength per unit area of muscle) with age (22).

Power (time-rate of doing work) decreases proportionally more than strength with age. Preferential type II muscle fiber atrophy accounts for some of the accelerated loss of power with age because the maximum velocity of shortening and power production are higher in type II than type I muscle fibers. Decreased strength or power production also probably results from impaired excitation-contraction coupling (23), given that calcium release and dihydropyridine receptor expression both decline with age (17). Adults lose only 5% to 10% of their muscle mass between the ages of 30 and 50 years, but they lose an additional 30% to 40% between the ages of 50 and 80 years. In addition, visceral fat increases with age. This increase is dramatic, quadrupling in women (24) and doubling in men between the ages of 25 and 65 years (25). Three main factors appear to be responsible for this visceral fat increase: weight gain, fat-free mass loss, and shift of fat away from the periphery toward the viscera.

INTERACTION OF FITNESS AND PHYSICAL ACTIVITY WITH MORTALITY AND RISK OF DISEASE

Debate surrounds the relative contributions of exercise fitness and physical activity to overall wellness and well-being. Both physical activity (contraction of skeletal muscle that increases energy expenditure) and cardiorespiratory fitness are inversely related to heart disease, diabetes, some cancers, and all-cause mortality in men and women (1, 26, 27).

A dose-response relationship exists, with the most physically active or fit individuals experiencing mortality rates less than half those of the least physically active or fit individuals (26). Whether the favorable effects of the physical activity are obtained entirely by increased energy expenditure or whether further favorable health-related effects can be obtained by participation in physical activity of sufficient intensity to create a training effect is unclear, however.

Several studies suggested that intense vigorous activity gives some advantage over light- to moderate-intensity physical activity (26). For example, reviews suggested that insulin insensitivity, dyslipidemia, and hypertension are more strongly affected by training that affects cardiorespiratory fitness (28).

The problem is complicated, however, because visceral adiposity is related to an adverse lipid profile, increased blood pressure, insulin insensitivity, cardiovascular disease, diabetes, and mortality (29) and because both more active and more fit individuals have less visceral fat (30, 31). Few studies have evaluated the independent effects of physical activity, aerobic fitness, and visceral adiposity on the risk of disease, although available population studies suggest that metabolic changes associated with weight loss may be primarily responsible for the decreased incidence of cardiovascular disease found in more active men (32). Hunter et al (24), using the best current techniques for measurement of physical activity (combination of doubly labeled water and indirect calorimetry), aerobic fitness ($\dot{V}O_{2max}$), and visceral fat (computed tomography) showed that visceral fat is adversely related to insulin sensitivity and blood lipids independent of physical activity and aerobic fitness. Although not as strongly related, physical activity was independently related to total cholesterol and low-density lipoprotein (LDL) cholesterol, whereas cardiorespiratory fitness was independently related to high-density lipoprotein (HDL) cholesterol and insulin sensitivity. Consistent with these results, Thompson et al (33) suggested that relatively high-intensity physical activity ($\geq 75\%$ $\dot{V}O_{2max}$) may be necessary to improve glucose metabolism and that prolonged exercise is necessary to produce changes in LDL cholesterol. In any event, both physical activity of low to moderate intensity and cardiorespiratory fitness training probably have positive independent effects on risk of disease. Some of the positive effects of participation in physical activity and cardiorespiratory training may be mediated through their effects on visceral adiposity, however (34, 35).

PHYSICAL ACTIVITY AND WEIGHT MAINTENANCE

Many studies have shown that total energy expenditure is related to obesity and subsequent weight gain. This is particularly problematic as we age because both resting energy expenditure and AEE decline with age. The decrease is even more pronounced in AEE (17). A review by Westerterp (36) indicated that daily AEE decreases from 35% of the total energy expenditure at age 20 years to 25% at age 90 years. Decreased AEE can have a major adverse effect on weight maintenance; studies showed that individuals who are physically active are more successful in maintaining weight than are those who are less physically active (17). In fact, in a doubly labeled water study, investigators demonstrated that 77% of the differences in weight gain between gainers and maintainers was accounted for by physical AEE (37). The rest of the weight gain was presumably caused by increased energy intake in the gainers. Exercise training can slow weight gain after weight loss (38). In addition, several studies showed that elevated aerobic fitness is associated with reduced visceral fat (39) and that visceral fat is preferentially lost with exercise training (40–43). More recently, exercise training was shown to prevent any gain in visceral fat for 1 year following a

25-lb weight loss, even though weight regain averaged approximately 7 lb (38).

HOW MUCH PHYSICAL ACTIVITY IS REQUIRED?

Studies using doubly labeled water to measure energy expenditure suggested that approximately 80 minutes/day would be needed to prevent weight gain (37, 44). The 2002 International Association for the Study of Obesity First Stock Conference consensus report on physical activity recommended 60 to 90 minutes/day of moderate-intensity exercise or lesser amounts of vigorous-intensity activity (45). Moderate-intensity exercise is defined as exercise that is 3 to 4 metabolic equivalents (METs; an increment of resting metabolic rate). For example, 4 METs would be an intensity that is 4 times resting. Significant increases in overall health can be obtained with as little as 30 minutes/day of moderate-intensity exercise. At least 80 minutes/day of moderate-intensity exercise (one study suggests as much as 101 minutes) may be needed to prevent weight gain if dietary restriction is not practiced (Fig. 112.2), however (17). Because many individuals do not have the time or motivation to participate in 100 minutes/day or even 80 minutes/day of physical activity, weight maintenance may entail dietary restraint as well

as an active lifestyle. The relationship between physical activity and well-being should be considered a continuum, with some physical activity better than none and more physical activity associated with increased health until some ceiling effect is reached, probably in excess of 80 to 100 minutes of moderate-intensity exercise.

It is obvious that increased energy expenditure, especially AEE, may be beneficial for weight maintenance. Because low- to moderate-intensity exercise is believed to be more easily tolerated, efforts to increase physical activity have focused on low- to moderate-intensity exercise (31). High-intensity exercise may be important to exercise programs, adding components that cannot be achieved with low- to moderate-intensity exercise. For example, Kraus et al (46) have shown that exercise equivalent to walking or jogging 12 miles/week was associated with some improvements in blood lipid profile and also found that higher levels (20 miles/week) of high-intensity exercise (jogging at 65% to 80 % peak $\dot{V}O_2$) was necessary to increase HDL cholesterol. In addition, relatively short-duration high-intensity exercise training is related to greater decreases in subcutaneous skinfolds than longer duration low-intensity exercise training that produced over 2 times greater energy expenditure (31).

HIGH-INTENSITY EXERCISE AND ENERGY EXPENDITURE

Besides the possible relationship between cardiorespiratory fitness and increased HDL cholesterol and insulin sensitivity, high-intensity exercise training appears to have several potential advantages for increasing total energy expenditure and decreasing the likelihood of gaining metabolically harmful visceral fat (31). First, the volume of work and thus of energy expended is much greater with high-intensity exercise during any similar exercise time. Second, as intensity of most exercise tasks increases, efficiency or economy decreases. Running is one of the few activities in which this does not seem to occur. The magnitude of the variation can be large, increasing more than 300% over a wide spectrum of exercise intensities. For example, 22% more energy is required to bicycle at 100 watts for 30 minutes than to bicycle at 50 watts for 60 minutes, whereas 12 times as much energy is required to complete 1 bench press at 80% maximum strength compared with 1 bench press at 20% of maximum (31). Although the reason is not definitively known, increased dependence on inefficient type II muscle fibers at higher intensities is probably a major contributor (47).

EXERCISE TRAINING AND RESTING ENERGY EXPENDITURE

High-intensity exercise may have some effect on resting energy expenditure. Cross-sectional studies demonstrated that athletes who participate in high-intensity exercise

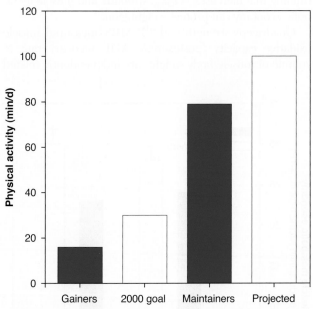

Fig. 112.2. Estimated time necessary to prevent weight gain (minutes/day). Based on difference in energy expenditure between groups of maintainers and gainers, maintainers would have to restrict energy intake to maintain weight. If no dietary restriction were present in maintainers (differences in activity-related energy expenditure accounting for all the difference in time spent in physical activity between the gainers and maintainers), 101 minutes instead of 79 minutes of moderate-intensity exercise would be needed to maintain weight (group labeled projected). (Adapted with permission from Weinsier RL, Hunter GR, Desmond RA et al. Free-living activity energy expenditure in women successful and unsuccessful at maintaining a normal body weight. Am J Clin Nutr 2002;75:499–504.).

training have resting energy expenditures that are 5% to 20% higher than nonathletes (31). In addition, a single bout of cardiorespiratory exercise of at least 70% of $\dot{V}O_{2max}$ increases resting energy expenditure for up to 48 hours (31). Increases in sympathetic nervous system activity (48) and in protein turnover (31) are likely factors in contributing to this transient rise in resting energy expenditure.

Bodybuilders have resting energy expenditures that are 5% to 31% higher than would be expected for young men and women of similar age and body mass (31). In addition, strength training programs of 4 to 6 months in untrained individuals result in increases in fat-free mass of between 2 and 6 lb (17). This increase in fat-free mass is associated with an increase in resting energy expenditure of 5% to 10%. The increase in fat-free mass and hence in resting energy expenditure can occur with an investment in time of as little as 30 minutes twice a week (31).

IMPROVED FUNCTION IN PHYSICAL ACTIVITY

A decline in both cardiorespiratory fitness and strength fitness begins at approximately 30 years. The decline cannot be prevented by being physically active, as evidenced by progressive declines in performance of highly trained athletes (17). Several factors probably cause this decrease, including reductions in lung function, maximal heart rate and cardiac output, muscle size, muscle quality, and metabolic capacity of skeletal muscle and increases in fat mass (2, 17). One half or more of the decline in fitness probably is caused by decreases in quantity and intensity of physical activity (2). This situation creates a positive feedback loop that can lead to progressively lower physical activity levels and weight gain: (a) decreased physical activity leads to reduction in functional fitness and weight gain; (b) decreased functional fitness and the increased work required to move additional weight (from weight gain) during physical activity lead to increased difficulty in being active and a reduction in physical activity; and (c) further reductions in physical activity lead to further reductions in functional fitness.

EXERCISE TRAINING AND WEIGHT LOSS MAY BREAK THIS FEEDBACK LOOP

Although diet-induced weight loss is associated with increased ease during walking and climbing stairs (49), most individuals who lose weight also regain it. It is obvious that other interventions are also required.

Training-induced improvements in functional fitness decrease the rate of weight gain (38). Cardiorespiratory fitness is negatively related to weight gain over 1 year. In addition, women who maintain weight over 1 year are stronger (Fig. 112.3) and have better muscle metabolic economy (produce more force per unit of ATP) (Fig. 112.4) than women who gain weight. Muscle metabolic economy, $\dot{V}O_{2max}$, and quadriceps strength all are independently related to rate of weight gain; these findings suggest that

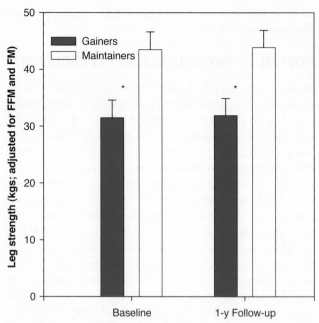

Fig. 112.3. Leg strength in premenopausal women who gained and maintained weight over 1 year. *FM*, fat mass; *FFM*, fat-free mass. (Adapted with permission from Weinsier RL, Hunter GR, Desmond RA et al. Free-living activity energy expenditure in women successful and unsuccessful at maintaining a normal body weight. Am J Clin Nutr 2002;75:499–504.)

training that increases $\dot{V}O_{2max}$, strength, and muscle metabolic economy can protect weight gain.

Quadriceps strength and ^{31}P MRS–measured muscle oxidative capacity (postexercise ADP recovery rate × volume of muscle/body weight) are independently related

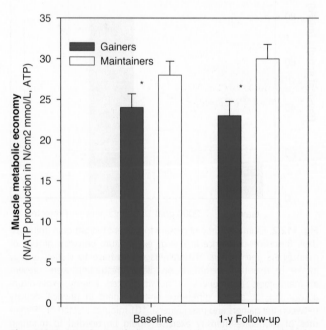

Fig. 112.4. Muscle metabolic economy (as measured by phosphorus-31 magnetic resonance spectroscopy) in women who gained and women who maintained weight over 1 year. *ATP*, adenosine triphosphate. (Unpublished data from our laboratory.)

to time to exhaustion on an endurance test (50). Both strength and aerobic capacity independently improve grade walking endurance. It is not unusual that oxidative capacity is related to an endurance task. Strength is independently related to endurance, however. One possible explanation for a relationship between physical strength and endurance performance is that less muscle activation is needed to perform a task when muscle is stronger (31), thus decreasing reliance on inefficient and fatigable fast-twitch muscle fibers and delaying fatigue.

Resistance training improves exercise economy, including running even in trained runners (17). Ease of performing daily tasks such as standing from a chair and carrying groceries is improved following 16 weeks of resistance training (17). This improvement can then assist in increasing physical activity and the likelihood of weight maintenance.

Existing data suggest that weight maintenance programs should include some combination of high- and low- to moderate-intensity physical activity. The low-intensity exercise, if preferred by the participant, may be done more frequently and will be the exercise in which most energy is expended. Much of the low-intensity exercise may not be formalized exercise training but may consist of efforts to increase daily free-living activity. Increasing use of stairs, walking or bicycling short to moderate distances rather than driving, and using a push lawn mower are examples of ways individuals may increase physical activity without large increases in time commitment. Some minimum amount of high-intensity exercise may be needed, however, to elevate energy expenditure, improve fitness, and thus decrease exercise difficulty. The combination of high- and low-intensity exercise that will be most productive is not known and probably varies depending on an individual's available time and tolerance for high-intensity exercise.

ACKNOWLEDGMENTS

In memory of Dr. Roland L. Weinsier, a good friend, colleague, and nutrition scientist.

REFERENCES

1. Blair SN, Yiling C, Holder JS. Med Sci Sports Exerc 2001;33(Suppl):S379–99.
2. McArdle WD, Katch FI, Katch VL. Exercise Physiology. Philadelphia: Lippincott Williams & Wilkins, 2001.
3. Rose MI, Himwich HE. Am J Physiol 1927;81:485–6.
4. Ford LE. Muscle Physiology and Cardiac Function. Traverse City, MI: Cooper Publishing Group, 2000.
5. Huxley AF. The Origin of Force in Skeletal Muscle: Energy Transfer in Biological Systems. New York: Ciba Foundation 1975:271–99.
6. Lifson N, Gordon GB, McClintock R. J Appl Physiol 1955;7:704–10.
7. Schoeller DA, van Santen E. J Appl Physiol 1982;53:955–9.
8. Pette D, Staron RS. Rev Physiol Biochem Pharmacol 1990;116:1–76.
9. Bergstrom J. Scand J Clin Lab Invest 1962;68:1–110.
10. Chance B, Eleff S, Leigh GS. Proc Natl Acad Sci U S A 1980;77:7430–4.
11. Howley ET. Med Sci Sports Exerc 2001;33(Suppl):S364–9.
12. Houston ME. Biochemistry Primer for Exercise Science. Champaign: Human Kinetics, 1995.
13. Larson DE, Newcomer BR, Hunter GR Am J Physiol 2004;282:E95–106.
14. Muoio DM, Leddy JJ, Horvath PJ et al. Med Sci Sports Exerc 1994;26:81–8.
15. Hargreaves M. Exerc Sport Sci Rev 1997;25:21–39.
16. Bassett DR Jr. Med Sci Sports Exerc 1994;26:957–66.
17. Hunter GR, McCarthy JP, Bamman MM. Sports Med 2004;34:329–48.
18. Wisloff U, Najjar SM, Ellingsen O et al. Science 2005;307: 418–20.
19. Brock DW, Irving BA, Gower BA et al. Int J Obes 2010; 18:982–86.
20. Roy JLP, Hunter GR, Fernandez JR et al. Am J Hum Biol 2006;18:454–60.
21. Lexell J. J Gerontol A Biol Sci Med Sci 1995;50(Spec No):11–6.
22. Lynch NA, Metter EJ, Lindle RS et al. J Appl Physiol 1999;86:188–94.
23. Lowe DA, Baltgalvis KA, Greising SM. Exerc Sport Sci Rev 2010;38:61–7.
24. Hunter GR, Lara-Castro C, Byrne NM et al. Int J Body Comp Res 2005;3:55–61.
25. Kekes-Szabo T, Hunter GR, Nyikos I et al. Obes Res 1994;2:450–457.
26. Lee IM, Paffenbarger RS Jr. Exerc Sport Sci Rev 1996;24: 135–71.
27. Michaud DS, Giovannucci E, Willett WC et al. JAMA 2001;286:921–9.
28. Shephard RJ. Med Sci Sports Exerc 2001;33:S400–18.
29. Despres JP, Lemarche B. Physical activity and the metabolic complications of obesity. In: Claude Bouchard, ed. Physical Activity and Obesity. Champaign, IL: Human Kinetics 2000:331–54.
30. DiPietro L. Exerc Sport Sci Rev 1995;23:275–303.
31. Hunter GR, Weinsier RL, Bamman MM et al. Int J Obes 1998;22:489–93.
32. Williams PT. Med Sci Sports Exerc 2001;33(Suppl): S611–21.
33. Thompson PD, Crouse SF, Goodpaster B et al. Medi Sci Sports Exerc 2001;33(Suppl):S438–45.
34. Hunter GR, Kekes-Szabo T, Snyder S et al. Med Sci Sports Exerc 1997;29:362–9.
35. Hunter GR, Kekes-Szabo T, Treuth MS et al. Int J Obes 1996;20:860–5.
36. Westerterp KR. Curr Opin Clin Nutr Metab Care 2000;3:485–8.
37. Weinsier RL, Hunter GR, Desmond RA et al. Am J Clin Nutr 2002;75:499–504.
38. Hunter GR, Brock DW, Byrne NM et al. Obesity 2010; 18:690–5.
39. Hunter GR, Chandler-Laney PJ, Brock DW et al. Obesity 2009;18:274–81.
40. Hunter GR, Bryan DR, Wetzstein CJ et al. Med Sci Sports Exerc 2002;34:1023–8.
41. Treuth MS, Hunter GR, Kekes-Szabo T et al. J Appl Physiol 1995;78:1425–31.
42. Kohrt WM, Obert KA, Holloszy JO. J Gerontol 1992;47: M99–105.
43. Oppert JM, Nadeau ATA, Despres JP et al. Am J Physiol 1997;272:E248–54.

44. Schoeller DA, Shay K, Kushner RF. Am J Clin Nutr 1997;66:551–6.

45. Saris WHM, Blair SN, van Baak MA et al. Obes Rev 2003;4:101–14.

46. Kraus WE, Houmard JA, Duscha BD et al. N Engl J Med 2002;347:1483–92.

47. Hunter GR, Newcomer BR, Larson-Meyer DE et al. Muscle Nerve 2001;24:654–61.

48. Poehlman ET, Danforth E. Am J Physiol 1991;261:E233–9.

49. Hunter GR, Weinsier RL, Zuckerman PA et al. Int J Obes 2004;28:1111–7.

50. Larew K, Hunter GR, Larson-Meyer EE et al. Med Sci Sports Exerc 2003;35:230–6.

SUGGESTED READINGS

Howley ET, Franks BD. Fitness Professionals Handbook. 5th ed. Champaign, IL: Human Kinetics, 2007.

Baechle TR, Earle RW, eds. Essentials of Strength and Conditioning. 3rd ed. Champaign, IL: Human Kinetics, 2008.

McArdle WD, Katch FI, Katch VL. Exercise Physiology. 6th ed. Philadelphia: Lippincott Williams & Wilkins, 2007.

113 SPORTS NUTRITION[1]

MELVIN H. WILLIAMS

Sport, an international phenomenon, is characterized by the pursuit of excellence; and for any given athlete, excellence in sports performance is dependent on the combination of nature (genetics) and nurture (environment). Genetic endowment with physical and mental attributes important to a specific sport is vital to sports success, but so too are common environmental effects such as appropriate training programs and sports nutrition (1).

Sports nutrition has evolved considerably over the course of 50 years and now is considered by many sports nutritionists to have several main objectives:

- To promote good health
- To promote adaptations to training
- To recover quickly after each training session
- To perform optimally during competition

These objectives include some applications to help optimize performance in specific sports, such as attaining an appropriate body mass and composition, providing appropriate amounts of energy substrate, preventing a nutrient deficiency that may impair performance, and preventing the premature onset of fatigue.

In general, the diet that is optimal for health is also optimal for performance for most athletes. However, in their joint position stand on *Nutrition and Athletic Performance,* the American Dietetic Association (ADA), Dietitians of Canada (DC), and American College of Sports Medicine (ACSM) (2) indicated that some athletes may benefit from increased intake of specific macronutrients, particularly carbohydrate and protein, whereas some may need specific micronutrients, including vitamins and minerals; others may benefit from specific sports supplements.

This chapter highlights some of the key findings of sports nutrition research with a focus on performance enhancement. The selected readings and references cited at the end of the chapter provide greater detail. The evidence-based ADA/DC/ACSM position stand (2) provides

---

[1]**Abbreviations: 2,3-DPG,** 2,3-diphosphoglycerate; **ACSM,** American College of Sports Medicine; **ADA,** American Dietetic Association; **AMDR,** Acceptable Macronutrient Distribution Range; **ATP,** adenosine triphosphate; **BCAA,** branched-chain amino acids; **CES,** carbohydrate-electrolyte solutions; **CLA,** conjugated linoleic acid; **DC,** Dietitians of Canada; **DHA,** docosahexaenoic acid; **EPA,** eicosapentaenoic acid; **FFA,** free fatty acid; **hGH,** human growth hormone; **HMB,** β-hydroxy-β-methylbutyrate; **IMTG,** intramuscular triglyceride; **ISSN,** International Society of Sports Nutrition; **MCT,** medium-chain triglyceride; **PCr,** phosphocreatine; **RDA,** recommended dietary allowance; **$\dot{V}O_{2max}$,** maximal oxygen uptake; **WADA,** World Anti-Doping Agency.

detailed recommendations for athletes 18 to 40 years of age, whereas other reviews provide recommendations for younger (3) and older (4) athletes. The previous version of this chapter (5) provides details of supplements not covered here. Additionally, for detailed information related to a specific macronutrient or micronutrient discussed in this chapter, please refer to the respective chapter in this text.

ENERGY AND SPORTS PERFORMANCE

The nutrients in the food we eat have three basic functions—to provide energy, regulate metabolism, and promote growth and development. Although all three functions are important to athletes, energy production and energy balance are the essential factors.

Energy production in the muscles provides movement for all sport activities. In brief, muscles contain various forms of energy stores whose contribution to muscle energy production is dependent primarily on the intensity of exercise; the following hierarchy presents muscle energy sources from highest to lowest exercise intensity:

- Adenosine triphosphate (ATP): Immediate source of energy for high-intensity exercise
- Phosphocreatine (PCr): Replaces ATP very rapidly during high-intensity anaerobic exercise
- Glycogen: Replaces ATP rapidly during high-intensity anaerobic exercise and moderately rapidly during endurance aerobic exercise
- Fatty acids: Replace ATP less rapidly during aerobic endurance exercise

Dietary carbohydrate and dietary fat provide glucose and fatty acids that, respectively, also may enter into muscle energy pathways and help to replenish muscle glycogen and fatty acid energy stores. Dietary protein provides amino acids that may be used as a source of muscle energy, although amino acids are not very important energy sources during exercise. Other dietary nutrients, such as creatine, also may help increase specific muscle energy stores. Energy balance is the key to weight control, and body mass and composition are important considerations for most athletes. Increasing body mass, primarily muscle mass, may enhance performance in a wide variety of sports, such as weightlifting competition, in which strength and power are main determinants of success. Decreasing body mass, primarily fat mass, also may enhance performance in sports, such as distance running, in which economy of motion is important. Discussion of body weight control is beyond the scope of this chapter, but methods used to determine energy requirements, increases muscle mass, and lose excess body fat for enhanced sport performance have been provided in ACSM position stands (2, 6, 7). All ACSM position stands discussed in this chapter may be accessed at http://www.acsm-msse.org.

DIETARY CARBOHYDRATE AND SPORTS PERFORMANCE

Carbohydrate use rises progressively with increases in exercise intensity and is the most important energy source for high-intensity anaerobic and moderately high- to high-intensity aerobic exercise. Fatigue during anaerobic exercise is associated with adverse effects of muscle cell acidity caused by increased lactic acid production during anaerobic glycolysis, whereas fatigue during prolonged aerobic exercise may be associated with low blood glucose (hypoglycemia), which may impair central nervous system functions, inducing muscular weakness and fatigue. Additionally, low muscle glycogen levels may reduce energy production from both anaerobic and aerobic glycolysis. Thus, adequate carbohydrate intake is an important nutritional concern for both aerobic endurance and high-intensity, intermittent sport athletes if it can help maintain optimal blood glucose and muscle glycogen levels (8, 9).

Carbohydrates in the Daily Diet

The slogan "train high and compete high" refers to the concept of training and competing with high carbohydrate intake. A high daily intake of carbohydrate during training helps sustain high levels of training intensity. The ACSM, ADA, and DC (2) note that during times of high physical activity, energy and macronutrient needs, especially carbohydrate, must be met. The carbohydrate recommendation for athletes ranges from 6 to 10 g/kg body weight daily, the amount depending on the athlete's total daily energy expenditure, type of sport, gender, and environmental conditions. For example, the amount of carbohydrate needed by an athlete exercising to lose weight is quite different than that by one in training to run a marathon. The recommended carbohydrate intake for athletes meets or exceeds the upper level of the acceptable macronutrient distribution range (AMDR) of 45% to 65% of daily energy intake.

In general, athletes should consume *healthy* carbohydrates, mainly whole grains and rice, legumes, fruits, and vegetables within an overall balanced diet. An excellent model is the OmniHeart (Optimal MacroNutrient Intake) diet based on consumption of healthy carbohydrates, healthy fats, and healthy protein. However, given total daily energy expenditure and increased dietary carbohydrate recommendations for many athletes, such diets may be complemented with some high–glycemic index foods to replenish muscle glycogen.

Carbohydrates before and during Exercise

Consuming carbohydrates before and/or during training or competition may or may not help enhance performance. If blood glucose and muscle glycogen levels are optimal, carbohydrate intake does not enhance exercise performance in activities lasting less than approximately 45 minutes. However, if blood glucose or muscle glycogen levels are low, or exercise performance is greater than approximately 45 minutes, then carbohydrate intake may improve performance. During training, athletes should experiment with various types and concentrations of carbohydrates, both before and during exercise, that may be used in competition. Ingesting excessive amounts of various forms of carbohydrates may lead to gastrointestinal distress (10).

If consumed approximately 4 hours before exercise, carbohydrate intake may approximate 4 to 5 g/kg body weight. Such preexercise meals should contain balanced macronutrient content, but the focus should be on carbohydrates because they are more readily digested and may help bolster muscle glycogen stores. Approximately 1 to 2 g/kg may be appropriate about an hour before exercise (10). Simple carbohydrates may be recommended, particularly sports drinks because preexercise hydration also be an important consideration.

Numerous studies support the efficacy of carbohydrate supplementation during prolonged aerobic exercise tasks to improve performance (10). For example, marathoners ingesting carbohydrate compared to placebo beverages were able to run at a higher intensity during a competitive marathon, and yet the psychological ratings of perceived exertion were similar in both groups of runners, suggesting that carbohydrates may have permitted them to run at a faster rate with similar psychological effort (11). Research also supports a beneficial role of carbohydrates for prolonged, intermittent high-intensity exercise tasks, such as multiple sprints in soccer (12).

A review (13) provides guidelines for carbohydrate intake during exercise tasks of varying duration.

- Maximal exercise for less than 45 minutes: None required
- Maximal exercise for approximately 45 to 60 minutes: Less than 30 g
- Team sports for approximately 90 minutes: 50 g/hour
- Submaximal exercise for more than 2 hours: Up to 60 g/hour
- Near maximal and maximal exercise for more than 2 hours: 50 to 70 g/hour
- Ultraendurance events: 60 to 90 g/hour

Glucose, sucrose, glucose polymers, and solid carbohydrates appear to be equally effective as a means of enhancing performance, but fructose may be more likely to cause gastrointestinal distress if used alone. Combinations of carbohydrates such as glucose, fructose, sucrose, and maltodextrins consumed during exercise appear to optimize the amount of exogenous carbohydrate that can be oxidized (10). Sports drinks contain carbohydrates and are discussed briefly in the section on fluids and electrolytes.

Carbohydrate loading involves a very-high-carbohydrate diet and exercise-tapering regimen several days before prolonged aerobic endurance competition and is designed to elevate endogenous muscle glycogen stores and postpone fatigue. Some sports nutritionists recommend consumption of approximately 10 to 12 g/kg body weight daily for 2 to 3 days before prolonged endurance events. Research findings are equivocal relative to its effectiveness. Although carbohydrate loading may be an effective technique to enhance performance in prolonged aerobic endurance sports, research suggests that the most effective protocol is to carbohydrate load and consume carbohydrates during the event (10).

Carbohydrates after Exercise to Promote Recovery

Athletes may train intensely on a day-to-day basis, or may even train several times daily, and may need to replenish muscle glycogen to sustain such high training loads. Reviews of dietary strategies to promote glycogen synthesis after exercise indicated that supplementing at 30-minute intervals at a rate of 1.2 to 1.5 g of carbohydrate/kg body weight/hour appears to maximize synthesis for a period of 4 to 5 hours after exercise (10). Carbohydrates with a high glycemic index may facilitate muscle glycogen replenishment when consumed immediately after exercise and every 2 hours thereafter.

Carbohydrate Metabolites and Exercise Performance

Several metabolites of carbohydrate have been theorized to possess ergogenic potential. Pyruvate, a three-carbon metabolite of glycolysis, is theorized to accelerate the Krebs cycle or use glucose more efficiently. However, limited research suggests that pyruvate supplementation is not ergogenic (5, 14). Ribose is a five-carbon monosaccharide that comprises the sugar portion of ATP. Supplementation is theorized to increase ATP resynthesis and promote faster recovery and exercise performance. However, reviews and studies (10, 15, 16) indicate that ribose supplementation has no effect on a wide variety of exercise and sport performance tasks.

DIETARY FAT AND SPORTS PERFORMANCE

Fat may be an important energy source during exercise. Although endogenous fat stores cannot produce energy anaerobically, free fatty acids (FFAs) can contribute significantly to muscular energy production via aerobic lipolysis during endurance exercise. FFA oxidation may be derived from intramuscular triglycerides (IMTGs) or delivered to muscles via blood FFAs derived from adipose cell triglycerides or the liver. Endurance exercise training, by enacting multiple mechanisms, enhances the use of fat for energy during aerobic exercise. Endurance athletes are better fat burners.

However, several reviews (17, 18) noted that despite considerable progress, our understanding of how lipid oxidation is controlled during exercise remains unclear. Research indicates that the rate of lipid oxidation reaches a peak at 50% to 60% of maximal oxygen uptake ($\dot{V}O_{2max}$), after which the contribution of lipids decreases both in relative and absolute terms. With exercise greater than 60% $\dot{V}O_{2max}$, metabolic byproducts of increased carbohydrate oxidation, among other factors, may impair lipid oxidation. Theoretically, it may be advantageous for endurance athletes to optimize the use of fat as an energy source to spare enough liver and muscle glycogen for the later stages of an aerobic endurance contest.

Fats in the Daily Diet

The ADA/DC/ACSM (2) position stand notes that fat, a source of energy, essential fatty acids, and fat-soluble vitamins, is important in the diets of athletes and recommends that athletes should obtain approximately 20% to 35% of total energy intake from fat, which is the AMDR. The position stand also notes that consuming less than 20% of energy from fat does not benefit performance. As with *healthy* carbohydrates, diets for athletes should focus on *healthy* fats, which are promoted in the OmniHeart diet. In general, the goal is to replace saturated fats, sugars, and refined starches with monounsaturated and polyunsaturated fats, such as olive oil, canola oil, and unsalted nuts such as almonds and pecans.

Increased Dietary Fat and Exercise Performance

Several sports nutritionists have challenged the dogma that endurance athletes need high-carbohydrate diets and suggest that endurance performance may benefit from high-fat diets, even one that comprises more than 50% of the daily energy intake as fat (19). Proponents of the high-fat diet suggest that athletes can adapt to high-fat, low-carbohydrate diets and maintain physical endurance capacity; high-fat diets can increase the muscle concentration of triglycerides; and high-fat diets increase use of fat as a fuel during exercise and decrease the use of carbohydrate, leading to enhanced endurance in prolonged aerobic exercise (19). The term "fat loading" has been used to describe both acute (1 to 2 days) and chronic (1 to 2 weeks) dietary techniques theorized to increase IMTG content and fat oxidation during exercise (10). Fat loading has been shown to increase IMTG content and increase fat oxidation during exercise (20), but as noted (5), its ability to enhance exercise performance has not been well documented. Fat-loading practices, either acute or chronic, may increase use of fat during endurance exercise, but do not appear to enhance exercise or sport performance. One study indicated that high-fat diets actually may impair some types of performance, such as sprint cycling stages during a 100-km cycling time trial (21). The ADA/DC/ACSM position stand does not recommend high-fat diets for athletes (2).

Fat Metabolites and Regulators and Exercise Performance

Several different types of fats, fatty acids, and regulators of fat metabolism have been theorized to enhance exercise performance. Omega-3 fatty acids, primarily eicosapentaenoic acid (EPA) and docosahexaenoic acid (DHA), have been theorized to enhance exercise performance in a variety of ways. As noted (5), omega-3 fatty acid supplementation does not promote muscle anabolism during resistance exercise, and more recent research with α-linolenic fatty acid, another omega-3, also reports minimal effect on muscle mass and strength during resistance training (22). Studies report that EPA and DHA supplementation could increase stroke volume and cardiac output (23) and reduce heart rate and oxygen consumption (24) during submaximal exercise. However, other exercise studies reported no effect of fish oil (EPA and DHA) supplementation on peak oxygen uptake or peak exercise workload (24), glucose or lipid energy metabolism (25), or 10-km time-trial performance in trained cyclists (26). Overall, current research suggests that omega-3 fatty acid supplementation does not enhance sports performance.

Medium-chain triglycerides (MCTs) have been theorized to be ergogenic because of their more rapid absorption into the portal circulation, facilitated entrance into muscle cell mitochondria, and an oxidation rate comparable with exogenous carbohydrate. MCT supplementation, either alone or combined with carbohydrate, has been investigated as a means to enhance endurance exercise performance. However, as noted here (5) and in a subsequent review (10), research indicates that MCT supplementation does not improve, and may impair, endurance exercise performance. Additionally, consuming an MCT-carbohydrate solution provides no additional benefits compared with a carbohydrate solution alone.

Conjugated linoleic acid (CLA) is a collective term for a group of isomers of linoleic acid, one of which is theorized to reduce lipid uptake by adipocytes. CLA supplementation is purported to have several health benefits but has been studied primarily for its potential to decrease body fat. Losing excess fat may be beneficial to some athletes. However, although studies with mice have shown significant effects on body fat reduction, research findings with humans have not been as strong. In two metaanalyses of 18 studies (27, 28), CLA supplementation was shown to produce a very modest loss of body fat, approximately 0.05 kg/week, and a small total increase (<1%) in lean body mass. Studies involving physically active subjects are limited. In one well-designed study, CLA supplementation resulted in minimal changes in body composition and no changes in strength tests in men and women involved in resistance training (29). Investigators indicate that the antiobesity mechanisms of action of CLA are unclear, and its use in humans is controversial (30). Additional research is merited, particularly with athletic subjects.

Phospholipids represent a class of lipids found in most cell membranes that contain a diglyceride (glycerol and two fatty acids), a phosphate group, and another molecule such as choline. Several phospholipid supplements—lecithin and phosphatidylcholine—have been studied for their ergogenic potential. Several older studies suggested that lecithin supplementation could increase strength and power, but the experimental design used was improper. Subsequent well-controlled research reported no ergogenic effects of lecithin supplementation (31). More recently, phosphatidylserine supplementation has been theorized to enhance exercise performance by various means, including direct effects on cell membrane transport and hormonal responses to exercise (32). Current research has emanated from one research laboratory, and several studies suggested that phosphatidylserine supplementation could increase running and cycling time to exhaustion (10). These findings are interesting, but research with phosphatidylserine supplementation and exercise performance is in its preliminary stages and additional research is merited.

Carnitine is synthesized from amino acids in the body. Two forms are produced, with L-carnitine being the most physiologically active. L-Carnitine is present in the muscles to help move fatty acids into the mitochondria for oxidation. Theoretically, increased L-carnitine levels would facilitate fatty acid oxidation and enhance endurance exercise performance. Major reviews relative to the effect of oral L-carnitine supplementation, as well as other forms of carnitine, have been published. The following are some of the key points of these reviews (10, 33).

- Supplementation increases plasma levels of carnitine but does not appear to increase muscle levels.
- Supplementation does not appear to increase fat oxidation during exercise.
- Neither acute nor chronic (6-day) oral supplementation enhances aerobic endurance exercise performance.
- Supplementation does not induce weight loss in obese individuals and is unlikely to do so in fit athletes.

Nevertheless, one review (33) suggested that elevated muscle carnitine may have some effects beneficial to exercise performance. The problem is finding a practical means by which the typical athlete may increase muscle carnitine content.

In general, various dietary strategies and supplements theorized to increase oxidation of fat during exercise and enhance prolonged aerobic endurance performance have not been shown to be effective (10).

DIETARY PROTEIN AND SPORTS PERFORMANCE

Protein always has been considered to be one of the main staples of an athlete's diet. Protein is required for a number of metabolic functions important to exercise performance, including promotion of growth and repair of muscle and other tissues and synthesis of hormones and neurotransmitters (10, 34). Both resistance and endurance training exercise induce protein catabolism during exercise, but protein synthesis predominates in the postexercise recovery period and the type of protein synthesized is specific to the type of exercise (10, 35). Such findings have stimulated research to evaluate the effect of protein supplementation on exercise performance.

Protein in the Daily Diet

The recommended dietary allowance (RDA) for protein is based on the body weight of the individual and the amount needed per unit body weight is greater during childhood and adolescence than during adulthood. The adult RDA for protein is 0.8 g/kg body weight. The AMDR for protein is 10% to 35% of daily energy intake.

Whether athletes require more than the RDA for protein is debated. The National Academy of Sciences (36), in establishing the RDA for protein, concluded that in view of the lack of compelling evidence to the contrary, no additional dietary protein is suggested for healthy adults undertaking resistance or endurance exercise. Furthermore, some scientists contend that physically active people probably could manage perfectly adequately on less protein (37). However, the ADA/DC/ACSM position stand (2) notes that recommending protein intakes in excess of the RDA to maintain optimum physical performance is commonly done in practice and cites recommendations of 1.2 to 1.4 g/kg daily for endurance athletes and 1.2 to 1.7 g/kg daily for strength athletes. In another position stand, the International Society of Sports Nutrition (ISSN) recommended that a protein intake of 1.4 to 2.0 g/kg may improve body adaptations to exercise training (38). Some researchers recommend that older individuals, including athletes, may help prevent the sarcopenia of aging by consuming approximately 25 to 30 g of high-quality protein at each meal (39), which over the course of the day will exceed the protein RDA.

Although these viewpoints are divergent, the available scientific data suggest it may be prudent for athletes, particularly those in weight-control sports who may be at risk for protein insufficiency, to consume more protein than the RDA as recommended by the ADA/DC/ACSM and ISSN. Moreover, meeting these recommendations may be achieved by consuming natural food sources. For example, 10% of energy intake from protein provides 75 g of protein, or 1.0 g/kg, to a 75-kg athlete consuming 3000 kcal/day. Increasing the percentage of protein intake to 15% or 20% provides 1.5 and 2.0 g/kg, respectively, meeting the amounts recommended by the ADA/DC/ACSM (2) and ISSN (38) and staying well within the AMDR recommendation of 10% to 35% of daily energy derived from protein.

As with *healthy* carbohydrates and *healthy* fats, diets for athletes should be composed of *healthy* protein foods. The OmniHeart diet may contain 15% to 25% of energy from protein. Animal sources provide high-quality protein but should be reduced in fat content, such as lean meat, fish, and poultry; fat-free and low-fat milk and dairy products; whole and high-protein grains (e.g., bulgur wheat, millet); and legumes, nuts, and seeds. Combining animal and plant proteins in one meal, such as milk and cereal or stir-fry vegetables and meat, increases the protein quality of the meal.

Protein Supplementation and Postexercise Recovery

Increased protein before, during, and after exercise has been studied as a means to facilitate recovery from exercise, promote muscle synthesis, and enhance both strength and endurance exercise performance. In most studies, protein supplements, such as whey protein, colostrum, or protein hydrolysate (a high-protein dietary supplement containing a solution of amino acids and peptides prepared from protein by hydrolysis), were added to the diet. In general, protein supplements contained all the essential amino acids. Reviews by several experts have indicated that the difference in anabolic response between preexercise and postexercise ingestion of protein is not apparent, and it is uncertain whether ingesting amino acids immediately before exercise further enhances the muscle protein buildup associated with protein intake during recovery (10). In general, research has shown that consuming protein supplements with all essential amino acids during the first few hours of recovery from heavy resistance exercise produces a transient, net positive increase in muscle protein balance (10).

Many studies also combined protein with carbohydrate, and the general recommendation is a carbohydrate-to-protein ratio of approximately 3 to 4 g of carbohydrate for each gram of protein, preferably in a highly digestible liquid form. Research from one prominent group (40) reported that ingestion of a protein/carbohydrate supplement increased markers of protein synthesis during recovery from aerobic exercise. However, one expert indicated that if adequate protein is available, there is no need for carbohydrates to promote muscle protein synthesis and also noted that because resistance exercise uses muscle glycogen, the carbohydrate could help replenish muscle glycogen (41).

In general, although consumption of adequate protein or protein/carbohydrate preparations during exercise training may provide a milieu conducive to muscle protein anabolism, some have contended that research is insufficient to support an ergogenic effect of such preparations on resistance or aerobic endurance exercise performance beyond that associated with training alone (5, 42). However, some research findings, particularly with whey and colostrum protein supplements, have revealed mixed but generally positive effects relative to the ergogenic potential for whey supplementation to resistance-trained individuals. Small gains in strength and lean body mass have been reported, but additional research is merited (10).

Protein Supplementation and Aerobic Endurance Exercise

Protein supplementation in aerobic endurance athletes has been studied for its effects on recovery when provided after exercise and for its effect on performance when provided during exercise, usually in combination with carbohydrate. As for recovery, one review concluded that consumption of protein/carbohydrate solutions has been associated with reduced markers of muscle damage and less muscle soreness (43). However, other reviewers contend that advantages of added protein with carbohydrate in reducing true muscle damage from endurance exercise remains to be verified (44).

As for aerobic endurance performance enhancement, some early studies reported improved aerobic endurance performance with protein/carbohydrate solutions, but one reviewer (43) cited limitations to these studies, the main factor was that in the studies showing improved performance, the protein supplied in the beverage was in addition to the carbohydrate, thus providing more energy. In one review, an expert (45) indicated that no established mechanism exists by which protein intake during exercise should improve acute endurance performance, and a review of well-controlled studies supports this viewpoint (10). Moreover, replacing carbohydrate with protein during prolonged aerobic endurance exercise actually may impair performance by approximately 1%, as documented in one study (46). High-protein and moderate-carbohydrate diets, with equal energy content, consumed over the course of a week may impair cycling endurance performance by almost 20% when compared with a high-carbohydrate diet (47).

For endurance athletes, carbohydrates are their main energy source. Adding protein to a feeding strategy that provides adequate carbohydrates during or after exercise does not enhance performance or glycogen resynthesis during recovery (10, 40, 45).

Protein Metabolites, Amino Acids, and Exercise Performance

Individual amino acids, or combinations of several, as well as various protein metabolites, may induce metabolic responses that may enhance exercise performance. Details are provided elsewhere (10, 48), but the following represents a brief summary of the research findings.

Arginine supplementation may induce a number of metabolic processes theorized to be ergogenic, such as increased blood flow and decreased accumulation of lactic acid (49–51). However, current research does not support a beneficial effect on blood flow during resistance exercise, performance in intermittent anaerobic exercise by well-trained male athletes, or performance in a maximal cycling time trial (52–54). Arginine, combined with other amino acids (ornithine, lysine, citrulline, aspartate), also has been studied to promote vasodilation or increase human growth hormone (hGH) production. However, a review of related studies revealed no ergogenic effect of such supplementation (10).

β-Alanine is a naturally occurring amino acid, but unlike the normal form of alanine, it is not used in protein formation. However, it may be used in the muscle to increase the amount of carnosine, a peptide that may help buffer lactic acid and enhance anaerobic exercise capacity (10). A study reported no ergogenic effect of β-alanine supplementation, but the exercise task does not appear to be dependent on anaerobic glycolysis and lactic acid production (55). On the other hand, a review concluded that chronic oral ingestion of β-alanine can substantially elevate the carnosine content of human skeletal muscle, may act as a buffer, and may lead to improved performance in high-intensity exercise in both untrained and trained individuals and also noted that additional research is needed to document any potential side effects (56).

Potassium and magnesium aspartates are salts of aspartic acid, an amino acid. They have been used as ergogenics, possibly by mitigating the accumulation of ammonia during exercise. A review noted that the effect of aspartate supplementation on endurance generally seems favorable in humans, but the underlying mechanism for performance enhancement has not been confirmed (57).

L-Tryptophan is a precursor for serotonin, a brain neurotransmitter theorized to suppress pain. Free tryptophan enters the brain cells to form serotonin. Thus, tryptophan supplementation has been used to increase serotonin production in attempts to increase tolerance to pain during intense exercise. However, well-controlled research indicates that L-tryptophan supplementation does not enhance high-intensity running or cycling performance or aerobic endurance performance at 70% to 75% of VO_{2max} (10).

Branched-chain amino acids (BCAAs; leucine, isoleucine, valine) are important components of muscle tissue, and BCAA supplementation has been studied as a means to promote recovery or enhance exercise performance. As noted in a review, BCAA supplementation before or after exercise, comparable with protein supplementation, may have beneficial effects for decreasing exercise-induced muscle damage, promoting muscle–protein synthesis, and improving immune functions (58). However, little evidence supports a performance-enhancement effect of BCAA supplementation (10, 58). Leucine supplementation alone has been studied, but when added to a complete protein supplement had no additional anabolic effect (59).

Glutamine has been theorized as an anabolic, either by increasing hGH levels or increasing muscle cell volume and stimulating protein synthesis, promoting increased strength. Glutamine is also an important fuel for some cells of the immune system and supplementation has been

recommended as a means for enhanced immune function for quicker recovery, decreased frequency of respiratory tract infections, and prevention of overtraining. However, two reviews indicated that such claims are not supported by well-controlled scientific studies in healthy, well-nourished humans (60, 61).

β-Hydroxy-β-methylbutyrate (HMB) is a byproduct of leucine metabolism in the human body and is currently marketed as calcium-HMB-monohydrate. Although the ergogenic mechanism is unknown, investigators speculate that HMB may be incorporated into cell components or may influence cellular enzyme activity, in some way inhibiting the breakdown of muscle tissue during strenuous exercise and facilitating the response to training (62). Studies with HMB supplementation have focused primarily on strength and lean body mass responses to resistance training. Over the course of almost 20 years, research findings have been equivocal regarding the ergogenic potential of HMB supplementation, with one major point being different responses in trained versus untrained individuals. An earlier review concluded that HMB use in athletes involved in regular high-intensity exercise has not been proven to be beneficial when multiple variables are evaluated (63). A more recent metaanalysis (64) of nine qualifying studies revealed that the overall average strength increase was trivial, although uncertainty allows for a small benefit. Effects on fat and fat-free mass were trivial. Results also reveal that supplementation with HMB during resistance training incurs small but clear overall and leg strength gains in previously untrained men, but effects in trained lifters are trivial. The HMB effect on body composition is inconsequential. The authors conclude that an explanation for strength gains in previously untrained lifters requires further research.

Overall, although several interesting hypotheses have been proposed, individual amino acid supplements and related protein metabolites currently are not considered to be effective as a means of improving exercise performance. However, several, such as β-alanine and aspartates, merit additional research.

VITAMINS AND MINERALS AND SPORTS PERFORMANCE

Vitamins and minerals are classified as micronutrients because their requirement is measured in milligrams or micrograms, and RDA have been established for approximately 25 essential micronutrients. Numerous vitamins and minerals are needed for a wide variety of physiologic processes underlying exercise and sports performance, including muscle contraction, oxygen transport, coenzyme functions necessary for energy production from the macronutrients, formation of neurotransmitters and hormones, prevention of oxidative damage associated with exercise, immune functions, and growth and development of bone tissue. Sports nutritionists indicate that exercise may stress many of the metabolic pathways requiring vitamins and minerals, and also note that exercise training may increase micronutrient requirements (2, 65).

A healthy, balanced diet containing a wide variety of foods (e.g., the OmniHeart diet) and providing adequate energy, carbohydrate, fat, and protein should meet the vitamin and mineral needs of most athletes; athletes should concentrate on foods with a high density of micronutrients (10). However, some athletes, particularly those involved in weight-control sports, may consume diets restricted in specific micronutrients or energy intake and thus may suffer from micronutrient deficiencies that could impair exercise performance. In such cases, vitamin/mineral supplementation may be beneficial.

Moreover, because specific vitamins and minerals play important metabolic roles during exercise, supplementation has been theorized to enhance performance. Researchers disagree as to whether or not athletes need more micronutrients, but one authority indicates that the intensity, duration, and frequency of the sport or exercise training and the overall energy and nutrient intakes of the individual all have an impact on whether or not micronutrients are required in greater amounts (65). Nearly every essential vitamin, eight essential minerals, and even several nonessential minerals have been studied for their ergogenic potential.

Vitamins and Sports Performance

Most exercise nutrition research has focused on the B vitamins, multivitamins or multivitamin/mineral supplements, and antioxidant supplements, particularly vitamins C, E, and β-carotene. Some research with vitamin D may have application to older athletes.

A vitamin B deficiency may impair physical performance, usually by interfering with some phase of the energy-producing process. In some cases, impairment may be seen in 2 to 4 weeks on a deficient diet (10, 66). Older athletes, those more than 50 years old, may experience decreased absorption of dietary vitamin B_{12}, which is essential for red blood cell production, and may benefit by consuming it from fortified foods or supplements (10). However, although a B vitamin deficiency may impair exercise performance, athletes who obtain adequate energy intake, particularly from high-quality carbohydrate and protein foods, should not experience such deficiency (66).

Multivitamin supplements, including B vitamin combinations and multivitamin/mineral preparations, have been studied for their effects on exercise performance. The overall review of the literature supports the viewpoint that multivitamin/mineral supplements are unnecessary for athletes or other physically active individuals who are on a well-balanced diet with adequate energy intake. Several well-controlled studies have provided multivitamin/mineral supplements over prolonged peri-

ods (up to 8 months) and reported no significant effects on both laboratory and sport-specific tests of physical performance (67, 68).

Antioxidant vitamins (e.g., β-carotene, vitamin C, vitamin E) have been studied individually or collectively (often with selenium) in attempts to enhance exercise performance by various means, mitigate adverse effects of strenuous exercise on immune system functions, or reduce indices of muscle tissue damage after exercise. An earlier review of antioxidant supplementation studies with either individual or combined antioxidant vitamins found little evidence of enhanced exercise performance (69). Studies confirm these findings and report no effect of 6 months of vitamin E supplementation on indices of physical performance and body composition in older sedentary adults undergoing aerobic training (70) and no effect of 3 months of vitamin C and E supplementation on strength, speed, or aerobic capacity in professional soccer players (71). One possible exception involves vitamin E supplementation and aerobic endurance exercise enhancement at high altitudes, a finding that needs confirmation with additional research (5). Antioxidants, particularly vitamin C, also have been claimed to strengthen the immune system and prevent upper respiratory tract infections in physically active individuals. However, studies indicate that vitamin C supplementation or combined antioxidant vitamin supplementation are not effective countermeasures to exercise-induced immunosuppression (72, 73). Antioxidant supplements also have been studied as a means to prevent muscle tissue damage during strenuous exercise. As noted (5), expert reviewers were divided on the therapeutic effects of antioxidant supplements, and some concluding studies have not provided clear evidence for their prophylactic effect on various types of muscle damage following exercise and others concluding favorable effects on lipid peroxidation and exercise-induced muscle damage. More recently, reviewers have concluded that although vitamins C and E, either alone or in combination, can reduce indices of oxidative stress, little evidence supports a role for vitamin C and/or vitamin E in protecting against muscle damage (74). Moreover, several studies and reviews suggest that antioxidant supplementation actually may interfere with some beneficial cellular effects of radical oxygen species, impairing muscle recovery and thereby adversely affecting muscle performance (74–76). Some contend that because the potential for long-term harm does exist, the casual use of high doses of antioxidants by athletes and others perhaps should be curtailed (74).

Vitamin D supplementation may be of interest to older athletes. Research suggests vitamin D supplementation may lower the risk of bone fractures in older people by increasing strength, which helps maintain balance and prevent falls. One metaanalysis reported a trend toward a reduction in the risk of fall among patients treated with vitamin D_3 (77). Vitamin D supplementation also may be recommended for athletes who live in northern latitudes or train primarily indoors throughout the year, such as gymnasts (2).

Minerals and Sports Performance

A mineral deficiency could impair exercise performance. The primary minerals low in the diets of athletes who have a low energy intake and those who restrict or avoid animal products are calcium, iron, zinc, and magnesium (2). Correcting a mineral deficiency via supplementation could enhance exercise performance or provide other health benefits to physically active individuals. However, various mineral supplements have been used by well-nourished athletes in attempts to enhance a variety of sports performances, including aerobic endurance, strength, and power.

Calcium is used in the body primarily for bone formation, but calcium is also involved in numerous metabolic processes, including muscle contraction. Most research involving calcium supplementation and exercise has focused on bone health, and physical exercise has been shown to improve bone mass, particularly at load-bearing bone cites (78). The National Institutes of Health (79) indicated that supplementation with calcium, along with vitamin D, may be necessary for optimal bone health in persons not achieving the recommended dietary intake. Thus, calcium supplements may be recommended for some athletes, particularly those involved in strenuous exercise in weight-control sports. Increased calcium intake has also been theorized to promote weight loss (80), which may be of interest to some athletes. Early research, primarily from one research laboratory, reported beneficial effects of foods rich in calcium on weight loss (10). However, a metaanalysis of 13 studies concluded that calcium supplementation has no statistically significant association with a reduction in body weight (81). Research involving calcium supplementation and exercise performance is almost nonexistent, but one study reported no effect of an acute calcium supplement (500 mg) on metabolism during a 90-minute run or performance in a subsequent 10-km run (82).

Phosphates are found as components of various compounds in the body, including 2,3-diphosphoglycerate (2,3-DPG), which is essential for oxygen release from hemoglobin. An increased 2,3-DPG level is the prevalent theory underlying phosphate supplementation to endurance athletes. Although not all studies have shown ergogenic effects following phosphate supplementation, remarkably similar increases in $\dot{V}O_{2max}$ and aerobic endurance exercise performance have been documented in four studies with sodium phosphate supplementation conducted in the 1990s (10). In support of these previous findings, a more recent study found that sodium phosphate loading had a tendency to increase oxygen uptake and significantly improved mean power output in trained cyclists under laboratory conditions. Performance also was significantly faster for a 16.1-km time-trial compared with the placebo, but not the control condition (83). However, some confounding variables in this and previous research have been identified, and additional research is merited.

Magnesium supplementation has been theorized to play a significant role in promoting strength and cardiorespiratory function in healthy persons and athletes. Strenuous exercise apparently increases urinary and sweat losses that may increase magnesium requirements by 10% to 20% (84). Magnesium supplementation or increased dietary intake of magnesium has beneficial effects on exercise performance in magnesium-deficient individuals. However, a review and a metaanalysis concluded that magnesium supplementation of physically active individuals with adequate magnesium status has not been shown to enhance physical performance, including aerobic, anaerobic-lactic acid, and strength activities (84, 85).

Iron is one of the most critical minerals with implications for sports performance, particularly for aerobic endurance athletes. Iron is a component of hemoglobin, myoglobin, cytochromes, and various enzymes in the muscle cells, all of which are involved in the transport and metabolism of oxygen for aerobic energy production. Iron losses can result from various mechanisms during exercise, such as hematuria, sweating, and gastrointestinal bleeding, and iron deficiencies are commonly observed among athletes, especially women (2). Many female athletes are diagnosed as iron deficient; however, contrasting evidence exists as to the severity of deficiency and the effect on performance (86). Some sport nutritionists contend that iron deficiency, with or without anemia, can impair muscle function and limit exercise capacity (2). Curing iron deficiency anemia improves exercise performance. Although some debate exists on whether iron supplementation may enhance performance in athletes who are iron deficient but do not have anemia (10), sports nutritionists recommend that female athletes be tested periodically for iron status and suggest it may be advantageous to begin nutrition intervention before iron deficiency anemia develops (2). Such intervention may include increased iron in the diet as well as supplementation. In one study, iron supplementation, as compared with a placebo, provided to female soldiers during 8 weeks of intense basic military training improved performance in a 2-mile run (87). Endurance athletes who initiate training at altitude increase red blood cell production, and thus may benefit by increasing dietary iron intake or taking iron supplements (10). Doses of 100 mg have been effective (2). The typical multivitamin/mineral supplement contains 0 to 18 mg.

Zinc, chromium, vanadium, boron, and selenium also have been studied for their ergogenic potential. Zinc is required for the activity of more than 300 enzymes, several involved in the major pathways of energy metabolism. Chromium is an insulin cofactor, and its theorized ergogenic effect is based on the role of insulin to facilitate

BCAA transport into the muscle. It has been advertised for strength-type athletes to gain muscle and lose fat. Vanadium also has been advertised for its anabolic potential, purportedly by enhancement of insulin activity. Boron has been marketed as an anabolic mineral as well, theoretically by increasing serum testosterone. Selenium serves as an antioxidant and is theorized to prevent muscle tissue damage during intense exercise (5). Although a deficiency of any of these minerals could possibly impair exercise performance, reviews indicate that there does not appear to be much valid scientific evidence to support an ergogenic effect of zinc, chromium, vanadium, boron, or selenium supplementation to well-nourished athletes (5, 10, 88, 89).

In summary, use of vitamin and mineral supplements does not improve performance in individuals consuming nutritionally adequate diets (2). Moreover, excessive intake of some vitamins and minerals may pose serious health risks.

FLUIDS AND ELECTROLYTES AND SPORTS PERFORMANCE

Environmental heat may affect exercise performance in various ways, including dehydration caused by excessive sweat losses (10). Fluid replacement is critical during prolonged exercise, particularly under warm environmental conditions, and is one of the most studied areas in sports nutrition. Electrolyte replacement, particularly sodium, is also an important consideration during very prolonged exercise. As mentioned, carbohydrate intake during exercise may enhance endurance performance, and carbohydrate-electrolyte solutions (CESs), or sports drinks, have been developed to help meet the needs of athletes.

Significant scientific evidence documents the deleterious effects of hypohydration, or reduced total body water, on endurance exercise performance, and a critical review also indicates that hypohydration may limit strength, power, and high-intensity endurance exercise performance (90). Thus, sustaining euhydration, or optimal body water status, is the major goal of hydration strategies. Exercise under warm environmental conditions also may predispose athletes to exertional heat illnesses, such as muscle cramps, heat exhaustion, and exertional heat stroke. The ACSM developed position stands on exercise and fluid replacement (91) and exertional heat illness during training and competition (92); and, along with other relevant reviews and studies, the following sections highlight the key points of those position stands. However, it is important to note that athletes need to develop a personalized hydration strategy that takes account of preexercise hydration status and of fluid, electrolyte, and substrate needs before, during, and after a period of exercise (93). Individual sweat rates can be estimated by measuring body weight before and after exercise (10).

Hydration Strategies before Training or Competition

The goal of the ACSM guidelines is to start in a state of euhydration with normal plasma electrolyte levels. The following key points are from the ACSM position stand (91) and other sources (10).

- Drink enough the day before competition to be sure you are adequately hydrated.
- Slowly drink approximately 5 to 7 mL of fluid/kg (0.08 to 0.11 oz/lb) body weight at least four 4 hours before exercise.
- Drink another 3 to 5 mL/kg (0.05 to 0.08 oz/lb) body weight approximately 2 hours before exercise if no urine is produced or the urine is dark or highly concentrated.
- Drink CES with carbohydrate (6% to 8%) to help increase body stores of glucose and glycogen for use in prolonged exercise bouts.
- Drink CES with sodium (20 to 50 mEq/L) and/or salty foods or snacks to help stimulate thirst and retain fluids.
- Do not drink excessively, which may increase the risk of dilutional hyponatremia if fluids are aggressively replaced during and after exercise.

Glycerol added to water has been studied as a hyperhydration technique, and some sport scientists indicate that, compared with water alone, the technique clearly has the capacity to enhance body fluid retention (94, 95), but documented benefits as a means to enhance exercise performance remain inconsistent (96). Guidelines for glycerol use in hyperhydration have been developed (96, 97).

Hydration Strategies during Training or Competition

The goal of the ACSM guidelines is to prevent excessive (>2% body weight loss from water deficit) dehydration and excessive changes in electrolyte balance to avert compromised performance. The amount and rate of fluid replacement depends on individual sweating rate, exercise duration, and opportunities to rehydrate. The following are essential points from the ACSM position stand (91) and other sources (10):

- Determine your sweat loss for a given intensity and duration of exercise in the heat. This will provide you with an estimate for fluid intake during exercise.
- Rehydrate early in endurance events because thirst does not develop until approximately 1% to 2% of body weight has been lost.
- Drink ad libitum approximately 0.4 to 0.8 L of fluids per hour, which is approximately 3.5 to 7.0 oz every 15 minutes. Amounts may be adjusted to individual preferences.
- Drink cold water if carbohydrate intake is of little or no concern, for example, in endurance events of less than 50 to 60 minutes.

- Drink a CES with 6% to 8% carbohydrates, or fluids with sport gels, during prolonged endurance or high-intensity intermittent exercise, consuming enough to provide approximately 30 to 80 g of carbohydrate per hour.
- Use a CES containing multiple sources of carbohydrate, including glucose, sucrose, fructose, or maltodextrins, to facilitate absorption.
- Drink a CES containing small amounts of electrolytes, approximately 460 to 690 mg/L of sodium and 78 to 195 mg/L of potassium, amounts present in many commercial sports drinks. Some recommend a range of approximately 700 to 1150 mg/L of sodium and 120 to 225 mg/L of potassium for athletes involved in ultraendurance competition.

Hydration Strategies after Training or Competition

The goal of the ACSM guidelines is to replace any fluid and electrolyte deficit. If time is short to the next exercise session, aggressive rehydration is important. The following are essential points from the ACSM position stand (91) and other sources (10, 98, 99).

- Rapid replacement
  - Drink 1.5 L of fluid for every kilogram of body weight loss, or approximately 1.5 pints for each pound loss.
  - Consume approximately 1.0 to 1.5 g/kg body weight of carbohydrate (~0.5 to 0.7 g/lb body weight) each hour for 3 to 4 hours.
  - Consume adequate sodium. Salty carbohydrate snacks, such as pretzels, may provide both sodium and carbohydrate.
  - Drinking a hypertonic glucose-sodium drink may be more effective at restoring and maintaining hydration.
  - Using glycerol hydration strategies also has been recommended in recovery.
- Leisurely replacement (24-hour recovery)
  - Eat a diet rich in wholesome, natural foods, adhering to healthy eating practices to help replenish needed carbohydrate and electrolytes.
  - Add extra salt to meals when sodium losses are high, or consume salty foods and snacks. Sodium is needed to ensure fluid balance.
  - Consuming a sports drink with protein may help promote muscle recovery, according to some research.

The Gatorade Sports Science Institute (100) provides very useful information on a wide variety of topics in sports nutrition, especially information relative to proper hydration practices to help enhance performance and prevent heat illness when exercising in the heat.

DIETARY SUPPLEMENTS AND SPORTS PERFORMANCE

Dietary supplements, known as sports supplements, are used by athletes worldwide as part of training and competition, and may be used by approximately 85% of elite athletes in some sports (101). As noted in previous sections of this chapter, various dietary supplements, including vitamins, minerals, and metabolites of carbohydrate, fat, and protein, have been purported to enhance sports performance. This section briefly highlights the effects of other dietary supplements marketed to athletes, primarily food ingredients that also may be classified as drugs, herbal products, and related supplements.

Caffeine is classified as a food, a drug, and a dietary supplement. Caffeine use by athletes was restricted at one time but was removed from the World Anti-Doping Agency (WADA) list in 2004. However, other athletic governing agencies, such as the National Collegiate Athletic Association, prescribe limits. Caffeine is now a very popular sport supplement, and it may be found in sports drinks, sports bars, sports gels, and sports candy. Many specific mechanisms have been proposed to underlie the ergogenic effect of caffeine, but little evidence supports the original hypothesis that caffeine has ergogenic effects as a result of enhanced fat oxidation (102). One reviewer noted that caffeine may affect both the central nervous system and the excitation-contraction coupling of skeletal muscle, suggesting that the ergogenic effects of caffeine are mediated partly by enhanced contractile force and partly by a reduction in perceived exertion, possibly though a blunting of effort or pain (103). However, currently, the mechanism underlying improved performance has not been determined (104). Although not all studies have shown ergogenic effects of caffeine supplementation, the following essential points presented in position stands by the ISSN (105) and the ADA/DC/ACSM (2), as well as several comprehensive reviews and metaanalyses (104, 106–109) do support an ergogenic effect.

- Caffeine doses of approximately 3 to 6 mg/kg body weight are effective, but more does not add to the ergogenic effect.
- Caffeine can enhance sustained maximal endurance exercise, including time-trial performance to simulate competitive events, in exercise tasks up to 60 minutes or more.
- Caffeine may enhance performance in speed endurance exercise ranging in duration from 60 to 180 seconds but appears to have minimal effect on maximal 30-second tasks such as the Wingate test.
- Caffeine may enhance performance in prolonged high-intensity, intermittent anaerobic exercise tasks, such as those found in team sports like soccer and rugby.
- Caffeine has shown a small beneficial effect on both maximal voluntary contraction strength and muscular endurance in a metaanalysis of 34 resistance exercise studies, but some other reviewers consider the findings equivocal and recommend additional research.
- Caffeine-induced diuresis does not appear to have adverse effects on body temperature regulation during exercise.
- Caffeine use may cause adverse effects, such as anxiety, jitteriness, and gastrointestinal distress, in some individuals and actually may impair performance.

Ephedrine is found in Chinese *Ephedra*, or *Ma Huang*, an herbal preparation that has been marketed as a dietary supplement for weight loss and increased energy. Ephedrine, like caffeine, is a stimulant and has been studied as a performance-enhancing drug. As noted, some research has shown positive ergogenic effects of ephedrine alone and also an additive effect when combined with caffeine, but no trial of herbal ephedra and athletic performance has been reported (5, 10). Ephedrine use is prohibited by WADA. Moreover, ephedrine misuse may be associated with significant health risks, such as hypertension, heart palpitations and tachycardia, stroke, and death in some individuals (110).

Ethyl alcohol (ethanol) has been studied for possible ergogenic effects since the 1890s and was used by Olympic marathon runners in the 1900 Paris games (10). Alcohol, which is produced from carbohydrates, is theorized to enhance performance by several means. First, alcohol contains 7 kcal/g and has been alleged to be a source of energy during aerobic endurance exercise. Second, it is also thought to exert favorable effects on metabolic processes during exercise. Third, alcohol is thought to cause the release of dopamine, a neurotransmitter associated with the pleasure center of the brain that may modify psychological perceptions of fatigue (10). However, a review (10) indicated that although alcohol contains substantial energy, the available evidence suggests it is not used to any significant extent during exercise. Moreover, research supports the finding that alcohol in small amounts does not beneficially affect $\dot{V}O_{2max}$ or other major physiologic variables associated with energy production during aerobic exercise (111) but may decrease the use of glucose and amino acids by skeletal muscles and impair the metabolic process during exercise (112). Small amounts of alcohol do not seem to enhance or impair aerobic endurance performance. However, larger amounts may impair performance, including aerobic endurance and, particularly, sports performance involving intricate motor skills (10). Moreover, in its position statement on fluid replacement, the ACSM indicated that alcohol consumption can increase urine output and delay full rehydration (91).

Sodium bicarbonate is an alkaline salt described as an antacid in the United States Pharmacopeia, but also may be used as baking soda, and has been studied since the 1930s as a nutritional ergogenic. Supplementation with sodium bicarbonate (0.3 g/kg body weight) may increase the alkaline reserve and help buffer lactic acid in the muscle cell, possibly preventing fatigue by preventing deleterious changes in muscle cell acid-base balance (113). Sodium citrate in a slightly larger dose also has been studied for similar reasons. Using these buffers to enhance exercise performance has been referred to as *buffer boosting* or *soda loading*, and they are theorized to improve athletic performance in anaerobic type events that depend primarily on anaerobic glycolysis. Over the years, not all studies have reported beneficial effects on performance, and that trend continues today with

evidence of enhanced performance in 200-m swim performance (114) and no improvement in a maximal 3-minute cycling test (115). Overall, however, research indicates that buffer salt supplementation increases the serum pH and may enhance performance in exercise tasks, particularly repetitive exercise tasks that maximize energy production for 1 to 6 minutes (2, 10). Ingestion of such buffer salts generally is regarded as safe, but may cause acute gastrointestinal distress and diarrhea. Supplementation with smaller doses over a longer time frame may be effective and less likely to cause intestinal problems (2, 10).

Creatine supplementation, usually as creatine monohydrate, may be an effective means to increase muscle levels of both PCr and free creatine. Consuming approximately 20 g daily, in four equal doses of 5 g each, for 4 to 5 days has been shown to be an effective loading protocol. Increased muscle creatine levels may be maintained with a dose of 2 to 5 g daily. Performance enhancement has been associated with enhanced ATP resynthesis from the increased PCr and a higher rate of PCr resynthesis from the free creatine (10). Creatine supplementation has been the subject of a position stand by the ISSN (116), discussed in the position stand by the ADA, DC, and ACSM (2) and critically analyzed in reviews (10, 117, 118). The following are key points from these resources:

- Creatine supplementation may improve performance in repetitive, short-duration, high-intensity, short-recovery exercise tasks such as isotonic and isokinetic resistance tests, cycle ergometer sprint protocols, sprint running, and simulated match play in sports with intermittent sprinting, that are primarily dependent on PCr.
- Creatine supplementation consistently appears to increase body mass; short-term gains may be primarily water, but long-term gains associated with resistance training may be lean muscle mass, including prevention of sarcopenia in the elderly.
- Creatine supplementation does not enhance aerobic endurance performance, such as distance running.
- Creatine supplementation with the recommended dosage does not hinder the body's ability to dissipate heat, does not negatively affect the athlete's body fluid balance during exercise in the heat, and does not cause muscle cramps.
- Creatine supplementation, with recommended doses, appears to be safe and no adverse effects have been associated with long term use in healthy subjects. Excess intake may cause diarrhea. Moreover, individuals with kidney or liver diseases should consult with their health care professionals regarding supplementation.

Additionally, creatine supplementation may have beneficial effects on the central nervous system (119) and affect energy metabolism in various neurodegenerative diseases, possibly playing a therapeutic role in several diseases characterized by muscle atrophy and weakness, such as muscular dystrophy (120, 121).

Herbal and botanic dietary supplements may be theorized to induce ergogenic effects in various ways, including enhanced energy production, increased myocardial activity, increased hemoglobin concentration, increased muscle mass, and decreased fat mass. Ginseng supplements have been available for many years and have been researched rather extensively as a potential ergogenic aid. However, as indicated (5) and as concluded in a review (122), enhanced physical performance after ginseng administration in well-designed investigations remains to be demonstrated. More recently, quercetin, a dietary flavonol found in many plants, has been studied for its ergogenic potential. It may function as an antioxidant, may be anti-inflammatory, may promote mitochondria formation, and has been studied for its immune effects during exercise. Several studies reported that quercetin supplementation in untrained, young adult males was associated with small improvements in endurance capacity (123, 124), with one of the studies also reporting modest but insignificant increases in markers of mitochondrial biogenesis (124). In contrast, another study concluded that quercetin supplementation was not ergogenic in untrained men, having no effect on muscle oxidative capacity, perceptual determinants of performance in prolonged exercise, or cycling performance (125). Moreover, research with exercise-trained individuals is limited, and that which is available does not provide evidence of significant ergogenic effects on fuel use, exercise efficiency, or perceived effort, even during ultramarathon events (126–128). Additional research is merited to evaluate the ergogenic effects of quercetin supplementation.

Numerous other dietary supplements have been studied for their ergogenic potential, but discussion of each is beyond the scope of this chapter. The selected readings at the end of this chapter provide detailed information on specific supplements, and the position stand of the ADA/DC/ACSM (2) provides a list of dietary supplements that (a) perform as claimed; (b) may perform as claimed but for which evidence is insufficient; (c) do not perform as claimed; or (d) are dangerous, banned, or illegal. Relative to the last point, some sports supplements, particularly those marketed to increase muscle mass, may contain substances, either added intentionally or contaminated inadvertently, that may lead to a positive doping test (129). Examples of contaminants include hGH, androstenedione, dehydroepiandrosterone, and other anabolic, androgenic steroids (2). Other ingredients, such as ephedrine and some herbals, may pose serious health risks to some individuals (10). Reliable information on the safety of dietary supplements is available on the Internet from the National Institutes of Health (130). When it comes to sports supplements, caveat emptor.

SUMMARY AND CONCLUSIONS

Athletes benefit most from consumption of a balanced and varied healthful diet, but use of some dietary strategies and supplements may benefit athletes involved in certain types of athletic endeavors. Individuals may respond differently to various nutritional strategies or dietary supplements, so athletes and their advisors must be prepared to experiment with specific strategies and supplements to optimize both training and performance.

REFERENCES

1. Brutsaert TD, Parra EJ. Med Sport Sci 2009;54:11–27.
2. American College of Sports Medicine. Med Sci Sport Exerc 2009;41:709–31.
3. Nemet D, Eliakim A. Curr Opin Clin Nutr Metab Care 2009;12:304–9.
4. Tarnopolsky MA. Clin J Sport Med 2008;18:531–8.
5. Williams MH. Sports nutrition. In: Shils ME, Shike M, Ross AC et al. Modern Nutrition in Health and Disease. 10th ed. Baltimore: Lippincott Williams & Wilkins, 2006:1723–40.
6. Donnelly JE, Blair SN, Jakicic JM et al. Med Sci Sports Exerc 2009;41:459–71.
7. American College of Sports Medicine. Med Sci Sports Exerc 2009;41:687–708.
8. Bangsbo J, Mohr M, Krustrup P. J Sports Sci 2006;24:665–74.
9. Coyle E. 2007. Sports Med 2007 37:306–11.
10. Williams MH. Nutrition for Health, Fitness, and Sport. New York: McGraw-Hill, 2010.
11. Utter AC, Kang J, Robertson RJ. Med Sci Sports Exerc 2002;34:1779–84.
12. Welsh RS, Davis JM, Burke JR. Med Sci Sports Exerc 2002;34:723–31.
13. Jeukendrup A. Sports Sci Exchange 2007;20:1–6.
14. Koh-Banerjee PK, Ferreira MP, Greenwood M et al. Nutrition 2005;21:312–9.
15. Dunne L, Worley S, Macknin M. Clin J Sport Med 2006;16:68–71.
16. Kerksick C, Rasmussen C, Bowden R et al. Int J Sport Nutr Exerc Metab 2005;15:653–64.
17. Sahlin K, Harris RC. Acta Physiol 2008;194:283–91.
18. Sahlin K, Sallstedt EK, Bishop D et al. J Physiol Pharmacol 2008;59(Suppl):19–30.
19. Brown R, Cox C. Am J Med Sports 2001;3:75–86.
20. Shaw CS, Clark J, Wagenmakers AJ. Annu Rev Nutr 2010;30:13–34.
21. Havemann L, West SJ, Goedecke JH et al. J Appl Physiol 2006;100:194–202.
22. Cornish SM, Chilibeck PD. Appl Physiol Nutr Metab 2009;34:49–59.
23. Walser B, Stebbins CL. Eur J Appl Physiol 2008;104:455–61.
24. Peoples GE, McLennan PL, Howe PR et al. J Cardiovasc Pharmacol 2008;52:540–7.
25. Bortolotti M, Tappy L, Schneiter P. Clin Nutr 2007;26:225–30.
26. Nieman DC, Henson DA, McAnulty SR et al. Int J Sport Nutr Exerc Metab 2009;19:536–46.
27. Whigham LD, Watras AC, Schoeller DA. Am J Clin Nutr 2007;85:1203–11.
28. Schoeller DA, Watras AC, Whigham LD. Appl Physiol Nutr Metab 2009;34:975–8.
29. Pinkoski C, Chilibeck PD, Candow DG et al. Med Sci Sports Exerc 2006;38:339–48.
30. Kennedy A, Martinez K, Schmidt S et al. J Nutr Biochem 2010;21:171–9.
31. Williams MH. Nutritional Aspects of Human Physical and Athletic Performance. Springfield, IL: Charles C Thomas, 1985.

32. Kingsley M. Sports Med 2006;36:657–69.

33. Stephens FB, Constantin-Teodosiu D, Greenhaff PL. J Physiol 2007;581:431–44.

34. Kreider RB, Campbell B. Phys Sportsmed 2009;37:13–21.

35. Fielding RA, Parkington J. Nutr Clin Care 2002;5:191–6.

36. Food and Nutrition Board, Institute of Medicine. Dietary Reference Intakes for Energy, Carbohydrates, Fiber, Fat, Protein and Amino Acids (Macronutrients). Washington, DC: National Academy Press, 2002.

37. Rennie MJ. Int J Sport Nutr Exerc Metab 2001;11:S170–76.

38. Campbell, B., Kreider, RB, Ziegenfuss T et al. J Int Soc Sports Nutr 2007;4:8.

39. Paddon-Jones D, Rasmussen BB. Curr Opin Clin Nutr Metab Care 2009;12:86–90.

40. Howarth KR, Moreau NA, Phillips SM et al. J Appl Physiol 2009;106:1394–402.

41. van Loon L. Int J Sport Nutr Exerc Metab 2007;17:S104–S117.

42. Gibala MJ. Sports Sci Exchange 2002;15:1–4.

43. Saunders M. Int J Sport Nutr Exerc Metab 2007;17:S87–S103.

44. Millard-Stafford M, Childers WL, Conger SA et al. Curr Sports Med Rep 2008;7:193–201.

45. Gibala, M. Sports Med 2007;37:337–40.

46. Toone RJ, Betts JA. Int J Sport Nutr Exerc Metab 2010;20:34–43.

47. Macdermid, P, Stannard, S. J Sport Nutr Exerc Metab 2006;16:65–77.

48. Williams MH. Int J Soc Sports Nutr 2005;2:63–67.

49. Wu G, Bazer FW, Davis TA et al. Amino Acids 2009;37:153–68.

50. Liu TH, Wu CL, Chiang CW et al. J Nutr Biochem 2009;20:462–8.

51. McConell G. Curr Opin Clin Nutr Metab Care 2007;10:46–51.

52. Fahs CA, Heffernan KS, Fernhall B. Med Sci Sports Exerc 2009;41:773–9.

53. Liu TH, Wu CL, Chiang CW et al. J Nutr Biochem 2009;20:462–8.

54. McConell GK, Huynh NN, Lee-Young RS et al. Am J Physiol Endocrinol Metab 2006;290:E60–E66.

55. Sweeney KM, Wright GA, Glenn Brice A et al. J Strength Cond Res 2010;24:79–87.

56. Derave W, Everaert I, Beeckman S et al. Sports Med 2010;40:247–63.

57. Trudeau, F. Sports Med 2008;38:9–16.

58. Negro M, Giardina S, Marzani B et al. J Sports Med Phys Fitness 2008;48:347–51.

59. Tipton KD, Elliott TA, Ferrando AA et al. Appl Physiol Nutr Metab 2009;34:151–61.

60. Gleeson M. J Nutr 2008;138:2045S–49S.

61. Phillips G. Curr Sports Med Rep 2007;6:265–68.

62. Nissen S, Sharp R, Ray M et al. J Appl Physiol 1996;81:2095–2104.

63. Palisin T, Stacy J. Curr Sports Med Rep 2005;4:220–23.

64. Rowlands DS, Thomson JS. J Strength Cond Res 2009;23:836–46.

65. Volpe S. Clin Sports Med 2007;26:119–30.

66. Woolf K, Manore M. Int J Sport Nutr Exerc Metab 2006;16:453–84.

67. Singh A, Moses DM, Deuster PA. Med Sci Sports Exerc 1992;24:726–32.

68. Telford R, Catchpole EA, Deakin V et al. Int J Sport Nutr 1992;2:135–53.

69. Powers SK, Hamilton K. Clin Sports Med 1999;18:525–36.

70. Nalbant O, Toktaş N, Toraman NF et al. Aging Clin Exp Res 2009;21:111–21.

71. Zoppi CC, Hohl R, Silva FC et al. J Int Soc Sports Nutr 2006;13:37–44.

72. Nieman DC. Can J Appl Physiol 2001;26:S45–55.

73. Nieman DC, Henson DA, McAnulty SR et al. J Appl Physiol 2002;92:1970–7.

74. McGinley C, Shafat A, Donnelly AE. Sports Med 2009;39:1011–32.

75. Teixeira VH, Valente HF, Casal SI et al. Med Sci Sports Exerc 2009;41:1752–60.

76. Close GL, Ashton T, Cable T et al. Br J Nutr 2006;95:976–81.

77. Jackson C, Gaugris S, Sen SS et al. QJM 2007;100:185–92.

78. Maïmoun L, Sultan C. Calcif Tissue Int 2009;85:277–86.

79. National Institutes of Health. Ann Intern Med 2006;145:364–71.

80. Zemel M. J Am Coll Nutr 2005;24:537S–46S.

81. Trowman R, Dumville JC, Hahn S et al. Br J Nutr 2006;95:1033–8.

82. White KM, Lyle RM, Flynn MG et al. Int J Sport Nutr Exerc Metab 2006;16:565–79.

83. Folland JP, Stern R, Brickley G. J Sci Med Sport 2008;11:464–8.

84. Nielsen F, Lukaski H. Magnes Res 2006;19:180–9.

85. Newhouse IJ, Finstad EW. Clin J Sport Med 2000;10:195–200.

86. Peeling P, Dawson B, Goodman C et al. Eur J Appl Physiol 2008;103:381–91.

87. McClung JP, Karl JP, Cable SJ et al. Am J Clin Nutr 2009;90:124–31.

88. Lukaski HC. Can J Appl Physiol 2001;26:S13–22.

89. Volpe SL. Curr Sports Med Rep 2008;7:224–9;

90. Judelson DA, Maresh CM, Anderson JM et al. Sports Med 2007;37:907–21.

91. American College of Sports Medicine, Sawka MN, Burke LM et al. Med Sci Sports Exerc 2007;39:377–90.

92. American College of Sports Medicine, Armstrong LE, Casa DJ et al. Med Sci Sports Exerc 2007;39:556–72.

93. Maughan RJ, Shirreffs SM. Int J Sport Nutr Exerc Metab 2008;18:457–72.

94. Nelson JL, Robergs RA. Sports Med 2007;37:981–1000.

95. Goulet ED, Aubertin-Leheudre M, Plante GE et al. Int J Sport Nutr Exerc Metab 2007;17:391–410.

96. van Rosendal SP, Osborne MA, Fassett RG et al. Nutr Rev 2009;67:690–705.

97. Goulet ED. J Strength Cond Res 2010;24:74–8.

98. Evans GH, Shirreffs SM, Maughan RJ. Nutrition 2009;25:905–13.

99. van Rosendal SP, Osborne MA, Fassett RG et al. Sports Med 2010;40:113–29.

100. Gatorade Sports Science Institute. Available at: http://www.gssiweb.com. Accessed May 10, 2010.

101. Maughan RJ, Depiesse F, Geyer H et al. J Sports Sci 2007;25(Suppl):S103–13.

102. Graham TE, Battram DS, Dela F et al. Appl Physiol Nutr Metab 2008;33:1311–8.

103. Tarnopolsky MA. Appl Physiol Nutr Metab 2008;33:1284–9.

104. Davis JK, Green JM. Sports Med 2009;39:813–32.

105. Goldstein ER, Ziegenfuss T, Kalman D et al. J Int Soc Sports Nutr 2010;7:5.

106. Burke LM. Appl Physiol Nutr Metab 2008;33:1319–34.

107. Astorino TA, Roberson DW. J Strength Cond Res 2010;24:257–65.

108. Ganio MS, Klau JF, Casa DJ et al. J Strength Cond Res 2009;23:315–24.

109. Warren GL, Park ND, Maresca RD et al. Med Sci Sports Exerc 42:1375–87.

110. Haller CA, Benowitz NL. N Engl J Med 2000;343:1833–8.
111. Coiro V, Casti A, Saccani Jotti G et al. Neuro Endocrinol Lett 2007;28:145–8.
112. El-Sayed MS, Ali N, El-Sayed Ali Z. Sports Med 2005;35:257–69.
113. McNaughton LR, Siegler J, Midgley A. Curr Sports Med Rep 2008;7:230–6.
114. Lindh AM, Peyrebrune MC, Ingham SA et al. Int J Sports Med 2008;29:519–23.
115. Vanhatalo A, McNaughton LR, Siegler J et al. Med Sci Sports Exerc 2010;42:563–70.
116. Buford TW, Kreider RB, Stout JR et al. J Int Soc Sports Nutr 2007;30;4:6.
117. Lopez RM, Casa DJ, McDermott BP et al. J Athl Train 2009;44:215–23.
118. Dalbo VJ, Roberts MD, Stout JR et al. Br J Sports Med 2008;42:567–73.
119. Adhihetty PJ, Beal MF. Neuromol Med 2008;10:275–90.
120. Andres RH, Ducray AD, Schlattner U et al. Brain Res Bull 2008;76:329–43.
121. Gualano B, Artioli GG, Poortmans JR et al. Amino Acids 2010;38:31–44.
122. Bahrke MS, Morgan WP, Stegner A. Int J Sport Nutr Exerc Metab 2009;19:298–322.
123. Davis JM, Carlstedt CJ, Chen S et al. Int J Sport Nutr Exerc Metab 2010;20:56–62.
124. Nieman DC, Williams AS, Shanely RA et al. Med Sci Sports Exerc 2010;42:338–45.
125. Cureton KJ, Tomporowski PD, Singhal A et al. J Appl Physiol 2009;107:1095–104.
126. Dumke CL, Nieman DC, Utter AC et al. Appl Physiol Nutr Metab 2009;34:993–1000.
127. Utter AC, Nieman DC, Kang J et al. Res Sports Med 2009;17:71–83.
128. Quindry JC, McAnulty SR, Hudson MB et al. Int J Sport Nutr Exerc Metab 2008;18:601–16.
129. Geyer H, Parr MK, Koehler K et al. J Mass Spectrom 2008;43:892–902.
130. National Institutes of Health. Available at: http://nccam.nih.gov/health/supplements. Accessed May 25, 2010.

SUGGESTED READINGS

Burke L, Deakin V. Clinical Sports Nutrition. New York: McGraw-Hill, 2009.
Clark N. Nancy Clark's Sports Nutrition Guidebook. Champaign, IL: Human Kinetics, 2008.
Dunford M, ed. Sports Nutrition. Chicago: American Dietetic Association, 2005.
Jeukendrup A, Gleeson M. Sport Nutrition. Champaign, IL: Human Kinetics, 2010.
Williams MH. Nutrition for Health, Fitness, and Sport. New York: McGraw-Hill, 2010.

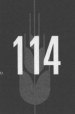

114

THE EVOLVING SCIENCE OF DIETARY SUPPLEMENTS[1]

CHRISTINE A. SWANSON, PAUL R. THOMAS, AND PAUL M. COATES

Dietary supplements are a heterogeneous group of products that contain one or any combination of nutrients, herbs, and various other ingredients derived primarily from natural sources, from which they are extracted or chemically synthesized and then manufactured into finished products. Widely available for purchase without a prescription, dietary supplements are sold as capsules, tablets, liquids, and myriad other forms. Supplements and, increasingly, conventional foods containing supplement ingredients are often promoted as providing potential health benefits beyond basic nutrition.

Supplementation of the diet is not a new concept. By the early part of the twentieth century in the United

States, cod liver oil and its concentrates were a marketed source of supplemental vitamins A and D. Supplements providing these and other nutrients became available in grocery stores in the mid-1930s, and the first multivitamin tablets were introduced in the early 1940s (1, 2). The number and diversity of dietary supplement products have grown enormously to include nonnutrients, so that today, tens of thousands of products are estimated to be available, with total sales exceeding $30 billion in 2011 in the United States alone (3).

In the United States, dietary supplements are primarily overseen by the Food and Drug Administration (FDA), as are drugs and most foods. The Dietary Supplement Health and Education Act (DSHEA) of 1994 created the first regulatory structure for this class of products. Dietary supplements were legally defined as products containing vitamins, minerals, herbs or botanicals, amino acids, "a dietary substance . . . to supplement the diet by increasing the total dietary intake [e.g., enzymes or tissues from organs or glands]," or "a concentrate, metabolite, constituent, extract, or combination" of any of these ingredients (4). They are further described as being intended for ingestion, not to be represented as a conventional food or as a sole item of a meal or diet, and must be labeled as a dietary supplement. Further details about FDA's responsibilities for regulating dietary supplements and manufacturers' responsibilities for marketing them are available at http://www.fda.gov/Food/DietarySupplements/default.htm (5).

Under the DSHEA, dietary supplements are considered to be foods and therefore require no formal preapproval by FDA. However, manufacturers proposing to use a "new dietary ingredient" must notify FDA before marketing. Because they are not drugs, dietary supplement products may not be promoted as a preventive, treatment, or cure for any specific diseases or conditions (6). Once purchased, however, consumers may use them for such purposes. The Federal Trade Commission regulates and monitors the advertising of dietary supplements in the marketplace (7).

In the United States, dietary supplements are often used as part of personal, proactive health care practices to ensure adequate intake of nutrients, maintain health, prevent illnesses, and in some cases to treat or manage various health problems and diseases, some minor (e.g., mild

---

[1]**Abbreviations: AER**, adverse event report: **AMRM**, Analytical Methods and Reference Materials; **ATBC**, Alpha-Tocopherol, Beta-Carotene Cancer Prevention Study; **CAM**, complementary and alternative medicine; **DSHEA**, Dietary Supplement Health and Education Act; **FDA**, Food and Drug Administration; **NCCAM**, National Center for Complementary and Alternative Medicine; **NHANES**, National Health and Nutrition Examination Survey; **NHIS**, National Health Information Survey; **NIH**, National Institutes of Health; **NVNMS**, non-vitamin nonmineral supplements; **ODS**, Office of Dietary Supplements; **RCT**, randomized controlled trial; **SRM**, standard reference material.

indigestion) and others that require medical supervision. The use of dietary supplements is considered by some consumers and health practitioners to be essential for achieving optimal health, together with attention to nutrition, fitness, stress management, and emotional and spiritual development. Supplements are often recommended to patients by practitioners of conventional medicine and complementary and alternative medicine (CAM). The latter group tends to emphasize holistic health care and often includes naturopaths—medical doctors who emphasize "natural" remedies.

Many of today's dietary supplements contain ingredients derived from medicinal plants that have been used for millennia by people throughout the world, particularly in medical systems such as traditional Chinese medicine, Indian Ayurveda, and Arabic Unani medicine (8). Garlic (*Allium sativum* L.), for example, has been eaten as a food, used as a spice, and in more recent times taken as a supplement by consumers in the hope of reducing blood pressure and blood cholesterol levels. The world's poorest populations still rely on herbs as medicines in primary health care (9).

Health care providers should ask their patients what dietary supplements they are taking, including herbal products. Unfortunately, most conventional medical practitioners and naturopaths in the United States have inadequate knowledge of the history, evidence base, and appropriate use of herbal medicines. The application of this practice, once embraced by eminent pharmacologists with an appreciation of pharmacognosy, involves expertise in a diverse and challenging array of disciplines ranging from ethnobotany to contemporary methods of natural products chemistry. Other indispensible skills include plant biochemistry, including an appreciation of the role and function of secondary plant metabolites and their pharmacology when administered to humans (10). Many of these secondary plant metabolites have been developed into pharmaceuticals widely used today (11). Plants with potential medicinal properties contain numerous bioactive constituents and can have beneficial, adverse, or no observable health effects. By emphasizing a multidisciplinary scientific framework for studying phytomedicinals, it is feasible that "rationale phytotherapy" as described by Varo Tyler (12) may someday reemerge as a well-respected discipline in the United States and also return to western European countries, where it once flourished.

DIETARY SUPPLEMENT USE IN THE UNITED STATES

Dietary supplement use in the United States is assessed by large, nationally representative, cross-sectional surveys. The gold standard of surveys into the health status and health-related behaviors of the US civilian, noninstitutionalized population is the National Health and Nutrition Examination Survey (NHANES). It incorporates assessment methods designed to measure exposure to dietary supplement ingredients and has

monitored supplement use since the 1970s. Prevalence data are collected to assess exposure of populations to nutrient and nonnutrient ingredients. Although sales data suggest increased use of specific ingredients, survey data provide the only means of quantifying supplement exposures and describing use by various population groups (e.g., children, pregnant women, elderly people).

National Surveys

The first comprehensive information about supplement use by the US population after the DSHEA came from NHANES data collected from 1999 to 2002 (13, 14). Interviewers asked about supplement use (prescription and nonprescription) in the previous month, and most participants provided their supplement containers, from which ingredient and dosage information was taken from the label. Prevalence of use of any supplement among infants, children, and adults is shown in Figure 114.1.

Use of supplements was lowest among infants, increased through age 5 years, and then declined throughout adolescence. Nearly one-third of children took at least one dietary supplement, and most used multivitamins with or without minerals. Supplement use likely contributed substantially to total nutrient intakes (14). Use of supplements containing single botanical ingredients (e.g., echinacea) was minimal, similar to findings of another population-based survey of children (15).

The increasing linear trend in supplement use among adults aged 19 to 65 years was followed by a plateau (13). Fifty-two percent reported supplement use in the following rank order: multivitamins with or without minerals (35%), calcium plus calcium-containing antacids (35%), vitamins E and C (12% to 13%), and B-complex vitamins (5%). Among supplement users, the majority reported daily intake, and about half reported taking only one product. Compared with the 1988 to 1994 NHANES, supplement use among adults increased substantially. The use of botanic products containing single herbs was minimal.

The National Health Information Survey (NHIS), another periodic survey of a nationally representative sample of the civilian, noninstitutionalized population of the United States, is a primary source of information about use of CAM. It, like NHANES, is conducted by the National Center for Health Statistics at the Centers for Disease Control and Prevention. Since 1988, NHIS has included questions about use of nonvitamin nonmineral supplements (NVNMS), defined as products without vitamins or minerals. The 2007 survey found that almost 18% of adults and 4% of children had used NVNMS over the previous 30 days (16). Among adults, the five most commonly used NVNMS were fish oil/omega-3 fatty acids, followed by glucosamine, echinacea, flaxseed, and ginseng. Children most commonly took echinacea, fish oil/omega-3 fatty acids, combination herbal pills, and flaxseed products. Use of herbal products decreased between the 2002 and 2007 surveys, but the exposure periods differed

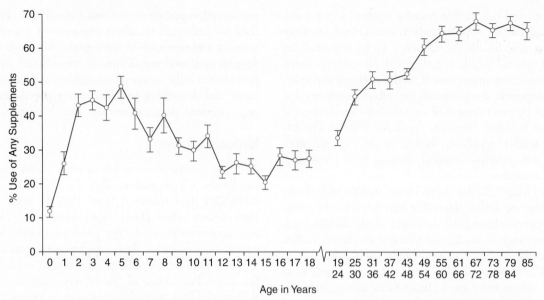

Fig. 114.1. Prevalence and standard error of dietary supplement use in the past 30 days by age, NHANES 1999–2002. (Reproduced with permission from Picciano MF, Dwyer JT, Radimer KL et al. Dietary supplement use among infants, children, and adolescents in the United States, 1999–2002. Arch Pediatr Adolesc Med 2007;161:978–85.)

in the two surveys, thus adding some uncertainty about the observed change over time.

Supplement Contributions to Total Nutrient Intake

The use of nutrient-containing dietary supplements will help some individuals obtain recommended intakes of vitamins and minerals while leading others to consume more than needed amounts (or do both to the same individual, depending on the nutrient). Both these situations have been observed (17, 18). Although estimates of intake depend on the quality of food and dietary supplement databases, assessments of adequacy and excess intake also reflect the validity of the nutrient reference values used.

Exposure Assessment Methods

As is the case with dietary assessment methods for food intake, no standard approach exists for obtaining either qualitative or quantitative information about dietary supplement use. Accurate reporting of usual intake can be a complicated cognitive task (19). Given the variation in questions about supplement use, it is unlikely that respondents describe their supplement use in a standardized manner, so cross-study comparisons are difficult. Researchers themselves differ considerably in their approach to supplement classification, particularly for botanicals. In addition, many investigators fail to address the quantitative uncertainty associated with supplement exposure assessment (20, 21). Exposure is based on marketed products, which vary in composition across brands. Some researchers do not clarify whether default values or supplement-specific composition data have been used. Even when label information is obtained directly, accurate quantitative assessment is not ensured, because

the label declarations are not usually based on validated methods of chemical analysis. The impact of these errors depends on how the data are used and interpreted. More recently, several federal agencies have collaborated to improve methods to assess dietary supplement use and measure exposure to ingredients in specific products more accurately (22).

Characteristics of Supplement Users

Surveys find that adult supplement users differ from nonusers in various demographic characteristics, lifestyle, and health status. Users are more likely to be female, older, more educated, of non-Hispanic white race or ethnicity, physically active, of normal weight or underweight, and more likely to report excellent or very good health (13, 23). Users of herbal supplements may differ from those who take only nutrient-containing supplements. Some evidence indicates, for example, that use of botanicals is associated with lack of insurance coverage and limited access to conventional health care (24).

DIETARY SUPPLEMENT QUALITY AND SAFETY

Consumers and regulatory agencies expect that contents listed on supplement labels should accurately reflect the contents of marketed products and that they are safe when used as directed. ConsumerLab.com, a company that has tested more than 2400 dietary supplement products for more than 11 years, finds approximately 1 in 4 with a quality problem, mostly because of an inadequate amount or substandard ingredients followed by contamination with heavy metals (25). In a similar vein, agencies funding research relevant to dietary supplements expect grant applicants to have the capacity to characterize proposed interventions used in preclinical and clinical research properly. These expectations are defined by product quality, which is also essential for product safety.

Natural Product Quality

Product quality is largely determined by identity, purity, and chemical composition of the ingredients. The assessment of these properties is inherently linked to the availability of qualitative and quantitative analytic methods. The background and challenges associated with the development of an analytic methods program are beyond the scope of this chapter, but they have been summarized (22, 26). The progress of the National Institutes of Health (NIH) Office of Dietary Supplements (ODS) Analytical Methods and Reference Materials (AMRM) Program is regularly updated on the ODS website (http://ods.od.nih.gov).

In 2003, the pace of the ODS analytic methods program was rapidly accelerated because of a confluence of events involving multiple stakeholders with interests in dietary supplements. When the FDA provided notice of its intent to institute good manufacturing practices (GMP) for dietary supplements, the supplement industry recognized and expressed a need for suitable analytic methods to facilitate their compliance with the new FDA regulations (27). At about the same time, NIH applicants pursuing natural products research relevant to dietary supplements found it increasingly difficult to secure funding because they could not meet product integrity guidelines, specifically those of the National Center for Complementary and Alternative Medicine (NCCAM). The purpose of the NCCAM integrity guidelines, which eventually became policy (http://nccam.nih.gov/research/policies/naturalproduct.htm) (28), was to improve the quality of proposed research and better ensure that funded studies could be interpreted and reproduced. Similar guidelines have been proposed by various journals interested in natural products research (29–31). The NIH sponsored a workshop to address clinical research involving various soy interventions. Several concerns, including heterogeneity and poor characterization of soy interventions were addressed. Guidelines for future clinical research involving soy interventions were published (32).

The ODS was directed to lead the effort to satisfy the analytic needs of multiple dietary supplement stakeholders and facilitate collaborations across a wide range of scientific and other professional groups. Progress of the AMRM program is perhaps best highlighted by the publication of more than 100 validated official analytic methods for dietary supplement ingredients, most published in the *Journal of the American Organization of Analytical Chemists International*. No articles of this type appeared in the journal before the program. One of the first, and perhaps most challenging, tasks was the development of validated methods for multivitamin-mineral products. The list of publicly available methods also includes various nutrients and nonnutrient phytochemicals in both raw materials and finished products. Additional validated analytic methods are needed to continue the development of a dietary supplement ingredient database based on chemical analysis (33).

The AMRM Program also funds research organized by scientists at the US National Institutes of Standards and Technology to develop standard reference materials (SRMs). SRMs are used for several purposes, including developing accurate methods of analysis by research laboratories and ensuring the long-term performance and adequacy of measurement quality assurance programs. SRMs relevant to dietary supplements are currently available for the product most widely used by consumers (e.g., multivitamins and minerals), for dietary supplement ingredients used as test materials or intervention agents by the research community (e.g., carotenoids in extract form), and for analytes (e.g., 25-hydroxyvitamin D) in matrices relevant to nutrition monitoring of populations (34) and in clinical practice.

Dietary Supplement Safety

By law, a dietary supplement manufacturer is responsible for ensuring that its products are safe before marketing them. The FDA is responsible for taking action against supplements found to pose significant or unreasonable risks to health after they are marketed. The FDA conducts postmarketing surveillance by tracking and evaluating adverse event reports (AERs) and by reviewing the scientific safety literature. Health care providers and consumers may voluntarily report any adverse event to the FDA by phone, email, letter, or online through its MedWatch system. In addition, since 2008, supplement companies are required to notify the FDA of any serious adverse events about which they receive information (35).

AERs do not prove that an ingredient is dangerous, because such reports vary in comprehensiveness, quality, and supporting medical detail, and there may be confounding factors associating the product with the AERs (e.g., concomitant use of medications). Nevertheless, AERs help the agency identify early signals that a product may present safety risks to consumers. In 2011, the FDA received 1777 AERs for dietary supplements (36). Using AERs and the scientific literature, the FDA has identified problematic dietary supplements and taken various actions. For example, it banned the sale of products containing ephedrine alkaloids in 2004. Ephedra was a popular stimulant used for weight loss and to improve energy levels and athletic performance, but it is related to amphetamines in its pharmacologic action. Its use, particularly in combination with caffeine-providing herbs such as guarana, led to deaths, strokes, seizures, and other harms to the heart and central nervous system. The FDA has also issued advisories warning against the use of supplements containing kava (liver injury), aristolochic acid (nephropathy), and comfrey (damage to liver and other organs).

DIETARY SUPPLEMENTS AND CHRONIC DISEASE

In the United States and several other Westernized countries, the shift in emphasis has been from prevention and treatment of nutrient deficiency diseases to nutrition interventions aimed at prevention of chronic disease. This trend has been largely generated by prospective cohort studies, many of which have identified dietary patterns or individual nutrients as modifiable risk factors with significant potential to reduce disease burden.

Randomized controlled trials (RCTs) are widely regarded as a level of evidence above observational studies, because of the advantage of randomization of study participants to placebo and treatment groups to eliminate sources of bias. Of all the RCTs of diet and chronic disease, the study of cancer has received the most attention. In contrast to the promising results from observational studies, RCTs designed to examine efficacy of dietary modification and nutrient supplementation for cancer prevention have been disappointing.

Nutrient Supplementation

Efficacy of supplementation with various antioxidant nutrients was one of the first topic areas to be addressed in large clinical trials with cancer outcomes. The link to antioxidant nutrients and reduced cancer risk was inferred from diet patterns associated with risk reduction noted in observational studies and also supported by preclinical data. In retrospect, it was premature to attribute beneficial effects of diet patterns rich in fruit and vegetables to specific antioxidant constituents.

The Alpha-Tocopherol, Beta-Carotene Cancer Prevention Study (ATBC study) (37) provided important lessons about the potential for unexpected consequences of supplementation. The trial was designed to assess the efficacy of supplementation with α-tocopherol and β-carotene for risk reduction of lung cancer among Finnish men who were smokers. Unexpectedly, intervention with β-carotene was associated with increased, rather than decreased, risk of lung cancer. Soon thereafter, the combination of β-carotene and retinol was also found to be associated with increased risk of lung cancer among male past or current smokers (38). Subsequent studies in experimental animals provided a possible biochemical basis for enhanced risk of β-carotene supplementation combined with exposure to cigarette smoke (39). The ATBC study was subject to considerable criticism, but this well-conducted study was done, in part, to address an important issue directly related to proposed clinical practice, because serious consideration was being given to recommending antioxidant supplements to smokers in the absence of any evidence of efficacy.

Other investigators (40–43) have provided commentary about potential flaws and pitfalls associated with RCTs involving diet modification and nutrient supplementation. A common criticism of supplementation studies is the reductionist approach of the use of nutrients versus diet modification. Although the criticism is reasonable, the superiority of holism is not firmly established in the prevention of chronic disease in populations. Baseline nutritional status may be an important determinant of response, as indicated by results of nutrient intervention in a population of Chinese adults with documented malnutrition and high rates of both esophageal and gastric cancer (44). Total mortality was reduced among adults randomized to selenium, vitamin E, and β-carotene, at doses not more than two times the 1980 recommended dietary allowance values. Reduced risk of death was attributed primarily to a reduction in cancer.

Herbal Supplementation

Studies of herbs as phytomedicines do not easily lend themselves to observational studies for various reasons, including lack of adequate exposure assessment methods. The results of the limited number of NIH-funded RCTs of herbal interventions for prevention and treatment of chronic disease have been disappointing but instructive. NIH sponsorship of RCTs of herbal interventions is relatively new, and these interventions present an entirely different set of research challenges. This topic is illustrated here by a single RCT with a treatment focus.

One of the first NIH-supported RCT relevant to dietary supplements involved the herb St. John's wort (*Hypericum perforatum* L.). Sponsorship of the trial by the NCCAM and ODS was largely motivated by increased availability of dietary supplement products after the DSHEA and a perception of growing use of St. John's wort products for the treatment of depression, usually without medical supervision. *H. perforatum* L. had a long history of prescribed use of well-characterized products in Europe. The NIH determined that the efficacy and safety of St. John's wort for treatment of major depression needed to be evaluated in a supervised patient population in the United States.

NIH investigators and collaborators from academic institutions designed and conducted a RCT (45) to study the efficacy of a well-characterized extract of *H. perforatum* L. reported to be effective in clinical studies in Germany. Patients were randomized to receive a placebo, the St. John's wort extract, or an active comparator drug (sertraline) for 8 weeks. An allowance for variable dosing of the herbal extract and sertraline was incorporated into the study design to allow for the possibility of dose escalation. The chemical composition of plants, particularly secondary metabolites, can be highly variable and influenced by numerous factors including climate, growing conditions, and initial processing steps. In contrast to isolated nutrients or chemically synthesized single agent pharmaceuticals, precise replication is not possible for herbal extracts because they tend to be complex chemical mixtures. This is important, given that synergism of multiple active constituents within an herbal extract may be the key to efficacy (46). The challenges associated with standardization of herbal products are described elsewhere (47).

Similar to initial studies of large RCTs with nutrients, the herb *H. perforatum* L. showed no benefit compared with the placebo. The study was widely interpreted to mean that St. John's wort was ineffective, despite the observation that the active comparator drug (sertraline) was also similar to the placebo for two primary outcome measures. Another criticism of the study was the failure to have identified the mechanism of action of the herbal extract before conducting the RCT. It is not widely appreciated that the precise mechanism of action associated with efficacy of most pharmaceuticals is not usually known with certainty when a pivotal RCT is launched or at the time of marketing. Aspirin (salicylic acid) and its other over-the-counter relatives, for example, are widely used to treat pain and inflammation and are regarded as effective, yet their mechanism of action remains uncertain (48, 49).

It is not unusual for initial RCTs with drugs to fail and then be repeated with modifications in the hope of demonstrating benefit and obtaining FDA drug approval. A second NIH-funded RCT to study the efficacy of *H. perforatum* L. for treatment of minor depression has been completed, but it is not yet published (ClinicalTrials. gov identifier: NCT00048815).

ADVANCING DIETARY SUPPLEMENT RESEARCH

Improving Clinical Trials

The Women's Health Initiative, the largest and most expensive RCT ever conducted, tested the efficacy of estrogen replacement therapy, diet modification, and dietary supplements on chronic disease risk reduction in postmenopausal women. Neither a low-fat diet pattern nor supplementation with calcium and vitamin D reduced the risk of incident breast cancer or hip fracture, respectively (50, 51). Following publication of these results, the NIH held a meeting to discuss methods for improving clinical trials (52). The expense and complexity of RCTs were noted, as were their advantages. Among its conclusions, prospective cohort studies of diet were encouraged because of the potential of well-designed observational studies to complement and inform future RCTs. However, current dietary assessment methodologies with their associated measurement error (53) may remain the greatest impediment to achieving this goal.

Biomarkers

Although challenges are inherent in conducting clinical research to investigate the role of nutrition (including dietary supplements) in reducing chronic disease risk, they are not unique to these interventions. Whenever end points of interest result from a slowly evolving disease process (e.g., cancers, heart disease, cognitive decline), the time needed to study them can be very long. Thus, attempts have been made to identify markers along the path to disease development that could be used to indicate whether an intervention is having an impact on the disease end point. Examples that have been used include adenomatous polyps for colorectal cancer and low-density lipoprotein cholesterol for coronary heart disease.

Surrogate biomarkers could enable faster, more efficient clinical trial designs and may be useful in guiding health choices, but the use of biomarkers depends on the quality of the data supporting them and the context in which they are applied (54). The Institute of Medicine has developed a framework for evaluating biomarkers that includes validation (demonstration of the analytic validity of the measured biomarker), qualification (assessment of evidence on associations between biomarkers and disease states, including data showing the effects of interventions on both biomarkers and clinical outcomes), and use (contextual analysis based on the specific use proposed) (54).

Qualification of surrogate biomarkers is a major research challenge, particularly in studies of diet and nutrient interventions, given that the effect size is expected to be relatively modest. For a biomarker to serve as a true surrogate, a test of the intervention and the surrogate end point must give the same result as carrying the study to the true end point (55); a costly qualification procedure, indeed. In addition, qualification of a surrogate for one exposure does not imply qualification of all exposures (56). This has been amply demonstrated for drugs used to treat heart disease (54). No evidence indicates that this issue does not apply to other exposures, including diet patterns, nutrients, phytochemicals, or herbal extracts. Finally, the working assumption that diet or nutrient interventions are likely to travel through a single biologic pathway to a chronic disease end point is expedient but undoubtedly naive (57).

Evidence-Based Reviews of Dietary Supplement Efficacy and Safety

In the United States, the NIH funds most of the research on dietary supplements, investing $250 to $300 million per year on basic botany and chemistry, preclinical and clinical research, and population surveys to explore patterns of use. In 2002, the ODS implemented an evidence-based approach to better inform the development of research agendas for these products. It has sponsored the systematic review of more than a dozen topics, including ephedra for weight loss and athletic-performance enhancement (58) and multivitamins and multiminerals in chronic disease prevention (59).

A systematic review is a powerful tool for evaluating literature on the health effects of an intervention. It involves several standard steps (60), the first being to organize a research team. Topics for systematic review are framed by a set of precisely and carefully crafted questions. Eligibility criteria for studies that will bear on these questions are selected. Reviewers locate, synthesize, and evaluate evidence from available studies that meet these criteria. Evidence and summary tables are constructed, and assessments of methodologic quality are made. Meta-analyses are performed when appropriate. Results are synthesized, and the resulting report is reviewed by a technical evaluation panel and external reviewers.

Several systematic reviews of dietary supplements have been invaluable in informing subsequent research (e.g., soy, omega-3 fatty acids). In the case of ephedra, products containing this botanical were removed from the US market not long after the release of an NIH-sponsored evidence report. Systematic reviews have been more broadly applied to the development of dietary reference intakes (61), the Dietary Guidelines for Americans (62), and clinical practice guidelines by the American Dietetic Association (63).

Concerns raised about the systematic review approach, as applied to nutrition topics, include the paucity of clinical trial data in many cases, small effect sizes that are often masked by heterogeneity of the study populations, difficulty in generalizing results from a patient group to a healthy population, and the fact that noninterventional studies are rarely included. These concerns, however, do not diminish the value of approaching the study of dietary (and dietary supplement) interventions in a systematic and transparent way.

SUMMARY

It is somewhat ironic that increased availability to a wider variety of dietary supplement products resulted in increased research to establish or reassess the potential health benefits and risks of nutrients already used for decades in supplements. Unexpectedly, the DSHEA also stimulated research to study ingredients with relatively limited use in the United States (e.g., herbals) and promoted research on supplement ingredients of interest to the research community, clinicians, and consumers (e.g., glucosamine, omega-3 fatty acids, vitamin D).

To begin to develop a science base relevant to dietary supplements, various government agencies recognized a need to establish research priorities, and much of that activity was initially focused on identifying research gaps. The ODS, for example, was charged with developing an analytic methods and reference materials program. Validated analytic methods and laboratory quality control are indispensible to research efforts related to supplements. They allow researchers to monitor nutritional status of populations and assess trends over time. Supplement databases used to assess exposures should be based on validated methods for chemical determinations, and that work is in progress. To evaluate, interpret, compare, and replicate studies, all test materials must be adequately characterized. The requirements for adequate characterization of test materials is not unique to research relevant to dietary supplements; but in this arena, the activity is helpful to funding agencies, grant applicants, to those who conduct evidenced-based reviews, supplement manufacturers, and eventually consumers.

The efficacy of dietary supplement ingredients to reduce risk of chronic diseases remains unclear, in large part because of difficulties associated with the design and conduct of RCTs. Additional randomized clinical trials of supplement interventions are needed, but the number will be limited. In the meantime, prospective cohort studies could serve to inform RCTs, but only if the issue of measurement error associated with dietary assessment methods is resolved; this is a tremendous challenge. Perhaps there should be less discussion about which dietary assessment method gives the expected answer and more concern about which method or combination of methods gives the correct answer.

In the United States, botanicals or constituents derived from them have received mixed reception in scientific circles. Many chemical constituents derived from plants regarded as foods or spices are generally regarded as relatively benign but with the potential to improve health. Medicinal herbs or phytomedicines, in contrast, are widely dismissed as being either ineffective or unsafe. This criticism could have been tempered considerably if, in the United States, pharmacognosy had remained as a discipline within pharmacology. The importance of synergy of constituents within medicinal plants or from the combination of herbs is often noted, but the science base is difficult to document, as is the concept of holism in nutrition. Resolving these issues is fundamental to advancing the science in both areas and seems a topic well suited to a research effort involving both disciplines.

ACKNOWLEDGMENTS

We would like to acknowledge the contributions of the staff of the ODS and particularly the work of the late Mary Frances Picciano, PhD, Senior Nutrition Research Scientist with the ODS from 1999 to 2010. We have no disclosures to report.

REFERENCES

1. NIH State-of-the-Science Panel. Am J Clin Nutr 2007; 85:257S–64S.
2. Apple RD. Vitamania: Vitamins in American Culture. New Brunswick, NJ: Rutgers University Press, 1996.
3. Anonymous. Nutr Bus J 2012;17:5.
4. Dietary Supplement Health and Education Act of 1994. Public Law 103–417. Available at: http://ods.od.nih.gov/About/DSHEA_Wording.aspx. Accessed September 14, 2012.
5. US Food and Drug Administration. Dietary Supplements. Available at: http://www.fda.gov/Food/DietarySupplements/default.htm. Accessed September 14, 2012.
6. US Food and Drug Administration. Overview of Dietary Supplements. Available at: http://www.fda.gov/Food/DietarySupplements/ConsumerInformation/default.htm. Accessed September 14, 2012.
7. Federal Trade Commission. Dietary Supplements: An Advertising Guide for Industry. Available at http://business.ftc.gov/documents/bus09-dietary-supplements-advertising-guide-industry. Accessed September 17, 2012.
8. World Health Organization. WHO Traditional Medicine Strategy 2002–2005. Geneva: World Health Organization, 2002.
9. Fowler MW. J Sci Food Agr 2006;86:1797–804.
10. Barnes S, Prasain J. Curr Opin Plant Biol 2005;8:324–8.
11. Newman DJ, Cragg GM. J Nat Prod 2007;70:461–77.
12. Robbers JE, Tyler VE. Tyler's Herbs of Choice: The Therapeutic Use of Phytomedicinals. New York: Haworth Herbal Press, 1999.

13. Radimer K, Bindewald B, Hughes J et al. Am J Epidemiol 2004;160:339–49.
14. Picciano MF, Dwyer JT, Radimer KL et al. Arch Pediatr Adolesc Med 2007;161:978–85.
15. Briefel R, Hanson C, Fox MK et al. J Am Diet Assoc 2006;106:S52–65.
16. Barnes PM, Bloom B, Nahin RL. Natl Health Stat Report 2008:1–23.
17. Murphy SP, White KK, Park SY et al. Am J Clin Nutr 2007;85:280S–4S.
18. Bailey RL, Dodd KW, Gahche JJ et al. Am J Clin Nutr 2010;91:231–7.
19. Subar AF, Thompson FE, Smith AF et al. J Am Diet Assoc 1995;95:781–8.
20. Park SY, Murphy SP, Wilkens LR et al. J Nutr 2006;136:1359–64.
21. Yetley EA. Am J Clin Nutr 2007;85:269S–76S.
22. Dwyer JT, Holden J, Andrews K et al. Anal Bioanal Chem 2007;389:37–46.
23. Rock CL. Am J Clin Nutr 2007;85:277S–9S.
24. Gardiner P, Graham R, Legedza AT et al. Altern Ther Health Med 2007;13:22–9.
25. Cooperman T. Third party dietary supplement testing: ConsumerLab.com. In: Bonakdar RA. The H.E.R.B.A.L. Guide: Dietary Supplement Resources for the Clinician. Philadelphia: Lippincott Williams & Wilkins, 2010:126–30.
26. Betz JM, Fisher KD, Saldanha LG et al. Anal Bioanal Chem 2007;389:19–25.
27. Food and Drug Administration. Current Good Manufacturing Practices (CGMPs): Dietary Supplements. Available at: http://www.gpo.gov/fdsys/pkg/FR-2003-03-13/html/03-5401.htm. Accessed September 17, 2012.
28. National Center for Complementary and Alternative Medicine, NIH. NCCAM Policy: Natural Product Integrity. Available at: http://nccam.nih.gov/research/policies/natural product.htm.
29. Swanson CA. Am J Clin Nutr 2002;75:8–10.
30. Williamson EM. Phytomedicine 2001;8:401–9.
31. Gagnier JJ, Boon H, Rochon P et al. Ann Intern Med 2006;144:364–7.
32. Klein MA, Nahin RL, Messina MJ et al. J Nutr 2010;140:1192S–204S.
33. Dwyer JT, Picciano MF, Betz JM et al. J Food Comp Anal 2008;21:S83–S93.
34. Looker AC, Pfeiffer CM, Lacher DA et al. Am J Clin Nutr 2008;88:1519–27.
35. Food and Drug Administration. Dietary Supplements. Adverse Event Reporting. Available at: http://www.fda.gov/Food/GuidanceComplianceRegulatoryInformation/GuidanceDocuments/DietarySupplements/ucm171383.htm. Accessed September 17, 2012.
36. Kux L. Federal Register 2012;77:31622–4.
37. The Alpha-Tocopherol, Beta-Carotene Cancer Prevention Study Group. N Engl J Med 1994;330:1029–35.
38. Omenn GS, Goodman GE, Thornquist MD et al. J Natl Cancer Inst 1996;88:1550–9.
39. Russell RM. Pure Appl Chem 2002;74:1461–7.
40. Byers T. CA Cancer J Clin 1999;49:353–61.
41. Byers T. Am J Epidemiol 2010;172:1–3.
42. Prentice RL. Am J Clin Nutr 2007;85:308S–13S.
43. Gann PH. JAMA 2009;301:102–3.
44. Blot WJ, Li JY, Taylor PR et al. J Natl Cancer Inst 1993;85:1483–92.
45. Hypericum Depression Trial Study Group. JAMA 2002;287:1807–14.
46. Kinghorn AD. J Pharm Pharmacol 2001;53:135–48.
47. Barrett M, Koetter U. Standardization of botanical preparations: what it does and does not tell us. In: Barrett M, ed. The Handbook of Clinically Tested Herbal Remedies. New York: Haworth Press, 2004:37–48.
48. Weissmann G. Sci Am 1991;264:84–90.
49. Amann R, Peskar BA. Eur J Pharmacol 2002;447:1–9.
50. Prentice RL, Caan B, Chlebowski RT et al. JAMA 2006;295:629–42.
51. Jackson RD, LaCroix AZ, Gass M et al. N Engl J Med 2006;354:669–83.
52. Kramer BS, Wilentz J, Alexander D et al. PLoS Med 2006;3:e144.
53. Prentice RL. J Natl Cancer Inst 2010;102:583–5.
54. Institute of Medicine. Evaluation of Biomarkers and Surrogate Endpoints in Chronic Disease. Washington, DC: National Academies Press, 2010.
55. Schatzkin A, Gail M. Nat Rev Cancer 2002;2:19–27.
56. Fleming TR, DeMets DL. Ann Intern Med 1996;125:605–13.
57. Heng HH, Bremer SW, Stevens JB et al. J Cell Physiol 2009;220:538–47.
58. Shekelle PG, Hardy ML, Morton SC et al. JAMA 2003;289:1537–45.
59. Huang HY, Caballero B, Chang S et al. Am J Clin Nutr 2007;85:265S–8S.
60. Lichtenstein AH, Yetley EA, Lau J. J Nutr 2008;138:2297–306.
61. Yetley EA, Brule D, Cheney MC et al. Am J Clin Nutr 2009;89:719–27.
62. 2010 Dietary Guidelines Advisory Committee. NEL Evidence-Based Systematic Reviews. 2010. Available at: http://www.nutritionevidencelibrary.com/category.cfm?cid=21. Accessed September 14, 2012
63. American Dietetic Association. ADA Method of Creating Evidence-Based Nutrition Practice Guidelines. 2010. Available at: http://www.adaevidencelibrary.com/category.cfm?cid=16&cat=0&library=EBG. Accessed September 14, 2012

SUGGESTED READINGS

Dwyer JT, Picciano MF, Betz JM et al. Progress in developing analytic and label-based dietary supplement databases at the NIH Office of Dietary Supplements. J Food Compos Anal 2008;21:S83–S93.

Prentice RL, Anderson GL. The Women's Health Initiative: lessons learned. Annu Rev Public Health. 2008;29:131–50.

Lichtenstein AH, Yetley EA. Application of systematic review methodology to the field of nutrition. J Nutr 2008;138:2297–2306.

Looker AC, Pfeiffer CM, Lacher DA et al. Serum 25-hydroxyvitamin D status of the US population: 1988–1994 compared with 2000–2004. Am J Clin Nutr 2008;88:1519–27.

Ross AC, Russell RM, Miller SA et al. Application of a key events dose-response analysis to nutrients: a case study with vitamin A (retinol). Crit Rev Food Sci Nutr 2009;49:708–17.

INDEX

Page numbers followed by *f* denote figures; those followed by *t* denote tables.